SURGERY OF THE FOOT AND ANKLE

Sixth Edition

Volume 2

Surgery of the Foot and Ankle

Sixth Edition

Volume 2

ROGER A. MANN, M.D.
Director, Foot Fellowship Program
Chief of Foot Surgery and Staff Orthopaedic Surgeon
Samuel Merritt Hospital
Oakland, California
Associate Clinical Professor
Department of Orthopaedic Surgery
University of California at San Francisco School of Medicine

MICHAEL J. COUGHLIN, M.D.
Staff Orthopaedic Surgeon
St. Alphonsus Regional Medical Center
Boise, Idaho

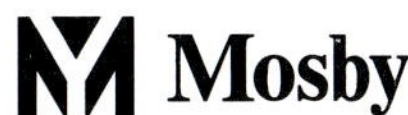

St. Louis Baltimore Boston Chicago London Philadelphia Sydney Toronto

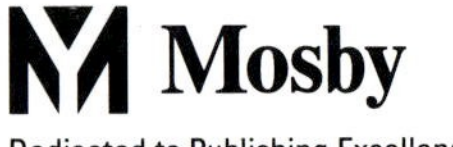

Dedicated to Publishing Excellence

Sponsoring Editor: James D. Ryan
Assistant Editor: Joyce-Rachel John
Developmental Editor: Kathryn H. Falk
Assistant Director, Manuscript Services: Frances M. Perveiler
Production Supervisors: Karen Halm, Kathryn Solt
Proofroom Manager: Barbara M. Kelly

Mosby–Year Book, Inc.
11830 Westline Industrial Drive
St. Louis, MO 63416

1 2 3 4 5 6 7 8 9 0 CL/MV 97 96 95 94 93

Library of Congress Cataloging-in-Publication Data

Surgery of the foot and ankle.—6th ed. / [edited by] Roger A. Mann, Michael J. Coughlin.
p. cm.
Rev. ed. of: Surgery of the foot / editor, Roger A. Mann. Ed. 5. 1986.
Includes bibliographical references and index.
ISBN 0-8016-6683-X
1. Foot—Surgery. 2. Ankle—Surgery. I. Mann, Roger A., 1936–
II. Coughlin, Michael J. III. Surgery of the foot.
[DNLM: 1. Ankle—surgery. 2. Foot—surgery. WE 880 S9602]
RD563.S87 1992
617.5′85059—dc20 92-19174
DLC CIP
for Library of Congress

To our parents for the opportunities presented to us.
To our wives, Joan and Kirsten, for their patience and understanding.

CONTRIBUTORS

Donald E. Baxter, M.D.
Clinical Professor of Orthopaedics
Baylor College of Medicine
Houston, Texas

R. Luke Bordelon, M.D.
Clinical Assistant Professor of Orthopaedics
Louisiana State University
New Orleans, Louisiana
Director, Foot Clinic
Doctors Hospital of Opelousa
Opelousa, Louisiana

James W. Brodsky, M.D.
Clinical Assistant Professor of Orthopaedic Surgery
University of Texas Southwestern Medical School
Director, Orthopaedic and Diabetic Foot Clinic
Veteran's Administration Hospital
Baylor University Medical Center
Dallas, Texas

Michael W. Chapman, M.D.
Professor and Chairman
Department of Orthopaedic Surgery
University of California at Davis
Chief, Department of Orthopaedic Surgery
University of California Medical Center at Davis
Davis, California

Thomas O. Clanton, M.D.
Clinical Associate Professor of Orthopaedic Surgery
University of Texas Medical School at Houston
Chief, Foot and Ankle Service
Hermann Hospital
Houston, Texas

Michael J. Coughlin, M.D.
Staff Orthopaedic Surgeon
St. Alphonsus Regional Medical Center
Boise, Idaho

Jesse C. DeLee, M.D.
Associate Professor
Department of Orthopaedics
University of Texas Health Science Center
San Antonio, Texas

Earl N. Feiwell, M.D.
Associate Clinical Professor
Orthopaedic Surgery
University of Southern California School of Medicine
Los Angeles, California
Orthopaedic Consultant, Spina Bifida Program
Rancho Los Amigos Medical Center
Downey, California

Richard D. Ferkel, M.D.
Clinical Instructor of Orthopaedic Surgery
Division of Orthopaedics
UCLA School of Medicine
Los Angeles, California
Chief, Arthroscopy Service
Wadsworth Veteran's Administration Hospital
West Los Angeles, California

J. Gordon Frierson, M.D.
Clinical Professor
Department of Medicine and Epidemiology
University of California Medical Center at San Francisco
San Francisco, California
Samuel Merritt Hospital
Oakland, California

William G. Hamilton, M.D.
Assistant Clinical Professor of Orthopaedic Surgery
Columbia University College of Physicians and Surgeons
Senior Attending Orthopaedic Surgeon
St. Luke's-Roosevelt Hospital Center
New York, New York

M. Mark Hoffer, M.D.
Professor of Orthopaedics
University of California at Irvine
Irvine, California
Rancho Los Amigos Medical Center
Downey, California

John D. Hsu, M.D., C.M.
Clinical Professor of Orthopaedics
University of Southern California School of Medicine
Chairman, Department of Surgery
Chief of Orthopaedics
Rancho Los Amigos Medical Center
Downey, California

Walter W. Huurman, M.D.
Associate Professor of Orthopaedics and Pediatrics
University of Nebraska
Director, Children's Orthopaedics
University of Nebraska Medical Center
Children's Memorial Hospital
Omaha, Nebraska

James O. Johnston, M.D.
Professor of Orthopaedic Oncology
University of California School of Medicine at San Francisco
San Francisco, California

Roger A. Mann, M.D.
Director, Foot Fellowship Program
Chief of Foot Surgery and Staff Orthopaedic Surgeon
Samuel Merritt Hospital
Oakland, California
Associate Clinical Professor
Department of Orthopaedic Surgery
University of California at San Francisco School of Medicine

Thomas J. Moore, M.D.
Assistant Professor
Department of Orthopaedics
Emory University School of Medicine
Atlanta, Georgia

Mark S. Myerson, M.D.
Chief, Foot and Ankle Service
Assistant Professor
The Johns Hopkins University
The Union Memorial Hospital
Baltimore, Maryland

Landrus L. Pfeffinger, M.D.
Assistant Clinical Professor
University of California at San Francisco
San Francisco, California

Paul Plattner, M.D.
Private Practice
Summit Medical Center
Oakland, California

G. James Sammarco, M.D.
Volunteer Professor of Orthopaedics
Department of Orthopaedics
University of Cincinnati Medical Center
Cincinnati, Ohio

Lew C. Schon, M.D.
Associate Director of Foot and Ankle Center
Director, Dance Medicine Clinic
Union Memorial Hospital
Baltimore, Maryland

Francesca M. Thompson, M.D.
Assistant Clinical Professor of Orthopaedic Surgery
Columbia University College of Physicians and Surgeons
Chief, Adult Orthopaedic Foot Clinic
St. Luke's-Roosevelt Hospital Center
New York, New York

Paul D. Traughber, M.D.
Clinical Assistant Professor
University of Utah Medical Center
Staff Radiologist
Saint Alphonsus Regional Medical Center
Boise, Idaho

PREFACE TO THE SIXTH EDITION

The sixth edition of *Surgery of the Foot and Ankle* has undergone extensive revision. The change in the title of the book reflects the expanded coverage of the ankle. Michael J. Coughlin, M.D., my first foot Fellow, has joined me as co-editor. Dr. Coughlin brings to the book his extensive knowledge of foot and ankle surgery gleaned from his private practice in Boise, Idaho. Several new contributing authors also have been added. These authors with extensive knowledge in their specific areas of interest enhance the depth and scope of the book.

This edition has been designed to be user-friendly. The text has been reorganized into nine sections. Every major aspect of the foot and ankle is presented to the reader (whether he or she is a practicing surgeon, resident, general practitioner, or medical student) in a clear, concise manner. Surgical techniques are described and illustrated in detail to enable the reader not only to understand, but also to gain insight about how to perform each procedure. Although the authors may present several treatment modalities, at the conclusion of each section they present their recommended treatment plan for each clinical entity. Some topics are presented by more than one author. Rather than eliminating these sections, we have elected to leave them in place to give the reader varying points of view.

In the clinical chapters written by the editors, the treatment protocol we present is the result of our continuing evaluation and updating of our techniques. With the help of my foot Fellows, we have carefully reassessed the clinical results of most of the major surgical procedures about the foot and ankle since publication of the last edition. Patients have been recalled, carefully examined, and new radiographs obtained. We have identified and evaluated recurring problems with specific procedures and made necessary technical changes where appropriate. By carefully evaluating our cases in this manner, we believe we can provide the reader the most accurate assessment of the surgical procedures we present. Thus we are able to present our most current thinking regarding diagnosis, treatment, and specific surgical techniques.

In the section on general considerations, biomechanics and principles of examination of the foot and ankle have been enhanced by a comprehensive evaluation of imaging of the foot and ankle. Anesthetic techniques and conservative office treatment also are covered in this section.

In the section on the forefoot an extensive discussion of the deformities of the great toe, along with the complications associated with bunion surgery, are presented in the chapter on adult hallux valgus. This chapter has been updated to point out the pitfalls of specific bunion procedures in order to make the reader aware of complications that may result. Because of the anatomic characteristics of the juvenile bunions and its requirement for surgical decision based upon the underlying pathophysiology, a new chapter has been added on the evaluation and treatment of juvenile hallux valgus. The chapter on lesser toes has been updated to present the reader with a fuller understanding of the clinical problems associated with these often complex forefoot deformities. The chapter on sesamoids and accessory bones has been completely rewritten to aid the physician in gaining a fuller understanding of accessory bones and their evaluation and treatment. Keratotic disorders of the forefoot again is designed to provide the clinician with a clearer understanding regarding the differential diagnosis and appropriate treatment for these sometimes difficult problems.

Neuromuscular diseases that affect the foot and ankle are presented in an in-depth fashion, with chapters on congenital neurologic disorders (such as myelodysplasia, cerebral palsy, and motor unit disease), and acquired neurologic disorders resulting from cerebrovascular accidents, as well as head trauma. Static nerve disorders and impingement syndromes also are discussed in this section.

The section on arthritic conditions presents our current knowledge and treatment of systemic arthritis, traumatic arthritis, and osteoarthritis. A separate chapter on arthrodesis techniques about the foot and ankle, detailing the surgical indications and technical aspects of each procedure is included.

An in-depth evaluation of flatfoot in children and its treatment is presented in the section on postural disorders of the foot. Clinical entities that result in acquired flatfoot in adults are discussed, their etiology and treatment carefully outlined. Another chapter in this section provides an in-depth review of the evaluation and treatment of the cavus foot deformity.

In the section on miscellaneous conditions of the foot, chapters on tumors and metabolic conditions of the foot, toenail disorders, and dermatologic abnormalities have been completely revised. In addition, the chapter on diabetes has been completely revised to provide the reader with a better understanding of the conservative and surgical management of the diabetic foot. A separate chapter on amputations about the foot and ankle has been added.

A section on sports medicine is introduced in this edition. Included in this section is a comprehensive chapter on athletic injuries to the soft tissues. The specific problems associated with the foot in running and dancing have been greatly expanded and divided into individual chapters. Ankle arthroscopy about the foot and ankle also has been expanded and placed in a separate chapter to familiarize the reader with this exciting new, evolving technique.

Pediatrics has been updated with the preferred method of treatment for the various clinical entities brought up to date.

Trauma has been expanded to include an in-depth chapter on the management of soft tissue trauma to accompany the updated chapters on fractures and dislocations about the foot and ankle.

We believe this new edition of *Surgery of the Foot and Ankle* will greatly enhance one's knowledge of this dynamic field whether they are students or practicing surgeons.

Roger A. Mann, M.D.
Michael J. Coughlin, M.D.

PREFACE TO THE FIRST EDITION

This book has been written in response to a continuing request by my students and colleagues that I draw together into one place of reference the fundamentals and the recommendations contained in my lectures and clinical demonstrations over a span of 30 years. As Frederic Wood Jones commented, "It is probably the experience of most teachers of anatomy that the student is generally better acquainted with the intimate structure of the hand than with that of the foot."* My friends among orthopaedic surgeons agree that the teaching of their specialty does not allot sufficient time to problems of the foot. They will forgive, therefore, and perhaps welcome as an adjunct to teaching, the elementary portions of the contents and the didactic approach.

Extreme disabilities of the foot, such as the talipes deformities, have received studious attention in published reports. They have on that account been given only a cursory nod of recognition here. This book is directed toward the commoner disabilities, which have been sparsely considered in medical writing and which have been widely neglected in teaching and practice.

The expanding awareness of the diversity of pathologic changes in the feet and of the complexities of treatment represents an advance since the days when all foot disabilities were always attributed to so-called fallen arches and when a prescription of arch supports satisfied the diagnostician that nothing further could be done about the patient whose feet continued to hurt.

This far from definitive effort of mine has reached the printed page through the encouragement and helpfulness, advice, and direction of so many of my friends and colleagues that I hesitate to name them lest by inadvertence one should be overlooked. If that happens, my deepest regret! Certainly I must mention my friends of long standing, Dr. August F. Daro; Dr. William M. Scholl, who turned his collection of photographs and anatomic models over to me for study and selective use and who has been otherwise helpful in so many ways; Dr. Ernest Nora, Sr., a constant friend since our medical school days, who reviewed the chapter on Tumors, Cysts, and Exostoses; so many on the Staff of Columbus Hospital; Dr. Carlo Scuderi, who reviewed the first rough material and then introduced me to my patient and cooperative publishers; Dr. Edwin Hirsch, who made the photographic facilities of St. Luke's Hospital† available to me; Dr. Karl A. Meyer, my former professor in medical school, who wrote the Foreword as a final expression of years of encouragement. Dr. Edward L. Compere crowned my effort by writing the Introduction, having first reviewed some of the material in its early stages and, later, all in its final form.

Special credit should be given to Miss Ethel H. Davis for superbly editing and organizing the manuscript.

It is tempting to list those who gave me direction in one way or another: Dr. Peter A. Rosi, Dr. Charles N. Pease, Dr. Joseph P. Cascino, Dr. Steven O. Schwartz, Dr. Caesar Portes, Dr. Abe Rubin, and Dr. Harold Wheeler. The skill of my artists, Miss Edith Hodgson, Miss Gloria Jones, and Dr. Allen Whitney, must not go unsung. And to all, mentioned or not, in the measure of their interest, my gratitude!

Only wives whose husbands have attempted the writing of books and the husbands who have known the stamina of their wives during the process can appreciate how much meaning there is in my dedication to Frances DuVries.

Henri L. DuVries, D.P.M., M.D.
1959

**Jones FW:* Structure and function as seen in the foot, London, 1944, Baillière, Tindall & Cox, Ltd, p 3.

†Now Presbyterian-St. Luke's Hospital.

ACKNOWLEDGMENTS

We would like to acknowledge those who have assisted us in the preparation of this revision: Claudia Smith (data processing and editing); Penny Dunlap, R.N. (word processing); Craig Schonhardt (illustrations); Jerry Jones, Director, St. Alphonsus Media Services (photography); and Judy Balcerzak, Librarian, St. Alphonsus Library (research).

Roger A. Mann, M.D.
Michael J. Coughlin, M.D.

CONTENTS

Volume 2

Preface to the Sixth Edition *ix*
Preface to the First Edition *xi*

SECTION VI: MISCELLANEOUS CONDITIONS OF THE FOOT

19 / Disorders of Tendons *805*
Paul Plattner and Roger Mann

20 / Heel Pain *837*
R. Luke Bordelon

21 / Infections of the Foot *859*
John G. Frierson and Landrus L. Pfeffinger

22 / The Diabetic Foot *877*
James W. Brodsky

23 / Amputations of the Foot and Ankle *959*
James W. Brodsky

24 / Tumors and Metabolic Diseases of the Foot *991*
James O. Johnston

25 / Toenail Abnormalities *1033*
Michael J. Coughlin

26 / Dermatology *1073*
Landrus Pfeffinger

SECTION VII: SPORTS MEDICINE

27 / Athletic Injuries to the Soft Tissues of the Foot and Ankle *1095*
Thomas O. Clanton and Lew C. Schon

28 / The Foot in Running *1225*
Donald E. Baxter

29 / Foot and Ankle Injuries in Dancers *1241*
William G. Hamilton

30 / Arthroscopy of the Ankle and Foot *1277*
Richard D. Ferkel

SECTION VIII: PEDIATRICS

31 / Congenital Foot Deformities *1313*
Walter W. Huurman

SECTION IX: TRAUMA

32 / Soft-Tissue Trauma—Acute and Chronic Management *1367*
Mark Myerson

33 / Miscellaneous Soft-Tissue Injuries *1411*
G. James Sammarco

34 / Fractures and Fracture-Dislocations of the Ankle *1439*
Michael W. Chapman

35 / Fractures and Dislocations of the Foot *1465*
Jesse C. DeLee

Index *xvii*

Volume 1

SECTION I: GENERAL CONSIDERATIONS

1 / Biomechanics of the Foot and Ankle *3*
Roger A. Mann

2 / Principles of Examination of the Foot and Ankle *45*
Roger A. Mann

3 / Imaging of the Foot and Ankle *61*
Paul D. Traughber

4 / Conservative Treatment of the Foot *141*
Roger A. Mann

5 / Peripheral Anesthesia *151*
Michael J. Coughlin

SECTION II: THE FOREFOOT

6 / Adult Hallux Valgus *167*
Roger A. Mann and Michael J. Coughlin

7 / Juvenile Bunions *297*
Michael J. Coughlin

8 / Lesser Toe Deformities *341*
Michael J. Coughlin and Roger A. Mann

9 / Keratotic Disorders of the Plantar Skin *413*
Roger A. Mann and Michael J. Coughlin

10 / Sesamoids and Accessory Bones of the Foot *467*
Michael J. Coughlin

SECTION III: NEUROLOGIC CONDITIONS

11 / Diseases of the Nerves *543*
Static Nerve Disorders *544*
Roger A. Mann
Functional Nerve Disorders *559*
Donald E. Baxter

12 / Congenital Neurologic Disorders of the Foot *575*
Motor Unit Disease *575*
John D. Hsu
Myelodysplasia *580*
Earl N. Feiwell
Cerebral Palsy *594*
M. Mark Hoffer

13 / Acquired Neurologic Disorders of the Adult Foot *603*
Thomas J. Moore

SECTION IV: ARTHRITIC CONDITIONS

14 / Arthritides *615*
Francesca M. Thompson and Roger A. Mann

15 / Arthrodesis of the Foot and Ankle *673*
Roger A. Mann

SECTION V: POSTURAL DISORDERS

16 / Flatfoot in Children and Young Adults *717*
R. Luke Bordelon

17 / Flatfoot in Adults *757*
Roger A. Mann

18 / Pes Cavus *785*
Roger A. Mann

Index *xvii*

SECTION

VI

MISCELLANEOUS CONDITIONS OF THE FOOT

CHAPTER

19

Disorders of Tendons

Paul Plattner, M.D.
Roger Mann, M.D.

Anatomy of tendons
Etiology of injuries to muscles and tendons
Pathology of injuries to muscles and tendons
Peritendinitis
Tendon rupture
Bursae
Bursitis
  Bursitis associated with intermetatarsal phalangeal bursa
  Intermetatarsal bursitis
  Bursitis about the posterior aspect of the heel
  Achilles tendon bursitis and retrocalcaneal bursitis
Achilles tendon
Physical findings
Radiographic examination
Treatment
  Peritendinitis
  Ruptured Achilles tendon
Results
Peroneal tendons
Anatomy
Peritendinitis
  Clinical Findings
  Treatment
Rupture
  Diagnosis
  Treatment
Traumatic dislocation
  Classification
  Clinical findings
  Treatment
Flexor hallucis longus
Stenosing tenosynovitis
Stenosis at the posteromedial ankle
  Clinical Findings
Stenosis at the great toe
  Clinical findings
  Treatment
Extensor tendons
Peritendinitis
Rupture
  Tibialis anterior tendon
  Extensor hallucis longus and extensor digitorum longus
Tibialis posterior tendon
Tendon transfers about the foot and ankle
Biomechanical principles
Principles of muscle function
Patient evaluation
  Natural history of the muscle imbalance
  Age of the patient
Diagnosis
Treatment
  Surgical principles

ANATOMY OF TENDONS

All of the tendons crossing the ankle joint have true synovial sheaths except for the Achilles and plantaris tendons.[80, 189] The tibialis anterior, extensor hallucis longus, extensor digitorum longus, and peroneus tertius tendons pass beneath a tight fibro-osseous canal formed by bands of the superior and inferior retinaculum. Along the medial aspect of the ankle the tibialis posterior, flexor digitorum longus, and flexor hallucis longus each lie in separate compartments behind the malleolus deep to the retinaculum. The medial malleolus serves as a pulley for the tibialis posterior and flexor digitorum longus, whereas the flexor hallucis longus passes beneath the posterior process of the talus and sustentaculum tali. Laterally, the peroneus brevis and longus tendons pass behind the fibula and are restrained by the superior and inferior peroneal retinacula. The peroneus longus has an added fulcrum at the peroneal trochlea (tubercle) and the undersurface of the cuboid. Posteriorly, the Achilles and plantaris tendons insert into the posteroinferior aspect of the calcaneus and are separated from it by a bursa.

ETIOLOGY OF INJURIES TO MUSCLES AND TENDONS

The etiology of muscle and tendon dysfunction is multifactorial (Table 19–1). Most injuries are probably the result of a combination of factors.[42, ,66, 77, 94, 142] A classification of injury based on causative factors, contributing factors, and relative frequency is presented in Table 19–2. Generally speaking, a tendon may become inflamed or subluxed, dislocate, or rupture.

TABLE 19–1.
Causes of Muscle and Tendon Dysfunction*

- Aging and degeneration
- Pathologic changes
  - Peritendinitis
    - Nonspecific
    - Arthritic
    - Infectious
    - Neoplastic
  - Myositis
  - Calcinosis
  - Vascular changes
- Bony changes
  - Fractures
  - Rough bone
  - Spurs/exostoses
- Tethering
  - Partial constriction
    - Trigger toes, tarsal tunnel
    - Peroneal constriction with a fractured os calcis
  - Complete tethering
    - Incarceration
    - Adhesive, including checkrein deformity
- Contractures
- Occupation
- Fatigue/stress
- Trauma
  - Direct
  - Indirect
- Iatrogenic conditions
- Congenital conditions

*From Plattner PF, Johnson KA: Tendons and bursae. In Helal B, Wilson D, editors: *The foot,* London, 1988, Churchill Livingstone, pp 581–613. Used by permission.

TABLE 19–2.
Classification of Muscle and Tendon Injuries*

- Direct injury
  - Laceration (open wound)
  - Blow or crush (closed wound)
- Indirect injury
  - Stretching force applied to contracting muscle
  - Unusually forceful contraction
- Spontaneous rupture (partial or complete)
  - Posttraumatic
    - Single injury (catastrophic failure)
    - Repetitive injury (fatigue failure)
  - Pathologic (disease of the tendon)
    - Degenerative
- Dislocation/subluxation of tendons
  - Acute
  - Chronic
- Iatrogenic (corticosteroids?)[104]

*From Plattner PF, Johnson KA: Tendons and bursae. In Helal B, Wilson D, editors: *The foot,* London, 1988, Churchill Livingstone, pp 581–613. Used by permission.

PATHOLOGY OF INJURIES TO MUSCLES AND TENDONS

In order to appreciate the pathology, a knowledge of the anatomy and physiology of tendons, tendon sheaths, and bursae is required.[80, 94, 192] A tendon consists of connective tissue composed of densely packed collagen fibers and protein mucopolysaccharides. These components are formed by the tenocyte and are grouped into bundles surrounded by the endotenon, which is a woven mesh of loose connective tissue. These bundles that make up the tendon are surrounded by a fine connective tissue sheath, the epitenon (paratenon), that is continuous with the endotenon. The entire tendon is surrounded by the paratenon, which is a loose, fatty areolar tissue. The paratenon is replaced by a synovial sheath or bursa when the tendon is subjected to increased local pressure or friction and therefore lies contiguous to the joints. The mesotenon, which is also called the vinculum, in some areas is a mesentery-like structure on the nonfriction side of a tendon that carries blood vessels.

The blood supply to the tendon is at its musculotendinous junction, at the tendo-osseous junction, and along its length by means of the paratenon, mesotenon, and tendon sheath. These structures are responsible for the segmental blood supply to most tendons.[34, 64, 111, 192, 210]

Following a tendon injury there is a standard sequence of histologic changes that occur. The inflammatory process involves multiple reactions at the site of injury, including a cellular reaction and humoral, vascular, and neurologic response. The characteristics of the inflammatory response depend upon the intensity

TABLE 19–3.
Sequential Changes of Tendon Healing*

Stage	Histologic Change	Time (Days)
I	Sparse inflammatory cellular infiltrate	0–1
II	Diffuse infiltration of leukocytes	1–4
III	Abundant granulation tissue	4–14
IV	Formation of undifferentiated connective tissue	>14

*From Plattner PF, Johnson KA: Tendons and bursae. In Helal B, Wilson D, editors: *The foot,* London, 1988, Churchill Livingstone, pp 581–613. Used by permission.

and duration of the insult; the type of injury, e.g., mechanical, bacterial, or chemical; the degree of cell degeneration and death, which ultimately influences the extent and progress of the inflammatory response; and the types of cells and tissues involved.[110]

An inflammatory response is usually designated as acute or chronic, depending upon the duration and type of cells that predominate in the inflamed tissue. In an acute inflammation the dominant changes are vascular and exudative, associated with the immigration and accumulation of leukocytes. Chronic inflammation is characterized by proliferative changes as the tissue attempts to repair and heal itself. The undifferentiated connective tissue that is formed may have changes of mucoid, fatty, hyaline, myxoid, or fibrinoid degeneration; cartilage metaplasia; calcification; or bone metaplasia.* A classification of healing following a rupture of the Achilles tendon and its sequence of histologic changes are presented in Table 19–3.[9, 10]

Using a classification based upon temporal considerations, Clancy classified the inflammatory response as acute, subacute, or chronic. An acute response is when the symptoms have been present for less than 2 weeks; subacute, between 2 and 6 weeks; and chronic, for greater than 6 weeks.

Peritendinitis

Peritendinitis is defined as an inflammatory process about tendons or portions of tendons that possess no sheath, as compared with tenosynovitis, which refers to an inflammatory process about tendons with sheaths.[125] Peritendinitis is an inclusive term denoting either tenosynovitis or paratendinitis. The term *tendinosis* is used to define a degenerative lesion in tendon tissue with no evidence of alteration of the paratenon.[175] By utilizing this classification, tendon disease could be a pure peritendinitis, peritendinitis with tendinosis, or tendinosis alone.

**References 10, 11, 29, 38, 39, 46, 59, 72, 129, 175, 224.*

TABLE 19–4.
Classification of Tendon Inflammation*

Peritendinitis: An inflammatory process involving peritendinous structures
- Paratendinitis: No synovial sheath
- Tenosynovitis: Synovial sheath

Peritendinitis with tendinosis: An inflammatory process involving peritendinous structures with a degenerative lesion of tendon tissue

Tendinosis: An asymptomatic degenerative process of tendon tissue without inflammation

*From Plattner PF, Johnson KA: Tendons and bursae. In Helal B, Wilson D, editors: *The foot,* London, 1988, Churchill Livingstone, pp 581–613. Used by permission.

Peritendinitis with tendinosis or tendinosis alone may eventually result in a rupture. This classification of tendon inflammation is presented in Table 19–4.

Lipscomb[125] analyzed 651 cases of nonspecific peritendinitis, 36% of which involved the foot and ankle. The anatomic distribution about the foot and ankle was as follows: tibialis anterior, 24%; Achilles tendon, 20%; tibialis posterior, 16%; peroneals, 16%; and others, 24%. The types of peritendinitis described are presented in Table 19–5. In looking at a series of running-associated injuries, Brody[21] noted that 30% involved the knee, 20% involved the Achilles tendon, 15% involved shin splints and stress fractures, and 10% involved plantar fasciitis.

Tendon Rupture

In his classic experiments with tendon rupture, McMaster[142] observed that a rupture does not occur when a normal muscle-tendon system is subjected to severe strain. He noted that approximately half of the fibers of a tendon had to be severed to permit immediate

TABLE 19–5.
Types of Peritendinitis*

Nonspecific	Infectious
Stenosing	Suppurative
Crepitans	Nonsuppurative
Hypertrophica	Tuberculous
Serosa chronica	Fungal
Arthritic	Syphilitic
Hypertrophic	Gonococcal
Rheumatoid	Neoplastic
Sarcoid	Xanthomatous
Gout	Lipomatous
Reiter's syndrome	Hemangiomatous
Collagen-vascular disease	Neurofibromatous
Scleroderma	

*From Plattner PF, Johnson KA: Tendons and bursae. In Helal B, Wilson D, editors: *The foot,* London, 1988, Churchill Livingstone, pp 581–613. Used by permission.

rupture when subjected to a severe strain and that even with 75% of the fibers severed, normal activity did not cause rupture. He concluded that true rupture of normal tendon does not occur and that rupture can take place only through diseased tendon substance. When rupture occurs, it does so at one of four sites: the insertion of the tendon into bone, the musculotendinous junction, the muscle belly, or the tendinous origin from bone.

Spontaneous ruptures in association with systemic and local disease have been reported. Patients with lupus erythematosus.[232] hyperparathyroidism,[37] or chronic acidosis because of lead neuropathy[154] have had tendon ruptures with and without trauma.

If the disease process is mild, microscopic changes, as one would expect, are minimal, but more extensive inflammation may lead to gross thickening of the peritendinous sheath with enlargement and fraying of the tendon. The final event in this process may result in a degenerated fibrotic tendon that ultimately will rupture. Clancy et al.[38, 39, 61] classified these chronic inflammatory changes as interstitial microscopic failure, central necrosis, frank partial rupture, and acute complete rupture. Microscopic damage to portions of the vascular supply of the tendon substance is an important factor in pathologic ruptures,[111, 192] as is aging, degeneration, and recurrent microtrauma.[46] Clancy et al.[38, 39] hypothesized that repetitive mechanical stress results in disruption of the collagen fibrils and that subsequent chronic inflammatory changes permanently alter the capacity of fibroblasts to synthesize collagen, thus setting up a vicious cycle, and rupture finally ensues.

In a study of 1,014 disruptions of muscles or tendons, Anzel et al.[8] noted that the upper extremity was involved six times more frequently than the lower. Males were afflicted more often than females. The average age of the patient was 40.5 years. The anatomic distribution of the 143 injuries to the lower extremity is presented in Table 19–6.

TABLE 19–6.
Location of 143 Tendon Disruptions in the Lower Extremity*

Muscle/Tendon	No.	Percentage
Quadriceps	54	38
Achilles tendon	22	15
Triceps surae	21	15
Extensors of the toes	16	11
Tibialis anterior	10	7
Tibialis posterior	3	2
Flexor hallucis longus	3	2
Peroneus longus	2	1.5
Peroneus tertius	2	1.5
Others	10	7
Total	143	100

*From Plattner PF, Johnson KA: Tendons and bursae. In Helal B, Wilson D, editors: *The foot,* London, 1988, Churchill Livingstone, pp 581–613. Used by permission.

BURSAE

A synovial bursa is a potential space with a secretory endothelial-type lining. Bursae are usually associated with joint cavities and are present at birth. They function to reduce friction and are usually located between the skin and bony projections and between tendons and prominences over which they must move (deep or subfascial).[31, 36, 100] Adventitial bursae are acquired after birth in response to repeated trauma (friction) to soft tissue over a bony prominence.[23, 107] They are most often subcutaneous or superficial and have no true endothelial lining. The lining almost appears to be a myxomatous or mucoid change in the connective tissue. Jahss'[95] classification of bursae according to location and type is presented in Table 19–7. Anatomic depictions and descriptions of numerous bursae about the foot have been described by Sarrafian[189] and Hartmann.[80]

Bywaters[30] believed that synovial bursae were a neglected group of anatomic structures of considerable importance, "subject to the same ills that joints are heir to." Roberts[175, 181] believed that bursitis was a neglected cause of disability. Although afflictions of these various bursae about the foot were described in the early literature, they appear to be less important in recent publications.[84, 180, 181]

Bursitis

Although various classifications of bursitis have appeared in the literature, the workable classification of pathologic bursae presented by Jahss is presented in Table 19–8. Probably the most common cause of bursitis about the foot and ankle is increased pressure or friction

TABLE 19–7.
Types of Bursae*

- Anatomic
  - Subfascial
    - Between tendon and bone
    - Between tendon or muscle and a bony prominence
    - Between tendons
  - Between tendons and ligaments
  - Subcutaneous
- Adventitial
  - Usually subcutaneous

*From Plattner PF, Johnson KA: Tendons and bursae. In Helal B, Wilson D, editors: *The foot,* London, 1988, Churchill Livingstone, pp 581–613. Used by permission.

TABLE 19–8.
Classification of Bursal Irritation*

Noninflammatory
Pressure-induced
Traumatic
Spontaneous
Inflammatory
Gout
Rheumatoid arthritis
Suppurative
Calcified or ossified

*From Plattner PF, Johnson KA: Tendons and bursae. In Helal B, Wilson D, editors: *The foot,* London, 1988, Churchill Livingstone, pp 581–613. Used by permission.

over a bony area that leads to an adventitial bursa, usually due to ill-fitting shoes. Layfer[116] referred to this condition as a "last bursitis." Bony prominences and tendons about the malleoli, calcaneus, and metatarsophalangeal and interphalangeal joints make the foot particularly susceptible to this condition. Usually symptomatic relief is obtained by removing the pressure. This would consist of modification of the shoe wear such as use of a wider and deeper toe box, stretching of the shoe at localized areas, a softer heel counter, or various types of orthoses and pads. At times, aspiration of the inflamed bursa is useful in decompressing the area and ruling out a metabolic, rheumatoid, or infectious cause.[144, 157, 167, 187] A steroid preparation can be injected locally, provided that there is no contraindication, e.g., sepsis.[6, 82] If conservative management fails, there are numerous surgical procedures that can be utilized to relieve pressure by removing the underlying exostosis or bony prominence or correcting an underlying deformity.

Bursitis Associated With an Intermetatarsal Phalangeal Bursa

This bursa lies between the metatarsophalangeal joints dorsal to the transverse metatarsal ligament, whereas the neurovascular bundle passes plantar to the ligament. The bursae in web spaces 1, 2, and 3 are constant, whereas the bursa in the fourth web space is absent in 80% of cases.[80] The bursae extend about 1 cm distal to the transverse metatarsal ligament in the second and third web spaces, whereas it is at the same level as the distal margin of the transverse metatarsal ligament in the fourth web space.[16]

Intermetatarsal Bursitis

Inflammation of the intermetatarsal phalangeal bursa, regardless of the cause, may be a source of pain in the forefoot in the region of the metatarsal heads. Bossley and Cairney[16] pointed out that because of the close proximity of the plantar digital nerve and the intermetatarsal bursa in the second and third web spaces, the classic symptoms of Morton's metatarsalgia could be caused not only by a neuroma but also by an intermetatarsal phalangeal bursitis with pressure on a normal nerve. Shepherd[198] believed that bursal swelling could be a cause of divergence of the toes bordering on the affected web space. Lateral compression of the metatarsal head squeezes the inflamed bursa, thereby reproducing the pain, and may cause a click. Since the bursa is of synovial origin, its inflammation may be one of the first manifestations of rheumatoid arthritis in the foot.[165, 198] Bursae in patients with rheumatoid arthritis are often thick-walled, with lymphocytic infiltration, villous proliferation, fibrinoid necrosis, and the presence of rice bodies.[16, 98, 198] Radiographs of the foot should be closely inspected for evidence of erosion of the metatarsal heads.

Injection of a steroid preparation into the bursa may affect relief. If symptoms persist, surgical excision of the bursa can be carried out.

Bursitis About the Posterior Aspect of the Heel

The Achilles tendon at its insertion is between the superficial subcutaneous bursa of the Achilles tendon and the deep subfascial retrocalcaneal bursa.[80, 189] The superficial adventitial bursa forms in response to chronic trauma. The retrocalcaneal bursa is a synovial-lined structure that is constantly present and is situated between the posterosuperior end of the calcaneus and the deep surface of the Achilles tendon.

Achilles Tendon Bursitis and Retrocalcaneal Bursitis

Irritation at the posterosuperior aspect of the heel has various causes and has been referred to by many terms in the literature, as indicated in Table 19–9. After observing the many causes for inflammation in this region, it becomes obvious that it is important to anatomically distinguish between inflammatory lesions involving the subcutaneous and subfascial bursal structures at the insertion of the Achilles tendon (bursitis) and those of the peritendinous lining of the Achilles tendon (peritendinitis).

When one is dealing with inflammation of the superficial, subcutaneous, adventitial bursa of the Achilles tendon, tenderness is palpable over the calcaneus at the tendon insertion. The formation of superficial bursitis seems to be related to mechanical factors, mainly chronic irritation from friction between the shoe and a prominence of the posterosuperior aspect of the calcaneus. It is more common in women than men.[45, 102]

TABLE 19–9.

Terms Used for Inflammation of Heel Bursae in the Literature*

Achillodynia[4, 30, 76]
Albert's disease[4]
Retrocalcanean bursitis[103, 157, 234]
Bursitis retrocalcanea Achilli (Steffensen and Evensen, 1958)[209]
Bursitis retrocalcanearis[65]
Inflammation of the deep calcaneal bursa[85]
Bursitis of the posterior part of the heel[103]
Bursitis Achillea[76]
Achillobursitis (Zadek, 1939)[239]
Tendo-Achilles bursitis[48, 103]
Winter heel (Nisbet, 1954)[159]
Pump bumps[48, 168]
Prow-beak deformity (Ruch, 1974)[184]
High prow heels (Miller & Buhr, 1969)[148]
Heel tuberosities[19]
Haglund's disease, syndrome[15, 76, 83, 168]
Sever's disease (apophysitis of the os calcis) (Sever, 1912; Ferguson and Gingrich, 1957)[57, 196]
Knobby heels (Miller & Buhr, 1969)[147]
Calcaneus altus (Miller & Buhr, 1969)[147]
Cucumber heels (Miller & Buhr, 1969)[147]

*From Plattner PF, Johnson KA: Tendons and bursae. In Helal B, Wilson D, editors: *The foot,* London, 1988, Churchill Livingstone, pp 581–613. Used by permission.

The physical examination demonstrates a noticeable bursal thickening over the bony prominence lateral to the tendon attachment.

If the deep subfascial synovial retrocalcaneal bursa is inflamed, the tenderness is usually palpable anterior to the tendon. Men are usually more afflicted than women.[102] Since the bursa has a synovial lining, inflammation may be a prodrome of rheumatoid arthritis or one of its variants such as Reiter's syndrome.* Lateral radiographs of the calcaneus should be critically assessed to look for the presence of erosions, which would be suggestive of an inflammatory articular disorder. According to Keck and Kelly,[103] there is no conclusive evidence to implicate a prominence of the superior portion of the calcaneal tuberosity as a major factor in producing retrocalcaneal bursitis. See Chapter 20 for a discussion of the prominent posterior superior surface of the calcaneus.

ACHILLES TENDON

Physical Findings

Disease of the Achilles tendon is probably a spectrum of manifestations on a continuum from peritendinitis to tendinosis to rupture.[38, 39, 72, 121, 175] Clinically, it is important to differentiate between bursitis at the posterior aspect of the heel, Achilles peritendinitis, Achilles peritendinitis with tendinosis, and partial rupture. The distinction between these clinical entities is not always easy from clinical findings, but it is important if one is to prevent a partial rupture from becoming complete.* As a rule, the diagnosis of an acute, complete rupture is not difficult to make because the history is very characteristic, although most published series estimate that the diagnosis is missed in 20% to 25% of cases since it is unfamiliar to many physicians.[9, 115, 158, 177] The physician may be misled because the patient may minimize the symptoms after the acute pain has subsided, and by the time of physical examination some plantar flexion is maintained because of the remaining plantar flexors. If the patient presents late, the swelling and hemorrhage about the rupture may obscure the ends of the tendon and make it more difficult to make a precise diagnosis.[88, 115, 177] Rupture of the Achilles tendon usually occurs 2 to 6 cm proximal to the insertion, where the vascularity has been demonstrated to be decreased[91, 111] (Fig 19–1). When a chronic rupture is present, the defect in the tendon becomes more difficult to palpate, although a defect in the tendon can often be noted. Weakness in plantar flexion, particularly brought out by having the patient attempt to stand on the tiptoes of one foot, is a constant finding brought about by the lengthening of the tendon. A summary of the differentiating factors of peritendinitis, partial rupture, and complete rupture is presented in Table 19–10.

The Thompson "squeeze test" is very useful in diagnosing a complete rupture.[221, 222] This test is performed by having the patient in a prone position and squeezing the calf muscle just distal to its maximum girth. This will bring about plantar flexion of the ankle joint. The test is positive when there is no plantar flexion of the ankle, which indicates a complete rupture of the Achilles tendon.

Radiographic Examination

Although several different types of radiographic studies have been advocated for diagnosing a ruptured Achilles tendon, computed tomography (CT) and magnetic resonance imaging (MRI) are probably the most effective tests in the diagnosis of ankle and foot tendon injuries. MRI is the preferred study because of its supe-

**References 19, 31, 32, 83, 102, 135, 165, 233.*

**References 38, 39, 47, 68, 72, 109, 121, 130, 175, 202, 203.*

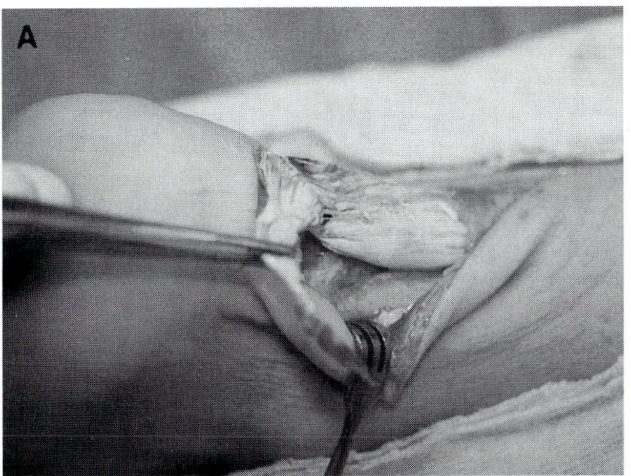

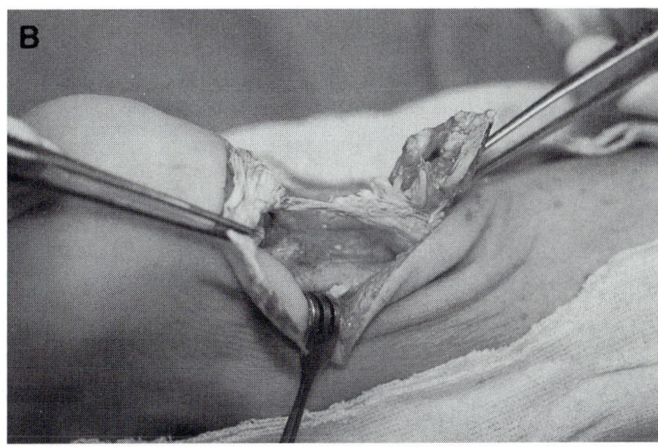

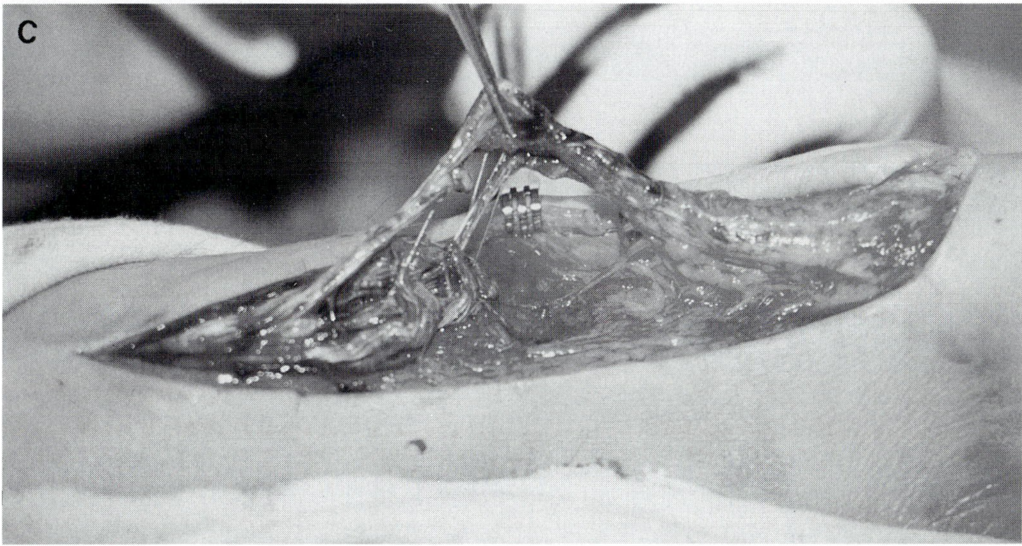

FIG 19–1.
Examples of acute Achilles tendon ruptures. **A,** complete rupture with minimal fraying of the tendon. **B,** separation of the fragments, demonstrating lack of fraying of the tendon. **C,** Achilles tendon rupture with marked fraying of the tendon.

rior soft-tissue contrast resolution, multiplanar capabilities, and lack of ionizing radiation.

MRI has been shown to be useful in classifying Achilles tendon injuries and distinguishing between peritendinitis, tendinosis, incomplete rupture, and complete rupture.[231] This diagnostic technique is most useful in differentiating inflammatory reactions about the tendon from degenerative changes affecting the structural integrity of the tendon itself. This distinction is an important one that may affect treatment in select groups of highly motivated individuals such as athletes (especially runners) for whom surgical treatment may be suggested for chronic posterior heel pain. The vast majority of patients, however, can be treated successfully by nonoperative measures, so the routine use of MRI in patients with posterior heel pain probably would not influence the initial conservative management or prove to be cost-effective.

Treatment

Peritendinitis

The initial treatment of the inflammatory process should be nonoperative. Nonoperative treatment is outlined in Table 19–11.

Surgery is generally indicated only in the patient who has not responded to nonoperative treatment for several months.* The surgical management of peritendinitis usually consists of exploration with excision of

**References 38, 39, 47, 109, 117, 120, 194, 202, 203.*

TABLE 19–10.

Differentiating Factors of Peritendinitis, Peritendinitis With Tendinosis and Partial Rupture, and Tendinosis With Acute, Complete Rupture*

Factor	Peritendinitis	Peritendinitis With Tendinosis and Partial Rupture	Tendinosis With Acute, Complete Rupture
Symptoms	Acute	Subacute, chronic	Immediate
Audible snap	No	Maybe	Yes
Weakness	Yes	Yes	Yes
Limp	Yes	Yes	Yes
Swelling	Yes	Yes	Yes
Tenderness	Yes	Yes	Yes
Defect in tendon	No	Maybe	Yes
Crepitus	Maybe	Maybe	No
Passive dorsiflexion	Decreased	Decreased	Increased
Thompson test	Negative	Negative	Positive
Atrophy	No	Yes	Proximal calf belly retraction
Ability to stand on tiptoes	Probably	Possibly	No

*From Plattner PF, Johnson KA: Tendons and bursae. In Helal B, Wilson D, editors: *The foot,* London, 1988, Churchill Livingstone, pp 581–613. Used by permisison.

the involved peritendinous structures and resection of any diseased or degenerated tissue. If tendinosis is present and resection of diseased tendon tissue is performed, some type of surgical reconstruction of the tendon may be necessary. In that select patient population of highly motivated or competitive athletes who have failed nonoperative treatment, surgical management produces good or excellent results in 70% to 90% of cases.[120, 194]

Ruptured Achilles Tendon

Nonoperative vs. Operative Treatment.—There is a great deal of controversy concerning the proper treatment of this condition, with more than 400 articles published on treatment of the ruptured tendon.[13, 52] The controversy centers around those that favor surgical repair with postoperative casting* and those that advocate only cast immobilization.† For many years the technique of casting in an equinus position to minimize tension at the site of rupture was an accepted method of treatment, but questions have been raised regarding this technique. In one report, selective atrophy of the soleus muscle has been reported if tension is not kept on the musculotendinous unit during healing.[75]

The proponents of closed treatment believe that the success of their method is based upon the ability of the Achilles tendon to reconstitute itself when it is ruptured. This trait has been demonstrated both experimentally and clinically.[122, 128, 129, 190, 223] They believe that the functional differences in strength, power, and endurance are not statistically significant when groups of operated and nonoperated patients are compared.[117, 118, 160] Obviously, the nonoperative approach avoids the risks of anesthesia and the many complications of open surgery. In a review of 25 reports documenting 2,647 ruptures, the following major complications were noted: fistulas, 3%; necrosis of the skin and tendon, 2%; rerupture, 2%; and deep infection, 1%.[160]

**References 53, 91, 96, 120, 170, 183, 196.*
†References 67, 117–119, 160, 161, 210, 211.

TABLE 19–11.

Types of Nonoperative Treatment of Peritendinitis*

- Patient education
  - Proper warm-up, cool down
  - Reduction or cessation of athletic activity
    - No running on hills
    - No interval training
    - Avoidance of training on hard surfaces
- Proper equipment
  - Good running shoes (flexible, cushioned soles)
  - Orthoses (heel lifts, University of California Biomechanics Laboratory [UCBL] inserts, inlays)
- Physical therapy
  - Massage
  - Stretching exercises
  - Ultrasound, heat, ice
- Immobilization
  - Taping
  - Crutches
  - Casting
- Medication
  - Nonsteroidal anti-inflammatory drugs
  - Corticosteroid injections?[103]

*From Plattner PF, Johnson KA: Tendons and bursae. In Helal B, Wilson D, editors: *The foot,* London, 1988, Churchill Livingstone, pp 581–613. Used by permission.

Minor complications included hematoma, superficial infection, granulomas, and skin adhesions in another 5% of cases. The major drawback of closed treatment is stated to be the higher incidence of rerupture and questionably inferior dynametric data.*

Nonoperative treatment consists of a gravity equinus cast for 8 to 12 weeks with cast changes at monthly intervals to gradually increase the amount of dorsiflexion.[117–119] Following removal of the cast, heel elevations and sometimes a double upright ankle/foot orthosis with a stop at the neutral position for an additional 4 to 8 weeks are utilized.[215]

Those who advocate open surgical treatment do so on biomechanical grounds and state that immediate repair allows for closure of the gap, which maintains the musculotendinous unit at its proper physiologic length: tension ratio.[133, 134] By maintaining the proper physiologic length: tension ratio this treatment method should provide optimal strength, power, and endurance. In theory, the site of repair may contain less scar tissue and therefore have greater mechanical strength and lead to a decreased rate of rerupture. Whether this technique is advantageous for the patient with a delayed diagnosis is less clear.[122] In the patient with a delayed diagnosis, often the gap cannot be closed without lengthening the tendon; therefore, the biomechanical advantage of the immediate repair is compromised.[2, 58] Rather than performing a repair procedure in such cases, one is sometimes faced with a rather difficult reconstruction to close the gap.

It has been suggested that an acute rupture of the Achilles tendon can be satisfactorily treated with nonoperative casting when the diagnosis is made within 48 hours of injury but that surgical management is the treatment of choice when the diagnosis has been delayed for more than a week.[33] Patients who were treated more than 1 week after the injury with nonoperative treatment had inferior results with respect to the power of plantar flexion. Although Achilles tendon ruptures have been successfully treated at 4 weeks or more without surgery,[67] operative intervention for such neglected ruptures can significantly improve the strength and function of the triceps surae.[14]

The literature abounds with methods of repair and reconstruction.†

For acute, complete injuries, open direct suturing with buried stitches is preferred if surgical treatment is selected (Figs 19–2 and 19–3). A percutaneous method

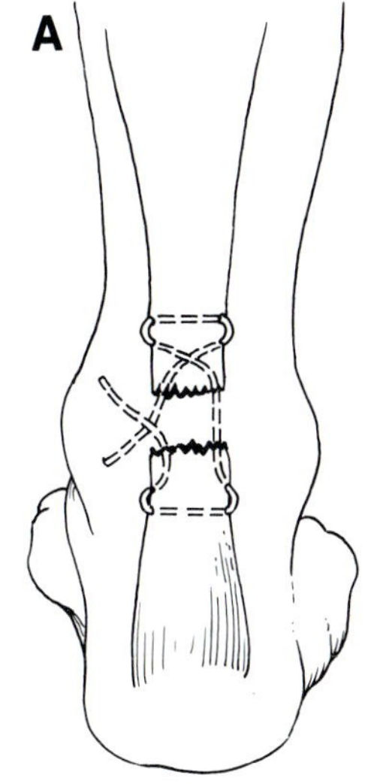

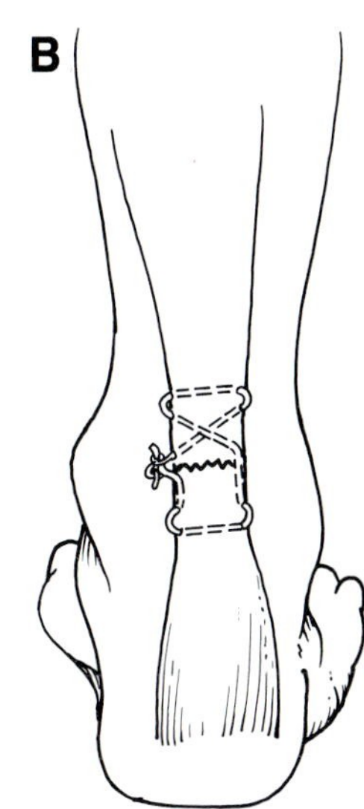

FIG 19–2.
A and **B,** a Bunnell or box-type suture technique may be used to approximate the ruptured Achilles tendon. The repair is reinforced with interrupted sutures.

of repair in which the strength of the repair compares favorably with the standard open repair has been described.[133] This technique presumably bridges the gap between nonsurgical treatment and surgical treatment; excellent results have been reported with closed percutaneous repairs of acute Achilles ruptures, and many risks of open surgical treatment are avoided with virtually no complications. In a series of 18 patients, minor wound infection developed in only 2 patients, and there were no reruptures. This procedure has received enthusiastic reports; however, some investigators who have attempted to duplicate this procedure have met with technical difficulties, and one report had a 12% rerupture rate.[18] The disadvantage of this technique is that the tendon ends cannot be opposed under direct vision, so it is difficult to check the tendon length, apposition, and tension and to assess the adequacy of fixation. Therefore, the results of percutaneous repair are acceptable, with recovery of motion and strength essentially equal to open surgery. The rate of rerupture is higher than with open procedures, but probably better than with closed treatment.

Neglected or undiagnosed Achilles tendon ruptures represent a difficult problem in surgical repair due to retraction of the proximal tendon and excessive scar formation at the rupture site. End-to-end anastomosis is virtually impossible since contracture of the muscle occurs quickly. Various methods of reconstruction to span the gap between the ruptured tendon and posterosuperior surface of the calcaneus have been described: procedures that turn down a strip of tendon or have bridged

---

**References 22, 53, 91, 93, 160, 196, 199.*

†References 1, 5, 9, 17, 24, 27, 35, 58, 89, 123, 124, 132–134, 136, 156, 164, 176, 193, 215, 219, 226.

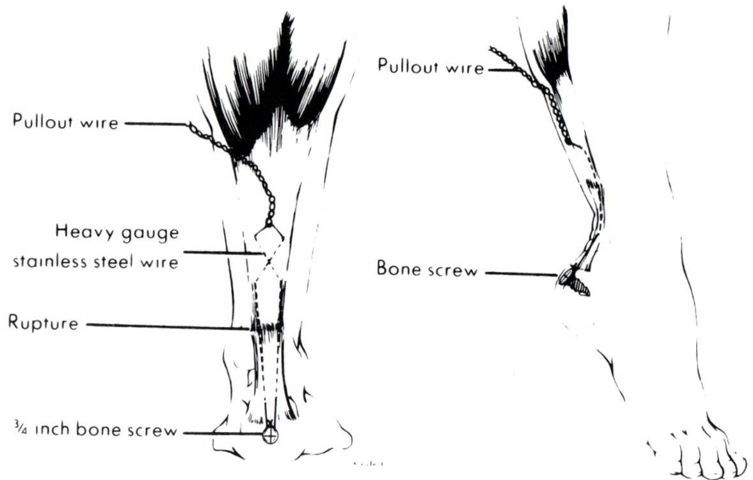

FIG 19–3.
L. D. Howard technique for repair of Achilles tendon. Utilizing a pull-out wire technique. (Courtesy of J. B. Hann III.)

the defect with a graft of fascia lata; lengthening of the tendon at the musculotendinous junction in a V-Y manner; resection of diseased tendon with direct suturing; transfer of nearby tendons such as the peroneus brevis, plantaris, or flexor digitorum longus; and the use of synthetic materials such as carbon fiber or Dacron polyester (Fig 19–4).

For a chronic, neglected, or undiagnosed rupture of the Achilles tendon in a patient with pain, weakness, and a gap between the ruptured portions of the tendon, transfer of the flexor digitorum longus as an autogenous graft to span the gap is an ideal choice.[168] This transfer utilizes a viable, readily available tendon structure with an intact vascular supply and suitable biomechanical characteristics. Transfer of the flexor digitorum longus retains its function as a plantar flexor of the foot without running the potential risk of upsetting the balance between the evertors and invertors of the foot, which may occur if the peroneus brevis muscle is used for transfer instead. After surgery, immobilization is similar to that used in the nonoperative approach (Fig 19–5).

Complications following reconstruction of a neglected rupture of the Achilles tendon are the same as those following primary repair of an acute Achilles tendon rupture. Because of a significant amount of scar tissue present, the possibility of a sural nerve injury is increased. Likewise, wound healing problems may be higher owing to the extensive dissection necessary for reconstruction. Nevertheless, the marked lack of endurance and strength with a neglected Achilles tendon rupture and the impairment of gait make reconstruction of the neglected Achilles tendon rupture a definite consideration.

Results

At this time the best study assessing the results of surgical and nonsurgical treatment is that presented by Nistor.[160] This study was prospective and randomized

FIG 19–4.
Various methods of reconstruction for untreated Achilles tendon ruptures. **A,** one or two strips of fascia from the gastrocnemius-soleus complex may be turned down and used to reinforce the repair. **B,** repair utilizing fascia lata strips *a,* Rupture with gap, *b,* three fascial strips used to bridge the gap; *c,* a sheet of fascia used to cover and reinforce the repair. (**B** redrawn from Bugg EI Jr, Boyd BM: *Clin Orthop* 56:73–75, 1968.) **C,** repair utilizing fascial strip from proximal gastroc-soleus complex. *a,* distally based fascial strip is passed transversely through proximal tendon fragment. *b,* the strip is woven across the gap. *c,* enlarged diagram of *b.* (**C** from Bosworth DM: *J Bone Joint Surg [Am]* 38:111–114, 1956. Used by permission.) **D,** repair using V-Y gastroplasty. *a,* a V-shaped incision is made in the aponeurosis. The limbs of the V should be one and a half times longer than the width of the gap in the Achilles tendon. *b,* the intermediate segment is advanced distally and the gap is closed and repaired. The proximal incision is closed as a Y in the lengthened position. (**D** redrawn from Abraham E, Stirnaman JE: *J Bone Joint Surg* [Am] 57:253–255, 1975.) **E,** repair utilizing peroneus brevis tendon. The peroneus brevis is isolated and detached from its insertion into the fifth metatarsal. *a,* a transverse drill hole is placed in the calcaneus. *b,* the peroneus brevis is transferred through the drill hole. *c,* the tendon is sutured to itself and to the Achilles tendon proximally and distally.

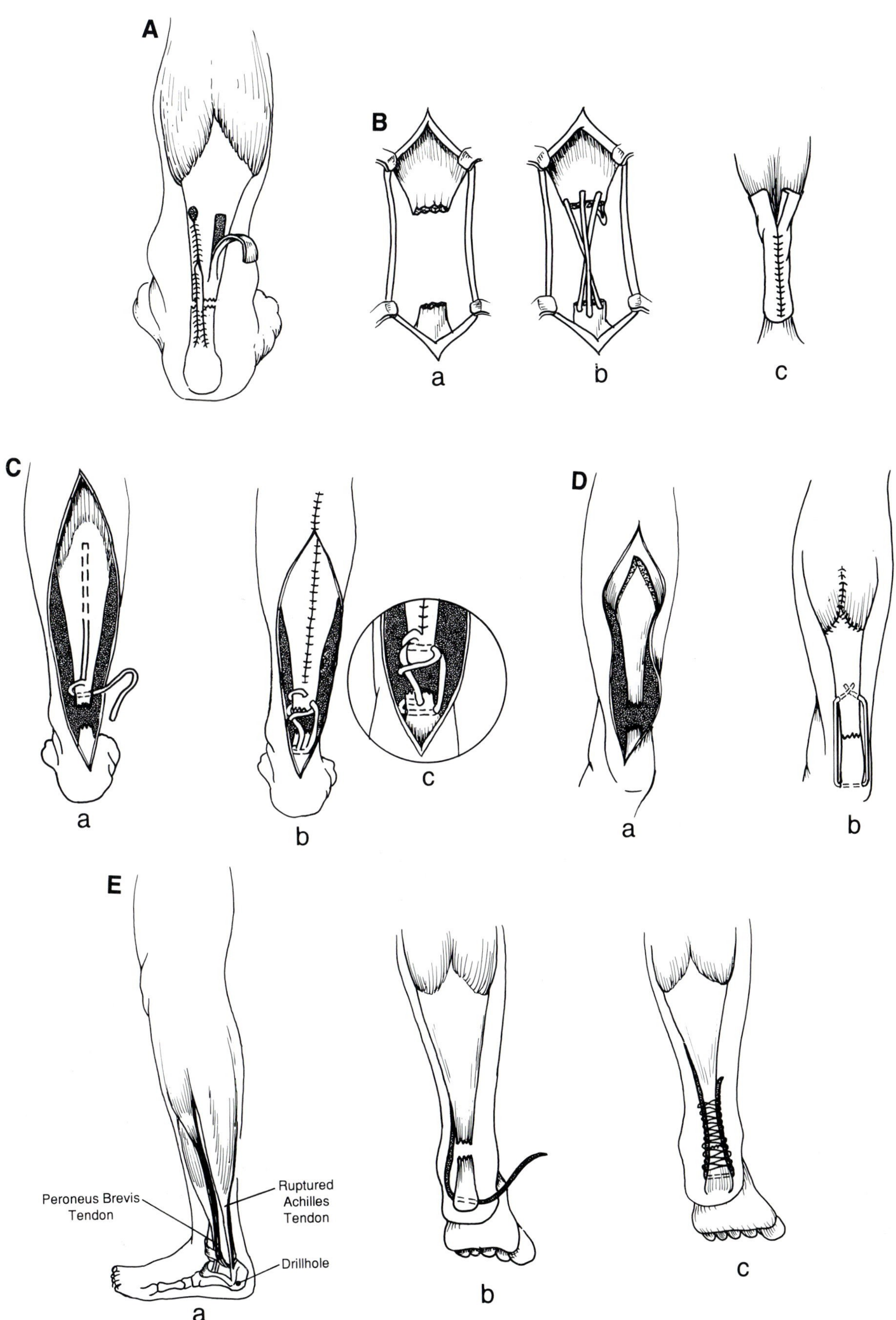
A
B
a
b
c
C
a
b
c
D
a
b
E
Peroneus Brevis Tendon
Ruptured Achilles Tendon
Drillhole
a
b
c

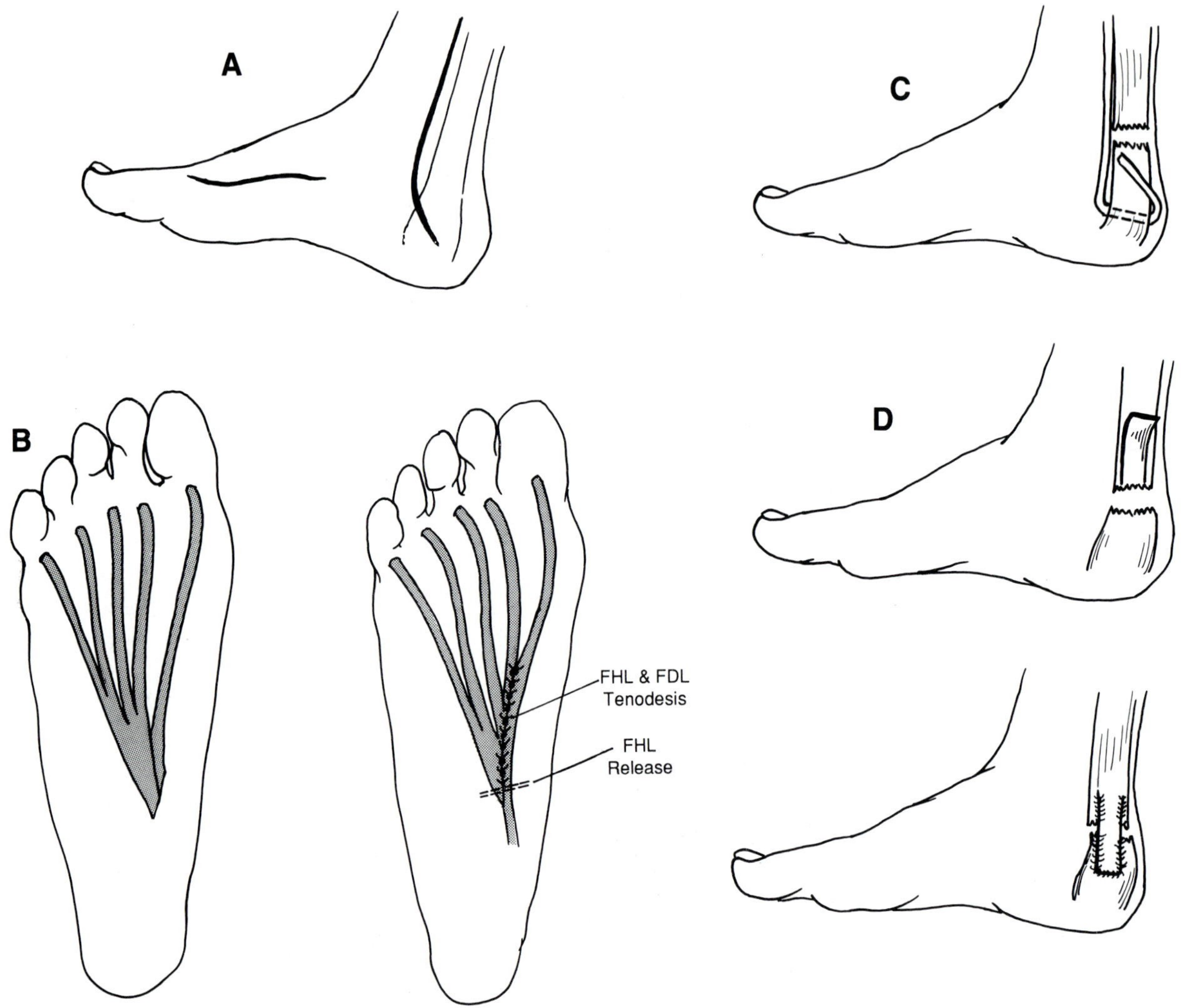

FIG 19–5.
Delayed repair of ruptured Achilles tendon using flexor digitorum longus transfer. **A,** operative technique demonstrating incisions. **B,** tenodesis of the flexor digitorum longus stump to the flexor hallucis longus. **C,** flexor digitorum longus pulled through drill hole in calcaneus. **D,** augmentation of spanned gap by turndown of fascial strip from gastroc-soleus complex. (Redrawn from Mann RA, Holmes GB, Seale KS, et al: *J Bone J Surg [Am]* 73:214–219, 1991.)

and therefore avoided a bias in selecting which patients would receive a particular type of treatment. He concluded that nonoperative treatment offers advantages over operative treatment (see Table 19–12). The major problems of nonoperative treatment are (1) the higher incidence of tendon rerupture following cast removal and (2) the persistent relative weakness and lengthening of the cast-treated triceps surae that sometimes occurs. The main problems with operative treatment are (1) the operative risk and complications inherent to surgery in this area and (2) the time and cost of hospitalization.

A more recent review of the literature comparing surgical treatment with nonsurgical treatment found a 1.54% rate of rerupture (12/777) for surgically treated patients vs. a 17.7% (40/226) rate of rerupture for nonsurgically treated patients.[237] These authors concluded that the difference in cost between surgical and nonsurgical treatment, including the cost of rerupture treatment, may not be significant.

The ultimate decision as to which form of treatment to use must be individualized and depends upon the physician, the patient, and the circumstances involved. Probably the persons who benefit most from operative treatment are the young, active individuals or high-performance athletes, where the increased risk of rerupture (10% to 17%) following nonoperative treatment is unacceptable.

TABLE 19–12.
Considerations in the Choice of Treatment of Acute Rupture of the Achilles Tendon*

Consideration	Type of Treatment: Nonoperative (Casting Alone)	Type of Treatment: Operative (Operation and Casting)
Morbidity	Decreased	Increased
Surgical risk	None	Increased
Hospital stay (cost)	Decreased	Increased
Dynametric data	Inferior	Superior
Rerupture	10%	2%
Compliance with rehabilitation	Less	More

*From Plattner PF, Johnson KA: Tendons and bursae. In Helal B, Wilson D, editors: *The foot,* London, 1988, Churchill Livingstone, pp 581–613. Used by permission.

PERONEAL TENDONS

A spontaneous rupture of the peroneal tendons is rare, although peritendinitis and traumatic dislocations are probably more common than recognized. Recently, peroneal involvement with peritendinitis rupture and dislocation is receiving more attention in the literature. Any of these conditions may be a cause for persistent lateral ankle pain and swelling, which are commonly believed to be residuals of disruption of the lateral ligaments and ankle instability. The diagnosis of "chronic residual from lateral ankle ligament sprain" is nonspecific and can include the following:

1. Ligamentous instability
2. Peroneal tendon subluxation
3. Longitudinal attrition of the peroneus brevis tendon
4. An anomalous peroneus quartus causing impingement
5. Stenosing peritendinitis or pseudotumors in the peroneal tendon sheath
6. Valgus hindfoot with lateral impingement at the subtalar joint
7. Subtalar joint arthritis

Anatomy

The peroneal tendons pass within a common synovial sheath that begins approximately 4 cm proximal to the lateral malleolus where they are restrained by the superior retinaculum. As the tendons pass behind the lateral malleolus along its distal margin, a fibrocartilaginous ridge lends increased stability.[138] The retromalleolar sulcus was noted to be very shallow in 82% of cases and not well formed in 18% according to Edwards.[54] After leaving the fibro-osseous tunnel inferior to the lateral malleolus, each tendon enters a separate sheath. The sheath about the peroneus brevis ends just proximal to the insertion of the tendon into the tuberosity at the base of the fifth metatarsal. The sheath about the peroneus longus tendon ends as the tendon passes beneath the cuboid, after which a second tendon sheath envelops the peroneus longus as it exits the canal formed by the long plantar ligament and cuboid groove.

The anatomy of additional peroneal muscles, i.e., peroneus quartus, the peroneus accessorius, and the peroneus digiti minimi, is nicely described in the study by Sobel et al.[204, 206] The most important of these is the peroneus quartus, present in 21.7% of cadaver specimens. The size, origin, and insertion of this muscle varied, but in 63% of the specimens the muscle took its origin from the muscular portion of the peroneus brevis in the lower third of the leg and inserted on the peroneal tubercle of the calcaneus. The clinical relevance of this tendon is that it can be used for reconstructive procedures about the lateral aspect of the ankle such as anterior dislocation of the peroneal tendons and reconstruction of the lateral ankle ligaments.[147] Its use in these applications, when present, can avoid problems related to sacrificing the peroneus brevis tendon, which can result in restricted inversion of the foot or compromised eversion of the foot associated with loss of the peroneus brevis muscle.

Peritendinitis

Nonspecific and posttraumatic peroneal tenosynovitis has been discussed in numerous articles.* The most common type of tenosynovitis is a stenosis of the peroneal tendon at three anatomic sites: posterior to the lateral malleolus (peroneal sulcus), at the level of the peroneal trochlea (tubercle) of the calcaneus, and at the undersurface of the cuboid.[25] It is believed that trauma is the major factor attributed to precipitating tenosynovitis and may include a fractured fibula, inversion ankle injuries, direct trauma to the peroneal tubercle, and calcaneal fractures with or without calcaneofibular impingement of the peroneal tendon sheath.[92] A congenitally enlarged peroneal tubercle or sesamoid bone in the peroneus longus as well as a compressive tenosynovitis has also been implicated.[28]

Clinical Findings

Pain and swelling distal to the lateral malleolus over the peroneal tendon sheath are suggestive of peritendinitis. The symptoms are aggravated by bringing the

**References 7, 25, 43, 60, 166, 224, 230.*

foot into plantar flexion and inversion. Physical examination often reveals an antalgic gait, tenderness and swelling along the peroneal tendon sheath, and limitation, particularly of subtalar joint inversion. Injection of a local anesthetic into the tendon sheath will usually relieve the patient's symptoms. Peroneal tenography may demonstrate a complete block or constriction of the sheath at the inferior peroneal retinaculum.[60, 218] A pseudotumor of the peroneal tendons may be palpable along the course of the tendons. It should be kept in mind that this may represent the os peroneum, which is located in the peroneus longus tendon at about the level of the cuboid.

Treatment

Conservative management is determined by the severity of the symptom complex. Nonoperative measures include anti-inflammatory medications, immobilization, stretching exercises, physical therapy such as ice and/or heat, a cloth or neoprene anklet, and occasionally an injection of a steroid preparation into the tendon sheath. Shoe modifications may include a medial heel wedge to roll the calcaneus away from the peroneal tendons, a wider heel for increased stability, a rocker-bottom sole, or elevation of the heel. If conservative measures fail, surgical exploration with tenolysis or debridement may be necessary. If the main problem involves the subtalar joint, a subtalar arthrodesis may be indicated.

Rupture

Chronic longitudinal attrition or rupture of the peroneus brevis tendon at or distal to the fibular groove of the lateral malleolus is a more common degenerative defect than previously recognized.[113, 185, 204–207] This lesion was noted in 11.3% of specimens, and the longitudinal rupture averaged 1.9 cm in length.[206] The significance of this finding is that chronic lateral ankle pain disability may be related to attritional changes of the peroneus brevis tendon in the fibular groove. The etiology of this defect is felt to be secondary to the compressional wedgelike frictional force of the overlying peroneus longus tendon against the splayed-out peroneus brevis tendon as it passes around the lateral malleolus in the fibular groove with tendon excursion.

Diagnosis

In a clinical series of 47 ankle ligament reconstructions, peroneus brevis tendon lesions were observed in 11 ankles of 10 patients.[225] All patients had a history of chronic recurrent ankle sprains with symptoms of pain more disabling than instability. At the time of surgery there was gross evidence of chronic inflammation associated with through-and-through defects on the deep aspect of the tendon. None of the patients had any evidence of rheumatoid or seronegative arthritis, gout, steroid injections, infections, or connective tissue disorders. The common thread that frequently occurred was a history of significant trauma to the ankle with abnormal repetitive stress to the peroneus brevis tendon over a long period of time.

The possibility of chronic longitudinal attritional rupture of the peroneus brevis tendon should be considered in patients with chronic lateral ankle pain, swelling, instability, or symptoms suggestive of stenosis. MRI is the diagnostic test of choice both to assess longitudinal attrition of the peroneus brevis tendon as well as to identify the presence of the peroneus quartus tendon, which may be useful in lateral ankle ligament reconstruction.[207]

Closed, subcutaneous rupture of one or both of the peroneal tendons is rare when compared with the more common attritional or longitudinal rupture of the peroneus brevis tendon.[2, 28, 57, 169, 212, 217, 220] Rupture of the peroneus longus tendon through a fracture of the os peroneum sesamoid or distal to the sesamoid bone adjacent to the cuboid tunnel has been surgically documented only a few times.[169, 220] Several mechanisms have been offered to account for this lesion: rupture of the tendon associated with peritendinitis, a crush injury due to a direct blow to the area of the os peroneum on the lateral aspect of the foot, failure of the tendon or bone under tension in an attempted forced eversion of the supinating foot, pushing off with the foot in inversion, or increased stress where the tendon changes direction at the cuboid tunnel.

Careful examination of the radiographs with multiple views to distinguish an avulsion fracture of the cuboid from the os peroneum, as well as differentiate an os peroneum fracture from a congenitally multipartite os peroneum, is important. Serial radiographs, especially with opposite comparison views, are extremely helpful in identifying an abnormal position of the sesamoid bone or migration.

Treatment

Initially most patients with chronic lateral ankle pain and swelling are treated nonoperatively with nonsteroidal anti-inflammatory medication, restricted activity, and immobilization or strapping. If symptoms persist and are disabling enough in spite of casting for 6 to 8 weeks, surgical intervention may be suggested. Most articles suggest that when surgical intervention is suggested, it has been for a presumptive diagnosis of chronic lateral ligamentous instability or tenosynovitis of the peroneal sheath. In the cases described where surgery took place, either a partial or complete rupture of the peroneal tendon(s) was discovered with pathologic changes suggestive of peritendinitis, tendinosis, or both.

Surgical repair consisted of tenolysis, excision of diseased tendon tissue, end-to-end repair if possible, or tenodesis of the peroneus longus and brevis tendons. Follow-up revealed satisfactory results.

These reports emphasize the importance of considering peritendinitis and rupture of the peroneal tendons in the differential diagnosis of any patient with chronic lateral ankle pain.

Traumatic Dislocation

As a general rule, dislocations of tendons about the ankle are uncommon. The peroneal tendons are most frequently involved and are usually associated with athletic endeavors such as skiing, soccer, ice skating, and, less frequently, basketball or football.* Traumatic dislocation of the posterior tibial tendon is a rare occurrence.[114]

The acute peroneal dislocation is frequently unrecognized and misdiagnosed as an ankle sprain, particularly if the examining physician is unaware of the clinical entity. This lack of treatment may result in chronic dislocations. Most of the literature regarding this problem deals with operations designed to stabilize the peroneal tendons.†

Classification

Eckert and Davis described their experience with 73 acute anterior dislocations of the peroneal tendon with injury to the retinaculum and divided the injury into three specific types.[51] Oden, in 1987,[163] modified the classification of Eckert and Davis by adding a rare type IV tear of the posterior retinaculum (Table 19–13 and Fig 19–6).

After examination of the groove present in 178 fibulas, Edwards, in 1928, observed that it was usually very shallow (2 to 3 mm) in 82% of specimens. He also noted an absence of the posterior fibular groove in 11%, a convex posterior fibula surface in 7%, and laxity of the retinaculum.[54]

Clinical Findings

Acute traumatic dislocation of the peroneal tendons is believed to be due to a sudden forceful passive dorsiflexion of the inverted foot with reflex contraction of the peroneal tendons and plantar flexors.[51, 155, 213] This may occur while skiing if the ski tip digs in and the skier falls forward and sustains an inversion-type injury. Others believe that the forceful contraction of the peroneal tendons that occurs as the inner border of the ski digs into the snow while turning may cause dislocation of the tendons. Not infrequently, the patient will give a history of snapping over the posterolateral aspect of the ankle with twisting movements. Physical examination demonstrates swelling and tenderness about the peroneal tendon sheath behind the lateral malleolus.[12, 51, 55, 141, 155, 230] It should not be difficult to differentiate an acute ankle sprain of the anterior talofibular ligament from an acute peroneal dislocation if one carefully examines the ankle since the pain in the former will be anterior to the fibula and the latter posterior to the fibula. Asking the patient to dorsiflex the foot when it is held in a plantar-flexed, everted position will usually cause pain about the posterior aspect of the malleolus and possibly result in a dislocation of the peroneal tendons. The findings of a grade III injury and a rim avulsion fracture of the lateral malleolus are considered to be pathognomonic of tendon dislocation.[151, 155, 213] If lateral instability of the ankle is of concern, a stress view looking for talar tilt would be indicated. The combination of lateral ankle instability with peroneal tendon injury is rare but has been reported. When present, use of the Chrisman-Snook procedure for lateral ankle instability with dislocation of the peroneal tendons has been reported.[207]

Radiographic techniques utilized for diagnosis include peroneal tenograms, which may show leakage of the contrast dye anteriorly, and the use of a CT scan may be of some value.[214] Unless the dislocation is observed when the patient is first examined or it is reproduced at the time of the examination, the diagnosis of an acute anterior peroneal dislocation is uncertain and only suspected.

TABLE 19–13.
Gradations of Dislocations of the Peroneal Tendons*

Type	Characteristics
I	The retinaculum is still attached to the periosteum on the posterior aspect of the fibula; however, the periosteum is elevated from the underlying malleolus by the dissecting tendons that are displaced anteriorly
II	The retinaculum is torn free from its anterior insertion on the malleolus, and the periosteum of the tendons dissects through at this level
III	The retinaculum is avulsed from the insertion on the malleolus with avulsion of a small fragment of bone
IV	The retinaculum is torn from its posterior attachment as the tendon dissects through, with the retinaculum lying deep to the dislocating peroneal tendon

*Adapted from Oden RF: *Clin Orthop* 216:63–69, 1987.

References 41, 138, 141, 155, 188, 191, 213, 240.

†*References 12, 45, 71, 79, 97, 104, 140, 146, 149, 156, 188, 207, 209, 240.*

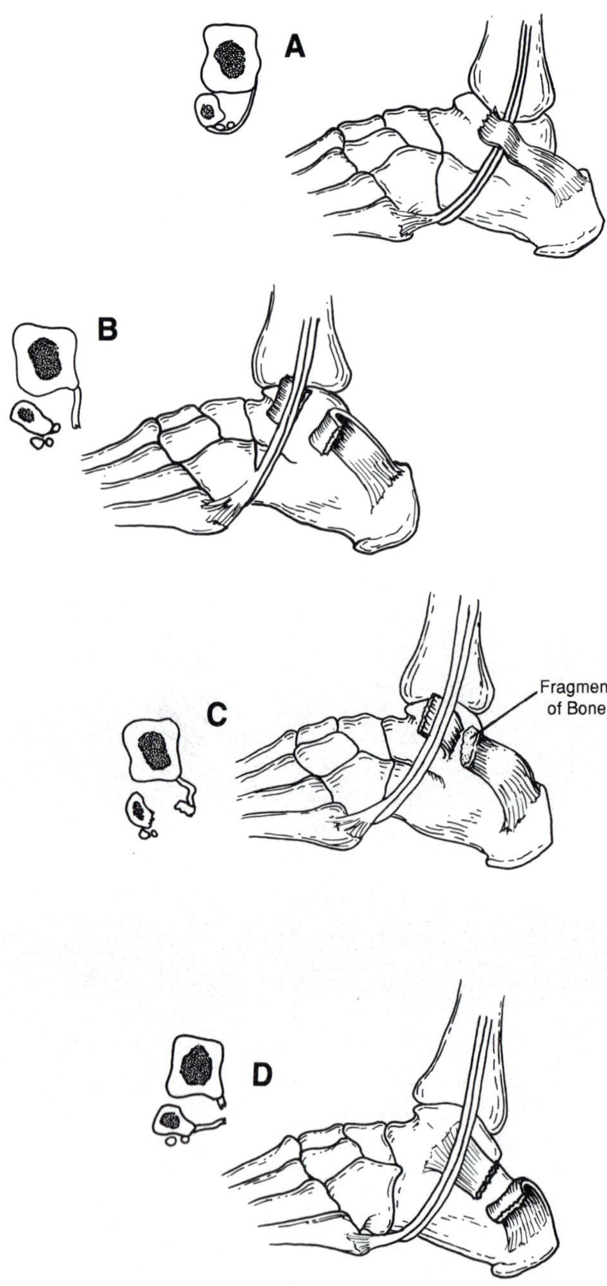

FIG 19–6.
Gradations of dislocations of the peroneal tendons. **A,** retinaculum is still intact, although it is elevated from the underlying malleolus. **B,** retinaculum is torn from its anterior insertion on the malleolus, permitting dislocation of the peroneal tendons. **C,** retinaculum is avulsed from the insertion on the malleolus with a small fragment of bone. **D,** retinaculum is torn from its posterior attachment, permitting the tendons to dislocate over the retinaculum. (Redrawn from Oden RF: *Clin Orthop* 216:63–69, 1987.)

Chronic dislocations, on the other hand, may present less diagnostic difficulty. The patient will often give a history of a sense of apprehension that the ankle is going to "give way" or the tendons are going to "dislocate" when carrying out physical activities. Physical examination will frequently demonstrate that the retinacular structures are lax secondary to recurrent dislocations; in this case the peroneal tendons can be noted to dislocate anteriorly along the side of the fibula. It is important to always compare the injured side with the uninjured side since some people normally have some laxity of their retinaculum.

Treatment

Conservative management of an acute injury is somewhat controversial.* Treatment consists of strapping techniques or a well-molded, non–weight-bearing cast

**References 12, 51, 55, 138, 141, 191, 213.*

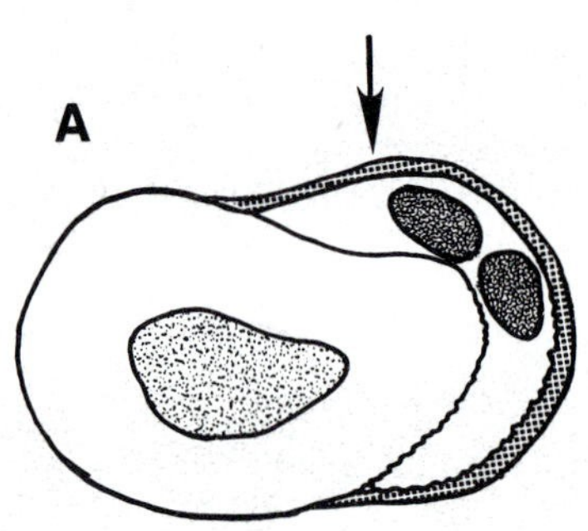

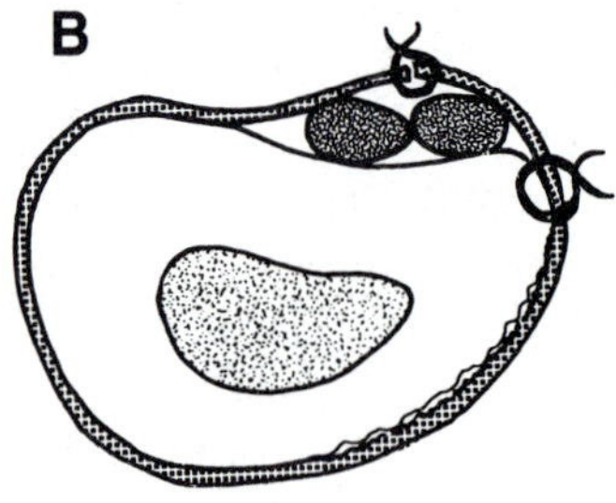

FIG 19–7.
Diagram of a transverse section of the distal end of the left fibula viewed from above. **A,** false pouch formed by stripping of the periosteum from the lateral malleolus in continuity with the superior peroneal retinaculum. *Arrow* denotes the site for incision in the retinaculum. **B,** normal anatomy is restored by obliteration of the false pouch and closing the incision in the peroneal retinaculum. (Redrawn from DasDe S, Balasubramanium P: *J Bone J Surg [Br]* 67:585–587, 1985.)

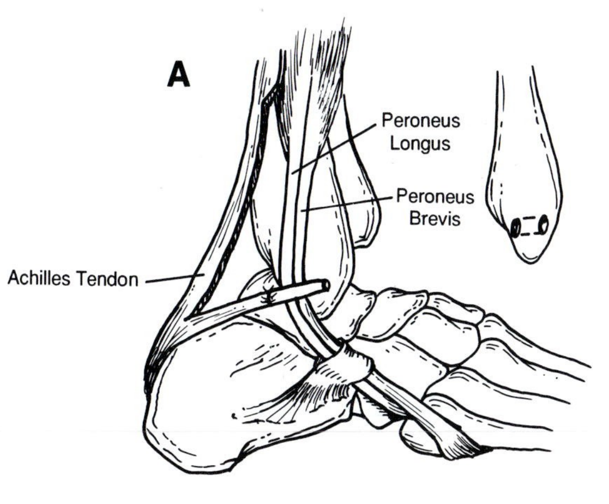

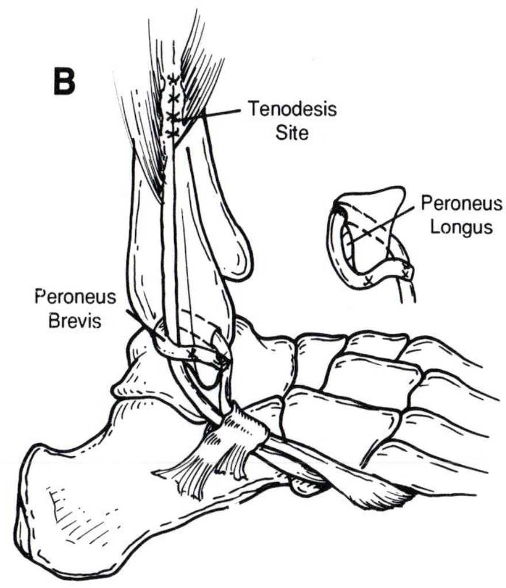

FIG 19–8.
Reconstruction of peroneal retinaculum. **A,** Ellis-Jones reconstruction of peroneal retinaculum employing the Achilles tendon. **B,** Allmans' modification of the Evans lateral ankle reconstruction. (Redrawn from Arrowsmith SR, Fleming LL, Allman FL: *Am J Sports Med* 11:142–146, 1983.)

in an attempt to hold the tendons in a reduced anatomic position to permit the superior peroneal retinaculum to heal. When the cast is applied, the foot is left in mild plantar flexion to relax the peroneal tendons. A report by Stover and Bryan[213] of 19 patients with acute injuries demonstrated that the 5 patients treated with a non–weight-bearing cast had excellent results and no evidence of recurrent dislocation. Of the 10 patients treated with a strapping technique, 6 had recurrent dislocations, 4 of which subsequently required surgery. They concluded that a well-molded, non–weight-bearing cast for 4 to 5 weeks was the treatment of choice. Eckert and Davis[51] were disappointed with closed treatment and recommended operative treatment for all acute injuries except when a lesion was determined to be type I, in which case closed treatment might be adequate. Oden[163] believed that type I and III injuries should be treated with cast immobilization for 6 weeks to allow primary healing.

A series of both acute and chronic dislocations reported by McLennan[141] demonstrated a 56% satisfaction rate with cast immobilization. He believed that

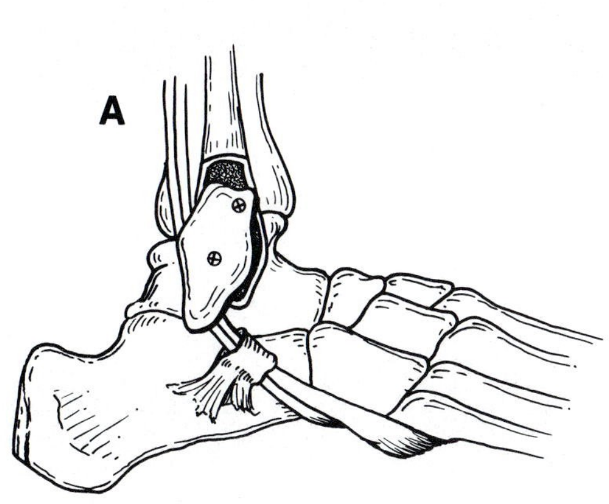

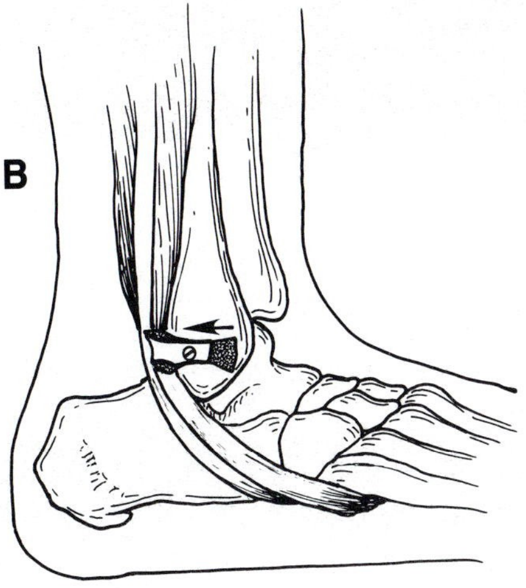

FIG 19–9.
Bone block procedures for repair of subluxing peroneal tendons. **A,** Kelly's first technique for deepening the retromalleolar sulcus. **B,** DuVries modification of Kelly's second technique, employing dovetail cuts to stabilized the siding graft. (Redrawn from Arrowsmith SR, Fleming LL, Allman FL: *Am J Sports Med* 11:142–146, 1983.)

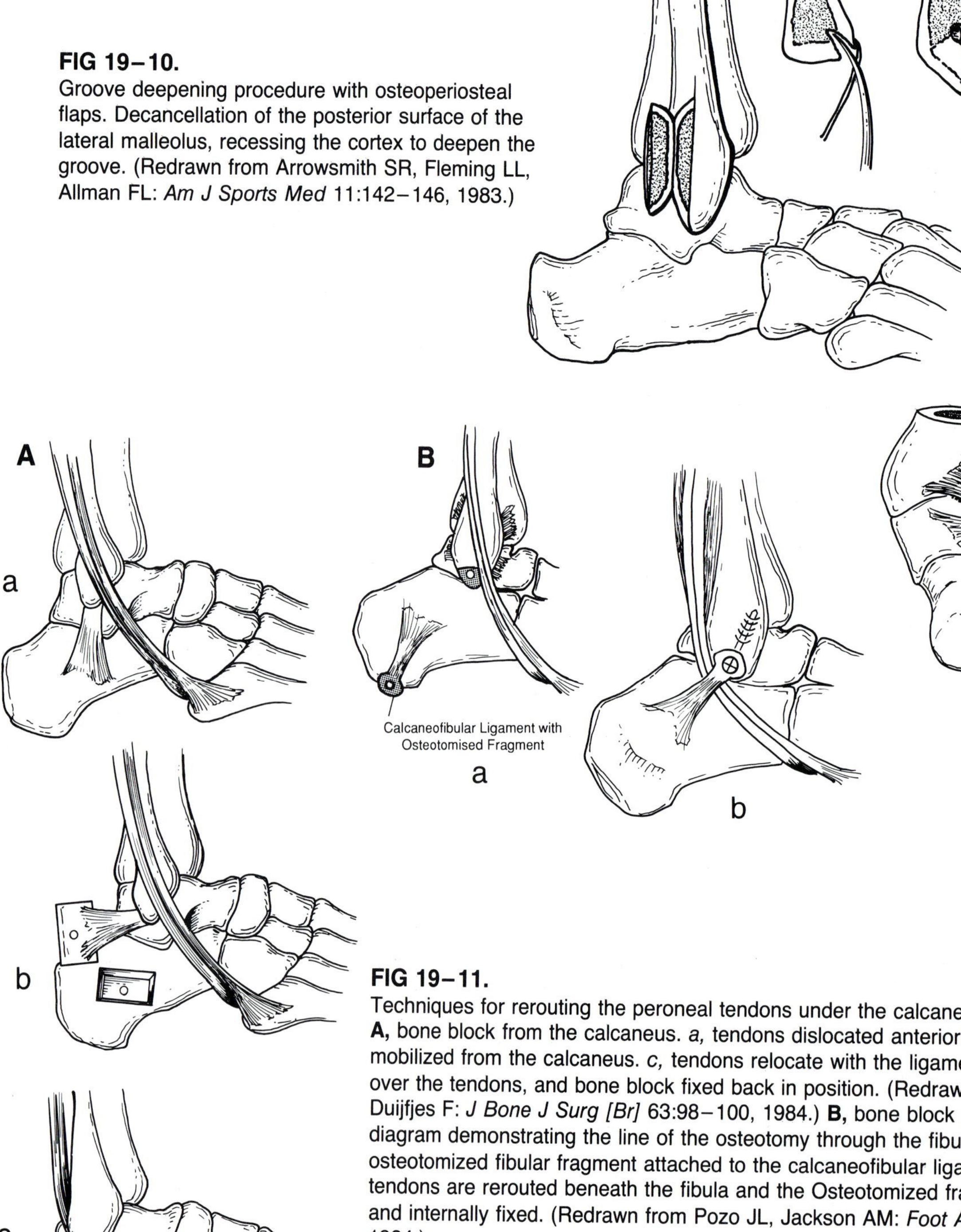

FIG 19–10.
Groove deepening procedure with osteoperiosteal flaps. Decancellation of the posterior surface of the lateral malleolus, recessing the cortex to deepen the groove. (Redrawn from Arrowsmith SR, Fleming LL, Allman FL: *Am J Sports Med* 11:142–146, 1983.)

FIG 19–11.
Techniques for rerouting the peroneal tendons under the calcaneofibular ligaments. **A,** bone block from the calcaneus. *a,* tendons dislocated anteriorly. *b,* bone block mobilized from the calcaneus. *c,* tendons relocate with the ligament transposed over the tendons, and bone block fixed back in position. (Redrawn from Pöll RG, Duijfjes F: *J Bone J Surg [Br]* 63:98–100, 1984.) **B,** bone block from the fibular. *a,* diagram demonstrating the line of the osteotomy through the fibula. *b,* osteotomized fibular fragment attached to the calcaneofibular ligament. *c,* peroneal tendons are rerouted beneath the fibula and the Osteotomized fragment reduced and internally fixed. (Redrawn from Pozo JL, Jackson AM: *Foot Ankle* 5:42–44, 1984.)

TABLE 19–14.

Types of Surgical Treatment of Dislocations of the Peroneal Tendons as Described in the Literature

Direct repair or reattachment of peroneal retinaculum.[45]
Reconstruction of peroneal retinaculum.
  Achilles tendon sling[97]
  Plantaris sling[149]
  Peroneus brevis sling[12, 209]
  Anomalous muscle[79, 147]
Bone block
  Lateral malleolar osteotomy[104]
  Sliding graft (lateral malleolus)[50, 146]
Groove deepening with an osteal-periosteal flap[12, 240]
Rerouting procedure beneath the CF* ligament
  CF ligament mobilized from a bone block from the calcaneus[173]
  CF ligament mobilized by osteotomizing the lateral malleolus[174]
  Peroneal tendons divided and rerouted under the CF ligament[137, 188]

*CF = calcaneofibular.

nonoperative treatment was effective in cases that he felt were stable against dislocation after the acute injury, but that operative treatment may be indicated for acute injuries in the athlete.

Operative treatment of a symptomatic, well-documented, recurrent peroneal dislocation is advocated by most authors.* The types of operations described for reconstruction consist of soft-tissue procedures that reconstruct the peroneal retinaculum, bony procedures to deepen the retromalleolar groove, or a combination of soft-tissue and bony procedures.

The various techniques of surgical treatment for subluxing peroneal tendons are described in Table 19–14 and include the following:

1. Direct repair or reattachment of the peroneal retinaculum (Fig 19–7)
2. Reconstruction of the peroneal retinaculum (Fig 19–8)
3. Bone block procedures (Fig 19–9)
4. Groove-deepening procedures with osteo-periosteal flaps (Fig 19–10)
5. Rerouting procedures of the peroneal tendons under the calcaneofibular ligaments (Fig 19–11)

FLEXOR HALLUCIS LONGUS

If a laceration of the flexor hallucis longus tendon occurs, the literature supports primary repair.[61, 63, 179, 235, 238] If both the flexor hallucis brevis and flexor hallucis longus were divided and the proximal portion of the longus could not be retrieved, it has been suggested that the distal stump of the flexor hallucis longus be sutured to the flexor hallucis brevis.[63] Patients should be told that after repair of the flexor hallucis longus tendon, active flexion of the interphalangeal joint may not be present. This does not seem to presentany serious inconvenience or functional problem. Although the studies are small and not conclusive in favor of either surgical or conservative treatment, attempts to repair the flexor hallucis longus tendon in cases of laceration or rupture seem justified.

Rupture of the flexor hallucis longus tendon as a complication after hallux valgus surgery has only recently been described.[20] It seems that this rare complication is the iatrogenic result of either partial or complete laceration of the flexor hallucis longus tendon at the time of initial surgery.

Although uncommon, closed ruptures of the flexor hallucis longus tendon have been reported. Two cases were reported of partial rupture of the central fibers of the flexor hallucis longus in classical ballet dancers,[186] another case involved traumatic rupture of the flexor hallucis longus in combination with an Achilles tendon rupture in a diving accident,[107] complete rupture of the flexor hallucis longus tendon in the midfoot of a long-distance athlete following a tenosynovitis caused by overuse of a foot with increased pronation has been reported,[87] and an acute rupture has been described in a 34-year-old male who twisted his foot without falling while lifting a minor object.[178] This rupture occurred distally and was felt to be caused by forceful extension against a contracted flexor hallucis longus muscle. All five patients underwent surgical repair.

STENOSING TENOSYNOVITIS

Stenosing tenosynovitis occurs when a tendon, along with its surrounding peritendinous structure, passes through a fibro-osseous canal. Stenosing tenosynovitis of the flexor hallucis longus tendon has been reported to occur at three anatomic sites: (1) at the beginning of the fibro-osseous tunnel on the posterior aspect of the talus, (2) within the flexor tendon sheath behind the medial malleolus, and (3) distally as the tendon passes through the sesamoid bones and inserts into the distal phalanx of the hallux.[70, 78, 139, 186, 225] As a result of stenosis at the origin of the fibro-osseous tunnel and within the flexor tendon sheath, triggering of the great toe may occur.

Stenosis at the Posteromedial Ankle

Possibly due to the unnatural position of the foot and ankle of dancers while in the pointe position, a tenosyn-

**References 12, 97, 104, 137, 141, 146, 149, 155, 188, 240.*

ovitis at the posteromedial aspect of the ankle may occur and result in stenosis at the posterior process of the talus or sustentaculum tali.[78, 186] This stenosis may result in triggering due to entrapment of the flexor hallucis longus tendon within the flexor tendon sheath posterior to the malleolus.[139]

Clinical Findings

The patient will usually experience pain, swelling, tenderness, and crepitation behind the area of the medial malleolus. Triggering and locking of the great toe in association with a pop or snap in the region of the posteromedial aspect of the ankle is noted as the foot is brought into plantar flexion and the hallux is actively flexed. One must keep in mind, however, that if the pain is present on forced plantar flexion of the ankle, a possible posterior impingement or block of the ankle joint caused by an os trigonum, a large posterior tubercle of the talus, or prominence on the posterior part of the os calcis may be the cause of the pain.[78, 90] As a rule, pain from a posterior impingement syndrome is most commonly located posterolaterally, but it should not be confused with peroneal tendinitis.[25, 60, 153, 224] Radiographs obtained with the foot and ankle in maximum plantar flexion may demonstrate the posterior impingement.

Hamilton[78] described a pseudo–hallux rigidus caused by the flexor hallucis longus tendon becoming adherent within its sheath and restricting movement of the hallux. He also described a functional hallux rigidus that he believed was due to abnormal distal insertions of muscle fibers of the flexor hallucis longus, which, due to its bulk, cannot pass into the fibro-osseous tunnel at the posterior aspect of the talus. As a result of this, when the knee is in full extension and the ankle is in maximum dorsiflexion, the hallux is unable to dorsiflex, and "functional hallux rigidus" results.

Stenosis at the Great Toe

As the flexor hallucis longus tendon passes beneath the sesamoid bones, it is subject to repetitive impact loading, particularly in runners, that may result in stenosis of the sheath.[70] Following a laceration, scarring of the flexor hallucis longus may occur in this area as well.[63] Injury to the sheath in this area may result in constriction about the tendon and limit its excursion.

Clinical Findings

Pain beneath the first metatarsophalangeal joint along with a decreased ability or an inability to flex the interphalangeal joint of the hallux when the metatarsophalangeal joint is stabilized in neutral position is suggestive of stenosis. Radiographs, which should include a sesamoid view, may be helpful in demonstrating fracture of a sesamoid.

Treatment

Conservative management consists of immobilization until the acute inflammatory process subsides, along with the use of nonsteroidal anti-inflammatory medicines and occasionally a steroid injection into the sheath. Following this, the patient should undergo physical therapy consisting of stretching of the toe. For distal stenosis it has been suggested that in order to break adhesions in the sesamoid area, the tendon sheath can be infiltrated with 1% lidocaine.[70] If conservative management fails, operative management from a medial approach in order to carry out a tenolysis of the tendon and early motion may be beneficial.

EXTENSOR TENDONS

Peritendinitis

The most frequently affected tendon is the tibialis anterior and occasionally the extensor digitorum longus.[124] The tenosynovitis is usually brought about secondary to irritation by shoes, boots, and, in particular, ski boots. As a rule, relief of pressure by modification of the footwear results in satisfactory resolution of the problem. On rare occasions, release of the synovial sheath in the front of the ankle may be necessary.

Rupture

Rupture of the extensor tendons about the dorsum of the foot and ankle is usually due to an open wound or laceration.[8, 61, 74, 126] Closed rupture of the tibialis anterior and extensor hallucis longus tendons has been reported.

Tibialis Anterior

Fewer than 20 reports of closed subcutaneous rupture of the tibialis anterior tendon have been described.* As a rule, ruptures occur in males over the age of 45 years. The rupture usually occurs after minimal or insignificant trauma consisting of forced plantar flexion against actively contracting dorsiflexors.

Open injuries causing disruption of the tibialis anterior tendon are not common occurrences.[44, 61] With traumatic wounds about the foot and ankle, the motion and strength of these tendons must be assessed so as to not overlook a tendon laceration. The patient should be

---

**References 26, 27, 49, 101, 112, 143, 145, 150, 152.*

carefully followed and surgical exploration of the traumatic wound considered if there is any hint of weakness, deformity, or gap in the underlying tendon.

Clinical Findings.—The patient will usually complain of weakness of the ankle associated with swelling over the anteromedial aspect of the ankle in the more recent cases, but in an old rupture, pain may be minimal, and the patient may complain of a gait abnormality. Three cases of rupture of the tibialis anterior tendon have been reported that were initially believed to be due to an underlying neurologic lesion: a peroneal palsy in two cases and an acute L5 radiculopathy in one case.[145, 152]

Physical examination reveals weakness of dorsiflexion of the foot against resistance. The patient is usually unable to walk on his heels. Active dorsiflexion of the ankle may result in some eversion, and there may be weakness of inversion. The patient may be unable to actively dorsiflex the foot with the toes plantar-flexed. At times, a gap in the tendon may be observed.

Treatment.—In an active patient who presents within 3 to 4 months following the injury, surgical repair of the tibialis anterior tendon has been recommended.[49, 143]

Several methods of operative treatment have been described. A sliding tendon lengthening using the proximal intact tibialis anterior tendon to span the ruptured site and anastomose the proximal and distal intact stumps of the tendon has been described.[101] If the tendon avulses from its insertion at the medial cuneiform and there has not been too much proximal retraction, the tendon can be advanced and reinserted through a drill hole back into bone. Suturing the proximal stump to the adjacent extensor hallucis longus tendon, which is then severed at the level of the metatarsophalangeal joint of the great toe and rerouted to the site of the insertion of the tibialis anterior tendon, has also been advocated.[49] The remaining distal portion of the extensor hallucis longus is then sutured to the extensor hallucis brevis tendon.

In patients who are treated nonoperatively, the tendon usually becomes adherent proximally and results in some loss of ankle dorsiflexion and diminished strength. In the elderly patient leading a sedentary life, the gait pattern may be functionally normal, and nonoperative treatment is justified.[49, 145]

Extensor Hallucis Longus and Extensor Digitorum Longus

In a review of 143 injuries to the lower extremity (see Table 19–6) by Anzel et al. at the Mayo Clinic in 1959,[8] disruptions of the extensor tendons occurred in 16 patients, or 11% of the injuries. These were all secondary to an open laceration. In a report of 20 patients with tendon injuries about the ankle, 9 had involvement of the extensor hallucis longus or extensor digitorum longus tendons.[74] In that series only 1 patient had a closed disruption, and that was due to erosion by rheumatoid tissue.[74] In a review of 46 patients with various tendon injuries, 13 had lacerations of the extensor hallucis longus, and 8 had lacerations of the extensor digitorum longus.[61] Only scattered reports of closed subcutaneous rupture or dislocation of the extensor hallucis longus or extensor digitorum longus have been reported.[3, 201]

Clinical Findings.—Physical examination demonstrates weakness of extension of the great toe or lesser toes. At times the proximal or distal end of the tendon is palpable subcutaneously.

Treatment.—Aggressive surgical repair is advocated for open lacerations of tendons about the foot, particularly in children.[61, 74, 126, 235] This would include thorough exploration, debridement, and anatomic restoration of the tendon. Others have advocated that since extensor tendons tend to heal spontaneously, formal repair of the extensor hallucis longus tendon may not be necessary.[74, 235] Others, however, did not believe that conservative management was supported in the literature and recommended surgical repair for both the extensor hallucis longus and extensor digitorum longus tendons, when feasible.[61]

TIBIALIS POSTERIOR TENDON

See Chapter 17.

TENDON TRANSFERS ABOUT THE FOOT AND ANKLE

A tendon transfer is utilized to help reestablish balanced muscle function about the foot and ankle in order to create a plantigrade foot. The plantigrade foot may also secondarily enable the patient to obtain a better gait pattern by allowing the hip and knee to once again begin to establish a normal range of motion.

There are many factors that need to be considered with tendon transfers.

Biomechanical Principles

The main biomechanical principles that need to be considered in contemplating a tendon transfer is that of the axes of the ankle and subtalar joint and the relationship of the tendon to the axes. Other factors that need to be considered are the muscle strengths and their phasic activity (stance vs. swing phase).

The axes about the foot and ankle are demonstrated in Figure 19–12. Those muscles that are located anterior to the ankle axis produce dorsiflexion, while those posterior to it produce plantar flexion. When looking at the subtalar joint axis, those muscles lying medial to the axis produce inversion, while those lateral to the axis produce eversion. Since motion occurs about both of these axes simultaneously, muscles lying posterior to the ankle axis and medial to the subtalar axes produce plantar flexion and inversion, those posterior to the ankle axis and lateral to the subtalar joint axes produce plantar flexion and eversion, and those anterior to the ankle axis and lateral to the subtalar axes produce dorsiflexion and eversion. By keeping an illustration like this in mind, one can then often plot out which muscles are deficient and the resultant deformity. It also enables one to visualize the muscles that are still available for transfer and where they may be placed in order to correct the deformity.

Principles of Muscle Function

Although we tend to view muscle function about the foot and ankle as a balance of strength between dorsiflexors and plantar flexors and invertors and evertors, Silver et al.[200] have demonstrated that this concept is not quite that simple. In looking at the relative strengths of the muscles about the ankle, they point out that an "imbalance" exists between the dorsiflexors and plantar flexors. Utilizing a numbering system based upon fiber length and muscle mass, they pointed out that the relative strength of the dorsiflexors is 9.4 units and that of the plantar flexors is 69 units. The evertors were assigned 11.9 units and invertors, 60.9 units (Table 19–15).

In view of this obvious "imbalance," clearly the control of muscle balance about the foot and ankle is not based upon one muscle group balancing another but, rather, the fact that a central nervous system mechanism is functioning to maintain muscle balance about the foot and ankle. When this cerebral balance has been upset as a result of cerebral palsy, stroke, or a head injury, the effects of this imbalance become painfully apparent. It is for this reason that following the loss of this central balancing mechanism we observe an equinovarus deformity about the foot and ankle in response to the relative strength of the plantar flexors and invertors in relation to the dorsiflexors and evertors.

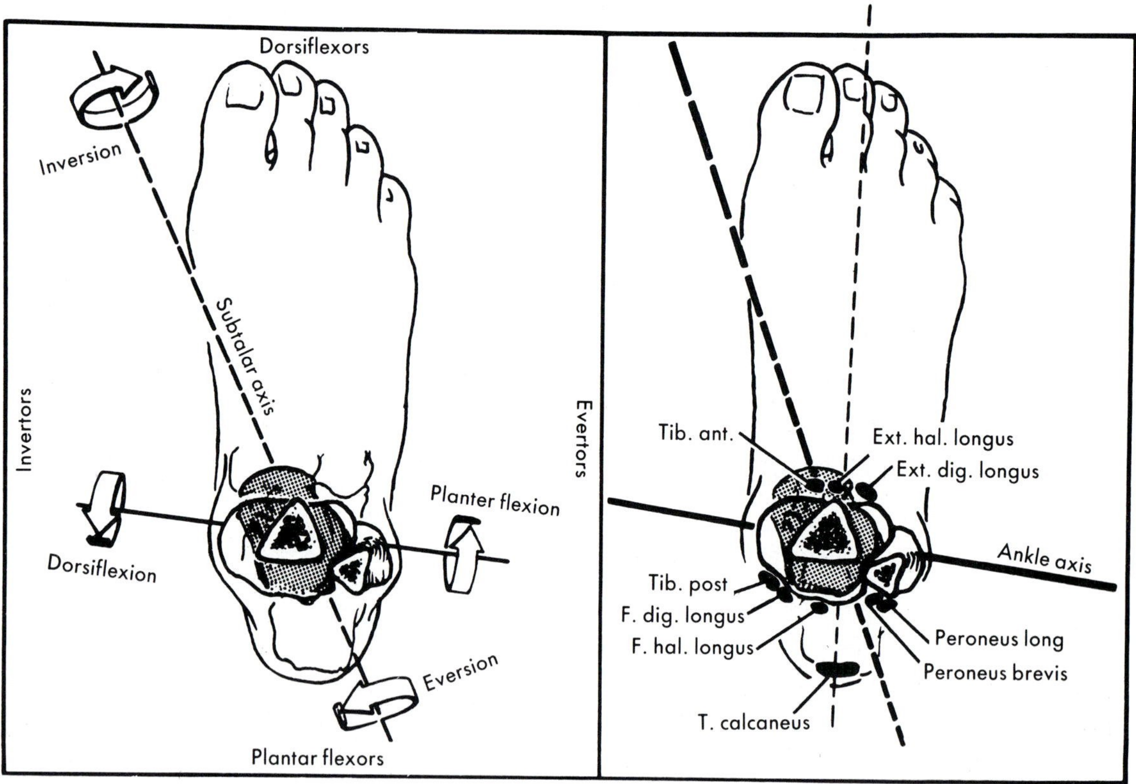

FIG 19–12.
Left diagram demonstrates rotation that occurs about the subtalar and ankle axes. *Right* diagram demonstrates relationship of various muscles about the subtalar and ankle axes. (From Mann RA: Biomechanics of the foot, in American Academy of Orthopedic Surgeons, *Atlas of orthotics,* St Louis, 1975, Mosby–Year Book.)

TABLE 19–15.
Relative Strengths of Muscles

Plantar Flexion		Dorsiflexion	
Soleus	29.9	Tibialis Anterior	5.6
Gastrocnemius—medial	13.7	EDL*	1.7
Gastrocnemius—lateral	5.5	EHL*	1.2
FHL*	3.6	Peroneus tertius	0.9
FDL*	1.8	Total	9.4
Tibialis posterior	6.4		
Peroneus longus	5.5		
Peroneus brevis	2.6		
Total	69.0		

Inversion		Eversion	
Tibialis posterior	6.4	Peroneus longus	5.5
FHL	3.6	Peroneus brevis	2.6
FDL	1.8	EDL	1.7
G-S*	49.1	EHL	1.2
Total	60.9	Peroneus tertius	0.9
		Total	11.9

*FHL = flexor hallucis longus; FDL = flexor digitorum longus; G-S = gastrocnemius-soleus; EDL = extensor digitorum longus; EHL = extensor hallucis longus.

The next consideration when looking at muscles is their phasic activity. Muscle function about the foot and ankle is generally divided into those muscles that function during the swing phase and those that function during the stance phase. The swing-phase muscles consist of those in the anterior compartment, bring about dorsiflexion of the ankle joint, and control the initial plantar flexion following heel strike. The stance-phase muscles, which include the posterior and lateral compartments, function during the period of midstance and control the forward movement of the tibia over the fixed foot and then initiate plantar flexion of the ankle joint.

The question that is frequently raised is whether a stance-phase muscle can convert its phase to become a swing-phase muscle. Most people agree that on a voluntary basis the patient with a lower motor neuron lesion can usually bring about active dorsiflexion following transfer of the stance-phase posterior tibial or toe flexor muscles. When this individual walks and concentrates on using the transferred muscle again, the stance-phase muscle will usually function as a swing-phase muscle. Over time, however, Waters[229] questions whether or not true phase conversion persists. As a general principle, one should attempt to transfer a swing-phase muscle to replace a lost swing-phase muscle and conversely for the plantar flexors, but this may not be possible. More than likely, the nonphasic transfers usually tend to function more as a tenodesis than an active transfer.

One always has to be mindful of the consequences of moving a muscle from one part of the foot to another. It has been well documented that moving the peroneus longus in the presence of a normal tibialis anterior results in dorsiflexion of the first metatarsal and produces a dorsal bunion. This is because the normal agonist-antagonist relationship between these two muscles has been disrupted and as a result the deformity occurs. The same problem has been encountered if the tibialis anterior is moved too far laterally or the tibialis posterior muscle is moved, particularly in the immature foot; here a pronation deformity results.

The type of muscle imbalance that is present also plays an important role in tendon transfers. A lower motor neuron lesion that produces a flaccid paralysis is significantly easier to evaluate and treat than an upper motor neuron lesion that results in spasticity. In flaccid paralysis it is relatively simple to evaluate which muscles are present and their relative strength as compared with the upper motor neuron injury in which spasticity is present. When spasticity is present, it is often difficult for the patient to cooperate sufficiently to permit an adequate muscle examination due to a lack of selective voluntary control. Under these circumstances, release, lengthening, or transfer of a muscle may result in a new deformity because of a change in the balance present in the foot. It is for this reason that dynamic electromyographic analysis is often important in evaluating the patient with spasticity.[171]

The overall posture of the foot needs to be evaluated to be sure that a plantigrade foot is present. If a deformity is present and the foot cannot be placed flat on the floor, it is essential that corrective measures be taken to create a plantigrade foot prior to a tendon transfer. A tendon transfer is unable to function if passive motion is not present in the direction that the transfer is expected to function.

Patient Evaluation

Natural History of the Muscle Imbalance

A thorough understanding of the type of muscle imbalance that is present and its natural history is critical in determining treatment. It is important to appreciate whether the muscle imbalance is progressive or nonprogressive and whether it represents an upper or a lower motor neuron lesion. Both types of motor deficiencies can bring about a progressive deformity, but only the lower motor neuron lesion can at times result in a nonprogressive deformity. Typically, the patient who has sustained a lower motor injury presents with a nonprogressive deformity (e.g., a peroneal and sciatic nerve injury). Other types of lower motor neuron disease such as myopathies or peripheral neuropathies may demonstrate a progression of their deformity. Although we tend to look at upper motor neuron lesions as resulting in spasticity, which is usually the case when they are present at the spinal cord level such as in myelodysplasia, a flaccid paralysis may be present or sometimes a mixed picture.

Age of the Patient

When faced with a child with a muscle imbalance, the surgeon must carefully consider the possible bony deformity secondary to the effects of growth. In the young child one must be concerned as to what may occur following the tendon transfer, such as the development of a dorsal bunion or flatfoot deformity, and in the older child one must be concerned that the presence of a long-standing muscle imbalance has resulted in distortion of the foot so that it is no longer plantigrade. As a rule, in the adult there usually is no significant bony distortion since the muscle imbalance occurred after skeletal maturity has been achieved. There may be fixed contractures present that need to be corrected by release or possibly arthrodesis, but the overall bony architecture is normal.

Diagnosis

Diagnostic evaluation of the patient begins with a careful history of the problem, the types of bracing that have been utilized, and whether or not the patient's overall gait pattern seems to be stable or deteriorating. A detailed analysis of the range of motion of the joints and the relative muscle strengths needs to be determined. A determination needs to be made as to whether or not the patient has a plantigrade foot and, if not, what is preventing the foot from becoming plantigrade, i.e., muscle imbalance, fixed contracture, or abnormal bony architecture. Once this part of the evaluation has occurred, a determination needs to be made as to what type of gait evaluation is necessary. This may be as simple as observing the patient walking or, more sophisticated, with the use of motion analysis of the lower extremity and dynamic electromyographic data.[9]

Treatment

Surgical Principles

In order to create a satisfactory tendon transfer, the following basic principles need to be considered.

1. A plantigrade foot must be present prior to the transfer. This can be created by carrying out a tendon lengthening, release of a joint contracture, or, if necessary, bony stabilization. The tendon lengthening may be a tendo Achillis lengthening, posterior tibial lengthening, etc; the release of the joint contracture may consist of a posterior capsulotomy; and the bony stabilization may consist of a subtalar or triple arthrodesis or occasionally an osteotomy of the first metatarsal to alleviate plantar flexion.
2. The muscle or muscles that are to be transferred should be of adequate strength and, if possible, of similar fiber length and the same phasic activity to provide an optimal transfer. It is important to keep in mind that a transferred muscle usually loses one grade of strength, i.e., from normal to good, and, therefore, if the muscle strength is only good to fair, the transfer may not be successful.
3. Technical considerations when carrying out a tendon transfer are as follows:
   a. The tendon transfer should be carried out through adequate soft-tissue coverage. If dense scar is present, it needs to be resected and possibly some type of resurfacing carried out to provide adequate soft-tissue coverage and a gliding surface for the tendon transfer.
   b. If the tendon is brought through the interosseous membrane, a window of adequate size should be utilized.
   c. The line of pull of the tendon between the muscle and its insertion should be as straight a line as possible to provide maximum efficiency.
   d. The tendon transfer should preferably be implanted into bone and sutures placed between the periosteum and the tendon so as to prevent failure of the site of implant.
4. Adequate postoperative immobilization and subsequent retraining should be undertaken.

Tendon transfers are generally grouped as follows: anterior transfer, split-tendon transfer, posterior transfer, lateral transfer, and distal transfers. Only a brief, general discussion of each type will be presented in this section, and the reader is referred to Chapters 12 and 13 for more specific details regarding tendon transfers.

Anterior Transfer.—Anterior tendon transfers are carried out in order to reestablish dorsiflexion power. For this transfer to be successful it is imperative that adequate passive dorsiflexion be present prior to surgery. If it is not, release of the contracture is essential prior to the transfer.

When the transfer is carried out for flaccid paralysis, a tibialis posterior transfer through the interosseous septum is frequently utilized.[127] At times this may be reinforced by use of the flexor hallucis and/or flexor digitorum longus muscles. It should be kept in mind that the excursion of the tibialis posterior tendon is about 2 cm due to the shape of its muscle fibers, whereas the overall excursion of the long flexor tendons is about 3 cm, which enables them to move the ankle through a greater range of motion. It is imperative, however, that when multiple tendons are transferred through the interosseous septum, an adequate window be created in order to minimize the possibility of adhesions following the transfer.

If there is instability of the subtalar joint due to a loss of more than just dorsiflexors, it may be necessary to stabilize the subtalar joint or to carry out a triple arthrodesis prior to the tendon transfer.

At times the extensor digitorum longus tendon may be utilized to provide increased dorsiflexion power at the ankle joint. This is a phasic transfer and may provide just enough extra dorsiflexion power to permit the patient to become brace free. It is usually transferred into the second or third cuneiform.

Following a transfer in the patient with spasticity, even with the addition of the long flexor tendons to the toes, the following problems may result:

1. Persistence or recurrence of the original deformity.[195]
2. Alteration of the original deformity resulting in a calcaneus or valgus deformity.[195, 227]
3. Lack of phase conversion during gait, although the patient has the ability of selective voluntary control.[40, 195]

Split-Tendon Transfer.—The split anterior tibial tendon transfer (SPLATT) has been performed to provide a yoke-type of tendon configuration to the dorsum of the foot.[86] It is based on the principle that by tightening the lateral aspect of the yoke a more plantigrade foot posture can be achieved while utilizing a muscle of the same phase to achieve it. This transfer is most useful in the patient with spasticity and overpull of the invertors of the foot. It is important, however, that when this procedure is performed, adequate dorsiflexion be present, and if not, a tendo Achillis lengthening and possible posterior tibial tendon lengthening be added to the procedure. It is also imperative that the lateral band of the yoke be tightened sufficiently to pull the foot into an everted position; otherwise the procedure will fail.

The tibialis posterior split-tendon transfer has been utilized to correct a varus deformity of the hindfoot. The split posterior tibial tendon transfer has the advantage that when carried out in the younger individual a flatfoot deformity will not result, and again, an in-phase muscle is used to provide improved muscle function.[73, 102, 106]

A further modification of the split-tendon transfers has been utilized in the treatment of footdrop. A recent modification by Rodriguez[182] has been described for footdrop in which the tibialis posterior tendon is passed through a hole created in the tibialis anterior tendon and is subsequently inserted into the second cuneiform. The peroneus longus tendon is then rerouted in front of the lateral malleolus and tightened in order to help provide medial-lateral balance to the foot as well. The advantage of this procedure is that by tightening the medial and lateral bands a plantigrade foot is created along with reestablishment of dorsiflexion strength.

Posterior Transfer.—Posterior tendon transfers into the Achilles tendon or calcaneus are utilized to prevent or retard the development of a calcaneal deformity and to restore plantar flexion power. Even if only weak plantar flexion is achieved following this transfer, it is more desirable and easier to brace a foot that is in equinus than to manage a calcaneal deformity.

Depending upon the muscle function that is present, posterior transfer of the tibialis anterior through the interosseous septum or posterior transfer of the peroneus longus or tibialis posterior are utilized most frequently. If possible, a phasic transfer is more desirable, although it appears as though the tibialis anterior tendon can undergo phase conversion and function as a plantar flexor during gait.[40, 227]

Lateral Transfer.—A lateral tendon transfer is usually utilized for loss of peroneal muscle function. It should be kept in mind that the peroneus brevis is a powerful evertor of the subtalar joint, whereas the peroneus longus functions mainly to plantar-flex the first metatarsal and is a weak evertor. In the patient who has selectively lost the function of the peroneus brevis, possibly due to attritional changes of the tendon or a laceration, one may consider utilizing the peroneus longus as a transfer to help reestablish eversion function. The split anterior tibial tendon transfer can likewise be utilized for this situation. Since most of these muscles involve phasic transfers, uniformly good results can usually be expected.

Distal Tendon Transfer.—The Jones tendon transfer[99] is utilized to correct the cock-up deformity of the first metatarsophalangeal joint that is brought about by weakness of dorsiflexion by the tibialis anterior and subsequent use of the extensor hallucis longus as a secondary dorsiflexor of the ankle joint. In these circumstances the extensor hallucis longus tendon is transferred into the neck of the first metatarsal in order to provide increased dorsiflexion power of the foot and, at the same time, usually correct the chronic plantar flexion posture of the first metatarsal. A fusion of the interphalangeal joint of the great toe is always added to offset the unopposed pull of the flexor hallucis longus tendon, and occasionally an osteotomy at the base of the first metatarsal is utilized to bring the first metatarsal out of plantar flexion. See Chapter 18 for detailed surgical technique.

The Girdlestone-Taylor flexor tendon transfer is utilized when a dynamic deformity of the lesser toes is present and results in hammering of the lesser toes. This transfer involves detachment of the long flexor tendon from its insertion and transfer to the extensor hood mechanism on the dorsum of the proximal phalanx. When this procedure is carried out, it is imperative that there be no contracture of the proximal interphalangeal joint or spasticity, which may result in a swan-neck–like deformity. See Chapter 8 for detailed surgical technique.

REFERENCES

1. Abraham E, Pankovich AM: Neglected rupture of the Achilles tendon: treatment by V-Y tendinous flap, *J Bone Joint Surg [Am]* 57:253–255, 1975.
2. Abraham E, Stirnaman JE: Neglected rupture of the peroneal tendons causing recurrent sprains of the ankle: case report, *J Bone Joint Surg* 61:1247–1248, 1979.
3. Akhtar M, Levine J: Dislocation of extensor digitorum longus tendons after spontaneous rupture of the inferior retinaculum of the ankle: case report, *J Bone Joint Surg [Am]* 62:1210–1211, 1980.
4. Albert E: Achillodynie, *Weiner Med Presse* 34:41–43, 1893.
5. Aldam CH: Repair of calcaneal tendon ruptures: a safe technique, *J Bone Joint Surg [Br]* 71:486–488, 1989.
6. Altman D: Managing bursitis in podiatry, *J Am Podiatr Assoc* 56:408–410, 1966.
7. Andersen E: Stenosing peroneal tenosynovitis symptomatically simulating ankle instability, *Am J Sports Med* 15:258–259, 1987.
8. Anzel SH, Covey KW, Weiner AD, et al: Disruption of muscles and tendons: an analysis of 1,014 cases, *Surgery* 45:406–414, 1959.
9. Arner O, Lindholm Å: Subcutaneous rupture of the Achilles tendon: a study of 92 cases, *Acta Chir Scand Suppl* 239:1–51, 1959.
10. Arner O, Lindholm Å, Lindvall N: Roentgen changes in subcutaneous rupture of the Achilles tendon, *Acta Chir Scand* 116:496–500, 1958.
11. Arner O, Lindholm Å, Orell SR: Histologic changes in subcutaneous rupture of the Achilles tendon: a study of 74 cases, *Acta Chir Scand* 116:484–490, 1958.
12. Arrowsmith SR, Fleming LL, Allman FL: Traumatic dislocations of the peroneal tendons, *Am J Sports Med* 11:142–146, 1983.
13. Barfred T: Achilles tendon rupture: aetiology and pathogenesis of subcutaneous rupture assessed on the basis of the literature and rupture experiments on rats, *Acta Orthop Scand Suppl* 152:1–126, 1973.
14. Barnes MJ, Hardy AE: Delayed reconstruction of the calcaneal tendon, *J Bone Joint Surg [Br]* 68:121–124, 1986.
15. Berlin D, Coleman W, Nickamin A: Surgical approaches to Haglund's disease, *J Foot Surg* 21:42–44, 1982.
16. Bossley CJ, Cairney PC: The intermetatarsophalangeal bursa—its significance in Morton's metatarsalgia, *J Bone Joint Surg [Br]* 62:184–187, 1980.
17. Bosworth DM: Repair of defects in the tendo Achillis, *J Bone Joint Surg [Am]* 38:111–114, 1956.
18. Bradley JP, Tibone JE: Percutaneous and open surgical repairs of Achilles tendon ruptures: a comparative study, *Am J Sports Med* 18:188–195, 1990.
19. Brahms MA: Common foot problems, *J Bone Joint Surg [Am]* 49:1653–1664, 1967.
20. Brand JC, Smith RW: Rupture of the flexor hallucis longus after hallux valgus surgery: case report and comments on technique of adductor release, *Foot Ankle* 11:407–410, 1991.
21. Brody DM: Running injuries, *Clin Symp* 32:2–36, 1980.
22. Brown TD, Fu FH, Hanley EN Jr: Comparative assessment of the early mechanical integrity of repaired tendo Achillis ruptures in the rabbit, *J Trauma* 21:951–957, 1981.
23. Buck RM, McDonald JR, Ghormley RK: Adventitious bursas, *Arch Surg* 47:344–351, 1943.
24. Bugg EI Jr, Boyd BM: Repair of neglected rupture or laceration of the Achilles tendon, *Clin Orthop* 56:73–75, 1968.
25. Burman M: Stenosing tendovaginitis of the foot and ankle: Studies with special reference to the stenosing tendovaginitis of the peroneal tendons at the peroneal tubercle, *Arch Surg* 67:686–698, 1953.
26. Burman MS: Subcutaneous rupture of the tendon of the tibialis anticus, *Ann Surg* 100:368–372, 1934.
27. Burman M: Subcutaneous strain or tear of the dorsiflexor tendons of the foot, *Bull Hosp Jt Dis Orthop Inst* 4:44–50, 1943.
28. Burman M: Subcutaneous tear of the tendon of the peroneus longus: its relation to the giant peroneal tubercle, *Arch Surg* 73:216–219, 1956.
29. Burry HC, Pool CJ: Central degeneration of the Achilles tendon, *Rheumatol Rehabil* 12:177–181, 1973.
30. Bywaters EGL: Bursae of the body (editorial), *Ann Rheum Dis* 24:215–218, 1965.
31. Bywaters EGL: Heel lesions of rheumatoid arthritis, *Ann Rheum Dis* 13:42–51, 1954.
32. Canoso JJ, Wohlgethan JR, Newberg AH, et al: Aspiration of the retrocalcaneal bursa, *Ann Rheum Dis* 43:308–312, 1984.
33. Carden DG, Noble J, Chalmers J, et al: Rupture of the calcaneal tendon: the early and late management, *J Bone Joint Surg [Br]* 69:416–420, 1987.
34. Carr AJ, Norris SH: The blood supply of the calcaneal tendon, *J Bone Joint Surg [Br]* 71:100–101, 1989.
35. Cetti R, Christensen SE: Surgical treatment under local anesthesia of Achilles tendon rupture, *Clin Orthop* 173:204–208, 1983.
36. Cherry JH, Ghormley RK: Bursa and ganglion, *Am J Surg* 52:319–330, 1941.
37. Cirincione RJ, Baker EB: Tendon ruptures with secondary hyperparathyroidism: a case report, *J Bone Joint Surg [Am]* 57:852, 1975.
38. Clancy WG Jr: Tendinitis and plantar fasciitis in runners. In D'Ambrosia R, Drez D Jr, editors: *Prevention and treatment of running injuries*, Thorofare, NJ, 1982, Charles B Slack, pp 77–87.
39. Clancy WG Jr, Neidhart D, Brand RL: Achilles tendonitis in runners: a report of five cases, *Am J Sports Med* 4:46–56, 1976.
40. Close JR, Todd FN: The phasic activity of muscles of the lower extremity and the effect of tendon transfer, *J Bone Joint Surg [Am]* 41:189–208, 222, 1959.
41. Cohen I, Lane S, Koning W: Peroneal tendon disloca-

tions: a review of the literature, *J Foot Surg* 22:15–20, 1983.
42. Conwell HE, Alldredge RH: Ruptures and tears of muscles and tendons, *Am J Surg* 35:22–33, 1937.
43. Cox D, Paterson FWN: Acute calcific tendinitis of peroneus longus, *J Bone Joint Surg [Br]* 73:342, 1991.
44. Crosby LA, Fitzgibbons TC: Unrecognized laceration of tibialis anterior tendon: a case report, *Foot Ankle* 9:143–145, 1988.
45. DasDe S, Balasubramaniam P: A repair operation for recurrent dislocation of peroneal tendons, *J Bone Joint Surg [Br]* 67:585–587, 1985.
46. Davidsson L, Salo M: Pathogenesis of subcutaneous tendon ruptures, *Acta Chir Scand* 135:209–212, 1969.
47. Denstad TF, Roaas A: Surgical treatment of partial Achilles tendon rupture, *Am J Sports Med* 7:15–17, 1979.
48. Dickinson PH, Coutts MB, Woodward EP, et al: Tendo Achillis bursitis: report of twenty-one cases, *J Bone Joint Surg [Am]* 48:77–81, 1966.
49. Dooley BJ, Kudelka P, Menelaus MB: Subcutaneous rupture of the tendon of tibialis anterior, *J Bone Joint Surg [Br]* 62:471–472, 1980.
50. DuVries HL: *Surgery of the foot*, St. Louis 1965, Mosby–Year Book, pp 256–257.
51. Eckert WR, Davis EA Jr: Acute rupture of the peroneal retinaculum, *J Bone Joint Surg [Am]* 58:670–673, 1976.
52. Editorial: Achilles tendon rupture, *Lancet* 1:189–190, 1973.
53. Edna T-H: Non-operative treatment of Achilles tendon ruptures, *Acta Orthop Scand* 51:991–993, 1980.
54. Edwards ME: The relations of the peroneal tendons to the fibula, calcaneus, and cuboideum, *Am J Anat* 42:213–253, 1928.
55. Escalas F, Figueras JM, Merino JA: Dislocation of the peroneal tendons: Long-term results of surgical treatment, *J Bone Joint Surg [Am]* 62:451–453, 1980.
56. Evans JD: Subcutaneous rupture of the tendon of peroneus longus: report of a case, *J Bone Joint Surg [Br]* 48:507–509, 1966.
57. Ferguson AB Jr, Gingrich RM: The normal and abnormal calcaneal apophysis and tarsal navicular, *Clin Orthop Rel Res* 10:87–95, 1957.
58. Fish JB: Ruptured Achilles tendon: A method of repair, *Contemp Orthop* 5:21–25, 1982.
59. Fisher TR, Woods CG: Partial rupture of the tendo calcaneus with heterotopic calcification: report of a case, *J Bone Joint Surg [Br]* 52:334–336, 1970.
60. Fitzgerald RH Jr, Coventry MB: Post-traumatic peroneal tendinitis. In Bateman JE, Trott AW, editors: *The foot and ankle: a selection of papers from the American Orthopaedic Foot Society Meetings*, New York, 1980, Brian C Decker, pp 103–109.
61. Floyd DW, Heckman JD, Rockwood CA Jr: Tendon lacerations in the foot, *Foot Ankle* 4:8–14, 1983.
62. Fox JM, Blazina ME, Jobe FW, et al: Degeneration and rupture of the Achilles tendon, *Clin Orthop* 107:221–224, 1975.
63. Frenette JP, Jackson DW: Lacerations of the flexor hallucis longus in the young athlete, *J Bone Joint Surg [Am]* 59:673–676, 1977.
64. Frey C, Shereff M, Greenridge N: Vascularity of the posterior tibial tendon, *J Bone Joint Surg [Am]* 72:884–888, 1990.
65. Fuglsang F, Torup D: Bursitis retrocalcanearis, *Acta Orthop Scand* 30:315–323, 1961.
66. Gilcreest EL: Ruptures and tears of muscles and tendons of the lower extremity: report of fifteen cases, *JAMA* 100:153–160, 1933.
67. Gillies H, Chalmers J: The management of fresh ruptures of the tendo Achillis, *J Bone Joint Surg [Am]* 52:337–343, 1970.
68. Gillström P, Ljungqvist R: Long-term results after operation for subcutaneous partial rupture of the Achilles tendon, *Acta Chir Scand Suppl* 482:78, 1978.
69. Girdlestone GR: Physiotherapy for hand and foot, *J Chartered Soc Physiother* 32:167, 1947.
70. Gould N: Stenosing tenosynovitis of the flexor hallucis longus tendon at the great toe, *Foot Ankle* 2:46–48, 1981.
71. Gould N: Technique tips: footings repair of dislocating peroneal tendons, *Foot Ankle* 6:208–213, 1986.
72. Gould N, Korson R: Stenosing tenosynovitis of the pseudosheath of the tendo Achilles, *Foot Ankle* 1:179–186, 1980.
73. Green NE, Briffin PP, Shiavi R: Split posterior tibial tendon transfer in spastic cerebral palsy, *J Bone Joint Surg [Am]* 6:748–754, 1983.
74. Griffiths JC: Tendon injuries around the ankle, *J Bone Joint Surg [Br]* 47:686–689, 1965.
75. Häggmark T, Eriksson E: Hypotrophy of the soleus muscle in man after Achilles tendon rupture: discussion of findings obtained by computed tomography and morphologic studies, *Am J Sports Med* 7:121–126, 1979.
76. Haglund P: Contribution to the diseased conditions of tendo Achillis (abstract), *Acta Chir Scand* 63:292–294, 1928.
77. Haldeman KO, Soto-Hall R: Injuries to muscles and tendons, *JAMA* 104:2319–2324, 1935.
78. Hamilton WG: Stenosing tenosynovitis of the flexor hallucis longus tendon and posterior impingement upon the os trigonum in ballet dancers, *Foot Ankle* 3:74–80, 1982.
79. Hammerschlag WA, Goldner JL: Chronic peroneal tendon subluxation produced by an anomolous peroneus brevis: case report and literature review, *Foot Ankle* 10:45–47, 1989.
80. Hartmann: The tendon sheaths and synovial bursae of the foot, *Foot Ankle* 1: 247–269, 1981.
81. Håstad K, Larsson L-G, Lindholm Å: Clearance of radiosodium after local deposit in the Achilles tendon, *Acta Chir Scand* 116:251–255, 1958.
82. Helfand AE, Hirt PR, Madresh AC, et al: Triamcinolone acetonide in the treatment of bursitis and other foot disorders, *J Am Podiatr Assoc* 61:174–179, 1971.
83. Heneghan MA, Pavlov H: The Haglund painful heel syndrome: experimental investigation of cause and therapeutic implications, *Clin Orthop* 187:228–234, 1984.
84. Hertzler AE: Bursitides of the plantar surface of the foot (painful heel, gonorrheal exostosis of the os calcis, metatarsal neuralgia), *Am J Surg* 1:117–126, 1926.
85. Hertzler AE: Inflammation of the deep calcaneal bursa, *JAMA* 81:8–9, 1923.
86. Hoffer MM, Reiswig JA, Garrett AM, et al: The split anterior tibial tendon transfer in the treatment of spastic varus hindfoot of childhood, *Orthop Clin North Am* 5:31–38, 1974.
87. Holt KWG, Cross MJ: Isolated rupture of the flexor

hallucis longus tendon: a case report, *Am J Sports Med* 18:645–646, 1990.

88. Hooker CH: Rupture of the tendo calcaneus, *J Bone Joint Surg [Br]* 45:360–363, 1963.
89. Howard CB, Winston I, Bell W, et al: Late repair of the calcaneal tendon with carbon fiber, *J Bone Joint Surg [Br]* 66:206–208, 1984.
90. Howse AJG: Posterior block of the ankle joint in dancers, *Foot Ankle* 3:81–84, 1982.
91. Inglis AE, Scott WN, Sculco TP, et al: Ruptures of the tendo Achillis: an objective assessment of surgical and non-surgical treatment, *J Bone Joint Surg [Am]* 58:990–993, 1976.
92. Isbister JF St C: Calcaneo-fibular abutment following crush fracture of the calcaneus (abstract) *J Bone Joint Surg [Br]* 56:567–568, 1974.
93. Jacobs D, Martens M, Van Audekercke R, et al: Comparison of conservative and operative treatment of Achilles tendon rupture, *Am J Sports Med* 6:107–111, 1978.
94. Jahss MH: *Disorders of the foot*, vol 1, Philadelphia, 1982, WB Saunders, pp 828–868.
95. Jahss MH: Spontaneous rupture of the tibialis posterior tendon: clinical findings, tenographic studies, and a new technique of repair, *Foot Ankle* 3:158–166, 1982.
96. Jessing P, Hansen E: Surgical treatment of 102 tendo Achillis ruptures—suture of tenotoplasty? *Acta Chir Scand* 141:370–377, 1975.
97. Jones E: Operative treatment of chronic dislocation of the peroneal tendons, *J Bone Joint Surg* 14:574–576, 1932.
98. Jones HT: Cystic bursal hygromas, *J Bone Joint Surg* 12:45–89, 1930.
99. Jones R: An operation for paralytic calcaneocavus, *Am J Orthop Surg* 5:371, 1908.
100. Kaplan L, Ferguson LK: Bursitis, *Am J Surg* 37:455–465, 1937.
101. Kashyap S, Prince R: Spontaneous rupture of the tibialis anterior tendon: a case report, *Clin Orthop* 216:159–161, 1987.
102. Kaufer H: Split tendon transfers, *Orthop Trans* 1:1991, 1977.
103. Keck SW, Kelly PJ: Bursitis of the posterior part of the heel: evaluation of surgical treatment of eighteen patients, *J Bone Joint Surg [Am]* 47:267–273, 1965.
104. Kelly RE: An operation for the chronic dislocation of the peroneal tendons, *Br J Surg* 7:502–504, 1920.
105. Kleinman M, Gross AE: Achilles tendon rupture following steroid injection: report of three cases, *J Bone Joint Surg [Am]* 65:1345–1347, 1983.
106. Kling TF, Kaufer H, Hensinger RN: Split posterior tibial-tendon transfers in children with cerebral spastic paralysis and equinovarus deformity, *J Bone Joint Surg [Am]* 67:186–191, 1985.
107. Krackow KA: Acute, traumatic rupture of a flexor hallucis longus tendon: a case report, *Clin Orthop* 150:261–262, 1980.
108. Kuhns JG: Adventitious bursas, *Arch Surg* 46:687–696, 1943.
109. Kvist H, Kvist M: The operative treatment of chronic calcaneal paratenonitis, *J Bone Joint Surg [Br]* 62:353–357, 1980.
110. Kvist MH, Lehto MUK, Jozsa L, et al: Chronic Achilles paratenonitis: an immunohistologic study of fibronectin and fibrinogen, *Am J Sports Med* 16:616–623, 1988.
111. Lagergren C, Lindholm Å: Vascular distribution in the Achilles tendon: an angiographic and microangiographic study, *Acta Chir Scand* 116:491–495, 1958.
112. Lapidus PW: Indirect subcutaneous rupture of the anterior tibial tendon: report of two cases, *Bull Hosp Jt Dis Orthop Inst* 2:119–127, 1941.
113. Larsen E: Longitudinal rupture of the peroneus brevis tendon, *J Bone Joint Surg [Br]* 69:340–341, 1987.
114. Larsen E, Lauridsen F: Dislocation of the tibialis posterior tendon in two athletes, *Am J Sports Med* 12:429–430, 1984.
115. Lawrence GH, Cave EF, O'Connor H: Injury to the Achilles tendon: experience at the Massachusetts General Hospital, 1900–1954, *Am J Surg* 89:795–802, 1955.
116. Layfer LF: "Last" bursitis—a cause of ankle pain (letter), *Arthritis Rheum* 23:261, 1980.
117. Lea RB: Achilles tendon rupture: results of closed management. In Moore M, editor: *Symposium on trauma to the leg and its sequelae*, St Louis, 1981, Mosby–Year Book, pp 353–357.
118. Lea RB, Smith L: Non-surgical treatment of tendo Achillis rupture, *J Bone Joint Surg [Am]* 54:1398–1407, 1972.
119. Lea RB, Smith L: Rupture of the Achilles tendon: nonsurgical treatment, *Clin Orthop* 60:115–118, 1968.
120. Leach RE: Achilles tendon ruptures. In Mack RP, editor: *Symposium on the foot and leg in running sports*, St Louis, 1982, Mosby–Year Book, pp 99–105.
121. Leach RE, James S, Wasilewski S: Achilles tendinitis, *Am J Sports Med* 9:93–98, 1981.
122. Lennox DW, Wang GJ, McCue FC, et al: The operative treatment of Achilles tendon injuries, *Clin Orthop* 148:152–155, 1980.
123. Lieberman JR, Lozman J, Czajka J, et al: Repair of Achilles tendon ruptures with Dacron vascular graft, *Clin Orthop* 234:204–208, 1988.
124. Lindholm Å: A new method of operation in subcutaneous rupture of the Achilles tendon, *Acta Chir Scand* 117:261–270, 1959.
125. Lipscomb PR: Tendons: number 1. Nonsuppurative tenosynovitis and paratendinitis. *Instr Course Lect* 7:254–261, 1950.
126. Lipscomb PR, Kelly PJ: Injuries of the extensor tendons in the distal part of the leg and in the ankle, *J Bone Joint Surg [Am]* 37:1206–1213, 1955.
127. Lipscomb PR, Sanchez JJ: Anterior transplantation of the posterior tibial tendon for persistent palsy of the common peroneal nerve, *J Bone Joint Surg [Am]* 43:60–66, 1961.
128. Lipscomb PR, Wakim KG; Further observations in the healing of severed tendons: an experimental study, *Proc Staff Meet Mayo Clin* 36:277–282, 1961.
129. Lipscomb PR, Wakim KG: Regeneration of severed tendons: an experimental study, *Proc Staff Meet Mayo Clin* 36:271–276, 1961.
130. Ljungqvist R: Subcutaneous partial rupture of the Achilles tendon, *Acta Orthop Scand Suppl* 113:1–86, 1968.
131. Ljungqvist R, Eriksson E: Partial tears of the patellar

tendon and the Achilles tendon. In Mack RP, editor: *Symposium on the foot and leg in running sports*, St Louis, 1982, Mosby–Year Book, pp 92–98.
132. Lynn TA: Repair of the torn Achilles tendon, using the plantaris tendon as a reinforcing membrane, *J Bone Joint Surg [Am]* 48:268–272, 1966.
133. Ma GW, Griffith TG: Percutaneous repair of acute closed ruptured Achilles tendon: a new technique, *Clin Orthop* 128:247–255, 1977.
134. Ma GWC, Griffith TG: Percutaneous repair of acute closed ruptured Achilles tendon: a new technique. In Moore TM, editor: *Symposium on trauma to the leg and its sequelae*, St Louis, 1982, Mosby–Year Book, pp 358–370.
135. Mann RA: Acquired flatfoot in adults, *Clin Orthop* 181:46–51, 1983.
136. Mann RA, Holmes GB, Seale KS, et al: Chronic rupture of the Achilles tendon: a new technique of repair, *J Bone Joint Surg [Am]* 73:214–219, 1991.
137. Martens MA, Noyez JF, Mulier JC: Recurrent dislocation of the peroneal tendons: results of rerouting the tendons under the calcaneofibular ligament, *Am J Sports Med* 14:148–150, 1986.
138. Marti R: Dislocation of the peroneal tendons, *Am J Sports Med* 5:19–22, 1977.
139. McCarroll JR, Ritter MA, Becker TE: Triggering of the great toe: a case report, *Clin Orthop* 175:184–185, 1983.
140. McConkey JP, Favero KJ: Subluxation of the peroneal tendons within the peroneal tendon sheath: a case report, *Am J Sports Med* 15:511–513, 1987.
141. McLennan JG: Treatment of acute and chronic luxations of the peroneal tendons, *Am J Sports Med* 8:432–436, 1980.
142. McMaster PE: Tendon and muscle ruptures: clinical and experimental studies on the causes and location of subcutaneous ruptures, *J Bone Joint Surg* 15:705–722, 1933.
143. Mensor MC, Ordway GL: Traumatic subcutaneous rupture of the tibialis anterior tendon, *J Bone Joint Surg [Am]* 35:675–680, 1953.
144. Meyerding HW: The treatment of bursitis, *Surg Clin North Am* 18: 1103–1117, 1938.
145. Meyn MA Jr: Closed rupture of the anterior tibial tendon: a case report and review of the literature, *Clin Orthop* 113:154–157, 1975.
146. Micheli LJ, Waters PM, Sanders DP: Sliding fibular graft repair for chronic dislocation of the peroneal tendons, *Am J Sports Med* 17:68–71, 1989.
147. Mick CA, Lynch F: Reconstruction of the peroneal retinaculum using the peroneus quartus, *J Bone Joint Surg [Am]* 69:296–297, 1987.
148. Miller BF, Buhr AJ: Pump bumps or knobby heals, *Nova Scotia Med Bul* 48:191–192, 1969.
149. Miller JW: Dislocation of peroneal tendons—a new operative procedure: a case report, *Am J Orthop* 9:136–137, 1967.
150. Moberg E: Subcutaneous rupture of the tendon of the tibialis anterior muscle, *Acta Chir Scand* 95:455–460, 1947.
151. Mortiz JR: Ski injuries, *Am J Surg* 98:493–505, 1959.
152. Moskowitz E: Rupture of the tibialis anterior tendon simulating peroneal nerve palsy, *Arch Phys Med Rehabil* 52:431–433, 1971.
153. Munk RL, Davis PH: Longitudinal rupture of the peroneus brevis tendon, *J Trauma* 16:803–806, 1977.
154. Murphy KJ, McPhee I: Tears of major tendons in chronic acidosis with elastosis, *J Bone Joint Surg [Am]* 47:1253, 1965.
155. Murr S: Dislocation of the peroneal tendons with marginal fracture of the lateral malleolus, *J Bone Joint Surg [Br]* 43:563–565, 1961.
156. Nada A: Rupture of the calcaneal tendon: treatment by external fixation, *J Bone Joint Surg [Br]* 67:449–453, 1985.
157. Nielson AL: Diagnostic and therapeutic point in retrocalcanean bursitis, *JAMA* 77:463, 1921.
158. Nillius SA, Nilsson BE, Westlin NE: The incidence of Achilles tendon rupture, *Acta Orthop Scand* 47:118–121, 1976.
159. Nisliet NW: Tendo achillis bursitis ("winter heal"), *Br Med J* 2:1934–1935, 1954.
160. Nistor L: Conservative treatment of fresh subcutaneous rupture of the Achilles tendon, *Acta Orthop Scand* 47:459–462, 1976.
161. Nistor L: Surgical and non-surgical treatment of Achilles tendon rupture: a prospective randomized study, *J Bone Joint Surg [Am]* 63:394–399, 1981.
162. O'Brien T: The needle test for complete rupture of the Achilles tendon, *J Bone Joint Surg [Am]* 66:1099–1101, 1984.
163. Oden RF: Tendon injuries about the ankle resulting from skiing, *Clin Orthop* 216:63–69, 1987.
164. Ozaki J, Fujiki J, Sugimoto K, et al: Reconstruction of neglected Achilles tendon rupture with Marlex mesh, *Clin Orthop* 238:204–208, 1989.
165. Palmer DG: Tendon sheaths and bursae involved by rheumatoid disease of the foot and ankle, *Australas Radiol* 14:419–428, 1970.
166. Parvin RW, Ford LT: Stenosing tenosynovitis of the common peroneal tendon sheath: report of two cases, *J Bone Joint Surg [Am]* 38:1352–1357, 1956.
167. Patterson RL Jr, Darrach W: Treatment of acute bursitis by needle irrigation, *J Bone Joint Surg* 19:993–1002, 1937.
168. Pavlov H, Heneghan MA, Hersh A, et al: The Haglund syndrome: initial and differential diagnosis, *Radiology* 144:83–88, 1982.
169. Peacock KC, Resnick EJ, Thoder JJ: Fracture of the os peroneum with rupture of the peroneus longus tendon, *Clin Orthop* 202:223–226, 1896.
170. Percy EC, Conochie LB: The surgical treatment of ruptured tondo Achillis, *Am J Sports Med* 6:132–136, 1978.
171. Perry J. Hoffer MM: Preoperative and postoperative dynamic electromyography as an aid in planning tendon transfers in children with cerebral palsy, *J Bone Joint Surg [Am]* 54:531–537, 1977.
172. Plattner PF, Johnson KA: Tendons and bursae. In Helal B, Wilson D, editors: *The foot*, London, 1988, Churchill Livingstone, pp 581–613.
173. Pöll RG, Duijfjes F: The treatment of recurrent dislocation of the peroneal tendons, *J Bone Joint Surg [Br]* 63:98–100, 1984
174. Pozo JL, Jackson AM: A rerouting operation for dislo-

cation of peroneal tendons: operative technique and case report, *Foot Ankle* 5:42–44, 1984.
175. Puddu G, Ippolito E, Postacchini F: A classification of Achilles tendon disease, *Am J Sports Med* 4:145–150, 1976.
176. Quigley TB, Scheller AD: Surgical repair of the ruptured Achilles tendon: analysis of 40 patients treated by the same surgeon, *Am J Sports Med* 8:244–250, 1980.
177. Ralston EL, Schmidt ER Jr: Repair of the ruptured Achilles tendon, *J Trauma* 11:15–19, 1971.
178. Rasmussen RB, Thyssen EP: Rupture of the flexor hallucis longus tendon: case report, *Foot Ankle* 10:288–289, 1990.
179. Reinherz RP: Management of flexor hallucis longus tendon injuries, *J Foot Surg* 23:366–369, 1984.
180. Roberts PW: Bursitis of the foot: a neglected cause of disability, *Am J Surg* 6:313–317, 1929.
181. Roberts PW: Fifty cases of bursitis of the foot, *J Bone Joint Surg* 11:338–344, 1929.
182. Rodriguez RP: The bridle procedure in the treatment of paralysis of the foot, *Foot Ankle* 13(2):63–69, 1992.
183. Rubin BD, Wilson HJ Jr: Surgical repair of the interrupted Achilles tendon, *J Trauma* 20:248–249, 1980.
184. Ruch JA: Haglund's disease, *J Am Podiatr Med Assoc* 64:1000–1003, 1974.
185. Sammarco GJ, DiRaimondo CV: Chronic peronus brevis tendon lesions, *Foot Ankle* 9:163–170.
186. Sammarco GJ, Miller EH: Partial rupture of the flexor hallucis longus tendon in classical ballet dancers: two case reports, *J Bone Joint Surg [Am]* 61:149–150, 1979.
187. Sarma PJ: The injection treatment of ganglions and bursae: indications and limitations, *Surg Clin North Am* 20:135–140, 1940.
188. Sarmiento A, Wolf M: Subluxation of peroneal tendons: case treated by rerouting tendons under calcaneofibular ligament, *J Bone Joint Surg [Am]* 57:115–116, 1975.
189. Sarrafian SK: *Anatomy of the foot and ankle: descriptive, topographic, functional,* Philadelphia, 1983, JB Lippincott, pp 251–259.
190. Saunders DE, Hochberg J, Wittenborn W: Treatment of total loss of the Achilles tendon by skin flap cover without tendon repair, *Plast Reconstr Surg* 62:708–712, 1978.
191. Savastano AA: Recurrent dislocation of the peroneal tendons. In Bateman JE, Trott AW, editors: *The foot and ankle: a selection of papers from the American Orthopaedic Foot Society Meetings,* New York, 1980, Brian C Decker, pp 110–115.
192. Schatzker J, Brånemark P-I: Intravital observation on the microvascular anatomy and microcirculation of the tendon, *Acta Orthop Scand Suppl* 126:1–23, 1969.
193. Schedl R, Fasol P: Achilles tendon repair with the plantaris tendon compared with repair using polyglycol threads, *J Trauma* 19:189–194, 1979.
194. Schepsis AA, Leach RE: Surgical management of Achilles tendinitis, *Am J Sports Med* 15:308–315, 1987.
195. Schneider M, Balon K: Deformity of the foot following anterior transfer of the posterior tendon and lengthening of the Achilles tendon for spastic equinovarus, *Clin Orthop* 125:113–118, 1977.
196. Scott WN, Inglis AE, Sculco TP: Surgical treatment of reruptures of the tendo Achillis following nonsurgical treatment. *Clin Orthop* 140:175–177, 1979.
197. Sever JW: Apophysitis of the os calcis, *N Y Med J* 95:1025–1029, 1912.
198. Shephard E: Intermetatarso-phalangeal bursitis in the causation of Morton's metatarsalgia, *J Bone Joint Surg [Br]* 57:115–116, 1975.
199. Shields CL Jr, Kerlan RK, Jobe FW, et al: The Cybex II evaluation of surgically repaired Achilles tendon ruptures, *Am J Sports Med* 6:369–372, 1978.
200. Silver RL, DeLa Garza J, Rang M: The myth of muscle balance: a study of relative strengths and excursions of normal muscles about the foot and ankle, *J Bone Joint Surg [Br]* 67:432–437, 1985.
201. Sim FH, DeWeerd JH Jr: Rupture of the extensor hallucis longus tendon while skiing, *Minn Med* 60:789–790, 1977.
202. Skeoch DU: Spontaneous partial subcutaneous ruptures of the tendo Achillis: review of the literature and evaluation of 16 involved tendons, *Am J Sports Med* 9:20–22, 1981.
203. Snook GA: Achilles tendon tenosynovitis in long-distance runners, *Med Sci Sports Exerc* 4:155–158, 1972.
204. Sobel M, Bohne WHO, Levy ME: Longitudinal attrition of the peroneus brevis tendon in the fibular groove: an anatomic study, *Foot Ankle* 11:124–128, 1990.
205. Sobel M, Bohne WHO, Markisz JA: Cadaver correlation of peroneal tendon changes with magnetic resonance imaging, *Foot Ankle* 11:384–388, 1991.
206. Sobel M, Levy ME, Bonhe WHO: Congenital variations of the peroneus quartus muscle: an anatomic study, *Foot Ankle* 11:81–89, 1990.
207. Sobel M, Warren RF, Brourmans: Lateral ankle instability associated with dislocation of the peroneal tendons treated by the Chrisman-Snook procedure: a case report and literature review, *Am J Sports Med* 18:539–543, 1990.
208. Steffensen JCA, Evensen A: Bursitis retrocalcanean achilli, *Acta Orthop Scand* 27:228–236, 1958.
209. Stein RE: Reconstruction of the superior peroneal retinaculum using a portion of the peroneus brevis tendon: a case report, *J Bone Joint Surg [Am]* 69:298–299, 1987.
210. Stein SR, Luekens CA: Methods and rationale for closed treatment of Achilles tendon ruptures, *Am J Sports Med* 4:162–169, 1976.
211. Stein SR, Luekens CA Jr: Closed treatment of Achilles tendon ruptures, *Orthop Clin North Am* 7:241–246, 1976.
212. Stiehl JB: Concomitant rupture of the peroneus brevis tendon and bimalleolar fracture, *J Bone Joint Surg [Am]* 70:936–937, 1988.
213. Stover CN, Bryan DR: Traumatic dislocation of the peroneal tendons, *Am J Surg* 103:180–186, 1962.
214. Szczukowski M Jr, St Pierre RK, Fleming LL, et al: Computerized tomography in the evaluation of peroneal tendon dislocation. A report of two cases, *Am J Sports Med* 11:444–447, 1983.
215. Taylor LW: Achilles tendon repair: results of surgical management. In Moore M, editor: *Symposium on trauma to the leg and its sequelae,* St Louis, 1981, Mosby–Year Book, pp 371–384.
216. Taylor RG: The treatment of claw toes by multiple transfers of flexor into extensor tendons, *J Bone Joint Surg [Br]* 33:539–542, 1951.
217. Tehranzadeh J, Stoll DA, Gabriele OM: Open-quiz solution: case report 271, *Skeletal Radiol* 12:44–47, 1984.

218. Teng MMH, Destouet JM, Gilula LA, et al: Ankle tenography: a key to unexplained symptomatology. Part 1: Normal tenographic anatomy, *Radiology* 151:575–580, 1984.
219. Teuffer AP: Traumatic rupture of the Achilles tendon: reconstruction by transplant and graft using the lateral peroneus brevis, *Orthop Clin North Am* 5:89–93, 1974.
220. Thompson FM, Patterson AH: Rupture of the peroneus longus tendon, *J Bone Joint Surg [Am]* 71:293–295, 1989.
221. Thompson TC: A test for rupture of the tendo Achillis, *Acta Orthop Scand* 32:461–465, 1962.
222. Thompson TC, Doherty JH: Spontaneous rupture of tendon of Achilles: a new clinical diagnostic test, *J Trauma* 2:126–129, 1962.
223. Toygar O: 1947. Cited by Arner et al, 1958–1959.
224. Trevino S, Gould N, Korson R: Surgical treatment of stenosing tenosynovitis at the ankle, *Foot Ankle* 2:37–45, 1981.
225. Tudisco C, Puddu G: Stenosing tenosynovitis of the flexor hallucis longus tendon in a classical ballet dancer: a case report, *Am J Sports Med* 12:403–404, 1984.
226. Turco VJ, Spinella AJ: Achilles tendon ruptures–peroneus brevis transfer, *Foot Ankle* 7:253–259, 1987.
227. Turner JW, Cooper RR: Anterior transfer of the tibialis posterior through the interosseous membrane, *Clin Orthop* 83:241–244, 1972.
228. Turner JW, Cooper RR: Posterior transposition of tibialis anterior through the interosseous membrane, *Clin Orthop* 79:71–74, 1971.
229. Waters RL: Acquired neurologic disorders of the adult foot. In Mann RA, editor: *Surgery of the foot*, ed 5, St Louis, 1986, Mosby–Year Book, p 339.
230. Webster FS: Peroneal tenosynovitis with pseudotumor, *J Bone Joint Surg [Am]* 50:153–157, 1968.
231. Weinstabl R, Stisical M, Neuhold A, et al: Classifying calcaneal tendon injury according to MRI findings, *J Bone Joint Surg* 73:683, 1991.
232. Werner JA, Shein AJ: Simultaneous bilateral rupture of the patellar tendon and quadriceps expansion in systemic lupus erythematosus: a case report, *J Bone Joint Surg [Am]* 56:823, 1974.
233. Weston WJ: The bursa deep to tendo Achillis, *Australas Radiol* 14:327–331, 1970.
234. White CS: Retrocalcanean bursitis, *N Y Med J* 98:263–265, 1913.
235. Wicks MH, Harbison JS, Paterson DC: Tendon injuries about the foot and ankle in children, *Aust N Z J Surg* 50:158–161, 1980.
236. Williams R: Chronic non-specific tendovaginitis of tibialis posterior, *J Bone Joint Surg [Br]* 45:542–545, 1963.
237. Wills CA, Washburn S, Caiozzo V, et al: Achilles tendon rupture: a review of the literature comparing surgical versus nonsurgical treatment. *Clin Orthop* 207:156–163, 1986.
238. Yancey HA Jr: Lacerations of the plantar aspect of the foot, *Clin Orthop* 122:46–52, 1977.
239. Zadak I: An operation for cure of archillobursitis, *Am J Surg* 43:542–546, 1939.
240. Zoellner G, Clancy W Jr: Recurrent dislocation of the peroneal tendon, *J Bone Joint Surg [Am]* 61:292–294, 1979.

C H A P T E R

20

Heel Pain

R. Luke Bordelon, M.D.

Subcalcaneal pain syndrome (heel spur syndrome/plantar fasciitis)
Anatomy
Diagnosis
History
Physical examination
Diagnostic and roentgenographic studies
Treatment
Treatment of subcalcaneal pain syndrome in athletes
Other causes of inferior heel pain
Authors method of treatment
Superior heel pain (retrocalcaneal bursitis, Haglund's disease, enlargement of the superior tuberosity of the os calcis, insertional Achilles tendinitis)
Anatomy
Diagnosis
Physical examination
Radiographic studies
Etiology and diagnostic tests
Treatment
Author's method of treatment

SUBCALCANEAL PAIN SYNDROME (HEEL SPUR SYNDROME/PLANTAR FASCIITIS)

Pain in the region of the medial tuberosity of the heel along with increased pain upon activity and sometimes related to a spur of the os calcis has been described for many years.

In reviewing the literature, apparently many different theories exist regarding the etiology of the pain, and different methods of treatment have been suggested for subcalcaneal pain.* It has been said that although it is familiar to all orthopaedic surgeons, it is probably fully understood by none.[4]

The pain has been attributed to pull of the plantar fascia,[3–5, 33, 34, 38] perhaps associated with microtrauma to the plantar fascia near its attachment, which leads to attempted repair and chronic inflammation. This syndrome has been attributed to nerve entrapment. Freeman[13] and others[3, 50] have attributed the pain to irritation of the medial calcaneal nerve, which is the sensory nerve to the heel. Przylucki and Jones[43] and Baxter and Thigpen[2] have attributed the pain to entrapment of the nerve to the abductor digiti quinti, which arises from the lateral branch of the plantar nerve. Bordelon[3, 4] has described this as a clinical syndrome. He suggested that the condition be considered in light of the structures that are present in the area, with specific treatment being directed toward those structures that are inflamed with the thought that irritation and inflammation of one structure may produce abnormalities of other structures.[3, 4]

There has been much discussion regarding the relationship of the calcaneal spur to subcalcaneal pain, but the relationship has not been definitely established. The heel spur lies in the origin of the short-toe flexors and

*_References 1–11, 13, 14, 19, 20, 23, 24, 27, 29–33, 35–39, 41–45, 47, 50, 54–57, 59, 61–63._

not in the plantar fascia.[33, 34, 52, 59] (Fig 20–1). Heel spurs are noted in about 50% of cases of subcalcaneal pain syndrome.[6, 57, 59]

Shmokler et al.[55] reviewed 1,000 random patients with radiographs of the foot. They found that there was a 13.2% incidence of heel spurs and only 5.2% of the total patients with heel spurs reported any history of subcalcaneal heel pain. They believed that this tended to support the premise that the presence of a heel spur did not mandate pain. Williams et al.,[64] in evaluating 45 patients with 52 painful heels, found that 75% of the patients had a heel spur as compared with 63% of the opposite nonpainful heels. With a comparison of 63 heels in 59 age- and sex matched controls, the incidence of heel spur was 7.9%.

A heel spur may be present or absent with the subcalcaneal pain syndrome. It probably cannot be considered the etiology but has to be considered in the context of the entire syndrome.

Anatomy

The plantar aponeurosis arises from the os calcis and is composed of three segments[18, 21, 22, 48] (Fig 20–2). Clinically when referring to the plantar aponeurosis, especially in regard to the subcalcaneal pain syndrome, one is generally referring to the central portion that originates from the medial tuberosity of the os calcis and inserts in the toes. It passes to the proximal phalanges of the lesser toes through the longitudinal septa, to the big toe through the sesamoids, and into the skin of the ball of the foot through the vertical fibers.[19] Hyperextension of the toes and the metatarsophalangeal joints tense the plantar aponeurosis, raise the longitudinal arch of the foot, invert the hindfoot, and externally rotate the leg. This mechanism depends entirely on the bony and ligamentous stability and is passive. It has been classified as the "windlass mechanism" by Hicks.[25]

The posterior tibial nerve is located on the medial side of the foot behind the medial malleolus and beneath the flexor retinaculum (Fig 20–3). The medial calcaneal nerve arises at the level of the medial malleolus or below and passes superficial to innervate the skin of the heel. It may consist of one or two branches. The most important anatomic reference point is that this nerve passes in the subcutaneous tissue between the plantar aponeurosis and the skin. The nerve to the abductor digiti quinti comes off the lateral plantar nerve and passes deeper beneath the plantar aponeurosis and underneath the spur if present to innervate the abductor digit quinti. It is important to differentiate the medial calcaneal nerve from the nerve to the abductor digiti quinti[3–5] (Fig 20–4). This can be done by the position because the medial calcaneal nerve is in the subcutaneous tissue and passes superficial to the plantar aponeurosis whereas the nerve to the abductor digiti quinti is deeper and passes beneath the plantar aponeurosis.

Rondhuis and Huson[46] noted that the entrapment of the nerve to the abductor digiti quinti may be located between the abductor hallucis and the medial margin of the medial head of the quadratus plantae muscle (Fig 20–5,A and B). They did not find a perforation of the fascia as described by Baxter and Thigpen,[2] nor did they find any bursa in the origin of the plantar aponeurosis. They concluded that fibers were present that innervate the perichondrium and that sensory fibers are present that form free endings and produce pain sensation. Motor branches to the flexor digitorum brevis and abductor digiti quinti muscles were present.

The medial and lateral plantar nerves pass through

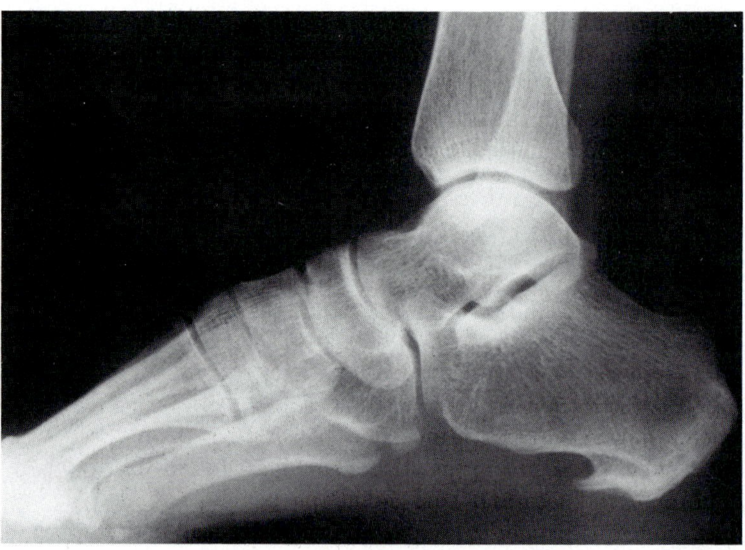

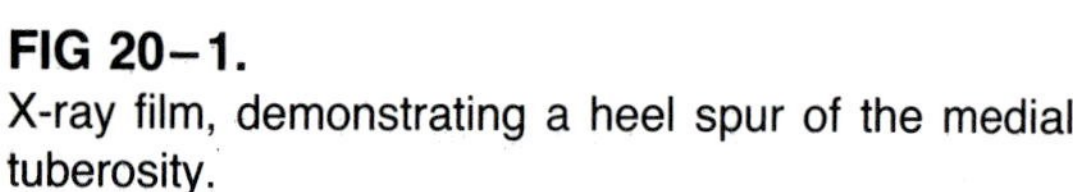

FIG 20–1.
X-ray film, demonstrating a heel spur of the medial tuberosity.

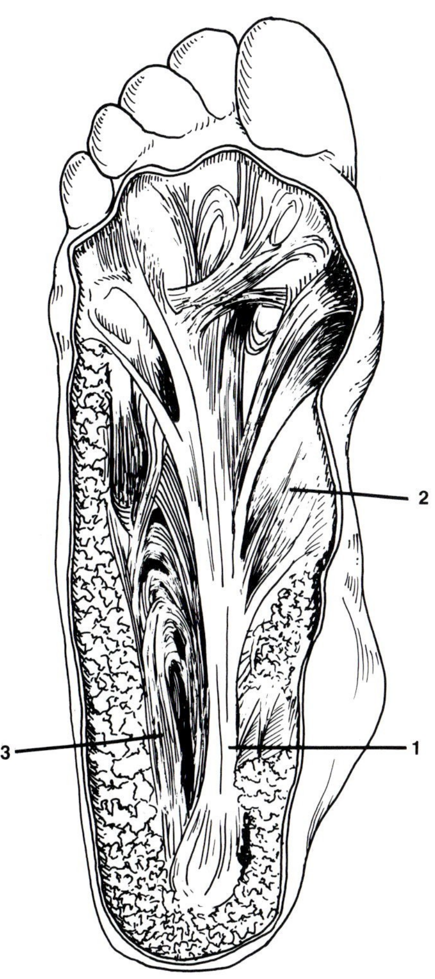

FIG 20–2.
The plantar aponeurosis consists of three parts: *(1)* central component of the plantar aponeurosis, *(2)* medial component of the plantar aponeurosis, and *(3)* lateral component of the plantar aponeurosis. From a clinical standpoint, the central portion is considered to be in the plantar aponeurosis. (Adapted from Sarrafian SK: *Anatomy of the foot and ankle,* Philadelphia, 1983, JB Lippincott, pp 127–142.)

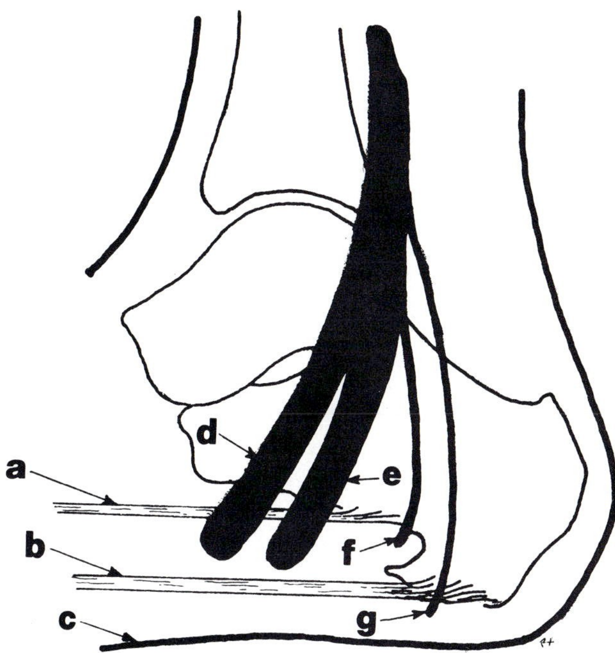

FIG 20–3.
Relationships of structures commonly associated with heel pain: *a,* long plantar ligament: *b,* plantar fascia; *c,* skin; *d,* medial plantar nerve; *e,* lateral plantar nerve; *f,* nerve to the abductor digiti quinti; and *g,* medial calcaneal nerve. (From Bordelon RL: *Instr Course Lect* 33:283–287, 1984. Used by permission.)

the respective foramina of the abductor muscle. When entrapment of the posterior tibial nerve is considered, it is important to note that this nerve may be trapped beneath the flexor retinaculum at the level of the medial malleolus or may be trapped at these foramina as the medial and lateral plantar nerves exit.

Diagnosis

History

The history usually reveals that there is a gradual onset of pain along the inside of the heel.[3–5] Occasionally, the pain may be associated with a foot injury producing an abrupt onset of pain.[34] However, the clinical course is generally similar regardless of the onset. The pain is usually described as being along the medial side of the foot at the bottom of the heel and worse upon first arising in the morning with some abatement upon increased activity. However, it may increase after prolonged activity. Periods of inactivity are generally followed by an increase in pain as activity is started again. Numbness of the foot is usually not present. When severe pain is present, the patient is unable to bear weight on the heel.

Physical Examination

Physical examination is performed to ascertain what specific type of foot is present.[5]

The type of foot will influence the mechanics of the foot and thus the function of the plantar fascia.

A supple foot with a tendency toward a flatfoot deformity will place increased strain upon the origin of the plantar fascia and the calcaneus with ambulation because of the increased dependence of the windlass mechanism in maintaining a stable arch during the propulsive phase of gait. With this type of plantar fascial strain, efforts to decrease the strain on the plantar fascia with strapping, a University of California Biomechanics

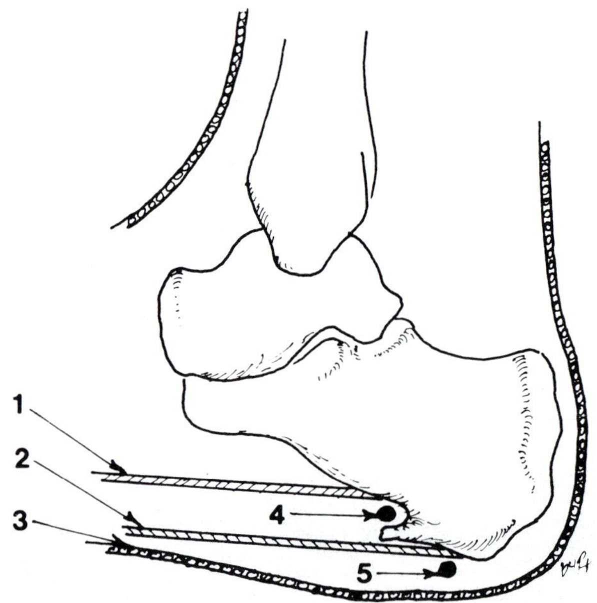

FIG. 20–4.
Sagittal section of os calcis with relationships of the nerves to the abductor digiti quinti and the medial calcaneal nerve as described by Baxter[2] and Przylucki and Jones:[43] *(1)* long plantar ligament, *(2)* plantar fascia, *(3)* skin, *(4)* nerve to the abductor digiti quinti, and *(5)* medial calcaneal nerve. (From Bordelon RL: *Instr Course Lect* 33:283–287, 1984. Used by permission.)

Laboratory (UCBL) type of insert, and orthotic devices to correct the biomechanical deformity may be helpful.

When a cavus foot is present, there may be excessive pressure on the heel area because of a lack of ability to evert to allow the foot to absorb shock and adapt to the ground. With a cavus foot a cushioning material may be used to decrease the shock and increase the area of contact.

As with any examination of the foot, the examination must include the entire lower extremity. One must be aware of the relationship of the foot to the body.

Specific examination of the foot will usually reveal that there is acute tenderness along the medial tuberosity of the os calcis. This tenderness may be at the origin of the central slip of the plantar fascia, or the tenderness may be deep and perhaps may represent deep inflammation with involvement of the nerve to the abductor digiti quinti.

The plantar fascia is palpated to determine whether the plantar fascia is tender solely at its origin or throughout its course. The plantar fascia is also palpated for nodules. Sometimes the plantar fascia is most tender when placed under stress and should be palpated with both the toes and ankle extended and flexed.

The tarsal tunnel is palpated and percussed to elicit any tenderness, inflammation, or a Tinel sign of the posterior tibial, medial or lateral plantar, or the medial calcaneal nerves. Sensation of the foot is evaluated by light touch and pinprick to ascertain the status of the sensory nerves. The subtalar joint complex and ankle joint are examined for motion and mobility, both actively and passively to rule out referred pain from these areas. Active motor power of the muscles that cross or affect this area such as the posterior tibial, anterior tibial, peroneus longus and brevis, and toe flexors and extensors are checked to determine the motor power and also to see whether there is any pain produced with active motor function. Neurologic examination of the remainder of the lower extremities and back is performed as indicated.

Diagnostic and Roentgenographic Studies

Roentgenograms are taken of the heel, including the foot in the anteroposterior (AP) and lateral standing projections. Radiographs taken in this manner will provide information concerning the osseous structures of the foot as well as specific details of the os calcis. The standing roentgenograms will also provide information regarding the biomechanical status of the foot if they are taken in the standing position with the foot in the base and angle of gait. X-ray films taken in this manner will help to classify the feet as to whether they are normal, flat, or cavus-type feet. These x-ray films will demonstrate whether there is a spur or calcification along the medial tuberosity. Axial non–weight-bearing views of the os calcis may be taken to provide information in a second plane if necessary.

A technetium 99 bone scan may be performed. If results are positive, it will provide evidence of an inflammatory abnormality in this area (Fig 20–6).

Sewell et al.[51] studying five patients with heel pain, interpreted the bone scans to show that the uptake is increased at the site of insertion of the long plantar tendon into the calcaneus in patients with a clinical picture of plantar fasciitis and that this may occur in the absence of any radiologic change. Changes in intensity of tracer uptake reflected symptomatic improvement. They suggested that radiologic imaging allowed a quantitative assessment of inflammation of the "enthesis" and allowed therapy to be evaluated. Vasavada et al.[60] reported on obtaining early blood pool images to detect soft-tissue inflammation (plantar fasciitis) when delayed images are normal.

Williams et al.[64] reported on 45 patients with painful heel syndrome without evidence of associated inflammatory arthritis. They were studied with technetium 99 isotope bone scans and lateral and 45-degree medial oblique radiographs of both feet. Of the 52 painful heels

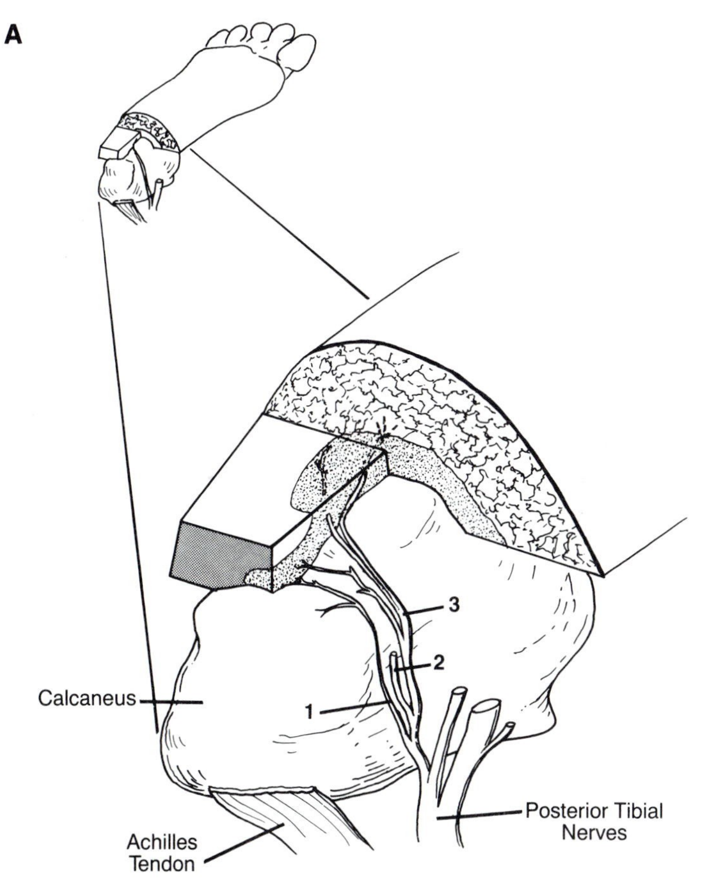

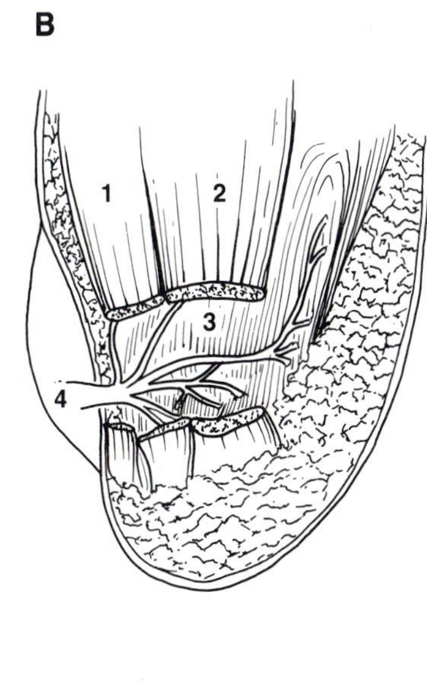

FIG 20–5.
A, illustration of the nerve to the abductor digiti quinti: *(1)* branch running to the medial process of the calcaneal tuberosity and bifurcating into a branch covering the perichondrium of the medial process and another one running to a more lateral part of the calcaneal perichondrium, *(2)* branch to the flexor digitorum muscle, and *(3)* branches to the abductor digiti minimi muscle. **B,** drawing of the nerve to the abductor digiti quinti as dissected in an adult foot. Parts of the abductor hallucis *(1)* and flexor digitorum *(2)* muscles have been removed with the nerve running across the quadratus plantae muscle *(3)* in a plantar direction and then turning into a horizontal plane to proceed lateralward. Also shown is the nerve to the abductor digiti quinti *(4)*. (Adapted from Rondhuis JJ, Huson A: *Acta Morphol Neer Scand* 24:269–279, 1986.)

in these 45 patients, 59.6% showed increased uptake at the calcaneus. They found that patients with scans showing increased uptake tended to have more severe heel pain and responded more frequently to local hydrocortisone injection. These findings suggested that patients with normal scan results may have had some noninflammatory lesion such as simple trauma or entrapment of the medial calcaneal nerve. They did not find any evidence of a stress fracture in contrast to the report by Graham.[20]

Laboratory studies in most cases of subcalcaneal pain syndrome show normal findings. However, when the subcalcaneal pain syndrome is present and especially if it is persistent and severe, consideration must be given to the diagnosis of a severe systemic disorder such as seronegative arthropathy. It has been reported that patients presenting with the subcalcaneal pain syndrome may have an incidence as high as 16% of subsequent development of a systemic arthritic disorder.[4]

Eastmond et al.[12] reported 26 patients with seronegative pauciarticular arthritis and positive HLA-B27. They noted that low back and buttock pain, Achilles tendinitis, and dactylitis of the toes were more frequent in HLA-B27–positive patients. They believed that these tests should be part of a workup for chronic, recurrent, incapacitating heel pain.

Gerster[15] reported on the painful heel syndrome with plantar fasciitis and/or Achilles tendinitis in 33 of 150 patients suffering from a seronegative spondarthritis. An HLA-B27 antigen was found in 91% of the patients. He contrasted this to a study of 220 cases of rheumatoid arthritis and found that Achilles tendinitis was not encountered and plantar fasciitis was exceptional in these patients. Gerster and Piccinin[16] reported

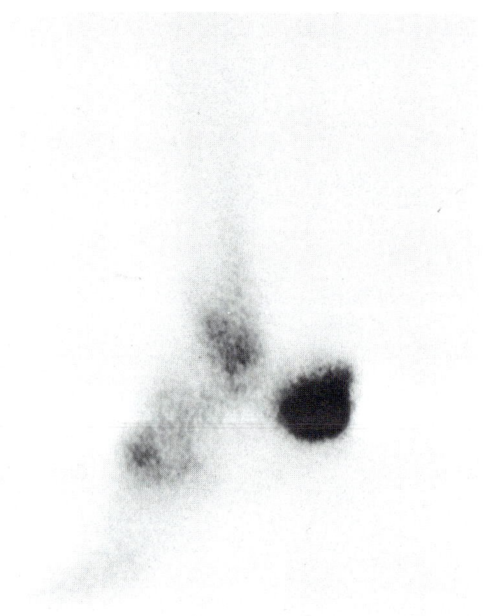

FIG 20–6.
A bone scan for subcalcaneal pain demonstrates intense activity in the calcaneus.

that severe heel pain was present in 4 of 18 cases of juvenile-onset seronegative spondyloarthropathy. Four other patients had mild heel pain. The overall prognosis for the disease was poor in patients with severe heel pain. Gerster et al.[17] also reported 30 cases of severe heel pain with seronegative spondyloarthropathy in which four patients underwent surgical intervention with either release of the plantar aponeurosis or rasping of the calcaneal spur upon failure of the surgery. They stated that surgery is contraindicated in severe heel pain associated with seronegative spondarthritis.

Proximal neurologic causes of heel pain should also be considered. Tarsal tunnel entrapment may be present with referred pain to the heel and sole of the foot. A positive Tinel sign should suggest this diagnosis. Electromyographic (EMG) and nerve conduction studies should be utilized to rule out this condition.[5]

Heel pain may also be referred proximally from the lumbar spine. If a spinal or proximal etiology appears to be a possibility, then appropriate laboratory and radiographic studies are performed as indicated.

Treatment

Callison[6] reviewed 400 consecutive patients with heel pain seen in his office during a 40-month period from October 1985 to February 1989. All underwent radiographic studies. Forty-five percent had heel spurs and 53% had no heel spurs. Sixty-five percent were women, and 35% were men. Thirty percent of the women were obese, while only 10% of the men were obese. Seven percent were involved in active sports. Patients were treated with steroid injections, orthoses, calf stretching, and nonsteroidal anti-inflammatory medication. Plaster immobilization was occasionally used. Seventy-three percent improved significantly within 6 months. Twenty percent failed to improve, and 7% did not return and were lost to follow-up. Of the 81 patients who failed to improve, 36 patients were offered surgery with a cautious prognosis. Sixteen patients declined for various reasons, and 20 patients (5%) underwent surgery. Eighteen patients had release of the plantar aponeurosis alone through a transverse, slightly oblique incision distal to the heel pad. A short-leg cast was applied for 3 weeks postoperatively. Of the 18 patients who underwent a plantar fasciotomy alone, 15 patients experienced a very good result. Fourteen of the 15 were pain free within 6 months postoperatively. One patient described occasional soreness in the arch. Three patients experienced a poor result. Two patients underwent plantar fasciotomy with release of the medial and lateral plantar nerves and medial calcaneal nerve because of symptoms of intermittent burning of the heel with occasional paresthesia in the foot and toes. Neither of these patients had Tinel signs and had normal nerve conduction studies. Both of these patients were pain free 3 months postoperatively.

Snook and Chrisman[57] reported on 22 patients with 25 painful heels. Sixteen of the 18 patients obtained relief of pain with a variety of conservative measures. Seven of the patients with 8 painful heels required surgery consisting of excision of the medial and inferior tuberosity of the os calcis. All obtained relief during a follow-up period ranging from 2 to 7 years.

O'Brien and Martin[41] studied the results of conservative care of 58 painful heels in 41 patients. Seventy were classified as being in the excellent category (no remaining symptoms). Twenty-six were classified as good (50%) or fewer of the symptoms remaining), and only 3.5% were symptomatic and classified as poor. In heels responding best to orthotic therapy, the duration of preceding symptoms was an average of 2.5 years. From this an assumption can be made that the most acute duration cases respond better to injection therapy while more chronic cases respond better to the use of orthoses.

Shikoff et al.[54] reported a retrospective study of 195 patients with heel pain. They found that the typical patient was middle-aged and overweight. Approximately 50% of patients continued to take oral medication, wear padding, or both for months after the initial visit. Thirty percent experienced only marginal relief or an unsatisfactory result.

Goulet[19] reported on the use of a soft orthosis in treating plantar fasciitis.

Surgical care has been reported by the following authors.

Ward and Clippinger[61] reported on the use of a curved oblique plantar incision in the proximal aspect of the medial longitudinal arch to release the plantar fascia in eight feet with recalcitrant plantar fasciitis. Seven feet became pain free, and the eighth was 75% improved. Normal sensation was preserved in all cases. There were no painful scars or neuromas.

Contompasis[8] reported on 129 patients who had surgery through a medial horizontal incision with exostosectomy and fasciotomy, fasciotomy only, or exostosectomy only. The majority of heels underwent more exostosectomies than fasciotomies. This was in 115 cases. Overall, there was complete improvement in 43%, some improvement in 38%, no improvement in 17%, but no worsening of symptoms in any patient.

DuVries[11] reported on 37 cases treated by a medial incision and fasciotomy and rasping of the spur with good results and no recurrence of symptoms.

Jay et al.[27] reported calcaneal decompression for chronic heel pain through a lateral approach in four patients, with pain relief in three of the four patients. One patient had immediate relief, two had relief of symptoms several weeks postoperatively, and the fourth patient did not become pain free.

Lester and Buchanan[35] reported on ten patients who underwent stripping of the plantar fascia and superficial plantar muscles from the calcaneus. These patients had been treated for an average of 12.4 months prior to surgery and were followed for 24 months after the operation. Complete symptomatic relief was obtained in all patients, although hypoesthesia of the heel was present in five feet after the operation. Three patients were receiving workmen's compensation but returned to work within 16 weeks of surgery.

Kenzora[30] reported on exploration of the nerve to the abductor digiti quinti and release of the nerve through a midline plantar incision of the heel. He submitted a preliminary report on six patients with only a short follow-up, none of whom were dissatisfied, although two patients had temporary numbness along the medial aspect of the incision. He considered the procedure experimental.

Ali[1] reported in his series that steroid injections provided relief in 13% of the patients treated. Plantar fasciotomy provided permanent relief in 75%. Plantar fasciotomy with excision of the calcaneal spur produced a cure in 85%.

Hassab and El-Sherif[23] reported on drilling of the os calcis for relief of recalcitrant heel pain. They performed 68 operations on 60 patients, with excellent results in 62, good in 2, and bad in 4.

Treatment of Subcalcaneal Pain Syndrome in Athletes

McBryde[39] followed 100 patients with plantar fasciitis in his running clinic. He found that plantar fasciitis accounted for 9% of total running injuries seen. The conservative (nonoperative) approach consisted of (1) ice massage for 2 minutes, four to six times daily including before and after runs; (2) heel cord stretching for 3 to 5 minutes, three to four times daily; (3) posterior tibial and peroneal strengthening; (4) heel cushioning and control, and (5) anti-inflammatory medication. He found this regime to be usually successful in treating plantar fasciitis seen within the first 8 weeks. In cases with symptoms lasting longer than 6 weeks, a period of absolute rest with casting was usually required. Five percent of the patients in this series underwent surgery consisting of plantar fascial release through a short 1-in. longitudinal incision in the medial arch. All embarked on a successful running program within 6 to 12 weeks after surgery. Overall, of the 100 patients with plantar fasciitis, 82 recovered with conservative treatment; 11 stopped running; 5 underwent surgery, all of whom returned to running; and 2 refused surgery and continued to be symptomatic.

Lutter[37] outlined decision making in athletes with subcalcaneal pain. He reported on 182 patients with heel complaints related to sports injuries with running producing the greatest number of complaints (76%). Approximately 20% of these patients required 3 to 4 months of conservative treatment before returning to sports activity. Five percent had chronic heel pain and did not recover within 9 to 12 months. A surgical approach was considered for these. He stated that the decision to operate on an athlete is based on six specific tenets: (1) correct diagnosis, (2) approximately 12 months of conservative treatment, (3) EMG for diagnosis and appropriate nerve blocks, (4) thorough knowledge of the anatomy, (5) the patient's understanding that even successful surgery may not allow him to return to high-performance athletics, and (6) correct and appropriately directed surgery. The procedure used depended upon the preoperative diagnosis and varied from release of the nerves, to release of the fascia, to complete exploration of the posterior tibial nerve and its branches. Cycling or swimming was begun 2 weeks postoperatively. Gentle walk/dash run training and a gradual escalation up to running at approximately 6 weeks postoperatively were allowed. The patient was asked to refrain from running until he was pain free and without tenderness. If there was pain upon increased activity, the workout was cut by 50% until the patient could tolerate the workout without pain.

Sammarco[47] divided heel pain into three clinical classifications and provided a treatment algorithm for these conditions. First, calcaneodynia, produced by a stress fracture, was treated with a foot orthosis and decrease in running. Second, plantar fasciitis was treated with a foot orthosis, anti-inflammatory medication, a flexibility program, and occasional injection of corticosteroids. Recalcitrant plantar fasciitis (with symptoms greater than 1 year in duration) was treated by release of the plantar fascia and bone spur if one was present. Finally, calcaneodynia involving entrapment of the medial calcaneal nerve and/or the nerve to the abductor digiti quinti was diagnosed by a positive Tinel sign and treated with an orthosis or release of the nerve.

Clancy[7] reported on treating patients conservatively with a medial heel wedge and flexible leather support, heel cord stretching, and rest for 6 to 12 weeks, with a gradual return to running while wearing an orthotic and medial heel wedge for 10 weeks. In those patients who did not respond, surgery consisting of release of the plantar fascia and the fascia over the abductor hallucis longus was performed. He performed surgery in 15 cases in a 2-year period at the University of Wisconsin, with all of the patients returning to running within 8 to 10 weeks.

D'Ambrosia et al.[9, 10] used the conservative measures of anti-inflammatory medication, physical therapy, orthotic devices, and shoe modifications, with orthotic devices seeming to be the most useful modality of treatment.

Jørgensen[28] reported on a diagnostic method to evaluate the shock absorbing ability of the heel pad by a visual compressible index calculated on the basis of x-ray films of the heel, loaded and unloaded by body weight. He reported on three athletes with unusually soft and fat heel pads who were heel strikers. These were treated successfully with external heel shock absorption pads.

Kwong et al.[32] treated fasciitis as produced by an excessive amount and/or a prolonged duration of pronation, with temporary relief being obtained by anti-inflammatory drugs and therapy. Long-term relief was obtained by adequate control of pronation by a semi rigid custom-molded orthosis to reduce plantar fascial strain by supporting the first metatarsal and controlling the calcaneal position in conjunction with a shoe with a firm posterior counter.

Leach et al.[33] stated that most patients would respond well to conservative therapy consisting of decreased activity, stretching, heel cups, and occasional local steroids. They reported on 15 competitive athletes who had 16 operations performed. The surgery consisted of plantar fascial release at the insertion of the os calcis from an incision along the medial side of the heel. In 1 instance the medial calcaneal nerve was described as being involved in the inflammatory process. The quickest return to running activity was at 6 weeks. The majority of patients returned to running within 9 weeks after surgery. Most patients continued to improve up to 6 months after the surgical procedure. Of the 15 operations, 14 were successful in that the athletes returned to their previous level of activity. There was 1 failure in a marathon runner who improved but was unable to train at the level he desired. There were no complications.

Snider et al.[56] reported 11 plantar fascial releases for chronic fasciitis in nine distance runners who had symptoms for an average of 20 months and who had not responded to non surgical treatment. The results of the operations were excellent in 10 feet and good in 1 foot with an average follow-up time of 25 months. Eight out of 9 patients returned to their desired full training at an average time of 4.5 months.

Baxter and Thigpen[2] performed 34 operative procedures in 26 patients with recalcitrant heel pain. The procedure consisted of isolated neurolysis of the nerves supplying the abductor digiti quinti muscle as it passed beneath the abductor with release of the deep fascia of the abductor hallucis longus and removal of the spur if it impinged or produced entrapment of the nerve. Of the 34 operated heels, 32 had good results, and 2 had poor results.

Henricson and Westlin[24] reported on 11 heels in 10 athletes with chronic heel pain unrelieved by conservative therapy and with compression of the calcaneal branch of the tibial nerve. They said that there was entrapment of the anterior calcaneal branch where the nerve passed between the tight and rigid edges of the deep fascia of the abductor hallucis and the medial edge of the os calcis. Surgery consisted of identification and release of the tibial nerve and both calcaneal branches and release of the deep fascia of the abductor hallucis. Follow-up of 58 months after surgery revealed that 10 of the 11 heels were asymptomatic. The patients had resumed athletic participation after an average of 5 weeks. It seems to this author that both the nerve to the abductor digiti quinti and the medial calcaneal nerve were released.

Other Causes of Inferior Heel Pain

Calcaneal apophysitis, or Sever's disease, is a common cause of heel pain in the young child.

Micheli and Ireland[40] reported calcaneal apophysitis in 137 heels in 85 children, with both heels being affected in 61% of the patients. Soft orthotics or heel cups were used in 98% of the patients along with proper athletic footwear, physical therapy consisting of stretching, and ankle dorsiflexion strengthening. All patients improved and were able to return to the sport of their choice 2 months after the diagnosis; only 2 patients had recurrent difficulty.

Sullivan[58] reported that radiographic irregularity of the calcaneal apophysis was the rule rather than the exception. He found no treatment that altered the radiographic picture. He wondered whether Sever's disease was even a true entity.

This author believes that calcaneal apophysitis of the heel is a true entity. The tenderness is along the posterior portion of the heel rather than along the medial tuberosity as with plantar fasciitis. Treatment consisting of heel elevation, anti-inflammatory medication, stretching, and decreased activity is generally successful.[5]

Rask[44] has reported on an unusual cause of heel pain that he described as medial plantar neurapraxia. He termed this *jogger's foot*. It was thought that there was some probable entrapment of the medial plantar nerve behind the navicular tuberosity in the fibromuscular tunnel formed by the abductor hallucis, with the inciting factor being eversion of the foot. These three patients were treated successfully with conservative measures consisting of a change in running posture of the foot, anti-inflammatory medication, and proper footwear.

Satku et al.[49] reported heel pain produced by the unusual cause of an osteocartilaginous nodule found within the heel. This was a glistening, circumscribed, lobulated, ovoid mass measuring 1.6 by 2.5 by 1.4 cm. The pain was relieved with excision of the nodule.

Shaw et al.[53] called attention to the fact that heel pain can occur in sarcoidosis. They reported seven cases of sarcoid-related heel pain as a major characteristic of the sarcoid disease process. They stated that bilateral heel pain can be a presenting symptom of sarcoidosis and can accompany or precede sarcoid arthritis.

Hoffman and Thul[26] reported on two cases of fracture of the os calcis following surgical procedures for excision of the calcaneal exostosis and plantar fasciotomy.

In summary, conservative treatment of the subcalcaneal pain syndrome consists of anti-inflammatory medication, orthoses, heel cups, injections, physical therapy, and a decreased activity level. This will be effective in 95% of cases of the subcalcaneal pain syndrome. In those patients who have not responded to an adequate trial of these conservative measures, surgery may be performed that consists of release of the plantar fascia and/or release of the nerve to the abductor digiti quinti or the sensory medial calcaneal nerve with the expectation that a good result will occur (Fig 20–7). Heel spurs, if present, are removed. Although the reports are good from the literature, this author has noted in his practice that there are problems with decreased sensation and persistent pain in some patients.

Author's Method of Treatment

The subcalcaneal pain syndrome with plantar fasciitis arising at the medial tuberosity probably represents a traction periostitis with degeneration and tears of the plantar fascia and subsequent secondary involvement of the adjacent structures such as the medial calcaneal nerve and the nerve to the abductor digiti quinti. Occasionally, there will be primary entrapment of the nerve of the abductor digiti quinti and the sensory branch of the medial calcaneal nerve. A calcaneal spur is present in 50% of the cases and may be part of the inflammatory process. Treatment should be directed initially toward reducing the inflammatory process by the use of medication, decreased activity level, orthotics, injection of corticosteriods, and physical therapy modalities.

Conservative Treatment.—The patient with subcalcaneal pain syndrome and associated proximal plantar fasciitis is evaluated to determine the foot type and also whether there is any associated abnormality of the lower extremity or body. If there is none, treatment is begun that consists of anti-inflammatory medication and an orthotic device that will cushion the heel and relieve pressure on the tender area of the heel. There are many types of off-the-counter heel cups and cushioning devices that may be used. If these do not suffice, then a custom-made insert will usually suffice that is made of a medium-density polyethylene closed cell foam thermoplastic material (Plastazote) molded so that there is a slight medial elevation and support beneath the heel and with a relief area cut out at the bottom so that there is no pressure on the medial tuberosity. The orthosis goes only to the metatarsal heads and thus can be worn in the patient's regular shoes (Fig 20–8). Activities are restricted according to the patient's symptomatic tolerance. If a specific, acutely tender area is located, one to three corticosteroid injections may be used. The injection generally used is 1.0 cc of betamethasone sodium phosphate/betamethasone acetate suspension with 3 cc of bupivacaine hydrochloride and 3 cc of mepivacaine hydrochloride. The amount of this injection depends upon the area injected and the amount required to obtain relief of pain. When an injection is performed, it should be directed into a specific area and this serves as a therapeutic and diagnostic endeavor. Utilizing a long-acting local anesthetic allows one to ascertain whether injection in this area will produce relief of pain. It is important not to inject the corticosteroids into the fat septa

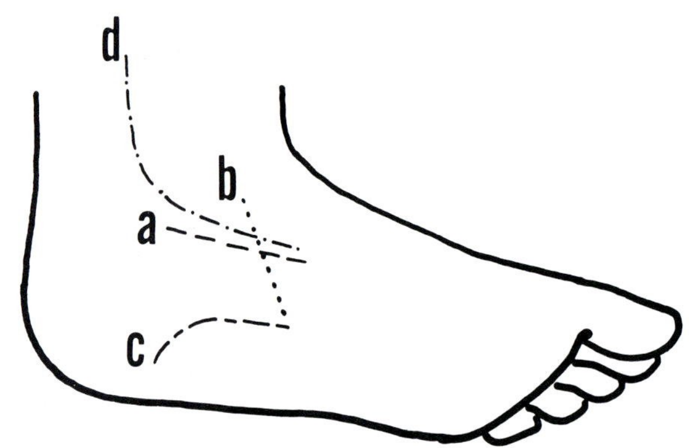

FIG 20–7.
Incisions for subcalcaneal pain surgery: *a,* medial incision; *b,* oblique incision; *c,* incision of Ward and Clippinger; *d,* incision for complete release and exploration. (From Drez D, DeLee J: *Orthopaedic sports medicine: principles and practice,* Philadelphia, WB Saunders (in press). Used by permission.)

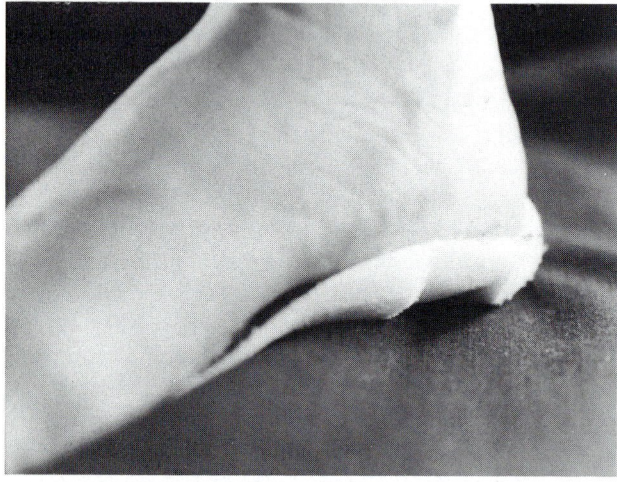

FIG 20–8.
A custom-molded orthosis for subcalcaneal pain made of medium-density Plastazote incorporates the features common to orthoses for this condition: (1) cushions for the heel, (2) arch support, (3) medial heel elevation, and, (4) relief area for a tender medial tubercle.

of the plantar surface of the heel because this may produce fat necrosis and increased vulnerability to pressure periostitis.

Physical therapy consisting of stretching, strengthening, ultrasound, and at times iontophoresis and/or phonophoresis might be utilized. A night splint may be utilized to maintain the foot in dorsiflexion and prevent contracture of the plantar fascia. Complete rest in a short-leg weight-bearing cast for 4 weeks is used if other measures fail.

If the patient responds to conservative treatment and becomes asymptomatic and the tenderness disappears, the anti-inflammatory medication and decreased activity level may be continued for 4 to 6 weeks. Then a gradual increase in activity is allowed. The orthosis is used for several months unless the patient has biochemical abnormality of the foot, in which case the orthosis is continued for an indefinite period of time.

The previous methods of conservative therapy will be continued for approximately 9 to 12 months. If the patient still has sufficient symptomatology to interfere with the performance of the activities of daily living or the desired athletic activity, then surgical intervention may be considered.

Surgical Treatment.—Prior to a surgical endeavor, nerve conduction and EMG studies are usually performed. Laboratory studies to exclude systemic arthritis and/or spondyloarthropathies are considered. A bone scan with technetium 99 may be considered if one suspects a fatigue fracture or if the exact localization of the pain is not clear.

There are two types of heel pain surgery that are performed. The first type is that of release of the offending structures with the least amount of surgery. The second type is that of complete exploration of all of the structures that might produce symptomatology.

Minimal Surgical Release

Surgical Technique.

1. For the patient who has the subcalcaneal pain syndrome and localized pain along the plantar fascia, the medial tubercle, and the area of the nerve to the abductor digiti quinti and/or medial calcaneal nerve, an incision is made along the medial side of the heel with a curve into the arch just distal to the weight-bearing area of the heel. Loop magnification is used.
2. The sensory branch of the medial calcaneal nerve is located, inspected, and preserved. It may be trapped as it comes through the fascia.
3. The central slip of the plantar fascia is released at its origin.
4. The spur, if present, is removed by using a small rongeur after stripping the muscle.
5. The fascia of the abductor hallucis and the fascia of the quadratus plantae are divided to release the nerve to the abductor digiti quinti as it passes laterally. An attempt is made to visualize this nerve, if possible.
6. The wound is irrigated and closed with plain subcutaneous catgut sutures and interrupted mattress sutures.

Postoperative Care.—The patient is placed in a short-leg cast and may be weight bearing if comfortable after 4 to 7 days. A weight-bearing cast or an off-the-counter brace is used for 3 weeks. If the patient is comfortable at 3 weeks, weight bearing with a shoe is permitted, with full activity started at 6 to 12 weeks if the symptomatology will allow this. If the patient has a biochemical foot abnormality, an orthotic device is used postoperatively.

If the patient did not have any entrapment of the medial calcaneal nerve and did not have a spur that one wished to excise, then an oblique incision just distal to the medial tuberosity may be utilized to release the plantar fascia and the nerve to the abductor digit quinti. The same post operative regimen is followed.

In the patient who has symptomatology involving the posterior tibial nerve along with pathology of the medial tuberosity or who has recurrent or failed surgery, an operation of greater magnitude may be considered with the understanding that whereas this operation may relieve the pain, the operation may produce more morbidity with a decreased chance of recovery.

Complete Surgical Exploration

Surgical Technique.

1. A long incision is made from the posterior malleolus to the medial tubercle and distally.
2. The posterior tibial nerve is explored from behind the medial malleolus while at the same time exploring, inspecting, and releasing, if trapped, the medial calcaneal nerve, the nerve to the abductor digiti quinti, and the medial and lateral plantar nerves as they pass through the foramina of the abductor musculature.
3. The central portion of the plantar fascia is released.
4. The spur is excised if present, and the wound is closed.

Postoperative Care.—The patient is maintained non–weight bearing in a cast for 2 weeks and then weight bearing in a short-leg cast for 2 more weeks. Increased activity is started at 12 weeks. This operation involves a great deal of dissection. It is utilized only in recalcitrant conditions and without any guarantee that the patient will be able to return to preinjury status.

SUPERIOR HEEL PAIN (RETROCALCANEAL BURSITIS, HAGLUND'S DISEASE, ENLARGEMENT OF THE SUPERIOR TUBEROSITY OF THE OS CALCIS, INSERTIONAL ACHILLES TENDINITIS)

Symptomatology and pain located in the posterosuperior portion of the calcaneus can be produced by a retrocalcaneal bursitis, enlargement of the superior bursal prominence of the calcaneus, Achilles tendinitis, or inflammation of an adventitious bursa between the Achilles tendon and the skin* (Fig 20–9). There is usually some enlargement of the superior bursal promi-

**References 65, 69, 70, 79, 81, 82, 85, 86, 88–90, 92.*

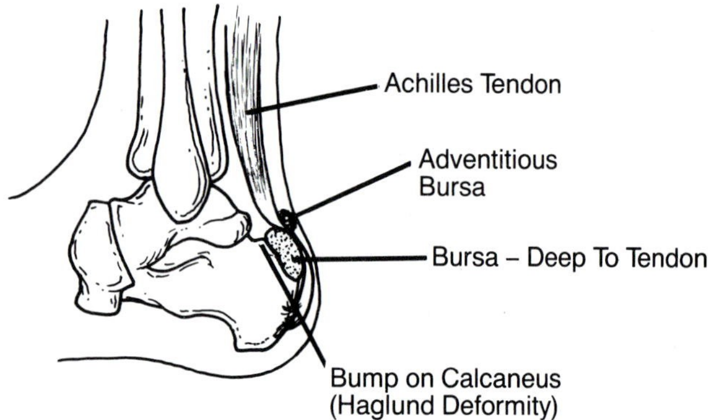

FIG 20–9.
Illustration of Haglund's deformity with (1) a retrocalcaneal bursa between the Achilles tendon and the superior bursal prominence and (2) an adventitious bursa between the Achilles tendon and the skin.

nence of the os calcis. Achilles tendinitis and adventitious bursitis may be associated with this, although each of these entities may exist as an isolated condition.

Anatomy

The superior tuberosity of the os calcis may be hyperconvex, normal, or hypoconvex[86] (Fig 20–10). The roentgenographic appearance of the os calcis has been described by Heneghan and Pavlov[79, 88] as having the following anatomic landmarks on the lateral projection (Fig 20–11). The superior aspect of the talar articulation marks the most proximal portion of the posterior facet. The bursal projection is the area of the superior tuberosity of the os calcis. The tuberosity of the posterior surface marks the site of the most proximal portion of insertion of the Achilles tendon. The medial tubercle is the site in which the central portion of the plantar aponeurosis is inserted.

The Achilles tendon inserts into the middle of the posterior surface of the calcaneus.[77] A retrocalcaneal bursa between the Achilles tendon and the superior tuberosity of the calcaneus is a constant finding[73, 77, 78] (Fig 20–12). Anatomically, the retrocalcaneal bursa has an anterior bursal wall composed of fibrocartilage laid over the calcaneus, while the posterior wall is indistinguishable from the thin epitenon of the Achilles tendon.[73] Dorsiflexion of the foot and ankle will produce increased pressure in the retrocalcaneal bursa. Plantar flexion will decrease the pressure in the retrocalcaneal bursa.[67, 89] The bursa and the prominence probably function to maintain a relatively constant distance between the axis of the ankle joint and the insertion of the Achilles tendon.[67, 89]

An adventitious bursa may be present between the Achilles tendon and the skin. This is generally produced by irritation from the counter of a shoe.

Retrocalcaneal pain syndrome may be commonly associated with the high-arch cavus foot and a varus heel, with these factors producing prominence of the heel and also a foot that does not dorsiflex readily.[69, 89]

Diagnosis

The symptoms are usually pain in the area of the retrocalcaneal bursa that is aggravated by activity and certain shoewear. There may be a slow or sudden onset of pain. When the condition is due primarily to an acutely swollen retrocalcaneal bursitis, the pain is usually constant with some aggravation with activity. If the pain is of acute origin and associated with a traumatic incident, the initiating factor may be a tear or calcification of the Achilles tendon.

Physical Examination

Physical examination reveals that there is swelling in the area of the retrocalcaneal bursa between the Achilles tendon and the calcaneus.[65] The swelling in the retro-

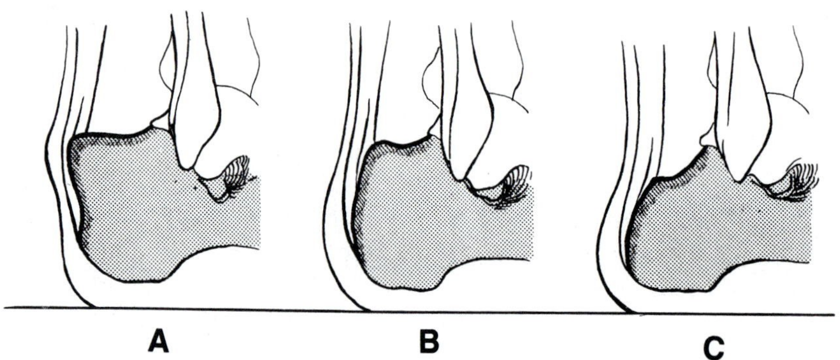

FIG 20–10.
Variations in the shape of the superior tuberosity of the os calcis. The *left* illustrates hyperconvexity. The *middle* is normal. The *right* illustrates hypoconvexity.

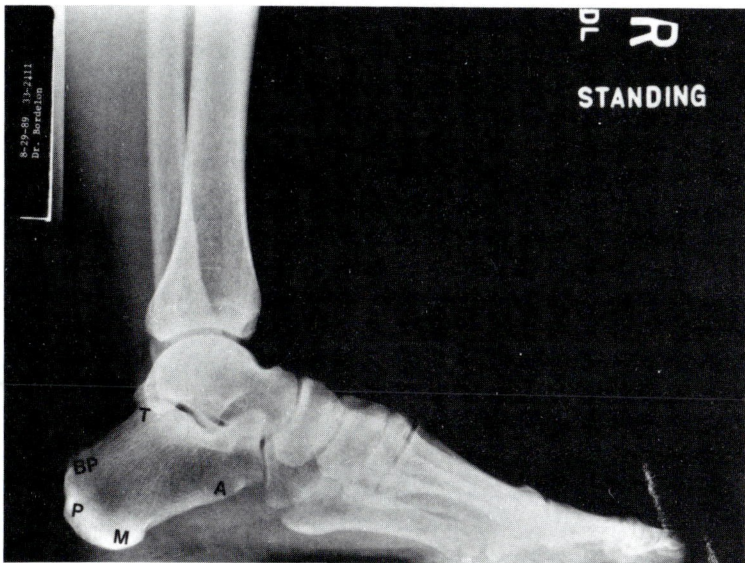

FIG 20–11.
Important radiographic landmarks of the os calcis: *T* = superior aspect of the talar articulation; *BP* = bursal projection; *P* = posterior tuberosity indicating attachment of the Achilles tendon; *M* = medial tuberosity attachment of the plantar aponeurosis; *A* = anterior tubercle.[88]

calcaneal bursa will be just anterior to the Achilles tendon. By palpating medially and laterally at the same time or with ballottement, one can sometimes feel fluid within the bursa. With careful and discreet palpation, differentiation can usually be made between swelling in the retrocalcaneal bursa and the Achilles tendon. There is generally some increase in bony prominence of the superior tuberosity of the os calcis. When there is swelling of the Achilles tendon in association with retrocalcaneal bursitis or perhaps with degeneration and inflammation of the attachment of the tendon itself, this is usually at the level just proximal to the insertion. This tenderness is different from the tear with degeneration of the tendon, primarily due to vascular insufficiency that is more proximal.

An adventitious bursa is located between the skin and the os calcis. It is usually located along the lateral side of the Achilles tendon and usually in the foot with the varus heel. It is produced by pressure from a shoe counter.

Radiographic Studies

A lateral view of the foot is taken with the patient standing to allow biomechanical evaluation of the foot

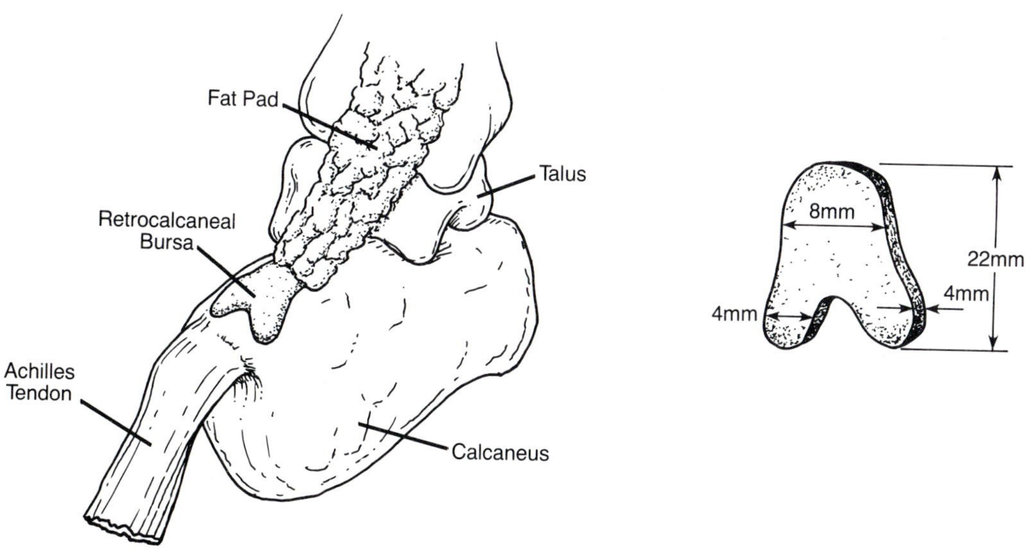

FIG 20–12.
Demonstration of the disk-shaped retrocalcaneal bursa. (From Frey C, Rosenberg Z, Shereff MJ: The retrocalcaneal bursa, American Orthopaedic Foot and Ankle Society, Las Vegas, Feb 1989. Used by permission.)

as well as evaluation of the specific points of the os calcis. The shape and appearance of the superior bursal prominence are noted. The specific points identified are the posterior margin of the posterior facet, the superior bursal projection, tuberosity indicating the site of Achilles tendon insertion, the medial tubercle, and the anterior tubercle.[66, 88] Radiographic evaluation may be performed by the method of Fowler and Philip for measuring the posterior calcaneal angle[71] (Fig 20–13). An angle of greater than 75 degrees is significant.

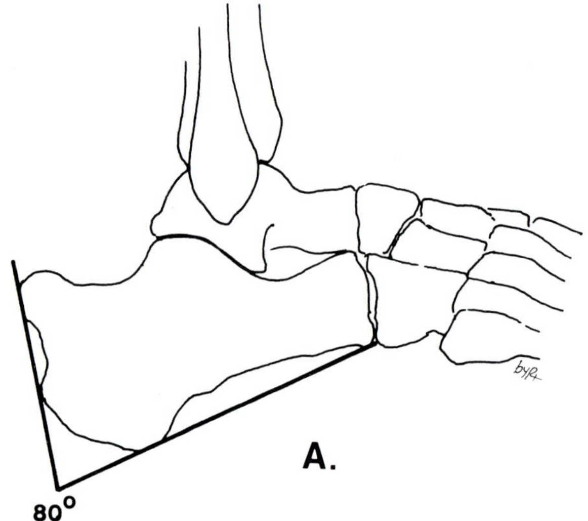

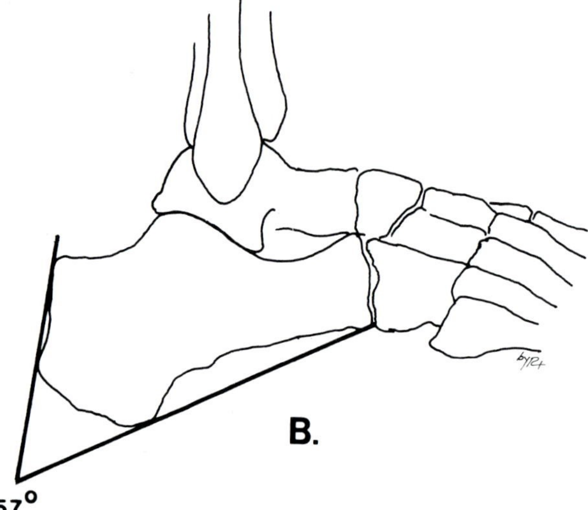

FIG 20–13.
Measurement of the Fowler and Philip angle. Normal is considered to be less than 69 degrees. **A,** an abnormal angle of 80 degrees. **B,** normal angle of 57 degrees. (From Drez D, DeLee J: *Orthopaedic sports medicine: principles and practice,* Philadelphia, WB Saunders (in press). Used by permission.)

Ruch[89] and Vega et al.[92] have concluded that a combination of the Fowler angle and the angle of calcaneal inclination are more important in correlating the x-ray appearance with symptomatology than the Fowler and Philip angle alone. They stated that the combined angle was greater than 90 degrees in patients with symptomatic Haglund's disease.

Heneghan and Pavlov[79] have used parallel pitch lines to determine the prominence of the bursal projection.

Etiology and Diagnostic Tests

In all cases of retrocalcaneal bursitis, one should always be aware that this may represent a focal manifestation of other conditions such as systemic arthritis or gout.[78, 80]

Gerster et al.[74–76] reviewed cases of painful heel syndrome with plantar fasciitis and/or Achilles tendinitis. They found that heel pain was frequently seen in seronegative arthritis. However, it was not common in rheumatoid arthritis.

Canoso et al.[68] reported bursal fluid findings in cadavers without rheumatoid disease, in three with Reiter's syndrome, and in one with pseudogout. The presence of pain in the retrocalcaneal and Achilles tendon area should always be considered as a possible manifestation of a general systemic disorder. Examination and laboratory studies should be performed to rule these out. However, most of the time retrocalcaneal bursitis is idiopathic. Many times it presents with a tense and swollen retrocalcaneal bursa.

Frey et al.[73] have described the retrocalcaneal bursa. Their studies indicate that the bursae of symptomatic patients accepted less contrast material and were more irregular than those in the asymptomatic group.

Treatment

Heneghan and Pavlov[79] experimentally investigated the effects of plantar osseous projections and shoe/heel height on the prominence of the bursal projection and the calcaneal pitch angle. They found that heel elevation decreased the pitch angle and allowed the prominence of the bursal projection and the foot to slip forward and displace the posterior calcaneus away from the shoe counter.

Fiamengo et al.[70] reviewed the charts of patients in whom a diagnosis of Haglund's disease, retrocalcaneal bursitis, or pump bumps had been made. They found 12 available for review. They also reviewed 104 controlled cases to look for the presence of calcaneal spurs, Achilles tendon calcification, and a posterior calcaneal step (horizontal ledge in the middle of the posterior portion of the os calcis corresponding to the level at which the Achilles tendon inserts into the calcaneus). The incidence of Achilles tendon calcification and posterior calcaneal steps was higher in patients who had chronic posterior heel pain as compared with the control population. The recommendation was that in cases of chronic posterior heel pain resection of the posterosuperior aspect of the calcaneus as well as excision of the degenerative and calcific soft tissue in and about the distal portion of the Achilles tendon should be performed.

Pavlov et al.[88] reported on the use of parallel pitch line measurements in 10 symptomatic feet and 78 control feet (Fig 20–14). They thought that the symptoms correlated statistically with a positive posterior pitch line but not with an abnormal posterior calcaneal angle. They concluded that radiographically the syndrome is characterized by (1) retrocalcaneal bursitis (loss of the lucent retrocalcaneal recess between the Achilles tendon and the bursal projection); (2) Achilles tendinitis (an Achilles tendon measuring over 9 mm, 2 cm above the bursal projection); (3) superficial tendo Achillis bursitis (a convexity of the soft tissues posterior to the Achilles tendon insertion); and (4) a cortically intact but prominent bursal projection with a positive parallel pitch line.

Vega et al.[92] reported on 20 cases of Haglund's deformity. They noted that the combination of the Fowler and Philip angle and the calcaneal angle when greater than 90 degrees correlated with the symptomatic findings.

Keck and Kelly[82] reported on 13 patients with 20 symptomatic heels that were treated surgically. Seventeen heels underwent excision of the superior bursa prominence. Three had dorsally based closing wedge cuneiform osteotomies. Good results were reported in 15 of the heels treated. The initial results were good in all but 2 patients. The final result was considered poor in these because of recurrence of pain as a manifestation of rheumatoid arthritis. Osteotomy was used to reduce the posterior prominence and was rated good in 2, fair in 1, and poor in 2 heels. The thought was that there were too few osteotomies to evaluate this method. The osteotomy had the disadvantage of requiring a longer convalescence.

Zadek[93] reported in 1939 on closing wedge osteotomy of the superior part of the os calcis in three patients for treatment of adventitious bursitis; all were relieved of their symptoms.

Ruch[89] reported on 65 patients, 17 of whom were operated upon and evaluated 6 months to 5 years postoperatively. The procedure used was resection of the posterosuperior portion of the os calcis, both medially and laterally, with sufficient bone being removed so as to remove the palpable prominence. Fifteen demonstrated good to excellent results with elimination of symptoms. Three of the patients required a second procedure to obtain a good result.

Clancy,[69] Schepsis and Leach,[90] Jones and James,[81] and Sullivan[91] have reported on the treatment of athletes with retrocalcaneal bursitis.

Clancy[69] noted that there was an articular-like surface lining the superior aspect of the calcaneus where it comes in contact with the Achilles tendon. He thought that from constant overuse, enlargement of the bony prominence, or external pressure a bursa may form. He noted that the majority of those requiring surgery had significant cavus deformities and recommended treatment by steroid injections behind but not through or

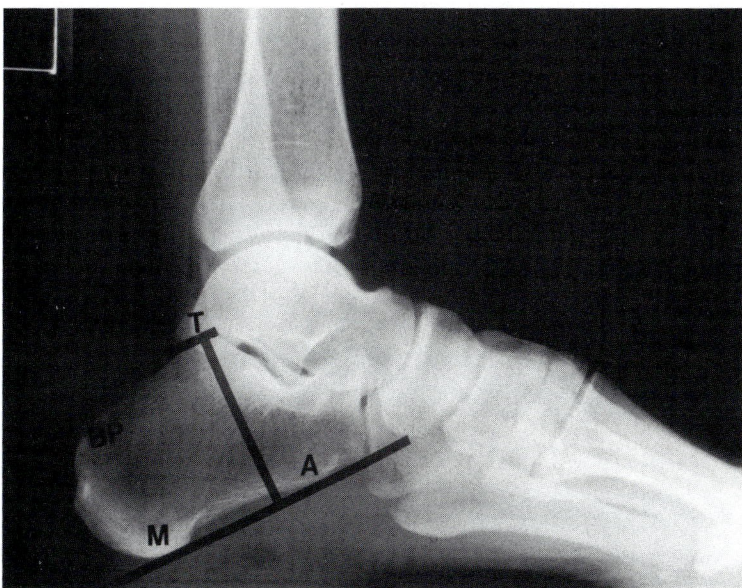

FIG 20–14.
Parallel pitch lines as used to determine the prominence of the bursal projection. A line is drawn from the medial tuberosity *(M)* and the anterior tuberosity *(A)*. A parallel is constructed from the superior prominence of the posterior facet. If the bursal projection *(BP)* is above the superior line, the projection is considered abnormally large.[88]

into the tendon. In those who did not obtain relief with conservative measures, ostectomy proved successful.

Schepsis and Leach[90] reported that the majority of athletes who presented were managed nonoperatively with a combination of (1) a decrease or cessation of weekly mileage, (2) a temporary termination of interval training and workouts on hills, (3) a change from a harder bank surface to a softer surface, (4) the addition of one-fourth- to one-half-inch lift inside the shoe or to the shoe, and (5) a program to stretch and strengthen the gastrocnemius-soleus complex. Oral anti-inflammatory medication and an occasional injection of corticosteroid injected into the retrocalcaneal bursa were utilized. Postural abnormalities were treated with orthoses. Retrospectively they studied 45 cases of chronic posterior heel pain treated surgically in 37 patients. All but 2 of these patients were competitive long-distance runners who averaged between 40 and 120 miles per week prior to the onset of symptoms, with their ages ranging from 19 to 56 years. The patients were divided into three groups—those with Achilles tenosynovitis/tendinitis, those with retrocalcaneal bursitis, and those with a combination of both. In the group of 24 cases of Achilles tendosynovitis/tendinitis, there were 63% excellent, 29% good, 4% fair, and 4% poor results. In the 14 cases of retrocalcaneal bursitis, there were 50% excellent, 21% good, and 29% fair results. In the group with combinations of both, there were 71% excellent and 29% good results. It was noted that 4 of the 6 unsatisfactory results occurred in the group with retrocalcaneal bursitis.

The surgical approach was with a longitudinal incision 1 cm medial to the Achilles tendon that was continued transversely to form a J-shaped incision if necessary (Fig 20–15). The surgical procedure addressed the pathology found. If Achilles tenosynovitis or tendinitis were found, the tendon sheath was excised. If the pathology was within the tendon itself, a longitudinal splitting incision was used, with the area of fibrotic degeneration excised. If an old partial tear was found, it was debrided and the tendon approximated with side-to-side sutures. If the retrocalcaneal bursa was inflamed, it was excised, and the superior bursal prominence of the os calcis was removed. Postoperative casting was 2 to 3 weeks, with weight bearing being permitted after 1 week. When there was pathology of the tendon that required excision and repair, immobilization was continued for 1 to 2 weeks longer. Range of motion was emphasized. A graduated program of swimming, stationary bicycling, and isometric, isotonic, and isokinetic strengthening of the calf muscles was prescribed. Jogging was permitted at 8 to 12 weeks, with full return to a competitive level usually requiring 5 to 6 months.

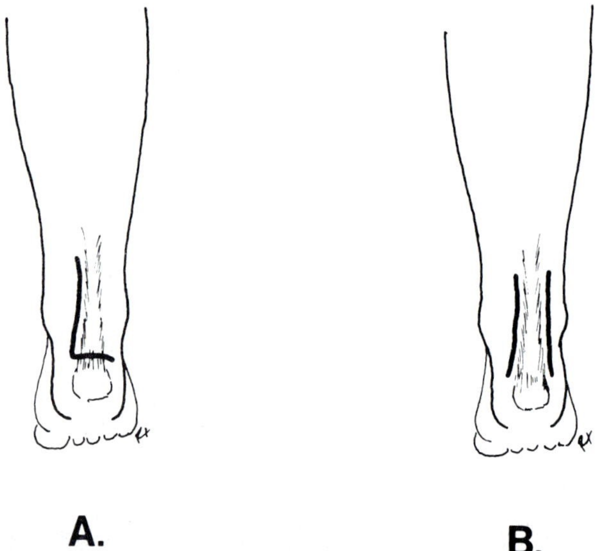

FIG 20–15.
Illustration of surgical incisions for retrocalcaneal bursitis. The drawing on the *left* depicts the medial approach with a J extension as per Schepsis and Leach.[90] On the *right* are medial and lateral incisions as per Jones and James.[81] (From Drez D, DeLee J: *Orthopaedic sports medicine: principles and practice,* Philadelphia, WB Saunders (in press). Used by permission.)

Jones and James[81] reported on ten patients who underwent partial calcaneal exostosectomies with excision of the retrocalcaneal bursa for retrocalcaneal bursitis. They said that conservative measures should be attempted prior to surgical intervention. These measures included a decrease in mileage, elevation of the heel, instruction in Achilles tendon strengthening, removal of external pressure from the heel, utilization of oral anti-inflammatory medication, and evaluation and treatment of postural foot deformities. In recalcitrant cases they suggested immobilization of the leg in a short-leg walking cast for a brief period of time while continuing cardiovascular maintenance on an exercise bicycle.

Steroid injection was used as the last resort prior to surgery. Over an 8-year period, ten patients with retrocalcaneal bursitis were operated upon: six were competitive distance runners, and four were avid recreational runners. The symptoms consisted of pain and tenderness in the retrocalcaneal area that developed either immediately or after running several miles. The age range was from 21 to 42 years. Surgery was performed through longitudinal incisions on both sides of the Achilles tendon with exostosectomy and excision of the bursa (see Fig 20–15). They emphasized that the ridge of bone at the insertion site must be carefully removed with a small curet and rongeur so that there is no prominence left beneath the Achilles tendon posteriorly. A short-leg walking cast was utilized for 8 weeks with partial weight bearing for the first 2 weeks and then full weight bearing. After removal of the cast a 1-in. heel elevation was used until the foot went into the neutral position easily. General muscular conditioning was carried out until Cybex testing revealed symmetric muscle strength. All of the patients returned to their desired level of activity within 6 months.

Sullivan,[91] regarding the problem of recurrent pain in the pediatric athlete, stated that heel pain may be due to osteochondrosis of the apophysis of the calcaneus (Sever's disease) or to Achilles tendinitis with pain on palpation just above the insertion of the tendon. He noted that in severe cases there was crepitation of the tendon. He recommended rest, aspirin, and other mild anti-inflammatory agents.

Kennedy and Willis[83] reported on the effects of local steroid injections in tendons. They found that actual collagen necrosis occurred and that the return to normal in the injected tendon occurred by 14 days. They concluded that local steroids placed directly in a normal tendon weakened it significantly for up to 14 days and said that in any patient with posterior heel pain the injection should be made in the retrocalcaneal area and not the tendon.

Lagergren and Lindholm[84] reported on the vascular supply of the tendon. They found that rupture of the tendon was usually limited to the segment of the tendon between 2 and 6 cm proximal to its insertion in the os calcis and that this was an area of decreased vascularity and nutrition. This is important relative to the retrocalcaneal bursal syndrome because this classic type of Achilles tendinitis is proximal to the area of tendinitis usually associated with the retrocalcaneal bursal syndrome.[72]

Nelimarkka et al.[87] have reported a soleus muscle anomaly in which a soft bulge due to a large mass of anomalous soleus muscle simulating a retrocalcaneal bursitis was present. This condition responded satisfactorily to excision of the anomalous muscle.

In summary, the retrocalcaneal bursitic syndrome is a condition characterized by enlargement of the superior tuberosity of the os calcis and inflammation of the retrocalcaneal bursa, the Achilles tendon just above its insertion, and at times the tissue between the Achilles tendon and the skin. It is generally managed by conservative measures consisting of anti-inflammatory medication, decreased activity, padding to prevent pressure on the affected area, orthoses or heel lifts, and strengthening and stretching exercises. If it does not respond to these modalities and the patient is incapacitated, then surgical intervention may be considered. This generally consists of excision of the exostosis, the retrocalcaneal bursa, and at times the adventitious bursa if present, with exploration and correction of the Achilles tendon pathology if present.

Author's Method of Treatment

The patient is first evaluated to ascertain the exact reason for the pathology and whether it is a retrocalcaneal bursitis in isolation or associated with an Achilles insertional tendinitis and/or an adventitious bursitis. Adventitious bursitis is usually seen in women and does not seem to be a prominent problem with athletes. It is generally treated conservatively by softening the shoe counter, utilization of a small U-shaped pad to relieve the pressure of the shoe or counter against the inflamed area, anti-inflammatory medication, and occasionally an injection of steroid directly into the inflamed area (Fig 20–16). It is unusual for surgical intervention to be performed solely for an adventitious bursitis.

Surgical procedures are usually performed for retrocalcaneal bursitis associated with the superior bony prominence. The retrocalcaneal bursa and the superior bursal prominence are excised. The adventitious bursa is excised if it is prominent.

If the adventitious bursa is excised, the surgeon must take care to excise it carefully and meticulously so as

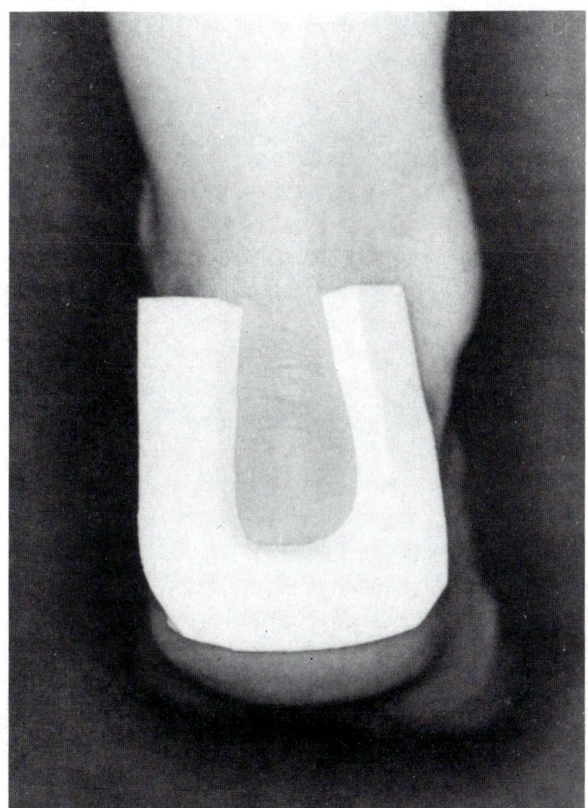

FIG 20–16.
Demonstration of the use of a U-shaped pad to remove pressure on the bony prominence of the heel.

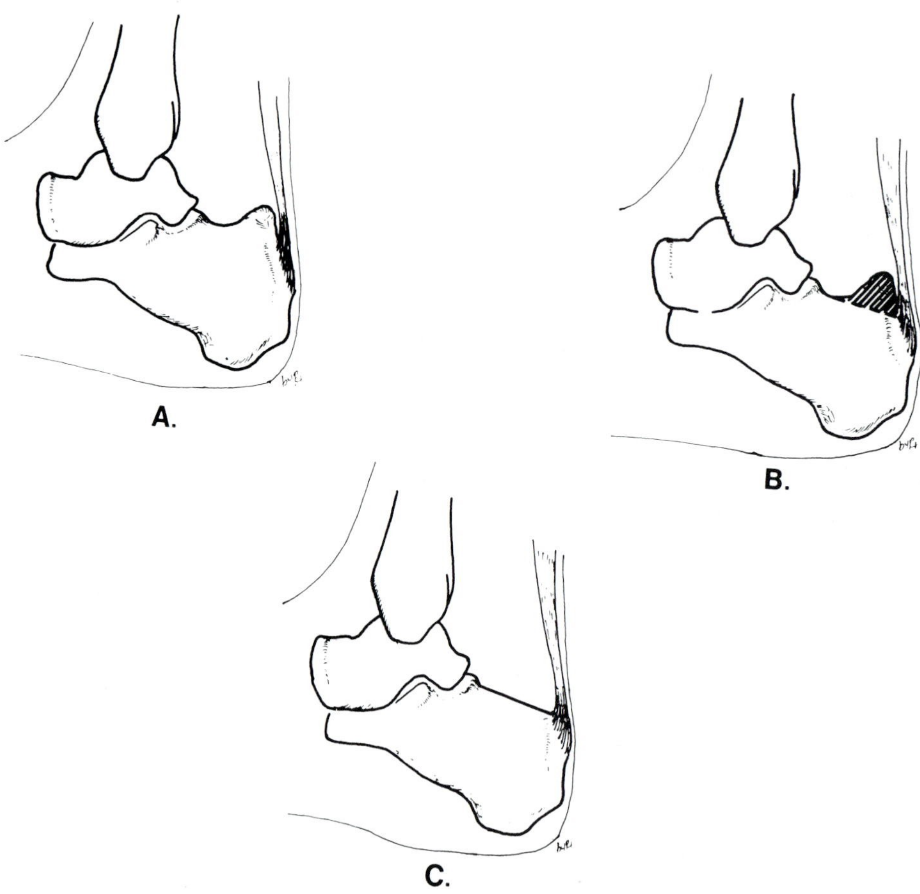

FIG 20–17.
A, Haglund's deformity with prominence of the posterosuperior portion of the os calcis. **B,** *shaded* bone to be resected. **C,** appearance of the os calcis after surgical resection of the posterosuperior prominence for symptomatic Haglund's deformity. (From Drez D, De Lee J: *Orthopaedic sports medicine: principles and practice,* Philadelphia, WB Saunders (in press). Used by permission.)

not to damage or adversely affect the blood supply or the skin overlying this area because skin slough would be a serious complication.

Surgical Technique.

1. The patient is operated upon in the prone position.
2. Medial and lateral incisions are made 1½ cm anterior to the Achilles tendon. The incision is carried directly to the subcutaneous tissue, and dissection is carried out deep to the subcutaneous tissue to avoid skin necrosis. Attention should be paid to the calcaneal branch of the sural nerve on the lateral side and the posterior branch of the medial calcaneal nerve on the medial side.
3. The Achilles tendon is inspected. If any scarring around the tendon is present, this is removed.
4. The retrocalcaneal bursa is excised.
5. An exostosectomy is performed by removing the bone from the area of insertion of the Achilles tendon to the superior portion of the posterior facet of the os calcis.
6. Adequate bone is removed (Fig 20–17).
7. The edges are smoothed with a rasp.
8. If an adventitious bursa is present, it is carefully dissected and removed. The skin must not be compromised.
9. The wound is irrigated and closed.

Postoperative Care.—A short-leg weight-bearing cast with the foot in the neutral position is used for 1 to 3 weeks. A heel lift of three eights of an inch is used for 3 more weeks. The patient is then started on a program of stretching and strengthening exercises. Return to full activity will probably require a period of time of about 3 months.

When Achilles tendinitis is present along with retrocalcaneal bursitis, surgery is performed as in the preceding paragraph except that the Achilles tendon is inspected even more proximally. Any scar tissue or tendosynovitis is removed. Any calcification or degenerative area within the tendon is removed by making a longitudinal incision into the tendon. The horizontal step is removed with a small curet. Care is taken to leave adequate insertion of the Achilles tendon, although this author has had the experience where the degeneration has been severe enough that the Achilles tendon had to be reinserted and reinforced.

The time of postoperative immobilization will depend upon the degree of pathology of the Achilles tendon. Generally, a short-leg non–weight-bearing cast with the foot slightly plantar-flexed or in the neutral position is utilized for 1 to 3 weeks. Then a short-leg weight-bearing cast with the foot slightly plantar-flexed and in the neutral position is utilized for another 2 to 3 weeks. Ambulation with a one-half-inch heel lift is utilized for several more weeks. Strengthening and stretching exercises are started at 6 to 9 weeks. Jogging and running are not allowed until 3 to 6 months.

REFERENCES

Subcalcaneal pain syndrome (heel pain syndrome/plantar fasciitis)

1. Ali E: Calcaneal spur in Guyana, *West Indian Med J* 29:175–183, 1980.
2. Baxter DE, Thigpen CM: Heel pain—operative results, *Foot Ankle* 5:16–25, 1984.
3. Bordelon RL: Subcalcaneal pain—a method of evaluation and plan for treatment, *Clin Orthop* 177:49–53, 1983.
4. Bordelon RL: Subcalcaneal pain: present status, evaluation and management, *Instr Course Lect* 33:283–287, 1984.
5. Bordelon RL: *Surgical & conservative foot care*, Thorofare, NJ, 1988, Charles B Slack 105–115.
6. Callison WJ: Heel pain in private practice. Presented at a meeting of the Orthopaedic Foot Club, Dallas, April 1989.
7. Clancy WG: Runners' injuries. Part two. Evaluation and treatment of specific injuries, *Am J Sports Med* 8:287–289, 1980.
8. Contompasis JP: Surgical treatment of calcaneal spurs: a three-year post-surgical study, *J Podiatr Assoc* 64:987–999, 1974.
9. D'Ambrosia RD: Conservative management of metatarsal and heel pain in the adult foot, *Orthopedics* 10:137–142, 1987.
10. D'Ambrosia RD, Richtor N, Douglas R: Orthotics. In D'Ambrosia RD, and Drez D, editors: *Prevention and treatment of running injuries*, ed 2, Thorofare, NJ, 1989, Charles B Slack, pp 245–258.
11. DuVries HL: Heel spur (calcaneal spur), *Arch Surg* 74:536–542, 1957.
12. Eastmond CJ, Rajah SM, Tovey D, et al: Seronegative pauciarticular arthritis and HLA B27, *Ann Rheum Dis* 39:231–234, 1980.
13. Freeman C: Heel pain. In Gould JS, editor: *The foot book*, Baltimore, 1988, Williams & Wilkins, 228–238.
14. Galinski AW: Calcaneodynia-herniation, *J Am Podiatr Assoc* 67:647–650, 1977.
15. Gerster JC: Plantar fasciitis and Achilles tendinitis among 150 cases of seronegative spondarthritis, *Rheumatol Rehabil* 19:218–222, 1980.
16. Gerster JC, Piccinin P: Enthesopathy of the heels in juvenile onset seronegative B-27 positive spondyloarthropathy, *J Rheumatol* 12:310–314, 1985.
17. Gerster JC, Saudan Y, Fallet GH: Talalgia. A review of 30 severe cases, *J Rheumatol* 5:210–216, 1978.
18. Goss CM: Gray's anatomy, ed 27, Philadelphia, 1959, Lea & Febiger, pp 545–559.
19. Goulet MJ: Role of soft orthosis in treating plantar fasciitis. Suggestion from the field, *Phys Ther* 64:1544, 1984.
20. Graham CE: Painful heel syndrome: rationale of diagnosis and treatment, *Foot Ankle* 3:261–267, 1983.
21. Hamilton WG: Surgical anatomy of the foot and ankle, *Clin Symp* 37:2–32, 1985.
22. Hartmann HO: The tendon sheaths and synovial bursae of the foot, *Foot Ankle* 1:247–296, 1981.
23. Hassab HK, El-Sherif AS: Drilling of the os calcis for painful heel with calcanean spur, *Acta Orthop Scand* 45:152–157, 1974.
24. Henricson AS, Westlin NE: Chronic calcaneal pain in athletes: entrapment of the calcaneal nerve? *Am J Sports Med* 12:152–154, 1984.
25. Hicks JH: The mechanics of the foot: the plantar aponeurosis and the arch, *J Anat* 88:25–31, 1954.
26. Hoffman SJ, Thul JR: Fractures of the calcaneus secondary to heel spur surgery. An analysis and case report, *J Am Podiatr Med Assoc* 75:267–271, 1985.
27. Jay RM, Davis BA, Schoenhaus HD, et al: Calcaneal decompression for chronic heel pain, *J Am Podiatr Med Assoc* 75:535–537, 1985.
28. Jorgensen U: Achillodynia and loss of heel pad shock absorbency, *Am J Sports Med* 13:128–132, 1985.
29. Katoh Y, Chao EY, Morrey BF, et al: Objective technique for evaluating painful heel syndrome and its treatment, *Foot Ankle* 3:227–237, 1983.
30. Kenzora JE: The painful heel syndrome: an entrapment neuropathy, *Bull Hosp J Dis Orthop Inst* 47:178–189, 1987.
31. Kopell HP, Thompson WAL: *Peripheral entrapment neuropathies*, Huntington, NY, 1986, Robert E Krieger, pp 25–29.
32. Kwong PK, Kay D, Voner RT, et al: Plantar fasciitis. Mechanics and pathomechanics of treatment, *Clin Sports Med* 7:119–126, 1988.
33. Leach RE, Dilorio E, Harney RA: Pathologic hindfoot conditions in the athlete, *Clin Orthop* 177:116–121, 1983.
34. Leach RE, Seavey MS, Salter DK: Results of surgery in athletes with plantar fasciitis, *Foot Ankle* 7:156–161, 1986.
35. Lester DK, Buchanan JR: Surgical treatment of plantar fasciitis, *Clin Orthop* 186:202–204, 1984.
36. Lin E, Ronen M, Stampler D, et al: Painful piezogenic heel papules. A case report, *J Bone Joint Surg [Am]* 67:601–604, 1985.
37. Lutter LD: Surgical decisions in athletes' subcalcaneal pain, *Am J Sports Med* 14:481–485, 1986.
38. Mann RA: *Surgery of the foot*, ed 5, St Louis, 1986, Mosby–Year Book, pp 244–247.
39. McBryde AM Jr: Plantar fasciitis, *Instr Course Lect* 33:278–282, 1984.

40. Micheli LJ, Ireland ML: Prevention and management of calcaneal apophysitis in children: an overuse syndrome, *J Pediatr Orthop* 7:34–38, 1987.
41. O'Brien D, Martin WJ: A retrospective analysis of heel pain, *J Am Podiatr Med Assoc* 75:416–418, 1985.
42. Paice EW, Hoffbrand BI: Nutritional osteomalacia presenting with plantar fasciitis, *J Bone Joint Surg [Br]* 69:38–40, 1987.
43. Przylucki H, Jones CL: Entrapment neuropathy of muscle branch of lateral plantar nerve: a cause of heel pain, *J Am Podiatr Assoc* 71:119–124, 1981.
44. Rask MR: Medial plantar neurapraxia (jogger's foot): report of 3 cases, *Clin Orthop* 134:193–195, 1978.
45. Riddle DL, Freeman DB: Management of a patient with a diagnosis of bilateral plantar fasciitis and Achilles tendinitis. A case report, *Phys Ther* 68:1913–1916, 1988.
46. Rondhuis JJ, Huson A: The first branch of the lateral plantar nerve and heel pain, *Acta Morphol Neerl Scand* 24:269–279, 1986.
47. Sammarco GJ: Prevention and treatment of running injuries. In D'Ambrosia RD, Drez D, editors: *Injuries to the foot*, ed 2, Thorofare, NJ, 1989, Charles B Slack, pp 155–183.
48. Sarrafian SK: *Anatomy of the foot and ankle*, Philadelphia, 1983, JB. Lippincott, pp 127–142.
49. Satku K, Pho RW, Wee A: Painful heel syndrome—an unusual cause. Case report, *J Bone Joint Surg [Am]* 66:607–609, 1984.
50. Savastano AA: Surgical neurectomy for the treatment of resistant painful heel, *Rhode Island Med J* 68:371–372, 1985.
51. Sewell JR, Black CM, Chapman AH, et al: Quantitative scintigraphy in diagnosis and management of plantar fasciitis (calcaneal periostitis): concise communication, *J Nucl Med* 21:633–636, 1980.
52. Shama SS, Kominsky SJ, Lemont H: Prevalence of nonpainful heel spur and its relation to postural foot position, *J Am Podiatr Assoc* 73:122–123, 1983.
53. Shaw RA, Holt PA, Stevens MB: Heel pain sarcoidosis, *Ann Intern Med* 109:675–677, 1988.
54. Shikoff MD, Figura MA, Postar SE: A retrospective study of 195 patients with heel pain, *J Am Podiatr Med Assoc* 76:71–75, 1986.
55. Shmokler RL, Bravo AA, Lynch FR, et al: A new use of instrumentation in fluoroscopy controlled heel spur surgery, *J Am Podiatr Med Assoc* 78:194–197, 1988.
56. Snider MP, Clancy WG, McBeath AA: Plantar fascia release for chronic plantar fasciitis in runners, *Am J Sports Med* 11:215–219, 1983.
57. Snook GA, Chrisman OD: The management of subcalcaneal pain, *Clin Orthop* 82:163–168, 1972.
58. Sullivan JA: Recurring pain in the pediatric athlete, *Pediatr Clin North Am* 31:1097–1012, 1984.
59. Tanz SS: Heel pain, *Clin Orthop* 28:169–178, 1963.
60. Vasavada PJ, DeVries DF, Nishiyama H: Plantar fasciitis—early blood pool images in diagnosis of inflammatory process, *Foot Ankle* 5:74–76, 1984.
61. Ward WG, Clippinger FW: Proximal medial longitudinal arch incision for plantar fascia release, *Foot Ankle* 8:152–155, 1987.
62. Warren BL: Anatomical factors associated with predicting plantar fasciitis in long-distance runners, *Med Sci Sports Exerc* 16:60–63, 1984.
63. Warren BL, Jones CJ: Predicting plantar fasciitis in runners, *Med Sci Sports Exerc* 19:71–73, 1987.
64. Williams PL, Smibert JG, Cox R, et al: Imaging study of the painful heel syndrome, *Foot Ankle* 7:345–349, 1987.

Superior Heel Pain (retrocalcaneal bursitis, Haglund's disease, enlargement of the superior tuberosity of the os calcis, insertional Achilles tendinitis)

65. Bordelon RL: *Surgical and conservative foot care*, Thorofare, NJ, Charles B Slack 1988.
66. Burhenne LJ, Connell DG: Xeroradiography in the diagnosis of the Haglund syndrome, *J Can Assoc Radiol* 37:157–160, 1986.
67. Canoso JJ, Liu N, Trail MR, et al: Physiology of the retrocalcaneal bursa, *Ann Rheum Dis* 47:910–912, 1988.
68. Canoso JJ, Wohlgethan JR, Newberg AH, et al: Aspiration of the retrocalcaneal bursa, *Ann Rheum Dis* 43:308–312, 1984.
69. Clancy WG: Runners' injuries. Part two. Evaluation and treatment of specific injuries, *Am J Sports Med* 8:287–289, 1980.
70. Fiamengo SA, Warren RF, Marshall JL, et al: Posterior heel pain associated with a calcaneal step and Achilles tendon calcification, *Clin Orthop* 167:203–211, 1982.
71. Fowler A, Philip JF: Abnormality of the calcaneus as a cause of painful heel: its diagnosis and operative treatment, *Br J Surg* 32:494–498, 1945.
72. Fox JM, Blazine ME, Jobe FW, et al: Degeneration and rupture of the Achilles tendon, *Clin Orthop* 107:221–224, 1975.
73. Frey C, Rosenberg Z, Shereff MJ: The retrocalcaneal bursa: anatomy and bursography, American Orthopaedic Foot and Ankle Society Specialty Day Meeting, Las Vegas, February 1989.
74. Gerster JC: Plantar fasciitis and Achilles tendinitis among 150 cases of seronegative spondarthritis, *Rheumatol Rehabil* 19:218–222, 1980.
75. Gerster JC, Piccinin P: Enthesopathy of the heels in juvenile onset seronegative B-27 positive spondyloarthropathy, *J Rheumatol* 12:310–314, 1985.
76. Gerster JC, Saudan Y, Fallet GH: Talalgia. A review of 30 severe cases, *J Rheumatol* 5:210–216, 1978.
77. Goss CM: *Gray's anatomy*, ed 27, Philadelphia, 1959, Lea & Febiger, 544–553.
78. Hartmann HO: The tendon sheaths and synovial bursae of the foot, *Foot Ankle* 1:247–296, 1981.
79. Heneghan JA, Pavlov H: The Haglund painful heel syndrome. Experimental investigation of cause and therapeutic implications, *Clin Orthop* 187:228–234, 1984.
80. Ippolito E, Ricciardi-Pollini PT: Invasive retrocalcaneal bursitis: a report on three cases, *Foot Ankle* 4:204–208, 1984.
81. Jones DC, James SL: Partial calcaneal osteotomy for retrocalcaneal bursitis, *Am J Sports Med* 12:72–73, 1984.
82. Keck SW, Kelly PJ: Bursitis of the posterior part of the heel: evaluation of surgical treatment of 18 patients, *J Bone Joint Surg [Am]* 47:267–273, 1965.
83. Kennedy JC, Willis RB: The effects of local steroid injections on tendons: a biomechanical and microscopic correlative study, *Am J Sports Med* 4:11–21, 1976.
84. Lagergren C, Lindholm A: Vascular distribution in the Achilles tendon: an angiographic and microangiographic study, *Acta Chir Scand* 116:491–495, 1958.

85. Leach RE, James S, Wasilewski S: Achilles tendinitis, *Am J Sports Med* 9:93–98, 1981.
86. Mann RA, editor: *(DuVries surgery of the foot)*, ed 5. St Louis, 1986, Mosby–Year Book.
87. Nelimarkka O, Lehto M, Jarvinen M: Soleus muscle anomaly in a patient with exertion pain in the ankle. A case report, *Arch Orthop Trauma Surg* 107:120–121, 1988.
88. Pavlov H, Heneghan MA, Hersh A, et al: The Haglund syndrome: initial and differential diagnosis, *Radiology* 144:83–88, 1982.
89. Ruch JA: Haglund's disease, *J Am Podiatr Assoc* 64:1000–1003, 1974.
90. Schepsis AA, Leach RE: Surgical management of Achilles tendinitis, *Am J Sports Med* 15:308–315, 1987.
91. Sullivan JA: Recurring pain in the pediatric athlete, *Pediatr Clin North Am* 31:1097–1112, 1984.
92. Vega MR, Cavolo DJ, Green RM, et al: Haglund's deformity, *J Am Podiatr Assoc* 74:129–135, 1984.
93. Zadek I: An operation for the cure of achillo-bursitis, *Am J Surg* 43:542–546, 1939.

CHAPTER

21

Infections of the Foot

John G. Frierson, M.D.
Landrus L. Pfeffinger, M.D.

Bacterial infections

- Soft-tissue infections
  - Technique for surgical treatment of felon
  - Puncture wounds
  - Trauma
  - Deep infections
- Joint infections
  - Diagnosis
  - Treatment
- Bone infections
  - Diagnosis
  - Treatment
- The infected diabetic foot
  - Diagnosis
  - Treatment
- Lyme disease

Mycobacterial infections

- Tuberculosis
  - Diagnosis
  - Treatment
- Atypical mycobacterial infections

Fungal infections

- Tinea pedis
- *Coccidioides immitis*
- *Cryptococcus neoformans*
- Mycetoma

Antibiotics

- The penicillins
- The cephalosporins
- Other β-lactam antibiotics
  - Aztreonam
  - Imipenem
- Other antibiotics
  - Clindamycin
  - Trimethoprim-sulfa
  - Aminoglycosides
  - Quinolones

The principles underlying the acquisition, diagnosis, and management of infections of the foot are much the same as those underlying infections elsewhere in the body. The foot however, both in health and disease, offers some particular features that color the presentation and management of infections. This is particularly evident in patients with diabetes and peripheral vascular disease. Foot infections may be subtle and chronic or quite aggressive, eventually leading to the loss of a foot—a major disability for the patient.

Infections can be classified according to tissues involved or by the infecting organism. A convenient classification might be as follows:

1. Bacterial infections
   a. Soft tissues (includes fat, fascia, lymphatics, tendons, bursae)
   b. Joint infections
   c. Bone infections
2. Mycobacterial infections (includes categories a, b, and c)
3. Fungal infections (includes categories a, b, and c)

Foot infections frequently present with various combinations of the above. However, the above outline is useful for organizational purposes and can be modified as the clinical situation warrants.

BACTERIAL INFECTIONS

Soft-Tissue Infections

The clinical presentation of soft-tissue infections will depend on causative factors as well as the organism(s) involved. Thus, infections stemming from superficial lesions such as infected blisters, scratches, or dermatologic afflictions usually present as cellulitis, lymphangitis, or both. The organisms most often responsible, in the uncompromised host, are the common skin organisms *Staphylococcus aureus* and β-hemolytic streptococci. *S. aureus* causes cellulitis and abscess formation, while hemolytic streptococci cause cellulitis and lymphangitis. The two organisms are frequently combined in soft-tissue infections, and it is wise to treat for both unless or until cultural data dictate otherwise.

A particular form of pure *S. aureus* infection is the *felon.* In this condition pus collects in the pulp space of the distal phalanx of a toe near a nail and causes considerable pain. Untreated, it may penetrate deeper and cause a local osteomyelitis. The presence of lymphangitic streaks suggests the presence of hemolytic streptococci, although occasionally gram-negative organisms (especially in diabetics and compromised hosts) may induce this. A variety of other organisms may be present in cellulitis and abscesses occurring after trauma and surgery and in immunocompromised hosts, in which case the clinical picture described above may be supplemented by varying degrees of necrosis, foul odor, and bullae.

The treatment of cellulitis and lymphangitis is primarily with antibiotics. If the infection has arisen from a superficial lesion, it can almost always be treated with an antibiotic directed against *S. aureus* and hemolytic streptococci. Such an agent would be dicloxacillin, cephalexin, clindamycin, as well as the newer more broad-spectrum cephalosporins and flouroquinolones (see the antibiotic section). In cases of more complicated cellulitis, antibiotic therapy should be based on culture data. Soaks and elevation are also helpful. An abscess or felon is treated by surgical drainage, soaks, and an antistaphylococcal antibiotic.

Technique for Surgical Treatment of Felon

1. Under digital or regional block and with a local anesthetic (without epinephrine), the pulp is widely opened with a "fish-mouth" incision extending from one side of the toe to the other.
2. If necrotic bone is present, it must be debrided (Fig 21–1).
3. The wound is left open to allow drainage.
4. Wound packing, if necessary, is done lightly and should be removed within 24 hours after surgery.
5. Delayed primary closure is performed once swelling and cellulitis have subsided and the wound appears clean and granulating—usually 5 to 7 days after incision and drainage in the nondiabetic patient.
6. If the infection progresses rapidly, as often occurs in the diabetic patient, with extensive soft-tissue and bony involvement, then partial (terminal Symes) or complete amputation is indicated. Again the wound is left open followed by delayed closure after appropriate time.

Puncture Wounds

Puncture wounds of the foot represent a challenging problem. They are most common in children and are frequently due to nails but can be due to splinters, tacks, glass, palm thorns, and other objects. Bits of clothing are often carried into the wound. Early complications include cellulitis and abscess formation, while late complications include osteomyelitis, osteochondritis and septic arthritis[21, 42] often due to *Pseudomonas aeruginosa.*[21] Osteomyelitis occurs in about 0.8% to 1.6% of cases and most often affects the metatarsals or calcaneus.[41] Retained foreign material is often found as a nidus for both the early and late complications.

If the patient is seen early, the wound should be cleansed with an iodophor solution and probed to be sure that there is no retained foreign material. The use of high-pressure syringe irrigation within the puncture wound is not fully studied but is recommended.[54] An attempt should be made to ascertain whether the puncture has penetrated to bone or cartilage. When a retained foreign body is suspected, radiographs should be obtained with a soft-tissue technique. The exact role of antibiotics is controversial.[12,54] If the wound is "clean," as in the case of a needle puncture, probably no antibiotic is indicated. If the wound is contaminated with dirt or clothing, if foreign material is possibly retained, or if the wound reaches bone, cartilage, or a joint, it is advisable to prescribe antibiotics. Drugs that cover *Staphylococcus* and *Streptococcus*, such as semisynthetic penicillins, cephalexin, or clindamycin, would be appropriate. It is tempting to recommend an antipseudomonal agent in cases where there is deep penetration (i.e., to bone), but this has not been studied.[8] Whether an antipseudomonal agent is used or not, it is important to observe these patients carefully and to obtain cultures (by aspiration if needed) if there is any sign of deep infection and treat accordingly. Tetanus prophylaxis should be given for all but the most superficial wounds, as outlined by the American College of Surgeons (ACS).

Trauma

In the case of trauma, the standard principles of cleansing the wound and debriding devitalized tissue are indicated. Antibiotics are recommended in most cases, especially when there has been foreign material introduced. Depending on the level and type of contam-

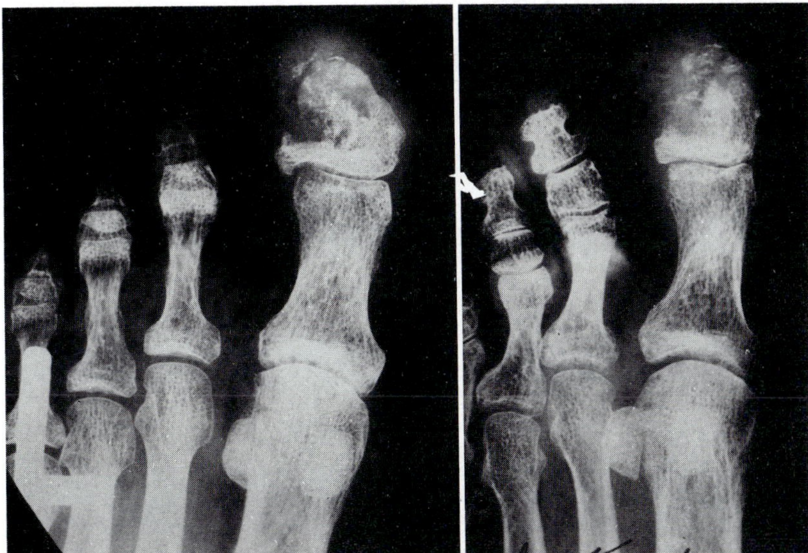

FIG 21–1.
Felon of the great toe with involvement of the distal tuft.

ination, a first-generation (to cover skin flora) or a third-generation cephalosporin might be used, the latter providing broader coverage in cases of dirtier wounds (see the antibiotic section). Coverage should include drugs effective against *Staphylococcus* and *Streptococcus.* The use of antibiotics in cases of trauma is not really a "prophylactic" use but rather a treatment directed at organisms already present. If an infection develops after trauma or puncture wounds, particularly if antibiotics have been used, then culture data are essential for rational use of antibiotics, and an assessment regarding the need for drainage is in order.

Deep Infections

Penetrating wounds and massive trauma to the foot can result in deep infection with abscess formation and, in later stages, osteomyelitis. The diabetic, immunosuppressed, or otherwise medically compromised patient is at greatest risk. Clostridial infections (gas gangrene) as a result of severe tissue trauma and contamination must be treated aggressively with surgical debridement of the involved tissue along with appropriate antibiotics, or else loss of the extremity or life will ensue (Fig 21–2).

Cat and dog bites can introduce an organism called *Pasteurella multocida*, which often behaves aggressively and can lead to cellulitis, tissue destruction, invasion of tendons and bone, and abscess formation.[27, 36] Such wounds are treated by debridement and irrigation and may be closed primarily. Prophylactic antibiotics should be administered. Penicillin, ampicillin, or amoxicillin will cover *Pasteurella multocida* as well as mouth flora, while cephalosporin and amoxicillin–clavulanic acid (Augmentin) has the advantage of also covering *Staphylococcus.* The penicillin-allergic patients can be given a combination of tetracycline and clindamycin. Tetanus toxoid should be administered as per ACS recommendations. Follow-up is needed because infection may occur in spite of these measures. If a patient is seen some days after a bite and infection has already set in, some form of debridement is usually needed along with antibiotics (which should be parenteral in severe cases).

Tenosynovitis and *bursa infections* can result from spread from adjacent cellulitis or from direct inoculation via trauma, puncture wounds, and the like. Tendinitis can be diagnosed by palpation of an enlarged, tender tendon sheath, by eliciting pain on stretching the tendon, by magnetic resonance imaging (MRI) or by direct visualization at surgery. The principles of treatment are the same: antibiotics and appropriate surgery.

Retrocalcaneal bursitis is an infection of the bursa situated between the Achilles tendon and the posterosuperior surface of the calcaneus. It generally arises by spread from a superficial infection that may relate to pressure and friction on the heel but can be metastatic. It is treated by antibiotics and soaks, followed by surgical drainage if needed.

Surgical Debridement of Deep Infections.—The plantar fascial spaces through which deep infections can spread need to be adequately drained. Loeffler and Ballard[31] have described an incision that allows exposure of the five plantar spaces (Figs 21–3 and 21–4) and heals without a sensitive scar.

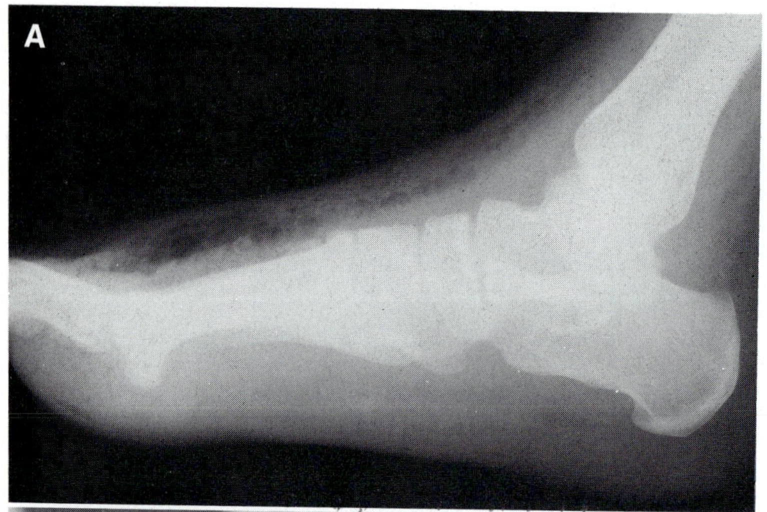

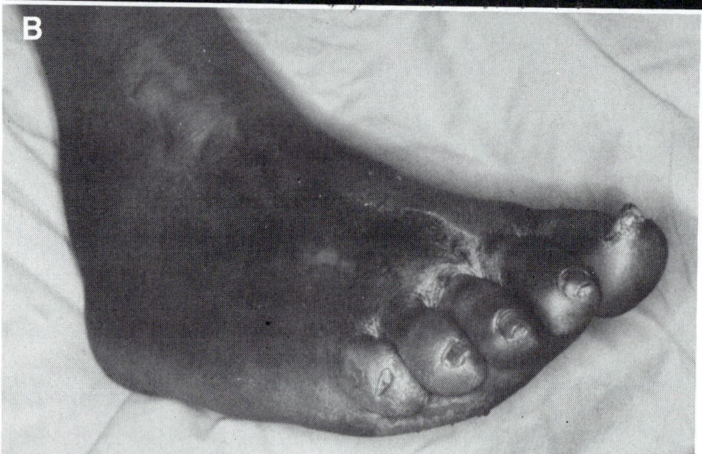

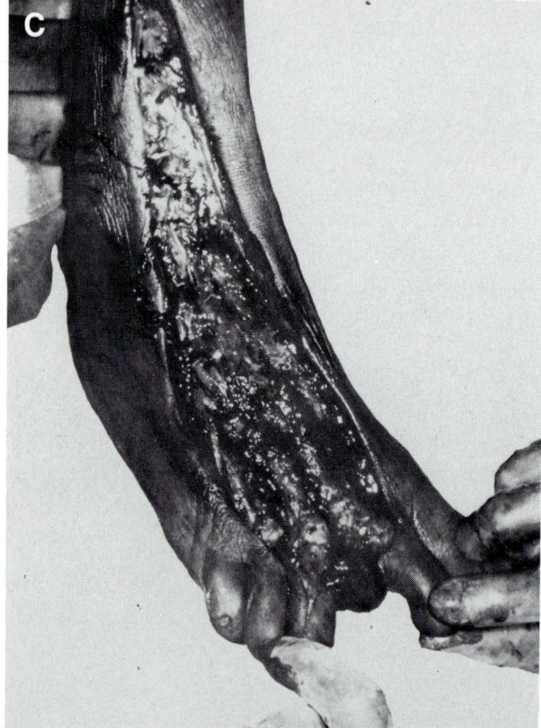

FIG 21–2.
Gas gangrene of the foot. **A,** Lateral view showing gas formation in subcutaneous tissue on the dorsum as result of clostridial cellulitis. **B,** clostridial cellulitis of the dorsum of the foot. Note the fluctuant swelling of subcutaneous tissue. **C,** after a wide incision and drainage, necrotic tissue is excised.

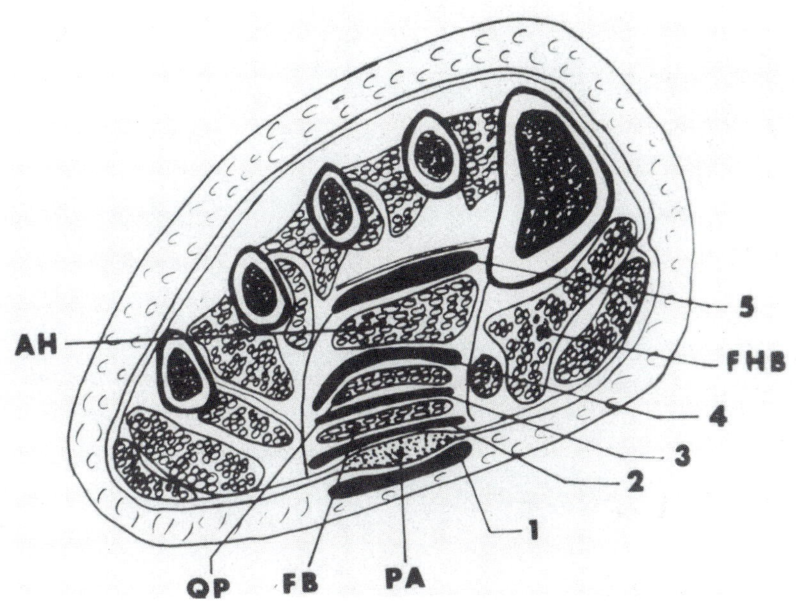

FIG 21–3.
Sagittal section of the foot. Fascial spaces 1 to 5 are identified by number. *AH* = adductor hallucis; *PA* = plantar aponeurosis; *FHB* = flexor hallucis brevis; *QP* = quadratus plantae. (From Loeffler RD, Ballard A: *Foot Ankle* 1:11–14, 1980. Used by permission.)

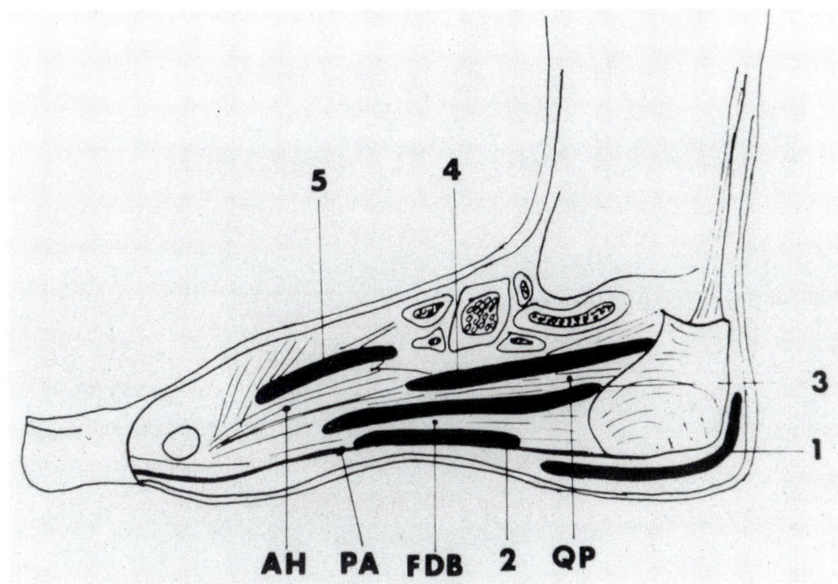

FIG 21–4.
Cross-sectional diagram of the foot (through the base of the metatarsals). Plantar spaces 1 to 5 are identified by number. *AH* = adductor hallucis; *QP* = quadratus plantae; *FDB* = flexor digitorum brevis; *PA* = plantar aponeurosis. (From Loeffler RO, Ballard A: *Foot Ankle* 1:11–14, 1980. Used by permission.)

Technique

1. The incision begins posterior to the medial malleolus (over the tarsal tunnel), extends medially and distally to the plantar midline of the midpart of the foot, and then extends distally to between the first and second metatarsal heads (Fig 21–5). All or any part of the incision is used.

2. Dissection is taken down through the thick plantar aponeurosis into plantar spaces 1 and 2.

3. From there dissection continues through the interval between the abductor hallucis and the flexor digitorum brevis entering plantar space 3 where the plantar nerves and arteries are located.

4. The abductor hallucis and flexor digitorum brevis are detached from the calcaneus and retracted anteriorly.

5. The quadratus plantae (or accessory flexor) muscle is now exposed. The flexor hallucis longus tendon is separated from the quadratus, and plantar space 4 is entered.

6. The dissection continues distally to visualize the plantar nerves, and now the fifth space is exposed.

7. The wound is left open in most cases and closed by secondary intention or delayed primary closure. A bulky dressing is applied, and progressive weight bearing is allowed once skin healing has occurred.

Joint Infections

Infections in foot joints can arise by spread from adjacent infection or by inoculation through various means or may arise from septicemic illness. The most common organism infecting joints is *Staphylococcus aureus*, which reaches the joint space either by extension from adjacent infection or from the bloodstream. *Haemophilus influenzae* is seen almost exclusively in children under 6 years of age and is generally blood-borne; blood cultures (as well as joint fluid cultures) are positive. *Neisseria gonorrhoeae* is the most common cause of septic arthritis in the young adult. It presents in two ways: the first is a bacteremic form in which one finds distinctive skin lesions on the extremities (pustules on a hemorrhagic base), frequently positive blood cultures, and involvement of multiple joints. The joints usually show periarticular inflammation and sometimes contain a sterile effusion.[25] The second form is a monarticular purulent arthritis where the aspirate fluid usually yields the organism. Arthritis due to *Streptococcus* and *Pneumococcus* tends to be secondary to foci elsewhere in the body and is associated with purulent effusions that yield the organism readily.

Diagnosis

The diagnosis of joint infection may be made clinically by appreciating redness, swelling, and tenderness of the joint, by needle aspiration, by direct vision at surgery, or by blood culture in the case of sepsis. Radiographs may show adjacent osteomyelitis or soft-tissue swelling, and computed tomography (CT) and MRI scans will show fluid in the joint and may also demonstrate adjacent soft-tissue or bone infection. Confirmation is by culture of an aspirate or at surgery. In the differential diagnosis such entities as gout, Reiter's syndrome, and neuropathic joints should be considered. The synovial fluid should be examined for cell count, bacteria (gram stain), sugar, urate crystals, and should be cultured.

Treatment

Joint infections that are acute can often be treated by parenteral antibiotics and repeated aspiration. Antibiotic levels in joint fluid approximate those found in

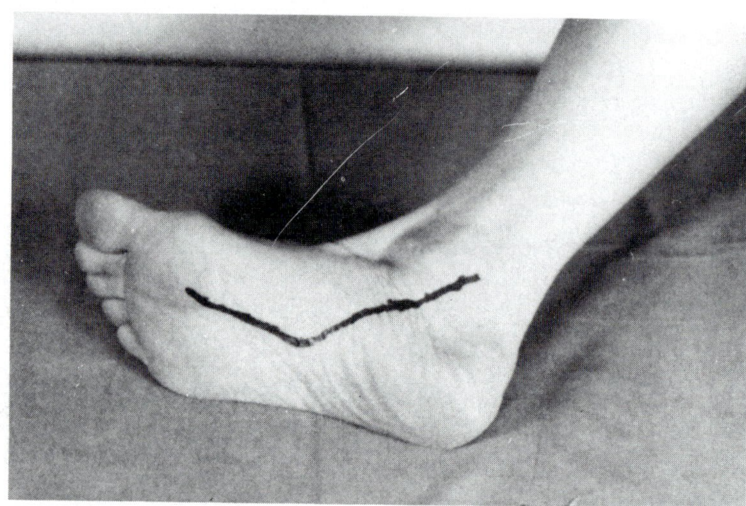

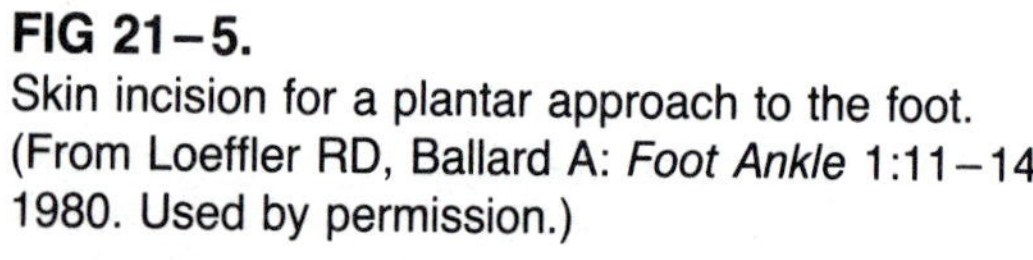

FIG 21–5.
Skin incision for a plantar approach to the foot. (From Loeffler RD, Ballard A: *Foot Ankle* 1:11–14, 1980. Used by permission.)

plasma,[29, 39] but because the antibiotic must act in an avascular space that may have some neutralizing properties, it is recommended that fairly liberal doses be given. Before culture results have returned, empiric antibiotic therapy may be instituted. Empiric therapy depends on the organism suspected and should promptly be adjusted to reflect culture results. *Staphylococcus* should be treated with nafcillin, a cephalosporin, clindamycin, or perhaps ciprofloxacin. Gonococci should be treated with ceftriaxone or, if the strain is known to be penicillin sensitive, with penicillin. Streptococci and pneumococci can be treated with penicillin or clindamycin. *Haemophilus* can be treated with ampicillin if it is known to be β-lactamase–negative or with third-generation cephalosporins, ampicillin-sulbactam, or aztreonam if β-lactamase–positive, while other gram-negative organisms can usually be treated with third-generation cephalosporins, aztreonam, imipenem, or others of the broad-spectrum drugs (for pharmacology and doses see the antibiotic section.) Several studies have shown that medical management will suffice for most joint infections.[7, 16, 43] Repeated aspiration will remove purulent and potentially destructive material and allow one to be sure of a therapeutic effect through examination and culture of the aspirate. If purulence does not improve or if effusions continue to form beyond 5 to 6 days, if it is a chronic infection, or if there is clinical or x-ray evidence of bone destruction, the joint should be opened surgically. The placement of tubes for intra-articular closed suction-irrigation is controversial and has not been subjected to controlled trials. Supportive measures such as rest are helpful. The affected joint does not need to be immobilized, but should be quiet, and weight bearing should be avoided until healing is progressing well.[19]

The prognosis of joint infections depends on the duration of infection before treatment, the organism involved (gram-negative infections generally have a worse prognosis,[17]) pre-existing joint disease, host competence, and the particular joint involved.[19]

Bone Infections

Osteomyelitis may arise through blood-borne transport of organisms, spread from adjacent soft-tissue or joint infection, or direct inoculation through trauma or surgery.

Primary blood-borne infections are most commonly due to *Staphylococcus aureus* and are more common in children. The upper portion of the tibia is the area most frequently involved, although other sites, including the lower part of the tibia and even the sesamoid bone[13] may be involved. Fever, local pain and swelling, tenderness, and elevation of the white blood cell (WBC) count would be the expected findings. X-ray findings can take 7 to 10 days to appear but are confirmatory when present. A particular form of subacute or chronic osteomyelitis usually found in the lower portion of the tibia is called Brodie's abscess (Fig 21–6). Radiographically it appears as a rounded lucent area surrounded by sclerotic bone, with nearby cortical and periosteal thickening. It can also be seen in the talus.[49] Osteomyelitis arising from trauma, surgery, or adjacent infection represents a heterogeneous group, whose clinical presentation will vary according to preceding events. Diagnosis is more difficult due to these complications. The principles of diagnosis and treatment are the same as for the blood-borne variety.

Diagnosis

It is important to diagnose correctly since the treatment consists of prolonged antibiotic administration, with or without surgery. A number of studies have been done on this subject with somewhat varying results, but a few helpful conclusions can be drawn. Diagnosis by direct vision or bone biopsy is conclusive. Needle aspirates are useful but should be interpreted with care if the needle is passed through an infected area. A number of imaging techniques are available. The plain radiograph may take 7 to 10 days to show changes of bone dissolution (especially at the cortex) that support the diagnosis, but its reliability once the changes are present is good. MRI and CT are able to visualize osteomyelitis earlier and provide more detail. CT scanning gives a little less detail than MRI, does not show the soft tissues as well, and is not multiplanar. MRI shows the greatest detail, can detect osteomyelitis early, can show soft-tissue detail (including nearby abscesses and sinus tracts), and can be viewed in the sagittal and coronal planes. However, the alterations in signal intensity are not specific for osteomyelitis and can be mimicked by anything that increases tissue water and replaces marrow, such as healing fractures and tumors.[46, 52, 56, 61] When used in conjunction with clinical data, however, MRI may be useful.

The use of radionuclide bone scans to diagnose osteomyelitis has also been studied. With the technetium 99m bone scan, the radioactivity concentrates in areas of increased vascularity and areas of increased osteoblastic activity. The commonly used procedure for diagnosing osteomyelitis of the foot is the "three-phase" bone scan.[46] The first phase, or flow phase, resembles an angiogram and consists of imaging over the suspect area in the first few seconds after injection of technetium. The second phase, the blood pool phase, is taken about 5 minutes after injection, and the third phase, or bone image, is taken 1 hour after injection. Bone infections

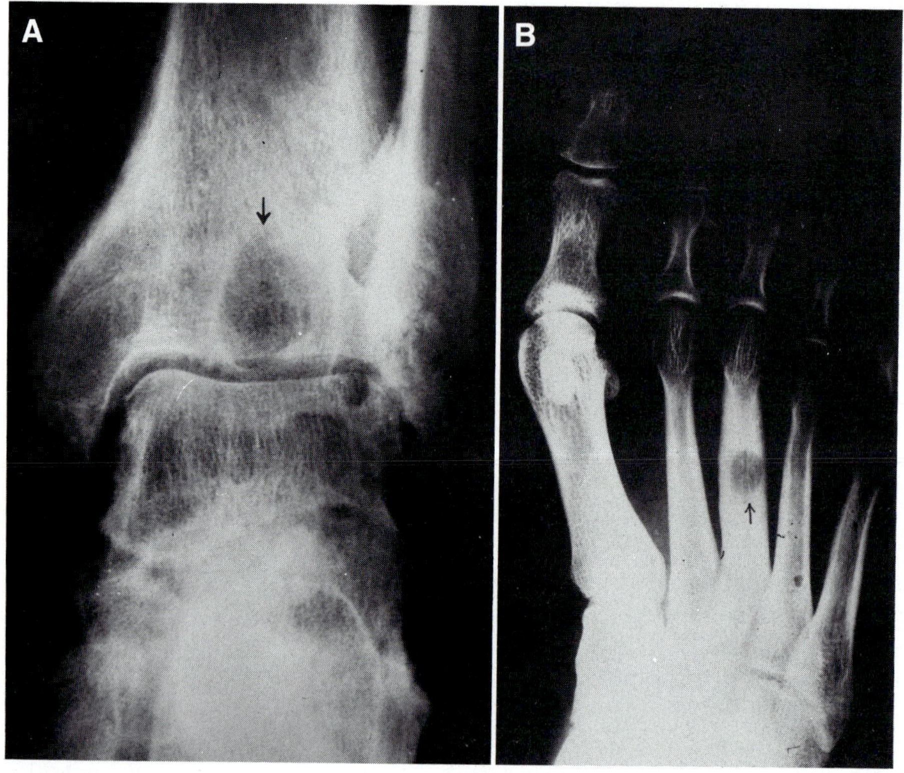

FIG 21–6.
Brodie's abscess. **A,** in the lower end of the tibia *(arrow)*. **B,** in the third metatarsal *(arrow)*. Note the increased density and periosteal thickening of the entire metatarsal shaft.

cause increased vascularity, and in stages 1 and 2 one sees focal radioactivity due to the extra technetium perfusion and pooling in this area. Later, as the circulatory pooling is washed out, radioactivity is concentrated in the active osteoblasts and "lights up" the infected bone in the third stage. In acute hematogenous osteomyelitis technetium scanning is very useful and will show the involved area before the radiograph. When it is used in conjunction with the clinical picture and blood culture results, a diagnosis of this condition can usually be made. False-negative bone scans occur most often in infants. Indium scanning, MRI, or follow-up radiographs may be used to confirm a diagnosis.

In trying to diagnose chronic osteomyelitis or osteomyelitis arising from adjacent infection, however, certain problems may arise. Soft-tissue infection often gives rise to local increases in vascularity and in periosteal reaction. These changes can produce changes in the bone scan that resemble those of osteomyelitis, thus producing a "false-positive" scan. This is particularly true of small bones of the foot since the anatomic detail in the scan is poor. False-positives can also result from surgery, fractures, and neuropathic osteopathy, while false-negatives can result from arterial insufficiency[23, 46, 48, 61] and are not uncommon in small infants.

Radionuclide scanning with gallium 67 and indium 111 has been studied in attempts to improve diagnostic accuracy. Gallium 67 is taken up by leukocytes, is bound to lactoferrin (a bacterial product), and concentrates in areas of infection. However, it lacks specificity and can be concentrated where there is surgery, trauma, etc. Additionally, it can take 2 to 3 days to complete. Comparison or subtraction studies using sequentially taken technetium and gallium scans has had limited success.[44] Indium 111 scanning is done by labeling the patient's own leukocytes with indium 111, reinjecting them, and scanning the suspect area the next day. The leukocytes travel preferentially to the infected area and are detected as increased radioactivity. This increases the specificity of the scan,[28, 37] but distinguishing bone from soft-tissue infection remains difficult, especially where small bones are involved. False-positives have also been reported with rheumatoid arthritis, healing fractures, metastatic carcinoma, and diabetic osteopathy. False-negative In^{111} scans may be seen with inadequate blood flow and sometimes after antibiotic therapy has been under way.

Given this multiplicity of techniques, how should

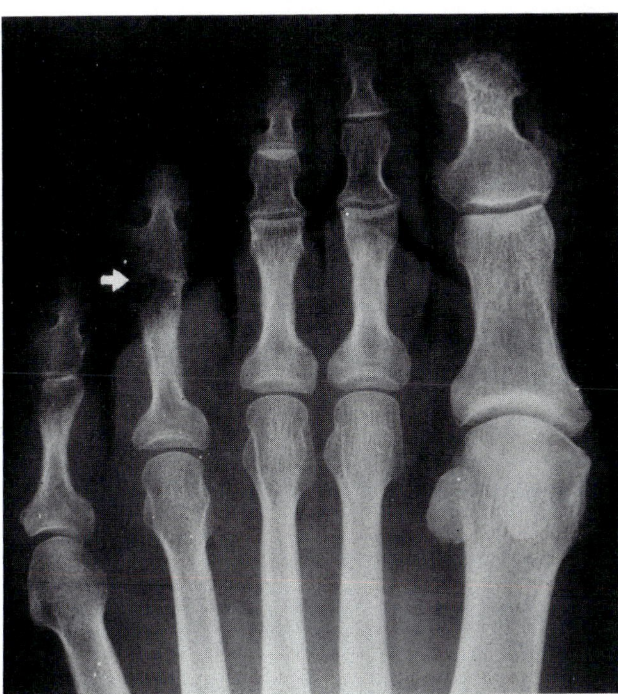

FIG 21–7.
Acute osteomyelitis of the head of the fourth proximal phalanx *(arrow)*.

one proceed? If the plain radiograph shows changes characteristic of osteomyelitis (Fig 21–7) (and it is suspected clinically), then further studies are not needed. If the radiograph is normal and infection is suspected, then one might select one or more of the imaging techniques described above, depending on the integrity of the circulation, the presence of fractures, etc. Alternatively, one can institute antibiotic treatment and take another radiograph in 2 weeks. If no changes of osteomyelitis have appeared, it is safe to stop treatment.[58]

Culture.—In addition to diagnosing osteomyelitis it is essential to determine the organism(s). In acute osteomyelitis this can be done through blood culture or by needle aspiration of the suspect bone. In osteomyelitis that is chronic or secondary to adjacent soft-tissue infection, culture of bone biopsy specimens is a gold standard but still an invasive technique. Needle aspirates are reliable if taken through otherwise sterile tissue. A culture of surface drainage believed to communicate with infected bone may be misleading.[34] If this technique is used, one should clean the surface well and then carefully culture a bead of expressed pus without touching the skin while keeping an open mind about the possibility of different flora in the bone itself. Material should always be sent for anaerobic as well as aerobic culture and mycobacterial and fungal culture if indicated.

Treatment

Acute Osteomyelitis.—The treatment of osteomyelitis of the foot usually involves a combined medical-surgical approach. In acute osteomyelitis, if the diagnosis is made early (before any radiographic changes), prompt administration of antibiotics will sometimes suffice to produce a cure.[47] More commonly surgical drainage will be needed along with parenteral antibiotics. Local irrigation of antibiotics postoperatively has not been shown in a controlled trial to be superior to parenteral antibiotics, and there is the potential danger of introducing infection by this route. Although there is no definitive study to prove their superiority, the bactericidal antibiotics are preferred (see the antibiotic section).

Intravenous treatment of gram-positive organisms should continue for 4 weeks and perhaps up to 6 weeks for gram-negative organisms. In this age of diagnosis-related groups (DRGs) and home treatment services, the intravenous treatment of osteomyelitis at home is more routine and less expensive than heretofore. Studies in children have shown that 2 weeks of intravenous antibiotics followed by 2 weeks of appropriate doses of oral antibiotics is satisfactory.[47]

In adults the issue of oral therapy is less well studied.[14] However, ciprofloxacin has been studied in some detail as oral therapy for osteomyelitis. Several studies have shown its effectiveness in this regard,[22, 24] and in one study using a randomized protocol, the results were comparable to parenteral therapy.[15] It must be remembered that the success of oral therapy is dependent on patient compliance.

Much debate has centered around the advisability of obtaining serum "bactericidal" levels. This is a measurement of the dilution of the patient's serum, while receiving antibiotics, that will kill the organism in vitro. A large multicenter trial examined this problem. The authors concluded that bactericidal levels of 1:2 in acute osteomyelitis and 1:4 in chronic osteomyelitis just before administration of the next dose of antibiotic were desirable.[57] However, the number of treatment failures was fairly small, which makes the predictive value of these numbers less certain. It has been recommended that these levels be used mainly as a guide to therapy while bearing in mind drug toxicity.[40]

Chronic Osteomyelitis.—In the management of more chronic osteomyelitis, surgical debridement or removal of involved bone is essential. The principles of antibiotic management are the same as for acute osteomyelitis. Where more than one organism exists, combinations of antibiotics may be needed, although the third-generation cephalosporins, imipenem, and the quinolones have broad spectrums that often allow their use as a single agent. Accurate culture data are essential. Recommendations for longer courses of antibiotics have been made in chronic osteomyelitis. This would apply only if the affected bone cannot be debrided appropriately. If such is the case, treatment intravenously for a month followed by oral therapy for 2 to 3 months can be recommended. Sometimes osteomyelitis of a phalanx, even though radiographically visible (Fig 21–8) and thus not very acute, can be treated successfully with antibiotics alone.

Surgical treatment of chronic osteomyelitis of the calcaneus presents a formidable challenge to the surgeon. Subtotal or total excision of the os calcis produces a loss of weight-bearing bone and violation or removal of the plantar soft tissue. Without appropriate treatment this may result in amputation of the foot. However, with successful free muscle transfer and overlying split-thickness skin grafts, amputation can be avoided.[2]

The Infected Diabetic Foot

Infections in the diabetic foot present particular features that are considered separately here. In one study, foot problems were responsible for 15% of admissions of diabetic patients and accounted for 23% of their hospital days.[30] One of 15 diabetics eventually requires a limb amputation. Diabetics often have a peripheral neuropathy that makes it difficult to perceive small abrasions and induces the formation of ulcers at pressure points. Arterial and renal insufficiency are often present, both of which impair healing and defenses against infection.

Infections in diabetics are usually introduced through foot ulcers or paronychia, although there are many possible routes of entry. *Staphylococcus aureus* is the most frequently encountered bacteria, but mixed infections containing gram-negative and anaerobic bacteria are common. One study showed that 30% of patients had a single organism, while 42% had as many as four organisms.[59] One cannot predict specific organisms by the size or appearance of the lesion, but certain correlations exist. Uncomplicated cellulitis is most often due to *Staphylococcus aureus* and hemolytic streptococci. A foul smell suggests anaerobes. Gas in the tissues suggest the presence of anaerobes, gram-negatives, or both. Gangrene suggests mixed infection, most commonly with anaerobes, but sometimes with gram-negative organisms.[45] Patients who have recently taken antibiotics often have more resistant flora such as *Pseudomonas*.

Diagnosis

Clinical evaluation should always include x-ray studies to look for gas in the tissues and osteomyelitis. Culture data can be obtained by aspiration of bullae, culture of drainage, needle aspiration, or at surgery. Flora in surface drainage may not reflect what is in the tissues,[34] and if in doubt an aspirate is preferred. However, there may be a reluctance to introduce a needle into an ischemic foot, in which case the relative risks must be balanced.

Treatment

Antibiotic Therapy.—Empiric antibiotic therapy should be started before culture data are returned. In case of mild or superficial infection a first-generation cephalosporin, dicloxacillin, or clindamycin may be used. In any infection that looks more complicated, broad-spectrum coverage for aerobes and anaerobes should be included. Many hospital laboratories do not

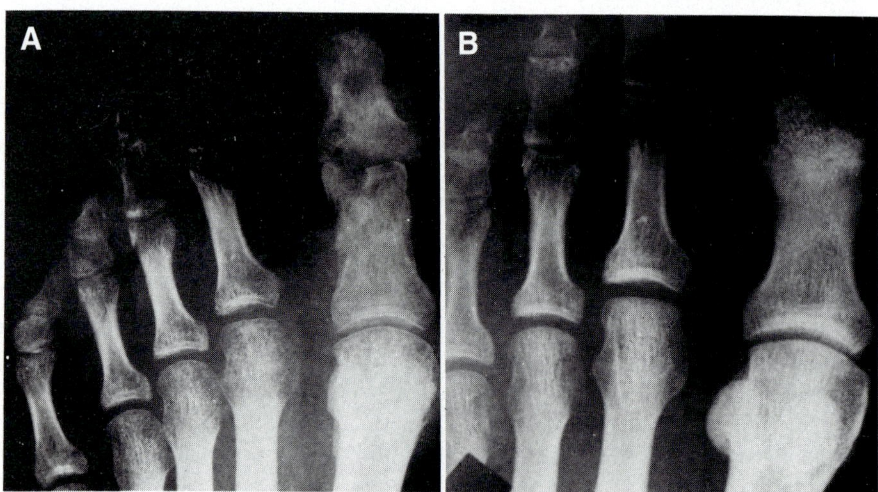

FIG 21–8.
A, osteomyelitis of the entire hallux. **B,** after healing.

test anaerobe sensitivities routinely. Antibiotics that can be given parenterally and are reliably effective against anerobes are metronidazole, clindamycin, imipenem, and piperacillin (see the section on antibiotics). Thus the broad-spectrum coverage could be accomplished by imipenem alone, combinations like third-generation cephalosporins (ceftriaxone, ceftazidime) and either clindamycin or metronidazole, or a combination of clindamycin and aztreonam for the penicillin-allergic patient. For a fuller discussion of antibiotics, see the antibiotic section. In any but the mildest infections, the intravenous route is preferred, and adequate doses should be given to overcome impaired delivery through arterial insufficiency. A recent study of osteomyelitis in diabetic feet suggests that in the absence of necrosis, aggressive antibiotic management carries a favorable prognosis.[3] The presence of necrosis, whether of ischemic or infectious origin, carries a worse prognosis for limb salvage.

Hyperbaric oxygen, even when anaerobes are present, has not been proven to be of additional benefit and should not replace proper surgical debridement.

Evaluation for Surgical Treatment.—In any but superficial infections surgical evaluation is required. Necrotizing fasciitis, abscesses, and osteomyelitis may coexist with cellulitis. Some infections, particularly necrotizing fasciitis, can progress quite rapidly, and prompt surgery can be decisive in saving a limb (see Fig 21–2).

Plain radiographs should always be obtained. MRI and nuclear scans may be of help. One study suggests that MRI is useful in distinguishing osteomyelitis from diabetes neuroarthropathy, a distinction that may be difficult or impossible on plain radiographs.[4]

An assessment of the circulatory status of the foot is essential. If arterial perfusion is poor, a decision regarding a revascularization procedure or amputation may be needed. If the arterial circulation is good, then debridement and drainage should be carried out as in any other infected foot.

Systemic pressure measurement is the most important and useful parameter for noninvasive screening of peripheral arterial occlusive disease. The Doppler ultrasound technique is simple, cost-effective, and comparatively accurate in comparison to other techniques. When combined with clinical and radiographic assessment, Doppler studies are invaluable to the surgeon in the diagnosis, prognosis, and choice of treatment.

There are considerable clinical and laboratory data to indicate that there are specific arterial pressures that result in successful healing. A toe pressure of at least 40 mm Hg is necessary for healing. Wagner's clinical experience with diabetic patients predicts that satisfactory healing can be obtained at any lower-extremity level if flow is pulsatile, the systolic pressure index (as compared with brachial systolic pressure) is greater than 0.45, and the systolic pulse is near 70 mm Hg.[55]

By carefully evaluating the clinical, radiographic, and Doppler studies one can in most cases avoid "whittling away at the foot," which is a disservice to the patient.

For example, with favorable Doppler systolic pressures a chronic recurring diabetic ulcer beneath a metatarsal head can be treated by simple excision of the metatarsal head. Subsequent to healing, appropriate shoe wear, padding, or inserts, with or without metatarsal bars or rocker-bottom shoes, as well as patient education, can help to avoid further ulcers.

Lyme Disease

Lyme disease, caused by the spirochete *Borrelia burgdorferi* and transmitted by ixodic ticks, was first recognized in 1975 because of joint involvement. The first manifestation of the illness is an annular skin lesion known as erythema chronicum migrans, often followed by fever and various systemic complaints. Anywhere from 1 week to 2 years from the onset there may be arthritic complaints in one or more joints.[51] These vary from migratory arthralgias, to intermittent arthritis, to chronic erosive joint disease. In those presenting with frank arthritis, only one or two joints are usually involved, most often the knee, with the ankle being the third most frequently involved joint. Heel pain may also occur.[51] The sedimentation rate is normal or mildly elevated, and synovial fluid findings, if present, are nonspecific. Radiographically there is soft-tissue swelling, and in more chronic cases there may be thinning of articular cartilage, erosions at the cartilaginous margins, osteoporotic changes, osteophytes, and subchondral cysts.[33]

The diagnosis is usually made by obtaining a history of erythema chronicum migrans and by serology. False-positive serologies may occur, however, particularly in patients with syphilis, and the results need to be integrated into the clinical and epidemiologic picture. The differential diagnosis includes rheumatoid arthritis, Reiter's syndrome, and gonococcemia. Treatment is with penicillin, tetracycline, or ceftriaxone.

MYCOBACTERIAL INFECTIONS

Tuberculosis

Mycobacterium tuberculosis infection of the foot is uncommon. Overall, bone and joint involvement accounts for 15 to 19% of all extrapulmonary tuberculosis,[1] and involvement of the hands and feet constitutes only 2% of skeletal disease.[6] Tuberculosis of the ankle is the most common presentation, while in the foot proper the talus, the subtalar joint, the tarsus, the talonavicular joint, the calcaneus, and the first metatarsophalangeal joint are the most frequently involved (Fig 21–9). The organism arrives there through the bloodstream and rarely by inoculation. A prior history of trauma is not uncommon, followed weeks or months later by indolent swelling and pain. Radiographs early in the process may show only soft-tissue swelling, but eventually subchondral osteoporosis, areas of bone destruction, thickening of periosteum, and cartilage destruction can appear. Often there is no active extra-skeletal tuberculosis.[18]

Diagnosis

The diagnosis should be suspected in cases of single lesions of bone or joints, especially in high-risk groups such as patients from developing countries. Synovial fluid analysis shows quite variable degrees of inflammation, with cell counts ranging from 40 to 136,000, but averaging about 20,000.[18] A biopsy of synovium or bone, depending on involvement, is almost always needed to make the diagnosis and also to obtain the organism. Culture of synovial fluid alone is said to yield the organism in 80% of cases of articular disease, the figure rising to 90% with culture of synovial tissue.[53] A positive skin test and evidence of tuberculosis elsewhere are helpful signs. Whenever possible the organism should be cultured and sensitivities determined since the incidence of drug-resistant tuberculosis in developing countries is high.

Treatment

With the advent of chemotherapy, surgery of bone and joint tuberculosis has assumed a secondary role. Therapy is with two or more drugs for at least 9 months, the precise regimen to be guided by sensitivity testing. Casting and immobilization measures are not needed except for relief of pain. Surgery is needed only when joint instability requires fusion, and this should be only after the results of chemotherapy are evaluated.

Atypical Mycobacterial Infections

Infection of bones and joints with nontuberculous mycobacteria is relatively rare. *Mycobacterium kansasii* has some propensity for joints, but almost always in the upper extremity. Patients with acquired immunodeficiency syndrome (AIDS) have a predilection for *Mycobacterium avium-intracellulare* infections that are usually generalized. Bones and joints are seldom involved, however. Patients exposed to tropical fish or marine life may be infected with *Mycobacterium marinum*. Soil-contaminated wounds may give rise to *Mycobacterium fortuitum*, a rapidly growing *Mycobacterium*.[10]

A mycobacterial infection should be suspected in patients with more indolent bone and joint infections, especially if routine cultures are unrevealing, if pathologic examination shows granulomas, or if the patient is immunocompromised. Synovial fluid resembles that seen

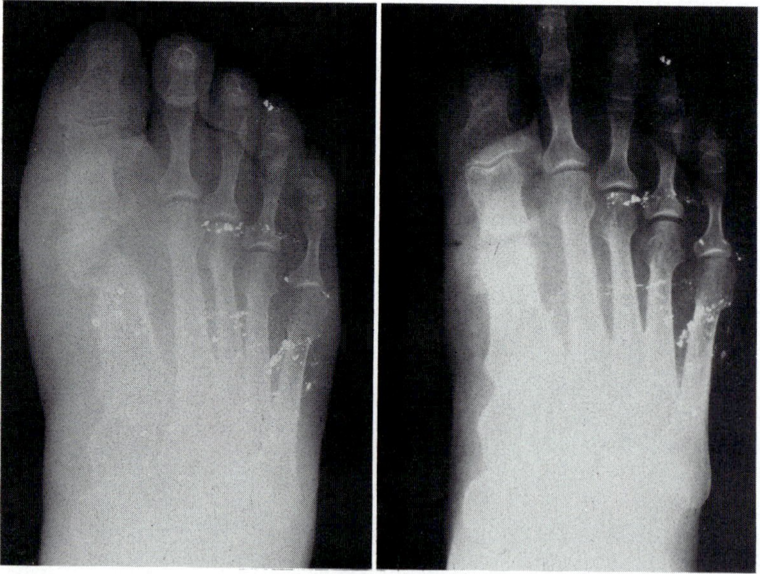

FIG 21–9.
Tuberculosis of the first metatarsal. Buckshot wounds antedated the onset of this involvement. Infection was proved by biopsy and guinea pig inoculation. (Courtesy of Dr. D.D. Dickson.)

in tuberculous arthritis, with cell counts ranging from 2,900 to 132,000 WBCs and polymorphonuclear cells ranging from 12% to 90%.[60] The sugar content is generally depressed. The diagnosis is made by a biopsy of synovium or bone, with appropriate cultures.

Treatment is primarily medical. Antituberculous drugs are used. Results with *M. avium-intracellulare* are poor, but other infections generally respond if sensitivities are taken into account. *M. fortuitum* has a tendency to form abscesses, and drainage and debridement may be indicated.

FUNGAL INFECTIONS

Tinea Pedis

Tinea pedis (athlete's foot) is a very common fungal infection of the skin and nails of the foot. Varying degrees of itching, cracking, scaling, and blister formation are seen. The soles and interdigital spaces are most frequently affected. *Trichophyton rubrum* and *Trichophyton mentagrophytes* are the most commonly encountered organisms. Treatment of skin infections is by a topical antifungal agent such as clotrimazole. Nail infections may be treated by oral griseofulvin, but it may require up to a year to clear, relapse is common, and it is probably best to advise against treatment. Skin lesions of tinea pedis may serve as a portal of entry for bacteria that can cause cellulitis, especially in diabetics.

Coccidioides Immitis

Deeper tissues can be infected by other fungi, although this is uncommon. In California and the southwestern United States *Coccidioides immitis* may be found. It is acquired through the respiratory tract, but after dissemination it may cause chronic ulceration of the skin and underlying soft tissue and, less commonly, may invade bone and joints. More than one skeletal site is involved in about 50% of cases. In one series, the talus, os calcis, fifth metatarsal, and the soft tissues were the pedal sites involved.[5] Symptoms may come on years after the initial exposure.[32] A bone scan can be helpful in screening patients for multiple skeletal sites. X-ray films show the expected lytic changes of bony destruction. Analysis of joint fluid shows variable numbers of white cells, but usually not the organism. Biopsy of the synovium or bone is the diagnostic procedure of choice.[5] Treatment depends on the type of involvement. Pure joint involvement usually requires synovectomy and amphotericin, while bone involvement may be treated by amphotericin alone or in conjunction with surgical debridement, depending on the extent of involvement.

Cryptococcus Neoformans

Skeletal affliction with *Cryptococcus neoformans* is uncommon. The organism is acquired through the respiratory tract, and preferentially involves the lungs and the cerebrospinal fluid. Dissemination may occur to any part of the body, with the skeleton being involved in fewer than 10% of cases. In one series, the foot and ankle were affected in 5 out of 117 sites in 59 cases of skeletal involvement.[9] Underlying disease, including lymphoma, sarcoidosis, and rheumatoid arthritis, is not uncommon. Radiographs usually show pure lytic lesions with little sclerosis. Diagnosis is made by culture of bone biopsy specimens or sometimes drainage.

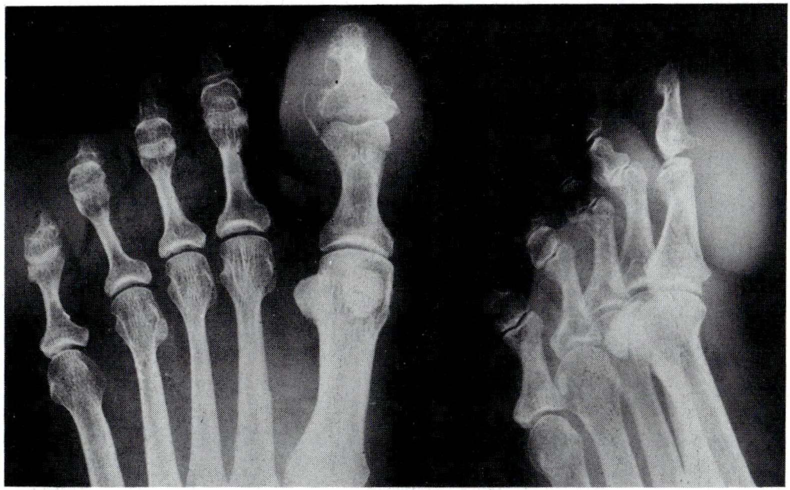

FIG 21–10.
Massive granuloma of the great toe as a result of mycotic infection acquired in a tropical country.

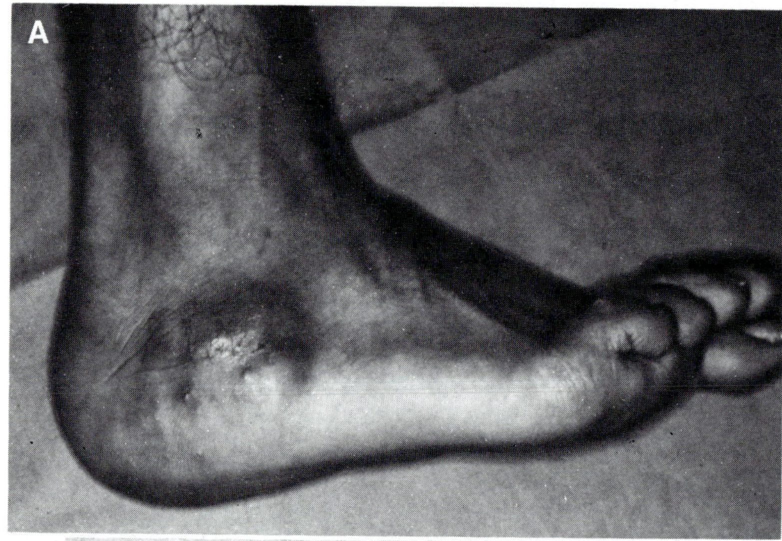

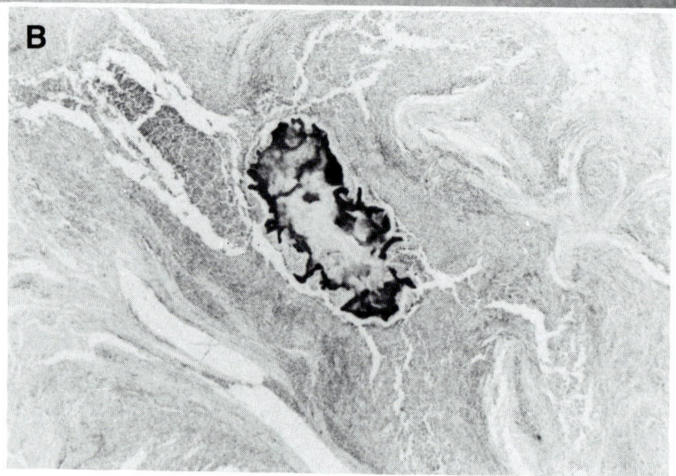

FIG 21–11.
A, draining sinus of the side of the heel. A biopsy specimen of an extensive nodular lesion revealed *Nocardia.* **B,** *Nocardia* colony with chronic inflammation; sulfur granule of the lesion in **A.**

Treatment is with local debridement or excision in association with amphotericin and often 5-flucytosine. If there is no other site of involvement, some have recommended local excision alone as adequate therapy.[20]

Mycetoma

Rare in the developed world but common in some developing countries, mycetoma, or Madura foot (Fig 21–10), is a chronic foot infection caused by a number of organisms that are classified as actinomycetes or as fungi. The organisms are introduced through puncture wounds. At first small nodules are formed, and then there is gradual spread along fascial planes and drainage through sinus tracts. In the drainage are little "sulfur granules" of coalesced organisms, which are characteristic. Eventually bone, muscle, and nerve destruction may occur, as well as secondary infection. If the infection is caused by actinomycetes such as *Nocardia* (Fig 21–11), response to drug treatment may be good, and surgery should be delayed until the response can be evaluated. If fungi are the culprits, drug treatment may still be effective but is less promising. In advanced cases, amputation may be needed.[35, 38]

Involvement of bone and joints of the foot by other fungi is very rare, but organisms such as *Blastomyces dermatitidis*, *Candida albicans*, *Histoplasma capsulatum*, and *Sporothrix schenckii* are occasionally encountered.[11]

ANTIBIOTICS

The rational use of antibiotics requires knowledge of the pharmacology and side effects of the agents and knowledge of the organisms to be treated. The proliferation of antibiotics has made their use a more complicated endeavor than before, sometimes requiring the help of a specialist. However, a brief review of the major classes and their properties should allow a nonspecialist to make proper use of these drugs in many situations.

Certain principles underlie the choice of a particular antibiotic:

1. Knowledge of the infecting organism and its habitat. Usually this is derived from culture data. It is important to know how a culture is obtained (preferably for the physician to obtain it himself) so as to assess its reliability. When using empiric therapy one must know the most likely flora for a given situation. Thus, in superficial cellulitis one is usually dealing with *Staphylococcus aureus* or β-hemolytic streptococci. Adjustments can then be made when culture results are available. (See the individual headings for specific recommendations.)

2. Antimicrobial sensitivities. This is as essential as organism identification but takes an extra day or two. When ordering antibiotics before sensitivity data are available or when empiric therapy is used, Table 21–1 will be useful. However it is only an outline and should not be considered a substitute for proper data from the laboratory. The list in Table 21–1 is not an exhaustive one. For example, the aminoglycosides are almost uniformly effective against gram-negative rods but are not always mentioned because of their toxicity and because safer alternatives are now available.

3. Knowledge of the patient. The age of the patient affects drug dosage. Elderly patients metabolize drugs more slowly even if creatinine and liver function tests give normal results. Impaired hepatic and renal function can affect both the dose and choice of antimicrobial agent, as can pregnancy. Age may also predispose to selective side effects. For instance, tetracycline should be avoided in children under 8 years of age and the quinolones in prepubertal children.

4. The need for bactericidal agents. The so-called bactericidal antibiotics are those that when incubated in vitro with susceptible bacteria, render them incapable of growing when subcultured onto fresh media. Exam-

TABLE 21–1.
Antimicrobial Sensitivities

Organism	Antibiotics Usually Effective
Group A streptococci	Penicillin and penicillin derivatives, all cephalosporins, erythromycin, clindamycin, vancomycin
Staphylococcus aureus	Cloxacillin, dicloxacillin, cephalosporins, clindamycin, imipenem, vancomycin, ciprofloxacin. For methicillin-resistant staphylococci use vancomycin
Streptococcus pneumoniae	Same as group A streptococci
Enterococci	Ampicillin, imipenem, vancomycin
Haemophilus influenzae	Cefamandole, cefuroxime, cefonicid, third-generation cephalosporins, aztreonam, ciprofloxacin, trimethoprim-sulfa, and (if β-lactamase–negative) ampicillin
Neisseria gonorrheae	Cefoxitin, cefuroxime, ceftriaxone, trimethoprim-sulfa, ciprofloxacin
Escherichia coli	Second- and third-generation cephalosporins, aztreonam, imipenem, trimethoprim-sulfa, ciprofloxacin, mezlocillin, azlocillin, piperacillin, ampicillin-sulbactam
Klebsiella pneumoniae	Second- and third-generation cephalosporins, imipenem, trimethoprim-sulfa, aztreonam, ampicillin-sulbactam, ciprofloxacin
Proteus mirabilis	Ampicillin, all cephalosporins, azlocillin, mezlocillin, piperacillin, ampicillin-sulbactam, aztreonam, imipenem, ciprofloxacin
Other *Proteus* sp.	Third-generation cephalosporins, azlocillin, mezlocillin, piperacillin, aztreonam, imipenem, ciprofloxacin
Enterobacter sp.	Third-generation cephalosporins, azlocillin, mezlocillin, piperacillin, imipenem, trimethoprim-sulfa, ampicillin-sulbactam, ciprofloxacin
Pseudomonas aeruginosa	Azlocillin, mezlocillin, piperacillin, ceftazidime, aztreonam, imipenem, ciprofloxacin, aminoglycosides
Anaerobes	
Anaerobic streptococci	Penicillins, clindamycin, cephalosporins, imipenem
Bacteroides sp.	Clindamycin, metronidazole, imipenem, azlocillin, mezlocillin, piperacillin, ampicillin-sulbactam
Clostridium sp.	Penicillin, clindamycin, metronidazole

ples of these agents are the penicillins and cephalosporins. The importance of this phenomenon for the foot is restricted to therapy for bone infections. Here, because of the local avascular (and hence immunocompromised) environment, bactericidal agents are preferred.

The following is a brief description of the major antibiotic classes.

The Penicillins

The penicillins share a common thiazolidine and β-lactam ring. They bind to the penicillin-binding proteins of bacterial cell walls and from this position exert an inhibitory effect on the assembly of the peptidoglycan chains of the cell wall, although in some cases there is rapid lysis of the cell wall by other mechanisms. This confers a bactericidal property. Many organisms produce β-lactamases, enzymes that catalyze the degradation of the penicillin ring, thus allowing resistance to penicillin. The penicillins with broader spectrum are, to a greater or lesser extent, resistant to this action. Penicillins are excreted by the kidney and metabolized by the liver in variable degrees, depending on the drug. The major obstacle to their use is the presence of allergic reactions. Examples of the penicillin class are penicillin, ampicillin, amoxicillin, the "semisynthetic" penicillins (cloxacillin, dicloxacillin, methicillin, nafcillin, oxacillin), carbenicillin, ticarcillin, azlocillin, mezlocillin, and piperacillin. The agents clavulanate and sulbactam, which are inhibitors of β-lactamase, have been combined with penicillins to make them more resistant to degradation by bacteria and thus broaden their spectrum. Examples of this combination are ampicillin-clavulanate (Augmentin), ticarcillin-clavulanate (Timentin), and ampicillin-sulbactam (Unasyn).

The Cephalosporins

The cephalosporins share a dihydrothiazine ring and the same β-lactam ring characteristic of penicillins. As with penicillins, they bind to penicillin-binding proteins in the cell wall, where they interfere with cell wall synthesis or may cause direct cell wall lysis. They are bactericidal but are susceptible to β-lactamases, although the agents with broader spectrums are more stable against these enzymes. Their pharmacokinetics revolve around excretion by the kidney and hepatic metabolism, and doses may need modification in the presence of renal insufficiency. Patients allergic to penicillin may also exhibit an allergy to cephalosporins, and they should be used with caution in this setting. Some may interfere with vitamin K synthesis and lead to hypoprothrombinemia and subsequent bleeding. This is preventable by prophylactic vitamin K administration. Moxalactam also interferes with platelet function and is the cephalosporin most associated with bleeding.

Cephalosporins are divided into first-, second-, and third-generation categories. First-generation drugs are most active against gram-positive organisms except enterococci and to some extent against *Escherichia coli*, *Klebsiella*, and *Proteus mirabilis*. Examples of parenteral agents are cephalothin and cefazolin. Second-generation drugs are more reliably effective against *E. coli*, *Klebsiella*, and other *Proteus* species, and some have anaerobic activity. Examples of parenteral agents are cefoxitin, cefotetan, cephamandole, cefuroxime, and cefonicid. Third-generation cephalosporins have the broadest spectrum, extending to most gram-negative organisms, although antipseudomonal activity is variable. Some also have activity against anaerobes. Enterococci are not affected. Examples of this generation are ceftriaxone, cefotaxime, ceftizoxime, cefoperazone, ceftazidime, cefpiramide, and moxalactam.

Other β-Lactam Antibiotics

Aztreonam

Aztreonam is a monobactam. It is of interest in that it binds only to penicillin-binding proteins of gram-negative organisms, thus producing a broad gram-negative spectrum, including *E. coli*, *Enterobacter*, *Klebsiella*, and many *Pseudomonas* species, but spares the gram-positives. It appears not to produce allergic reactions in penicillin-allergic patients. It is excreted primarily by the kidney, and doses need modification in renal failure. When it is used with clindamycin, one can provide broad gram-negative, gram-positive, and anaerobic coverage in a penicillin-allergic patient.

Imipenem

Imipenem is a carbapenem, similar to the penicillins in composition but stereochemically different. It has truly broad-spectrum activity, being effective against staphylococci, streptococci, enterococci, anaerobes, and most gram-negatives, including *Pseudomonas aeruginosa*. It is largely excreted by the kidneys, and doses must be modified in renal failure. Cross-reactions in penicillin-allergic patients may occur, and seizures may occur at higher doses (4 g daily) and/or in the presence of renal insufficiency. It can be used effectively as a single agent in mixed infections, especially where anaerobes are present.

Other Antibiotics

Clindamycin

Clindamycin is active against most gram-positive organisms, including streptococci, staphylococci, many clostridia, and some enterococci. It is effective against most anaerobes but not against gram-negatives. It is bactericidal, although more slowly than the penicillins. It is cleared by the liver, and doses are unchanged in renal failure. The principal serious side effect, pseudomembranous colitis, is relatively uncommon when given parenterally but may occur.

Trimethoprim-sulfa

Trimethoprim is combined in a ratio of 1:5 with sulfamethoxazole, a long-acting sulfonamide. These two drugs block sequential steps in the synthesis of folic acid, a precursor of DNA. The fixed combination has activity against most gram-positive aerobic organisms, with enterococci being variably sensitive. Most gram-negatives, except *Pseudomonas aeruginosa,* are sensitive, although resistance may be present in institutions where the drug is frequently used. Anaerobes are resistant. The drug is bactericidal. The most frequent side effects are allergic in nature, with rashes and fever being the most common. Leukopenia, thrombocytopenia, and hemolysis occur less commonly.

Metronidazole

Metronidazole is very active against anaerobes and is bactericidal against virtually all *Bacteroides* species and gram-positive and gram-negative anaerobic cocci as well as clostridia. Resistance seldom develops. It is metabolized by the liver and has a half-life of about 8 hours. Dosing every 8 to 12 hours is adequate. Larger doses may produce dizziness, tingling, other central nervous system symptoms (including seizures), nausea, and in time a peripheral neuropathy. Coingestion of alcohol may cause a disulfiram (Antabuse)-like reaction.

Aminoglycosides

The aminoglycosides gentamicin, tobramycin, and amikacin are all effective against a broad range of gram-negative organisms, including *Pseudomonas aeruginosa,* but are not effective against gram-positives or anaerobes. They all exhibit significant renal toxicity and ototoxicity, and with the recent availability of safer broad-spectrum agents, there is less need for these agents. They are generally now reserved for special situations such as the neutropenic patient or the patient who has highly resistant flora.

Quinolones

This relatively new class of drugs acts by inhibiting DNA synthesis and is bactericidal. The prototype drug was nalidixic acid, but the newer ones, norfloxacin, ofloxacin, and ciprofloxacin represent a new generation with more activity and broader spectrum. Ciprofloxacin as an oral agent is better absorbed than norfloxacin and is better suited for systemic infections. A parenteral form of ciprofloxacin has just been made available. These drugs are very broad spectrum and cover staphylococci, streptococci (including enterococci), and most gram-negatives, including most *Pseudomonas aeruginosa* organisms. Anaerobes are not affected, however. Oral ciprofloxacin has been shown to be effective in treating osteomyelitis and soft-tissue infections (see page 21–9), although the newly released parenteral form will allow more latitude in that context. Side effects are relatively light and include gastrointestinal problems, mild central nervous system effects (rarely severe with psychosis and seizures), and skin eruptions, including some sun sensitivity.

REFERENCES

1. Alvarez S, McCabe WR: Extrapulmonary tuberculosis revisited: a review of the experience at Boston City and other hospitals, *Medicine (Baltimore)* 63:25, 1984.
2. Anderson RB, Foster MD, Gould JS, et al: Free tissue transfer and calcanectomy as treatment of chronic osteomyelitis of the os calcis: a case report, *Foot Ankle* 11:168–71, 1990.
3. Bamberger DM, Gaus GP, Gerding DM: Osteomyelitis in the feet in the diabetic patients. Long term results, prognostic factors, and the role of antimicrobial and surgical therapy, *Am J Med* 83:653, 1987.
4. Beltran J, Campanini S, Knight C, et al: The diabetic-foot: magnetic resonance imaging evaluation, *Skeletal Radiol* 19:37, 1990.
5. Bisla RJ, Taber TH: Coccidioidomycosis of bone and joints, *Clin Orthop* 121:196, 1976.
6. Boulware DW, Lopez M, Gum OB: Tuberculous podagra, *J Rheumatol* 12:1022, 1985.
7. Broy SB, Schmid FR: A comparison of medical drainage (needle aspiration) and surgical drainage (arthrotomy or arthroscopy) in the initial treatment of infected joints, *Clin Rheumatol Dis* 12:501, 1986.
8. Chisholm CD: Plantar puncture wounds: controversies and treatment recommendations, *Ann Emerg Med* 18:1352, 1989.
9. Chleboun J, Nade S: Skeletal cryptococcosis, *J Bone Joint Surg [Am]* 59:509, 1977.
10. Colver GB, Chattopadhyay B, Francis RS, et al: Arthritis of the subtalar joint due to *Mycobacterium fortuitum, Br Med J* 283:468, 1981.
11. Espinoza L, editor: *Infection in the rheumatic diseases,* Orlando, Fla, 1988, Grune & Stratton, pp 173–213.
12. Fitzgerald RH, Cowan JDE: Puncture wounds of the foot, *Orthop Clin North Am* 6:965, 1975.
13. Freund KG: Hematogenous osteomyelitis of the first metatarsal sesamoid: a case report and review of the literature, *Arch Orthop Trauma Surg* 108:53, 1989.
14. Gentry LO: Antibiotic therapy for osteomyelitis, *Infect Dis Clin North Am* 4:485, 1990.
15. Gentry LO, Rodriguez GC: Oral ciprofloxacin compared with parenteral antibiotics in the treatment of osteomyelitis, *Antimicrob Agents Chemother* 34:40, 1990.
16. Goldenberg DL, Brandt KD, Cohen AS, et al: Treatment of septic arthritis: Comparison of needle aspiration

and surgery as initial modes of joint drainage, *Arthritis Rheu* 18:83, 1975.
17. Goldenberg DL, Cohen AS: Arthritis due to gram-negative bacilli, *Clin Rheumatol Dis* 4:197, 1978.
18. Goldenberg DL, Cohen AS: Arthritis due to tuberculous and fungal microorganisms, *Clin Rheumatol Dis* 4:211, 1978.
19. Goldenberg DL, Reed JI: Bacterial arthritis, *N Engl J Med* 312:764, 1985.
20. Govender S, Ganpath V, Charles RW, et al: Localized osseus cryptococcal infection: report of 2 cases, *Acta Orthop Scand* 59:720, 1988.
21. Green NE, Bruno J: *Pseudomonas* infections of the foot after puncture wound, *South Med J* 73:146, 1980.
22. Greenberg RN, Kennedy DJ, Reilly PM, et al: Treatment of bone, joint, and soft tissue infections with oral ciprofloxacin, *Antimicrob Agents Chemother* 31:151, 1987.
23. Gupta NC, Prezio JA: Radionuclide imaging in osteomyelitis, *Semin Nucl Med* 4:287, 1988.
24. Hessen MT, Ingerman MJ, Kaufman DH, et al: Clinical efficacy of ciprofloxacin therapy for gram-negative bacillary osteomyelitis, *Am J Med* 82(suppl 4A):262, 1987.
25. Holmes KK, Counts GW, Beaty HN: Disseminated gonococcal infection, *Ann Intern Med* 74:979, 1968.
26. Jackson RW, Parsons CJ: Distension-irrigation treatment of major joint sepsis, *Clin Orthop* 96:160, 1973.
27. Jarvis WR, Banko S, Snyder E, et al: *Pasturella multocida:* osteomyelitis following dog bites, *Am J Dis Child* 135:625, 1981.
28. Keenan AM, Tindel NL, Alavi A: Diagnosis of pedal osteomyelitis in diabetic patients using current scintigraphic techniques, *Arch Intern Med* 149:2262, 1989.
29. Kelley PJ: Bacterial arthritis in the adult, *Orthop Clin North Am* 6:973, 1975.
30. Lipsky BA, Pecoraro RE, Wheat LJ: The diabetic foot: soft tissue and bone infection, *Infect Dis Clin North Am* 4:409, 1990.
31. Loeffler RD, Ballard A: Plantar fascial spaces of the foot and a proposed surgical approach, *Foot Ankle* 1:11–14, 1980.
32. Koster FT, Galgiani JN: Coccidioidal arthritis. In Espinoza L, editor: *Infections in the rheumatic diseases,* Orlando, Fla, 1988, Grune & Stratton, p 165.
33. Lawson JP, Steere AC: Lyme arthritis: radiologic findings, *Radiology* 154:37, 1985.
34. Mackowiak PA, Jones SR, Smith JW: Diagnostic value of sinus tract cultures in chronic osteomyelitis, *JAMA,* 239:2772, 1978.
35. Mahgoub ES: Medical management of mycetoma, *Bull World Health Organ* 54:303, 1976.
36. Marcy SM: Infections due to dog and cat bites, *Pediatr Infect Dis* 1:351, 1982.
37. McCarthy K, Velchik AA, Mandell GA, et al: Indium-111 labeled white blood cells in the detection of osteomyelitis complicated by a pre-existing condition, *J Nucl Med* 29:1015, 1988.
38. McGinnis MR, Fader RC: Mycetoma: a contemporary concept, *Infect Dis Clin North Am* 2:939, 1988.
39. Nelson JD: Antibiotic concentrations in septic joint effusions, *N Engl J Med* 284:349, 1971.
40. Norden CW: Osteomyelitis. In Mandell GL, Douglas RG, Bennett JE, editors: *Principles and practice of infectious diseases,* ed 3, New York, 1990, Churchill Livingstone, p 929.
41. Patzakis MJ, Wilkins J, Brien WW, et al: Wound site as a predictor of complications following deep nail punctures to the foot, *West J Med* 150:545, 1989.
42. Riegler HF, Routson GW: Complications of deep puncture wounds of the foot, *J Trauma* 19:18, 1979.
43. Rosenthal J, Bole GG, Robinson WD: Acute nongonococcal infectious arthritis. Evaluation of risk factors, therapy, and outcome, *Arthritis Rheum* 23:889, 1980.
44. Rosenthal L, Kloiber R, Damtew B, et al: Sequential use of radiophosphate and radiogallium imaging in the differential diagnosis of bone, joint, and soft tissue infection: quantitative analysis, *Diagn Imaging* 51:249, 1982.
45. Sapico FL, Witte JL, Canawati HN, et al: The infected foot of the diabetic patient: quantitative microbiology and analysis of clinical features, *Rev Infect Dis* 6(suppl 1):171–176, 1984.
46. Schauwecker DS, Braunstein EM, Wheat LJ: Diagnostic imaging of osteomyelitis, *Infect Dis Clin North Am* 4:441, 1990.
47. Scott RJ, Christofersen MR, Robertson WW, et al: Acute osteomyelitis in children, a review of 116 cases, *J Pediatr Orthop* 10:649, 1990.
48. Segall GM, Nino-Murcia M, Jacobs T, et al: the role of bone scan and radiography in the diagnostic evaluation of suspected pedal osteomyelitis, *Clin Nucl Med* 14:255, 1989.
49. Skevis XA: Primary subacute osteomyelitis of the talus, *J Bone Joint Surg [Br]* 66:101, 1984.
50. Somerville EW, Wilkinson MC: *Girdlestone's tuberculosis of bone and joints,* revised, ed 3, London, 1965, Oxford University Press.
51. Steere AC, Schoen RT, Taylor E: The clinical evolution of Lyme arthritis, *Ann Intern Med* 107:725, 1987.
52. Unger E, Moldofsky P, Gatenby R, et al: Diagnosis of osteomyelitis by MR imaging, *AJR* 150:605, 1987.
53. Valdazo J, Perez-Ruiz F, Albarracin A, et al: Tuberculous arthritis. Report of a case with multiple joint involvement and periarticular tuberculosis, *J Rheumatol* 17:399, 1990.
54. Verdile VP, Freed HA, Gerard J: Puncture wounds to the foot, *J Emerg Med* 7:193, 1989.
55. Wagner FW Jr: The diabetic foot and amputations of the foot. In Mann RA, editor: *Mann's surgery of the foot,* St Louis, 1986, Mosby–Year Book, pp 422–423.
56. Wang A, Weinstein D, Greenfield L, et al: MRI and diabetic foot infections, *Magn Reson Imaging* 8:805, 1990.
57. Weinstein MP, Stratton CW, Hawley HB, et al: Multicenter collaborative evaluation of a standardized serum bactericidal test as a predictor of therapeutic efficacy in acute and chronic osteomyelitis, *Am J Med* 83:218, 1987.
58. Wheat J: Diagnostic strategies in osteomyelitis, *Am J Med* 78:218, 1985.
59. Wheat LJ, Allen SD, Henry M, et al: Diabetic foot infections, bacteriologic analysis, *Arch Intern Med* 146:1935, 1986.
60. Yangco BG, Espinoza CG, Germain BF: Nontuberculous mycobacterial joint infections. In Espinoza L, editor: *Infections in the rheumatic diseases,* Orlando, Fla, 1988, Grune & Stratton.
61. Yuh WTC, Corson JD, Baraniewski HM, et al: Osteomyelitis of the foot in diabetic patients. Evaluation with plain film, ^{99m}Tc-MDP bone scintigraphy, and MR imaging, *AJR* 152:795, 1989.

CHAPTER

22

The Diabetic Foot

James W. Brodsky, M.D.

Background and history
Pathophysiology
Neuropathy
Angiopathy
Metabolic control
Nutrition
Limited joint mobility syndrome
Diagnosis
Physical examination
Neurologic evaluation
Vascular evaluation
Imaging of the diabetic foot
Radiographs
Bone scans and MRI
Computed tomography
Gallium scans
Classification systems
Clinical problems and their treatment
Ulcers
The total-contact cast
Wound care
Nonhealing ulcers
Surgery for chronic and recurrent ulceration
Infections in the diabetic foot
Microbiology
Antibiotic regimens and selections
Gas in the soft tissue
Surgical principles in the treatment of diabetic foot infections
Cellulitis
Abscess
Osteomyelitis
Wound closure and foot reconstruction: principles
Charcot joints
Pathophysiology
Epidemiology
Clinical signs and symptoms of Charcot joints of the foot and ankle
Imaging and diagnosis of the Charcot foot
Anatomic classification of Charcot joints
Treatment techniques of the Charcot joint
Complications of Charcot joints of the foot and ankle
Surgical techniques in the Charcot foot
Skin and nail problems
Shoe wear and shoe insoles
Shoe wear
Shoe insoles
Nomenclature
The Team Approach

BACKGROUND AND HISTORY

Diabetes mellitus was described in the medical writings of the fifth century B.C. Greece; indeed, the name itself is Greek (*dia* = through, *banein* = to run, *mellitos* = honey). It was diagnosed by the sweet taste of the sufferer's urine, the patient's excessive thirst, and the agony of his inevitable death.[75] Although the method of diagnosis was slightly less crude at the beginning of this century, little else changed in the natural history or course of this disease for 2,500 years. Only with the discovery of insulin by Banting and Best in 1922 did the modern era of diabetes as a chronic disease begin, and only in the intervening 70 years since that landmark discovery has medicine learned of the myriad multisystemic complications by which this protean disease is now well known.

The American Diabetes Association currently estimates that the number of diabetics in the United States is approximately 14 million and is rising as our population's average age increases, since the incidence of diabetes increases with age.[33]

At least half of these diabetics are estimated to be undiagnosed. Foot problems, especially infections of the feet, are the most common problem necessitating hospital admission, and it is estimated that 25% of all diabetics' hospital admissions are for pathologic conditions of the feet.

Far from being an esoteric problem, the diabetic foot and its complications will be encountered by almost every orthopaedic surgeon because of its prevalence in the same population that, for example, requires total joint replacement. The complications of diabetes affect such "ordinary" orthopaedic problems as fractures of the foot and ankle. Figure 22–1,A depicts such a case of a 43-year-old diabetic lady who slipped and fell on a terrazzo floor in her home and sustained a nondisplaced bimalleolar fracture. The fracture was treated with cast immobilization of a duration that is usually appropriate to such an injury. One month following cast removal, the patient sustained the disastrous changes depicted in Figure 22–1,B and C in the process of ordinary walking. Because of the patient's undetected or, at least, unrecognized diabetic peripheral neuropathy, this seemingly simple fracture progressed to complete destruction of the ankle joint and Charcot joints of the rest of the hindfoot and midfoot as well, as shown in Figure 22–1,D and E. The enigmatic delay in healing of the diabetic extremity converted an ordinary orthopaedic lesion into an extraordinary one.

There is a major increase in the incidence of diabetes in people over the age of 40 years, with an estimated 15% of the population over the age of 65 years being affected. The cost in morbidity, mortality, and time lost from work and family is enormous, just in human terms. But the economic impact of diabetic foot problems and their sequelae on our health care system is mammoth in degree.

Greater than half of all nontraumatic amputations are done in diabetics, and diabetics have a higher risk of developing peripheral vascular disease, of having gangrene in an extremity, or of requiring a major amputation, and each of these carries a higher mortality rate than in nondiabetics. The risk of peripheral vascular disease increases with the duration of the diabetes.[75] The pathways to amputation are varied because of the multiplicity of pathologic changes that affect the diabetic lower extremity. One study identified 23 unique pathways to amputation, 22 of which were multifactorial, including ulceration (in 84%), neuropathy (in 64%), infection (in 59%), gangrene (in 55%), and ischemia (in 46%).[83] The incidence of pathologic changes in the foot is high and often precedes the onset of clinical problems or crises. A review of diabetic patients in a medical clinic showed a 68% incidence of some form of foot pathology: most were mild and showed early changes such as callus formation (51%) and hammer toes (32%), some were more apparent as sources of eventual injury and pathology such as sensory (34%) and autonomic (25%) neuropathy, but all represent the early requisites that can lead to later problems of ulceration and infection.[50]

The severity of the complications of diabetes in the foot is not necessarily related to the severity of the disease itself. The majority of complications occur in patients with milder forms of the disease, i.e., the non–insulin-dependent (type II) diabetics, who account for the large majority of the diabetic population. Despite all of the advances in the field of diabetic foot care including better control of hyperglycemia, the discovery of a multitude of new antibiotics, advanced techniques for vascular reconstruction, both surgical and nonsurgical, dissemination of knowledge on the relief of pressure to treat ulcerations, and new diagnostic modalities for evaluating tissue oxygenation in the extremities, the treatment of problems of the diabetic foot remain obscure if not puzzling to many physicians and surgeons. The chronicity of the disease, the occasional paradox of gangrene in the presence of palpable pulses, and the seeming indifference of the patient who is unable to be aware of impending disaster in a body part that he or she cannot feel and therefore does not recognize as "self" all contribute to the aura of mystery and defeat that have surrounded this subject for many years.

The effect of the diabetes, which is a multisystem disease crossing the boundaries of orthopaedic surgery, vascular surgery, endocrinology, neurology, infectious diseases, physical medicine and rehabilitation, orthotics, prosthetics, and other fields, is that it is difficult for any single practitioner in any one field to feel that he can manage the problem alone; it is aptly likened to the proverbial blind men feeling the different parts of the elephant. Since there is not yet a cure for diabetic neuropathy or for the disease itself, treatment efforts must be directed to managing, retarding, and it is hoped, preventing the complications of diabetes. An understanding of the pathophysiology of diabetic foot problems is an essential first step.

PATHOPHYSIOLOGY

Neuropathy

It is a common misconception that impaired circulation is the primary cause of diabetic foot problems. Quite the contrary, neuropathy, especially sensory neuropathy, is the preeminent source or initiating event of almost all ulcerations and most infections (Fig 22–2). Peripheral vascular disease often coexists with neuropathy and contributes to poor or delayed healing, but it is not the initiating event. Vascular insufficiency causes tissue ischemia and can produce gangrene, prevent healing due to marginal nutrition of tissue, or even cause

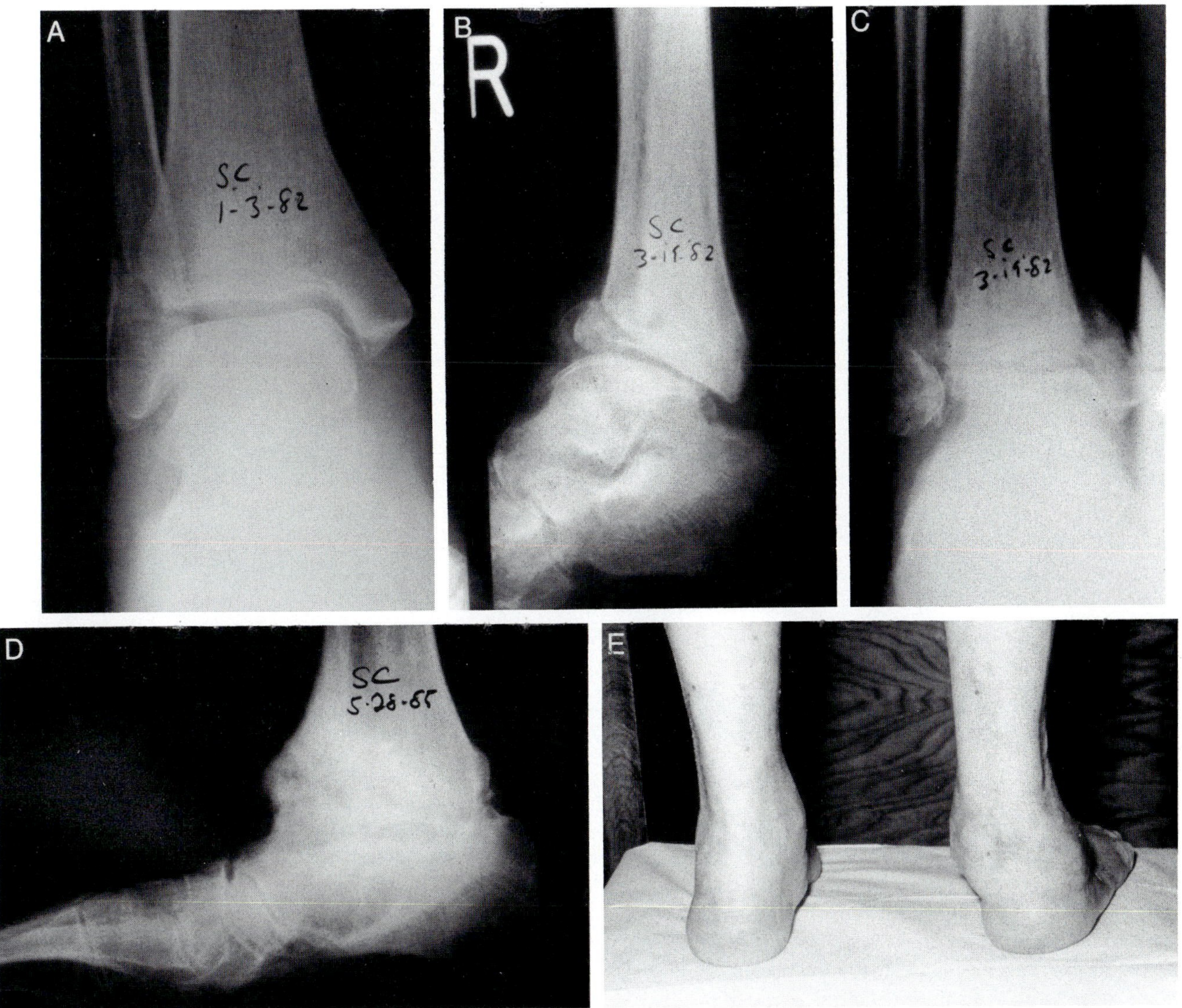

FIG 22–1.
A, nondisplaced bimalleolar fracture in adult-onset, non–insulin-dependent diabetes. **B** and **C,** sudden, subsequent displacement 3 months later in the absence of additional trauma. **D** and **E,** eventual severe Charcot changes of the ankle joint with valgus deformity and secondary collapse of the foot 3 years later.

ischemic pain. But the loss of protective sensation combined with acute trauma, recurrent trauma, repetitive trauma, or even microtrauma leads to most instances of breakdown in the diabetic foot.[3, 11, 31, 65] It is the absence of this basic protective mechanism that makes problems of the diabetic foot unique in their difficulty and frustrating for both the patient and physician. Almost every other problem for which the patient seeks medical care, especially orthopaedic consultation, is motivated by a chief complaint of pain or some related symptom. In contrast, the diabetic with peripheral neuropathy and, for example, a draining ulcer of the great toe, must somehow become aware or know that he or she should seek immediate medical attention because she has *no* pain. Neglect of the foot by the diabetic is not obstinate or willful but is caused by an absent or impaired sensory input that makes him or her unaware of the situation. This would be a problem for any of us because we are attuned only to things of which we can be aware, and we are only aware of things that we can *sense.* If one were asked "how do you know it is so?," the answer is always based on one's senses: "I saw it, I heard it, I felt it, I smelled it," etc. This gives rise to the usually unjustified stereotype of the diabetic patient as uncompliant, inattentive, and uncooperative, when in reality, the patient has not been adequately taught

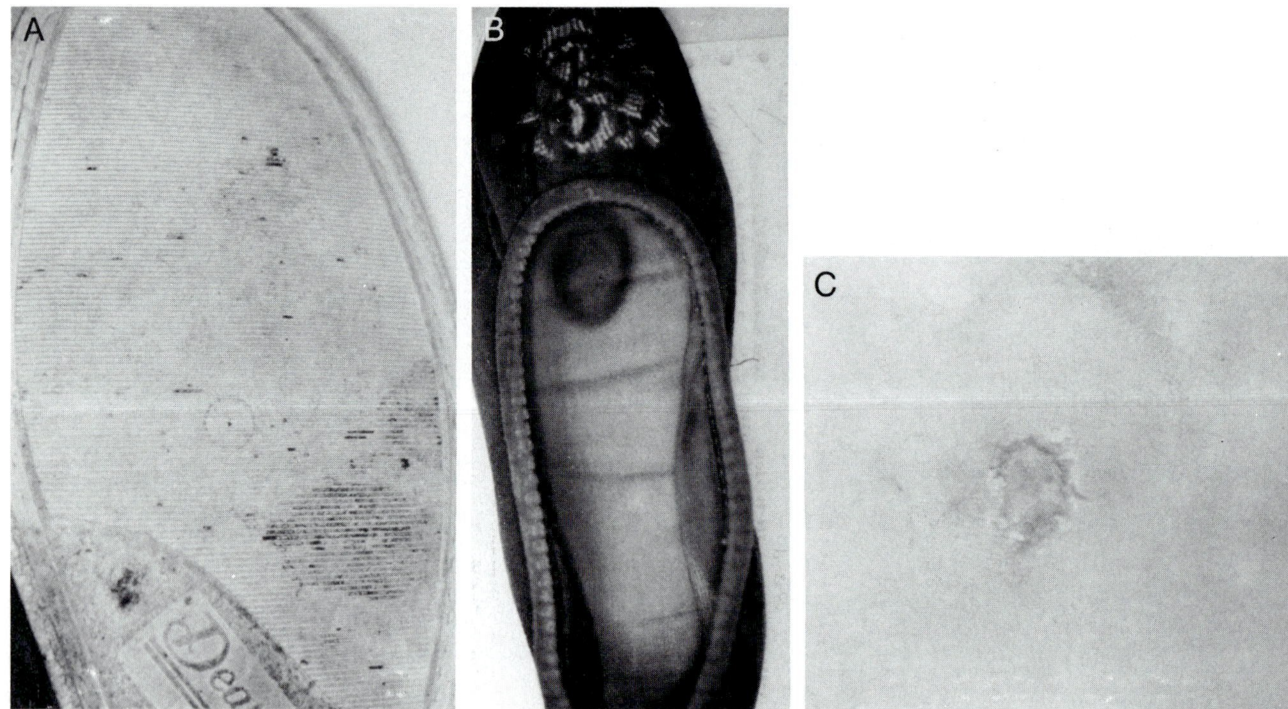

FIG 22–2.
A, insensitivity allows this patient to walk on a tack that protruded through the slipper and into her foot: the outline of the tack is seen on the sole of the shoe. **B,** the drainage from her ulcer is seen on the inside. **C,** the corresponding ulcer.

how to substitute vision (daily inspection) or the help of a family member for the absent or impaired sensation in the feet.

The exact etiology of diabetic neuropathy remains somewhat elusive; however, autopsy studies have indicated that changes in the *vaso nervorum* with resulting ischemia to the nerves are the major pathway. There are two theories regarding these microvascular changes in the nerves: one postulates the accumulation of sorbitol, and the other supposes intraneural accretion of advanced products of glycosylation. The only current possible treatment involves enzymatic blocking of the biochemical path toward sorbitol, but the efficacy of this treatment remains unproven.[2] For all practical purposes, at this time neuropathy remains an irreversible condition that tends to gradually and somewhat relentlessly progress and that lies at the heart of most foot pathology in the diabetic.

Sensory neuropathy alone does not cause breakdown but acts in combination with pressure. All neurotrophic ulceration is caused by these two factors combined. Brand elegantly demonstrated with animal models that repetitive trauma produces tissue inflammation that can then progress to tissue necrosis, even in the absence of ischemia.[13] The inflammation was confirmed histologically, as was the necrosis. This is mechanical breakdown of the tissue; repetitive trauma, which is not excessive for a given repetition but abnormal in the number of repetitions permitted (by abnormal sensation), causes tissue breakdown by eventually exceeding the threshold of soft-tissue tolerance.

Plantar ulcerations are caused by this type of repetitive trauma that occurs with standing and especially with walking. The animal models by Brand explain the cumulative effect of this repetitive trauma on the soft tissue.[13] Plantar ulcerations *almost always* correspond to areas of underlying bony prominence in the foot, which explains why most ulcers occur under the metatarsal heads, the medial sesamoid, and the base of the fifth metatarsal; over the proximal interphalangeal joint of clawtoes; etc (Figure 22–3). The orthopaedic surgeon must keep in mind this principle: whenever plantar ulceration occurs in the diabetic, it is the result of abnormal sensation together with underlying bony prominences that produce pressure. Therefore, the vast majority of both treatments for the diabetic foot as well as preventive interventions for the diabetic foot are for the purpose of relieving the pressure (since neuropathy cannot be changed). This formula (pressure + neuropathy = tissue breakdown) also represents the source of

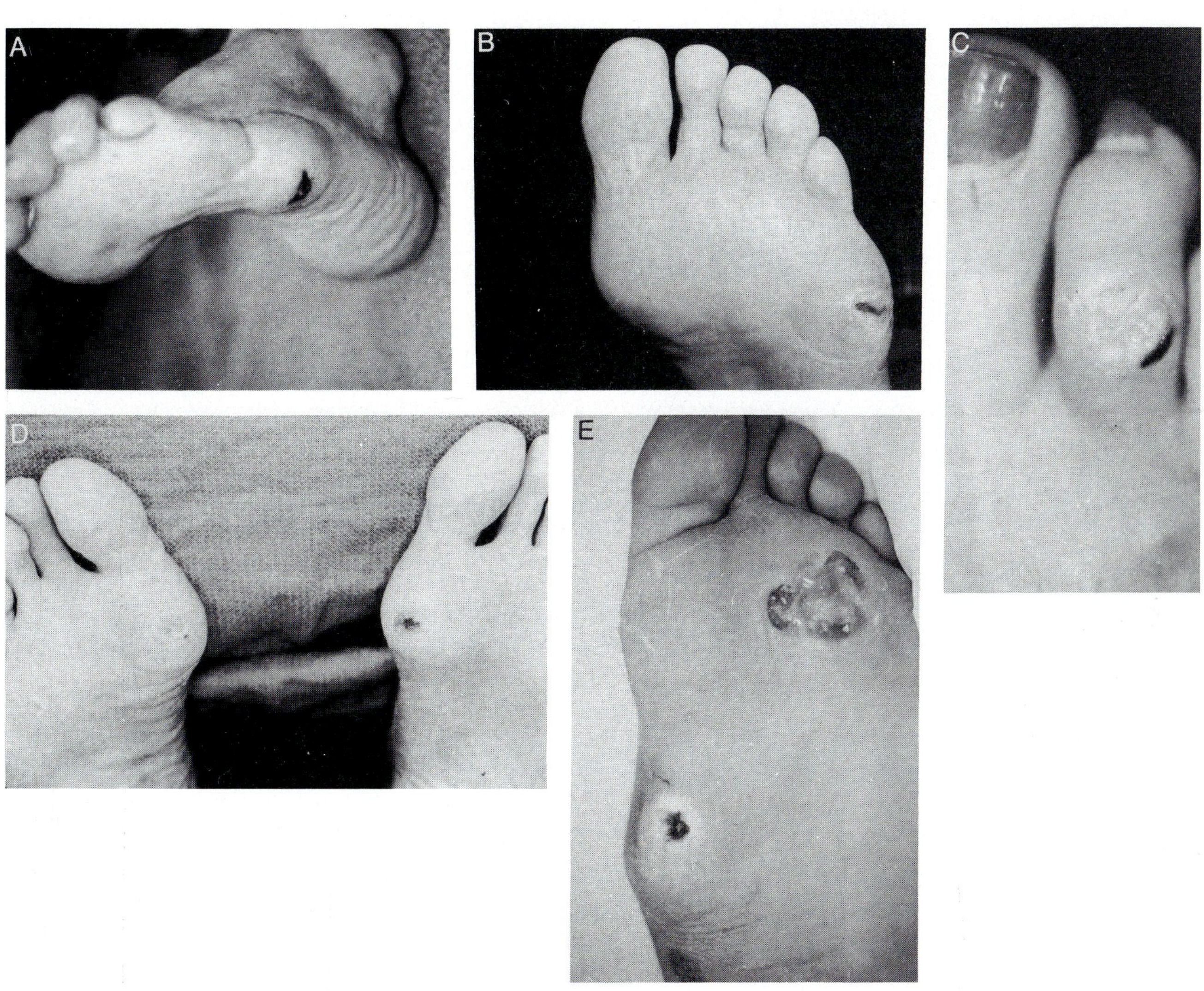

FIG 22–3.
Examples of pressure ulceration at various locations on bony prominences. **A,** fifth metatarsal base. **B,** fifth metatarsal head. **C,** dorsum of the proximal interphalangeal joint of a hammer toe. **D,** medial sesamoid/first metatarsal head. **E,** exostosis of a midfoot (type 1) Charcot joint, as well as intermediate metatarsal heads.

most diabetic foot infections since they begin with a break in the soft tissue produced by pressure combined with neuropathy.

In contrast to the plantar ulcerations caused by *intermittent* pressure, the ulcerations on the dorsum and medial and lateral sides of the foot are usually caused by *constant* pressure exerted by a shoe. This can produce an ulcer even more quickly, often within 1 hour of wearing a poorly fitting shoe. The surgeon must correctly recognize this as the cause of ulcers such as the one depicted in Figure 22–4 in order to address the issue of shoe wear. Once a break in the skin occurs, whether plantar or dorsal on the foot, the protective barrier of the dermis has been breached, and a portal for infection has been opened. The underlying insensitivity fosters and encourages the incipient infection. Not only is the patient only vaguely aware of the problem, if at all, but in the absence of the appropriate amount of pain, he or she continues to walk, and the continuing action of the muscles and motion of tendons in the foot and ankle can advance the infection proximally. In a person with normal sensation, the pain of the lesion would discourage such activity, and the normal splinting produced by inactivity would curtail such rampant advancement of the infection. The diabetic foot, like problems of spina bifida, is in striking contrast to most orthopaedic conditions because it illustrates the protective nature of pain. Recent advances in optically based[8, 9, 36, 41] and elec-

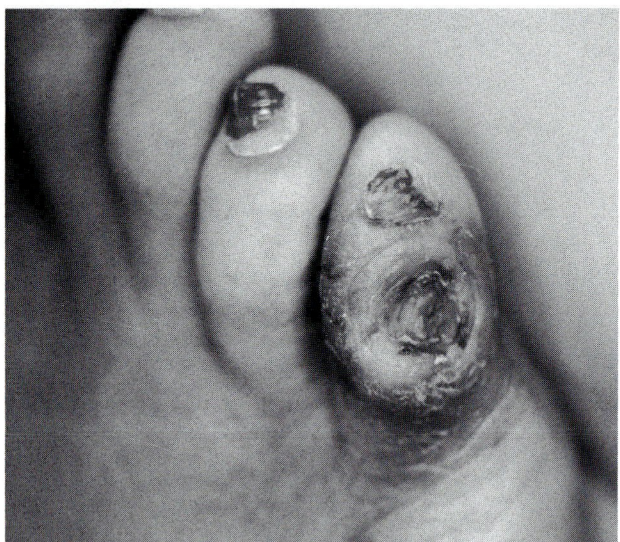

FIG 22–4.
Ulceration over the dorsolateral aspect of the fifth toe due to the pressure of a shoe.

tronically based[23] pressure measurement systems have opened a new frontier of information on the abnormal pressures under the diabetic foot that have been postulated for so long but could not be measured or quantified prior to these developments. One such study[8] utilized the optical pedobarograph to examine patients with neuropathy for abnormal plantar pressures, defined as pressures greater than 10 kg/cm.[2] The same patients, when examined 3 years later, showed that some of these pressure areas resolved while new ones appeared in others; 5 of 6 patients in the group of 39 who developed ulcers developed them in the areas identified previously as locations for abnormal pressure. Even more fascinating was a study by the same group[8] in which 14 patients in a group of 44 patients thought clinically not to have neuropathy were discovered to have abnormal plantar pressures. When tested for vibratory sensation and sensory nerve conduction, these patients showed significantly decreased function, which suggests that the pathologic pressures that lead to ulceration may occur in conjunction with neuropathy, but at a point before the neuropathy itself is apparent. A study comparing diabetic patients who have a history of ulcerations with diabetic controls without such a history revealed that both the severity of neuropathy and the peak pressures under the foot were greater in the group who had ulcerated.[97] Objective scientific methods have now corroborated the assertions that ulcerations are the result of a combination of pressure and neuropathy, such as the study comparing plantar pressures in a group of diabetics and a group of patients with rheumatoid arthritis. Each had abnormal pressures under the foot in about the same degree and incidence, but only the diabetics had plantar ulceration corresponding to the presence of neuropathy, whereas ulceration did not occur in the patients with arthritis.[73]

Much remains to be learned about these plantar pressures, as well as the new methods of investigating the pressures themselves, including the limitations and pitfalls of the methods. One study pointed out that there is a difference between static (standing) and dynamic (walking) pressures and that each identified some areas of increased pressure missed by the other in a program meant to prevent ulceration.[36] Cavanagh and Ulbrecht nicely summarized the (quickly evolving) state of the art in biomechanical testing methods in the diabetic foot, including some of the technical limitations and problems of the devices themselves.[24] All of the above studies are truly pioneering in nature, and much yet remains to be understood: Why are pressures similar in the two feet of diabetics with only a unilateral history of ulceration?[97] What is the meaning of the overlap in absolute pressure values between patients with and without ulceration?[30]

Although our attention has been focused primarily on sensory neuropathy, it is important to recognize that there are three types of neuropathy: sensory, autonomic, and motor neuropathy. Although the sensory component is the most prominent, all three have some part in the pathophysiology of diabetic foot lesions. Autonomic neuropathy produces a loss of normal sweating in the skin of the foot. This leads to stiff, dry, scaly skin that cracks easily due to its inflexible quality. Cracks in thickened skin and especially in the stiff calluses on the sole propagate into and through the dermis to open pathways for infection (Fig 22–5). Loss of nor-

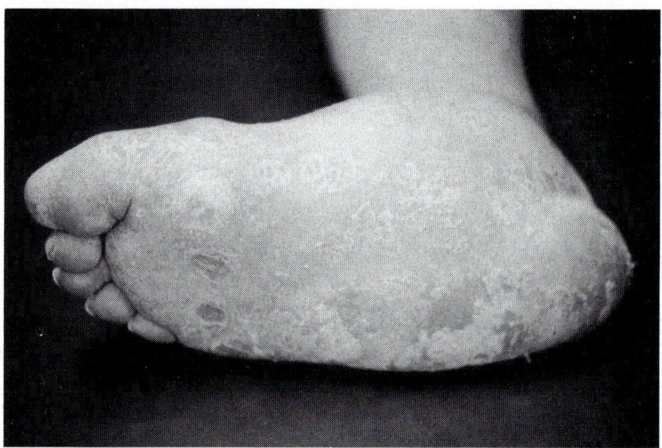

FIG 22–5.
Dry, scaly skin associated with the autonomic component of diabetic peripheral neuropathy.

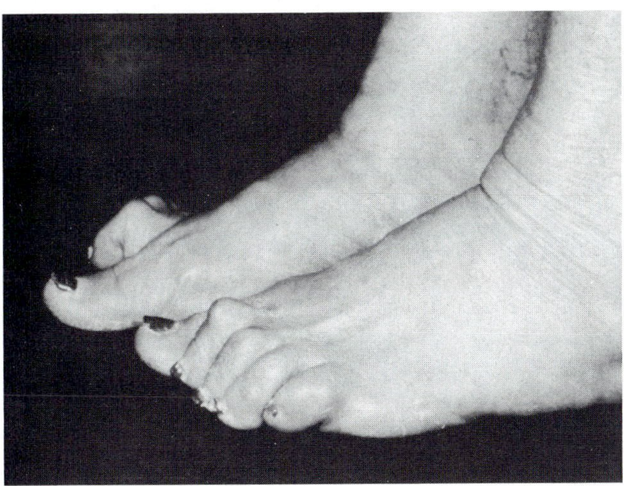

FIG 22–6.
Clawing of the toes associated with the motor component of diabetic peripheral neuropathy. The hyperextended metatarsophalangeal joint increases the pressure under the metatarsal heads, while the flexed proximal interphalangeal joint increases the risk of ulceration on the dorsum of the toes.

mal skin temperature regulation is a result of autonomic neuropathy. A blunted response in diabetic extremities to increased temperature demonstrates this "autosympathectomy" effect and is thought to contribute to infection and injury because of inhibition of the normal reactive hyperemia.[43]

Motor neuropathy is expressed as a loss of function and contracture of the intrinsic muscles of the foot that leads to the classic clawtoe deformities seen in Figure 22–6. These predispose to ulcerations on the dorsum of the digits. The clawtoe deformity contributes to a second area of ulceration as well because it increases pressure beneath the metatarsal head as the pressure of the base of the hyperextended proximal phalanx pushes down on the metatarsal head through its intact but contracted tendons. The decrease in pressure loading of the toes caused by intrinsic paresis has been documented to lead to commensurate increases in pressure under the first metatarsal head.[43] Mononeuropathy, most commonly affecting the peroneal nerve, can produce unilateral or bilateral foot drop, which is often unrecognized until such time as the patient has developed a fixed equinus deformity. This also predisposes to ulceration of the forefoot or the distal end of a partial foot amputation.

Angiopathy

Arteriosclerotic disease is more common and more severe in diabetics than in nondiabetics. It occurs earlier, is more diffuse, affects a higher percentage of women, is more often bilateral, and progresses more aggressively than in the nondiabetic. The calcification of atherosclerotic plaques in nondiabetics is patchy and occurs within the intimal layer of the vessel, while the characteristic calcification in diabetic arteries is circumferential and diffuse and occurs within the media of the arteries. This produces the typical "lead pipe" appearance of calcified arteries that can be seen in large and small vessels alike. It is often visible out to the vessels of the midfoot or even the toes; the orthopaedic surgeon will sometimes be the first to diagnose underlying diabetes based on the suspicion of these changes seen on a plain radiograph taken for a foot complaint. These calcified vessels are noncompliant and brittle. They produce artifactual changes on Doppler pressure measurement and make vascular reconstruction problematic at the time of anastomosis of a saphenous vein bypass graft into this stiff tissue. There is no evidence, however, that calcification *per se* rather than occlusion is directly responsible for decreased perfusion in the foot.[25]

Proximal occlusive vascular disease does occur in diabetics in the aortic, iliac, and femoral vessels, and vascular reconstruction of these proximal lesions is often required to salvage foot lesions. However, the vascular involvement in the distal part of the lower extremity of the diabetic is unusual and different from the nondiabetic because of the diffuse pattern of involvement that occurs below the popliteal artery trifurcation. The widespread, "ragged," multisegmental occlusion of these small arteries usually requires dilatation or bypass procedures down to the level of the ankle. The procedures are done to whichever, if any, of the anterior tibial, posterior tibial or peroneal arteries is patent and has adequate "runoff" at the ankle level. Furthermore, the diabetic limb is unusual because of the common involvement of the major arteries of the foot by the atherosclerotic process, unlike the nondiabetic. Occlusive changes may be variable at different levels of the limb, with significantly diminished toe pressures in a foot that has a reasonable dorsalis pedis or posterior tibial pulse.

Much has been made of the so-called small-vessel disease or microvascular changes of the diabetic foot. However, recent studies call into question the reality of "small-vessel disease" at the subarteriolar level. The occlusive nature of this supposed entity in the absence of large-vessel occlusion remains undocumented and unproven. In addition, there has not been adequate correlation proved between the known changes in capillary permeability and basement membrane thickening in the diabetic foot and the physiologic events of gangrene and infection.[72] Actual measurement of blood flow in diabetics with supposed "small-vessel disease" failed to show a difference when compared with controls with and without peripheral neuropathy from other causes; this led the investigators to conclude that toe lesions were due to changes of neuropathy and that the lesion of "microvascular disease" remains unproven.[14,52]

Metabolic Control

Blood glucose control is well known to be complicated or made more difficult, if not wildly unstable, in the presence of an acute infection. Once the foot abscess has been drained, for example, the patient often returns to his or her normal insulin requirements. The converse relationship may apply to some extent as well because recent studies have suggested that enhanced glucose control may improve healing or decrease the incidence of infection.[85]

Nutrition

Failure of lesions in the foot to heal (and successfully heal for that matter) is usually multifactorial, which is what makes it so difficult to evaluate studies whose criterion for successful outcome is simply healing of a lesion, unless the groups have been controlled—not just for the identifiable factors (glucose control, antibiotics, adequate surgical drainage, relief of mechanical pressure, etc.) but also for any *unidentified* factors. Some studies have indicated that one source of poor wound healing is poor nutrition. The surgical literature is replete with work in this area, and the orthopaedic literature has reflected this research in a more limited way. Simple indices of adequate surgical nutrition can be helpful or even predictive of successful wound or amputation healing.[34, 57] The most basic of these include total lymphocyte count, serum albumin, and serum total protein (see Table 22–1).

Limited Joint Mobility Syndrome

Biochemical changes in the periarticular tissues, especially of the small joints, e.g., the hand, have been noted to produce thickened skin, diminished range of motion, and joint contractures in diabetics.[62] Recent studies have demonstrated similar changes producing abnormal joint mechanics in the feet. Subtalar motion has been noted to be decreased in diabetics and to a greater degree in diabetic patients with a previous history of ulceration than in those who have not had foot ulcers.[32] It is not possible to state that this represents a cause-and-effect relationship between joint stiffness and the ulcerations; the two may simply be associated in patients who have more advanced complications of diabetes. There is a suggestion that the limited joint mobility syndrome *per se* leads to increased plantar pressures.[41] No doubt, much more will be learned about these effects of collagen glycosylation and the changes in joint mechanics over the next few years that will be helpful in the prevention of diabetic foot lesions.

TABLE 22–1.
Basic Indices of Surgical Nutrition

Total lymphocyte count: >1,500/µL
Albumin: >3.5 g/dL
Total protein: >6.2 g/dL
Hemoglobin: >11 g/dL; Hematocrit: >32%

DIAGNOSIS

Physical Examination

Orthopaedic physical examination of the diabetic, like all patients with foot complaints, should generally include an evaluation at least up to the level of the knee because this is the basic musculotendinous unit of the foot. Both lower extremities should *always* be examined. Pathology on the less severely affected limb is often overlooked simply from a failure to check both. On initial examination, the patient's gait should usually be observed and note made of abnormalities at the proximal limb and pelvic levels. The shoes should be inspected to observe patterns of wear and to look for and feel for foreign objects or protruding staples or nails, etc.

The examiner should record the palpable examination of the pulses, and the warmth and hair growth of the skin and should examine between the toes. Clinically significant skin and nail abnormalities should be noted, including erythema, edema, and breaks in the skin. Ulcerations should be either measured or preferably, traced out on a clear piece of acetate or unexposed x-ray film and copied onto the chart (Figs 22–7 and 22–8). Bony prominences and structural deformities such as clawtoes, bunions, hindfoot varus, collapse of the longitudinal arch, or gross change in shape of the foot such as is typical of a Charcot joint are important to note. Restriction of range of motion may be important information relative to present or future ulceration.

Sometimes a patient will present with a hot, red, swollen foot that is difficult to diagnose clinically; it may represent cellulitis, an abscess, or an acute and acutely inflamed Charcot joint. The swelling will not quickly recede, but there is a trick that can help to clinically distinguish between the erythema of cellulitis and the dependent rubor of a Charcot joint before resorting to a battery of tests. The dependent rubor of an inflamed Charcot joint will recede after 5 minutes of elevation of the foot higher than the level of the heart with

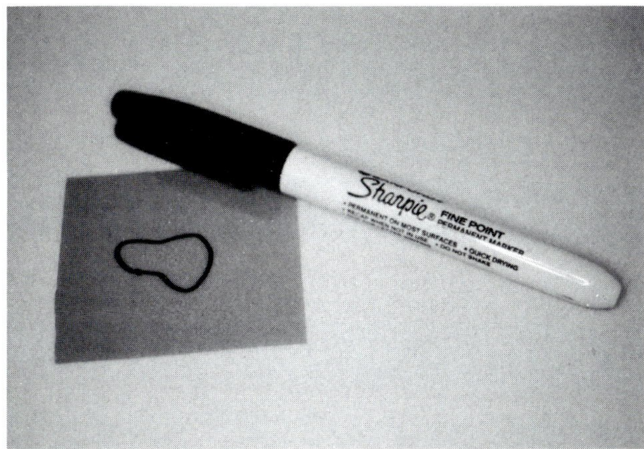

FIG 22–7.
Clear (unexposed and developed) x-ray film and an indelible felt marker used to trace out the patient's ulcer for recording on the chart.

the patient in the supine position, whereas the erythema of cellulitis will not. This is particularly helpful in the case of an early Charcot joint that has produced minimal or no discernible changes on plain radiographs.

Neurologic Evaluation

The effects of sensory, motor, and autonomic neuropathy, including toe deformity and dry, flaking, cracked skin, should be sought. It is reasonable to begin testing with pinprick, light touch, and position sense examinations. However, more reproducible are the objective threshold tests of neurologic function that can be done with monofilaments (Fig 22–9), temperature testing, or vibratory methods using a tuning fork and a biothesiometer. The latter is an electrically powered device that delivers a quantified, reproducible vibratory stimulus, although it is somewhat cumbersome. Studies done in different countries are not comparable if there is a difference in electrical current. (For example, the United Kingdom and the United States have currents with different numbers of cycles per second.)

A comparison of these three threshold methods has demonstrated approximately comparable sensitivity in identifying patients with advanced peripheral neuropathy that might lead to ulceration. However, the use of Semmes-Weinstein monofilaments is more specific and accurate.[98] Most importantly, the monofilaments are easy to use in an everyday clinic situation.

The monofilaments are a modern modification of the von Frey hairs[44, 69] and are supplied in a set of filaments of graduated size in which the amount of pressure applied by each monofilament is calculated, after factoring in the difference in filament thickness, stiffness, and the

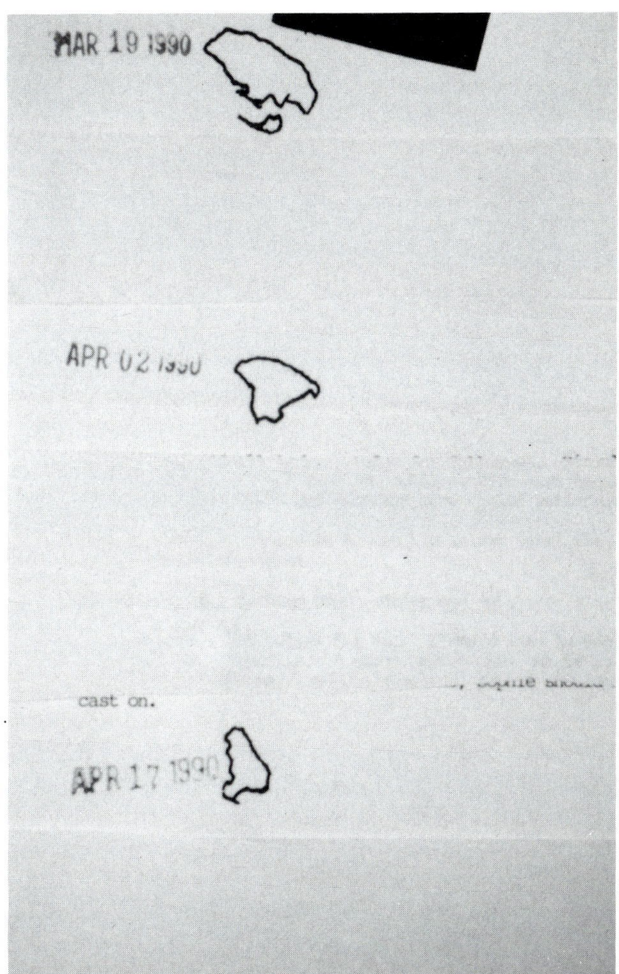

FIG 22–8.
An example of the visual record created on the chart to document the progressive shrinking (healing) of the ulcer.

area at the tip, and then labeled by pressure expressed on a logarithmic scale (see Fig 22–9). They are placed on the skin as perpendicular as possible to the surface, and pressure is applied until the filament begins to buckle slightly. The patient, with eyes closed, is asked to signal when she feels the stimulus. The monofilaments are not without problems: they can be affected by temperature, the amount of pressure applied can vary by large factors if applied obliquely to the skin, and the application of the filament to a callus or thickened rind around an ulcer may interfere with its perception. However, at this time, they are the most economical, most easily used and widely accepted, and generally most reproducible method for threshold neurologic testing of the insensitive foot.

Research on use of the monofilaments continues, but investigators have attempted to determine an absolute value of sensibility that represents the presence or ab-

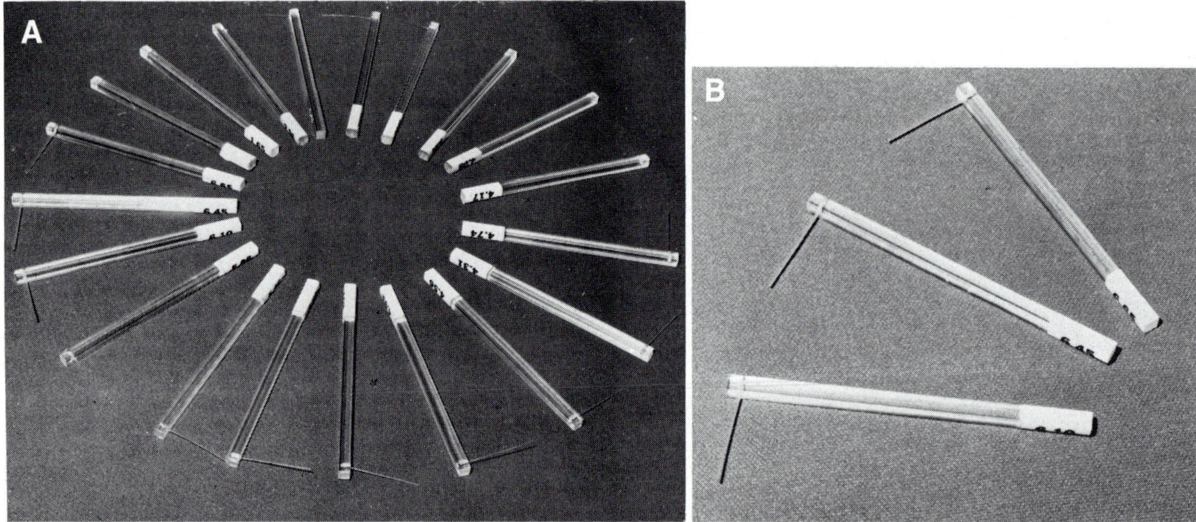

FIG 22–9.
Semmes-Weinstein monofilaments for sensory threshhold testing. The set of graduated filaments is seen from above **(A)** and from the side **(B).**

sence of "protective sensation" in the neuropathic foot. A number of sources have suggested that this is equivalent to the ability to feel the 5.07 monofilament, but this is extrapolated data[6] and has not been adequately tested in multiple centers to this date. Moreover, the monofilaments are still only an approximation, and most researchers in this area note that about 10% of patients who have sensation at the 5.07 level still develop neuropathic changes such as ulceration or a Charcot joint.

It is paradoxical but not uncommon that the diabetic patient with diminished sensibility in the lower extremities can still experience severe pain, and both are manifestations of peripheral neuropathy. The painful neuropathy of diabetes is described variably as a burning, searing, tingling, or lancinating dysesthesia, often unrelenting or excruciating in degree. It is frequently worse at night and is usually bilateral and symmetric. While the treatment of this disorder most often falls to the neurologist or primary-care physician, the orthopaedic surgeon needs to be aware of its source and its characteristic symptoms. The pain is often severe enough to prompt the use of narcotic analgesics, something that should be avoided if at all possible. Treatment is usually with oral medications such as imipramine, amitriptyline (Elavil), phenytoin (Dilantin), and carbamazepine (Tegretol), and all have been reported to have variable rates of success.[39, 56, 64, 77, 88] The drugs must usually be monitored for side effects. Another (new) treatment for painful diabetic peripheral neuropathy is the use of topical creams containing capsaicin, a nonprescription, naturally occurring substance. While these remain to be fully evaluated with regard to efficacy, some patients appear to be achieving relief. The lowest concentration should be used initially since the cream itself can cause a transient burning sensation and it must be continued for at least several days to a week to judge effectiveness.

Foot drop must be investigated to determine its origin, which could include peripheral nerve injury to the peroneal nerve, motor mononeuropathy, a spinal lesion, or other central nervous system abnormality. Treatment of a motor mononeuropathy that causes a foot drop usually requires a polypropylene ankle-foot orthosis (AFO) to hold the foot in neutral dorsiflexion. In the patient with sensory neuropathy, the AFO should be custom-made with additional depth in the foot plate to accommodate a cushioning, molded foot orthosis (Fig 22–10).

Vascular Evaluation

The purpose of vascular evaluation is to determine whether adequate local circulation is present to support primary healing either with or without surgical intervention. Patients without palpable pulses but with nonhealing wounds or ulcers and preoperative patients usually require vascular screening with arterial Doppler ultrasound pressure measurements. While previously published guidelines by Wagner and others[54, 78, 102, 104] have used the Doppler pressures as a criterion for wound and amputation healing, the Doppler measurements are best considered as estimations and screening tests rather than absolute criteria for healing. The Dop-

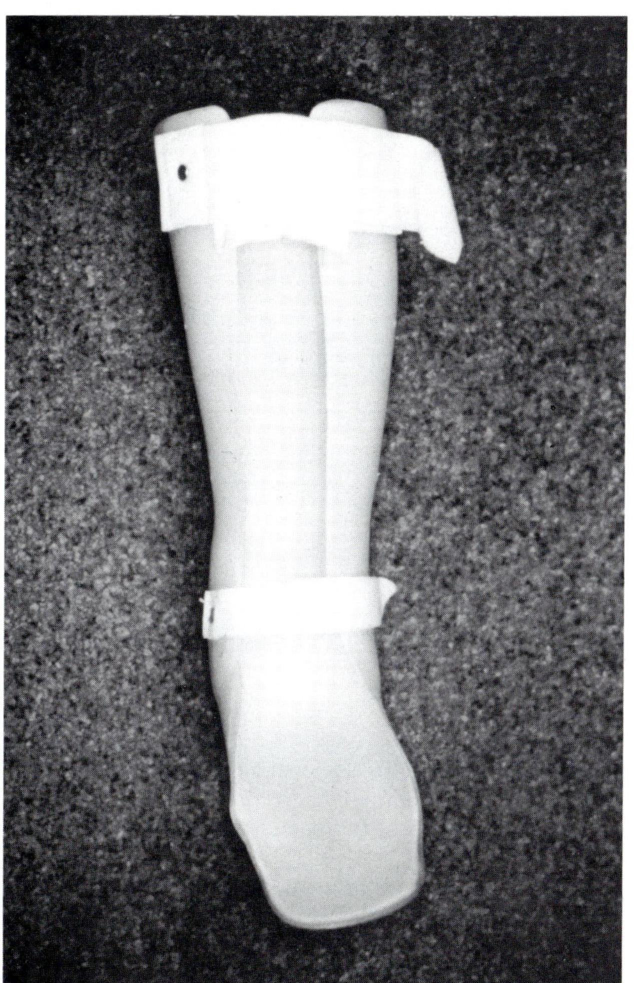

FIG 22–10.
Polypropylene AFO with a molded Plastazote lining.

pler data are expressed as absolute pressures and as the ratio of ankle or foot pressure to arm Doppler arterial pressure, where both are measured by using a pneumatic blood pressure cuff of appropriate size and readings are taken with the Doppler probe rather than a stethoscope. Wagner cites a ratio of 0.45 or greater as necessary to heal diabetic foot lesions and a ratio of 0.35 to heal lesions in the nondiabetic patient with peripheral vascular disease. However, these are only rough guidelines to relative perfusion of the foot and are not absolute measures of healing potential, especially since, as noted above, healing is a multifactorial phenomenon.

When ordering an arterial Doppler study, always specify that it be done bilaterally and include measurement of toe pressures, and copies of the waveforms or pulse-volume tracings should be provided together with the numeric pressure values (Fig 22–11,A).

Doppler arterial readings are subject to a number of potential distortions, the most common and most important one occurring as a result of arterial calcification. This calcification, discussed above, produces stiffening and loss of compliance of the arterial wall. Falsely elevated pressures are then observed because of the increased cuff pressure required to produce vessel occlusion in the process of taking the measurement. The Doppler pressures are intended to assess blood flow but do not directly measure flow itself. Flow is extrapolated by the assumption that greater pressure must be exerted in order to compress a vessel with greater flow. This assumption begins to lose validity as the artery becomes more and more calcified. Pressures are often obtained in the foot and ankle that are paradoxically greater than brachial artery pressures, thus producing a ratio greater than 1.0. Ratios greater than 1.0 are usually an indication of vessel calcification and should serve as a warning to the surgeon that the pressures obtained are falsely elevated. Of course, even pressures less than the arm pressure may still represent falsely elevated values due to calcification.

In this situation it is valuable to refer to the pulse-volume tracings to assess whether or not there is pulsatile flow in the foot and its quality. When the ratios and pressures are distorted by calcified vessels, at the very least, the tracings reveal the presence or absence of pulsatile flow, without which healing is unlikely to occur (see Fig 22–11,B and C).

Absolute pressures have recently been shown to be a more reliable predictor of healing than the more familiar ankle-arm ratios. Using ulcer healing rather than amputation healing as the criterion, Apelqvist et al. found that 85% of patients with toe pressures greater than 45 mm Hg achieved healing while none healed with an ankle pressure less than 40 mm Hg. Lower healing rates were seen in patients with incompressible arteries.[1]

Patients who complain of painful ulcers should be suspected of having severe distal ischemia. The pain of neuropathy should be excluded, but it is vital to remember that neurotrophic ulcers occur as a result of a *lack* of sensation; they are not painful. Another source of the pain must be identified, and most often if not almost always, it is peripheral vascular insufficiency. Similar admonitions are to be made regarding the not uncommon clinical situation of the diabetic patient with neuropathy who complains of an excruciatingly painful ingrown great toenail. Most often, the patient is experiencing rest ischemia, felt most severely at the most distal point in the extremity. The unsuspecting practitioner who trims the nail without first considering vascular

A

Sample Doppler Tracings

Normal Triphasic Pulse-Volume Recordings (Waveforms)

Posterior Tibial Art.

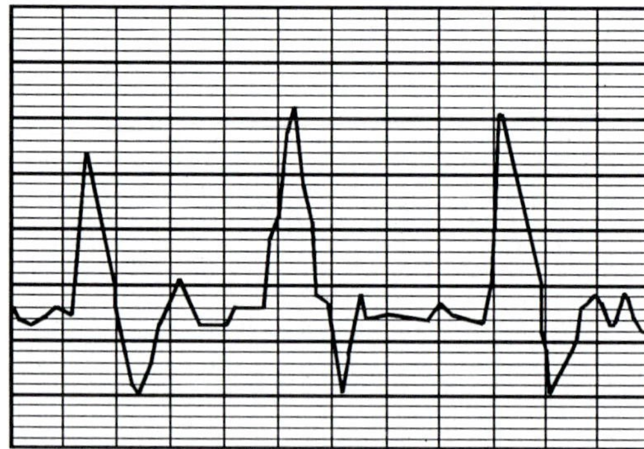

Dorsalis Pedis Art.

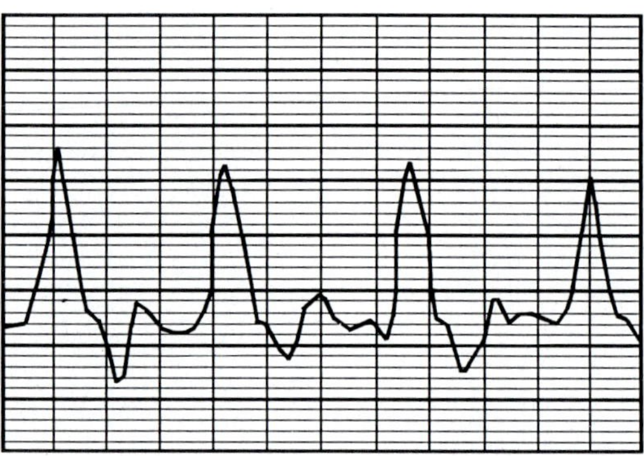

FIG 22–11.
Doppler arterial studies. **A,** normal pulse-volume recording ("waveforms") demonstrating a triphasic flow pattern. **B,** severe proximal and distal arterial occlusion. Toe pressures are unobtainable, and the waveforms demonstrate the absence of a recognizable pattern of pulsatile flow. **C,** diminished but adequate perfusion with greater flow on the left. Pulsatile flow is present; the ankle-arm ratio is greater than 1.0, and this indicates arterial calcification. **D,** distal gangrene of the toe following toenail trimming. (**B** courtesy of Baylor University Vascular Laboratory.)

evaluation may find that a below-knee amputation is required to complete the job. Evaluation, and if, necessary revascularization, should be considered prior to procedures, even a "minor" one, in order to prevent a calamitous outcome (Fig 22–11,D). Once it is determined that the patient has significant vascular impairment of the limb, a vascular surgery consultation is appropriate. The consultant will usually proceed with an arteriogram to determine the full extent of vascular occlusion, its levels, and the possible remedies. At some centers, the invasive radiologist or vascular surgeon can perform procedures to improve flow such as a balloon angioplasty of selected discrete lesions if there is adequate "runoff" distally. Vascular reconstruction in the form of a one-level or multilevel bypass operation is often the key to limb salvage.

It deserves emphasis that every diabetic foot with serious infection or ischemia needs a vascular evaluation. Aggressive use of vascular reconstruction coupled with thorough and complete debridement of infected and/or gangrenous tissue is the key to maximal salvage of limbs and feet.[59] Limbs that would otherwise require below-knee amputation may be converted to a Syme level; ankle disarticulation may be converted to a partial foot amputation; and nonhealing wounds can often close. Salvage rates are as high as three quarters of patients requiring emergent surgery.[100]

The importance of limb salvage has been scientifically demonstrated, thus reinforcing the intuitive notion that function is maximized by lowering the level of amputation. The level of work, as proven by oxygen consumption, increases with more proximal levels of amputation.[107] Syme amputations are preferable to below-knee amputations, which are preferable to above-knee procedures in terms of the likelihood of the patient ambulating independently postoperatively (Fig 22–12).[107]

Imaging of the Diabetic Foot

Radiographs

Although radiographs are still the mainstay of diagnosis of osseous disorders of the diabetic foot, they are limited in sensitivity, accuracy, and the range of disorders that they can detect. Roentgenograms have been demonstrated to have an accuracy and a sensitivity in the diagnosis of the diabetic foot of about 75%.[109] However, the radiograph is the first diagnostic test that is usually done, and the characteristic findings on plain films are worth summarizing and knowing. Osteolysis in the bones of a diabetic, especially in the distal seg-

B

Severe Proximal and Distal Arterial Occlusion No Pulsatile Flow on Waveforms

ARTERIAL STUDIES

Doppler Pressure

	R	L
Br	140	140
Thigh	180	185
Above Knee	115	130
Below Knee	75	80
Ankle	DP40 PT45	DP60 PT50
Ankle Ratio	.32	.43
Toe	X	X

CC: Vascular check.

IMPRESSION: Resting pressures as recorded. Severe bilateral superficial femoral and popliteal arterial occlusive disease. On the left there is below the knee arterial occlusive disease. No waveforms obtained at the right 1st, 2nd or 3rd toes. Waveform only obtained at left great toe without cuff.

Right Posterior Tibial

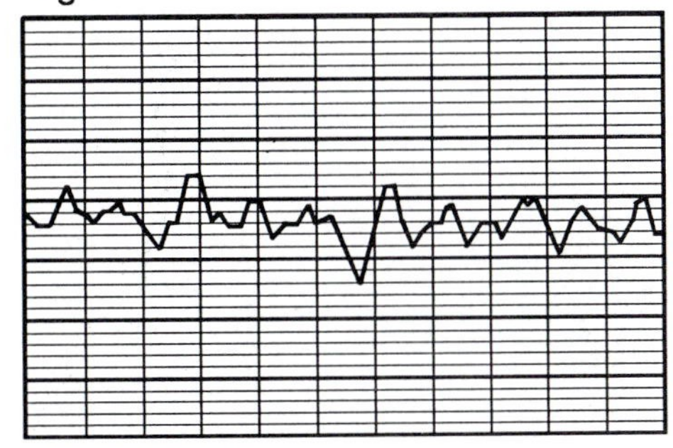

Left Posterior Tibial

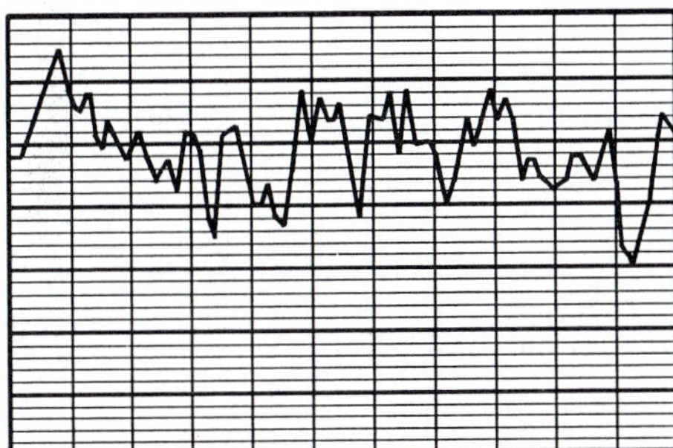

Right Dorsal Pedis

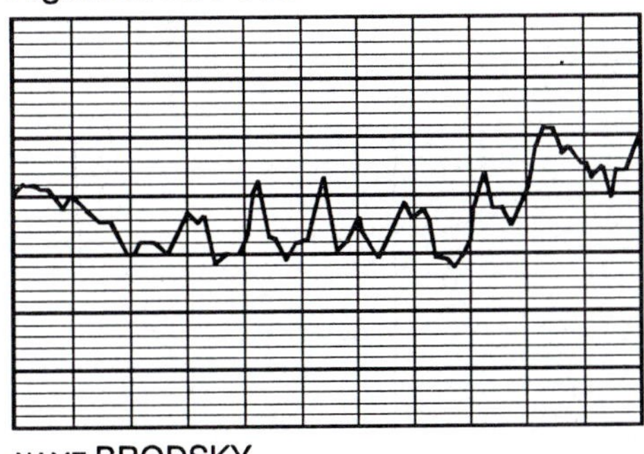

Left Dorsal Pedis

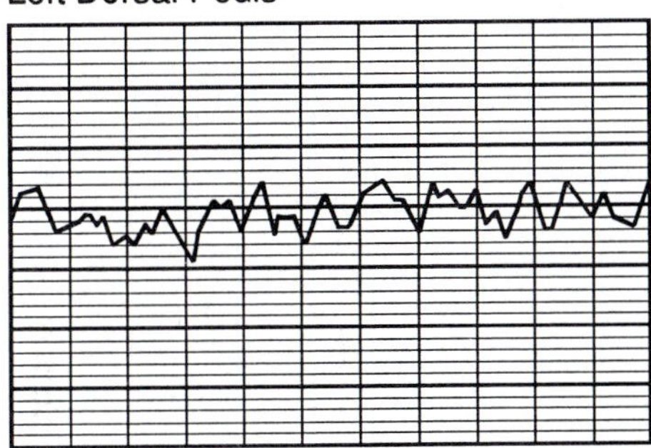

02/08/90

NAME BRODSKY

DOCTOR'S NAME

DIV. ______ ROOM NO. ________

DATE

BAYLOR UNIVERSITY MEDICAL PLAZA
DALLAS, TEXAS
VASCULAR LABORATORY
ROOM 254 PHONE: 820-3447

FIG 22–11 (cont.).

C

Diminished but adequate perfusion, left greater than right, pulsatile flow present. Ankle ratio greater than 1.0, indicating arterial calcification.

ARTERIAL STUDIES

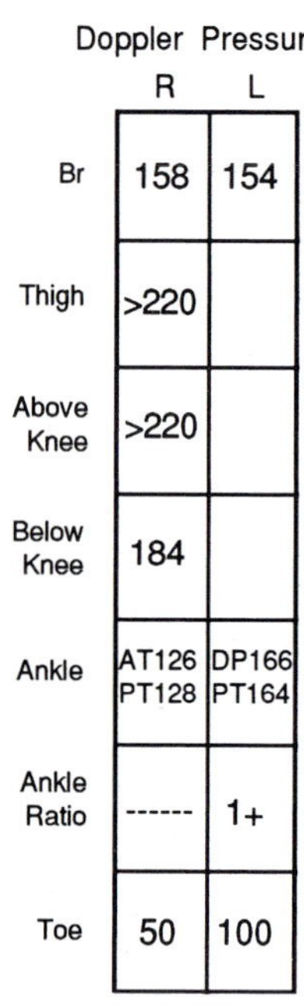

Doppler Pressure	R	L
Br	158	154
Thigh	>220	
Above Knee	>220	
Below Knee	184	
Ankle	AT126 PT128	DP166 PT164
Ankle Ratio	------	1+
Toe	50	100

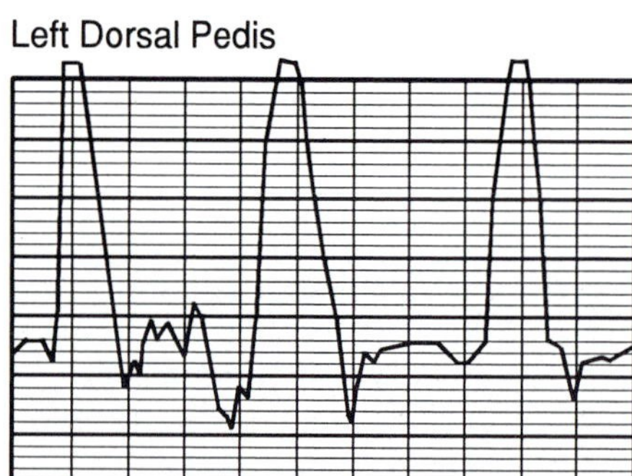

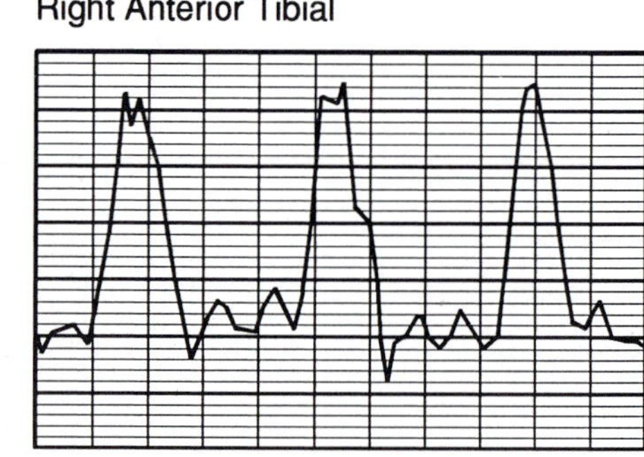

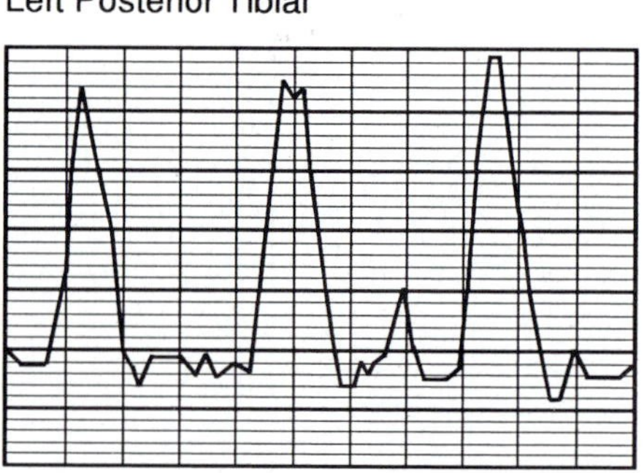

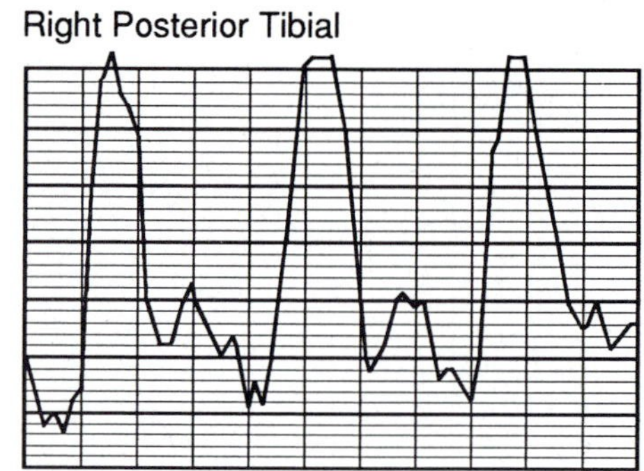

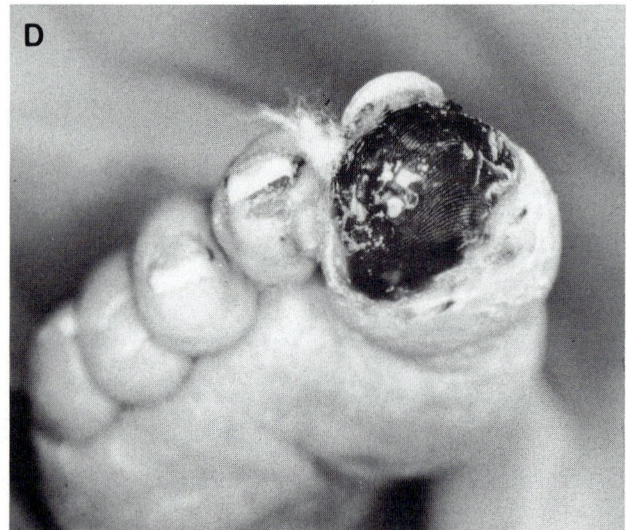

FIG 22–11 (cont.).

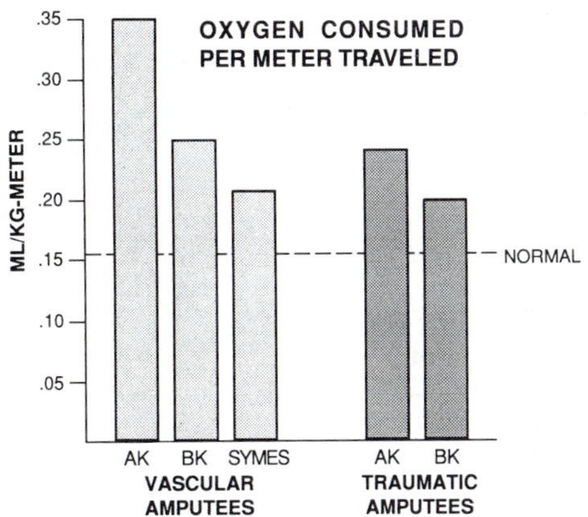

FIG 22–12.
Greater limb preservation results in enhanced function with lower oxygen consumption. (Adapted from Waters RL, Perry J, Antonelli D, et al: *J Bone Joint Surg [Am]* 56:44, 1976.)

ments such as the phalanges, is often mistaken for osteomyelitis, even in the absence of clinical signs and symptoms of infection. The characteristic "penciling" of a distal metatarsal or "vanishing phalanx" (Fig 22–13) is usually not associated with infection, although it is sometimes necessary to evaluate for associated infection, especially if there is an underlying ulcer. This can be a difficult task since the bone destruction itself can produce a positive technetium scan; therefore either magnetic resonance imaging (MRI) or an indium scan is required, preferably the latter. When osteolysis is neuropathic in origin in the absence of infection,[110] it occurs most often in the distal part of the forefoot, usually distal to the midmetatarsal level and involving the distal metatarsals and the phalanges. The mechanism is not clearly understood but is probably related to a neurally mediated hyperemia that resorbs the bone and is caused by a loss of sympathetic nervous functional control over vasoconstriction.[21]

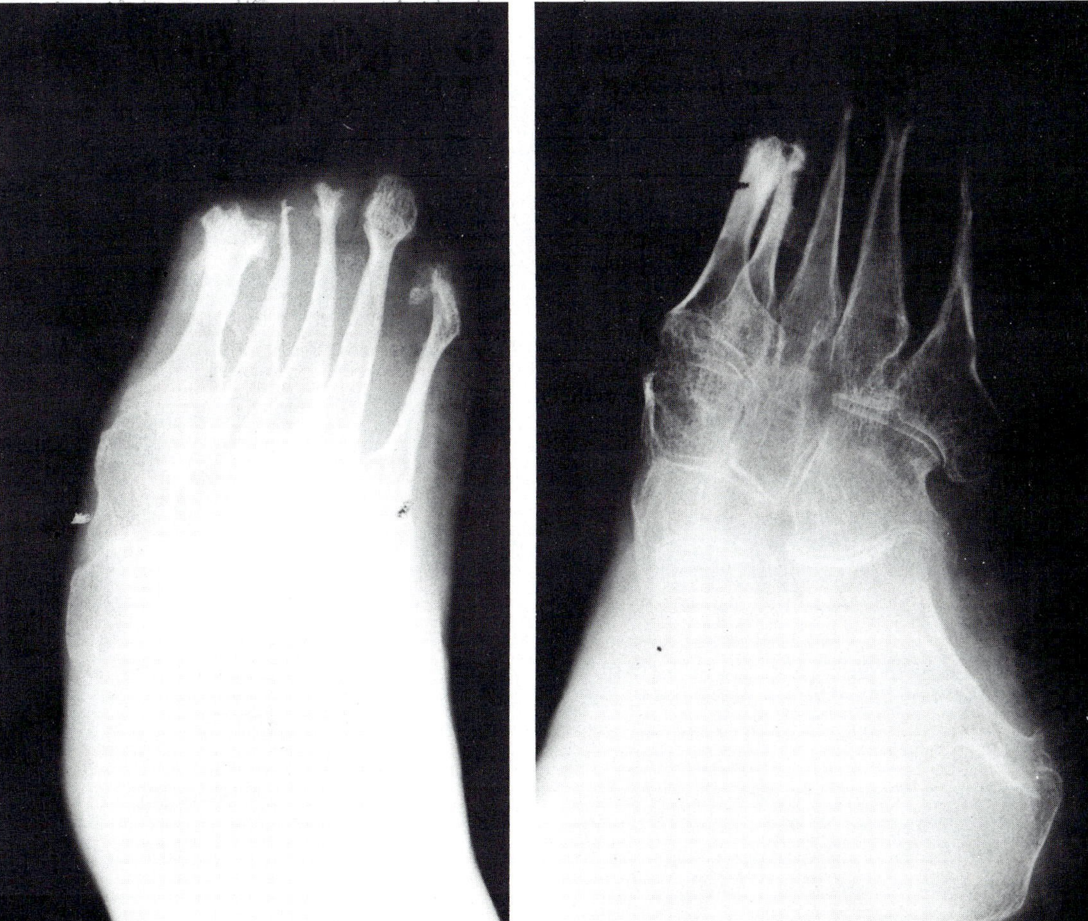

FIG 22–13.
Diabetic osteolysis in the absence of infection.

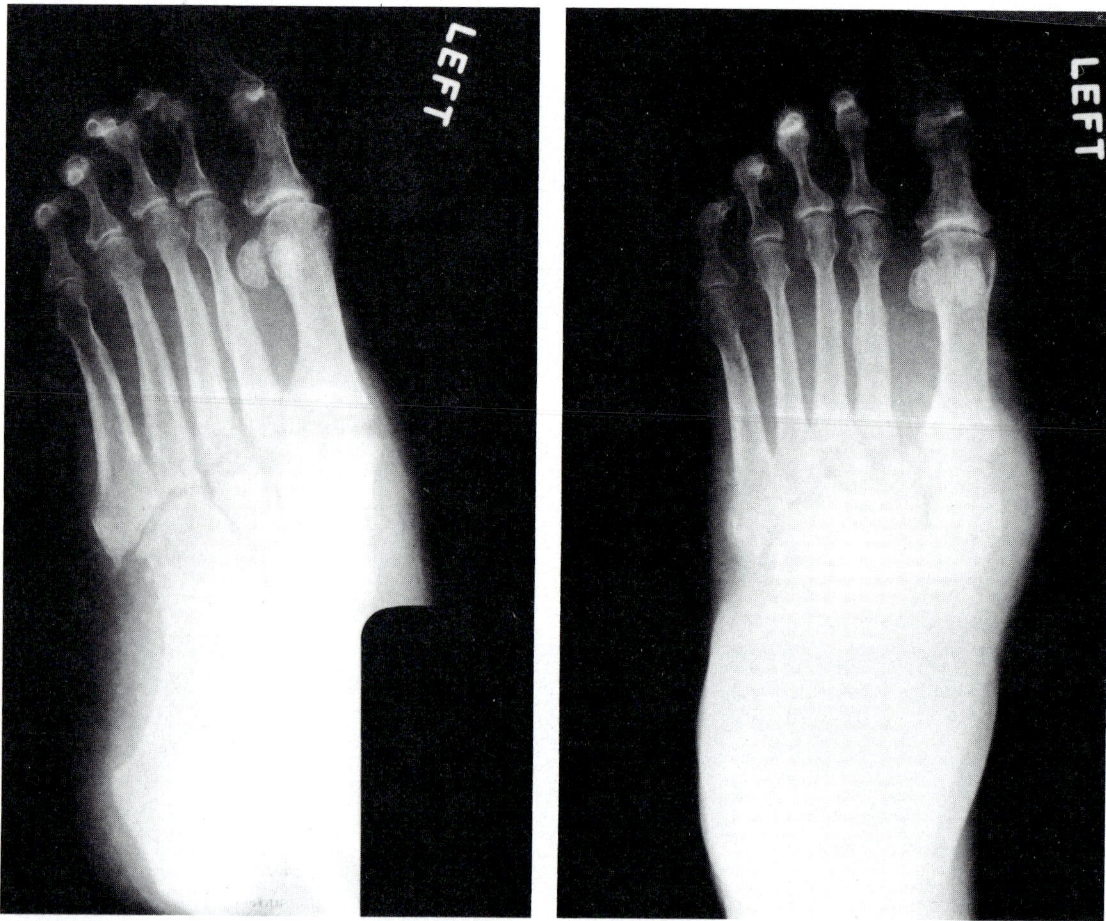

FIG 22–14.
Osseous destruction without surrounding osteopenia, characteristic of Charcot neuropathic arthropathy.

The changes of a Charcot joint, another form of osteoarthropathy, are possibly related in a pathophysiologic fashion but present a different radiographic appearance. Here the cardinal features are fractures, dislocations, bone destruction, multiple fragmentation, and an architectural disruption of one or multiple joints of the foot. The affected joint or joints may be partially or completely destroyed, not only through a loss of the articular surface and configuration but also because of a shift of the whole relationship of the bone to other surrounding bony structures. However, one of the cardinal features of neuropathic fractures and dislocations (Charcot foot) is the relative *absence* of surrounding and adjacent osteopenia when compared with an infectious process producing the same amount of bone destruction.[86] Subsequent healing is demonstrated by new bone formation, both periosteal and enchondral, and often extensive bony consolidation across several tarsal or metatarsal bones. This often produces a stable, although deformed, foot of different shape and wider proportions than before the neuroarthropathic process began (Fig 22–14).

Bone Scans and MRI

Technetium 99 bone scans and MRI are both very much more sensitive in detecting early bone changes of osteomyelitis and Charcot joints than plain radiographs are. However, MRI is significantly more sensitive than bone scans and detects osteomyelitis earlier than the bone scan.[109] The bone scan is still considerably less costly than an MRI study in most institutions and so still serves a purpose for screening; bone scan activity can persist for a year or longer after a fracture or other osseous change, and the pattern of positive uptake is entirely nonspecific. Negative bone scan results strongly exclude bone pathology such as osteomyelitis, but a positive study is highly nonspecific.[109] Although much has been made over the use of the "triple-phase" bone scan, there is *no* diagnostic advantage to making this study in three phases in regard to the diabetic foot, either in theory or by documentation in the literature. Images are taken in the injection or radionuclide angiography stage for the blood flow first phase, then in the first few minutes for soft-tissue images (blood pool), and then again for the usual delayed bone images at about 3 hours after injection. The first two phases indicate cellulitis or soft-tissue inflammation when they are positive and the late or third phase is negative. However, such soft-tissue inflammation or cellulitis is better or more easily diagnosed clinically than on technetium scans. If all three phases are positive, this is often consistent with bone pathology itself, which can cause accompanying soft-tissue inflammation, but the positivity or negativity of the first two phases adds nothing to the differentiation of osteomyelitis from neuropathic osteoarthropathy.

Neither the bone scan, radiographs, nor any other single study represents the *sine qua non* in diagnosing infection or arthropathy in the diabetic foot and must be combined with clinical examination, history, and other diagnostic modalities. Surgical follow-up studies have demonstrated the inaccuracy (both poor specificity and poor sensitivity) of single studies in making the diagnosis of osteomyelitis.[95]

Computed Tomography

Computed tomography (CT) is a valuable test for anatomic localization of infection and pathology such as an abscess in the deep structures of the foot. Prior to the advent of MRI it was the best technique for obtaining information on the nonosseous pathology of the foot and especially of the deep structures. The weakness of the CT scan is the poor differentiation or wide transition zone between normal and infected tissues.[91] It has since been surpassed by MRI, which is superior in its ability to differentiate a wider range of different tissues in their normal and abnormal states.

MRI has been a major advance in the treatment of the diabetic foot. Patients with acutely inflamed, swollen feet with an early Charcot joint and negative radiographic findings who were previously assumed to have a deep plantar abscess and then subjected to an inappropriate incision and drainage operation can now be spared this inaccurate treatment. MRI can reveal abnormalities of bone and soft tissue equally well. However, the differentiation of osteomyelitis from the marrow changes of Charcot joints is not necessarily easy or possible. All MRI changes are based on changes in proton activity, i.e., the presence or absence of water in the tissues. Most changes in the bone on MRI are based upon changes in the character of the marrow from a fat-type signal to a water signal due to the increased edema within the marrow. This edema can occur from injury, infection, or neuroarthropathy, alike. The distinction between a Charcot joint and osteomyelitis, while claimed to be possible by a few authors,[4] is disputed by most. These claims must be examined very carefully because there are major differences between acute and chronic Charcot changes and their appearance on MRI and radiographs. Most chronic changes can be diagnosed by simple radiographs, while the acute marrow changes of a Charcot joint are *not* pathognomonic on MRI.

Gallium Scans

Gallium scans are too non specific to be helpful in making the distinction between a Charcot joint and osteomyelitis and are usually not helpful in the diagnosis of a diabetic foot. By contrast, the use of indium-labeled white blood cells may be quite useful based on the greater specificity of this study for infection. A direct comparison of combined, simultaneous indium and technetium imaging may aid in detecting the rare but troublesome clinical problem of diagnosing a Charcot joint that might also have osteomyelitis.[62, 99] This is particularly problematic because this is the only imaging technique in which the characteristic changes of the two conditions do not almost entirely overlap. The key to this technique is to do both images at the same time and compare the spatial presentation of the positive areas on the two studies. If the location and size of the positive area on both scans are the same, then the infection resides in the bone. If one presumes that the Charcot process is active, the positive area on the scans represents infection in the Charcot joint. If the area of uptake in the indium 111 scan is in the soft tissue or superficial to the area of uptake on the technetium 99 bone scan, then osteomyelitis is most likely not present.

CLASSIFICATIONS SYSTEMS

The classification system developed in the 1970s at Rancho Los Amigos Hospital in California by Wagner and Meggitt, otherwise known as the "Wagner" classification has been the most widely used and accepted grading systems for lesions of the diabetic foot.[102] It has provided a basis for communication and comparison among physicians and investigators in this area. The system has six grades of lesions, the first four of which are related to the depth of the lesion through the soft

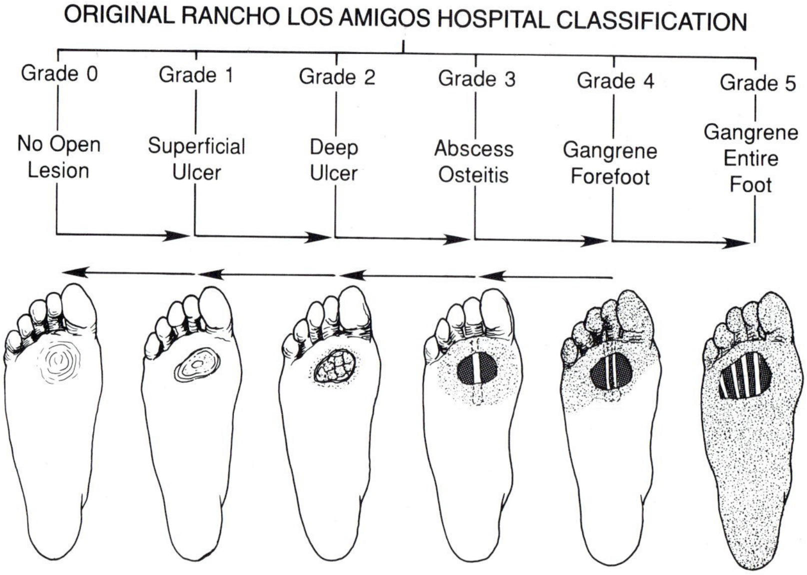

ORIGINAL RANCHO LOS AMIGOS HOSPITAL CLASSIFICATION

Grade 0 — No Open Lesion
Grade 1 — Superficial Ulcer
Grade 2 — Deep Ulcer
Grade 3 — Abscess Osteitis
Grade 4 — Gangrene Forefoot
Grade 5 — Gangrene Entire Foot

FIG 22–15.
The original Rancho Los Amigos classification by Wagner and Meggitt presented the first widely referenced classification of diabetic foot lesions. However, two concepts included in this classification are now in need of revision in light of further experience. The first is the concept that all lesions of the diabetic foot from grade 1 ulcers to grade 5 gangrene occur along a natural continuum. While this may often be true for the grade 1 ulcer, which progresses to the grade 3 lesion of osteomyelitis, this is not the case with grades 4 and 5. Grades 4 and 5 are vascular lesions or descriptions of the vascular status of the foot and are not necessarily related to the progression of the lesser grades. The ischemic lesions of grades 4 and 5 may exist separately from the lesser grades or coincide with any of them including a forefoot that is otherwise grade 1 (i.e., a superficial lesion). Vascular pathology can and should be graded also, but there is not a necessary relationship between the *depth* of ulcerative lesions, i.e., grades 0, 1, 2, and 3, and the dysvascularity of the foot, i.e., grades 4 and 5. Moreover, the grade 5 foot is truly no longer a foot problem but belongs in the domain of salvage of the proximal portion of the leg. The second concept that needs to be refined is that there are not necessarily pathways backwards and forwards from each grade of lesion, e.g., grade 4 feet (partial gangrene) cannot be reversed to grade 3.

tissue. The last two (grades 4 and 5) are entirely different and are related to the extent of the loss of vascularity in the foot (Fig 22–15). Most of the lesions fall within three grades: grades 1, 2, and 3. Of these, most outpatient treatments are applied to grade 1 lesions. The treatment of grades 4 (partial gangrene) and 5 (total gangrene) are rather straightforward, i.e., amputation with considerations of revascularization and treatment of infection as needed.

A modification of the Wagner classification is offered in Table 22–2, the two purposes of which are to simplify the task of correlating treatments to the appropriate grade of lesion and to clarify the distinctions among the grades, especially between grades 2 and 3. It is hoped that this revision will make the classification clearer and easier to apply to treatment regimens. Please refer to the text below for the appropriate details on treatment; this simplification, combined with the treatment flowchart (Fig 22–16) is meant to make the decision-making path more clear and to make this information more accessible than the old algorithms,[105] which contain a great deal of repetition of the basic diagnostic workup from one to the other.

While much attention has been given to the depth of the diabetic foot lesion, as expressed in old and new grading systems, relatively little has been investigated regarding the important issue of the anatomic location of the lesion. In general, lesions of the forefoot, especially distal to the distal third of the metatarsal, have a much lower associated mortality and much higher limb salvage than more proximal lesions of the foot, even though the actual healing time of the proximal and distal lesions may be similar.[60] This type of prognostic generalization puts into perspective the increased seriousness of lesions of the midfoot and hindfoot and should aid the orthopaedic surgeon in his counseling of the patients.

In general, hindfoot lesions are associated with a higher incidence of serious problems and a greater risk of amputation.

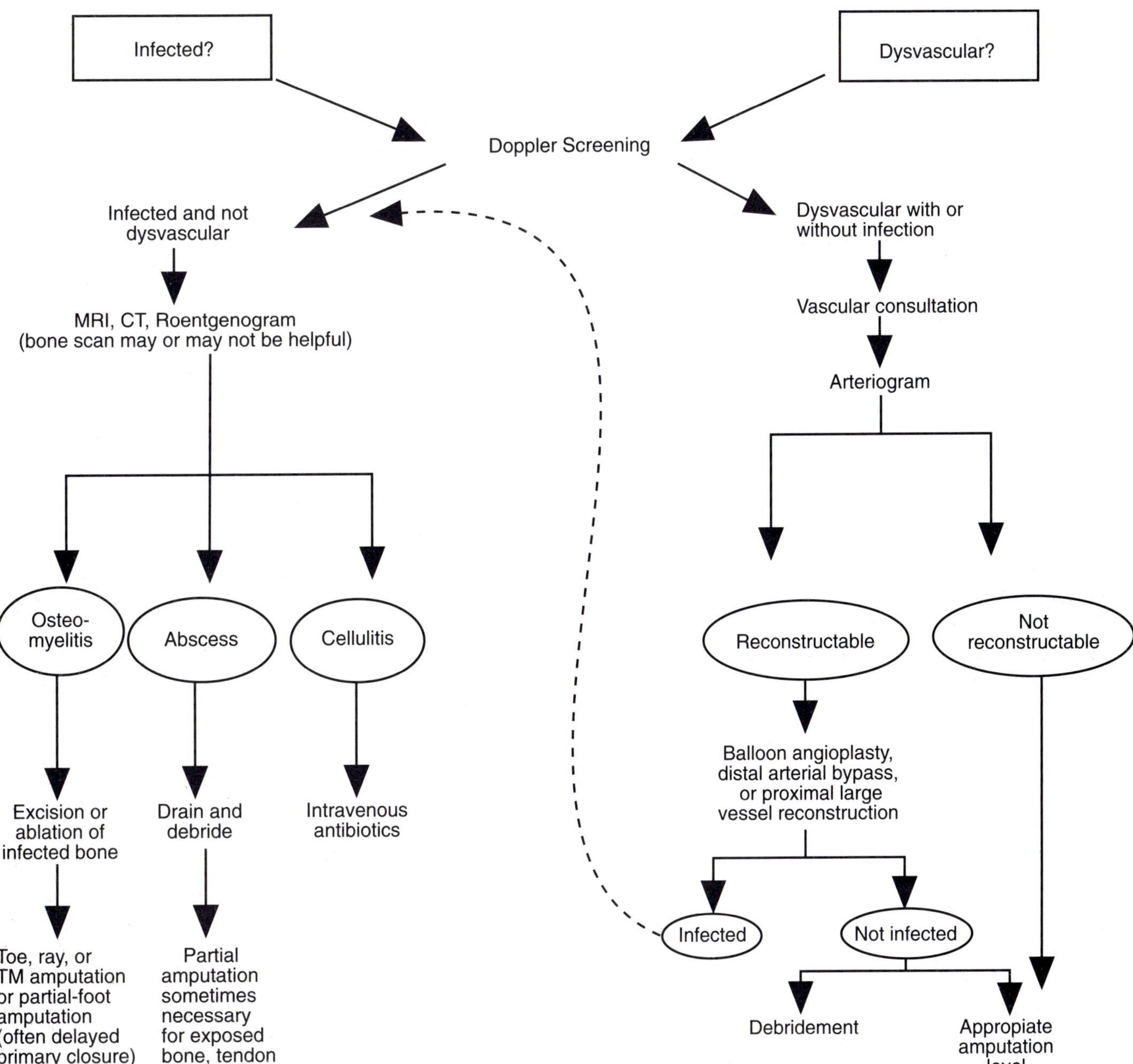

FIG 22–16.
Flowchart of the principles of care of the diabetic foot. Note the two columns representing the two major issues of infection and vascularity. Once the dysvascular limb has been revascularized, the level of infection is determined and treated.

TABLE 22–2.

The "Depth/Ischemia" Classification of Diabetic Foot Lesions

Grade	Definition	Treatment
Depth classification		
0	The "at-risk" foot: previous ulcer or neuropathy with deformity that may cause new ulceration	Patient education Regular examination Appropriate shoe wear and insoles
1	Superficial ulceration, not infected	External pressure relief: total-contact cast, walking brace, special shoe wear, etc.
2	Deep ulceration exposing a tendon or joint (with or without superfical infection)	Surgical debridement → wound care → pressure relief if the lesion closes and converts to grade 1 (prn antibiotics)
3	Extensive ulceration with exposed bone and/or deep infection, i.e., osteomyelitis, or abscess	Surgical debridements → ray or partial foot amputations → IV antibiotics → pressure relief if wound converts to grade 1
Ischemia classification		
A	Ischemia without gangrene	*Vascular evaluation* (Doppler, $TcPo_2$ arteriogram, etc.) → *vascular reconstruction* prn
B	Partial (forefoot) gangrene of the foot	*Vascular evaluation* → *vascular reconstruction* (proximal and/or distal bypass or angioplasty) → *Partial foot amputation*
C	Complete foot gangrene	*Vascular evaluation* → *major extremity amputation* (BKA, AKA)* with possible proximal vascular reconstruction

*BKA, AKA = below/above-knee amputation

CLINICAL PROBLEMS AND THEIR TREATMENT

There are four basic clinical orthopaedic problems that affect the feet of diabetics: ulcerations, infections, Charcot joints, and skin and nail problems. Although they not only can but commonly do coexist, the discussion of the treatment of each will follow sequentially.

Ulcers

Ulcerations of the diabetic foot are the single most common problem for which medical assistance is sought. The natural history of these lesions varies by location, size, and depth. Plantar ulcers are caused by weight-bearing pressure, while dorsal and side ulcers are usually caused by shoe pressure. Ulcers of greater size and especially of greater depth are more difficult to treat. However, the outcome of ulcerations and their treatment is often enigmatic and unpredictable. Why do some ulcers persist largely unchanged, with or without treatment, sometimes for years? Why do some ulcerations rapidly progress to deep infection and osteomyelitis? The answers to these questions are often elusive, but chronic ulcers should not be allowed to persist untreated out of concern that they may progress. Simply trimming the hyperkeratotic "rind" around the edges of the ulcer is insufficient and inadequate treatment unless something is additionally done to relieve the pressure or alter the weight-bearing characteristics of the lesion.

Many grade 1 ulcers can persist in an indolent state for years without either resolution or progression. When these patients are placed in a total-contact cast, the ulcer will usually heal within a matter of weeks, most likely because they *are* grade 1, i.e., there is enough underlying pressure to perpetuate the ulcer but not so much as to cause involvement of the deep tissues (Fig 22–17). Conversely, an ulcer may develop in a matter of days or even hours. Once breakdown occurs, there may be too much pressure to allow healing in spite of the fact that the pressure was mild enough to leave the previously undisturbed skin intact. Treatment methods that are adequate to maintain the condition of healed skin, such as a properly molded accommodative insole and an "extra-depth" shoe, are usually *not* adequate to achieve healing once breakdown has occurred (Fig 22–18).

The first question that must be answered in treating an ulcer in a diabetic foot is to determine whether it is infected or not. All ulcers are colonized, at least superficially, and a superficial swab will document some bacterial growth. An infected ulcer usually appears differently: it is draining and deep (greater than grade 1), may have surrounding erythema and/or cellulitis, and may have associated edema and possibly lymphangitis as well (Fig 22–19).

If the ulcer is significantly infected, the patient usually needs to be admitted to the hospital, started on

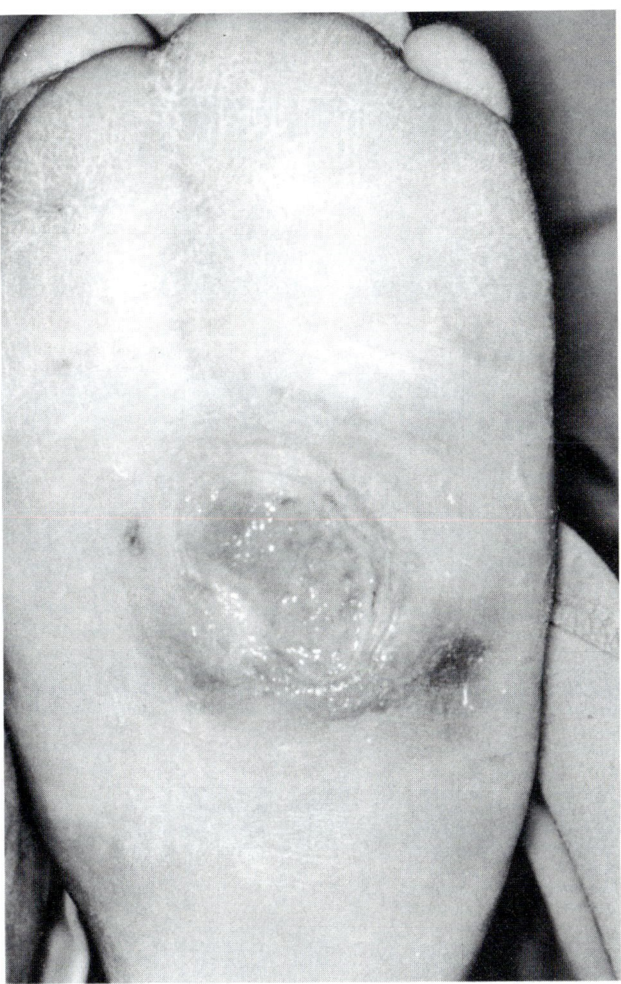

FIG 22–17.
A grade 1 ulcer. Note its superficial, granulating base.

intravenous antibiotics, have an internal medicine or endocrinology consultation for glucose control, and undergo debridement of the wound. Wound care must follow general principles until such time as the wound is converted to grade 1. The use of whirlpool treatment is satisfactory when wound care requires low-level daily debridement. Whirlpool, in other words, is simply one form of debridement. Once a clean, granulating wound has been achieved, there is no place for continued use of whirlpool baths. Outpatient whirlpool seldom has a place in the author's protocol for the treatment of ulcers. Once the wound is clean, then pressure-altering strategies are the key to healing, provided that adequate vascularity of the limb has been documented. At that time it can be treated with the array of outpatient pressure-relieving methods detailed below (see Fig 22–16). The second question to answer is what the grade of the ulcer is (see above, "Classifications" and Table 22–2). Most ulcers treated in an outpatient setting are grade 1. Lesions that are deeper than grade 1 usually require inpatient or surgical care, although there are exceptions. Third, it should be determined whether there is adequate vascularity to promote healing. One of the common causes for a nonhealing, persistent chronic wound, especially an ulcer, is peripheral vascular insufficiency. Patients with recalcitrant wounds and patients admitted for care of diabetic foot lesions are routinely screened with arterial Doppler studies for this purpose.

Once the questions of infection, ulcer grade, and vascularity have been satisfactorily addressed, the surgeon can address attention to the key to healing ulcer lesions, namely, relief of pressure. Several options for modification of weight-bearing pressure are pictured in Figure 22–20 and include a postoperative-type surgical shoe, a Plastazote shoe, a prefabricated walking brace, bed rest, or a total-contact cast. The choice depends upon the lesion, the particulars of each patient and their prior treatment, and the anatomic location of the ulcer. As noted above, ulcers on the dorsum and sides of the feet are usually caused by pressure from shoe wear and would most likely be treated with a surgical shoe or prefabricated walking brace. Total-contact casts are not as effective for these ulcers as they are for those caused by the pressure of standing and walking, i.e., plantar ulcers. Plantar ulcers, which constitute the majority of neuropathic ulcerations, might be treated in those devices as well but would often require a total-contact cast if the other methods were unsuccessful, as is often the case. Choosing the best pressure-relieving device is not always easy, and patients will sometimes resist a cast at first, especially in a hot climate. This rejection may be out of fear or disbelief or out of a rational comprehension of the inconvenience of the cast. It is important to set some kind of timetable for the progression of treatment from the simplest (surgical shoe) to the more rigorous (total-contact cast or surgery) techniques for relief of pressure so that the lesion is not allowed to persist indefinitely; this is important for the lesion as well as for the frame of mind of the patient so that he or she can perceive real progress. The insensitivity of the ulcer represents *the absence of sensory input* that caused the ulcer in the first place; problems exist only insofar as we perceive or are able to perceive them. All too often, this ostensible oblivion allows the diabetic with peripheral neuropathy to inexorably slide into disastrous complications of what were initially small, treatable problems. The doctor can also be lulled into accepting these chronic, persistent, or recurrent lesions. Thus a timetable for progression of treatment is important. Bed rest will certainly aid in or achieve healing of plantar neurotrophic ulcerations. Figure 22–21 illus-

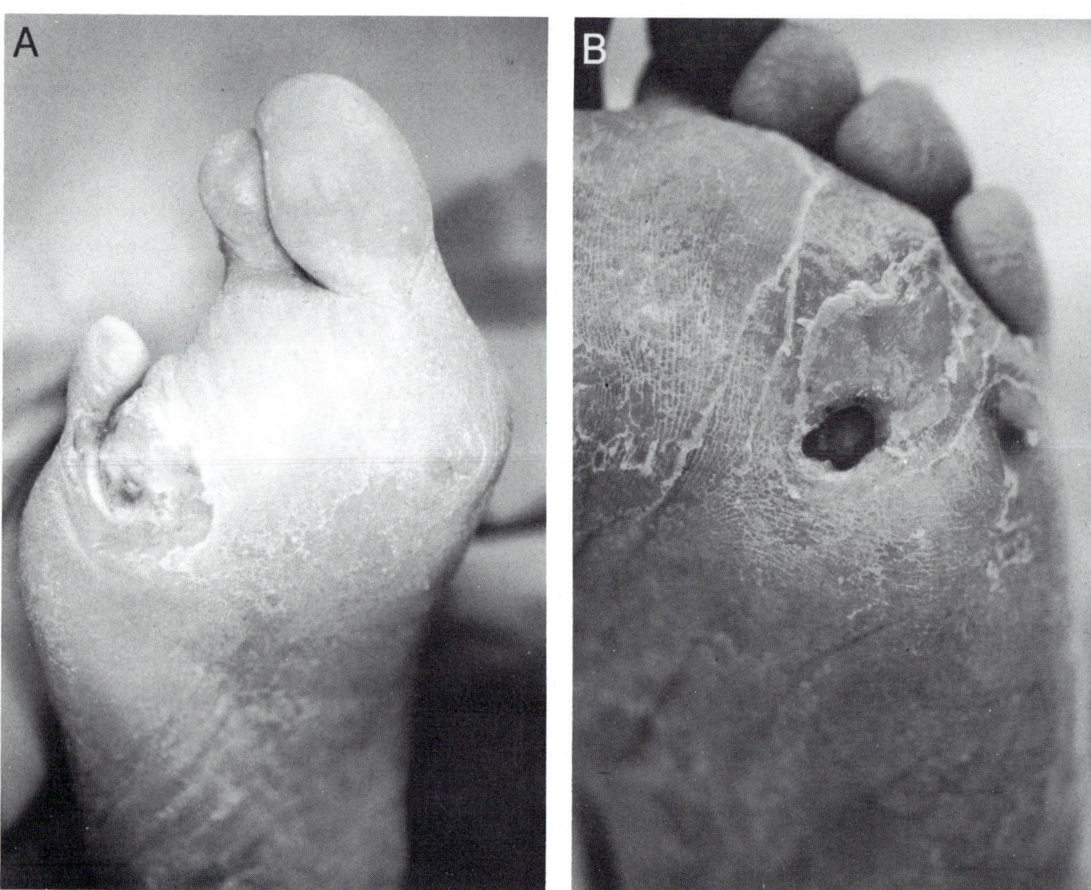

FIG 22–18.
Comparison of grade 1 **(A)** and Grade 2 **(B)** ulcers (new depth/ischemia classification; see Table 22—2). Note the exposed deep tissues of the grade 2 ulcer.

trates a patient with severe plantar ulcerations associated with bilateral Charcot joints and midfoot collapse who was bedridden because of other severe medical problems and healed her ulcers without surgery or any other external device. However, bed rest is not a prescribed treatment and is mentioned only to emphasize that the issue in healing the ulcerations is always relief of pressure. Bed rest has many deleterious effects and potential risks and is not routinely recommended for healing the ulcers. Unless the mechanical solution is more permanent, the ulcers will recur as soon as the patient is on her feet again.

Unloading the foot with crutch ambulation may be a helpful adjunct to the other mechanical methods and devices applied to the extremity. Non–weight bearing alone is not recommended. It is tiring, difficult, and impossible to monitor for compliance. The patient with neuropathy probably has difficulty complying with it because she cannot tell whether the foot is down on the floor or not and may inadvertently be bearing weight for turning, pivoting on the toilet, transfers, etc.

The progress of healing of the ulcer should be recorded in the patient's record by describing the ulcer depth and its characteristics but, most importantly, by tracing an outline of the ulcer onto the chart. The latter is the best record of change of an ulcer and is done with a piece of unexposed (but developed) x-ray film or clear acetate and an indelible felt-tipped marker. The ulcer is traced out on the film and then traced onto the patient's chart (see Figs 22–7 and 22–8). This has the added benefit of affording (visual) sensory input for the patient to perceive the improvement as the ulcer resolves.

The Total-Contact Cast

The total-contact cast is still the best and most widely used method for healing the most common type of plantar ulcerations (grade 1 ulcers). The method has been proven to be efficacious and cost-effective in the healing of plantar ulcers due to insensitivity.[7, 10, 49, 79, 106] There are any number of variations of technique, but the mystique that has apparently grown up around the total-contact cast is rather undeserved. The method is not unrea-

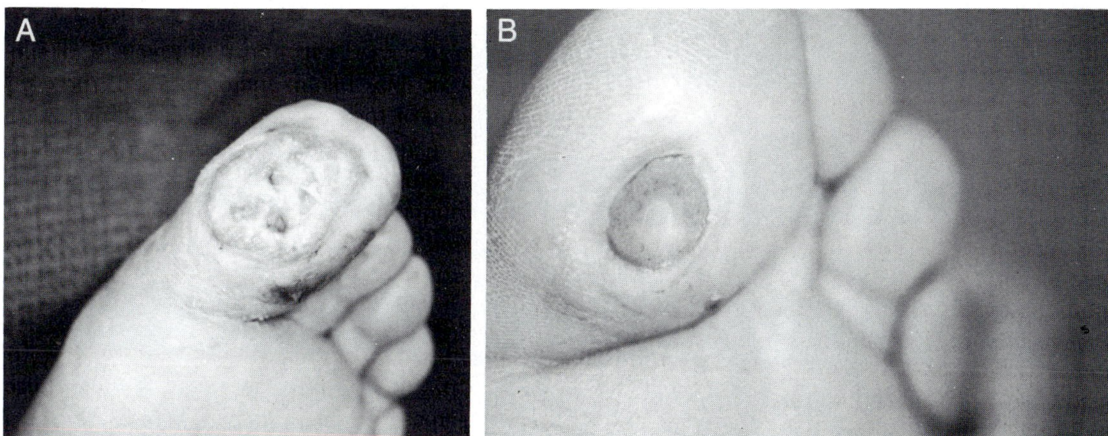

FIG 22–19.
Comparison of infected **(A)** and noninfected **(B)** ulcers of the hallux.

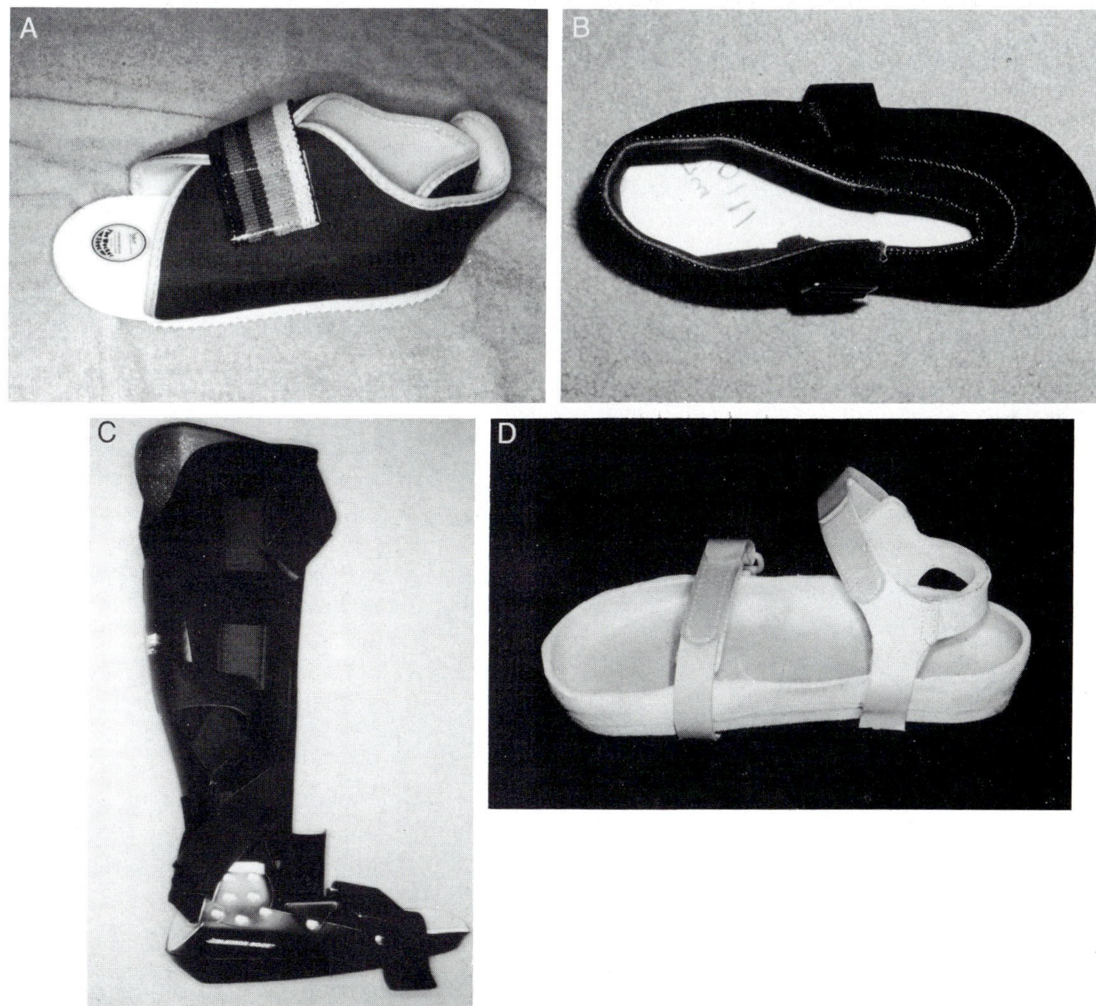

FIG 22–20.
Different types of weight-relieving devices for the diabetic foot. **A,** wooden-soled postoperative shoe. **B,** Plastazote "healing" shoe. **C,** prefabricated walking brace. **D,** Carville sandal.

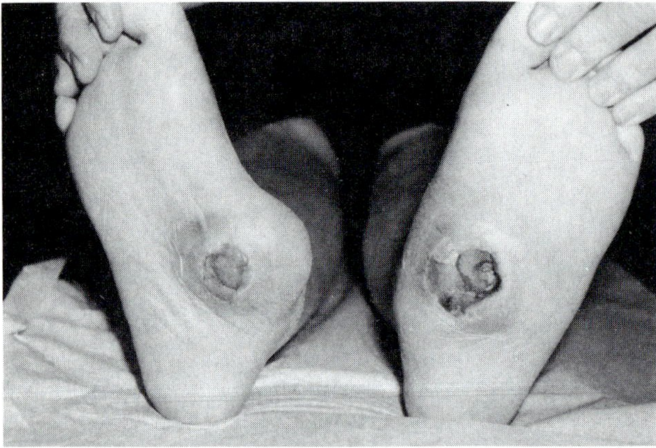

FIG 22–21.
Bilateral midfoot ulcerations over Charcot joints. These eventually healed with bed rest when the patient was bedridden due to other severe medical problems.

sonably difficult, but attention to details and principles is critical (see Appendix 22–2). The first important principle is that the cast must not be over padded; this leads to shifting of the limb within the cast as the padding compresses in the course of use and can lead to new pressure lesions. Second, the cast must limit toe motion, either by being of the closed-toe variety (Fig 22–22) or, in the open-toe variety, by careful molding in the dorsal-plantar direction to inhibit hyperextension of the metatarsophalangeal joints (Fig 22–23). This helps to diminish the accentuated pressure of the metatarsal heads that occurs as a result of the "clawed" (or hyperextended metatarsophalangeal joint) position and contributes to the persistence of the ulcer in that typical location. Third, the bony prominences and anticipated areas of high pressure should be padded with felt or foam to diminish the concentration of pressure on the anterior subcutaneous crest of the tibia, the malleoli, the dorsum of the toes, the protuberance of a Charcot joint, etc. Fourth, the first cast should generally be changed within 7 to 10 days because the cast functions to reduce edema, often dramatically, and the first cast frequently becomes loose and allows the limb to shift and slide within the cast, potentially causing new abrasions, blisters, or ulcers. Subsequent casts can be changed at longer intervals of 2 to 4 weeks. Fifth, if the cast is not promoting ulcer healing adequately, after checking the other principles listed above, one can consider stiffening the plantar walking surface of the cast by incorporating a wooden platform into the outer layers. The space between the cast and the board is filled in with casting material. There are published video demonstrations of different methods for applying the "total-contact" cast.[12, 16] Appendix 22–2 lists the materials and the step-by-step method for applying a total-contact cast.

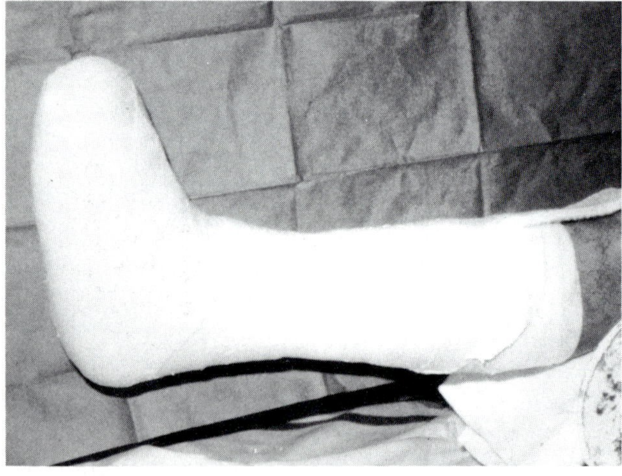

FIG 22–22.
Closed-toe type of total-contact cast.

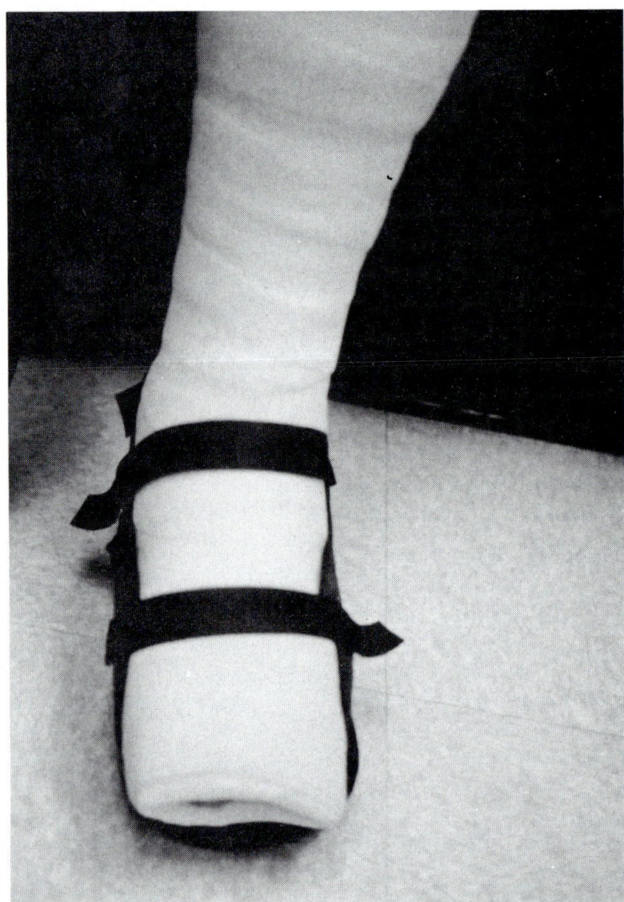

FIG 22–23.
Open-toe, total-contact cast with molding in a dorsal-plantar direction to limit toe extension.

Total-contact casts are not without complications, the most common of which is the production of a superficial abrasion, blister, or new ulcerations due to pressure of the cast or movement within the cast. The toes are the most frequently affected area, and the patient needs to be warned at the time of application that this can occur. It is usually mild and only a temporary setback, if that. The patient may be left out of the cast or placed in a removable walking brace (prefabricated type) that is open or adjustable over the lesion for a week or two until the new lesions heal, and then cast treatment can usually resume. The prefabricated walking braces, most of which are outfitted with Velcro straps, uprights medially and laterally, and a rockered sole, are not equivalent to a total-contact cast for several reasons. If a foot is misshapen by a Charcot joint or previous surgery, excess pressure can be applied by the rigid portion of the structure. The ability of the device to accommodate the area of excessive pressure that causes the ulcer is minimal when compared with the cast, which is always "custom-fitted" by its nature. Prefabricated braces cannot and do not exert the circumferential pressure of the cast and as such are not nearly as effective in relieving pressure concentration. Moreover, the prefabricated brace cannot control swelling like a cast can. These devices do indeed have a very beneficial role to play in the treatment of diabetic foot problems, but the nuances of their use must be understood.

Ulcerations that occur on the plantar surface of the midfoot in the longitudinal arch in the absence of trauma are almost invariably the result of a Charcot joint since there is usually not a normal bony prominence in the arch region and ulcers cannot develop where there is no bone pressure.

Ulcerations that occur on the heel are frequently among the most difficult to manage. The skin over the lateral and medial sides of the heel is immobile and thin and has little subcutaneous tissue. Ulcerations on the plantar or posteroplantar aspect of the heel, by contrast, have a thick layer of subcutaneous fat but have the disadvantage that this is relatively avascular tissue even in a normal foot (Fig 22–24). The effects of peripheral vascular disease in this area exacerbate this relative ischemia. Ulcers on the heel granulate especially slowly, if at all. They tend to be more recalcitrant, respond much less well to relief of mechanical pressure (such as the total-contact cast), and are frequently characterized by ischemia. If the ulcer is situated posteriorly over the heel, this can rapidly lead to osteomyelitis. Heel ulcers are among the most common to require surgical intervention (see the section below on surgery for ulceration) in the form of debridement, bony resection, or amputation.

The principle to remember is that once an ulcer occurs in the diabetic, it signifies that the patient has now reached a level of peripheral neuropathy at which the feet will always be at equal or greater risk in the future. The immediate goal is to follow the flowchart of increasingly extensive and aggressive treatment alternatives until healing is achieved, up to and including surgical resection of the bony prominences that perpetuate the problem. However, the long-term goal must be to prevent or at least minimize recurrence of this ulcer or other neuropathic lesions. This is accomplished in three ways: (1) patient education regarding care and daily inspection of the feet; (2) appropriate shoe wear; and (3) when applicable, molded insoles in the shoe to protect and unweight the high-pressure areas of the plantar surface. Specific recommendations are discussed below in the section on shoe wear and shoe insoles.

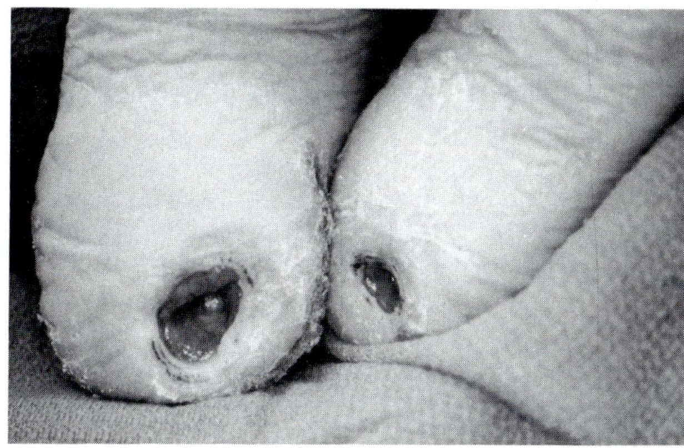

FIG 22–24.
Bilateral heel ulcerations in a diabetic. One healed with casts, and the other required partial calcanectomy.

Wound Care

The most important principle in wound care has already been emphasized, i.e. if the wound is pressure related, as the vast majority are (without a history of a specific traumatic incident), then the choice of wound dressing is often largely irrelevant unless the issue of pressure is addressed.

The number and quality of studies are inadequate to support advocating one wound care program over another or one type of dressing rather than another. The author generally prefers a moist-to-dry dressing, either with saline or povidone-iodine solution, for the effect of continuing debridement and for the drying effect on the wound. As the bandage is removed, the wound is debrided by the adherence of debris to the dried bandage, thus stimulating epithelialization from the wound margins. The key to the method is to lightly moisten the gauze (do not use cotton-filled gauze because it adheres poorly) but not to soak it. If the bandage has not dried out by the time of the next bandage change, it was applied too wet. Most moist-to-dry dressings should be changed two to three times a day. As noted above, there is no indication for daily whirlpool baths once a clean wound has been attained. At that point, the foot is only being exposed to a moist, warm environment that supports bacterial growth.

In general, the author advises against using occlusive type dressings or ointment because they prevent drainage and do not promote debridement of the wound.

Recently developed wound-healing agents derived from platelets and blood products have been suggested by their proponents to be beneficial in achieving healing of chronic wounds. In the opinion of experts in the field, these treatments not only remain controversial but are also unproven. Adequate, objective, nonproprietary, multicenter controlled studies remain to be performed to demonstrate the efficacy of these treatments. At the time of this writing, endorsement must be withheld from these treatments.

Nonhealing Ulcers

When ulcers fail to heal or if they recur after healing has been achieved once, this is an indication of excessive internal bony pressure that perpetuates the ulcer. If external relief of pressure cannot be achieved by shoe wear, insoles, or the cast treatments outlined above, then pressure relief must be obtained by internal methods of modifying the bony prominences within, i.e., surgery.

Surgery in the diabetic should never be done in a cavalier fashion, and the patient should be shown to have adequate vascularity to support healing; otherwise the surgery might produce further tissue necrosis. However, the presumed prohibition against any and all surgical procedures in the diabetic foot is unwarranted and incorrect. Failure to remove the source of the lesion is more dangerous than the judicious use of surgery to correct a deformity and relieve bony pressure. Surgical procedures for the relief of pressure are considered below by the anatomic region of the foot involved and by the type of lesions that occurs.

Surgery for Chronic and Recurrent Ulceration

Certain technical principles apply to this type of procedure. A separate incision should usually be made away from the area of the ulcer, if possible, along the medial or lateral border of the foot or dorsally. In most cases, excision of bone through the ulcer itself should be avoided. It is preferable to avoid plantar incisions if possible; in most instances it is best to leave the ulcer open to heal secondarily after it has been debrided. At surgery, the ulcer is debrided and opened up to enhance drainage by gravity; if anything is closed, it is the surgical incision, which is usually loosely closed, depending on the condition of the surrounding soft tissue and the presence or absence of infection. If uncertain whether to close the incision, it is best to leave it open and return the patient to the operating room for redebridement, irrigation, and delayed closure after several days. Once the surgical wounds have healed, the ulcer should be treated with the same type of external pressure relief noted above, such as a cast. Removal of the internal source of pressure should allow healing of the ulcer thereafter. Failure of the ulcer to heal signifies that either an insufficient amount of bone was resected (i.e., inadequate relief of pressure) or there is another factor responsible such as residual infection, ischemia, or poor nutrition.

Toe Ulcerations.—Many chronic toe ulcers lead to osteomyelitis; these typically occur over the dorsum of the proximal interphalangeal joint from shoe pressure against a hammer toe or at the tip of a clawed or hammered toe. Osteomyelitis in the phalanges is rarely cured by antibiotics alone and usually requires partial or complete toe amputation. (See Chapter 23 on amputations for the technique.)

Ulceration of the Hallux.—Most ulcerations of the great toe occur on the plantar-medial surface of the digit, underlying the bony prominences of the interphalangeal joint (Fig 22–25). This is the widest part of the toe, and the pressure is frequently accentuated by pronation of the digit, which is associated with a hallux valgus or pes planus deformity. If these ulcers are treated in a cast, care must be taken to extend the cast

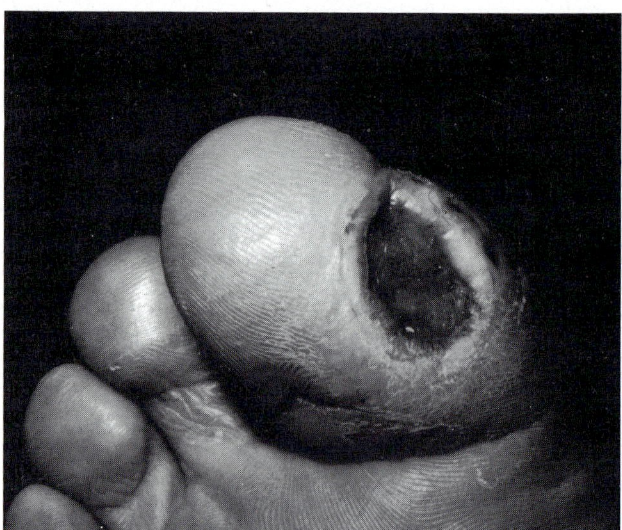

FIG 22–25.
Characteristic ulceration over the plantar-medial aspect of the interphalangeal joint of the hallux.

just past the tips of the toes (in an open-toe type). The cast is frequently made too thin at this distal edge and is flexible or breaks; reinforcement or application of a piece of ¼-in. plywood may be necessary if a closed-toe cast is not used. If this is unsuccessful, then surgery is considered.

There are four different procedures that can be used to alleviate the pressure in this location (Fig 22–26,A–D). The easiest and most commonly used is partial resection of the condyles of both the proximal and distal phalanges at the joint. Another choice is to resect the joint and excise the base of the distal phalanx and the head of the proximal phalanx all the way across the joint; however, this procedure is more frequently used in cases of osteomyelitis that has extended from an ulcer in this location. If condylar resection is unsuccessful or the ulcer recurs, the next choice is usually a dorsiflexion osteotomy done at the base of the proximal phalanx. These usually heal slowly and must be protected with a surgical shoe, walker, or cast postoperatively. The advantage of this procedure is that the function of the toe is relatively preserved and the toe is not floppy as it is with resection of the joint.

The fourth choice is to perform a modified Keller procedure, i.e., resection of the proximal half of the base of the proximal phalanx. This decompresses the toe and diminishes its function by rendering it rather floppy. This has a high success rate in terms of ulcer healing[35] but has the disadvantage of significantly weakening the toe. If it is too floppy, it may be subject to other pressures in the shoe and lead to ulceration in other locations. A mechanically incompetent (floppy) toe may retard weight transfer to the first metatarsal and can possibly contribute to a transfer of pressure lat-

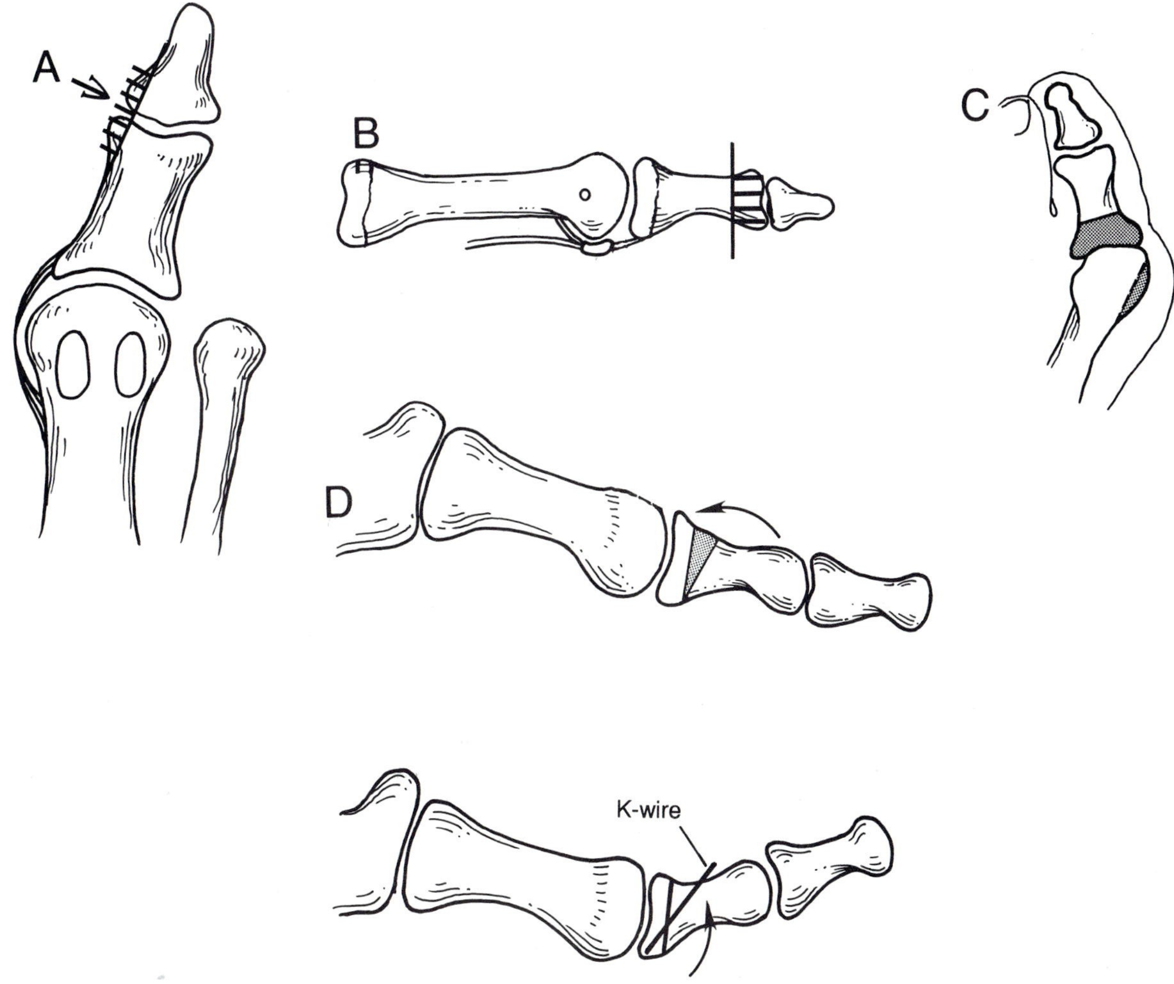

FIG 22–26.
Four procedures for recalcitrant ulceration over the condyles of the interphalangeal joint of the hallux. **A,** reduction of the condyles of the joint. **B,** resection of the interphalangeal joint. **C,** modified Keller procedure (resection of the base of the proximal phalanx. **D,** dorsiflexion osteotomy of the base of the proximal phalanx. (**C** from Mann RA, Coughlin MJ: *The video textbook of foot and ankle surgery,* St Louis, 1991, Medical Video Productions. Used by permission.)

erally, with development of lesions underneath the second metatarsal head.

First Metatarsal Head Ulcerations.—Ulcerations beneath the first metatarsal head are usually due to pressure from the two weight-bearing points of the sesamoids; the medial sesamoid is usually slightly larger, usually bears more weight, and is associated with ulceration much more often than the lateral sesamoid. Progression of ulcers in this area can rapidly lead to osteomyelitis of the sesamoids, exposure of the flexor hallucis longus tendon and/or the metatarsophalangeal joint, and osteomyelitis of the first metatarsal head with subsequent loss of the ray through amputation. There are two basic ways to unweight the area: resection of a sesamoid, either partially or completely, or a dorsiflexion osteotomy at the base of the first metatarsal.

Partial resection of the medial sesamoid is relatively easy and is done through a horizontal incision on the medial border of the foot just plantar to the midpoint of the metatarsal (Fig 22–27,A) (see Chapter 10). Scissors dissection is done to identify the plantar sensory nerve to the great toe. Rather than entering the metatarsal-sesamoid joint, dissection is made through the fibers of the abductor hallucis and periosteum and then reflecting these structures plantarward (Fig 22–27,B). The plantar half of the bone is then resected with an oscillating saw and smoothed with a rasp. This procedure can be combined with the metatarsal dorsiflexion osteotomy described below.

Complete resection of the medial sesamoid requires opening the metatarsal-sesamoid joint. The bone is meticulously shelled out of the fibers of the medial head of the abductor hallucis. Special care is necessary to avoid the flexor hallucis longus tendon, which lies between the sesamoids. The most critical task in the procedure is preservation of the intersesamoidal ligament. Following resection the latter is sutured to the fibers of the abductor hallucis and the defect closed as completely as possible in order to minimize postoperative hallux valgus deformity. The risk of postoperative deformity is higher in diabetics with insensitivity than in nondiabetics (Fig 22–28). Postoperative cast immobilization is frequently needed for 3 to 6 weeks.

Dorsiflexion osteotomy is done at the base of the metatarsal by making a dorsally based closing wedge osteotomy to raise the head of the metatarsal.[47] Fixation may be achieved with a compression screw. The patient is placed in either a surgical shoe or a cast postoperatively (Fig 22–29).

Ulceration Beneath the Middle Three Metatarsal Heads.—Recurrent or persistent ulcers beneath the middle three metatarsal heads are frequently associated with clawtoe deformities, i.e., metatarsophalangeal joint hyperextension and flexion of the interphalangeal joints. Surgical correction may require correction of the clawtoe as well as a surgical procedure on the metatarsal itself. This usually requires extensor tendon lengthening, extensive capsulotomy of the metatarsophalangeal joint, and proximal interphalangeal joint resection with retrograde pinning of the toe back to the metatarsal. If the clawtoe deformity is mild, the procedure can often be limited to the metatarsal itself. There are three options for metatarsal procedures: (1) metatarsal condylectomy, (2) metatarsal head resection, or (3) dorsiflexion osteotomy of the metatarsal. The often repeated caveat against resection of a metatarsal head is only partially correct. Although it can lead to transfer of pressure to an adjacent metatarsal and subsequent new ulcer formation, in the diabetic with advanced neuropathy, metatarsal head excision is generally preferable to an osteot-

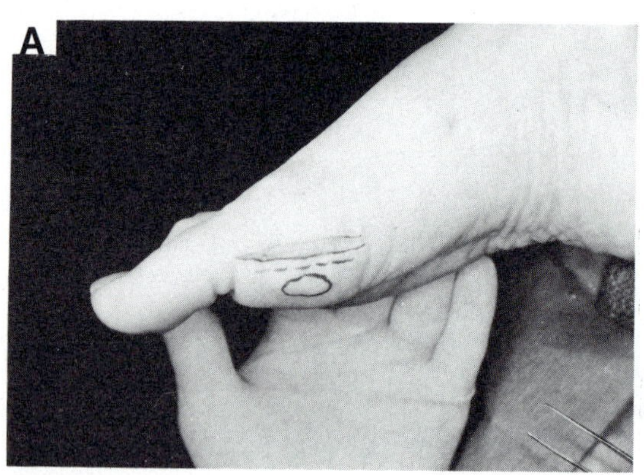

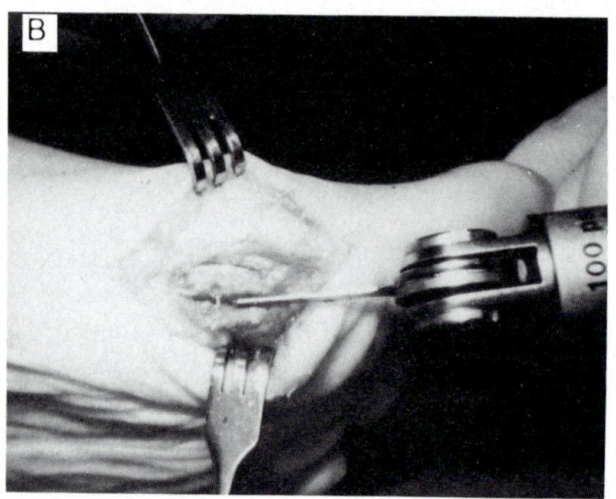

FIG 22–27.
A and **B,** partial excision of the medial sesamoid for plantar ulceration. The dissection remains extra-articular, and the plantar half of the bone is resected with a saw.

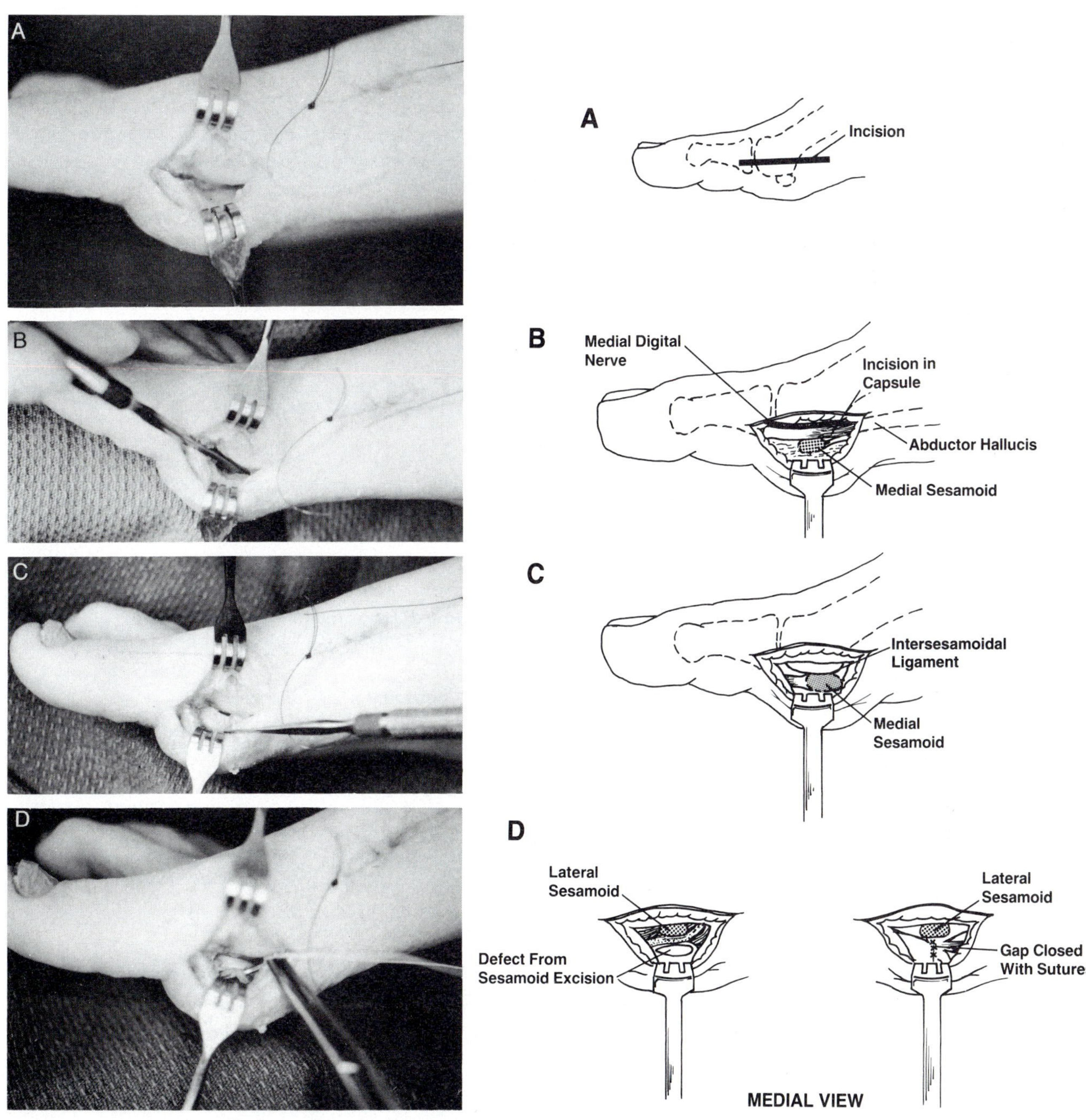

FIG 22–28.
Surgical technique for complete excision of the medial sesamoid. **A,** the sesamoid-metatarsal joint is exposed. **B,** the lateral edge of the medial sesamoid is demonstrated. This is where the intersesamoid ligament is preserved. **C,** the sesamoid is removed. **D,** reconstruction of the flexor hallucis brevis tendon. The flexor hallucis longus tendon is visualized.

omy of the metatarsal. An osteotomy requires time to heal, and failure of healing with development of a nonunion may occur because of the underlying neuropathy. Many patients with solitary metatarsal head excisions function well with proper shoe wear and insoles. The procedure should be done through a dorsal incision that is loosely closed; simultaneous resection of the ulcer is done if there is necrotic tissue or infection; otherwise the ulcer.is not resected if it is grade 1. If debrided, the ulcer should be excised in an elliptical shape down through the full thickness of soft tissue, including removal of exposed tendon and plantar plate, if necessary.

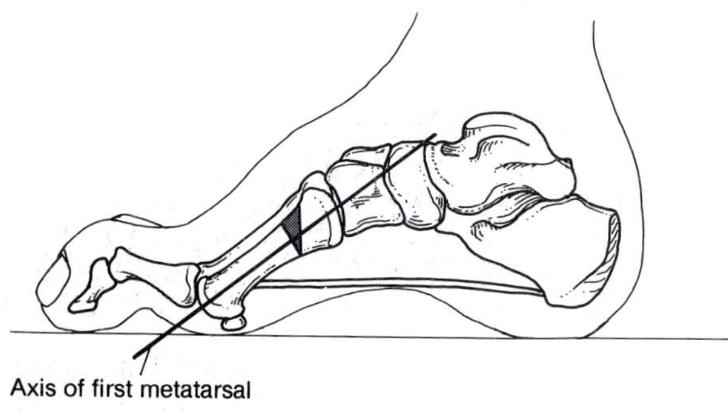

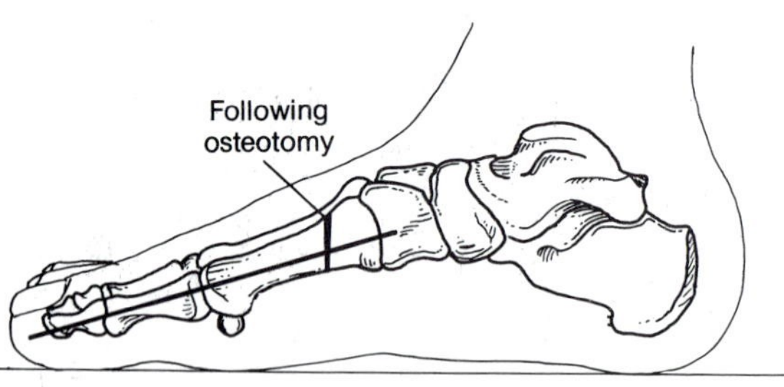

FIG 22–29.
Dorsiflexion osteotomy at the base of the first metatarsal for relief of chronic ulceration under the first metatarsal head. (From Mann RA, Coughlin MJ: *The video textbook of foot and ankle surgery,* St Louis, 1991, Medical Video Productions. Used by permission.)

The bone is resected with a saw because it splinters less than osteotomes, and the cut is beveled from the dorsal distal to the plantar proximal direction (Fig 22–30,A and B) in order to prevent a sharp plantar edge on the residual bone end.

A modified DuVries condylectomy is a reasonable intermediate solution between osteotomy and metatarsal head resection. There is a lower risk of transfer lesions because some of the weight-bearing function of the metatarsal head is preserved (see Chapter 9). Postoperative care requires protection in a surgical shoe, brace, or a cast until the ulcer is healed. The choice is somewhat empiric and depends upon the circumstances of the given patient.

When a patient has had multiple, recurrent ulcerations under several metatarsal heads, the surgeon is faced with two choices once it has been determined that conservative, nonoperative techniques will not work. These include either transmetatarsal amputation or a modified Hoffmann procedure (resection of all five of the lesser metatarsal heads). The latter has the advantage of preserving the toes. While they are largely nonfunctional in flexion and extension, they serve to preserve the length of the forefoot and make shoe fitting easier. A high-top shoe is less likely to be necessary after the metatarsal head resections than after a transmetatarsal amputation, where it is frequently required. The procedure is best done in a fashion similar to a rheumatoid foot reconstruction, but with resection of all five metatarsal heads. They are beveled as illustrated in Figure 22–30, with each metatarsal cut made at least 2 to 3 mm proximal to the level of resection of the metatarsal immediately medial to the one being cut. Good results have been reported.[53]

Fifth Metatarsal Head Ulcerations.—Fifth metatarsal head ulcerations are somewhat less difficult surgically because a condylectomy can be done from the lateral border of the foot (Fig 22–31). Resection of the metatarsal head or distal third of the bone can also be done through this approach if a condylectomy is unsuccessful or needs to be revised. Care must be taken to repair the capsule of the joint and to not detach the insertion of the capsule and plantar plate from the base of the prox-

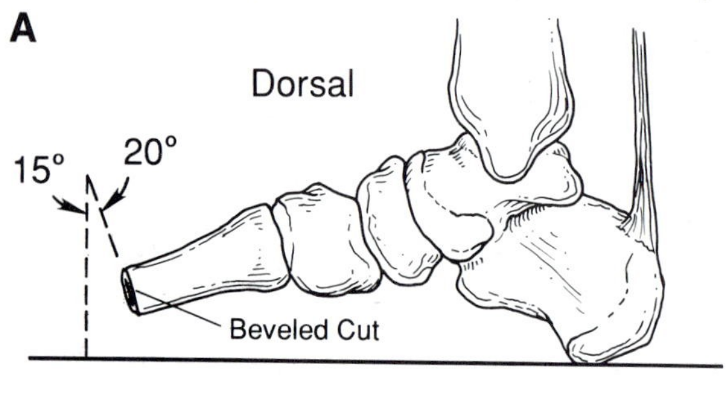

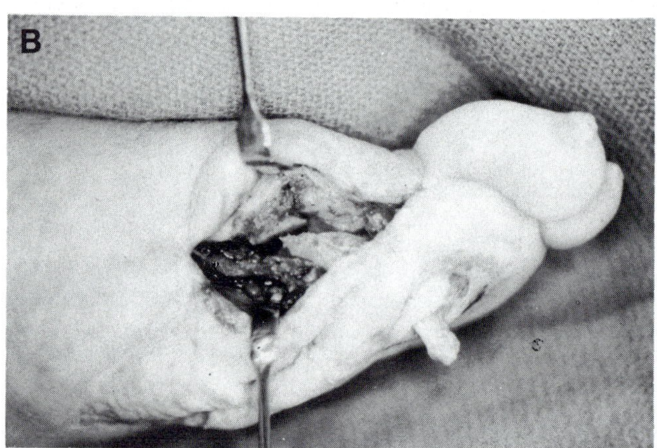

FIG 22–30.
A, beveled saw cut on the resected metatarsal angled from a dorsal-distal to a plantar-proximal direction in order to prevent a sharp corner on the distal plantar edge of the bone. **B,** resection of a metatarsal causing persistent ulceration in a patient with previous ray amputation. The relation of the ulcer to the distal metatarsal is shown by the bone protruding through the skin.

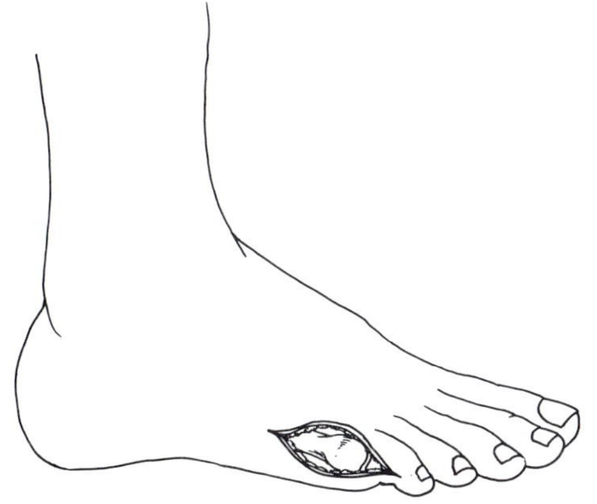

FIG 22–31.
Technique for fifth metatarsal condylectomy through a lateral incision.

imal phalanx because of the risk of dorsal or medial migration of the toe postoperatively (Fig 22–32).

Ulcerations Associated With Charcot Joints.—Ulcerations occur around Charcot joints as a result of the bony pressure caused by the structural disruption of the foot. Huge portions of the bone can migrate to the plantar surface or to the medial or lateral borders of the foot. The collapse of the arch, which produces the classic "rocker-bottom" foot, can concentrate pressure on the midtarsal bones that leads to pressure ulcerations. Initially these should be treated with the same wound care and external methods for relief of pressure as ulcers in the forefoot, i.e., using special shoes, walking braces, or total-contact casts. Surgical intervention takes two possible forms: resection of the bony protuberances that underlie the ulcer or surgical reconstruction and arthro-

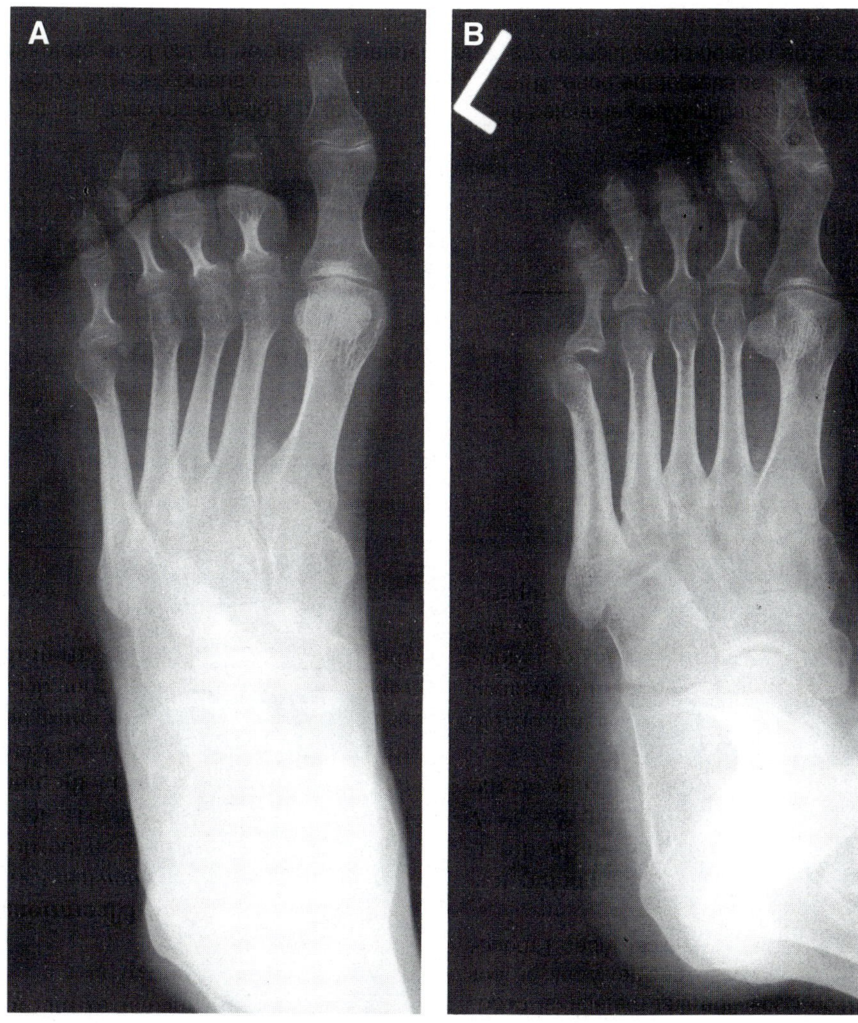

FIG 22–32.
Complication of condylectomy of the fifth metatarsal with subsequent dislocation of the metatarsophalangeal joint.

desis of the midfoot, hindfoot, or ankle, depending upon the area affected by the Charcot joint. The techniques, risks, and pitfalls of these procedures are discussed below in the section on Charcot joints.

Ulcers on the Lateral Border of the Foot.—Persistent ulcers on the lateral border of the foot occur most often at or over the base of the fifth metatarsal. There is almost always a pre-existing varus deformity of the hindfoot that predisposes to increased pressure in this area, and the examiner should suspect and document this (Fig 22–33). Resection of the prominent bone is only sometimes successful, depending in large measure on the severity of the varus position. If too much bone is removed, the function of the peroneus brevis may be lost. If a large amount of bone is removed, the peroneus brevis tendon must often be reattached. Oftentimes it is impossible to resect enough bone to allow healing of the ulcer because the force applied by the varus deformity is so great. In this case, external bracing with a custom polypropylene AFO can be considered, but the patient will sometimes require a triple arthrodesis to correct the hindfoot position. This is another procedure to be done with at least a modicum of circumspection in the face of the insensitivity of diabetic neuropathy. The risk for amputation from chronic osteomyelitis of the midfoot caused by the ulcer must be balanced against the risk of producing a Charcot-type foot if the arthrodesis fails and proceeds to nonunion.

Soft-Tissue Coverage.—Soft-tissue coverage under a plantar ulcer is almost always achieved by allowing granulation and healing by secondary intention once the bone resection or bone modification has been achieved. The principles underlying these procedures are adequate resection of bone followed by protected weight bearing. In addition to this traditional approach, a technique of soft-tissue coverage has been described in which muscle transposition has been used to cover soft-tissue defects on the sole by using the intrinsic flexor muscle bellies.[45]

Infections in the Diabetic Foot

Microbiology

The most important characteristic of infection of the diabetic foot is the frequency with which it is polymicrobial.[72, 108] In other orthopaedic infections, cultures that have more than one organism are generally considered to be contaminated since most major infections have a single or primary etiologic agent. In major infections of the diabetic foot, a failure to exercise the proper technique that would yield multiple organisms can significantly impair the outcome of treatment. The most common mistake is a failure to culture for anaerobic organisms. Proper technique is essential and requires the use of special culture swabs usually with a gel-like transport media designed for anaerobic specimens, without which anaerobic cultures are not reliable. Proper selection of an antibiotic regimen is based upon these culture results whenever possible (Fig 22–34). The presence of a foul odor in certain diabetic foot infections is attributable to the participation of anaerobic pathogens, which give rise to the classic "fetid foot" of diabetes.

The most typical combination of organisms includes gram-positive cocci (e.g., *Staphylococcus*, group B *Streptococcus*, group D *Streptococcus*, i.e., *Enterococcus*), gram-negative aerobic enteric rods (e.g., coliforms such as *Escherichia coli*, *Enterobacter*, *Proteus*, *Pseudomonas*), and anaerobes (e.g., *Bacteroides fragilis*, *Bacteroides* and

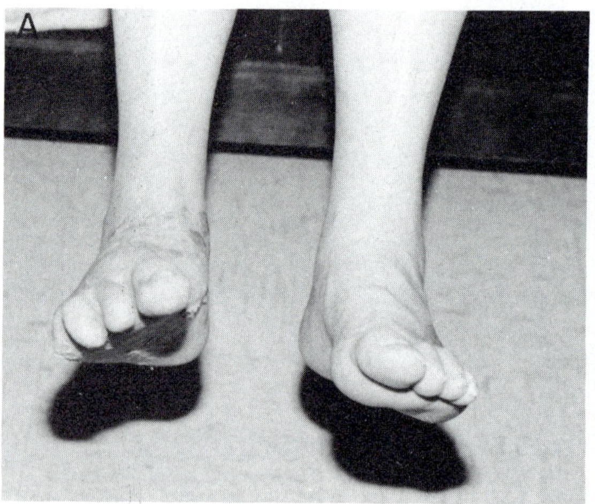

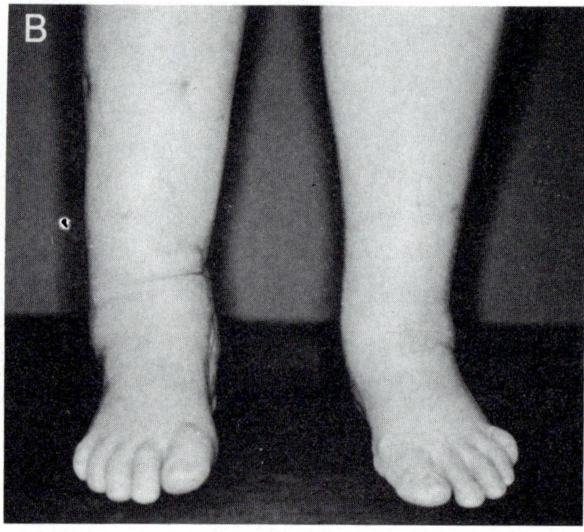

FIG 22–33.
Ulceration on the lateral border of the foot as a result of varus deformity of the hindfoot **(A)** and ankle **(B)**.

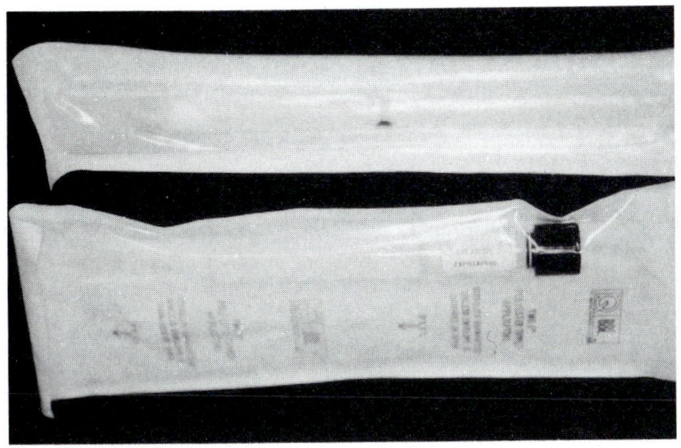

FIG 22–34.
Anaerobic and aerobic culture transport media.

Clostridium species, peptostreptococci). It is possible to have an infection caused by a single organism; when this occurs, it is usually a gram-positive bacterium, sometimes a gram-negative, but almost never an anaerobe alone.[94, 108] *Enterococcus* is a common but distinct organism that is important to distinguish from the other (group B) streptococci. It is virulent, can lead to bacteremia, and has a particularly resistant pattern of antibiotic sensitivity. Enterococcal species are known colonizers of the intestinal tract and include *Streptococcus faecalis* and others classified as group D streptococci. Unlike the nonenterococcal species of streptococci, these organisms are resistant to penicillin, aminoglycosides, and cephalosporins, although synergistic killing is obtained with certain combinations. They are usually sensitive to certain semisynthetic penicillins, imipenem, and vancomycin.

Not only is the proper culture technique important, but the quality of material from which the culture is obtained is crucial as well. Organisms obtained by taking superficial swabs from the surface of ulcers, sinus tracts, and the outside layer of a deep wound have been proved to correlate poorly with the microbiology of the deep tissues of the wounds.[89, 90, 94] Although some correlation often occurs, there is frequently a superficial colonization of organisms other than those responsible for the deep pathology below. For major wounds, especially those that will require surgical debridement, cultures must be obtained by techniques other than simple swabbing of the wound. The most reliable technique is to biopsy the tissue intraoperatively through a separate incision apart from the ulcer or wound. In the outpatient setting of the clinic or office, curettage and culture of the base of the ulcer have been shown to yield greater concordance with deep cultures as compared with simply swabbing the surface. Deep or even curetted cultures are not always possible or practical to obtain but should be especially considered in deep or difficult wounds.

The purpose of dwelling on the types of cultures and technique for gathering cultures is that the choice of antibiotic and the duration of therapy usually depend on this information. Antibiotic selection is initially empiric and based on the most likely combination of organisms. Once culture reports have been obtained, then the antibiotic regimen can usually be modified to the specific sensitivity patterns of adequately obtained specimens. A more detailed discussion of the selection of empiric and culture-specific antibiotics is below.

More the rule than the exception, patients who are admitted to the hospital for treatment of severe diabetic foot infections have already been treated as outpatients with oral antibiotics. This is often tantamount to partial antibiotic treatment such that the patient has received enough antibiotic to suppress the new cultures but not sufficient antibiotic to cure the infection.

This can lead to not inconsiderable confusion when the culture report returns as "negative," suggesting that there is no active infection at all, or the culture report reflects a superficial colonization unrepresentative of the smoldering infection below. Certainly this is a time when deep specimens are needed for culture. Sometimes it is additionally necessary to stop all oral antibiotics for 24 to 72 hours preoperatively in order to enhance the surgical cultures. Even with this measure, some of the cultures will be negative. In cases of suspected or known osteomyelitis, the surgeon must always submit a bone specimen for histologic examination as well as for aerobic and anaerobic cultures. These should be in addition to aerobic and anaerobic cultures of the soft tissue also. In fact, whenever bone is resected in the diabetic foot, it should undergo pathologic examination for microscopic evidence of infection within the bone. The surgeon should specifically request that the pathologist "examine the bone for histologic evidence of osteomyelitis." This is usually illustrated by the presence of inflammatory cells acutely and/or chronically within the marrow space. The histologic substantiation of the presence or absence of osteomyelitis is often the decisive basis for determining the length of treatment with intravenous antibiotics, as well as the choice of antibiotic regimens, especially given the frequency that cultures are affected by presurgical oral antibiotic regimens.

Antibiotic Regimens and Selections

As noted, an empiric antibiotic selection is necessary until specific culture and sensitivity information is available. In the patient who has been pretreated with oral antibiotics and negative cultures have resulted or in the

TABLE 22–3.

Useful Newer Antibiotics*

Antibiotics†	Class	Spectrum Covered	Usual Dose‡	Route
Ceftazidime (Fortaz) (Tazidime) (Tazicef)	Third-generation cephalosporin	Some gram-positive cocci, staphylococci, and streptococci *Pseudomonas aeruginosa* Not enterococci, methicillin-resistant *Staphylococcus aureus (MRSA),* or *Bacteroides fragilis* Poor against *S. aureus* and anaerobes	1–2 g q8–12h	IV
Ceftriaxone (Rocephin)	Third-generation cephalosporin	Similar to ceftazidime except for poor *Pseudomonas* coverage	1–2 g/day 1–2 g q12h	IV
Imipenem (Primaxin)	Carbapenem	Staphylococci, streptococci, gram-negative rods, *Pseudomonas,* and some anaerobes *Pseudomonas* resistance develops Not for MRSA and methicillin-resistant *Staphylococcus epidermidis* (MRSE)	500 mg q6–8h	IV
Ticarcillin-clavulanate (Timentin)	β-Lactam plus β-lactamase inhibitor	Gram-positive cocci, gram-negative rods, and some anaerobes Good for *enterococcus,* but not MRSA or MRSE	3.1 g q4–6h	IV
Ampicillin-sulbactam (Unasyn)	Same as ticarcillin-clavulanate	Same as ticarcillin-clavulanate (not for *Pseudomonas)*	3 g q6h	IV
Amoxacillin-clavulanate (Augmentin)	Same as ticarcillin-clavulanate	Same as ticarcillin-clavulanate (not for *Pseudomonas)*	500 mg q8h	PO
Clindamycin	Macrolide	Anaerobes and aerobic gram-positive cocci Not for gram-negative rods Complications of *Clostridium difficile* colitis	300–900 mg q4–8h	IV or PO
Aztreonam (Azactam)	Monobactam	Aerobic gram-negative rods Same spectrum as aminoglycosides, low nephrotoxicity	1–2 g q8–12h	IV
Ciprofloxacin (Cipro)	Quinolone	*S. aerus,* gram-negative rods including *Pseudomonas* Do not use in children under 16 years or in pregnant women Poor activity against anaerobes and streptococci Usually not as a single agent in major infections	500–750 mg bid	PO
Vancomycin	Macrolide	MRSA, MRSE, enterococci in penicillin-allergic patients Not gram-negative rods or anaerobes Nephrotoxic with aminoglycosides Oral form not absorbed	1 g q12–24h; must adjust according to serum levels	

*Adapted from Brodsky JW, Schneidler C: *Orthop Clin North Am* 22:473–489, 1991. Used by permission.

†Proprietary names (in parentheses) are noted as examples only and do not signify endorsement or recommendation. No outside financial support has been given to this article or authors.

‡Dosages may require adjustment according to renal function, which is often diminished in diabetics, and in the elderly.

patient in whom deep cultures cannot be obtained for whatever reason, then an empiric regimen is the only choice.

In the past, regimens of two and three drugs have been required to treat documented or suspected multiple organisms. Older regimens such as an aminoglycoside (e.g., gentamicin) and a β-lactamase–resistant penicillin have been adequate but raise the issue of possible nephrotoxicity, of special concern in the diabetic who may have pre-existing impairment of renal function. In general, the empiric regimen must be aimed at a broad spectrum of coverage.[20]

Newer third-generation cephalosporins have found a special place in these drug regimens. While most of these have an enhanced spectrum of coverage for gram-negative organisms, they are less effective than first-generation cephalosporins against gram-positive cocci such as *Staphylococcus* and *Streptococcus*. Examples include but are not limited to drugs such as ceftriaxone and cefotaxime. Another third-generation cephalosporin, ceftazidime, is unique in its applicability against *Pseudomonas aeruginosa*. Imipenem, a new carbapenem drug, is a penicillin-related drug that has activity against *Staphylococcus*, *Enterococcus*, anaerobes, and *Pseudomonas*, although resistance to the drug can develop in *Pseudomonas* infections.

Other newer drugs that can be used in combination in the treatment of diabetic foot infections include the β-lactams with β-lactamase inhibitors such as ticarcillin–clavulanic acid or ampicillin-sulbactam. Clindamycin has activity against both aerobic and anaerobic cocci, although it is not active against gram-negative rods. Aztreonam is a new monobactam antibiotic that functions with a spectrum similar to the aminoglycosides without the risks of nephrotoxicity of the latter. See Tables 22–3 to 22–5 for a summary of some of the useful newer antibiot-

TABLE 22–4.
Drug Regimen Alternatives*

Organism	Regimen†	Route
Bacteroides fragilis	Ticarcillin-clavulanate (emerging resistance)	IV
	Metronidazole	IV & PO
	Clindamycin (emerging resistance in some hospitals)	
Group D *Streptococcus (Enterococcus)*	Ampicillin	IV & PO
	β-Lactam–based inhibitor (sulbactam or ticarcillin-clavulanate)	IV
	Vancomycin	IV
	Imipenem	IV
	Use of aminoglycoside adjunctively may be considered	IV
Staphylococcus	First-generation cephalothin, cephalosporin (Cefazolin)	IV & PO
	β-Lactamase–resistant penicillins (oxacillin, nafcillin, methicillin)	IV & PO
	Vancomycin	IV
	β-Lactamase–resistant penicillin and rifampin for difficult cases	IV & PO
Methicillin-resistant *Staphylococcus aureus*	Vancomycin	IV
Methicillin-resistant *Staphylococcus epidermidis*	Vancomycin	IV
Anaerobes	β-Lactam with β-lactamase inhibitor (ampicillin-sulbactam or ticarcillin-clavulanate)	IV
	Clindamycin	IV or PO
	Metronidazole	IV or PO
Pseudomonas aeuroginosa	Ceftazidime	IV
	Imipenem	IV
	Piperacillin	IV
	Ciprofloxacin	PO

*Adapted from Brodsky JW, Schneidler C: *Orthop Clin North Am* 22:473–489, 1991. Used by permission.
†These regimens are given as examples and do not necessarily represent the best or only regimen for a given clinical situation.

TABLE 22–5.

Sample Empiric Combination Drug Regimens for Mixed Infection in the Diabetic Foot Based on Gram Stain*

Organisms	Examples of Possible Empiric Drug Regimens†
Gram-positive cocci and gram-negative rods	Third-generation cephalosporin (e.g., ceftriaxone or ceftazidine)
Gram-positive cocci and/or gram-negative rods plus *Enterococcus*	Ampicillin-sulbactam or ticarcillin-clavulanate
Gram-positive cocci and *Bacteroides*	Imipenem Clindamycin
Gram-negative rods and *Bacteroides*	β-Lactam with β-lactamase inhibitor
Gram-positive cocci, gram-negative rods, and *Bacteroides*	Imipenem Third-generation cephalosporins plus metronidazole β-Lactam with β-lactamase inhibitor

*Adapted from Brodsky JW, Schneidler C: *Orthop Clin North Am* 22:473–489, 1991. Used by permission.

†These regimens are given as examples and do not necessarily represent the best or only regimen for a given clinical situation. Regimens should be appropriately modified according to culture and sensitivity results.

ics and for examples of possible drug regimens. It is important to note that most surgeons will consider the assistance of the primary-care physician or an infectious disease specialist in the selection and monitoring of antibiotic therapy for serious diabetic foot infections as a part of the team approach to the care of the diabetic foot. The information here represents broad guidelines and principles for the surgeon.

A few other considerations are worth mentioning regarding the use of antibiotics in this situation. First, the use of antimicrobial agents, even when properly selected empirically or on the basis of specific culture and sensitivity information, are no substitute for proper wound care and surgical debridement. It is an adjunct therapy, and a combination of all of these is usually required to achieve a cure. This is particularly true in the case of osteomyelitis, where antibiotics alone are almost *never* sufficient to achieve a cure.

Second, although surgeons are highly aware of the complications that can occur with surgical therapy, complications of the antibiotic regimen can occur also. These include intravenous catheter infection or sepsis, especially if a patient is undergoing long-term intravenous therapy for osteomyelitis and has an indwelling central line. The complication of antibiotic-induced colitis, now known to be caused by a toxin-mediated response elaborated by *Clostridium difficile*, can occur after treatment with a number of different antibiotics. Stool assays for the toxin may be required in patients who develop severe diarrhea on the drug regimens.

Third, the surgeon should take into account factors regarding the onset of the infection that influence the likelihood of a given organism. For example, patients whose infections develop in the hospital or even in a nursing home may be more likely to have a *Staphylococcus* that is methicillin resistant, a most serious problem not only for the given patient but also with regard to nosocomial spread of the pathogen to others. This situation underscores the importance of obtaining the best possible culture material prior to beginning a protracted antibiotic regimen. In this situation, vancomycin is usually the drug of choice for *Staphylococcus*. Vancomycin must usually be infused intravenously slowly over about a period of an hour or more in order to reduce the risk of the "red man syndrome," a histamine flushing reaction, and requires monitoring of blood levels. Additional drugs would still be needed to cover anaerobes and gram-negative rods that coexisted in the wound.

Another example of specific organisms related to the method or place of acquisition is a puncture wound of the foot. These injuries, especially if they occur through a shoe, classically involve infection by *Pseudomonas aeruginosa*. The organism has been isolated in the inner sole glue in tennis shoes.[42] and must be suspected when this history is present.

Gas in the Soft Tissue

Gas in the soft tissue in diabetic foot infections is not uncommon. It is very seldom if ever caused by the *Clostridium perfringens* of classic gas gangrene. Most gas in the soft tissue is caused by aerobic organisms including gram-positive cocci such as group B streptococci or enterococci, or by mixed gram-negative rods.[5] When gas is demonstrated in the soft tissue either clinically and/or on radiographs, an immediate Gram stain of the exudate is the most expeditious way to find out whether this is true gas gangrene. True gas gangrene will demonstrate gram-positive rods on the Gram stain. Gas in the soft tissue also occurs in necrotizing fascitis, an extremely serious and often fatal disorder. This disorder produces rapidly progressive tissue necrosis that can extend proximally at an alarming rate. It is fortunately uncommon, and most gas in the soft tissue of diabetic foot infections is due to the more "ordinary" pathogens.

Surgical Principles in the Treatment of Diabetic Foot Infections

The basic philosophy in the surgical treatment of the diabetic foot is "foot salvage." This signifies the use of aggressive techniques of debridement and reconstruction of the vascularity and soft tissue and conservative preservation of any soft-tissue flaps that might survive the initial debridement. As noted in the earlier section of this chapter, one of the keys to saving the foot or converting a leg amputation into a partial foot amputation is aggressive revascularization of the limb prior to or accompanying debridement or amputation. This aggressive approach has proven to yield excellent results, i.e., the maximum amount of *functioning* foot, at centers such as Rancho Los Amigos Hospital and in other locations as well, with some authors reporting a salvage rate of almost three quarters of patients who require emergency surgery.[100]

Grossly infected wounds or severe acute abscesses usually do require early aggressive surgical treatment. In theory, excessive delay can lead to progression of the disease with resultant wider areas of involvement. However, pretreatment of an indolent osteomyelitis, abscess, or infected wound that has wide concomitant cellulitis with one to several days of preoperative intravenous antibiotics can produce better rates of healing and foot salvage.[46] Diminution of the cellulitis prior to making an incision through the infected skin and subcutaneous tissue has been documented to result in a better healing rate. This is particularly true if an amputation or partial foot amputation is necessary and primary or delayed primary closure is planned. Better tissue healing generally occurs when the acute cellulitis is resolved at the time that the skin and soft-tissue flaps are handled and sutured. Pretreatment includes medical management of the diabetes as well as treatment with antibiotics; advancement to the surgical procedure is considered ideal in these cases when fever, elevation of the white blood cell count, elevation of blood glucose levels, and skin erythema diminish.[46]

As noted above, when the diagnosis of osteomyelitis is sought in the midfoot or forefoot by biopsy through a separate incision, it is possible to close that incision primarily although loosely with a few full-thickness (skin and subcutaneous tissue) nonabsorbable sutures. Simultaneous debridement of the ulcer, after the biopsy sample has been taken, allows for drainage, usually dependent drainage, which is particularly important if the biopsy (or debridement) incision is closed.

Wagner has popularized the use of an irrigation system to be used in infected wounds that are loosely closed with either a primary or delayed primary closure.[63, 105] Although antibiotics can be added to the irrigant, there is some unquantified risk of absorption of the medication from a large wound, which is of concern, especially in the diabetic patient with impaired renal function.

The author's preferred technique is illustrated in Figure 22–35 where a no. 8 pediatric feeding tube is placed in the wound through a small, separate, proximal stab incision. The irrigant, usually normal saline or Ringer's lactate, is infused at a rate of 30 to 60 mL/hr, depending on the size of the wound. The inflow is allowed to efflux through the incision itself and out through the ulcer, if an ulcer is present, between the loosely placed sutures of nonabsorbable material. The irrigation must

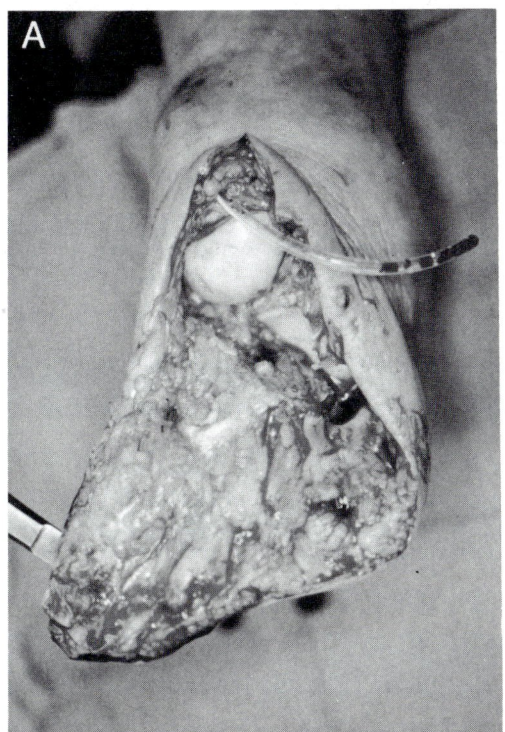

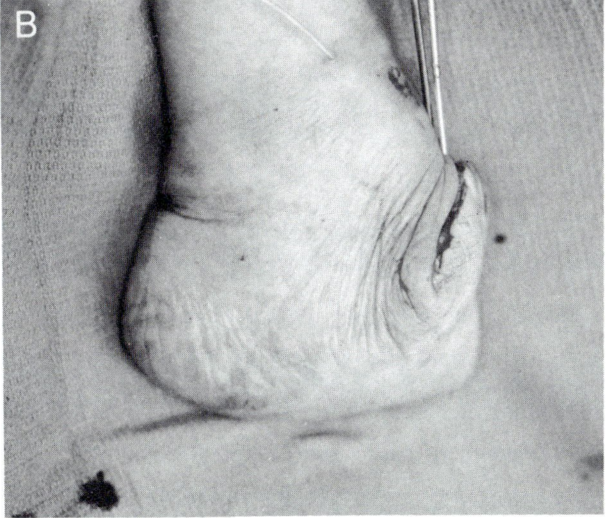

FIG 22–35.
Wound irrigation system made from a no. 8 pediatric feeding tube before **(A)** and after **(B)** wound closure.

be started prior to beginning the closure so that the holes in the catheter do not become immediately clogged with wound hematoma. Sterile intravenous extension tubing is connected intraoperatively. Additional holes are sometimes cut in the tube to increase flow. A bulky sterile dressing is applied in order to absorb the outflow from the wound. The bandage is reinforced postoperatively with towels, etc., as it soaks through. The tube is usually removed after overnight use or 24 hours, although it is occasionally left for 48 hours. Maceration of the surrounding skin is usually minimal, and a dry sterile dressing is applied after the irrigation tube is removed.

Cellulitis

Very early cellulitis can be treated on an outpatient basis with oral antibiotics if the patient is watched carefully and reexamined frequently. Once cellulitis has become established, intravenous antibiotics are the treatment of choice. Two tasks should be addressed: (1) the appropriate level of diagnosis and/or imaging to rule out a deeper infection that may be the source of the soft-tissue infection and (2) examination for clues to the onset of the infection, such as a break in the skin between the toes or a predisposing deformity that has resulted in soft-tissue breakdown. Rest and elevation are helpful adjuncts. Elevation of the red, hot, swollen foot, as noted earlier in this chapter, also helps to distinguish noninfective sources of an inflammed foot, i.e., the dependent rubor of an acute Charcot foot. Even experienced clinicians can be fooled when trying to make this distinction.

Abscess

There are three basic issues in the treatment of an abscess in the diabetic foot. The first is to delineate its location and extent and determine the method to obtain adequate material for culture and sensitivity (Fig 22–36,A and B). The second is the surgical approach for drainage and, usually, debridement of the surrounding tissues as well.[70] Third is to determine the involvement of the adjacent osseous structures and the most appropriate method of closure and foot salvage.

Preoperative imaging is especially important in the diagnosis of a suspected abscess. Prior to the development of MRI, CT afforded excellent anatomic localization. Now the former (MRI) is more sensitive and specific in visualizing an abscess because of its enhanced resolution among different soft tissues. These images should assist the surgeon in planning drainage, i.e., the closest location to the surface, the need for incisions plantarly, dorsally, or both, etc.

Most incisions for the drainage of abscesses should be made longitudinally rather than transversely because of the greater flexibility for extension that this affords (Fig 22–36,C). Plantar abscesses can involve the entire plantar fascia and/or deep compartment and require a long incision. If possible, abscesses should be drained through an incision along the lateral or medial border of the foot, depending on the location of the pathology. However, a plantar incision is often unavoidable. The author prefers straight rather than curvilinear incisions on the sole for these situations. While there is generally some reluctance to do wide exposures or radical debridements in a diabetic, as a rule, the patient is better served by and will heal sooner with a longer incision that affords adequate exposure than a small incision that forces the surgeon to leave necrotic material behind. Web space abscesses often require a web-splitting incision that wraps 270 degrees around dorsally to plantarly (Fig 22–36,C). The latter may be necessary for adequate debridement; if the adjacent metatarsophalangeal joints become dessicated, then they may have to be resected with resultant loss of one or more rays in order to achieve healing and closure of the soft tissue.

Osteomyelitis

As has been noted, osteomyelitis, once established, is seldom eradicated without surgical intervention. The principle is to resect the infected, involved bone and to do extensive debridement of the surrounding involved tissue as well. The surgeon must achieve a balance between resecting sufficient bone to allow a cure of the infection while saving as much bone as possible for the benefit of stability of the residual foot. The bone can be resected wholly or partially; transection of a bone, such as a metatarsal that has gross osteomyelitis in the metatarsal head, in the course of partial removal leads to the question of potentially leaving behind bone that still harbors microscopic medullary foci of infection. There are currently no adequate data to answer this question, but clinically, it is frequently possible to do a subtotal resection, especially of a metatarsal, and achieve resolution of the osteomyelitis provided that the patient is treated with appropriate antibiotics and thorough wound care.

The length of treatment with intravenous antibiotics that is truly "appropriate" is a matter of clinical judgment at this time. The classic fiat requiring 6 weeks of intravenous antibiotics for the entire spectrum of disease signified by the diagnosis of "osteomyelitis" is undocumented and ignores the variability of individual cases. If the infected area has been aggressively debrided and the bone or section of the bone with infec-

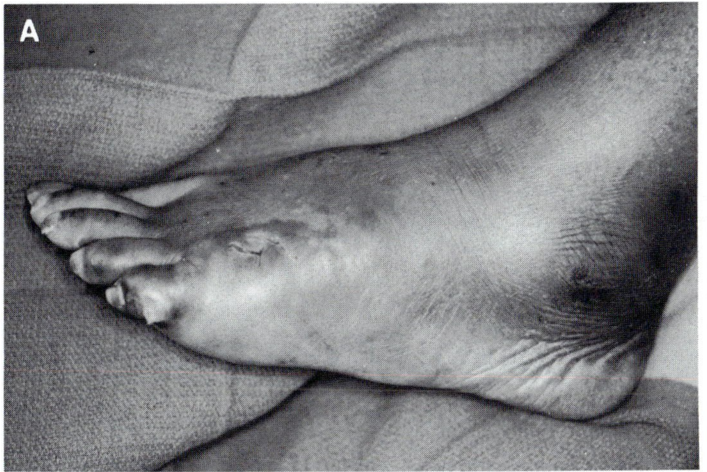

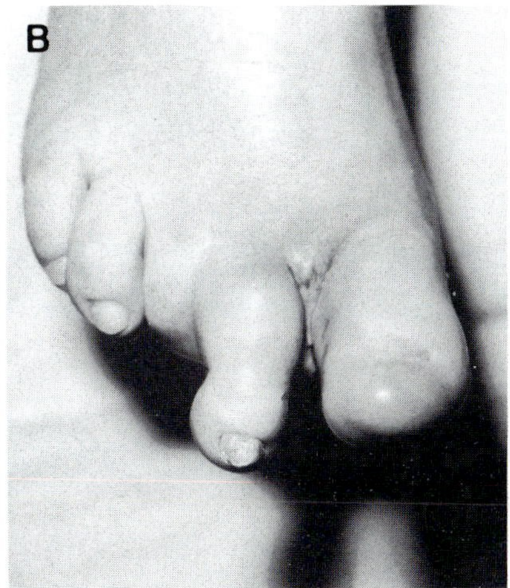

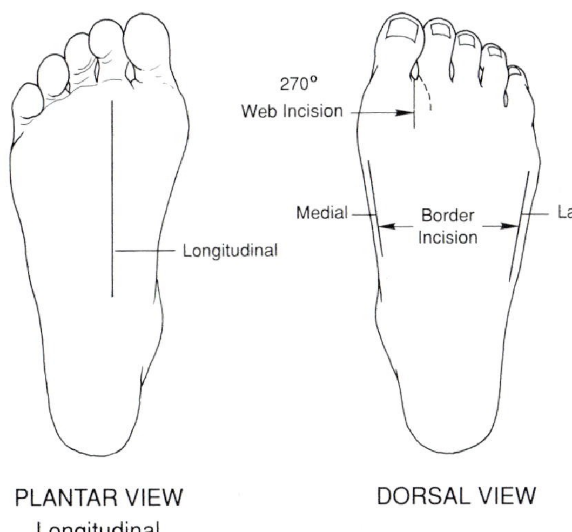

FIG 22–36.
Diabetic foot abscesses. **A,** dorsal, involving the fourth and fifth rays. **B,** a first web space abscess. **C,** incisions for drainage of abscesses.

tion has been removed in its entirety, a shorter course of antibiotics is often justified. An example would be the resection of an infected toe or distal phalanx or resection of a metatarsal head with early osteomyelitis. The decision is based upon the adequacy of the resection, and only the operating surgeon can decide this. On the other hand, when the residual bone is very close to the area of the resected osteomyelitic bone, longer treatment with intravenous antibiotics is justified. This may occur when it is too destructive or destabilizing to ablate the entire bone. An example would be retention of the base of a middle metatarsal when osteomyelitis involves the shaft, but resection of the base could lead to instability and breakdown of the entire midfoot through the tarsometatarsal joint, i.e., a Charcot joint. Another example would be osteomyelitis of the posterior portion of the tubercle of the calcaneus in which it is functionally desirable to retain as much of the bone as possible for walking, while the line delineating an adequate level of resection to eradicate the infection remains relatively indistinct.

Osteomyelitis of the Forefoot.—The majority of cases of osteomyelitis in the diabetic foot occur in the forefoot region and parallel the frequency of ulceration in this area, which in turn reflects the fact that ischemia and neuropathy generally increase in severity as they progress more distally in the limb. Many of the principles of surgical management of osteomyelitis in the diabetic foot are equally applicable to amputation surgery, and a number of techniques of amputation surgery, noted in the next chapter, apply to debridement as well.

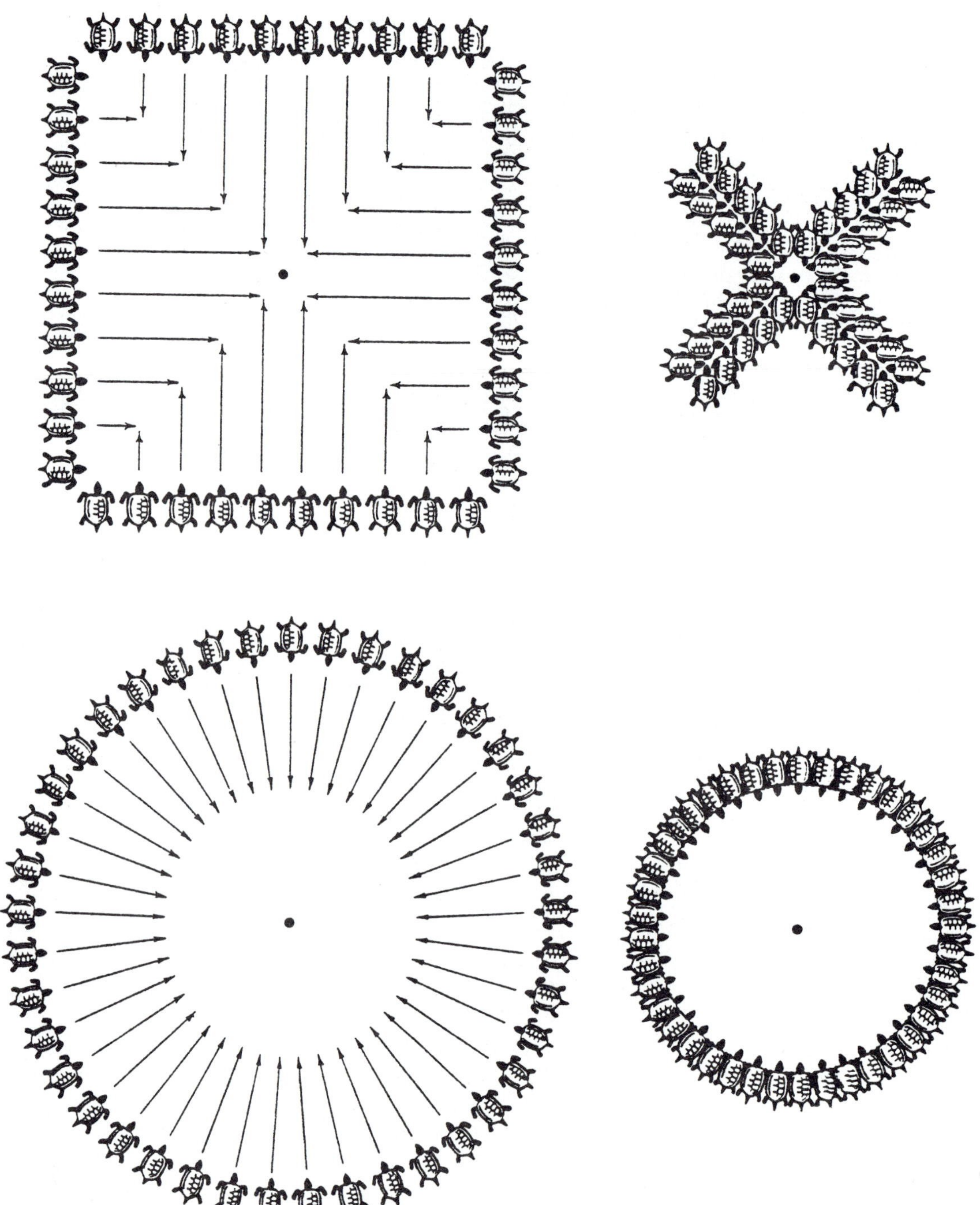

FIG 22–37.
Principles of wound contraction: round wounds do not heal until converted to another shape. (From Majno G: *The healing hand: man and wound in the ancient world,* Cambridge, Mass, Harvard University Press, 1975. Used by permission.)

The separation is somewhat artificial since amputations are commonly required to cure osteomyelitis; however, other forms of debridement and reconstruction are possible, and amputation surgery should not be construed as synonymous with surgery of the diabetic foot.

When osteomyelitis is present in the forefoot, it is best to do the debridement through an incision on the dorsum[48] or along the medial or lateral border of the foot. Most important is to keep the incision away from the area of the ulcer or draining wound in most instances, i.e., the debridement is usually approached through a separate surgical incision, not through the infected wound itself. This often allows loose primary closure of the wound with full-thickness nonabsorbable sutures in order to allow drainage, provided that the wound or ulcer is adequately debrided as well. The ulcer debridement must be aggressive and remove a generous layer of tissue, not just in the dermis, but through the full thickness of the soft tissue in order to allow adequate (and preferably, gravity) drainage. If an irrigation system is used as discussed in the preceding section, good flow allows early closure of the dorsal surgical incision. The ulcer debridement should be conceptualized as the removal of a cylinder of tissue in the dorsal-plantar direction. If the surgeon is reticent to aggressively widen the wound, the amount of tissue removed becomes less and less the deeper the debridement goes, and a wide hole is left in the skin but a narrow outlet to the wound in its deepest level (reverse funnel). This type of ulcer debridement drains poorly and impedes healing.

The ulcer will also heal more readily if, in the course of debridement, it is converted from a round shape to an ellipse (at all its levels) (Fig 22–37). Some authors advocate closing the ulcer and leaving the surgical incision open, but it makes sense to do the opposite, i.e., to close the cleaner, surgical wound and leave open the more contaminated of the two.

Osteomyelitis of the Toes.—Osteomyelitis of the toes can rarely be treated with long-term antibiotics alone, and this is the exception and not the rule. The few cases the author has witnessed have been in patients who could not undergo surgery because of other severe medical problems that required 2 months or greater of intravenous antibiotics, during which time the toe healed. Such a treatment primarily for osteomyelitis of the toe would be impossible to justify on a cost or risk basis routinely and, in most cases, would not result in a cure.

In general, osteomyelitis of the toes must be dealt with by an ablative procedure that transects or disarticulates all or part of the toe. Acral osteomyelitis in the distal phalanx of a toe in a diabetic is typically indolent and can persist without significant progression for months, oftentimes suddenly spreading or becoming more severe without warning. The indolent course of the osteomyelitis is, however, often marked by a huge, sausage-like enlargement of the entire digit, even when the infection appears confined to one small area on the radiograph (Fig 22–38). Many times the toe will enlarge to a volume double the normal size.

Not all toe amputations should be performed at the metatarsophalangeal joint level. There is a definite indication for partial toe amputations in the armamentarium of the orthopaedic surgeon. This procedure permits ablation of the infected portion of the digit while preserving enough of the toe to serve as a spacer between the two adjacent toes (Fig 22–39). In cases of amputation of the distal phalanx for osteomyelitis, it is often possible to do a primary closure, especially if pretreated with antibiotics to reduce the cellulitis and edema in the soft tissue. The technique must emphasize preservation of soft tissue for closure. The surgeon should save a maximum of skin and subcutaneous tissue, and it must be cut at a level at least 5 mm distal to the level of bone resection. Sometimes this requires cutting through the skin right up to the edge of the necrosis or ulcer; as is always the case in diabetic wound closure, a balance must be struck between the amount of bone preserved and the amount of soft tissue available to cover it. When there is insufficient soft tissue, the best technique is usually to remove more bone so that a primary closure can be achieved without skin tension.

Once the entire toe has been amputated, the pressure of even properly fitted prescription shoe wear will cause the two adjacent toes to drift into the defect from either side (Fig 22–40). As they drift into varus and valgus respectively, these toes touch as if to fill the void and leave a defect in which other toes can also drift in "domino" fashion.

It is often worthwhile to save just the base of the proximal phalanx, provided that the surgeon is relatively confident that it is free of infection. This is especially true in the great toe if a minimum of 1 cm can be preserved.[84] By preserving the base of the proximal phalanx in the hallux or the lesser toes, the attachment of and at least partial function of the plantar fascia is retained, thus enhancing the weight-bearing function of the corresponding metatarsal.

Osteomyelitis of the First Metatarsophalangeal Joint and Sesamoids of the Hallux.—The most plantar structures beneath the joint, which correspond to the pressure concentration that leads to ulcers and thus also to osteomyelitis, are the sesamoids. As noted above, the medial sesamoid is usually larger, exerts more pressure, and is more often involved with infection. Special sesamoid views are frequently required on plain radiographs to identify an erosion of the plantar cortex of the sesamoid bone, which represents osteomyelitis (Fig 22–41). Technetium bone scans can be helpful in localization only and do not distinguish infection from fracture or even severe sesamoiditis. If a bone scan is performed, it should be specified that the radionuclide camera be turned upside down and the feet placed directly on it in order to image the plantar surface of the

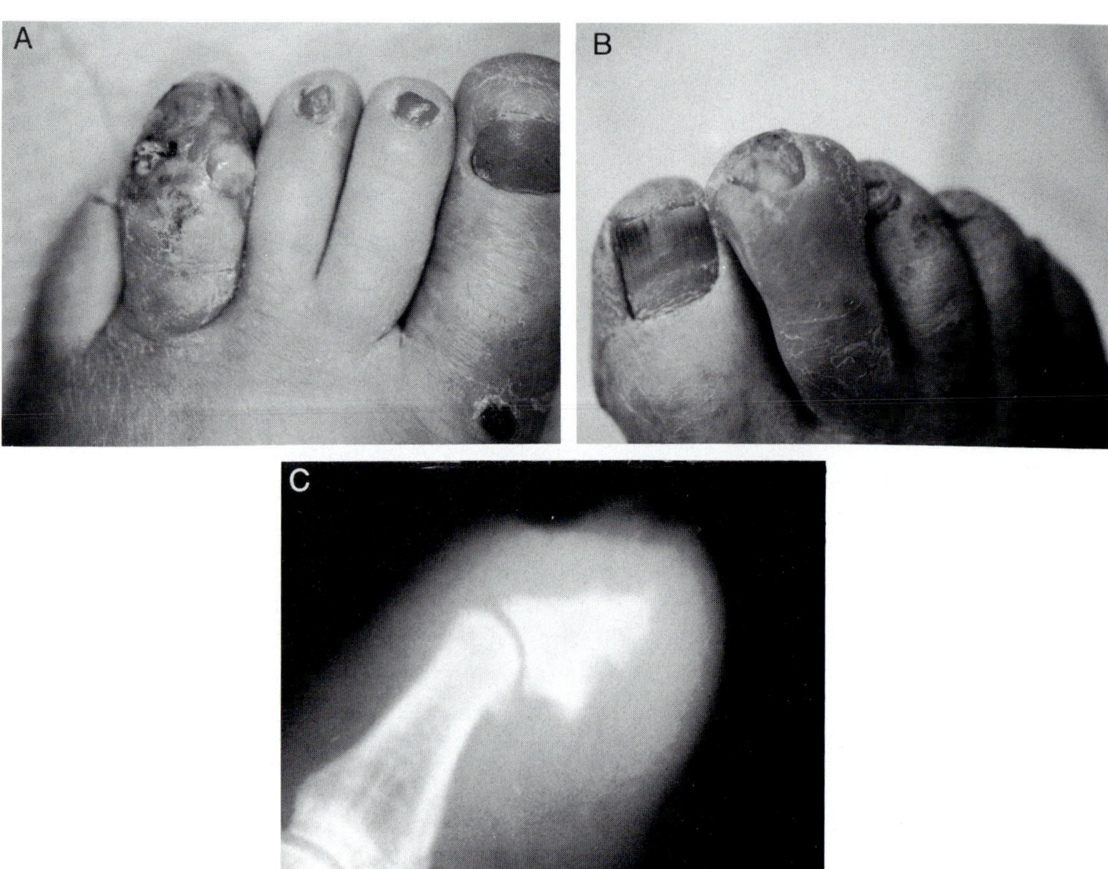

FIG 22–38.
Osteomyelitis of the toe. **A,** destruction of the proximal interphalangeal joint. **B,** involvement of the distal phalanx due to ulceration at the tip of a mallet toe deformity. **C,** erosion of the distal phalanx of the toe in **B.**

foot. Complete excision of a sesamoid may be required once osteomyelitis is established, with the attendant risks of a late hallux valgus deformity (see also Chapter 10). The surgical technique is described above in the section on ulcerations. Once a sesamoid has been resected, the problem of exposed articular cartilage of the plantar aspect of the first metatarsal head remains. There is no single answer to this dilemma; sometimes the soft tissue can be drawn together or covered with the muscle transposition noted above. Occasionally, resection of the articular cartilage and subchondral bone is necessary in order to expose bleeding cancellous bone to prompt the formation of granulation tissue, even though the barrier to metatarsal infection provided by the cartilage is removed. This remains a frequently problematic wound; therefore it is advisable to aggressively treat ulcers in this area in order to decrease the risk of progression to osteomyelitis.

Once osteomyelitis has progressed to involve the first metatarsal head, partial or complete first ray resection is usually the result (Fig 22–42). The technique is described in the following chapter on amputations. Although many feet with the first ray amputated function well, some develop problems of subsequent ulceration under the lesser metatarsal heads due to the transfer of weight-bearing pressure in a lateral direction in the forefoot. This can occur whenever the first metatarsal head is no longer bearing weight normally. The other alternative besides ray amputation is resection of the infected distal half of the metatarsal and retention of the great toe. To some patients this is cosmetically desirable and has the advantage of saving some length of the forefoot, which aids in holding onto the shoe. The disadvantage is that the toe is flail and usually drifts into a hyperextended position of variable severity; when severe, it can interfere with rather than assist in shoe fitting and lead to breakdown and further infection.

Many diabetics will require amputations of single or multiple rays (the latter being referred to as a partial forefoot amputation), and many function well. These

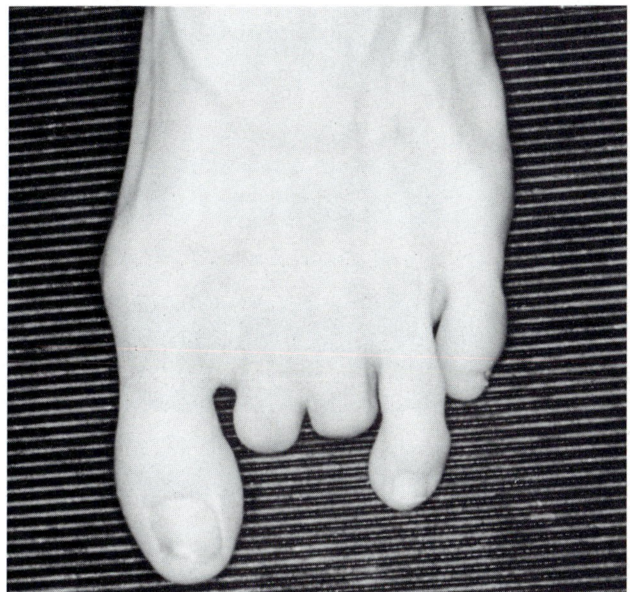

FIG 22–39.
Partial-toe amputations blocking later drift of the adjacent digits.

partial forefoot amputations frequently function well, especially if the absent ray or rays are the fifth ray alone or both of the lateral two rays. The function of medial ray amputations is more variable, but there is still a high success rate. Regardless of whether the feet have had single (or multiple) medial, lateral, or intermediate ray resections, almost all require the postoperative use of wide, deep shoes that accommodate the residual forefoot and a custom-molded cushioning insole, usually a combination of foamed polyethylene materials (Fig 22–43).

Osteomyelitis of the Lesser Metatarsal Heads.— This is one of the most common locations for the development of osteomyelitis in addition to corresponding to the most common location for ulcerations. Implied in this statement is that the vast majority of cases of osteomyelitis in the diabetic foot occur as the result of direct extension from wounds and lesions that begin locally in the overlying soft tissues. Although hematogenous osteomyelitis is not impossible, it is noticeably rare. Osteomyelitis in the lesser metatarsal heads presents a problem in view of the oft-quoted admonition against removal of a metatarsal head, as has been discussed in the section on ulcerations. However, it is often an excellent procedure not only for persistent ulcerations but also for localized bone infection. Once transfer lesions have occurred on more than one occasion, i.e., more than two metatarsal heads have been resected for osteomyelitis, then the patient should have one of two more definitive procedures: a transmetatarsal amputation or a modified Hoffmann procedure as described above in the section on ulcerations.

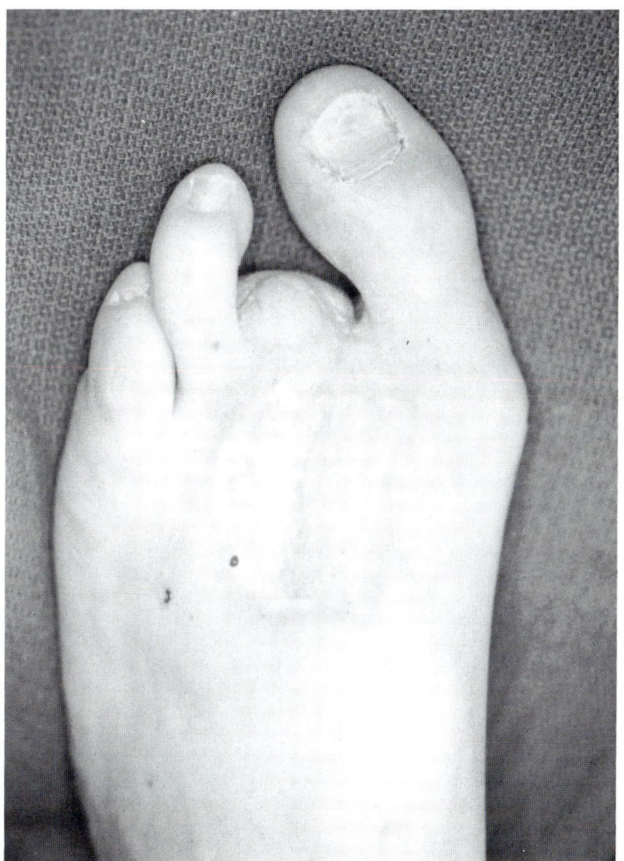

FIG 22–40.
Drift of the toes to fill the defect created by toe amputation.

As will be discussed in the chapter on amputations, one of the keys to successful ray resection is to determine whether the corresponding toe is viable or not. If the foot is relatively stiff and the toe will work to block migration of the adjacent digits and if it is clearly uninvolved by the infection, it can be saved. The other key is to maximally preserve the viable surrounding soft tissue. When the soft tissue is infected and/or necrotic as well as the bone, it must be vigorously debrided until the surgeon reaches a bleeding, viable margin of soft tissue. As noted above, regarding the principle of balancing the residual soft tissue and bone, it is often necessary to resect an additional ray that does not have osteomyelitis because there is insufficient soft tissue to cover; it is often better to sacrifice the additional ray and obtain a closed wound covered with durable plantar skin than have a slightly wider forefoot covered with an unstable skin graft that produces recurrent breakdown.

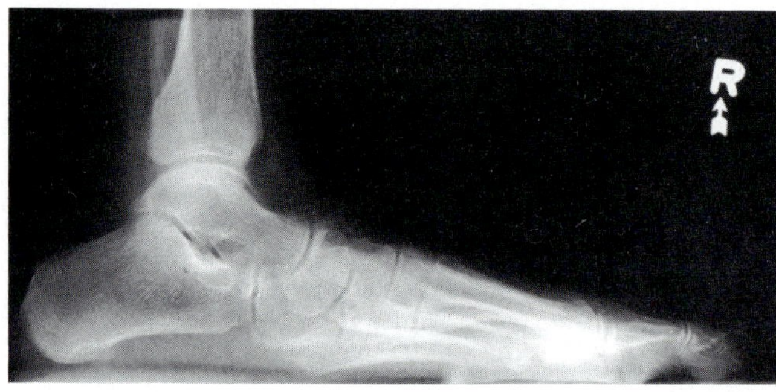

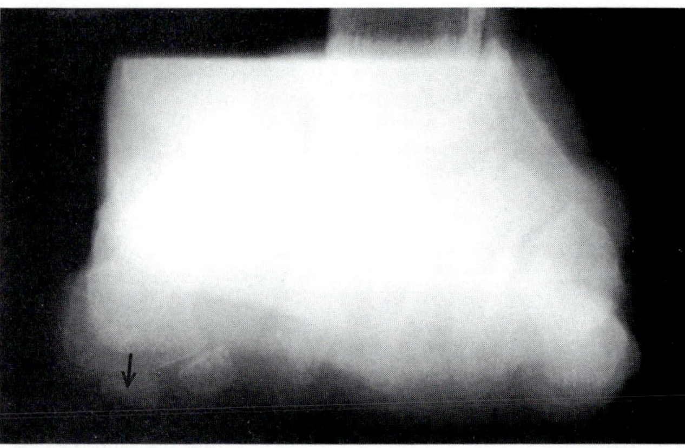

FIG 22–41.
Standing sesamoid radiographs demonstrating erosion of the plantar cortex of the medial sesamoid from osteomyelitis.

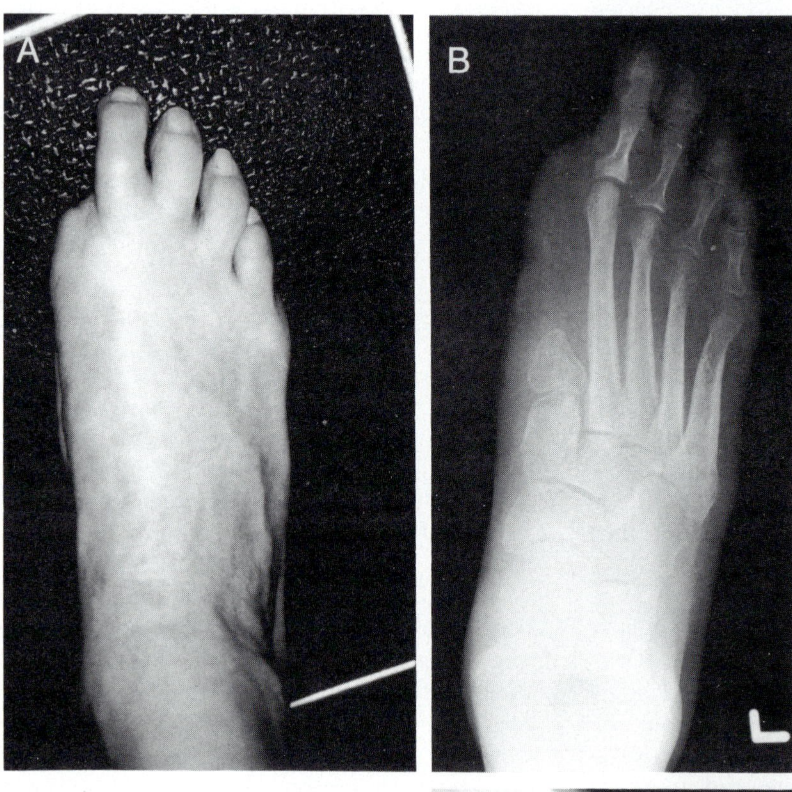

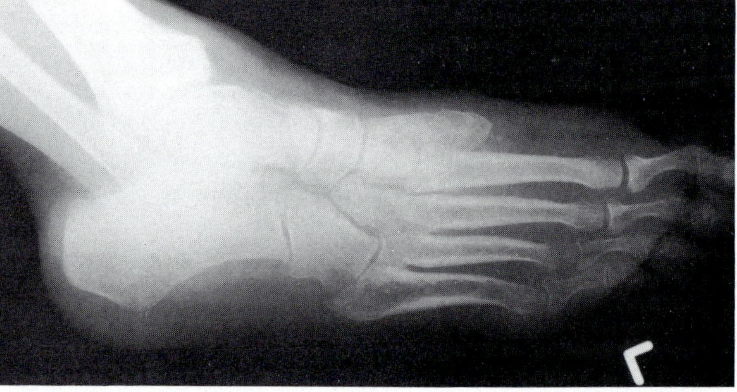

FIG 22–42.
A, first ray amputation. **B,** radiograph of the same patient's foot.

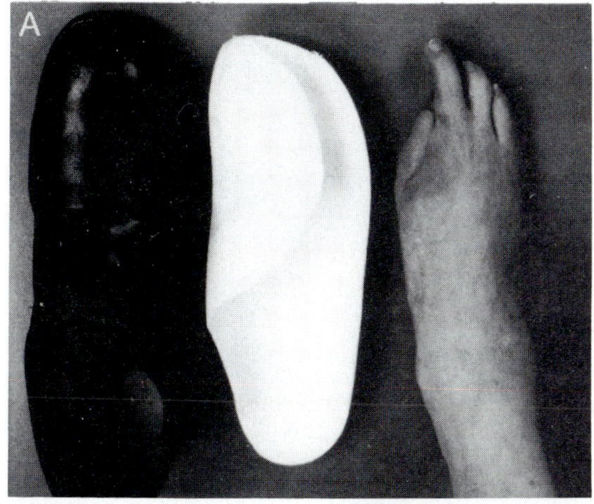

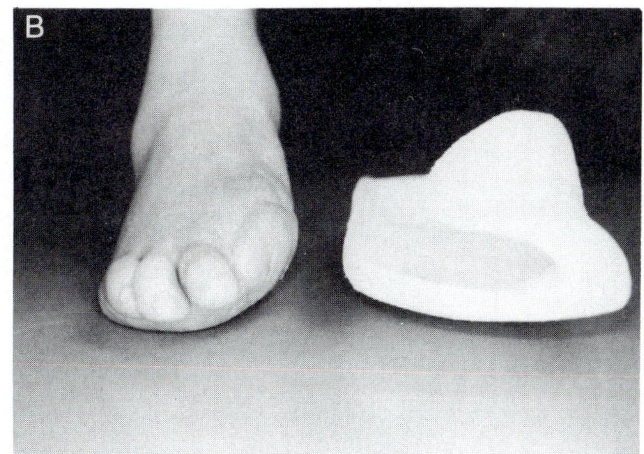

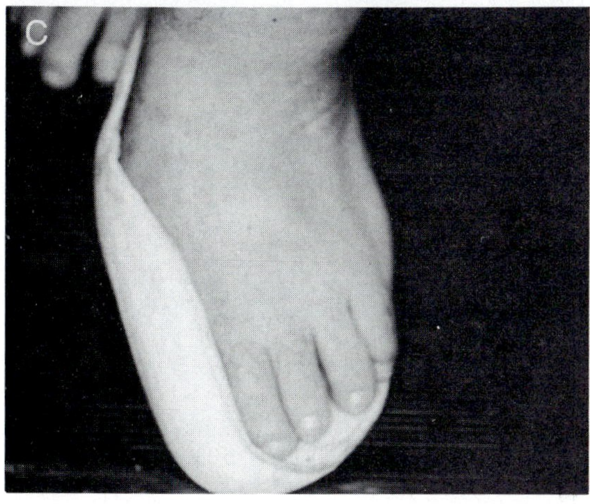

FIG 22–43.
A–C, examples of various shoe insoles with fillers or wraparound liners for partial amputation of the forefoot.

Single- or double-ray amputations are generally preferable to a transmetatarsal amputation in most but not all patients because it is easier to fit them in low-quarter, off-the-shelf, extra-depth shoes. Transmetatarsal amputations usually require a high-top shoe to hold the shoe on the shortened foot. Most patients with a transmetatarsal amputation have a shortened stride as well.

Osteomyelitis of the Midfoot.—Osteomyelitis of the midfoot is most often caused by the abnormal bony projections of a Charcot joint that has led to ulceration and then progressed. It can also occur in the midfoot over naturally occurring bony prominences that have sustained pressure from shoe wear. These prominences are the navicular tuberosity medially and the base of the fifth metatarsal laterally. Bone resection in these areas can lead to secondary deformities, and the patient must be warned of this possibility.

Osteomyelitis of the base of the fifth metatarsal should raise a proverbial warning flag to the examining physician because it is a hallmark of hindfoot varus deformity, just as is the case with ulceration in this area (see Fig 22–33). Shoe pressure can cause an ulceration here also, even without hindfoot varus. However, shoe modifications alone will seldom heal such an ulcer if the varus deformity is present. Once the osteomyelitis has become established, the surgeon must do two things: vigorously debride the infected bone and address the underlying deformity. If the base of the fifth metatarsal is resected, the function of the peroneus brevis is lost, and the varus tendency can be accentuated. The tendon can be reattached, but healing of the reattached tendon in the neuropathic foot can be difficult. The underlying varus should first be approached with a total-contact cast or posterior-shell polypropylene AFO (Fig 22–44). If it fails to be controlled with this, i.e., the ulcer continues, then in some cases a triple arthrodesis may be necessary; however, this is the exception rather than the rule. Arthrodesis can lead to a full-blown Charcot joint and must be approached with caution in a patient who has sufficient neuropathy to develop an ulceration.

Osteomyelitis of the Hindfoot.—Osteomyelitis of the hindfoot is particularly difficult because the skin is thin and there is very little subcutaneous tissue for coverage. Many times the issue is a choice between debridement

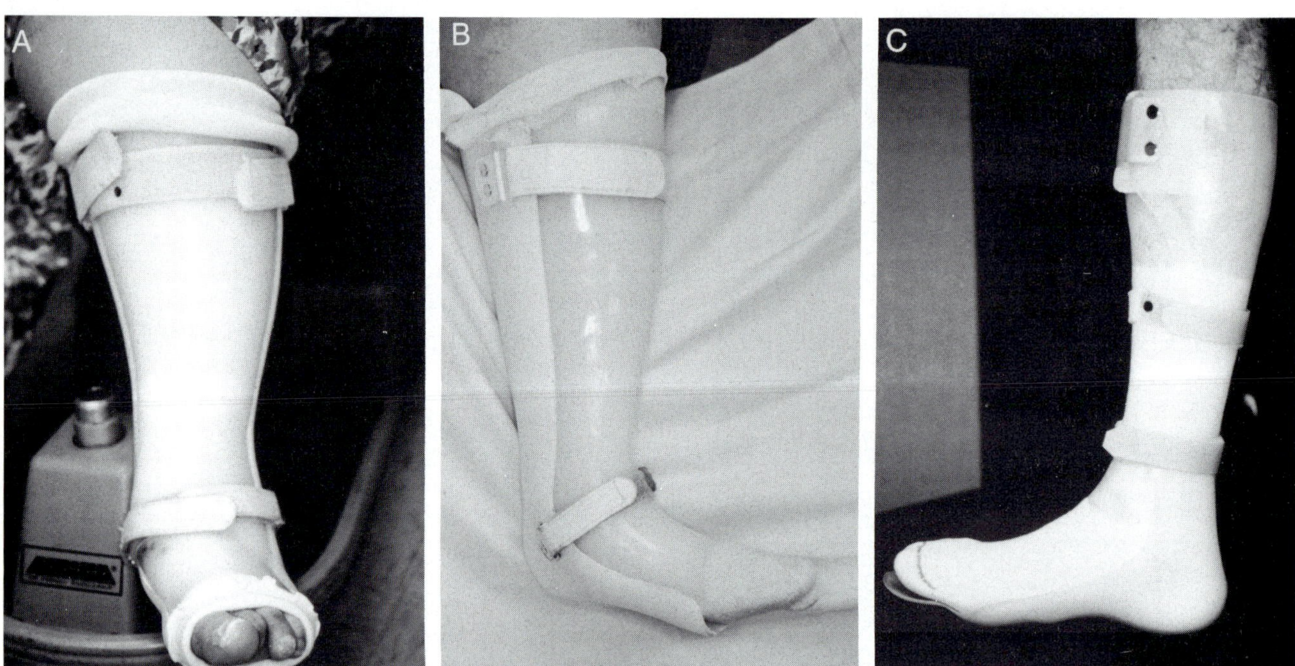

FIG 22–44.
A–C, examples of different styles of combined anterior- and posterior-shell total-contact AFOs.

and an amputation, and the latter is usually the more viable of the two alternatives. One exception to this is osteomyelitis in the posterior portion of the tubercle of the calcaneus. Most of these begin with a pressure ulceration caused by resting the heel in bed or in a chair coupled with the insensitivity of neuropathy, and many end up requiring a below-the-knee amputation. Any loss of the integrity of the heel, its skin, or the heel pad makes the patient no longer eligible for a Syme amputation. However, some of these can be salvaged by a partial calcanectomy.[56]

The procedure is illustrated in Figure 22–45. Most or all of the tubercle of the calcaneus is resected through a posterior midline incision. Exposure is obtained by splitting the Achilles tendon and reflecting it sharply off of the bone while preserving its attachments in the heel pad. The posterior ulcer in the soft tissue is debrided and freshened in an elliptical shape that aids in closure. The bone resection must be generous. It usually but not always spares the posterior facet of the subtalar joint. This procedure can result in ablation of the osteomyelitis; the wound is closed either primarily over an irrigation system as described above or left open and a delayed primary closure performed at another sitting after a number of days of wound care. Most (but not all) patients require the permanent use of a custom polypropylene AFO but still find this preferable to a below-knee prosthesis. The AFO brace must be fitted to a larger shoe with additional depth; a few patients func-

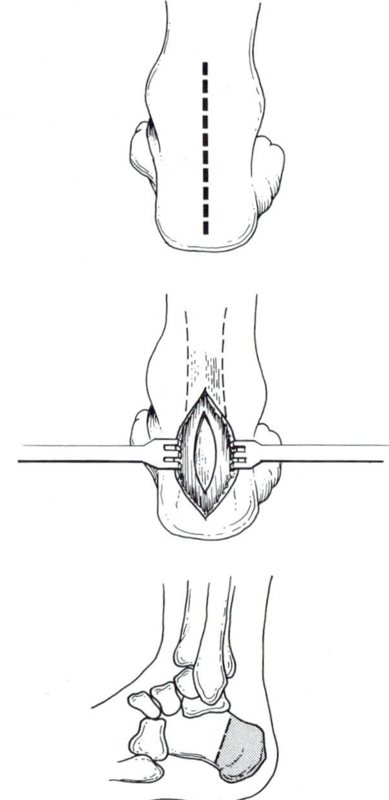

FIG 22–45.
Surgical technique for partial calcanectomy for recalcitrant ulceration of the heel.

tion and walk independently simply with the extra-depth shoe and the molded insoles alone. The published series of partial calcanectomies in diabetics report a significant failure rate.[29] However, if the calcanectomy fails, the patient seldom loses much except the time and morbidity of a second procedure, and treatment is revised to the inevitable below-knee amputation that she would otherwise have had (Fig 22–46).

Osteomyelitis of the Ankle.—Most cases of bone infection around the diabetic ankle are due to Charcot joints producing deformity that exposes the malleoli to pressure and subsequent ulceration. Local debridement and management of the deformity with casts and AFO braces are still the first order of treatment. Bone procedures such as arthrodesis are reserved for salvage of the most severe cases that would otherwise eventually require amputation (see the section below on Charcot joints).

Wound Closure and Foot Reconstruction: Principles

As has been noted in other parts of this chapter, the goal of surgery on the diabetic foot is to achieve healing of the foot while preserving as much of the foot as possible. Waters et al. emphasized that the greater the amount of limb that is salvaged, generally the greater the function of the patient.[107] The two caveats are that the foot must be plantigrade and it must have achieved full soft-tissue coverage with a stable wound. While forefoot amputations are generally preferable to hind-

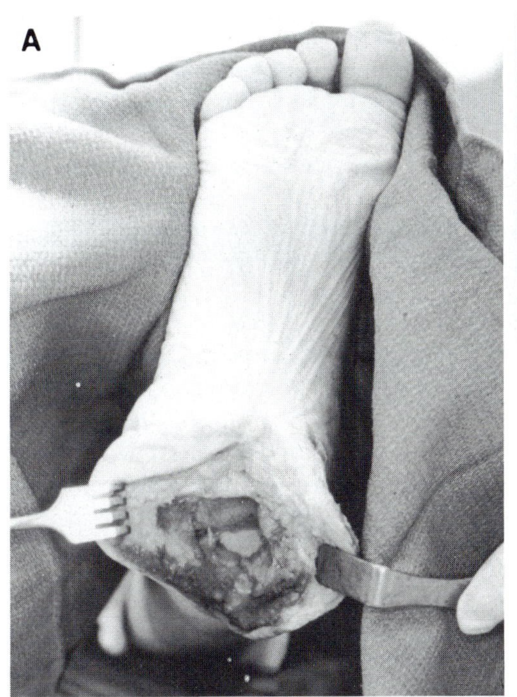

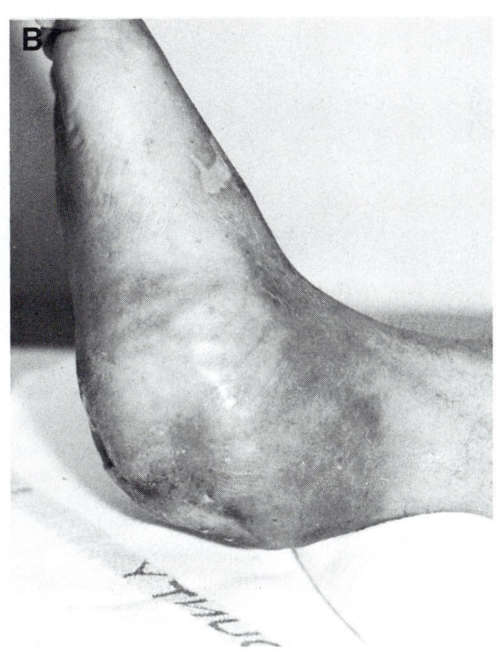

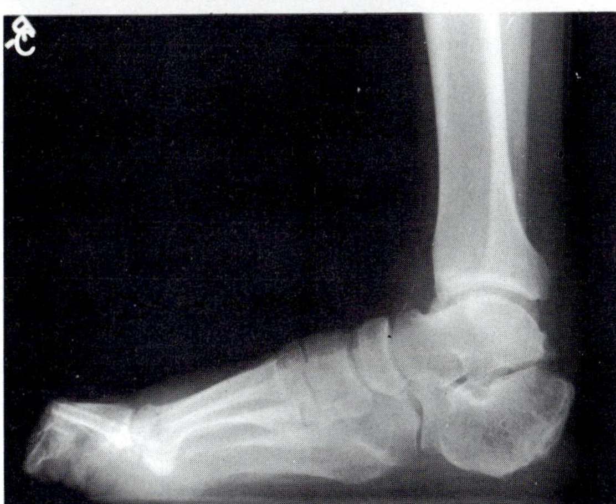

FIG 22–46.
Partial calcanectomy. **A,** heel-splitting incision. **B,** clinical appearance of a calcanectomy. **C,** radiograph of a partial calcanectomy. This patient did not require an AFO to walk but used a depth shoe with a molded insole.

foot amputations because they allow greater stability and ease of shoe fitting, a more proximal amputation may be better and more functional when taking into consideration the debilitation sustained by the patient as a result of unsuccessful prolonged treatment to save a toe, a metatarsal, the forefoot, etc. The patient is usually better served by a definitive and healed amputation that allows walking and resumption of most daily activities than if left incapacitated and debilitated by the continuing wound care required to save a marginally viable segment of the foot or limb. The goal of foot salvage must be tempered by the ability of the patient to participate in normal activities of daily life. Insufficient attention has been paid in the past to the physical, economic, and psychological losses incurred in the process of the disease and recuperation itself. A balance must be struck between limb salvage and ultimate function that is left to the patient. If the patient is totally or even frequently non–weight bearing, then the upper extremities are always occupied with the task of ambulation, thus limiting the ability to perform most activities of work and leisure.

There are a number of techniques that can maximize the success of wound healing and foot salvage. The most important is aggressive debridement of all infected tissue and bone while at the same time sparing the viable soft tissue for closure, especially plantar flaps. If the wound is grossly infected and/or the viability of the soft tissue cannot be determined at the initial debridement, the wound should be packed in an open manner and the patient returned to the operating room for repeat debridement in a few days. Debridements should be repeated every several days until the wound has responded and started to heal. Once a clean, granulating wound has been achieved, then the surgeon can consider a delayed primary closure. This is usually a loose closure, often over drains.

The closure wound, whether closed early or late, requires sculpting the soft-tissue coverage to achieve the balance between bone and soft tissue discussed earlier in the chapter. The surgeon must often use "creative" flaps, i.e., not the classic textbook closures, in order to salvage the foot. These flaps depend upon the peculiar pattern of residual viable soft tissue created by the configuration of tissue necrosis or infection. It is often necessary to modify a midfoot amputation such as a transmetatarsal, a Chopart, or a Syme to achieve a viable, albeit unorthodox closure in order to save a limb (Fig 22–47,A). In short, it is better for the patient to wear a "special" shoe than a "standard" prosthesis.

Leaving large wounds to heal by granulation and secondary intention, especially entire amputation wounds, is debilitating and may take 6 months or more to heal in some diabetics. The functional loss is tremendous, and this is undesirable. The surgeon should at least try to achieve closure; these slowly granulating, gaping wounds often represent the failure of the surgeon to commit and determine which tissue is viable and which is not. It is usually in the patient's best interest to determine the vascularity and healing potential of a wound and, if necessary, debride, revascularize, or amputate it in order to achieve primary closure. Wounds that are left open to granulate more often require skin grafting and more frequently produce unstable scars. Even if delayed primary closure is only partially successful and a portion of the wound still gapes or has to heal by secondary intention, it is worthwhile. It reduces the morbidity and expense of wound care by shortening the time required for wound healing. The volume of the wound that must heal by secondary intention is much smaller, an important consideration when the healing process can take many months.

However, there are some wounds that simply will not heal except by secondary intention, and this is one possible method of treatment when attempts at delayed primary closure are unsuccessful. The scars tend to be more irregular and more unstable (Fig 22–47,B).

If the wound is not ready to close, than it either needs further debridement, it requires revascularization, or it needs more time to granulate. Split-thickness skin grafts, while acceptable, are more liable to have recurrent breakdown, especially on the sole of the foot (Fig 22–48). Wherever possible, closure with local skin and soft tissue, especially on the plantar surface of the foot, is preferable to split-thickness skin grafts because skin grafts are thinner, less mobile, less durable, and totally insensate.

There is a limited place for the use of free tissue transfer ("free flaps") in wounds of the diabetic foot, but not as a part of routine amputations. The "free flap" is also insensitive but has the advantage of the transfer of soft tissue of greater thickness as well as the fact that it brings new vascularity to the wound. In the diabetic foot, a free tissue transfer is usually used to salvage the foot by achieving coverage of the heel or hindfoot, and the success of the flap eventually signifies the ability of the patient to wear a shoe instead of a knee-high prosthesis. Calcification of the vessels in this area often makes the required vascular anastomoses of the transfer difficult or precludes it altogether.

There are some exceptions to the principle of using local tissue for wound closure in the diabetic foot. One example is a plantar abscess that produces a large loss of plantar skin and intrinsic plantar musculature and ne-

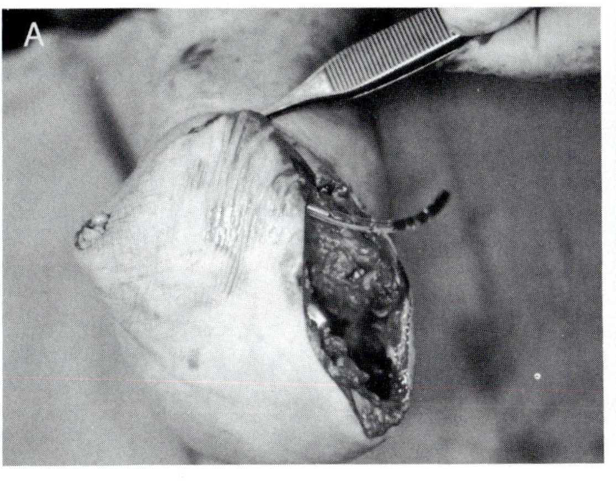

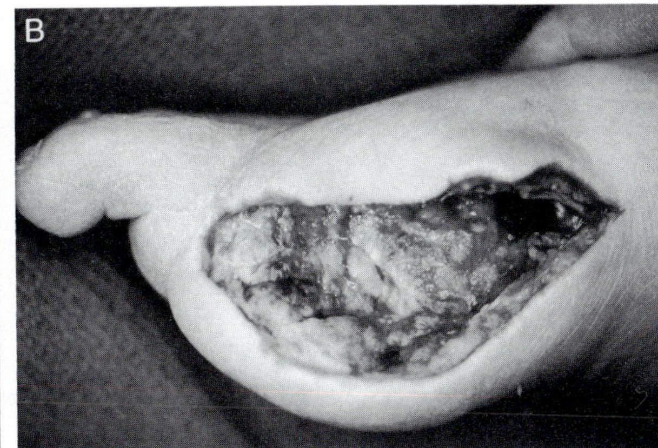

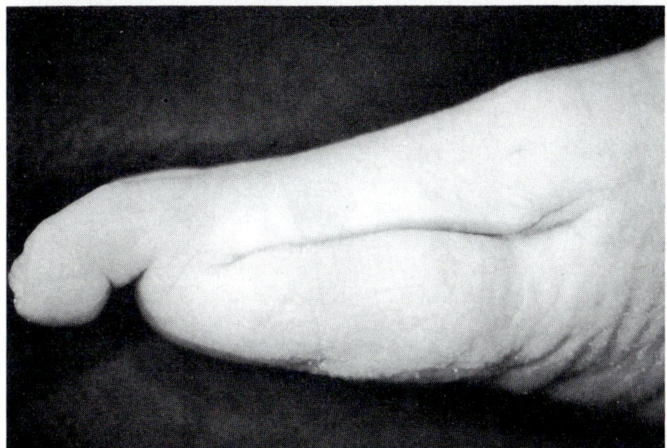

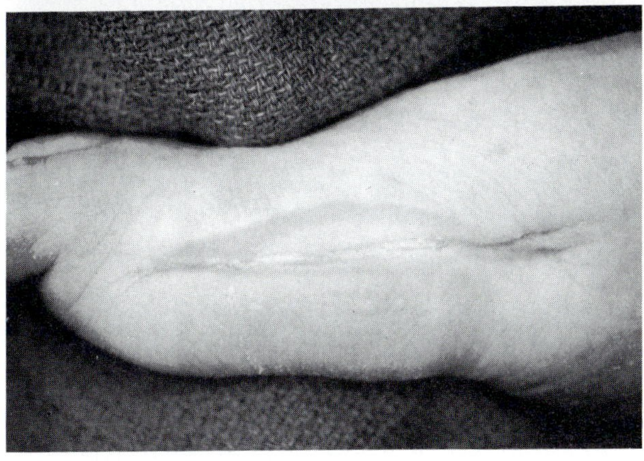

FIG 22–47.
A, irregular flap used to close a Chopart amputation. Note the asymmetry of the short medial and long lateral sides of the wound. **B,** irregular wound with infolded edges produced by slow healing by secondary intention after amputation of the great toe and its metatarsal. Healing took 5 months. The depth of the infolded edges can be seen in the third frame, where they are being spread apart.

crosis of the overlying plantar fascia. This is a situation in which delayed primary closure cannot be done because the immobility of the tissues in this area do not allow the edges of the wound to be drawn together. Closure depends primarily upon granulation tissue to fill in the defect; skin healing occurs through either skin grafting or gradual epithelialization. It is important to not skin-graft too soon because wound contracture occurs to a great extent (Fig 22–49). Once granulation tissue has filled in the defect, total-contact casting may accelerate epithelialization, just as occurs in forefoot plantar ulceration.

Charcot Joints

Diabetes is now the leading cause of Charcot joints in the developed world, having long surpassed syphilis, which was the original cause of neuroarthropathy at the time that it was first described by Jean Martin Charcot in 1868. The principle that he recognized was that joint

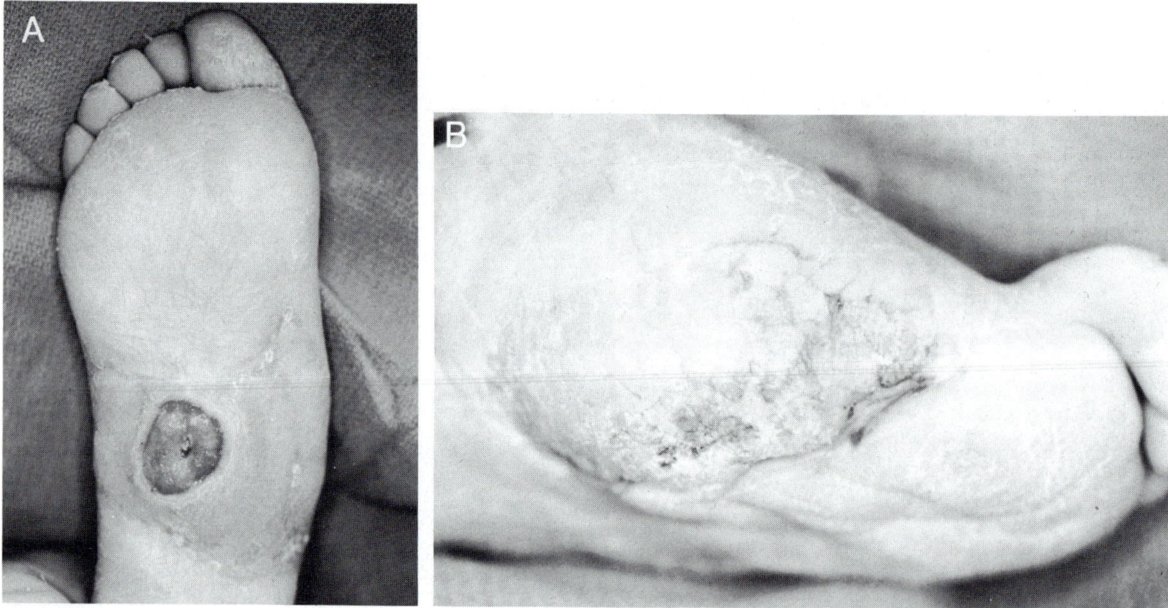

FIG 22–48.
Recurrent breakdown of split-thickness skin grafts. **A,** on the sole following a previous resection of a plantar abscess and Charcot exostosis. **B,** on the medial border of the foot after first ray amputation.

destruction could occur due to abnormalities extrinsic to the joint itself. This was acknowledged as coming from the nerves to the joint, but controversy arose (and exists even now) as to the specific effect (or lack thereof) that the nerves exerted on the joint. Charcot called it the "trophic" effect, but modern commentators have divided the theories into two major alternatives.[21] The first is the neurotraumatic theory and predicates that the joint destruction, fractures, and collapse of the foot occur as the result of cumulative mechanical trauma, usually unrecognized microtrauma in a joint that has been rendered insensitive to proprioception and pain. The second theory is neurovascular and postulates that the joint dissolution occurs due to bone resorption and ligamentous changes as a result of a neurally stimulated vascular reflex interpreted as an "autosympathectomy." There is reason to believe, at this time, that both theories may partially represent the reality of this disorder. Regardless of the proper explanation, Charcot joints remain the most enigmatic and at the same time most dramatic manifestation of the profound and ever-present danger of diabetic peripheral neuropathy. Despite the ever-increasing numbers of Charcot joints, this is a problem that is generally poorly recognized, underdiagnosed, and often poorly managed. Charcot joints are also known by the term *neuroarthropathy*. While this is technically a very correct term, it has, at times, been used almost interchangably in the literature[27, 96] as a synonym for the changes of diabetic osteopathy, some of which are Charcot joints and some of which are bone resorption or bone changes beneath or associated with neurotrophic ulcers. The latter raises the question whether many of these reported cases of "neuroarthropathy" may actually represent bone erosion due to infection, especially since the majority of the cases in those series involve changes in the phalanges and distal metatarsals.[27, 96] To make certain that this section deals with changes that are unquestionably neuropathic destruction of bones and joints, the illustrations and principles of Charcot joints will be centered on cases with fractures, dislocations, and subluxations proximal to the midmetatarsal shafts.

The first case of a Charcot joint associated with the peripheral neuropathy of diabetes was reported in 1936 by Jordan.[58] Since that time there have been a multitude of sporadic case reports or small groups of patients recorded in the literature. Only a few large series have been reported to date.[15, 18, 19, 27, 96] This adds to the impression of most practitioners that this is a rare and unusual condition. Unfortunately, the incidence is increasing, and it is becoming better recognized and appearing in even "ordinary" orthopaedic practice. Charcot joints can no longer be thought of as the domain of only a few subspecialists. Illustrated in Figure 22–1 is the kind of case that orthopaedic surgeons must be aware of in the future, for it demonstrates that the problem of the Charcot joint relates to everyday orthopaedic practice. As noted in the beginning of this chap-

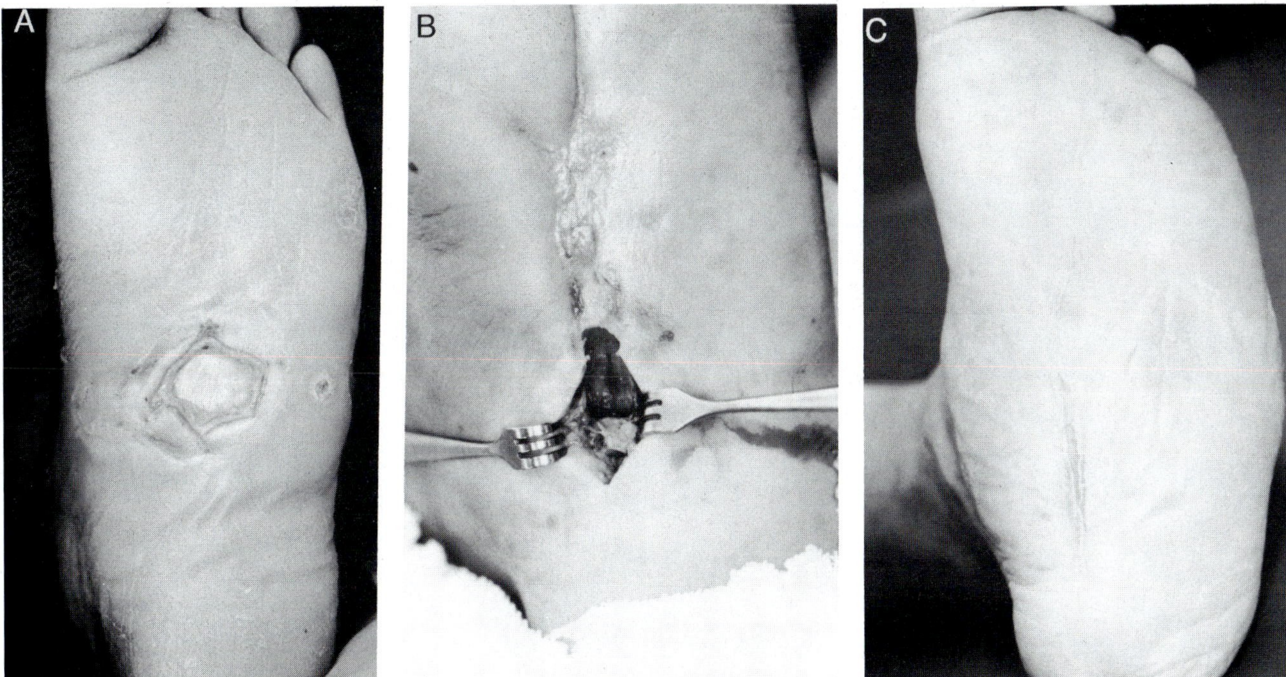

FIG 22–49.
Plantar abscesses. **A,** necrosis of the plantar fascia. **B,** a different patient with recurrent abscess. **C,** healing of the sole in the second patient.

ter, this is the case of a middle-aged woman with a short history of non–insulin-dependent diabetes whose non displaced bimalleolar fracture was properly treated with cast immobilization and a period of non–weight bearing on crutches. After a proper length of immobilization, the patient suddenly developed the severe displacement seen in Figure 22–1,B and C that subsequently progressed to a major Charcot ankle joint with secondary collapse of the foot and severe neuropathic pes planus deformity (see Fig 22–1,D and E). The patient required treatment for several years, primarily in the form of a cast and a total-contact AFO. The problems inherent in this illustrative case are several. The fact that the patient was a diabetic with a fracture should now alert physicians that there may be a problem with delayed healing, nonunion, or the development of a Charcot joint. Patients can be warned of this possibility. Testing the patient, even crudely, for the level of peripheral neuropathy, while not strictly dependable, may give some guidelines to the physician in advising a patient about this potential problem. The treating physician may wish to prolong the period of immobilization if significant neuropathy can be documented; the author usually recommends approximately doubling the period of immobilization if the neuropathy is very dense, but this is a clinical guideline, and there are no data at this time on which to compare various periods of immobilization for fractures in the diabetic with neuropathy. The frustrating and difficult nature of diabetic Charcot joints is emphasized by the above case because even recognizing the potential for this scenario would not necessarily have prevented it; even if one anticipates the problem and increases the already long immobilization and period of non–weight bearing, further collapse can occur within the cast as illustrated in Figure 22–50. The redeeming feature of the case illustrated in Figure 22–1 is that the patient did not lose his foot and that eventual healing occurred with nonsurgical treatment.

A similar case, not rare, of a Charcot joint occurring after a properly treated fracture of the ankle is demonstrated in Figure 22–51. This is a young man, 28 years of age, with juvenile-onset, insulin-dependent diabetes whose fracture was treated entirely appropriately. Splitting of the syndesmosis and collapse of the ankle, which occurred many months after the initial operation and surgery, included extensive disintegration of the body of the talus.

Pathophysiology

As noted above, there is probably both a vascular and a traumatic etiology of the Charcot joint. The vascular etiology is reflected in cases of patients who develop a Charcot joint or whose Charcot joint worsens

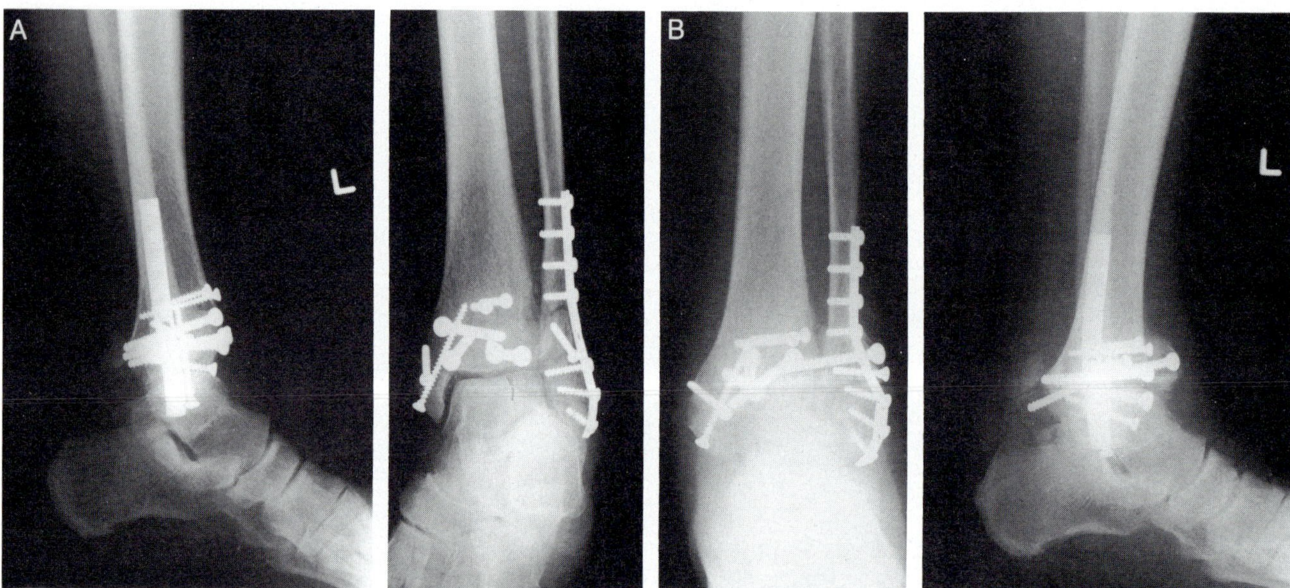

FIG 22–50.
A and **B,** Charcot joint following open reduction and internal fixation of a comminuted ankle fracture. This patient was in a cast at the time the plate broke and the joint disintegrated, almost 6 months postoperatively and after a prolonged period of non–weight bearing.

while at bed rest for some other serious medical condition such as heart disease associated with the patient's diabetes. These patients have been observed to develop the architectural changes in the foot simply by rolling over in bed. However, the majority of Charcot joints are the result of trauma and impaired sensation caused by the neuropathy. It is also important to remember that the density of the sensory neuropathy is not necessarily related to the severity of the diabetes, its duration, or whether it is insulin dependent (type I, or juvenile) or non–insulin dependent (type II, or adult). Some of the worst cases of Charcot joints occur in patients with mild, adult-onset diabetes treated with oral hypoglycemic agents or diet modification alone. In occasional patients, the Charcot joint may even be the very first manifestation of previously undiagnosed diabetes (Fig 22–52). The trauma may be microtrauma (such as an abnormal gait causing increased pressure with each footstep as a result of poor sensory feedback from the limb) or a minor trauma (such as bumping the foot) or a major traumatic event (such as a fall or a twisting injury to the ankle). The trauma may be recognized or unrecognized, subacute or chronic.

Experimental documentation of the relationship of neuropathic joint destruction and loss of normal sensation was first elucidated in a study by Eloesser in 1917[40] in which he selectively denervated single limbs of cats with otherwise normal sensation to produce Charcot joints in only those limbs.

The Charcot joint may present as a fracture,[26] subluxation, dislocation,[68, 81] or fracture-dislocation. In the earliest stages, it may simply present as a hot, red, swollen foot. It may also present as sudden or insidious bone destruction or collapse of the arch. There are numerous patients who have presented after having ground the tibia through the talus until they are bearing weight directly on the distal end of the tibia, which has subluxated off of the foot (Fig 22–53), or developed a pseudoarticulation between the calcaneus and the tibia (Fig 22–54).

Eichenholtz[38] described three stages of development of the Charcot joint that represent its course from the initial events to eventual healing. Stage I is characterized by an acute inflammatory process in which the primary radiographic finding is *fragmentation*, the synonym for stage I. It is associated with hyperemia, and it is typical for the joint to be swollen, hot, and erythematous. On radiographs, the bone evidences dissolution, fragmentation, and dislocation. Stage II, known as *coalescence*, is typified by the beginning of the reparative process, as signified by a diminution of the edema, warmth, and redness and the radiologic finding of new bone formation. This coalescing new bone forms at the site of the initiating fracture and bone destruction or even at the site of dislocation in the absence of a major fracture. Stage III is characterized by bony consolidation and healing, usually with residual deformity. It should be added that this is sometimes a confusing pic-

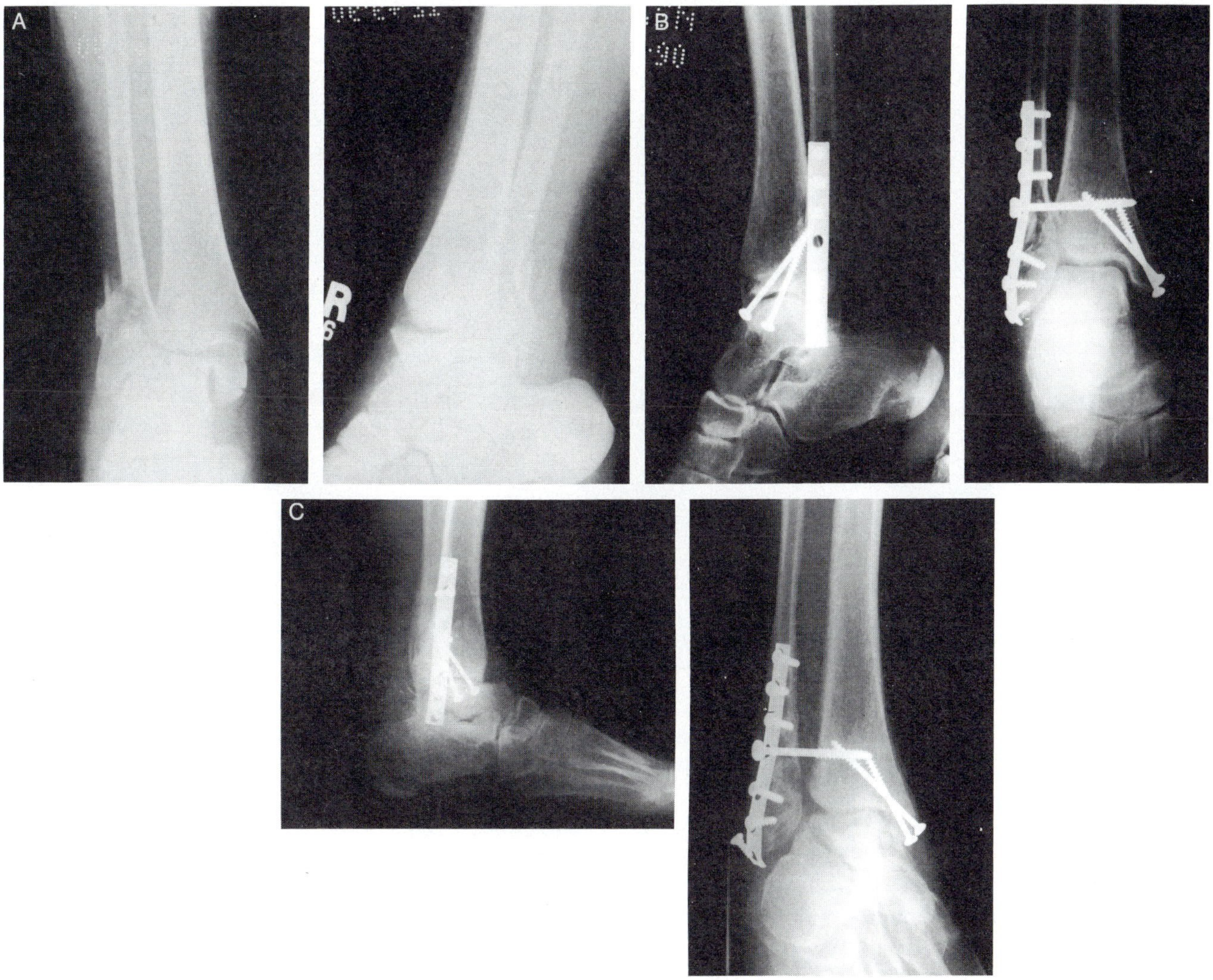

FIG 22–51.
A–C, another example of a diabetic patient with Charcot joint formation following open reduction and internal fixation of an unstable ankle fracture. In both cases, treatment was appropriate. This patient had simultaneous spontaneous splitting and collapse of the talus.

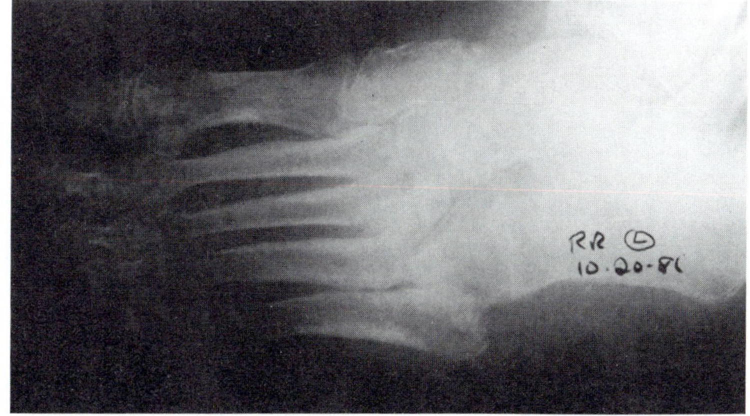

FIG 22–52.
A patient whose Charcot foot was the presenting symptom of her previously undiagnosed diabetes.

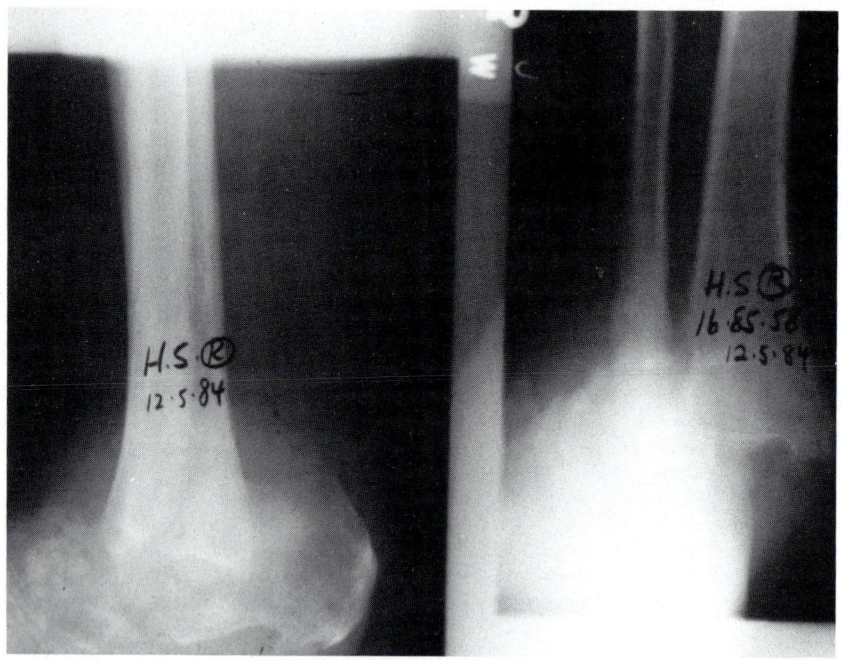

FIG 22–53.
Severe Charcot joint. This patient has fractured the talus and subluxed the entire foot lateral to the tibia. The patient refused all surgery and was weight bearing on the foot and the tibia in a custom shoe.

ture since the joint may be enlarged despite the resolution of edema in this last stage. While it is possible for the Charcot process to be reactivated in the same location, this is the exception rather than the rule and, when it occurs, usually does so in stage II rather than in Stage III when solid bony healing has occurred (Fig 22–55).

Epidemiology

The ratio of men and women is about equal, and the average duration of diabetes prior to the occurrence of the Charcot joint is over 10 years; however, the range of duration of diabetes is from zero to 45 years. Charcot joints of the feet occur bilaterally in approximately 30% of cases. There is *not* a preponderance of juvenile-onset

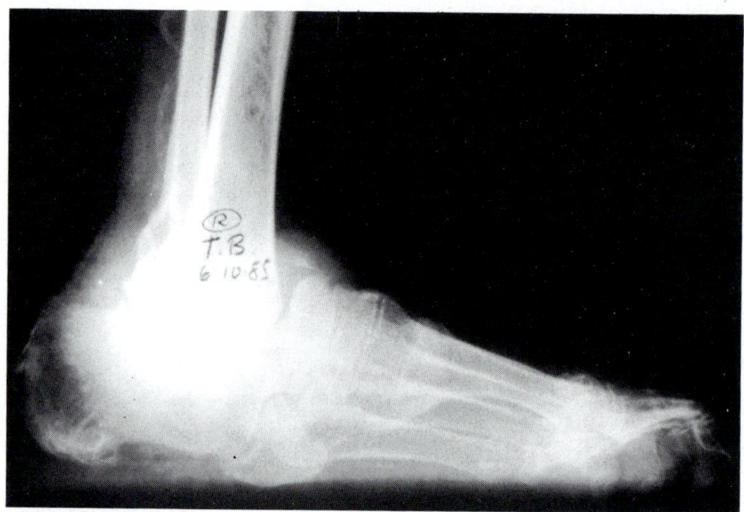

FIG 22–54.
Charcot joint in which the patient has ground the talus to detritus and is weight bearing with the tibia directly on the calcaneus.

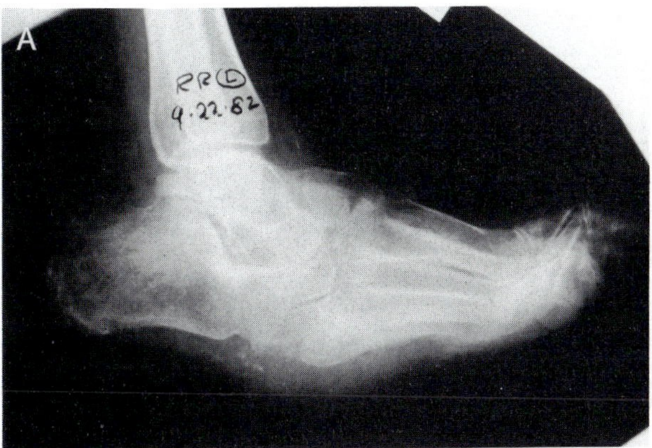

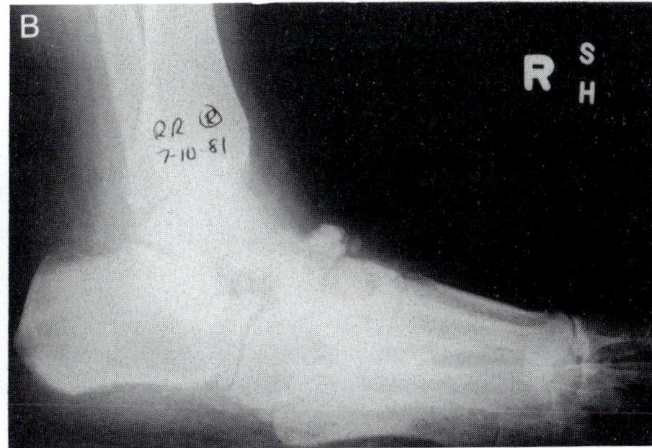

FIG 22–55.
A and **B**, stages I and III in the same Charcot foot. Note the new bone formation and mature osseous healing.

(insulin-dependent) diabetics, but the ratio of insulin-dependent diabetics (16%)[15, 18, 19] reflects a somewhat higher proportion of insulin-dependent patients than in the population as a whole (which is 5% to 10%).[33]

Clinical Signs and Symptoms of Charcot Joints of the Foot and Ankle

The clinical signs of presentation of a Charcot joint depend upon whether or not it is acute or subacute. The acute Charcot joint can mimic other causes of acute inflammation. The foot and or ankle are always swollen, with varying degrees of increased warmth and erythema. In the earliest stage, the inflammation and swelling may be remarkable, but the radiographs may still be negative. The patient may appear to have cellulitis, so intense is the erythema. Thus, the differential diagnosis for the acutely swollen, hot, red foot in a diabetic includes cellulitis, abscess formation, or an early Charcot joint prior to the radiographic changes. The clinical trick, noted in pages 884 to 885, of elevation of the limb to distinguish cellulitis from dependent rubor (which is present in the acute Charcot joint) is applicable here. If clinically uncertain, the use of CT and MRI can rule out the presence of an abscess.

The signs of a subacute or chronic Charcot joint are proportionately less than those of acute inflammation and proportionately more than those of deformity, with varying severity of radiographic changes. The *sine qua non* of the Charcot joint is architectural disruption of the structure of the foot, whether it is in a single joint surface or across half of the foot. The foot is usually widened, with bony prominences on the plantar surface and/or medial and lateral borders of the foot. In some cases, the longitudinal arch collapses or even reverses to produce the classic "rocker-bottom foot" (Fig 22–56). As the longitudinal arch collapses, the dynamic effect of the Achilles tendon is altered by loss of the normal calcaneal pitch, i.e., its relative plantar flexion as compared with normal (Fig 22–57). The bony protuberances are clinically important because they can cause neuropathic ulceration, either on the plantar surface due to the pressure of walking and standing or on the medial and/or lateral border of the foot due to the pressure of shoe wear. The change in the shape of the foot makes shoe fitting difficult. The most common problem of diabetic patients who need a custom shoe rather than an off-the-shelf additional-depth shoe with a custom insole is a Charcot joint.

Other cases exhibit more bulbous enlargement, depending upon the area most affected. This becomes a persistent form of the deformity when the extensive destructive process of stage I advances but fails to progress to stages II and III of healing. Severe proximal deformities can result, such as deviation of the foot on the leg into terrible and uncorrectable varus or valgus. The severe pressure on the malleoli, heel, or hindfoot can lead to ulceration, infection, osteomyelitis, and eventual amputation.

The symptoms of the Charcot joint are also affected by its acute or chronic nature. The classic Charcot joint has become well known by the epithet of "painless swelling." However, about half of the patients present with a chief complaint of pain.[15, 18, 19] The pain is generally not commensurate with the severe destruction seen in the limb. Most patients with Charcot joints are ambulatory when they first present; they frequently exhibit a severity of bone and joint destruction that would render a person with a sensate limb incapacitated and immobile.

The symptoms may be related to the patient suddenly or gradually noticing a change in the shape of a foot or a difficulty with shoes no longer fitting. Most of-

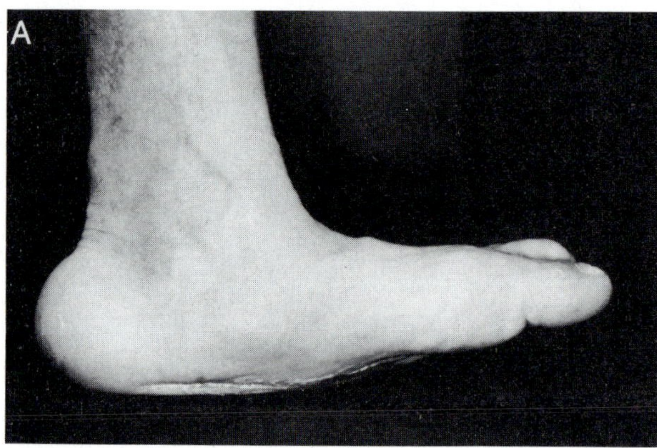

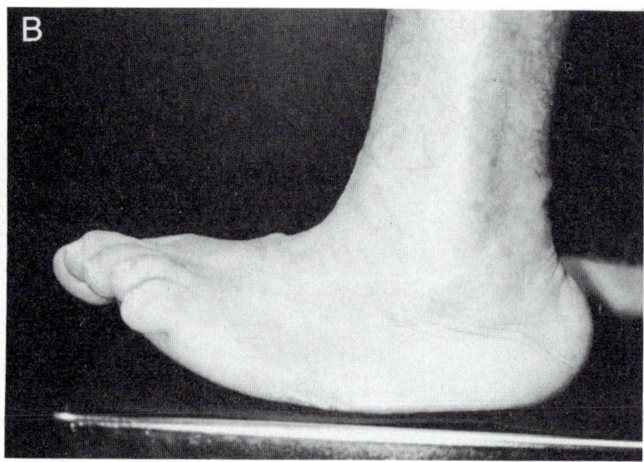

FIG 22–56.
A and **B,** the classic "rocker-bottom" Charcot foot, with collapse and then reversal of the longitudinal arch.

ten and more than any other symptom, patients note tenacious swelling made worse by weight bearing but usually never resolving entirely. Patients with severe bony destruction and instability seldom complain of "giving way" or other symptoms that relate to the loss of structural integrity of the ankle or hindfoot, the areas where this is most likely to occur (see the section on classification). The reason for this presumably is the absence of an adequate proprioceptive sense.

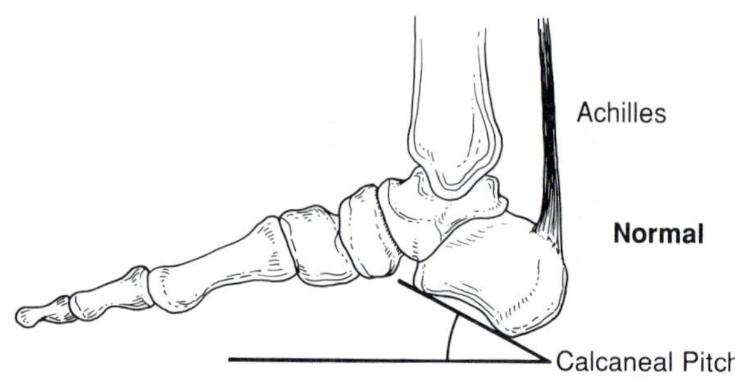

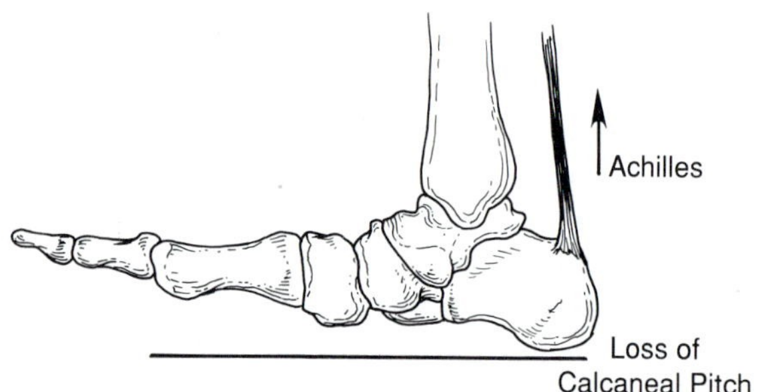

FIG 22–57.
Loss of the normal calcaneal pitch, or angle relative to the floor in patients with Charcot collapse of the arch. This leads to a mechanical disadvantage for the Achilles tendon.

Imaging and Diagnosis of the Charcot Foot

The radiographic appearance of the Charcot joint is usually distinct and easy to recognize once it has progressed to the point of significant architectural disruption of the foot. There are combinations of fractures and dislocations; separations of the bones; new bony projections on the plantar, medial, or lateral aspects of the foot; bone compressions or disintegrations; fluffy new bone formation; and gross alterations in the skeletal anatomy. However, in the early stages of the Charcot joint, the changes may be difficult to find or are at least subtle. As has been shown in the earlier sections some Charcot joints will exhibit negative radiographic findings initially, even though clinically the process of inflammation and swelling of the Charcot joint has begun. Changes may be subtle, such as a diastasis between the bases of the metatarsals (Fig 22–58) that subsequently progresses to further collapse.

Patients who are first seen by the physician in late stage I or early stage II may be tempted to diagnose the changes in the bone as osteomyelitis; indeed, the distinction may be difficult given the erosive changes diffusely through the bone, sometimes accompanied by new bone formation (Fig 22–59). One subtle but valuable hallmark of a neuropathic fracture is that it lacks the surrounding osteopenia that typically occurs in osteomyelitis.[86] When the distinction between osteomyelitis and Charcot bone changes cannot easily be made, the definitive study is biopsy of the bone through an incision away from any associated ulcer or skin breakdown. The specimen should be submitted to the laboratory for aerobic and anaerobic cultures; part of the bone specimen should be submitted to the pathologist for examination of histologic evidence of osteomyelitis or Charcot changes. Provided that the specimen was a sampling near or at a joint, the histology can reveal the

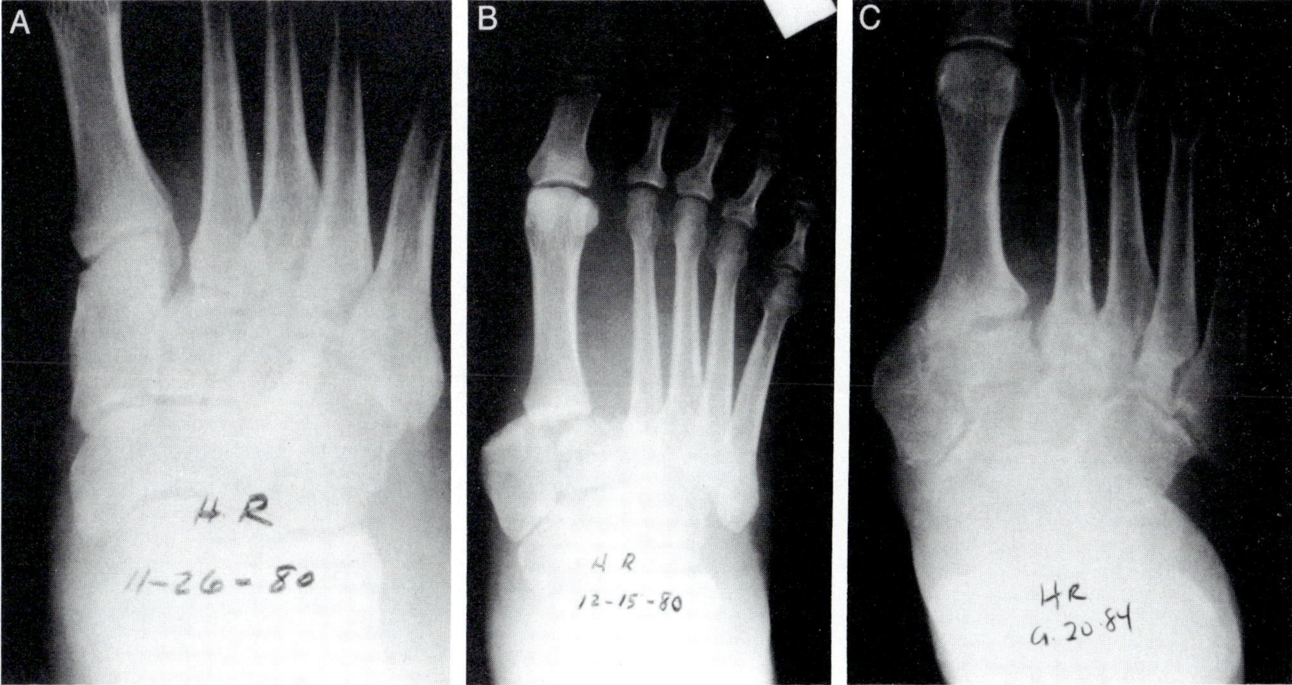

FIG 22–58.
A, subtle diastasis between the first and second metatarsal bases after minor trauma was missed on the initial examination. **B,** 19 days later, the foot underwent this catastrophic collapse during ordinary walking indoors. **C,** subsequent healing with deformity 3½ years later after cast and AFO treatment. The patient remained active and continued to work.

pathognomonic changes of Charcot joint destruction, i.e., bone particles embedded within the synovium (Fig 22–60). Osteomyelitis can be distinguished by the acute and chronic inflammatory cells within the marrow spaces, with or without associated osteonecrosis and fibrosis in the marrow.

Recent studies have shown that nuclear scintigraphy with ^{111}In-labeled leukocytes may be the study of choice to determine the presence of osteomyelitis in all lesions of the diabetic foot, including ulcers and Charcot joints.[66, 89, 92, 93, 99] Some authors have even suggested that the use of ^{111}In oxyquinoline scanning may even be accurate enough to be a substitute for bone biopsy.[82] Certainly the use of technetium 99 scanning is too nonspecific and persists too long to be useful in determining the presence of infection within the bone. The use of simultaneous scanning with technetium and indium may be extremely useful, however, since overlying cellulitis in the soft tissue may occur in both the swollen foot with neuropathic joint changes and in the foot with osteomyelitis. If the indium scan is positive, indicating the presence of infection, the evaluation proceeds with a technetium scan also. If the latter has negative findings, then it is clear that the positive indium scan is attributable to soft-tissue infection. If the technetium scan is positive, a comparison is made between the pattern of the two scans. If they coincide in the location of uptake, then the infection is most likely within the bone; if the indium scan can be clearly shown to be positive in a pattern superficial to or separate from the area of uptake on the technetium scan, then the patient most likely has a superficial soft-tissue infection concomitant with underlying, noninfected neuropathic arthropathy.

A word of caution is required to stave off a host of unnecessary tests: the clinical situations in which the radiographic changes of a Charcot joint are suspected to represent superimposed osteomyelitis are quite unusual. It is not justified to do nuclear medicine studies on every or even many patients with destructive changes in the bone when the clinical picture is clearly one of a Charcot joint. This is especially true if there has never been an associated ulcer or breakdown in the skin and soft tissue overlying the Charcot joint. The vast majority of cases of osteomyelitis in the diabetic foot occur through local extension from a breakdown and infection in the skin and soft-tissue envelope. There is little reason to suspect osteomyelitis in the Charcot joint if such a breakdown has not occurred. Although cases do exist of presumed hematogenous osteomyelitis that has set-

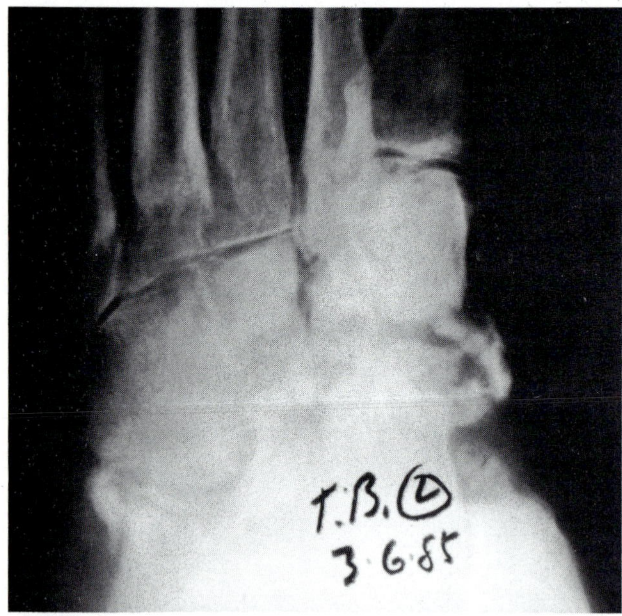

FIG 22–59.
The radiographic changes of osteomyelitis and Charcot disintegration of the joint are not always easily distinguished. This patient never had infection.

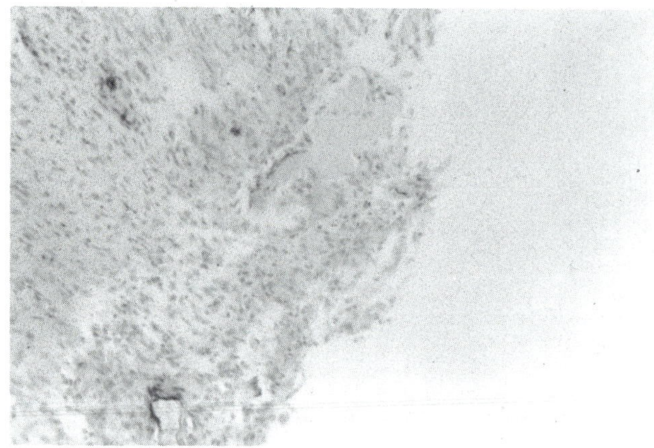

FIG 22–60.
Histologic section from a Charcot joint showing the bony detritus within the synovial tissue.

tled in such an area of Charcot bone dissolution, they are exceptionally rare.

Anatomic Classification of Charcot Joints

The classification of Charcot joints of the foot and ankle into anatomic categories is a simple but clinically useful mechanism for defining the broad categories of progression and natural history of this often-devastating disorder.[15, 18, 19] The classification is based upon which of the four anatomic areas is predominantly affected by the Charcot process, as judged by the findings on plain radiographs, which makes it easy to apply in the course of patient care (Table 22–6). Type 1 Charcot joints affect the midfoot area, i.e., the metatarsocuneiform and naviculocuneiform joints. Type 1 joints are the most common and represent about 60% of Charcot feet. Type 2 Charcot joints represent those in which the main changes are within the hindfoot, i.e., any or all of the triple joints of the subtalar complex, namely, the subtalar, calcaneocuboid, and talonavicular joints. Type 2 accounts for 30% to 35% of the Charcot joints. Types 3A and 3B are relatively minor groups numerically, although they behave quite differently. Type 3A joints represent those in which the predominant changes are within the ankle joint, and these produce serious, long-lasting changes. Type 3B Charcot feet are those that develop a pathologic fracture of the tubercle of the calcaneus with secondary deformity and collapse of the distal portions of the foot. The types of Charcot joints are illustrated in Figure 22–61. The vast majority of Charcot joints of the foot and ankle (90% to 95% approximately) are represented by type 1 ("midfoot" group) and type 2 ("hindfoot" group). The remaining two types are less

TABLE 22–6.
Classification of Charcot Joints

Type	Name	Description*	Major Problem
1	Midfoot type	Tarsometatarsal and naviculocuneiform joints	Symptomatic plantar and medial bony prominences
2	Hindfoot type	Subtalar, talonavicular, and/or calcaneocuboid joints	Instability and slow bony consolidation and healing
3A	Ankle type	Tibiotalar joint	Instability and the longest time required for bony healing
3B	Os calcis type	Pathologic fracture of the tubercle of the calcaneus usually with secondary pes planus	Pes planus, loss of normal calcaneal pitch, widened heel Special shoe wear required

*Based upon the joint or joints that are primarily affected as seen on plain radiographs.

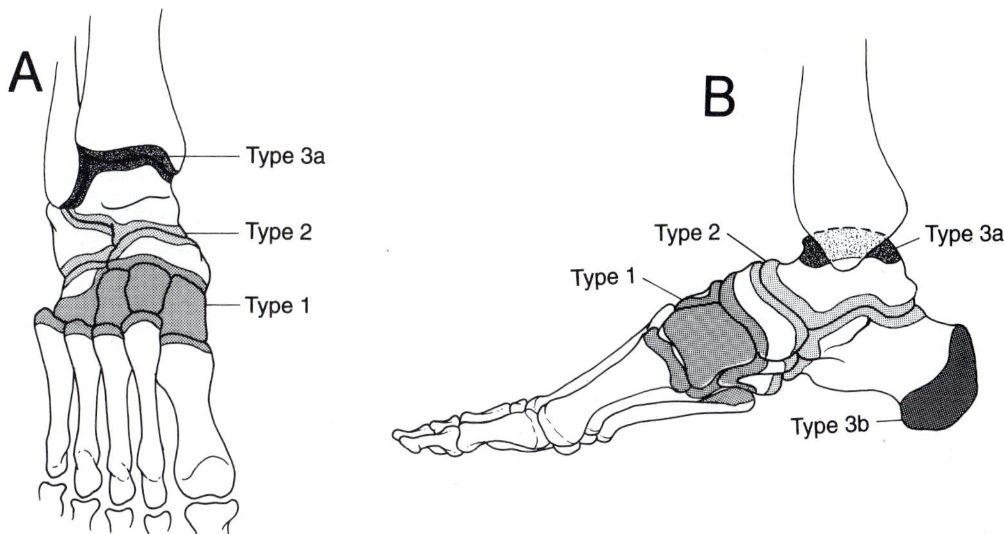

FIG 22–61.
A and **B,** the anatomic classification of Charcot joints of the tarsus: type 1 ("midfoot" involving the tarsometatarsal and naviculocuneiform joints); type 2 ("hindfoot" involving the subtalar, talonavicular, or calcaneocuboid joints); type 3A ("ankle" involving the tibiotalar joint); and type 3B ("os calcis" involving a pathologic fracture of the tubercle of the calcaneus).

common but more frequently associated with discrete traumatic incidents such as a major ankle fracture in the case of type 3A Charcot joints.

Although there is clearly quite a bit of overlap in the natural history of the different types of Charcot joints, there are clear patterns of behavior and progression of the different types of Charcot joints. It is useful to both physician and patient to know the most commonly expected course, problems, and outcomes that can be reasonably anticipated on the basis of the anatomic classification. As described above, the two major problems inherent in Charcot joints are the development of *bony prominences* caused by the structural shift or collapse of the foot and the development of extensive bone destruction with *persistent instability* due to the loss of skeletal integrity. While the two problems are not mutually exclusive, a study of 112 feet in 86 diabetics with major Charcot changes in the tarsus (from the tibiotalar joint down to and including the tarsometatarsal joint) revealed clear patterns of natural history.[18]

The type 1 or midfoot group was typified by the development of symptomatic bony prominences, a shorter average period of immobilization required for bony healing, and lower likelihood of requiring long-term immobilization (of a year or more) in a cast or brace (Fig 22–62). This group is typified by the occurrence of rocker-bottom feet and/or severe midfoot valgus deformity and bony protuberances that produce increased pressure leading to serious and persistent ulcerations on the medial and lateral borders and especially on the plantar surface of the foot. Other characteristics include a higher proportion of hypertrophic bony changes and a lower incidence of erosive bone changes than found in type 2 feet. Type 1 feet tend to settle into a stable, but deformed shape and thus are most likely to present late when the patient has already reached Eichenholtz stage 2 of osseous coalescence or even Eichenholtz stage 3 of bony healing, even without having been treated. This group of Charcot feet are most likely to require treatment of ulcerations, either with total-contact casts and AFO braces or by surgical resection of the underlying bony prominences that are causing the ulcers.

By contrast, the type 2 or hindfoot group was typified by the development of chronic, persistent skeletal instability, often associated with the anecdotal term "bag of bones" (Fig 22–63). These patients were less likely to develop ulcerations due to symptomatic bony prominences, but bony prominences did occur in about a third; they were more likely to require long periods of immobilization until Eichenholtz stages 2 and 3 of bony consolidation are finally reached. The average period of immobilization was also longer in type 2 feet than in type 1 feet, almost 2 years. The association of type 2 Charcot joints with long-term immobilization of 1 year or greater was also statistically significant. These patients are more likely to have persistent enlargement that cannot be easily contained in normal shoe wear and that produces a shift of the entire foot off of the weight-bearing axis of the leg.

Type 3 joints, in which the changes are in the ankle

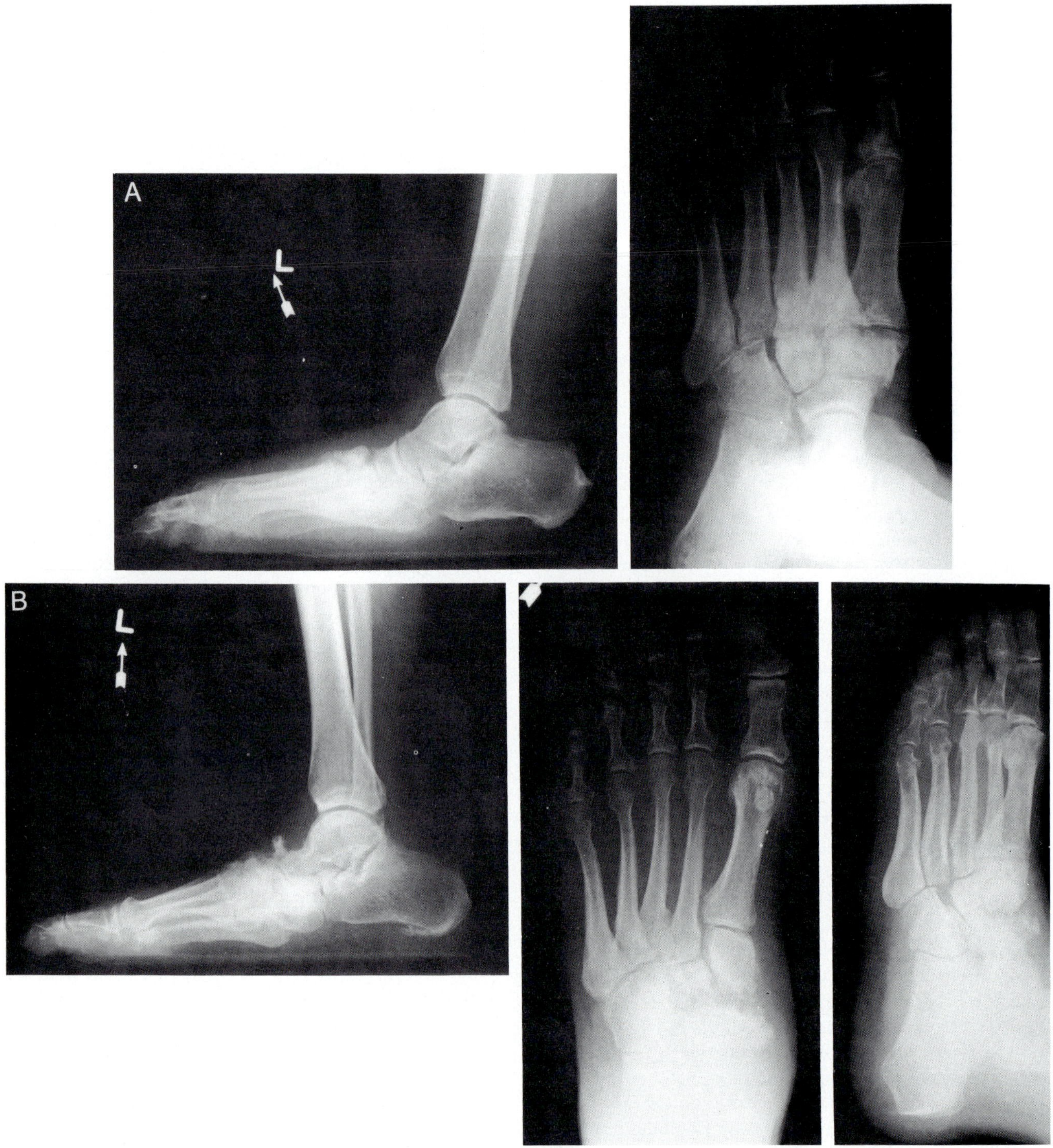

FIG 22–62.
Type 1 (midfoot) Charcot joints of the diabetic tarsus. **A,** primarily affecting the tarsometatarsal joints. Note the loss of the arch and the abduction through the midfoot. **B,** primarily affecting the naviculocuneiform joints with arch collapse.

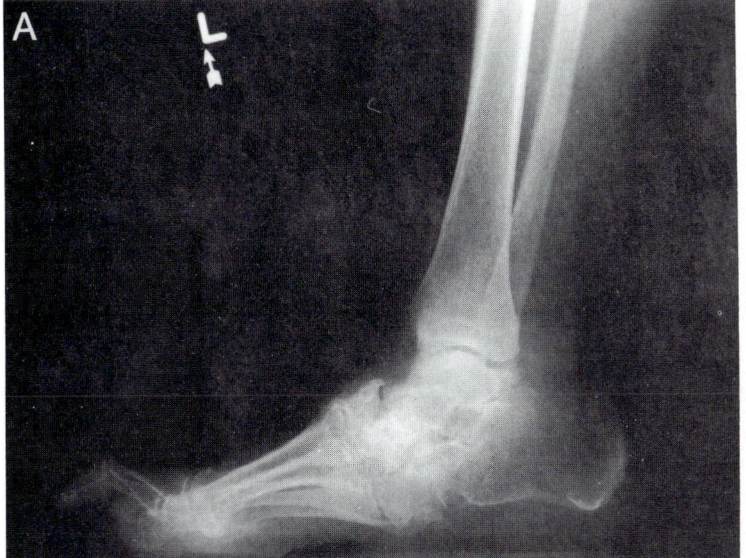

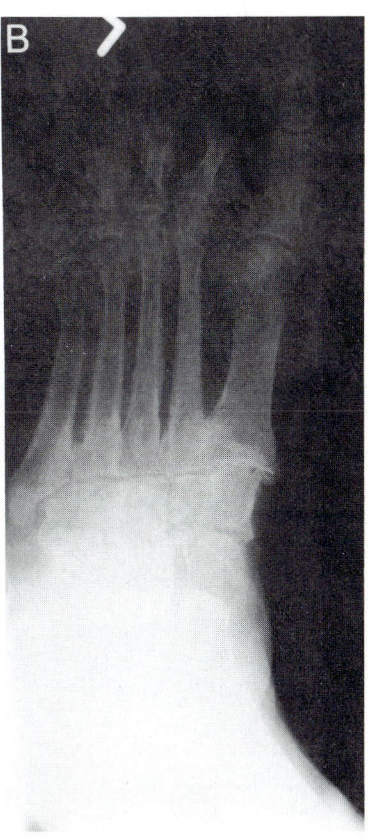

FIG 22–63.
A and **B,** type 2 (hindfoot) Charcot joint. The navicular is no longer interposed between the talus and the cuneiforms while the talar head is deviated downward and laterally.

itself, are similar to the hindfoot (type 2) group, with the formation of chronic swelling and instability requiring immobilization for an average of over a year in order to achieve bony healing. Type 3 joints develop chronic enlargement and shortening and can then drift into serious varus or valgus deformities and lead to pressure over the malleoli with subsequent ulcerations, infection, and osteomyelitis (Fig 22–64). Thus, type 3 (ankle) Charcot joints experience a combination of both of the major problems, bony prominences and instability.

The principle that was borne out by this study is that the closer the area of neuropathic joint destruction is to the axis of weight bearing in the limb, i.e., the more proximal the area of the Charcot change, the longer the immobilization and the greater the propensity for producing long-term instability.

Type 3B Charcot joints occurred in patients who developed a pathologic fracture in the tubercle of the calcaneus that later led to secondary collapse of the foot (Fig 22–65). In contrast to the three other types of Charcot joints in which the primary process was articular, in type 3B feet, the changes occurred primarily with a fracture whose mechanical effect led to secondary, more distal joint changes. These patients were treated with shoe modifications after relatively short periods of immobilization. Similar cases have been reported sporadically.[28] The association of the occurrence of symptomatic bony prominences with type 1 Charcot joints and the association of long-term instability (greater than 1 year) with type 2 Charcot joints are statistically significant.[18, 19]

Treatment Techniques of the Charcot Joint.—The goals of treatment of the Charcot foot are to achieve the third stage of bony healing, to minimize and treat soft-tissue breakdown and ulcerations, and to keep the patient as normally ambulatory as possible during the process. The inherently slow nature of the healing process needs to be emphasized both to the physician and the patient. Once expectations have been set for a treatment period that lasts from several months to several years, appropriate conservative measures can be instituted. It is important to note that the majority of Charcot feet can and should be treated by primarily nonsurgical regimens. Surgical reconstructions, even when correctly indicated, do not speed the healing of a Charcot joint, nor do they restore entirely normal size or configuration to the foot. In contrast, surgery may even temporarily delay the healing process by its effect of creating new "fractures" or additional instability through operative realignment or resection. The specific indications for surgical intervention will be discussed below.

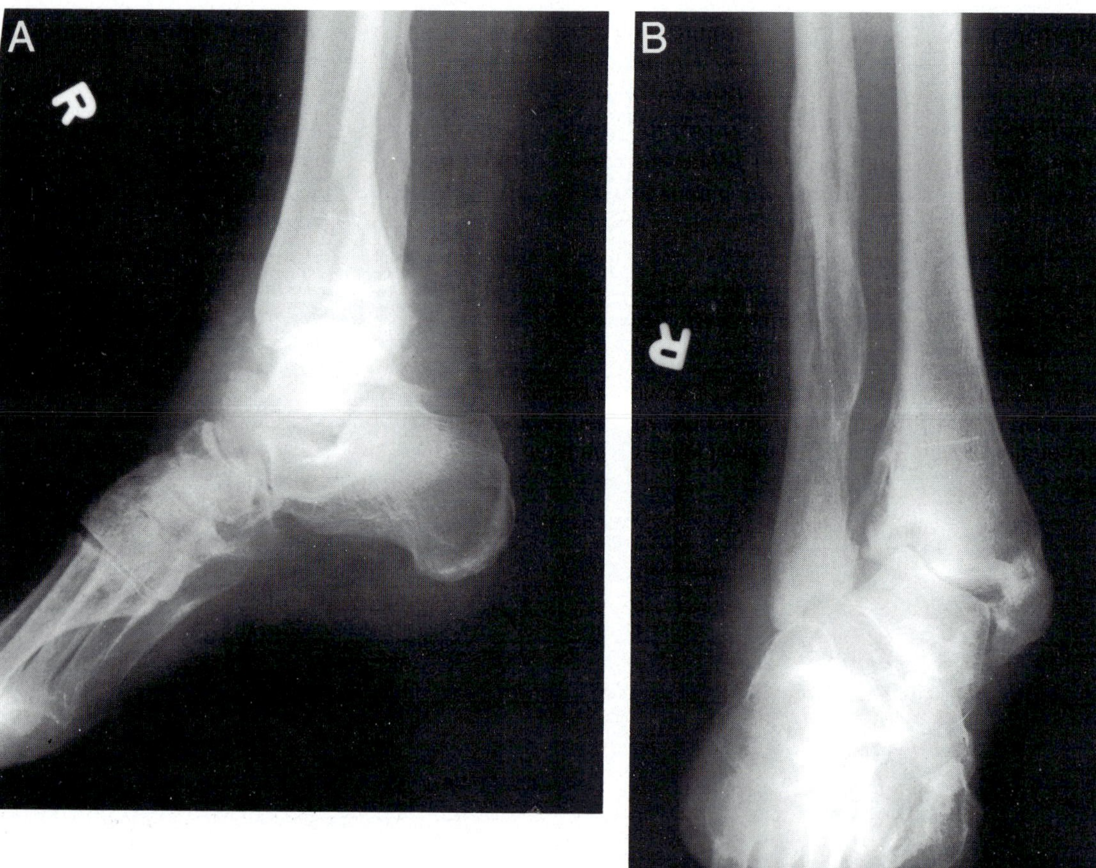

FIG 22–64.
A and **B,** type 3A (ankle) Charcot joint. Note the severe valgus. The patient presented in Figures 22–1 to 22–3 also has a type 3A joint.

Treatment of the Charcot joint begins with rest and elevation to diminish the swelling. Some centers use pneumatic devices to initially reduce swelling, but the most common and most effective measure is the use of a total-contact cast. The cast does not significantly differ from the cast used to treat neuropathic plantar ulcers. The first total-contact cast should be changed at approximately 1 week because it usually produces a dramatic reduction in swelling and thus effectively loosens the cast. If loose enough, the cast can slide on the limb and produce an increased risk of blisters and new ulcers, both of which are always a concern with use of the cast in any case. As noted in the previous section on the total-contact cast, two of the most important details of technique are not to overpad the cast, because this packs down with wear and increased subsequent loosening, and to use felt or foam on the bony prominences of the tibia, malleoli, etc. If the patient develops secondary blisters, abrasions, or ulcerations, the most common complication of the total-contact cast, then temporary discontinuation of the cast may be necessary for a brief period of non–weight bearing or the use of a prefabricated walking brace (see Fig 22–20,C). While some authors have suggested using these braces for all Charcot joints, this is clearly neither practical nor desirable. While there is a definite place for these devices as cast substitutes when other alternatives are not possible in certain cases, it has some distinct disadvantages and liabilities. Prefabricated walkers are not customized to the foot and leg like a cast and are often unable to accommodate bony prominences; this leads to soft-tissue breakdown itself, especially around the malleoli. Many Charcot feet are too deformed to fit into these prefabricated devices, especially if there is varus or valgus at the ankle or marked abduction and flattening at the midfoot. These devices also lack the very important effect of controlling edema, an effect of a cast made possible by its intimate fit and its circumferential nature, as well as the fact that it cannot be removed by the patient.

Thus, the first step in treatment of most Charcot

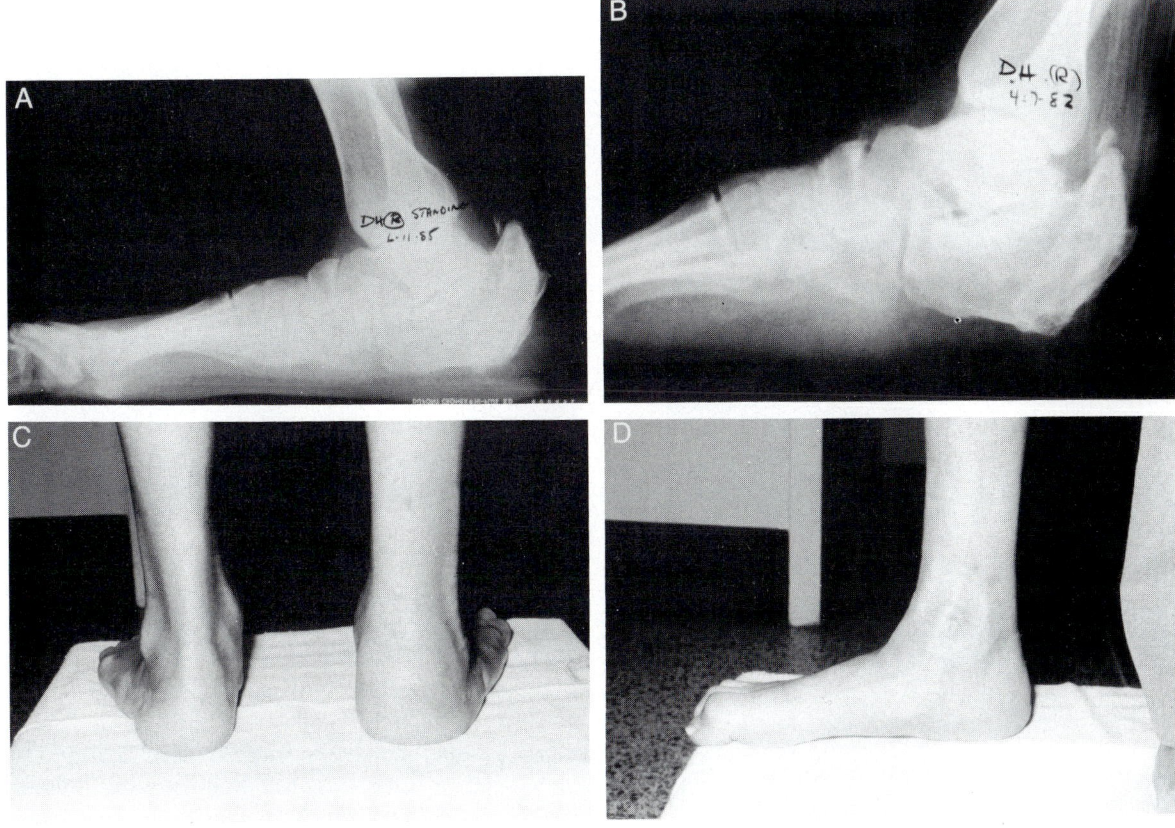

FIG 22–65.
A–D, type 3B (os calcis) Charcot joint. The pathologic fracture of the tubercle of the calcaneus has produced secondary collapse of the longitudinal arch and widening of the heel.

joints, presuming that they present in Eichenholtz stage I, is cast immobilization. This represents acute treatment of the acutely inflamed and swollen foot and ankle and continues until the inflammation begins to subside substantially. The interval for replacement of the casts gradually increases from 1 to several weeks as the process moves into the subacute phase. Various methods have been used to judge the subsidence of stage I (fragmentation, acute inflammation) and the onset of stage II (coalescence, diminished swelling, and inflammation). These include water displacement measurements (the Archimedes principle) of foot volume (Fig 22–66), measuring the temperature with an infrared thermometer (Fig 22–67), or simply examining the foot for diminished swelling and reduced warmth as judged by touching the foot with the back of the hand and fingers. Water displacement is accurate but cumbersome, even with a regular setup for its use, and is better if repeated at about the same time of day each session due to the fluctuations in swelling over the course of the day; infrared thermometers are expensive devices.

The exact timing of advancement to the second stage of treatment is not critical but should be marked by a reduction in the acute erythema and warmth and a substantial reduction in the daily fluctuations in swelling so that a removable AFO with anterior and posterior shells will be practical and not become excessively tight at the end of the day. The second stage of treatment is the use of a custom-made cast substitute, usually manufactured of polypropylene or similar thermoplastic material and made by an orthotist. The anterior and posterior shells should fit together in "clamshell" fashion (see Fig 22–44) with the device extending from just below the knee down onto the foot and ankle. One of the disadvantages in the second stage of treatment of a Charcot joint is that the total-contact AFO is bulky, thus necessitating a larger shoe to go around it, and it is uncosmetic, which is a source of unhappiness for some patients. The AFO can be lined with a heat-moldable polyethylene foam (such as Plastazote, Aliplast, Pelite, etc.) to function as a protective interface for cushioning and resistance to shear stress on the skin. Additional depth is sometimes built into the posterior half shell containing the foot plate in order to have room to place

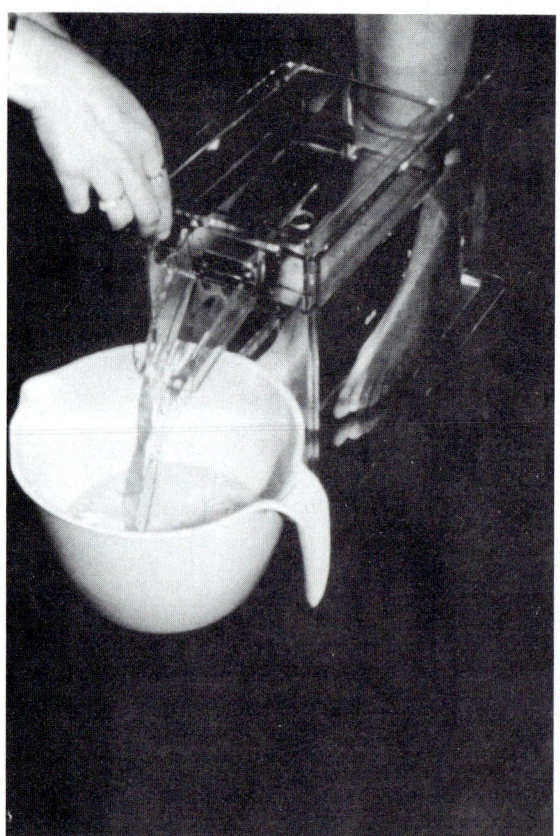

FIG 22–66.
The water-displacement technique for measuring Charcot foot edema. (Courtesy of Drs. J. Johnson and J. Gould.)

a removable (and replaceable) insole to further accommodate and pad the bony prominences of the foot. The AFO treatment is continued until the patient has reached the Eichenholtz stage III of bony consolidation and healing, a process that may take many, many months and a number of AFO modifications and refurbishments to accommodate changes in foot swelling and shape as well as wear of the brace.

Stage III of the Charcot joint is reached when the foot has stabilized clinically, achieved bony healing as judged by radiography, and does not have significant soft-tissue breakdown due to the underlying bony prominences. At this point, the patient is provided a custom-molded, dual-density accommodative insole (see the section on shoes and insoles below) and then fitted with appropriately large shoe wear to fit the combination of the foot and insole. The shoe wear may be a custom-made shoe, an additional-depth orthopaedic shoe, or even a well-fitted jogging or walking shoe, provided that it has enough room to accommodate the altered shape of the foot as well as the moderately bulky insole. Proper manufacture of the insole and selection of the correct shoe can be critical and requires professional input (see the section on shoe wear and insoles below). The physician must aid the patient in this last stage of treatment; it is not enough to shepherd the patient through the healing; provision must be made to treat the residual changes and try to prevent the recurrence of soft-tissue breakdown in a foot that is almost always deformed to some extent. Some patients, even though they have reached the third stage of healing, have sufficient deformity that for the purposes of support, they must permanently wear an AFO brace with the molded insole incorporated and with appropriate shoe wear, as needed. There are also some patients with very severe involvement of the hindfoot and ankle, especially if they have had surgery for the purpose of an arthrodesis, who achieve little or no bony healing, with the ankylosis being fibrous in nature. These patients usually require permanent use of an AFO brace as well.

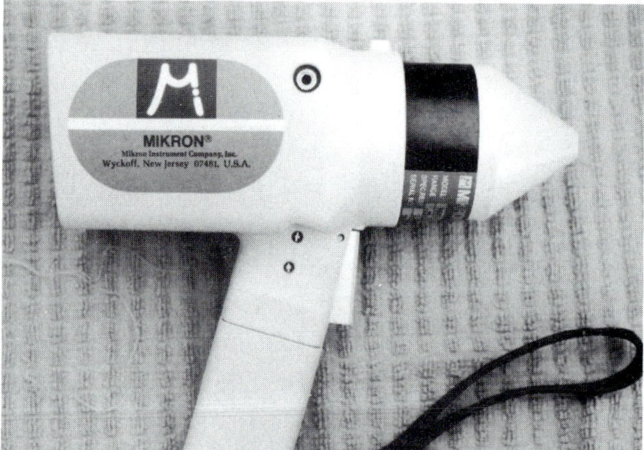

FIG 22–67.
Infrared thermometer for assessing reductions in local heat in the Charcot foot.

Some patients are first diagnosed or seen by the orthopaedic surgeon in a subacute or chronic stage rather than at the onset of their disease. A delay in the diagnosis of Charcot joints has been common in the past, and patients are often seen with a chief complaint of a suspected abscess or a "cellulitis" that is unresponsive to antibiotics. Treatment should be modified to the stage of the foot along the continuum of treatment at the time of presentation (Fig 22–68). As noted above, type 1 Charcot feet are the most likely to present at a later stage, and many will even be seen late in a stage II or even stage III when they have undergone autoarthrodesis.

Complications of Charcot Joints of the Foot and Ankle

Complications of the Charcot joint include deep infection as well as osteomyelitis, ulcerations due to Char-

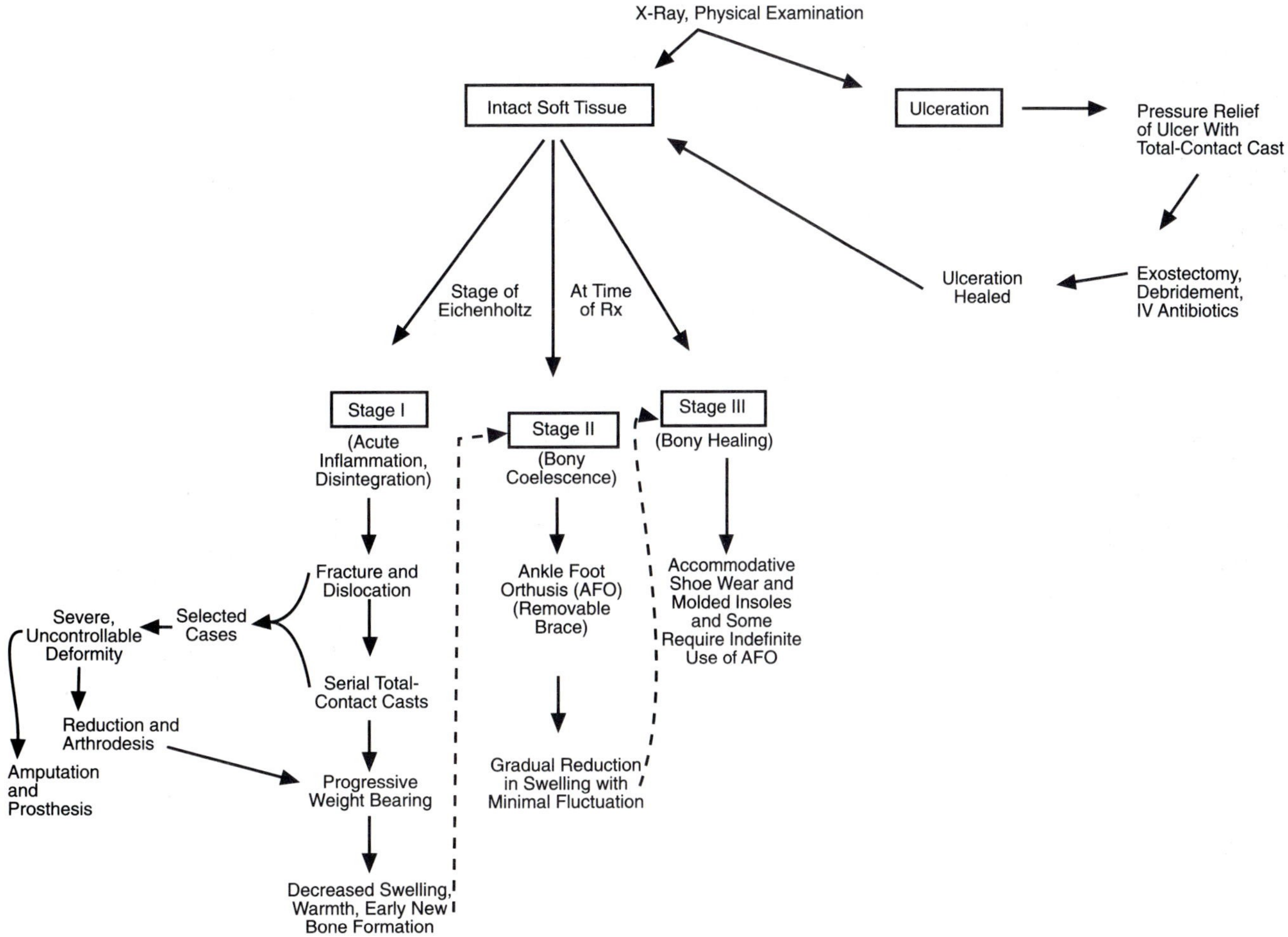

FIG 22–68.
Flowchart diagramming the basic treatment of a Charcot foot.

cot bony prominences, and severe uncontrollable deformity (not necessarily a discrete prominence) causing soft-tissue breakdown, even to the point of requiring amputation.

Deep Infection.—Osteomyelitis occurs in the Charcot foot as the result of extension from a soft-tissue focus, usually an ulcer. One type of deep infection that is particularly difficult to treat is osteomyelitis that occurs over the lateral border of the midfoot and hindfoot and is caused by a varus hindfoot or ankle deformity secondary to the Charcot joint. Once this proximal varus leads to deep infection, surgical intervention is required to deal with the osteomyelitis as delineated in the section on that subject, as well as to correct the predisposing varus deformity. As has been noted above, this is usually accomplished with a triple arthrodesis if not controllable with AFO bracing alone.

Ulcerations.—When the bony prominences produce plantar ulcerations, these ulcers should be treated with local wound care, antibiotics, and total-contact casts or other weight-modifying techniques, just as forefoot ulcers would be treated. This often coincides with the use of a cast for immobilization of the deep osseous dissolution. If the ulcer can be healed in the cast, then treatment proceeds according to the algorithm above. If the ulcer is the result of so much underlying bony pressure that it cannot heal or if it heals but recurs once casting is discontinued (provided that the patient is in stage II or III), then surgical intervention may be required. The goal of surgery at this stage is once again to relieve the bony prominence that is causing the ulcer either through exostectomy or, less often, arthrodesis.

Severe, Uncontrollable Deformity.—An excellent example of this is the patient depicted in Figure 22–69, an

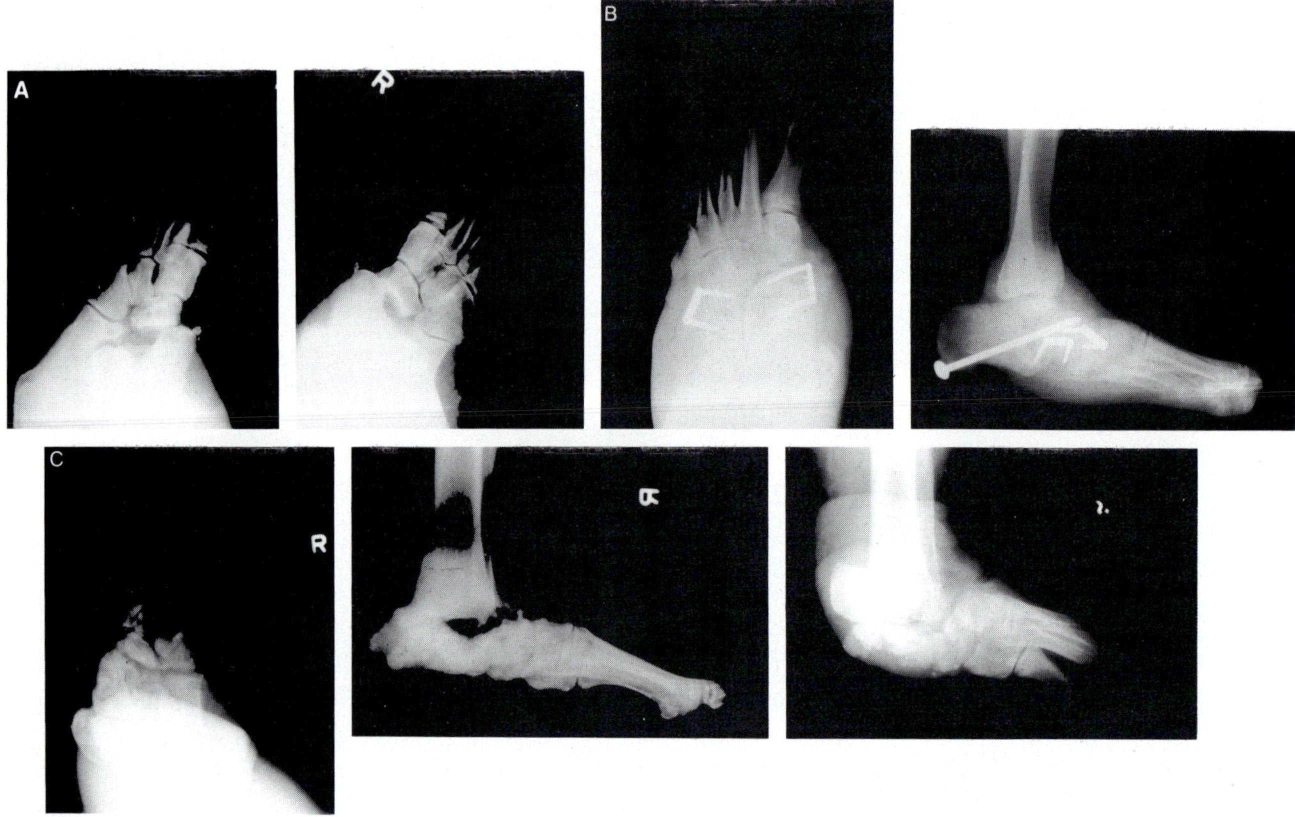

FIG 22–69.
A, acute atraumatic neuropathic subtalar dislocation with threatened soft-tissue breakdown over the talar head. **B,** triple arthrodesis with iliac bone grafting in an attempt to salvage the foot. **C,** loss of fixation accompanied by wound breakdown and infection. The hardware was removed, and the patient required a below-knee amputation.

obese patient with previous diabetic foot problems who presented with an acute subtalar dislocation. The deformity is too great to even simulate a plantigrade position for weight bearing, and thus, treatment in a total-contact cast or AFO is impossible. The foot is skewed off the end of the leg, and massive soft-tissue breakdown, infection, and amputation are imminent. This patient requires either amputation or one of the two other forms of surgical intervention.

Surgical Techniques in the Charcot Foot

There are two basic surgical techniques applicable to the Charcot foot. The first is excision of the bony prominences that cause ulceration and lead to infection. The second is arthrodesis to realign the deformed area and to reconstruct the architecture of the foot in order to produce a plantigrade foot and to relieve pressure on the soft tissue.

Exostectomy.—Excision of the bony prominences of a Charcot joint is similar to the technique used on the forefoot as described in the section on ulcers. Pretreatment of the ulcer with debridement, local wound care, and antibiotics is frequently necessary. Diagnostic studies such as biopsy or radionuclide imaging may be required to evaluate for underlying osteomyelitis. Documentation of the presence of infection in the bone would change therapy by leading to a longer period of treatment with intravenous antibiotics and possibly by causing the surgeon to do a more extensive bony debridement procedure.

Excision of the bony prominence is usually done through an incision on the medial or lateral border of the foot parallel to the sole; an incision on the sole that debrides and ellipses out the ulcer is used much less frequently. The soft tissue is dissected off of the bone as a full-thickness, single-layer flap until the bone projection has been exposed all around. A tourniquet is frequently used due to the hypervascular nature of most Charcot feet. Hemostasis is important but difficult, especially if there is much arterial calcification since the calcified vessels hold neither sutures nor electrocautery coagulates well. The bone is resected with osteotomes or an oscillating saw and the surface smoothed with rasps as needed (Fig 22–70). The surface should be made as level as possible over an area as wide as the exposure in order not to leave a new ridge or bony projection. A judgment must be made between resecting sufficient bone to relieve the pressure and preserving as much as possible to minimize further destabilization of the Charcot joints. Resection of prominences can also require a combination of removal of bone from the plantar surface and the medial and lateral borders of the foot. This is particularly common at the cuneiform-metatarsal joints if the forefoot is skewed into abduction. Resection of bone at the malleoli may be necessary for chronic ulceration, even if a more extensive realignment or arthrodesis is being performed simultaneously.

Exostectomy wounds usually require a postoperative suction drain or irrigation system. A loose closure is especially warranted if the latter is used. Swelling in these wounds is common, as is delayed healing of the skin and soft tissue whether a loose closure is used or not. Postoperative immobilization, usually in a total-contact cast, usually resumes once the healing of the wounds permits. Patients are usually kept non–weight bearing at least until the external support resumes, if not longer. Judgment on the part of the surgeon is necessary to determine the length of immobilization and depends on the maturity of the healing preoperatively (i.e., the Eichenholtz stage) and on the amount of instability produced by the surgical removal of bone.

Arthrodesis.—When severe deformity threatens the viability of a limb such that ulceration, infection, and amputation are the inevitable result, this is the clearest indication for arthrodesis of a Charcot joint. In most cases and in the hands of most surgeons, arthrodesis should be considered a salvage procedure only, without which the foot or limb would be sacrificed to amputation.

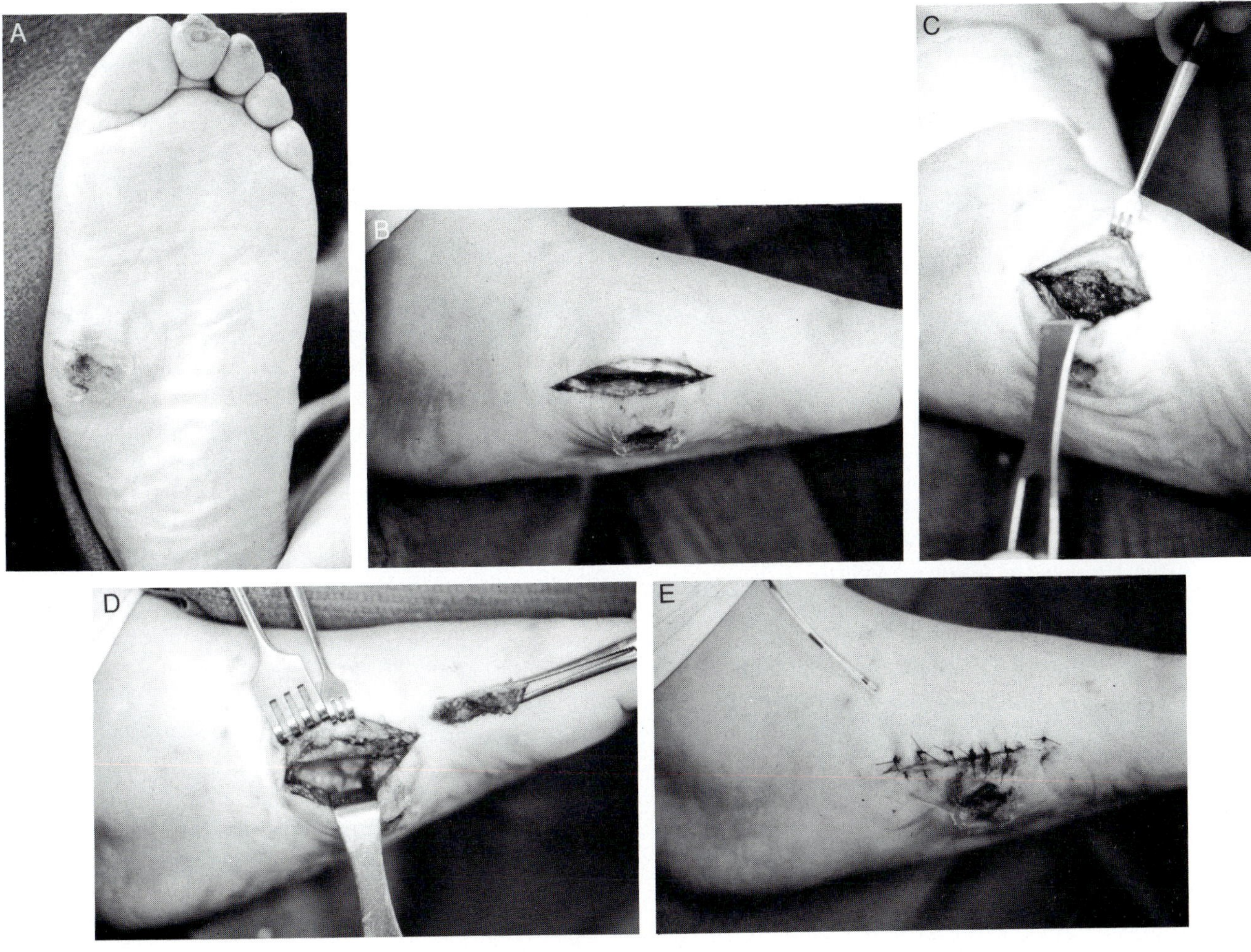

FIG 22–70.
Exostectomy for ulceration under a Charcot bony prominence. **A,** ulceration under a widened midfoot. **B,** straight medial incision with a full-thickness soft-tissue flap developed down to the bone. **C,** exposure of the bony prominence. **D,** resection of the exostosis and the excised piece of bone. **E,** closure over either an irrigation system or a suction drain.

While there are exceptions to this principle, arthrodesis of insensitive limbs is fraught with pitfalls and potentially horrendous complications and should be done by an orthopaedic surgeon with experience in this area. It is not to be considered nonchalantly because the frequent result of failed arthrodesis here is amputation. In a patient who would otherwise be doomed to amputation because of the severity of deformity in the limb, arthrodesis is an especially appropriate salvage procedure.

To achieve a solid arthrodesis in a Charcot foot can be a daunting task at best. The same forces that caused dissolution of the normal bone and joint structures still exist to cause breakdown of the surgical construct as well. It bears reiteration that arthrodesis is only occasionally necessary and the majority of Charcot feet proceed to solid bony healing, a form of autoarthrodesis that occurs with only immobilization and time. The technique for arthrodesis must be meticulous. Iliac or other extensive bone grafting is usually recommended. Timing of the surgery also has great bearing on the outcome. The surgery should be done either early in stage I, i.e., soon after the time of the acute dislocation and/or fracture, before the development of extensive osteopenia due to the local hyperemia and non–weight bearing, or delayed until stage II when new bone formation is occurring and the acute inflammatory stage has abated. The osteopenia of full-blown stage I is exemplified by its synonym fragmentation; fixation is difficult to achieve, and results are even more unpredictable.

Every attempt must be made to achieve as rigid an internal fixation construct as possible—although it must be said at the onset that it is not always possible. Screws and sometimes plates are required (Fig 22–71). Unfortunately, sometimes Steinmann pins are the best fixation that can be secured; these are usually cases when the limited goal of the procedure is to realign the foot on the leg, even if fibrous ankylosis is the result. This is a relatively common outcome, and a high percentage of attempted arthrodeses will not result in bony ankylosis.[80] Despite the fact that a large number of these relatively uncommon procedures will only achieve fibrous ankylosis, internal fixation, especially in the hindfoot (type 2) and ankle groups (type 3A), will serve to maintain alignment of the foot and achieve limited success. This success is converting the foot to a plantigrade one that is now "braceable." Such a foot may require permanent use of a posterior-shell or total-contact, anterior- and posterior-shell AFO, in the hope an amputation may be averted and the limb continue to function in weight bearing.

Illustrated in Figure 22–69 is a case that did not have such a fortunate outcome, a patient with acute, spontaneous, neuropathic subtalar dislocation. There was no associated trauma. Despite internal fixation and extensive bone grafting of the triple arthrodesis, the patient was simply unable to be non–weight bearing due to obesity and debilitation. Wound breakdown and infection developed and required removal of the hardware and debridement and, eventually, a below-knee amputation. Other patients with the same severe, spontaneous dislocation have chosen to have an amputation primarily and rapidly returned to work with the use of a Syme prosthesis.

The greatest challenge of the Charcot foot still lies in accurate recognition and early conservative treatment with proper immobilization in the majority of cases. Although approximately 10% to 12% develop a major complication that leads to amputation, the majority of patients continue to function and even work despite this permanent deformation of the foot or ankle. The well-informed physician needs to counsel the patient on both the serious nature of the problem and its protracted course of healing, as well as the reasonable outcome, albeit with deformity, that is the result of most cases.

Skin and Nail Problems

While care of the skin and nails is widely considered unglamorous at best and tedious at worst, it is an essential part of the routine care of the diabetic foot.[55] The loss of normal sweating that occurs as a result of autonomic neuropathy causes the skin to become excessively dry and thus more susceptible to cracks that propagate down into the dermis and lead to infection. The patient should be instructed, as a part of the once- or twice-daily routine inspections, to apply skin lotion to dry areas of the skin. Care should be taken to avoid moistening between the toes, where the skin is least likely to become scaly and where excessive moisture leads to maceration. Application of lotion or a very thin layer of petroleum jelly immediately after bathing can seal in the hydration absorbed by the skin during the bath or shower.

Care of the nails requires a few special instruments to be kept in the office or clinic. These are illustrated in Figures 22–72 and 22–73. (Appendix 22–3). It is usually most convenient to keep the instruments together in a sterile tray; extras of the most frequently used instruments can be wrapped separately. The double-action bone rongeur is, of course, a surgical instrument. It has many advantages for trimming the nails in diabetics, for whom nail pathology can be the initiating event of more serious foot problems. The rongeur can generate

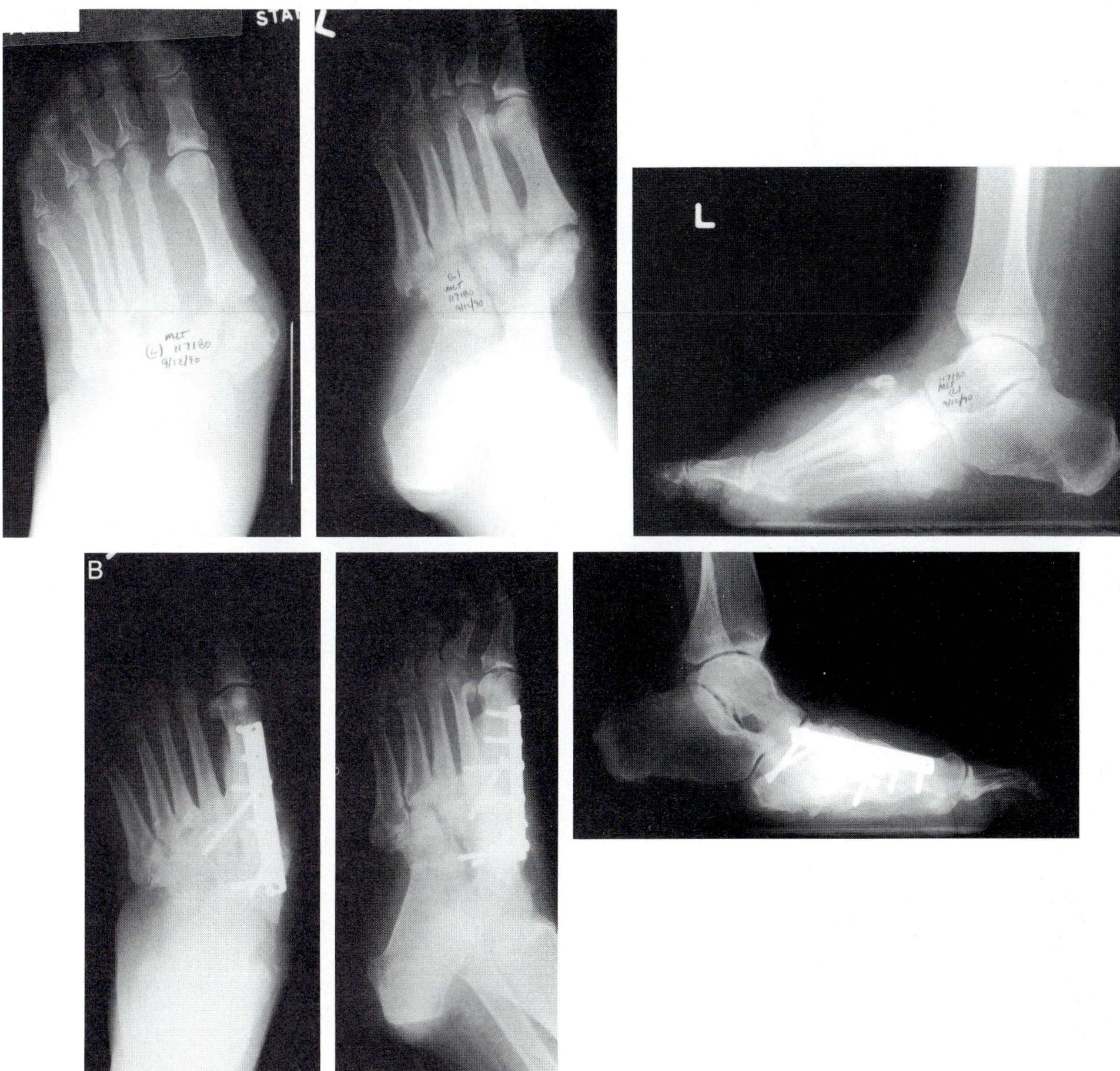

FIG 22–71.
A, patient with advanced midfoot Charcot deformity and soft-tissue breakdown over an extruded medial cuneiform. **B,** limited arthrodesis with internal fixation and iliac grafting to relieve pressure on soft tissue and reestablish first ray weight bearing.

enough force to clip thickened nails without twisting the nail on its attachments. The rounded beaks can be used to protect and push the soft tissue away from the cutting edges. Very hard nails should be "nibbled" away, a bit at a time.

The anvil-type nail splitter has a flat lower jaw that is pushed under the nail to separate it from the nail bed, while the sharp, triangular upper jaw splits the nail by coming together with the flat "anvil" portion. This is the safest way to remove a nail margin for an acutely infected and ingrown toenail while preventing cutting the nail bed below, which could lead to infection or inflammation of the underlying bone of the distal phalanx. The Freer elevator is useful for lifting up the split portion of the nail and for separating the nail from the overlying eponychial fold. The nail curet is used for de-

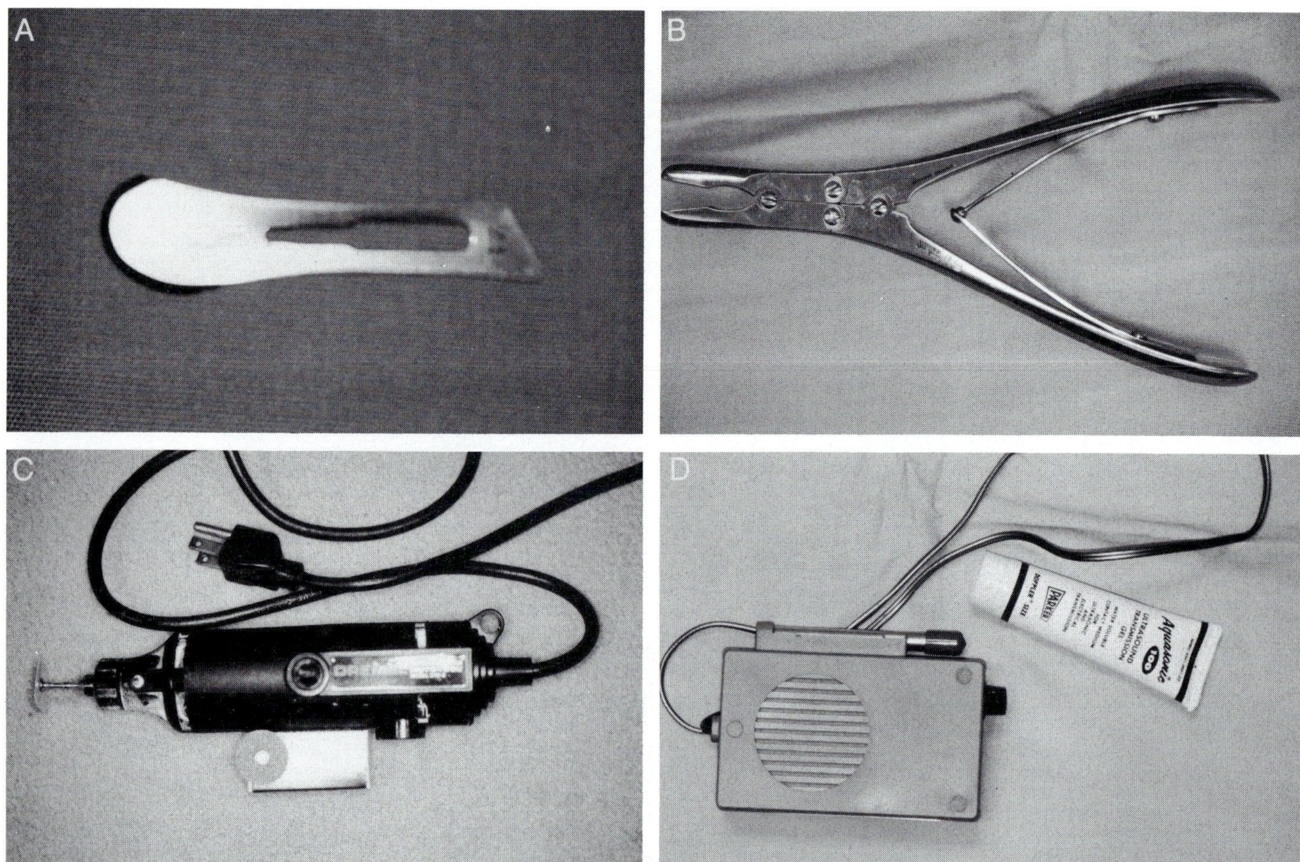

FIG 22–72.
Useful office instruments for skin and nail care of the diabetic foot. **A,** no. 17 blade for trimming calluses. **B,** a double-action bone rongeur for clipping thickened, onychomycotic toenails. **C,** a motorized hobby drill with sanding disks for filing and smoothing calluses and nails. **D,** a hand-held Doppler ultrasound device for auscultation of pedal pulses.

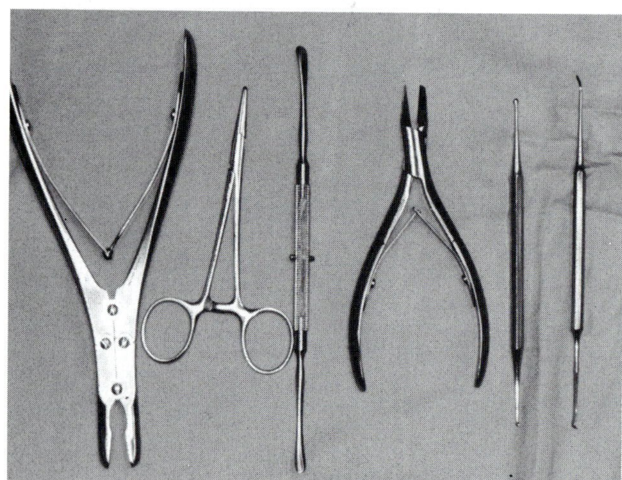

FIG 22–73.
Basic instruments to keep in a sterile tray for clinic care of nails. From *left to right,* double-action rongeur, hemostat, Freer elevator, anvil-type nail splitter, nail curette, and nail elevator. See Appendix 22–3.

briding a corner of the nail where it is compressing the adjacent soft tissue.

Shoe Wear and Shoe Insoles

The use of proper shoes and shoe insoles constitutes an important, actually crucial part of the care of the diabetic with foot problems. Even the patient with a "grade 0" foot, i.e., one without actual breakdown or infection but with risk of the same, needs correct and professional advice since ill-fitting shoes and areas of concentrated plantar pressure within shoes are the most common problems that initiate the sequence of events leading to ulceration, infection, and amputation of the diabetic's lower extremity.

Much scientific work remains to be done in the study of shoe and shoe insoles, but some of the principles of each will be elucidated here. Even greater and more arduous tasks await health professionals in the job of convincing their patients to modify their behavior and attitudes toward the fashion of footwear. Altering opinions on unhealthy behavior can be done, as has been shown in campaigns to change diet and smoking habits, for example, but is difficult at best. The gravity and immediacy of the threat from improper shoe wear to the health of the individual with insensitive feet can be even greater than the problems of diet and smoking and needs to be emphasized through education of diabetic patients.

Shoe Wear

The goal of shoe wear in the diabetic (or other patient with diminished sensitivity of the feet) is to help protect the foot by relieving or diminishing areas of potential pressure concentration that can lead to blistering or ulceration. It is well known that a diabetic with dense neuropathy can develop severe ulceration within the space of an hour or two of wearing a poorly fitting shoe. Shoes for the diabetic should not have to be "broken in," i.e., they should basically be fit to the proper size at the time they are dispensed and not depend upon stretching to achieve that fit; otherwise, soft tissues will usually break down before the shoe does. However, once a new pair of even correctly fitted shoes has been dispensed, during the first few days the shoes should be removed at intervals of gradually increasing length at first in order to inspect the skin of the feet for areas of abrasion, redness, or pressure. The shoe and/or insole can then be modified or replaced before major skin breakdown occurs.

The attributes of a "good" shoe for a diabetic include several characteristics. The toe box should be wide *and* deep enough to prevent pressure, especially against the dorsum of the proximal interphalangeal joint of hammered toes. The leather should be fairly soft and pliable so that it conforms to the foot; inelastic materials like plastic, canvas, or patent leather should be shunned because they will contribute to high-pressure areas. The shoe should usually have a lace-up or Velcro closure of a Blucher-type (not a Balmoral) eyelet lacing because it allows more adjustment of the shoe fit (Fig 22–74). A padded heel counter or heel backstay, especially of the "pillow" type, helps diminish pressure on the area of the Achilles tendon (Fig 22–75).

One of the most important features of a diabetic shoe is that it should have additional depth to allow for placement of a custom-molded protective shoe insole. This type of shoe is best known by one of its trade names, "The Extra Depth Shoe," manufactured by the P.W. Minor Shoe Company. Other companies make shoes with additional depth as well, including but not necessarily limited to the Alden Shoe Company, Drew Shoes, etc. This is particularly critical in patients with prior plantar ulcerations, and the physician and surgeon should insist on the immediate fitting of the patient with a newly healed ulcer in some type of special shoe wear.

The options include an additional-depth shoe with a molded insole, a Plastazote shoe, or a Carville sandal. The latter two represent temporary fitting solutions as a transition from the total-contact cast to definitive shoe wear. Both the Plastazote shoe and the Carville sandal are lined with a forgiving, molded or moldable surface of a cushioning polyelthylene foam such as Plastazote. Cosmetic acceptance of these two devices can be rather limited, and neither represents the final shoe wear to be dispensed. The Carville sandal is usually manufactured by an orthotist or a certified pedorthist. The technique was developed at the Gillis W. Long National Hansen's Disease Center in Carville, Louisiana, where a sizable population of patients with leprosy and the resulting insensitive limbs have been cared for over many years. The technique for manufacturing the sandal has been published.[12] Plastazote shoes are commercially available.

Definitive shoe wear for the diabetic is usually either an off-the-shelf, additional-depth shoe or a custom-made shoe. The former comes with a ¼-in. liner that can be removed and substituted with a custom-molded insole; this constitutes the "extra depth" that is required not only for the foot but also for the insole. Custom-made shoes are sometimes required, but most patients can be fit in stock shoes if seen and fitted properly by a professional shoe fitter. Custom-made shoes must also be made with additional depth so that the liner of the shoe can be changed periodically as it fatigues. This should be the same type of custom-molded insole that lines the stock shoe so that only the liner and not the whole shoe can be replaced to accommodate minor changes in the foot. Custom shoes are most frequently needed for patients with Charcot joints and gross disruption of the structure of the foot.

Patients are generally advised to have at least two pairs of properly fitted shoes and insoles so that they may be changed in the course of heavy wear, even in the middle of a day's activity. Although in theory this is an excellent idea, the cost of the shoe wear and insoles can be prohibitive for many patients, especially since most health plans do not cover the costs of therapeutic footwear. In response to the issues of both cost and cosmesis, many professional shoe fitters have added the athletic or "jogging" or walking type of shoes to their armamentarium. These have a higher level of cosmetic acceptance, especially with popular styles of causal dress, and many come with a premade liner that can be removed and substituted with the custom-molded insole

Anatomy of the Shoe

Illustrated below are the component parts of a Goodyear Welt. Most functional shoes are constructed the same, depending on the style and pattern.

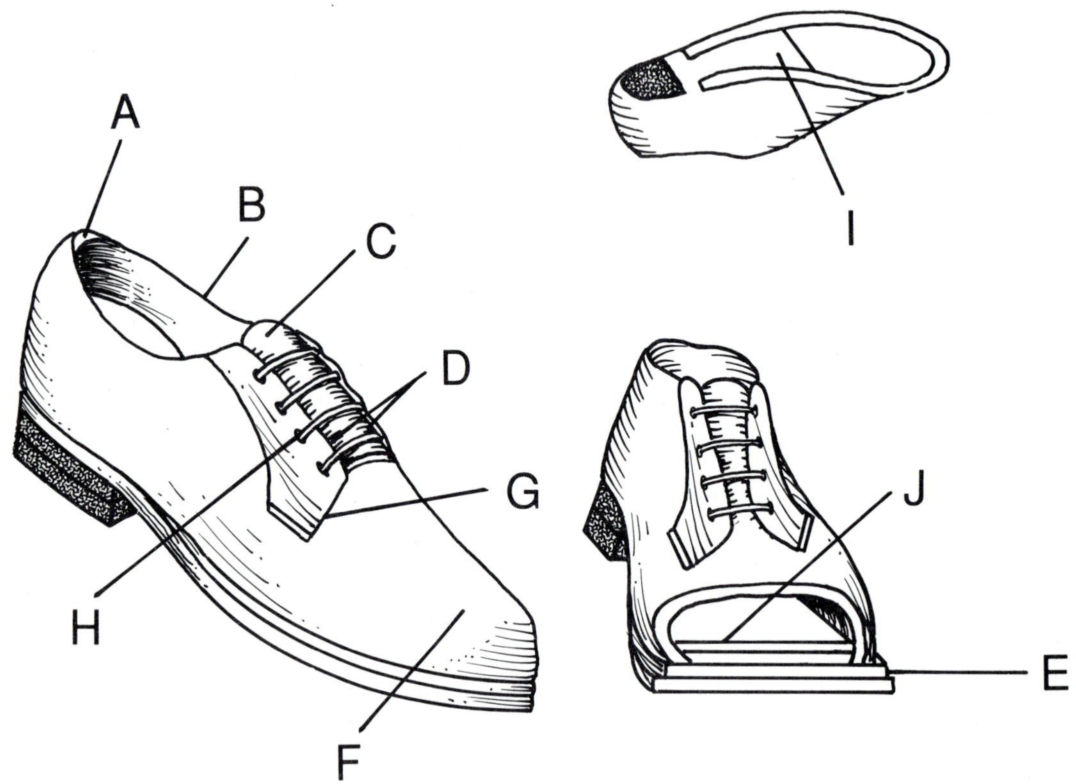

Legend:

A. Heel Counter
B. Top Line
C. Tongue
D. Vamp
E. Welt
F. Toe Cap
G. Throat Line
H. Eyelet Facing
I. Shank
J. Insole

FIG 22–74.
Basic anatomy of the shoe. This vocabulary is necessary for communicating shoe prescriptions.

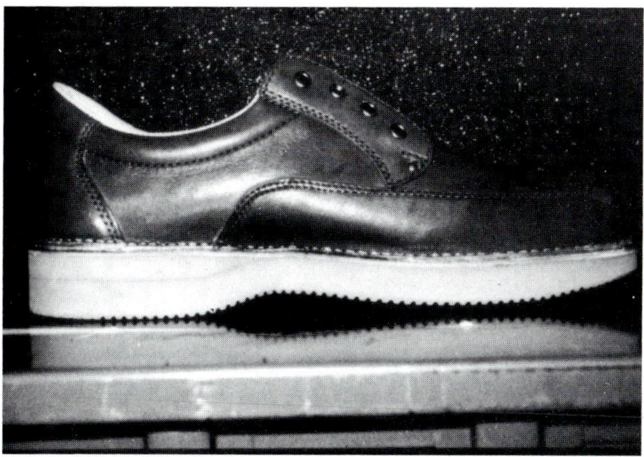

FIG 22–75.
"Pillow" or cushioned heel counter to protect the Achilles insertion in an insensitive limb.

to afford extra space within the shoe. Because women's shoes tend to be manufactured with narrower toes, some women are advised to purchase a man's athletic shoe because they usually come with a wider toe box for a given length. Even though these athletic shoes are widely available, patients should still be advised to be fitted by a professional shoe fitter, orthotist, or certified pedorthist who is trained not only in proper shoe fitting but also in the manufacture of the protective insoles since the foot must be fit to the combination of the shoe and the insole; the insole cannot be made as an afterthought because there will not be sufficient room in the shoe to accommodate it; the foot will be crowded, pressure created, and the problems made worse. The Professional Footwear Association (PFA) is the organization that offers education, training, and preparation for certification of pedorthists. **Appendix 22–7** lists this valuable resource; contact the PFA for a certified pedorthist in your area. In order to adequately communicate with professional shoe fitters and pedorthists, the basic glossary of shoe terms should be familiar for the purposes of writing prescriptions (see Fig 22–74).

Shoe Insoles

The use of shoe insoles in the patient with insensitive feet is a mainstay of both conservative management as well as a preventive measure in patients with deformity and neuropathy, especially those with a history of previous ulceration. There are myriad types of materials, combination of materials, and different devices that have been used in the shoes of diabetics and nondiabetics. Most of the prescribing rationale has been anecdotal or pseudoscientific, the latter representing an undocumented system of foot "biomechanics" without objective measurements or data. While some very fine work has been done recently and continues to be done in university settings on the mechanics of gait and the quantification of plantar pressures,* much remains to be learned about the effect of insoles and the materials of which they are composed. The following discussion is based on the current state of practice, which will no doubt rapidly advance in the near future.

Nomenclature

There has been a great deal of disservice done and misinformation spread by the use of the word "orthotic," meant in the sense of "a device to put into the shoe." In the first place, the word "orthotic" is an adjective, not a noun, and cannot be properly used in this context alone. It would be correct to say "orthotic device" or to delineate an "orthotic principle." The use of the term "orthotic" as a noun, usually meant to refer to a rigid or semirigid shoe insole of varying types, has been pseudoscientifically manipulated to infer that all such shoe devices exert a specific and predictable mechanical effect on the foot and as such are sophisticated and expensive medical devices. However, reliable, scientific data to support such claims or inferences simply do not exist for the majority of such devices that are currently sold in this country under the name "orthotics."

Second, the misuse of the word "orthotic" has led to an impression, held by the public at large, if not the medical community as well, that the discipline of the orthotist, i.e., the manufacture of orthoses, is strictly limited to the foot if not strictly limited to the manufacture of costly, rigid plastic devices to put into shoes. Of course, certified orthotists manufacture orthotic devices of many kinds pertaining to all parts of both the lower and upper limbs as well as the spine. This has unfortunately produced confusion and suspicion whenever the term "orthosis" is used in prescribing other kinds of external supports for the limbs and spines of our patients.

Because of the confusion over this common misnomer, it is more clear and concise to refer to the prescribed devices in the shoe as "shoe insoles," "shoe inserts," or "foot orthoses." The latter term is broader and could be construed to include other types of devices such as the University of California Biomechanics Laboratory (UCBL) device or the plastic AFO; the former term "shoe insole" is the most descriptive and will be used here for the devices prescribed to put into the shoe of diabetic patients with peripheral neuropathy and foot pathology.

**References 8, 9, 23, 24, 30, 36, 41, 73, 97.*

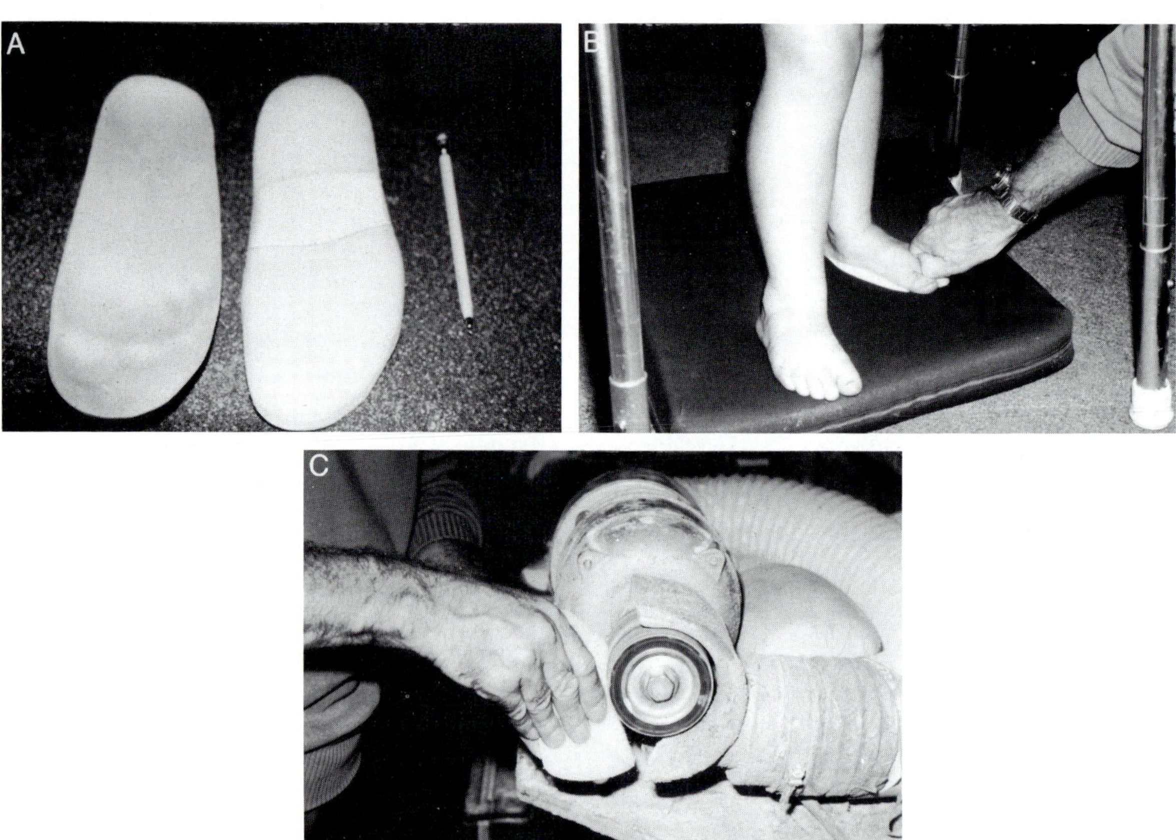

FIG 22–76.
Manufacture of custom-molded accommodative insoles from foamed polyethylenes (e.g., Plastazote, Aliplast, Pelite). **A,** dual-density design with softer material on top and firmer material underneath. **B,** molding of the heated material with weight bearing. **C,** grinding the edges of the molded insole to shape and fit it in a shoe.

Current practice is to use a custom-molded insole for diabetics that is made of two different densities of materials, at least one of which is a polyethylene foam that has been heated and molded to the foot of the patient. Examples of the most common combinations include soft or medium Plastazote on top of a firmer Pelite, Aliplast, or Plastazote, or the Plastazote on top of a nonmoldable material such as PPT, sorbothane, or PQ. The author's current preferred method may change in the near future but consists of using two layers of heat-moldable material that are first glued together and then heated in a convection oven at about 270°F for 60 to 90 seconds. The material is allowed to cool and then is molded by the weight-bearing pressure as the patient stands on the materials, which rest on top of a foam pillow. The block is then cut, shaped, and ground on a lathe to adjust its shape and thickness to fit it into the designated shoe. Additional modifications can be made on the undersurface such as adding a metatarsal pad or excavating the insole to provide relief for an area of high pressure (Fig 22–76).

The softer material is placed on the upper layer close to the foot so that it will compress and fatigue more easily than the skin of the foot. This is "backed" with a firmer material that maintains the shape and structural integrity of the device within the shoe. The insoles can be moved from shoe to shoe, depending upon the number of appropriately fitted shoes available. Studies of numerous insole materials have documented the general effectiveness of the materials in relieving pressures.[17, 67] Repetitive loading, as would occur in the course of walking, results in compression and loss of thickness of the materials that are made of polyethylene foam and are heat-molded.[22] This compression results in fatigue of the devices with loss of both the cushioning function and the custom-molded shape that distributes force over the plantar surface. For this reason, insoles do need to be replaced periodically; longer life can be attained by having two pair and alternating their use. The exact interval for replacement of diabetic insoles is highly variable, depending on the number of pairs of insoles used and the activity of the patient, but ranges from 4 to 12 months on average.

Presumably, the most important function of the insole materials is the attenuation of force in the areas of local pressure concentration that threaten to lead to soft-tissue breakdown. The diminution of pressure occurs as a result of the dissipation of the force of weight bearing over a wider area, the same concept that explains the function of the total-contact cast. The insole cannot reduce the absolute amount of force distributed through the patient's foot since that is a function of muscle action, the patient's mass, and the gravitational field of Earth. What the insole materials and shoe *can* do is to slow the rate of the impact and spread those forces over a wider area, thus attenuating the "hot spot" of extremely high pressure. A model of a bony plantar prominence with a force transducer below it to measure transmitted pressure (Fig 22–77) was devised and tested to measure the change in the forces relayed without and then with intervening insole materials. A variety of materials were placed between the pressure source and the projection of the model with its underlying transducer[17] in order to quantitate the amount of attenuation of force affected by the various materials. In this particular study, all of the materials were found to be effective in reducing pressures, with a moderate variability in effectiveness. The soft polyethylene foams (Plastazote and Pelite) were the most effective in force attenuation ("force distribution"), while the viscoelastic polymer (Sorbothane) was the most rigid and transmitted more of the applied forces. The materials were also tested for the effect of repetitive compression as well as the effect of combined shear and compression as analogues of the effects of standing and walking, respectively. Results were measured as the percentage of reduction in the thickness of the materials. The polyethylene foams were found to compress the most, followed by the neoprene rubber (Spenco) and the viscoelastic polymer (Sorbothane), with virtually no compression of the open-cell urethane foam (PPT or poron) (Fig 22–78). The attribute of compression of the foams is one, when viewed in a clinical perspective, that has both desirable and undesirable aspects. Greater compression means fatigue of the materials and is undesirable because of the need to replace the insole. However, it is desirable because the plantar skin will be protected better than by a rigid material since the compressible insole will give way and spare the skin of the sole.

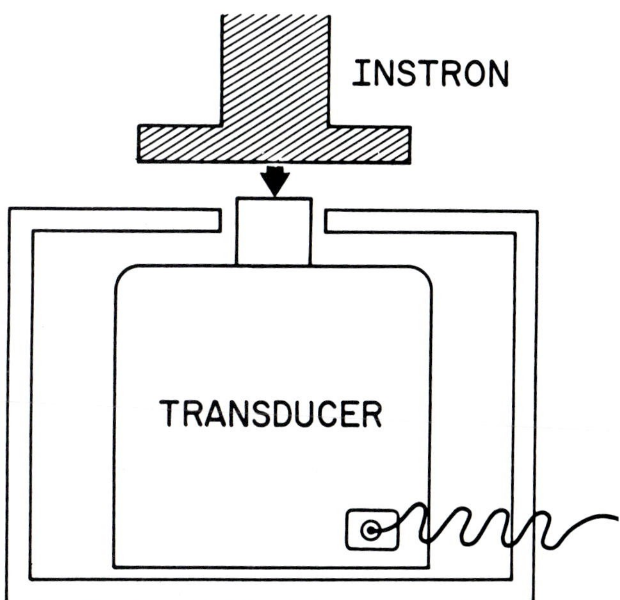

FIG 22–77.
Experimental model of a plantar bony prominence. This force attenuation jig with a transducer inside it was designed to test the properties of insole materials in relieving forces "felt" by the model. (From Brodsky JW, Kourosh S, Stills M: *Foot Ankle* 9:111–116, 1988. Used by permission.)

Other qualities of the materials must be considered as well, for example, the attribute or lack thereof of the material to be molded to the foot. For diabetic insoles, it is currently considered essential that at least the upper or closer layer be moldable. Some of the nonmoldable materials have the advantage of longer life after compression stress; the current concept is that a combination of materials probably affords the best compromise between a cushioning, molded insole and one that has durability and structural strength. One caveat that should be made is that the use of rigid orthoses, especially those made of hard plastics, "Rohadur," and the popular "sport orthotics" (Fig 22–79), are strictly contraindicated in the diabetic patient with neuropathy or a history of ulcerations. The use of rigid orthoses in the shoe of a patient with insensitivity is an invitation to disastrous consequences. The shoe insoles of the diabetic are meant to prevent or reduce the incidence of pressure-related problems and must, by definition, be made of accommodative materials. See Appendix 22–5 for examples of commonly used insert materials.

It is important to make a specific point to the patient who is prescribed a shoe insole for the first time that she will most likely need to be fitted for a different and larger-size shoe that has the appropriate last (shape) as well as room to fit the insole inside of it. Patients are not infrequently resistant to this since they may see shoes almost purely as an issue of cosmesis or style of dress rather than as a therapeutic device. In such an instance, it must be explained that the use of the insole in too small a shoe will exacerbate the pressure problems it is meant to deter by creating increased pressure in the shoe, especially in the toe box area.

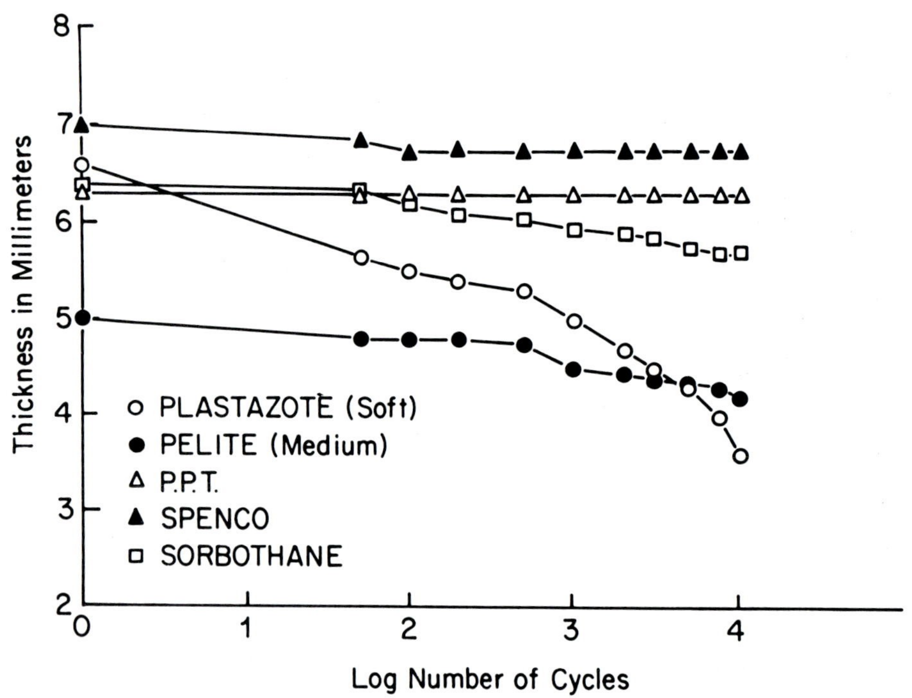

FIG 22–78.
Force attenuation properties of different insole materials. (From Brodsky JW, Kourosh S, Stills M: *Foot Ankle* 9:111–116, 1988. Used by permission.)

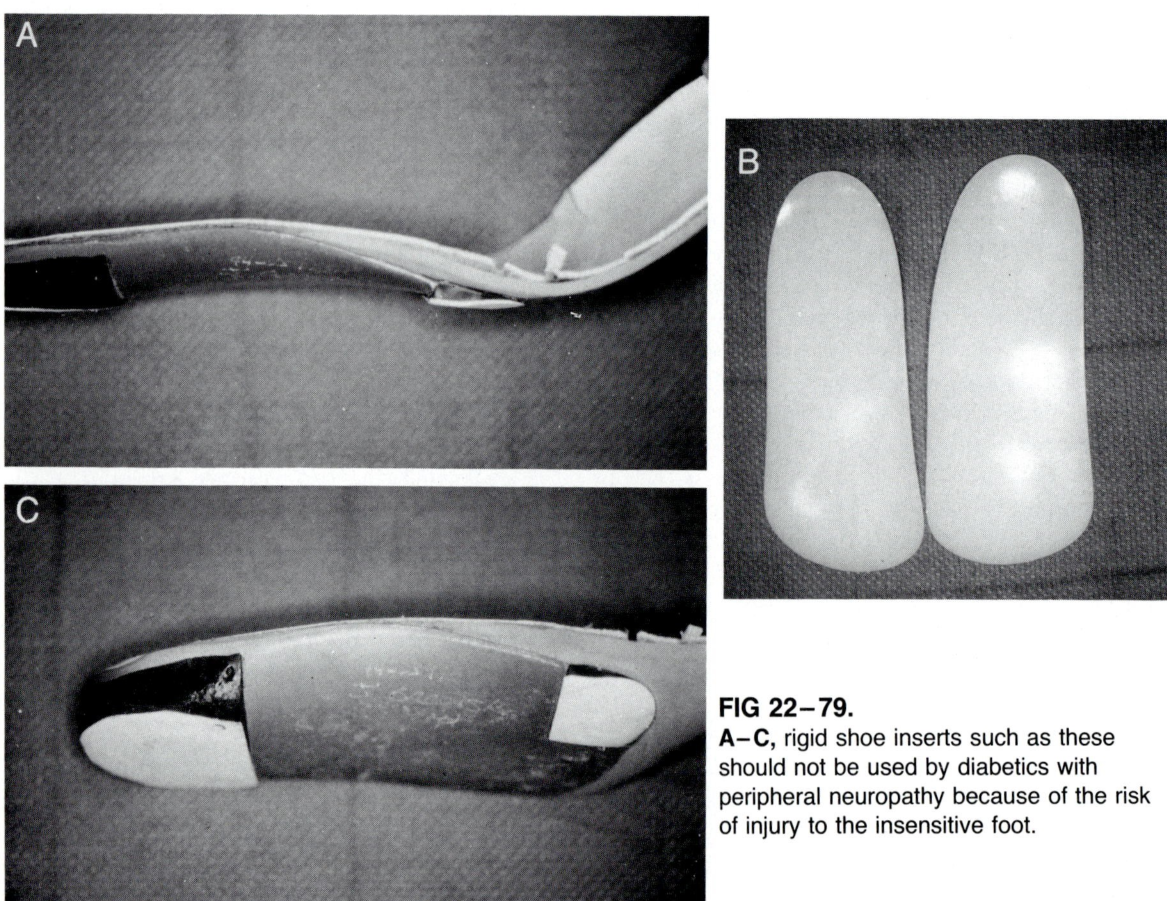

FIG 22–79.
A–C, rigid shoe inserts such as these should not be used by diabetics with peripheral neuropathy because of the risk of injury to the insensitive foot.

THE TEAM APPROACH

It is an often-repeated but an incontrovertible principle that the care of the diabetic foot is like no other area of orthopaedic care of the foot and ankle. The needs of the diabetic patient are many because the effects of the diabetes are multisystemic and thus require the expertise of many different medical specialists and subspecialists as well as those of many allied health professionals. The basic pathophysiologic problems of the disease often occur at the same time; to list the various members of the team of health care professionals who provide some aspect of the care of diabetic foot problems is risky since the number and range are so great. At the risk of an inadvertent omission, the team will include, at various times and according to need, orthopaedic surgeons, vascular surgeons, primary-care physicians, endocrinologists, physical medicine and rehabilitation specialists, radiologists, neurologists, nephrologists, infectious disease specialists, nurses, physical and occupational therapists, orthotists, prosthetists, certified pedorthists, professional shoe fitters, and others. In the complex and sometimes frustrating task of caring for the problems of the diabetic foot, the talents and knowledge of multiple disciplines are required. There have been studies that document the effectiveness of specific, multispecialty clinics for the care of the diabetic foot;[37] however, similar effectiveness can be achieved by use of the multiple disciplines, even when not all are physically housed in the same clinic location. The key is to consider the coordination of a team effort.

No doubt, great strides will be made in the next few years in futhering the cause of treatment and prevention of problems of the diabetic foot. Few efforts in the field of surgery of the foot and ankle have a more tangible, beneficial effect on the life and quality of life of patients with serious systemic disease.

REFERENCES

1. Apelqvist J, Castenfors J, Larsson J, et al: Prognostic value of systolic ankle and toe blood pressure levels in outcome of diabetic foot ulcer, *Diabetes Care* 12:373–378, 1989.
2. Asbury AK: Understanding diabetic neuropathy (editorial), *N Engl J Med* 319:577–578, 1988.
3. Bauman JH, Girling JP, Brand PW: Plantar pressures and trophic ulceration, *J Bone Joint Surg [Br]* 45:652–673, 1963.
4. Beltran J, Campanini S, Knight C, Mc Calla M: The diabetic foot: magnetic resona imaging evaluation. *Skeletal Radiol* 19:37–41, 1990.
5. Bessman AN, Wagner FW: Nonclostridial gas gangrene; report of 48 cases and review of the literature, *JAMA* 233:958–963, 1975.
6. Birke JA, Sims DS: Plantar sensory threshold in the ulcerative foot, *Lepr Rev* 57:261–267, 1986.
7. Birke JA, Sims DS, Buford WL: Walking casts: effect on plantar foot pressures, *J Rehabil Res* 22:18–22, 1985.
8. Boulton AJ, Betts RP, Franks CI, et al: Abnormalities of foot pressure in early diabetic neuropathy, *Diabetic Med* 4:225–228, 1987.
9. Boulton AJ, Betts RP, Franks CI, et al: The natural history of foot pressure abnormalities in neuropathic diabetic subjects, *Diabetes Res* 5:73–77, 1987.
10. Boulton AJM, Bowker JH, Gadia M, et al: Use of plaster casts in the management of diabetic neuropathic foot ulcers, *Diabetes Care* 9:149–152, 1986.
11. Boulton AJM, Kubrusly DB, Bowker JH, et al: Impaired vibratory perception and diabetic foot ulceration, *Diabetic Med* 3:335–337, 1986.
12. Brand PW: *Video lectures on the insensitive foot*, Carville, La, Gillis W Long Hansen's Disease Center.
13. Brand PW: The insensitive foot (including leprosy). In Jahss MH, editor: *Disorders of the foot and ankle*, Philadelphia, 1991, WB Saunders, pp 2171–2178.
14. Brodsky JW: Foot and ankle disorders in diabetes and arthritis, *Cur Opin Orthop* 1:147–153, 1990.
15. Brodsky JW: Management of Charcot joints of the foot and ankle in diabetes, *Semin Arthrop* 3:58–62, 1992.
16. Brodsky JW: The diabetic and insensitive foot, *Video J Orthop Surg* 3:1989.
17. Brodsky JW, Kourosh S, Stills M: Objective evaluation of insert material for diabetic and athletic footwear, *Foot Ankle* 9:111–116, 1988.
18. Brodsky JW, Kwong PK, Wagner FW, et al: Patterns of breakdown in the Charcot tarsus of diabetes and relation to treatment, American Orthopaedic Foot and Ankle Society 16th annual meeting, New Orleans, February 1986.
19. Brodsky JW, Kwong PK, Wagner FW, et al: Patterns of breakdown, natural history, and treatment of the diabetic Charcot tarsus, *Orthop Trans* 11:484, 1987.
20. Brodsky JW, Schneidler C: Diabetic foot infections, *Orthop Clin North Am* 22:473–489, 1991.
21. Brower AC, Allman RM: Neuropathic osteoarthropathy, *Orthop Rev* 14:81–88, 1985.
22. Campbell GJ, McLure M, Newell EN: Compressive behavior after simulated service conditions of some foamed materials intended as orthotic shoe insoles, *J Rehabil Res Dev* 21:57–65, 1984.
23. Cavanagh PR, Sims DS, Sanders LJ: Body mass is a poor predictor of peak plantar pressure in diabetic men, *Diabetes Care* 14:750–755, 1991.
24. Cavanagh PR, Ulbrecht JS: Biomechanics of the diabetic foot: a quantitative approach to the assessment of neuropathy, deformity and plantar pressures. In Jahss MH, editor: *Disorders of the Foot and Ankle*, Philadelphia 1991, WB Saunders, pp 1864–1907.
25. Chantelau E, Ma XY, Herrnberger S, et al: Effect of medial arterial calcification of O_2 supply to exercising diabetic feet, *Diabetes* 39:938–941, 1990.
26. Clohisy DR, Thompson RC: Fractures associated with neuropathic arthropathy in adults who have juvenile-onset diabetes, *J Bone Joint Surg [Am]* 70:1192–1200, 1988.
27. Cofield RH, Morrison JJ, Beabout JW: Diabetic neuroarthropathy in the foot. Patient characteristics and patterns of radiographic change, *Foot Ankle* 4:15, 1983.

28. Coventry MB, Rothacker GW: Bilateral calcaneal fracture in a diabetic patient, *J Bone Joint Surg [Am]* 61:462–464, 1971.
29. Crandall RC, Wagner FW: Partial and total calcanectomy, *J Bone Joint Surg [Am]* 63:152–155, 1981.
30. Ctercteko GC, Dhanendran MK, Hutton WC, et al: Vertical forces acting on the feet of diabetic patients with neuropathic ulceration, *Br J Surg* 68:608–614, 1981.
31. Delbridge L, Ctercteko G, Fowler C, et al: The aetiology of diabetic neuropathic ulceration of the foot, *Br J Surg* 72:1–6, 1985.
32. Delbridge L, Perry P, Marr S, et al: Limited joint mobility in the diabetic foot: relationship to neuropathic ulceration, *Diabetic Med* 5:333–337, 1988.
33. Diabetes: 1991 Vital Statistics, American Diabetes Assoc, *J Bone Joint Surg [Am]* 1991, Alexandria, Va.
34. Dickhaut SC, DeLee JC, Page CP: Nutritional status: Importance in predicting wound-healing after amputation, *J Bone Joint Surg [Am]* 66:71–75, 1984.
35. Downs D, Jacobs RL: Treatment of resistant ulcers in the plantar surface of the great toe in diabetics, *J Bone Joint Surg [Am]* 64:930–933, 1982.
36. Duckworth T, Boulton AJM, Betts RP, et al: Plantar pressure measurements and the prevention of ulceration in the diabetic foot, *J Bone Joint Surg [Br]* 67:79–85, 1985.
37. Edmonds ME, Blundell MP, Morris ME, et al: Improved survival of the diabetic foot: the role of a specialized foot clinic, *Q J Med* 232:763–771, 1986.
38. Eichenholtz SN: *Charcot Joints* Springfield, Ill, 1966, Charles C Thomas.
39. Ellenberg M: Treatment of diabetic neuropathy with diphenyhydantoin, *N Y State J Med* 68:2653, 1968.
40. Eloesser L: On the nature of neuropathic affectations of joints, *Ann Surg* 66:201–206, 1917.
41. Fernando DJS, Masson EQ, Veves A, et al: Relationship of limited joint mobility to abnormal foot pressures and diabetic foot ulceration, *Diabetes Care* 14:8–11, 1991.
42. Fisher WC, Goldsmith JF, Gilligan PH: Sneakers as a source of *Pseudomonas aeruginosa* in children with osteomyelitis following puncture wounds, *J Pediatr* 106:608–609, 1985.
43. Gaylarde PM, Fonseca VA, Llewellyn G, et al: Transcutaneous oxygen tension in legs and feet of diabetic patients, *Diabetes* 37:714–716, 1988.
44. Gelberman RH, Szabo RM, Williamson RV, et al: Sensibility testing in peripheral-nerve compression syndromes, *J Bone Joint Surg [Am]* 65:632–638, 1983.
45. Ger R: Muscle transposition in the management of perforating ulcers of the forefoot, *Clin Orthop* 175:186, 1983.
46. Goodman J, Bessman AN, Teget B, et al: Risk factors in local surgical procedures for diabetic gangrene, *Surg Gynecol Obstet* 143:587–591, 1976.
47. Hammerschlag WA, Harrelson JM, Isbell M et al: First metatarsal osteotomy for treatment of recalcitrant diabetic neuropathic plantar ulceration, American Orthopaedic Foot and Ankle Society 5th annual summer meeting, Sun Valley, Idaho, August 1989.
48. Harrelson JM: Management of the diabetic foot, *Orthop Clin North Am* 20:605–619, 1989.
49. Helm PA, Walker SC, Pullium G: Total contact casting in diabetic patients with neuropathic foot ulceration, *Arch Phys Med Rehabil* 65:691–693, 1984.
50. Holewski JJ, Moss KM, Stess RM, et al: Prevalence of foot pathology and lower extremity complication in a diabetic outpatient clinic, *J Rehabil Res* 26:35–44, 1989.
51. Hoogwerf FJ: Amitriptyline treatment of painful diabetic neuropathy: an inadvertent single-patient trial, *Diabetes Care* 8:526, 1985.
52. Irwin ST, Gilmore J, McGrann S, et al: Blood flow in diabetics with foot lesions due to "small vessel disease," *Br J Surg* 75:1201–1206, 1988.
53. Jacobs RL: Hoffman procedure in the ulcerated diabetic neuropathic foot, *Foot Ankle* 3:142–149, 1983.
54. Jacobs RL, Karmody AM: Diabetic-neurotrophic foot: diagnosis and treatment, American Academy Orthopaedic Surgeons, *Instr Cours Lect* 28:118–143, 1979.
55. Jacobs RL, Karmody AM: Office treatment of the insensitive foot, *Foot Ankle* 2:230, 1982.
56. Jacobs RL, Karmody AM: Salvage of the diabetic foot with exposed os calcis, *Foot Ankle* 3:173, 1980.
57. Jany RS, Burkus JK: Long-term follow-up of Syme amputations for peripheral vascular disease associated with diabetes mellitus, *Foot Ankle* 9:107–110, 1988.
58. Jordan WR: Neuritic manifestations in diabetes mellitus, *Arch Intern Med* 57:307, 1936.
59. Karmody AM, Jacobs RL: Salvage of the diabetic foot by vascular reconstruction, *Orthop Clin North Am* 7:957–977, 1976.
60. Kaufman J, Breeding L, Rosenberg N: Anatomic location of acute diabetic foot infection, *Am J Surg* 53:109–112, 1987.
61. Kennedy EJ, Johnson JE, Shereff MJ, et al: The role of nuclear imaging in the evaluation of the diabetic foot, American Orthopedic Foot and Ankle Society 7th annual summer meeting, Boston, July 1991.
62. Knowles HB: Joint contractures, waxy skin, and control of diabetes (editorial), *New Engl J Med* 305:217–218, 1981.
63. Kritter AE: A technique for salvage of the infected diabetic gangrenous foot, *Orthop Clin North Am* 4:21, 1973.
64. Kvinesdal B, Molin J, Froland A, et al: Imipramine treatment of painful diabetic neuropathy, *JAMA* 252:1727–1730, 1984.
65. Lang-Stevenson AI, Sharrard WJW, Betts RP, et al: Neuropathic ulcers of the foot, *J Bone Joint Surg Br* 67:438–442, 1985.
66. Larcos G, Brown ML, Sutton RT: Diagnosis of osteomyelitis of the foot in diabetic patients: value of in-leukocyte scintigraphy, *AJR* 157:527–531, 1991.
67. Leber C, Evanski PM: A comparison of shoe insole materials in plantar pressure relief, *Prosthet Orthot Int* 10:135–138, 1986.
68. Lesko P, Maurer RC: Talonavicular dislocations and midfoot arthropathy in neuropathic diabetic feet, *Clin Orthop* 240:226–231, 1989.
69. Levin S, Pearsall G, Ruderman RJ: Von Frey's method of measuring pressure sensibility in the hand: an engineering analysis of the Weinstein-Semmes pressure aesthesiometer, *J Hand Surg* 3:211–216, 1978.
70. Livingston R, Jacobs RL, Karmody A: Plantar abscess of the diabetic patient, *Foot Ankle* 5:205–213, 1985.
71. LoGerfo FW, Coffman JD: Vascular and microvascular

disease of the foot in diabetes. Implications for foot care, *N Engl J Med* 311:1615–1619, 1984.
72. Louie TJ, Bartlett JG, Tally FP, et al: Aerobic and anaerobic bacteria in diabetic foot ulcers, *Ann Intern Med* 85:461–463, 1976.
73. Masson EA, Hay EM, Stockley I, et al: Abnormal foot pressures alone may not cause ulceration, *Diabetic Med* 6:426–428, 1989.
74. Maurer AH, Millmond SH, Knight LC, et al: Infection in diabetic osteoarthropathy: use of indium-labeled leukocytes for diagnosis, *Radiology* 161:221–225, 1986.
75. Medvei VC: *History of Endocrinology*, Lancaster, UK, 1982, MTP Press.
76. Melton LJ, Macken KM, Palumbo PJ, et al: Incidence and prevalence of clinical peripheral vascular disease in a population-based cohort of diabetic patients, *Diabetes Care* 3:650–654, 1980.
77. Mendel CM, Klein RF, Chappell DA, et al: A trial of amitriptyline and fluphenazine in the treatment of painful diabetic neuropathy, *JAMA* 255:637, 1986.
78. Mooney V, Wagner FW Jr: Neurocirculatory disorders of the foot, *Clin Orthop* 122:53–61, 1977.
79. Mueller MJ, Diamond JE, Sinacore DR, et al: Total contact casting in treatment of diabetic plantar ulcers. Controlled clinical trial, *Diabetes Care* 12:384–388, 1989.
80. Myerson MS: Salvage of severe diabetic neuroarthropathy with arthrodesis, American Orthopaedic Foot and Ankle Society 5th annual summer meeting, Sun Valley, Idaho, August 1989.
81. Newman JH: Spontaneous dislocation in diabetic neuropathy, *J Bone Joint Surg [Br]* 61:484–488, 1979.
82. Newman LG, Waller J, Palestro CJ, et al: Unsuspected osteomyelitis in diabetic foot ulcers, *JAMA* 266:1246–1251, 1991.
83. Pecoraro RE, Reiber GE, Burgess EM: Pathways to diabetic limb amputation, *Diabetes Care* 13:513–521, 1990.
84. Quill GE, Myerson MS: Clinical, radiographic, and pedobarographic analysis of the foot after hallux amputation, American Association of Orthopaedic Surgeons 58th Annual Meeting, Anaheim, Calif, March 1991.
85. Rayfield IJ, Ault MJ, Keusch GT, et al: Infection and diabetes: the case for glucose control, *Am J Med* 72:439–450, 1985.
86. Resnick D: Neuropathy, in Resnick D, Niwayana, editors: *Diagnosis of bone and* joint disorders, Philadelphia, 1988, WB Saunders, p 3162.
87. Rosenbloom AL, Silverstein JH, Lezotte DC, et al: Limited joint mobility in childhood diabetes mellitus indicates increased risk for microvascular disease, *N Engl J Med* 305:191–194, 1981.
88. Rull JA, Quibrera H, Gonzales-Millan H, et al: Symptomatic treatment of peripheral diabetic neuropathy with carbamazepine (Tegretol): double-blind crossover trial, *Diabetologia* 5:215, 1969.
89. Sapico FL, Canawati HN, Witte JL, et al: Quantitative aerobic and anaerobic bacteriology of infected diabetic feet, *J Clin Microbiol* 12:413–420, 1980.
90. Sapico FL, Witte JL, Canawati HN, et al: The infected foot of the diabetic patient: quantitative microbiology and analysis of clinical features, *Rev Infect Dis* 6(suppl 1):171–176, 1984.
91. Sartoris DJ, Devine S, Resnick D, et al: Plantar compartmental infection in the diabetic foot. The role of computed tomography, *Invest Radiol* 20:772–784, 1985.
92. Schauwecker DS, Park HM, Burt RW, et al: Combined bone scintigraphy and indium-111 leukocyte scans in neuropathic foot disease, *J Nucl Med* 29:1651–1655, 1988.
93. Seabold JE, Flickinger FW, Kao SCS, et al: Indium-111-leukocyte/technetium-99m-MDP bone and magnetic resonance imaging: difficulty of diagnosing osteomyelitis in patients with neuropathic osteoarthropathy, *J Nucl Med* 31:549–556, 1990.
94. Sharp CS, Bessman AN, Wagner FW, et al: Microbiology of deep tissue in diabetic gangrene, *Diabetes Care* 1:289–292, 1978.
95. Shults DW, Hunter GC, Mcintyre KE, et al: Value of radiographs and bone scans in determining the need for therapy in diabetic patients with foot ulcers, *Am J Surg* 158:525–529, 1989.
96. Sinha S, Munichoodappa CS, Kozak GP: Neuroarthropathy (Charcot joints) in diabetes mellitus, *Medicine (Baltimore)* 51:191–210, 1972.
97. Smith L, Plehwe W, McGill M, et al: Foot bearing pressure in patients with unilateral diabetic foot ulcers, *Diabetic Med* 6:573–575, 1989.
98. Sosenko JM, Gadia MT, Natori N, et al: Neurofunctional testing for the detection of diabetic peripheral neuropathy, *Arch Intern Med* 147:1741–1744, 1987.
99. Splittgerber GF, Speigelhoff DR, Buggy BP: Combined leukocyte and bone imaging used to evaluate diabetic osteoarthropathy and osteomyelitis, *Clin Nucl Med* 14:156–159, 1989.
100. Taylor LM, Porter JM: The clinical course of diabetics who require emergent foot surgery because of infection or ischemia, *J Vasc Surg* 6:454–459, 1987.
101. Video series on the insensitive foot, Gillis W. Long Hansen's Disease Center, Carville, La.
102. Wagner FW: A classification and treatment program for diabetic, neuropathic and dysvascular foot problems, American Academy of Orthopaedic Surgeons, *Instr Course Lect* 28:143–165, 1979.
103. Wagner FW: The dysvascular foot: a system for diagnosis and treatment, *Foot Ankle* 2:64–122, 1981.
104. Wagner FW Jr: Amputation of the foot and ankle—current status, *Clin Orthop* 122:62, 1977.
105. Wagner FW Jr: The diabetic foot and amputations of the foot. In Mann RA, editor: *Surgery of the Foot* ed 5, St Louis, 1986, Mosby–Year Book, pp 421–455.
106. Walker SC, Helm PA, Pullium G: Total contact casting and chronic diabetic neuropathic foot ulcerations: healing rates by wound location, *Arch Phys Med Rehabil* 68:217–221, 1987.
107. Waters RL, Perry J, Antonelli D, et al: Energy cost of walking of amputees: the influence of level of amputation, *J Bone Joint Surg [Am]* 56:42–46, 1976.
108. Wheat LJ, Allen SD, Henry M, et al: Diabetic foot infections: bacteriologic analysis, *Arch Intern Med* 146:1935–1940, 1986.
109. Yuh WTC, Corson JD, Baraniewski HM, et al: Osteomyelitis of the foot in diabetic patients: evaluation with plain film,[99] Tc-MDP bone scintigraphy, and MR imaging, *AJR* 152:795–800, 1989.
110. Zlatkin MB, Pathria M, Sartoris DJ, et al: The diabetic foot, *Radiol Clin North Am* 25:1095–1105, 1987.

APPENDIX 22–1.

Neurovascular Testing Instrument*

Basic Kit

- Pinwheel or pin
- Reflex hammer
- Tuning fork, 128 cps.

Additional

Semmes-Weinstein monofilaments—these are graded by the logarithm of the pressure exerted. Method: Apply the tip of the filament perpendicular to the skin until it begins to bend and the patient answers that he does or does not feel it.

One source: Research Designs, Inc.
7520 Hillcroft
Houston, TX 77081
(713) 995-8591

A basic set requires numbers 4.17, 5.07, and 6.10.

Doppler Ultrasound

A small hand-held model such as no. 840 or no. 841 will do (about $250).

One source: Parks Medical Electronics
PO Box 5669
19460 SW Shaw
Aloha, OR 97007
(503) 649-7007

*Sources listed here are not exclusive and are only examples. No endorsement is given or intended. No benefits in any form have been received or will be received from a commercial party related directly or indirectly to the information included herein. No funds were received in support of this project.

APPENDIX 22–2.

Diabetic Total-Contact Cast

Purposes

- Redistribution to reduce high pressure under forefoot or midfoot ulceration.
- Edema control and structural protection of bone and joint disintegration in Charcot arthropathy.

Indications

- Ulcers must be plantar, grossly clean, and without cellulitis, abscess, or purulent drainage.
- Charcot joint: If acute, do the first cast change at 1 week because edema usually subsides quickly in a cast.

Materials

- Clear x-ray film
- Indelible felt-tipped marker
- 2 × 2-in. gauze
- Smooth cast padding
- Felt or adhesive foam
- 1-in paper tape
- Stockinette
- Elastic plaster (for example, Orthoflex by Johnson & Johnson, red & silver wrapper).
- Fast or extra-fast plaster—4- and 6-in. rolls
- Synthetic casting material—4- or 6-in. rolls
- Quarter-inch plywood pieces cut in a foot shape in several sizes

Instructions

- First measure and trace out the ulcer, and record the tracing in the chart by holding the paper and the tracing against the x-ray viewbox.
- Dress the wound with 2 × 2-in. gauze with or without saline or Betadine. Do not use ointment or an occlusive dressing.
- Apply a stockinette followed by felt or adhesive foam over the bony prominences including the malleoli and a strip down the anterior crest of the tibia. The padding may be applied to the bony prominences of a Charcot foot as well when necessary.
- Apply cast padding and overlap by half each time. In some of the traditional total-contact casts, padding is omitted, but this single-layer wrap has worked well.
- Apply elastic plaster as the first layer of the cast, followed quickly thereafter by the regular plaster, and mold it together well around the bony prominences and up into the arch of the foot. Make certain that the ankle is at neutral and the toes are not extended. Once this has hardened, apply a layer of synthetic cast material in order to allow immediate weight bearing. In recalcitrant ulcers, incorporate a plywood platform into the plaster portion of the cast, and use plaster to fill in the area beneath the arch; wrap with additional plaster prior to applying the fiberglass.
- A cast shoe rather than a walking heel is used.

Warnings

- Do not overpad the cast. The padding will compress and produce a loose cast that can cause ulceration.
- Extend the cast distally to the tips of the toes. Mold the cast in a dorsal-plantar direction over the toes in order to limit the excursion or extension of the toes. This reduces the risk of ulceration on the digits from the cast and decreases the pressure.
- Some prefer to make a totally closed-toe cast, but a well-molded cast that leaves the tips of toes visible usually produces a satisfactory result.

APPENDIX 22–3.

Nail Care Instruments*

Basic
- Double-action bone rongeur.
  - Example: Miltex no. 19-856 is a useful size and of sufficient strength.
- Anvil-type nail splitter.
  - Example: C.M.E.C.† catalog no. 253.
- Freer elevator.
- Straight hemostat for nail margin removal.

Additional
- Iris scissors and Adson's forceps.
- Nail curette and excavator.
  - Examples: C.M.E.C. catalog nos. 94 and 66.
- Straight, concave and convex nail clippers.
  - Also available from numerous instrument companies.

*Sources listed here are not exclusive and are only examples. No endorsement is given or intended. No benefits in any form have been received or will be received from a commercial party related directly or indirectly to the information included herein. No funds were received in support of this project.

†C.M.E.C. = Chicago Medical Equipment Co
300 Wainwright Dr
Northbrook, Il 60062
(708) 564-1000

APPENDIX 22–4.

Callus Trimming Instruments*

No.17 scalpel blades
- Example: H.L. Moore Co catalog no. 09275
  389 John Downey Dr
  New Britain, CT 06050
  1-203-225-4621

Dremel Moto-Tool with sanding discs and drums available at hobby shops.
- Suggest model no.370. Must have variable speed—set it at the lowest speed, and check the skin temperature with the fingertip intermittently.

*Sources listed here are not exclusive and are only examples. No endorsement is given or intended. No benefits in any form have been received or will be received from a commercial party related directly or indirectly to the information included herein. No funds were received in support of this project.

APPENDIX 22–5.

Selected Materials Used in Insoles for Insensitive Feet

Name	Description
Soft Plastazote	Open-cell polyethylene foam
Medium Plastazote	Firmer open-cell polyethylene foam
Pelite	Open-cell polyethylene foam
PPT (poron)	Closed-cell urethane foam
Spenco	Microcellular neoprene rubber with nylon covering
"P.Q." and sorbothane	Viscoelastic polymers

APPENDIX 22–6.

Patient Instructions for Diabetic Foot Care

Understand
- Understand that the loss or absence of normal, protective sensation is the cause of most diabetic foot problems. What you cannot feel will hurt you.
- Therefore, constant vigilance is required to exercise prevention, which is the best cure.

Inspect
- Inspect your feet twice daily.
- Use a mirror, or have a companion inspect the feet for you if you are unable to see each part of your foot due to poor vision and/or poor flexibility.
- Look all over the feet for cracks, blisters, reddened spots, cuts, and ulcers or for excessively moist skin between the toes.

Wash
- Bathe your feet daily with warm water and mild soap.
- Always test the temperature with, e.g., your elbow, i.e., an area unaffected by neuropathy, or have someone else test it—but remember you might burn your foot and not even feel it!
- Dry gently and carefully between the toes. Blot, do not rub.

Beware of burns
- Never use heating pads, hot water bottles, or any other heat source to warm your feet! Irreparable damage can be done in a minute.
- Wear socks in bed if your feet are cold at night.

Skin: calluses and corns
- Do not use chemical agents or "medicated" pads. These can cause burns.
- Do not do "bathroom surgery" with a razorblade!
- Use a pumice stone or foot file to gently reduce calluses at bath time.
- Keep the skin moist regularly to prevent cracking and infection by using a gentle skin lotion. A very thin layer of petroleum jelly can also be used to seal in moisture after the bath.
- Do not put creams, lotions, or ointments between the toes because excessive moisture can result.
- See your doctor for persistent or difficult skin problems. Some corns and calluses can only be removed professionally, especially if you have severely impaired circulation.

Nail problems
- Trim nails straight; do not attempt to "dig out" the corners.
- Filing the nails daily reduces the frequency of clipping; avoid rubbing the skin.
- Consult your doctor if the nails are too thickened or hard to trim.

Shoes
- Fashion is an unfortunate enemy of the diabetic with neuropathy. Many, many serious foot problems result from shoe pressure.
- Shoes should be long and wide enough and have enough room for the toes, especially if they are clawed.
- Synthetic materials that do not "breathe" are to be avoided. Leather is still generally the best material because it shapes and stretches.
- Avoid shoes of hard materials, e.g., plastic or patent leather.
- Inspect the feet frequently when new shoes are obtained. Wear new shoes no more than an hour the first day.
- Shoes should be professionally fitted (see Appendix 22–7, the PFA) if you have neuropathy or have had previous serious foot problems.
- Shop for a properly fitted shoe, not for what you remember as your size. Shoes vary, and feet change in width and shape.

Dressing
- Inspect the shoes, and turn them upside down to detect any foreign object each time before putting them on.
- Changing shoes during the day can reduce the risk of pressure problems.
- Do not use hard devices or rigid "orthotics" in the shoe. These can produce excessive pressures on the foot.

Stockings
- Avoid stockings with elastic tops or garters.
- Do not use socks or stockings with heavy seams.
- Wash and change stockings daily.
- Stockings made of absorbent, natural materials such as cotton and wool are best.

Inform!
- Inform all shoe fitters that you are diabetic.
- Be sure that your physician examines your feet periodically.

APPENDIX 22—7.

Resource for Certified

Contact: Prescription Footwear Association
9861 Broken Land Parkway
Columbia, MD 21046
(301) 381-7278

*Sources listed here are not exclusive and are only examples. No endorsement is given or intended. No benefits in any form have been received or will be received from a commercial party related directly or indirectly to the information included herein. No funds were received in support of this project.

CHAPTER

23

Amputations of the Foot and Ankle

James W. Brodsky, M.D.

General considerations

Surgical techniques

Tourniquets
Soft-tissue preservation
Wound closure
Drains
Skin grafting and flap coverage
Vascular reconstruction
Determination of amputation level

Specific amputation levels and techniques

Terminal amputation of the toe and nail (terminal syme)
  Surgical technique
  Aftercare
  Pitfalls and complications
Amputation of the great toe
  Surgical technique
  Aftercare
Amputation of the lesser toes
  Surgical technique
  Pitfalls and complications of toe amputations
Ray amputations and partial forefoot amputations
  Pitfalls and complications
Transmetatarsal amputations
  Surgical technique
  Aftercare
  Pitfalls and complications
Chopart amputations
  Surgical technique
  Aftercare
  Pitfalls and complications
Syme amputation
  Surgical technique
  Aftercare
  Pitfalls and complications
Below-knee amputations

Amputation of part or all of the foot is an ancient procedure, if not the oldest foot operation, and yet foot amputations are often abhorred by the surgeon. Perhaps the reason is the repugnance of removing a body part, perhaps because amputation is seemingly so unaesthetic or perhaps because amputation is seen, consciously or not, as an admission of failure, a form of surgical defeat. However, in the patient who has a foot that is no longer either viable or functional, an amputation is a positive procedure because it is the first step on the road to restored or renewed function. The amputation is therefore the beginning of rehabilitation of the patient, many of whom have become debilitated both physically and emotionally in the battle to save part or all of a foot, and in this process, the function and activities of normal daily life have been held hostage to the hopes and efforts to save the foot, oftentimes past the time of reasonable expectations for good function. To save a poorly functioning foot of marginal viability is to have won the battle and lost the war, for the goal is to enhance the function and quality of life for the patient, not the limb. Nevertheless, once a decision to do an amputation has been made as the joint effort of surgeon and patient together, a number of challenges remain. These include selection of the proper level of amputation, methods of maximal foot salvage to maximize function, proper surgical technique, postoperative management, and shoe wear modification and the use of prostheses.

The causes for partial or complete foot amputation are many. In decreasing order of frequency they are as follows:

1. Diabetes (many of whom also have peripheral vascular disease)
2. Peripheral vascular disease (in the absence of diabetes)
3. Trauma
4. Chronic infection (primarily osteomyelitis)
5. Tumors
6. Congenital abnormalities

Amputation of part or all of the foot is correctly viewed as a procedure of last resort and reflects the proper desire of the surgeon to save the foot. "Foot salvage" is a term that signifies the emphasis that has been placed in recent times on the shift from complete to partial foot amputations. The goal is to convert many of the operations that in the past would have been below-knee amputations to partial foot amputations and in the process, convert these patients to users of modified shoe wear rather than users of prosthetic limbs.

GENERAL CONSIDERATIONS

The goals of an amputation are fundamentally greater in the patient who requires ablative surgery as a result of trauma than the goals in patients requiring amputation for diabetic foot problems. The diabetic or the patient with insensitivity due to any cause needs to achieve a plantigrade foot with stable healing of the wounds. The patient with trauma needs the same, but also requires an extremity that does not hurt. This is compounded by an increased proclivity of traumatic amputations to develop symptomatic neuromas and reflex sympathetic dystrophy. The advantages and disadvantages, as always, are obverse sides of the same coin. The traumatic amputee is not subject to the same frequency of recurrent problems and multiple revisions of the amputation to a higher level as a diabetic because he has sufficient sensation to prevent neuropathic breakdown of the soft tissues.

One of the major goals in amputation surgery of the foot is to salvage as much of the foot as possible. The general principle holds true that preservation of a greater portion of the limb allows greater function. The experimental basis for limb preservation was documented in a study done at Rancho Los Amigos Hospital in which the authors showed increasing energy costs of walking, as evidenced by greater oxygen consumption, in patients who had higher levels of amputation.[18] The two qualifications of that principle are that (1) the salvaged foot must achieve complete healing with a stable soft-tissue envelope and (2) the foot be sufficiently plantigrade to be functional. Partial foot amputations such as the transmetatarsal or ray resections are worthwhile because they allow the use of fairly normal shoes, often with only minor modifications. However, a higher amputation level may be better for the patient and yield a more functional result if the patient becomes debilitated due to prolonged and unsuccessful treatment in an attempt to save a toe, one metatarsal, etc. If the patient is non–weight bearing, full-time or intermittently, the upper extremities are always occupied with ambulation, thereby limiting the ability of the patient to participate in most activities of work and daily living. Thus, the goal of foot salvage must be moderated by the functional result and the length of time that it takes to achieve the healing. The patient is usually better served with a more proximal but healed, definitive amputation that allows walking and resumption of daily routines than if rendered incapacitated with overly protracted wound care in an attempt to save a portion of the foot that is not viable.

SURGICAL TECHNIQUES

Tourniquets

Although the use of tourniquets in amputation surgery has oftentimes been proscribed in the past, the experimental basis for this prohibition is lacking. A controlled, randomized trial of tourniquet use in foot amputations in diabetic and dysvascular nondiabetic patients demonstrated that there was no difference in healing rates between patients with tourniquets and those who did not have non-tourniquets applied.[2] In this series the tourniquet was released once the amputated part was removed, prior to beginning the closure, in order to check for hemostasis and flap viability.

Soft-tissue Preservation

The most important first step in amputation surgery is aggressive debridement of infected and necrotic bone and soft tissue. This must be balanced by the need to maximally preserve viable skin and soft tissue, especially plantar flaps because they make the best possible soft-tissue coverage of weight-bearing surfaces. When the amputation is done for gangrene, the initial and preliminary line of resection should be quite close, usually less than 5 mm from the edge of the gangrene, in order to save the maximum soft tissue. If this proves not to be viable, the edge can be cut back further. Surprisingly, the skin is usually viable since the level of nonviability has already been demarcated. Taking too generous a margin of skin can often force the surgeon to go to the next higher level of amputation. There should be no hesitation to make irregular or asymmetric flaps and to then reevaluate the pattern of closure once a bleeding edge has been obtained all around the wound (Fig 23–1). The surgeon must make the best use of the available soft tissue and is encouraged to use "creative" local flaps. The principle is to make use of the areas of viable tissue that may not fit the pattern of a standard flap for the level of amputation. For example, the pattern of locally viable tissue may allow one to swing a local flap medially to laterally instead of the usual long posterior flap over a transmetatarsal amputation. The innovative use of local tissue in a situation like this will oftentimes be the only way to achieve closure at the level; otherwise, the patient has the disadvantage of receiving a more proximal amputation. This type of local flap is also preferable to a skin graft because it is more durable and more sensate. Ideally, flaps should be of a length no greater than half of the width of their bases. However, the real-life situation of patient care is not always ideal, and some allowance must be made for the vagaries of a given case if it affords a potential advantage to the patient. Residual local flaps often need to be thinned, especially where they form corners. This is true at all levels of amputations. As the excessively thick flap is folded over, it bunches up in the corner and pushes the skin edges away from each other. Thinning the flap excessively may disturb the vascularity of the skin edge; some residual thickness contributes to a natural eversion of the edges.

If there is doubt about the viability of an area, it can be preserved and observed and then further debrided at the next session in the operating room several days later. Especially in the infected wound, it is common to take the patient to the operating suite at least three times: the first time for initial, aggressive debridement, the second time for redebridement of residual areas of

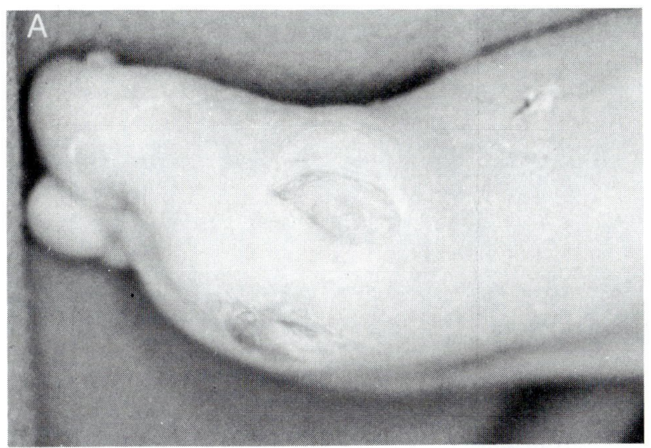

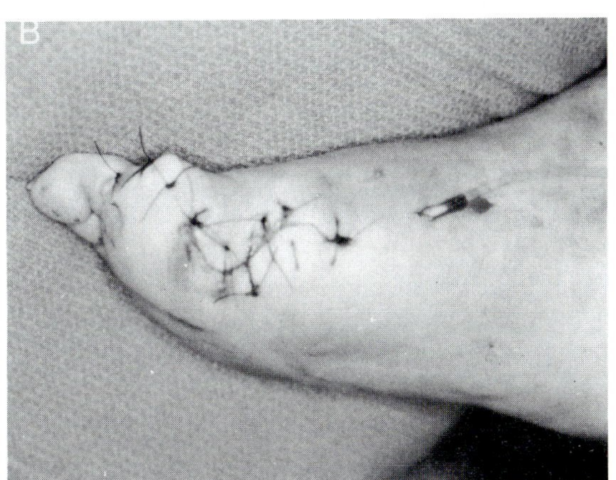

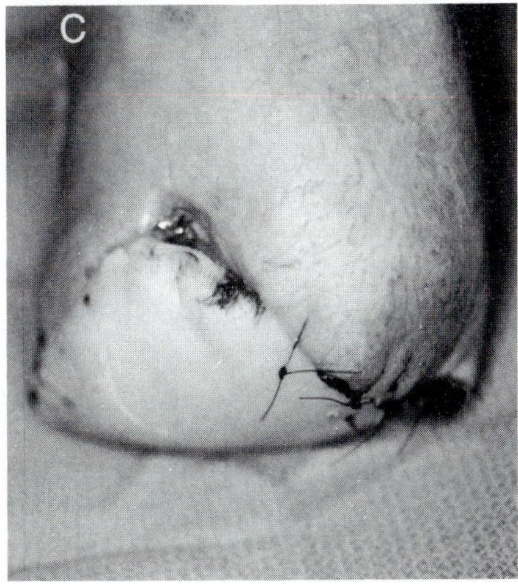

FIG 23–1.
A and **B,** amputation of the great toe. The remaining soft tissue was maximally preserved and the irregular flaps contoured to fit together. This healed, and the patient has excellent function. **C,** irregular and asymmetric flap used to successfully close a transmetatarsal amputation.

infection or necrosis after a period of intervening wound care, and the third time for the definitive closure. Sometimes it is necessary to expand the middle step to more than one secondary debridement. After the debridements, the wound is usually packed widely open with gauze bandages and these bandages changed after twice-daily wound care, for example, with intermittent whirlpool treatments. Redebridement in the operating room is repeated until the wound is clean and has a good granulating base (Fig 23–2).

Wound Closure

The final wound, especially in a partial amputation of the foot, must be fashioned to balance the length of preserved bone with the available soft tissue to cover it. In many cases it is necessary to sacrifice an additional portion of the osseous structure in order to achieve this balance. In the case of an infected diabetic foot, this may signify excision of an additional metatarsal that does not have osteomyelitis in order to achieve delayed primary closure of a partial forefoot amputation. This is a situation, for example, in which the metatarsal in question would have been partially exposed at surgery and with subsequent skin closure the surgeon finds it impossible to totally cover the wound with the remaining viable skin and soft tissue. Skin grafting would not result in a stable closure.

Once a clean, granulating wound is achieved, whether the procedure is a diabetic or a posttraumatic amputation, closure should be done. Although it cannot always be achieved, especially in the dysvascular or diabetic patient, the surgeon should strive for primary closure or delayed primary closure in foot amputations. Leaving large gaping wounds to granulate in as the main method of healing amputations, especially in diabetics, frequently condemns the patient to an unnecessarily long recovery. This technique often represents failure on the part of the surgeon to make a decision about the viability of the local tissue and the appropriate final level of healing. It is usually more effective and less debilitating to the patient (and more cost-effective) to establish knowledge of the vascularity and healing potential of the partial foot amputation wound and do a definitive procedure with good, viable local closure. If needed, the limb should be first revascularized by the vascular surgeon and then redebrided and eventually closed at the new level of viability.

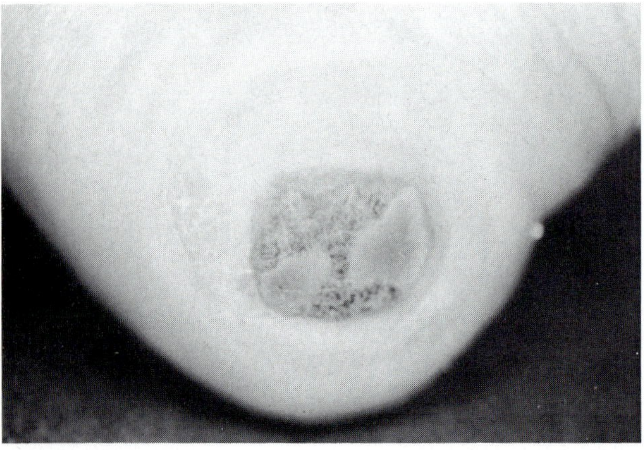

FIG 23–2.
A granulating ulcer with superficial necrotic material on the wound.

Allowing an entire amputation wound to granulate slowly is an extremely slow process in some but not all diabetic patients. The difference among them is probably based on the level of perfusion. Large wounds that are left to granulate are more likely to require skin grafting or produce an unstable scar. The process of wound contracture may be hindered by the shape of the wound and the amount of residual bony structure beneath. Delayed primary closure is best, even if it is only partially successful. In such cases, the wound adheres over part of its length, and a portion fails to close and/or continues to drain small amounts (Fig 23–3). This still reduces the morbidity since the residual wound that must be treated and that must granulate in is still only a fraction of the size of the original wound. A frequent pattern is adherence and closure of the two ends of the suture line, with a small dehiscence in the middle third. The sutures in the healing areas are usually left in place for a minimum of 6 weeks to 2 months while wound care and dressing changes on the middle third continue. This is an important consideration since a large wound in a diabetic or dysvascular patient may take 2 to 6 months to granulate in. If the wound does not appear ready for delayed primary closure, there are several possible explanations. There may have been inadequate debridement, and nonviable tissue remains; there may be inadequate vascularity of the wound; or there may have been insufficient time for the wound to begin granulating. Even if it is decided to cover the wound with a split-thickness skin graft, a good granulating base is necessary first.

In amputation closures, the skin edges should be handled as minimally as possible. Flaps should be tested at the time of closure by gently bringing them together manually. This should demonstrate an ability to close a wound without tension. If such a closure cannot be completed, more of the underlying bone must be resected in order to reduce the pressure on the flaps. The stump should be palpated through the flaps to make sure that no rough edges, sharp angles, or undesirable

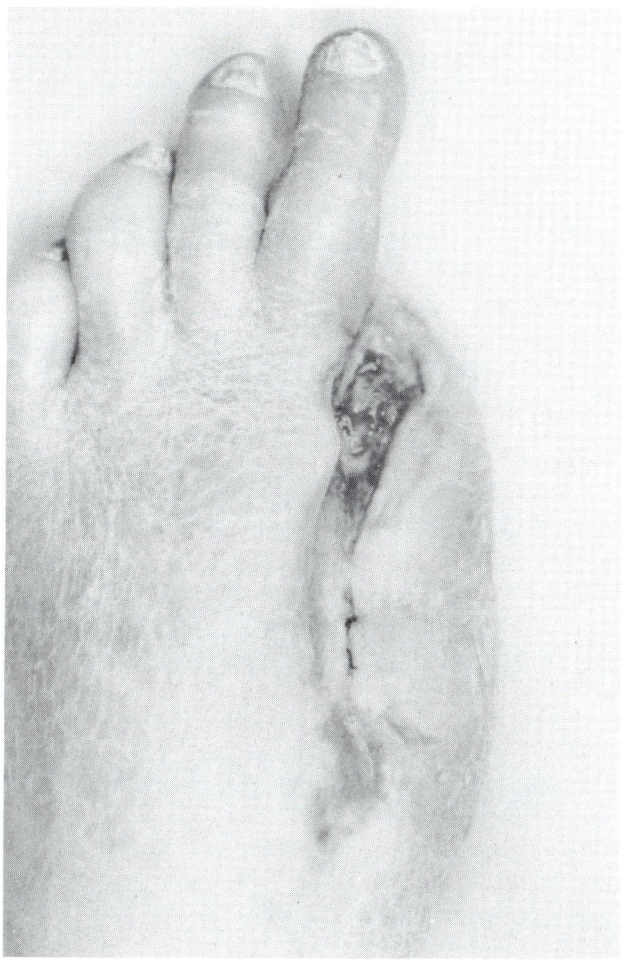

FIG 23–3.
A partially closed wound after delayed primary closure. While a small part of the wound has yet to close by secondary intention, this area has been greatly reduced in comparison to leaving the whole wound open.

bony prominences remain on the bone. At the time of closure, forceps should be used to hold the subcutaneous layer rather than the skin wherever possible. The balance of soft tissue to bone discussed above is most evident at closure because there should be no tension on the skin edges or suture line. The surgeon should inspect the skin for excessive blanching because this may indicate an overtight closure. In diabetic amputations, the sutures should be left in place a very long time, usually at least twice as long as in a nondysvascular patient.

Drains

Drains are usually used at the time of the delayed primary closure. These can be Penrose drains, suction drains, or an irrigation system (as described in Chapter 22, and in Fig 22–35). The choice is the surgeon's and depends upon the configuration of the wound and how loose or tight the wound closure is. If the amputation was done for infection or if there is a fair amount of bleeding at the time of closure, the surgeon may lean toward the use of the irrigation system. Drains are usually pulled at 1 to 2 days; most irrigation systems have their primary effect within the first 12 to 24 hours. Penrose drains, which exit between the sutures, tend to deter adherence of the wound edges in that location and are generally less desirable when compared with the other two drain types, which exit through small, separate stab wounds.

Skin Grafting and Flap Coverage

Skin grafting is an acceptable technique for obtaining coverage (as distinguished from closure) of amputation wounds. Split-thickness grafting is somewhat more successful in traumatic amputations than in those done in insensitive diabetic feet. Because of the loss of protective sensation, primary closure with local soft-tissue flaps is still preferable in diabetics. Skin grafts in diabetics often make the difference between salvage and loss of an amputation stump, but they have a higher rate of recurrent breakdown than local skin coverage does.

Free tissue transfer has been a valuable adjunct to limb salvage, especially in traumatic amputations of the foot. The greatest benefit has been in obtaining coverage over wounds of the ankle, heel, and hindfoot (see Chapter 32). These areas have relatively little subcutaneous tissue, and the skin, especially in the hindfoot, is fixed and immobile, which makes rotation of local flaps difficult. A free tissue transfer has the additional dramatic effect when saving the hindfoot or heel of converting the patient from a user of a prosthesis (Syme ankle disarticulation or below-knee amputee) to a user of a shoe.

Vascular Reconstruction

In an amputation in a diabetic or dysvascular limb, the skin edges should be checked once the final flaps have been fashioned. If there is no visible bleeding of at least a small amount, the flaps should probably be revised to a more proximal level. When the limb is dysvascular, a vascular consultation should be obtained early. Revascularization of the limb, either through angioplasty or distal bypass surgery, is frequently the key to salvage of the foot. Bypass is more common and more applicable than balloon angioplasty and, in the nondiabetic, usually takes the form of proximal bypass of a major occlusion at the iliac, femoral, or popliteal levels. In the dysvascular diabetic, similar proximal occlusions or stenoses occur and respond well to a vascular bypass. In addition, if not more common, are the distal, diffuse occlusions of the arteries distal to the trifurcation of the popliteal artery in the lower part of the leg. Unlike the situation in the nondiabetic, these are not discrete blockages, but usually atherosclerotic involvement of most or all of the vessel. Bypass is usually done down to the level of the ankle by using in situ or reversed saphenous vein grafts. The emphasis should be upon doing the revascularization first and then fashioning the amputation flaps and determining the final level once maximum tissue perfusion has been achieved.

The customary surgical techniques described here are basic guidelines, not absolute requisites for successful amputations. No matter what the conscientious surgeon does, some amputations will fail and will need to be revised to a higher level. If every amputation heals primarily, then the surgeon is probably doing some amputations at too proximal a level and not squeezing out enough salvaged cases from the feet. Multiple procedures and revisions are frequently needed before the final result is obtained, and the revisions do not prejudice the quality of the ultimate result; rather, they make the attempt at foot salvage worthwhile.[7] Healed amputations that are the result of revision procedures yield satisfactory results similar to those that heal after a single level of amputation. Once partial amputations of the foot heal, the reported rate of revision is as low as 10%, thus indicating that these function as definitive procedures.[10] The surgeon must use laboratory data, clinical experience, and surgical judgment to determine the proper level for initial attempts at partial foot amputation.

Determination of Amputation Level

A plethora of tests have been promulgated in the surgical and orthopaedic literature as the "best" method to determine the proper level of amputation. Most are based on statistical review of ultimate healing of the amputated limb and the correlation with predicted healing of the test. These procedures include arterial Doppler pressures, fluorescein angiography, transcutaneous oxygen tension, xenon clearance, and others.[12, 14, 19] The literature is replete with these reports, although most do not address the question of the proper level of amputation within the foot, i.e., the question of the correct level for a partial foot amputation procedure. For this reason, these studies are often difficult or impossible to apply to the decision-making process of foot salvage, which depends to a great degree on local wound factors of gangrene, infection, and general perfusion of the foot. Differences in vascularity between a transmetatarsal amputation and a Syme ankle disarticulation are difficult at best to determine on the basis of most of the noninvasive preoperative testing. Even when it may indicate differences, the reliability of these tests to differentiate levels of viability within the foot has not been widely accepted. Most of the studies on predictive tests for amputation healing levels have been aimed at assessment of the segmental vascularity of the limb, i.e., healing below the ankle, at the ankle, below the knee, or above the knee. None of the procedures has been demonstrated to have a clear hegemony in this battle to correctly forecast healing, at least not in the arena of widespread clinical practice. There are clear advantages to each of these procedures, and a few of these characteristics will be mentioned here, although this is by no means an exhaustive review of this very broad subject.

The most commonly used and widely available test is the arterial Doppler ultrasound. The Doppler is most useful as a guideline to general levels of perfusion and is the best initial screening test to determine whether the patient needs a vascular surgery consultation and an arteriogram. The Doppler is painless, quick, and relatively inexpensive and does not require extensive instrumentation. As discussed in the section on vascular evaluation in the preceding chapter, the pulse-volume recordings, ("waveforms") are often more reliable than pressure ratios, especially in the diabetic patient with noncompliant calcified vessels that give falsely elevated pressures (see Fig 22–11, A–C).

Transcutaneous oxygen measurements are much more accurate and clearly much more cumbersome and difficult to obtain. The readings must be obtained in an environment of controlled temperature because they are temperature-dependent, and they are time-consuming to perform. On a practical level, an adequate number of readings cannot be done efficiently without multiple simultaneous probes. The real question is to what degree the surgeon finds a correlation of these test results with wound edge bleeding at surgery and with the healing rate of amputation wounds in that particular institution.

SPECIFIC AMPUTATION LEVELS AND TECHNIQUES

Terminal Amputation of the Toe and Nail ("Terminal Syme")

This procedure, which has been described for severe deformity, onychomycosis, or recurrent infection of the great toenail, can be used for the same problems in a lesser toe as well. The key is to remove sufficient bone to allow closure without tension.

Surgical Technique

1. An elliptical incision is centered over the distal aspect of the distal phalanx encircling the toenail plate (Fig 23–4).

2. The dorsal soft tissue and nail plate are excised to expose the distal phalanx. (Depending upon the presence and magnitude of dysvascular tissue, varying skin incisions and soft-tissue resections may be necessary.)

3. The distal phalanx is transected with a bone-cut-

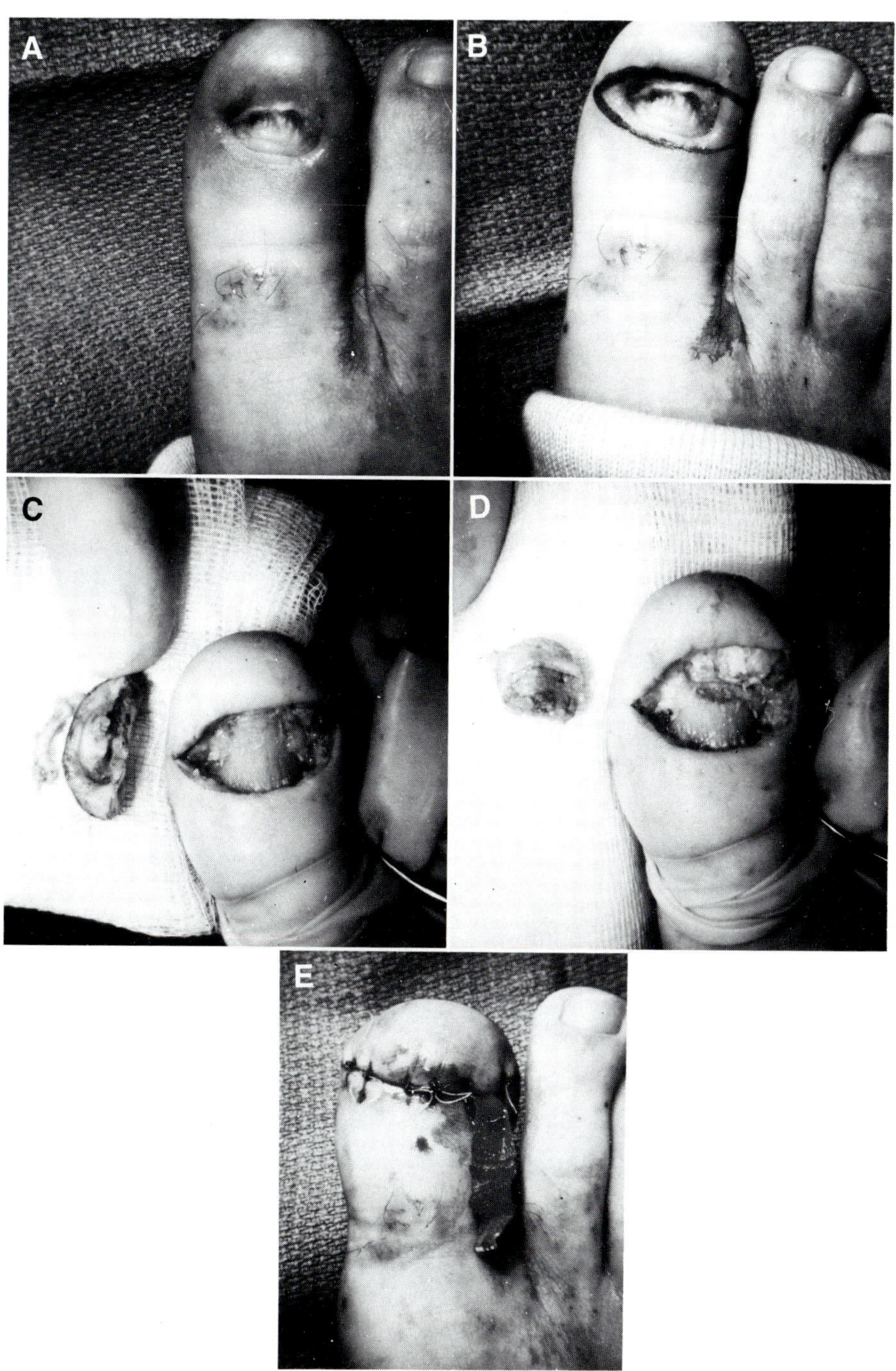

FIG 23–4.
Technique of terminal amputation of the hallux, toenail, and matrix. **A,** a chronic ingrown nail with fungal infection has been debrided. **B,** elliptical incision to remove the nail and matrix. **C,** nail and matrix removed. **D,** distal 1 cm of bone removed to allow closure of the wound. **E,** wound closed over an iodoform wick to allow escape of hematoma from raw bone.

ting forceps and the distal fragment removed. (Frequently it is necessary to remove more than 1 cm of bone.)

4. A drain may be used depending upon a surgeon's preference.

5. The skin flap is shaped to minimize medial and lateral "dog-ears."

6. A single interrupted layer of sutures is used to loosely approximate and evert the skin edges. (A loose skin closure will usually allow adequate drainage and obviate the need for a wick drain.)

7. A gauze and tape compression dressing is applied.

Aftercare

The dressing is changed 24 to 48 hours after surgery and then as frequently as necessary until adequate wound healing has occurred. Skin sutures are removed 4 to 8 weeks after surgery. Early suture removal is avoided because this may lead to wound dehiscence.

Pitfalls and Complications

Shaping of the excised ellipse of tissue is important; production of a bulbous end is not uncommon, and although it usually shrinks to some degree, flaps should be sculpted to minimize this. The main complication is dehiscence due to a tight closure caused by insufficient resection of bone. In diabetic or nondiabetic dysvascular patients, preoperative Doppler arterial studies should be done as a basic screening test of the vascularity of this most distal segment.

Amputation of the Great Toe

Although it is easier to amputate the great toe through a metatarsophalangeal disarticulation, it is very much preferable to save the base of the proximal phalanx. The minimum length of the base to save is about 1 cm (Fig 23–5). This recommendation is both intuitive and scientific; the benefits of preservation of the base of the phalanx on the subsequent gait of the patient and the pattern of pressure under the foot have been demonstrated in plantar pressure studies with the pedobarograph.[13] The intuitive basis is that by saving the base of the phalanx, the attachments and thus the functions of the plantar fascia and flexor hallucis brevis are preserved, at least partially. The independent plantar flexion mechanism of the first ray is not entirely lost; some of the weight-bearing function of the first ray is preserved, and transfer of excess pressure to the second and third metatarsal heads is reduced.

Surgical Technique

1. A curvilinear skin incision is used to encircle the dysvascular area and excise nonviable tissue.

2. Frequently sufficient skin is present on the dorsal/plantar aspect or medial lateral aspect of the hallux to enable the development of "fish-mouth" flaps (an alternative is a "racket-type" incision) (see Fig 23–7).

3. A power saw is used to transect the proximal phalanx at its base. Roughened surfaces are beveled with a rongeur.

4. Alternatively, if the great toe is disarticulated, the

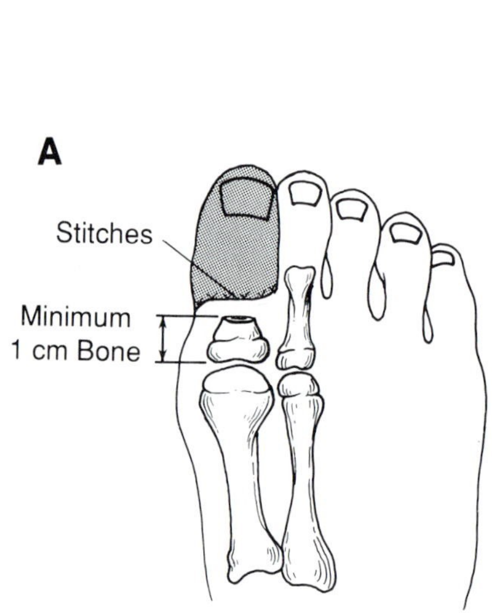

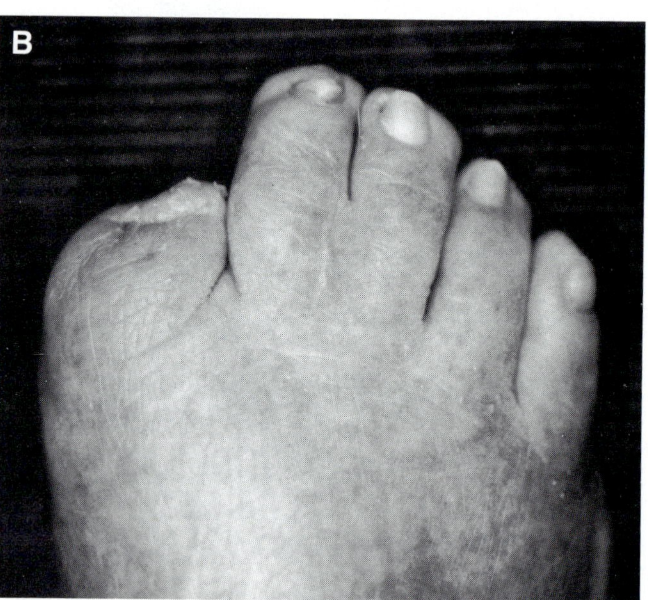

FIG 23–5.
A, preservation of at least 1 cm of the base of the proximal phalanx in amputations of the hallux is desirable to maximize the weight-bearing function of the first metatarsal. **B,** this patient has two thirds of the proximal phalanx preserved.

metatarsophalangeal capsular ligaments are severed, and the toe is removed. The sesamoids are not resected unless the removal is necessary. (The articular surface of the metatarsal head is left because its removal is unnecessary and probably undesirable since the cartilage and subchondral bone are barriers to infection of the cancellous bone of the metatarsal head.)

5. The capsule and extensor mechanisms are approximated with interrupted absorbable sutures.

6. The use of a drain is left to the surgeon's preference.

7. The skin is approximated with interrupted sutures.

8. A gauze and tape compression dressing is applied and changed 24 to 48 hours after surgery.

Aftercare

Routine dressing changes are continued until adequate healing has occurred. The patient is permitted to ambulate in a postoperative shoe with partial weight bearing on the heel and lateral aspect of the foot. Sutures are removed 4 to 8 weeks after surgery. Early suture removal should be avoided because wound dehiscence may occur.

Once a great toe has been amputated, a custom-molded filler in the shoe helps to compensate and diminish sliding of the foot inside the shoe (see Fig 23–15).[3]

Amputation of the Lesser Toes

Amputation of the lesser toes can be done as a disarticulation or by resecting through bone. If a toe requires amputation because of ischemia, necrosis, or sometimes infection, partial amputation is a good alternative, provided that there is adequate bleeding to support healing. The advantage of this over disarticulation at the metatarsophalangeal joint or transection of the proximal phalanx is that the residual partial toe serves to "maintain its space" and block migration of the two adjacent toes toward one another into the gap created by the absent digit (Fig 23–6).

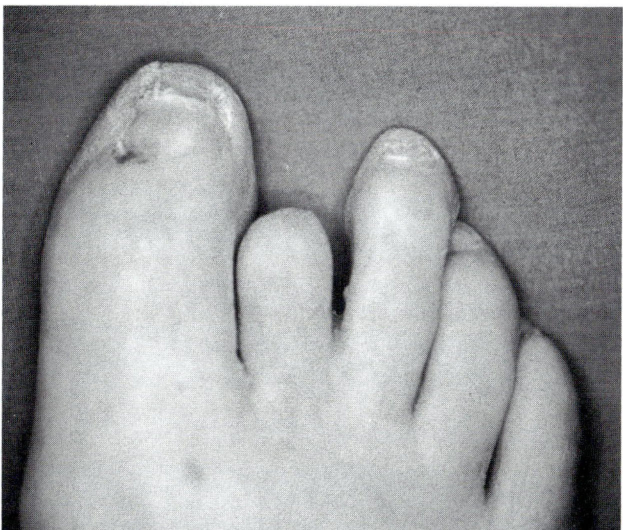

FIG 23–6.
Partial toe amputation. The residual portion of the digit blocks migration of the adjacent toes.

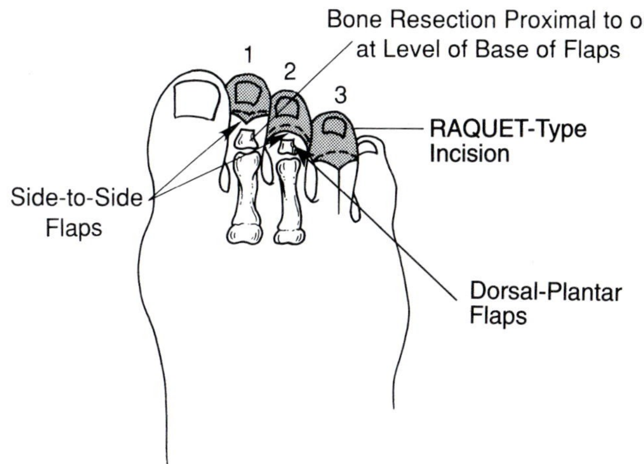

FIG 23–7.
Incisions for toe amputations: fish-mouth or medial-lateral side to side, dorsal-plantar flaps, and racquet-type incision.

Surgical Technique

A similar operative approach is used for resection of the lesser toes.

While preservation of the base of the phalanx in the lesser toes probably produces the same mechanical advantage, it is less important than in the hallux. "Fish-mouth" flaps can be fashioned side to side or dorsally to plantarly; the other alternative is the use of the "racquet-type" incision (Fig 23–7).

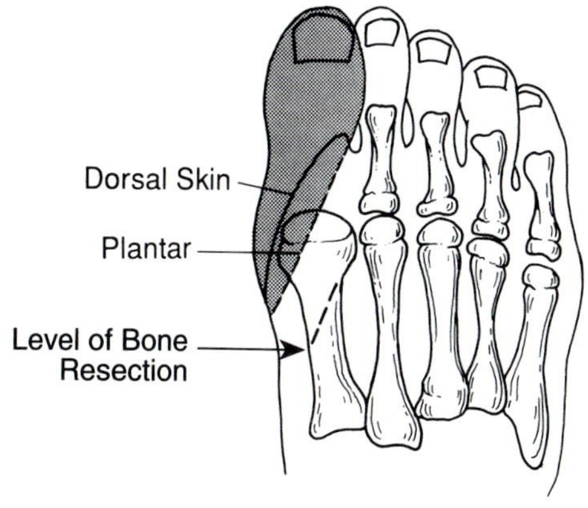

FIG 23–8.
A balance must be achieved between the level of soft-tissue and bone resection so that there is adequate coverage for wound closure without tension on the flaps.

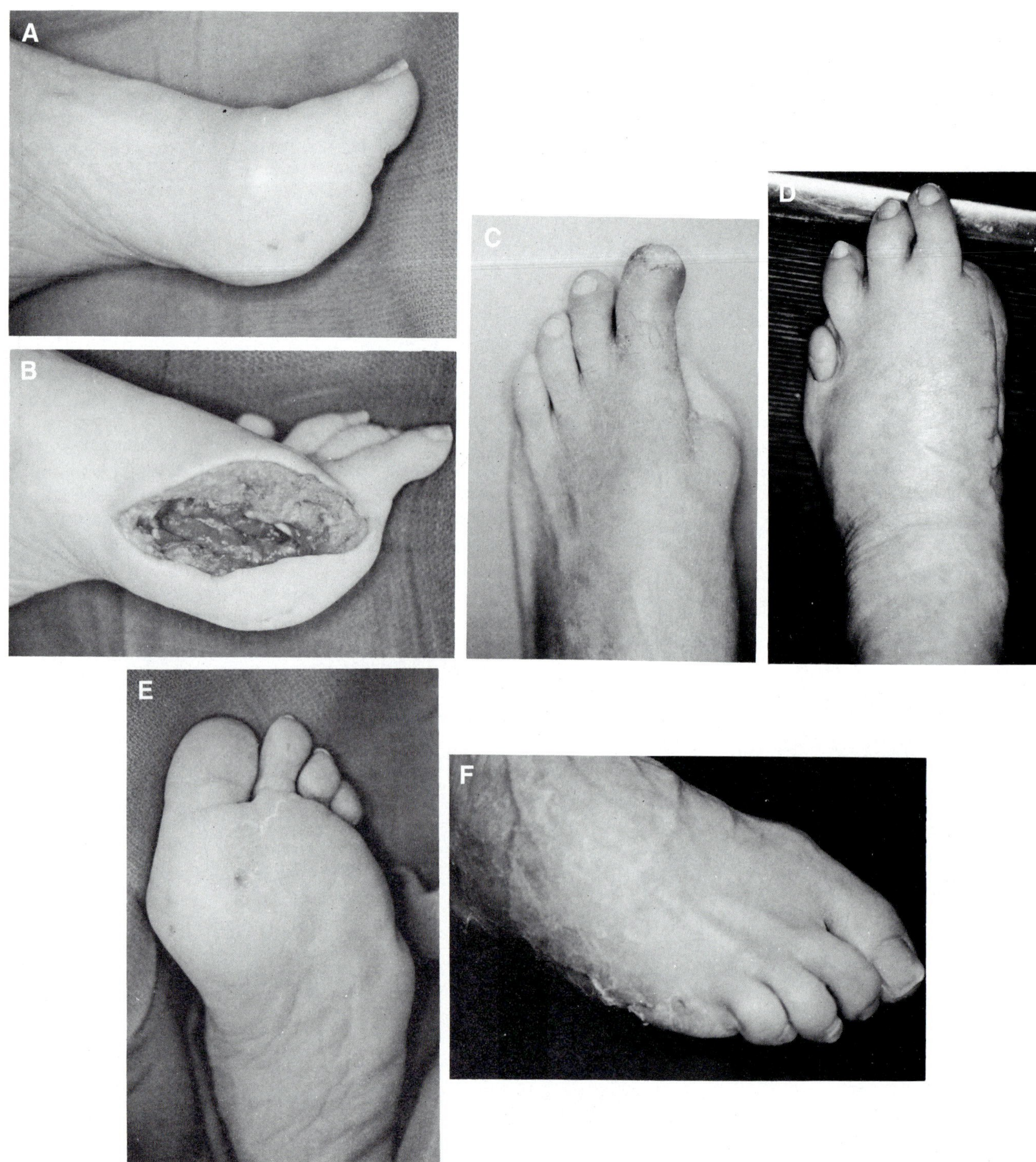

FIG 23–9.
A, prior to first ray resection, condition began with a plantar ulcer. **B,** surgical resection. **C,** following successful healing. **E** and **F**, following fifth ray resection.

Pitfalls and Complications of Toe Amputations

The most common complications are related to inadequate balance of soft tissue and bone. This leads to wound dehiscence caused by closure under tension. Other complications, mentioned above, include drift of the adjacent toes toward the defect created by the absent digit. This can be retarded by the use of a soft sponge or Plastazote filler worn inside the sock or stocking. A late deformity of a partial toe amputation is dorsal elevation of the stump caused by a hyperextension contracture at the metatarsophalangeal joint. In the lesser toes, this requires resection of the toe remnant back to the metatarsophalangeal joint or release of the

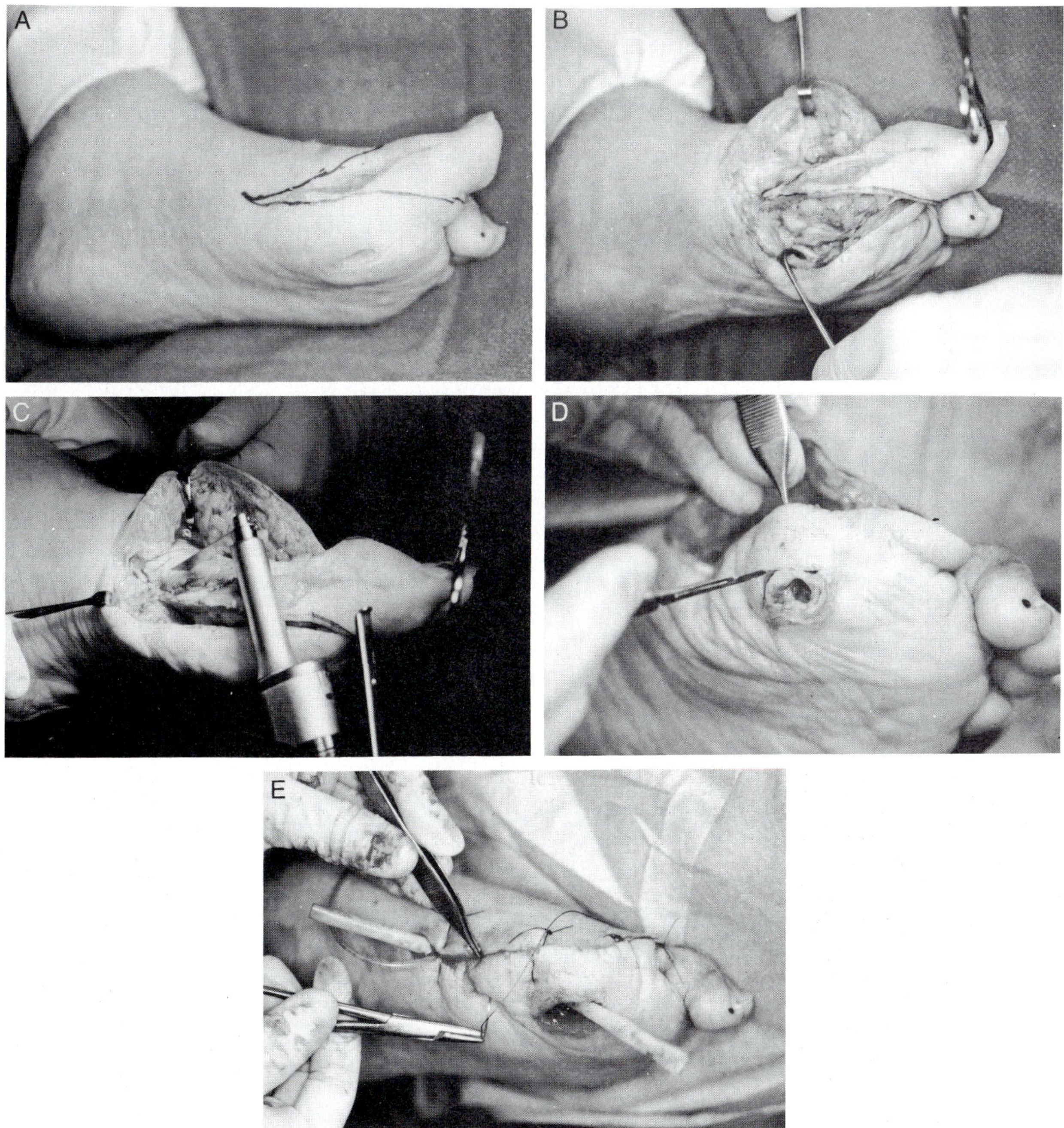

FIG 23–10.
Technique for a first ray amputation. **A** and **B** racquet incision. Edges are close to wound but wound is excised with bone and toe. **C,** note the difference in the level of the skin flaps and the level of resection of the bone. **D,** also note the way in which the ulcer is excised in elliptical fashion to enhance drainage and improve wound shape for healing. **E,** loose closure over drains.

extensor tendons and sectioning of the capsule of the metatarsophalangeal joint on three sides (medially, laterally, and dorsally).

Ray Amputations and Partial Forefoot Amputations

Amputations of a toe with all or part of its corresponding metatarsal (ray amputations) are more common than any other amputation of the foot except toe amputations. They are durable and, once they are healed, are relatively easy to fit in shoes with minor modifications. Ray amputations are commonly used to treat trauma in healthy individuals as well as infection and gangrene in the dysvascular and diabetic populations (Figs 23–8 and 23–9).

The easiest single rays to amputate are the border rays, i.e., the first and fifth. Straight medial and lateral incisions are used, respectively. When the corresponding toe is amputated along with the metatarsal, the distal end of the incision loops around the digit (the "racquet"). Specific operative techniques are so variable in this area that it is impossible to describe a routine operative approach. Surgical incisions and osseous resections

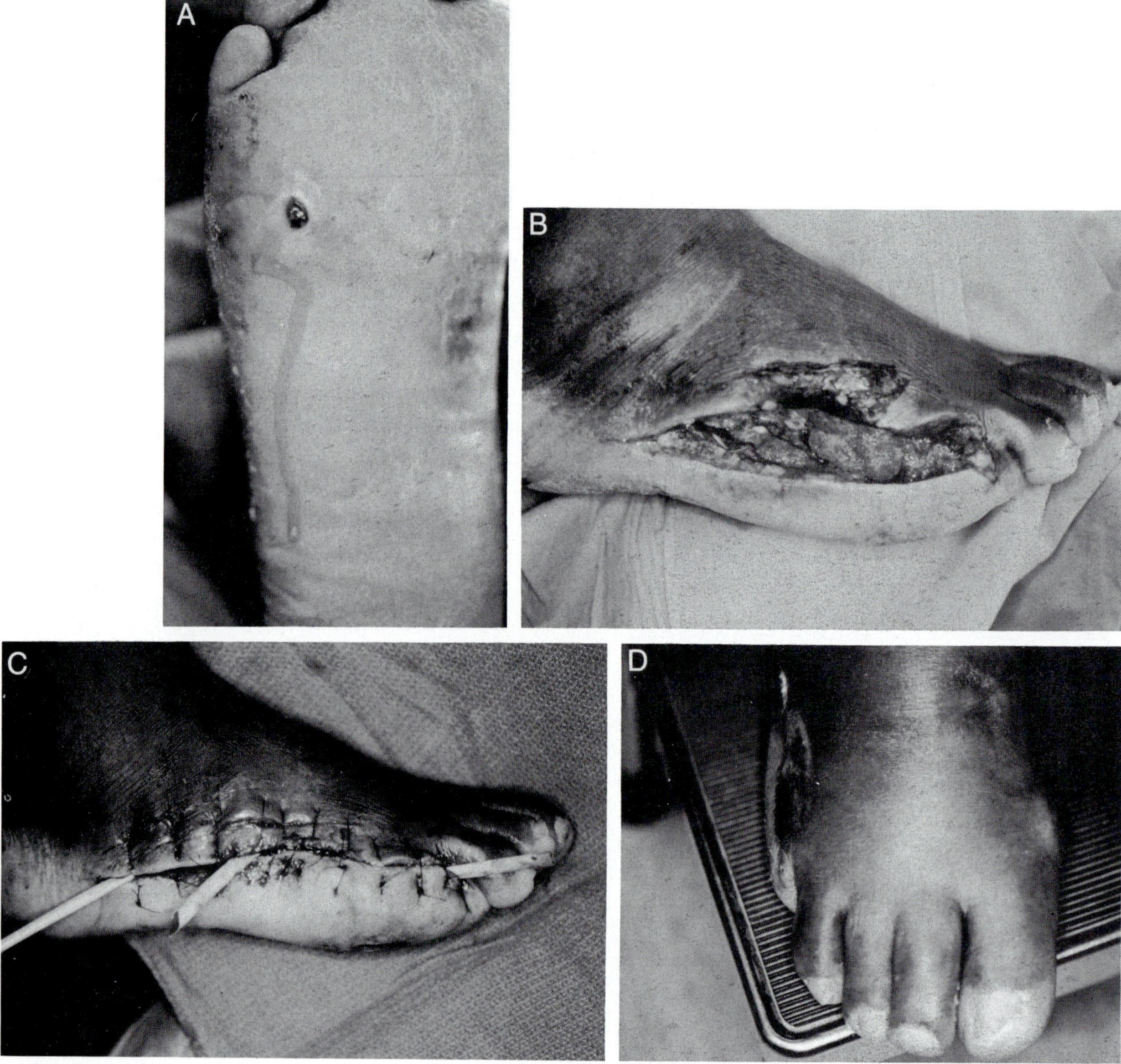

FIG 23–11.
Technique for fifth ray amputation for osteomyelitis that began with a fifth metatarsal ulcer **(A). B,** second procedure for closure, 1 week after amputation. Note the granulation tissue. **C,** closure over drains. **D,** healed amputation.

must be tailored to the individual problem area of infection, the magnitude of soft-tissue necrosis, and the extent of osteomyelitis. Care must be taken to save some of the skin that is over the digit itself and always save more skin than one would think necessary; it is obviously easy to trim away excess skin, but insufficient soft tissue for closure leads to closure under tension, dehiscence, or wound necrosis (Figs 23–10 and 23–11).

Single ray amputations of one of the three central rays is more difficult because the soft-tissue flaps cannot be approximated with as much mobility (Fig 23–12). Sometimes the gap created by the absent ray does close down when the incision is closed; other times the defect allows the two adjacent toes to drift into the space, as occurs in a simple toe disarticulation at the metatarsophalangeal joint. The key to successful central ray amputations in diabetics and dysvascular patients, in particular, is to incise the skin and soft tissue that is being saved right at the edge of necrosis and infection and then test the flaps for closure and trim thereafter as needed. When possible, the creation of a longer plantar flap when the procedure involves the border of the foot allows for an easier closure. A fillet flap can be created from the toe by removing the bone subperiosteally and preserving the full thickness of the soft tissue, which is then turned proximally to cover a defect and then trimmed appropriately (Fig 23–13). Fillet flaps can be done on border rays most easily.

Partial forefoot amputations can comprise the removal of two or occasionally three rays from the medial or lateral side of the foot; this occurs most often in the diabetic but is also the result of trauma (Fig 23–14). In most instances, once it becomes necessary to amputate three or more rays, it is easier and yields a better result to perform a transmetatarsal amputation instead. On the whole, partial forefoot amputations of the lateral side fare better than those on the medial side of the foot, although successful examples of both abound, even in diabetic and dysvascular patients. Loss of the first ray results in an effective foot somewhat less often because the foot does not balance as well and transferred pressure under the lesser metatarsals leads to further ulcerations.

Proper shoe wear after partial forefoot amputations is essential (Fig 23–15). The shoe must be wide toed and have extra depth in the toe box to accommodate the insole. A filler should be built as a part of the insole to block side-to-side motion of the remaining narrow forefoot (i.e., prevent the "windshield wiper" motion that can occur in walking). Deformity of the remaining toes is common and takes the form of clawing as well as medial or lateral drift toward the absent rays; shoe wear

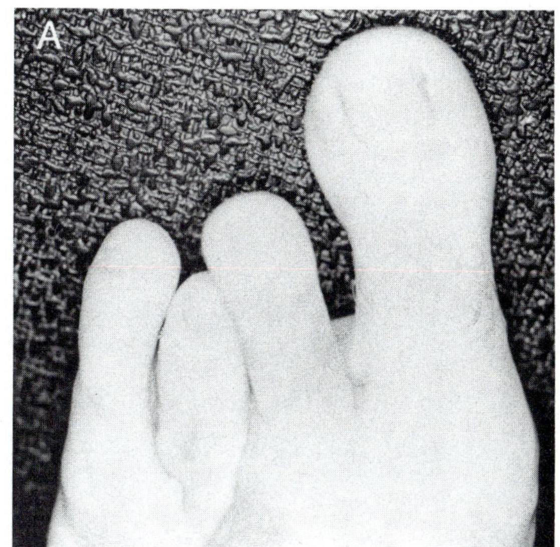

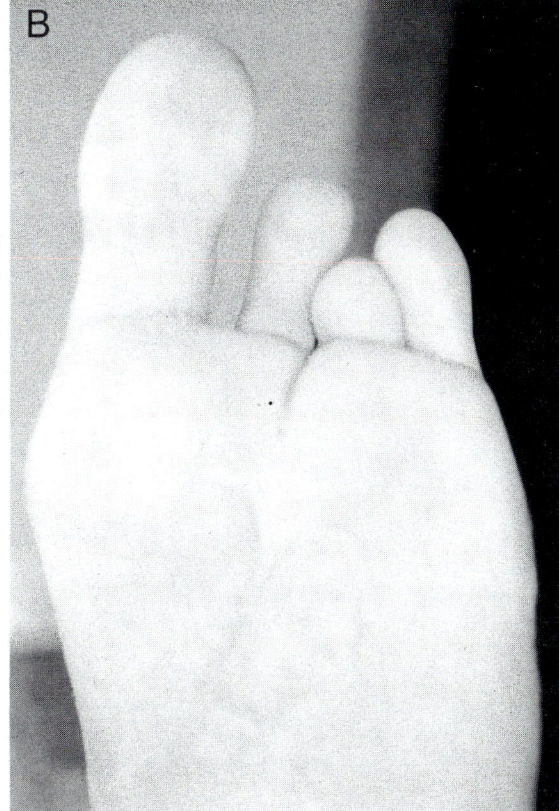

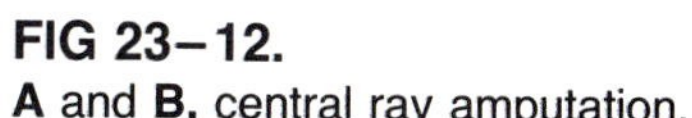
FIG 23–12.
A and **B,** central ray amputation.

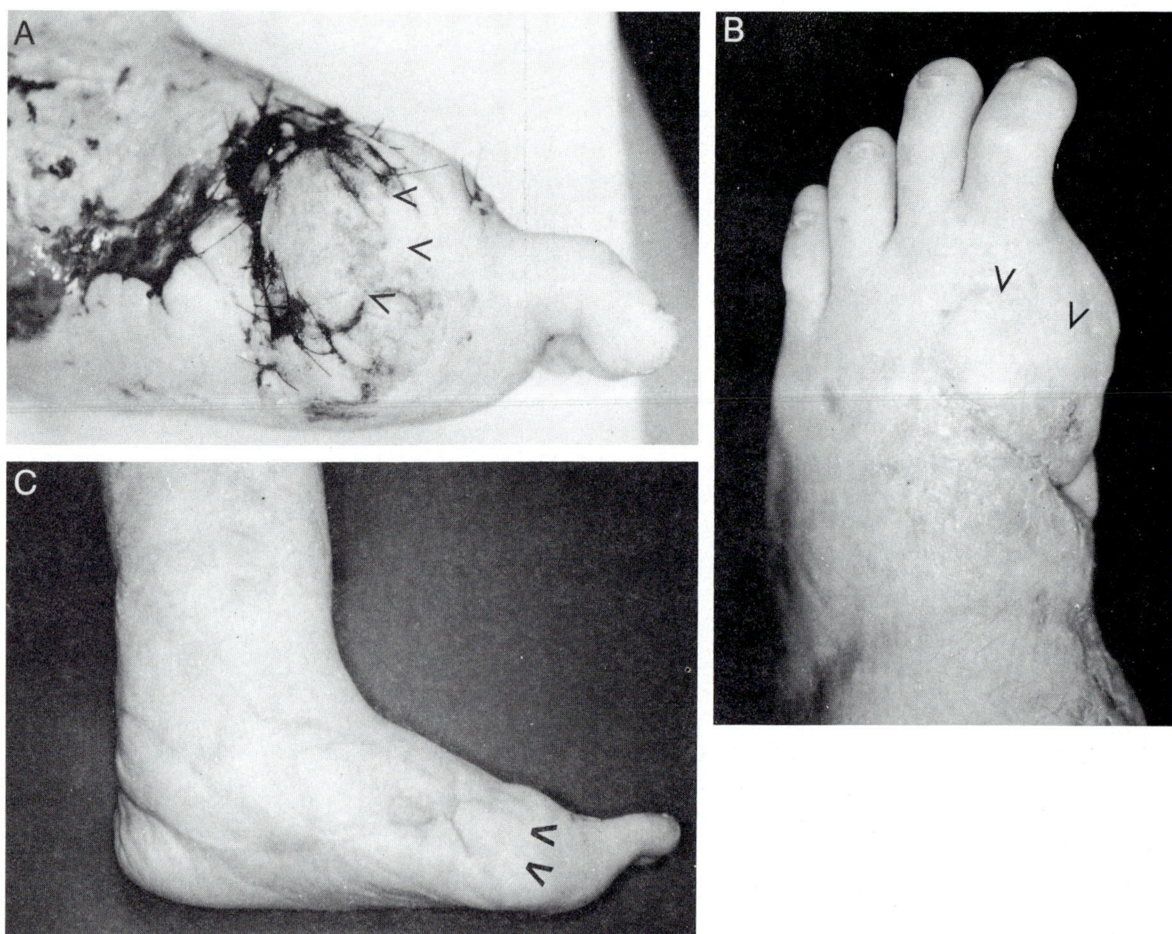

FIG 23–13.
Toe fillet flap. **A,** the great toe soft tissue has been turned proximally to cover a defect over the first metatarsal. **B** and **C,** healed flap.

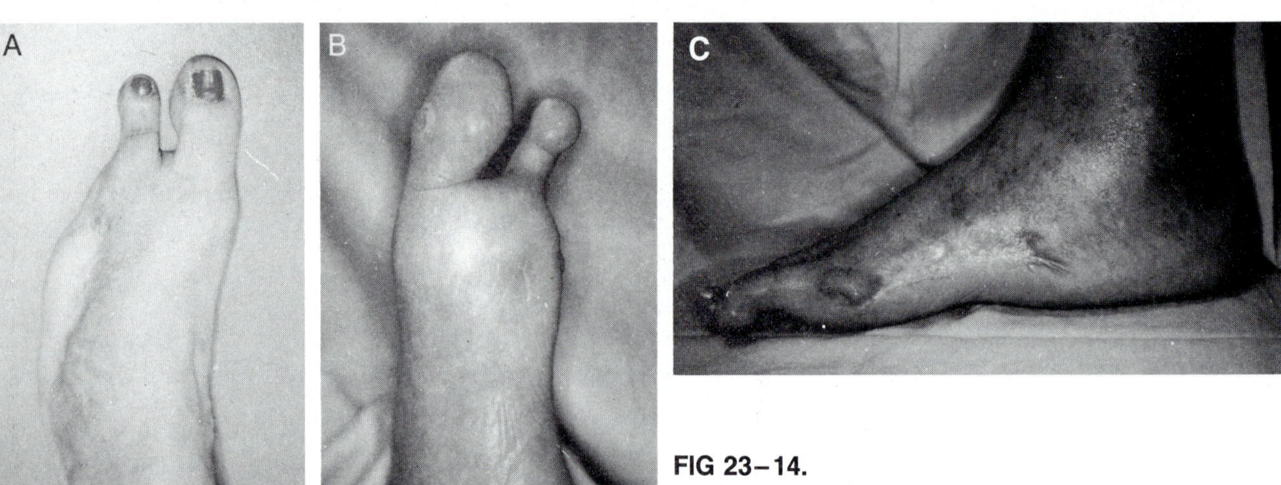

FIG 23–14.
A–C, an example of lateral partial forefoot amputation.

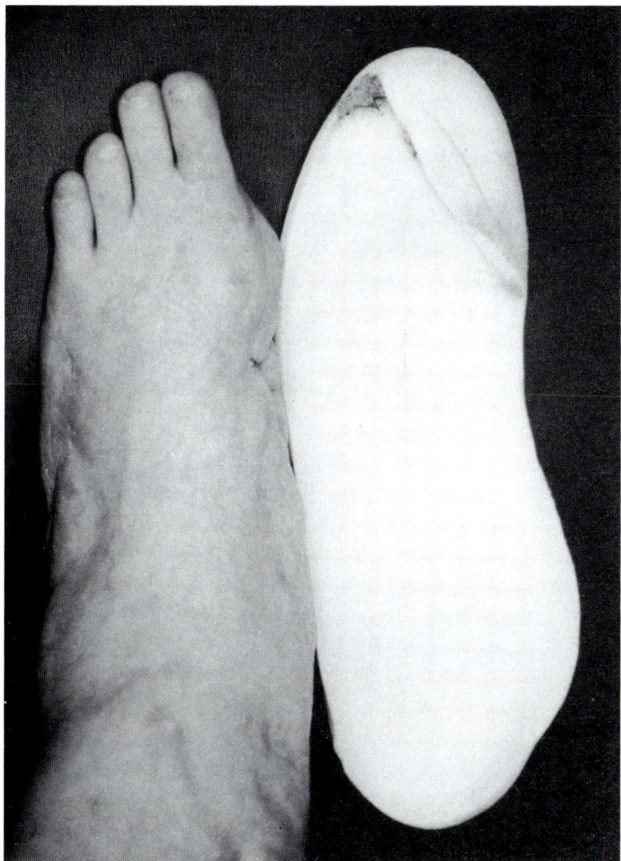

FIG 23–15.
Molded insole for healed partial forefoot amputations.

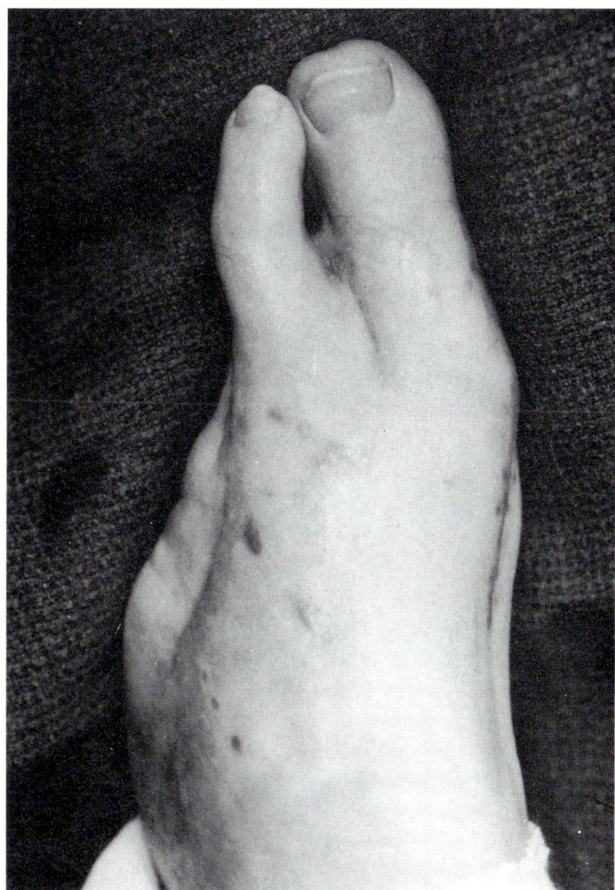

FIG 23–16.
Late clawtoe after a partial forefoot amputation.

must accommodate these problems as well. In some cases, it is necessary to surgically correct these secondary toe deformities several months after amputation (Fig 23–16).

Partial forefoot amputations and transmetatarsal amputations are the most common situation in which the surgeon may want to use "creative" flaps. This signifies utilization of whatever viable tissue is available to close the wound, with the goal of achieving primary closure over the maximum length of bone by using local tissues (Fig 23–17).

Pitfalls and Complications

The two main complications of the resection of one or more rays are delayed or poor wound healing and an unstable stump that bears weight unevenly and results in recurrent pressure ulceration under the residual metatarsal heads (Fig 23–18). In both cases, the best salvage is revision to a more proximal level, usually a transmetatarsal amputation. In the insensitive patient (usually diabetic), another complication is the development of Charcot midfoot joints caused by destabilization after resection of one or more rays. The midfoot collapses and produces a secondary deformity. This cannot always be prevented, but it can be retarded by preserving the base of the metatarsal whenever possible when a ray amputation is performed. In the case of a first ray amputation, an additional benefit is preservation of the entire attachment of the anterior tibialis tendon. In some cases that require resection of the base of the first metatarsal, if the residual insertion of the tendon on the medial cuneiform is attenuated, it is a good idea to reattach the tendon altogether.

Transmetatarsal Amputations

Transmetatarsal amputations are a sturdy, practical solution to severe gangrene, infection, or tissue loss in the forefoot (Fig 23–19). They are technically easy to perform and have as a primary advantage the preservation of the attachment of the anterior tibialis tendon. This not only is important for active dorsiflexion in walking but also serves to counteract the pull of the tri-

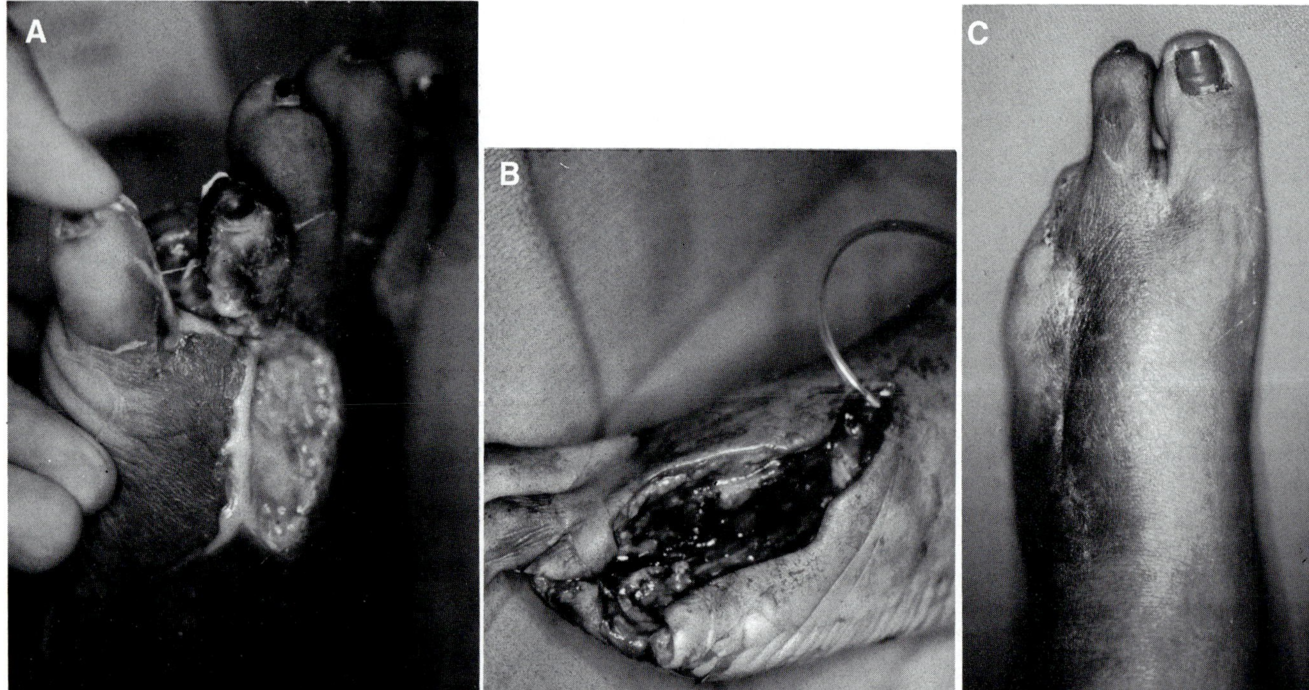

FIG 23–17.
A, partial forefoot amputation for abscess and osteomyelitis. **B,** the maximum amount of soft tissue has been preserved, right up to the edge of viable tissue, in order to achieve closure. **C,** healed wound. Patient resumed original job in mailroom.

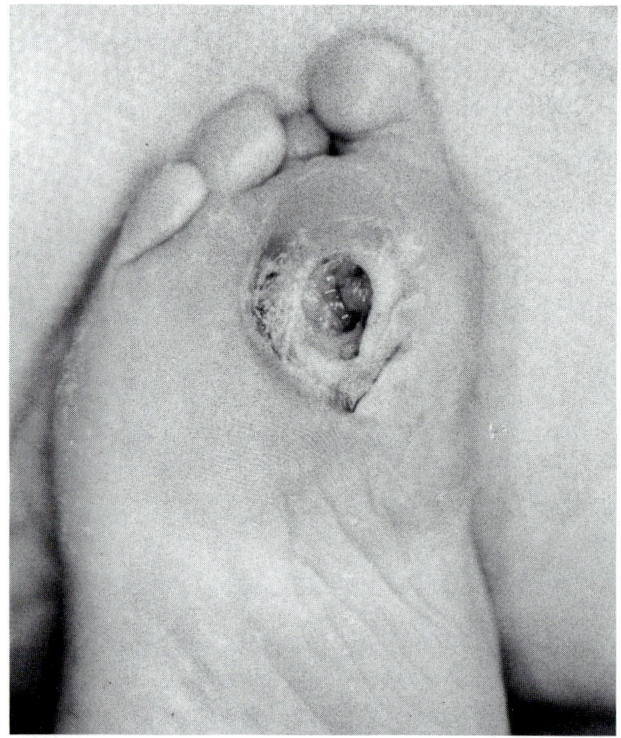

FIG 23–18.
Recurrent ulceration after a partial forefoot amputation due to transfer of pressure to the remaining rays. The patient required a transmetatarsal amputation.

ceps surae, which almost always produces an equinus contracture when unopposed. Sometimes it is necessary to do concomitant lengthening of the Achilles tendon with or without posterior ankle and subtalar joint capsulotomies for an equinus contracture that has developed over a long period of non–weight bearing prior to the time of the amputation.

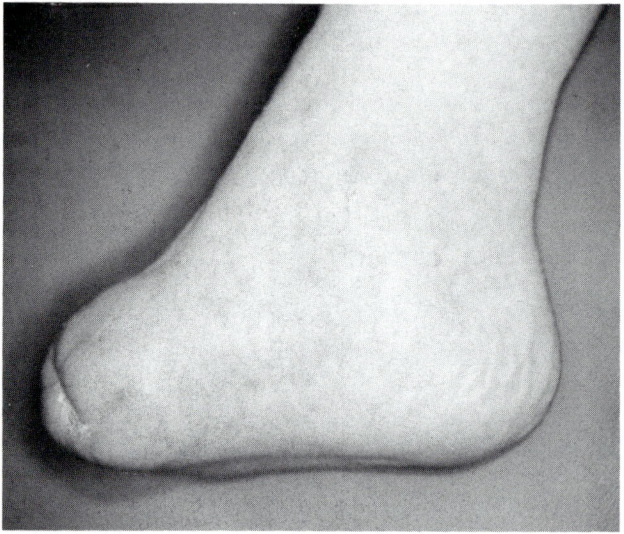

FIG 23–19.
Healed transmetatarsal amputation.

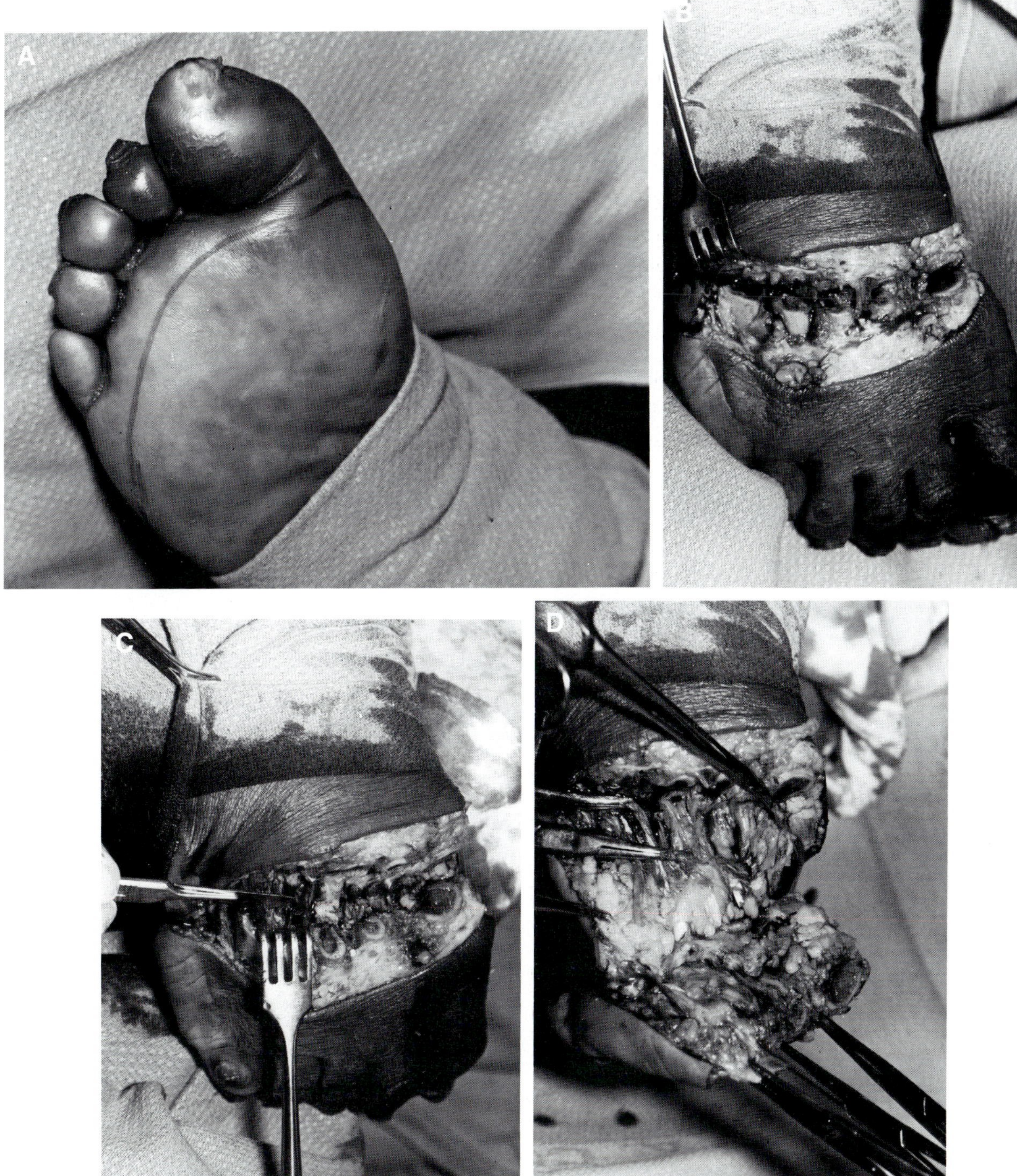

FIG 23–20.
Surgical technique for transmetatarsal amputation. **A,** plantar skin incision for transmetatarsal amputation. **B,** metatarsals divided about 15 degrees from the transverse axis. **C,** soft tissue divided from the metatarsal necks and heads. **D,** toes divided from the plantar flap. **E,** tendons drawn down and divided. **F,** inferior edges of the metatarsals rounded to relieve pressure. **G,** soft dressing is used until the wound has healed. *(Continued.)*

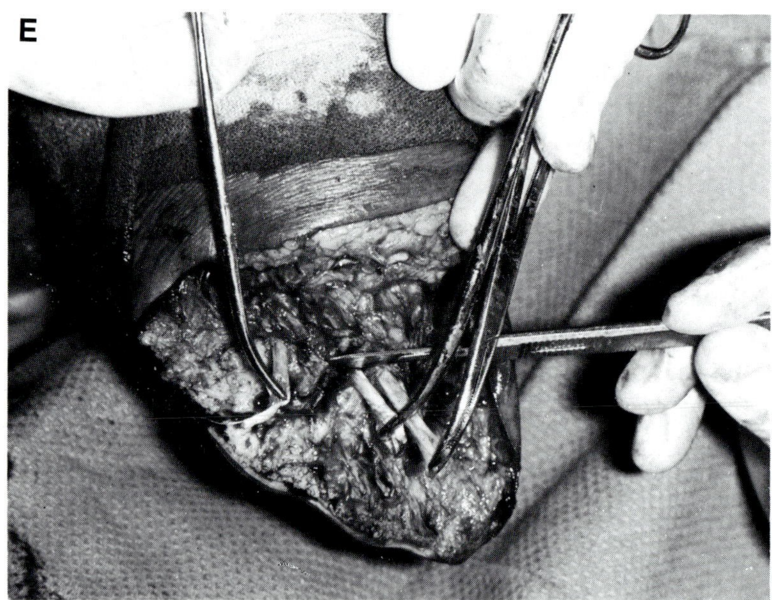

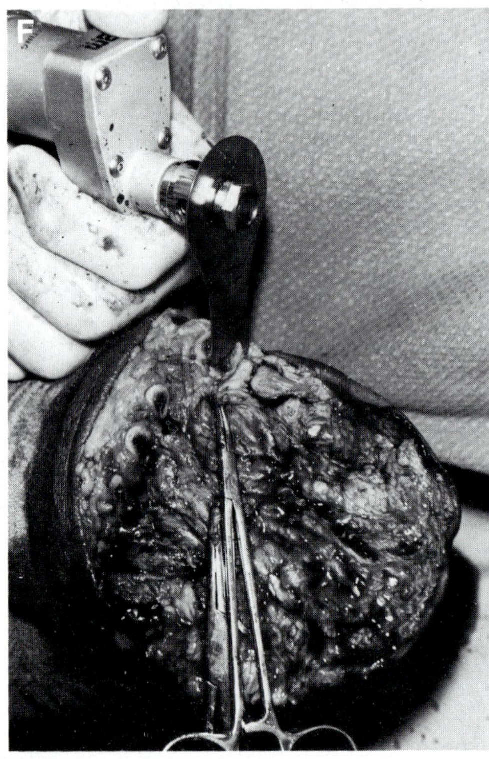

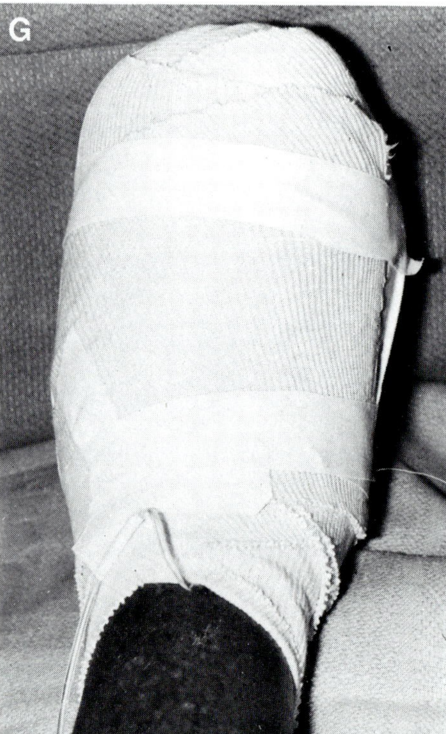

FIG 23–20. (cont.).

Surgical Technique

1. The proposed skin incision is marked preoperatively.

2. The skin incision, as in all amputations of the foot, is selected by the level at which good, viable skin is available. The incision is curved gently proximally from a medial to a lateral direction to match the length of the metatarsals (Fig 23–20, A).

3. A full-thickness flap is developed dorsally down to the bones.

4. The flap from the plantar surface is usually made longer so that it wraps around the bone ends; while this is not always possible, it is desirable (see Fig 23–20, A). (The use of local dorsal skin is still vastly superior to split-thickness skin grafting and should be used if the plantar skin is insufficient.)

5. The tendons are cut back to the proximal edge of

the wound while they are held under tension with a clamp (Fig 23–20, E).

6. When the metatarsals are resected, it is best to use a small power saw since osteotomes tend to splinter and split the cortical bone of the metatarsal shafts.

7. The bones should be beveled in a direction from dorsal distal to plantar proximal and at an angle of 15 to 20 degrees in order to prevent a sharp plantar edge of the bone that may lead to later pain or ulceration. The metatarsals are cut in a cascade of length: each successively lateral metatarsal is cut at least 2 to 3 mm shorter than the metatarsal immediately medial to it (Fig 23–21). The fifth metatarsal should be cut even shorter than this because it tends to produce symptoms since it is the most mobile of all the metatarsals (Fig 23–20, B and F).

8. Once the bones have been cut, the amputated forefoot is divided from the plantar flap by cutting just under the bones down to the plantar skin edge (Fig 23–20, D).

9. The plantar flap usually needs to be thinned in order to achieve closure without tension. Excessive or uneven "planing" of the plantar flap may jeopardize the viability of the flap.

10. The flaps tend to bulge at the medial and lateral edges in particular. Closure in diabetics is done in a single layer with interrupted nonabsorbable sutures.

11. In an infected foot, presuming that the infected area has been ablated, an irrigation system as described previously is used (see Chapter 22).

12. A compression dressing is applied as well as a carefully padded posterior splint with the ankle held in a neutral position.

13. The drainage system is discontinued 24 to 48 hours after surgery.

Aftercare

Sutures in diabetics are left in place a minimum of 4 weeks, but they are frequently kept more than twice this long. The patient is kept non–weight bearing for 2 to 4 weeks, depending on the wound healing. A postoperative cast may be used after the first week or so, depending on the wound healing.

The length of the transmetatarsal amputation can vary considerably, depending on the amount of soft tissue vs. the length of bone that can be retained. Longer stumps have the advantage of holding onto a shoe better, but a short stump that heals primarily is better than a longer one that fails to heal or must be left open to granulate.

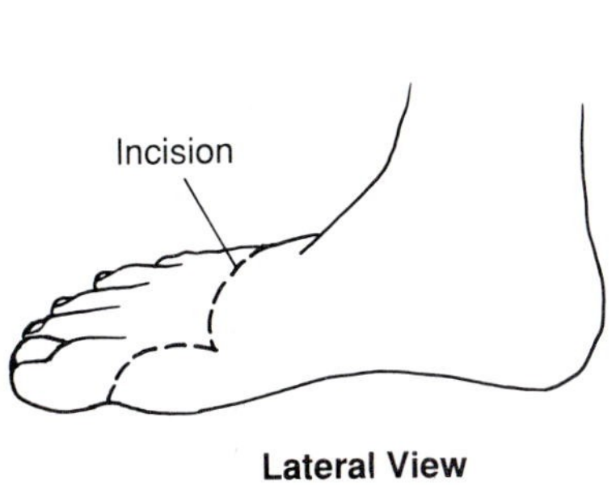

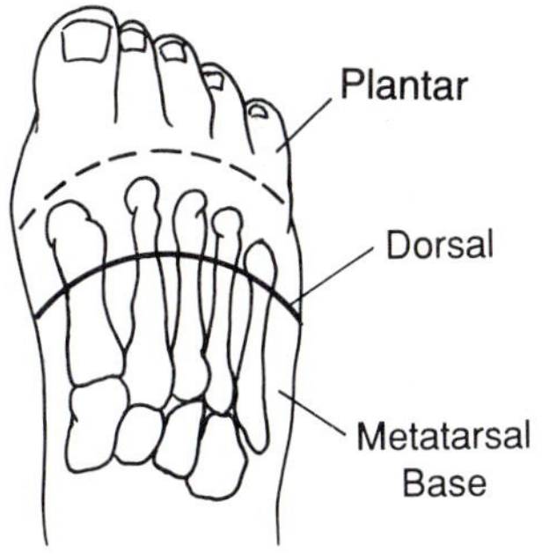

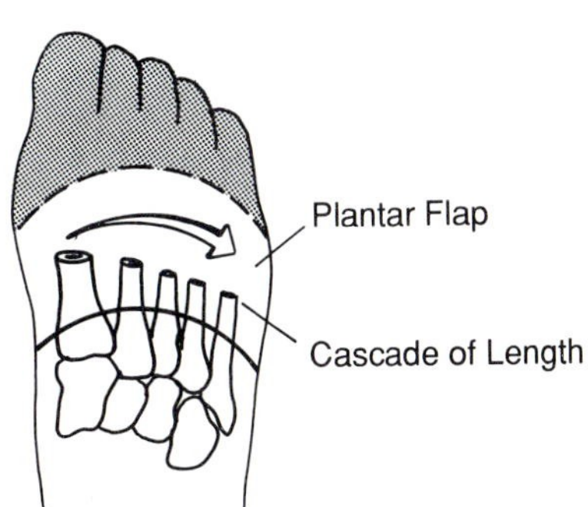

FIG 23–21.
Incisions and level of bone resection for transmetatarsal amputation.

Whenever possible, preservation of all five bases of the metatarsals is worthwhile. In the traumatic amputee, there is better balance of the midfoot. In the diabetic with neuropathy, removal of one or more metatarsal bases may increase the risk of Charcot breakdown of the midfoot and hindfoot, as has been mentioned above. This risk is still significant in any transmetatarsal amputation in a patient with severe neuropathy, even when all the bases of the metatarsals have been retained.

Most patients with transmetatarsal amputations can be fit in off-the-shelf shoe wear or at most, a high-top shoe because of its additional lacing. The shoes generally need to be either lace-up or Velcro closure types. The shoe should have additional depth for a dual-density molded insole to which is attached a block or toe filler that holds the shoe in the area of the missing forefoot (Fig 23–22).

Pitfalls and Complications

The most common complication of this amputation is development of recurrent and recalcitrant ulceration on the stump. Occasionally it is due to the plantar projection of one of the residual metatarsals, in which case it occurs on the plantar surface, requiring resection of the prominence. Most often, ulcerations occur on the distal edge of the stump and are due to an equinus contracture at the ankle and possibly to some extent the transverse tarsal joint. Treatment consists of Achilles lengthening, caspsulotomies of the ankle and subtalar joints, and treatment in a postoperative cast.

Chopart Amputations

This disarticulation through "Chopart's joint," i.e., the transtarsal joints of the talonavicular and calcaneocuboid joints combined, had fallen into disfavor but has been repopularized by Jacobs.[7] The failures of this procedure occurred because of late equinus deformities that developed as a result of the unopposed pull of the tendo Achillis. Therefore, it is necessary to lengthen or preferably completely release the Achilles tendon at the time of the amputation. Once healed the patient must be fitted into either a prosthesis or a polypropylene ankle-foot orthosis (AFO) so that the loss of Achilles function is more than compensated for by the absence of deformity together with the function of the fitted device. The advantages of the Chopart amputation vs. the Syme amputation are several. First, it is technically much easier to do. Second, when coupled with an AFO, it allows use of a shoe rather than a knee-high prosthesis (Fig 23–23). Third, it does not produce as much shortening of the limb. Unfortunately, the indications for its use are quite limited. Most patients who have an insufficient amount of viable soft tissue for a transmetatarsal amputation do not have enough for a Chopart amputation and require either a Syme or a below-knee amputation.

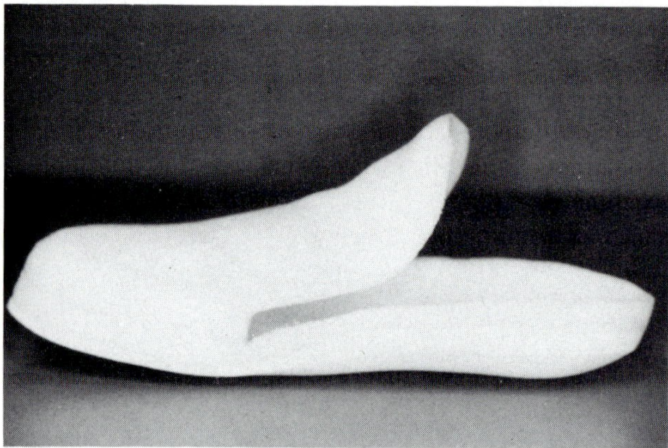

FIG 23–22.
Shoe insole with a toe filler for transmetatarsal amputation.

Surgical Technique

1. The skin incision is marked postoperatively.
2. Fashion the flaps dorsally and plantarly if possible; otherwise use the tissue that is available. Take care to resect the soft tissue sufficiently distal to the level of the disarticulation while remembering that the cross section of the foot at this level is wide (Fig 23–24).
3. The skin is retracted and the **resection** is carried down directly through the soft tissue, again leaving sufficient soft tissue to close over the amputation area.
4. The tendons are clamped and, with distal traction, are severed and allowed to retract.
5. The Chopart joint is located. The dorsal and plantar ligaments of the calcaneocuboid and **talonavicular** joints are released.
6. If a tourniquet has been used, it is released and adequate hemostasis achieved.
7. A peracutaneous Achilles tendon tenotomy is frequently performed to prevent the development of an equinus contracture.
8. A soft compression dressing is applied, and frequently a postoperative cast is used as well to hold the ankle in a neutral position.

Aftercare

The patient is maintained in a postoperative splint or cast that is changed frequently to monitor wound healing. Sutures are removed 4 to 8 weeks after surgery depending upon wound healing. Early suture removal should be avoided to prevent wound dehiscence. The patient is kept non–weight bearing during the healing

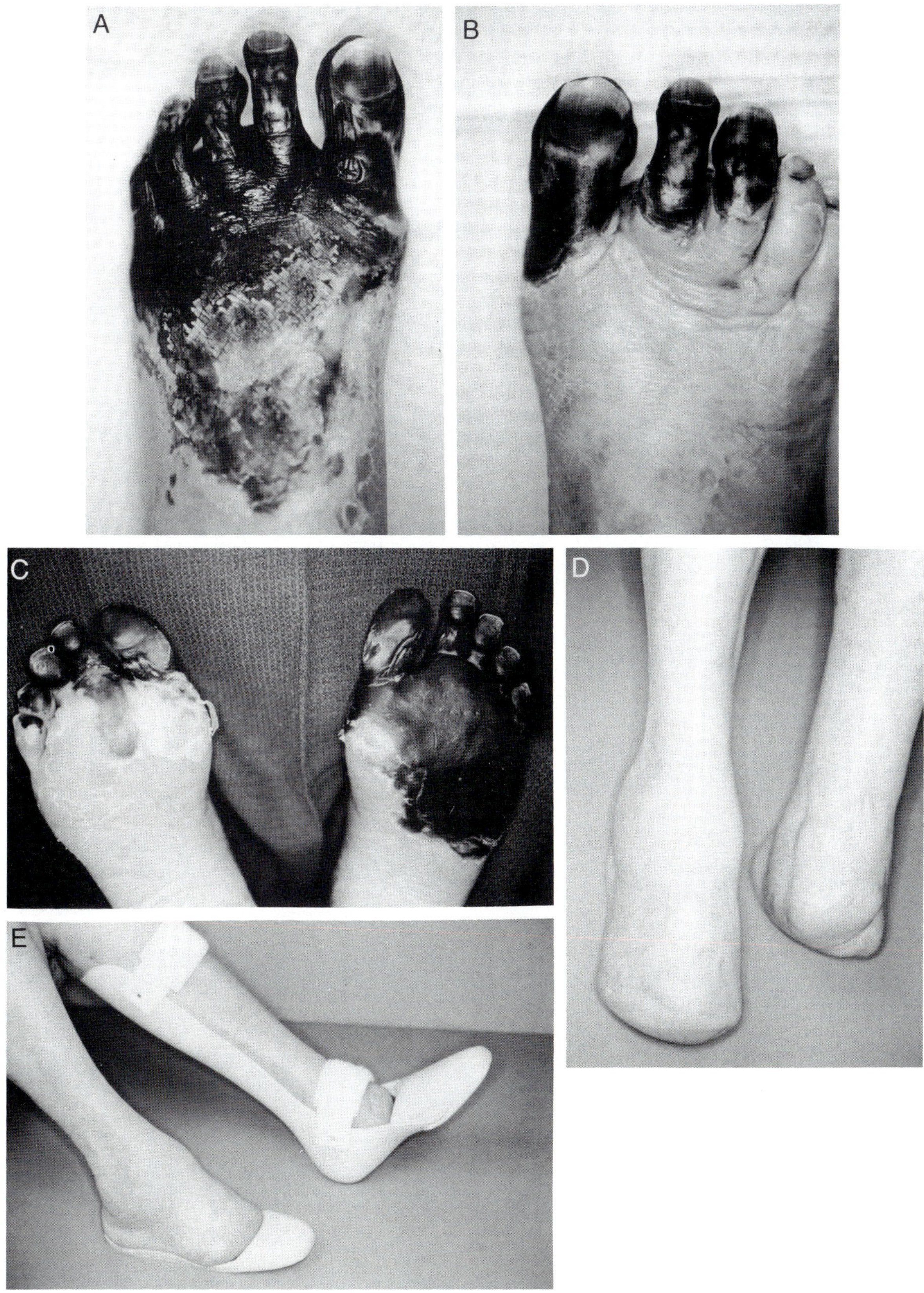

FIG 23–23.
Bilateral distal gangrene due to embolism. **A,** left foot with a more proximal level of gangrene. **B,** right foot with gangrene involving the toes. **C,** plantar views. **D,** right transmetatarsal and left Chopart amputation. **E,** a shoe insole with a toe filler on the *right* and an AFO with filler on the *left* allow the patient to wear low-counter laced shoes.

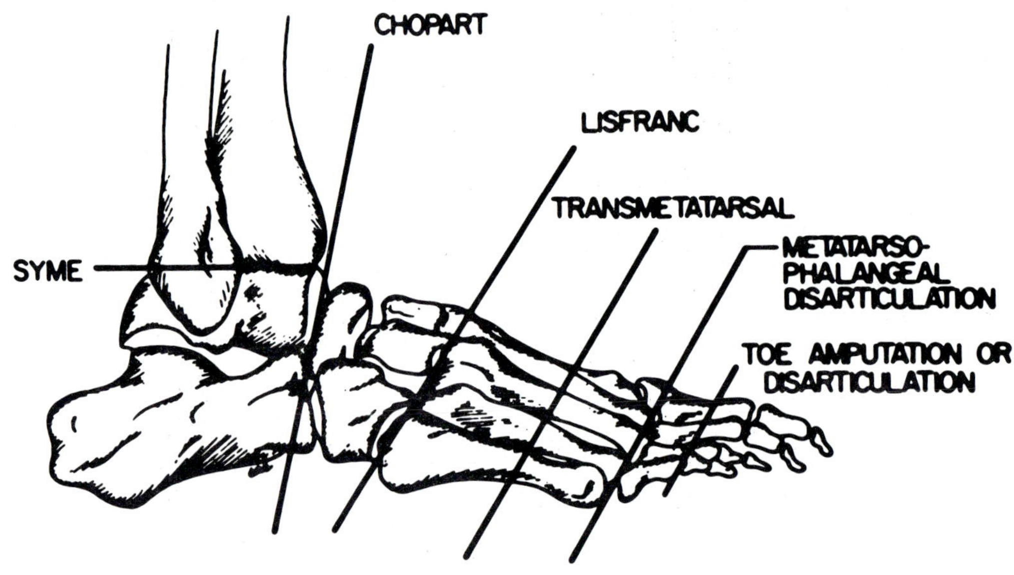

FIG 23–24.
Levels of partial foot amputation.

process. An AFO is fitted after completion of healing to stabilize the ankle joint and to assist with ambulation.

Pitfalls and Complications

The primary complication is the development of an equinus contracture leading to recalcitrant ulcerations and osteomyelitis; this is usually preventable by doing the Achilles tenotomy at the time of surgery; secondary procedures are occasionally necessary. Other problems arise when attempting to fit the patient in a shoe without the AFO.

Syme Amputation

The Syme amputation, or ankle disarticulation, is named for James Syme, Professor of Clinical Surgery, University of Edinburgh, who first described it in 1843. Although invented in an era before antisepsis, antibiotics, or anesthesia, its great advantage was that it did not have the 25% to 50% mortality of the below-knee amputation, which frequently became infected due to contamination in a large wound that contained the transected medullary cavities of the tibia and fibula. In our era, the procedure retains its other major advantage originally ascribed to it, i.e., a stump of "greater comfort and utility" when compared with the below-knee amputation. This advantage derives from the fact that the amputation is partially weight bearing on its end and because the end-bearing stump is covered with the special skin and pad of the heel, which withstand this weight well. The remainder of the weight is borne through the flare of the tibial metaphysis near the top of the prosthesis (Fig 23–25). Not only is this amputation indicated in trauma, gangrene, and infection, but it has

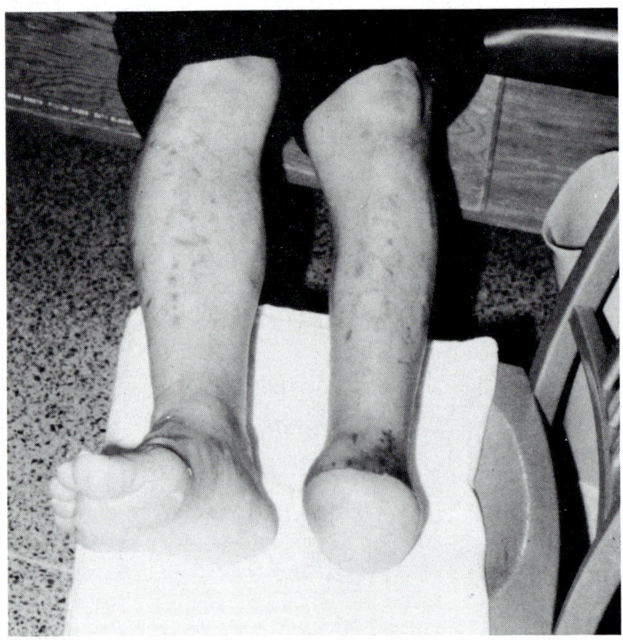

FIG 23–25.
Healed Syme amputation.

also been successfully used in patients with congenital limb deformities and deficiencies such as fibular hemimelia, proximal focal femoral deficiency, and congential pseudarthrosis of the tibia.[1, 4, 5, 8]

The Syme amputation can be done in one or two stages. There is very little difference except for a slight shift in the position of the initial skin incisions 1.5 cm more distally and anteriorly in the two-stage procedure in order to cover the malleoli, which are not resected in the first stage. The malleoli should not be resected in children unless severe pressure problems arise, and then they should be resected below the physeal line. In the one-stage procedure, the malleoli are cut at the time of the amputation itself.

While the two-stage method has been popularized by a number of authors, especially Wagner,[15] it is appropriate to use in cases of infection with possible spread near the level of the surgery. If the area of infection has been resolved or if the amputation is being done for trauma or distal gangrene, then it is usually not necessary to delay malleolar resection to a second stage.

Surgical Technique

1. The anterior incision is along a line that connects two points placed 1 to 1.5 cm below and 1 to 1.5 cm anterior to the midpoint of the tip of each malleolus. The two malleolar points are then connected by an incision across the sole and perpendicular to its plane (Fig 23–26, A).
2. The plantar incision is carried all the way down to bone, i.e., down to the calcaneus (Fig 23–26, B).
3. The dorsal incision is carried down to the dome of the talus.
4. The anterior tendons are pulled down with a clamp and divided so that they retract. The anterior tibial artery is ligated or electrocoagulated.
5. The collateral ligament attachments on the talus are divided by alternating back and forth medially to laterally while pulling the talus forward and down (Fig 23–26, C).
6. *Great care is taken to avoid the neurovascular bundle on the medial side.* This is one of the two critical points of

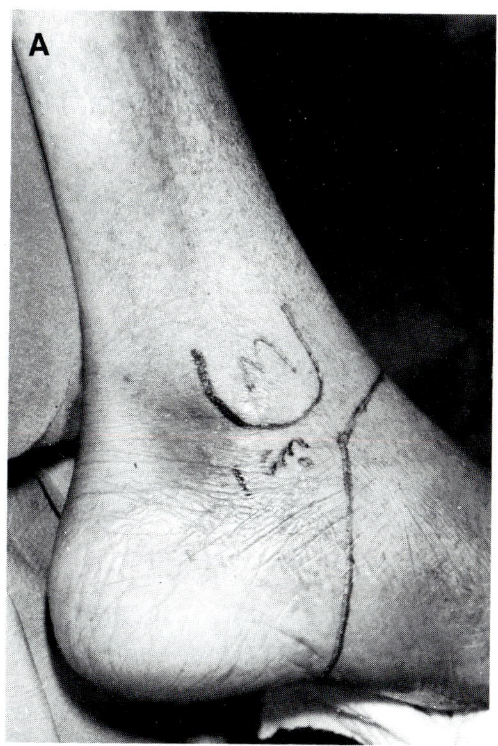

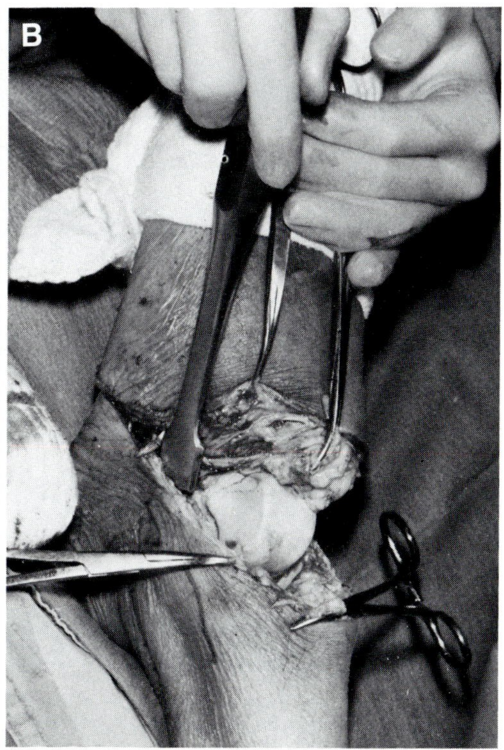

FIG 23–26.
Technique for Syme amputation. **A,** incisions for the Syme amputation. The two incisions connect points at 1 cm anterior and 1 cm distal to the tip of each malleolus. **B,** incision carried directly to bone; subperiosteal dissection of the os calcis is begun. **C,** bone hook in the talus for traction. Subperiosteal dissection to the os calcis continues. **D,** top of the os calcis dissected. A bone hook in the talus aids in peeling of the os calcis out of the soft-tissue envelope. **E,** the attachment of the Achilles tendon is carefully released with a scalpel; the dome of the ankle joint is just above the scalpel. **F,** avoid the neurovascular bundle on the medial side of the flap. **G,** closure of deep fascia to the plantar aponeurosis. **H,** skin closure with nylon or other nonabsorbable stuture. **I,** closed incision with dog-ears and a good base of the posterior skin. This would be sacrificed if the dog-ears were removed. *(Continued.)*

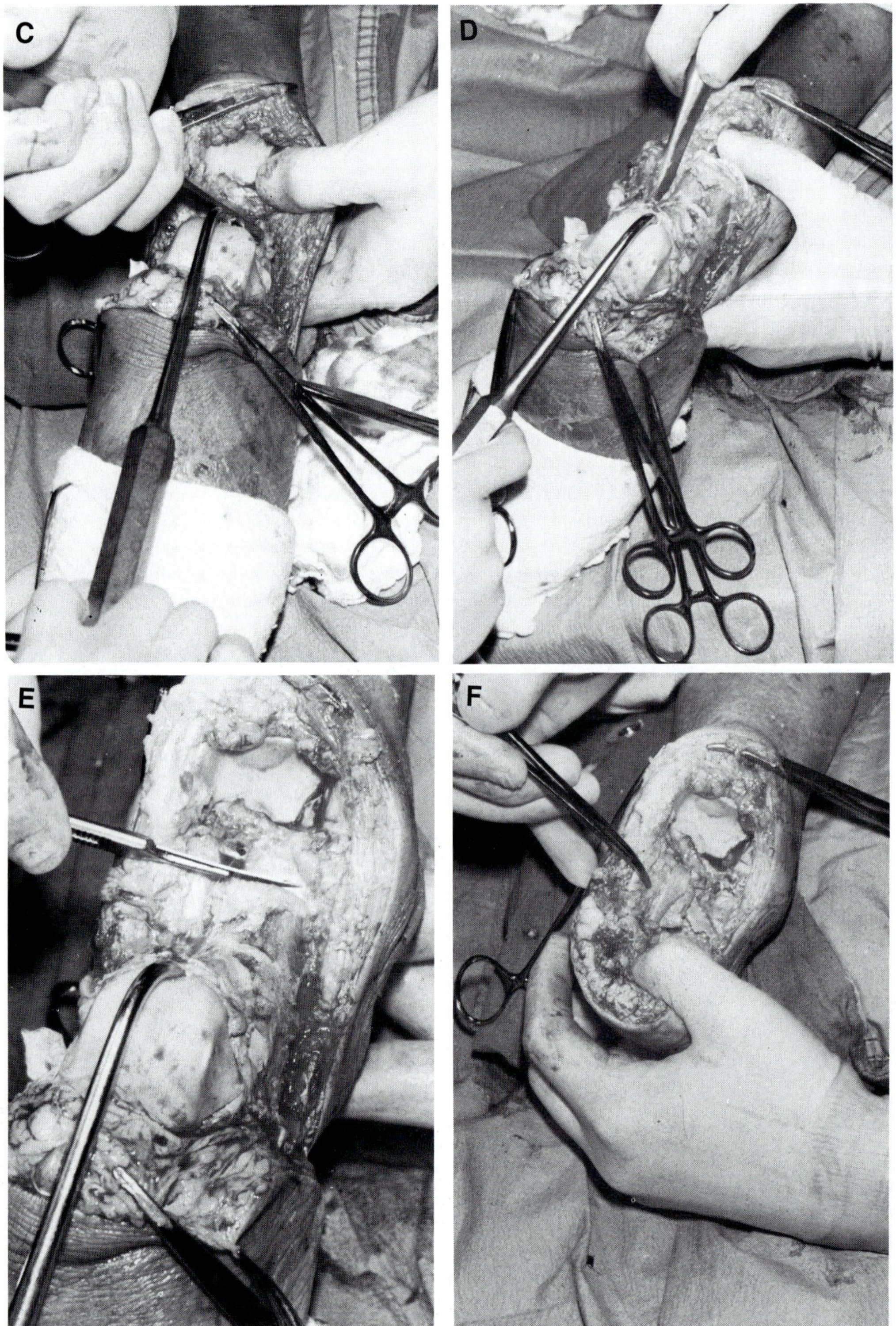

FIG 23–26. (cont.).

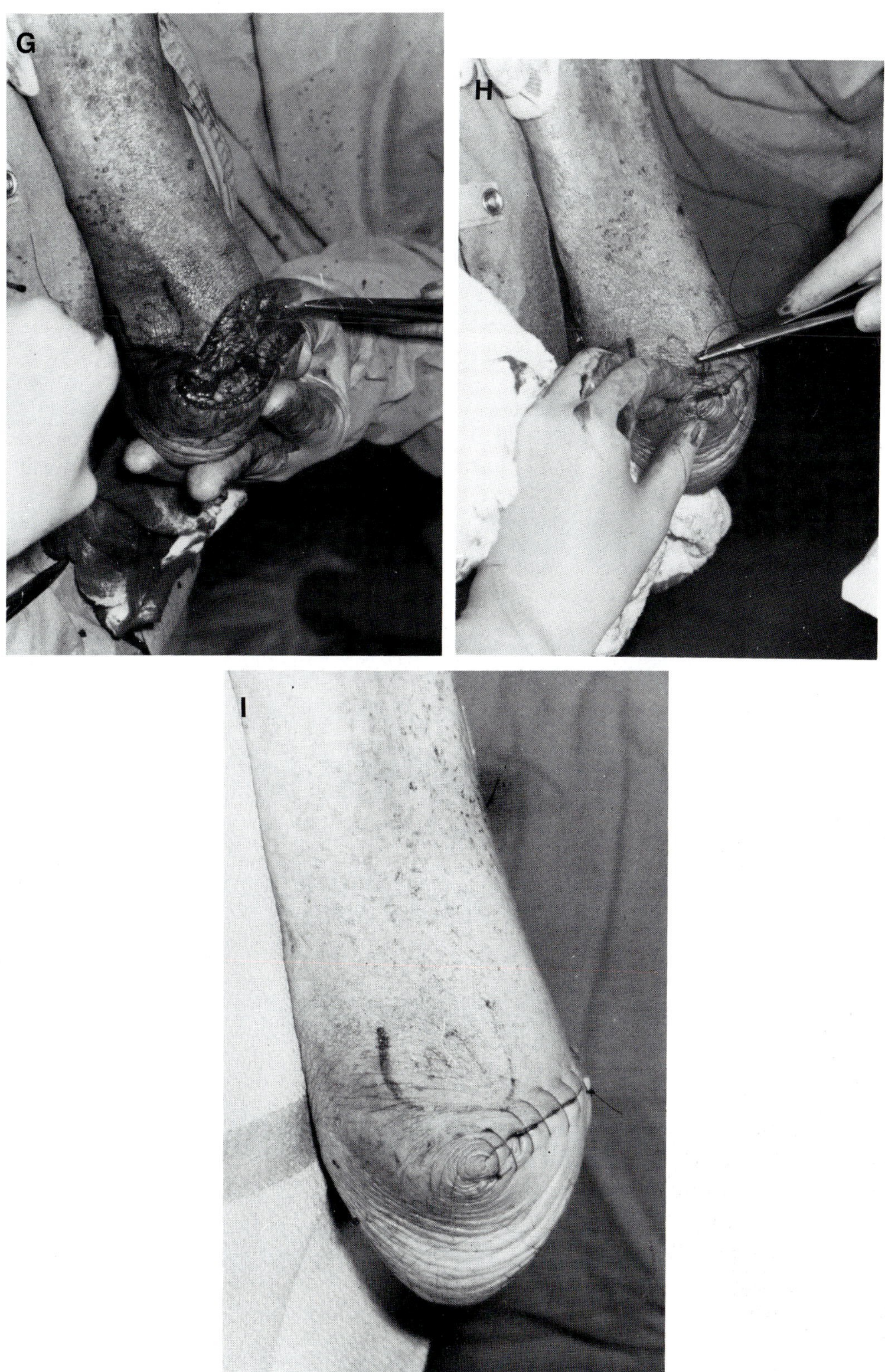

FIG 23–26. (cont.).

the operation, as was well described by Syme. The bundle lies between the flexor hallucis longus and the flexor digitorum longus and can be accidentally severed. The guide is the flexor hallucis longus tendon because the bundle lies just behind it (Fig 23–26, F).

7. Once it is seen, blunt dissection is used, e.g., with a broad Key elevator, to separate the bone from the entire soft-tissue envelope.

8. A bone hook in the talus assists in the dissection by applying traction to the interface of bone and soft tissue as the calcaneus is dissected out (Fig 23–26, D).

9. *This is the second major danger point in the operation: the subcutaneous attachment of the Achilles tendon.* Penetrating or "buttonholing" through the skin at this point will usually doom the procedure and lead to failure of the Syme stump due to damage to the heel pad. The alternating use of sharp and blunt dissection with scalpel and periosteal elevator works best (Fig 23–26, D and E). (It is this portion of the procedure that is responsible for making the Syme amputation the most technically difficult foot amputation.)

10. The subperiosteal dissection alternates from above at the Achilles tendon and from the undersurface and sides of the calcaneus until the bone is free from the soft tissue. (This then leaves the hollow of the stump ready for final shaping and closure.) Avoid the bundle within the flap as demonstrated in (Fig 23–26, F) in order to not damage the blood supply to the heel pad.

11. The closure is done in three layers over a suction drain that is brought out proximally through a separate tiny stab wound. The plantar fascia is either sutured to the deep fascia over the anterior portion of the tibia, or it can be sutured through drill holes in the anterior edge of the tibial plafond. This is followed by a subcutaneous closure with inverted interrupted absorbable sutures.

12. The skin is closed with nylon sutures or staples.

13. A soft dressing is applied.

Aftercare

After 7 to 10 days, a cast may be applied to protect the stump. If the patient is diabetic, non–weight-bearing ambulation is maintained for 4 to 6 weeks. Earlier ambulation in the cast can sometimes be allowed in nondiabetics, depending on the progression of wound healing.

In traumatic or uninfected cases, the points from which the incisions originate are the midpoints of the two malleoli. Prior to performing the closure the malleoli are cut off flush with the level of the tibial plafond. Although some authors have recommended narrowing the flare of the tibial metaphysis, it is better to preserve the flare because it gives a wider base to the bulbous stump and because the flare is the main structure that holds the prosthesis on and keeps it from slipping up and down (Fig 23–27). It is not necessary to remove the cartilage from the distal end of the tibia. If the pad appears to be too mobile at the time of closure, additional tissue should be resected from the distal (plantar) edge of the heel pad and the pad sutured to the bone.

In a two-stage procedure done for infected cases, the second stage is performed about 6 weeks after the initial amputation, provided that satisfactory healing has occurred. At the second stage, the "dog-ears" of soft tissue are removed both medially and laterally and the malleoli resected through these elliptical incisions (Fig 23–28). If the pad is excessively mobile at this stage, correction is obtained by taking larger wedges of soft tissue. It is usually not necessary to suture the pad to the bone at this time, although it can be done.

The reported success rate of Syme amputations has varied from 50% to 90%.[15–17] At this time, most centers report about a 70% success rate for healing of Syme amputations in diabetic and dysvascular patients. The vast majority of failures in this population occur *early* as the result of failure to achieve primary wound healing, usually due to vascular insufficiency of the heel pad, which is supplied by branches of the posterior tibial artery (Fig 23–29).

Late failure of the Syme amputation is usually due to progression of peripheral vascular disease that results in gangrenous changes of the entire lower-limb segment rather than complications inherent within the Syme stump. Occasionally, mobility of the stump together with soft-tissue shrinkage can lead to pressure areas over the residual distal and of the fibula (Fig 23–30). The treatment is resection of the fibula more proximally and in a diabetic, excision of the ulcer as well, with care

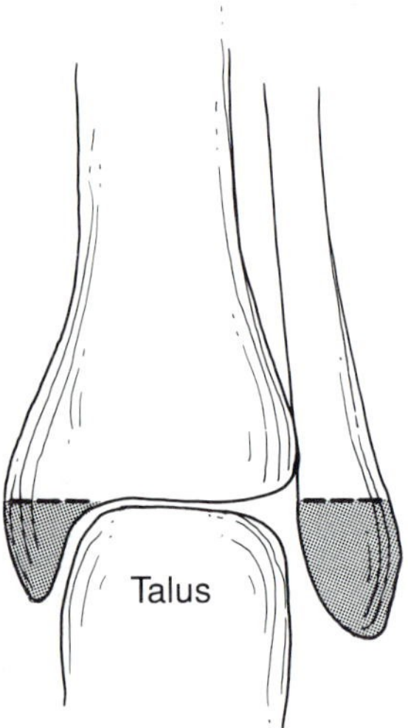

FIG 23–27.
Drawing of the bone cuts for a Syme amputation.

taken to resect enough bone in either case to relieve pressure and tension on the skin.

Prosthetic fitting of the Syme stump requires an experienced prosthetist. The challenge lies in the fact that a snug fit is required but the wide, bulbous end of the stump must pass through a very narrow portion of the prosthesis corresponding to the width of the distal end of the tibia. This fitting problem has been handled in a number of different ways, including placing a hinged window in the prosthesis, placing a wraparound filler above the bulb (Fig 23–31), or using an elastic double-wall construction for the distal part of the prosthesis. Most prostheses are fit with a "SACH" (solid-ankle cushion-heel) heel that aids gait. A minor disadvantage and the only drawback of the Syme amputation vs. a below-knee amputation is that the cosmesis of a Syme stump is poorer due to the wide "ankle" portion of the prosthesis.

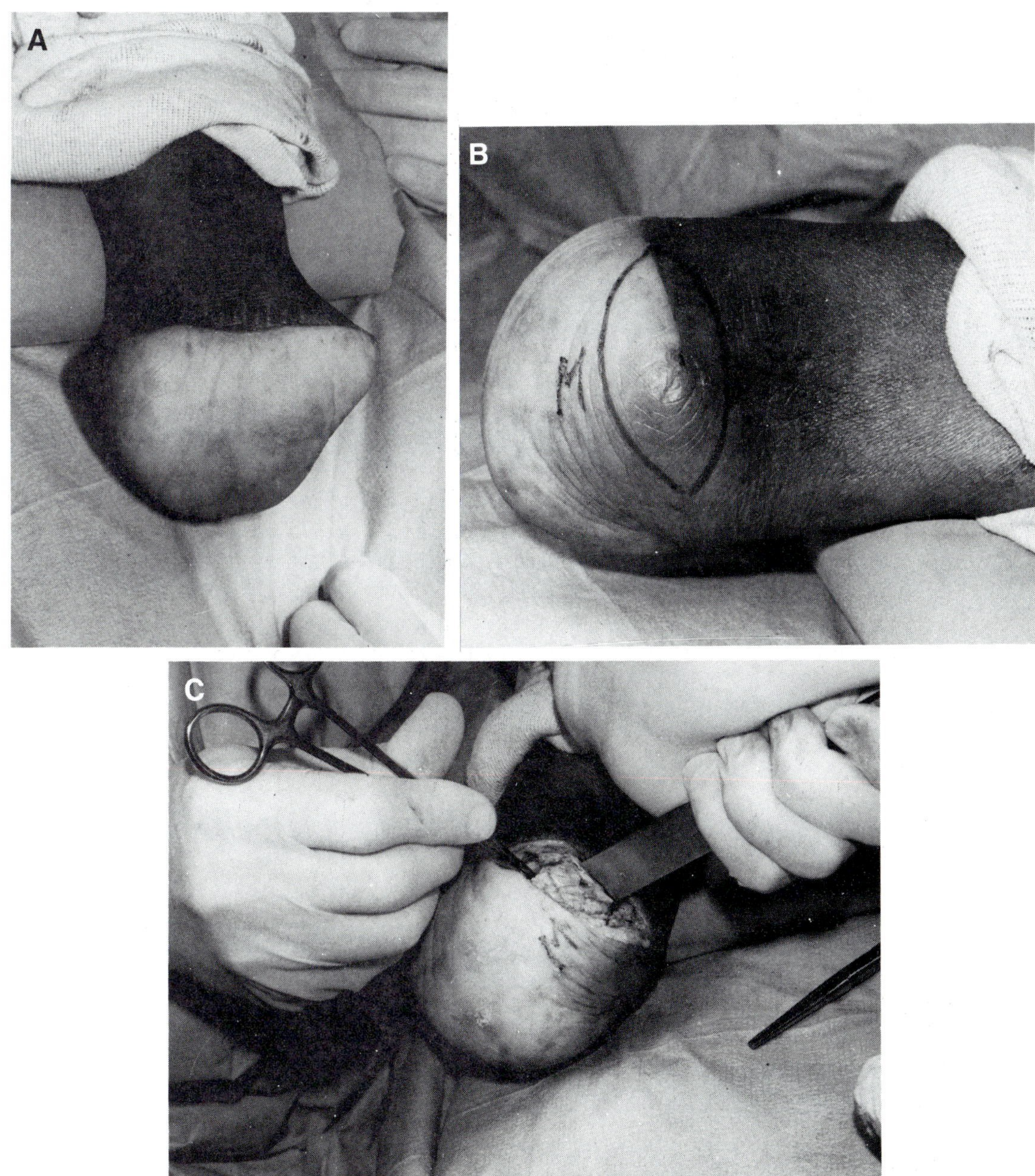

FIG 23–28.
A–F, technique for a second-stage Syme amputation. **A,** note medial and lateral "dog ears." **B,** these excised with an ellipse of skin and soft tissue. **C** and **D,** the malleoli are trimmed with osteotomes. **E,** deep soft tissue closure stabilizes pad. **F,** skin closure. *(Continued.)*

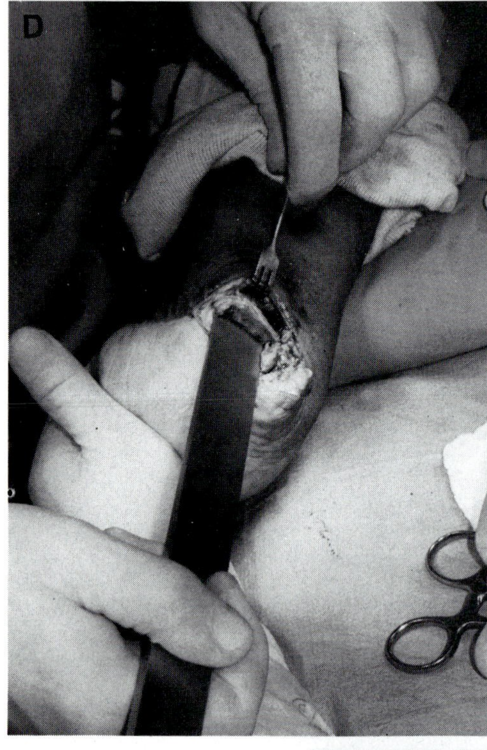

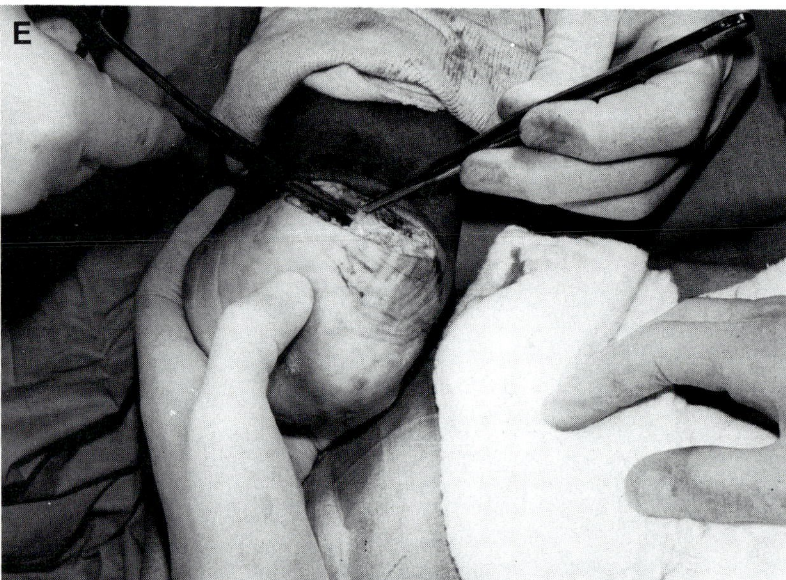

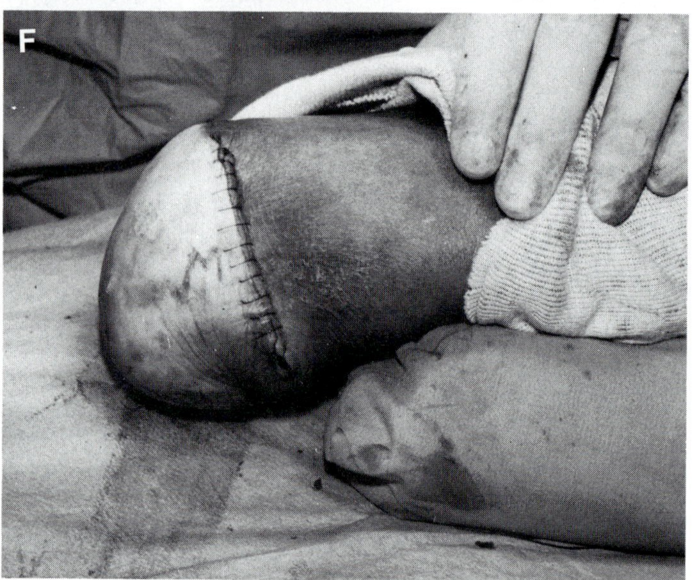

FIG 23–28. (cont.).

However, in every other way, the Syme prosthesis is preferable to a below-knee amputation. The Syme stump is partially end bearing, as noted above, and has fewer problems with skin breakdown over the proximal portion of the leg, even in diabetics. The mechanical advantage of a full lower-leg segment is enormous and gives great leverage to the quadriceps. Even more importantly most patients with Syme amputations need little or no prosthetic training since functionally the Syme procedure is a partial foot amputation and prosthetic walking is similar to the use of a cast, which most of the patients have used previously. The Syme amputation is superior in function to more proximal procedures such as below- and above-knee amputations because it has lower energy cost (oxygen consumption per meter) and allows higher velocity and stride length.[19]

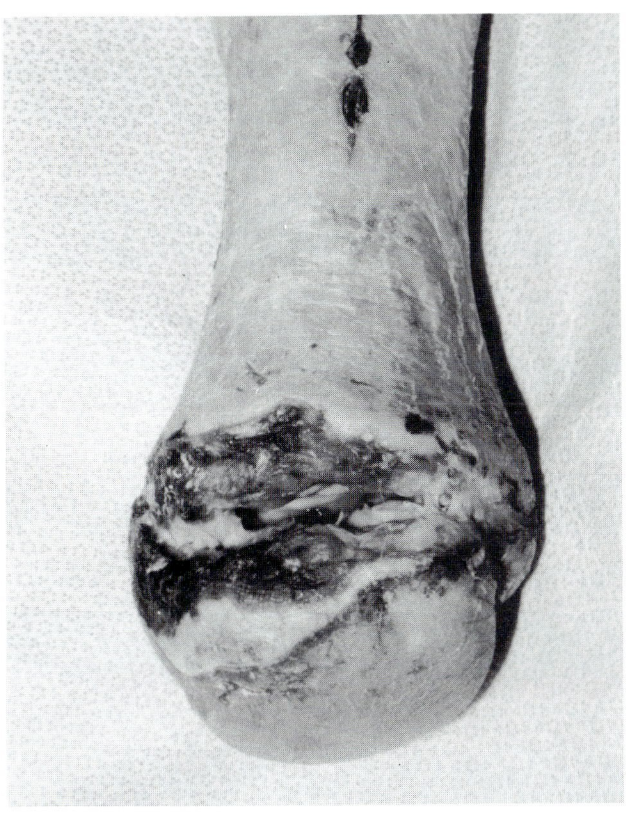

FIG 23–29.
Failed Syme amputation due to early gangrene and failure of the soft tissue to heal. This was revised to a below-knee amputation.

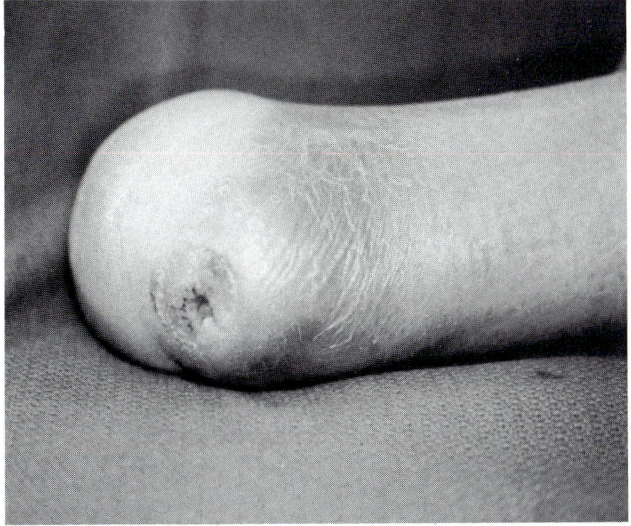

FIG 23–30.
Ulceration over the distal portion of the fibula due to stump mobility 6 years after a Syme amputation. The ulcer healed after resection of the bony prominence.

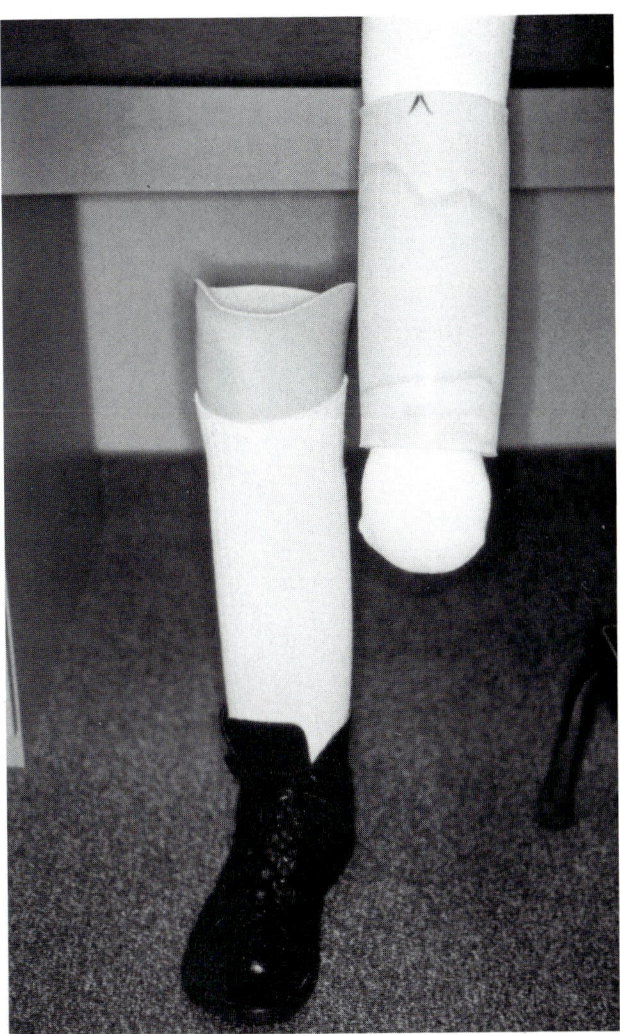

FIG 23–31.
One type of Syme prosthesis using a wraparound Plastazote sleeve for the narrow part of the leg above the distal bulb.

Pitfalls and Complications

The most common complication of the Syme procedure in diabetic and dysvascular patients is a failure of healing. Some of these cannot be prevented if the goal of salvaging as much of the limb as possible is to be pursued. However, the key to keeping a low incidence of this complication is the vascular evaluation of the patient both preoperatively and at the time of surgery. In the latter case, if the wound edges do not bleed adequately once the disarticulation is completed, it is usually best to proceed to an amputation at a more proximal level.

The second most common problem with this procedure is hypermobility of the stump. As noted above, this is corrected through resection of soft tissue and su-

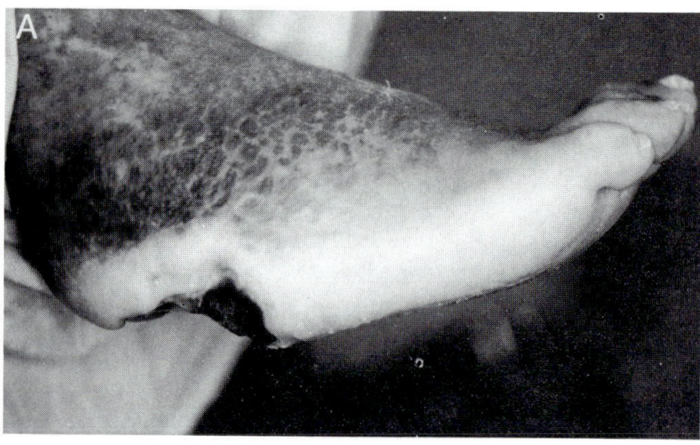

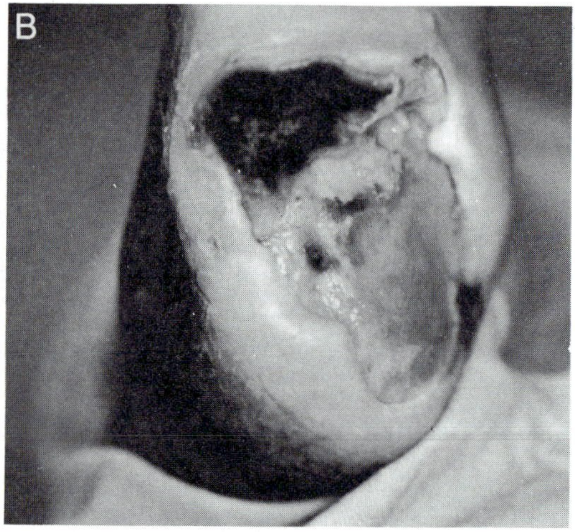

FIG 23–32.
A and **B,** this patient has the absolute contraindication for a Syme amputation, i.e., soft-tissue breakdown over the heel.

turing of the heel pad to drill holes in the distal end of the tibia.

In Syme amputations done for trauma, there are a moderate number of failures due to pain of two kinds. The first cause is neuroma formation at or above the level of the ankle joint, where the major nerves have been transected. Selective injection is helpful in diagnosis prior to surgical excision or burying of the neuromas. The second cause is recalcitrant heel pain, seen in patients who have sustained crushing trauma to the heel and hindfoot at the time of the original accident, most of which are industrial in nature. These frequently need to be revised to a long below-knee amputation.

The absolute contraindication to the use of a Syme amputation is the lack of an intact and viable heel pad. Patients with ulceration or even small gangrenous spots

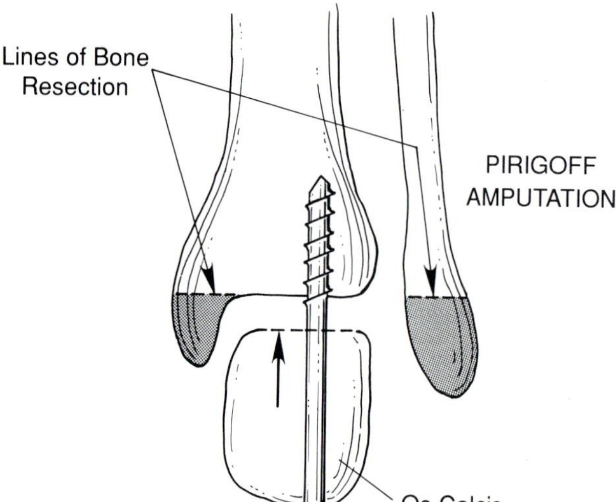

FIG 23–33.
Technique for a Pirigoff amputation.

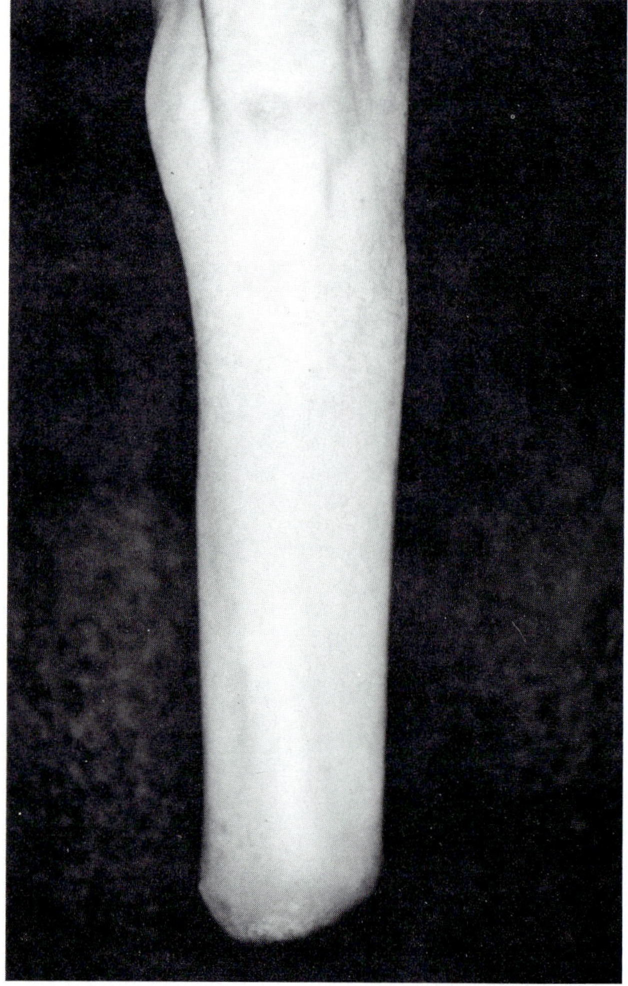

FIG 23–34.
A long below-knee amputation has mechanical advantages and is frequently possible when done for foot pathology that does not extend above the ankle.

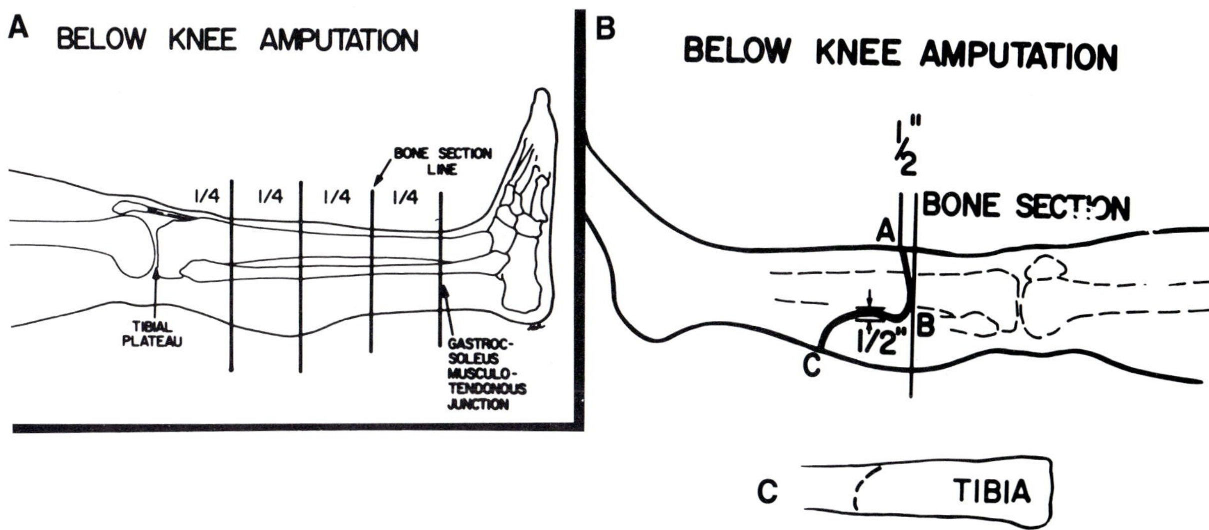

FIG 23–35.
Technique for below-knee amputation. **A,** the leg is divided into fourths from the knee joint to the musculotendinous junction of the triceps surae with a surgical towel. **B,** the long posterior flap is not square, which produces dog-ears, but oval in cross section by making it curve anteriorly in its midportion. Point *B* is proximal to *A* to produce a tapered stump. **C,** beveled cut on the tibia.

on the heel are not candidates for this procedure and should have a long below-knee amputation instead (Fig 23–32).

The Pirigoff amputation is a variation on the Syme procedure in which varying amounts of the tubercle of the calcaneus are preserved and then internally fixed to the distal cut end of the tibia (Fig 23–33). Longer soft-tissue flaps are required. The advantage of this operation is its longer length since the Syme procedure does result in some mild shortening that must be accommodated in the prosthesis. The thought of some surgeons is that it is technically easier since the Achilles tendon does not have to be dissected off of the calcaneus. On the other hand, fixation of the calcaneal tubercle to the distal end of the tibia is not without its own technical difficulties; moreover, symptomatic nonunions can be created and pose further problems.

Below-Knee Amputations

Below-knee amputations are sometimes the necessary treatment when foot salvage amputations fail. When a below-knee amputation is done for foot pathology, consideration should be given to the level of the below-knee resection. Whenever allowed by the vascularity of the limb, the below-knee amputation should be done as distally as possible. This usually equates to the level of the musculotendinous junction of most of the leg muscles. The longer stump has the same advantages of the long stump of the Syme amputation. At times, the only reason that a Syme procedure cannot be performed is a concomitant lesion at the level of the heel; this is the ideal patient for a long below-knee amputation (Fig 23–34).

The amputation stump can be closed with either a longer posterior flap or side-to-side flaps.[10] Proper shaping of the flaps for a posterior flap closure allows the surgeon to make an amputation that is tapered. This allows earlier prosthetic fitting since less shrinkage of the stump is necessary. The key is rounding the flaps; a square posterior flap leads to a stump with larger dog-ears that fits poorly within a temporary prosthesis (Fig 23–35).

While amputation of the foot is an unfortunate necessity for some of our patients, attention to detail, both in diagnostic evaluation and in surgical technique, improves our ability to successfully assist our patients in this major step toward rehabilitation of function and ambulation.

REFERENCES

1. Anderson L, Westin GW, Oppenheim WL: Syme amputation in children: indications, results, and long-term follow-up, *J Pediatr Orthop* 4:550–554, 1984.
2. Brodsky JW, Chambers RB: Effect of tourniquet use on amputation healing in diabetic and dysvascular patients, *Perspect Orthop Surg* 2:71–76, 1991.
3. Due TM, Jacobs RL: Molded foot orthosis after great toe medial ray amputation in diabetic feet, *Foot Ankle* 3:150–152, 1985.
4. Fergusson CM, Morrison JD, Kenwright J: Leg-length

inequality in children treated by Syme's amputation, *J Bone Joint Surg Br* 69:433–436, 1987.

5. Herring JA, Barnhill B, Gaffney C: Syme amputation, *J Bone Joint Surg [Am]* 68:573–578, 1986.
6. Hodge MJ, Peters TG, Efird WG: Amputation of the distal portion of the foot, *South Med J* 82:1138–1142, 1989.
7. Jacobs RL: The diabetic foot. In Johns MH, editor: *Disorders of the foot and ankle*, Philadelphia, 1991, WB Saunders, pp 1908–1936.
8. Jacobsen ST, Crawford AH, Millar EA, et al: The Syme amputation in patients with congenital pseudarthrosis of the tibia, *J Bone Joint Surg [Am]* 65:533–537, 1983.
9. Jany RS, Burkus JK: Long-term follow-up of Syme amputations for peripheral vascular disease associated with diabetes mellitus, *Foot Ankle* 9:107–110, 1988.
10. Kwong *Foot Ankle* 81–84.
11. Larrson U, Andersson GBJ: Partial amputation of the foot for diabetic or arteriosclerotic gangrene, *J Bone Joint Surg [Br]* 60:126–130, 1978.
12. Moore WS: Determination of amputation level measurement of skin blood flow with xenon (Xe133), *Arch Surg* 107:798, 1973.
13. Oishi CS, Fronek A, Golbranson FL: The role of noninvasive vascular studies in determining levels of amputation, *J Bone Joint Surg [Am]* 70:1520–1530, 1988.
14. Quill GE, Myerson MS: Clinical, radiographic, and pedobarographic analysis of the foot after hallux amputation, American Association of Orthopaedic Surgeons 58th annual meeting, Anaheim, Calif, March 1991.
15. Wagner FW: The dysvascular foot: a system for diagnosis and treatment, *Foot Ankle* 2:64–122, 1981.
16. Wagner FW Jr: Amputations of the foot and ankle: current status, *Clin Orthop* 122:62–69, 1977.
17. Wagner FW Jr: The diabetic foot and amputations of the foot. In Mann RA, editor: *Surgery of the foot*, ed 5, St Louis, 1986, Mosby–Year Book, pp 421–455.
18. Waters RL, Perry J, Antonelli D, et al: Energy cost of walking of amputees: the influence of level of amputation, *J Bone Joint Surg [Am]* 56:42–46, 1976.
19. Wyss CR, Harrington RM, Burgess EM, et al: Transcutaneous oxygen tension as a predictor of success after an amputation, *J Bone Joint Surg [Am]* 70:203–208, 1988.

Additional Readings

Burgess EM, Marsden FW: Major lower extremity amputation following arterial reconstruction, *Arch Surg* 108:655, 1974.

Francis H III, Roberts JR, et al: The Syme amputation: success in elderly diabetic patients with palpable ankle pulses, *J Vasc Surg* 12:237–240, 1990.

Goldner M: The fate of the second leg in diabetic amputees, *Diabetes* 9:100, 1960.

Harris RI: Syme's amputation, *J Bone Joint Surg [Br]* 38:614–632, 1956.

Harris WR, Silversten EA: Partial amputations of the foot: a follow-up study, *Can J Surg* 7:6, 1964.

Kritter AE: A technique for salvage of the infected diabetic gangrenous foot, *Orthop Clin North Am* 4:21, 1973.

McElwain JP, Hunter GA, English E: Syme's amputation in adults: a long-term review, *Can J Surg* 28:203–205, 1985.

McKittrick LS, McKittrick JB, Risley TS: Transmetatarsal amputation for infection of gangrene in patients with diabetes mellitus, *Ann Surg* 130:826, 1949.

Nakhgevany KB, Rhoads JE: Ankle-level amputation, *Surgery* 95(5):549–552, 1984.

Scher KS, Steele FJ: The septic foot in patients with diabetes, *Surgery* 104:661–665, 1988.

Spittler AW, Brenner JJ, Payne JW: Syme amputation performed in two stages, *J Bone Joint Surg [Am]* 36:37, 1954.

CHAPTER

24

Tumors and Metabolic Diseases of the Foot

James O. Johnston, M.D.

Tumorous conditions of the soft tissues and bones of the foot

General considerations and the staging process
- History and physical examination
- Radiographic evaluation
- Diagnostic studies
- Tumor classification

Benign tumors of the soft tissues
- Fibroma
- Keloid
- Plantar fibromatosis
- Dermatofibrosarcoma protuberans
- Neurilemoma
- Neurofibroma
- Lipoma
- Ganglion
- Giant-cell tumor of the tendon sheath
- Pigmented villonodular synovitis
- Vascular tumor
- Glomus tumor
- Ectopic ossification

Malignant tumors of soft tissue
- Fibrosarcoma
- Synovial cell sarcoma
- Kaposi sarcoma (angiosarcoma)
- Malignant melanoma

Benign tumors and cysts of bone
- Solitary bone cysts
- Epidermoid cyst
- Aneurysmal bone cyst
- Giant-cell tumor
- Osteochondroma
- Bone spur
- Subungual exostosis
- Osteoid osteoma
- Osteoblastoma
- Enchondroma, periosteal chondroma, and juxtacortical chondroma
- Chondroblastoma
- Fibroma of bone
- Sarcoidosis
- Melorheostosis
- Tarsoepiphyseal aclasis
- Stippled epiphysis
- Bone islands

Malignant tumors of bone
- Osteosarcoma
- Ewing's sarcoma
- Chondrosarcoma
- Fibrosarcoma
- Metastatic tumors to the foot

Metabolic bone disease

Osteoporosis
Osteomalacia
Paget disease
Gout
Acromegaly
Hypercholesterolemia

The osteochondroses

Kohler's disease
Freiberg's infraction
Sever's disease
Avascular necrosis of the talus

TUMOROUS CONDITIONS OF THE SOFT TISSUES AND BONES OF THE FOOT

In this discussion of tumor and tumorlike conditions occurring in the foot and ankle area, it should first be stated that malignant tumors of the foot (and incidentally of the hand) are rare conditions and that soft-tissue tumors are more common. Therefore when one is uncertain whether a lesion is benign or malignant, it is better to assume the benign condition and treat accordingly rather than perform an unnecessary amputation for a pseudomalignant condition.

Generally most of the neoplastic conditions occurring in the foot are seen more typically in other parts of the body and are not specific problems of the foot. There is, however, an important difference in clinical prognostication of like tumors located in different parts of the body. For example, when one considers cartilaginous tumors in the pelvis or proximal large bones of the extremity, one must be extremely cautious because of the known potential of these tumors for malignancy and a tendency to metastasize. By contrast, the same type of cartilaginous tumor located in the foot is almost always benign. This has a direct bearing on treatment: cartilaginous tumors in the proximal part of the body should be aggressively resected, whereas smaller lesions in the hand or foot can usually be handled by conservative resection. The giant-cell tumor is another good example of a tumor with variable prognosis depending on its location. Surgical treatment for the giant-cell tumor can therefore also vary.

General Considerations and the Staging Process

When a surgeon is faced with the clinical problem of a tumorous process in the foot and ankle area, he must first set upon a logical course of diagnostic or staging studies that will lead to an accurate diagnosis and precise anatomic location of the tumor. Then, based on this preoperative study, a course of treatment will follow in proper fashion.

History and Physical Examination

Even today with all our modern diagnostic modalities, there is still an important place for a careful history and physical examination. The history should reveal important information regarding the onset of the problem and related etiologic factors such as occupational and sports activities. Look for a history of prior illness that might result in local manifestations in the foot. The stress fracture seen in Figure 24–42 is a classic example of a bone-forming lesion in a metatarsal bone that could be interpreted as a tumor until the history reveals the patient to be a cross-country runner working out early in the season. Likewise, the surfer's knobs seen in Figure 24–2 would have escaped diagnosis without a careful history.

Still important as well is the physical examination of the foot. Look for color changes in the overlying skin such as the purplish discoloration of a cavernous hemangioma or a Kaposi's sarcoma. Look for inflammatory changes that would suggest infection instead of a neoplasm. Feel for tenderness and the degree of firmness in a tumor mass. A low-grade tumor such as a fibroma or chondroma will be firm and nontender, whereas a high-grade lesion such as Ewing's sarcoma will be soft and more tender to touch.

As a foot surgeon looking at an isolated lesion, the complete staging process should include the examination of other body parts such as the hand and chest to look for systemic manifestations of a more generalized disease process such as one would see in polyostotic fibrous dysplasia or in malignant tumors of the foot that have a high risk factor for metastatic lung disease.

Radiographic Evaluation

Next in order for a proper staging workup would be a routine radiographic examination of the involved part based on the physical findings. This simple and inexpensive examination will shed light as to the tissue of origin and its anatomic location. Even with soft-tissue tumors, the standard radiograph may reveal calcific patterns characteristic of lesions such as the hemangioma, soft-tissue chondroma, or synovial cell sarcoma. In most cases, further imaging studies will not be needed. However, in certain situations, better detail may be necessary for precise localization of a lesion prior to a surgical approach for either a biopsy or excision.

Computed tomography (CT) was the first major breakthrough in imaging technology that gave the clinician a transverse image of the extremity in sequential planes. This allows for exact localization of small bone lesions, especially in cortical locations. The osteoid osteoma is the typical situation where CT is still the best imaging study for diagnosis and exact localization purposes. CT is the study of choice in any situation where cortical detail or calcification in soft tissue is of importance for diagnostic reasons.

In most situations the newer magnetic resonance imaging (MRI) studies have surpassed the CT examination, especially in the case of soft-tissue detail. MRI not only affords a transaxial view of the extremity but also allows for coronal and sagittal views as well. The T1-weighted image is ideal for the marginal determinations of intramedullary bone lesions, whereas the T2-weighted image is ideal for defining the margin of a soft-tissue tumor. When a surgical resection with safe oncologic margins is considered MRI is extremely valuable in imaging the relation of the tumor margin to nearby vessels, nerves, and tendons. Prior to the MRI, arteriograms were used for this purpose. Presently, arteriograms are rarely indicated when staging tumors except perhaps for vascular tumors such as atrioventricular (AV) malformations.

Another imaging study that is helpful, especially for bone tumors, is the isotope bone scan. This is still a good survey study for the entire skeleton when looking for multicentric bone involvement such as metastatic conditions. The isotope study will often help differentiate between a benign dysplastic process such as a bone island and the painful osteoid osteoma that is always hot as seen with an isotope scan.

Diagnostic Studies

Upon completion of the noninvasive staging studies, it is frequently necessary to perform a tissue biopsy to obtain a histologic diagnosis. In the case of the foot where most lesions are small and benign, a simple excisional biopsy is the best approach. However, if one suspects a malignant condition, in a larger lesion it is best to perform either a needle biopsy or a small incisional biopsy. In the latter situation, one must be careful to not contaminate uninvolved surrounding compartments or vital and adjacent neurovascular structures that could eliminate the possibility of a limb salvage reconstruction.

Tumor Classification

With all the above information, one is then prepared to classify the tumor by the Enneking staging system that has been adopted by the American Musculoskeletal Tumor Society for both bone and soft-tissue sarcomas. This is a very simple system designed for surgeons that looks at two factors only: the histologic-biologic behavior of the tumor and its anatomic orientation to surrounding structures. Stage I refers to low-grade sarcomas such as a low-grade chondrosarcoma. Stage II includes high-grade sarcomas such as the typical osteosarcoma, and Stage III is used for metastatic tumors to regional lymph nodes or the lung. Stage A refers to a sarcoma located in a bony or fascial compartment as defined by CT or MRI studies, whereas a stage B lesion refers to an extracompartmental sarcoma such as one sees typically in the midfoot and hindfoot areas where tumors are frequently adjacent to neurovascular and tendinous structures passing through this portion of the foot. The Ewing's sarcoma seen in Figure 24–44 would be staged as a II-B lesion.

The purpose of a staging system is to aid the surgeon in the decision process concerning the choice of amputation vs. limb salvage. In the situation of the foot, most malignant tumors are seen in the midfoot and hindfoot areas, are extracompartmental, and usually require a below-knee amputation in order to obtain an oncologically acceptable wide margin.

Benign Tumors of the Soft Tissues

Fibroma

Fibromas are benign soft-tissue lesions seen in all parts of the body, in soft tissue and in bone. They are well-localized lesions in most cases with well-defined borders. Fibromas are frequently subcutaneous in location and firm to palpation. They grow very slowly and are usually asymptomatic and nontender to palpation.

Figure 24–1 shows a typical, firm, well-circumscribed subcutaneous fibroma resected from the tarsal sinus area of the foot. The lesion can be cut like a piece of hard rubber, and the exposed surfaces are white with the gross appearance of a cut Achilles tendon.

Microscopically this tumor is composed of well-differentiated fibroblasts producing large amounts of dense collagen fiber that contributes to its physical characteristics.

A fibroma can be easily resected, and there is very little chance of local recurrence.

Figure 24–2 shows a patient with surfer's knobs. These fibromatous lesions are found on the dorsum of the foot as the result of repeated physical trauma to this area (e.g., many hours spent on a surfboard).

Keloid

Keloid is the clinical name given to dense hypertrophic dermal fibrous tissue that forms in excess as a response to skin lacerations or surgical incisions. Keloids are familial and are firmly fixed in the genetic makeup of fibroblasts all through the body. It is therefore difficult to avoid keloid formation in certain patients when making surgical wounds for reconstructive purposes.

To reduce the chance of a disfiguring or disabling scar, one should at least be aware of this potential be-

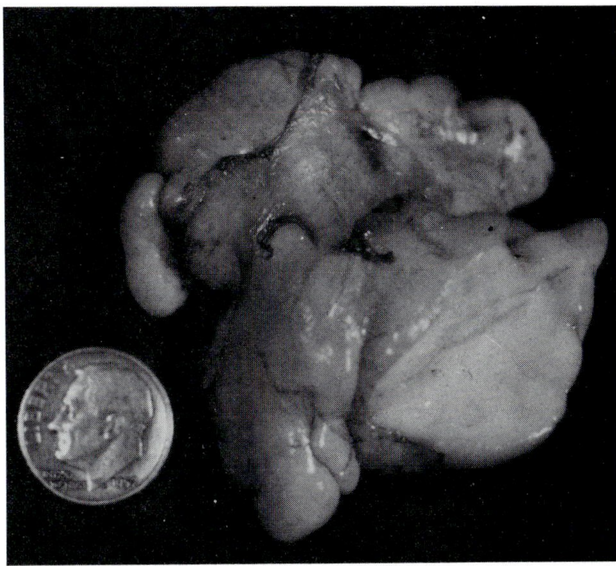

FIG 24–1.
Well-circumscribed firm subcutaneous fibroma removed from a foot.

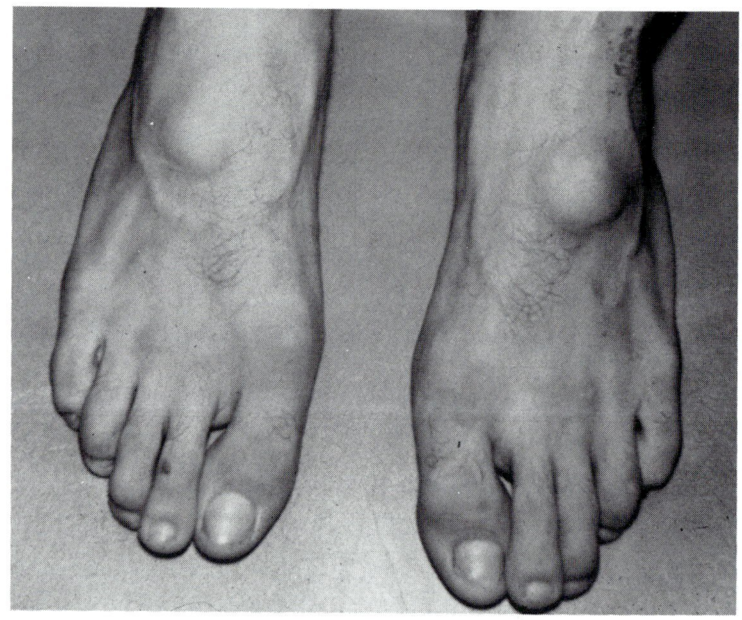

FIG 24–2.
Surfer's knobs.

fore performing surgery. It is well known that dark-skinned people are generally more prone to keloid formation whereas light-skinned races or individuals with hyperelastic skin rarely form keloids but instead tend to form flat scars that spread.

The best treatment for keloid formation is prevention if possible. For this reason it is best to make surgical incisions parallel with skin creases or skin lines (in the extremities, a transverse incision). It is also wise to use good subcutaneous closures and avoid surface stitches completely. Skin tapes left in place for several weeks and splinting of wounds near joints are helpful. The use of γ-irradiation or steroids to inhibit fibrosis is considered controversial and is probably best left in the hands of a plastic surgeon who has experience with these modalities.

Figure 24–72 is a classic picture of a keloid scar formed as the result of a longitudinal incision made along the heel cord and across the ankle joint.

Plantar Fibromatosis

Plantar fibromatosis is a locally aggressive idiopathic proliferative fasciitis of the plantar aponeurosis that is usually bilateral and frequently seen in children and young adults.[34] In older people it is often associated with Dupuytren's contracture of the palmar fascia of the hand. The basic microscopic pathology of Dupuytren's contracture and plantar fibromas is about the same. However, in children the microscopic picture is much more worrisome and can be misdiagnosed as a malignant fibrosarcoma. Figure 24–3 shows the typical nodularity of this fibroma in the long plantar ligament.

If the nodules are small and cause little trouble, they can be left alone. If they grow large and cause pain or pressure on an adjacent nerve, however, it is best to perform aggressive resection. Pedersen and Day[44] advised a longitudinal incision along the medial-plantar aspect of the first metatarsal proximally to the tarsal navicular. Skin flaps are developed to expose the fibroma and plantar fascia. The fibrotic lesion is aggressively ex-

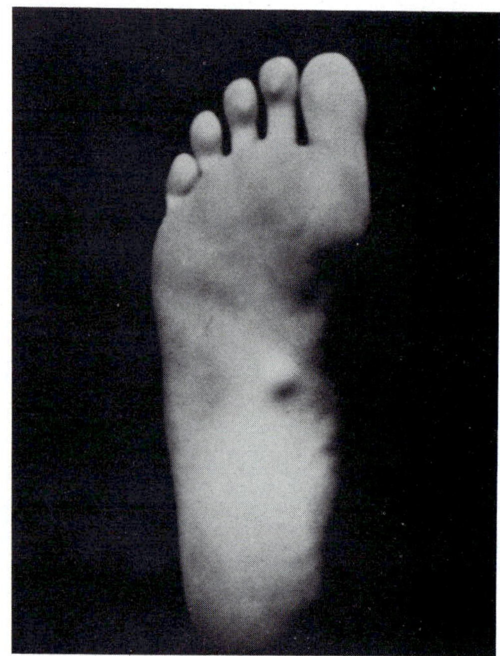

FIG 24–3.
Fibromatosis of the plantar fascia in an adolescent.

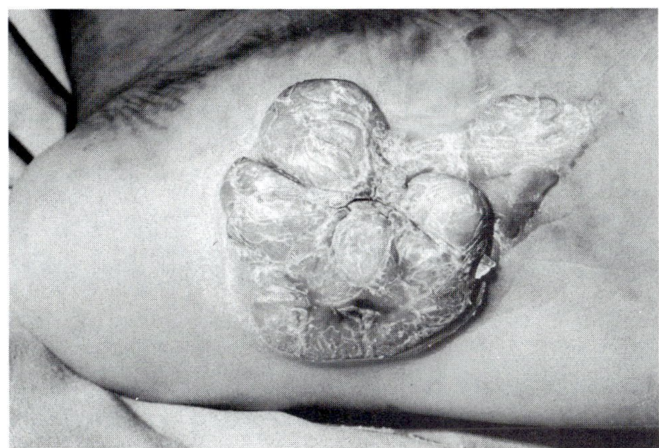

FIG 24–4.
Dermatofibrosarcoma seen on the plantar aspect of the heel of a young adult male.

cised, with removal of much of the normal-appearing adjacent plantar fascia. It is important to perform aggressive resection because of the high incidence of local recurrence when only the fibroma is removed. The skin flaps are then tacked down to prevent hematoma, and Hemovac suction tubes are placed beneath the skin as well. A firm compression dressing is also helpful in preventing hematoma formation.

Dermatofibrosarcoma Protuberans

Dermatofibrosarcoma protuberans is felt to be a fibrohistiocytic tumor of intermediate malignancy.[11] It is seen as a very slow-growing subcutaneous mass on the trunk of a young adult male patient. However, 20% will be found in the lower extremity such as the one seen in Figure 24–4 which had grown slowly over the past 5 years. The biologic and histologic behavior of this tumor lies halfway between the benign and malignant fibrous histiocytoma and for this reason has a 50% chance for local recurrence following simple resection, but very rarely does it metastasize to regional lymph nodes or the lungs. Because of the high local recurrence rate, it is advisable to perform a fairly wide resection initially, which in most cases at the foot level will require skin grafting. In the case illustrated here, it would be wise to consider a free vascularized myocutaneous graft.

Neurilemoma

The neurilemoma is a benign neurogenic tumor of nerve sheath origin that is well encapsulated, usually solitary, and found on the surface of a peripheral nerve. Figure 24–5 shows a typical lesion resected from the surface of the medial plantar nerve. This tumor is easy to resect and rarely causes damage to its nerve of origin because of its eccentric location. It rarely recurs or becomes malignant.

Neurofibroma

The most common neurogenic tumor is the neurofibroma. This tumor can be solitary (Fig 24–6) or multicentric and quite diffusely invasive, as in the plexiform

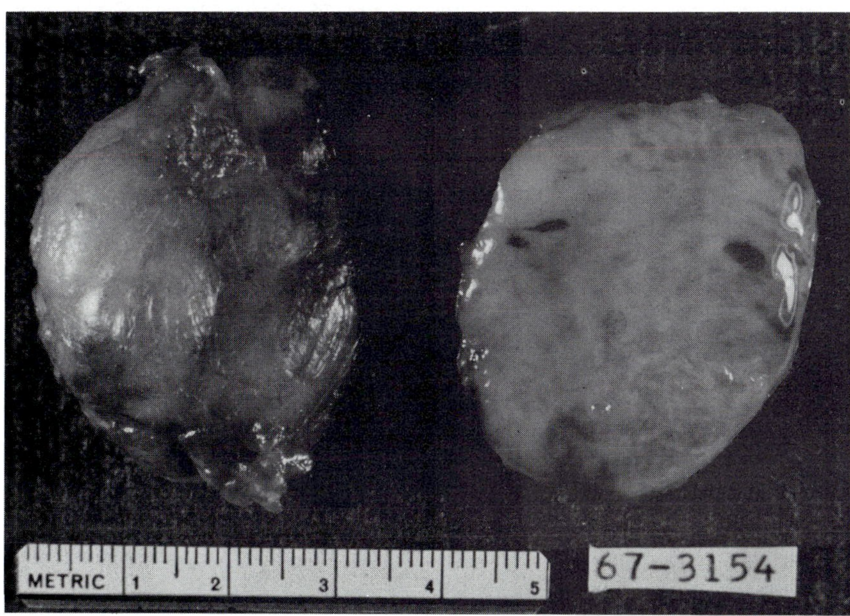

FIG 24–5.
Neurilemoma shelled off the surface of the medial plantar nerve.

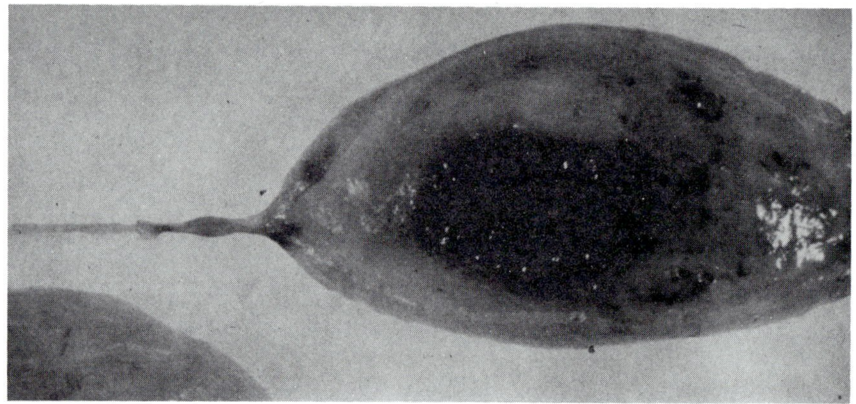

FIG 24–6.
Localized neurofibroma of a small peripheral nerve.

type seen in the dysplastic condition known as von Recklinghausen's disease (neurofibromatosis) with associated tan-pigmented café au lait spots on the skin. The neurofibroma is more disabling because of its central location in a peripheral nerve. As a result it interferes with nerve function, and if resected, the entire nerve is frequently removed with the tumor. A neurofibroma, by contrast with a neurilemoma, is more prone to become malignant. This usually occurs in larger more proximal nerves, however, and not in the hand or foot.

In *neurofibromatosis* many peripheral nerves are involved. Associated with the dysplastic condition, severe deformity of the subadjacent bones of the feet is not unusual (Fig 24–7). One may also find extensive soft-tissue hypertrophy and localized gigantism in neurofibromatosis.

Lipoma

In the extremities the subcutaneous lipoma is a common tumor. It can also be found in muscle bellies and, on rare occasion, in medullary bone. In the foot, however, lipomas are usually located just beneath the skin. These are soft nontender lesions that are asymptomatic. They are usually well encapsulated and easy to excise surgically, with very little chance for local recurrence or malignant transformation.

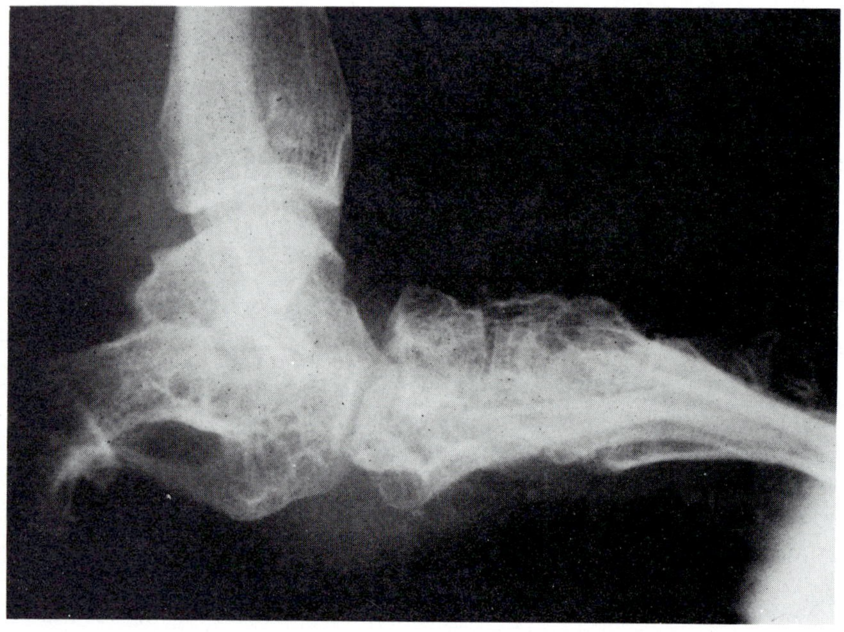

FIG 24–7.
Associated bone defect seen in a foot affected with neurofibromatosis.

Ganglion

Another common tumorous condition of the extremities is the ganglion cyst.[26] This lesion should not really be considered a tumor, mainly because it is not the product of proliferating cells. In fact, the ganglion is the product of mucoid cystic degeneration in the area of a dense collagen structure such as a joint capsule or thick collagenous tendon sheath. Ganglions are usually located in an area where such structures are under continuous physical stress, for example, around the wrist and ankle joints. With repeated activity across these areas, the collagen tissue undergoes mucoid degeneration with the formation of amorphous gelatinous material. If its point of origin is near the skin surface, as is usual around the ankle and dorsal aspect of the foot, the gelatinous material may form a firm subcutaneous nodule. In the case of a ganglion arising from a joint capsule, the cyst can rupture into the joint space and thus be converted to a synovial cyst filled with synovial fluid instead of gelatinous material.

Many small ganglions may appear spontaneously and grow gradually for a time and then rupture internally into subcutaneous tissues and be absorbed, without many symptoms or disability to the patient. If the cyst becomes unsightly or causes pain because of pressure against a shoe, the treating physician may elect to aspirate it and thus solve the immediate problem. However, there is a 70% chance of local recurrence with this conservative approach. If one wishes a more definitive cure, surgical excision is required. Then the surgeon must remove the entire cyst wall. Perhaps even more important, to prevent local recurrence the surgeon must excise most of the surrounding degenerative capsular or tendon sheath collagen tissue, which frequently contains small microscopic foci for potential additional lesions.

At times one will see a patient with multiple ganglion-like lesions involving multiple tendon sheaths across the dorsum of the ankle. In this case the diagnosis of a rheumatoid process should be strongly suspected and the appropriate studies begun to confirm the impression.

Giant-cell Tumor of the Tendon Sheath

Along with the ganglion cyst and lipoma, the so-called giant-cell tumor of the tendon sheath is a common tumor found subcutaneously in the hand and foot.[23] It has been named because of its common relations to tendon sheaths and tenosynovial tissues but can also be located in subcutaneous areas far removed from a synovial membrane. In this case it should probably be assigned a different name such as "benign fibrous histiocytoma."

These lesions are well circumscribed and relatively easy to resect.[33] They are considered by most surgeons to be a benign neoplastic process composed histologically of giant cells, reticulum cells, and cholesterol-laden histiocytes (foam cells) dispersed throughout a fairly dense fibrotic stroma. In the early stages these lesions take on a reddish-brown coloration because of the

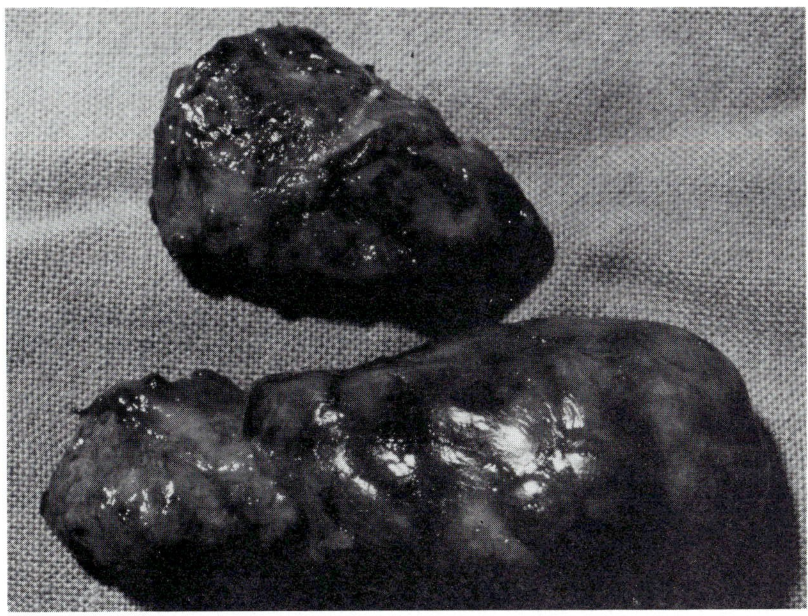

FIG 24–8.
Giant-cell tumor of a tendon sheath from the ankle area.

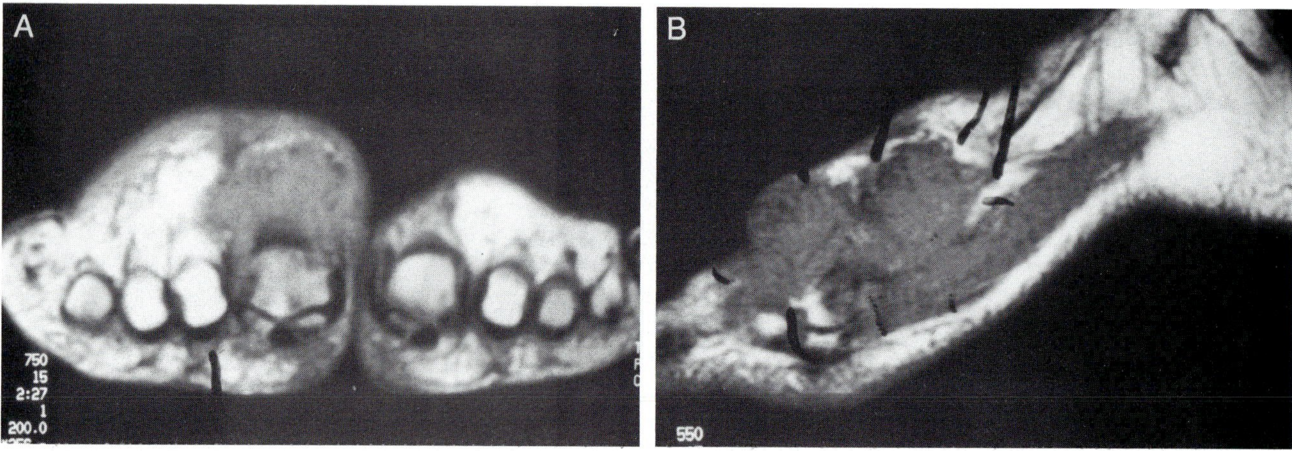

FIG 24–9.
A, MRI study of a giant-cell tumor of the tendon sheath in the transverse plane. **B,** MRI study of a giant-cell tumor of the tendon sheath in the sagittal plane.

large amount of hemosiderin found in the tissue. At this time they are usually growing in size and may be painful. As time passes, they tend to involute spontaneously and become more xanthomatous and fibrotic, which accounts for another pathologic name frequently assigned these lesions—xanthofibroma.

The giant-cell tumor of the tendon sheath can assume a considerable size around the ankle area and usually originates from a major tendon sheath such as the one seen in Figure 24–8 that measured 3 in. in length. This ankle lesion demonstrates the well-circumscribed and nodular appearance of the tumors, which may recur locally after resection but rarely if ever become malignant.

Another example of a large giant-cell tumor of the tendon sheath is seen by using MRI technology, which allows imaging in a transverse plane (Fig 24–9,A) as well as in a sagittal plane (Fig 24–9,B).

Pigmented Villonodular Synovitis

The same basic pathologic condition just described can also occur in subsynovial tissues of joints, and then the histology is identical to that of a giant-cell tumor of the tendon sheath. This condition usually occurs in the

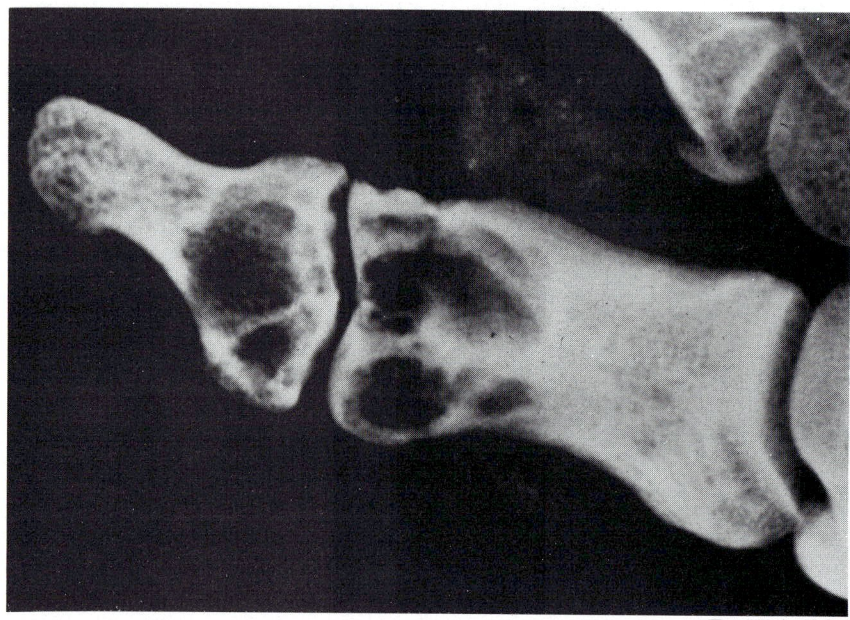

FIG 24–10.
Juxta-articular erosion in the interphalangeal joint of the great toe secondary to pigmented villonodular synovitis.

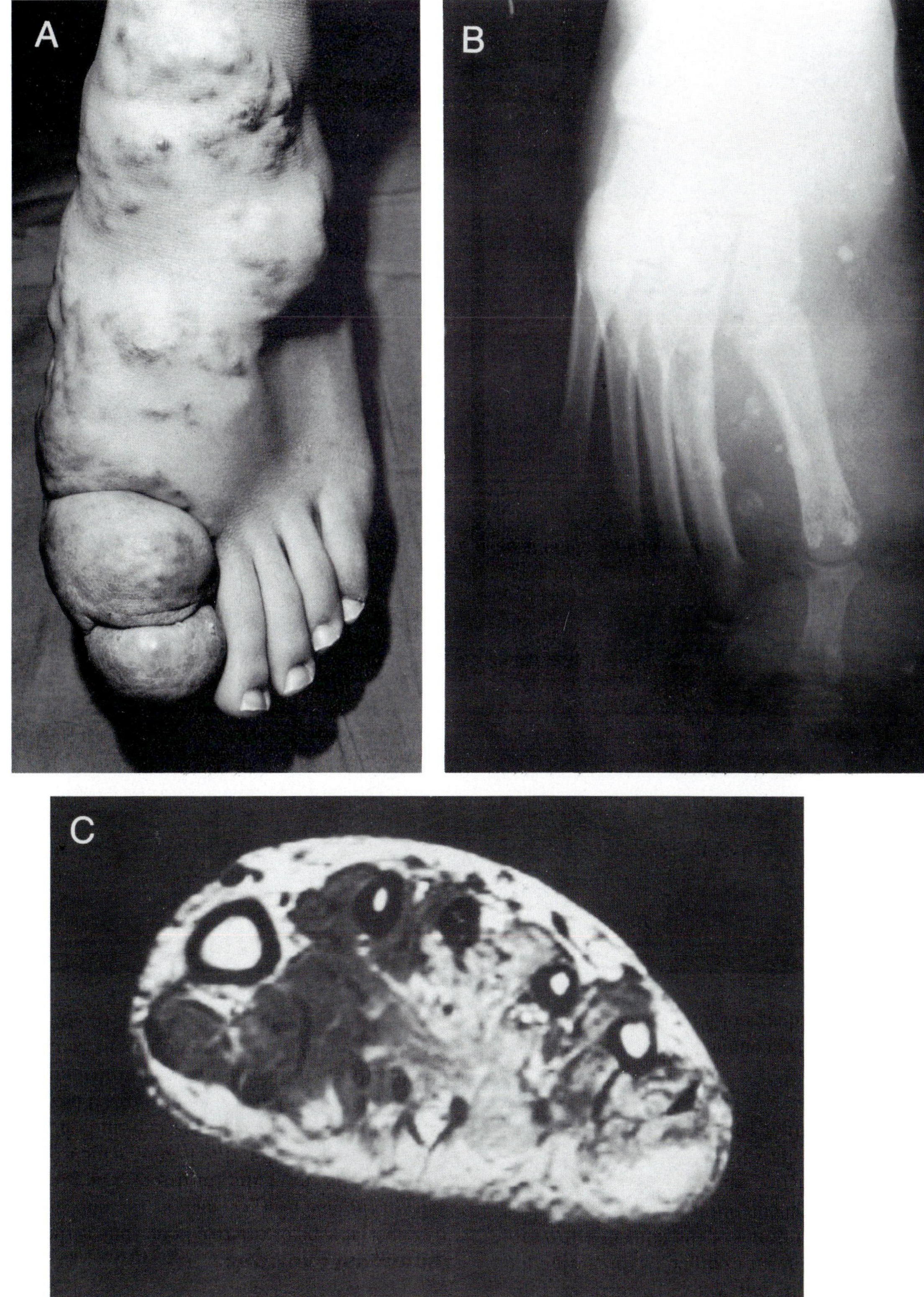

FIG 24–11.
A, large subcutaneous cavernous hemangioma of the foot. **B,** radiographic appearance with diagnostic calcific phleboliths. **C,** MRI study of a deep intramuscular hemangioma.

knee joint or the major joint of the lower extremity in young men as a monarticular form of hemorrhagic synovitis. The joint synovium has a characteristic brown discoloration and is thickened with a coarse villonodular pattern. The treatment for the benign process is to perform as complete a synovectomy as possible. Recurrences are not unusual, and occasionally low-dosage radiotherapy will be called for to combat multiple recurrences.

Sometimes these synovial lesions, and tenosynovial lesions as well, will invade adjacent bony structures (Fig 24–10).

Vascular Tumor

The most common vascular tumor seen in the extremity is the port wine capillary type of hemangioma.[25] These hamartomatous dysplastic lesions of a benign nature rarely cause clinical problems. They can result in localized erosive ulcerations that occasionally require surgical excision.

More extensive lesions of the cavernous type can present with large subcutaneous masses as seen illustrated in Figure 24–11,A. In Figure 24–11,B one sees the characteristic radiographic finding of many small spherical calcific phleboliths. In the case of deeper intramuscular hemangiomas, the tumor may not be visible on simple observation. In these cases MRI is of great value as seen in Figure 24–11,C. This is a diffuse dysplastic condition similar to neurofibromatosis insofar as it can cause subadjacent bony deformity and even disappearance of the bone (disappearing bone disease). Also, as seen in neurofibromatosis, there may be associated localized gigantism of adjacent bone and soft tissue (Fig 24–12), e.g., enlargement and deformity of the second and third toes. Treatment for these larger lesions is surgical, and whether one resects locally or amputates for severe local mechanical disability will depend on the extensiveness of the tumor. These lesions never become malignant.

Glomus Tumor

Another benign vascular tumor found in the hand or foot is a very small but frequently very painful one, the glomus tumor.[55] The glomus tumor is usually located in a subungual location in the hand or foot but may also arise in subcutaneous locations such as the one seen in Figure 24–13 in the web space between the toes. These tumors are usually bright red and assume the size of a small pea. Simple surgical excision brings on a dramatic relief of symptoms.

Ectopic Ossification

Areas of soft-tissue calcification or ossification in the hand or foot are usually the result of ischemia of tissues caused by either an old injury with scar formation or a generalized disease process associated with vasculitis such as scleroderma or Raynaud's disease.

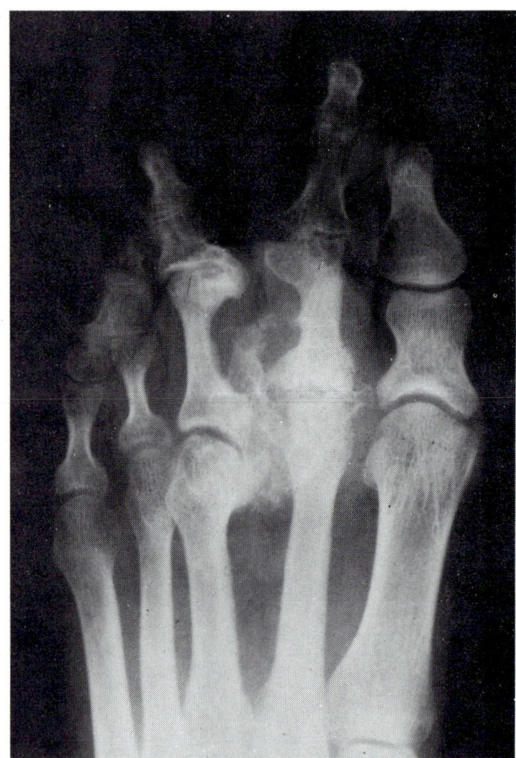

FIG 24–12.
Hemangioma of the foot with associated enlargement and deformity of the second and third toes.

Figure 24–14 shows an example of heterotopic bone formation in the heel cord as the very late sequelae of an old heel cord rupture. This resulted in fibrosis and ischemia that progressed to calcification. Then with gradual vascular ingrowth, bone was formed in the dense traumatized scar tissue.

Malignant Tumors of the Soft Tissues

Fibrosarcoma

The soft-tissue fibrosarcoma is an extremely rare tumor of the hand or foot.[53] One should always consider a benign diagnosis for this tumor. It does occur, it will do so in older individuals. The lesion may be slow growing with a fairly well differentiated fibroblast as the tumor cell, which forms a fair amount of collagen fiber. In this case the tumor might be resected by a radical en bloc resection without amputation. However, if the tumor is quite anaplastic with poorly differentiated fibroblasts and minimum collagen formation, amputation is usually best. An example of the latter situation is seen in Figure 24–15,A and B.

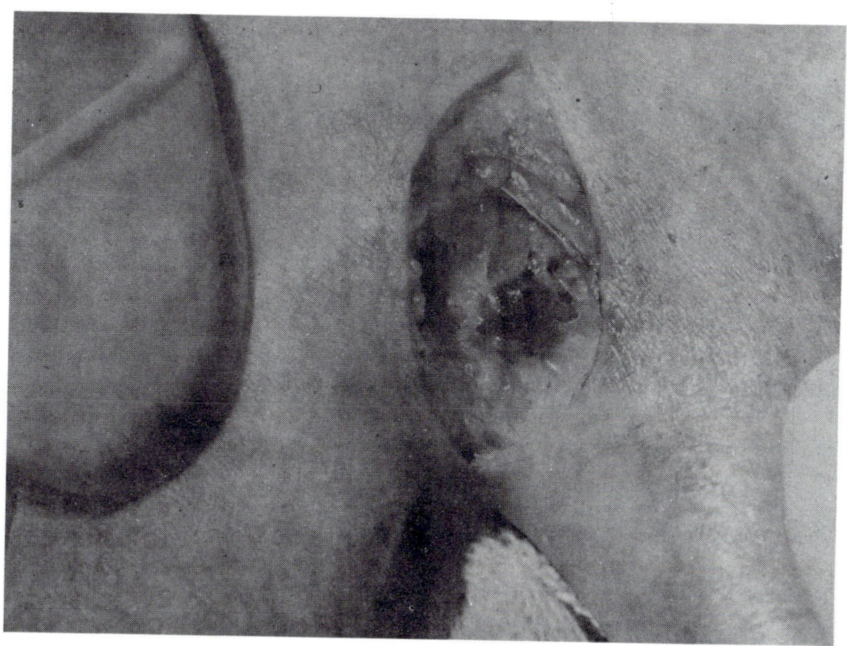

FIG 24–13.
Glomus tumor in a subcutaneous location in the dorsal web space between the toes.

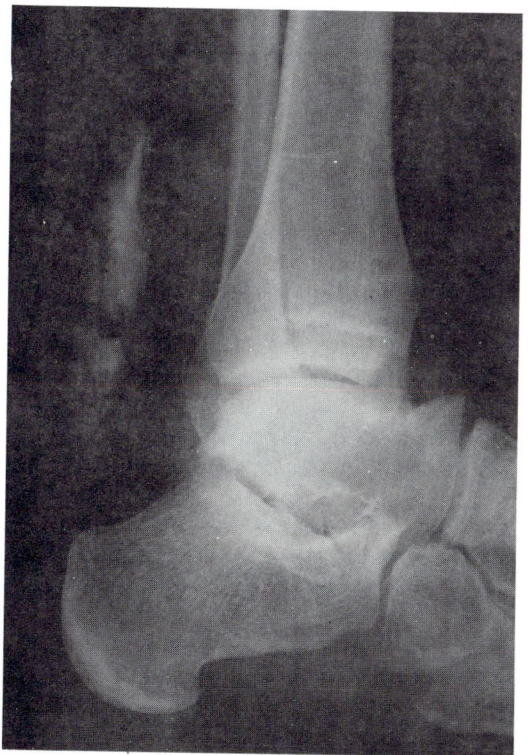

FIG 24–14.
Heterotopic bone formation in the heel cord as a late result of trauma.

Synovial Cell Sarcoma

The synovial cell sarcoma is also a rare tumor of the foot. It is most commonly seen about the knee area in young adults. Stening[57] pointed out the frequency of its occurrence about the ankle and tarsal area. Figure 24–16,A and B are T2-weighted MRI studies of a 28-year-old male with synovial cell sarcoma who had vague midtarsal foot pain for several years. Routine radiographs were normal appearing. These tumors grow slowly at first and may initially be confused with a benign process such as the ganglion cyst or lipoma. They are firm on palpation and may have mild symptoms of pain. The cell of origin is the synovioblast, which produces proteoglycan (hyaluronic acid).

Synovial cell sarcoma rarely occurs inside a joint cavity. It may calcify, as do fibrosarcomas. The most characteristic feature of the lesion, which is almost necessary to make a microscopic diagnosis, is the presence of a pseudoglandular epithelium that gives the tumor the appearance of an adenocarcinoma. However, there is no basement membrane beneath this pseudoepithelium as there would be in a true adenocarcinoma. The tumor is bimorphic (i.e., composed of fibroblastic cells as well). Both cell populations are felt to be of synovioblastic origin.

The tumor carries about the same prognosis as a malignant fibrosarcoma, with a 25% chance of 5-year survival.[15] The treatment of choice is amputation. Lymph-node metastasis often occurs, so a careful examination of the inguinal area is necessary before surgery. How-

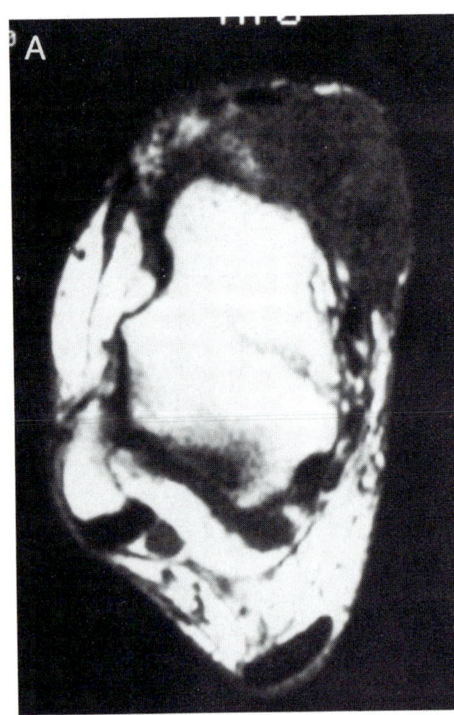

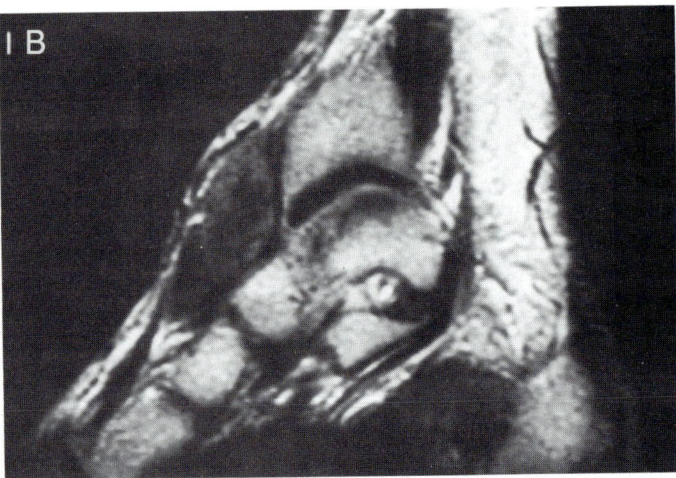

FIG 24–15.
A, MRI study of an aggressive fibrosarcoma anterior to the ankle joint in a 50-year-old female. **B,** MRI in the same patient in the sagittal plane.

ever, during the past decade[22] there has been an increase in the use of adjuvant chemotherapy following either a wide local resection or amputation for high-grade soft-tissue sarcomas of the extremity that has increased the survival rate of patients to 74%.

Kaposi's Sarcoma (Angiosarcoma)

The angiosarcoma of Kaposi deserves attention because of its predilection for the skin of the hands and feet, particularly of the great toe.[37] This tumor initially appears as multiple painful red or purple subcutaneous nodules that measure up to 1 cm in diameter (Fig 24–17). The lesions may be telangiectatic or verrucose. The tumor enlarges slowly and may cause lymphatic obstruction and edema. Because of the slow growth of this tumor, wide resection with grafting and radiotherapy successfully arrests it.

Recently there has been an increased interest in Kaposi's sarcoma because of its increased incidence in young homosexual males with a condition known as acquired immunodeficiency syndrome (AIDS).[26]

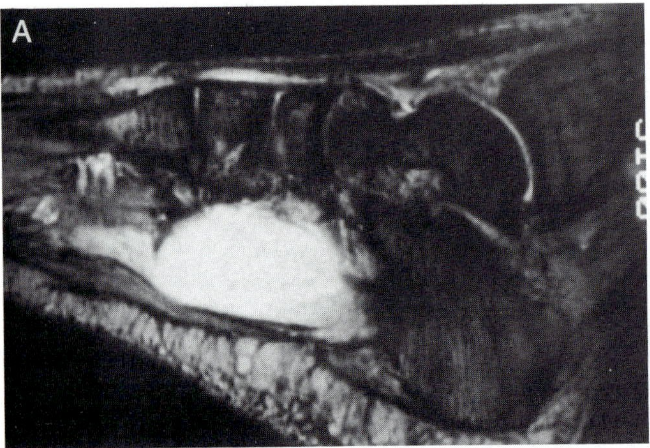

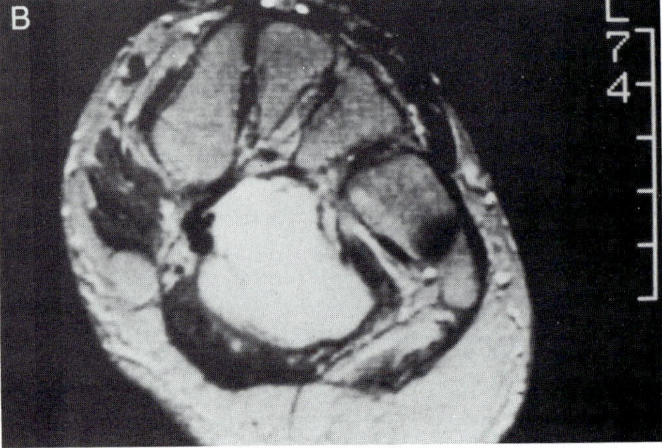

FIG 24–16.
A, T2-weighted MRI study in the sagittal plane of a synovial cell sarcoma in a 28-year-old male. **B,** same study in the transverse plane.

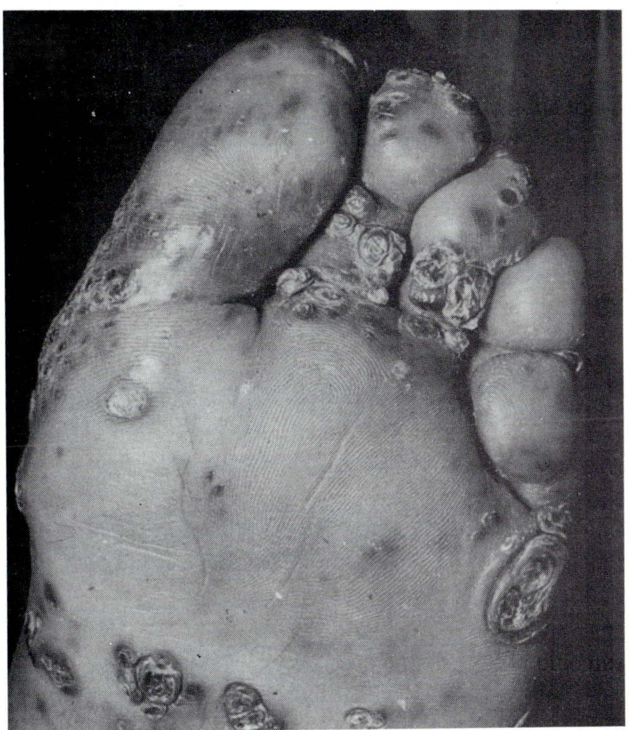

FIG 24–17.
Kaposi's sarcoma of the foot. (Courtesy of Dr. Marcus Caro.)

Malignant Melanoma

A malignant melanoma is an adult skin tumor that frequently occurs in the lower extremity, especially on the plantar surface of the foot. Nearly 50% of these lesions arise out of benign junctional nevi.[10] The junctional nevus is usually flat, tan, and nonhairy. Signs to alert the surgeon to a malignant transformation from a junctional nevus to malignant melanoma include enlargement, deepening pigmentation, ulceration, and halo pigmentation in the skin around the nevus. Fewer than 1% of junctional nevi on the sole of the foot become malignant, so routine prophylactic removal of all junctional nevi in this location is not justified. An ulcerating neoplasm on the plantar surface of the foot, however, is almost certain to be a truly malignant melanoma, even if not pigmented.

The *subungual melanoma* (seen in Fig 24–18) is another localized clinical entity that usually requires early amputation of the toe. A blue nevus, that is very dark and flat and can easily be confused with melanoma is, in fact, usually benign and rarely metastasizes.

Treatment of malignant melanomas of the foot other than the toe usually consists of widely excising the entire lesion and surrounding skin with a cold knife (noncautery). In some cases removal of the inguinal lymph nodes and even the deeper iliac nodes is advised. With this proper therapy the 5-year survival rate is 30%. Radiation treatment is of no value, however.

Benign Tumors and Cysts of Bone

Solitary Bone Cyst

The simple or unicameral bone cyst is a common defect found typically in growing bone on the diaphyseal side of the growth plate.[18] It is a cystic lesion, usually filled with serous liquid and lined by a thin membrane containing fibrous tissue and giant cells. It may be asymptomatic until an acute painful pathologic fracture occurs such as seen in the third metatarsal in Figure 24–19.

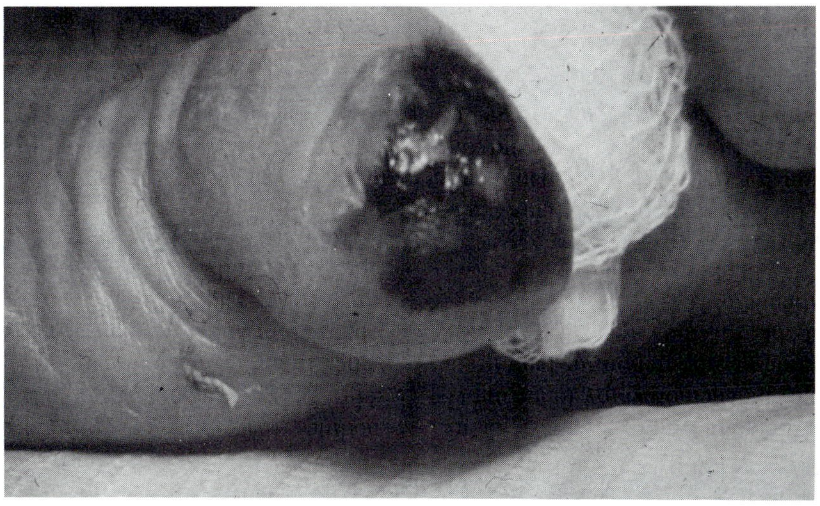

FIG 24–18.
Subungual melanoma of the fifth toe.

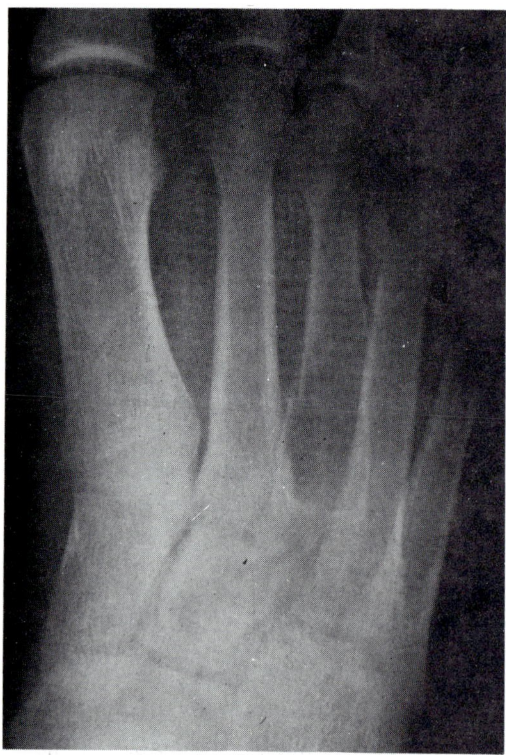

FIG 24–19.
Pathologic fracture through a solitary bone cyst at the base of the third metatarsal.

A common location for the simple cyst is the larger tarsal bones such as the os calcis or talus. An example of a lesion in the os calcis is seen in Figure 24–20,A by radiographic technique and in Figure 24–20,B by MRI technique. This 16-year-old patient was treated by local curettage and bone grafting. In younger patients under 15 years of age, the recurrence rate is quite high following bone grafting. For this reason, if possible, it is best to wait until the patient is 14 years old before a definitive graft is performed.

For the past 15 years the Italians have suggested a new and simple nonoperative technique for the management of solitary cysts.[18] This consists of injecting 80 to 200 mg of methylprednisolone acetate directly into the cyst through a large percutaneous needle every 2 months until the cyst resolves. The success rate with this technique is about 80%.

Epidermoid Cyst

The epidermoid cyst is seen typically in the distal phalanx of the finger or toe, beneath the nail bed. It is manifested as a bulbous enlargement of the tip of the digit; on radiographs a geographic cystic lesion in the subungual area of the terminal phalanx is seen. The cyst will transilluminate and is filled with serous fluid, like the solitary cyst, but its lining is made up of nail bed matrix and contains keratin. The cyst is usually the product of an old crushing injury to the tip of the toe that drives nail matrix down into the phalanx, where it continues to grow in an ectopic location to form a keratin-lined cyst. The treatment is simple curettage and grafting.

Aneurysmal Bone Cyst

A benign cystic lesion of bone that may occur in the foot is the hemorrhagic or aneurysmal bone cyst. It is a lesion seen in growing metaphyseal bone of children and is characterized by its dilated and thin-shelled appearance on radiographs (as viewed in the third metatarsal bone in Fig 24–21). This lesion is in a quiescent stage as compared with the cyst seen in Figure 24–22,A and B in which there is advanced hyperemic destructive

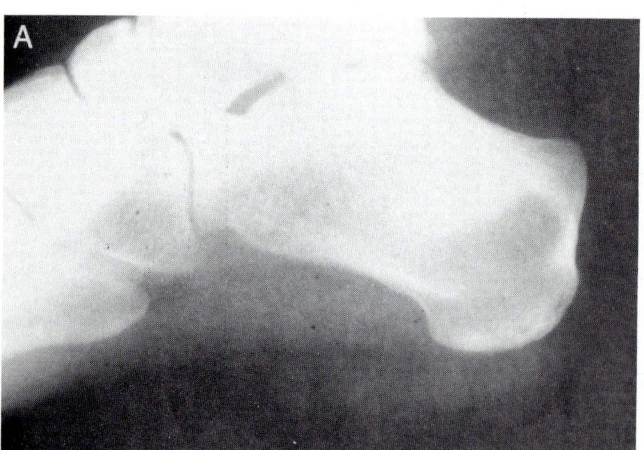

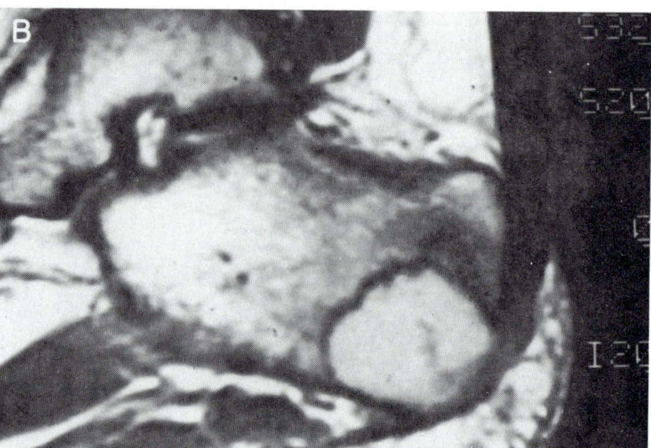

FIG 24–20.
A, radiographic appearance of an os calcis bone cyst in a 16-year-old male. **B,** same lesion seen by MRI.

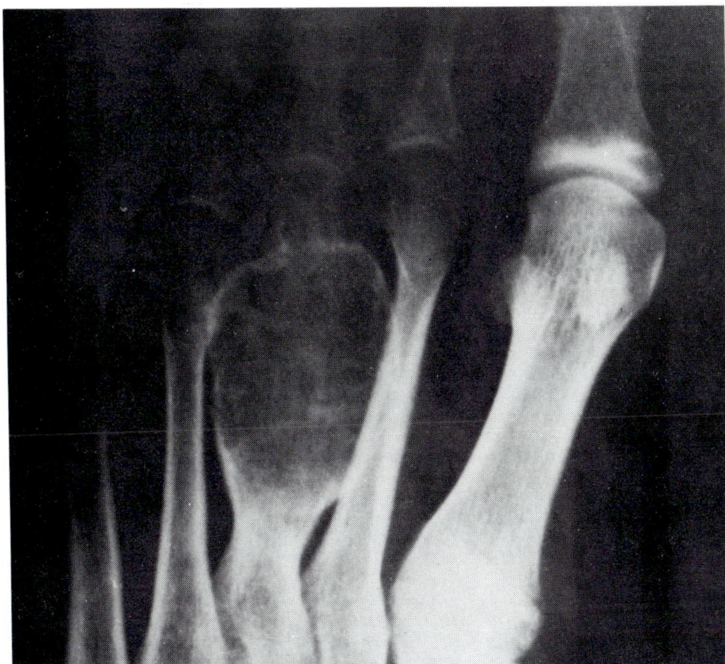

FIG 24–21.
Aneurysmal bone cyst of the third metatarsal.

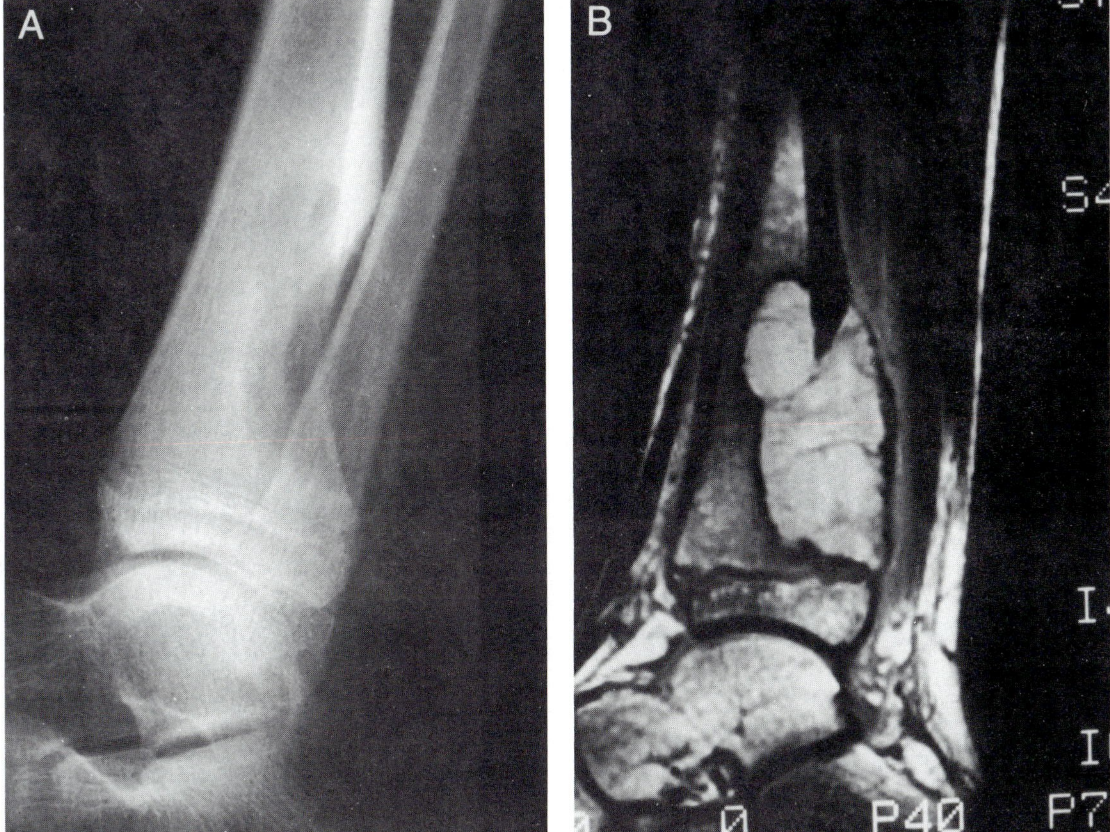

FIG 24–22.
A, radiographic appearance of an aneurysmal bone cyst in the distal tibial metaphysis in a 14-year-old boy. **B,** same lesion seen by MRI in the sagittal plane.

change in the posterior aspect of the distal tibial metaphysis in a 14-year-old boy that might suggest a malignant process or infectious disease.

At the time of biopsy, the cyst was filled mainly by unclotted blood and lined with a mossy friable layer of reddish-brown material. Microscopically the cyst was loaded with large giant cells that might suggest the diagnosis of a giant-cell tumor. A giant-cell tumor can also be aneurysmal in nature and fairly hemorrhagic. However, it is a more solid, fleshy tumor of bone, with more malignant potential. In the case of a foot lesion, the prognosis is very good following simple curettage and bone grafting, the same treatment used for a simple bone cyst.

Giant-cell Tumors

Giant-cell tumors are benign but aggressive tumors of bone that rarely involve the hand or foot.[17] Campanacci et al. recorded only 4 cases in the foot in his large series of 327 cases. The usual treatment in the past has been curettage and bone grafting with a 45% recurrence rate. Of late a new technique of aggressive curettage and packing the defect with bone cement has resulted in good function and a 10% recurrence rate. Figure 24–23,A and B is an example of this technique used to treat a giant-cell tumor of the talus in a 16-year-old female with an excellent result after 6 years. Most experts agree that radiation therapy for giant-cell tumors is contraindicated for extremity lesions because of the potential for irradiation sarcoma 8 to 25 years later.

Osteochondroma

Osteochondromas are common benign tumors located in the metaphyseal area of long bones in children. They may be solitary or multiple and probably result when small peripheral portions of the growth plate separate from the main plate and continue as separate localized growth centers on the surface of the metaphyseal cortex. Osteochondromas do not usually occur in the hand or foot. Figure 24–24 shows a typical sessile osteochondroma in the distal end of the part of the tibia, where it has interfered with the normal development of the adjacent fibula. Treatment consists of simple resection at the base of the bony stock while making sure to remove the entire cartilaginous cap, which on rare occasion can slowly develop into a secondary chondrosarcoma.

Bone Spur

A bone spur is a reactive lesion that commonly occurs in the foot. It is usually a result of repeated irritation of the foot bone at the point of attachment of a ligament or joint capsule. The spurs forming from the tuberosity of the os calcis are typical examples of reactive bone spurs and should not be confused with an osteochondroma, which has a cartilaginous cap and is never present at the tip of a spur.

Subungual Exostosis

A special type of reactive bone spur is the type found beneath the nail of a toe such as the one seen in Figure 24–25 on the tip of the third toe. The great toe is the most common site for this lesion, which on rare occasion will have a cartilaginous cap and, in fact, represents a very small osteochondroma. The pearly mass growing through the nail may be misdiagnosed as a malignant tumor. All these benign lesions can be easily resected. However, in the case of a reactive spur, one

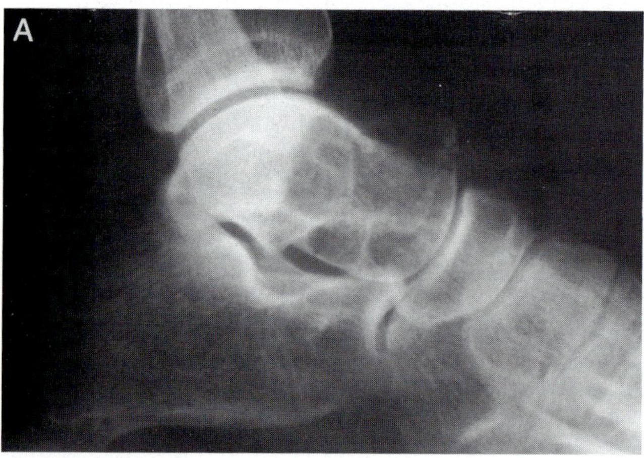

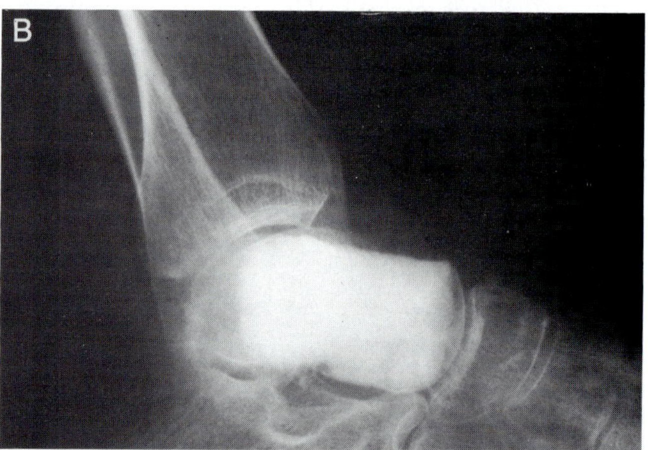

FIG 24–23.
A, radiographic appearance of a giant-cell tumor of the talus in a 16-year-old female. **B,** appearance 6 years later after curettage and cementation.

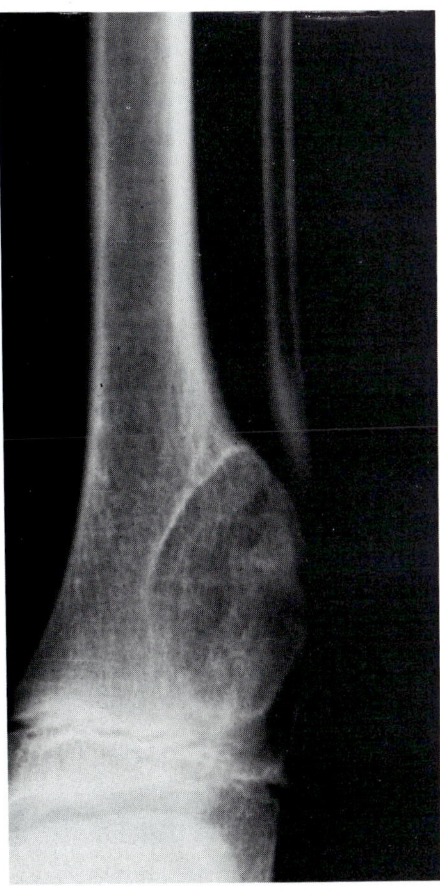

FIG 24–24.
Sessile osteochondroma of the distal end of the tibia.

might anticipate a recurrence unless the sources of irritation were removed.

Osteoid Osteoma

An osteoid osteoma is a small but painful neoplasm of the bone that occurs in children and is frequently observed in the lower extremities. The metaphyses of the long bones are the most frequent location; however, the tarsal bones of the foot are not unusual locations for this benign osteoid-forming lesion. The radiograph (Fig 24–26) of a typical lesion in the cuboid area shows a dense osteoblastic reaction surrounding the small osteolytic nidus that takes on the appearance of an inflammatory granuloma such as a Brodie abscess.

Osteoid osteomas will spontaneously resolve over several years as the nidus is gradually replaced by dense reactive bone similar to that seen in Figure 24–27 where there remains only a thin shell of inflammatory tissue around a centrally dense osteoma. When the lytic portion is completely filled in, the pain will stop. If pain necessitates an early operation, the critical portion of the lesion to remove is the hyperemic and painful nidus.

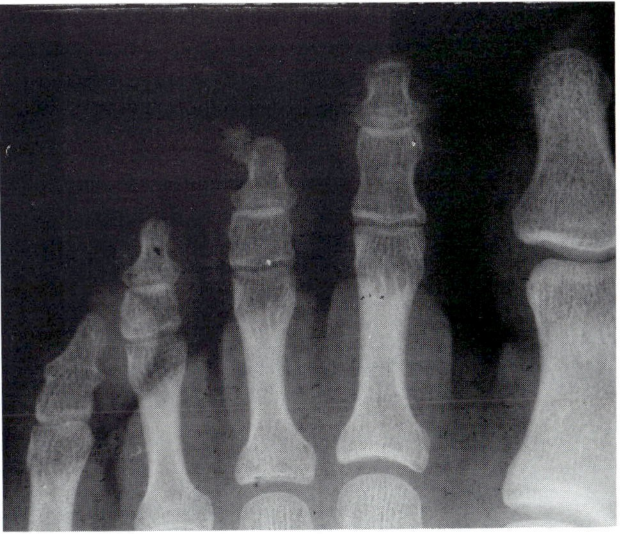

FIG 24–25.
Exostosis of the third distal phalanx.

The surrounding dense bone may be left intact. Local recurrence is almost nonexistent.

It has been shown by Makely[39] that there is a great increase in prostaglandins in the nidus of an osteoid osteoma. For this reason the use of nonsteroidal pros-

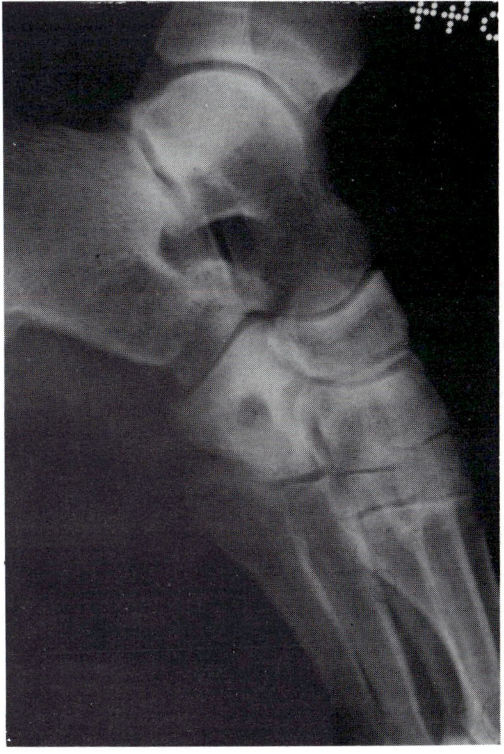

FIG 24–26.
Typical appearance of an osteoid osteoma of the cuboid.

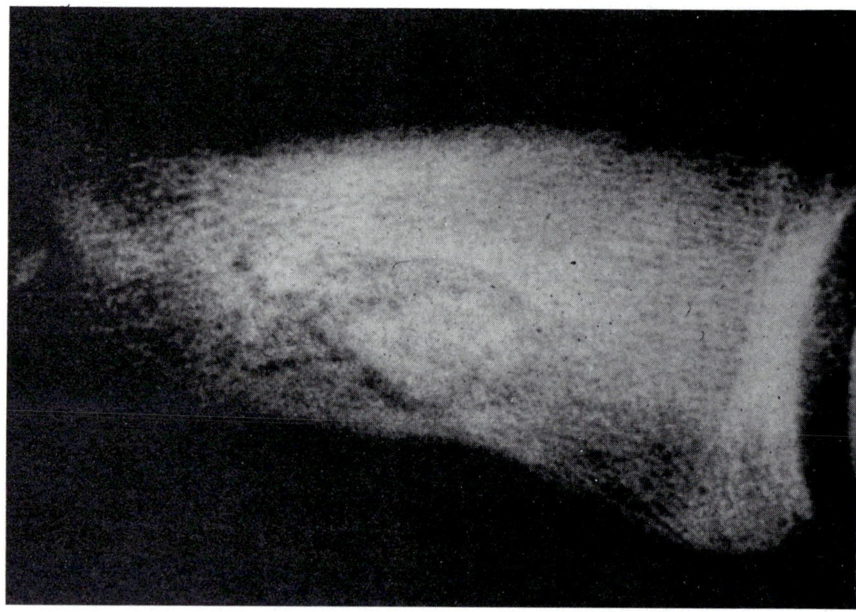

FIG 24–27.
Dense osteoid osteoma in the proximal phalanx of the great toe.

taglandin-inhibitory drugs can be considered in the nonsurgical management of these painful lesions.

Osteoblastoma

The large form of the osteoid osteoma is the osteoblastoma, also called the "giant osteoid osteoma."[59] It is found in the same locations as the osteoid osteoma, including the tarsal bones. Its central nidus must be larger than 1 cm, and it is a great deal more hemorrhagic in nature. The radiograph and MRI seen in Figure 24–28,A and B show a typical lesion protruding from the posterior aspect of the talar body in a 22-year-old male that required treatment by curettage and bone grafting.

Enchondroma, Periosteal Chondroma, and Juxtacortical Chondroma

A common benign tumor of bone in the hand or foot is the well-known enchondroma. This dysplastic, hamartomatous, cartilaginous lesion—like the simple bone cyst—is asymptomatic unless a pathologic fracture occurs through it. Figure 24–29 shows the typical appearance of a pathologic fracture through an enchondroma of the fifth metatarsal. Note the geographic punched-

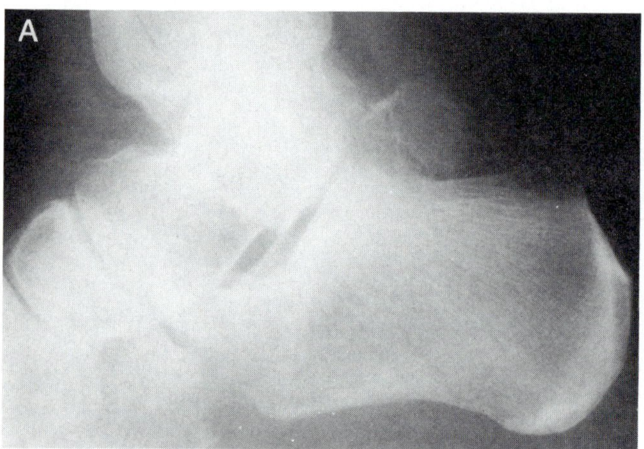

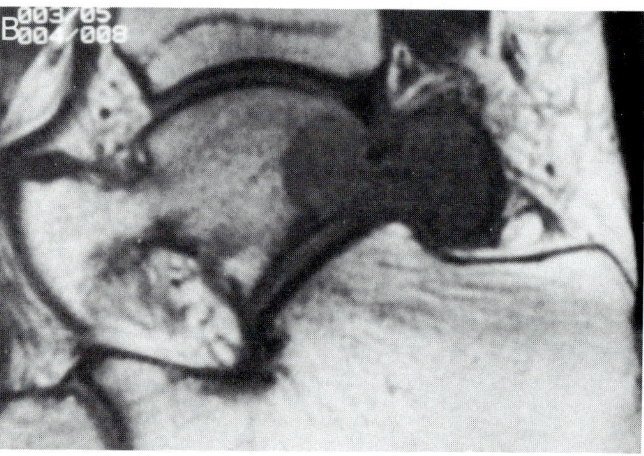

FIG 24–28.
A, radiographic appearance of an osteoblastoma of the talus in a 22-year-old male. **B,** same lesion with sagittal T1-weighted MRI.

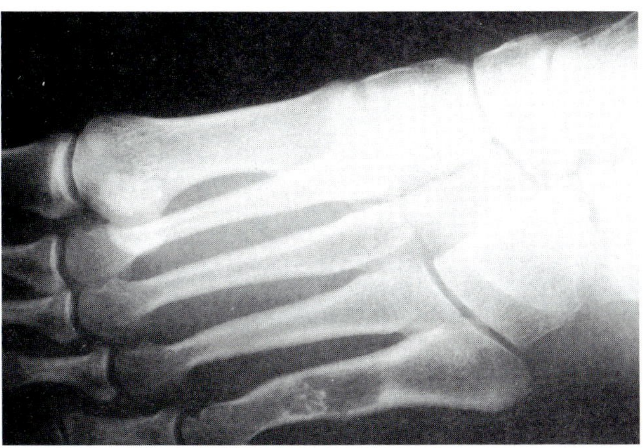

FIG 24–29.
Enchondroma in the fifth metatarsal with a pathologic fracture.

out appearance, a sharp reactive edge, and characteristic flocculated calcification in its central area. These lesions may be treated by simple curettage and bone grafting, but after the fracture has healed. Only on rare occasion do they turn malignant.

Dysplastic cartilaginous lesions can occur on the cortical surface of bone as seen in Figure 24–30, in which case it is referred to as a periosteal chondroma.

Even more unusual is the occurrence of a dysplastic cartilaginous lesion in the lining of a joint or tendon sheath. Figure 24–31 presents an example of a benign tumor of cartilage arising from the anterior capsule of the ankle joint. In this case the lesion is referred to as a juxta-articular chondroma, and treatment is by simple surgical excision.

Chondroblastoma

A chondroblastoma is a benign giant-cell lesion found typically in the epiphyseal areas of long bones in children. Figure 24–32 shows the radiographic appearance of a lesion located in the distal fibular epiphysis of a 12-year-old boy. Notice the characteristic flocculated calcification in the lytic lesion, which suggests chondroid elements. This tumor is sometimes referred to as an epiphyseal giant-cell tumor of adolescence. However, its prognosis is much better than for the adult giant-cell tumor. Treatment consists of simple curettage and possible grafting. The os calcis and talus are targets for this tumor in the foot.

Fibroma of Bone

Dysplastic fibroma of bone is a common condition of the skeletal system and can be found in all parts of the body including the foot. These fibromas have a similar radiographic appearance to the solitary cyst and may in fact have a similar pathologic origin. Figure 24–33 is a radiograph of a typical fibroma of bone seen in the os calcis. Notice the sharp geographic appearance, which suggests a benign condition. These lesions are usually asymptomatic until the time of a possible pathologic fracture. They are frequently seen in children and young adults in metaphyseal bone. If treatment is necessary because of recurrent fracture or a threat of fracture, it consists of simple curettage and grafting.

At times a patient is found to have multiple bony involvement with fibromas of bone in the feet; this condition is referred to as *polyostotic fibrous dysplasia* (Fig 24–34). There is chronic dilation of the first and fourth metatarsal shafts. The condition tends to amplify on one side of the body more than on the other, with a resultant leg length discrepancy caused by bowing of the femur.

Another benign variation of fibrous defects in bone is the so-called *chondromyxoid fibroma* (Fig 24–35). This tumor has about the same radiographic appearance as the nonossifying fibroma and can be treated the same way, i.e., with simple curettage and possible grafting. The distinguishing histologic characteristic of this rare lesion is the presence of myxoid and chondroid tissue.

Sarcoidosis

Sarcoidosis is a generalized systemic granulomatous disease of unknown cause that acts in many ways like a low-grade lymphoma. It involves structures of the lymphoid system (including bone marrow), especially in blacks. Bones most typically involved are located in the hands and feet. Figure 24–36 is a typical radiograph of a sarcoid foot with granulomatous changes in the distal first metatarsal that might suggest gout. However, the smaller, more centrally located lesions in the phalanges

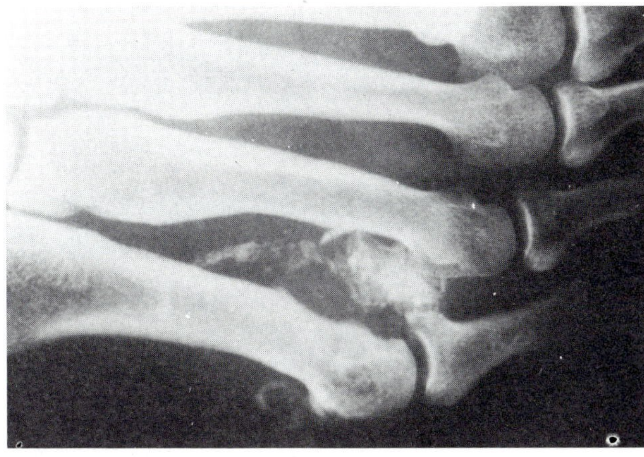

FIG 24–30.
Periosteal chondroma on the cortical surface of the fifth metatarsal.

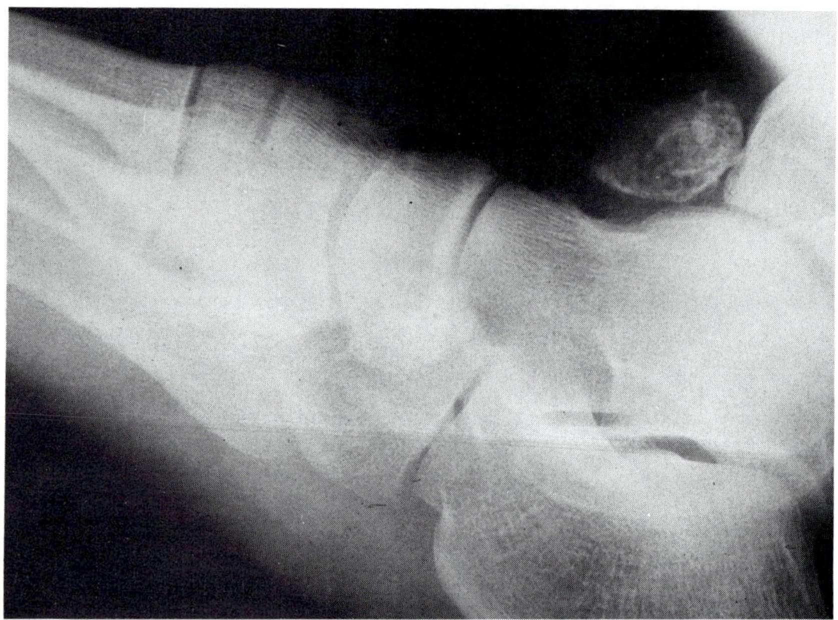

FIG 24–31.
Typical juxta-articular chondroma in the anterior ankle joint capsule.

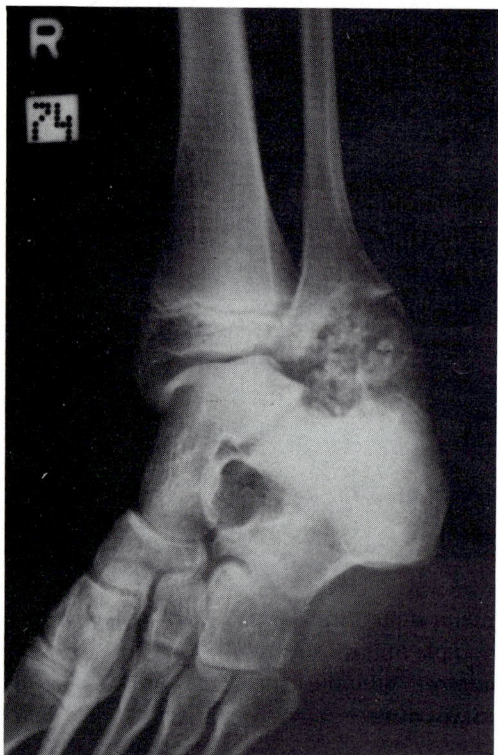

FIG 24–32.
Chondroblastoma in the distal fibular epiphysis of a 12-year-old boy.

suggest sarcoidosis. These patients have subcutaneous nodularities overlying the bony changes that could suggest a rheumatoid process.

Melorheostosis

Melorheostosis is an idiopathic condition seen typically in the bones of the lower extremities. It is usually picked up as an incidental finding from a radiograph obtained for some other reason. Figure 24–37 provides an example of this abnormality of enchondral ossification involving the tibia, talus, and first ray to the tip of the great toe. The flowing appearance on the radiograph accounts for the name given this condition, which can sometimes occur across joints and result in stiffening.

Tarsoepiphyseal Aclasis

Tarsoepiphyseal aclasis is a rare and localized epiphyseal dysplasia of a hypertrophic nature that is usually seen in bones about the ankle of one leg only. Its characteristic deformed enlargement of the talus is well demonstrated in Figure 24–38, where it might suggest other conditions such as fibrous dysplasia or neurofibromatosis. The talus is the most common place to find this defect, but it can occur in a growing child on the medial side of the knee with enlargement of the medial femoral condyle. Early recognition should lead to early surgical treatment.

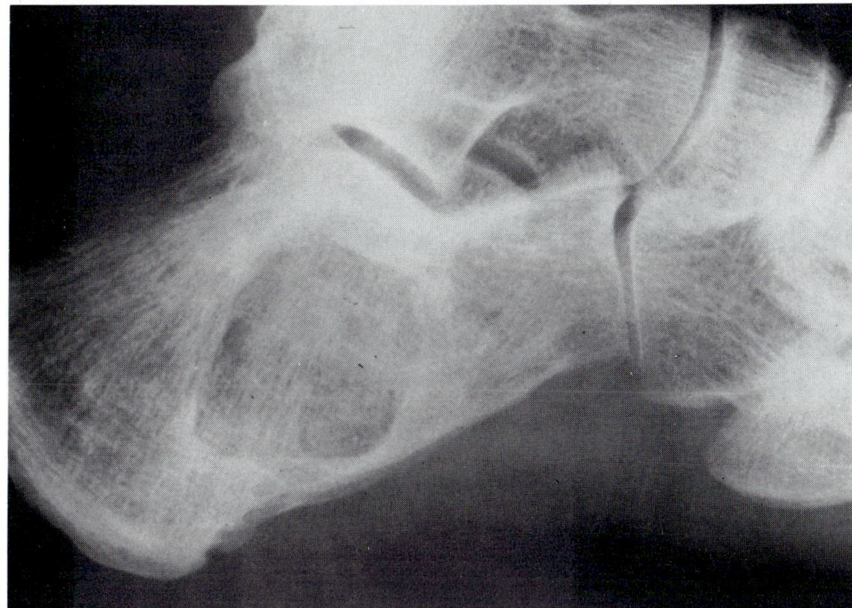

FIG 24–33.
Fibroma of the os calcis.

Stippled Epiphyses

Conradi's disease (chondrodysplasia punctata) is a rare form of congenital dwarfism seen at birth with the clinical manifestations of achondroplastic dwarfism. However, on radiographic examination, the diagnostic features of stippled epiphyses appear (Fig 24–39). There is extensive calcific stippling around the major epiphyseal ossification centers in the tarsal region of the foot. This is a dystrophic form of calcification in the germinal cartilage that gradually disappears with time and growth. In many cases the dwarfism clears up, and the older child may enjoy a fairly normal physical appearance.

Bone Islands

Bone islands are common findings on bone radiographs. These represent small, well-circumscribed areas of increased bone density secondary to a failure of

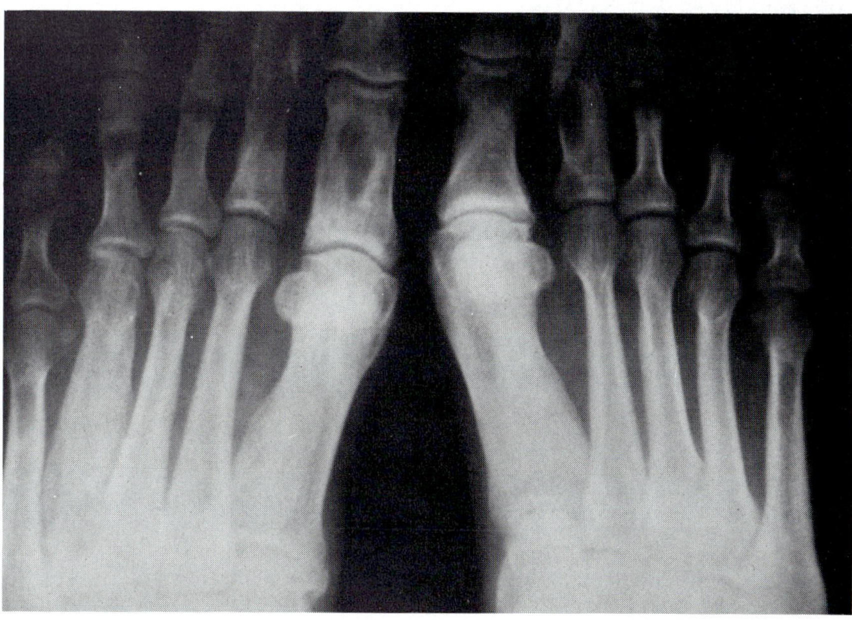

FIG 24–34.
Polyostotic fibrous dysplasia involving both feet.

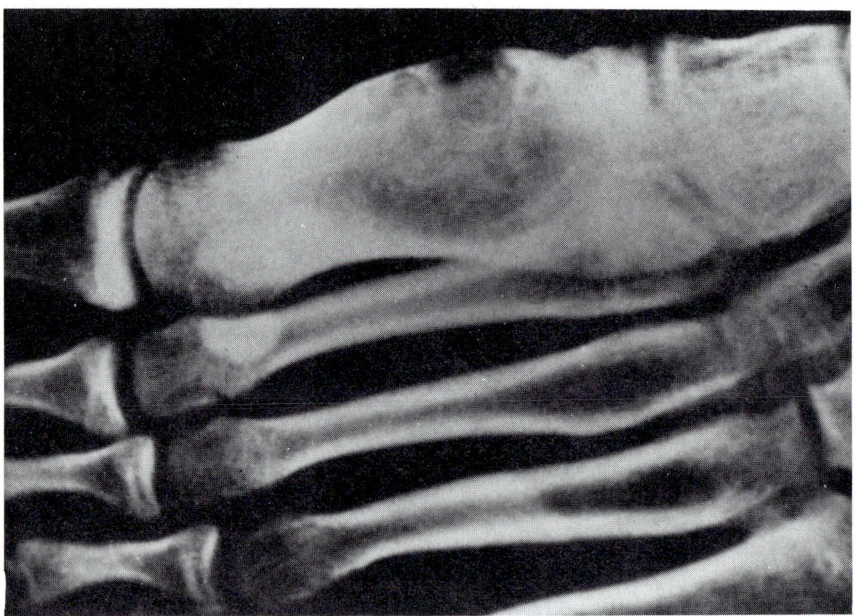

FIG 24–35.
Benign chondromyxoid fibroma of the first metatarsal.

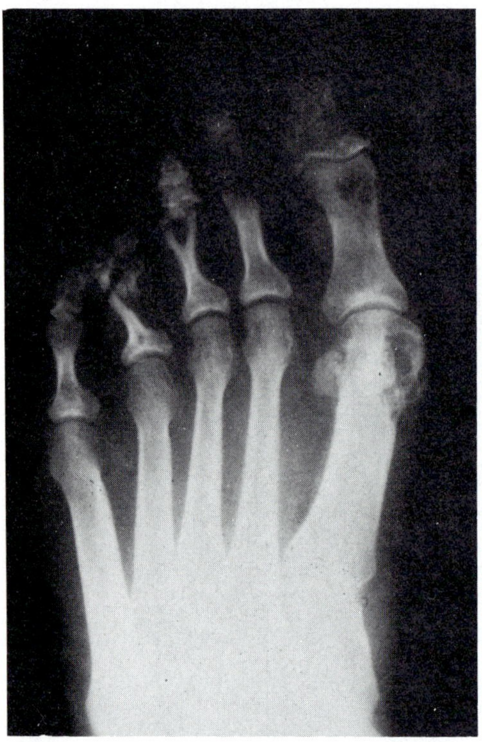

FIG 24–36.
Lytic-appearing granulomas in sarcoidosis of the foot.

proper remodeling of bone in the metaphyseal areas of the growing skeleton. If multiple lesions are seen (Fig 24–40), the condition is referred to as osteopoikilosis; it is usually observed in radiographs of asymptomatic hands and feet. Lesions located more proximally may suggest the possibility of osteoblastic metastatic disease. An isotopic bone scan can help clear this differential diagnostic point in most cases.

Malignant Tumors of Bone

Malignant tumors of the hand or foot are unusual; when they do occur, they tend to behave less aggressively than the same tumor in a more proximal portion of the extremity in larger bones. For this reason, when the pathologist is uncertain as to the exact nature of a lesion of the hand or foot at biopsy, it is frequently good judgment on the part of the clinician to assume a benign diagnosis and elect conservative local resection. The general statement can also be made that malignant tumors of the hand and foot will tend to metastasize rather late in the course of the disease.

Osteosarcoma

An osteogenic sarcoma is a highly malignant tumor, usually seen in the metaphyseal areas of fast-growing bones in children such as the tibia or femur. Most of these are seen in boys, and they are common about the knee joint. Bones of the feet are involved in fewer than

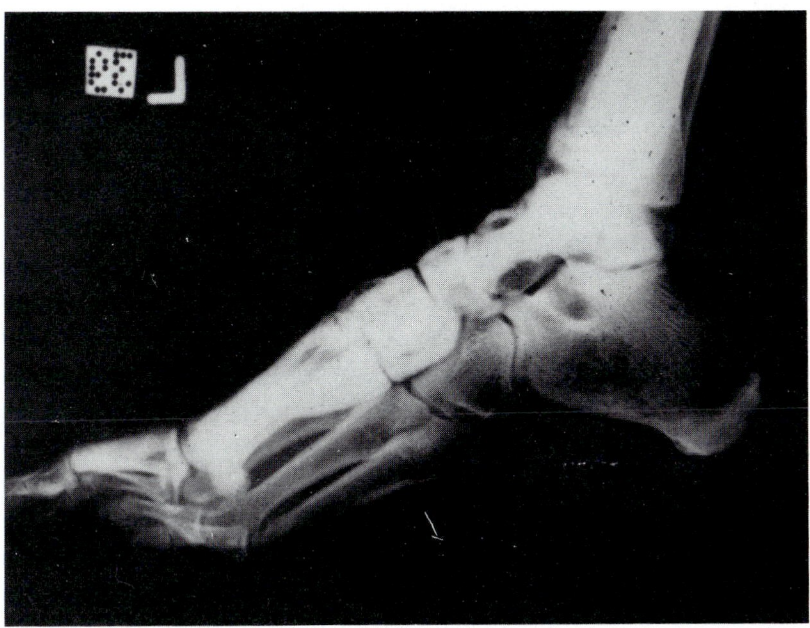

FIG 24–37.
Melorheostosis: flowing hyperostosis down the inner aspect of the foot and ankle.

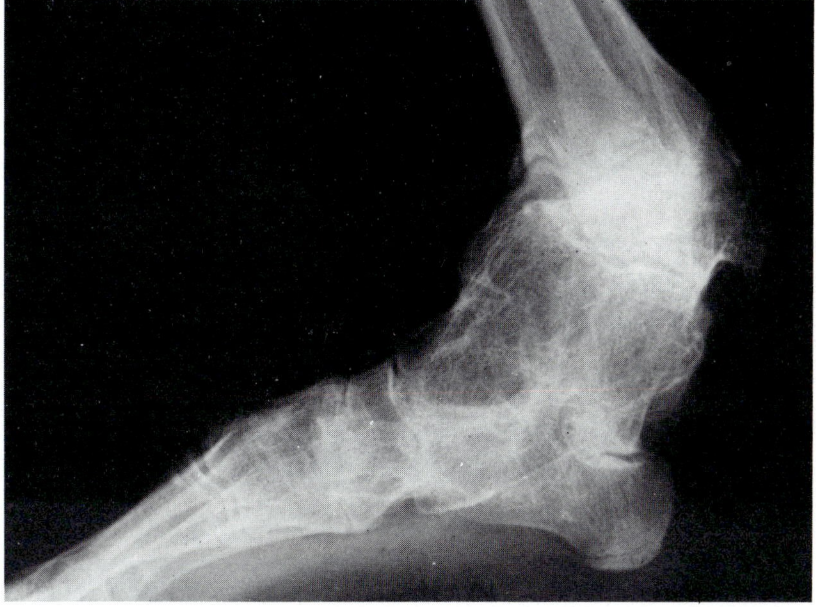

FIG 24–38.
Tarsoepiphyseal aclasis involving the entire talus and localized gigantism.

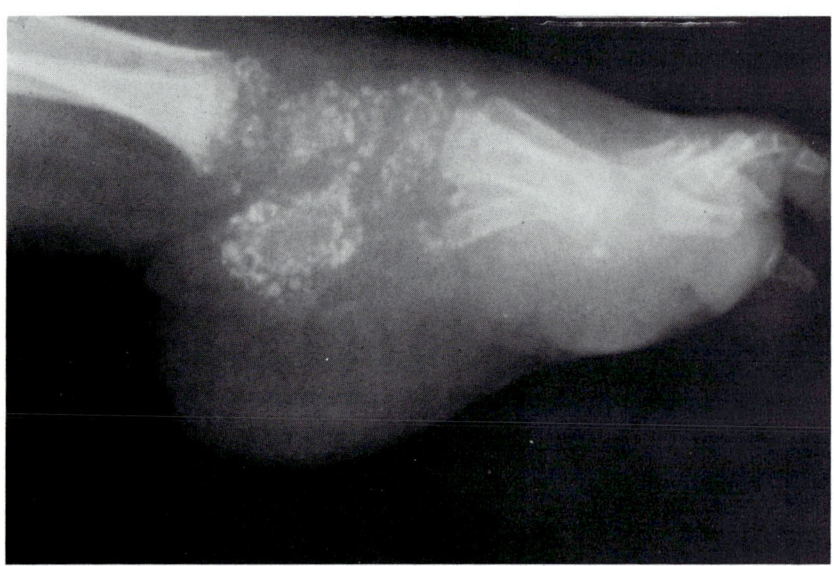

FIG 24–39.
Stippled epiphyses seen in a newborn dwarf.

1% of all cases, which makes this diagnosis rare. Figure 24–41 shows one of these rare cases of an osteosarcoma in the first metatarsal of a young man. The combination of lytic destruction of the subadjacent cortex and exuberant and chaotic production of neoplastic osteoid around the entire shaft of the metatarsal points strongly toward a malignant diagnosis of a bone-forming sarcoma.

At the present time in the case of the foot or ankle, the best surgical treatment is still a below-knee amputation. Over the past 20 years the prognosis for survival has improved dramatically with the advent of neoadjuvant multidrug chemotherapy. The drugs commonly used include doxorubicin (Adriamycin), high-dosage methotrexate, and cisplatin. They are given cyclically for 2 to 3 months prior to either an amputation or limb

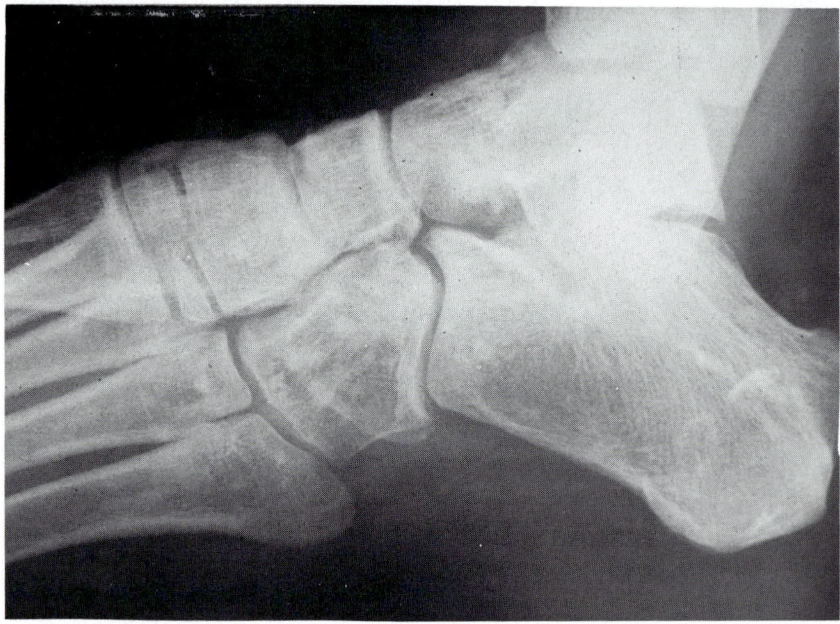

FIG 24–40.
Osteopoikilosis or multiple bone islands in the foot.

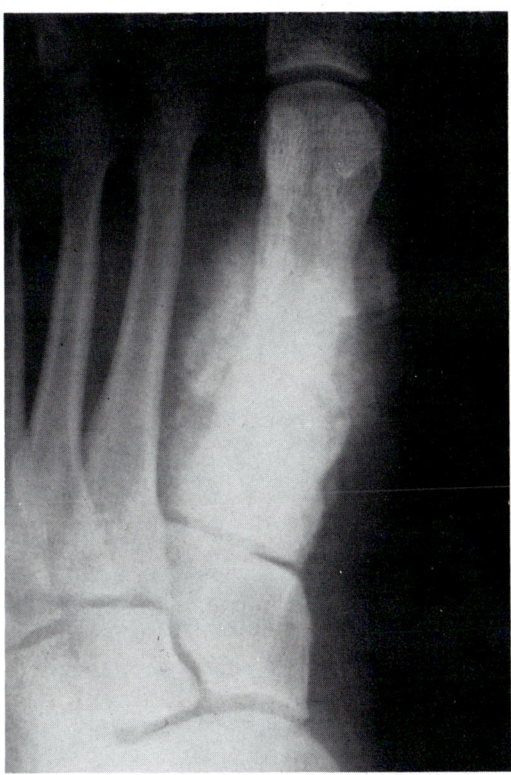

FIG 24–41.
Malignant osteosarcoma in the first metatarsal of a young man.

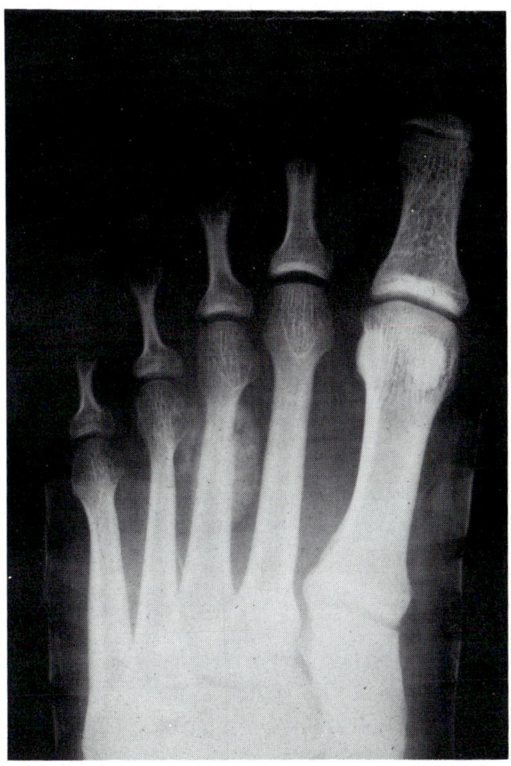

FIG 24–42.
Stress fracture in the third metatarsal presenting as pseudotumor.

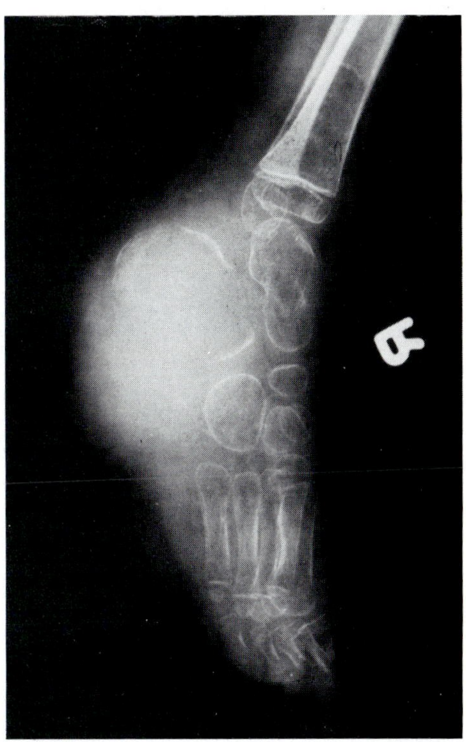

FIG 24–43.
Pseudotumor of hemophilia in the os calcis of a young boy.

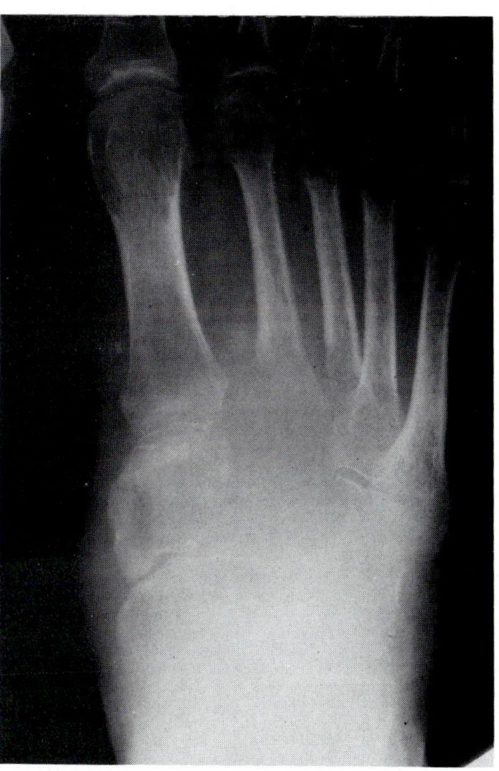

FIG 24–44.
Ewing's sarcoma in the midtarsal area of a young man.

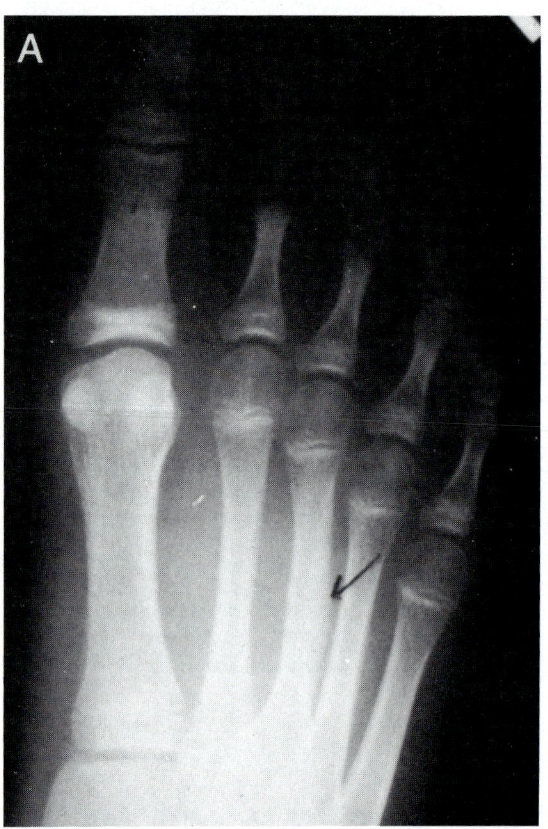

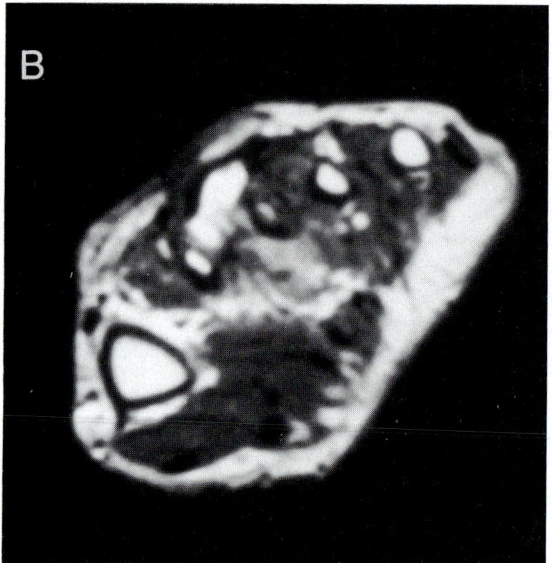

FIG 24–45.
A, periosteal new bone formation *(arrow)* in the third metatarsal of a 14-year-old female with Ewing's sarcoma. **B,** MRI of the lesion with extensive soft-tissue abnormality about the third metatarsal.

salvage procedure and continued for 4 to 6 months postoperatively. With this combined program the current 5-year survival rate ranges between 60% and 70%.

Pulmonary metastasis from this tumor was at one time considered a fatal condition, and nothing further was done for the patient. However, Spanos et al.[56] have presented encouraging results with resection of metastatic lesions. They report a 28% 5-year survival rate without recurrence. The new chemotherapy programs may well improve this figure.

It should be mentioned that radiotherapy has been dropped as a therapeutic modality for this tumor. Immunotherapy may hold some promise for the future.

Because the osteosarcoma is such a rare lesion in the foot, it might be wise to include a few pseudotumors that masquerade as malignant lesions. Figure 24–42 is a radiograph of such a pseudotumor in the third metatarsal of a 19-year-old track runner that demonstrates the typical callus formation seen in a stress fracture. These lesions frequently show no fracture line across the involved bone, and the patient may give no definite history of any single injury to the foot. Biopsy generally shows aggressive osteoid production that might suggest to the pathologist a malignant diagnosis. Such a mistaken diagnosis could then tragically lead to treatment by amputation for a benign process.

Another example of a pseudotumor is seen in Figure 24–43 in a young patient with factor VIII–type hemophilia. This occurs in the form of a highly lytic and aneurysmal lesion of the os calcis that could easily pass for an aggressive sarcoma of some type.

Ewing's Sarcoma

Ewing's sarcoma is also a childhood tumor seen more typically in the long bones of the lower extremities or in the pelvis. However, according to Pritchard et al.[47] at the Mayo Clinic, about 5% are located in the foot area. It carries the worst prognosis for survival of any of the primary sarcomas of bone. It probably is a very primitive mesenchymal tumor of the round cell variety, similar to the histiocytic lymphoma seen in adults.

Figure 24–44 shows the typical radiographic appear-

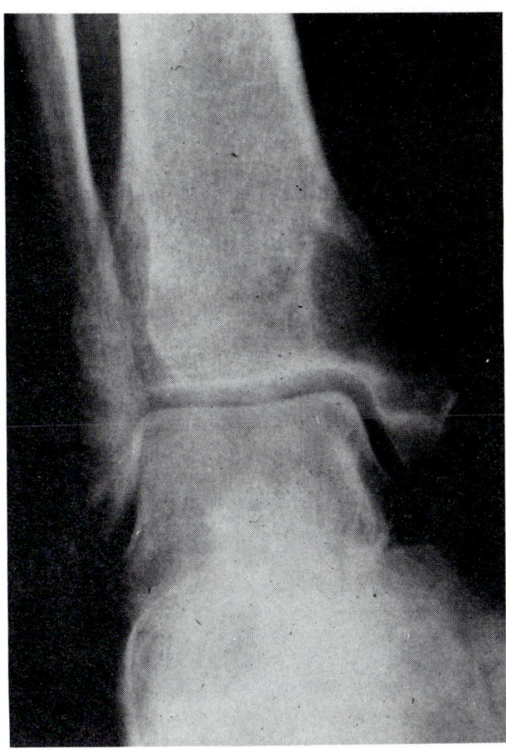

FIG 24–46.
Chondrosarcoma in the medial malleolus of a middle-aged man.

ance of Ewing's sarcoma seen in the midtarsal area of a young man. This lesion is purely lytic in nature, and its high degree of bony permeation suggests an infectious process such as tuberculosis. It is also quite necrotic and, when cut into, may drain a liquid necrotic material that suggests purulence to the operating surgeon.

Figure 24–45,A and B illustrates another Ewing's sarcoma of the third metatarsal in a 14-year-old female. The radiograph in Figure 24–45,A suggests the clinical diagnosis of a stress fracture. However, the MRI seen in Figure 24–45,B demonstrates extensive soft-tissue abnormality on the T1-weighted image that strongly suggests a neoplastic process.

In the past the traditional treatment for Ewing's sarcoma has been combined irradiation and multidrug chemotherapy with an expected 5-year survival rate of 60%. Currently there is a trend for more aggressive surgical resection with wide margins when possible. In the case of the foot, this usually requires an aggressive wide resection or below-knee amputation with the hope that the prognosis for survival may climb ever higher.

Chondrosarcoma

Like osteosarcoma, chondrosarcoma is rare in the foot. About 1% of all cases are seen in the foot or tarsal area and usually occur as primary lesions in middle-aged adults. The usual site for this tumor is the pelvis.

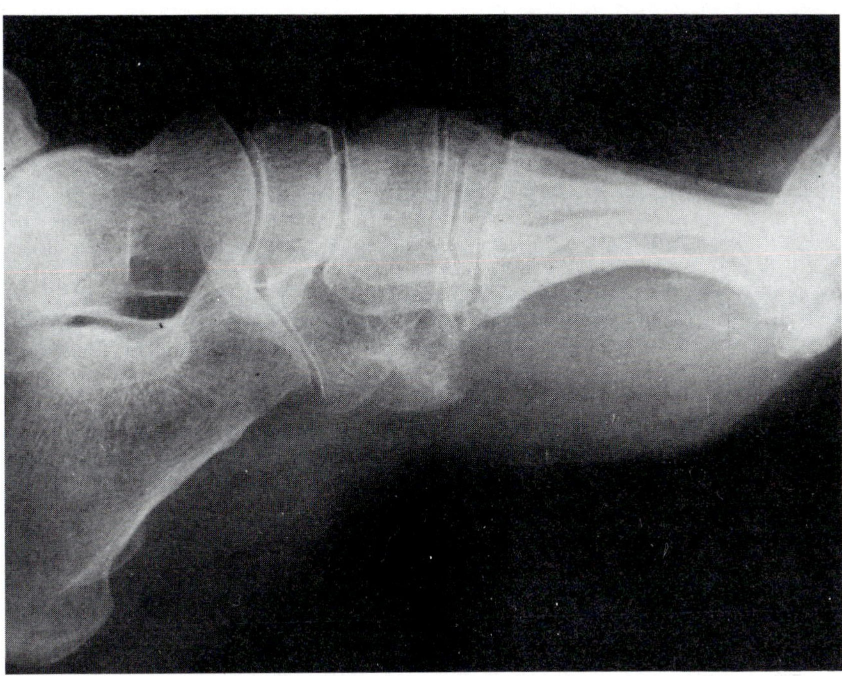

FIG 24–47.
Fibrosarcoma of the fifth metatarsal in a young man.

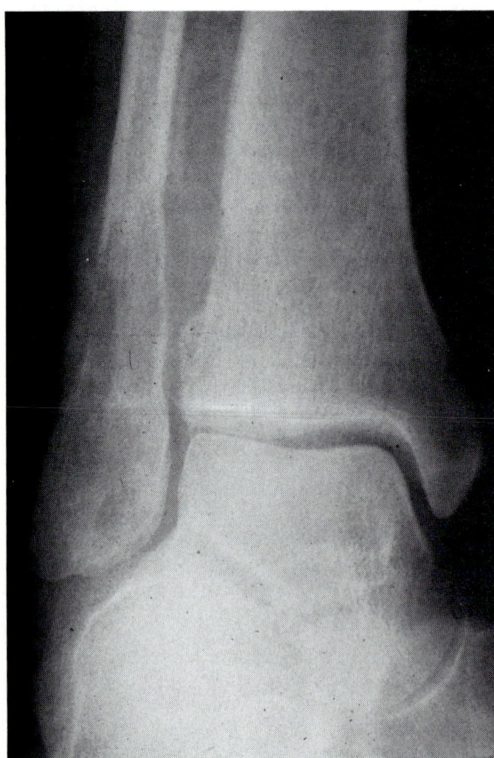

FIG 24–48.
Metastatic lung carcinoma to the lateral malleolus.

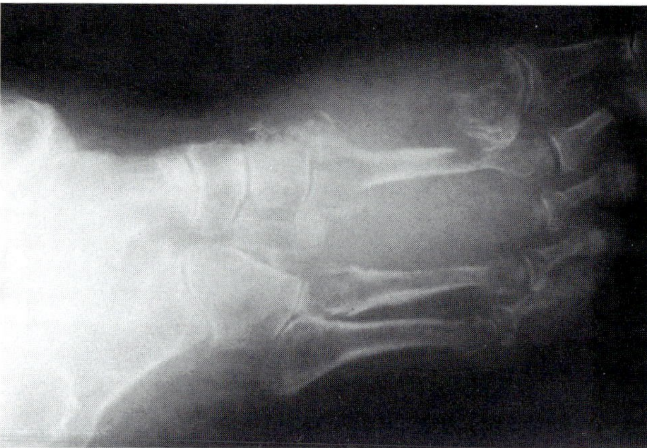

FIG 24–49.
Extensive colon metastasis to the metatarsal area of a 74-year-old female.

The tumor is slow growing and late to metastasize to the lung. Figure 24–46 is a radiographic film of a chondrosarcoma seen in the medial malleolus of a 50-year-old man. Unlike benign cartilage tumors, a malignant chondrosarcoma usually involves symptoms of pain. In the large study of these tumors of the foot by Dahlin and Salvador,[21] it was shown that local curettage is not beneficial. Treatment is by excision of the entire bone involved with the tumor. This gives very little chance of recurrence or metastasis.

Fibrosarcoma

Fibrosarcoma as a primary bone tumor of the foot is extremely rare.[36] Figure 24–47 is an example of a fibrosarcoma seen in the fifth metatarsal of a young adult man. This tumor occurs in about the same locations as osteosarcomas and the recommended treatment is amputation of the entire foot. Adjuvent chemotherapy could be considered for grade 3 to 4 lesions.

Metastatic Tumors to the Foot

It is generally unusual to find a metastatic carcinoma in the bones of the hand or foot or even distal to the elbow or knee. Of the metastatic group in this rare location, the bronchogenic carcinoma of the lung is perhaps the most common. Figure 24–48 is a radiograph of a metastatic carcinoma of the lung to the lateral malleolus with lytic destructive changes and periosteal lifting that might well suggest a primary sarcoma such as Ewing's tumor seen more typically in this location. Another example of a metastatic lesion in the foot is seen in Figure 24–49, where a carcinoma of the colon has metastasized to the metatarsal area with extensive lytic destructive changes noted. In this advanced situation an amputation is indicated in this 74-year-old female.

METABOLIC BONE DISEASE

Just as an internist looks at the chest radiograph for evidence of a generalized disease process, a physician who deals with hand or foot problems should become familiar with generalized radiographic changes in the structure of bone. Much can be learned about the general metabolic state of the entire patient from the various changes that take place in bone for one reason or another. This section will introduce some of the major categories of metabolic bone disease and present examples of these disease states as recognized on routine radiographs of the foot.

Osteoporosis

Osteoporosis is not a disease state but, in fact, is a condition of bone seen in many diseases in which there occurs a total decrease in bone volume that results in a decreased bone density and an increased bone porosity associated with decreased physical strength.

The most common cause for an osteoporotic change in normal bone is through the simple process of disuse. Just as muscle loses its volume with lack of exercise, so too does bone decrease in volume and weight if not physically stressed with activity. A good example of disuse osteoporosis is seen in Figure 24–50, a radiograph of a foot that had been in a non–weight-bearing cast for 6 weeks. The greatest degree of bone loss occurs in the metaphyseal-epiphyseal areas, where metabolic changes are seen early, as opposed to cortical bone, in which more time is needed to show thinning or increased porosity. The simple solution to this form of osteoporosis is removal of the cast as soon as possible to begin stressing the bone once again. Even weight bearing in a cast will help avoid unnecessary osteoporosis from inactivity.

Another example of osteoporosis related to the disuse

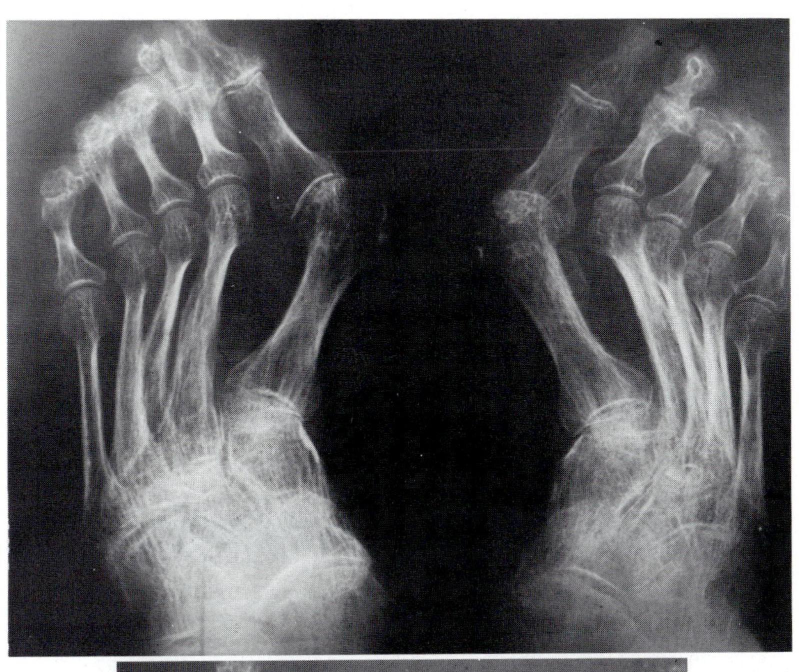

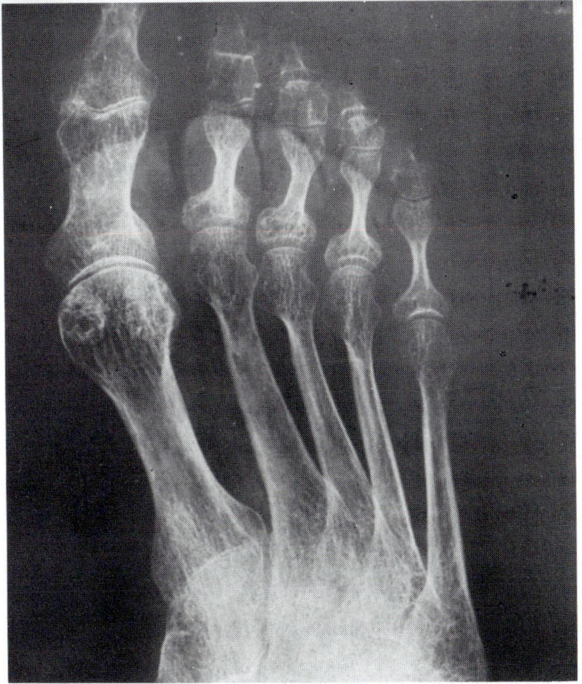

FIG 24–50.
Extensive osteoporosis; generalized decalcification.

type is *Sudeck's atrophy* (reflex sympathetic dystrophy),[12] sometimes referred to as sympathetic dystrophy of bone. This is a painful type of osteoporosis frequently seen in (often neurotic) women who sustain a minor injury to their foot that causes them to overreact to their injury by not using the foot for a prolonged period. The result is a radiographic picture like that seen in Figure 24–51, with characteristic spotty porosis throughout the midtarsal area. At first, the radiograph might suggest the infiltrative process of an inflammatory disease such as osteomyelitis. The foot may look cold and sweaty or at other times hot and swollen. These appearances have been attributed to some reflex instability of the autonomic system controlling the capillary flow of blood through the tissues of the foot. The best treatment for this chronic painful condition is to motivate the patient to exercise the foot and begin bearing weight as soon as possible. Sometimes lumbar sympathetic blocks are useful in decreasing the pain so that weight bearing can begin.

There are several hormonal abnormalities associated with osteoporosis. In *hypothyroidism* the general body metabolism slows down, and as a result, bone volume decreases. Figure 24–52 is a radiograph of the foot of a hypothyroid patient. Note the relative accentuation of the major stress trabeculae as a result of excessive loss of the finer transverse trabeculae. The bone takes on a coarsened vertical trabecular pattern, and there is thinning of the cortical anatomy of the tibia. The enlarged calcaneal spur is the by-product of any long-standing osteoporotic or osteomalacic process of bone. Other well-known hormonal causes of osteoporosis include *hyperthyroid osteoporosis* (high-turnover disease) and *steroid osteoporosis* (low-turnover disease); both diseases have a similar radiographic appearance (Fig 24–52). The most common of all porotic states in the hormone class is *postmenopausal osteoporosis*, which results from decreased blood estrogens at menopause and is seen mainly in white women. The treatment is aimed primarily at correction of the underlying hormone defect, if possible, and an attempt to stress the bone through exercise as much as possible.

It is well known that at least 30% of bone volume must be lost before osteoporotic changes can be detected on a simple clinical x-ray examination of the foot. Currently there are several commercial γ-emitting bone scanners with the technical capacity to detect a 3% or 4% loss in bone density. This can be helpful in early detection of osteoporosis or for following a given patient under treatment. Figure 24–53 is a photograph of the ^{125}I bone scanner used in our laboratory to determine

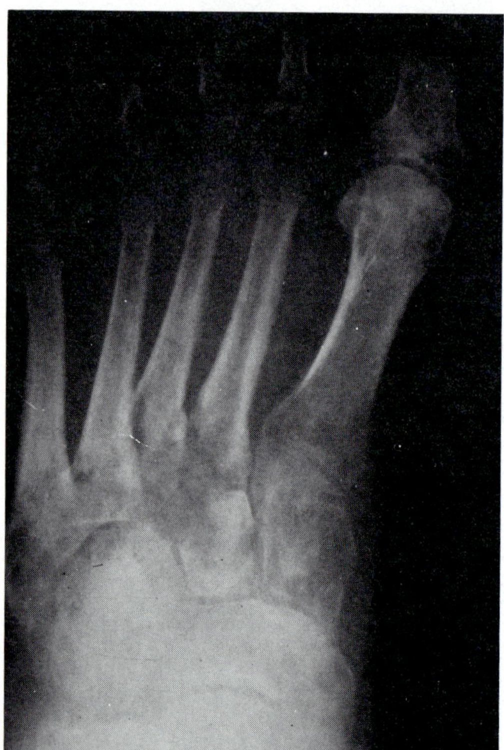

FIG 24–51.
Sudeck's atrophy in a foot as manifested by spotty osteoporosis.

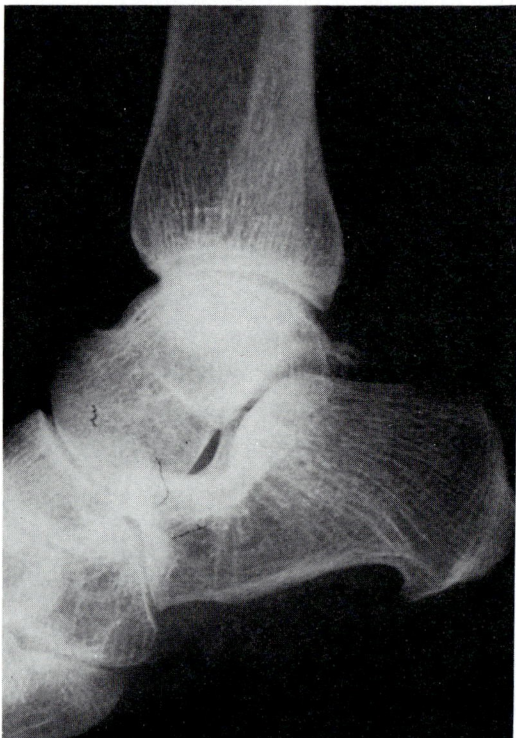

FIG 24–52.
Hypothyroid osteoporosis.

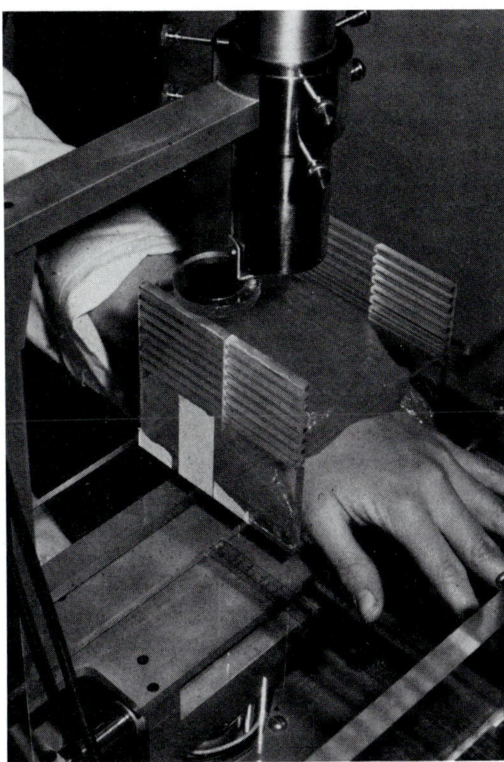

FIG 24–53.
^{125}I γ-emitting scanner to detect minute changes in bone density.

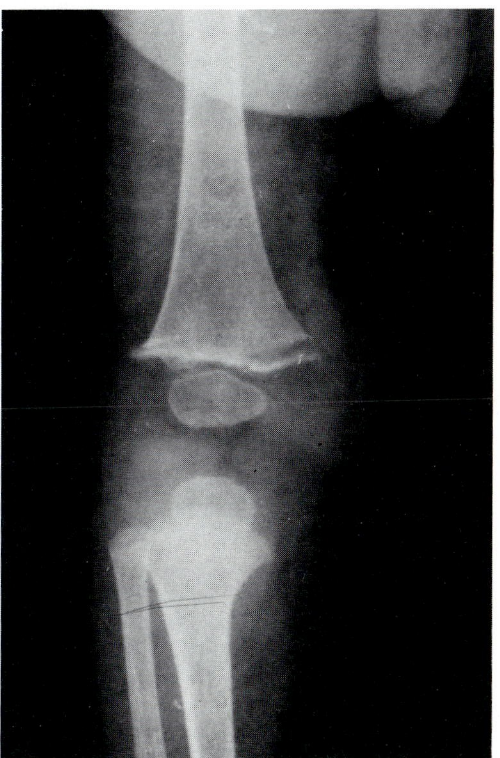

FIG 24–54.
Osteoporosis in a child with scurvy.

bone density at the wrist. Similar units are designed to scan the os calcis in the foot.

A well-known cause of osteoporosis in children is scurvy. Vitamin C is required by the body to produce collagen fiber needed to form osteoid by osteoblasts on the surface of bony trabeculae. When this vitamin is deficient, the radiograph is like Figure 24–54, which shows a child with scurvy. The thinned femoral cortex and the radiolucent scorbutic band running across the distal femoral metaphysis just above the increased radiodense markings of the zone of provisional calcification are characteristic.

Osteomalacia

Osteomalacic bone differs from osteoporotic bone insofar as there is a disproportionate loss of bone mineral as compared with bone osteoid. The result is a decrease in bone rigidity: the bone becomes more like hard rubber. In the early stages, the bone volume is affected only slightly, but if the condition persists, bone volume also decreases, and osteoporosis results as a terminal state. Numerous disease states exist that produce osteomalacia. The major ones include any intestinal disease in which there is a failure to transport calcium, phosphorus, or vitamin D across the gut wall into the bloodstream or renal disease in which there is a failure to activate vitamin D or there is a loss of too much calcium or phosphorus in the urine. Figure 24–55 is the radiograph of a typical osteomalacic ankle in an adult patient with a chronic malabsorptive syndrome of the intestinal tract. The coarsened trabecular pattern is similar to that seen in osteoporosis. Figure 24–56 is another example of the radiographic appearance of osteomalacia in an adult with chronic pancreatic insufficiency. Characteristic Looser's zones in the proximal areas of both first metatarsals are apparent. These transverse radiolucent bands have been attributed to vessels circumventing the malacic bone. Other physicians, including me, believe that the bands represent stress fractures or fatigued areas from ordinary activity on weakened bone.

The osteomalacic state in children is referred to as *rickets*, which is also a mineral-deficient state of bone created by many diseases affecting the intestinal tract or kidneys. Figure 24–57 is a radiograph of a child's foot that demonstrates severe rachitic changes resulting from a disease state known as *renal osteodystrophy*. In osteodystrophy, there are severe osteomalacic changes in bone as well as slipping of the epiphyses and calcification of the plantar ligaments not usually seen in ordinary vitamin D–deficient rickets; in ordinary rickets there is merely a

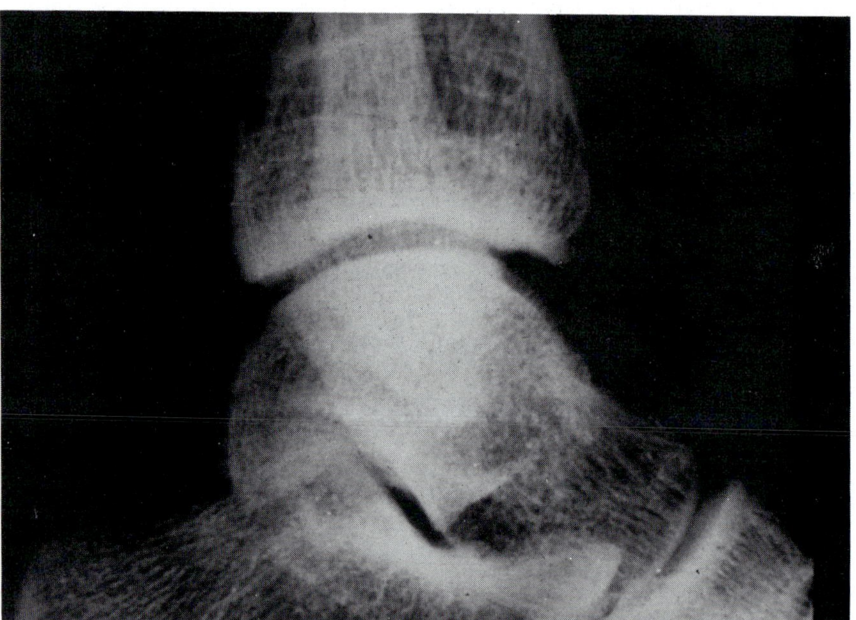

FIG 24–55.
Osteomalacia in an adult ankle.

widening of the growth plate. Renal osteodystrophy is another name for rickets following renal failure and is usually the end result of severe tubular glomerulonephritis in children. The ultimate cure for this condition is to have a renal transplant performed.

A familial condition with the physical and radiographic appearance of rickets in children is the *Schmid form* of metaphyseal chondrodysplasia (previously called metaphyseal dysostosis). Figure 24–58 is the radiograph of a child with the Schmid form of this heritable growth dysplasia, which has a widened and cupped growth plate but no evidence of the decreased bone density seen in rickets. The serum phosphorus level is normal in the Schmid syndrome and depressed in most rachitic states.

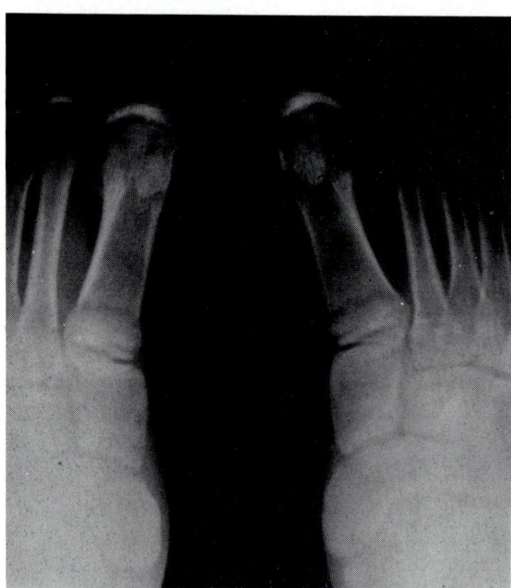

FIG 24–56.
Looser's zones in the first metatarsals of an osteomalacic bone.

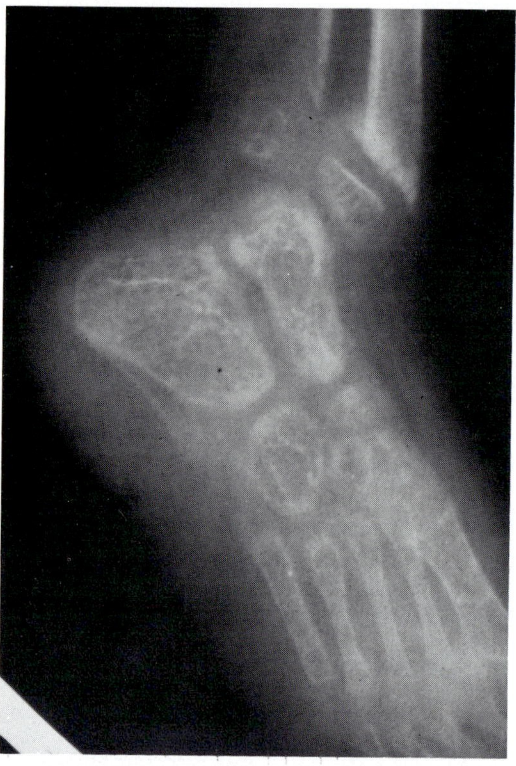

FIG 24–57.
Severe rachitic state in a child with renal osteodystrophy.

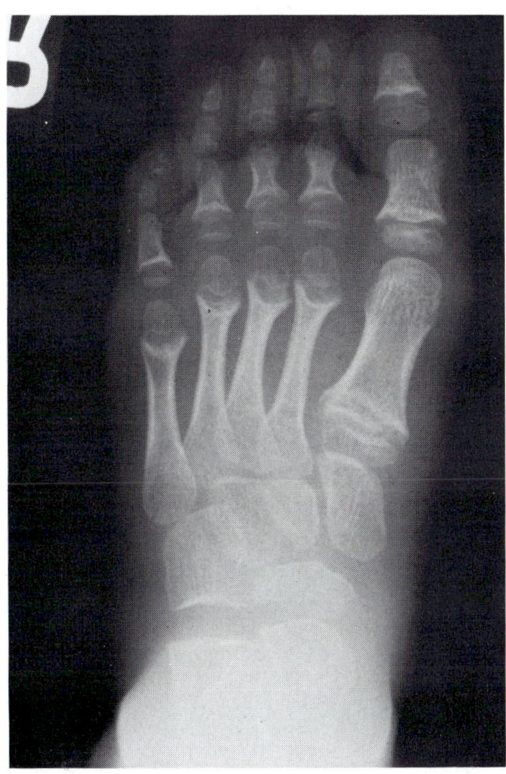

FIG 24–58.
Schmid form of metaphyseal chondrodysplasia that mimics rickets.

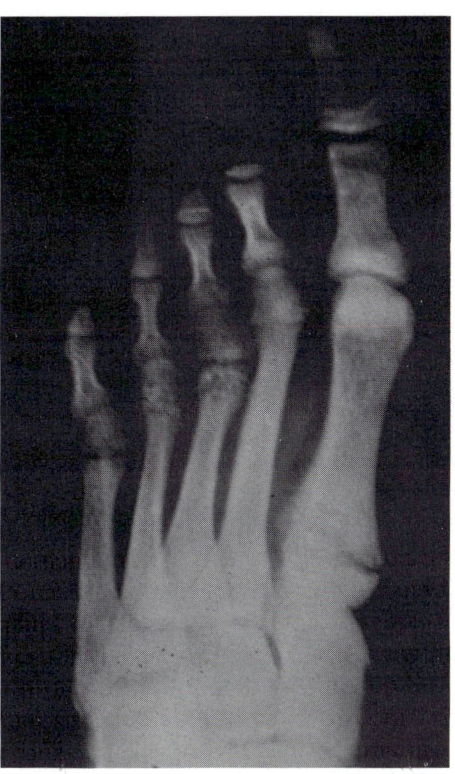

FIG 24–59.
Osteomalacic bone in an adolescent with primary hyperparathyroidism.

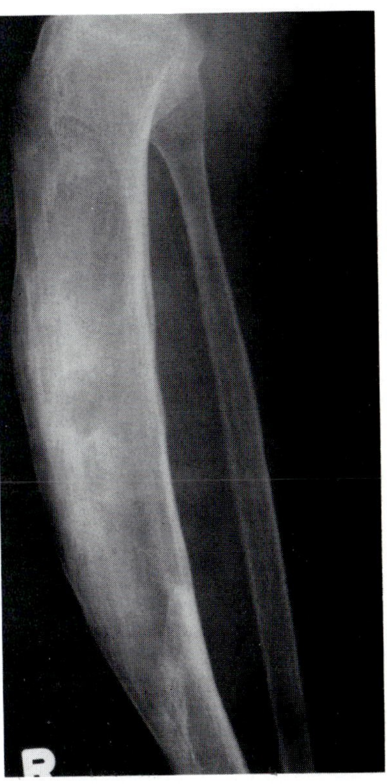

FIG 24–60.
Brown tumor of hyperparathyroidism giving the appearance of Paget disease.

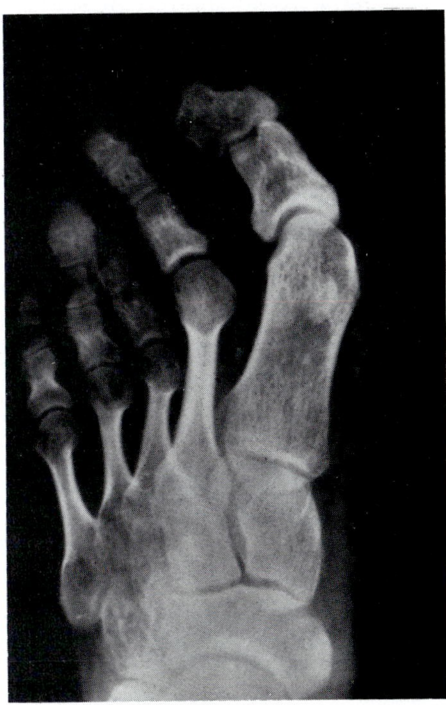

FIG 24–61.
Pseudohypoparathyroidism.

Because of a chronically suppressed serum calcium level, many forms of rickets demonstrate secondary states of hyperparathyroidism. However, there is a primary form of *hyperparathyroidism* seen following an adenoma of the parathyroid gland that causes it to put out excessive amounts of parathormone. Parathormone stimulates bone cells to destroy bony structure to mobilize large amounts of calcium into the bloodstream. If this metabolic state continues for a long time, the bones take on an osteomalacic appearance like those in Figure 24–59, which is a 14-year-old girl with a parathyroid adenoma. The bones look washed out, and there is a very specific tapering of the terminal tufts of the distal phalanges. One of the secondary complications of hyperparathyroidism is the production of pseudotumors of bone called brown tumors. These lytic aneurysmal lesions of bone are loaded with giant cells and can appear much like a giant-cell tumor of bone but are not neoplastic in any way. Figure 24–60 is a typical radiograph of a large brown tumor of the tibia that gives the appearance of Paget disease of the tibia.

Another interesting parathyroid disease of bone that frequently presents the radiographic appearance of hyperparathyroidism but exhibits low serum calcium levels is a disease known as *pseudohypoparathyroidism*. Figure 24–61 is the radiograph of a patient with this disease. Metatarsals 2 through 5 are short, with hypoplastic dis-

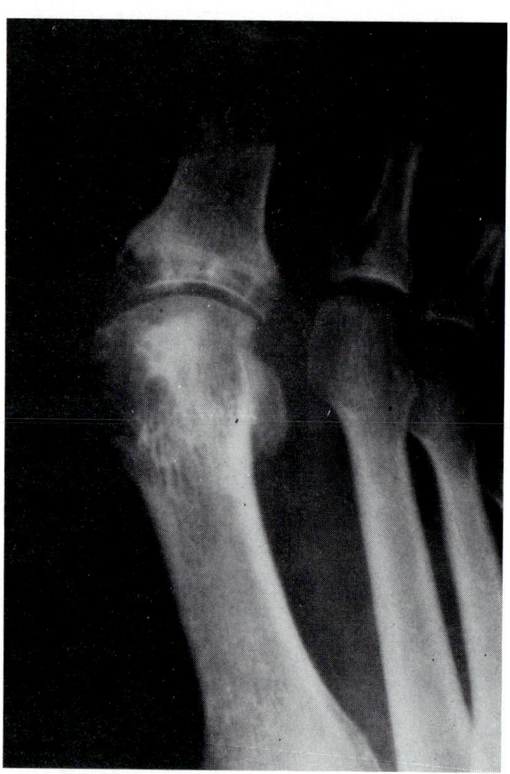

FIG 24–63.
Gouty arthropathy of the first metatarsophalangeal joint.

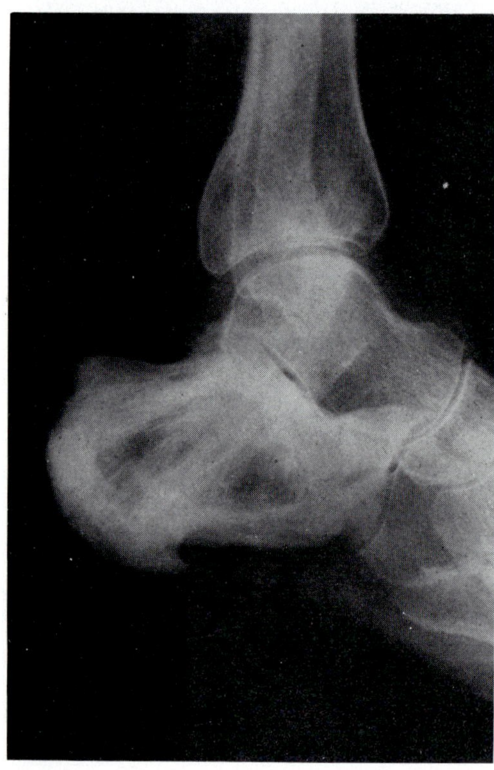

FIG 24–62.
Paget disease of the os calcis.

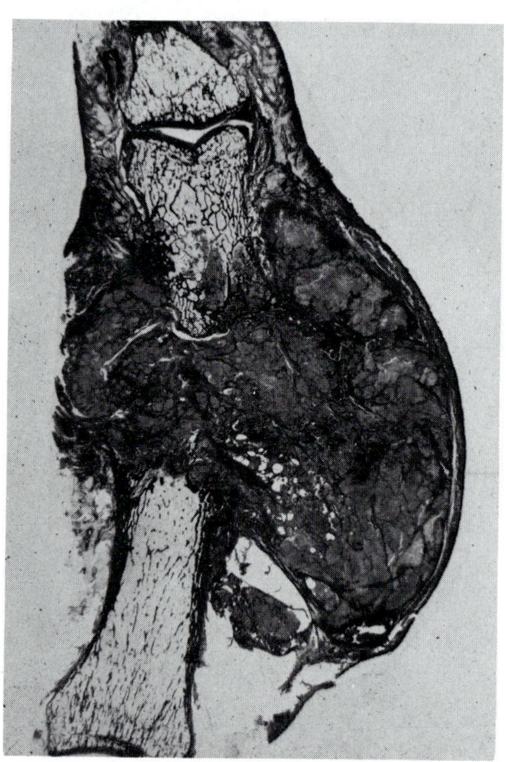

FIG 24–64.
Tophaceous gouty arthropathy of the first metatarsophalangeal joint.

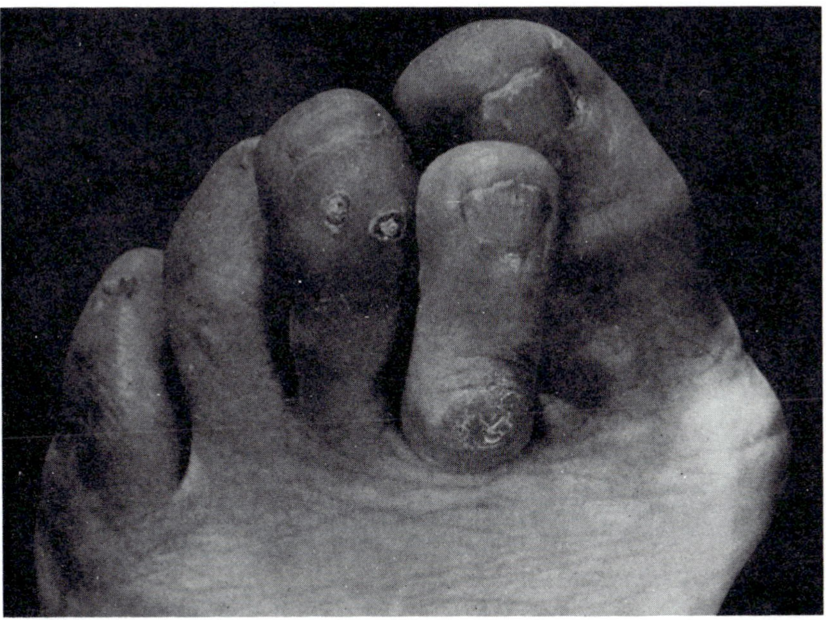

FIG 24–65.
Gouty ulcerations on the dorsum of the third toe.

tal phalanges. Subcutaneous ectopic bone is also seen. This disease results because of a heritable defect in the renal tubule that is resistant to the normal or elevated levels of parathormone in these patients.

Paget Disease

Most people still consider Paget disease of bone to be an idiopathic inflammatory disease state that initially produces a spotty hyperemic osteolysis associated with pain and an elevated alkaline phosphatase level in the blood. The bone becomes weakened because of the lytic process, and deformity results (e.g., bowing of the legs and widening of the skull). Then as a healing response by the patient, osteoblastic activity occurs, and the involved bones become very dense-appearing on x-ray examination. Figure 24–62 shows a good example of the late blastic changes seen in a pagetoid os calcis. The coarsened trabecular pattern and the chronic external enlargement of the bone shell are evident, as is the prominent calcaneal spur following the early softening phase of this disease that is similar to osteomalacia. This disease has been known to progress into a sarcoma; in the case of the hand or foot, such progression would be very unusual.

Gout

Gout is a heritable disease seen mostly in older men with a clinical picture of hyperuricemia associated with synovitis and the presence of urate deposits in soft tis-

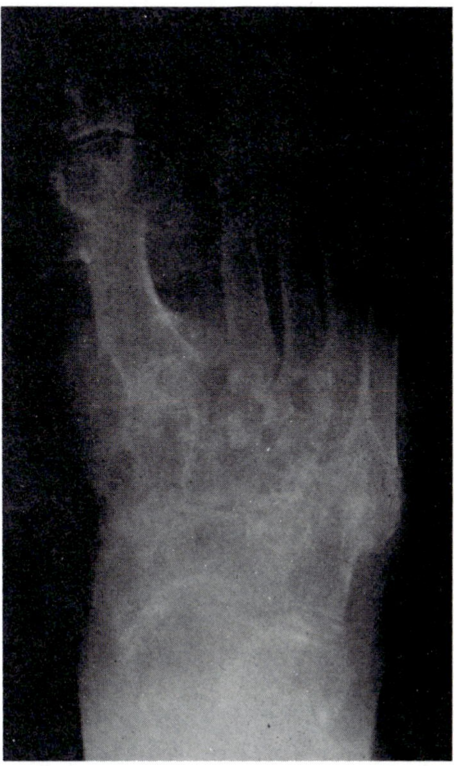

FIG 24–66.
Extensive gouty arthropathy of the midtarsal area.

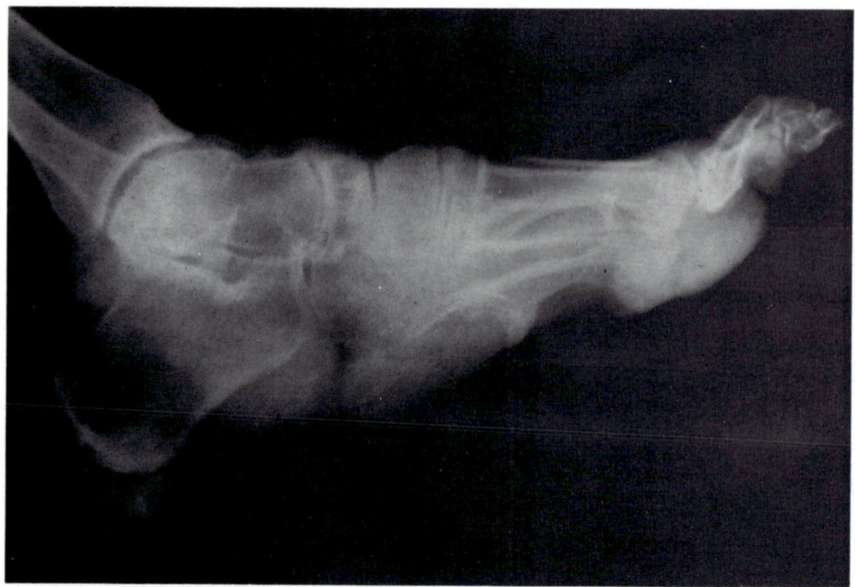

FIG 24–67.
Early tophaceous gout involving mainly subcutaneous tissues.

sue. The exact cause for the peripheral tissue production of excessive uric acid is still unknown. The condition frequently appears for the first time in the area of the first metatarsal heads with an acute intermittent cellulitis that eventually turns into a granulomatous process involving the juxta-articular structures about the first metatarsophalangeal joint (Fig 24–63). There is geographic erosion on the medial aspect of the first metatarsal head and on the base of the proximal phalanx. As time progresses, the arthritic process develops into a tophaceous condition with accumulation of urate deposits around the joint like those seen in the macroscopic section (Fig 24–64). Extensive destructive changes can be seen in the first metatarsophalangeal joint. Sometimes the presence of small cutaneous ulcerations with uric acid crystals at the center that can be scraped with a knife and viewed under the microscope confirm the clinical diagnosis of gout. Figure 24–65 shows a gouty foot with two diagnostic ulcers on the dorsum of the third toe. Figure 24–66 shows more extensive gouty arthritic changes throughout the entire midtarsal area and first ray. Tophaceous gout can produce extensive soft-tissue tumor masses beneath the skin that might suggest neurofibromatosis (as seen in Fig 24–67 in a 45-year-old with minimum arthritic changes). However, as time passes, the joints also become involved, and the tophaceous material calcifies as seen in Figure 24–68 in a much older patient. This radiograph takes on the appearance of the radiograph of a neuropathic foot. Balasubramanian and Silva[13] suggest

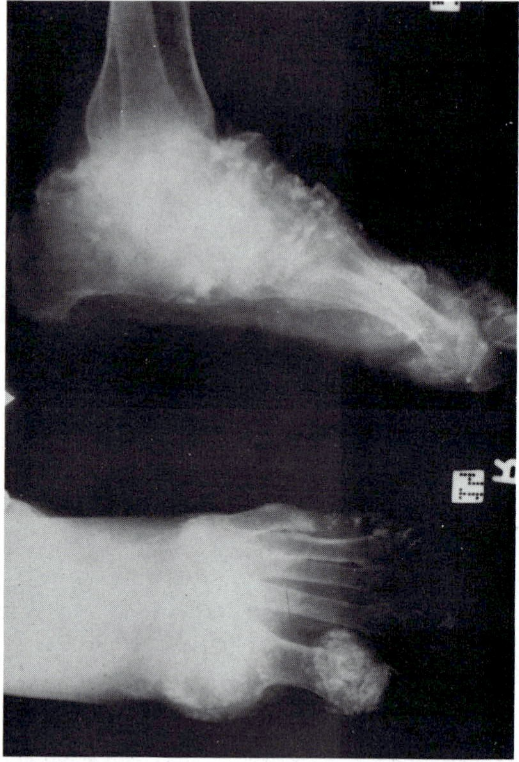

FIG 24–68.
Advanced calcific tophaceous gout in an elderly patient.

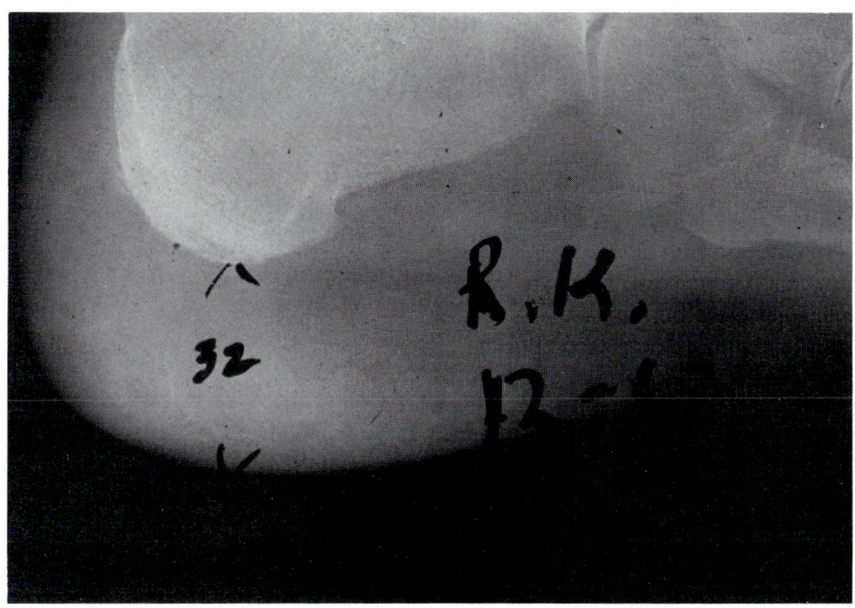

FIG 24–69.
Thickened heel pad in an acromegalic patient.

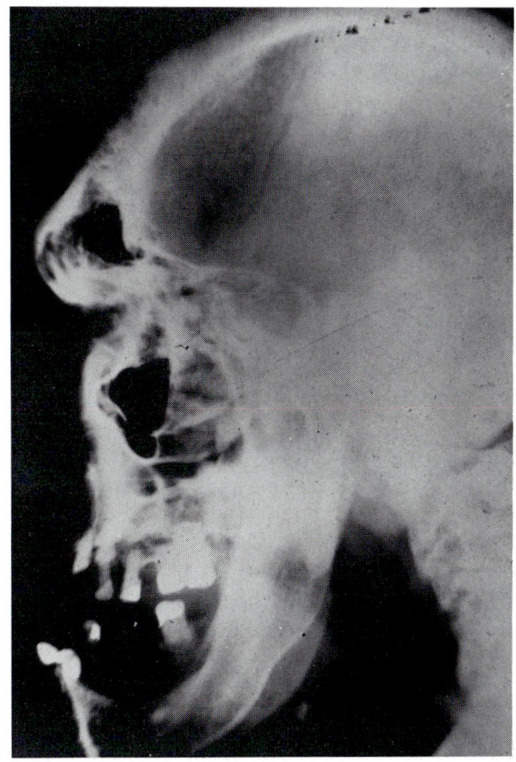

FIG 24–70.
Typical acromegalic skull and face.

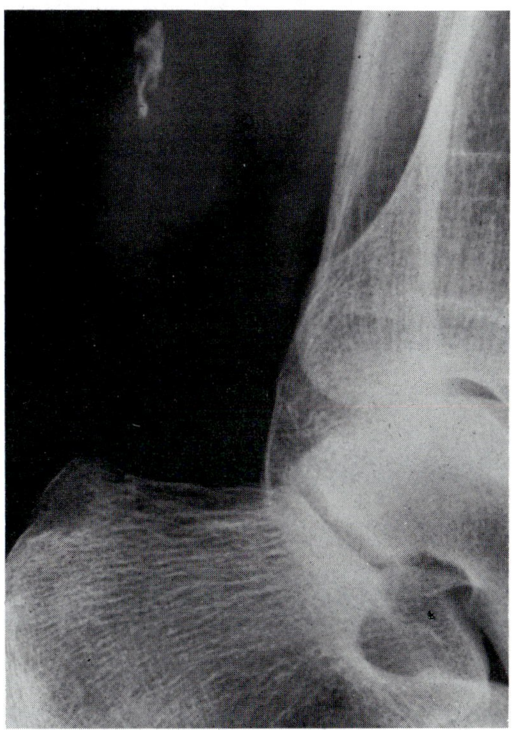

FIG 24–71.
Dystrophic calcification in the heel cord of a patient with hypercholesterolemia.

debridement of the tophi and bone grafting, if necessary.

Acromegaly

In acromegaly there is an overproduction of pituitary hormone after adult life is reached. This produces generalized hypertrophy of all somatic tissues including bone and soft tissues overlying the bones. Figure 24–69 shows an example of the thickening seen in the heel pad of such a patient. More characteristic of this disease state is the generalized hypertrophy of bone about the face and jaw (Fig 24–70). Large air sinuses and a "Dick Tracy" mandible are evident, and the sella turcica is enlarged as a result of the pituitary adenoma.

Hypercholesterolemia

Another metabolic disease state relating to the foot and ankle area is hypercholesterolemia, which can lead to the life-threatening problems of coronary artery disease and myocardial infarction. In the ankle area, however, one commonly sees evidence of dystrophic calcification in the heel cord associated with weakening of the cord, pain, and microscopic tearing in the weakened structure. Figure 24–71 shows the typical radiographic appearance of the calcification seen in a patient's heel cord associated with a fusiform enlargement of the cord that could even suggest a tumor mass.

These tendons should never be injected with cortisone, for this could increase the possibility of the pathologic rupture that occurs in a fair number of such patients. In one of my own patients both heel cords ruptured, and large deposits of cholesterol requiring multiple debridements were found in and around the area. It was eventually necessary to completely remove both heel cords because of advanced degenerative changes that frustrated any attempt at a reconstructive approach to her mechanical problem. Figure 24–72 is a photograph of this patient's heels after multiple surgical procedures.

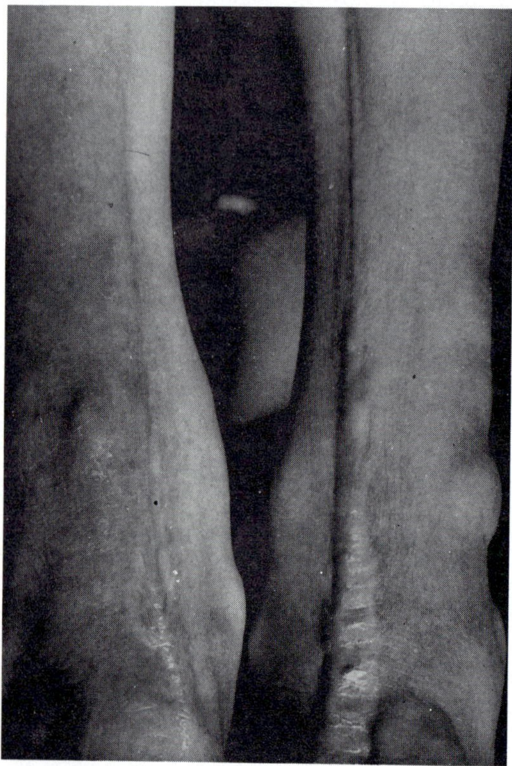

FIG 24–72.
Heel area in a hypercholesterolemic patient after complete debridement of both heel cords.

THE OSTEOCHONDROSES

The so-called osteochondroses are a wide selection of various painful conditions seen typically in growing children or young adults with associated radiographic changes in the epiphyses or apophyses adjacent to the painful area. Initially it was felt that avascular necrosis was the underlying etiology for all these conditions. However, with the passage of time and careful pathologic evaluation of these various conditions, it became apparent that many of these conditions demonstrated no evidence of bone necrosis and in some cases represented nothing more than normal variations of enchondral bone formation. The osteochondroses that do seem to have osteonecrosis as part of the clinical picture include Perthes' syndrome, Freiberg's infraction, Kienböck's disease and, perhaps, Köhler's and Panner's disease. The osteochondroses that result from repetitive stress injury to growth plates but have no evidence of bone necrosis include Osgood-Schlatter disease, Blount's disease, Scheuermann's disease and Sinding-Larsen disease. Sever's disease and ischiopubic osteochondroses are probably normal variations of ossification in which physical stress may play a role in the cause of pain. In this section special attention will be paid to the osteochondroses seen in the foot.

Köhler's Disease

Köhler first described this specific osteochondrosis of the tarsal navicular in 1908. It is felt by most that osteonecrosis occurs in this syndrome, but pathologic specimens to prove this theory are scarce because surgery is rarely required for treatment. It is seen typically in boys between the ages of 3 and 7 years. Twenty percent are bilateral and can be seen with Perthes' syndrome. Pain is frequently mild and precipitated by trauma in 35% of cases. Soft-tissue swelling about the midtarsal area is associated with a mild limp that clears spontaneously with a short period of rest and perhaps a short-leg walking cast. The characteristic radiographic changes are seen in Figure 24–73 with sclerotic flattening of the tarsonavicular ossification center. Within a period of 2 to 4 years the radiographic appearance returns to normal, and the patient is left with no disability, which would suggest the lack of any significant osteonecrosis in the early stages of this disease.

Freiberg's Infraction

Freiberg in 1914 described a syndrome of metatarsalgia associated with crushing or collapse of the metatarsal head.[28] This osteochondrosis is seen typically in the second metatarsal head in females between the ages of 13 and 18 years. It is felt to be a stress fracture through the head that results in osteonecrosis. The higher incidence in the second head is probably related to the greater length and increased rigidity of the second metatarsal. However, the third, fourth, and first heads have been involved as well. Pain and swelling is associated with a typical radiographic flattening of the involved metatarsal head, which may produce a loose osteochondral fragment that may require surgical intervention. Figure 24–74 demonstrates the typical radiologic flattening of the third metatarsal head in an 18-year-old female.

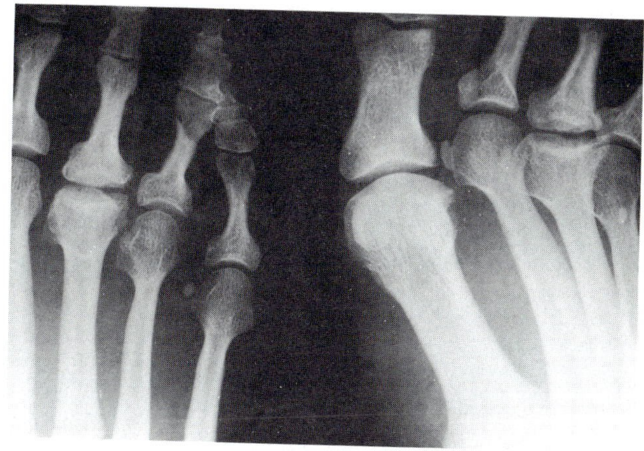

FIG 24–74.
Freiberg's infraction of the third metatarsal head in an 18-year-old female.

Sever's Disease

Sever in 1912 first described radiographic irregularities in the os calcis apophyseal center that he felt were inflammatory changes that could result in pain in a growing child.[52] Since then, others have described these same radiographic changes in asymptomatic children between the ages of 9 and 11 years that would suggest a normal variation of enchondral bone formation. The pain is probably related to a traction stress injury to the apophysis that may reflect changes in the subchondral bone as we see in Figure 24–75,A and B. This 10-year-old boy remained painful with push-off activity for 4 months and then became asymptomatic with no residual disability.

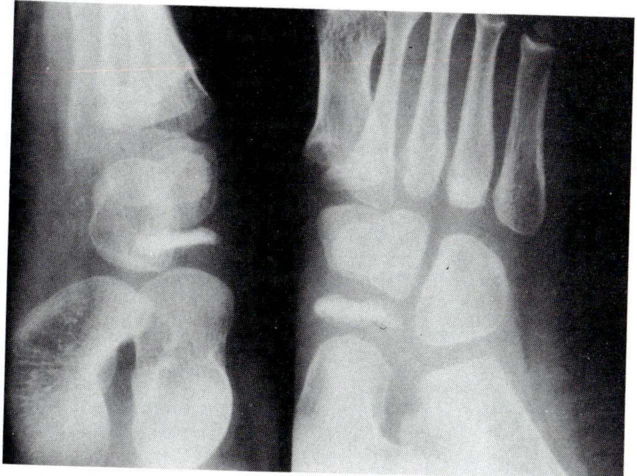

FIG 24–73.
Köhler's osteochondrosis of the tarsal navicular of a 5-year-old male.

Avascular Necrosis of the Talus

There is no specific osteochondrosis involving the talus. However, avascular necrosis of the body of the talus is a well-known complication of talar neck fractures associated with subtalar joint disruption. Trueta[43] in 1970 was the first to shed light on this problem with his classic work on the talar blood supply. He found the major blood supply enters through the medial entrance of the tarsal canal as a branch off the posterior tibial artery and named the tarsal canal artery. The tarsal canal artery then anastomoses with branches of both the dorsalis pedis and peroneal arteries that enter the tarsal canal laterally at the base of the tarsal sinus. A rich arcade of vessels then exits the tarsal canal artery to supply the major circulation to the talar body. Of great clinical importance to the trauma surgeon is the small deltoid branch coming off the tarsal canal artery just before entering the tarsal canal. This vessel courses through the lower deltoid ligament on its way to supply blood to the medial wall of the talus. It is well known that injuries to the talus with an associated subtalar dislocation will result in a 40% to 50% incidence of avascular necrosis of

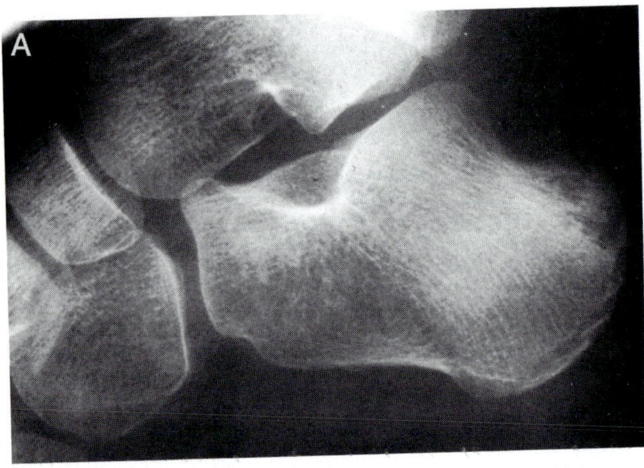

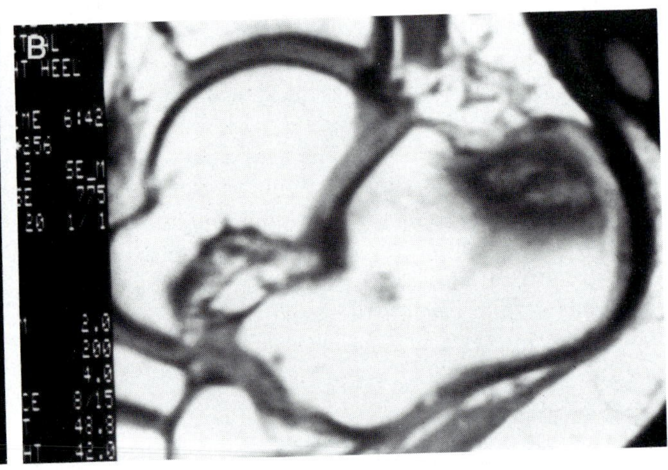

FIG 24–75.
A, Sever's disease in a 10-year-old male with subchondral changes beneath the os calcis apophysis. **B,** MRI evidence of traction injury to subchondral bone near the attachment of the heel cord.

the talus. This high incidence can be reduced if the subtalar joint anatomy is restored without damage to the deltoid branch, which is usually still preserved after significant subtalar disruption. This is best accomplished by a careful medial malleolar osteotomy for exposure of the ankle and subtalar joint without disrupting the deltoid ligament with its contained and functional deltoid branch to the medial portion of the talar body.

REFERENCES

General

1. Ackerman LV, Spjut HJ: *Tumors of bone and cartilage*, Washington, DC, 1962, Armed Forces Institute of Pathology.
2. Aegerter E, Kirkpatrick JA Jr: *Orthopedic diseases*, ed 4, Philadelphia, 1975, WB Saunders.
3. Dahlin DC: *Bone tumors*, ed 2, Springfield, Ill, 1967, Charles C Thomas.
4. Enzinger FM, Weiss SW: *Soft tissue tumors*, St Louis, 1982, Mosby–Year Book.
5. Geiser M, Trueta J: Muscle action, bone rarefaction and bone formation, *J Bone Joint Surg [Br]* 40:282, 1958.
6. Greenfield GB: *Radiology of bone diseases*, Philadelphia, 1969, JB Lippincott.
7. Jaffe HL: *Tumors and tumorous conditions of the bones and joints*, Philadelphia, 1958, Lea & Febiger.
8. Spjut HJ, Dorfman HD, Fechner RE, et al: *Tumors of bone and cartilage*, *Atlas of tumor pathology*, ser 2, fasc 5, Washington, DC, 1971, Armed Forces Institute of Pathology.
9. Stout AP, Lattes R: *Tumors of the soft tissues. Atlas of tumor pathology*, ser 2, fasc 1, Washington, DC, 1967, Armed Forces Institute of Pathology.

Specific

10. Ackerman LV: *Surgical pathology*, ed 4, St Louis, 1968, Mosby–Year Book.
11. Anderson M, Hall KV: Dermatofibrosarcoma protuberans, *Scand J Plast Reconstr Surg* 16:211, 1982.
12. Arieff AJ, Bell JL, Tigay EL, et al: Reflex physiopathic disturbances, *J Bone Joint Surg [Am]* 45:1329, 1963.
13. Balasubramanian P, Silva JF: Tophectomy and bone-grafting for extensive tophi of the feet, *J Bone Joint Surg [Am]* 53:133, 1971.
14. Bertini F, Capanna R, Biagini R, et al: Malignant fibrous histiocytoma of soft tissue, *Cancer* 56:356, 1985.
15. Cameron HU, Kostuik JP: A long-term follow-up of synovial sarcoma, *J Bone Joint Surg [Br]* 56:613, 1974.
16. Campanacci M: *Bone and soft tissue tumors*, New York, 1991, Springer-Verlag.
17. Campanacci M, Baldini N, Boriani S, et al: Giant cell tumor of bone, *J Bone Joint Surg [Am]* 69:106, 1987.
18. Capanna R, Dal Monte H, Gitelis S, et al: The natural history of unicameral bone cysts after steroid injection, *Clin Orthop* 166:204, 1982.
19. Chen KTK, Van Dyne TA: Familial plantar fibromatosis, *J Surg Oncol* 29:240, 1985.
20. Cowie RS: Benign osteoblastoma of the talus, *J Bone Joint Surg [Br]* 48:582, 1966.
21. Dahlin DC, Salvador AH: Chondrosarcoma of bones of the hands and feet; a study of 30 cases, *Cancer* 34:755, 1974.
22. Das Gupta TK, Patel MR, Chaudhuri PK, et al: The role of chemotherapy as an adjuvant to surgery in the initial treatment of primary soft tissue sarcomas in adults, *J Surg Oncol* 19:193, 1982.
23. Eisenstein R: Giant-cell tumor of tendon sheath, *J Bone Joint Surg [Am]* 50:476, 1968.
24. Enneking WF, Spanier SS, Goodman MA: A system for surgical staging of musculoskeletal sarcomas, *Clin Orthop* 153:106, 1980.
25. Enzinger FM, Weiss SW: Benign tumors and tumorlike lesions of blood vessels. In *Soft tissue tumors*, St Louis, 1983, Mosby–Year Book, p 379.
26. Enzinger FM, Weiss SW: Benign tumors and tumorlike lesions of uncertain histogenesis. In *Soft tissue tumors*, St Louis, 1983, Mosby–Year Book, p 771.
27. Enzinger FM, Weiss SW: Benign tumors of peripheral

nerve. In *Soft tissue tumors*, St Louis, 1983, Mosby–Year Book, p 580.

28. Freiberg AH: Infraction of the second metatarsal bone; a typical injury, *Surg Gynecol Obstet* 19:191, 1914.
29. Genant HK, Kozin F, Beckerman C, et al: The reflex sympathetic dystrophy syndrome, *Radiology* 117:21, 1975.
30. Hawkins L: Fractures of the neck of the talus, *J Bone Joint Surg [Am]* 52:991, 1970.
31. Hughes ESR: Painful heels in children, *Surg Gynecol Obstet* 86:64, 1948.
32. Johnston JO: Treatment of giant cell tumor of bone by aggressive curettage and packing with bone cement. In Enneking W, editor: *Limb salvage in musculoskeletal oncology*, New York, 1987, Churchill Livingstone.
33. Jones FE, Soule EH, Coventry MD: Fibrous xanthoma of synovium (giant-cell tumor of tendon sheath, pigmented nodular synovitis), *J Bone Joint Surg [Am]* 51:76, 1969.
34. Keller RB, Baez-Giangreco A: Juvenile aponeurotic fibroma: report of three cases and a review of the literature, *Clin Orthop* 106:198, 1975.
35. Köhler A: Ueber eine haufige bisher anscheinend unbekannte Erkrankung einzelner Kindlicherkernochen, *Munchen Med Wochnschr* 55:1923, 1908.
36. Larsson SE, Lorentzon R, Boquist L: Fibrosarcoma of bone: a demographic, clinical and histopathological study of all cases recorded in the Swedish Cancer Registry from 1958 to 1968, *J Bone Joint Surg [Br]* 58:412, 1976.
37. Lewis GM: *Practical dermatology*, ed 3, Philadelphia, 1967, WB Saunders.
38. Lewis RJ, Marcove RC, Rosen G: Ewing's sarcoma—functional effects of radiation therapy, *J Bone Joint Surg [Am]* 59:325, 1977.
39. Makely J: Personal communication, 1982.
40. McCauley RGK, Kahn PC: Osteochondritis of the tarsal navicular. Radioisotopic appearances, *Radiology* 123:705, 1977.
41. McNeill TW, Ray RD: Hemangioma of the extremities: a review of 35 cases, *Clin Orthop* 101:154, 1974.
42. Merkow RL, Lane JM: Metabolic bone disease and Paget's disease in the elderly: Part II. Paget's disease, *Clin Rheumatol Dis* 12:70–96, 1986.
43. Mulfinger GL, Trueta J: The blood supply of the talus, *J Bone Joint Surg [Br]* 52:160, 1970.
44. Pedersen HE, Day AJ: Dupuytren's disease of the foot, *JAMA* 154:33, 1954.
45. Pettersson H, Gillespy T III, Hamlin DJ, et al: Primary musculoskeletal tumors: Examination with MRI compared with conventional modalities, *Radiology* 164:237–241, 1987.
46. Pritchard DJ: Small round-cell tumors, *Orthop Clin North Am* 20:367–375, 1989.
47. Pritchard DJ, Dahlin DC, Dauphine RT, et al: Ewing's sarcoma: a clinicopathological and statistical analysis of patients surviving five years or longer, *J Bone Joint Surg [Am]* 57:10, 1975.
48. Raisz LG: Local and systemic factors in the pathogenesis of osteoporosis, *N Engl J Med* 318:808–828, 1988.
49. Riggs BL, Wakner HW: Bone densitometry and clinical decision-making in osteoporosis (editorial), *Ann Intern Med* 108:293–295, 1988.
50. Rosen G, Caparros B, Huvos AG, et al: Preoperative chemotherapy for osteosarcoma: selection of postoperative adjutant chemotherapy based on the response of the primary to preoperative chemotherapy, *Cancer* 49:1221, 1982.
51. Rosen G, Caparros B, Nirenberg A, et al: Ewing's sarcoma: 10-year experience with adjuvant chemotherapy, *Cancer* 47:2204, 1981.
52. Sever JW: Apophysitis of the os calcis, *N Y Med J* 95:1025, 1912.
53. Simon MA, Enneking WF: The management of soft tissue sarcomas of the extremities, *J Bone Joint Surg [Am]* 58:317, 1976.
54. Smillie IS: Freiberg's infarction, *J Bone Joint Surg [Br]* 39:580, 1955.
55. Smyth M: Glomus-cell tumors in the lower extremity: report of two cases, *J Bone Joint Surg [Am]* 53:157, 1971.
56. Spanos PK, Payne WS, Ivins JC, et al: Pulmonary resection for metastatic osteogenic sarcoma, *J Bone Joint Surg [Am]* 58:624, 1976.
57. Stening WS: Primary malignant tumors of calcaneal tendon, *J Bone Joint Surg [Br]* 50:676, 1968.
58. Tepper J, Glaubiger D, Lichter A, et al: Local control of Ewing sarcoma of bone with irradiation therapy and combined chemotherapy, *Cancer* 46:1969, 1980.
59. Tonai M, Campbell CJ, Ahn GH, et al: Osteoblastoma: classification and report of 16 cases, *Clin Orthop* 167:222, 1982.
60. Winkler K, Beron G, Delling G, et al: Neoadjuvant chemotherapy of osteosarcomas, *J Clin Oncol* 6:329–337, 1988.
61. Wright PH, Sim FH, Soule EH, et al: Synovial sarcoma, *J Bone Joint Surg [Am]* 64:112, 1982.

CHAPTER

25

Toenail Abnormalities

Michael J. Coughlin, M.D.

Anatomy

Dermatologic and systemic nail disorders

Psoriasis
Eczema and contact dermatitis
Pyodermas
Systemic diseases

Genetic disorders with nail changes

Trauma

Tumors

Glomus tumor
Subungual exostosis
  Treatment
Melanotic whitlow, malignant melanoma
Other tumorous conditions

Onychopathies and other common nail abnormalities

Common nail plate disorders
  Onychocryptosis
  Onychauxis/onychogryphosis
  Onychomycosis
  Onychia
  Onycholysis/onychomadesis
Nail bed disorders
  Subungual exostosis
  Subungual tumors
  Subungual clavus
  Subungual hematoma
  Subungual verruca
Nail fold disorders
  Paronychia
  Onychophosis
  Pyogenic granuloma
  Herpetic whitlow
  Periungual verruca
Nail matrix disorders
  Anonychia
  Pterygium
  Atrophy/hypertrophy of the nail matrix
  Pathologic keratinization

Conservative and surgical treatment of toenail problems

Digital anesthetic block
Partial nail plate avulsion
Complete toenail avulsion
Plastic reduction of the nail lip
Partial onychectomy (Winograd or Heifetz procedure)
Complete onychectomy (The Zadik procedure)
Syme's amputation (Thompson-Terwilliger procedure)
Phenol/alcohol matrisectomy

Diseases and deformities of the toenails are among the most common and disabling of foot problems. While a small percentage of toenail abnormalities result from systemic diseases such as psoriasis and endocrine disorders, the majority are accounted for by intrinsic factors and are directly or indirectly related to tinea infections. The remaining deformities stem from mechanical problems and constitute some of the most common yet difficult foot problems for the treating physician.

Krausz, during 41 years of practice,[45, 59] reported on 7,670 patients displaying one or more nail disorders. While little exists regarding reports on the documented frequency of the occurrence of nail disorders by physicians, Krausz reported on the incidence of nail disorders in his practice (Table 25–1).

Diseases of the nail may be local or systemic affections or may be the result of a congenital malformation. The nails are special cutaneous appendages, the primary function of which is protection of the distal phalanx. The nail has only a few pathologic responses to disease and may demonstrate abnormalities as a manifestation of either systemic or dermatologic diseases. However, before examining specific examples of nail

TABLE 25–1.
Frequency of Pathologic Nail Conditions*

Condition	Frequency
Onychocryptosis	26%
Onychogryphosis/onychauxis	23%
Onychophosis	19%
Onychomycosis	8%
Onychotrophia	4%
Onychorrhexis	4%
Miscellaneous	6%

*Data from Krausz CE: *Br J Chir* 35:117, 1970; and Nzuzi SM: *Clin Podiatr Med Surg* 6:273–294, 1989.

disorders, an understanding of the anatomy and physiology of the toenail and supporting structures is advantageous in understanding pathologic conditions.

ANATOMY

The toenail or nail plate is composed of several layers of dense, overlapping keratinized cells. The nail plate consists of three layers, each originating from a different area of the nail unit. The relatively thin dorsal layer is stiff and brittle and covers the relatively thick middle layer. The deep layer is believed to be in part derived from the nail bed itself.[34] The nail plate differs from hair or skin in that it does not desquamate skin cells. The hardness of the nail plate can be attributed to the paucity of water within the nail plate as compared with that in the skin. While the nail plate is ten times more permeable to water than the skin, the nail plate, because of its low fat content, is unable to retain water.[5] The hardness of the nail plate is attributed to its high sulfur content.[22]

The normal nail plate advances distally approximately 0.03 to 0.05 mm day, and it has a thickness of between 0.5 and 1 mm.[57] The nail plate is supported by the nail unit,[25] an area of epithelial tissue that is divided into four components[87] (Fig 25–1):

1. Nail bed
2. Hyponychium
3. Proximal nail fold
4. Nail matrix

The toenail plate lies on the nail bed, a roughened epithelial surface that consists of longitudinal grooves that interdigitate with corresponding grooves on the undersurface of the toenail. This creates a firm bonding of the nail plate to the nail bed. The nail bed does not typically contain basal cells, the germinative cell that produces the nail plate. At the distal end of the nail bed, as the nail bed and nail plate separate, a smooth border of skin called the hyponychium is found. The hyponychium forms a seal between the distal end of the toenail and the toenail bed.

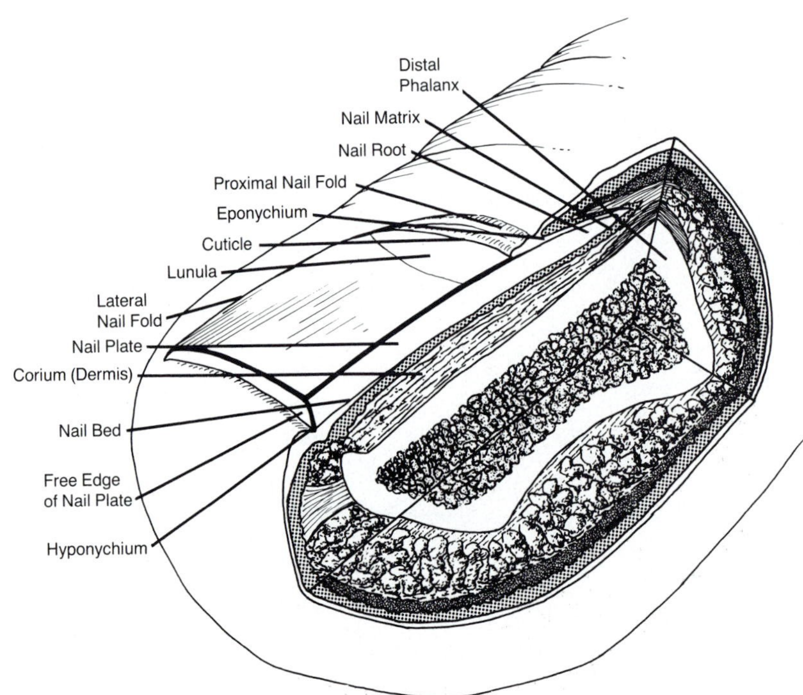

FIG 25–1.
Longitudinal section of the distal end of the toe demonstrating the components of the nail unit.

On the tibial and fibular borders of the toenail, the nail plate is surrounded by epidermal skin folds called "lateral nail folds." The base of the toenail is covered by the proximal nail fold, a complex structure that does participate in the germination of the nail plate. The dorsal surface of the nail fold is composed of skin on the dorsal surface of the toe. On the plantar surface of this fold, the eponychium forms a thin surface that attaches to the nail plate. The distal surface of these two components of the proximal nail fold composes the cuticle.

The toenail matrix is the main germinal area for the toenail. The toenail matrix extends from a point just distal to the lunula and as far laterally as the entire width of the nail plate.[21] The matrix extends 5 to 6 mm proximal to the edge of the cuticle and closely borders on the insertion of the long extensor tendon and the interphalangeal joint.[34] The nail matrix is seen beneath the nail plate as the lunula, the opaque crescent-shaped area at the base of the nail. Distally the toenail matrix is contiguous with the toenail bed. The germinal matrix is covered by a small epidermal surface and does not have the epidermal ridges characteristic of the nail bed. At the distal end of the lunula, the nail matrix terminates. At the proximal margin of the matrix, there appears to be a small area on the plantar surface of the proximal nail fold that contributes to nail plate growth.[34, 50, 70]

The major area of matrix germination occurs between the apex of the matrix and the distal border of the lunula. The area covered by the proximal nail fold forms the thin dorsal layer of the toenail plate.[34] The area of the lunula produces the thicker and softer area of the middle portion of the nail plate and joins with the dorsal area to form the toenail plate.[34] While the toenail matrix is the major germinal area for toenail growth, microscopic toenail matrix may be contained within the nail folds and the distal nail bed.[47] This produces a thin layer of the ventral toenail plate, a factor that may occasionally cause postoperative recurrence.[21, 34, 50]

The orientation of the matrix cells of the nail plate is in a longitudinal fashion. Because of pressure from the proximal nail fold, the nail plate grows in a distal rather than an elevated position. However, if the nail matrix is injured or altered because of trauma or surgery, the nail plate may grow in an abnormal direction. Likewise, the nail plate gives a certain rigidity to the soft tissue of the distal part of the toe. If the toenail is removed or ablated, the distal nail bed and soft tissue may become elevated due to upward pressure on these soft tissues (Fig 25–2). As the new nail plate begins to grow distally, it may abut against these soft tissues and lead to a club nail or an ingrown toenail.

Common diseases involving the nail include infection, psoriasis, contact dermatitis and eczema, tumor,

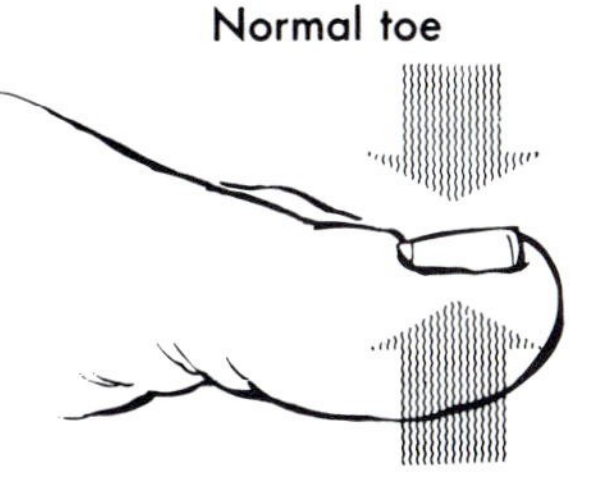

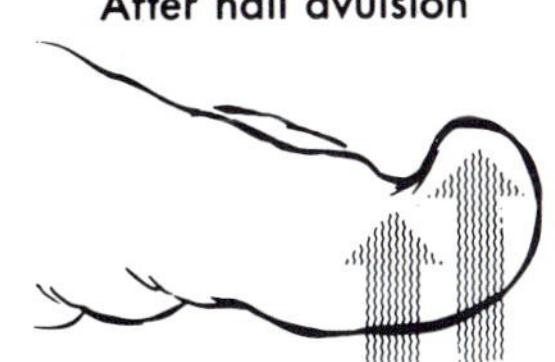

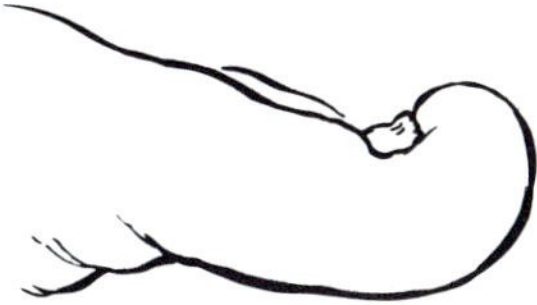

FIG 25–2.
Deformity of the distal end of the toe following nail plate avulsion. Due to a lack of soft-tissue support, clubbing may result along with impingement of the distal nail plate upon regrowth. (Adapted from Lloyd-Davies RW, Brill GC: *Br J Surg* 50:592, 1963.)

trauma, as well as general or systemic diseases.[79] Pardo-Castello[64] published a systematic review of nail disorders. This work classifies nail disorders and provides a useful means to categorize both common and less common nail abnormalities. The classification included the following:

1. Dermatologic and systemic diseases
2. Congenital and genetic nail disorders
3. Common nail affectations and onychodystrophies

Traumatic affectations and neoplasia are also considered within this generalized discussion.

Nzuzi[60] presented a logical classification of onychopathies based upon the anatomic structures primarily involved:

1. Nail plate disorders
2. Nail bed disorders
3. Nail fold disorders
4. Nail matrix disorders

Using Pardo-Castello's general classification for an overview of nail disorders and Nzuzi's classification for common nail affectations (onychopathies) provides a complete and systematic approach to a discussion of toenail disorders.

DERMATOLOGIC AND SYSTEMIC NAIL DISORDERS

Skin disorders involving the nails are usually within the province of the dermatologist. Systemic disorders involving nails may present to the treating physician but are typically within the scope of practice of the internist. Few of these entities require localized or systemic treatment. Nonetheless, an awareness of the underlying pathology as well as an understanding of the nail changes associated with specific dermatologic and systemic disorders helps to make a consulting physician aware of the myriad of generalized signs and symptoms associated with toenail abnormalities and assists in making a definitive diagnosis. Pathologic conditions of the toenail are defined in Table 25–2.

Psoriasis

Psoriasis of the toenails is a frequent accompaniment of the cutaneous disease and is often mistaken for fungal

TABLE 25–2.

Terms for Pathologic Conditions of the Nail

Anonychia.—Anonychia is the absence of nails. When the absence is congenital, it usually involves all of the nails, and the condition is permanent. This condition may also occur temporarily due to trauma or as a result of systemic or local disease. It is also seen in the nail-patella syndrome.

Beau's lines.—Beau's lines are transverse lines or ridges marking repeated disturbances of nail growth. They may be associated with trauma or a systemic disease process.

Clubbing.—Clubbing of the nail is associated with chronic pulmonary disease as well as cardiac disease.

Hapalonychia.—Hapalonychia refers to extremely soft nails that may be prone to splitting. This is associated with endocrine disturbances and malnutrition as well as contact with strong alkali solutions.

Hemorrhage.—Hemorrhage beneath the toenail may be associated with vitamin C deficiency, subacute bacterial endocarditis, as well as dermatologic disorders. Subungual hematoma follows trauma to the toenail bed.

Hyperkeratosis subungualis.—Hypertrophy of the nail bed that may be associated with onychomycosis, psoriasis, and other dermatologic disorders.

Koilonychia.—Concavity of the nail plate in both the longitudinal and transverse axis that is associated with nutritional disorders, iron deficiency anemia, and endocrine disorders.

Leukonychia.—White spots or striations in the nail resulting from trauma and systemic diseases such as nutritional and endocrine deficiencies.

Onychotrophia.—Atrophy or failure of development of a nail caused by trauma, infection, endocrine dysfunction, or systemic disease.

Onychauxis.—A greatly thickened nail plate caused by persistent mild trauma and/or onychomycosis.

Onychia.—Inflammation of the nail matrix causing deformity of the nail plate. Trauma, infection, and systemic diseases such as exanthemas are causes.

Onychitis.—Inflammation of the nail.

Onychoclasis.—Breakage or fracture of the nail plate.

Onychocryptosis.—Ingrowing of the nails or more specifically hypertrophy of the nail lip. Also referred to as hypertrophied ungualabia, it is one of the most frequent pathologic conditions of the toenail.

Onychogryphosis.—Claw nail or ram's horn nail. Extreme hypertrophy of the nail gives the appearance of a claw or horn. The condition may be congenital or a symptom of many chronic systemic diseases such as tinea infections. See onychauxis, synonym.

Onycholysis.—Loosening of the nail plate beginning along the distal or free edge when trauma, injury by chemical agents, or diseases loosen the nail plate. This condition is associated with psoriasis, onychomycosis, acute fevers, and syphilis.

Onychoma.—A tumor of the nail unit.

Onychomadesis.—Complete loss of the nail plate.

Onychomalacia.—Softening of the nail.

Onychomycosis.—Fungal infection of the nail associated with fungal disease of the foot.

Onychorrhexis.—Longitudinal riding and splitting of the nails caused by dermatoses, nail infections, systemic diseases, senility, or injury by chemical agents.

Onychoschizia.—Lamination and scaling away of the nails in thin layers caused by dermatoses, syphilis, or injury by chemical agents.

Onychosis.—Disease or deformity of the nail plate.

Pachyonychia.—Extreme thickening of all the nails. In this condition the nails are more solid and more regular than in onychogryphosis. Usually this is a congenital condition associated with hyperkeratosis of the palms and soles.

Paronychia.—Inflammation of the soft tissues about the nail margin. It may occur after infection or trauma. The infectious agent may be either bacterial or fungal.

Pterygium.—The cuticle appears to grow distal to the nail plate and splits the nail into two or more portions that gradually reduce in size as the pterygium widens. This may result from trauma as well as decreased circulation in the toes.

involvement of the nail by the lay population (Fig 25–3,A and B). The most severe form of nail involvement with psoriasis, which sometimes involves shedding of the nail (onychomadesis), is associated with psoriatic arthritis; however, many patients without arthritic changes who have psoriasis show the following abnormal findings[86]:

1. Stipling or geographic pitting (tiny, often grooved depressions in the surface of the nail plate) (Fig 25–3,C and D). This change is not unique for psoriasis but can also be seen in alopecia areata.
2. Onycholysis, especially lateral and distal (sometimes with yellowing and opacity of the nail plate, which becomes separated from the nail bed) (Fig 25–4,A).
3. Crumbling of the nail plate.
4. Subungual keratosis (Fig 25–4,B and C).

These changes may frequently be confused with onychomycosis. Scrapings of the nails for microscopic examination and fungal cultures should be made before therapy is instituted.

Treatment of psoriatic nail changes of the feet are generally unsatisfactory. Intralesional injection of corticosteroids may be effective for treating fingernails af-

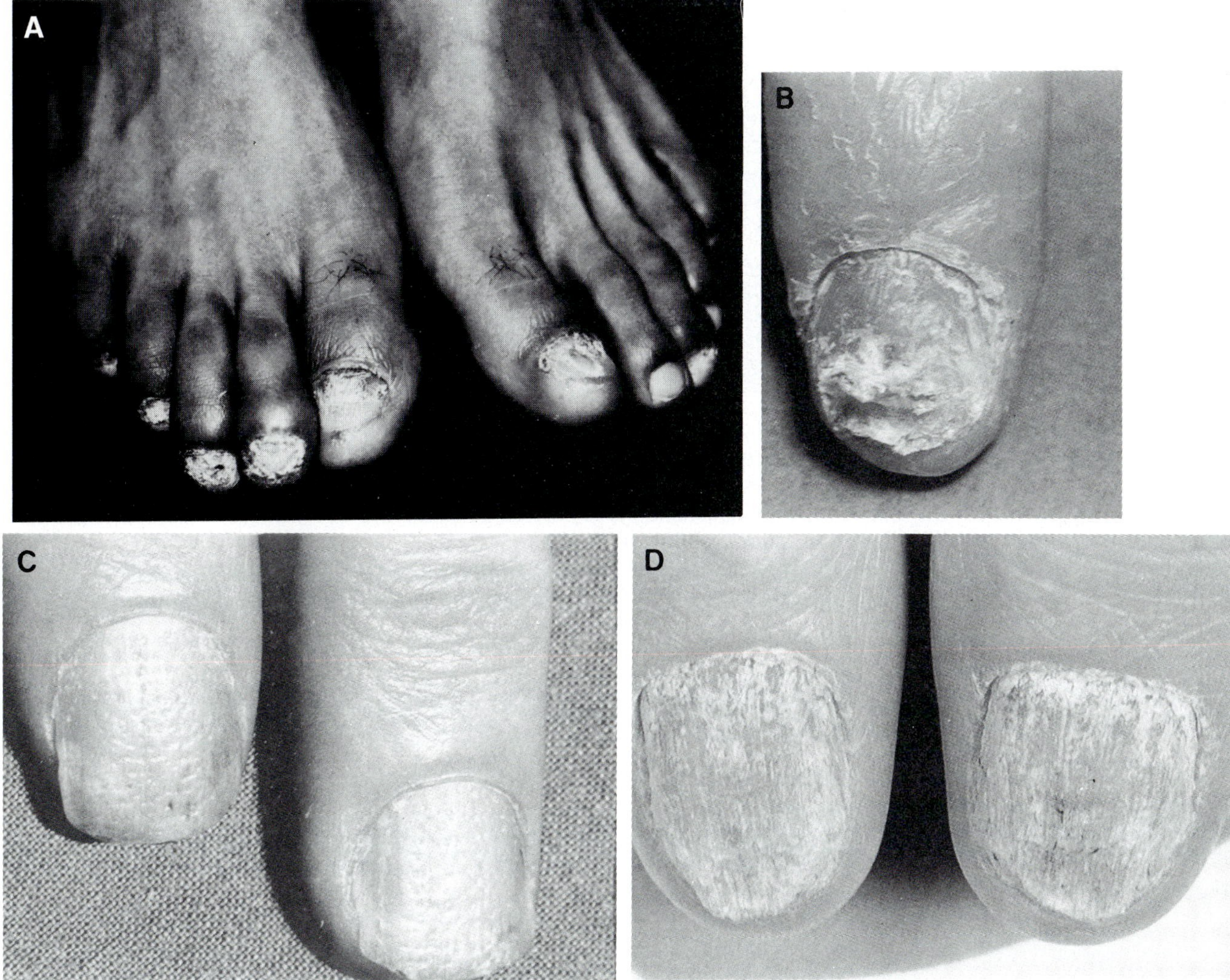

FIG 25–3.
A, psoriatic toenail dystrophy. Severe destruction of the nail plates is occasionally seen in psoriasis associated with arthritis. The crumbly appearance of the nails may be identical to that of onychomycosis, which should be ruled out by appropriate tests. **B,** psoriasis may cause gross deformation of the nail plate. **C,** Psoriasis may lead to pitting and onycholysis of the nail plate. **D,** pitting may occur in a linear fashion and produce longitudinal lines with chronic psoriatic disease. (**B–D** from duViver A: *Atlas of clinical dermatology,* ed 2, London, 1992, Gower Medical Publishing. Used by permission.)

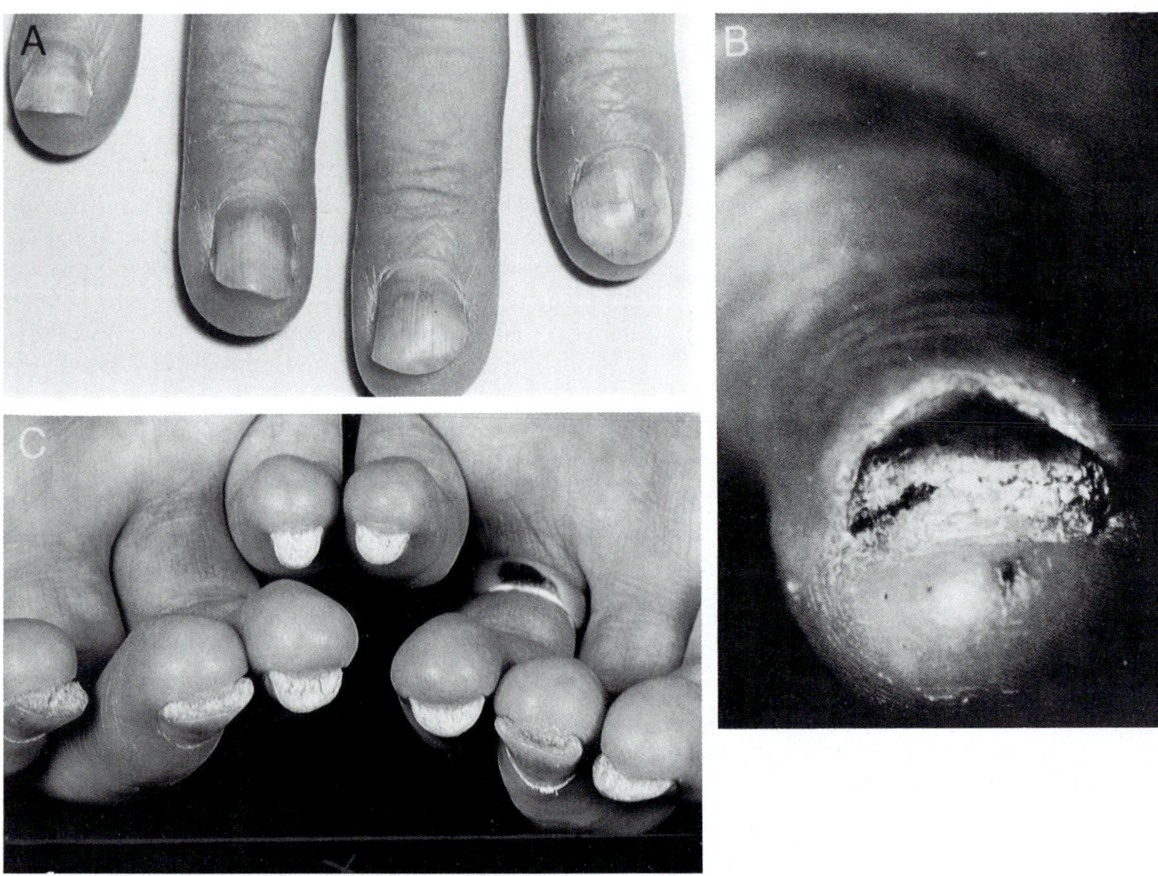

FIG 25–4.
A, extensive onycholysis may develop with psoriasis. This development may occur in the absence of psoriatic findings elsewhere, which makes the clinical diagnosis difficult. This patient developed cutaneous psoriasis 1 year later. **B,** subungual hyperkeratosis is a frequent finding of psoriasis. **C,** symmetric hyperkeratotic psoriasis may develop beneath the nails and lead to onycholysis. (**A** and **C** from duViver A: *Atlas of clinical dermatology,* ed 2, London, 1992, Gower Medical Publishing. **B** from Moschella SL, Hurley H, editors: *Dermatology,* ed 2, Philadelphia, 1986, WB Saunders, p 1411. Used by permission.)

flicted with psoriasis,[8] but similar therapy on involved toenails is less often performed.

Eczema and Contact Dermatitis

Eczema and contact dermatitis frequently involve not only the skin on the dorsum of the toes but also the lateral and proximal nail folds. With chronic inflammatory changes of a long-standing duration, abnormalities of the nail plate may occur. Transverse ridging and scaling as well as discoloration of the nail plate may develop. Accumulation of serous fluid may lead to detachment of the nail plate (onycholysis) and subsequent loss of the nail (onychomadesis). Allergic reaction to nail polish, resins, dyes, solvents, detergents, and other chemicals may cause eczema. Atopic dermatitis with no known cause may lead to the development of similar nail changes. With the resolution of acute inflammation, the chronic changes of fissuring and dryness may be treated with topical corticosteroids. The major objective with eczema and contact dermatitis is resolution of the acute inflammatory process surrounding the toenail unit.

Pyodermas

Bacterial infections occur frequently in the feet and are divided into primary and secondary pyodermas. Impetigo is a superficial skin infection that is frequently caused by *Staphylococcus*, *Streptococcus*, or both and usually affects younger children. The typical lesion consists of a thin-walled vesicle on an erythematous base. The vesicles form yellow crusts, and peripheral extension results in irregular serpiginous lesions. The lesions are common on the face but can occur everywhere on the body except the palms of the hands and the soles of the feet. Ecthyma is a form of pyoderma that begin as small vesicles or pustules on an erythematous base and quickly develops a purulent, irregular ulcer. These lesions are common on the lower extremities and, like impetigo, readily respond to systemic antibiotics. Burow's compresses are helpful in removing the crusts, and topical antibiotic ointment is usually applied several times a day.

Secondary pyodermas that may affect the feet can be grouped into the following categories:

1. Infectious eczematoid dermatitis results from a discharge of wet drainage seeping over the skin from an underlying cellulitis or pyodermic infection. Autoinoculation often occurs, and the infection spreads by contiguous drainage.
2. Infected intertrigo results from the effects of friction, moisture, and sweat retention and is common between the toes where it is often diagnosed as a tinea infection. Treatment consists of promoting dryness by cool, drying compresses and a bland absorbant powder. Secondary infection is treated by an appropriate topical antibiotic.
3. Miscellaneous pyogenic infections of the web space by gram-negative bacteria such as *Pseudomonas* and *Proteus* produce clinical pyodermic infections that are resistant to the usual forms of antibacterial therapy. The organisms and antibiotic therapy should be determined by culture and sensitivity.

Careful investigation to determine the presence of any underlying systemic disorders such as diabetes, lymphoma, or an immune deficiency syndrome that could predispose to the establishment of such cutaneous infections should be made. Amonette and Rosenberg[1] found topical management with a combination of bed rest, exposure to air, and the application of silver nitrate solution, Castellani's paint, and gentamicin sulfate cream to be the best treatment regimen. Erythrasma is frequently seen in the intertriginous areas such as the web spaces. The causative organism is *Corynebacterium minutissimum*, which produces a well-demarcated reddish brown fine desquamation that fluoresces orange-red or coral-pink under a Wood's lamp. The wearing of loose stockings and shoes and the use of antibacterial soaps will usually prevent this infection or eliminate it once it has been established. On occasion treatment will require appropriate oral antibiotics.

Not every form of intertrigo of the web space is linked to infection by a fungal or bacterial organism. With psoriasis, there can be extensive involvement of the skin involving the feet, and usually the web space area is involved as well. A therapeutic trial of a topical steroid cream may be effective in eliminating this form of intertrigo.

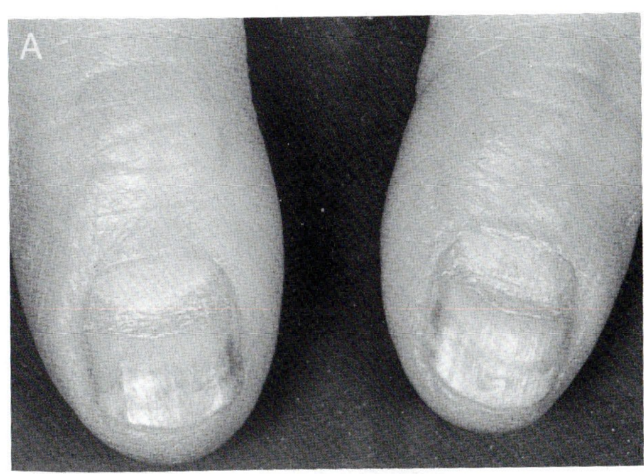

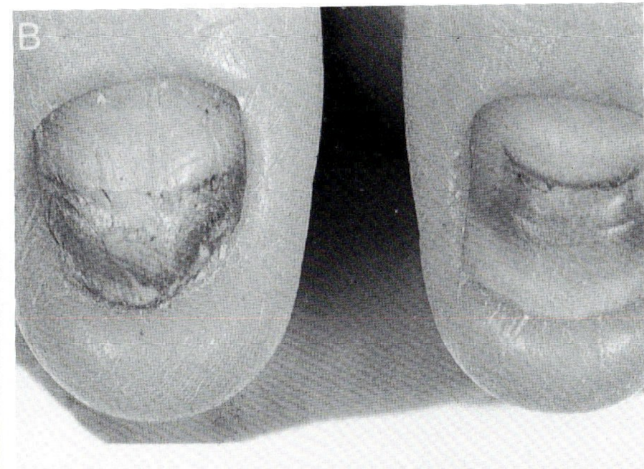

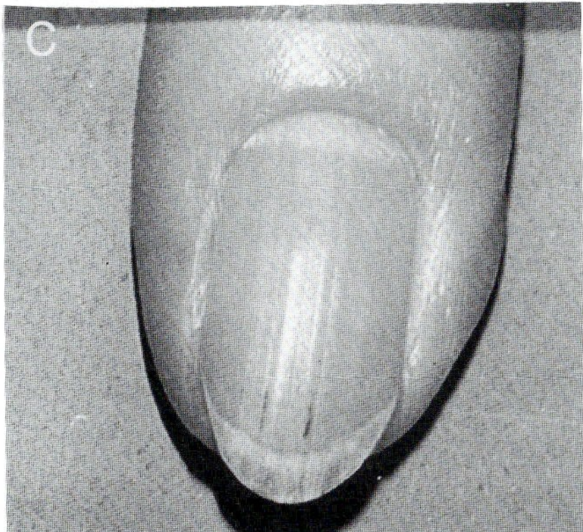

FIG 25–5.
A, Beau's lines are manifested as transverse lines in the nail plate. **B,** yellow nail syndrome is characterized by deformity and discoloration of the nail. **C,** splinter hemorrhages are tiny, subungual hemorrhages that result in hyperpigmentation visualized through the nail plate. While trauma is the most common cause, certain systemic diseases can also cause splinter hemorrhages. (From duViver A: *Atlas of clinical dermatology*, ed 2, London, 1992, Gower Medical Publishing. Used by permission.)

TABLE 25–3.
Cardiovascular Disorders*

Disease Entity	Pathologic Changes
Arterial emboli	Splinter hemorrhages
Arteriosclerosis obliterans	Leukonychia partialis
Bacterial endocarditis	Clubbing, splinter hemmorhages
Hypertension	Splinter hemorrhages
Ischemia	Onycholysis, pterygium
Mitral stenosis	Splinter hemorrhages
Myocardial infarction	Mee's lines, yellow nail syndrome
Vasculitis	Splinter hemorrhages

*Adapted from Kosinski M, Stewart D: *Clin Podiatr Med Surg* 6:295–318, 1989.

Systemic Diseases

Diseases of the toenail may accompany many systemic disease processes. The nail is an underutilized means with which diagnoses can be made. Often a provisional diagnosis of a fungal infection or trauma may be made when in reality a systemic disease process may cause changes in the color, shape, rate of growth, or texture of the toenail. While many of these changes are nonspecific, they can give a diagnostician reason to suspect the presence of a systemic disease.

The consistency and color of the nail plate may change with systemic disease. Several eponyms have been associated with these changes and, while confusing, have come into general use in the description of specific pathology.

1. *Beau's lines.*—With the sudden arrest in longitudinal nail growth, a transverse sulcus 0.1 to 0.5 mm in depth develops (Fig 25–5,A). With further growth of the nail plate, a Beau's line will progress distally. This is associated with severe febrile episodes, peripheral vascular disease, diabetes, trauma, Hodgkin's disease, and infection such as malaria, rheumatic fever, syphilis, leprosy, typhoid fever, and various parasitic infections.

2. *Mee's lines.*—Also associated with growth arrest of the nail plate, Mee's lines are horizontal striations involving typically more than one nail. They are usually 1 to 3 mm in width and are associated with Hodgkin's

TABLE 25–4.
Hematologic Disorders*

Disease Entity	Pathologic Changes
Cryoglobinemia	Splinter hemorrhages
Hemochromatosis	Brittleness of nails, koilonychia, leukonychia, longitudinal striations, splinter hemorrhages
Histocytosis X	Onychylosis, pitting of nails, splinter hemorrhages
Hodgkin's disease	Leukonychia partialis, Mee's lines, yellow nail syndrome
Hypochromic anemia	Koilonychia
Idiopathic hemochromatosis	Brittleness of nails, koilonychia, longitudinal striations, splinter hemorrhages
Osler-Weber-Rendu disease	Splinter hemorrhages, telangiectasia
Polycythemia rubra vera	Clubbing, koilonychia
Porphyria	Onycholysis
Sickle cell anemia	Leukonychia, Mee's lines, splinter hemorrhages
Thrombocytopenia	Splinter hemorrhages

*Adapted from Kosinski M, Stewart D: *Clin Podiatr Med Surg* 6:295–318, 1989.

TABLE 25–5.
Endocrine Disorders*

Disease Entity	Pathologic Changes
Addison's disease	Appearance of brown bands, diffuse hyperpigmentation, leukonychia, yellow nail syndrome, longitudinal pigmented bands of deep yellow color
Diabetes mellitus	Beau's lines, koilonychia, leukonychia, onychauxis, onychomadesis, paronychia, pitting of the nail plate, proximal nail bed telangiectasia, pterygium, splinter hemorrhages, yellow nail syndrome
Hyperthyroidism	Clubbing, increased nail growth, onycholysis, splinter hemorrhages, yellow nail syndrome
Hypothyroidism	Onycholysis, koilonychia, yellow nail syndrome
Thyroiditis	Yellow nail syndrome
Thyrotoxicosis	Koilonychia, onychomadesis, splinter hemorrhages, yellow nail syndrome

*Adapted from Kosinski M, Stewart D: *Clin Podiatr Med Surg* 6:295–318, 1989.

TABLE 25–6.
Connective Tissue Disorders*

Disease Entity	Pathologic Changes
Alopecia areata	Leukonychia partialis, nail pitting
Atopic dermatitis/eczema	Onycholysis, onychorrhexis
Lichen planus	Atrophy of the nail plate, onycholysis, onychorrhexis, pterygium
Psoriasis	Beau's lines, leukonychia, Mee's lines, nail pitting, onycholysis, splinter hemorrhages
Raynaud's syndrome	Koilonychia, yellow nail syndrome
Reiter's syndrome	Onycholysis, nail pitting
Rheumatoid arthritis	Splinter hemorrhages, yellow nail syndrome
Scleroderma	Absent lunula, koilonychia, leukonychia, onycholysis, onychorrhexis, pterygium
Systemic lupus erythematosus	Clubbing, hyperpigmented periungual tissue, nail pitting, onycholysis, subungual petechiae, yellow nail syndrome

*Adapted from Kosinski M, Stewart D: *Clin Podiatric Med Surgery* 6:295–318, 1989.

TABLE 25–7.
Systemic and Localized Infections*

Disease Entity	Pathologic Changes
Bacterial endocarditis	Clubbing, splinter hemorrhages
Leprosy	Disappearance of the lunula, nail plate dystrophy, onychogryphosis, onychauxis, onycholysis, onychodesis, onychomadesis, onychorrhexis
Malaria	Grayish nail bed, leukonychia
Measles	Onychomadesis
Recurrent cellulitis	Yellow nail syndrome
Scarlet fever	Onychomadesis
Syphilis	Koilonychia, leukonychia partialis, onychauxis, onychia, onycholysis, onychomadesis, onychorrhexis, paronychia
Trichinosis	Splinter hemorrhages, leukonychia
Tuberculosis	Leukonychia partialis, yellow nail syndrome
Typhoid fever	Leukonychia, Mee's lines
Yaws, pinta	Hypopigmentation, nail atrophy, onychia, onychauxis, paronychia, pterygium

*Adapted from Kosinski M, Stewart D: *Clin Podiatr Med Surg* 6:295–318, 1989.

TABLE 25–8.
Tumors*

Disease Entity	Pathologic Changes
Breast carcinoma	Yellow nail syndrome
Bronchogenic carcinoma	Clubbing, Muehreke's lines, onycholysis
Hodgkin's disease	Leukonychia partialis, Mee's lines, yellow nail syndrome
Laryngeal carcinoma	Yellow nail syndrome
Metastatic malignant melanoma	Clubbing, yellow nail syndrome
Multiple myeloma	Onycholysis

*Adapted from Kosinski M, Stewart D: *Clin Podiatr Med Surg* 6:295–318, 1989.

TABLE 25–9.
Hepatic, Renal, Pulmonary, and Gastrointestinal*

Disease Entity	Pathologic Changes
Hepatic	
Chronic hepatitis	Half-and-half nails, leukonychia
Cirrhosis	Clubbing, Muehreke's lines, splinter hemorrhages, Terry's nails
Renal	
Nephritis	Leukonychia
Nephrotic syndrome	Half-and-half nails, Muehreke's lines, yellow nail syndrome
Renal failure	Brown lunula, half-and-half nails, Mee's lines
Pulmonary	
Asthma	Yellow nail syndrome
Bronchiectasis	Clubbing, inflammation of the nail fold and nail bed, onychauxis, onycholysis, yellow nail syndrome
Chronic bronchitis	Clubbing, yellow nail syndrome
Interstitial pneumonia	Clubbing, yellow nail syndrome
Pleural effusion	Clubbing, onycholysis, yellow nail syndrome
Pneumonia	Leukonychia, Mee's lines
Pulmonary fibrosis	Clubbing, yellow nail syndrome
Pulmonary tuberculosis	Cyanosis, multiple paronychia, nail pitting, onychauxis
Gastrointestinal	
Peptic ulcer disease	Splinter hemorrhages
Plummer-Vinson syndrome	Koilonychia
Postgastrectomy	Koilonychia
Regional enteritis	Clubbing
Ulcerative colitis	Clubbing, leukonychia

*Adapted from Kosinski M, Stewart D: *Clin Podiatr Med Surg* 6:295–318, 1989.

disease, myocardial infarction, malaria, and arsenic and thalium poisoning.[59, 60]

3. *Muehreke's lines.*—Muehreke's lines are white lines occurring in a paired fashion, parallel to the lunula, that do not progress distally with nail plate growth. They occur with hypoalbuminemia and nephrotic syndrome as well as chronic liver disease.

4. *Half-and-half nail.*—Biphasic discoloration of the nail occurs in which the distal portion is brown, red, or pink while the proximal portion is more normal in appearance. Half-and-half nails are associated with both chronic liver and renal diseases.

5. *Blue nail, blue-gray nail.*—A bluish discoloration of the nail is associated with subungual hematoma, melanotic whitlow, as well poor oxygen profusion in methemoglobinemia, pulmonary disease, and cyanosis.

6. *Terry's nail.*—Characteristic changes involve opacification of the nail plate with a 1- to 3-mm pinkish band located at the distal edge of the nail plate. This condition may frequently be associated with chronic changes associated with diabetes mellitus and liver disease.

Nail changes may be manifested in cardiovascular (Table 25–3) and hematologic diseases (Table 25–4), endocrine disorders (Table 25–5), connective tissue diseases (Table 25–6), local and systemic infection (Table 25–7), neoplasia (Table 25–8), as well as renal, hepatic, pulmonary, and gastrointestinal disorders (Table 25–9). Kosinski and Stewart[44] have reported the frequent pathologic nail conditions associated with these systemic disease entities (Fig 25–5,B and C).

GENETIC DISORDERS WITH NAIL CHANGES

Heritable traits may influence the appearance of toenails. There are many genetic diseases with collagen abnormalities in which dermatologic abnormalities and hair and nail disorders are present.

Darier's disease (Darier-White disease)[56] (Table 25–10), an autosomal dominant disease, is characterized by distal subungual wedge-shaped keratoses, red and white longitudinal striations (Fig 25–6,A), splinter hemorrhages, notching of the distal nail plate, subungual hyperkeratosis, and thinning of the nail plate with splintering along the edge.

Pachyonychia congenita (Jadassohn-Lewandowsky syndrome),[46, 58] another autosomal dominant genetic disorder, is characterized by hypertrophy of the nail plate with severe thickening and a yellowish brown discoloration of the nail plate (Fig 25–6,B and C). The extreme thickening is more solid and more regular than with onychogryphosis and is accompanied by palmar and plantar keratoses. The thickening of the nail plate may lead to elevation of the distal nail plate and an incurved and elevated toenail. Tauber and associates[73] reported a case of pachyonychia congenita and reviewed published reports of this disease.

The *nail-patella syndrome* (onycho-osteodysplasia),[58, 71] an autosomal dominant disease, is characterized by a triangular lunula and total atrophy or hemiatrophy of the nail plate (Fig 25–6,D). Other orthopaedic conditions associated with this disease include subluxation or dislocation of the radial head, iliac horns, joint hypermobility, and a subluxated or dislocated hypoplastic patella.

Dyskeratosis congenita[58] can be transmitted as an autosomal dominant or X-linked recessive trait and is characterized by ridging and thinning or atrophy of the nail plate. *DOOR syndrome*[58] is an autosomal recessive trait characterized by mental retardation and deafness and may also be associated with absent or atrophic nails and curved fifth digits.

Congenital nail abnormalities are errors of development that can produce other anomalies such as anony-

TABLE 25–10.
Heritable Disorders of the Nail*

Disease or Syndrome	Genetic Inheritance	Pathologic Nail Findings
Darier's disease	Autosomal dominant	Longitudinal red/white striations, atrophy or hypertrophy of the nail plate, splinter hemorrhages, distal subungual wedge-shaped keratoses
Pachyonychia congenita	Autosomal dominant	Massive hypertrophy of the nail plates, brown or yellow discoloration
Nail-patella syndrome	Autosomal dominant	Atrophy, hemiatrophy of the nail, triangular-shaped lunula
Dyskeratosis congenita	X-linked recessive or autosomal dominant	Atrophy of the nail plate, ridging, fusion of the proximal nail fold
DOOR† syndrome	Autosomal recessive	Anychia or atrophic nails

*Adapted from Norton LA: *J Am Acad Dematol* 2:451–467, 1980.
†DOOR = deafness, onycho-osteodystrophy, mental retardation.

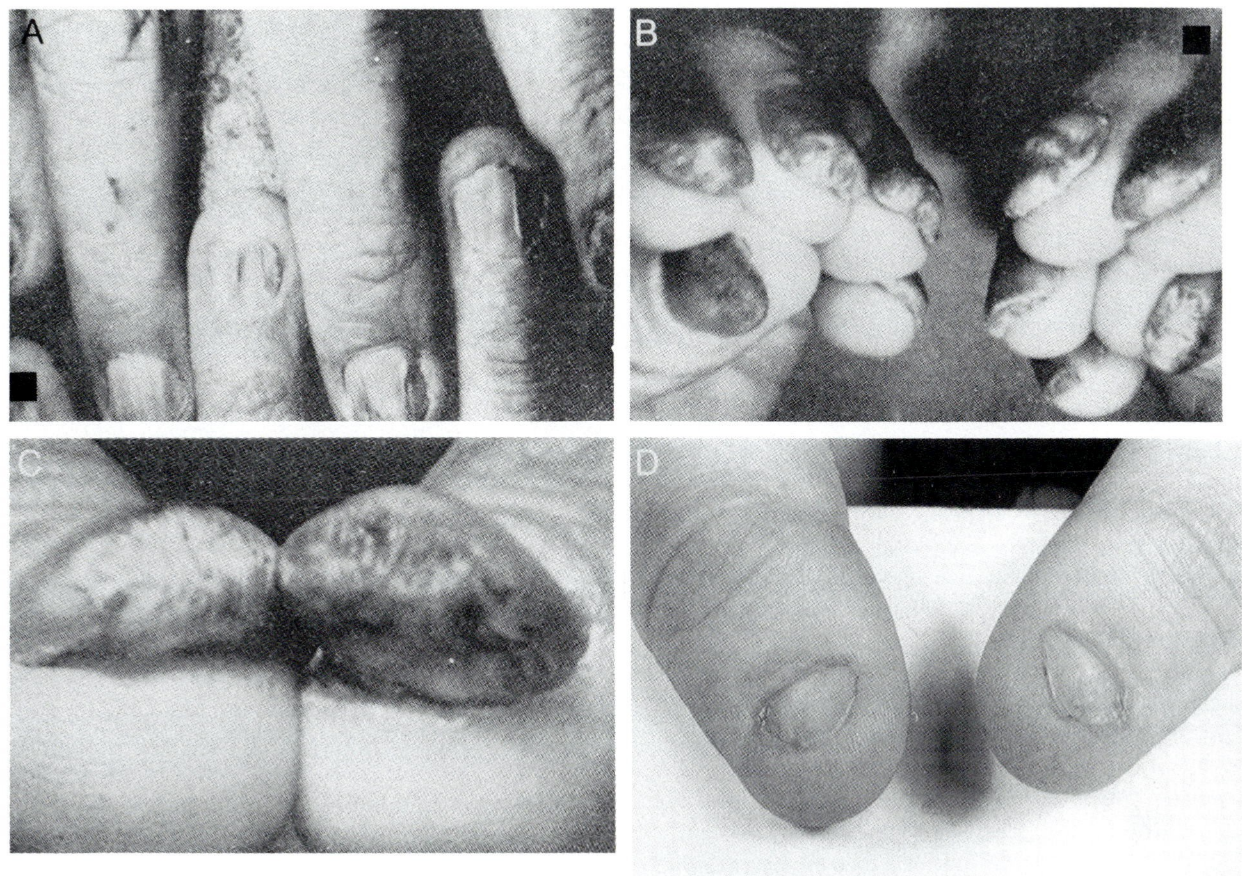

FIG 25–6.
A, Darier's disease demonstrating characteristic longitudinal striations in the fingernails. **B,** severe dystrophic thickening of the fingernails as seen in pachonychia congenita. **C,** severe dystrophic thickening of the toenails. **D,** deformities of many of the nails including nail absence may occur with nail-patella syndrome. (**A–C** from Moschella SL, Hurley H, editors: *Dermatology,* ed 2, Philadelphia, WB Saunders, p 1405. **D** from duViver A: *Atlas of clinical dermatology,* ed 2, London, 1992, Gower Medical Publishing. Used by permission.)

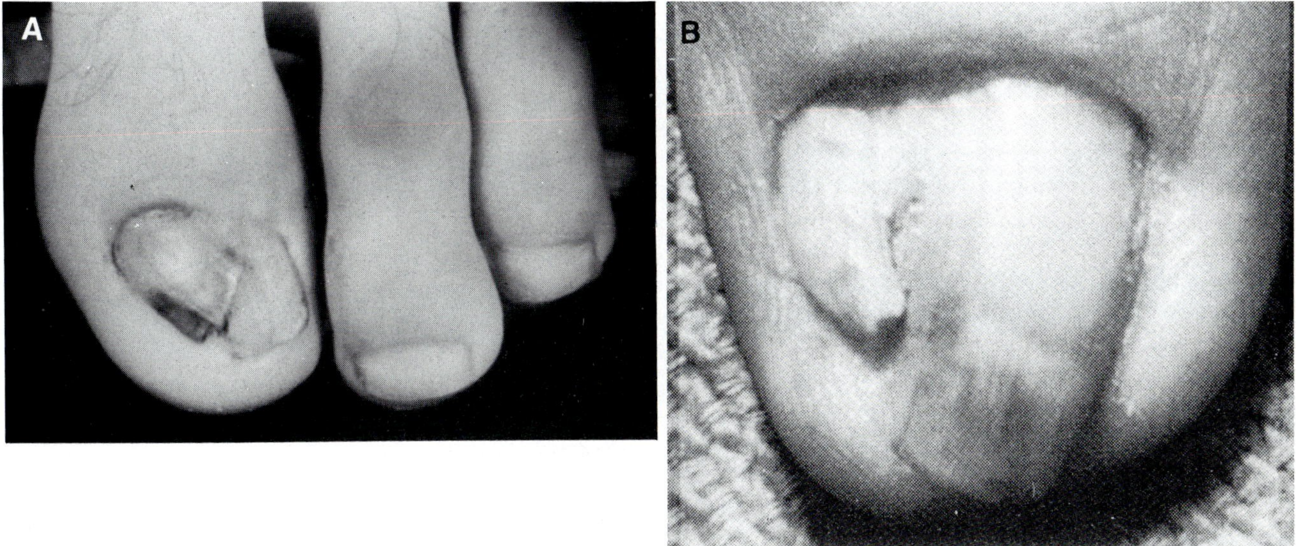

FIG 25–7.
A, polyonychia or congenital duplication of the nail plate of the great toe. (Courtesy of Dr. C.E. Krausz.) **B,** a split nail may appear to be a congenital deformity, but in fact in this case is secondary to trauma to the nail matrix. (From Moschella SL, Hurley H, editors: *Dermatology,* ed 2, Philadelphia, 1986, WB Saunders, p 1419. Used by permission.)

chia (absence of the nails) and polyonychia (the presence of more than one nail on a digit) (Fig 25–7,A).

TRAUMA

The nail plate and nail bed can be damaged by trauma (Fig 25–7,B). Injury to the nail matrix may cause abnormalities such as ridging, pitting, or grooving. A toenail may be lost, and a new nail plate may grow in an abnormal or normal fashion. An injury to the toenail may cause regrowth of a thickened, discolored nail. An osseous injury to the distal phalanx may cause callus formation that may affect the new toenail. A subungual exostosis is believed by some to develop secondary to trauma to the distal phalanx and often causes a deformity of the nail plate. Thickening of the distal phalanx may cause an incurved toenail that pinches the underlying soft tissue.

Trauma to the nail plate may be caused by biomechanical abnormalities as well. The lateral nail fold adjacent to the second toe may be compressed by the second toe and cause an overgrowth of soft tissue with secondary infection. On the medial aspect of the nail plate, with excessive pronation, hypertrophy of the ungualabia may result in an ingrown toenail. Constricting foot wear and snug-fitting stockings and hosiery may also lead to incurvation of the medial nail border with subsequent inflammation and infection.

TUMORS

Tumors of the soft tissue adjacent to the toenails or involving the nail unit itself can be of a benign or malignant nature. Periungual and subungual warts (verruca) are one of the more common types of soft-tissue growths. Fibromas[69] (see Fig 25–21,A). and fibrokeratomas may result from trauma to the toes with resultant nodule formation impinging on the nail plate (Table 25–11). These lesions may also develop beneath the nail plate itself and cause elevation and deformity. They respond readily to excision or cauterization. Glomus tumors, pyogenic granuloma, and keratocanthomas must all be considered in the differential diagnosis.

Glomus Tumor

A glomus tumor is most frequently encountered on the acral portions of the extremities. This lesion is often in the subungual area and consists of a purplish nodule measuring only a few millimeters in diameter. It is tender and gives rise to severe paroxysmal pain. Glomus tumors rarely ulcerate or bleed, and excision usually results in a cure, although subungual lesions are more difficult to eradicate. The differential diagnosis includes hemangioma as well as neuroma, Kaposi's sarcoma (see Fig 25–12,B), hemangiopericytoma and granuloma telangiectaticum. Another type of glomus tumor is characterized by multiple painless hemangiomas and frequently has a familial pattern.[19] These multiple lesions are usually asymptomatic.

Subungual Exostosis

A subungual exostosis is a reactive bony growth commonly occurring on the dorsomedial aspect of the distal phalanx of the hallux.[11, 16] Although the lesser toes may occasionally develop a subungual exostosis, there is a definite predilection for this to occur in the great toe. A subungual exostosis is typically a slow-growing unilateral growth that rarely exceeds 0.5 cm in size. On rare occasion the exostosis develops a cartilage-capped surface, and in this situation a diagnosis of osteochondroma may be made. An osteochondroma characteristically occurs in the proximity of the epiphyseal line[11] (Table 25–12). It occurs more frequently in the adolescent male (ratio, 2:1) than in the female. On the other hand, the diagnosis of a subungual exostosis is more frequently made in young adults between the second and fourth decades. Ippoloito et al.[39] found subungual exostoses to occur more frequently in the female population (2:1 ratio), while Breslow and Dorfman[11] reported an equal distribution between males and fe-

TABLE 25–11.
Tumors of the Nail*

Benign nail tumors
Verruca
Fibroma
Fibrokeratoma
Neurofibroma
Myxoid cyst
Pyogenic granuloma
Glomus tumor
Pigmented nevus
Keratocanthoma
Malignant nail tumors
Squamous cell carcinoma
Malignant melanoma
Basal cell carcinoma
Metastatic carcinoma
Bowen's disease
Tumors of the bone
Bone cysts—solitary or aneurysmal
Enchondroma
Osteochondroma
Subungual exostosis

*Adapted from Gunnoe RE: *Postgrad Med* 74:357–362, 1983.

TABLE 25–12.
Differentiation of Subungual Exostosis From Osteochondroma*

Condition	Age (yr)	Sex Ratio	Trauma?	Growth Rate	Radiographic Appearance
Exostosis	20–40	F, 2:1	Occasionally	Moderate	Osseous growth with an expanded cap, often trabeculated (fibrocartilage cap)
Osteochondroma	10–25	M, 2:1	Often	Slow	Sessile bone lesion, often with a trabeculated pattern (hyaline cartilage cap)

*Adapted from Norton LA: *J Am Acad Derm* 2:457, 1980.

males. Grisafi et al.[32] suggested that subungual osteochondromas are congenital in origin while the etiology of a subungual exostosis is felt in general to be traumatic in origin.[61]

In differentiating between a subungual exostosis and a subungual osteochondroma, the histologic differentiation of the cartilage cap is the main difference. A subungual exostosis is characterized by a cartilaginous cap that is a reactive fibrous growth with cartilage metaplasia.[11] Jahss[40] noted that the histology of a subungual exostosis consists of chronic fibrosis due to irritation. A trabecular bony pattern connecting with the distal phalanx may underlie the fibrocartilaginous cap.[11] However, the distal tuft of the phalanx is usually not involved. In a subungual osteochondroma, a hyaline cartilage cap may overlie a trabeculated bony pattern.

Ippoloito et al.[39] in reporting on 21 cases of subungual exostosis, noted 12 of 21 to be in athletes involved in such activities as dancing, gymnastics, or football. It is believed that increased pressure against the dorsal aspect of the nail plate by a constricting toe box may cause irritation that leads to the development of a subungual exostosis. The connection between a specific traumatic incident and the later development of a subungual exostosis may also explain the increased incidence of this abnormality in the athletic population. Many patients describe a history of pain that is aggravated by activities such as running or walking. This is most likely due to pressure of an expanding lesion against a toe box. It is not uncommon for a subungual exostosis to be misdiagnosed or confused with other toenail abnormalities[39] (Fig 25–8). Elevation of the nail plate (Fig 25–9,A and B) and discoloration may resemble chronic onychomycosis (Fig 25–9,C) or a subungual hematoma. The differential diagnosis includes subungual verruca, pyogenic granuloma, glomus tumor, keratocanthoma, carcinoma of the nail bed, subungual nevus, and subungual melanoma.

The diagnosis of a subungual exostosis is determined by radiographic demonstration of the exostosis (Fig 25–9,D). While a dorsoplantar radiograph may not demonstrate the exostosis, a lateral or oblique radiograph will frequently help to identify the lesion. On the radiograph, the exostosis typically arises from the dorsomedial aspect of the distal phalanx. It is often oval shaped and irregular in density. While the cartilage cap may be quite large, the appearance of the exostosis on the radiograph may be smaller than the physical size of the growth.

Treatment

While a small asymptomatic lesion may be observed, surgical resection of a subungual exostosis or subungual osteochondroma is the most frequent treatment for a symptomatic lesion.

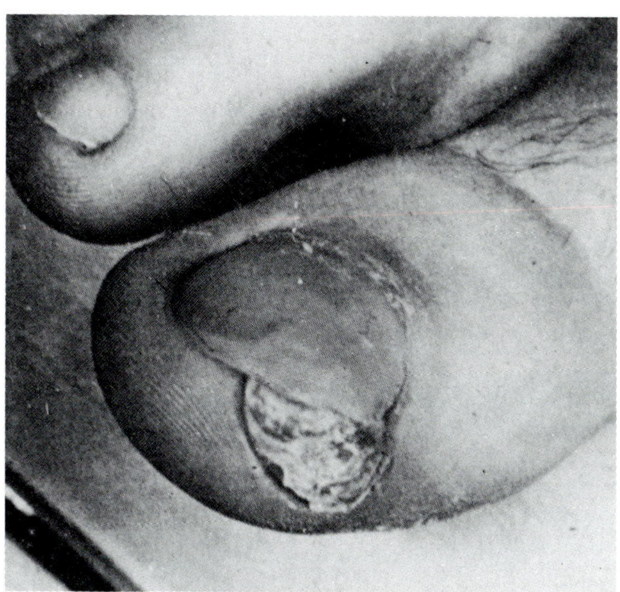

FIG 25–8.
Easily confused with a periungual wart, this keratotic lesion has developed in association with a subungual exostosis. (From Yale I: *Podiatric medicine,* Baltimore, Williams & Wilkins, p 172. Used by permission.)

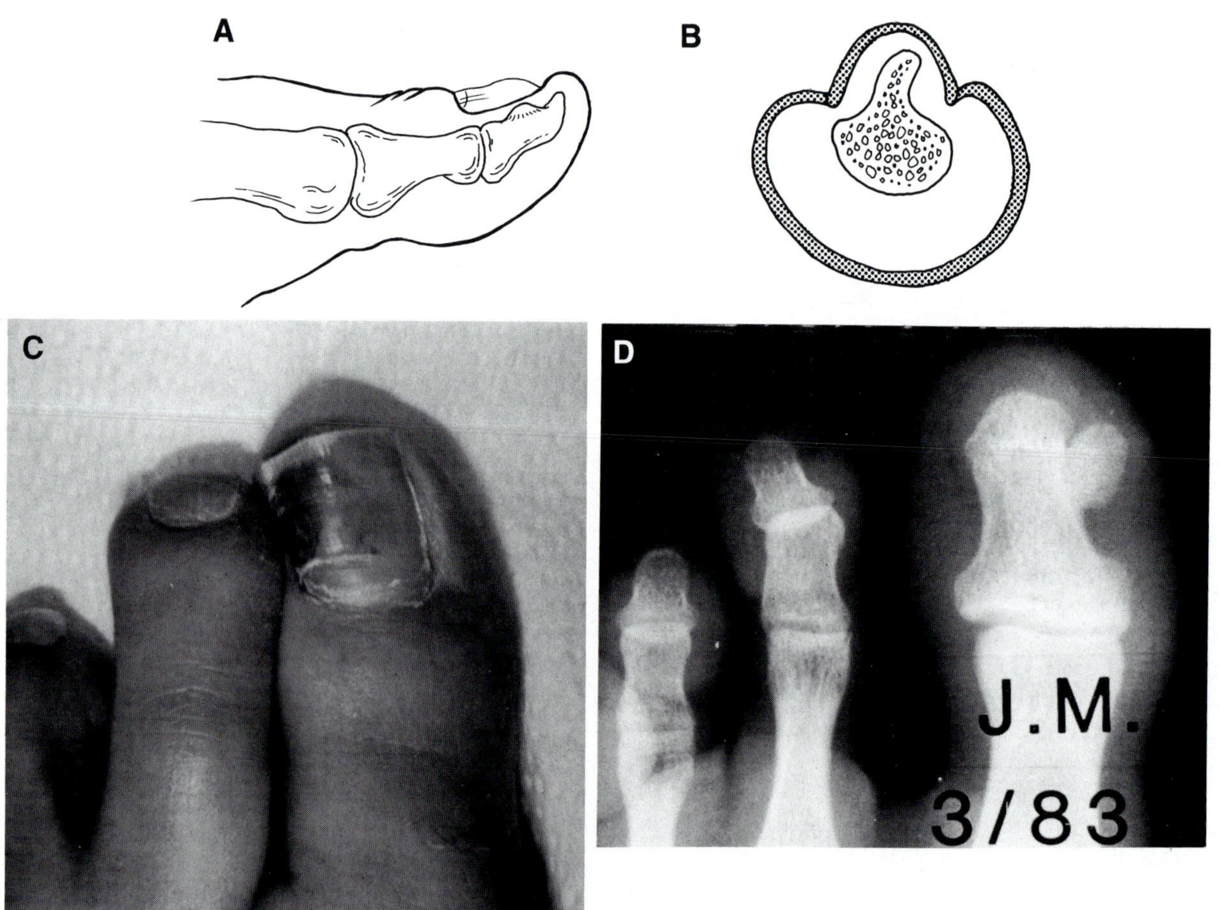

FIG 25–9.
Subungual exostosis. **A,** a lateral view of the toe demonstrates the effect of a subungual exostosis on the configuration of the nail plate. **B,** a cross section of the distal phalanx demonstrates deformation of the nail plate by the subungual exostosis. **C,** onycholysis or elevation of the nail plate due to an underlying subungual exostosis. **D,** radiograph of the same patient demonstrating a subungual exostosis. (**C** and **D** from Mann RA, Coughlin MJ: *The video textbook of foot and ankle surgery.* St Louis, 1990, Medical Video Productions. Used by permission.)

Technique.

1. A digital anesthetic block is administered and a ¼-in. Penrose drain applied.
2. A partial or complete toenail avulsion is performed (Fig 25–10,A).
3. A longitudinal incision is made in the nail bed (Fig 25–10,B). The nail bed is reflected off of the exostosis with care taken to avoid damage to the nail matrix (Fig 25–10,C).
4. The exostosis is resected with an osteotome or bone cutter (Fig 25–10,D). The base of the lesion is curetted.
5. The nail bed is relocated and closed with absorbable suture.
6. A compression dressing is applied and changed 24 hours postoperatively. Dressing changes are continued until drainage subsides. The nail bed is protected with a plastic strip bandage until tenderness resolves.

Recurrence of an exostosis is uncommon but may develop if an incomplete resection is performed. Recurrence may be a continuing source of irritation to the toenail. Breslow and Dorfman[11] reported a 53% incidence of recurrence when a subtotal excisional biopsy was performed. However, following wide local excision with curettage of the base, a 5% to 6% rate of recurrence can be expected.[61]

Melanotic Whitlow, Malignant Melanoma

Melanomas that involve the nails are termed melanotic whitlows.[30] Blackish discoloration develops, especially in the nail bed. These malignant tumors are more

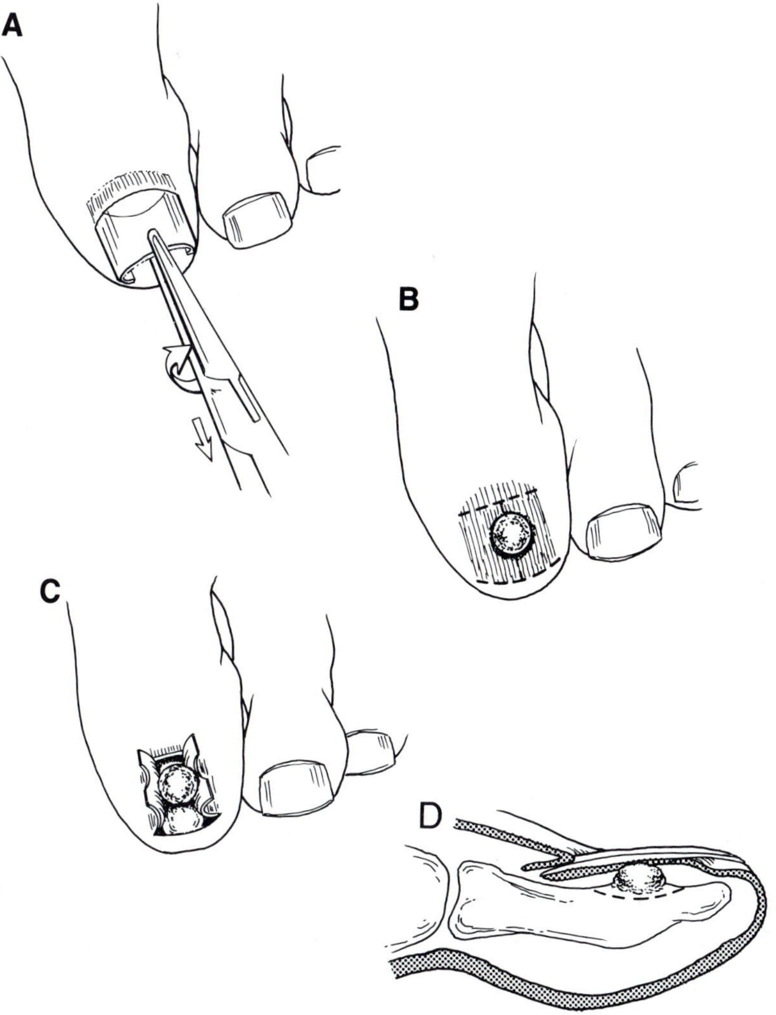

FIG 25–10.
Technique of surgical excision of subungual exostosis. **A,** a complete toenail avulsion is performed to expose the exostosis. **B,** a longitudinal incision is made in the nail bed with care taken to avoid injury to the nail matrix. **C,** the nail bed is retracted. **D,** a generous excision of the exostosis is performed, and the nail bed is then repaired.

common on the fingers than on the toes. Trauma is the most frequent cause of darkening of the nails, but other causes are Addison's disease and Peutz-Jeghers syndrome. The diagnosis of malignant melanoma may also be confused with a glomus tumor, benign nevus, paronychia, and pyogenic granuloma. However, with a malignant melanoma, the discoloration does not change as the nail grows distally and does not improve with time. A malignant melanoma may not damage the overlying nail plate, whereas a subungual hematoma may cause elevation of the nail plate. A malignant melanoma is usually deep black in color (Fig 25–11) as compared with the less distinct color of a subungual hemorrhage. Many patient with subungual melanoma give a history of trauma that makes an early diagnosis difficult. Welvaart and Koops[78] reported that in a series of 25 patients diagnosed with subungual melanoma, only 36% of patients remained alive at 5 years' follow-up. Leppard et al.[48] noted that 30% of their patients had distant lymph node metastasis at the time of surgery.

Other Tumerous Conditions

Basal cell carcinoma is very uncommon.[3] Squamous cell carcinoma,[4, 9, 20] Bowen's disease[31, 68] (Fig 25–12, A), Kaposi's sarcoma (Fig 25–12,B), and metastatic disease are relatively rare malignant lesions. Patients

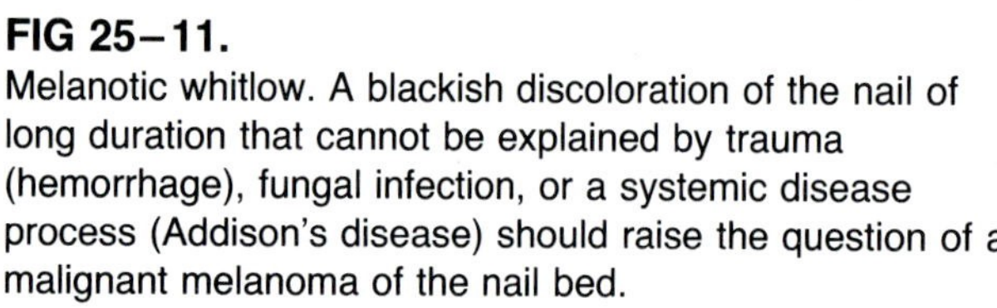

FIG 25–11.
Melanotic whitlow. A blackish discoloration of the nail of long duration that cannot be explained by trauma (hemorrhage), fungal infection, or a systemic disease process (Addison's disease) should raise the question of a malignant melanoma of the nail bed.

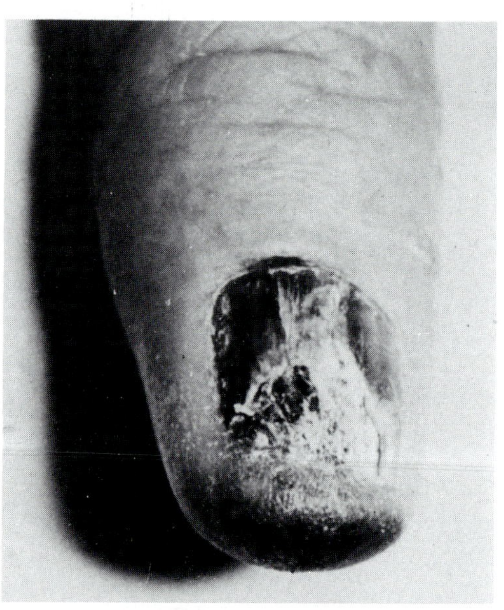

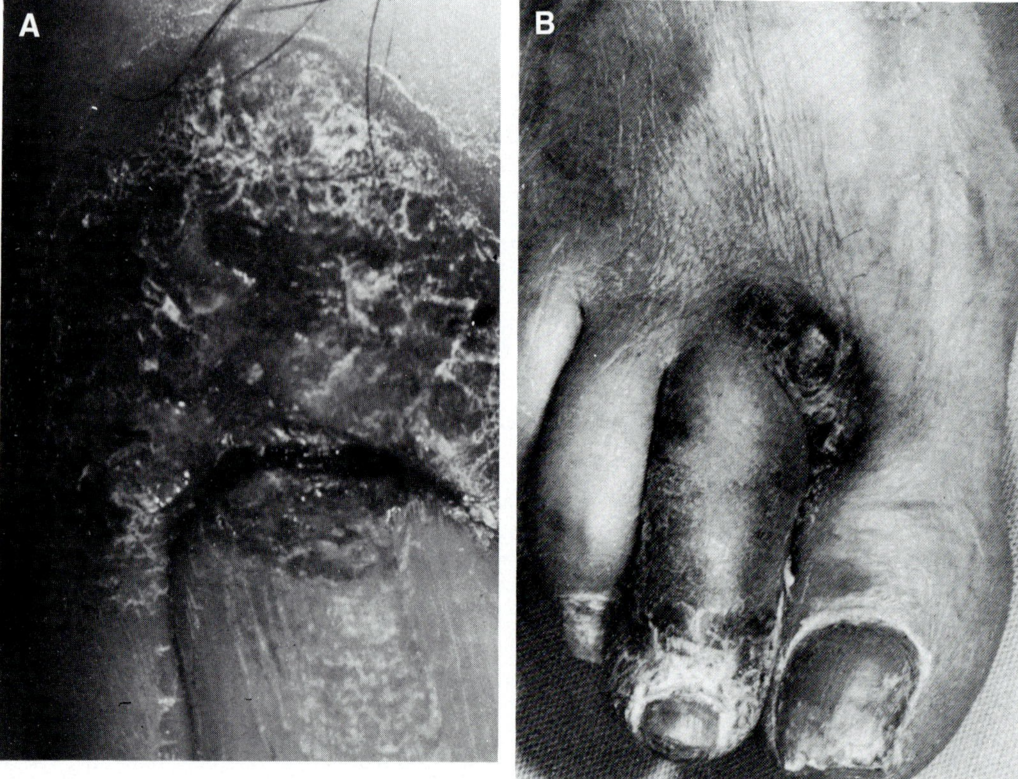

FIG 25–12.
A, Bowen's disease. This carcinoma in situ is frequently mistaken for a tinea infection or eczema and presents as a reddish, scaling, oozing, persistent patch of abnormal skin on the toes. **B,** an early lesion of Kaposi's sarcoma. A biopsy is necessary to establish the diagnosis. (**B** from Jahss M, editor: *Disorders of the foot and ankle,* ed 2, Philadelphia, 1991, WB Saunders, p 1549. Used by permission.)

with either abnormal x-ray findings or chronic pain, swelling, inflammation, infection, or persistent splitting of the nail plate should be evaluated for the possibility of an underlying tumor of the distal phalanx. A specific diagnosis is essential. Once the diagnosis of a malignant tumor has been made by biopsy, amputation of the digit is a common treatment.

ONYCHOPATHIES AND OTHER COMMON NAIL ABNORMALITIES

Onychopathy[59] (Tables 25–13 and 25–14) or abnormalities of the toenails are most easily discussed by dividing them into abnormalities of the nail plate, nail bed, nail fold or, nail matrix. Congenital and genetic nail disorders, traumatic nail disorders, tumors, and dermatologic and systemic nail disorders have been discussed elsewhere in this chapter.

TABLE 25–13.
Onychopathies and Other Common Toenail Abnormalities*

Nail plate
Onychocryptosis
Onychauxis
Onychogryphosis
Onychomycosis
Onychia
Onycholysis/onychomadesis
Nail bed
Subungual exostosis
Subungual tumor
Subungual clavus
Subungual hematoma
Subungual verruca
Nail fold
Paronychia
Onychophosis
Pyogenic granuloma
Herpetic whitlow
Periungual verruca
Matrix
Anychia
Pterygium
Atrophy/hypertrophy (onychauxis)
Keratinization disorders
Psoriasis
Mycotic infections
Onychoschizia
Koilonychia
Leukonychia
Onycholysis
Onychorrhexis

*Adapted from Nzuzi SM: *Clin Podiatr Med Surg* 6:273–294, 1989.

Common Nail Plate Disorders

Within this section onychocryptosis, onychauxis, onychogryphosis, onychomycosis, onychia, and onychomadesis are discussed.

Onychocryptosis

Onychocryptosis occurs when the border of the nail plate penetrates the adjacent soft tissue of the nail fold (Fig 25–13). Synonyms for this condition include ingrown toenail, unguis incarnatus, as well as hypertrophy of the ungualabia.[23, 24] The term *ingrown toenail* is misleading because it implies that the side of the nail plate grows laterally and extends further into the nail groove. All evidence points to the fact that the growth of nails in vertebrates depends upon the matrix width and that the width of the nail is directly related to the width of the matrix.[6, 7, 64] There is no evidence supporting the fact that the matrix becomes wider in a per-

TABLE 25–14.
Causes of Nail Deformities*

External pressure
Footwear
Excessive tightness
High heels
Pointed toe box
Short toe box
Stockings—excessive tightness
Casts extending beyond the nail
Hallux rigidus
Hallux valgus
Hallux varus
Lesser toes
Impingement on the hallux
Hammer toes
Overlapping or underlapping toes
Soft-tissue neoplasm
Pronation of the feet
Internal pressure
Subungual exostosis/osteoma
Subungual keratosis
Subungual hematoma
Subungual neoplasm
Onychia/paronychia
Trauma
Systemic conditions
Cardiac disorders
Circulatory disorders
Endocrine disorders
Renal disorders
Metabolic disorders
Infection
Genetic disorders
Geriatric nail changes
Obesity

*Adapted from Johnson KA: *Surgery of the foot and ankle,* New York, 1989 Raven Press, p 84.

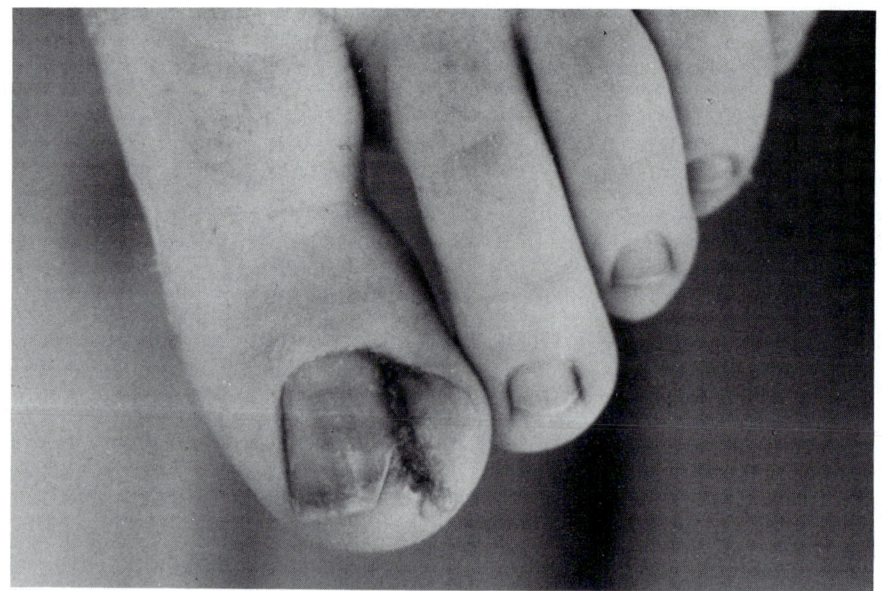

FIG 25–13.
Onychocryptosis. The lateral portion of the nail penetrates the adjacent soft tissue of the lateral nail fold.

son suffering from an ingrown toenail. The term ingrown toenail was chosen on the assumption that an ingrowth of the nail or a downward growth of the nail into the nail groove was caused by an increasing width in the convexity of the nail. Thus, initial attempts by surgeons at treating this disease were aimed at narrowing the nail margin. Frost[27] described three types of ingrown toenails:

1. A normal nail plate that with improper nail trimming develops a fish hook or spur in the lateral nail groove (Fig 25–14,A and B)
2. An inward distortion of one or both of the lateral margins of the nail plate (incurved nail) (Fig 25–14,C).
3. A normal nail plate with soft-tissue hypertrophy of the lateral border (Fig 25–15).

Lloyd-Davies and Brill[51] proposed that avulsion of the nail plate, which is commonly practiced as a treatment for an ingrown toenail, probably leads to hypertrophy of the distal lip of the nail and causes the entire nail to become embedded and clubbed (Fig 25–16). Unlike the fingernails, if the nail of the great toe has been removed, the new nail frequently becomes deformed as

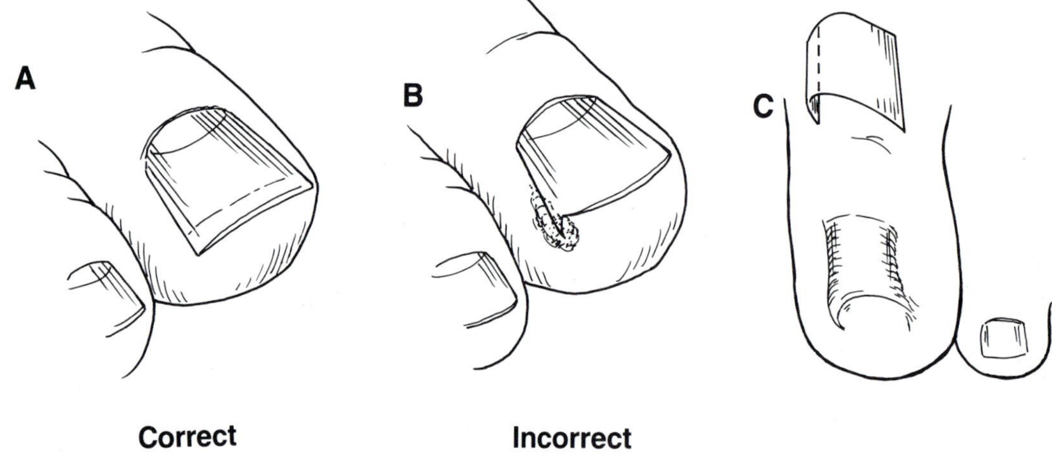

FIG 25–14.
A, correct nail trimming avoids "ingrowth" into the adjacent nail fold. **B** and **C,** incorrect nail trimming may lead to a "fish-hook spur" in the lateral nail fold with subsequent infection.

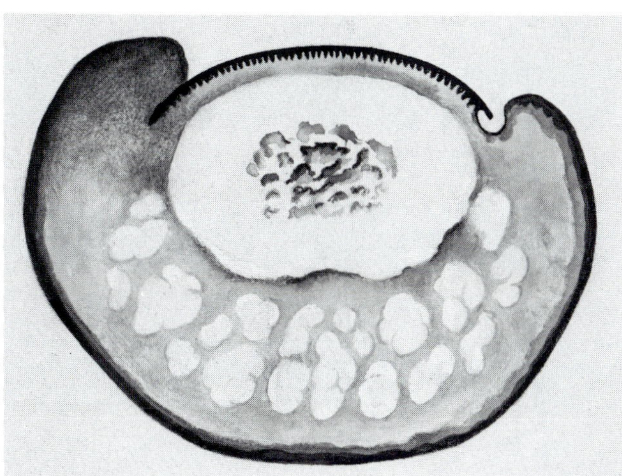

FIG 25–15.
Left, hypertrophy of the nail lip leads to occlusion of the nail groove. *Right,* a normal relationship is maintained between the nail margin and the lateral nail groove.

it grows distally because of upward pressure placed on it during weight bearing (see Table 25–2).

The main conditions that produce symptoms of onychocryptosis are primary hyperplasia of the nail groove, which occurs in approximately 75% of cases, and a deformity of the nail plate, which occurs in approximately 25% of cases. The latter is caused by an osseous malformation of the dorsum of the distal phalanx[49] or by hypertrophy and irregular thickening of the nail bed often as a result of a tinea infection. The normal nail plate and its bed are 2 to 3 mm thick. The contour is largely determined by the dorsal shape of the distal phalanx. The shape and contour of the dorsum of this bone may vary widely because of secondary changes in the distal phalanx from irritation and pressure. Such variations often produce nail deformities whose symptoms may all be grouped as an ingrown toenail. The most common type is incurvation of the nail margin.

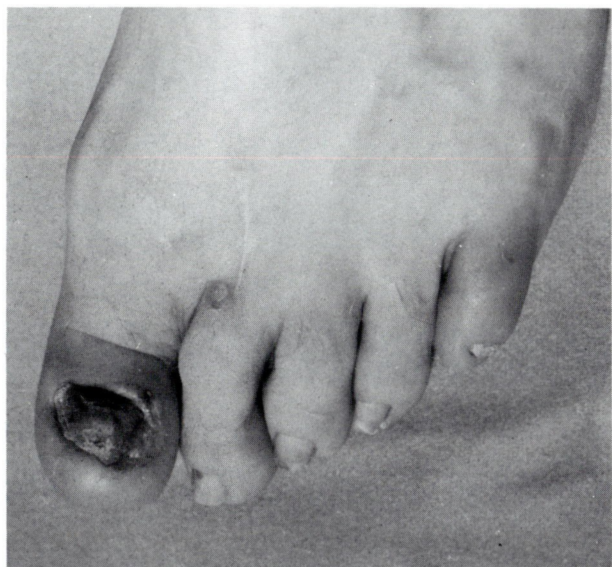

FIG 25–16.
Following avulsion of the nail plate, a club nail may form with impingement of the distal part of the nail against the distal soft tissue.

Normally the space between the nail margin and the nail groove is approximately 1 mm. The groove is lined with a thin layer of epithelium that lies immediately under and on the sides of the nail margins. Under normal conditions this space is sufficient to protect the groove from irritation. With a narrow toe box or tight-fitting stockings, downward pressure on the nail plate, the nail lip, or the lateral nail fold may occur. This pressure obliterates the space between the nail plate margin and the nail groove and produces constant irritation. The reactive swelling in the groove creates a cycle leading to gradual hyperplasia of the adjacent soft tissue and ultimately to permanent hypertrophy. As this process continues, the nail groove is finally incised by the nail margin, often with ensuing secondary infection. To relieve the acute symptoms, the surgeon may excise a triangular section of the nail margin (Fig 25–17,A).[17] However, the area left by the excision can often then develop into a thick fish-hook deformity of the lateral nail plate (Fig 25–17,B). Hypertrophy of the adjacent soft tissue fills the space of the excised nail margin. Then as the nail continues its distal growth, it impinges on the elevated nail groove and gives rise to recurrent episodes of infection and formation of granulation tissue.

A congenitally thick lateral nail margin predisposes to an ingrown toenail. This congenital factor explains why ingrown toenails sometimes occur in infants or even in neonates who have thick nail lips and/or an absence of a free margin between the nail groove and nail margin. In adults the condition is typically acquired.

A subungual exostosis may cause nail deformities with subsequent incurvation, infection, and pain (Fig 25–18,A and B).

The size, shape, and contour of the nail plate and bed are usually normal. Hyperplastic changes of the nail groove and lip are accompanied by the formation of granulation tissue on the lip and groove. The granulation tissue bleeds freely with slight provocation. Hypertrophy may mask a large part or even most of the nail. Heifetz[35] proposed a classification of ingrown toenails into three distinct stages.

Stage 1: Swelling and erythema along the lateral nail fold. The edge of the nail plate may be embedded in an irritated nail fold.

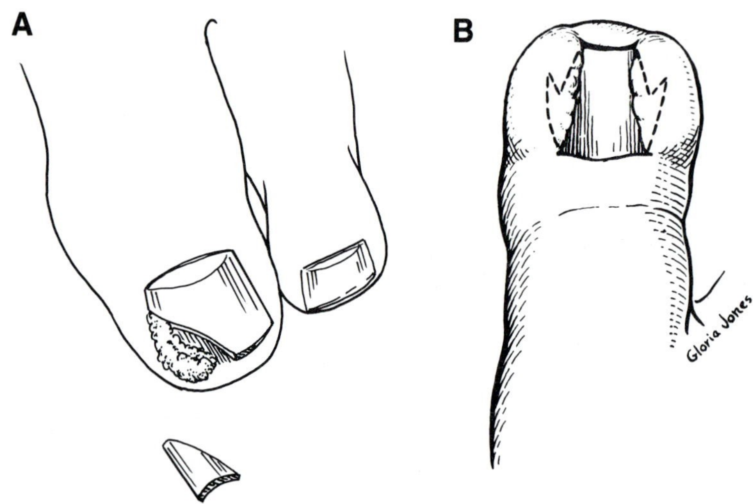

FIG 25–17.
A, symptoms of an acute infection may be relieved with diagonal trimming of the nail plate. **B,** as the nail plate regrows, recurrent infection may result.

Stage 2: Increased pain characterized by acute or active infection. Drainage is present.

Stage 3: With chronic infection, development of granulation tissue in the lateral nail fold. Hypertrophy of the surrounding soft tissue is present.

The differential diagnosis includes:

1. Trauma
2. Paronychia
3. Subungual exostosis
4. Onycholysis
5. Onychophosis

Treatment.—A variety of procedures have been reported for the cure of an ingrown toenail. Postoperative recurrence is frequent. Procedures generally practiced include (1) simple avulsion of the border of the nail plate (this may temporarily resolve the infection, but

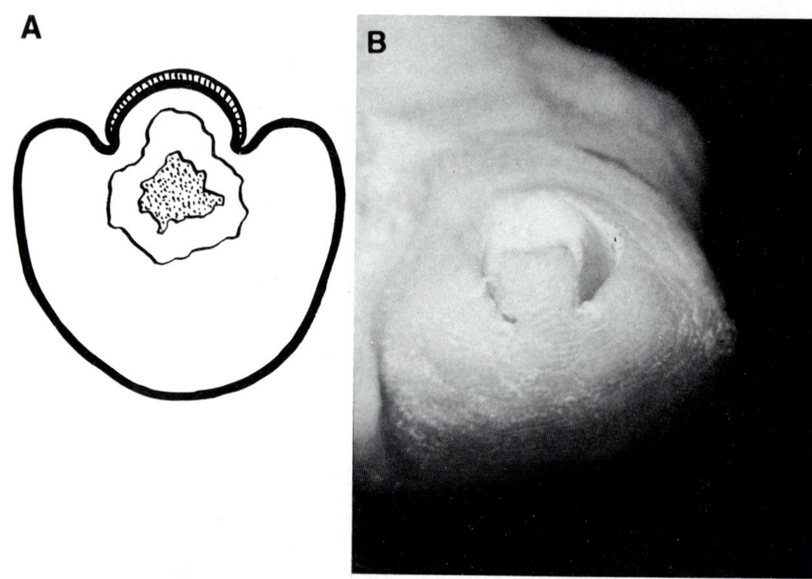

FIG 25–18.
A, subungual exostosis may cause deformity of the nail plate. **B,** clinical example of nail incurvation associated with subungual exostosis. In an elderly patient, incurvation may result without a subungual exostosis. (**B** from Mann RA, Coughlin MJ: *The video textbook of foot and ankle surgery,* St Louis, 1990, Medical Video Productions. Used by permission.)

there is a strong tendency for recurrent infection unless definitive treatment is later performed), (2) reduction of the hypertrophied lip, and (3) partial or total ablation of the nail plate (surgical, chemical, laser).

There is no question that patient education is necessary in the treatment of an ingrown toenail both acutely and to prevent a recurrence of infection. The patient should be instructed in proper shoe wear, the use of loose-fitting stockings or hose, and proper nail-cutting procedures. Patients with excessive pronation may be treated with an orthotic device to decrease axial pressure on the border of the hallux. (Specific surgical procedures are discussed later in this chapter.)

Onychauxis/Onychogryphosis

Onychauxis (club nail) refers to a hypertrophied nail plate. For the most part this involves the great toenail, but the lesser toes may be affected as well (Fig 25–19,A and B). The deformity may be caused by systemic problems such as nutritional deficiencies or psoriasis. The toenail may be yellow, brown, gray, or black. Most cases are a result of local conditions such as trauma to the nail matrix or nail bed and tinea infection. Indeed, tinea infection is the most frequent cause. The undersurface of the nail can become tremendously thickened from the accumulation of debris from a chronic mycotic infection.[85]

The affected nail and its bed are thickened and deformed. When the disorder is caused by tinea gypsum, the surface of the nail may have white streaks or patches that can readily be excised. When the undersurface of the nail contains a yellowish or brown powdery substance, destruction of the nail bed has been caused by tinea purpureum. In approximately 10% of cases of club nail, the nail bed and dorsal distal surface of the distal phalanx undergo hypertrophic changes.

Onychogryphosis refers to hypertrophy of the nail plate, especially of the hallux. The nail appears like a

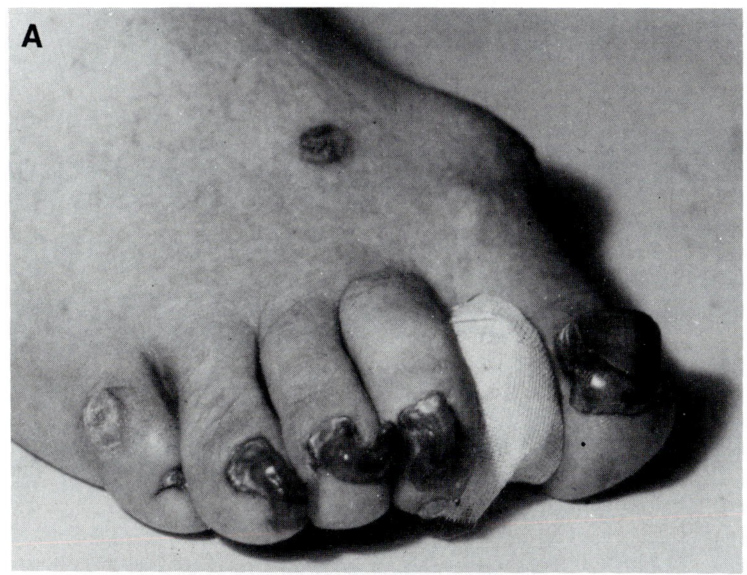

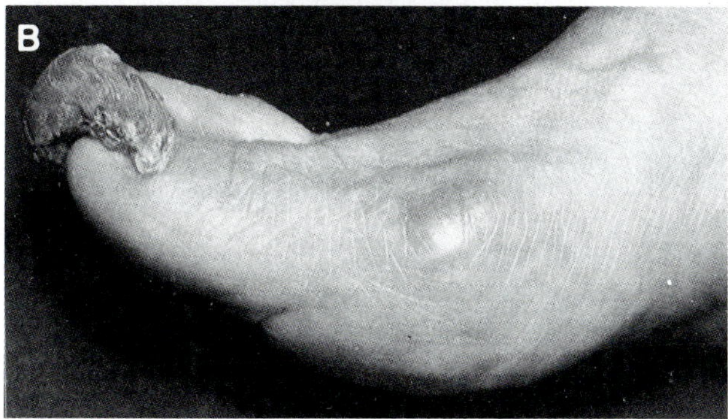

FIG 25–19.
A, Onychogryphosis of multiple nails. **B,** with onychogryphosis, a nail may become grossly thickened and excessively curved. (**B** from duViver A: *Atlas of clinical dermatology,* ed 2, London, 1992, Gower Medical Publishing. Used by permission.)

claw or horn, and while it is uncommon, its frequency in men who have tended horses has led to the appellation hostler's toe. It has also been referred to as ram's horn nail as well. The massive growth of the nail plate overlies the dorsal surface of the toe and often terminates on the plantar surface of the toe. This condition does not appear to have any relationship to a tinea infection. In most cases it is the result of a congenital or repeated trauma to the nail matrix along with poor hygiene. In some extreme cases, the nail measures several centimeters in length and curves upon itself to resemble a ram's horn.

Treatment.—With onychogryphosis, the entire nail horn up to where the nail is attached securely to the nail bed may be removed with a strong pair of nail clippers. Subsequent trimming and debridement will help the nail to become asymptomatic.

For a club nail, the hypertrophied nail and bed are gradually reduced by grinding with a motorized tool. Antifungal medication may be applied either topically or beneath the nail plate. In the case of severely deformed club nails, avulsion of the nail is advised. Later or concurrently, the nail matrix may be ablated with either a surgical ablation technique, chemical nail plate destruction, or a terminal Syme's procedure.

Onychomycosis

A mycotic infection of the toenails frequently accompanies tinea pedis (athlete's foot) or on occasion involves one or more of the toenails.[62] Zaias[85] has classified onychomycoses into four categories:

1. Distal subungual onychomycosis primarily involving the distal nail bed and hyponychium with secondary involvement of the undersurface of the nail plate.
2. White superficial onychomycosis. This is an invasion of the toenail plate on the surface of the nail by such organisms as *Trichophyton mentagrophytes*, *Cephalosporium*, and *Aspergillus*.
3. Proximal subungual onychomycosis, which is quite rare.
4. *Candida* onychomycosis involving the entire nail plate.

Onychomycosis is a very common disorder of the nail and infects possibly 20% of the population. The incidence may be much higher than this, but it is uncommon for a culture or biopsy to be taken on a regular basis. In patients over 60 years of age, involvement may approach 75% of the population. Infection with dermatophytes such as *Trichophyton rubrum*, *T. mentagrophytes*, and *Epidermophyton floccosum* is much more common than is infection due to *Candida*. Nondermatophytes account for fewer than 1% of cases of onychomycosis.[59, 60] *Candida* more typically is the cause of infection in children.

With chronic infection, the nail plate thickens and becomes discolored, brittle, and deformed. A buildup of chronic debris beneath the nail plate occurs with time. The thickened nail plate may become detached from the underlying nail bed and becomes painful when compressed by tight stockings or a constricting toe box (Table 25–15).

Distal subungual onychomycosis is the most common of all four types of mycotic infections (Fig 25–20,A). This deeply seated form of onychomycosis is demonstrated by yellowish, longitudinal streaks within the nail plate. The infectious organism invades insidiously from the free edge toward the base of the nail plate, with the end result being a thickened and deformed nail plate. The initial infection occurs in the stratum corneum. As the inflammation continues, the nail bed responds by cellular accumulation, nail elevation, and discoloration. With the accumulation of debris beneath the nail, further fungal and microorganism growth occurs. After invading the nail bed, the fungus penetrates the nail plate and causes delamination of the toenail. A number of der-

TABLE 25–15.
Common Organisms Cultured in Onychomycosis*

Distal subungual onychomycosis
Dermatophytes
Trichophyton rubrum
Trichophyton mentagrophytes
Epidermophyton floccosum
Yeasts and molds
Candida parapsilosis
Scopulariopsis brevicaulis
Aspergillus
Cephalosporium, Fusarium
Proximal subungual onychomycosis
Dermatophytes
Trichophyton rubrum
Trichophyton megninii
Trichophyton schoenleinii
Trichophyton tonsurans
Superficial white onychomycosis
Dermatophytes
Trichophyton mentagrophytes
Yeasts and Molds
Cephalosporium
Aspergillus
Fusarium
Candida onychomycosis
Yeasts and molds
Candida parapsilosis
Candida albicans

*Adapted from Norton LA: *J Am Acad Dermatol* 2:451–467, 1980.

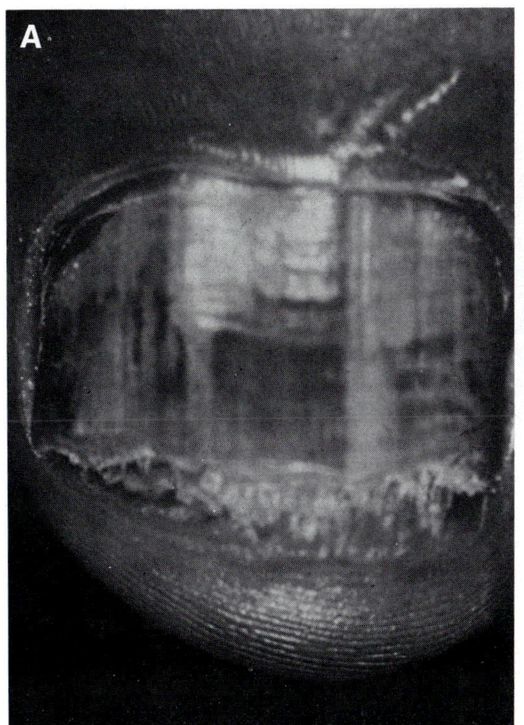

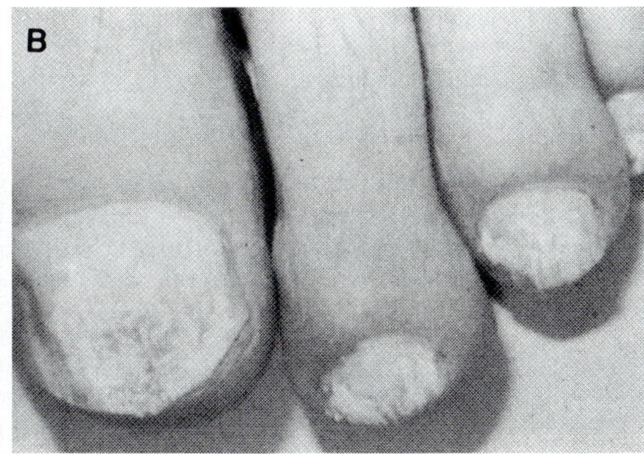

FIG 25–20.
A, onychomycosis. In this advanced case of distal subungual onychomycosis, the involved nail is thickened and opaque with distal crumbly material. In the toe web spaces, interdigital psoriasis appears to be whitish in color and is frequently mistaken for a fungal infection. **B,** superficial white onychomycosis (leukonychia trichophytica) infection confined to the nail plate. (**B** from Moschella SL, Hurley H, editors: *Dermatology,* ed 2, Philadelphia, 1986, WB Saunders, p 1406. Used by permission.)

matophytes are associated with subungual onychomycosis. *Trichophyton*, *Epidermophyton*, and *Microsporum* are the most common dermatophytes, with *T. rubrum* being the most common. *Trichophyton interdigitale* and *T. mentagrophytes* are also noted. *E. floccosum* as well nondermatophytes (*Scopulariopsis*, *Aspergillus*, *Fusarium*, and *Candida*) are also reported.[52] *T. rubrum* is considered to be the most common infectious organism. It is not felt that this is a contagious disease entity.

White superficial onychomycosis appears as opaque, white, well-demarcated islands on the surface of the nail plate (Fig 25–20,B). In this situation, the infectious organism invades the superficial dorsal aspect of the nail plate, which results in the development of white plaques. These plaques are localized fungal growth that may progress to more diffuse involvement invading the entire surface of the nail plate. The toenail may turn a brownish color and become roughened and pitted due to chronic infection. The most common infectious organism is *T. mentagrophytes*. Other agents include *Cephalosporium*, *T. interdigitale*, *Aspergillus*, and *Fusarium*.[52] Typical antiseptics may be an effective early treatment for this type of onychomycosis.

Proximal subungual onychomycosis is uncommon and is typified by whitish discoloration extending distally from underneath the proximal nail fold. *T. rubrum* is the most frequent infectious organism.

Candida onychomycosis, the fourth type of onychomycosis, is characterized by generalized thickening of the nail plate and is due to an infection of *Candida albicans* or *Candida parapsilosis*. Initially longitudinal white striations appear within the nail plate. The nail bed thickens, and the distal end of the digit appears bulbous and clubbed. Opacification of the nail plate may result as well.

Early signs of mycotic infection are thickening of the distal and lateral borders of the nail plate. Opacity may develop, and discoloration may be present with chronic infection. Erosion of the edges of the nail plate and partial loss or complete loss of the nail plate may occur. As time passes in advanced onychomycosis, it is difficult for the clinician to distinguish between the patterns of mycotic penetration of the nail plate.

When a fungal infection is suspected, an attempt at diagnosis is made by examining a specimen under light microscopy. Vigorous scraping of the nail may produce debris that may be moistened with a few drops of 10%

potassium hydroxide solution. Hyphae may be seen under microscopic examination. A culture on an appropriate medium may aid in the diagnosis.

Treatment.—Treatment of onychomycosis may be divided into systemic, local, and topical therapy.

Systemic.—The most aggressive treatment of onychomycosis involves systemic treatment with oral griseofulvin. Usually 1 g of griseofulvin is given daily for 8 to 12 months. In spite of this, there is a high failure rate. Ketoconazole,[13] a newer medication, has a broader spectrum than griseofulvin and has been reported to have a higher success rate in the treatment of chronic fungal infections. Patients should be advised of the systemic side effects. A pregnant patient should avoid treatment with systemic antifungal medication. In a report on 32 patients given 200 mg/day, Holub and Hubbard[37] reported a 56% success rate at 6 months, an 81% success rate at 8 months, and a 100% success rate following 12 months of systemic treatment. A 12.5% recurrence rate was also noted. Cure rates appear to be directly related to the duration of pharmacologic treatment. Adverse effects include nausea and vomiting, 3%; pruritus, 1.5%; and abdominal pain, 1%. Idiosyncratic liver dysfunction has been reported with an increase in liver enzymes and hepatocellular damage (severe reactions occur rarely—1:12,000). Patients should be informed of symptoms, side effects, and drug reactions.

Local.—Local therapy includes mechanical grinding and debridement of the thickened nail plate with a motorized device, curettage of the necrotic subungual tissue, and adequate trimming of the thickened nail plate. For many patients, this simple debridement technique may adequately relieve pain and discomfort without the need for surgical or pharmacologic intervention.

Topical.—Topical treatment may achieve success as well. Glutaraldahyde solution (10% buffered to a final pH of 7.8) has been used for topical treatment. One percent haloprogin (Halotex) solution applied twice daily beneath the toenail and ciclopirox olamine (Loprox), 1% cream applied to the dorsal aspect of the toenail, may also be applied on a twice daily-basis. Some clinicians prefer avulsion of the thickened nail plate, debridement of necrotic tissue, and treatment of the matrix and nail bed twice daily with Loprox cream.

Chemical nail plate destruction, surgical ablation, or a terminal Syme's amputation may be considered. These techniques will be discussed elsewhere.

Onychia

Onychia, also known as onychitis, occurs with inflammation of the nail matrix and the superficial soft tissue surrounding the toenail. This may be associated with ill-fitting footwear or tight stockings or may occur following trauma to the distal phalanx such as stubbing the toe or dropping an object onto the toe. On occasion osteomyelitis or osteitis may occur and cause painful symptoms.

Treatment.—Initial treatment requires removal of the causative agent. Minimizing trauma or pressure over the toenail may alleviate symptoms. In the presence of an acute bacterial or fungal infection, a culture and sensitivity should be obtained. Appropriate antibiotic therapy may be instituted. Radiographs are obtained to diagnose any osseous involvement. Local surgical care includes an incision and drainage in the presence of acute infection. Toenail avulsion may be necessary and, on occasion, surgical ablation of the toenail as well. Localized treatment with antifungal agents such as clotrimazole (Lotrimin) or nystatin cream may be helpful in the presence of a fungal infection. The simultaneous use of roomy footwear or sandals may help remove pressure from the painful toenail. Frequently symptoms will subside with time and aggressive conservative treatment.

Onycholysis/Onychomadesis

Onycholysis occurs when the nail plate becomes separated from the nail bed along the lateral and distal borders. Onychomadesis occurs with separation of the entire nail plate beginning proximally and ending distally. Onychomadesis may be associated with drug reaction, eczema, scarlet fever, leprosy, lead poisoning, or trauma.[60] A nail ablation procedure may be necessary to treat a chronic condition.

Onycholysis, which occurs more frequently in females than in males, seems to be associated with local trauma as well as drug and allergic reactions, eczema, hypothyroidism, hyperthyroidism, lichen planus, bacterial and fungal infections, and vascular insufficiency. *Candida albicans* and *Pseudomonas* are the most frequent infectious organisms. Trimming of the separated nail plate and the application of topical antifungal medication may be helpful in treating this condition. For more severe symptomatology, a toenail ablation procedure may be necessary.

Nail Bed Disorders

The structure and function of the nail bed may be altered by subungual exostosis, subungual tumor, subungual clavus, subungual hematoma, or a subungual verruca.

Subungual Exostosis

Abnormalities of the underlying bone can be diagnosed with the aid of a radiograph. Typically these will involve the distal phalanx. A subungual exostosis must be differentiated from an osteochondroma (see the discussion of subungual exostosis under "Tumors"). Likewise, when a lytic lesion in the distal phalanx occurs, usually a benign tumor such as an enchondroma or solitary bone cyst should be considered.

In a patient with complaints of pain, swelling, inflammation, and even chronic paronychia, consideration of a radiograph should be given to evaluate the patient for an underlying bony tumor. The development of chronic subungual ulceration should alert the clinician to the possibility of squamous cell carcinoma, probably the most common malignant tumor seen in the area of the toe.

Subungual Tumors

Subungual and periungual fibromas (Fig 25–21,A), exostoses, mucous cysts, glomus tumors, enchondromas, keratocanthomas, pyogenic granuloma, and other benign lesions can occur in the area of the distal phalanx. Likewise, malignant tumors such as squamous cell and basal cell carcinomas and malignant melanomas may be demonstrated as well in this area (see the section "Tumors").

Subungual Clavus

A hyperkeratotic lesion in the subungual region is characterized by the accumulation of debris beneath the nail plate. The development of a callus in this area may be due to pressure from a confining toe box or the chronic use of tight stockings. Likewise, vascular insufficiency, psoriasis, diabetes, localized fungal infection, as well as various systemic diseases may be the cause of a subungual clavus. As the amount of debris accumulates, a yellowish gray cast will occur in the toenail. Typically a patient will complain of pain due to external pressure from a closed toe shoe. The differential diagnosis includes subungual exostosis, subungual osteochondroma, trauma, subungual verruca, and a glomus tumor.

Treatment.—Debridement of the hyperkeratotic clavus is the treatment of choice. Trimming of the detached nail plate will make debridement of the necrotic tissue easier.

Subungual Hematoma

The accumulation of hemorrhage between the nail bed and the nail plate is referred to as a subungual hematoma. Typically this occurs with trauma to the nail bed and the rupture of small capillaries in this region. Crushing or shearing trauma to the nail produces a painful subungual hemorrhage manifested by a dusky swelling of the nail plate. Within hours pressure builds up following trauma because of bleeding beneath the nail, and a throbbing pain typically brings the patient to

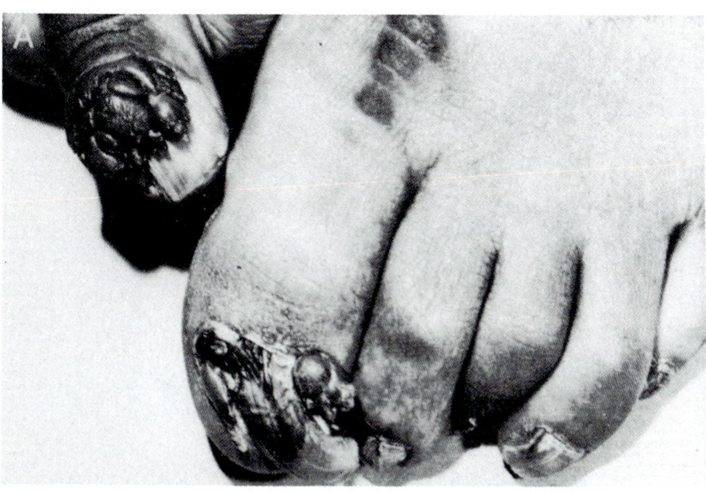

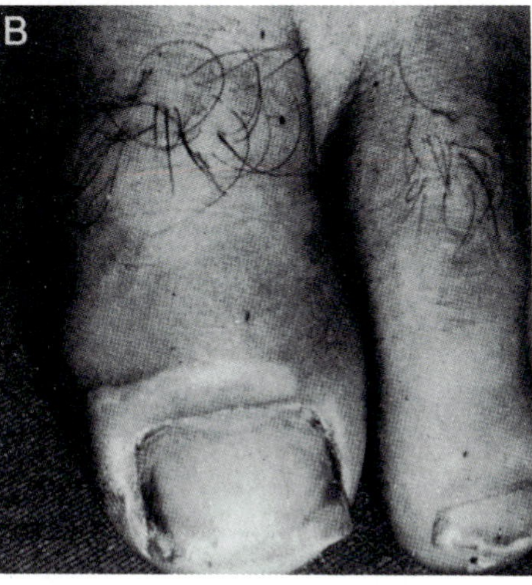

FIG 25–21.
A, a periungual fibroma as seen in epiloia, a syndrome characterized by epilepsy, mental retardation, angiomas, and fibromas. (From Jahss M, editor: *Disorders of the foot and ankle,* ed 2, Philadelphia, WB Saunders, p 1572. Used by permission.) **B,** acute paronychia of the hallux with extension to the proximal and lateral nail folds. (From Yale I: *Podiatric medicine,* Baltimore, Williams & Wilkins, p 170. Used by permission.)

the physician for relief. The use of a nail drill or burning through the nail plate with a red-hot paper clip is effective in releasing any increased pressure. Radiographs may be necessary to rule out a fracture. Further therapy may include oral antibiotics.

Subungual Verruca

A subungual or periungual verruca may occur beneath the nail plate or in the nail groove. The appearance of a verruca is similar to that of a wart on any other part of the foot. When a verruca involves the subungual tissue, care must be taken in the treatment plan in order to avoid damage to the nail matrix. Usually the wart can be ablated with chemical treatment, excision, electrocautery, or a combination of these treatments.

Nail Fold Disorders

Nail fold disorders include paronychia, onychophosis, pyogenic granuloma, herpetic whitlow, and periungual verrucae.

Paronychia

Paronychia is an inflammation of the nail groove that commonly affects the hallux, although it may affect the lesser toes as well (Fig 25–21,B). This cellulitis of the nail fold is characterized by swelling, erythema, pain, tenderness, and often a purulent discharge from beneath the nail fold. Secondary dystrophic changes of the nail are frequently seen, and chronic paronychia involvement with *Candida* may occur. At times, the infection extends to the nail matrix, in which case it is termed *onychia*. Unlike onychia, a paronychia by itself is rarely caused by the skin disorders. Paronychia may vary in severity. It may present as a mild cellulitis. When extrinsic pressure from a confining toe box crowds the tissue on the medial aspect of the nail, a severe infection may result. Granulation tissue and extensive ulceration in the nail groove are characteristic of chronic changes. Paronychia is either accompanied by or is a forerunner of an ingrown toenail.

Treatment.—Treatment consists of the following steps:

1. Relieving extrinsic pressure from shoe wear.
2. Excising a linear portion, about 2 mm of the nail margin, to relieve the cutting effect of the edematous nail groove.
3. Painting the granulation tissue with a silver nitrate stick.
4. Applying a fungicidal ointment and covering with a sterile dressing.

Onychophosis

Onychophosis occurs with accumulation of callus within the lateral nail groove. It more commonly occurs in the great toe than in the lesser toes. This may occur secondary to extrinsic pressure from a tight-fitting toe box but may also occur with pronation of the foot and abduction of the hallux or with an incurved nail plate. Typically erythema and swelling occur in the nail groove, and this may develop into an ingrown toenail. Pain is frequently associated with this condition. The differential diagnosis includes subungual clavus, onychia, paronychia, and onychocryptosis.

Treatment.—The initial treatment involves shaving or debridement of the callus. With a purulent infection, a partial avulsion of the nail and even eventual nail matrix ablation may be necessary. Radiographs may be helpful in ruling out a subungual exostosis, which may present with similar symptomatic findings.

Pyogenic Granuloma

A pyogenic granuloma[9, 26] is a vascular lesion that develops from connective tissue. Its color may vary from red to dark blue or black, and commonly this lesion varies from 2 to 10 mm in size. It may be pedunculated or sessile in appearance and is frequently complicated by a staphylococcal infection. It may develop secondary to trauma along the lateral nail fold. The differential diagnosis includes onychia, Kaposi's sarcoma, glomus tumor, periungual verruca, melanoma, fibroma, hemanigoma, and basal cell carcinoma.

Treatment.—Typical treatment involves cauterization with silver nitrate, electrocautery, or a laser technique. Following treatment, the application of moist dressings and the use of antibiotics may be indicated.

Herpetic Whitlow

Herpetic whitlow[41] is a primary infection with a herpetic virus. It often presents symptomatically as a painful group of vesicles on one or more swollen toes. The vesicles are often surrounded by an erythematous base. Regional lymphangitis may be associated with this condition, and the infection may be confused with bacterial infection or impetigo. Herpetic whitlow should be differentiated from a bacterial infection, which may require systemic antibiotics and incision and drainage. A typical antibiotic regimen is not effective with a viral infection. The use of oral antiviral medication (acyclovir) may be successful in decreasing symptoms.

Periungual Verruca

A periungual wart is located on the margin of the nail plate and resembles warts found elsewhere on the

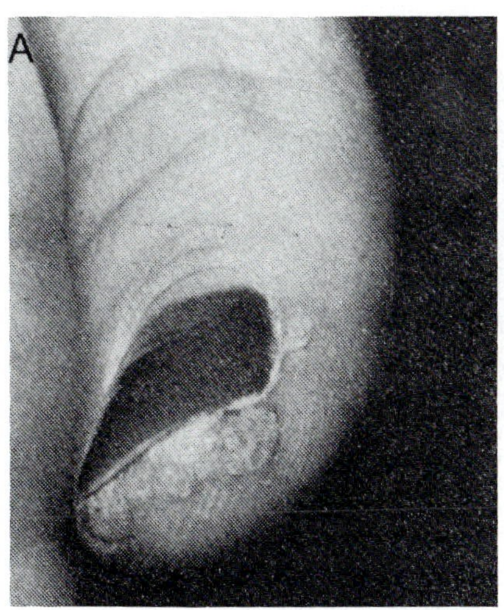

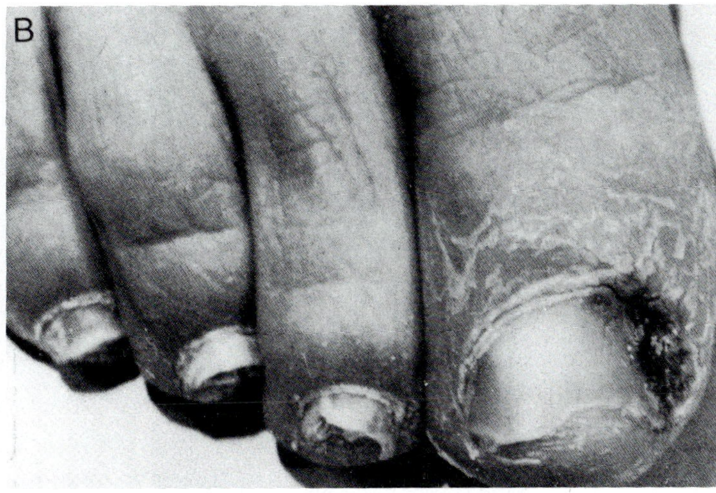

FIG 25–22.
A, periungual verruca of the distal nail plate and hyponychium. (From Moschella SL, Hurley H, editors: *Dermatology,* ed 2, Philadelphia, 1986, WB Saunders, p 690. Used by permission.) **B,** a periungual wart may suggest a periungual fibroma. A biopsy is necessary to establish a definitive diagnosis. (From Jahss M, editor: *Disorders of the foot and ankle,* ed 2, Philadelphia, 1991, WB Saunders, p. 1571. Used by permission.)

foot (Fig 25–22,A and B). Of viral origin, careful treatment is necessary to avoid trauma to the nail matrix, which may cause a permanent nail deformity. Treatment may vary from chemical ablation of the wart to electrocautery or cryotherapy. Surgical excision may also be considered.

Nail Matrix Disorders

Disorders of the nail matrix may result in an abnormality of the nail plate. Ridging, atrophy, partial or complete anonychia, and pterygium formation can occur following trauma.

Anonychia

Anonychia (Fig 25–23), or the absence of toenails, may be an inherited condition[77] or may follow destruction of a nail matrix after surgery. It may also occur with systemic illnesses. Vascular insufficiency, Raynaud's disease, and frostbite may also lead to the loss of nails. Typically there is no treatment warranted for acquired or congenital anonychia. Often the destruction of the nail matrix that leads to anonychia is surgically induced as a treatment for chronic nail conditions.

Pterygium

With pterygium (Fig 25–24,A), the cuticle grows forward on the nail plate and splits it into two or more portions. Zaias[87] has noted that this occurs more commonly in the fourth and fifth digits. Pardo-Castello[64] has reported that this occurs more commonly in association with leprosy and peripheral neuritis. Other disease entities that may present with pterygium include vascular insufficiency, Raynaud's disease, scleroderma, and lichen planus.

Atrophy/Hypertrophy of the Nail Matrix

The nail matrix may hypertrophy with resultant increased thickness of the nail plate and nail bed. The nail plate may become grooved, abnormally raised, and even

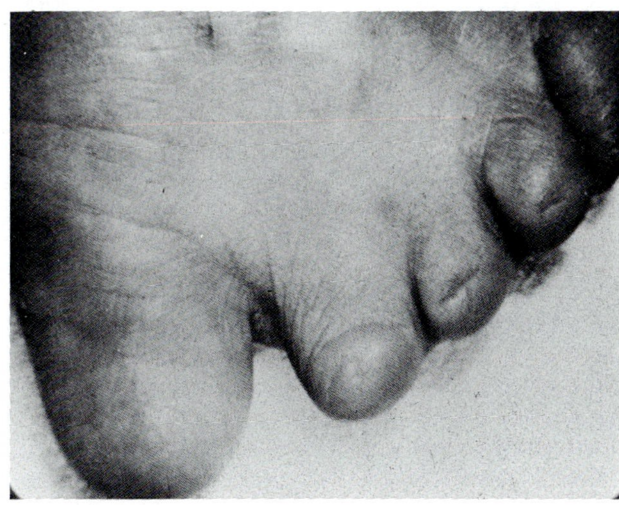

FIG 25–23.
Anonychia: congenital absence of the nails with associated absence of the distal phalanges. (From Yale I: *Podiatric medicine,* Baltimore, Williams & Wilkins, p 176. Used by permission.)

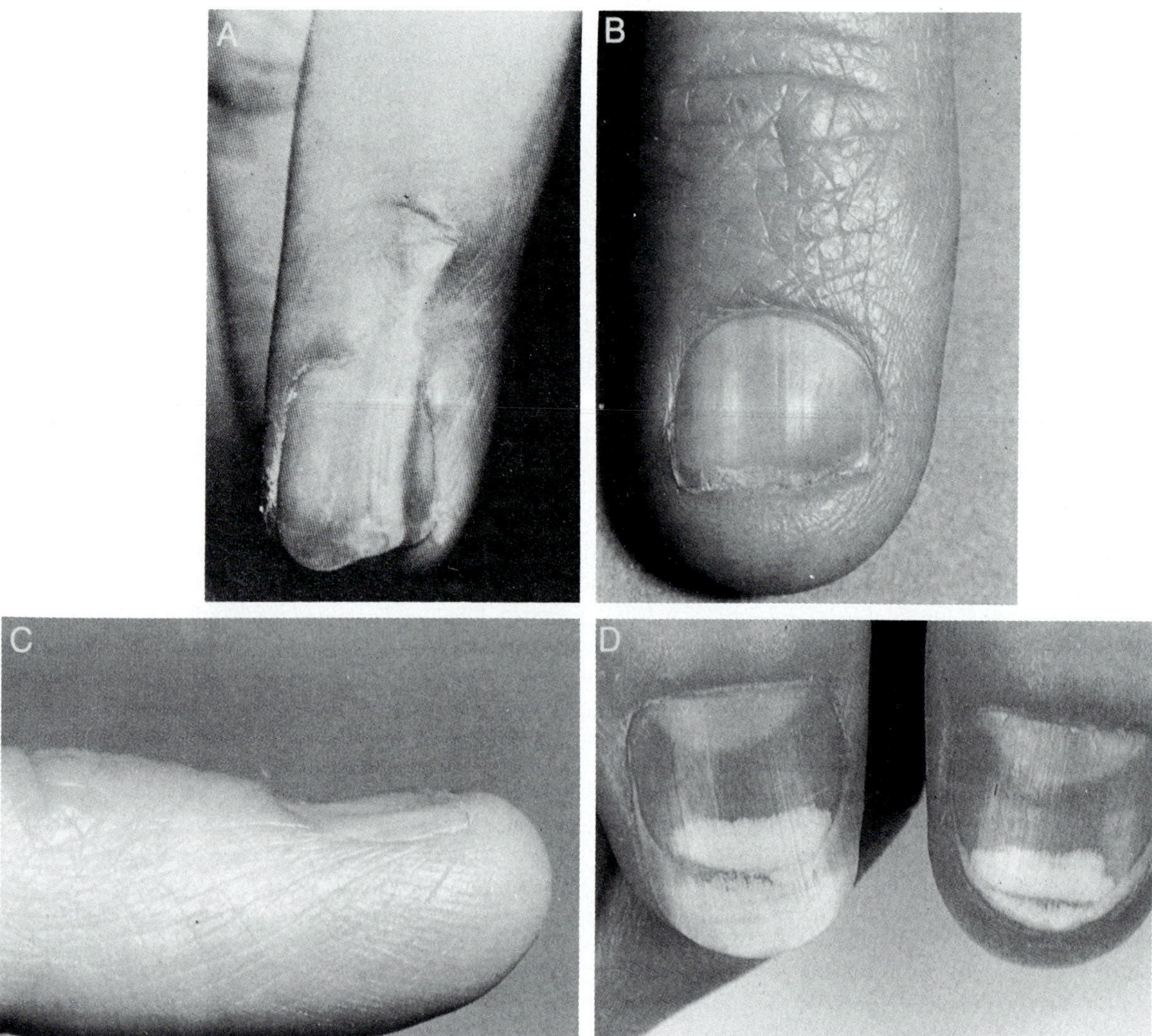

FIG 25–24.
A, pterygium formation in association with lichen planus. Attachment of adherent cuticle to the underlying nail bed is associated with the deformity. **B** and **C,** koilonychia is the development of a concave rather than a convex nail plate. It resembles a spoon shape. **D,** with leukonychia, a whitish discoloration of the nail plate is common. (**A** from Moschella SL, Hurley H, editors: *Dermatology,* ed 2, Philadelphia, 1986, WB Saunders, p 1412. **B** and **C** from duViver A: *Atlas of clinical dermatology,* ed 2, London, 1992, Gower Medical Publishing, Used by permission.)

elongated. With the occurrence of this abnormality the condition of onychogryphosis or onychauxis develops. At the other end of the spectrum, atrophy of the matrix may develop temporarily with resultant transverse ridges or lines in the nail plate referred to as Beau's lines. These occur with sudden arrest in the growth of the nail matrix. As regrowth occurs, a more normal nail plate develops that leaves the transverse line. This appears to be associated with increased fever, infection, and arthritis. Thinning of the nail plate may occur with anemia and lichen planus.

Pathologic Keratinization

The cells of the nail matrix may become involved with abnormal differentiation as associated with a systemic disease such as psoriasis when there is increased keratin formation in the nail bed. An abnormal rate of keratinization may occur with fungal infection and may be associated with onychoschizia, koilonychia, and leukonychia.

Onychoschizia describes a distal fissuring or splitting of the nail plate. Delamination may occur with longitudinal separation of the layers of the nail plate. Hematologic disorders, trauma, infection, hypovitaminosis, and dermatologic disorders may lead to onychoschizia.

Koilonychia describes a concavity of the nail plate or "spoon-shaped" nail (Fig 25–24,B and C). Genetic causes, endocrine disorders, thyroid disease, infection, hematologic abnormalities, Raynaud's disease, and nail bed tumors are all causes of koilonychia. The thickness of the nail plate may vary. The nail plate, however, retains a smooth surface, although it frequently opacifies.

Leukonychia describes the appearance of a whitish discoloration or spot on the nail plate (Fig 25–24,D). Multiple nails may become involved. Variations of leukonychia include punctate discoloration or transverse striations 1 to 2 mm in width that resemble Mee's lines. Opacification may be partial (Hodgkin's disease), complete (leprosy), or longitudinal (Darier-White disease).

CONSERVATIVE AND SURGICAL TREATMENT OF TOENAIL PROBLEMS

Conservative treatment is a frequent regimen used in stage I infections of the toenail as well as when there is a prominent and painful toenail edge. Typical treatment utilizes elevation of the lateral toenail plate from an inflamed or impinged nail fold. A wisp of cotton is carefully inserted beneath the edge of the nail plate (Fig 25–25,A and B).[17, 35, 54] With elevation of the nail plate, care must be taken to not fracture the toenail when the cotton is inserted. A digital anesthetic block may be used to reduce pain when the nail plate is elevated. Collodion may be added to the cotton wisp for longevity.[38] The patient is encouraged to soak the toe twice daily in a tepid salt solution. The toenail region is then dried and the inflamed area coated with a dessicating solution such as gentian violet or alcohol. When the cotton wisp is to be removed, usually the patient will return for a further visit. As the erythema diminishes, the patient is instructed to replace the cotton wisp. Dessicating agents are utilized until inflammation has subsided. The cotton packing must be replaced until the nail plate has grown beyond the distal extent of the nail fold. Usually the rate of nail growth is approximately 2 mm/month, so the estimated duration of treatment can be calculated for the patient. Once adequate length of the nail plate has developed, the patient is then instructed in proper trimming of the nail plate in a transverse fashion. Care is taken to not pick or tear the nail plate because this may cause recurrent infection.

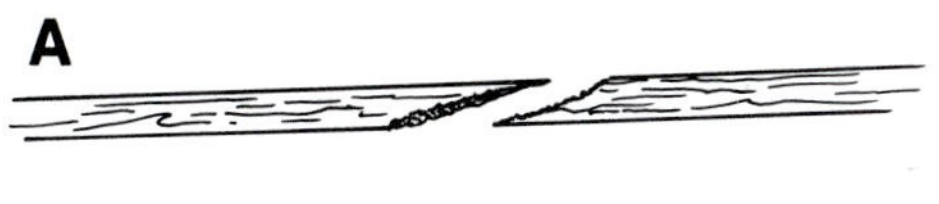

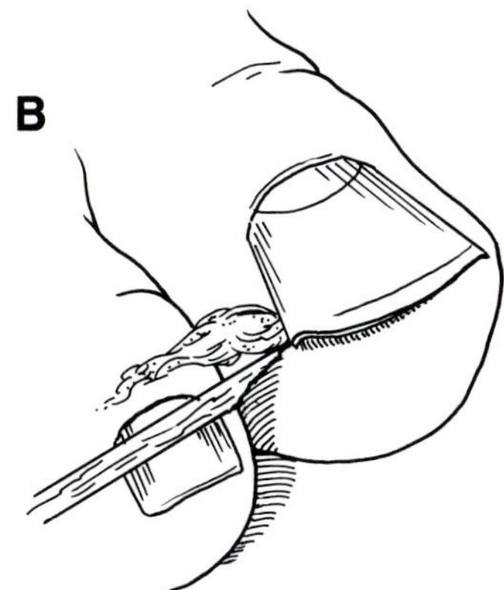

FIG 25–25.
Method of elevating the lateral margin of the nail plate. **A,** a cotton-tipped applicator is broken to create a sharp tipped point. **B,** a wisp of cotton is placed under the impinging edge of the nail plate.

Diagonal trimming of the nail may initially decrease the inflammation associated with acute infection, but it tends to temporize treatment; Dixon[21] has noted that "the nail fold tissue will quickly exploit the absence of the nail and can result in recurrence."

Treatment of ingrown toenails is individualized for each patient. Heifetz[35] observed that only during stage I can conservative methods be adequately used. When conservative care has been unsuccessful or where acute (stage II) or chronic (stage III) infection has occurred, aggressive nail care is necessary. Alternatives include the following:

1. Partial nail plate avulsion
2. Complete nail plate avulsion
3. Plastic nail wall reduction
4. Partial onychectomy
5. Complete onychectomy
6. Syme's amputation of the toe

Digital Anesthetic Block

A digital anesthetic block is usually sufficient anesthesia for any of the toenail procedures performed (Fig 25–26,A–B, C).[53] A small skin wheal is raised on the dorsomedial aspect of the hallux. The needle is directed in a dorsoplantar direction to anesthetize the dorsal and plantar digital sensory nerves. Once this is completed, the needle is turned horizontally and the dorsal aspect of the great toe infiltrated. The needle is then withdrawn and placed at the lateral base of the great toe, and the dorsolateral and lateral plantar digital nerves are anesthetized.

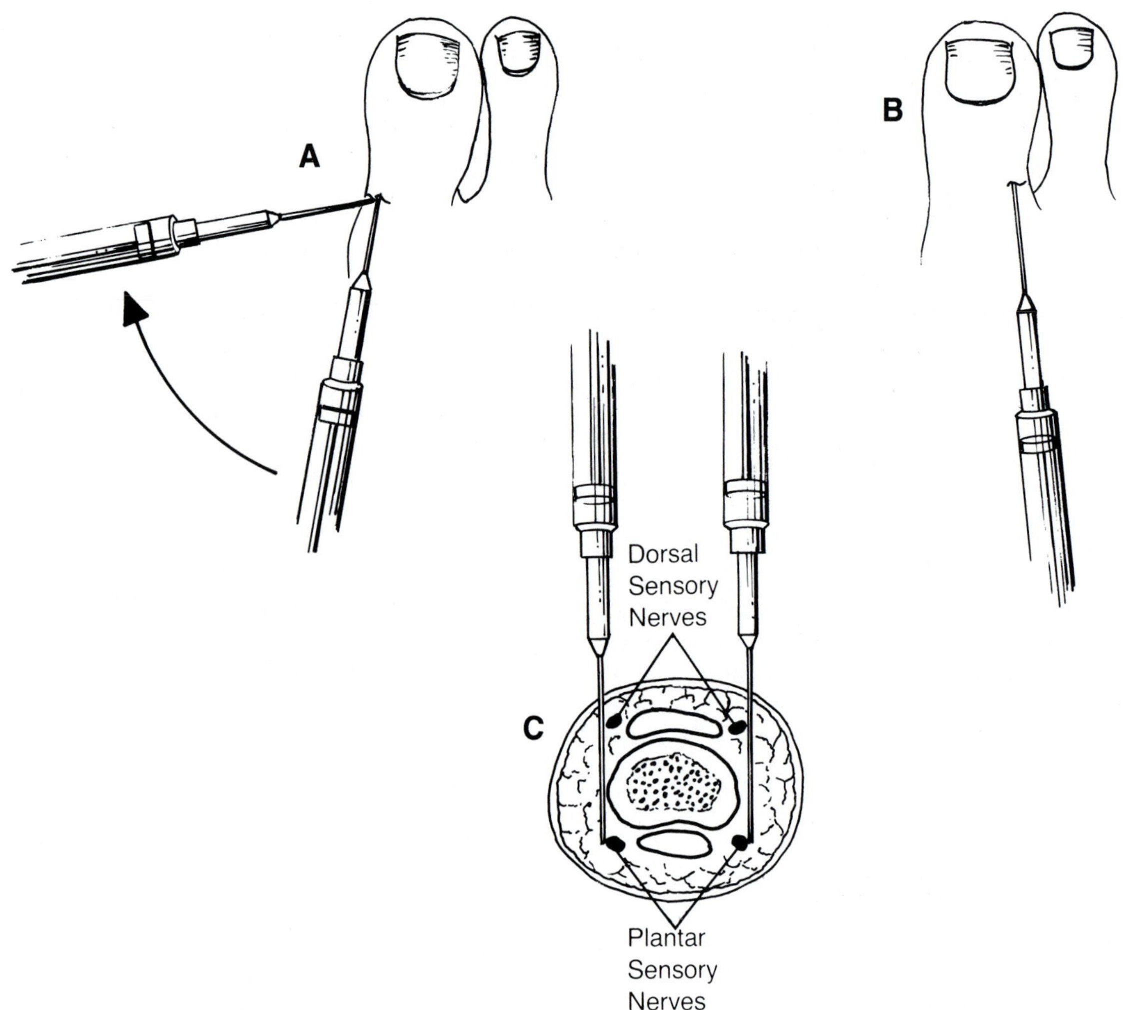

FIG 25–26.
Technique of digital anesthetic block with 1% lidocaine hydrochloride. **A,** initially, a medial wheal is raised and the needle advanced in a dorsoplantar direction. The needle is then turned horizontally and the dorsum of the toe blocked. **B,** a second injection is then done to anesthetize the lateral aspect of the toe. **C,** a cross section demonstrates the path of the needles. (From Mann RA, Coughlin MJ: *The video textbook of foot and ankle surgery,* St Louis, 1990, Medical Video Productions. Used by permission.)

Partial Nail Plate Avulsion

After the placement of a digital anesthetic block, the toe is cleansed in a routine fashion.

1. A ¼-in. Penrose drain is used as a tourniquet.
2. The outer edge of the toenail plate is elevated proximally to the cuticle (Fig 25–27,A and B).
3. Scissors or small bone cutters are used to section the nail longitudinally (Fig 25–27,C and D).
4. Care is taken to remove only as much nail as is necessary. The nail is then grasped with a hemostat and avulsed (Fig 25–27,E and F), and the nail bed is examined to ensure that no spike of nail tissue remains.
5. A gauze compression dressing is applied and changed as needed until drainage subsides, usually within a few days.

Following removal of the nail plate edge, acute or chronic infection ordinarily subsides. Antibiotics may be used depending upon the severity of the infection.

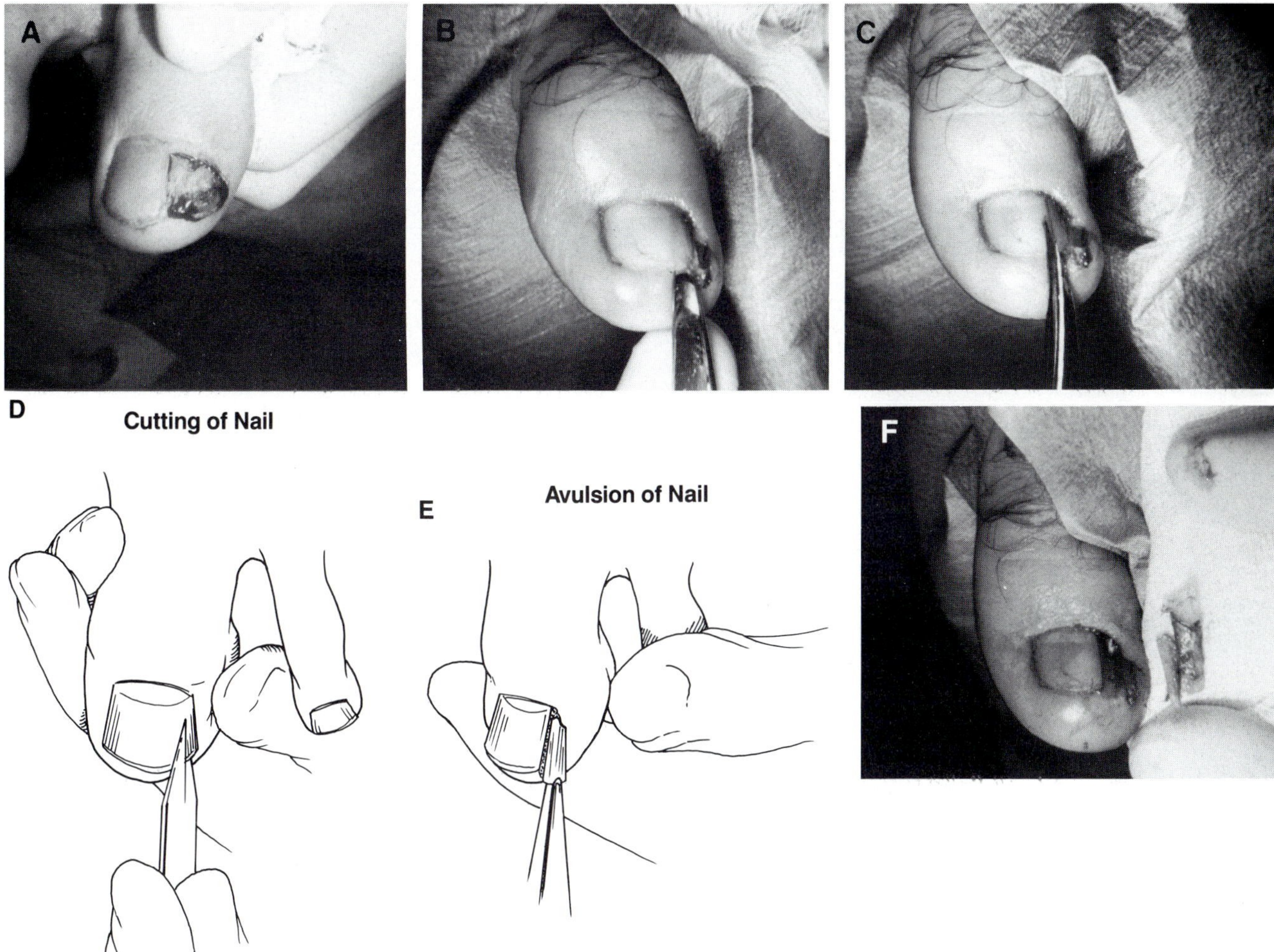

FIG 25–27.
A, an acute stage 3 infection with purulent drainage. **B** and **C,** the lateral edge of the nail plate is elevated and then longitudinally sectioned. The freed edge of the nail is grasped and avulsed with a hemostat. **D,** the nail plate is elevated along the border. **E,** the nail plate is sectioned longitudinally. **F,** the edge of the nail plate is avulsed. (**A–C** and **F** from Mann RA, Coughlin MJ: *The video textbook of foot and ankle surgery.* St Louis, 1990, Medical Video Productions. Used by permission.)

Aftercare is important for a successful outcome following partial toenail avulsion. With distal growth of the nail plate, the advancing edge is at risk for recurrent infection. A cotton wisp is placed beneath the advancing edge in order to elevate the nail plate. A digital block may be necessary to replace subsequent packs. The patient is instructed in the technique of packing the toenail plate edge with a cotton wisp, and packing is continued until the nail edge is advanced past the distal extent of the nail groove.

Lloyd-Davies and Brill[51] reported a 47% recurrence rate following partial nail plate avulsion. Another 33% reported residual symptoms following partial nail plate avulsion. Keyes[43] reported a 77% incidence of recurrence following partial nail plate avulsion.

Complete Toenail Avulsion

In the presence of more extensive infection, complete toenail avulsion may be performed. A digital anesthetic block is used and the toe cleansed in the usual fashion.

1. A ¼-in. Penrose drain is used as a tourniquet.
2. The nail plate is elevated from the nail bed and matrix (Fig 25–28,A).
3. The cuticle is incised and elevated from the nail plate (Fig 25–28,B).
4. The toenail is avulsed by grasping it with a hemostat (Fig 25–28,C and D). (Usually this is associated with fairly brisk bleeding, and a compression dressing is applied. Hemostasis is usually fairly prompt.)

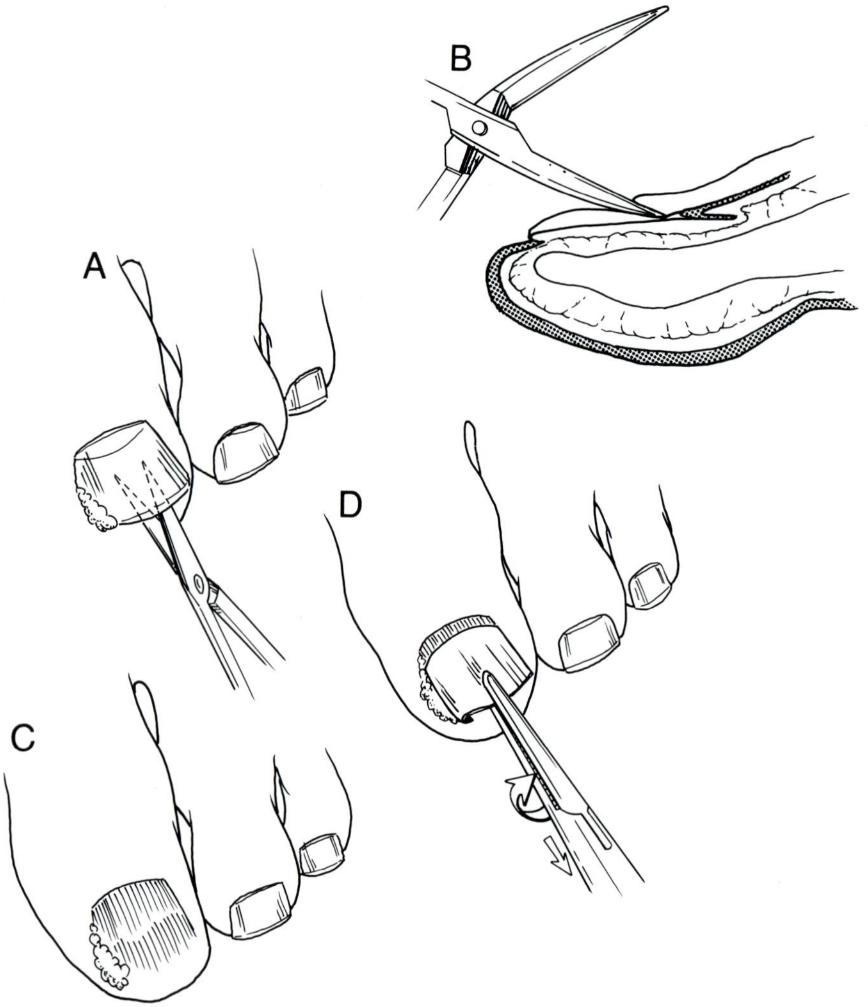

FIG 25–28.
Technique of complete toenail avulsion. **A,** the nail plate is elevated from the nail bed. **B,** lateral view demonstrating freeing of the dorsal soft-tissue attachments of the nail plate. **C,** the nail plate is grasped with a hemostat and avulsed **(D).**

5. After 24 hours, soaking is started on a daily basis in a tepid salt solution.
6. The bandage is replaced and changed daily until drainage has subsided.

Antibiotics may be prescribed depending upon the severity of the infection. Reepithelialization of the nail bed occurs over a 2- to 3-week period. As the nail regrows, the advancing edges should be elevated with a cotton wisp to prevent recurrence of a toenail infection.

Murray and Bedi[55] reviewed a series of 200 patients who underwent toenail procedures. Of the 145 patients who underwent a simple toenail avulsion, 64% experienced recurrent symptoms following the initial procedure, 86% experienced recurrence following a second procedure, and 80% had recurrence following more than two avulsions.

While toenail avulsion may give dramatic relief of not only infection but also symptoms, the rate of cure following toenail avulsion is quite low. Ordinarily a secondary procedure must be performed. Dixon[21] has noted a much higher recurrence rate of infection in cases where multiple avulsions of a single toenail have been performed. Lloyd-Davies and Brill[51] reported that within 6 months 31% of patients required further treatment following total nail plate avulsion. Palmer and Jones[63] reported a 70% recurrence of symptoms following total nail plate avulsion.

Plastic Reduction of the Nail Lip

A plastic nail lip reduction may be used for a younger patient with mild to moderate disease. In the presence of an acute infection, a partial toenail avulsion is initially performed. Following resolution of the acute infection, a plastic nail lip reduction is performed. A digital anesthetic block is applied and the toe cleansed in the usual fashion.

1. A ¼-in. Penrose drain is used for hemostasis.
2. A spindle-shaped section approximately 3 mm wide by 1 cm long is excised from the site of the nail lip. This is triangular in cross section (Fig 25–29,A and B).
3. The incision extends from the distal portion of the toe to approximately 5 mm proximal to the nail fold and is located about 2 mm from the lateral nail groove.
4. Excess subdermal fat is excised.
5. The skin margins are coapted with interrupted 3–0 nylon sutures. The closure will draw the nail groove lateralward and downward (Fig 25–29,C and D).
6. A sterile dressing is applied and changed as needed until drainage has subsided.
7. Sutures are removed 3 weeks following the procedure.

Keyes[43] in a small series of four patients reported a 25% recurrence rate with this procedure.

Partial Onychectomy (Winograd or Heifetz Procedure)

This procedure is only performed after an acute infection has resolved, usually following a partial nail plate avulsion.[35, 36, 80, 81]

A digital anesthetic block is applied.

1. A ¼-in. Penrose drain is used for tourniquet hemostasis after the toe has been cleansed in the usual fashion.
2. A vertical incision is made along the lateral edge of the toenail (usually at the edge of a previous nail plate avulsion).
3. With the Heifetz procedure, the resection is carried just distal to the terminal extent of the lunula. With the Winograd procedure, not only is the nail matrix excised, but the nail bed is resected as well.
4. An oblique incision is made at the apex of the nail bed (Fig 25–30,A). The proximal nail matrix and edge of the cuticle are excised. (Care is taken to not injure the extensor tendon insertion as well as to not violate the interphalangeal joint).
5. The germinal matrix is characterized by a "pearly white" color and texture. It extends into the nail fold laterally and must be completely excised.

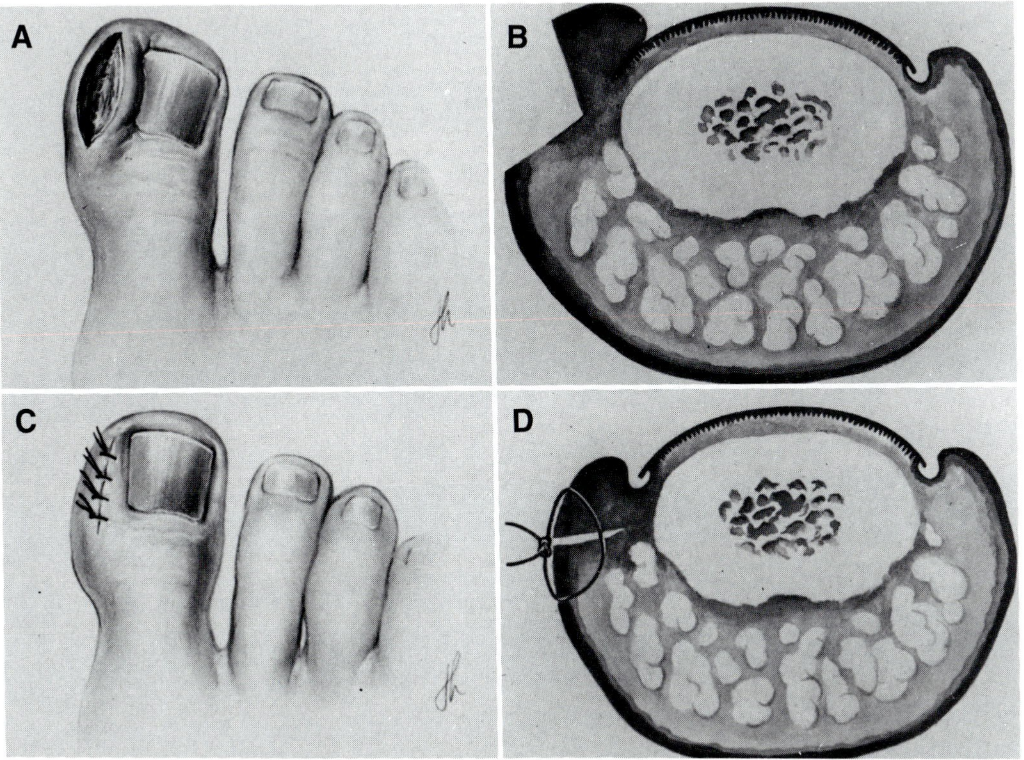

FIG 25–29.
Soft-tissue wedge resection for an ingrown toenail. **A,** a triangular section is removed from the lateral aspect of the nail groove. **B,** cross section after excision. **C,** the nail lip and groove are pulled down after suturing of the nail margins. **D,** cross section after suturing.

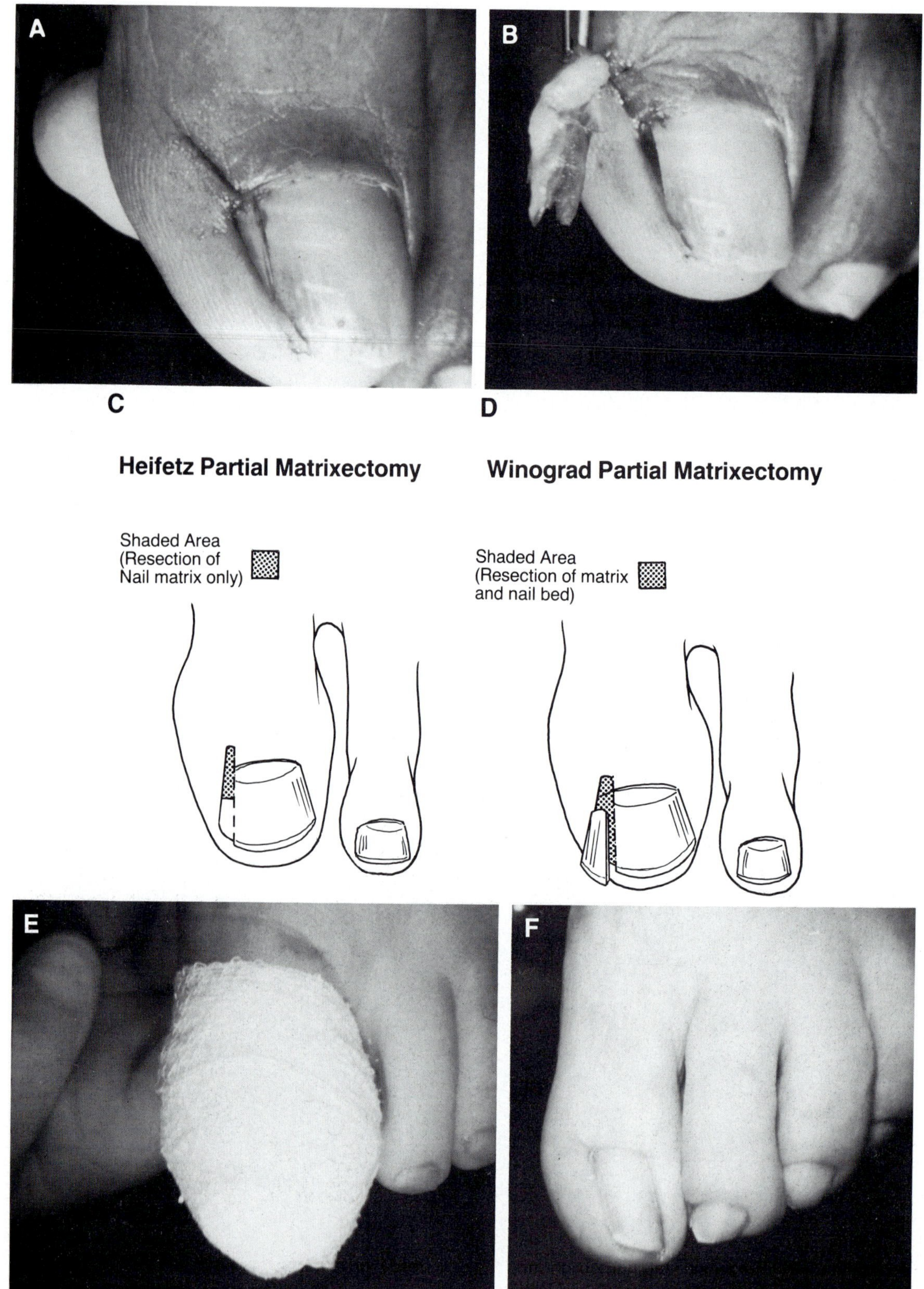

FIG 25–30.
A, a longitudinal vertical and oblique incision is used to incise the nail matrix and bed. **B,** following avulsion of the nail plate edge, the nail matrix and bed are excised. **C** and **D,** diagram of proposed soft-tissue excision. (With the Heifetz procedure, the

6. Remaining matrix is excised from the cortex of the distal phalanx. In the case of the Winograd procedure, the nail bed is resected as well (Fig 25–30,B–D).
7. The skin edges are coapted with an interrupted nylon suture.
8. A compression dressing is applied and changed at 24 hours (Fig 25–30,E).

Subsequent dressings are changed weekly until resolution of drainage.

Prophylactic antibiotics may be prescribed depending upon the surgeon's preference or if the patient is at high risk for infection. Sutures are removed 2 weeks following surgery (Fig 25–30,F).

Murray and Bedi[55] in their review of 200 patients reported a 27% recurrence rate after a Winograd procedure, and when a double Winograd procedure was performed, a 50% recurrence rate was experienced. Clarke and Dillinger[18] reported their experience with the Winograd procedure. Of 29 procedures evaluated, one third had unsatisfactory results. There were 9 recurrences and 2 patients who reported continued discomfort at follow-up ranging from 8 to 18 months. Palmer and Jones[63] reported a 29% recurrence rate following a Winograd resection. Gabriel et al.,[28] in a series of 528 patients who had an ablation of the lateral matrix, reported a 1.7% recurrence rate and a 79% satisfaction rate. Winograd[81] reported a 15% recurrence rate in a follow-up of 20 patients. Pettine et al.[65] reported the Heifetz procedure to have a 90% satisfaction rate with a 6% recurrence rate. Keyes[43] reported a 12% recurrence rate with the Heifetz procedure.

Complete Onychectomy (the Zadik Procedure)

On occasion, the patient may require a complete and permanent toenail removal.[84] This procedure is not performed in the face of acute infection, but usually after an initial toenail avulsion. It is wise to delay surgery until infection and inflammation have subsided.

A digital anesthetic block is applied and the toe cleansed in the usual fashion.

1. A ¼-in. Penrose drain is used for hemostasis.
2. An oblique incision is made at the medial and lateral apex of the toenail (Fig 25–31,A), and the toenail is avulsed (Fig 25–31,B and C).
3. The cuticle, eponychium, and proximal nail bed are completely excised.
4. The matrix is excised proximal to the cuticle, laterally into the nail folds, and distally as far as the distal extent of the lunula (Fig 25–31,D).
5. The nail matrix is curretted and remaining tissue excised.
6. The skin edges are closed with interrupted 3–0 nylon. Excess tension should be avoided along the suture line because it may lead to sloughing of the skin (Fig 25–31,E).
7. A compression dressing is applied and changed 24 hours postoperatively. Further dressing changes are performed as needed depending upon the amount of drainage.

Sutures are removed 2 to 3 weeks following surgery. The patient should be informed that minor recurrence of the toenail tissue may occur (Fig 25–31,F). The etiology of recurrent nail tissue growth may be from germinal cells within the nail bed.

Murray[54] reported a 16% recurrence rate with the Zadik procedure. Palmer and Jones[63] reported a 28% failure rate following the Zadik procedure. Townsend and Scott[75] reported a 50% failure rate with the Zadik procedure. Eighty-nine percent of patients reported acceptable results in spite of the small recurrence typically in the central region.

The use of a carbon dioxide laser for matrisectomy has had variable success. Apfelberg et al.[2] reported a 22% recurrence rate. Wright[83] reported a recurrence rate of 50% following laser toenail ablation and recommended that it not be used for either partial or complete toenail ablation.

Syme's Amputation (Thompson-Terwilliger Procedure)

For symptomatic recurrence of toenail tissue or when a patient requires a more reliable excision, a Syme's amputation of the distal phalanx may be considered.[74]

A digital anesthetic block is applied and the toe cleansed in the usual fashion.

1. A ¼-in. Penrose drain is used as a tourniquet after the toe has been cleansed in the usual fashion.
2. An eliptical incision is used to resect the nail bed, matrix, and proximal and lateral nail folds. The cuticle and proximal border of skin are excised as well (Fig 25–32,A).
3. Any remaining toenail matrix and toenail bed is

shaded area is excised; with Winograd procedure, the *stipled* area is excised). **E,** a compression dressing is applied. **F,** cosmetic result after the Winograd procedure following excision of the medial and lateral border of the matrix. (**A, B, D,** and **E** from Mann RA, Coughlin MJ: *The video textbook of foot and ankle surgery,* St Louis, 1990, Medical Video Productions. Used by permission.)

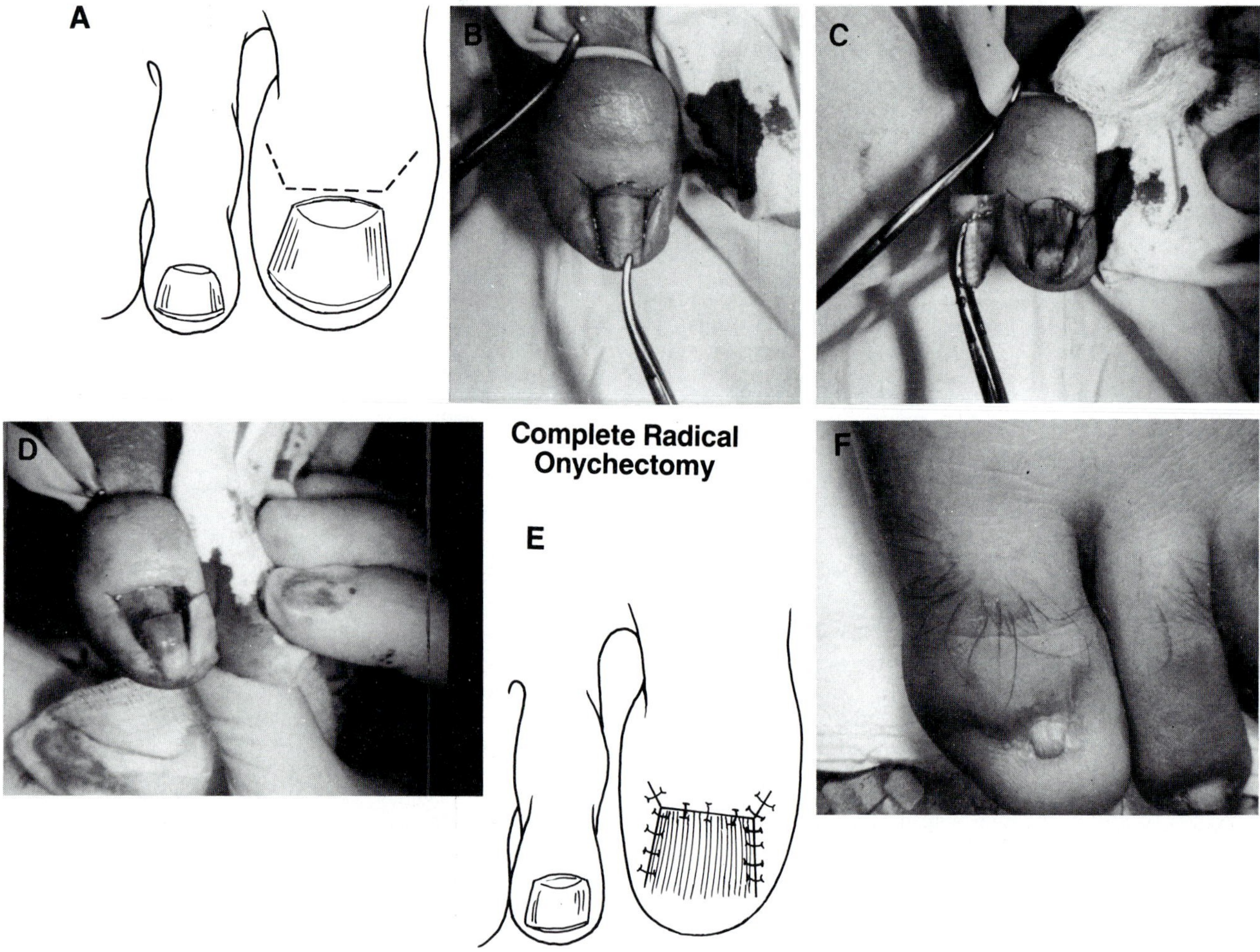

FIG 25–31.
Zadik procedure. **A,** proposed incision for complete toenail ablation. **B,** the toenail is grasped and avulsed **(C). D,** the nail matrix is excised. **E,** the soft tissue is approximated where possible. **F,** regrowth of some nail plate tissue may occur due to the presence of germinal tissue in the area of the nail bed. (**B–D** and **F** from Mann RA, Coughlin MJ: *The video textbook of foot and ankle surgery.* St Louis, 1990, Medical Video Productions. Used by permission.)

curretted from the dorsal surface of the distal phalanx.

4. Approximately half of the distal phalanx is removed, and the remaining edges of bone are beveled with a rongeur (Fig 25–32,B).
5. Excess skin is removed and the skin edges approximated with a nylon suture (Fig 25–32,C).
6. A compression dressing is applied and changed 24 hours after surgery.

Dressing changes are performed as needed until drainage has subsided. Prophylactic antibiotics may be used depending upon the surgeon's preference. Sutures are removed 3 weeks following surgery (Fig 25–32,D).

Murray[55] concluded that in the face of recurrent nail plate growth following repeated ablation procedures, the terminal Syme's procedure was the definitive technique. Thompson and Terwilliger[74] reported on a series of 70 Syme's procedures. They reported excellent results with a 4% recurrence rate (Fig 25–32,E). Pettine et al.[65] reported a 12% recurrence rate following a Syme's amputation.

Phenol/Alcohol Matrisectomy

A phenol and alcohol matrisectomy may be utilized as opposed to a surgical resection. Burzotta et al.[12] advised that this procedure could be performed in the presence of concurrent infection.

A digital anesthetic block is applied and the toe cleansed in the usual fashion.

1. A ¼-in. Penrose drain is applied for hemostasis.
2. The nail plate edge is avulsed as previously de-

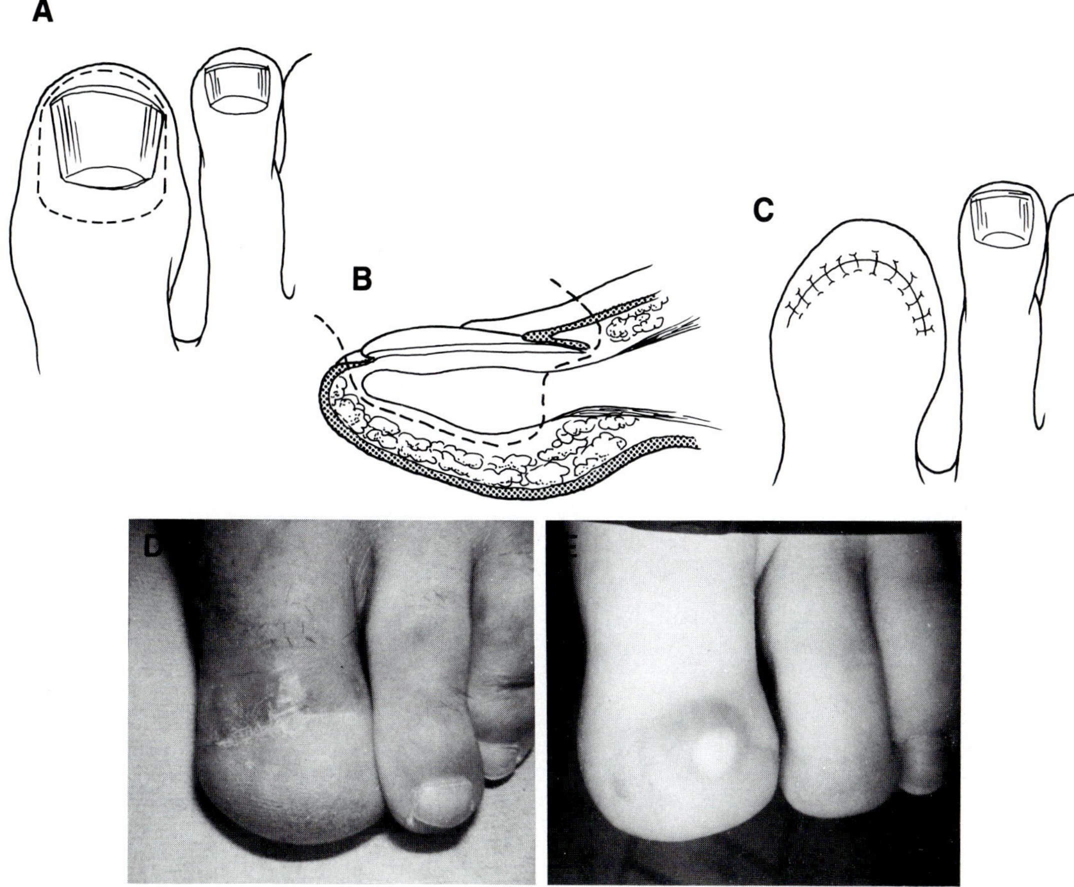

FIG 25–32.
Terminal Syme's procedure. **A,** an eliptical incision is used to excise all adjacent soft tissue as well as the toenail bed and matrix. **B,** one half of the distal phalanx is excised. **C,** excess skin is excised, and the skin edges are then approximated. **D,** appearance 3 months following surgery. **E,** recurrence following a Syme's amputation may present as a cyst formation. (**D** and **E** from Mann RA, Coughlin MJ: *The video textbook of foot and ankle surgery.* St Louis, 1990, Medical Video Productions. Used by permission.)

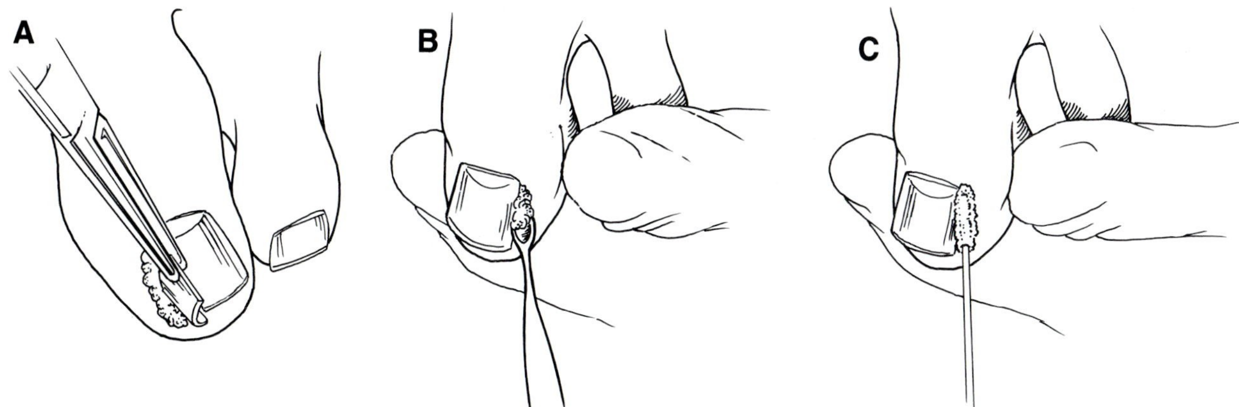

FIG 25–33.
Phenol matrixectomy. **A,** the edge of the nail plate is avulsed and curettage is performed on the lateral toenail groove and matrix **(B). C,** phenol is applied to cauterize the matrix (see the text).

scribed (Fig 25–33,A). The lateral toenail groove and nail matrix are curretted (Fig 25–33,B).

3. A cotton-tipped applicator from which most of the cotton has been removed is used to apply the phenol solution (Fig 25–33,C).

4. Fresh 88% carbolic acid (phenol) is used.

5. The skin area around the matrisectomy is coated with petroleum jelly to prevent injury to the surrounding soft tissue.

6. The cotton-tipped applicator is moistened with the phenol and the excess phenol blotted on a gauze pad. The applicator is inserted into the nail groove and matrix area for 1 to 2 minutes. Gallocher[29] prefers to rub the phenol into the tissue for 2 minutes.

7. The applicator is removed and the area flushed with alcohol to neutralize and free the phenol.

8. Two subsequent half-minute phenol applications are performed.

9. Following each application of phenol, alcohol is used to flush the nail groove and matrix region.

10. A sterile dressing is applied and changed daily until drainage has subsided.

11. The patient is allowed to soak his foot in a tepid salt solution on a daily basis.

REFERENCES

1. Amonette RA, Rosenberg EW: Infection of toe webs by gram negative bacteria, *Arch Dermatol* 107:71–73, 1973.
2. Apfelberg DB, Rothermel E, Widtfeldt A, et al: Progress report on use of carbon dioxide laser for nail disorders, *Curr Podiatr* 32:29–31, 1983.
3. Ashby BS: Primary carcinoma of the nail bed, *Br J Surg* 44:216–217, 1956.
4. Attiyeh FF, Shah J, Booher RJ, et al: Subungual squamous cell carcinoma, *JAMA* 241:262–263, 1979.
5. Baden H: Physical properties of nails, *J Invest Dermatol* 55:115–122, 1970.
6. Bean WB: Nail growth: A twenty-year study, *Arch Intern Med* 111:476–482, 1963.
7. Bean WB: Nail growth: 30 years of observation, *Arch Intern Med* 134:497–502, 1974.
8. Bedi TR: Intradermal triamcinolone treatment of psoriatic onychodystrophy, *Dermatologica* 155:24–25, 1977.
9. Berlin SJ, Block LD, Donick I: Pyogenic granuloma of the foot, a review of the literature and report of four cases, *J Am Podiatr Assoc* 62:94–99, 1972.
10. Berlin SJ, Stewart RC, Margolies MC, et al: Squamous cell carcinoma of the foot with particular reference to nail bed involvement: a report of three cases, *J Am Podiatr Assoc* 65:134–141, 1975.
11. Breslow AM, Dorfman HD: Depuytren's (subungual) exostosis, *Am J Surg Pathol* 12:368–378, 1988.
12. Burzotta JL, Turri RM, Tsouris J: Phenol and alcohol chemical matrixectomy, *Clin Podiatr Med Surg* 6:453–468, 1989.
13. Cacciaglia GB, Tenczar AJ, Kanat IO: A review of the literature of ketoconazole therapy in the treatment of tinea pedis and onychomycosis, *J Foot Surg* 23:420–423, 1984.
14. Cameron PF: Ingrowing toenails: an evaluation of two treatments, *Br J Med* 283:821–822, 1981.
15. Cangiolosi CP, Schnall SJ: A comparison of the phenol-alcohol and Suppan nail techniques (onychectomy/matrixectomy). *Curr Podiatr* 30:25–26, 1981.
16. Cavolo DJ, D'Amelio JP, Hirsch AL, et al: Juvenile subungual osteochondroma. Case presentation, *J Am Podiatr Med Assoc* 71:81–83, 1981.
17. Ceh SE, Pettine KA: Treatment of ingrown toenail, *J Musculoskel Med* 7:62–82, 1990.
18. Clarke BG, Dillinger KA: Surgical treatment of ingrown toenail, *Surgery* 21:919–924, 1946.
19. Conant MA, Wiesenfeld SL: Multiple glomus tumors of the skin, *Arch Dermatol* 103:481–485, 1971.
20. Dale SJ, Simmons J: Subungual squamous cell carcinoma, *J Am Podiatr Assoc* 70:421–425, 1980.
21. Dixon GL: Treatment of ingrown toenail, *Foot Ankle* 3:254–260, 1983.
22. Dockery GL: Nails, fundamental conditions and procedures. In McGlamary ED, editor: *Comprehensive textbook of foot surgery*, Baltimore, 1987, Williams & Wilkins, pp 3–37.
23. DuVries HL: Hypertrophy of ungual labia, *Chirop Rec* 16:11, 1933.
24. DuVries HL: Ingrown toenail, *Chirop Rec* 27:155, 164, 1944.
25. Dykyj D: Anatomy of the nail, *Clin Podiatr Med Surg* 6:215–228, 1989.
26. Estersohn HS, Stanock JF: Pyogenic granuloma, a literature review of two cases. *J Am Podiatr Assoc* 73:297–301, 1983.
27. Frost L: Root resection for incurvated nail, *J Am Podiatr Assoc* 40:19, 1950.
28. Gabriel SS, Dallos V, Stevenson DL: The ingrown toenail: a modified segmental matrix excision operation, *Br J Surg* 66:285–286, 1979.
29. Gallocher J: The phenol/alcohol method of nail matrix sterilization, *N Z Med J* 86:140–141, 1977.
30. Gibson HG, Montgomery H, Woolner LB, et al: Melanotic whitlow (subungual melanoma), *J Invest Dermatol* 29:119–129, 1957.
31. Graham J, Helwig E: Bowen's disease and its relationship to systemic cancer, *Arch Dermatol* 80:133–159, 1959.
32. Grisafi PJ, Lombardi CM, Sciarrino AL, et al: Three select subungual pathologies: subungual exostosis, subungual osteochondroma, and subungual hematoma, *Clin Podiatr Med Surg* 6:355–364, 1989.
33. Gunnoe RE: Disease of the nails: how to recognize and treat them, *Postgrad Med* 74:357–362, 1983.
34. Hashimoto K: Ultrastructure of the human toenail. Cell migration, keratinization, and formation of the intercellular cement, *Arch Dermatol Res* 240:1–22, 1971.
35. Heifetz CJ: Ingrown toenail: a clinical study, *Am J Surg* 38:298–315, 1937.
36. Heifetz CJ: Operative management of ingrown toenail, *J Missouri Med Assoc* 42:213–216, 1945.
37. Holub PG, Hubbard ER: Ketoconazole in the treatment of onychomycosis, *J Am Podiatr Med Assoc* 77:338–339, 1987.
38. Ilfeld FW: Ingrown toenail treated with cotton collodion insert, *Foot Ankle* 11:312–313, 1991.

39. Ippoloito E, Falez F, Tudisco C, et al: Subungual exostosis: histological and clinical considerations on cases, *Ital J Orthop Traumatol* 13:81–87, 1987.
40. Jahss MJ: *Disorders of the foot and ankle*, Philadelphia, 1982, WB Saunders, pp 937, 1548–1572.
41. Jarrat M: Herpes simplex infection, *Arch Dermatol* 119:99–102, 1983.
42. Johnson KA: *Surgery of the foot and ankle*, New York, 1989, Raven Press, p 84.
43. Keyes EL: The surgical treatment of ingrown toenails, *JAMA* 102:1458–1460, 1934.
44. Kosinski MA, Stewart D: Nails changes associated with systemic disease and vascular insufficiency, *Clin Podiatr Med Surg* 6:295–318, 1989.
45. Krausz CE: Nail survey (1942–1970), *Br J Chir* 35:117, 1970.
46. Langford JH: Pachyonychia congenita, *J Am Podiatr Assoc* 68:587–591, 1978.
47. Lapidus PW: The ingrown toenail, *Bull Hosp J Dis* 33:181–192, 1972.
48. Leppard B, Sanderson KV, Behan F: Subungual malignant melanoma: Difficulty in diagnosis, *Br Med J* 1:310–312, 1974.
49. Lerner LH: Incurvated nail margin with associated osseous pathology, *Curr Podiatr* 11:26–28, 1962.
50. Lewis BL: Microscopic studies of fetal and mature nail and surrounding soft tissue, *Arch Dermatol* 70:732–747, 1954.
51. Lloyd-Davies RW, Brill GC: The etiology and outpatient management of ingrowing toenail, *Br J Surg* 50:592–597, 1963.
52. Lundeen GW, Lundeen RO: Onychomycosis. Its classification, pathophysiology, and etiology, *J Am Podiatr Assoc* 68:395–401, 1978.
53. Mann RA, Coughlin MJ: Toenail abnormalities. In Mann RA, Coughlin MJ, editors: *The video textbook of foot and ankle surgery*, St Louis, 1990, Medical Video Productions, pp 56–66.
54. Murray WR: Onychocryptosis, *Clin Orthop* 142:96–102, 1979.
55. Murray WR, Bedi BS: The surgical management of ingrowing toenail, *Br J Surg* 62:409–412, 1975.
56. Nagata F, Chu C, Phipps R: Nail involvement in Darier's disease, *J Am Podiatr Assoc* 70:635–636, 1980.
57. Norton LA: Disorders of the nail. In Moschella SL, Pillsbury DM, Hurley HH, editors: *Dermatology*, Philadelphia, 1975, WB Saunders, pp 1222–1236.
58. Norton LA: Nail disorders, a review, *J Am Acad Dermatol* 2:451–467, 1980.
59. Nzuzi SM: Common nail disorders, *Clin Podiatr Med Surg* 6:273–294, 1989.
60. Nzuzi SM: Nail entities, *Clin Podiatr Med Surg* 6:253–271, 1989.
61. Oliviera ADS, Picoto ADS, Verde SF, et al: Subungual exostosis: Treatment as an office procedure, *J Dermatol Surg Oncol* 6:555–558, 1980.
62. Page JC, Abramson C, Lee W, et al: Diagnosis and treatment of tinea pedis, *J Am Podiatr Med Assoc* 81:304–316, 1991.
63. Palmer BV, Jones A: Ingrowing toenails: the results of treatment, *Br J Surg* 66:575–576, 1979.
64. Pardo-Castello V: *Diseases of the nails*, ed 3, Springfield, Ill, 1960, Charles C Thomas.
65. Pettine KA, Cofield RH, Johnson KA, et al: Ingrown toenail: results of surgical treatment, *Foot Ankle* 9:130–134, 1988.
66. Ramsay G, Caldwell D: Phenol cauterization for ingrown toenails, *Arch Emerg Med* 3:243–246, 1986.
67. Robb JE, Murray WR: Phenol cauterisation in the management of ingrowing toenails, *Scott Med J* 27:236–239, 1982.
68. Rubin L: Intraepidermal squamous cell carcinoma (Bowen's disease) of the nail bed, *J Am Podiatr Assoc* 63:195–202, 1973.
69. Saltzman BS: Periungual fibroma, *J Am Podiatr Assoc* 68:696, 1978.
70. Samman PD: The human toenail: its genesis and blood supply, *Br J Dermatol* 71:296–302, 1959.
71. Silverman ME, Goodman RM, Cuppagea FE: The nail patella syndrome, *Arch Intern Med* 120:68–74, 1967.
72. Stone DA: Suggestions for elimination of failures in chemosurgery of the nails, *Curr Podiatr* 11:14–15, 1962.
73. Tauber EB, Goldman L, Claassen H: Pachyonchia congenita, *JAMA* 107:29–30, 1936.
74. Thompson TC, Terwilliger C: The terminal Syme operation for ingrown toenail, *Surg Clin North Am* 31:575–584, 1951.
75. Townsend AC, Scott PJ: Ingrowing toenail and onychogryphosis, *J Bone Joint Surg, [Br]* 48:354–358, 1966.
76. Wee GC, Tucker GL: Phenolic cauterization of the matrix in the surgical cure of ingrown toenails, *Mo Med* 66:802–803, 1969.
77. Weiner AL: Alopecia areata with nail changes, *Arch Dermatol* 72:469, 1955.
78. Welvaart K, Koops HS: Subungual malignant melanoma: a nail in the coffin, *Clin Oncol* 4:309–315, 1978.
79. White CJ, Laipply TC: Disease of the nails: 792 cases, *Indiana Med Surg* 27:325, 1958.
80. Winograd AM: A modification in the technique for ingrown nail, *JAMA* 92:229–230, 1929.
81. Winograd AM: Results in operation for ingrown toenail, *Illinois Med J* 70:197–198, 1936.
82. Wolf WB, Cohen LS: Intra-epidural squamous cell carcinoma, Bowen's disease of the dorsum of the foot, *J Am Podiatr Assoc* 68:688–690, 1978.
83. Wright G: Laser matrisectomy in the toes, *Foot Ankle* 9:246–247, 1989.
84. Zadik FR: Obliteration of the nail bed of the great toe without shortening of the terminal phalanx, *J Bone Joint Surg [Br]* 32:66–67, 1950.
85. Zaias N: Onychomycosis, *Arch Dermatol* 105:263–274, 1972.
86. Zaias N: Psoriasis of the nail: a clinical pathologic study, *Arch Dermatol* 99:567–579, 1969.
87. Zaias N: *The nail in health and disease*, New York, 1980, *SP Medical*, pp 1–43.

C H A P T E R

26

Dermatology

Landrus Pfeffinger, M.D.

Inflammatory skin problems of the feet
Autoimmune diseases
Common infections of the feet
Bacterial infections
Tinea
Specific discrete skin lesions of the feet
Benign pigmented nevus
Glomus tumor
Eccrine poroma
Epidermal inclusion cyst
Pyogenic granuloma
Dermatofibroma
Foreign body of the sole
Keloids
Black heel
Arteriovenous fistula
Chromoblastomycosis and mycetoma
Malignant discrete skin lesions of the feet
Malignant melanoma
Kaposi's sarcoma
Kaposi's sarcoma associated with AIDS
Squamous cell carcinoma
Corns, calluses, keratoses, and warts
Calluses
Corns
Keratoses of the soles
Plantar warts
Differential diagnosis
Treatment

The skin is often a reflection of underlying bony abnormalities or systemic or localized disease processes. Successful treatment is obviously dependent on determining the underlying etiology. The practitioner needs to differentiate between *primary* lesions and *secondary* lesions.

Primary lesions are those caused by the disease process itself, as opposed to secondary lesions, which may be the result of scratching, infection, or trauma. Primary lesions can be described by size, color, and skin elevation, e.g., papule, plaque, macule, etc. If fluid is present, the terms *vesicle* or *bulla* are used. If a hemorrhagic appearance is present, then petechiae, purpura, and ecchymosis are descriptive.

Secondary lesions such as scars, ulcerations, and crusts are not as helpful diagnostically and can confuse the clinical picture.

The difference between plantar skin and dorsal skin must be recognized. The plantar skin has a very thick layer of stratum corneum, whereas this layer is normal in thickness on the dorsum of the foot. There are no sebaceous glands or hair on the sole of the foot in contrast to the dorsal skin.

If the clinical presentation is not clear then further consultation may be required with dermatologists, neurologists, vascular surgeons, and other specialists. Biopsy specimens 3 to 6 mm in size may be necessary. These need to be carefully planned, particularly on the weight-bearing areas. Wood's light examination of web space dermatoses can be helpful in the case of mycotic infections.

INFLAMMATORY SKIN PROBLEMS OF THE FEET

Eczema (dermatitis) is a common inflammatory cutaneous condition in which the rash shows vesicles, erythema, and subsequent fissuring, crusting, and marked itching. It can be manifested by a hyperpigmentation and hyperkeratinization of the skin that is sometimes referred to as lichenification.

Atopic dermatitis may involve both the palms and the soles. (Fig 26–1). A familial history of atopic diseases such as allergic rhinitis, asthma, urticaria, or migraine headaches is often associated. These patients have a tendency to develop brisk allergic reactions to various chemicals and biologic materials. These patients have an increased tendency toward allergic reactions to penicillin. Serologically they are known to develop eosinophilia and a flat glucose tolerance curve.

Patients with atopic dermatitis are often misdiagnosed as having a fungal infection and treated unsuccessfully with antifungal agents. Lichenification involving the distal part of the foot is a common manifestation. Scratching of the lesions leads to thickening of the skin.

Atopic dermatitis affecting the feet is generally successfully treated with topical corticosteroids, usually three times per day with 0.5%, 1%, or 2.5% hydrocortisone preparations in acute cases. Fluorinated preparations are also available. Generally ointments are used for dry lesions, and lotions are used for wet lesions.

Pompholyx, or dyshidrotic eczema, is an eczematoid reaction affecting the soles and palms and is manifested by deep-seated vesicles or even large bullae. It may be associated with symptoms of hyperhidrosis. The differential diagnosis includes vesicular-type tinea pedis, pustular psoriasis, and epidermolysis bullosa.

Treatment of pompholyx includes soaking in saline or Burrow's solution followed by application of a steroid cream. In chronic conditions systemic corticosteroid treatment is sometimes necessary.

Contact dermatitis is of two different types: a primary irritant, e.g., soaps and acids, or an allergic variety, e.g., topical antibiotics and antihistamines. Shoe dermatitis, another form of allergic contact dermatitis is the most common allergen in the rubber or glue used in shoe lining (Fig 26–2).

Treatment of contact or shoe dermatitis, as with all forms of eczema of the feet, usually involves the application of corticosteroid creams and lotions and cool astringent compresses or foot soaks when the process is in the acute vesicular stage. Oral steroids may be required

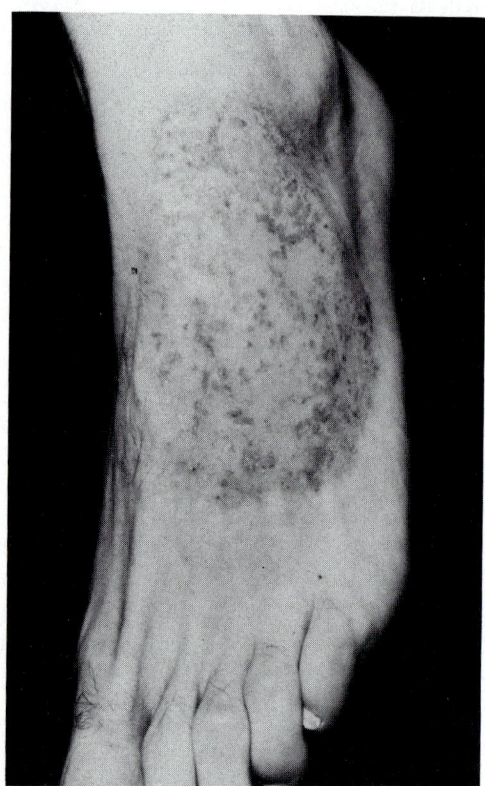

FIG 26–1.
Atopic dermatitis. This patch of eczematoid rash could be confused with tinea or contact dermatitis from shoes. Involvement of flexural folds along with a chronic history supports the diagnosis of atopic dermatitis.

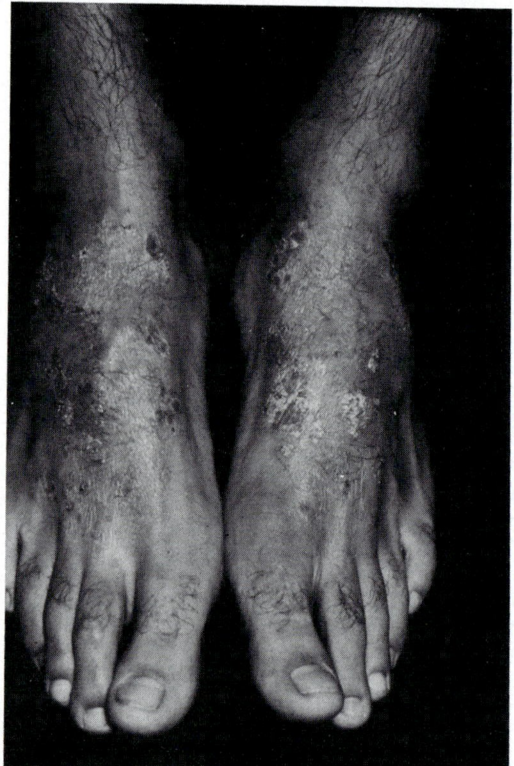

FIG 26–2.
Shoe dermatitis: two examples of allergic contact dermatitis, a reaction to one ingredient of new shoes. The clinical picture is of bilateral rash involving the dorsa of the feet.

in severe conditions. If secondary infection occurs, antibiotics must also be administered.

Psoriasis is a generalized skin disease affecting approximately 1% to 2% of people. In all forms, there may be psoriatic lesions on the feet (Fig 26–3) usually characterized by an erythematous plaque covered by a white silvery scale that is adherent and bleeds when removed. Pustular psoriasis can also occur. Frequently psoriasis of the foot is mistaken as "eczema." White psoriasis is simply macerated interdigital psoriatic plaques. It is often misdiagnosed as tinea pedis, soft corns, or monilial infection (other sites of psoriatic lesions, however, help in differentiation).

Treatment of psoriasis of the feet is similar to that elsewhere on the body, i.e., potent topical steroid creams usually with occlusive dressings at night to promote greater absorption. Treatment of interdigital psoriasis is difficult and requires periodic intralesion injec-

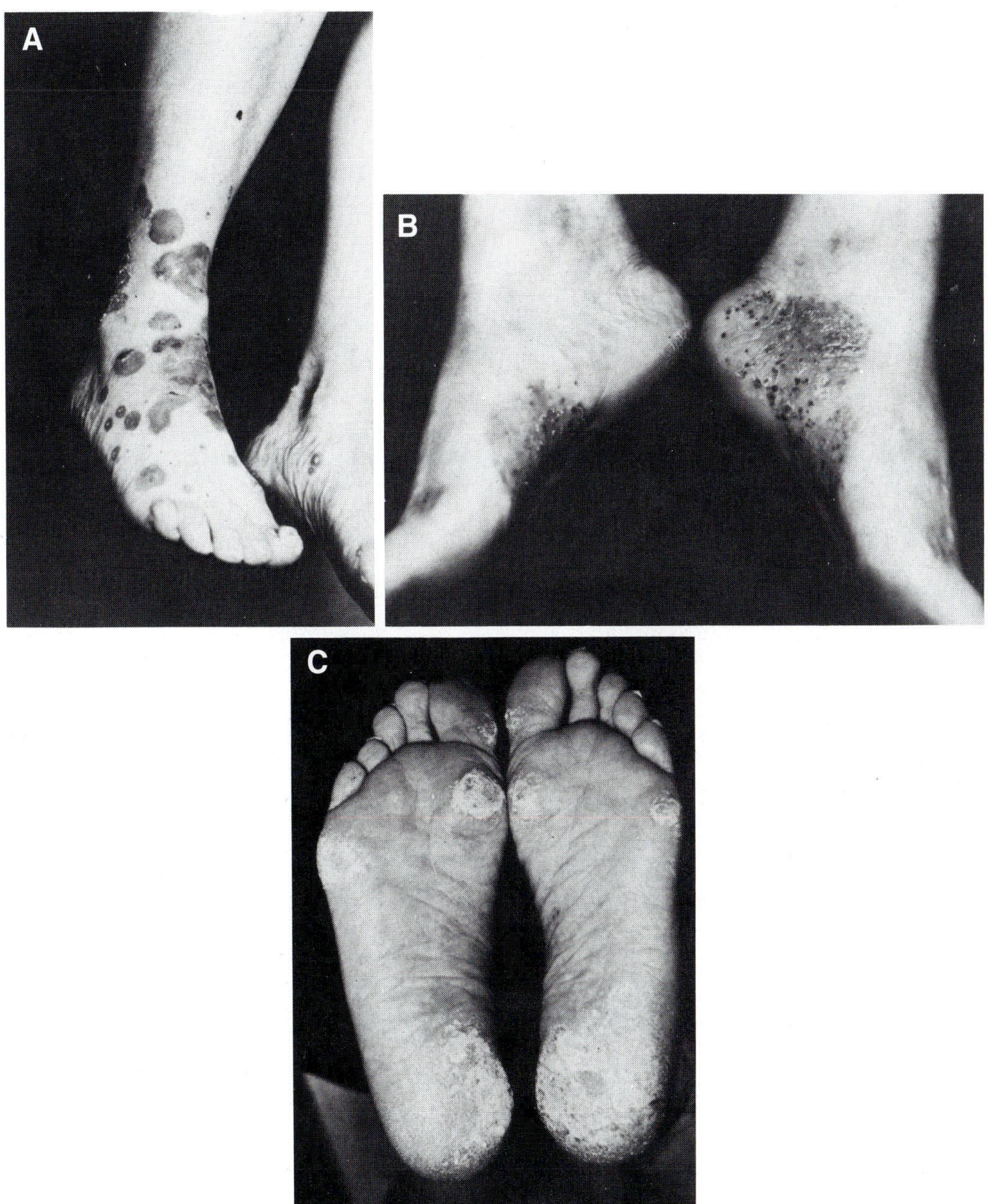

FIG 26–3.
Three variations on the theme of psoriasis. **A,** discrete red plaques on the right foot. There were also similar typical psoriatic lesions on the elbow and knees. **B,** pustules characteristically involving the soles. The rash consists of confluent erythematous patches with scaling and pustules. **C,** marked discrete keratoderma on the weight-bearing surfaces of the feet.

tions of diluted triamcinolone. Pustular psoriasis may be improved by periodic intramuscular injections of triamcinolone acetonide. Immunosuppressive and cytotoxic drugs such as methotrexate and cyclosporine are used in severe, resistant cases.

Lichen planus of the skin is characterized by flat-topped shiny violaceous papules that are usually distinctive in their location (Fig 26–4). The volar aspect of wrists, sacral area of the back, and mucous membranes such as the mouth, vulva, or penis are involved. It is usually pruritic, yet one does not see many excoriations due to scratching. The cause is unknown, although flare-ups can occur with nervous tension.

The disease is quite variable in its presentation. Diagnosis of lichen planus is usually characterized by topical polygonal violaceous skin lesions with a slight scale called Wickham's striae; however, on occasion, skin biopsy may be necessary to substantiate the diagnosis. In the differential diagnosis of lichen planus one must consider localized neurodermatitis showing a marked hyperkeratation element, Kaposi's sarcoma, drug reaction, and secondary lues.

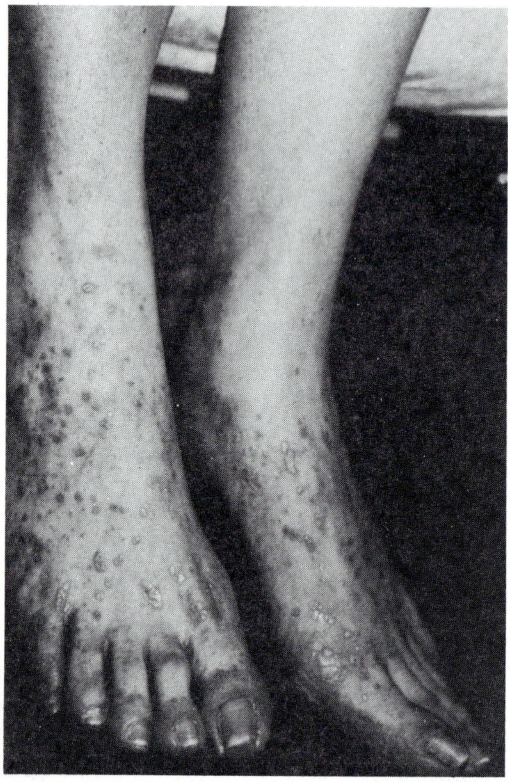

FIG 26–4.
Lichen planus: papulosquamous eruption showing flat, polygonal, shiny violaceous papules. Linear lesions resulting from scratch marks, the so-called Koebner phenomenon, are frequently seen.

Treatment consists of topical corticosteroids combined with occlusive dressings. Sometimes intralesional or even short low-dosage courses of systemic steroids are necessary.

Granuloma annulare is an idiopathic, invariably asymptomatic disease commonly affecting the dorsum of the feet. Other sites include the extensor aspects of the extremities. Children and women are more affected than their counterparts.

The lesion has a doughnut-shaped pink area with discrete papules composing the ring (Fig 26–5). The papules do not ulcerate, and occasionally they coalesce.

In the differential diagnosis one considers annular lichen planus, erythema multiforme, larva migrans, rheumatoid nodules, sarcoidosis, and tinea pedis. Inflammation and lack of scaling distinguish granuloma annulare from tinea. Biopsy of the skin reveals noncaseating granuloma.

Treatment is essentially the same as that for lichen planus. Interestingly, biopsy may also result in resolution of the condition.

Epidermolysis bullosa is an older term used to describe blistering caused by splits in the skin secondary to trauma. Classification is dependent on hereditary factors, location of the lesion, and the presence or absence of scarring.

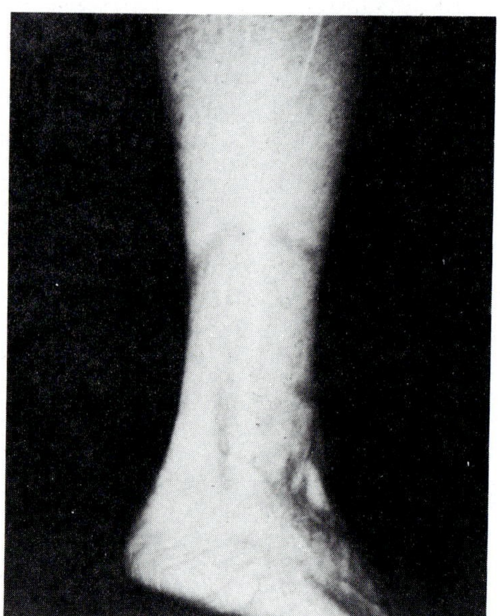

FIG 26–5.
Granuloma annulare with an unusually large plaque on the right foot that extends up the lower part of the leg. The lesion had been present for years. Its raised nonscaly annular border is fairly typical. A more typical case is represented by the faint, round, barely perceptible patch on the posterior aspect of the foot. The border of this lesion is raised, but there was no scaling.

A diagnosis of epidermolysis bullosa disease is made by biopsy, immunofluorescent tests (usually negative), and clinical appearance. Prednisone, moist dressings, and incision and drainage of large lesions are therapeutic for many acute lesions. In chronic forms, topically applied corticosteroids may be helpful. Trauma is to be avoided. Scarring with subsequent contracture of the toes may require surgical release.

Erythema multiforme is a generalized skin disease that may be caused by drugs or infection. There are multiple lesions composed of macular or patchlike papules and plaques. The soles are usually devoid of lesions.

The differential diagnosis includes tinea pedis or keratolysis exfoliativa in early stages. Later the annular lesions become more obvious. Immunofluorescent tests and biopsy assist in establishing the diagnosis. Orally administrated or topical steroids are given when the disease is severe.

AUTOIMMUNE DISEASES

Discoid lupus erythematosus causes red, atrophic irregular plaques and occurs rarely on the feet. It may resemble psoriasis and tinea pedis, but the skin atrophy distinguishes it from psoriasis. Negative fungal tests distinguish it from tinea pedis.

Systemic lupus erythematosus lesions can be seen on the feet particularly as ulcerations on the dorsum of the foot. The differential diagnosis include dermatomyositis, erythromelalgia, and drug eruptions. Serologic tests can assist in the diagnosis.

Dermatomyositis is rarely seen on the foot. It can appear as shiny, glazed, reddish coalescent papules forming plaques about the bony prominences of the ankle and great toes. Biopsy of the muscle and skin along with blood tests assists in the diagnosis.

Treatment of these autoimmune diseases is usually with topically applied and/or orally administered corticosteroids.

COMMON INFECTIONS OF THE FEET

Bacterial Infections

Streptococcal infection of the feet is usually secondary to fungal infections that form cracks and fissures in the web spaces of the toes. The toes become edematous and erythematous, and if the infection develops proximally, lymphangitis can occur and subsequently form bullae or erythematous nodules in plaques on the dorsal aspect of the feet or shins. Patients usually develop a high fever with recurrent bouts of erysipelas. With chronic recurring bouts of erysipelas, the affected limb may eventually develop elephantiasis. Clinically the infection is that of a typical streptococcal infection with cellulitis and erythema. Classic elephantiasis is unmistakable. Mycologic and bacteriologic studies are diagnostic.

Treatment is directed to both bacterial as well as fungal infections by the use of oral penicillin and griseofulvin.

Gram-negative bacteria may cause ulceration in the toe web spaces. Overhanging epidermis on the rim of the ulcer is characteristic of gram-negative bacterial infection. Patients will often provide a history of prolonged use of antimicrobial soaps. The erosions may suggest tinea pedis, but tests for fungal infection will be negative.

Treatment is directed at the offending organism and by the use of silver nitrate soaks (0.5%) locally.

Pitted keratolysis on the plantar aspect of the foot is a common disease caused by elaboration of a keratolytic enzyme. Clinically it appears as though the sole of the foot is dirty because the superficial pits are rapidly filled with debris. This is a pathognomonic clinical presentation. The disease is diagnosed by bacterial culture of the pits or by argyrophilic staining of the organism and biopsy specimens.

Treatment consists of oral erythromycin, 1 g daily in divided doses for a period of 2 weeks, together with 0.5% silver nitrate soaks daily followed by applications of erythromycin ointment if the skin becomes too dry.

Tinea (Superficial Fungal Infections, Tinea Pedis)

Athlete's foot, or superficial fungal infections of the feet, is frequently misdiagnosed and mistreated. It is a chronic infection that is more common in American men than women. A warm, moist environment and conditions that lead to increased maceration and penetration are the cause of infection by fungal organisms. The two most common organisms causing tinea pedis are *Trichophyton rubrum* and *Trichophyton mentagrophytes*.

The scaling and maceration often involve the fourth and fifth interdigital web space. *T. rubrum* infections tend to be chronic and often show a low-grade, dry, salmon-colored scaling inflammation on the sole of the foot such as in the instep and on the sides and sometimes enveloping the foot like a moccasin (Fig 26–6). *T. mentagrophytes* infection frequently shows clusters of blisters about the toes or in the area of the transverse arch (Fig 26–7). The diagnosis is made by performing a 10% potassium hydroxide examination of skin scrapings. Fungal cultures can pinpoint the pathogen but require 2 to 4 weeks for a final diagnosis. Fungal infections affecting the dorsum of the foot assume a more

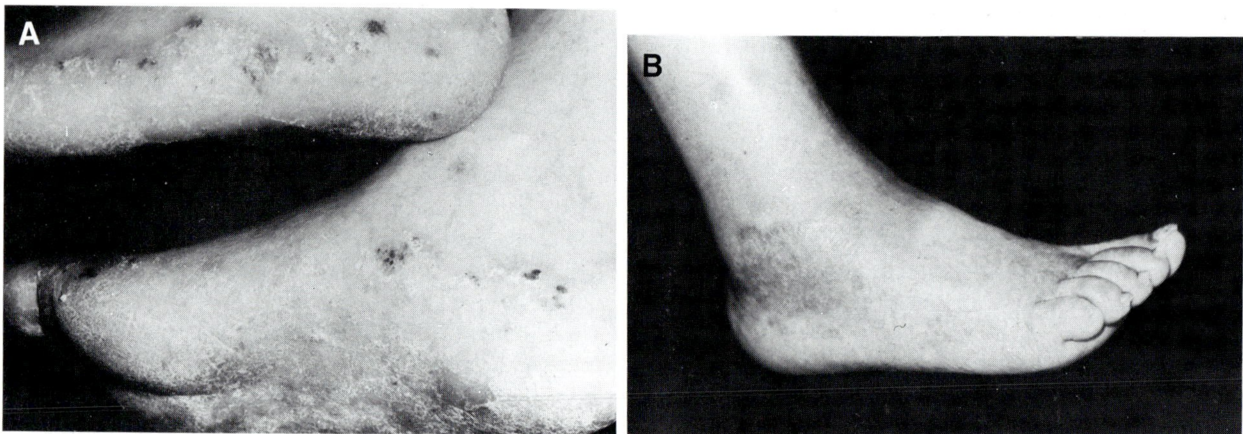

FIG 26–6.
Tinea pedis: two patterns of chronic *Trichophyton rubrum* infection of the feet. **A,** diffuse, red, scaly pattern of a mocassin that had been present for two decades. **B,** note the annular serpiginous character of the fungus on the side of the foot.

typical "ringworm" pattern with central clearing and extension of the lesions in an annular configuration. It is noteworthy that fungal infections of the feet are rare in children before puberty.

As to the differential diagnosis of tinea of the feet one must consider eczema (e.g., atopic, contact, dyshidrotic) as well as psoriasis and soft corns. Incumbent streptococcal infections can also occur.

Treatment of fungal infections depends upon the type of infection. For the acute blistering tinea pedis caused by *T. mentagrophytes*, one should not overtreat with antifungal agents, but should first treat the raw oozing surface of the skin as an acute dermatitis with antiseptic soaks like Burrow's solution and soothing ointments such as Vioform-HC cream. Local fungistatic agents, for example, Miconazole nitrate cream and Clotrimazole cream, are also beneficial. The patient should also be advised to keep the skin dry and exposed to air. Griseofulvin is not routinely used for most tinea pedis infections.

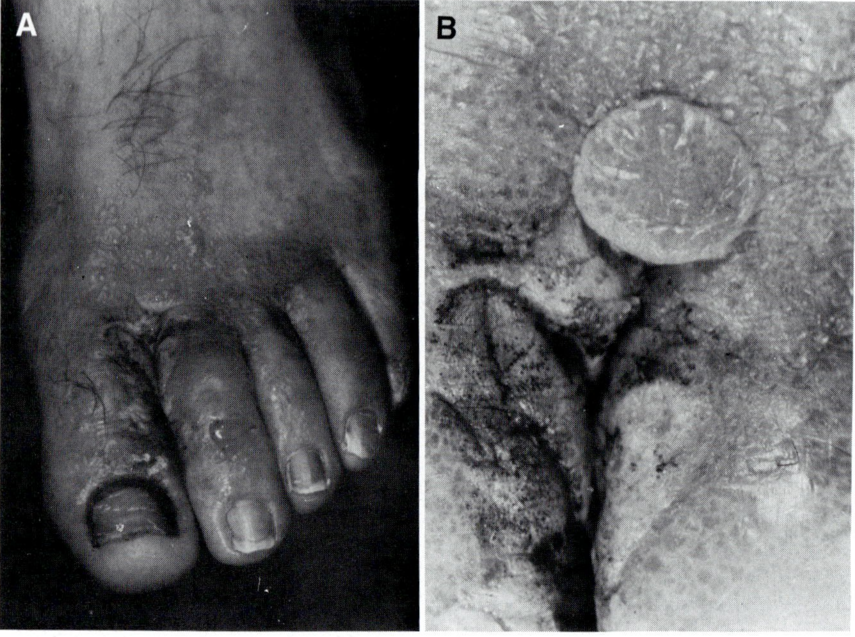

FIG 26–7.
Tinea pedis. **A,** vesicular form, most often caused by the organism *Trichophyton mentagrophytes.* **B,** close-up of a vesicle.

SPECIFIC DISCRETE SKIN LESIONS OF THE FEET

Benign Pigmented Nevus

Melanocytic nevi are the most common "skin tumor" in human beings, an estimated average of 20 or more nevi occurring per adult,[5] although for various reasons this count may be inaccurate. Suffice it to say that everyone has several nevi. More nevi occur on the upper part of the body than on the lower, but some appear on the foot, and hence the physician may be asked his opinions for management of a particular lesion. Most people have no pigmented lesions at birth; fewer than 3% of infants are born with pigmented nevi, the nevi appearing a few years after birth like small dark dots that gradually enlarge as the person grows. The varieties of nevi, named for the histologic appearance of their "nevus cells," fall into three general types—junctional, intradermal, and compound. Since 50% of melanomas arise from pre-existing nevi, it is important to know which nevi should be excised. Junctional and compound nevi are subjected to constant rubbing or trauma and should be excised. Small, flat, light brown lesions on the palms and soles should be left alone. Approximately 12% of people have pigmented lesions on their palms and soles, and it is not practical to excise all these lesions. The infrequently encountered large, elevated, dark nevus of the palm or sole, however, should be removed. An increase in size, darkening in color, itching, inflammation, and trauma are events that arouse concern in the patient regarding previously ignored nevi. In children and young adults nevi enlarge as the person grows. Bleeding into a nevus results in a blue to black discoloration. Changes vary according to the depth and extent of the bleeding. Most bleeding occurs following trauma. The injury may have been mild and is often forgotten by the patient. At times the examiner cannot tell whether the darkening is a result of melanin or blood; hence the lesion must be excised.

The blue nevus is another variety of melanocytic nevus that is so called because of the dark blue-black color of the lesion that results from the melanin pigment deep in the dermis. These nevi may be distributed anywhere on the body and not infrequently appear on the feet. Although generally benign, blue nevi can show malignant transformation, so they have to be evaluated with regard to change in size, irritation, etc., as discussed earlier (Fig 26–8).

Glomus Tumor

Glomus tumors are most frequently encountered on the acral portions of the extremities. The lesion is often subungual and consists of a purplish nodule measuring only a few millimeters in diameter. It is tender and gives rise to severe paroxysmal pains. Glomus tumors rarely ulcerate or bleed, and excision usually results in a cure, although subungual lesions are more difficult to eradicate. The differential diagnosis includes ordinary hemangiomas as well as neuroma, Kaposi's sarcoma, he-

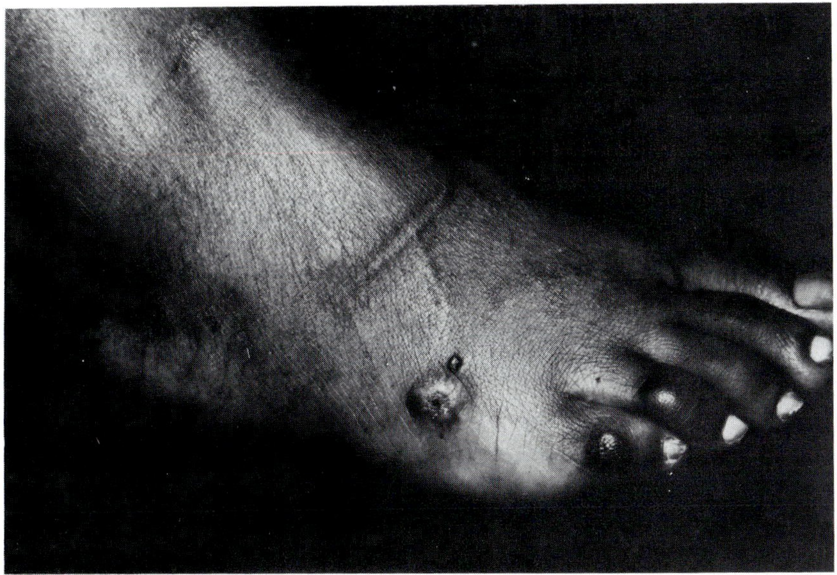

FIG 26–8.
Nevi of the feet. A blue nevus is not an uncommon lesion and is found on the dorsum of the foot. It is characterized by a dark blue-black color and often simulates melanoma.

mangiopericytoma, and granuloma telangiectaticum. There is another type of glomus tumor characterized by multiple painless hemangiomas and frequently a familial pattern.[1] The multiple lesions are usually asymptomatic.

Eccrine Poroma

Eccrine poroma was first described by Pinkus et al. in 1956[7] as a fairly common solitary tumor, two thirds of which occur on the soles or sides of the feet. This benign tumor is derived from the eccrine sweat ducts and usually arises in young or in middle-aged adults. It is rather firm, is often raised and slightly pedunculated, is usually asymptomatic, and measures less than 2 cm in diameter (Fig 26–9). Treatment by excision is curative in any location.

Epidermal Inclusion Cyst

Epidermal cysts are common skin lesions on the scalp, face, trunk, and extremities; infrequently they occur on the palms and rarely on the soles. When an epidermal cyst arises on the sole, it is probably a result of traumatic implantation of the epidermis. The lesions are often misdiagnosed as callus or verrucae and appear as an elevated nodule of up to 2 cm in diameter that is movable and tender. The differential diagnosis includes synovial lesions, fibroma, xanthoma, and tumors of the appendages. Surgical removal is usually curative.[4]

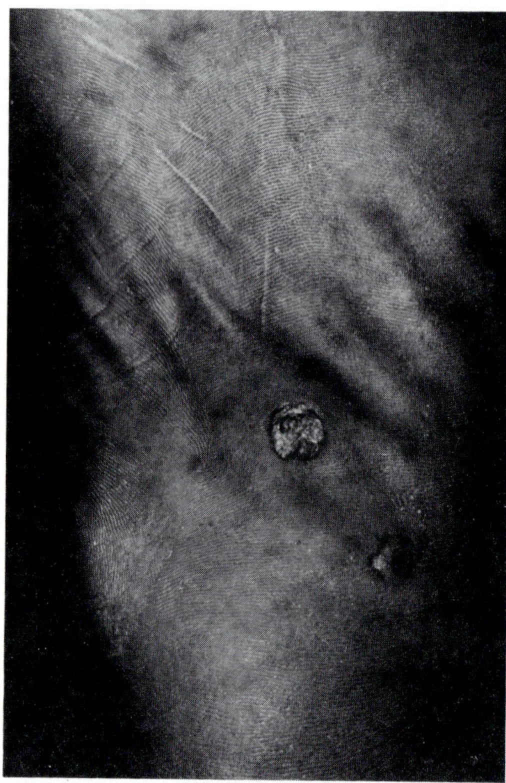

FIG 26–9.
Eccrine poroma, an adnexal papillomatous tumor frequently arising on the feet. Here, two poromas near the heel appear almost like verrucae. They are pedunculated friable lesions that bleed easily.

Pyogenic Granuloma

A pyogenic granuloma, sometimes called granuloma telangiectaticum, resembles proud flesh and occurs as a single lesion dull red in color that is soft to moderately firm, raised, and slightly pedunculated. It usually grows rapidly to 0.5 cm; occasionally, however, it reaches a size of 2 cm and remains unchanged. The surface of the lesion shows ulceration and crusting, and the patient relates that the lesion bleeds easily when only slightly touched. It may appear on the foot but most commonly is located on the fingers and face. Staphylococcal infection appears to have a role in the development of pyogenic granulomas, and they not uncommonly are seen on the lateral nail folds of the toes in conjunction with ingrown toenails. The differential diagnosis includes hemangioma, epithelioma, eccrine poroma, malignant melanoma, or foreign-body granuloma. Treatment is surgical by excision, although on the soles simple electrodesiccation and curettage can be relied on to effect a consistent cure.

Dermatofibroma

Dermatofibromas occur in the skin as firm, indolent, single or multiple nodules usually situated on the extremities, but they may occur anywhere. There are several synonyms of this lesion: nodular subepidermal fibrosis, sclerosing hemangioma, and histiocytoma; basically the lesion represents a reactive fibrosis consequent to some idiopathic inflammatory process.

The firm papules measure a few millimeters in size but may be as large as 2 to 3 cm. Most have a reddish brown color but occasionally become bluish black and even suggest a malignant melanoma. In histiocytomas, because of the cellular composition of the tumor, frequently the color is yellow because of lipid composition. Treatment is by surgical excision, although if the lesions are asymptomatic and not enlarging, they may be merely observed.

Foreign Body of the Sole

Foreign bodies of the sole are mistaken for warts or corns because of the protective callus that has formed. When this covering is pared away, some pus may exude, and further shaving will reveal a foreign body such as a stiff hair, a rose thorn, a piece of glass, a shell particle, or anything that may have invaded the skin. Once it has been extracted, a cure quickly results. When confronted with small calluses of the feet not overlying bony prominences, the physician should always consider the possibility of the presence of an embedded hair.

Keloids

Of the three types of scar—the ordinary flat scar, an elevated hypertrophic scar, and keloid—only the keloid shows extension of the scarring process beyond the borders of the initial injury; the hypertrophic and ordinary scars conform almost exactly to the area of injury. There is probably a predisposing genetic factor in the production of keloids and certainly a racial factor since blacks are more susceptible. Moreover, certain areas such as the V area of the chest and the earlobes, especially in women, are prone to develop keloids.

The keloid presents as a brawny elevated lesion that is usually hyperemic or hyperpigmented in the early stages and later becomes hard and stony white. Hypertrophic scars and keloids are frequently pruritic and sensitive to pressure. Because they may regress spontaneously, hypertrophic scars have a better prognosis than do keloids. Treatment of keloids involves intralesional injection with corticosteroids or radiotherapy; plastic surgery may be necessary with concomitant medical therapy including the administration of systemic corticosteroids.

Black Heel

Black heel, which usually affects the sole, was first described by Crissey and Peachey in 1961 under the title of "calcaneal petechiae."[2] The lesion presents as an irregular black or bluish black plaque, oval or circular in shape, on the posterior or posterolateral aspect of one or both heels (Fig 26–10).

Usually only a single lesion is present, and at first glance, it may resemble a melanoma or a large verruca with capillary tufts. However, paring the lesion with a scalpel reveals successive layers of reddish brown punctate specks of dry blood that arise because of a sudden shearing force such as that encountered in active sports (e.g., weightlifting, basketball, jogging, tennis). This condition, which is completely asymptomatic, almost invariably affects adolescents and young adults; after a diagnosis has been made, no treatment is required, although paring can remove the entire lesion.

Arteriovenous Fistula

An uncommon skin lesion usually on the foot or ankle that simulates Kaposi's sarcoma, the arteriovenous

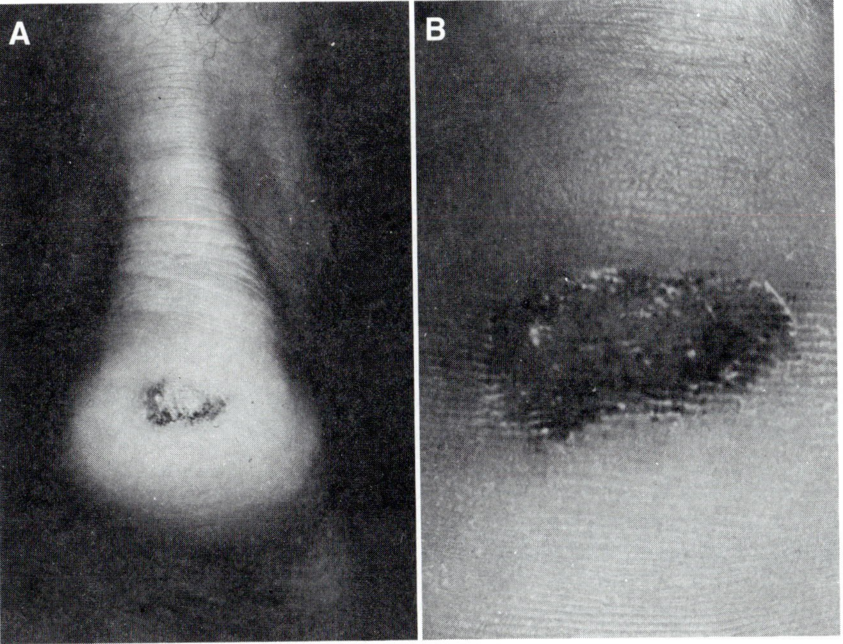

FIG 26–10.
Black heel. **A,** keratotic and wartlike lesions with pinpoint dark specks of dry blood, usually situated on the posterior of the heel, characterize the black heel (seen in athletes). **B,** close-up of the lesion.

fistula is seen in patients who are young (under 30 years of age) as opposed to the older age of patients affected by Kaposi's sarcoma.

The skin lesions are soft, reddish purple nodules and plaques that frequently ulcerate. Other characteristics include hyperpigmentation and a fibrous verrucoid eruption. The lesion results because of arteriovenous communication without an intervening capillary bed. Such fistulas are either traumatically acquired or congenital in origin. Other manifestations include enlargement of the limb, pain, bruit, increased warmth, stasis changes, edema, paresthesia, and increased sweating. The diagnosis is made by appreciation of the clinical signs and symptoms along with skin biopsy. Therapy, of course, is surgical.

Chromoblastomycosis and Mycetoma

Chromoblastomycosis and mycetoma are included in the present discussion because, although uncommon clinically, they characteristically and typically affect the foot. Chromoblastomycosis is caused by several morphologically similar fungi, the chief offenders of which are *Fonsecaea pedrosoi*, *Fonsecaea compactum*, and *Phialophora verrucosa*.

The lesion is slow growing and wartlike, occasionally developing an ulcerative papilloma with a tendency to spread along the lymphatic channels. Lymphedema and secondary infection may occur later. There is a high incidence of this infection among workers who are exposed to injury with wood. Usually the infection remains localized without dissemination. To be considered in the differential diagnosis are other verrucoid ulcerative diseases such as blastomycosis, Madura foot, and bromoderma. Treatment depends on the organism; amphotericin B has been recommended for some cases.

Also called maduromycosis or Madura foot, mycetoma, a deforming deep fungal infection, usually affects the foot but may involve the hand and invade the skin, subcutaneous tissue, and bone. Again, several organisms are involved, and the type of infection depends on the geographic area.

The infection starts as a small indurated subcutaneous papular nodule presumably from the site of trauma on the foot. The overlying skin breaks down to form a sinus tract; then exudate appears that contains the characteristic white, yellow, red, pink, or black granules according to the particular fungus involved. The "granules" are actually small hyphae produced by species of *Nocardia* or *Streptomyces;* granules with larger hyphae are produced by *Allescheria boydii* or other fungi. The infection continues for months or years and penetrates into the deep fascia, muscle, or bone with abscess and sinus formation and overgrowth of granulation tissue. The result is a grotesque enlargement of the foot and deformity that is usually relatively painless (Fig 26–11). Therapy depends on the organism. Some of the myocy-

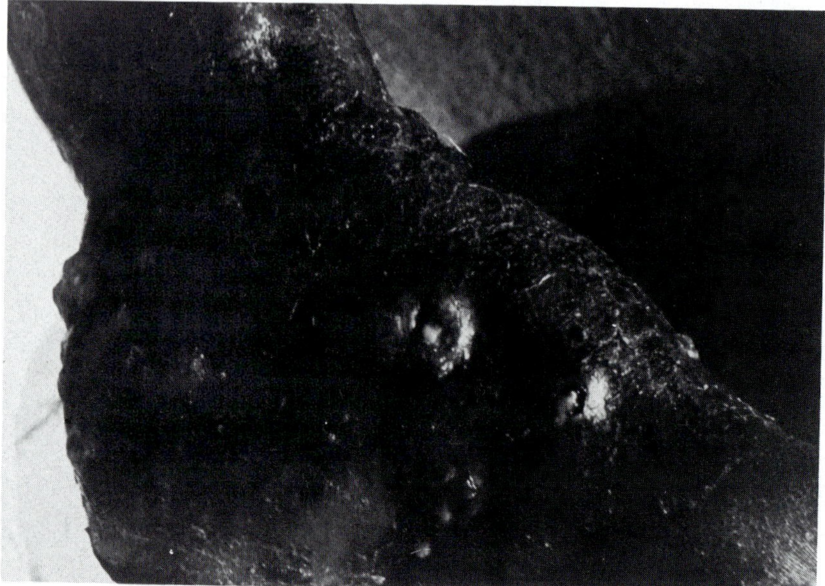

FIG 26–11.
Maduromycosis. This long-standing deep fungal infection of subcutaneous tissues results in marked deformity of the foot with sinus tracts, fibrosis, and papulonodules. Exudates containing characteristic "granules" drain from multiple sinuses and abscesses.

tomas caused by the actinomycetes respond to large doses of penicillin. Other drugs are being used including the sulfas, but sometimes myocytomas are unresponsive, and amputation of the foot becomes necessary.

MALIGNANT DISCRETE SKIN LESIONS OF THE FEET

Malignant Melanoma

Also called melanocarcinoma or the black cancer, malignant melanoma can occur anywhere on the cutaneous surface or mucous membranes but is frequently encountered on the soles. The majority of cases frequently evolve from a pre-existing nevi or pigmented lesions. This disease is rarely seen in blacks, but when it does occur, it usually occurs on the soles of the feet (Fig 26–12). Clinically, the lesion presents as a jet black mottled junctional nevus with the following history.

1. Increase in size
2. Increase in pigmentation
3. Formation of crusts
4. Formation of nodules within the lesion
5. Bleeding and ulceration

There is a wide range of clinical appearances of melanomas since almost any color change can be seen. Even the amelanotic melanomas are deadly. The differential diagnosis of melanoma includes very active junctional nevi prickle cell epithelioma, pyogenic granuloma, Kaposi's sarcoma, seborrheic keratosis, and angiokeratoma. Treatment includes wide surgical excision, and possible lymph node dissection, depending on the type of melanoma, either superficial spreading or nodular, and its depth of penetration.

Kaposi's Sarcoma

Multiple idiopathic hemorrhagic sarcoma, or Kaposi's sarcoma, characteristically involves the skin of the feet and affects predominantly men, especially those in the fifth to seventh decades (Fig 26–13). It has been noted to occur with greater frequency in those people who have immigrated from eastern Europe who are of Jewish or Italian extraction. The disease is rarely seen in American blacks, although it is endemic in certain areas of Africa.

The earliest clinical lesion appears as a pyogenic granuloma-like papule usually on the soles of the feet. Sometimes the bluish, violaceous, semihard small tumor gradually occurs with a tendency to coalesce; other times it seems to form verrucoid plaques resembling those of lichen planus. Ulceration can occur. This sarcoma is very slowly progressive in its cutaneous course, but eventually lymphedema of the affected tissue occurs and results in a brawny edema of the leg. In advanced cases, the disease is systemic with involvement of the gastrointestinal tract and other internal organs. This often leads to death.

The differential diagnosis includes stasis dermatitis, hypertrophic lichen planus, malignant melanoma, arte-

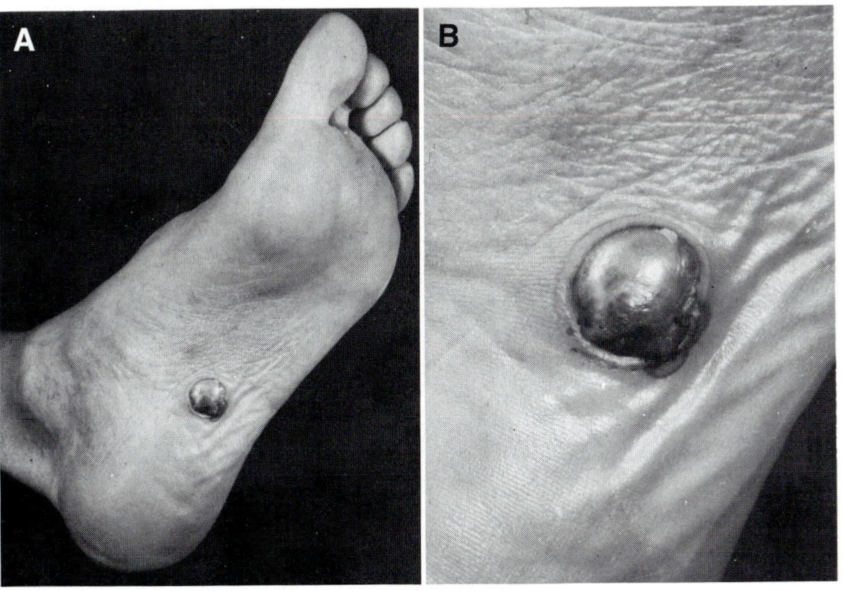

FIG 26–12.
A, malignant melanoma on the plantar surface of the foot. **B,** close-up of the lesion.

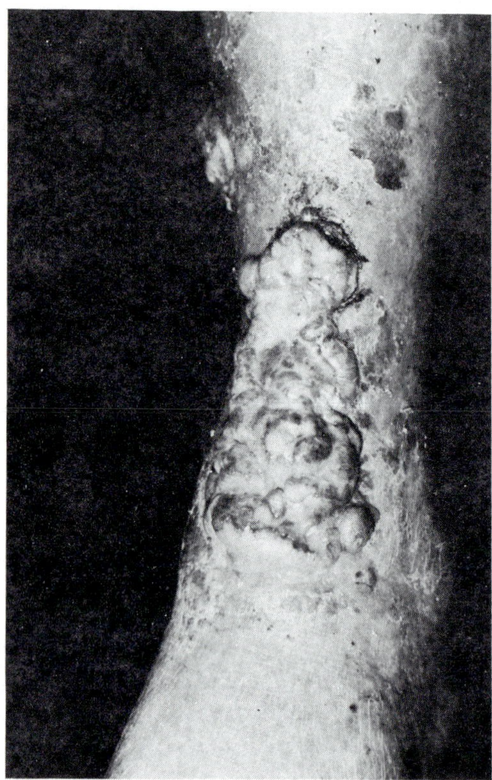

FIG 26–13.
Kaposi's sarcoma: advanced case with ulceration and beginning fungating tumors.

riovenous fistula, and deep mycoses. The diagnosis is made by biopsy. A complete internal examination should be done after diagnosis is established by biopsy because other organs can be involved.

Treatment includes several modalities such as chemotherapy, radiotherapy, electrocautery, surgical excision, and cryosurgery. Profusion with radioactive elements has also been employed.

Kaposi's Sarcoma Associated With AIDS

Acquired immunodeficiency syndrome (AIDS), as we know, is caused by the human immunodeficiency virus (HIV). The disease affects principally homosexuals (and bisexuals), intravenous drug users, and hemophiliacs and others who have received blood transfusions.

The viremia can cause skin changes resulting in lesions of Kaposi's sarcoma. This is often noted late in the course of the disease; however, it does suggest a better prognosis. Exacerbations characterize the infectious diseases of the feet in patients with AIDS. Thus fungal infections, interdigital bacterial infections, and viral infections such as warts are more difficult to treat. An atypical appearance of a lesion should also make one suspicious of AIDS.

Bacillary angiomatosis may resemble Kaposi's sarcoma. It is the same organism that causes cat-scratch fever. One may see underlying bony involvement by radiography. The disease does respond to erythromycin.

Squamous Cell Carcinoma

Squamous cell carcinoma, a malignant tumor of the skin, uncommonly affects the feet but is important because of its tendency to metastasize. Sometimes called "prickle cell epithelioma," squamous cell carcinoma develops on the feet in association with previously damaged or diseased skin (Fig 26–14). It may arise on the sites of burned out lupus vulgaris or discoid lupus erythematosus after a long period of time; it is also seen on skin that is chronically scarred or ulcerated by a previous injury such as a severe burn, the malignant ulceration being called a Marjolin ulcer.

The squamous cell carcinoma itself is not distinctive and appears as a friable ulcerated tumor with a granular surface. It may be mistaken for a pyogenic granuloma, basal cell carcinoma, eccrine poroma, verruca, foreign-body granuloma, or deep fungal infection such as chro-

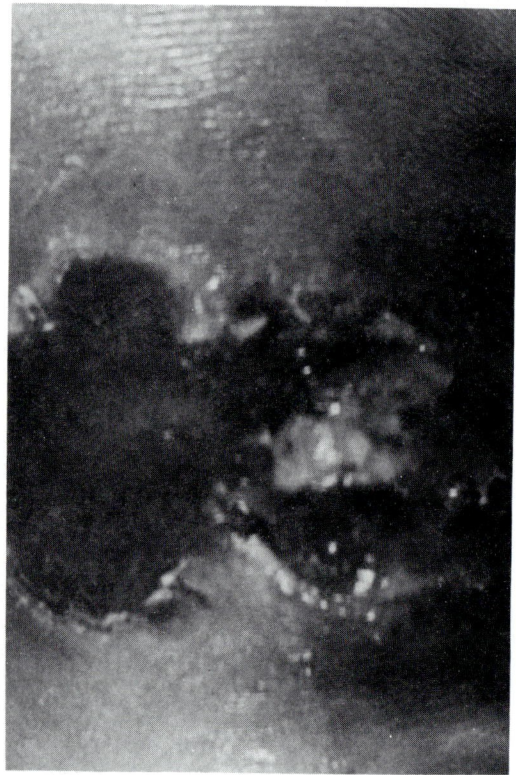

FIG 26–14.
Squamous cell carcinoma. This friable persistent ulceration developed on the foot of a 65-year-old man who also had multiple arsenical keratoses on his palms and soles.

moblastomycosis. Keratoacanthoma is another lesion that mimics squamous cell carcinoma, but it develops quickly, in a matter of weeks or months, whereas a squamous cell carcinoma usually develops slowly. Differentiation between these two lesions histologically is often difficult. Early treatment by surgical excision or, if small, by electrodesiccation and curettage prevents further complications.

Bowen's disease is a form of squamous cell carcinoma that because of its histology is often referred to as intraepithelial epithelioma or squamous cell carcinoma in situ. (Fig 26–15). The tumor is not usually a growth but more often resembles a plaque of psoriasis, eczema, or even tinea. It is usually erythematous and scaly, and the patient will remark that this "sore does not heal" but persists and enlarges. There is an association of Bowen's disease with internal malignancies, especially carcinoma of the respiratory and gastrointestinal tract.[3] Management of Bowen's disease consists of diagnosis and biopsy followed by local excision. An alternate surgical technique, if the lesion is very small, is destruction of the superficial tumor by electrodesiccation and curettage.

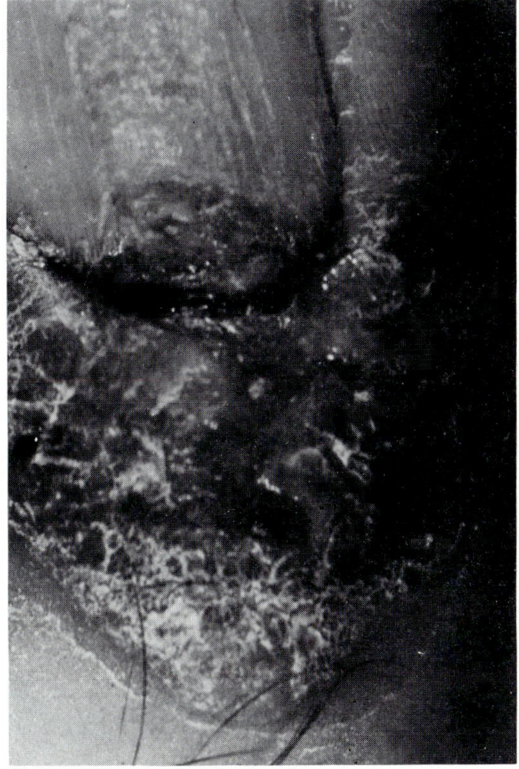

FIG 26–15.
Bowen's disease. This carcinoma in situ is frequently mistaken for tinea infection or eczema and presents as a red, scaly, oozing, persistent patch of abnormal skin on the digits.

Epithelioma cuniculatum is another variant of squamous cell carcinoma; it occurs on the sole and is very rare. This malignant lesion consists of a bulbous mass that is deeply involuted and perforated by numerous sinus tracts. Undoubtedly its appearance is influenced by the pressure effects of weight bearing. Metastases are not seen, for the tumor is only locally malignant. Treatment consists of surgical excision. In some cases, because of the extent of the lesion, amputation of the foot has been required.

Arsenic introduced into the body through industrial chemicals, medicine or hidden sources may be the cause of squamous cell carcinoma on the skin of the feet and on other portions of the integument. Inorganic arsenic in such medications as Fowler's solution, from sources like insecticides, and through industrial exposure as in mining and paints constitutes another form of this poisoning. There is a long latent period after introduction of the heavy metal into the system. Decades later discrete keratoses develop on the palms and soles along with epitheliomas on the torso and extremities. A peculiar diagnostic hyperpigmentation may occur in chronic arsenic poisoning and is seen as a "raindrop" form on the back or chest. Bowen's disease develops in cases of arsenic intoxication on the palms and soles as well as the extremities and torso. If the earlier squamous cell lesions are ignored, frank invasive squamous cell carcinomas may be seen on the acral areas of the extremities. Treatment consists of surgical excision of the carcinoma.

Basal cell carcinoma also goes by the terms basal cell epithelioma or "rodent ulcer." This tumor, which is the most common malignant tumor usually affecting the exposed areas of the body where sunlight hits, is extremely rare on the sole of the foot. Basal cell carcinoma is locally malignant and as a rule does not metastasize. The lesion may show a pearly border, although on the foot it appears more like a pyogenic granuloma. Treatment is by surgical excision.

CORNS, CALLUSES, KERATOSES, AND WARTS

Discrete hyperkeratotic skin lesions on the feet are perhaps the most common complaint. It is important to distinguish the exact identity of the lesion for successful therapy.

Calluses

Calluses develop at sites of pressure usually under the bony prominences of the feet. They tend to be the largest, whereas corns are the smallest of the hyperkeratotic lesions. To differentiate these plantar lesions, one must pare away the hyperkeratotic covering so that the distinguishing clinical characteristics are evident. Calluses have wide papillary lines that do not diverge from the normal direction. The margins of calluses are rather diffuse, whereas those of corns and warts are sharply demarcated. Corns and warts have deviating papillary lines or lines that are interrupted by a sharply marginated lesion (Fig 26–16). Calluses have no cores and no visible blood vessels. Corns have papillary lines diverging around a sharply marginated translucent cord devoid of blood vessels. Warts, on the other hand, have the fine capillaries that diagnostically rise perpendicularly to the surface. The pain may be a distinguishing feature with the various lesions. Calluses are usually not painful until they become large and extensive. Corns, particularly the neurovascular and soft types are quite painful. Warts may be painful, depending upon the type and location (Fig 26–17). Lateral pressure elicits pain in the wart; direct pressure causes pain in the corn.

Treatment of a callus usually requires the pressure causing it to be removed. This requires the patient to

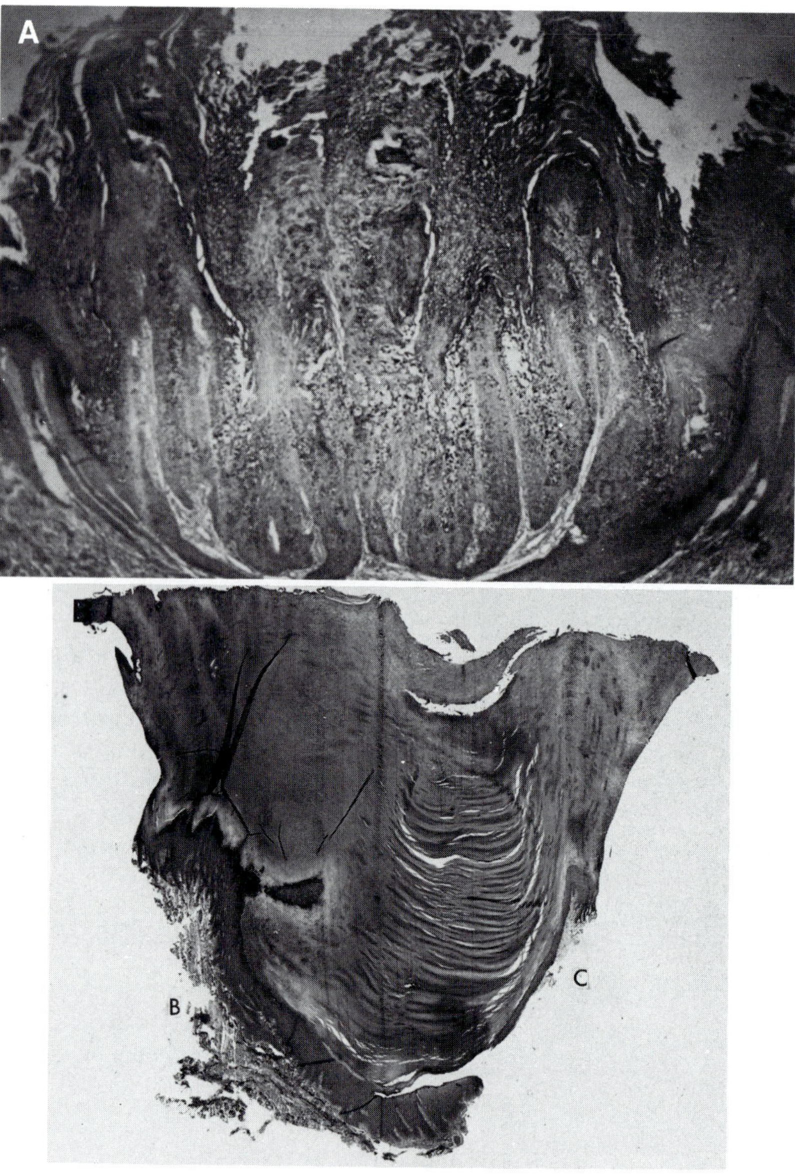

FIG 26–16.
Microscopic sections of verruca. **A,** typical mushrooming of the entire epidermis. Note the thickening of rete pegs with some fusion at the base and degeneration at the top. **B,** compression of subdermal living epithelium. Hyperkeratinization of the uppermost layers of epidermis with flushing of rete Malpighi (**B** and **C**) is shown.

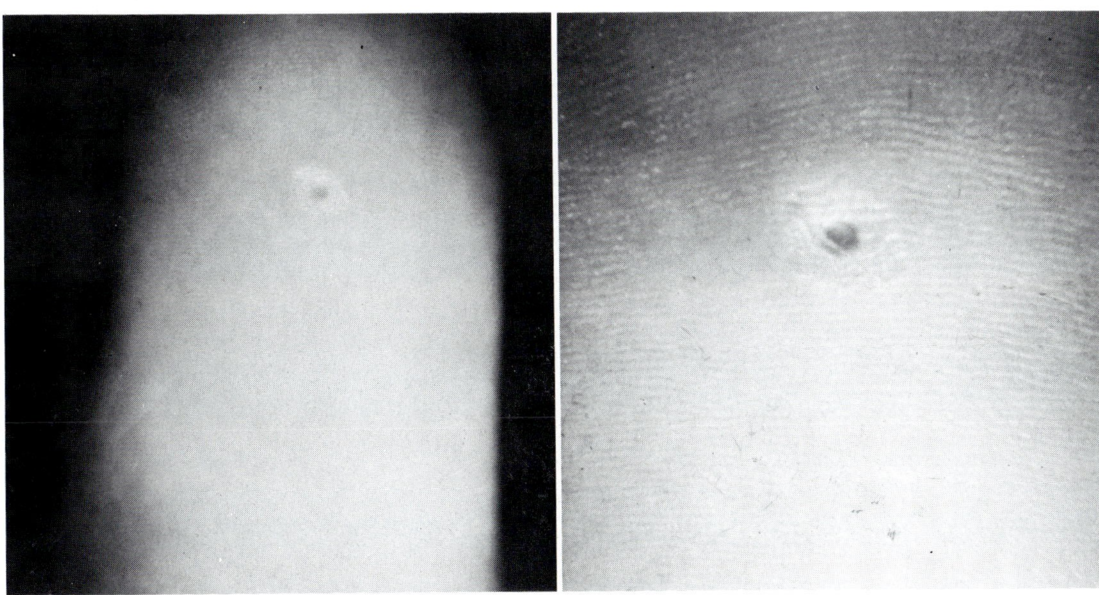

FIG 26–17.
Plantar clavus (corn). This painful lesion developed on the heel of an adolescent girl who suspected a wart. Inspection of her "everyday shoes" revealed a protruding nail at the site of the hyperkeratosis.

wear correctly fitted shoes or use corrective protective pads to distribute the body weight evenly over the weight-bearing portions of the foot. To reduce the callus formation, periodic paring plus the use of 40% salicylic acid plaster is effective.

Corns

Corns also result from friction and localized pressure, especially on the bulb of the great toe or on the sides, tips, and tops of other toes, under bony prominences, and in the metatarsal area. Treatment consists of paring periodically, plus application of a 40% salicylic acid plaster with a felt pad fashioned to fit around the corn to relieve the pressure. Protective padding is required to keep the corn from recurring; the padding or cushion can be incorporated into a supportive insole in the shoe. Again, it is important to emphasize that properly fitted shoes should be worn to prevent recurrences. Too narrow a shoe squeezes the toes together and may cause soft corns; too short a shoe may causes corns to form on the tips and tops of the toes; too high a heel interferes with the proper distribution of body weight across the foot and may cause painful calluses, corns, or warts.

The second type of corn, neurovascular corn, is usually painful and frequently mistaken as a verruca. It is usually situated on the plantar aspect of the foot under the first or fifth metatarsal head and appears as a small (1 to 3 mm) lesion with a diffuse translucent core that fades into the surrounding tissues. At the periphery of the corn, small dried up capillaries appear, some of which lie parallel with the skin rather than perpendicular as do the vessels in warts. Treatment of neurovascular corns consists of weekly paring and application of caustic agents such as 50% silver nitrate. Further thinning by applications of keratolytic agents such as 40% salicylic acid plaster can further thin down this tissue. Surgically excising these corns is inadvisable as it may result in a painful scar located on the weight-bearing portion of the foot. Orthopaedic surgery is sometimes required for removal of the plantar condyle of the metatarsal head for resistant cases (see Chapter 9).

A third type of corn affects the intertriginous aspects of the toes and is sometimes misdiagnosed as tinea pedis. The soft corn is painful and appears as a flat white soggy area on the opposing surfaces of adjacent toes usually in the fourth interdigital web space. Other interdigital spaces may be involved. The condition occurs whenever the condyle of a phalanx of one toe presses against the condyle of the head of the adjacent metatarsal. Paring away the superficial material leaves two small cores opposing each other. Sometimes for chronic cases, a sinus tract with purulent exudate will be present. Treatment of the soft corn may require simply separating the toes with a cushion such as lambs wool or a thin piece of foam rubber, or other measures may be tried such as keeping the corn thin by paring and the application of keratolytic agents such as salicylic acid plaster. Properly fitting shoes are also important. If conservative measures fail, then excision of the prominent condyle will effect a cure.

Keratoses of the Soles

Keratosis implies a hyperkeratosis not induced by friction as occurs with calluses and corns. Keratosis is frequently inherited, although trauma may cause secondary thickening. In addition, keratosis can frequently involve the palm of the hand. Keratoses occur in three morphologic varieties: diffuse, punctate, or guttate.

Diffuse keratoses are dominantly or recessively inherited and are the *most common variety*, so-called *Unna-Thost* disease or *keratosis palmaris et plantaris hereditarium.* The more severe type occurs in mal de Meleda. With time, the skin of the soles becomes yellowish white, atrophic, and thickened.

The *most frequent type, noninherited diffuse keratosis*, occurs without a specific underlying internal disease. In a rare situation, an underlying malignancy may be present. Many of these patients have associated skin diseases such as psoriasis, pachyonychia congenita, lichen planus, pityriasis rosea, and others to name a few.

Punctate (very small) or *guttate* (slightly larger) keratoses are inherited either dominantly or recessively. There is usually no history of hereditary or internal disease. In blacks, the lesions are best called pits, where they cluster in creases on the soles of the feet. In the basal cell nevus syndrome, reddish pathognomonic pits are found in association with abnormalities of bone, including cysts of the mandible, bifid ribs, and shortening of the fourth metacarpal and metatarsal.

Therapy for most keratoses is generally unsuccessful because of the rapid recurrence following treatment. Attempts must be made to debulk the thickened lesion on the soles, particularly in the diffuse types of keratoses, because this may interfere with walking, especially when fissuring occurs. Shaving of the keratoses and using softening agents are the mainstays of conservative treatment. Plasters with 40% salicylic acid are especially useful, and antimicrobial ointments may be required if fissuring occurs with secondary infection. While corticosteroid ointments are not helpful in trimming a keratosis, they may be of help in reducing peripheral inflammation.

In occasional cases, skin grafting has been performed with limited success.

Plantar Warts

Plantar warts, or "papillomas of the sole," are very common. They can occur on any part of the foot, but when localized under areas of pressure, for example, the heel or metatarsal head region, they give rise to tenderness and localized pain. Warts are caused by a DNA virus belonging to the papovavirus group.

The incidence of plantar warts is 1% to 2% in the general population and rises to as much as 25% in institutionalized children. Areas where young adults and adolescents live together and bathe in common areas such as boarding school, public baths, and military dwellings have the highest rates. Usually by 2 years, the warts will resolve spontaneously in 60% of the cases. Others have found a 20% spontaneous resolution rate. Warts are transmissible from location to location on a given patient and from person to person.

Plantar warts are usually grouped into one of three types:

1. A single or solitary wart surrounded by callus tissue with the papillary lines diverging around it. Depending upon location, i.e., if located under a bony prominence (in 80% of cases), it may be painful (Fig 26–18).
2. Multiple warts, a second type, are characterized by a larger "mother" wart surrounded by "daughter warts" that appear as blister satellites nearby (Fig 26–19). When these tiny lesions are pared, a minute capillary is usually found.
3. The mosaic wart is usually painless and is commonly mistaken for a callus. These warts may be quite large, "several centimeters in diameter," and may be present for years and appear as patches of individually coalescent cords resembling a mosaic (Fig 26–20).

Clinically, patients present because of pain caused by the plantar warts which in approximately 80% of the

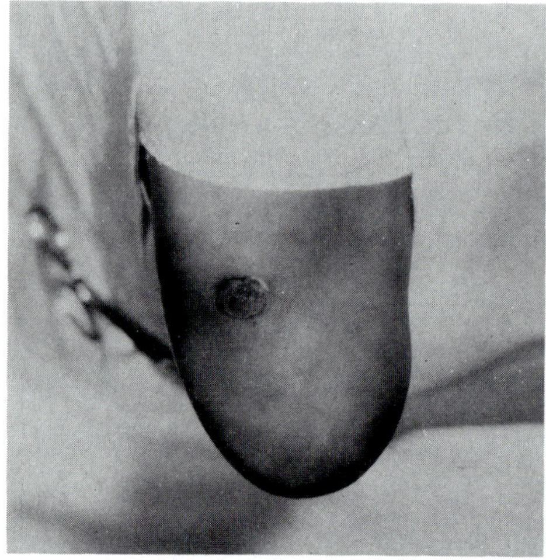

FIG 26–18.
Typical verruca plantaris on the heel.

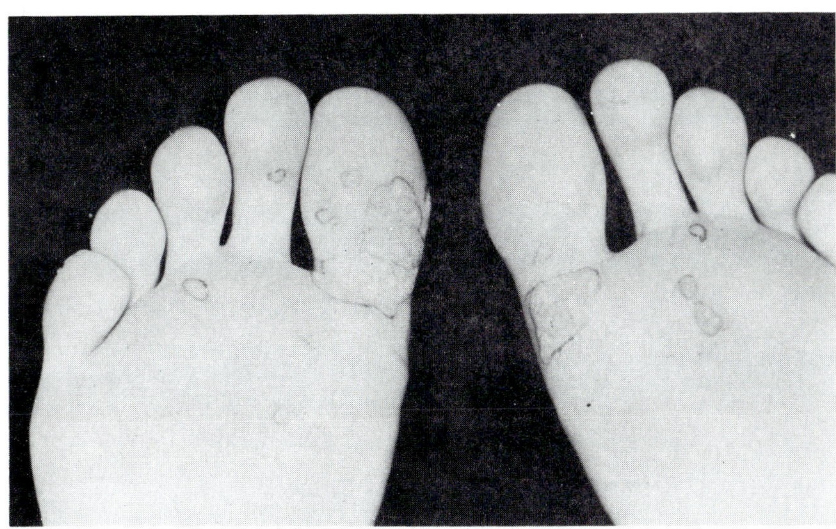

FIG 26–19.
Verrucae: larger "mother" warts and their satellite smaller "daughter" warts.

cases are found about bony prominences. This relates to areas that are subjected to trauma and result in small skin breaks that allow inoculation of the virus. Similar to calluses, pressure stimulates growth of the virus. Pain is directly proportional to the degree of hyperkeratoses overlying and surrounding the plantar wart. Single lesions are thick hyperkeratotic lesions. As opposed to the callus, papillary lines diverge around the lesion. After paring the lesion, one will note either thrombosed capillary tips, which appear as small punctate black dots at the base of the wart, or upon further paring, punctate bleeding will occur. Clinically this will make the diagnosis.

Laboratory studies are not of much use because they lack specificity and/or sensitivity to the virus. When the diagnosis is unclear, a biopsy will usually establish the diagnosis if microscopically the lesions are found to be *endophytic and hyperplastic hyperkeratotic.* Furthermore,

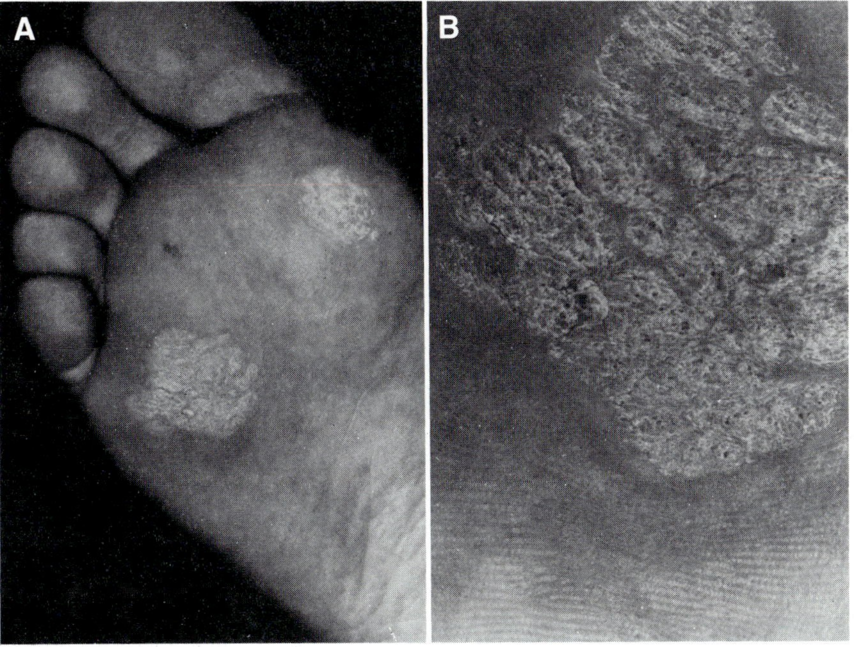

FIG 26–20.
Mosaic verrucae. **A,** large colonies of wart tissue on the sole. **B,** mosaic pattern of this viral lesion.

parakeratotic stratum corneum cells show nuclei filled with crystalline rays of compacted virus. Keratinocytes have many viruses in the nucleus, and the cytoplasm is filled with giant keratohyaline-like granules.

Differential Diagnosis

As to the differential diagnosis, the following can be considered: lichen planus, *acrokeratosis verruciformis*, epidermolytic hyperkeratosis, *acrochordons*, clavi, squamous cell carcinoma, keratoma, and callus. Usually the diagnostic dilemma is between a *keratoma*, callus, and a wart. Unlike a wart, the keratoma has a much more diffuse border after trimming it, and the skin ridges usually go over rather than around the lesion. Additionally, the keratoma may appear as a round homogeneous yellow growth about the size of a large pinhead that is covered with callous yellow epidermis. It is difficult to differentiate this lesion from a wart without paring the lesion. A *callositas* may have a similar clinical picture, but unlike the wart it will be insensitive to a pinprick and semitranslucent and may not have deep keratomas or "seeds." The usual problem in diagnosis is often not missing a wart but calling a nonviral lesion a wart. As indicated above, if the diagnosis is uncertain, biopsy will show that the lesion has viral particles, and the diagnosis is then made clear. Unfortunately, however, the morbidity of a biopsy of the plantar wart is greater than the morbidity of either treating or neglecting the lesion, and therefore biopsy is rarely performed.

Treatment

A myriad of treatments have been used by both the lay population and the medical community with varying degrees of success. In general, it is safe to say that all treatments work in some cases but no treatment works in all cases.

The following studies have dealt with plantar warts alone, and the treatments are presented as follows:

1. *Novocain (1%).*—The warts are pared, and then 2 to 3 mL of 1% procaine (Novocain) is injected with a 26-gauge needle under the wart until the wart blanches. This has resulted in a 73% resolution of the wart, and 95% had relief of their pain symptoms.
2. *Procaine (1%).*—Others have injected the wart with procaine without paring the wart first. This has resulted in a 48.5% cure rate; however, many patients objected to the pain and indicated that they would not undergo this form of treatment again.
3. *SAL paint.*—SAL paint (one part salicylic acid, one part lactic acid, and four parts flexible collodion) resulted in 84% of patients cured by 3 months and an 89% cure rate in children. Mosaic warts responded at a lower rate, with only a 45% cure rate.
4. *Glutaraldehyde.*—A 10% buffered solution of glutaraldehyde resulted in a 40% cure rate in patients with mosaic plantar warts. Others found that soaking the soles of the feet in a 2% aqueous solution of glutaraldehyde for 15 minutes per day resulted in a 75% cure rate.
5. *Benzalkonium chloride dibromide (40%).*—A 30% cure rate for mosaic plantar warts was found when this compound was used.
6. *5-Fluorouracil in dimethyl sulfoxide (5%).*—A 53% success rate for mosaic warts was noted when this compound was used.
7. *Sulfarsphenamine.*—When administered intramuscularly, there is a 68.8% response in plantar warts with this compound.
8. *Bismuth salicylate.*—When administered intramuscularly, bismuth salicylate resulted in a 58% response rate.
9. *Trichloroacetic acid with 40% salicylic acid plaster.*—By paring the lesion and applying this compound, there is a 65% cure rate over a period of four to five treatments. However, a 14% recurrence rate was noted by the end of 5 months. Because of pain after the use of this treatment, however, patients compliance was difficult.
10. *Electrocautery.*—Sixty-four percent of patients were cured, but all patients complained of pain. The recurrence rate was 29% at 3 months and 37.5% at 9 months.
11. *Liquid nitrogen.*—Liquid nitrogen is held against the plantar wart with a cotton-tipped application for 30 to 90 seconds. Pain was noted during and after the treatment, and a subsequent inflammatory reaction with edema was also noted. The wart was then scooped out approximately 36 to 48 hours later with a scalpel. Any scarring that occurred was usually soft and pliable. In one study, 27 of 62 patients required one treatment, 20 required two treatments, and 1 required three treatments. Overall the cure rate was 78.7%. Fourteen patients did not respond after five treatments. The use of procaine prior to freezing did not alter the cure rate.
12. *X-ray therapy.*—Radiotherapy was given in one or two doses totaling 1,200 rads. There was a 6.7% rate of recurrence at the same site, and the potential serious consequences of radiotherapy seem to outweigh the advantages.
13. *CO_2 laser.*—Use of the CO_2 laser was found to be between 50% and 95% effective.

In general, mosaic warts are more difficult to treat than solitary warts, and care must be taken as to type of treatment so that a diffuse painful scar will not result. Using various milder outpatient chemical agents is the best way to approach this type of wart.

The author's preferred treatment is the use of daily salicylic acid patches applied to a pared wart. Cantharone solution along with wart paring has also been utilized, and in both treatment forms an overall success rate of 70% to 80% can be expected within a 3-month period of time. The recurrence rate should be less than 1%.

In terms of prevention, personal as well as shoe wear hygiene is probably helpful although no studies have shown their effectiveness. Hyperhidrosis needs to be controlled by either chemical drying agents or ultrasound techniques to keep the feet dry.

REFERENCES

1. Conant MA, Wisenfeld SL: Multiple glomus tumors of the skin, *Arch Dermatol* 103:481, 1971.
2. Crissey JT, Peachey JC: Calcaneal petechial, *Arch Dermatol* 83:501, 1961.
3. Graham J, Helwig E: Bowen's disease and its relationship to systemic cancer, *Arch Dermatol* 80:133, 1959.
4. Greer KE: Epidermal inclusion cyst of the sole, *Arch Dermatol* 109:251, 1974.
5. Lerner AB: Pigmented nevi, *Mod Med* 1972, 131.
6. Morrell JF: "Pilonidal" sinus of the sole, *Arch Dermatol* 75:269, 1957.
7. Pinkus H, Rogin JR, Goldman P: Eccrine poroma, *Arch Dermatol* 74:511, 1956.

ADDITIONAL READINGS

Amonette RA, Rosenberg EW: Infection of toe webs by gram-negative bacteria, *Arch Dermatol* 107:71, 1973.

Ashby BS: Primary carcinoma of the nail-bed, *Br J Surg* 44:216, 1956.

Bartlett RW: A conservative operation for cure of so-called ingrown toenail, *JAMA* 108:1257, 1937.

Bean WB: Nail growth: a twenty-year study, *Arch Intern Med* 111:476, 1963.

Beneke ES: *Scope monograph on human mycoses*, ed 6, Kalamazoo, Mich, 1976, Upjohn.

Bloom W, Fawcett DW: *A textbook of histology*, Philadelphia, 1968, WB Saunders.

Bluefarb S: *Kaposi's sarcoma*, Springfield, Ill, 1964, Charles C Thomas.

Brown SM, Freeman RG: Epithelioma cuniculatum, *Arch Dermatol* 112:1295, 1976.

Caravati CM, Hudgins EM, Kelly LW: Tinea pedis in children, *Cutis* 17:313, 1976.

Cohen HJ, Frank SB, Minkin W, et al: Subungual exostoses, *Arch Dermatol* 107:431, 1973.

Costello M, Gibbs R: *The palms and soles in medicine*, Springfield, Ill, 1967, Charles C Thomas.

Dabrowa N, Landau JW, Newcomer VD: Antifungal activity of glutaraldehyde in vitro, *Arch Dermatol* 105:555, 1972.

DuVries HL: Hypertrophy of ungual labia, *Chiropody Rec* 16:11, 1933.

DuVries HL: Ingrown nail, *Chiropody Rec* 27:155, 164, 1944.

Fisher A: *Contact dermatitis*, Philadelphia, 1966, Lea & Febiger.

Frost L: Root resection for incurvated nail, *J Natl Assoc Chiropody* 40:19, 1950.

Gibbs R: *Skin diseases of the feet*, St Louis, 1974, Warren H Green.

Gibson HG, Montgomery H, Woolner LB, et al: Melanotic whitlow (subungual melanoma), *J Invest Dermatol* 29:119, 1957.

Glover MG: Plantar warts, *Foot Ankle*, 2:172–177, 1990.

Graham HF: Ingrown toe nail, *Am J Surg* 6:411, 1929.

Jansey F: Etiologic therapy of ingrowing toe nail, *Q Bull Northwest Univ Med School* 29:358, 1955.

Keyes EL: The surgical treatment of ingrown toenails, *JAMA* 102:1458, 1934.

Krausz CE: Nail survey: 28th October 1942, to 3rd April 1970, *Br J Chiropody* 35:117, 1970.

Lanthrop RG: Ingrowing toenails: causes and treatment, *Cutis* 20:119, 1977.

Lloyd-Davies RW, Brill GC: The aetiology and outpatient management of ingrowing toe-nails, *Br J Surg* 50:592, 1963.

Mann RA, DuVries HL: Intractable plantar keratosis, *Orthop Clin North Am* 41:67, 1973.

Montgomery RM: Painful plantar problems, *Consultant*, Oct 1977, p 45.

Ney GC: An operation for ingrowing toe nails, *JAMA* 80:374, 1923.

Pardo-Castello V: *Diseases of the nails*, ed 3, Springfield, Ill, 1960, Charles C Thomas.

Pringle WM, Helms DC: Treatment of plantar warts by blunt dissection, *Arch Dermatol* 108:79, 1973.

Raque CJ, Stein KM, Lane JM, et al: Pseudoainhum constricting bands of the extremities, *Arch Dermatol* 105:434, 1972.

Resnik SS, Lewis LA, Cohen BH: The athlete's foot, *Cutis* 20:353, 1977.

Rosin LJ, Harrell ER: Arteriovenous fistula, *Arch Dermatol* 112:1135, 1976.

Tauber EB, Goldman L, Claassen H: Pachyonychia congenita, *JAMA* 107:29, 1936.

Tromovitch TA, Kay DM: Plantar warts, *Cutis* 12:87, 1973.

White CJ, Laipply TC: Diseases of the nails: 792 cases, *Indiana Med Surg* 27:325, 1958.

Winograd AM: A modification in the technique of operation for ingrown toe-nail, *JAMA* 92:229, 1929.

Zaias N: Onychomycosis, *Arch Dermatol* 105:263, 1972.

SECTION

VII

SPORTS MEDICINE

CHAPTER

27

Athletic Injuries to the Soft Tissues of the Foot and Ankle

Thomas O. Clanton, M.D.
Lew C. Schon, M.D.

Etiology of injury in sports
Historical perspective
Epidemiology
Etiologic factors in athletic injury
  Biomechanical abnormalities
  Flexibility
  Strength
  Shoe wear and orthoses
  Playing surfaces

Chronic leg pain in athletes
Differential diagnosis
Incidence
Chronic compartment syndrome
  Definition
  Incidence
  Clinical features
  Diagnosis
  Treatment
  Results
Medial tibial stress syndrome
  Definition
  Classification
  Clinical features
  Diagnosis
  Treatment
Stress fractures of the tibia and fibula
  Clinical features
  Diagnosis
  Treatment
Gastrocnemius-soleus strain
  Definition
  Clinical features
  Treatment
Nerve entrapment syndromes
  Clinical features
  Treatment
Vascular problems
  Popliteal artery entrapment syndrome
  Femoral or external iliac arterial occlusion
  Venous disease
Exercise-induced muscle pain

Lateral ankle sprain
Anatomy
Biomechanics
Pathology
Diagnosis
  Clinical evaluation
  Radiographic evaluation
  Classification
Treatment of acute sprain
  Nonoperative treatment
  Surgical treatment
  Postoperative care
  Complications
Chronic lateral sprains and instability
  Diagnosis
  Treatment

Medial ankle sprain
Anatomy
Biomechanics
Diagnosis
  Clinical evaluation
  Radiographic evaluation
Treatment
  Technique of operative repair
  Postoperative care

Chronic medial instability
  Diagnosis
  Treatment

Syndesmosis sprain of the ankle

Definition
Incidence
Anatomy
Biomechanics
Mechanism of injury
Diagnosis
  Clinical evaluation
  Radiographic evaluation
  Classification
Treatment
  Acute injury
  Subacute injury
  Chronic injury
  Results

Subtalar sprains

Historical perspective
Anatomy
Diagnosis
  Clinical evaluation
  Radiographic evaluation
Treatment
  Historical perspective
  Acute vs. chronic treatment
  Nonoperative treatment
  Surgical treatment
  Results

Sinus tarsi syndrome

Historical perspective
Diagnosis
  Clinical evaluation
  Radiographic evaluation
Treatment
  Results

Peroneal tendon subluxation and dislocation

Etiology
Historical perspective
Anatomy
Mechanism of injury
Diagnosis
  Clinical evaluation
  Radiographic evaluation
Treatment
  Acute treatment
  Chronic treatment

Peroneal tendinitis and ruptures

Etiologic factors
Diagnosis
  Clinical evaluation
  Radiographic evaluation
Treatment
  Nonoperative treatment
  Surgical treatment

Posterior tibial tendinitis and tendon rupture

Incidence
Treatment

Achilles tendinitis and ruptures

Epidemiology
Etiology
Diagnosis and treatment
  Clinical evaluation
  Nonoperative treatment
  Surgical treatment

Midfoot sprains

Definition of injury
Incidence
Mechanism of injury
Diagnosis
  Anatomic considerations
  Clinical findings
  Radiographic evaluation
Treatment
  Acute injury
  Chronic injury

Forefoot sprains

Historical perspective
Epidemiology
Severity
Mechanism of injury
Anatomy and biomechanics
Etiologic factors
Diagnosis
  Clinical evaluation
  Radiographic evaluation
Treatment
  Nonoperative treatment
  Surgical treatment
  Results

Bunions in athletes

Definition
Etiology
Diagnosis
  Clinical evaluation
  Radiographic evaluation
  Differential diagnosis
Treatment
  Nonoperative treatment
  Surgical treatment

ETIOLOGY OF INJURY IN SPORTS

Given the emphasis that our society places on sports and recreation, it is not surprising that a new section would be devoted to this topic. As one views this multidisciplinary field, it quickly becomes evident that economics have become as much of a factor as the health and well-being of the athlete. With society's advancement have come both increasing leisure time for recreation and increasing knowledge of medicine among the general public. There has been a growth in the numbers of athletically related injuries coincident with an enlarging search by the public for specialists to provide the necessary treatment. What was once a secondary interest of the physician/sports enthusiast has now become a marketable commodity—expertise in sports medicine. Whether the expertise is more in sports or in medicine may at times create a conflict. Ideally, there is a marriage between knowledge and experience in the athletic setting with similar medical traits to allow the best possible medical treatment for the patient. This section will attempt to do just that.

Historical Perspective

Sports medicine has a long history dating back to the first recorded "athletic injury" in Genesis 32:24–25. "So Jacob was left alone, and a man wrestled with him till daybreak. When the man saw that he could not overpower him, he touched the socket of Jacob's hip so that his hip was wrenched as he wrestled with the man."[57] Although there is no record of treatment for this injury, it can safely be assumed that there was little that was unique in the treatment of athletic injuries during this period in history. Snook has attributed the first use of exercise as a therapeutic treatment to the Hindus and Chinese in approximately 1000 B.C. Herodicus recorded the first Western use of exercise as a treatment modality in the fifth century B.C.[132]

The first date recorded on a Western calendar relates to a sports event—the Olympiad of 776 B.C.[137] Track and field events were an integral part of the religious festivals held at Olympia, Delphi, Nemea, and Corinth, and the Greeks placed such an emphasis on the former that events were dated with reference to the year of the Olympiad.[7, 52, 100] The second-century Roman physician Galen has been credited as being the "Father of Sports Medicine" based upon his writings and his position as physician to the gladiators.[131] Others who are credited with major contributions to this field include Aurelianus, Avicenna, de Feltre, Veginus, Mercuriale, Joubert, and Paré.[132] Paré was the first to point out that exercise of the limbs was essential to recovery after the treatment of a fracture. As a physician treating an athlete, this appears to have a bearing on the essence of sports medicine. For the most part, the care of an athletic injury is little different from the care of a similar injury occurring to a nonathlete. The primary difference is in the more aggressive rehabilitative approach taken with the athlete. As we look at the soft-tissue injuries of the foot and ankle in athletes, it is important to remember that most of these injuries also occur in nonathletes and to patients who are not young and vigorous sports figures. Many of these injuries are discussed elsewhere in this textbook from a different perspective. It should be emphasized that the aggressive treatment and rehabilitation techniques described in this chapter are not always suitable to all patients in every situation.

Epidemiology

Sports participation has become a fundamental characteristic of our society. Just by surveying a few of the more popular sports one can find over 12 million playing football, 8 million playing soccer, 13 million playing baseball, 23 million playing basketball, and 20 million playing softball.[137] Injuries to the lower extremities constitute the majority of injuries for most sports. This is particularly true for the running, jumping, and kicking sports. If one takes injury rates calculated for the foot and ankle from studies done for various sports (Table 27–1), one can quickly perceive the magnitude of the athletic injury problem by multiplying these rates by the number of participants in the sport. While it is somewhat naive to view the incidence of injury in this manner, it does allow a general impression of the scope of this problem in terms of both numbers and health care costs.

Virtually all sports and recreational activities carry some intrinsic risk for injury. It is a natural consequence of pushing against the body's physical limitations and being involved in challenging competition. Nevertheless, one of the goals of sports medicine is to reduce the health risk of athletic participation through recognition and control of the risk factors. From the vantage point of careful epidemiologic study, it is possible to identify and quantify risk along with the incidence and prevalence of injury for a given set of conditions.[112]

In order to properly analyze epidemiologic data it is critical that the population being analyzed be assiduously defined. Many studies of athletic injuries that have engendered prejudicial thinking about the causes for injuries are flawed because of the methodology of the study. Most of the existing information on observed causes of athletic injury come from reports of cases studied. While many of these case series report an injury rate, they have often failed to accurately define the population at risk for injury. A good example of this is the prevalent idea that runners who pronate (or perhaps more precisely, overpronate) are at a greater risk for a running injury. The 1978 article by James and colleagues fostered this idea by noting that 58% of their 180 patients had a pronated foot configuration.[61] This study does not take into consideration the total number of people in the running population from whom this select group was derived who also pronate but do not have an injury problem.

Another problem with many studies is the failure to provide an accurate definition of the factor being analyzed. In sports injury studies this is frequently related to variations in the definition of what constitutes an injury from one study to the next. As an example, it is difficult to compare studies such as that of Rowe, where an injury is anything that causes an athlete to require medical attention and lose time from participation, with studies with much stricter definitions and classifications such as that of Torg and Quedenfeld.[120, 144] These are both studies of football injuries to the ankle and knee in

TABLE 27–1.

Injury Rates Calculated for the Foot and Ankle in Various Sports From a Review of the Literature

First Author	Skill Level	Ankle Injury	Foot Injury
Aerobics			
Rothenberger[118]	Recreational	12%	5%
Garrick[45]	Recreational	11%	18%
Ballet			
Garrick[44]	Professional and non professional	17%	22%
Sohl[134]	Review of literature	14%	15%
Baseball			
Garfinkel[43]	Professional	10%	4%
Basketball			
Zelisko[154]	Professional	19%	4%
Henry[55]	Professional	18%	6%
Moretz[90]	High school	31%	8%
Cycling			
Davis[32]	NA†	F&A†	8%
Kiburz[67]	Club	F&A	14%
Dance (general)			
Washington[151]	Various levels	17%	15%
Rovere[119]	Student	22%	15%
Equestrian			
Bernhang[12]	Top class	F&A	13%
Bixby-Hammett[15]	Top class	F&A	6%
Football			
Blythe[18]	High school	15%	2%
Culpepper[31]	High school	11%	4%
DeLee[33]	High school	18%	2%
Zemper[155]	College	16%	4%
		AE † = 1	0.25
Canale[24]	College	11%	2%
Golf			
McCarroll[81]	Professional	2%	3%
McCarroll[82]	Amateur	3%	2%
Gymnastics			
Caine[22]	Club	21%	3%
Garrick[41]	High school	10%	8%
Ice hockey			
Sutherland[141]	Amateur	0%	0
	High school	0%	0%
	College	7%	10%
	Professional	0%	0%
Park[101]	Junior	4%	1%
Lacrosse			
Mueller[91]	College	15%	4%
Nelson[93]	College	14%	4%
Mountaineering			
McLennan[83]	NA	41%	8%
Tomczak[143]	NA	40%	35% of subjects
Parachuting			
Petras[106]	Military	7%	0.3%
Rodeo			
Meyers[85]	College	6%	1%
Rollerskating			
Ferkel[41]	College	10%	NA
Perlik[102]	NA	8%	2%
Rugby			
Micheli[86]	College/club	8%	2%
Running			
Gottlieb[48]	Recreational	19%	11%
Walter[150]	Recreational	15%	16%
Temple[142]	NA	26%	26%
Marti[80]	NA	30%	10%

Ice skating			
Brown[21]	National males	8%	8%
Smith[129]	Age 11–19 yr	29%	8%
Skiing			
Downhill			
Johnson[64]	Various	9%	NA
Blitzer[17]	Youth	F&A	8%
Freestyle			
Dowling[35]	USSA	8%	NA
Snowboarding			
Pino[108]	Recreational	26%	3%
Soccer			
Ekstrand[36]	Swedish senior male division	17%	12%
Nielson[95]	Various	36%	8%
Berger-Vachon[11]	Amateur leagues (France)	20%	NA
Squash/raquetball			
Berson[13]	Recreational	21%	2%
Soderstrom[133]	NA	20%	7%
Tennis			
Winge[152]	Elite	11%	9%
Volleyball			
Schafle[122]	National amateur	18%	6%
Water skiing			
Hummel[60]	NA	4%	15%
Weight training			
Kulund[71]	Elite/olympic	2%	0%
Wrestling			
Roy[121]	College	10%	3%
Lok[74]	Olympic	10%	0%
Snook[130]	College	4%	0%
Requa[110]	High school	3.8/100 wrestlers	

*Adapted from Clanton TO: Etiology of injury to the foot and ankle. In Drez D Jr, DeLee JC, editors: *Orthopaedic sports medicine,* Philadelphia, 1992. WB Saunders.
†NA = not available; F&A = foot and ankle; AE = number of injuries per athletic exposure.

high school players. The comparison difficulties are magnified further when the comparison extends across sports and across levels of participation since an injury to a peewee football participant may have no relationship to what a professional rugby player considers an injury.

Finally, the homogeneity of the population being studied is important. This relates to such considerations as exposure to injury, age differences, gender differences, pre-existing injury, and other confounding variables that may significantly influence injuries. As an example, the third-string center who seldom practices or plays in games has a much different risk for a turf toe injury as compared with the starting running back.

With these factors in mind, one can appreciate the differences between studies and the number of variables that are involved.[27] The risk factors for injury can be divided into intrinsic and extrinsic varieties. The individual's physical and personality traits constitute the intrinsic factors, while training techniques, playing environment, and equipment are among some of the extrinsic risk factors. In this regard it has been demonstrated in several studies that weekly running mileage is the single most critical factor in the risk of injury in the running population.[16, 75, 80, 109, 150] When weekly mileage surpasses 64 km (40 miles), the risk of injury increases logarithmically. Other risk factors of significance are few and include a history of injury in the recent past, having run for 3 years or less, or a recent major change in the training regimen or environment. Even some of these risk factors have not been confirmed by all studies.

Etiologic Factors in Athletic Injury

As mentioned in the preceding section, there are both intrinsic and extrinsic factors that have a potential role in the etiology of injury to the athlete.[27] By analysis of these factors it is sometimes possible to intervene in a way to reduce or eliminate the risk factor and thereby lower the risk for injury. This is the heart of preventive sports medicine. Examples of such intervention include rule changes in football to eliminate the crackback block and improved generations of synthetic grass and underpadding brought about by research into the relationship between artificial turf and injury.[73, 103–105, 128] An even more profound example is the study by Janda and coworkers that showed a reduction in softball injuries from 1 in every 14 games when stationary bases are used to 1 in every 317 games when breakaway bases are used.[63] Since 56% of the injuries that occurred on stationary bases were to the foot and ankle, this is the type of research of which we should be cognizant.

Although it would be far beyond the scope of this section to discuss all the potential risk factors involved in athletic injuries to the foot and ankle, the investigation of a few of the more important ones will suffice for this section's overall educational purpose. The factors most often mentioned in association with foot and ankle injuries in sports include anatomic or biomechanical abnormalities, lack of flexibility, poor strength or muscle imbalance, shoes and/or orthoses, and the playing surface.

Biomechanical Abnormalities

Certain underlying anatomic conditions are frequently related to athletic injuries. The majority of runners and their coaches would place abnormal foot biomechanics in this category in the belief that the runner who overpronates has an innately higher risk for sustaining a running-related injury. This belief is probably held by most dancers and their instructors as well. Interestingly, there has been no reliable study to support this. One of the most comprehensive studies of running injuries is the Ontario cohort study, which included 1,680 runners. Anthropometric measurements were made on 1,000 of these runners, including femoral neck anteversion, pelvic obliquity, knee and patella alignment, rearfoot valgus, pes cavus/planus, somatotype, and running shoe wear pattern. "None of the anthropometric variables measured was significantly related to risk."[150] Although dance medicine specialists have related lower-extremity injury to poor technique and malalignment,[54, 59, 79] two independent studies failed to confirm such an association. McNeal and coworkers studied 350 dancers, while Solomon and coworkers looked at 40 professional ballet and modern dancers; neither research group found a significant relationship between alignment and injury rate for the knee, ankle, or foot.[84, 135] One could argue that by this stage the dancers with more severe biomechanical abnormalities have already undergone a rather strict selection process that has eliminated those with more severe biomechanical problems.

Studies of military recruits have provided much useful epidemiologic information due to the controlled nature of the population and their training regimen. A common injury among military trainees is the stress fracture. While flat feet have been a disqualifying factor for military service in the past, more recent studies have shown that those recruits with flat or pronated feet had no greater incidence of stress fracture than the remaining population.[10, 34, 47] A more recent study of the relationship between arch height and stress fractures was reported in 1989 and showed an increased incidence of metatarsal stress fractures in Israeli military recruits with a low arch.[127] However, they had fewer tibial and femoral stress fractures than did those recruits who had a higher arch. It appears that all the answers are not yet available concerning this relationship between biomechanical differences and injury. Clinically, it appears that biomechanical alterations are causally related to injury in some situations but not to the degree that some sports gurus have suggested.

Our personal experience in this area is that fewer than 10% of running injuries are specifically the result of a biomechanical problem with overpronation. Nevertheless, approximately 70% to 80% of injured runners who are treated with orthoses will improve.[61] If they continue to use the orthoses after the cessation of symptoms from the original problem, a substantial number will often present in short order with an entirely different set of symptoms. We believe that these are the result of the continued use of the orthoses. Therefore, in the majority of circumstances where we prescribe an orthosis for the treatment of a specific condition, we will have the patient discontinue its use once the symptoms have resolved. Only if the symptoms recur will we prescribe an orthosis on a more prolonged basis.

Flexibility

A lack of flexibility has often been cited as the factor responsible for any number of sports-related complaints. Indeed, a lack of flexibility is one of the critical components in the diagnosis of certain conditions such as hallux rigidus, where there is a characteristic loss of dorsiflexion in the first metatarsophalangeal joint.[77] By the same token, an aberrant increase in flexibility has been targeted as the etiologic factor in some injury situations. Since a discussion of flexibility and stretching can evolve into an expansive section of its own, the present discussion will be confined to relevant comments specific to the foot and ankle.

A lack of flexibility about the ankle and foot or limitation in motion of certain joints can be seen in association with certain disease processes or conditions (Fig 27–1). While this Figure 27–1 illustrates the dramatic spontaneous fusion that can occur in certain rheumatologic conditions, the more common situation for the

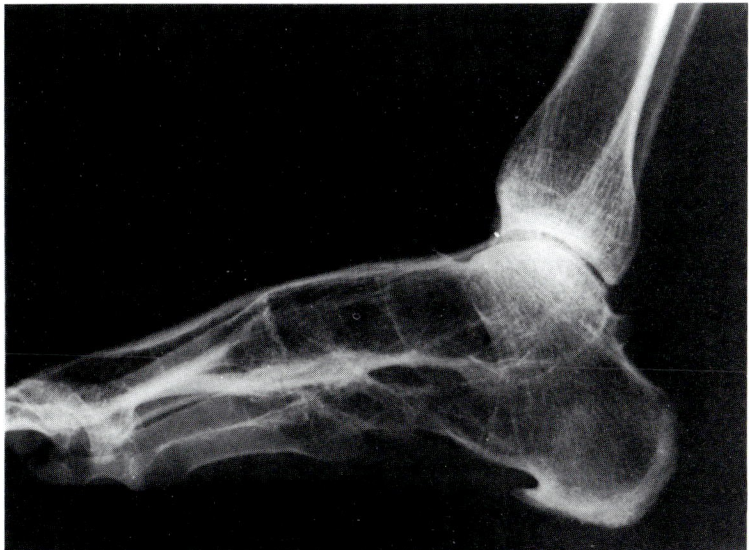

FIG 27–1.
Spontaneous fusion of the tarsal bones can be seen in certain rheumatologic conditions and creates remarkable stiffness in the foot.

sports medicine setting is the single-joint involvement seen in tarsal coalition. Athletes may have reached quite competitive levels of participation before the coalition limits them to the extent that they seek medical attention. There is commonly a history of frequent ankle sprains, and the limitation in subtalar motion seen with the talocalcaneal coalition may have been overlooked in the past. This is a common example where restricted motion is associated with athletic injury.

Restricted ankle motion in dorsiflexion is a factor in the anterior ankle pain seen in skiers and in runners who do hill work. This is commonly associated with anterior tibial osteophytes seen at the ankle joint and will be discussed in more detail later. Limited dorsiflexion of the ankle has been blamed for a multitude of other problems around the foot and ankle, including bunions,[78] turf toe,[117] midfoot strain and plantar fasciitis,[66, 72, 136] ankle sprains,[149] Achilles tendinitis,[26] calf strains,[38, 89] and hyperpronation (including all the problems that it can allegedly produce).[19, 20, 28, 76] All of these conditions have been related to a tight Achilles tendon and its consequent effect of limiting ankle dorsiflexion, but there have been no studies to unequivocally document this relationship.

Limited motion in the toes rarely receives much attention as an etiologic factor in injury or symptoms. The connection between hallux rigidus and limited dorsiflexion of the great toe metatarsophalangeal joint has already been noted. While it was originally thought that there was an association between limited first metatarsophalangeal joint motion and turf toe injury, our more recent work has not confirmed this.[29]

Limitation in motion in the other metatarsophalangeal joints is rarely seen. When the interphalangeal joints of the toes are involved in loss of motion, there is seldom a problem unless there is an associated deformity such as a hammer toe or mallet toe (Fig 27–2). These conditions can be seen in athletes and produce sufficient symptomatology to require surgical treatment.

At the opposite end of the mobility spectrum, hypermobility is infrequently mentioned as the source of problems in the foot and ankle in athletes. This dates back some 2,400 years to its first mention as a source of difficulty for athletes by Hippocrates in the fourth century B.C.[50] Certain connective tissue disorders are known for the hyperlaxity that they produce, including Ehlers-Danlos syndrome, Marfan's syndrome, Larsen's syndrome, Down's syndrome, hyperlysinemia, homocystinuria, and osteogenesis imperfecta.[50, 58, 139] The hypermobility syndrome, unassociated with known connective tissue disease, has been described as a potential source of musculoskeletal symptoms and signs including ankle joint effusions.[27]

In certain sports such as ballet and gymnastics there is some degree of selectivity for the more flexible performer. Ballet dancers are particularly noted for the tremendous mobility in their feet and ankles. The same could be said for divers and gymnasts, who are awarded for having greater ability in achieving maximum plantar flexion so that the foot is parallel to the lower part of the leg. While there are obvious advantages to this increased flexibility, there may be a negative side as well. Klemp et al. have found an increased incidence of injury in those ballet dancers who have greater mobility.[68, 69] While attempting to achieve the desired flexibility in ankle plantar flexion, it is not unusual to see the ballet student develop posterior ankle pain from im-

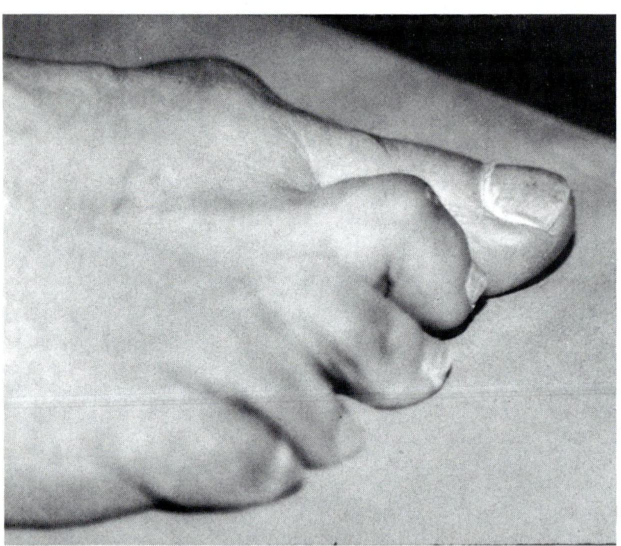

FIG 27–2.
The stiff proximal interphalangeal joint caused by a hammer toe in a college athlete can be a source of both pain and shoe-fitting problems.

pingement with a large posterior talar process or an os trigonum. These problems will be discussed in more detail later.

When there is a pathologic increase in joint laxity, it is termed *instability*.[27] Patients with instability in their joints are at increased risk for further injury. Ekstrand and Gillquist found that a history of a previous ankle sprain made a senior soccer player twice as likely to have a new ankle sprain as players without injury.[37] Instability in the ankle joint, whether the result of a proprioceptive deficit, loss of ligamentous integrity, or some other factor, is a major factor in recurrent injuries to the ankle. On the other hand, physiologic laxity has shown no similar trend. The difficulty from the clinical standpoint is in differentiating between these two conditions. This will be further clarified in the ankle ligament section.

Strength

It is a commonly held belief that weak musculature predisposes an individual to injury in sports. For example, it is often stated that weak peroneal muscles are a factor in inversion sprains of the ankle, and this is one of the goals of rehabilitation following an ankle sprain—to strengthen the peroneal muscles. It has been shown in several studies that improving strength can reduce the risk for reinjury.[1, 2, 25, 39, 52] Upon investigation it is evident that the majority of work in this area is related to strength in the thigh musculature about the knee. Similarly, muscle strength imbalances, which are viewed as creating a propensity for injury, have primarily been studied with reference to the quadriceps-to-hamstring ratio (ideally around 5:4 depending upon the test method and test speed).[6, 70, 94, 138, 153] Other studies have concluded that strength differences of more than 10% between the right and left legs increased the injury risk.[9, 22] This figure was used by Ekstrand and associates in their classic study on the prevention of soccer injuries wherein they reduced the incidence of injury by 75% with the institution of a prophylactic program that included rehabilitation to the point that 90% of muscle strength had been regained.[39]

There is no similar ratio found in the lower portion of the leg to guide rehabilitation or expose a greater potential for injury to the leg, ankle, or foot. Silver and coworkers have reported the ratio of plantar flexors to dorsiflexors as being 11 to 2, or stated conversely, the dorsiflexors are normally only 18% of the plantar flexors in terms of strength. The peroneals have a strength percentage of only 8.6 in comparison to the dorsiflexors at 9.4% and the plantar flexors at 54.5%. The peroneus brevis has a mean strength of 2.6 and the peroneus longus has a mean strength 5.5 in comparison to the strongest muscle, the soleus, at 29.9.[125] As yet there are no studies that demonstrate a relationship between an alteration in these ratios and injury risk in the lower part of the leg, foot, or ankle.

The relationship between weakness and potential for injury in sports has been further corroborated by studies of soccer players. Backous et al. performed a prospective study of boys and girls aged 6 through 17 years who were attending a summer soccer camp.[8] Among 1,139 youths there were 216 injuries, with the ankle being the most frequent site of involvement. The highest incidence of injury occurred in boys who were tall and had a weak grip strength, which led the authors to conclude that skeletally mature but muscularly weak boys were at increased risk for injury as compared with their peers. Ekstrand and Gillquist found that soccer players who sustained a minor injury during the preceding 2-month period had a 20% increase in their risk for developing a more serious subsequent injury.[36, 37] They attributed this to inadequate rehabilitation and poor muscle strength. While proof of the association between a lack of muscle strength and injury still awaits further study, the weight of empiric evidence supports this association and is the basis for working on strength as part of the rehabilitation process following injury or surgery. Furthermore, it is the foundational precept upon which colleges base their conditioning programs, including weight training.

Shoe Wear and Orthoses

In the field of sports medicine, shoes have been blamed for athletic injuries primarily from the standpoint of foot fixation on a playing surface resulting in abnormal torque. This is the most commonly cited etiologic factor for the noncontact injuries to the knee and ankle. Because of the obvious interdependency on the playing surface, these particular injuries are often attributed to the shoe-surface interface. While this section will deal with these two factors separately, the reader should keep in mind the relationship.

Torque generated by the body at the shoe-surface interface is an important factor in sports injuries, but there are other factors that are just as important. One of the most neglected but commonplace causes is improper fit of the athletic shoe. Just as this has been shown to be a prime cause of foot complaints in the general population, it is likewise a common source of relatively minor, although annoying problems for athletes.

When the athletic shoe is improperly fitted, the overly tight shoe causes pressure-related pain at the site of bunions and bunionettes or metatarsalgia. When the athletic shoe is too loose, it allows the foot to slide, and blisters result. When the shoe is too short, the toes jam into the end, and nail problems or the black toes of long distance runners occur (Fig 27–3). A more novel fitting-related problem occurs with tightly fitting ski boots, where excessive pressure at the ankle causes a neurapraxia of the posterior tibial nerve. Similarly, one can see a posterior tibial tendinitis or aggravation of an accessory navicular from an ice skating boot and irritation of the Achilles tendon and production of a retrocalcaneal bursitis from many varieties of shoe wear. Careful fitting of the athlete can generally avoid or alleviate these types of problems rather than having to resort to surgical intervention (Fig 27–4).

The shoe can be a source of problems in other ways as well, such as a lack of cushioning or lack of support. Load on the human body has been implicated as a specific etiologic factor in sports injuries.[96–98] Since a significant component of this load is the vertical impact force or ground reaction force, cushioning or shock absorption by the shoe is considered to be an important property. The ability of shoes to prevent injury through improved cushioning properties has had mixed reviews in the studies of this subject. Greaney et al. showed a reduction in calcaneal stress fractures in military recruits by switching to tennis shoes.[51] A study of South African military recruits reported a reduction in overuse injuries by incorporating a neoprene insole into the shoes used in training.[124] A recent report on aerobic dance injuries included a mention of the beneficial effects of cushioned shoes in reducing injuries.[113] Other studies have been less conclusive or have been shown no benefit from increased shock absorption either in shoes or insoles.[42, 65, 87, 88]

An interesting counterproposal to the idea that improved cushioning in the shoe is protective to the body is the Robbins and Hanna hypothesis.[116] They have proposed that increased cushioning can actually be an etiologic factor in injury by dampening the body's own sensory feedback mechanism coming from the plantar surface of the foot—a "pseudoneuropathic" condition.[114, 115] While this is a thought-provoking concept and there does appear to be some benefit from barefoot existence or performance, little support has been forthcoming for this idea.

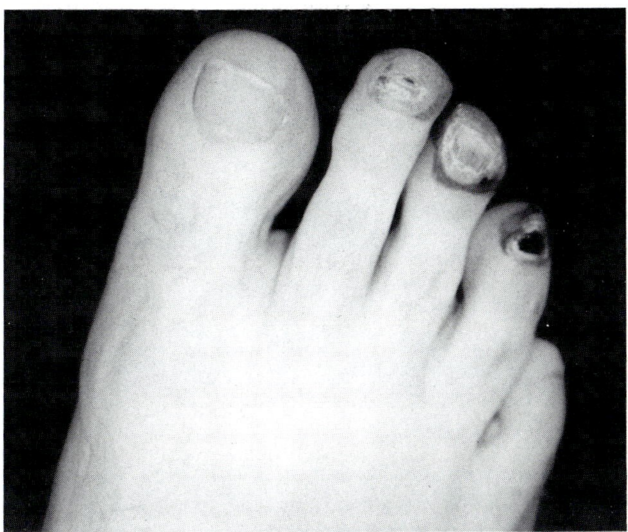

FIG 27–3.
Jamming the toes into the end of new shoes caused the black toes of this marathon runner.

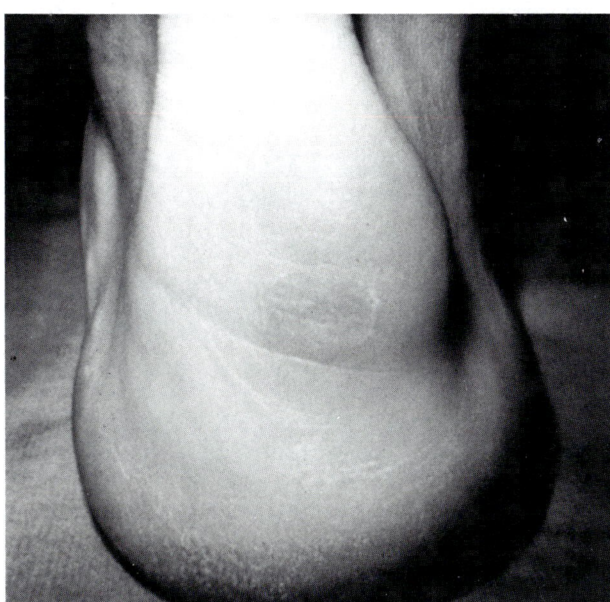

FIG 27–4.
A Haglund deformity can create a shoe-fitting problem for athletes.

Torque, as mentioned previously, is one of the most dangerous forces to which the body is subjected in sports. Cleating of the athletic shoe is designed to improve traction for more efficient performance but can significantly contribute to rotational load. Load on the body related to traction has been studied with reference to both torque and friction.[4, 30, 107, 123, 148]

Several components contribute to traction in shoe wear design analysis. These include the outsole material, sole pattern, and the presence of cleats as well as their number, length, and pattern. Torg and associates' studies of football shoes demonstrated precariously high torque when the shoes had ¾-in.-long cleats. Other shoe-surface combinations were also considered potentially unsafe.[144–147] Softer outsole materials are also associated with increasing torque when used on artificial or clean hardwood court surfaces, but the presence of dust on the floor can alter this effect.[111]

Research has clearly documented the relationship between cleating of the athletic shoe and sports injuries.[27] In one study of high school football injuries, the number of ankle injuries was halved by changing from the traditional seven-cleated conventional grass shoe to a soccer-style shoe.[120] Further support for this came from a study by Torg and Quedenfeld that found a reduction in ankle injuries from 0.45 per team per game while using conventional cleats to 0.23 in soccer-style shoes.[144] Similar reductions have been reported in other studies evaluating other cleating patterns and surfaces[18] (Fig 27–5). From the opposite standpoint, a lack of traction

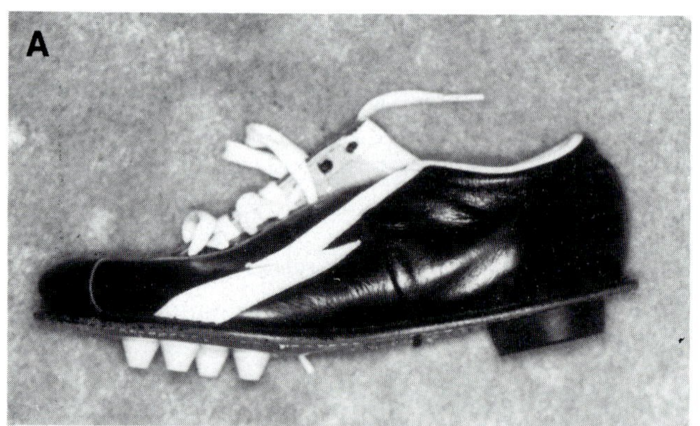

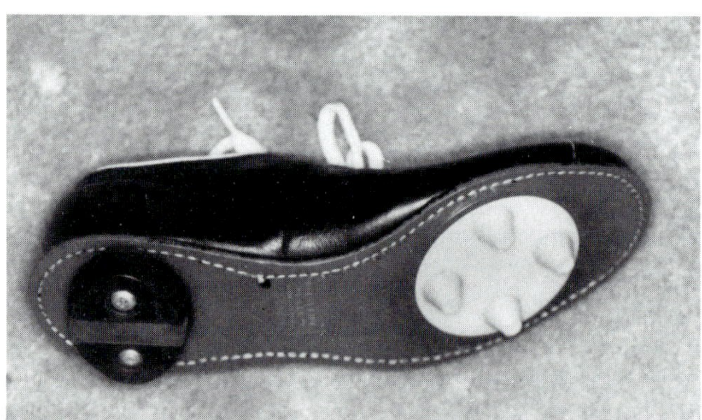

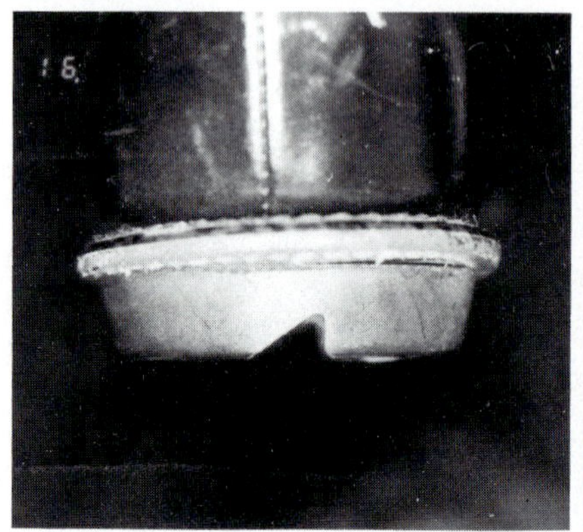

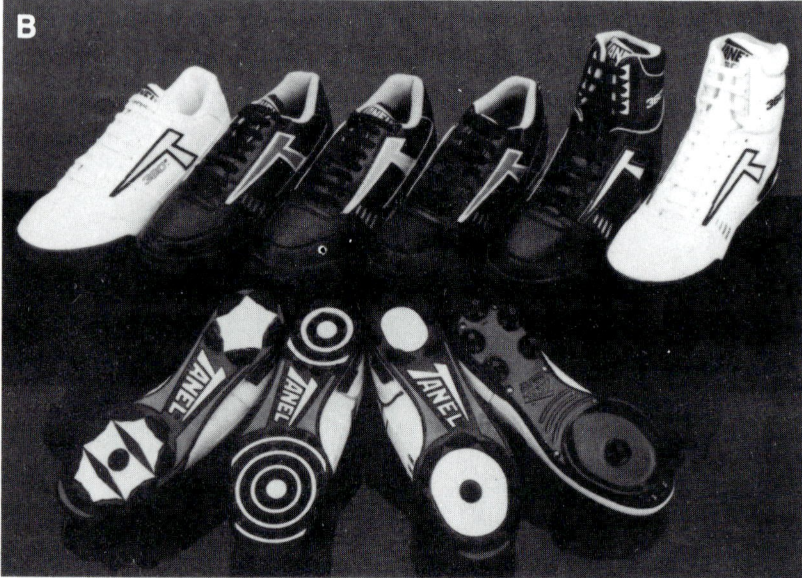

FIG 27–5.
Alternate cleating patterns in football shoes have been introduced in order to reduce injuries. **A,** Swivel shoe designed by Bruce Cameron, M.D., in the 1960s: **1,** side view demonstrating a unique heel disk; **2,** sole view showing four traditional cleats at the forefoot mounted on a rotating plastic component; **3,** heel view showing an unusual design of the heel disk to reduce foot fixation on the playing surface. **B,** alternate cleating patterns introduced in Tanel shoes in the late 1980s. (Courtesy of Tanel Shoe Corp.)

can potentially cause injury by increasing the frequency of slippages and falls. Biener and Calvori reported that slipping on wet tennis surfaces was a factor in injury in 21% of injuries.[14] Clearly, there are potential problems from both too much or too little traction. Athletes and coaches demand maximum traction for superior performance, but there comes a point where this can exceed the body's ability to handle the load. Perhaps future research in this field can define the limits of frictional and torsional forces to which the body should be subjected in the sports environment.

Playing Surfaces

Load on the athlete as a factor in injury has led to a critical analysis of playing surfaces during the past 20 years. This has primarily been stimulated by the introduction of artificial playing surfaces and particularly by the allegations against artificial grass as a cause of increasing injury rates. While there has been substantial attention given to this subject in both the lay and medical communities, the final proof has not been presented despite over 20 specific works on this issue.[27]

Although artificial surfaces have received the majority of the attention, there has been evidence against natural grass as a factor in injuries also. This is particularly true when the field is not well maintained. The classic study of high school injuries by Mueller and Blyth reported a 30% reduction in the injury rate by resurfacing and maintaining the grass practice and game fields.[92] Several studies of soccer, dance, and even ice hockey injuries have also indicated the playing surface as a factor.* Perhaps the most important study on the relationship between injuries and playing surfaces is that of Janda and coworkers, who found 70% of recreational softball injuries to be related to sliding into fixed bases.[62] The follow-up to this study was even more impressive in finding a 98% reduction in serious injuries with the use of breakaway bases; a potential savings of $2 billion in medical care costs would result if this were instituted nationwide.[63]

In running, it is a widely held opinion that hard surfaces and hills are big factors in injuries. Despite this, there have been very few confirmatory studies. The Ontario cohort study was one of the better epidemiologic studies of running injuries and found no relationship between surface and injury.[150] A simultaneously reported study from South Carolina noted the only significant relationship between injuries and training surface to be in females running on concrete.[75] Powell and associates have examined the multiple etiologic factors involved in running injuries, including the running surface, and found little correlation.[109] These studies have primarily examined injury from the standpoint of surface hardness. An alternate viewpoint is found in the European literature, where "eigen-frequencies" or vibrational forces from synthetic tracks are seen as a major factor in overuse problems in track athletes.[5, 53] Haberl and Prokop have described this as "Tartan syndrome"—a surface-related problem from "long-term nonphysiological stress, resulting in acute, chronic or periodical irritant states."[53] These considerations are quite important in analyzing running injuries, but the degree to which they contribute to the problem has not been established as yet epidemiologically.

**References 27, 40, 45, 54, 56, 126, 140.*

CHRONIC LEG PAIN IN ATHLETES

Leg pain in athletes is a common complaint seen by those who treat foot and ankle injuries. Those athletes who have foot and ankle complaints frequently have concurrent leg pain that the health care provider must address. Many in the sports medicine field have proposed foot and ankle abnormalities as the underlying cause of leg pain. In order to properly evaluate these athletes with leg pain, it is critical to have an understanding of the biomechanics of the lower extremity, the anatomy of this region, and the pathomechanics of athletic injury. With this as a background, it is possible to review the differential diagnosis of leg pain in athletes together with methods of evaluating this complaint.

Differential Diagnosis

A multitude of conditions must be considered when evaluating chronic leg pain in athletes, including chronic compartment syndrome, medial tibial stress syndrome, stress fractures, gastrocnemius strain, nerve entrapment syndromes, venous disease, arterial occlusion, fascial herniations, tendinitis, and radiculopathies. From these many potential etiologies, the clinician must narrow the diagnosis through the use of focused history taking and physical examination coupled with the selection of appropriate diagnostic tests. As in most circumstances in orthopaedics, a knowledge of anatomy and physiology forms the background for understanding these diverse causes for leg pain in the athlete.

Incidence

Although it is difficult to assess the relative incidence of these conditions, in our retrospective review of 150 patients evaluated for exercise-related leg pain, 33% had chronic compartment syndromes, 25% had stress fractures, 14% had muscle strains, 13% had medial tibial stress syndrome, 10% had nerve entrapments, 4% had venous pathology, and 1 patient had spinal stenosis. Styf reviewed 98 patients with recurrent anterior leg pain who were thought to have chronic compartment syndrome.[253] In his series, 25% had chronic anterior compartment syndrome, 25% had periostitis involving the anterior portion of the tibia with an associated medial tibial stress syndrome, 13% had superficial peroneal nerve entrapment, 7% had sequelae of previous fractures, 5% had muscle herniations without chronic compartment syndrome or nerve entrapment, 1 patient had a herniated nucleus pulposus, 1 patient had deep venous insufficiency, and 3 patients had muscular hypertension syndrome.

In another report, Styf identified periostitis in 40% of patients with anterior leg pain and in 30% to 50% of patients with chronic anterior compartment syndrome.[252] Patients with muscle strains, myositis, tendinitis, compartment syndrome, and stress fractures may all have periostitis as well. According to Styf, medial tibial syndrome was the most common cause of posterior medial leg pain, but it also occurred concurrently with chronic anterior compartment syndrome in 25% of his patients.

Although *shin splints* is a vague term implying nonspecific exertional leg pain, it has been diagnosed in 10% to 15% of all running injuries.[194, 203] The leg pain that has been called shin splints seems to correspond closely to the more descriptive "periostitis" described by Styf. Another study reported that shin splints accounted for 60% of painful conditions in athletes' legs.[232] In another study of 4,358 male joggers, severe injuries were noted in 877.[212] Of these, Achilles tendinitis was the source in 92, strained calf muscles in 71, and shin splints in 41. Obviously, exertional leg pain is the source of considerable symptomotology in the athletic population.

Chronic Compartment Syndrome

Definition

Chronic compartment syndrome is caused by elevated compartment pressures that result in ischemia of muscles and nerves. The noncompliant boundaries of the fascial compartments in the leg (Fig 27–6) when coupled with increased muscle bulk secondary to muscle contraction, intracellular and extracellular fluid accumulation, and muscle microtears are responsible for the increasing pressures (Fig 27–7). Often there is venous and lymphatic compromise that contributes to the vicious cycle of increasing tissue pressure resulting in further vascular compromise.[227]

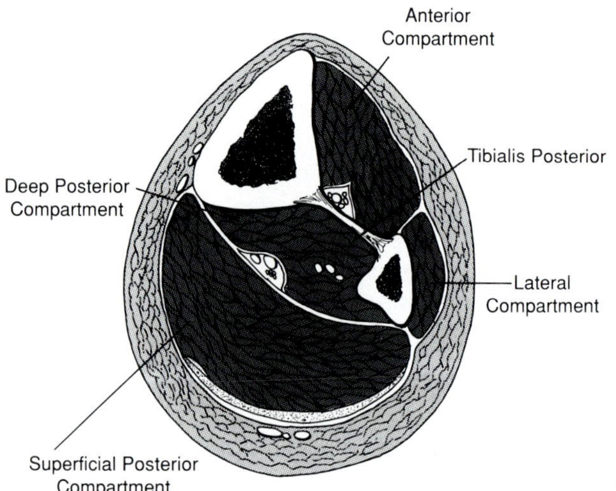

FIG 27–6.
Illustration of the compartments of the leg.

Incidence

Although the actual incidence of this condition is unclear, an approximation may be derived from one center that diagnosed 3 cases per year out of a university population of 40,000 students.[179] In this study of 100 patients treated operatively for chronic compartment syndrome, approximately 70% were runners. Ball and puck sports accounted for 20% followed by racquet sports (9%), skiing (6%), golf (4%), crew (3%), gymnastics (2%), boxing (2%), fencing (1%), and figure skating (1%).

Clinical Features

Athletes with chronic compartment syndrome complain of pain during exercise that begins after a certain distance, duration, or speed. The pain has an insidious onset and only gradually reaches a level where it restricts further performance. In the earlier stages of involvement, the pain completely or partially resolves with rest after a few minutes to several hours. Aching, cramping, or stabbing pain and a sensation of fullness over or distal to the involved compartment are characteristic. At times there are associated neurologic symptoms such as shooting pains, numbness, tingling, or burning along the course of the nerves traversing the involved compartment. Simultaneous bilateral involvement is common, but an asynchronous presentation is more frequent. Several compartments may be affected simultaneously, most commonly the anterior and the deep posterior compartments (Fig 27–8 and Table 27–2). Lateral and superficial posterior compartments are much less commonly involved.[166, 179, 212, 243] A history of previous or concurrent stress fracture has been noted in 17% of the patients in one series and is con-

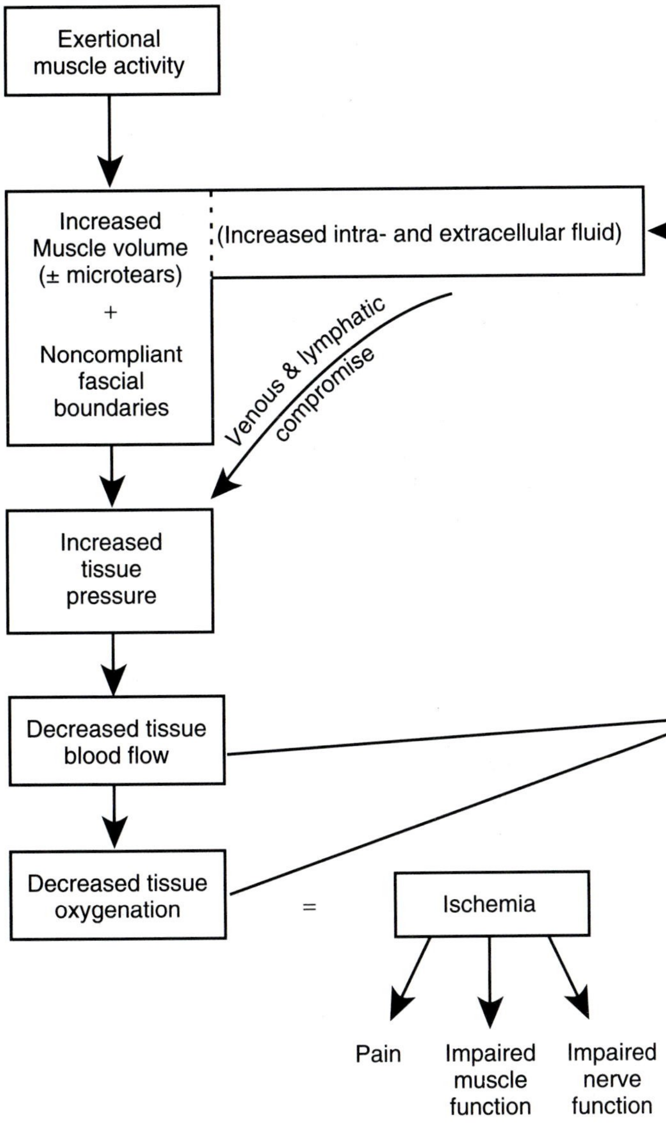

Exertional muscle activity
Increased Muscle volume (± microtears)
+
Noncompliant fascial boundaries
(Increased intra- and extracellular fluid)
Venous & lymphatic compromise
Increased capillary permeability
Increased tissue pressure
Increased metabolic byproducts
Decreased tissue blood flow
Decreased tissue oxygenation
=
Ischemia
Pain
Impaired muscle function
Impaired nerve function

FIG 27–7.
Flowchart depicting how compartment syndrome develops.

firmed by our own experience, although not to the same extent.[179]

Diagnosis

Physical Examination.—Physical examination performed with the patient at rest is typically unremarkable. There is usually some degree of tenderness over the mid to lower third of the tibia that is consistent with associated periostitis. Examination immediately following a period of exercise is frequently required to provoke the symptoms as well as to more clearly expose the signs to physical examination. Muscle herniations through fascial defects are often noted in this setting—a 20% to 60% incidence has been reported.[227, 238] It

Anterior Compartment
n=73
Deep Posterior Compartment
Lateral Compartment
n= 22
n=63
Superficial Posterior Compartment
n=9

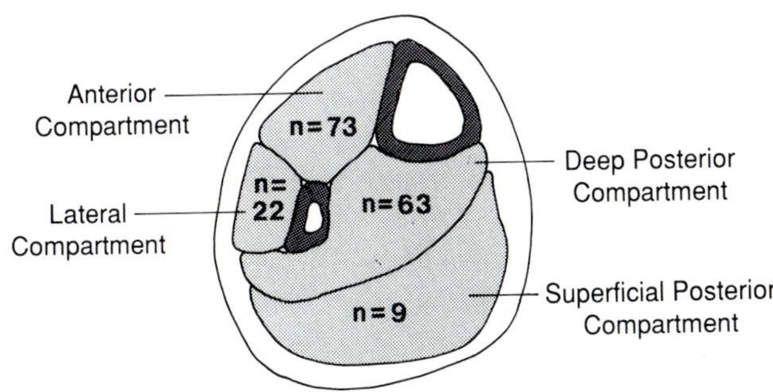

FIG 27–8.
Drawing showing the relative frequency of compartment involvement in the leg in 120 patients (Adapted from Martens MA, Moeyersoons JP: *Sports Med* 9:62–68, 1990.)

TABLE 27–2.

Number of Patients With Various Compartment Involvement (*N* = 120)*

Compartment	No. of Patients
Anterior	41
Deep posterior	40
Lateral	4
Anterior and lateral	12
Anterior and deep posterior	14
Deep posterior and superficial posterior	3
All compartments	6
Total compartments involved	167

*From Martens, MA, Moeyersoons JP: Acute and recurrent effort-related compartment syndrome in sports, *Sports Med* 9:62–68, 1990. Used by permission.

should be noted that muscle herniation through fascial defects without chronic compartment syndrome or nerve compression syndromes has also been described as a cause of chronic leg pain.[223, 231, 253] The neurologic examination is usually uneventful, but signs of deep peroneal nerve compression may occur when the anterior compartment is affected. Concurrent superficial peroneal nerve entrapment is common with anterior or lateral compartment syndrome.

Radiologic Evaluation.—Radiologic evaluation is warranted in all these cases since stress fractures may mimic these symptoms and it is possible to discover an occult tumor even in an unlikely setting (Fig 27–9). The lack of specific localized uptake on the technetium bone scan effectively rules out a stress fracture, but it is common to see a mild to moderate diffuse uptake in the tibia that is consistent with the periostitis noted clinically.[179, 253] Recent reports have documented the effectiveness of magnetic resonance imaging (MRI) in the evaluation of chronic compartment syndromes.[158] While this may have value in certain circumstances, it has not been necessary in our experience.

In general, the diagnosis of chronic exertional compartment syndrome can be made on clinical grounds.[157, 238] Confirmation of the syndrome can be achieved by obtaining compartment pressure recordings with any one of several available methods.[242] Mubarak's criteria for diagnosis using wick catheter measurement of the compartment pressure are as follows: resting pressures greater than 15 mm Hg are suggestive (normal pressure, 0 to 8 mm Hg), exercise pressures greater than 75 mm Hg are diagnostic (normal, less than 50 mm Hg), and postexercise pressures greater than 30 mm Hg that do not return to baseline within 5 minutes are confirmatory.[227] This has recently been modified to the following: (1) a pre-exercise pressure ≥ 15 mm Hg, (2) a 1-minute postexercise pressure ≥ 30 mm Hg, or (3) a 5-minute postexercise pressure ≥ 20 mm Hg.[233] A slight variation of these criteria is presented in Table 27–3.

TABLE 27–3.

Criteria for the Diagnosis of Chronic Exertional Compartment Syndrome

Mandatory
- Appropriate clinical findings

Secondary (at least 1)
- Compartment pressure ≥ 15 mm Hg preexercise
- Compartment pressure ≥ 30 mm Hg at 1 min postexercise
- Compartment pressure ≥ 15 mm Hg at 5–10 min postexercise

Several investigators have suggested that exercise pressures are the most critical value in making the diagnosis.[156, 227, 237] Other authors have disputed this and recommend the use of postexercise pressure determined by a microcapillary infusion technique.* Their criteria for diagnosis is a postexercise pressure greater than 30 to 35 mm Hg that does not return to normal resting pressure for more than 6 minutes. More recently Rorabeck et al. have suggested that the most valuable finding is postexercise pressure greater than 15 mm Hg at 15 minutes after an exercise that produced the patient's typical symptoms.[243] The importance of symptom reproduction during a stress test performed prior to the tissue pressure measurement has also been emphasized by Pedowitz and coworkers.[233]

Pressure Measurements.—For those who are going to perform these pressure measurements, certain factors should be taken into consideration. The device that one uses is not nearly as important as the user's familiarity with the device (Fig 27–10,A and B). Therefore, it is helpful to gain an appreciation for normal and abnormal values by using the traumatic situation to test patients for elevation in their compartment pressure. The testing of patients for exertional compartment syndrome can be quite tedious and time-consuming. There are numerous potential sources for error, particularly with systems such as the slit catheter connected through long tubing to a digital pressure recorder that must be calibrated prior to each use. For this reason, it may be preferable to have a technician trained in the performance of the test or to send the patient to a facility where the testing is performed routinely.

Treatment

Nonoperative Treatment.—Treatment of a chronic compartment syndrome largely depends on the goals of the athlete. If the patient is able to diminish activities

**References 163, 233, 241, 246, 255, 256.*

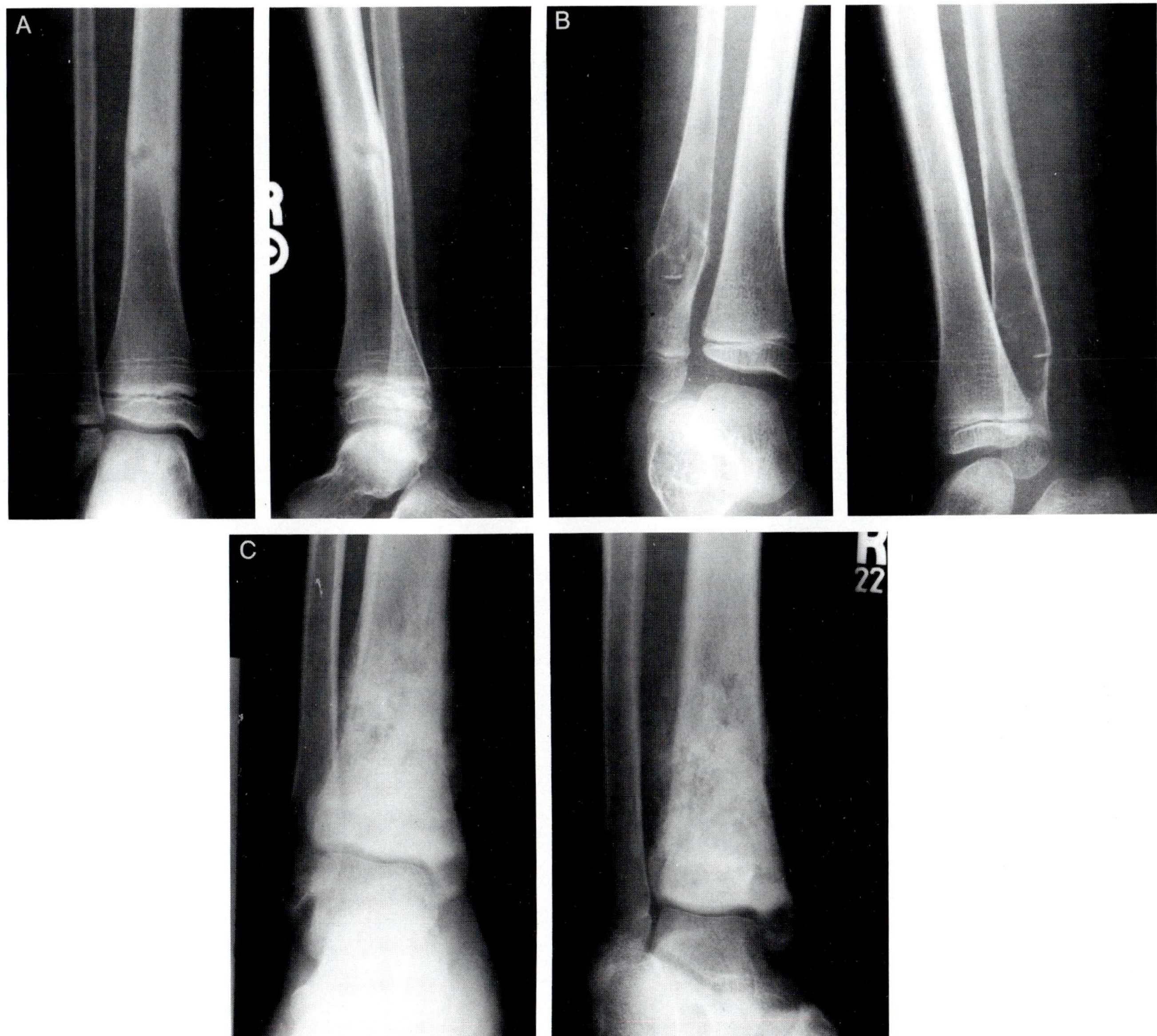

FIG 27–9.
Radiographs are essential in evaluating leg pain in an athlete since a rare surprise such as these tumors may be discovered. (Courtesy of John Murray, M.D.) **A,** radiographs of a stress fracture through a benign cartilage tumor of the tibia in a 9-year-old soccer player. **B,** radiograph of an aneurysmal bone cyst of the fibula in a 7-year-old child. **C,** radiographs of an osteosarcoma of the distal end of the tibia in an active 16-year-old.

and become comfortable, surgery is not warranted. Rest followed by a gradual increase in exercise in conjunction with ice, nonsteroidal anti-inflammatory medication, and cushioned insoles or orthoses may be tried but are often of little benefit. Definitive treatment requires fasciotomy of the involved compartment.

Surgical Treatment.—In *anterior compartment syndrome* the incision is made directly over the tibialis anterior muscle 2 to 4 cm lateral to the lateral border of the tibia (Fig 27–11). The incision begins just below the level of the tibial tubercle and extends for 5 to 10 cm longitudinally down the leg depending on the size of the patient. The procedure can be performed in the properly prepared patient under local anesthesia and a tourniquet is not used in this circumstance. Bleeding is carefully controlled with electrocautery, and great care is taken to avoid the superficial peroneal nerve as it exits the fascia between the anterior and lateral compartments in the lower third of the leg. Because of its variable course and

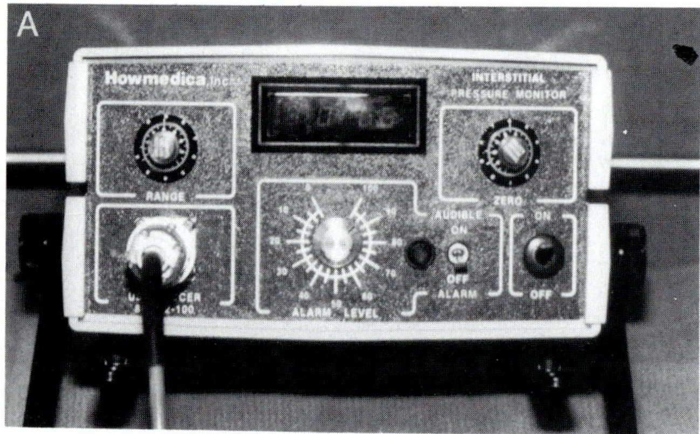

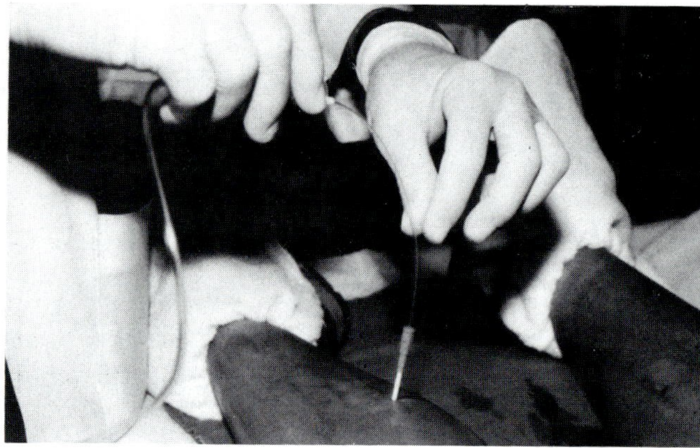

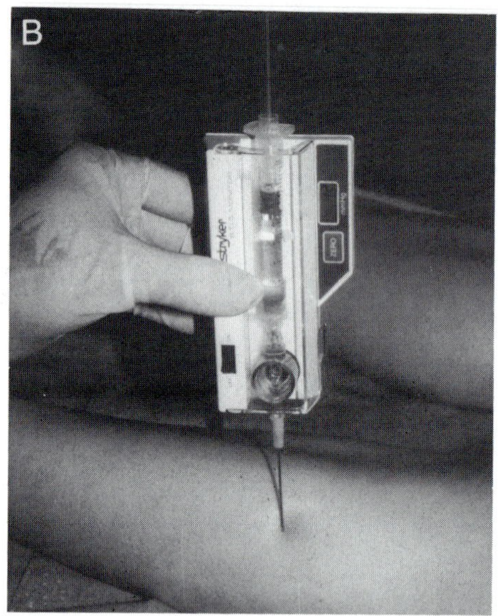

FIG 27–10.
Different methods have been advocated for determining tissue pressure within the muscle compartments. **A,** Howmedica slit catheter system: **1,** monitor; **2,** slit catheter in the leg. **B,** Stryker hand-held digital device.

its position immediately adjacent to the fascia, this nerve represents the most vulnerable structure during this procedure. The fascia is released distal and proximal to the skin incision with this in mind. It is beneficial to use loupe magnification and a headlight for better visualization. If a tourniquet is used, it is released prior to subcutaneous tissue closure and subcuticular skin closure. It is important to control the bleeding prior to closure and application of compressive dressing. Postoperatively, patients begin range-of-motion exercises immediately and may resume running or other sports activities approximately 3 weeks following an anterior or lateral compartment release.

The technique for the *lateral compartment syndrome* release is little different from the anterior fasciotomy except that the incision is moved more lateral and is longer to allow better visualization of the superficial peroneal nerve (Fig 27–12). It is essential to determine the interval between the anterior and the lateral compartments since it is in this area where the superficial peroneal nerve is located. It is found most often just under the fascia of the lateral compartment as this compartment abuts the anterior compartment. Once located, the nerve can easily be protected during the fasciotomy. Also, its exit from the fascia to the superficial tissues in the lower part of the leg can be isolated and included in the fasciotomy to preclude any possibility of postoperative entrapment as a source of persistent symptoms.

The *deep posterior compartment* fasciotomy is performed through a longitudinal incision that parallels the posterior medial border of the tibia, starts at the midtibia level, and ends about a handsbreadth above the ankle (Fig 27–13). The saphenous vein and nerve are immediately below the skin incision, and the surgeon must identify them and carefully retract them throughout the operation. The soleus muscle covers the deep posterior compartment in the midcalf, and it has a strong fascial insertion at the mid/distal third of the posteromedial aspect of the tibia. This must be released in the course of opening the deep posterior compartment. Dissection continues along the medial border of the

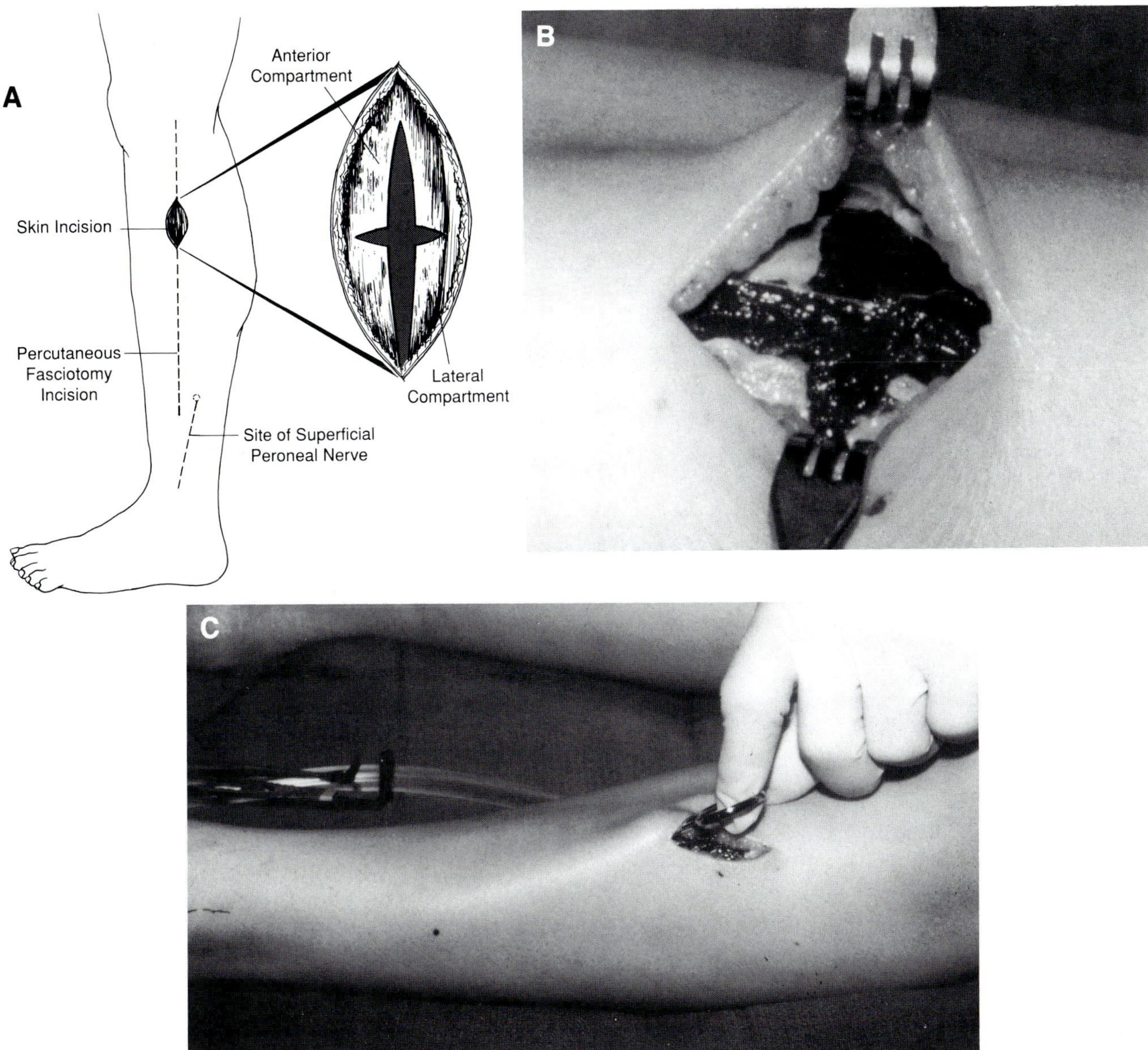

FIG 27–11.
Anterior compartment fasciotomy is performed through a relatively short incision in a partially percutaneous fashion. **A,** illustration of the technique. **B,** clinical photograph of fasciotomy of the anterior compartment. **C,** photograph demonstrating the technique of percutaneous release of the anterior compartment fascia.

tibia until the fascia enclosing the tibialis posterior muscle at the posterior border of the tibia is reached. Rorabeck and coauthors have brought attention to the compartment of the tibialis posterior muscle as a separate entity responsible for persistent symptoms following release of the deep posterior compartment.[176, 240] Our habit is to expose the tibialis posterior and to release its fascia. Whether or not this has improved our results is entirely speculation at this point. The postoperative course differs slightly since patients with a deep posterior compartment fasciotomy usually require a more prolonged recovery of about 6 weeks.

Results

Good results are to be expected when the procedure is carefully performed in the properly selected patient. Reneman's study of 40 patients undergoing anterior or lateral compartment fasciotomies found that 36 of the 40 had resumed sports in which they had been unable to participate preoperatively.[238] One patient was unim-

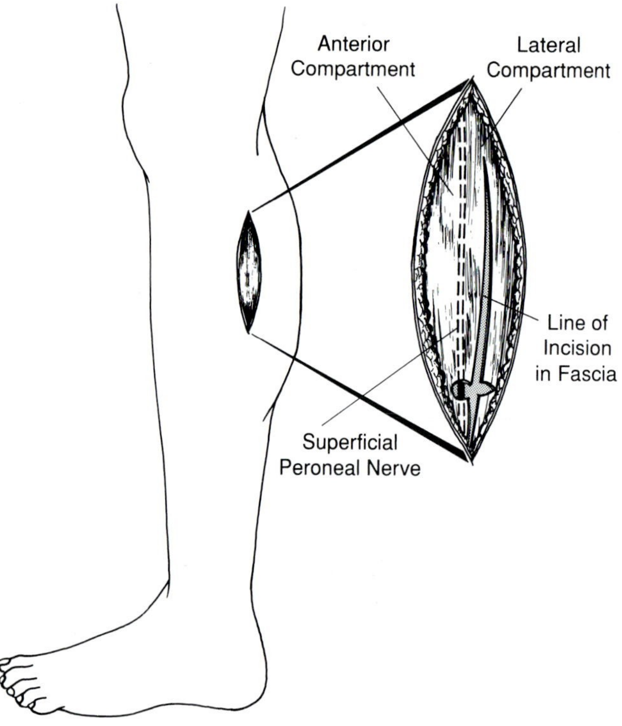

FIG 27–12.
Lateral compartment fasciotomy is performed through a longer incision to allow exposure of the superficial peroneal nerve.

proved, and 3 did not return for follow-up. In another study, Davey et al. described 12 patients with exertional compartment syndrome involving one or all compartments in both legs.[176] They found complete relief of symptoms in the 7 patients who had fasciotomies performed for anterior or lateral compartment syndrome only. One of the 3 patients with isolated deep posterior compartment syndrome had a recurrence of symptoms, and 1 of the 2 patients with anterior and deep posterior involvement had a recurrence in the deep posterior compartment (possibly related to a persistent tibialis posterior compartment problem). Puranen and Alavaikko reported on 32 patients with anterior compartment syndrome or medial tibial syndrome which appears to correspond to deep posterior compartment syndrome).[237] They stated that fasciotomy had a normalizing effect on the intracompartmental pressure but noted at least 5 cases with persistent pain after fasciotomy. They attributed this to incomplete release of the fascia. Martens reported a similar experience with 43 involved compartments in 29 patients.[211] Twenty patients underwent fasciotomy, with 16 patients having excellent results and no residual symptoms and 1 patient greatly improved. Two patients had considerable residual symptomotology, and 1 patient was unimproved. While fasciotomy is often successful in relieving pain, there has been some concern that strength may be impaired. Two studies have reported up to 20% decrease in strength in the affected compartment following fasciotomy.[188, 225] However, due to the relief of pain, the negative effect on strength is offset, and performance generally improves. The more significant potential complications include persistent swelling, hematoma formation, superficial infection, fascial herniation, nerve entrapment, residual low-grade pain, and recurrence of the compartment syndrome. We have even seen one case of postoperative reflex sympathetic dystrophy. Any of these can lead to patient dissatisfaction.[233]

Medial Tibial Stress Syndrome

Definition

Although the etiology of medial tibial stress syndrome remains the subject of debate, it is a well-established clinical entity that defines a constellation of symptoms and signs that have previously been attributed to stress fractures,[180] deep posterior compartment syndrome,[236] and shin splints.[159, 201, 249] Whether it is an insertional fasciitis of the soleus as it inserts on the posteromedial portion of the tibia or a periostitis underneath the tibialis posterior muscle, most authorities agree that the syndrome is caused by a stress reaction of fascia, periosteum, and/or bone along the posteromedial aspect of the tibia.[168, 178, 219, 231] More recently, Garth and Miller have proposed that overuse of the flexor digitorum longus muscle in association with a mild clawtoe deformity is the etiology in some patients.[190]

Classification

The various pathologic conditions that contribute to medial tibial stress syndrome are accommodated by Detmer's subclassification of the syndrome into three types.[178] Type I represents a stress fracture or stress reaction of bone. Type II denotes a chronic periosteal reaction secondary to overpull of the soleus fascia. Type III is the group with a deep posterior or tibialis posterior compartment syndrome. The syndrome is most prevalent in runners but also occurs in tennis, volleyball, basketball, and long jumping as well as most other running and jumping sports. Järvinnen et al. claim that it is the most common specific overuse injury among all athletes in Finland.[202]

Clinical Features

Complaints are recurrent pain along the medial border of the middle and distal aspects of the tibia that is

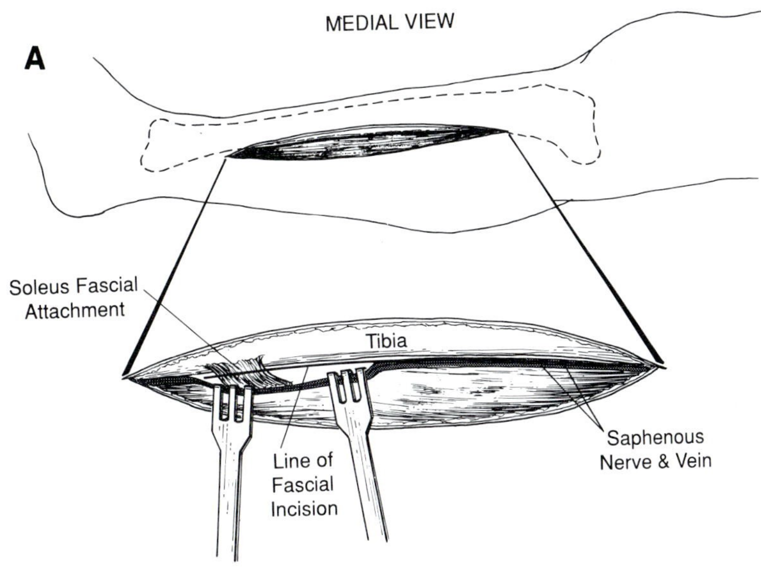

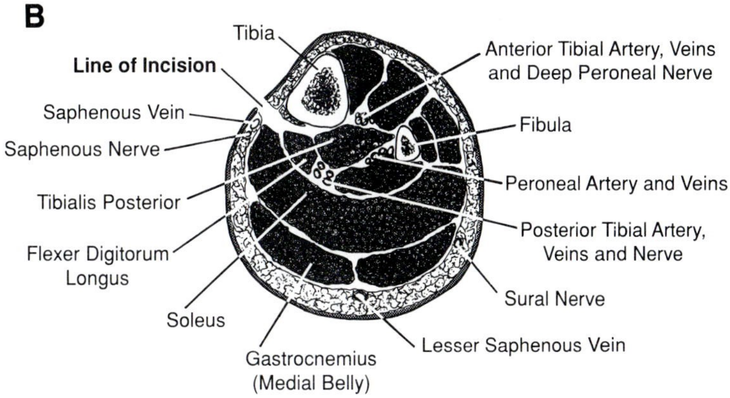

FIG 27–13.
Posterior compartment fasciotomy is performed through a medial incision at the posterior border of the tibia. **A,** medial view. **B,** cross-sectional view.

exacerbated by exercise and partially relieved by rest. The discomfort can range from a dull ache to intense pain and often worsens following exercise. Running on an indoor track with banked surfaces may induce the syndrome. Physical examination reveals tenderness along the posteromedial border of the tibia. Occasionally there is local induration in this region. The syndrome itself does not cause any neurologic or vascular findings. Several authors have remarked on a correlation between abnormal pronation and excessive posteromedial muscle or fascial stresses.[219, 235, 259] In one study comparing normal male athletes and 35 affected male athletes, excessive angular displacement in the subtalar joint was noted to be more common in the symptomatic group.[259]

Diagnosis

Other studies can assist in establishing this diagnosis. Radiographs should exclude other sources of tibial pain. Bone scan findings may be normal or may demonstrate diffuse linear uptake along the posteromedial border of the tibia that involves as much as one third of the bone's length[199] (Fig 27–14).

There has been some debate regarding the value of compartment pressure measurements in this syndrome. Some authorities have suggested that the medial tibial

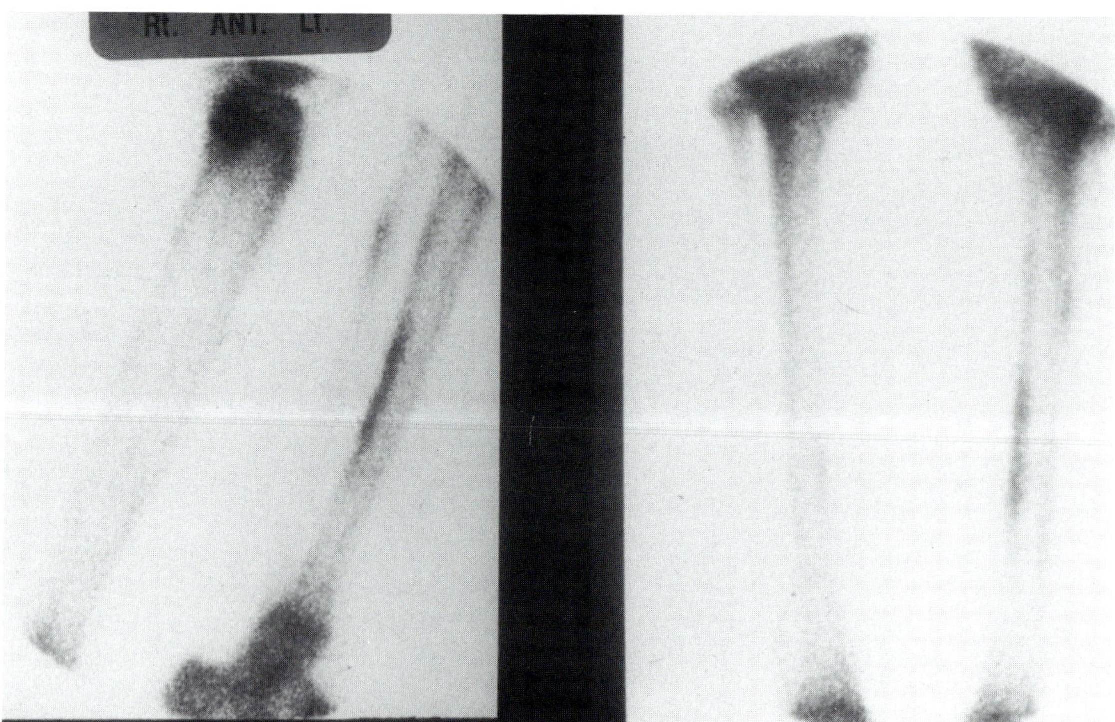

FIG 27–14.
This bone scan of medial tibial stress syndrome shows a linear area of increased uptake.

stress syndrome is actually due to a superficial posterior, deep posterior, or isolated posterior tibial compartment syndrome and have reported higher pressures in the affected compartments.* At the other extreme are studies demonstrating completely normal pressures before, during, and after exercise.[174, 228, 260, 261] Despite this dichotomy, the possible concurrence of anterior compartment syndrome with the medial tibial stress syndrome, reported by Allen and Barnes to be 50%, makes measurement of compartment pressures a valuable adjunct in these cases.[156]

Diagnosis is based on the characteristic history and physical examination coupled with negative x-ray findings and either a normal or characteristic bone scan pattern. Relief of pain following the injection of a local anesthetic agent may also help in establishing the diagnosis.

Treatment

Nonoperative Treatment.—Conservative treatment can be successful and relies heavily on rest followed by the gradual resumption of activity. Other methods of treatment, such as stretching, use of moist heat, cast application, local steroid injection, and taping, may offer temporary symptomatic relief but do not appear to change the overall course.[159, 201] A short course of nonsteroidal anti-inflammatory medication and crutch walking during the acute inflammatory phase followed by a program of progressive isometric and isotonic exercises is beneficial.[172] In patients with excessive pronation or abnormal subtalar mobility, orthotic devices may be tried.[204] When this syndrome occurs in the runner, we have recently begun using barefoot running in the retraining program following a short period of rest to allow the more severe symptoms to resolve. Barefoot running on grass seems to revitalize these legs to a certain extent.

Surgical Treatment.—The role of surgery in the treatment of medial tibial syndrome has been debated. While one report has found no benefit from fasciotomy, the majority opinion favors the use of surgery in the right circumstance.† Järvinnen and coauthors reported on 48 fasciotomies performed in 34 patients during a 10-year period.[202] Seventy-eight percent of these athletes had good to excellent results, 15% had fair results, and

**References 176, 205, 236, 237, 240, 250.*

†References 178, 202, 219, 236, 260, 261.

7% (2 patients) had poor results. Postoperative complaints included pain with exercise, hyperesthesia, or tenderness to palpation of the operative site. The two treatment failures underwent reoperations with good results. Our own experience with surgery in 15 cases is favorable. There have been 2 failures, 1 of whom improved with a more complete release at reoperation. Fasciotomy is offered to patients only after they have failed a well-supervised nonoperative program and have reached the point of ending their athletic career unless something is done. In this situation the potential risks and benefits are discussed, and the athlete is allowed to participate in the choice of proceeding with surgery or not. At the time of surgery, a posteromedial fasciotomy is performed with release of the soleus fascial bridge and the deep posterior compartment fascia.

Stress Fractures of the Tibia and Fibula

Stress fractures of the foot and ankle are covered in more detail elsewhere in this textbook, but their occurrence in the legs of athletes is of particular interest when chronic leg pain is the issue. Stress fractures result from abnormal repetitive loads on the bone that cause an imbalance of bony resorption over formation. As in the other conditions causing leg pain, running is the most common sport in patients who sustain tibia and fibula stress fractures. Other sports where tibial stress fractures have been frequently reported are basketball, soccer, aerobics, and ballet. Dancers and basketball players are particularly vulnerable to anterior midtibia stress fractures.[165, 167, 230, 239] Fibular stress fractures occur commonly in running, skating, and aerobics. Athletes with diminished mineral content (amenorrheic females) may be especially vulnerable to stress fractures.

Clinical Features

Those patients who have stress fractures typically report a recent change in their workout routine such as increased mileage, different shoes, altered terrain, or change of speed. Symptoms usually present gradually over the course of several weeks as the runner tries to "run through" the pain. Rarely, there will be a more rapid onset without the usual prolonged prodromal symptomatology. Examination confirms well-localized pain with tenderness over a rather confined area on the tibia or fibula. Swelling, erythema, and warmth may also be appreciated. One-legged hopping usually elicits pain, as will percussion of the bone. When patients with a stress fracture are treated with ultrasound, their pain is often aggravated, and they may be referred to the physician secondarily from the physical therapist or athletic trainer. Once the fracture is established, there is usually a palpable fibrous or bony mass.

Diagnosis

In most cases radiographs are initially normal, but by 2 to 3 weeks they will demonstrate a small cortical lucency or, more typically, a mild local radiodense haze. With time, a more defined periosteal reaction with cortical thickening may be appreciated. Occasionally a transverse cortical lucency occurs and indicates a more foreboding type of stress fracture. The presence of normal x-ray findings even after several months of symptoms does not rule out a stress fracture, and the technetium bone scan is the more sensitive and definitive study. In the presence of a stress fracture, the scan will show intense localized uptake (Fig 27–15).

Treatment

Nonoperative Treatment.—Treatment is largely symptomatic and should consist primarily of rest and

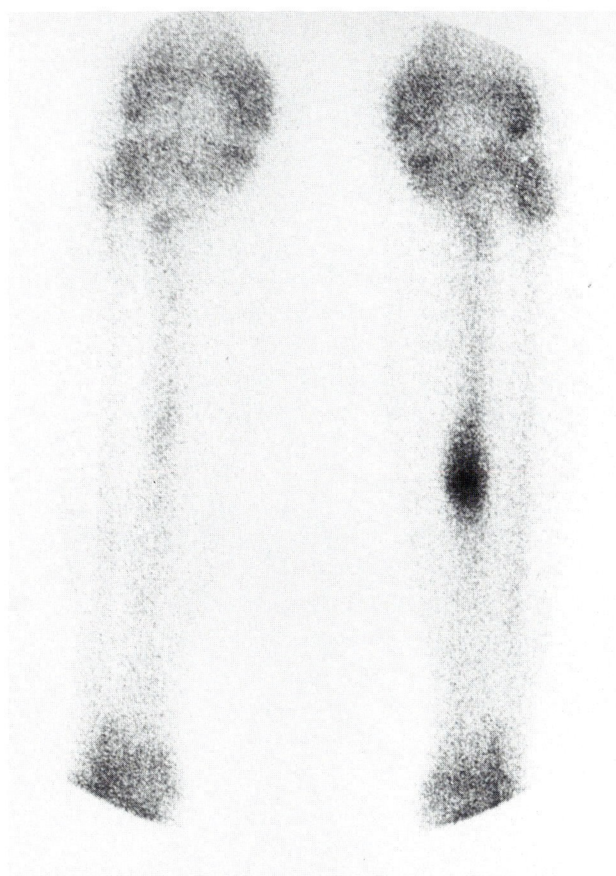

FIG 27–15.
This bone scan in a stress fracture of the tibia shows a well-localized area of increased uptake.

avoidance of the offending activity. During recovery from tibia or fibula stress fractures, immobilization is seldom necessary. Non–weight bearing may be utilized during the first few days to get control of the acute symptomatology but is quickly replaced with protected weight bearing and progression to normal walking as soon as symptoms allow. Normal athletic activities are replaced by swimming, pool running, and stationary cycling. As symptoms resolve, the athlete gradually resumes training at a level that is below the threshold for producing a worsening of the symptoms. The athlete resumes competition when he has full motion and strength and the injury is no longer tender to palpation. The use of a long Aircast brace has been valuable in protecting some of our basketball players who resumed play with the brace. The player who has a mild fibula fracture may be out only 2 to 10 weeks, while the athlete with an anterior tibial fracture may be out of competition for a considerably longer period of time, from 4 months to several years.

Surgical Treatment of Anterior Tibial Stress Fracture.—The special nature of the anterior tibial stress fracture deserves further discussion since it represents the most challenging management problem. Once this fracture develops a radiolucency, there is an increased risk of delayed union or complete fracture (Fig 27–16). Lack of uptake on the bone scan is also an ominous sign. Green and coworkers recommended excision and bone grafting if no healing occurs in 4 to 6 months since five of six athletes in their study went on to a complete fracture.[192] Rettig et al. proposed treatment with pulsing electromagnetic fields (PEMF) used for 10 to 12 hr/day for 3 to 6 months either with or without associated immobilization prior to considering surgery for bone grafting.[239] In their series only one of eight patients ultimately received a bone graft, and the average interval from the onset of symptoms to activity was 8.7 months. Another alternative is percutaneous drilling of the defect under fluoroscopic control to stimulate a healing response. This was the treatment used in the single patient whom we have seen with this unique form of stress fracture.

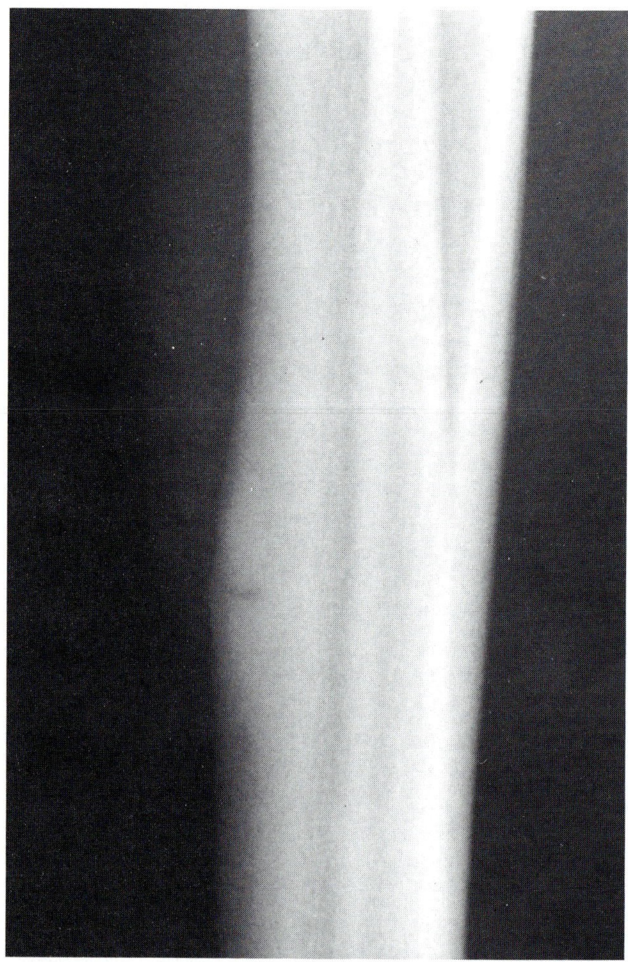

FIG 27–16.
Transverse anterior tibial stress fracture is an ominous finding.

Gastrocnemius-soleus Strain

Definition

A strain or rupture of the gastrocnemius-soleus muscle complex is a common injury in sports and is seen frequently in racquet sports, basketball, running, or skiing. Previously, there was some confusion over whether or not this entity represented a rupture of the plantaris muscle or tendon. Since this lesion was demonstrated in only one or two of the surgical cases in the literature, it is safe to assume that the majority of cases represent injury to the gastrocnemius and/or soleus muscles.[218, 247]

Clinical Features

The prevalence of the problem in middle-aged tennis players has resulted in this condition being labeled as "tennis leg."[187] It occurs when the player suddenly extends the knee while in the crouched position with the ankle dorsiflexed. There is a sudden sharp calf pain followed in some but not all cases by swelling and ecchymosis. The patient's gait is affected, and this makes it difficult to complete the toe-off portion of the stance phase. An aching or cramping pain may last for a variable duration of time depending on the severity of the initial injury, the effectiveness of initial treatment to limit the degree of hemorrhage, the use of treatment to prevent contracture of the muscle, and the compliance of the patient with the rehabilitation program.* Even in the best of circumstances, it is not unusual to see disability lasting several months and occasionally years.

Treatment

If the strain is mild, a program of rest, ice, compression, and elevation (RICE) in conjunction with passive stretching should be instituted. Once the pain decreases, standing calf stretches should be added to the regimen.[206] In the moderate strain, there is more swelling and ecchymosis and at times a palpable knot or defect. The patient is usually unable to stand on the toes secondary to pain and muscle spasm. A short-leg cast or brace with the ankle in equinus has been recommended in the acute stage to relieve symptoms, but it has been our experience that symptomatic treatment with crutches allowing weight bearing as tolerated and early institution of active dorsiflexion and gentle passive stretching results in the most rapid recovery of function. Surgical intervention is rarely indicated but may be warranted in the patient with a massive rupture and loss of muscle function.[222, 224]

*References 162, 187, 206, 221, 222.

Nerve Entrapment Syndromes

Various nerve entrapment syndromes that are responsible for exercise-induced leg pain have been described.* These are covered in some detail in Chapter 28 and will be discussed only briefly here. In our experience, the most common entrapment syndrome in the athlete (which must be differentiated in the evaluation of leg pain) is entrapment of the superficial peroneal nerve (Fig 27–17). The other entrapment syndromes include a high tarsal tunnel with entrapment of the posterior tibial nerve, entrapment of the common peroneal nerve at the neck of the fibula, saphenous nerve entrapment as it pierces Hunter's canal, and sural nerve entrapment in the posterior portion of the calf.

Clinical Features

Patients typically complain that the pain has a neuritic quality with burning, tingling, or radiation. Localized tenderness over the area of the nerve compression is characteristic on physical examination. Evaluation should exclude the possibility of a coexisting chronic compartment syndrome (as is often the case in entrap-

*References 196, 207, 213–216, 224, 226, 245, 248, 254, 263.

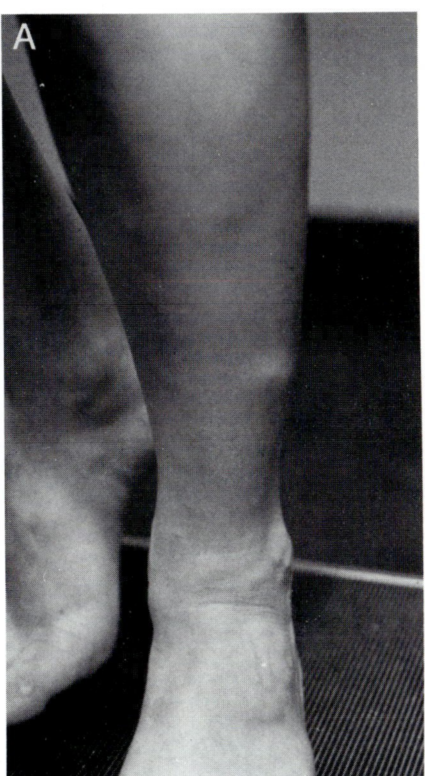

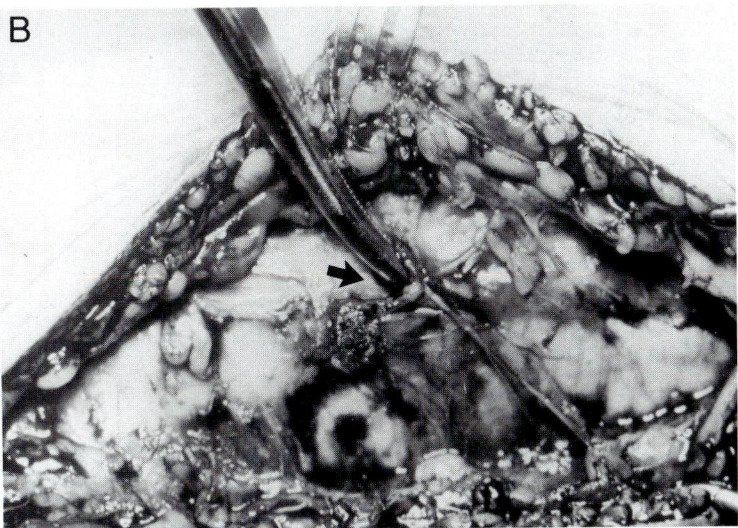

FIG 27–17.
Entrapment of the superficial peroneal nerve as it exits the fascia of the lower portion of the leg is one of the causes of chronic leg pain in athletes. **A,** clinical photograph demonstrating the commonly associated muscle herniation. **B,** intraoperative photograph showing the superficial peroneal nerve *(arrow)* exiting through a hole in the lateral compartment fascia of the leg in a case of entrapment.

ment of the superficial peroneal nerve) or a more proximal nerve entrapment (double-crush syndrome). In the double-crush syndrome, a clinical or subclinical proximal neurologic lesion diminishes the tolerance for compression of the nerve distally. Thus, a patient with a nerve entrapment syndrome or chronic compartment syndrome may manifest more pronounced neurologic symptoms if the syndrome is associated with an ipsilateral herniated nucleus pulposus or neuropathy than would be expected with an isolated ("single-crush") lesion.[245]

Treatment

Treatment consists of conservative modalities including injections (for both diagnostic and therapeutic purposes), massage, thermogesic or counterirritant creams, nonsteroidal anti-inflammatory medicines, amitriptyline, and shoe modifications. When these fail, surgical release of the nerve with associated fasciotomy may be warranted with the realization that reflex sympathetic dystrophy is a risk in nerve-related cases.

Vascular Problems

Popliteal Artery Entrapment Syndrome

Definition.—Popliteal artery entrapment syndrome (PAES) is a relatively rare entity that causes calf pain in young, athletic individuals. As a result, it is occasionally encountered primarily by the sports medicine specialist or the orthopaedist. If one is unaware of this problem as a potential source of pathology, the condition may be undiagnosed or misdiagnosed initially with devastating results—amputation of the leg below the knee.[183, 251] Since the condition closely mimics the leg pain seen in chronic exertional compartment syndrome, the physician should be particularly cautious in the patient in whom this is the suspected diagnosis.[164] When PAES is suspected on the basis of the clinical evaluation, further diagnostic procedures can confirm the diagnosis and lead to appropriate treatment.

Historical Perspective.—Popliteal artery entrapment was first described in 1879 by an Edinburgh medical student named Stuart.[251] He discovered an entrapped popliteal artery when examining the amputated leg of a 64-year-old man treated for gangrene. It was not until 1959 that Hamming reported the first clinical case treated surgically in a 12-year-old boy with intermittent claudication.[197] Love and Whelan were the first to describe this entity by the name popliteal artery entrapment syndrome.[208]

Classification.—Delaney and Gonzalez described four anatomic variants of this anomaly, which they classified as types I to IV, with type I being the most common.[177] In the type I anomaly, the popliteal artery courses medial to the medial head of the gastrocnemius muscle, which is inserted in its normal position on the posterior aspect of the medial femoral condyle (Fig 27–18). In the type II condition, the artery is entrapped by the medial gastrocnemius inserting abnormally on the posterior aspect of the femoral metaphysics, superior and lateral to its normal attachment. In type III entrapment, there is an accessory band of the medial head of the gastrocnemius. The type IV variant is caused by the artery looping medial to the medial gastrocnemius and beneath the popliteus muscle compressing the artery. Other variations have since been described (ten by di Marzo et al.[182]), which makes a classification system primarily an academic exercise.

Prevalence.—Although very little has been written on PAES in the orthopaedic literature,* it is a well-recognized and well-described entity in the general surgery and vascular literature.† Once considered exceedingly rare, there have now been over 300 cases reported.[182] It has been seen in professional athletes and nonathletes and in such sports as football, basketball, soccer, and running.‡ With the increasing involvement of the general population in sports, it can be expected that PAES will be seen with increasing frequency.

---

*References 164, 170, 175, 183, 209, 244, 257.

†References 169, 173, 177, 181, 182, 185, 190, 200, 208, 217, 220, 234, 258, 262.

‡References 169, 175, 182, 183, 209, 244.

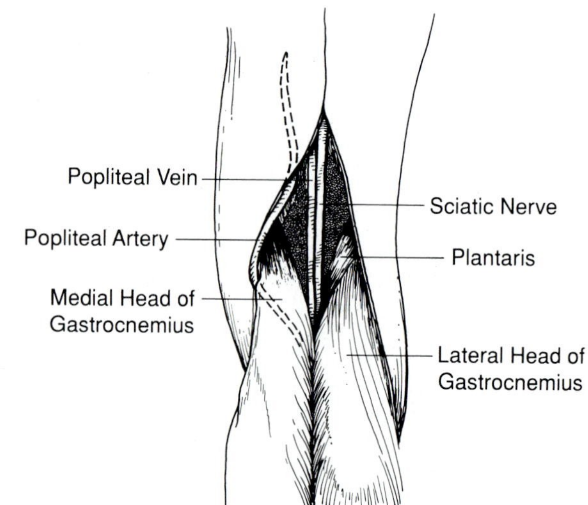

FIG 27–18.
Illustration of an anatomic variation in type I popliteal artery entrapment with the popliteal artery medial to the medial head of the gastrocnemius muscle.

Diagnosis.—*Clinical Evaluation.*—Patients with PAES are usually young athletic men who present with cramping pain in the calf with exercise.[200] This can be very typical intermittent claudication, or it may be quite atypical. The condition can be seen bilaterally in up to 67% of patients.[169, 173] A sensation of tingling in the toes may be described, but objective neurologic findings are rare.

Physical findings are surprisingly limited in the early stages of this condition, and provocative testing may be required. Pulses may be diminished or absent, particularly after exercise or with the knee in hyperextension and the foot dorsiflexed.[220, 244] The knee is sometimes warm to the touch from increased collateral circulation, and the foot may be cool.[170] Signs of ischemia are usually caused by thrombosis of the artery subsequent to damage of the intimal lining or aneurysm formation.[185] A palpable popliteal mass with pulsation or a bruit suggests an aneurysm.[195] Distal embolization can produce ischemic gangrene.[185] In the false variant of PAES, hypertrophy of the gastrocnemius in and of itself provides the compressive force on the artery to produce the entrapment.[183] Therefore, this possibility should be considered when the gastrocnemius is particularly large.

Diagnostic Studies.—In the patient presenting with exertional leg pain, further studies are often indicated in order to make a definitive diagnosis. As discussed earlier in this section, provocative testing with treadmill walking or running is frequently helpful.[234] This is the usual sequence of evaluation in chronic compartment syndrome as well, so the physician should keep the possibility of PAES in mind and examine the patient post exercise for absent pulses. If compartment pressure measurements are performed, there may be a reduction in compartment tissue pressure in PAES.[164] Doppler pressure measurement will usually show a reduction in pulse pressure, and this can be seen visually with pulse volume tracings before and after exercise.[175, 220] di Marzo and coauthors have described the use of continuous-wave Doppler and duplex scanning studies at rest and with active contraction of the calf muscles to detect decreased flow in this condition.[181] Ultrasonography can confirm the deviation in the course of the popliteal artery and demonstrate an aneurysm.[220] Other potentially useful noninvasive studies include computerized axial tomography (CAT) and MRI.[229, 262]

The definitive diagnostic study is biplanar arteriography performed after exercise[173, 193, 217, 234, 244] (Fig 27–19). The characteristic findings are medial deviation of the popliteal artery, segmental occlusion of the popliteal artery, poststenotic dilatation of the popliteal artery, stenosis of the popliteal artery with hyperextension of the knee and passive dorsiflexion of the ankle, and/or active plantar flexion of the ankle.[244] These findings are usually indicative of permanent changes to the artery.

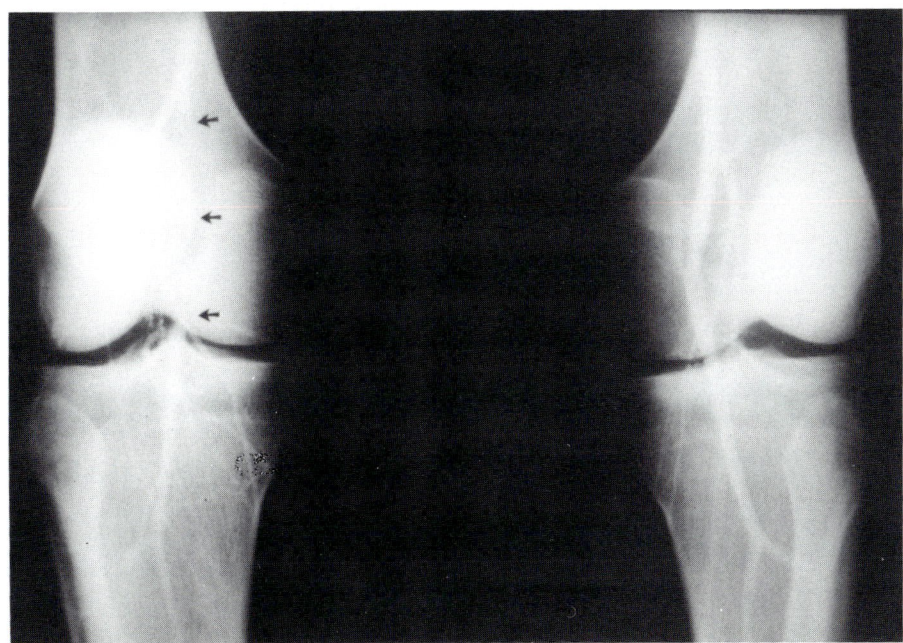

FIG 27–19.
Arteriogram is definitive in demonstrating popliteal artery occlusion *(arrows)* as in this young male runner who had pain with exercise. (Courtesy of Donald C. Jones, M.D.)

Treatment.—If the patient's symptoms are entirely exercise related and not severe, nonoperative treatment with avoidance of symptom-producing activity is a consideration. However, the vast majority of these patients require surgical treatment. This is obvious when there are ischemic changes present. When the patient has only symptoms of intermittent claudication with sports activity, the decision to intervene surgically is more thought provoking. Nevertheless, the potential risks in this condition are such that surgery should be performed in almost all circumstances. When PAES is diagnosed early and there is no damage to the artery, release of the artery from the entrapping structure may be adequate. When there are changes in the artery, these must be addressed with the appropriate vascular procedure including excision and reanastomosis, saphenous vein bypass grafting, or endarterectomy.[170, 182, 183, 217]

The best results occur when the condition is diagnosed early and can be treated by simple division of the musculotendinous structure that is compressing the popliteal artery. di Marzo et al. have reported a 94.4% long-term patency rate at a 46-month average follow-up in this situation.[182] When arterial grafting becomes necessary, the long-term patency rate decreases to 58.3%.

Femoral or External Iliac Arterial Occlusion

Definition.—A very rare syndrome of endofibrosis of the external iliac artery has been described in bicycle racers.[171] We have never seen this condition, although an occasional patient will present with leg pain following exercise that is a true intermittent claudication originating from atherosclerotic disease.

Diagnosis.—Symptoms described in cyclists with endofibrosis of the external iliac artery include paralyzing pain in the lower extremity occurring at the time of maximal effort. Descending painful muscular contraction in the calf and a subsequent sensation of motor palsy with a lack of responsiveness of the extremity is characteristic. Once the cyclist returns to less than maximal effort, the syndrome resolves within a few minutes. Physical examination performed at rest is generally unremarkable. Thigh and calf circumferences may be greater in the affected extremity. A systolic bruit may be noted with the thigh minimally flexed. Ergometric bicycle stress tests with Doppler systolic pressures at the ankle should reveal a reduction in flow at the onset of symptomatology. Angiography may demonstrate a stenotic lesion in the external iliac artery that is associated with arterial lengthening.[171]

Treatment.—Although avoidance of the activity will prevent the symptomatology, Chevalier and coauthors have shown that surgical treatment may be necessary in those individuals desiring to continue at a high level of competition.[171] In their study, endarterectomy and shortening of the artery were performed in seven racers, with four returning to competition 2 months after the surgery without a recurrence of symptoms. Referral to a knowledgeable vascular surgeon is clearly indicated when arterial disease is suspected as the source of the athlete's leg pain.

Venous Disease

Effort thrombosis is a recognized condition affecting the upper extremity and is called Paget-Schroetter syndrome.[191] The condition is quite rare in the lower extremity but has been reported.[191, 198, 264] Pain and swelling in the lower extremity associated with distended superficial veins and discoloration should alert one to the diagnosis, which is confirmed by venography. Treatment is hospital admission for anticoagulation with intravenous heparin followed by oral warfarin (Coumadin).

Thrombophlebitis may accompany either acute or chronic injury to the leg and can be a factor in prolonging recovery. Several factors increase the likelihood of development of phlebitis related to the athletic setting: immobilization after injury, inactivity during prolonged bus or air transportation following an event, high altitude, dehydration, alcohol or drug abuse, estrogen-based oral contraceptives, and hemoglobinopathies (e.g., sickle cell trait). Two patients in our series of gastrocnemius ruptures had serious venous sequelae. One patient who was a smoker developed a superficial femoral thrombosis and required anticoagulation. Another patient who had negative Doppler findings for venous disease subsequently developed a pulmonary embolism. Effort thrombosis or thrombophlebitis should be considered a potential source of symptoms in the athletic patient and should be investigated with noninvasive studies or venography when suspicion is aroused.[189, 191]

Exercise-Induced Muscle Pain

It is well known that exercise can produce muscle pain and even damage to the muscle, particularly in the case of unaccustomed strenuous activity.[160, 161] This is especially true for eccentric muscle contractions and is based on microinjury to the muscle, with the initial lesions occurring at the subcellular level.[160, 186] As a consequence of this injury, the muscle is temporarily unable to generate maximum force. Metabolic changes are evident, including elevation of muscle-derived enzyme, myoglobin, and metabolite levels. Muscle soreness can vary from being very mild to quite severe.

Symptoms include not only muscle soreness and pain but also fatigue, stiffness, and a certain loss of performance that develops 24 to 48 hours following exercise and subsides by 5 to 7 days.[184] The most common source of this pain is downhill running, which involves an eccentric contraction of the muscles. treatment is symptomatic, and the patient is cautioned to avoid repetition of the overly strenuous muscle activity during the recovery period since this may result in delayed recovery and more significant damage.

LATERAL ANKLE SPRAIN

Lateral ankle sprains are the most common specific injury in sports, especially in basketball, soccer, cross-country running, dance, and ballet.* Studies in Norway and Finland reported that acute ankle sprains accounted for 16% and 21% of all athletic injuries, respectively, in those countries.[354, 374] In basketball, ankle sprains account for 45% of all injuries, and in soccer, 17% to 31% of all injuries are ankle sprains.[302, 308, 374] In an injury that is so prevalent, an understanding of the anatomy and biomechanics of the lateral ligamentous complex is essential for proper treatment. Since it is the authors' belief that these lateral ankle sprains often include injury to the ligamentous structures of the subtalar joint, the ensuing discussion will include pertinent anatomic and biomechanical information for the subtalar joint as well as the tibiotalar joint and will be referred to collectively as the lateral ligamentous complex of the ankle and hindfoot. Further discussion of subtalar sprains and instability is included as a separate section later in this chapter.

Anatomy

The lateral ligamentous complex of the ankle consists of three ligaments: the anterior talofibular, the calcaneofibular, and the posterior talofibular (Fig 27–20,A–C). The lateral ligamentous complex of the subtalar joint consists of five important structures: the calcaneofibular ligament, the inferior extensor retinaculum, the lateral talocalcaneal ligament, the cervical ligament, and the interosseous talocalcaneal ligament (Fig 27–20,A–D). The calcaneofibular ligament is included with both joints because it spans both the tibiotalar and talocalcaneal joints and is integral to the proper biomechanics of both joints.

The anterior talofibular ligament blends with the anterior lateral capsule of the ankle. There are usually two bands with a small cleft permitting the penetration of vessels. The ligament is approximately 15 to 20 mm long and spans the anterior lateral ankle joint. It originates at the distal anterior tip of the fibula and inserts on the body of the talus just anterior to the articular facet. It does not insert on the talar neck. The ligament is approximately 6 to 8 mm wide and approximately 2 mm thick.[375]

The posterior talofibular ligament takes origin from the medial surface of the lateral malleolus and courses medially in a horizontal fashion to the posterior aspect of the talus. The ligament is approximately 3 cm long, 5 mm wide, and 5 to 8 mm thick. The insertion is broad and involves nearly the entire posterior lip of the talus. The ligament is confluent with the joint capsule and is well vascularized by vessels going to the talus and the fibula via the digital fossa.[375]

The calcaneofibular ligament originates from the anterior border of the distal lateral malleolus just below the origin of the anterior talofibular ligament. Contrary to popular belief, it does not originate from the apex of the tip of the lateral malleolus. The ligament courses medially, posteriorly, and inferiorly from its fibular origin to the calcaneal insertion. The superficial aspect of the ligament provides a surface over which the peroneal tendons glide as they begin their descent toward the fifth metatarsal. The calcaneofibular ligament is confluent with the peroneal tendon sheath just as the anterior talofibular ligament blends with the anterior capsule of the ankle joint. The calcaneofibular ligament is 2 to 3 cm long, 4 to 8 mm wide, and 3 to 5 mm thick. It typically runs 10 to 45 degrees posterior to the longitudinal axis of the fibula. The angle of the ligament in relationship to this axis can be quite variable. It may be directly in line with the longitudinal axis or may be as much as 80 to 90 degrees off this line.[373, 375] The ligament inserts on a small tubercle posterior and superior to the peroneal tubercle of the calcaneus.

Continuing with the hindfoot complex, the inferior extensor retinaculum is composed of three distinct components.[288, 318, 378, 386] These include the lateral, intermediate, and medial roots (Fig 27–20,D). The lateral root originates superficial to the extensor tendons, and the intermediate and medial roots come from the deep fascial layer below the short extensors. The superficial layer arises from the enveloping fascia of the foot, and the lateral root inserts on the lateral aspect of the anterior superior process of the calcaneus. Together with the calcaneofibular and lateral talocalcaneal ligaments, the lateral root of the inferior extensor retinaculum constitutes the superficial ligamentous support of the subtalar joint.[318] The intermediate root runs from beneath the extensor tendons alongside and slightly posterior to the cervical ligament, while the medial root courses

**References 281, 308, 310, 317, 347, 354, 355, 388.*

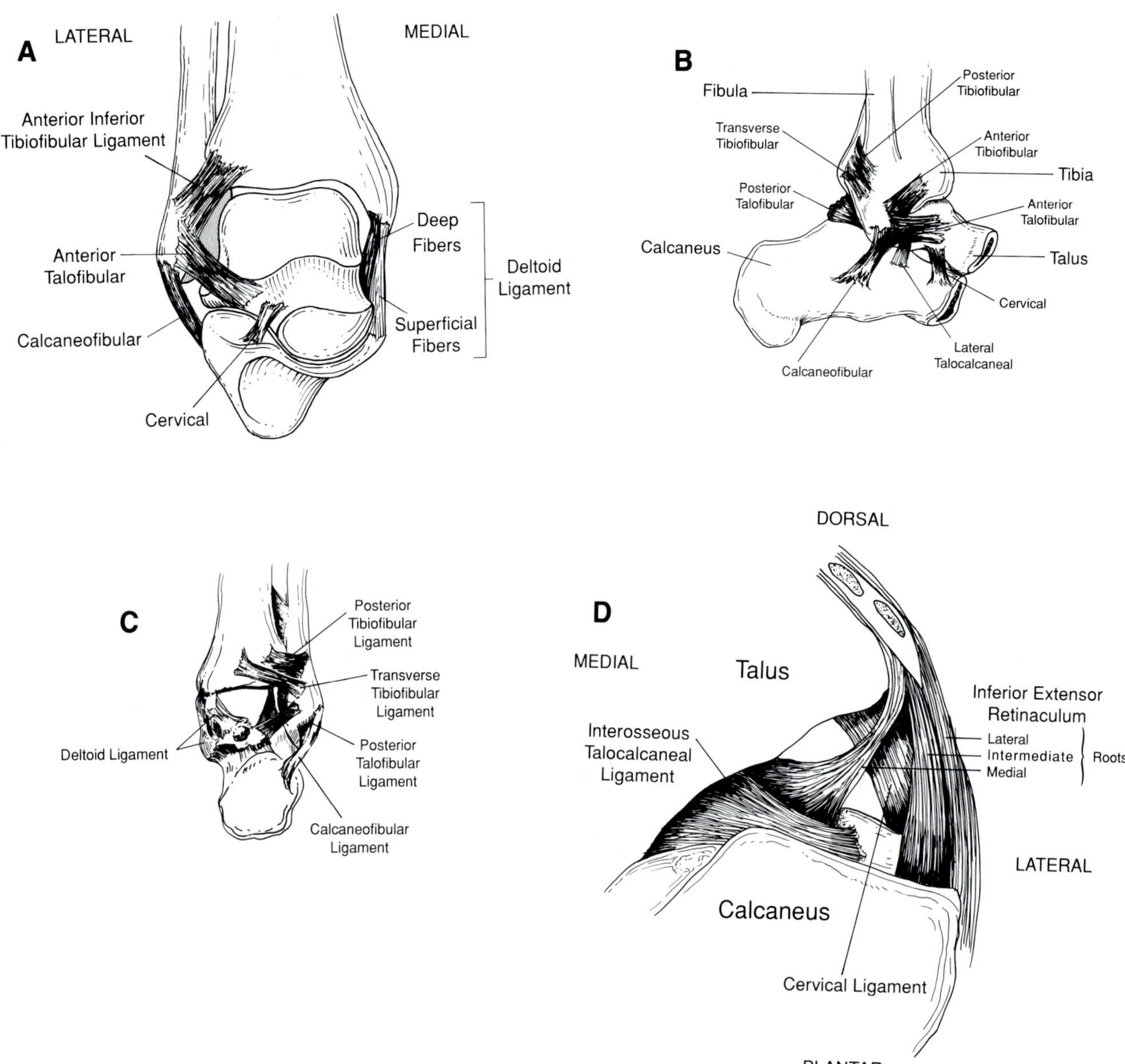

FIG 27–20.
Anatomic relationships at the lateral aspect of the ankle and subtalar joints. **A,** the ligamentous support of the lateral aspect of the ankle and hindfoot—anterior view. **B,** the ligamentous support of the lateral aspect of the ankle and hindfoot—lateral view. **C,** the ligamentous support of the lateral aspect of the ankle and hindfoot—posterior view. **D,** the ligamentous support of the lateral aspect of the ankle and hindfoot—medial view. **E,** the ligaments of the subtalar joint in a frontal-section view.

more deeply within the sinus tarsi and sends attachments to both the talus and calcaneus adjacent to the talocalcaneal ligament in the canalis tarsi.

The lateral talocalcaneal ligament originates from the lateral wall of the calcaneus just anterior to the calcaneal origin of the calcaneofibular ligament and inserts on the body of the talus just inferior to the anterior talofibular ligament. Often, this ligament can be seen as an arcuate complex blending with the calcaneofibular ligament and anterior talofibular ligament. It is variable in the extent of its development.[318]

The cervical ligament lies within the sinus tarsi and forms a strong and distinct band of collagenous tissue that connects the neck of the talus with the superior surface of the calcaneus. The ligament runs in an oblique direction from the talus above to the calcaneus below and makes about a 45-degree angle with the horizontal. It is approximately 2 cm in length, 12 mm in width, and 3 mm thick.[288]

Although it is not truly a lateral structure, the interosseous talocalcaneal ligament is important to the overall function of the lateral ankle and hindfoot complex. The talocalcaneal ligament measures approximately 15 mm in length, 5 to 6 mm in width, and 1 to 2 mm in thickness.[288] It is located at the most medial aspect of the sinus tarsi within the canalis tarsi and extends from a ridge at the sulcus tali. There is a large vascular foramen posterior to the ligament's origin, and the middle facet joint of the sustenaculum is anterior. The ligament then courses downward and lateral to the sulcus calcanei, where it blends with the most medial fibers of the cervical ligament.[386] On the other hand, the talocalcaneal ligament blends into the deep portion of the deltoid ligament on its medial side.[400]

Biomechanics

Each of the ligaments has a role in stabilizing the ankle and/or subtalar joint, depending on the position of the foot and ankle. In dorsiflexion, the anterior talofibular ligament is loose, while the calcaneofibular ligament is taut. In plantar flexion, the converse occurs: the anterior talofibular ligament is taut, and the calcaneofibular ligament becomes loose. Some variation to this is allowed by the different patterns of divergence between these two ligaments. The posterior talofibular ligament is maximally stressed in the dorsiflexed position.[295, 368, 375]

In biomechanical studies, the anterior talofibular ligament has a lower load to failure than does the calcaneofibular ligament.[385] According to Attarian et al., the maximum load to failure for the anterior talofibular ligament is 138.9 ± 23.5 newtons, and for the calcaneofibular ligament, it is 345.7 ± 55.2 newtons.[268] Conversely, the anterior talofibular ligament is capable of undergoing the greatest strain in comparison to the calcaneofibular ligament and the posterior talofibular ligament.[268, 295] These observations help to explain the greater frequency of injuries to the anterior talofibular ligament and the relative infrequency of injuries to the posterior talofibular ligament.

Sequential sectioning of the lateral ligaments have demonstrated the function of these ligaments in different positions and under various loading conditions. According to the studies of Rasmussen, the anterior talofibular ligament functions primarily in restricting internal rotation of the talus in the mortise.[368] When the ankle is plantar-flexed, the anterior talofibular ligament also inhibits adduction. The calcaneofibular ligament primarily prohibits adduction and acts almost independently in the neutral and dorsiflexed positions. In plantar flexion, it restricts adduction in conjunction with the anterior talofibular ligament. The posterior talofibular ligament prevents external rotation with the ankle in a dorsiflexed position. Although the medial ligaments are primarily responsible for restriction of ankle dorsiflexion, the posterior talofibular ligament assists in this function. There is also some role for the short fibers of the posterior talofibular ligament in restricting internal rotation after the anterior talofibular ligament has been ruptured. Following disruption of the calcaneofibular ligament, the posterior talofibular ligament inhibits adduction with the ankle in dorsiflexion. In unloaded ankle specimens, Rasmussen demonstrated ligamentous rupture in extreme positions. During forced dorsiflexion, the posterior tibiotalar ligament ruptures. In forced internal rotation, anterior talofibular ligament rupture was followed by injury to the posterior talofibular ligament. Extreme external rotation induced disruption of the deep deltoid ligament on the medial side. Adduction forces in the neutral and dorsiflexed positions caused disruption of the calcaneofibular ligament, while in plantar flexion the anterior talofibular ligament was primarily injured.[368]

The joint-stabilizing function of the ligaments is most critical in the unloaded ankle joint since in a loaded ankle the bony configuration of the mortise contributes to its stability.[355, 397] It can therefore be implied that many ankle ligamentous injuries occur while the extremity is being loaded or unloaded.

The ligaments of the hindfoot complex also act to constrain movement with the foot and ankle in certain positions. Smith claimed that the cervical ligament functions to limit inversion while the talocalcaneal ligament limits eversion.[386] This has been disputed by others who have found that the talocalcaneal ligament lies very close to the axis of rotation of the subtalar joint and functions primarily to maintain the bones in close apposition with no role in controlling inversion or eversion.[288, 400] Regardless, there is general agreement that the cervical ligament is the primary restraint and guide within the sinus and canalis tarsi to inversion movement occurring at the subtalar joint. Its greater degree of innervation suggests a role in proprioception and reflex activity that is not found in the less well innervated talocalcaneal ligament.[400]

Experimental work on the relative contribution of the different ligaments within the hindfoot complex to stability have shown that the calcaneofibular ligament plays a major role in the stability of the talocalcaneal joint.[336, 338] The cutting studies of Kjaersgaard-Andersen and coworkers showed a 20% increase in rotation of the talocalcaneal joint and a 61% to 77% increase in talocalcaneal adduction after sectioning the calcaneofibular ligament.[336, 338] They also found increases in rotation, adduction, and sagittal-plane motion (dorsiflexion and plantar flexion) in the tibiotalocalcaneal and talocalcaneal joints with section of the the cervical or interosseous talocalcaneal ligaments. The largest percent increase in motion was 43% at the talocalcaneal joint and occurred in dorsiflexion after section of the talocalcaneal ligament.[337] Heilman and coworkers performed a similar cutting study with sequential section of the calcaneofibular ligament, the lateral capsule, and the interosseous talocalcaneal ligament.[320] They documented a 5-mm opening between the posterior facets of the talus and calcaneus with a stress x-ray after the calcaneofibular ligament was sectioned and an increase to 7 mm when sectioning of the talocalcaneal ligament was added. The relationship between these studies and the clinical conditions of ankle and subtalar instability and sinus tarsi syndrome will be explored in the section on subtalar sprains and instability.

Pathology

From a literature review, laboratory studies, clinical experience, and operative findings, the most common ligament disruption involves the anterior talofibular ligament. Most of these disruptions are midsubstance, but bony avulsions of the talus and fibula can occur. Indeed, Berg has recently suggested that the symptomatic os subfibulare is a nonunion of an avulsion fracture of the anterior talofibular ligament.[273] The second most common injury is a combination rupture of the anterior talofibular and calcaneofibular ligaments. Again, in these injuries, midsubstance rupture is most common, but a considerable number also involve avulsion of the calcaneofibular ligament from the fibula or calcaneus. Isolated tears of the calcaneofibular ligament are uncommon lesions but have been reported and may be important in late subtalar instability.[306, 320] Next in the descending order of frequency are disruptions of the anterior talofibular, calcaneofibular, and posterior talofibular ligaments. Isolated injuries of the posterior talofibular and isolated combinations of calcaneofibular and posterior talofibular ligaments are exceedingly rare.

Various injuries are noted in association with lateral ligamentous sprains: partial or complete tears of the peroneus longus and brevis tendons, chondral fractures of the talus, osteochondral fracture of the talocrural joint, medial ligamentous injuries, syndesmotic injuries, and bifurcate ligament injuries. Displaced or nondisplaced avulsion fractures of the fifth metatarsal and calcaneocuboid compression injuries or ligament avulsions have also been noted. Although complete nerve disruption has not been reported, it is common to see a post-sprain neuritis of the sural nerve, superficial peroneal nerve, deep peroneal nerve, or posterior tibial nerve if the clinician takes the time to check for this.[358, 364, 379] The majority of these go unrecognized.

Diagnosis

Clinical Evaluation

Patients with a lateral ankle sprain sometimes describe a popping or tearing sensation in the ankle. Occasionally, there is an audible noise. Frequently they remember only the pain and loss of support. The injuries occur during running, while cutting, or while landing from a jump (often by landing on another athlete's foot). Patients who can remember the specifics describe an inversion, plantar flexion, or internal rotation mechanism. Swelling and pain occur immediately following the injury. Depending on the severity of the tear, the athlete may or may not be able to walk on the ankle. Typically, patients with a complete ligamentous tear and those with ligament tears of two or more ligaments will have difficulty in weight bearing, although this is not always the case. Many athletes give a past medical history of multiple ankle sprains.

On physical examination, there is swelling and tenderness over the affected ligaments. The range of motion of the ankle is limited in dorsiflexion, plantar flexion, and inversion. An anterior drawer maneuver frequently elicits pain in patients with an anterior talofibular ligament injury, although the patient with complete rupture may have less pain than in the sprained or partially ruptured case. In a relaxed patient with a complete anterior talofibular ligament tear, anterior subluxation of the talus may be appreciated, and a "suction sign" may be apparent at the anterolateral joint (Fig 27–21). An inversion stress on the calcaneus will induce pain or demonstrate instability in patients with calcaneofibular disruption. It can be quite difficult to differentiate tibiotalar from talocalcaneal opening on this maneuver in the acutely injured patient. In fact, it may be impossible to perform this maneuver in the acutely injured patient without some type of anesthesia. Despite these difficulties, meticulous examination with fingertip palpation of all structures potentially involved in an ankle sprain will often lead the examiner to the correct clinical diagnosis. With a thorough examination, one may find involvement of the peroneal or posterior tibial tendons. Avulsion or hairline fractures of the fibula, tibia, calcaneus, fifth metatarsal, cuboid, or talus

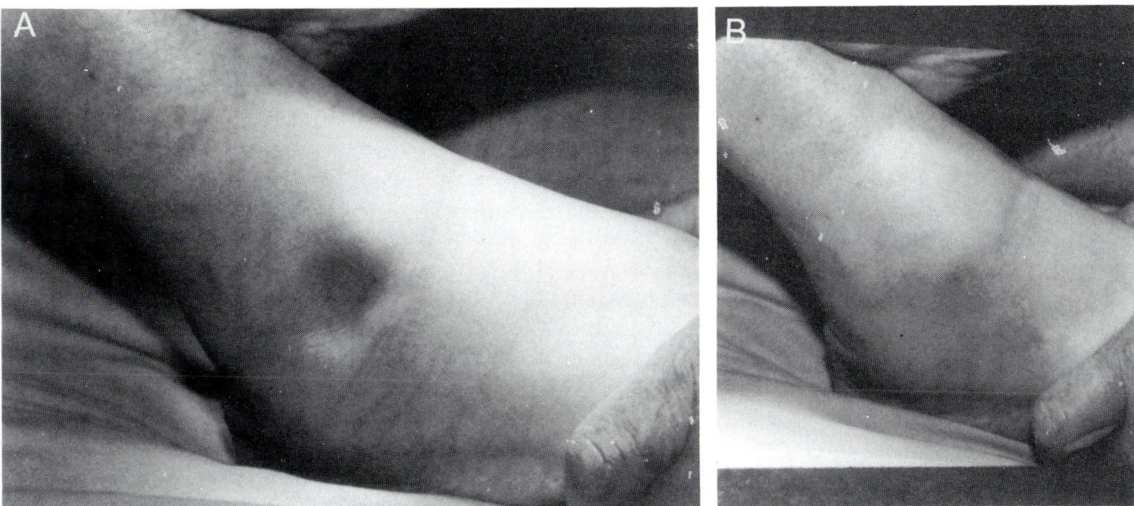

FIG 27–21.
Clinical photograph of positive anterior drawer test findings demonstrating a positive "suction sign." **A,** stressed. **B,** unstressed.

and subtle neurologic injuries can also be detected. Predisposing factors such as varus hindfoot alignment, hypermobile joints, and tarsal coalition should be appreciated.

Radiographic Evaluation

Once a concise clinical impression has been reached, radiographic evaluation can be utilized to confirm the presence of bony lesions as directed by the physical examination. In most situations, it is advisable to obtain three views of the ankle: anteroposterior (AP), lateral, and mortise views. As mentioned, it is important to analyze the routine x-ray films critically for avulsion fractures, osteochondral injuries involving the joint surface, and occult fractures. In the proper setting, stress radiographs are valuable.

Talar Tilt.—The talar tilt view is an AP view of the ankle while an inversion force is applied. The methods of obtaining this test vary greatly in the literature. Some authorities perform the test manually, while others use a jig with specifically defined stresses (Fig 27–22). Laurin and coauthors have demonstrated similar results in comparing both methods.[348] Local anesthesia, no anesthesia, or general anesthesia may be used for this test. Different authors recommend dorsiflexion, neutral, or plantar flexion of the foot during the stress maneuver. Finally, the position of the knee with either a straight knee or a flexed knee has also been disputed. We perform the test with the foot in relaxed plantar flexion, the knee slightly bent, and without the use of a foot-holding apparatus.

In analyzing the results of the talar tilt view, it should be recalled that there is a great deal of variability

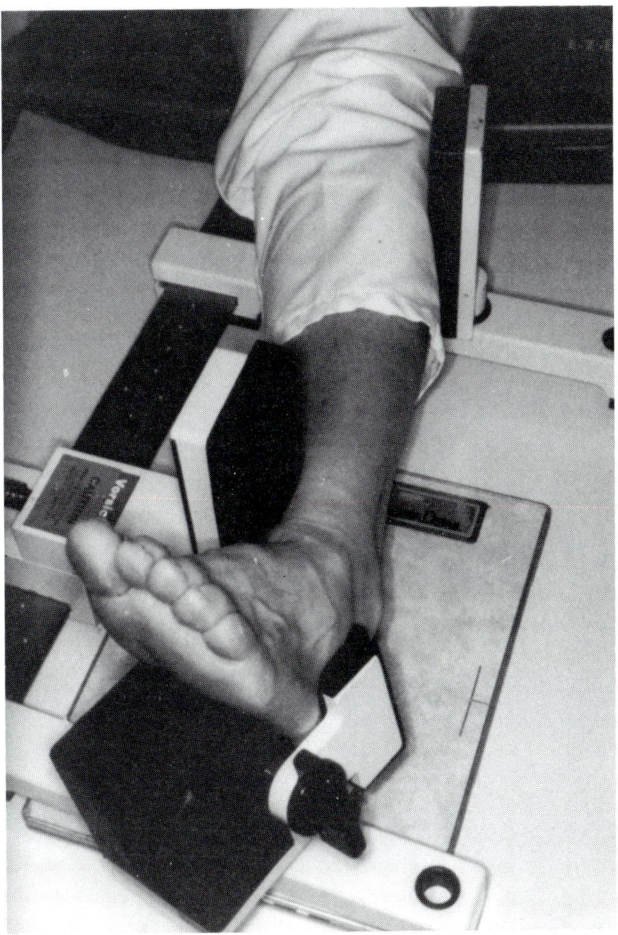

FIG 27–22.
Commercially available jig stressing the ankle for a talar tilt.

in what is considered to be normal or abnormal. Ruben and Witten's oft-quoted study analyzed 152 normal ankles with the talar tilt view and found a range extending up to 23 degrees. However, only 2 ankles were over 20 degrees, and only 6 were over 15 degrees.[372] A similar study by Sedlin of 155 patients subjected to stress x-ray studies found a talar tilt of less than 14 degrees in all normal ankles with a maximum side-to-side difference of 10 degrees.[383] Berridge and Bonnin confirmed that up to 5% of uninjured ankles could have a talar tilt as high as 25 degrees.[275] Bonnin classified those individuals with no history of an ankle injury but talar tilt angles from 5 to 15 degrees as having a "hypermobile ankle."[279] For the nonhypermobile ankle, Bonnin felt that a tilt of 5 to 15 degrees indicated a rupture of only the calcaneofibular ligament, whereas a 15- to 30-degree tilt meant that both the anterior talofibular and calcaneofibular ligaments were disrupted, and angles greater than 30 degrees indicated rupture of the anterior tablofibular, calcaneofibular and posterior talofibular ligaments.[279] Other authors emphasize the importance of side-to-side comparison and state that a difference of 3 to 5 degrees on side-to-side comparison is significant[289, 344] (Fig 27–23). A greater difference from side to side or a greater absolute number may have some relationship with the extent of the pathology. Ruben and Witten noted little benefit in side-to-side comparison since 22% of their uninjured subjects had differences of 3 to 19 degrees.[372] Cox and Hewes reviewed this controversial topic of the talar tilt angle in 1979 and noted that the vast majority of authors have stated that the normal talar tilt angle is under 5 degrees. In their own study of 404 ankles, they found that 90% of the tested ankles had no talar tilt and 8% had a tilt between 1 and 5 degrees. Only 7 ankles (1.7%) in 5 subjects had a tilt greater than 5 degrees. The maximum tilt in these normal ankles was 17 degrees, and only 2 ankles had angles over 10 degrees.[296] We have used 15 degrees as our cutoff for the talar tilt angle and consider this to indicate a high probability of a complete tear of the calcaneofibular ligament (and most often the anterior talofibular ligament as well). This is particularly true when the test is performed in more dorsiflexion (as shown in Fig 27–23). We do not generally perform comparison x-ray studies.

Anterior Drawer Test.—Just as the talar tilt test is designed primarily to evaluate a calcaneofibular ligament injury, the anterior drawer test mainly evaluates the anterior talofibular ligament. This test involves a lateral x-ray performed while the ankle is undergoing an anterior displacement stress. The stress may be applied manually or by a jig (Fig 27–24). Various studies have calculated the normal value for anterior subluxation to range from 2 to 9 mm, with the majority being under 4 mm* (Fig 27–25). When the anterior translation is greater than 5 mm, we consider it indicative that the anterior talofibular ligament is ruptured.

Other Radiographic Techniques (Ankle Arthrography, Peroneal Tenography, CAT, and MRI).—Although most authors feel that stress radiographs have largely replaced arthrograms, a recent study of 563 arthrograms following ankle injuries indicated that the diagnostic accuracy of arthrography is higher than that of stress radiography.[305] Perhaps the best indication for use of this test is in an athlete who is suspected of having a severe complete sprain of the lateral ankle complex. If the test is performed within the first 24 hours, the diagnostic accuracy appears to be quite high. Some feel that the test can still be valuable up to 4 or 5 days.[276, 277, 286, 334] The arthrogram is performed by using local anesthesia infiltration followed by injection of water-soluble radiographic contrast dye into the joint. The total amount of fluid will usually be less than 10 mL. If the ankle accepts a volume greater than this, it is very likely that there has been a rupture of the joint capsule. According to Broström et al. extra-articular dye in the peroneal tendon sheath is caused by a rupture of the calcaneofibular ligament, and extra-articular dye anterior to the lateral malleolus is indicative of an anterior talofibular ligament rupture. Dye penetration into the subtalar joint, flexor hallucis longus tendon sheath, and flexor digitorum longus sheath is not pathologic.[287] Peroneal tenography may also be done to help diagnose tears of the calcaneofibular ligament.[278] The test is most useful when a peroneal tendon injury is suspected in conjunction with a calcaneofibular ligament injury.

The CAT scan and MRI are both useful in cases of lateral ankle sprain when there is some question of involvement of the surrounding bone or tendons. Visualization of the ligaments is possible, but interpretation requires the experience of a skilled orthopaedist or radiographer.[359, 399]

Classification

Sprains of the lateral ligaments of the ankle have been classified by numerous methods. The most common methods grade lateral sprains from I to III or from mild to severe.[269, 270, 300, 327, 348] Unfortunately, the use of these methods can be confusing since some grade the injury by the severity of clinical signs and symp-

---

* *References 309, 312, 319, 331, 349, 352.*

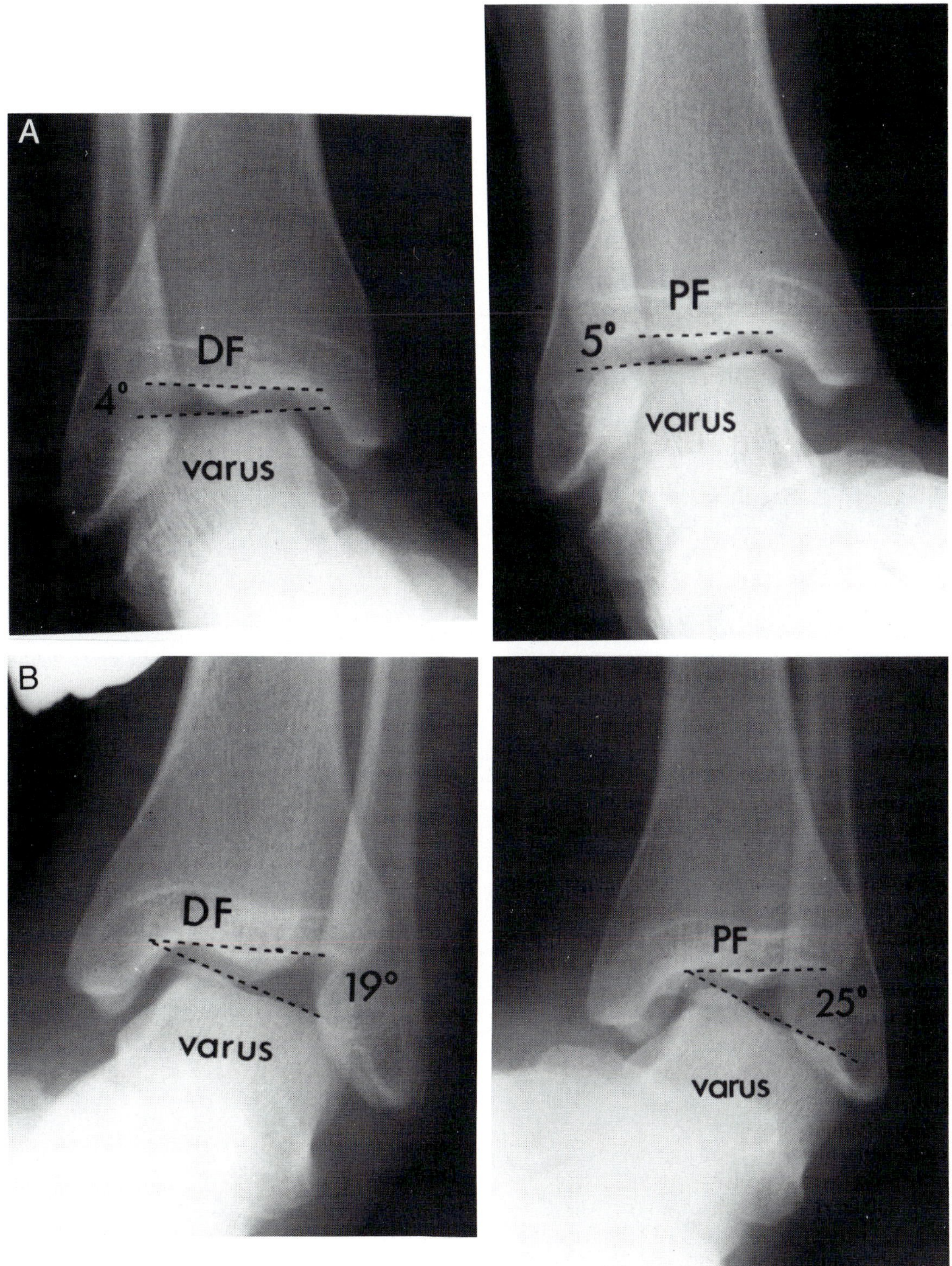

FIG 27–23.
Stress radiograph demonstrating significant talar tilt with the ankle held in slight dorsiflexion (*DF*). *PF* = plantar flexion. **A,** uninjured side. **B,** injured side.

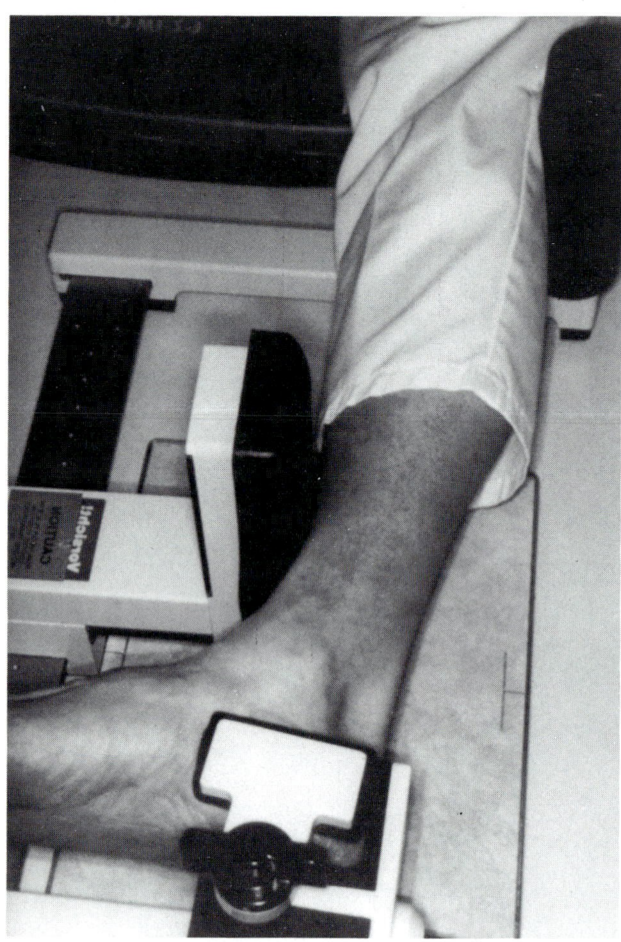

FIG 27–24.
Commercially available jig stressing the ankle in an anterior drawer test.

toms. Others correlate the grade with the degree of injury to the ligament(s), i.e., grade I sprain being a stretch and grade III being a complete ligament rupture. Finally, still others grade by the number of ligaments ruptured, grade I being a tear of the anterior talofibular ligament and grade III involving the anterior talofibular, calcaneofibular, and posterior talofibular ligaments.

Some of this quandary can be attributed to correlating sprains at the ankle with sprains elsewhere in the body (e.g., the knee). This analogy fails at the ankle since three separate ligaments compose the lateral collateral ligament complex rather than just a single isolated structure. A further complication is seen when one tries to impose the American Medical Association Standard Nomenclature of Athletic Injuries to this situation.[394] Here, a first-degree sprain is a mild injury with stretching of the ligament. A second-degree sprain is moderate and indicates a partial tear of the ligament, and a third-degree sprain is severe with complete rupture of the ligament. This could perhaps be used for classifying injury to a single ligament of the lateral ankle complex but fails when all of the structures are taken into consideration. Nevertheless, this has been the system used in classifying ankle sprains in some studies.[388]

The classification system proposed by Leach and Schepsis[350] and used in the previous edition of this text is primarily an anatomic classification based upon the number of ligaments involved in the injury as determined by physical examination: (1) first degree involves a partial or complete anterior talofibular ligament tear, (2) second degree includes partial and/or complete tears of the anterior talofibular and calcaneofibular ligaments, and (3) third degree equals partial or complete tears of the anterior talofibular, calcaneofibular, and posterior talofibular ligaments.[272] While this system seemingly bears more significance in terms of the anatomic lesion and severity, it is relatively impractical in terms of clinical application. Furthermore, it does not take into account the isolated calcaneofibular ligament tear.

In a clinically oriented classification system such as the widely used method of Jackson et al.,[327] a grade I, or mild, sprain is an intraligamentous tear with minimal swelling and tenderness. There is no instability and minimal functional disability. A grade II, or moderate, sprain is an incomplete tear of the ligament with mild to moderate instability. In these injuries there may be a fair amount of pain, swelling, tenderness, and loss of motion. Following grade II injuries, patients can walk, but with a limp and quite a bit of discomfort. Grade III injuries are complete ruptures of the ligament(s) associated with instability of the joint. There is marked swelling, pain, tenderness, and loss of motion. Most patients will need assistance with ambulation and only for a brief duration will be able to walk on the ankle. While this classification system is relatively straightforward, it does not correspond to the clinical situation or the operative findings in every situation. We have seen injuries with no instability that were quite painful and incapacitating for certain patients, while others have pronounced instability with very little pain.

In our opinion, a more practical classification system from the viewpoint of treatment is based on whether the ankle is stable or unstable as determined by the anterior drawer test and the talar tilt test (see Table 27–4). In the majority of circumstances, this can be determined clinically by careful examination shortly after the injury and without the need for anesthesia. Side-to-side comparison is useful but not foolproof. When there is excessive anterior translation and internal rotation on the anterior drawer test *and* an absence of a firm end point, this is considered to be a positive test. The ankle

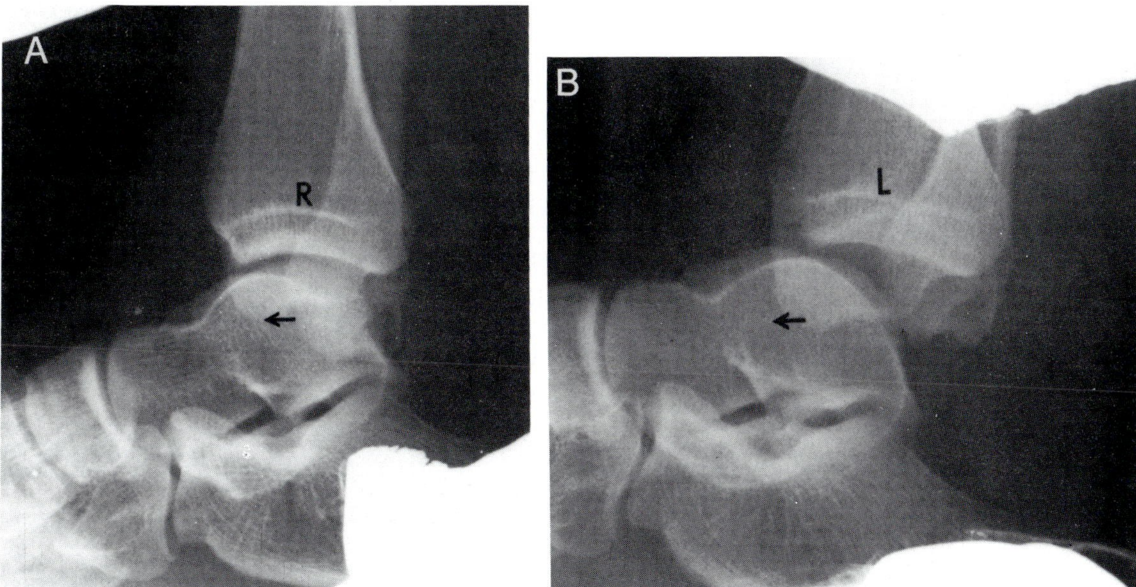

FIG 27–25.
Stress radiograph demonstrating positive anterior drawer test findings *(arrows)*. **A,** uninjured side. **B,** injured side.

is classified as unstable—a type II injury. When the ankle has excessive inversion or adduction movement as determined by the talar tilt maneuver, the ankle is also classified as unstable (type II) even in the absence of positive anterior drawer test findings, although this is admittedly unusual. If the tests are negative, the ankle is considered to be stable—a type I injury—and treatment can proceed in a symptomatic fashion by any method with which the clinician is comfortable. If there is instability, then more aggressive treatment is warranted (whether operative or nonoperative). In an ankle that cannot be adequately examined due to pain or a lack of patient cooperation, consideration is given to examination under anesthesia for the young athlete in order to classify the injury and provide proper treatment. This can be performed following an ankle block in the office or emergency room setting. When the ankle is determined to be unstable (type II) by clinical examination, then stress x-ray studies are performed *only* in the situation where operative intervention is contemplated (e.g., the competitive athlete). When the stress radiographs show a talar tilt greater than 15 degrees and an anterior drawer over 10 mm, we consider both ligaments to be torn. This is a type IIB injury, which we repair surgically in the competitive athlete. During evaluation of the stress radiographs, attention is also directed to the talocalcaneal relationship for any evidence of instability in that location. When it is present, we classify this as a type IIC injury. This system of classification is simple since there are only two main categories of injury—those that are stable and those that are unstable. The unstable group is further subdivided by stress radiographs only for those young athletic patients in whom surgery is a consideration. Stable injuries are treated symptomatically. The vast majority of unstable injuries are treated by functional treatment, with good results expected.[332]

Treatment of Acute Sprain

Nonoperative Treatment

Nonoperative treatment is the mainstay of management for the vast majority of ankle sprains, even in the athletic population. Certainly, in athletes with traditional grade I (mild) and II (moderate) injuries (i.e., stable ankle sprains), the conservative approach is associated with good or excellent results.*

Conservative treatment is also indicated for most cases of grade III (severe) ankle sprains (type II or unstable ankle sprains in our classification scheme). Currently, there is still some controversy regarding the optimal method of treatment for these injuries in the competitive athlete. A satisfactory subjective and objective result can certainly be achieved with primary repair.† However, proponents of conservative treatment have shown comparable results.‡

**References 269, 270, 283, 299, 300, 314, 315, 327, 347, 367, 377.*

†References 266, 282, 329, 341, 363, 369, 370, 373, 395.

‡References 265, 292, 301, 316, 322, 325, 327, 328, 340, 351, 357, 361.

TABLE 27–4.
Classification Systems for Lateral Ankle Sprains

I. Anatomical system (Leach)*
   Grade I = ATF sprain
   Grade II = ATF and CF sprains
   Grade III = ATF, CF, and PTF sprains
II. AMA standard nomenclature system
   Grade 1 = ligament stretched
   Grade 2 = ligament partially torn
   Grade 3 = ligament completely torn
III. Clinical system (Jackson et al.[327])
   Mild sprain = minimal functional loss, no limp, minimal or no swelling, point tenderness, pain with reproduction of the mechanism of injury
   Moderate sprain = moderate functional loss, unable to toe-rise or hop on the injured ankle, limp when walking, localized swelling, point tenderness
   Severe sprain = diffuse tenderness and swelling, crutches preferred by the patient for ambulation
IV. Authors' system (related to treatment)
   Type I = stable ankle by clinical testing (with anesthesia if necessary)—symptomatic treatment
   Type II = unstable ankle with positive anterior drawer and/or positive talar tilt test results by clinical examination
      Group 1: Nonathlete or older patient—functional treatment
      Group 2: Young athlete
         Type A = negative stress x-ray findings—treat functionally
         Type B = positive tibiotalar stress x-ray findings (talar tilt > 15 degrees; anterior drawer > 1 cm)—treat by surgical repair
         Type C = positive talocalcaneal stress x-ray findings (loss of parallelism on stress Brodén view and/or 2 mm or more anterior displacement of the calcaneus on the talus on the anterior drawer test)—treat by surgical repair

*ATF = anterior talofibular; CF = calcaneofibular; PTF = posterior talofibular.

In a recent review of 12 prospective randomized studies, Kannus and Renström reported that 75% to 100% of patients have a good or excellent outcome regardless of whether the treatment is operative or nonoperative. Late symptoms such as subjective ankle instability, swelling, pain, stiffness, or muscle weakness occurred with a similar frequency in the nonoperative and operative cases. In general, functional treatment provided the most rapid recovery, with earlier return to work and physical activity. In the nonoperative groups, there was a markedly lower incidence of total complications and no serious complications. Based on their review, the authors advocated functional treatment as the method of choice for grade III injury and cited the lower cost and lower complication rate with equally good results as the rationale for this approach. Furthermore, they emphasized that a secondary operative repair or reconstruction could be performed in the 10% to 20% of patients who have persistent problems. They concluded that operative management may be considered in the acute phase when there are large avulsion fractures or severe medial and lateral ligamentous damage or if the acute grade III injury is particularly severe or recurrent.[333] We have followed this practice of functional treatment in the large majority of our own patients and had equally good results.

The first phase of functional treatment includes rest, ice, compression, and elevation (RICE). This form of treatment is usually initiated by athletic trainers on site. The next phase may be instituted by the trainer or the orthopaedist and involves mobilization in either an elastic brace, lace-up ankle brace, plastic stirrup brace, or taping. During this time, the patients are allowed to bear weight to tolerance based on their swelling and discomfort. Crutches are discontinued as quickly as the athlete can tolerate full weight on the ankle. The athletes are instructed to avoid plantar flexion and inversion and to elevate the leg intermittently to reduce swelling. The next phase involves physical therapy (either personally performed or professionally supervised) with range-of-motion exercises, peroneal strengthening, and Achilles stretching. Once pain and swelling allow, proprioceptive training with a wobble board, tilt board, or minitrampoline is instituted. For type I (stable) injuries, the ankle is protected for approximately 3 to 4 weeks with a brace or taping during athletic activity, and for a type II (unstable) injury, a brace or taping is worn for the duration of the athletic season and indefinitely thereafter since it has been shown that those athletes with prior ankle sprains are at increased risk for reinjury.[302]

The compression component of the RICE formula is combined with various techniques of immobilization from ankle taping to ankle stirrups, Unna boots, plaster splinting, or casting. Ankle strapping requires a knowledgeable trainer or therapist and is infrequently applied by orthopaedic surgeons. Although many taping techniques exist, the most popular technique for the acute sprain is the open basket weave technique[270] (Fig 27–26,A). Once the risk of swelling has decreased, closed basketweave strapping may be instituted to permit reconditioning while supporting the ankle (Fig 27–26,B). The goal behind all these techniques is to control swelling and support the ankle in neutral dorsiflexion and slight eversion. Stirrup braces such as the Aircast (Aircast, Inc., Summit, NJ) are currently the most popular technique of immobilizing ankle sprains acutely. This type of brace consists of a medial and lateral splint beginning at the heel and extending over the lower third of the leg (Fig 27–27). These stirrup braces are designed to be worn in a shoe and are fairly easy to apply, remove, and adjust. Unfortunately, the brace is not foolproof, and oftentimes, the brace is put on without adequate patient instruction. At follow-up, the patient presents wearing the brace without a shoe and the foot held in plantar flexion. This is almost as bad as wrapping the ankle with an elastic bandage and placing the patient on crutches and non–weight bearing. Such treatment is seen all too commonly from emergency rooms and combines the untoward effects of unloading the extremity with improper positioning of the ankle. This method of treatment almost guarantees poor ligamentous healing and inevitably prolongs the recovery. For the most part, when worn properly, the stirrup brace is an effective and user-friendly means of treating lateral sprains whether stable or unstable.

Nonathletic patients who have more swelling, pain, and difficulty in ambulating may be best treated with an Unna boot, soft cast, or plaster immobilization wrapped so that the ankle is held in neutral to slight dorsiflexion. If there is greater potential for swelling, a U-shaped splint and posterior plaster splint should be applied with the foot in neutral to maximum dorsiflexion.[387] Once the swelling resolves, if the patient continues to have pain and difficulty in walking, a short-leg cast or removable walking boot can be used. When the Unna boot, plaster splint, or cast is used, it is probably best to switch to taping or the stirrup brace after 1 to 3 weeks. Longer periods of immobilization can be associated with increased stiffness, swelling, and disability. Once the patient is in a removable device, therapy with its obvious benefits can be instituted. Immobilization treatment, as opposed to functional treatment, has the benefit of relative safety, immediate pain relief, and a feeling of security for the patient and requires little instruction. However, it also means that muscle atrophy and stiffness will be greater and recovery more prolonged. We use this form of treatment only in selected nonathletic patients.

The authors do not recommend injection of cortisone or enzyme into the ankle joint or ligaments. Anti-inflammatory medication may be used within the first week or two of injury to decrease the pain and stiffness.[356] The use of liniments and creams is of no value for ankle sprains. Aspiration of the joint is of little value and carries an element of risk. For the next 6 months following their ankle sprain, athletes are advised to wear high-top shoes, with or without taping or bracing, to increase proprioceptive awareness of the ankle.[274]

Surgical Treatment

Operative treatment of a grade III ankle sprain, as mentioned previously, is a controversial topic. Of the

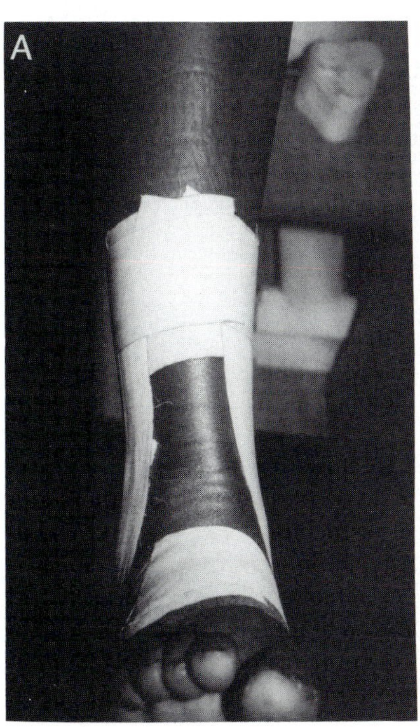

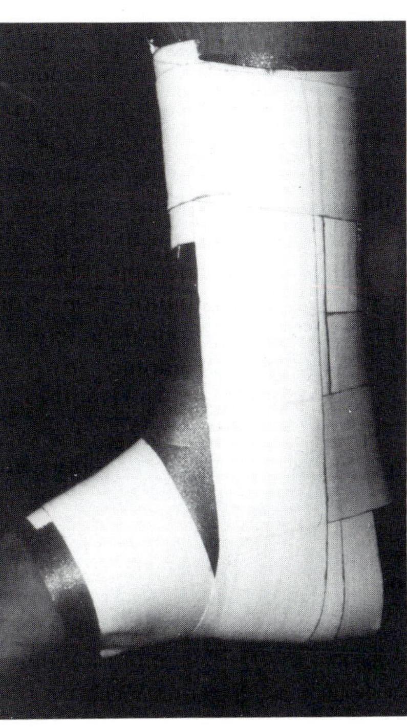

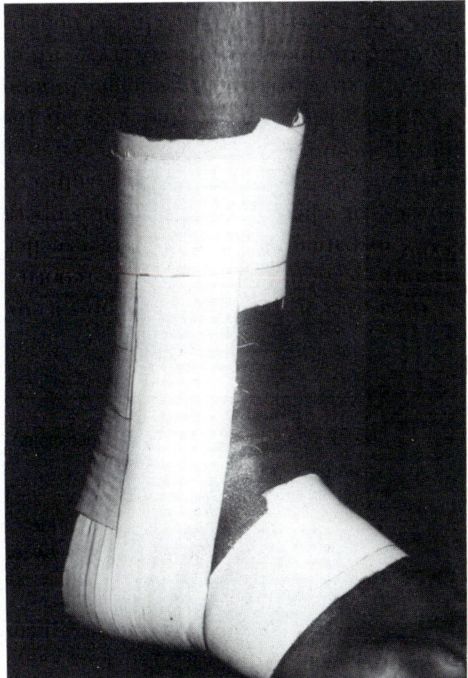

FIG 27–26.
Ankle-taping methods for use in lateral ankle sprains. **A,** Open method for use in acute injury with potential for swelling: **1,** anterior view; **2,** medial view; **3,** lateral view.

(Continued.)

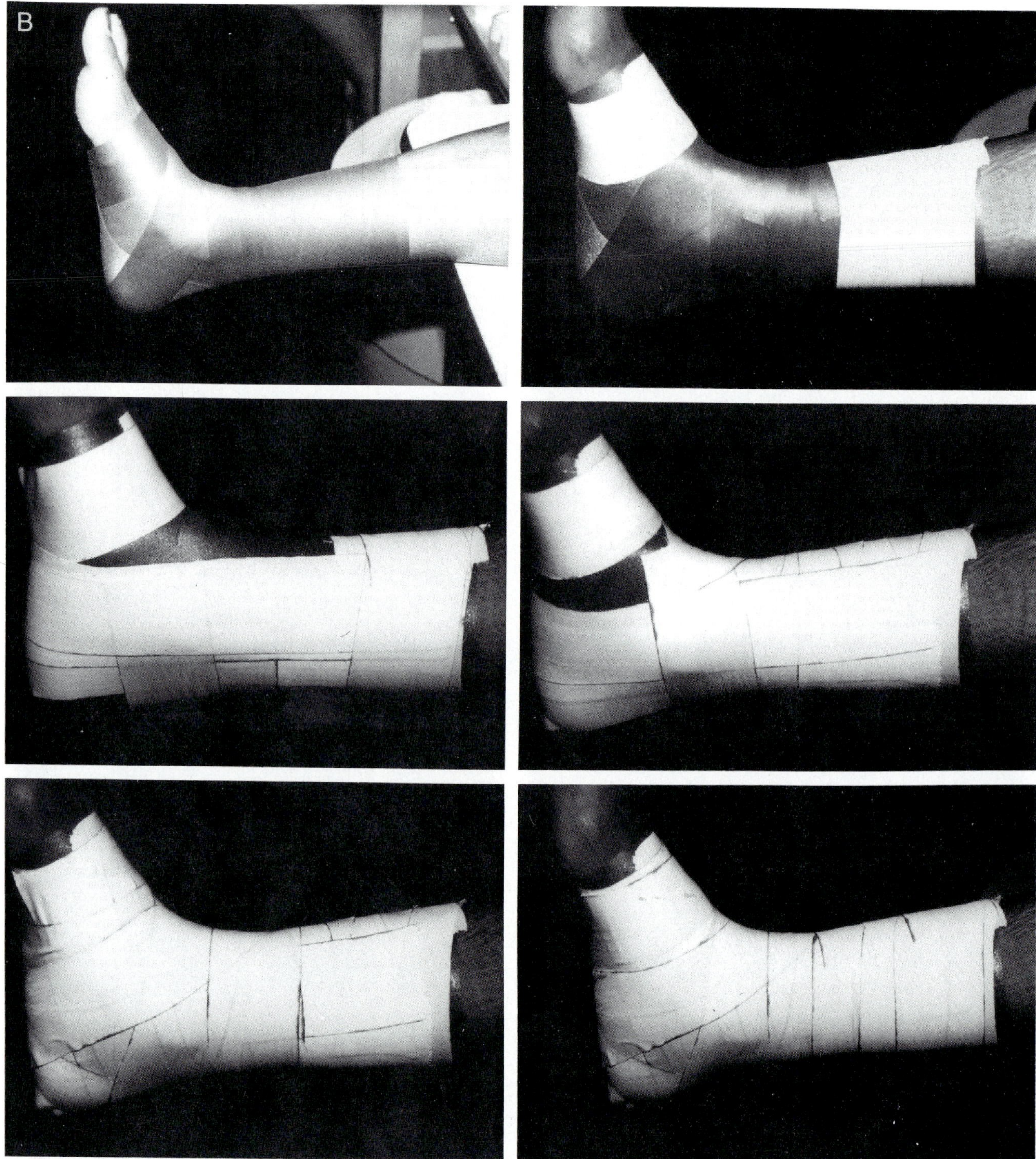

FIG 27–26 (cont.).
B, closed basketweave taping for a subacute ankle sprain. The taping sequence begins with the underwrap through completed taping of the ankle.

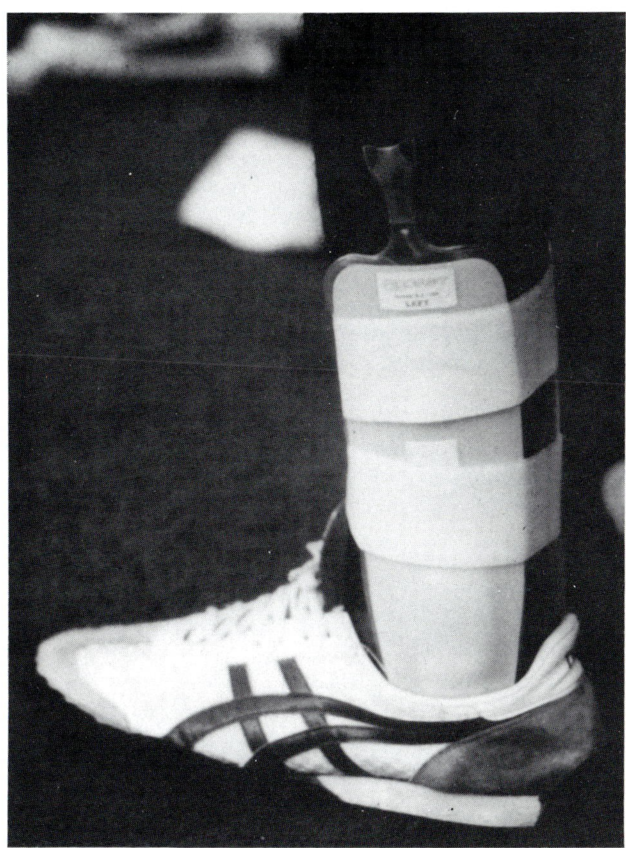

FIG 27–27.
Athlete wearing an Aircast ankle brace following a lateral ankle sprain.

12 studies reviewed by Kannus and Renström that compared operative and nonoperative treatment, 5 of these studies recommend operative treatment for the young athlete with a severe injury.* Clark and coworkers recommend operative repair in a young athlete with a talar tilt of more than 15 degrees.[294] The other four authors recommended operative repair in the young, active athlete.[285, 313, 342, 367] In these patients, the need for more guaranteed mechanical stability and reassurance that bench time is not for naught makes a more convincing argument for repair. Leach and Schepsis recommend acute repair in athletes, especially if there is (1) a history of momentary talocrural dislocation with complete ligamentous disruption, (2) the presence of a clinical anterior drawer sign, (3) a stress inversion test with 10 degrees more tilt on the affected side, (4) clinical or radiographic suspicion of tears of *both* the anterior talofibular and calcaneofibular ligaments, or (5) the presence of an osteochondral fracture.[350] Widening of the mortise is also an indication for repair, as indicated in the later section on syndesmosis sprains.

**References 283, 294, 313, 333, 342, 367.*

Acute Operative Repair.—Several authors have presented a detailed description of the operative technique, and for the most part, all are quite similar.†

Technique

1. For acute ruptures, we recommend an incision beginning above the level of the tibial plafond approximately 1 cm in front of and paralleling the anterior border of the fibula.
2. The incision is carried distally past the tip of the fibula by about 2 cm. Care must be taken during the subcutaneous dissection to spare the intermediate dorsal cutaneous nerve (a branch of the superficial peroneal nerve) and the lateral dorsal cutaneous nerve (a branch of the sural nerve). Oftentimes, the sural nerve is encountered at the most distal end of the incision.
3. One is always impressed by the degree of disruption of the ligaments and capsule that is encountered upon incising the skin. With an inversion or anterior drawer stress, the injury can be more easily identified. A formal arthrotomy is usually unnecessary for inspecting the joint for chondral or osteochondral fragments due to the extensive capsular disruption that is already present. Distally, the peroneal sheath is also open and permits visualization of the tendons and the calcaneofibular ligament. The posterior talofibular ligament is more easily identified by applying an anterior drawer stress and noting its presence on the medial side of the fibular tip running toward the posterior aspect of the talus.
4. After irrigation and appropriate debridement, nonabsorbable sutures are placed in the ligaments but not tied. We repair the posterior talofibular ligament when feasible but do not make an extended effort to do so since it is technically challenging and does not appear to influence the outcome when the other two ligaments are appropriately repaired.
5. If the ligamentous tissue is inadequate for a repair, a periosteal flap from the fibula can be raised and turned down over the remaining anterior talofibular ligament.
6. If a bony avulsion has occurred, an attempt is made to reduce and stabilize this fragment into proper position with the assistance of suture tunnels drilled with a Kirschner wire. If the fragment is too small, it is

†References 285, 314, 315, 350, 367, 398.

excised and the remaining ligament secured into the bony trough through suture tunnels created with a Kirschner wire.

7. Once the calcaneofibular and anterior talofibular ligament sutures have been placed, sutures are also placed in the anterior lateral capsule. The sutures are tied from posterior to anterior only after all have been placed. The ankle is held in neutral dorsiflexion and eversion.

8. The peroneal sheath is repaired with absorbable suture, and the skin is reapproximated by using a subcuticular or nylon mattress closure.

Postoperative Care

Postoperatively, the patient is placed in a U-shaped splint and posterior plaster splint with the foot in neutral dorsiflexion and slight eversion. The patient is non–weight bearing for 1 week and is instructed to elevate the extremity as much as possible during this time. Isometric calf contractions may be performed while in the splint. After a week the splint is changed, and a removable walking boot is applied for another 3 weeks. During this second phase, the patient begins weight bearing to tolerance and starts dorsiflexion and eversion motion. At approximately 4 weeks, the boot is removed, and the patient is placed in an ankle stirrup brace. Active dorsiflexion and plantar flexion are begun along with peroneal strengthening from the neutral position. Gentle active inversion is begun at 4 weeks in association with Achilles stretching. At the same time proprioceptive training and resistive exercises with Theraband or isokinetic equipment are begun. The patient is gradually allowed to progress from walking to straight-line running. As long as the patient shows no pain or undue swelling, rehabilitation continues as tolerated with figure-of-8 running in progressively smaller loops, and ultimately, cutting is instituted. The athlete is then allowed to resume activities specific to his sport with return to competition once each task of the sport can be accomplished. For 6 months following the repair, the patient is instructed to use a protective ankle brace and/or taping to protect the repair.

Complications

The most common complication following operative repair of the lateral ankle ligaments is trauma to the nerves. The incidence of hypersensitivity or hyposensitivity, with or without dysesthesias, ranges from 7% to 19%.[284, 304, 339, 362, 367] Wound problems and infection, postoperative stiffness, deep venous thrombosis, and wound necrosis have all been reported following acute repair. The importance of proper handling of the soft tissues and avoidance of the superficial nerves cannot be overemphasized, particularly for an injury that has infrequent disability and essentially no complications with nonoperative treatment.

Chronic Lateral Ankle Sprains and Instability

Diagnosis

Chronic symptoms following ankle sprain require very careful evaluation to detect bony, tendinous, ligamentous, cartilaginous, and/or neurologic pathology. Evaluation should always include routine radiographs (Table 27–5). Stress views (talar tilt and anterior drawer) including subtalar stress views are usually required, and when indicated, a CAT scan or MRI should be obtained.[298] The bone scan can be particularly useful in differentiating between bony and soft tissue problems, and we will usually have this done prior to choosing between a CAT scan or MRI for further information when the pathology remains unclear despite the prior studies. We find a very limited role for arthrograms, tomograms, or tenograms, but they may be indicated depending on the clinical situation.

Patients with chronic lateral ankle sprains and lateral instability most commonly present in one of two ways. Either they will be seen following an acute ankle sprain, which they relate to be a recurrent problem, or they

TABLE 27–5.
Sources of Chronic Pain or Instability After Ankle Sprain

Articular injury
Chondral fractures
Osteochondral fractures
Nerve injury
Superficial peroneal
Posterior tibial
Sural
Tendon injury
Peroneal tendon (tear or dislocation)
Posterior tibial tendon
Other ligamentous injury
Syndesmosis
Subtalar
Bifurcate
Calcaneocuboid
Impingement
Anterior tibial osteophyte
Anterior inferior tibiofibular ligament
Miscellaneous conditions
Failure to regain normal motion (tight Achilles)
Proprioceptive deficits
Tarsal coalition
Meniscoid lesions
Accessory soleus muscle
Unrelated ongoing pathology masked by routine sprain
Unsuspected rheumotologic condition
Occult tumor

will present to the office complaining of the feeling of looseness in the ankle and its propensity to turn under or give way. Rarely, their presenting complaint will be pain. The examination may reveal lateral tenderness, but the most common feature is the presence of a positive anterior drawer test and/or a positive inversion stress test result. The examination must be thorough enough to rule out other sources of symptomotology. More than one office visit is often necessary to allow an understanding of the patient and the dynamics of the particular situation and pathology. During this familiarization process, treatment can be started with an aggressive physical therapy program. Correction of the deficits in proprioception, strength, and flexibility is occasionally sufficient to relieve the patient of the disabling symptoms. If not, the physician can be more comfortable with the recommendation of surgical stabilization.

Treatment

Once the evaluation is complete and a working diagnosis formulated, treatment alternatives are explored. Nonoperative methods are discussed as noted above. When nonoperative treatment has failed, the risks and benefits of surgery are discussed. If there is any doubt as to the presence of intra-articular pathology, diagnostic arthroscopy may be warranted. This is particularly useful in cases of chondral fracture and talar impingement by the anterior inferior tibiofibular ligament since these lesions may be overlooked in routine diagnostic studies. Nevertheless, if surgical treatment for chronic ligamentous instability is clearly necessary, there is little benefit in arthroscopy of the ankle since all these conditions can be effectively addressed simultaneously with the reconstruction with little additional morbidity.

When chronic lateral ligamentous instability remains despite conservative treatment, the surgeon must choose between a multitude of operative methods for surgical stabilization. For nearly all the procedures described in the literature, the reported success rate is greater than 80%.* This includes secondary ligamentous repair and imbrication as well as ligamentous reconstructions with free tendon grafts or tendon transfers. In order to facilitate a choice of treatment, it is valuable to recognize the goals of a reconstruction or repair procedure. The ligaments should be repaired or imbricated whether or not a reconstructive procedure is performed. Associated pathology must be identified and addressed at the time of the surgery. An augmentation of the ligament repair may be indicated when the tissues are weak or the demands on the ankle are particularly unusual. Athletes who have undergone previous repairs are also candidates for ligamentous reconstruction. Whenever possible the surgeon should avoid sacrificing or weakening tendons that provide eversion stability. This is especially true in dancers, who rely on their peroneal tendons for performance. Finally, subtalar as well as ankle motion must be preserved during a reconstructive or repair procedure. Once subtalar motion is restricted beyond 50% of normal, there is an increasing likelihood that the athlete's performance and even the ability to return to play will be affected.

To simplify matters, procedures for treating chronic lateral ankle instability can be categorized into anatomic procedures and checkrein or tenodesis procedures. The most popular of the anatomic techniques is that presented by Broström and modified by others.* An anatomic augmentation of these repairs may be performed by using the plantaris tendon reconstruction as advocated by Kelikian, Anderson, and Schon and Hansen.[267, 335, 381] By using this technique, surgical trauma to the peroneal tendons is avoided, and an isometric reconstruction of the anterior talofibular and calcaneofibular ligaments is possible. Drawbacks are the technical difficulty of performing the procedure and the absence of a plantaris tendon as a donor source in approximately 7% to 10% of the the population.[297, 375] The procedure also requires two or more medial incisions to harvest the tendon in addition to the lateral incision. Augmentation procedures can also utilize a tendon graft from the fascia lata, a strip of Achilles tendon, or an extensor tendon of the third toe or peroneus brevis. More recently, the use of allograft tissue has been described in lateral ligament reconstruction of the ankle.[323]

Checkrein or tenodesis procedures are also useful. Four major procedures have been described and are used extensively: the Watson-Jones procedure (Fig 27–28), the Evans procedure (Fig 27–29), the Larsen procedure (Fig 27–30), and the Chrisman-Snook modification (Fig 27–31) of the Elmslie procedure (Fig 27–32). These reconstructive techniques require harvesting all or part of the peroneus brevis and routing the tendon through various bone tunnels to perform tenodesis on the ankle or reconstruct the anterior talofibular and/or the calcaneofibular ligament. While all these procedures can stabilize the lateral aspect of the ankle, their ability to do so varies considerably from report to re-

---

**References 267, 271, 276, 286, 289, 290, 293, 303, 307, 312, 324, 330, 343–345, 349, 353, 360, 361, 365, 371, 376, 382, 384, 389, 390, 392, 396, 401–403.*

**References 286, 313, 315, 316, 334, 401.*

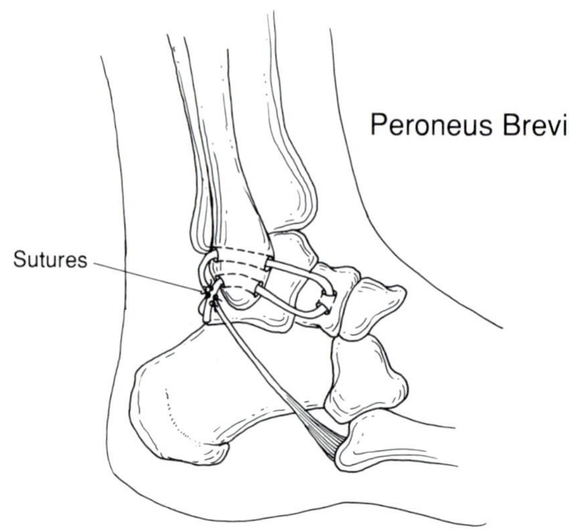

FIG 27–28.
Watson-Jones procedure.

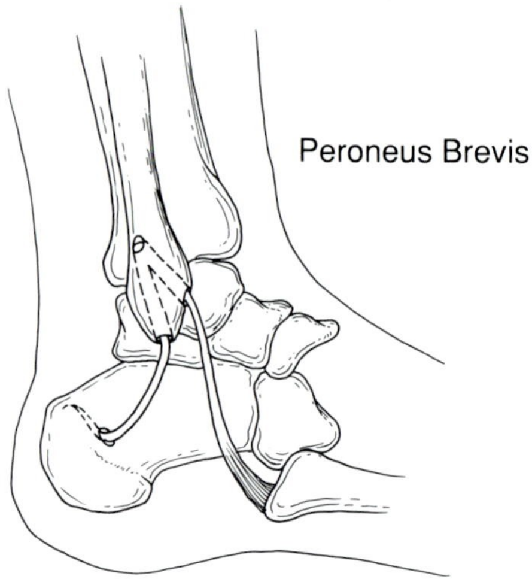

FIG 27–30.
Larsen procedure.

port. Importantly, these procedures vary greatly in their ability to correct any associated subtalar instability. In a review of the literature, the Watson-Jones procedure is associated with persistent subjective instability 20% to 90% of the time. The Evans procedure results in persistent subjective instability 20% to 33% of the time. Furthermore, with the Evans procedure, a persistent anterior drawer is found in 45% to 60% of the cases. The Chrisman-Snook procedure resulted in 13% to 30% subjective persistent instability, but does not have an associated high incidence of objective instability. In all of these procedures, decreased inversion is common (if not essential for a successful result). As previously mentioned in the section on acute ankle ligament repair, neurologic damage and wound complications are not infrequent.

Direct Ligament Repair (Modified Broström Procedure).—For most cases of chronic lateral ankle instability in the athletic population, we prefer to use a modified Broström technique. The procedure is performed through an anterior lateral incision paralleling the border of the fibula (Fig 27–33).

Technique

1. The incision begins at the level of the plafond and extends distally to the level of the peroneal tendons. The intermediate dorsal cutaneous nerve and sural nerve are protected.

2. Dissection is carried down to the capsule. In order to isolate the remaining portion of the anterior

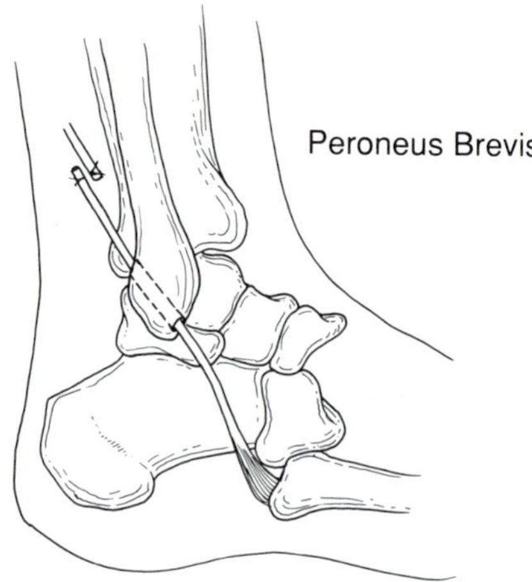

FIG 27–29.
Evans' procedure.

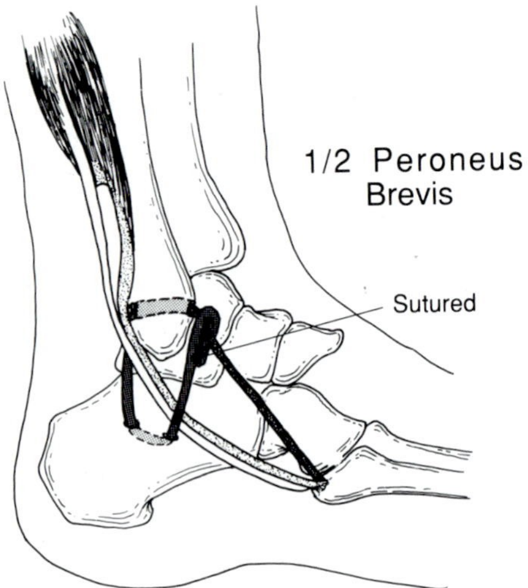

FIG 27–31.
Chrisman-Snook procedure.

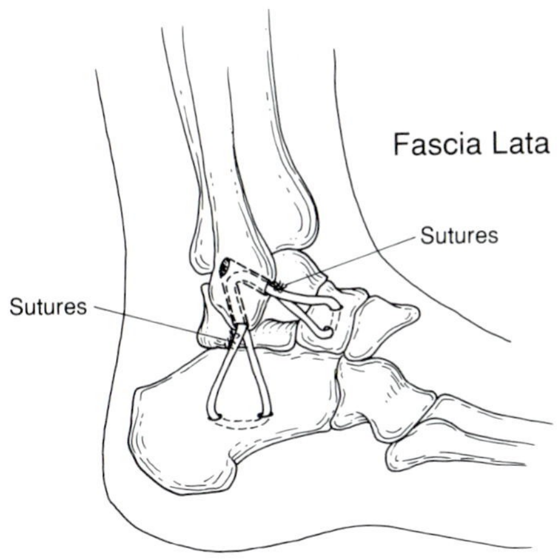

FIG 27–32.
Elmslie procedure with a fascia lata graft.

talofibular ligament, it is helpful to enter the anterolateral capsule at the plafond level and carefully dissect distally to expose the anterior talofibular fibers. If the ligaments appear stretched and there is no obvious rupture, the capsule and ligament are divided a few millimeters from their fibular origin and imbricated.

3. To address the calcaneofibular ligament, the peroneal sheath is opened and the quality of the calcaneofibular ligament is determined. A ligament that is simply stretched can be divided and imbricated. The previously ruptured anterior talofibular or calcaneofibular ligament is often scarred down to capsule and tendon sheath and requires dissection to disclose their location and character. For the calcaneofibular ligament, it is necessary to determine whether the remaining tissue can be used in the secondary repair. A distal avulsion from the calcaneus can be reattached with suture an-

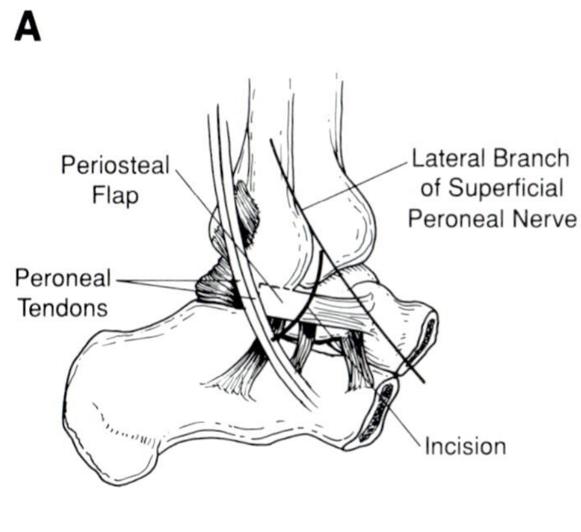

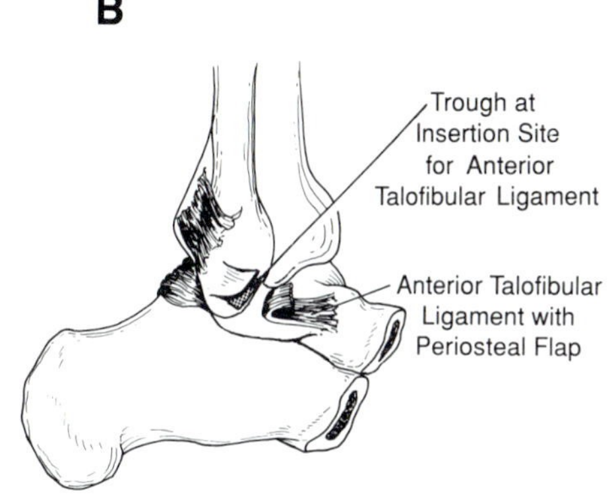

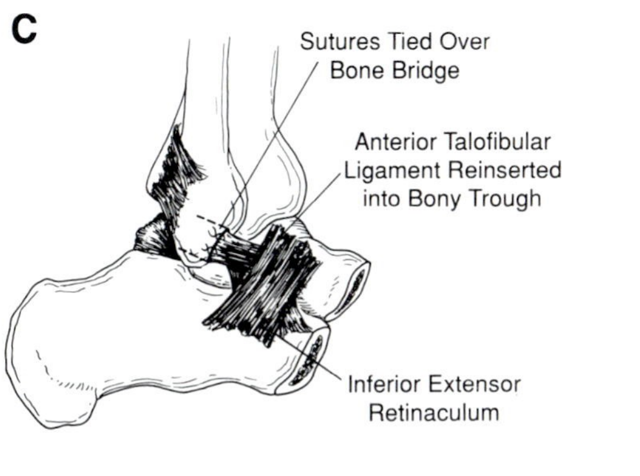

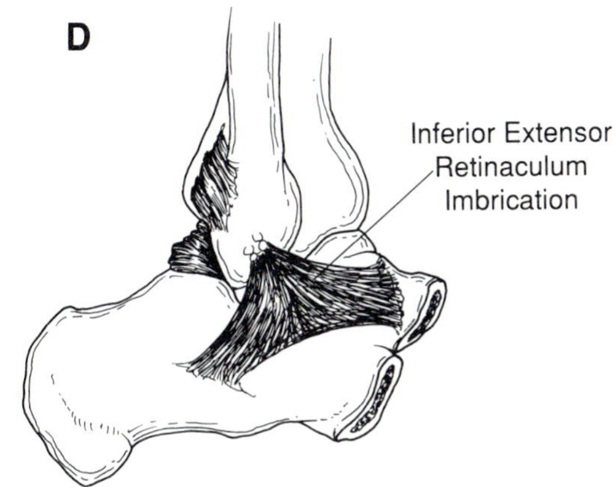

FIG 27–33.
Modified Broström direct repair with imbrication. **A,** lateral exposure and creation of a lateral periosteal flap continuous with the anterior talofibular ligament. **B,** Creation of a trough in the anterior part of the fibula for insertion of the anterior talofibular ligament. **C,** insertion of the anterior talofibular ligament into the fibular trough and sutures tied over the bony bridge. **D,** imbrication of the inferior extensor retinaculum to reinforce the repair.

chors. A proximal avulsion can be reattached with sutures through drill holes in the fibula (being careful to consider the anterior talofibular reconstruction) or with a suture anchor.

The greatest difficulty arises with a midsubstance tear that has extensively scarred to the surrounding tissue. Careful dissection will usually define a ligamentous remnant that can be imbricated. In the case where this remnant cannot be located, we have used the posterior talofibular ligament to reconstruct the calcaneofibular ligament. This is done by releasing the posterior talofibular ligament from its talar insertion and swinging it distally to insert at the calcaneal insertion site for the calcaneofibular ligament. In our experience, this has only been necessary in two cases of Broström repair with no identifiable ill effects.

4. To be certain of sufficient tissue for the anterior talofibular ligament reconstruction, a periosteal flap that is continuous with the capsule and the anterior talofibular scar can be created (Fig 27–33,A).

5. Next, nonabsorbable or slowly absorbable sutures are placed in the ligament. A small bony trough is created above the anterior and inferior border of the distal end of the fibula, and several drill holes are made with a small drill bit or Kirschner wire (Fig 27–33,B). This permits imbrication of the ends of the cut ligament and capsule, as well as anchoring of the ligament into bone.

6. The sutures are tied over a bony bridge on the lateral aspect of the fibula with the ankle held in neutral dorsiflexion and slight eversion (Fig 27–33,C). The surgeon must be careful to ensure that there is no anterior displacement force on the ankle while the sutures are being tied. To prevent this, we use a bump under the calf to relieve any anteriorly directed force on the calcaneus.

7. After securing the repair, the stability is checked and further imbrication performed as needed.

8. Prior to closure, attention is directed to the inferior extensor retinaculum, which is imbricated or sutured to the periosteum over the fibula (Fig 27–33,D). Whether this provides any real stability to the subtalar area or adds some proprioceptive feedback is unclear, but we believe that it is an important addition to the Broström technique as noted by Gould and coauthors.[312]

9. The subcutaneous tissues are reapproximated with absorbable sutures, and the skin is closed with a subcuticular technique.

10. A U-shaped splint and a posterior splint are applied.

Postoperative Care.—The postoperative protocol in athletes is the same as that used for treatment of the acute lesion. In nonathletes, a 12-week period of protection is warranted, with the first 4 to 6 weeks in a cast and the second 6 weeks in a removable brace or sometimes a cast.

Lateral Ligament Reconstruction (Modified Chrisman-Snook Procedure).—The Chrisman-Snook procedure is probably the most common lateral ligament reconstructive procedure. We recommend this technique for athletes who have generalized ligament laxity, in cases of a failed prior imbrication or tenodesis procedure, or in certain athletes with particularly long histories of severe recurrent instabilities. Also, athletes with combined ankle and subtalar instability are candidates for this procedure.[380] Most of the time it is sufficient to use half the peroneus brevis tendon to perform this procedure. Nevertheless, there are patients who have an inadequate peroneus brevis tendon or concurrent peroneus brevis pathology that requires harvesting the entire tendon. Slight and probably insignificant weakness may result, but overall ankle function is good without an intact peroneus brevis.[323] It is important in those cases where the whole tendon is harvested that the peroneus brevis muscle be sutured to the peroneus longus muscle tendon complex.[346]

Technique

1. In order to harvest sufficient tendon, a long lateral incision is required. A 16-cm incision is made beginning 11 cm proximal to the tip of the fibula over the peroneus brevis. The incision is continued distally to the vicinity of the calcaneocuboid joint.

2. Sharp dissection is performed proximally to expose the peroneal retinaculum, while distally, blunt dissection should be used to identify any branches of the sural nerve.

3. The peroneal retinaculum is split the entire length of the incision and 2 cm of the tissue left intact where the tendons curve anteriorly underneath the fibula. This will obviate repair of the superior peroneal retinaculum and prevent peroneal subluxation.

4. Next, the dorsal anterior flap is raised to expose the anterior talofibular ligament. A small arthrotomy is made just proximal to the superior border of the anterior talofibular ligament. This serves as entry point for a small curved hemostat that is passed along the anterior border of the fibula to facilitate identification of the anterior talofibular ligament.

5. Distal to the tip of the fibula, the peroneal sheath should be opened to prepare the tendons for transfer

and also permit visualization of the calcaneofibular ligament.

6. Subperiosteal dissection is performed along the lateral wall of the calcaneus beginning just outside the peroneal sheath. In this manner, the site for the calcaneal drill holes is exposed.

7. Half of the peroneus brevis tendon is harvested, beginning distally. The harvesting of the tendon graft is continued as proximally as possible, with the dissection proceeding into the belly of the peroneus brevis muscle where the tendon fans out. In this manner, an extra 2 to 3 cm of tendon length can be obtained. If the entire tendon is taken (e.g., cases where the tendon is abnormally small or torn), the muscle should be secured to the peroneus longus.

8. Once the tendon is harvested, it is passed underneath the intact peroneal retinaculum and drawn out to the distal part of the incised peroneal sheath. The tendon is wrapped in moist saline gauze while the drill holes are prepared.

9. With a 4.5-mm drill bit, bone tunnels are drilled in the following manner. The first hole is drilled approximately 2.5 cm above the tip of the fibula in an anterior-to-posterior direction and perpendicular to the axis of the fibula. The graft is threaded through this hole anteriorly to posteriorly. The hole is enlarged as necessary to allow passage of the graft. Next, two tunnels are created in a "V-like" fashion to span the insertion point of the calcaneofibular ligament. These two calcaneal holes are joined by using a curved curette.

10. The tendon graft is then passed into the most posterior calcaneal tunnel and out the anterior calcaneal tunnel.

11. The tendon is next routed toward the anterior aspect of the fibula, where it is secured to itself.

12. It is important to secure each limb of the reconstruction in the taut position and avoid slack with each passage of the tendon. At the anterior limb of the graft, the tendon is secured to the residual anterior talofibular ligament. There should be no anterior forces on the talus (caused frequently by the heel resting against the operating table) during the securing and tightening of the limbs of the reconstruction. The foot should not be placed into forced eversion, however, while securing the graft. This can produce a painful limitation of subtalar motion.[389] An imbrication of the anterior talofibular and calcaneofibular ligaments should also be performed in addition to the tendon reconstruction.

Postoperative Care.—Postoperatively, the patient is placed in a U-shaped splint and posterior splint. The ankle is protected for 12 weeks, with a removable walking boot used for approximately 6 weeks and an ankle stirrup brace for the second 6 weeks. After 2 weeks gentle dorsiflexion and eversion can be instituted. At 4 weeks peroneal strengthening from the neutral position and Achilles stretching are begun. Active inversion, plantar flexion, and proprioceptive training are begun at 6 to 8 weeks. Thereafter, the athlete is allowed to progress from walking, to jogging, to running, to figure-of-8 running, to cutting, and then to sports-specific activity. The ankle must be protected by using tape or a functional ankle brace for 6 months after the reconstruction.

MEDIAL ANKLE SPRAIN

The medial collateral ligaments are a strong fan-shaped or deltoid-shaped ligamentous complex that provides stability to the medial talocrural joint. Typically, deltoid injuries occur in association with lateral ligamentous injuries or bony injuries. Infrequently, isolated deltoid sprains may occur. It is rare to have chronic medial collateral ligament insufficiency, but subtle cases may be overlooked.

Anatomy

The deltoid ligament is divided into two portions: the superficial and the deep layers (Fig 27–34,A and B). The superficial deltoid ligament takes origin off the anterior colliculus of the medial malleolus. The superficial deltoid is most properly thought of as one structure with one origin and many insertions. There are no discreet bands of the superficial deltoid. The most anterior part of the superficial deltoid inserts onto the naviculum, both medially and plantarly. As it travels plantarly, the ligament acts as a strut for the spring ligament or plantar calcaneonavicular ligament. The next most posterior portion of the superficial deltoid begins at the anterior colliculus and inserts onto the sustentaculum tali. The deep deltoid takes origin from the intercollicular groove and the posterior colliculus. This shorter and thicker ligament inserts onto the medial wall of the nonarticular surface of the talus. The deep deltoid is confluent with the medial capsule of the ankle joint and the medial portion of the interosseous talocalcaneal ligament.[420, 421, 423]

Biomechanics

The deltoid ligament as a whole and specifically the talocalcaneal ligament primarily prohibit abduction. Following division of both the deep and superficial lay-

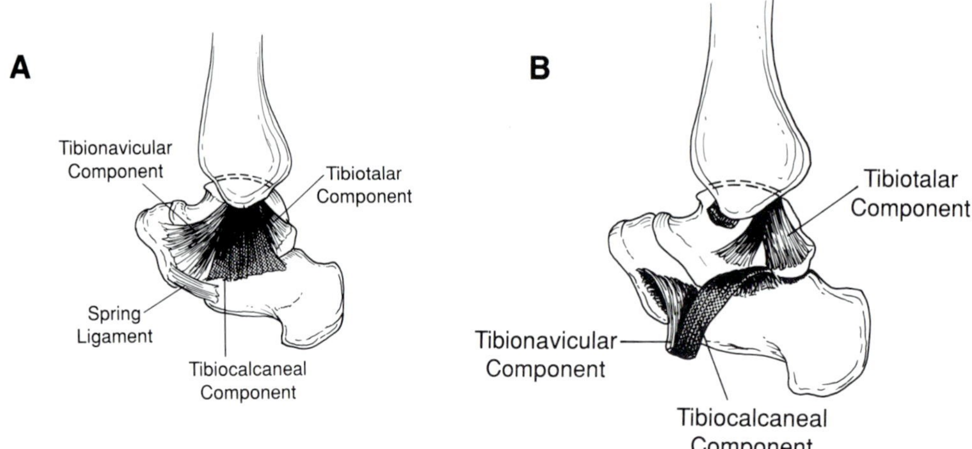

FIG 27–34.
Anatomy of the medial part of the ankle to show the deltoid ligament. **A,** superficial; **B,** deep.

ers of the deltoid, there is no increased anterior instability of the ankle.[413] Once the lateral ligaments are cut, the deltoid does act as a secondary restraint against anterior translation. Lateral translation of the talus is primarily inhibited by the fibula. With resection of the lateral malleolus, an intact deltoid allows up to 3 mm of lateral talar shift.[407, 408, 411–414, 417] The deep deltoid is responsible for the greatest restraint against lateral translation.[411, 413] Valgus tilting of the talus within the mortise requires rupture of both the superficial and the deep deltoid.[412] Rasmussen found that in forced abduction injuries, isolated rupture of the superficial deltoid, particularly the talocalcaneal band, occurs first followed by disruption of the deep deltoid. Deltoid ligament rupture can occur following pronation-eversion, forced plantar flexion, or forced dorsiflexion.[406, 422] The deltoid is a strong ligament that requires considerable force for disruption. Attarian and coworkers found that the deep deltoid ligament has the highest load to failure in comparison to the lateral collateral ligaments.[404]

Diagnosis

Clinical Evaluation

Most patients with deltoid ligamentous injuries will have either lateral ligamentous injuries, fibula fractures, syndesmotic injuries, or all of the above. In one study of lateral ligament ruptures, 2.8% were associated with medial ligamentous injury.[406] Isolated rupture of the deltoid ligament without lateral ligamentous or fibula injury is rare.[424] Patients with this injury usually have a more violent mechanism, typically an eversion injury of the ankle. Landing from a triple jump or a broad jump with the foot in abduction and the heel in valgus may result in deltoid injury. The patient hears or feels a pop on the medial side of the ankle that is usually accompanied by immediate swelling and pain.

In all cases, physical examination must exclude syndesmotic injury, lateral ligamentous injury, and high fibula fractures or proximal tibiofibular joint injury. Evaluation of the posterior tibial tendon, flexor digitorum longus, and flexor hallucis longus must also be performed. Tibial nerve and saphenous nerve traction injuries should be identified.

Radiographic Evaluation

The diagnosis may be suggested by radiographs, especially when there is an associated syndesmotic injury or fibula fracture. When there is an isolated deltoid injury, a valgus AP stress radiograph may show a talar tilt (Fig 27–35). It is not uncommon, however, for these studies to be normal. The diagnosis of an acute deltoid ligament tear may only be objectively confirmed by MRI or arthrography.

Treatment

Treatment of deltoid ligament injuries depends on the associated injuries. If the fibula fracture is reduced and stabilized or the syndesmosis is reduced and stabilized, there is no need to repair the deltoid, although this is a controversial topic. Casting these injuries for 8 to 10 weeks will typically result in sufficient healing of the deltoid.[405, 409, 416, 419] The authors do not recommend suturing the deltoid ligament in association with the other injuries unless there is difficulty in obtaining or maintaining reduction following the lateral syndesmotic repair or fibular fracture fixation. In the literature, there have been very few cases of deltoid ligament sprain without lateral bone or ligament injury.[415, 424]

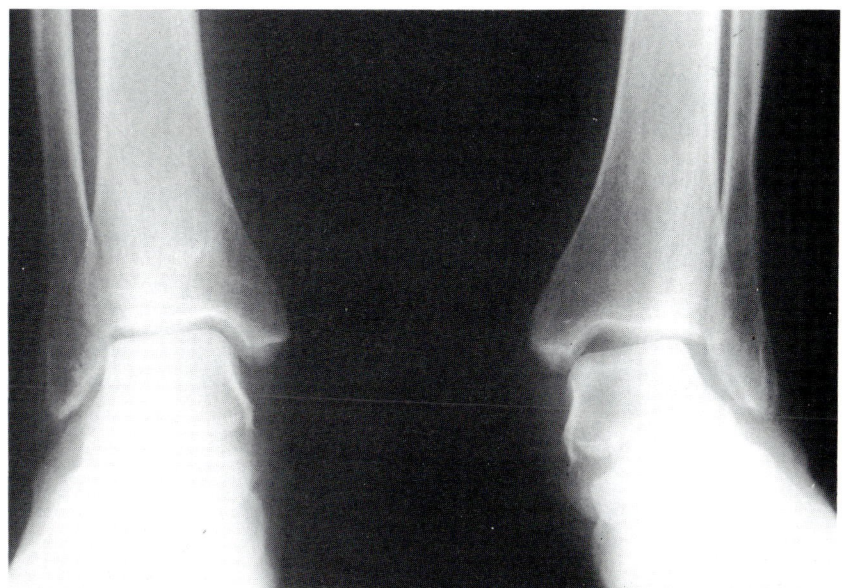

FIG 27–35.
Valgus tilt of the talus in an AP weight-bearing radiograph.

The authors recommend functional management in an Aircast for most of these cases of isolated deltoid ligament sprain in recognition of the fact that medial injuries heal more slowly than lateral injuries (at least from the standpoint of the athlete's ability to return to play). In a complete ligament disruption in an athlete, operative repair may be entertained, although we have not found this to be necessary in our experience.

Technique of Operative Repair

1. A longitudinal incision is made over the tip of the medial malleolus and extends anteriorly toward the talonavicular joint.

2. The superficial and deep fibers of the deltoid are inspected, and the posterior tibial and flexor digitorum longus tendons are also evaluated.

3. The joint is inspected for any loose bodies, and the articular surface is evaluated as well as possible.

4. Absorbable sutures are placed in the deltoid to permit an anatomic apposition of the ligament.

Postoperative Care

Postoperatively, the patient is in a cast for 4 weeks, followed by a brace for another 6 weeks. For the first 6 months following the injury, the patient should wear a brace during sports.

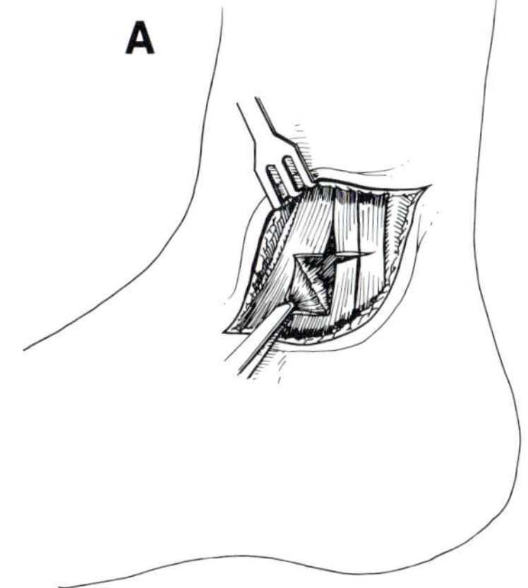

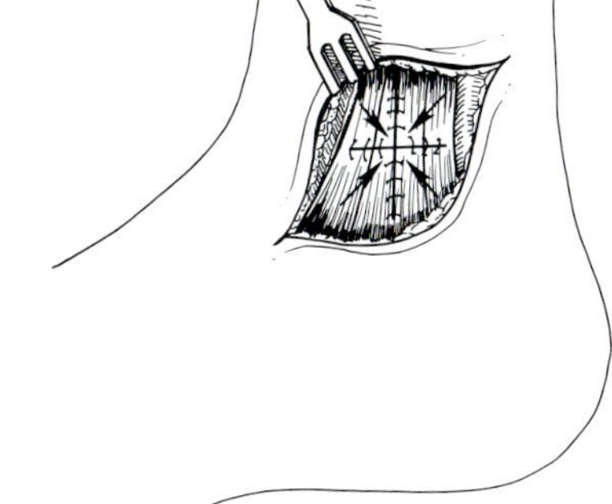

Medial Side

FIG 27–36.
DuVries technique for deltoid imbrication.

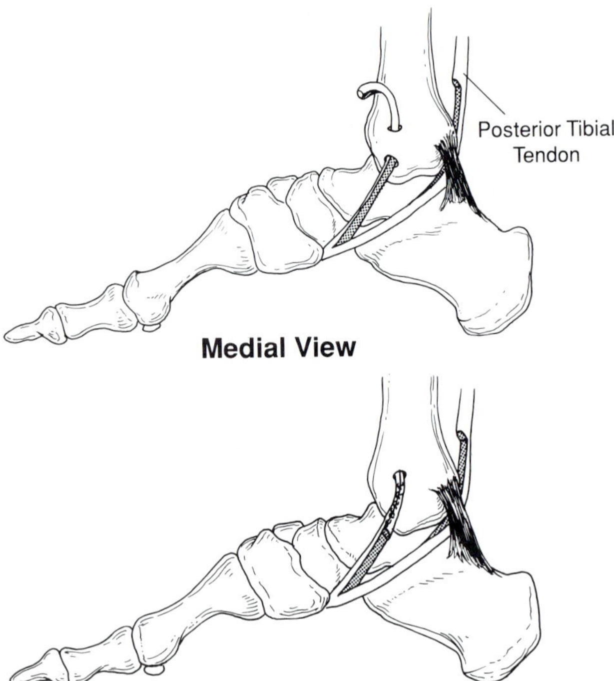

FIG 27–37.
Wiltberger and Mallory procedure for chronic medial ankle ligamentous insufficiency.

Chronic Medial Ligament Instability

Diagnosis

Chronic deltoid insufficiency is extremely uncommon.[415, 416, 418] Patients who complain of medial instability usually note discomfort on the medial side of the ankle and have slight valgus and abduction of the ankle with each step. Stress radiographs may show valgus instability of the ankle or medial clear space widening. If there is medial clear space widening, it is imperative to rule out a fibular fracture nonunion or malunion or prior syndesmotic injury. Occasionally, MRI will be helpful in identifying the pathology. An arthrogram adds little significant information.

Treatment

Conservative treatment of chronic medial ligamentous insufficiency includes taping, an ankle stirrup brace, casting, physical therapy, and orthoses. If these measures fail to achieve satisfactory results, surgical intervention is the next step. Two approaches may be used depending on the availability and quality of tissue apparent at the time of surgery. If the tissues are of good quality, direct imbrication may be performed[410] (Fig 27–36). On the other hand, if the tissues are inadequate, a free flexor digitorum longus graft or split posterior tibial tendon graft can be used by going from the tibia into the talus or naviculum to reconstruct the deltoid.[415, 416, 418, 425] (Fig 27–37). Other potential sources of graft material to rebuild the deltoid ligament are the plantaris tendon, the Achilles tendon, the peroneus brevis tendon, the semitendinosis tendon, or an allograft.

SYNDESMOSIS SPRAINS OF THE ANKLE

Sprains of the ligamentous structures about the ankle have already been established as one of the most common injuries in sports and the source of significant lost playing time for the athlete. Included among these sprains, but a source of considerably greater impairment than the lateral sprain, is the sprain of the syndesmotic ligaments of the ankle.[435] While much has been written about injury to the syndesmosis in connection with fractures about the ankle (a subject that is thoroughly covered in Chapter 34), there is very little literature devoted specifically to sprains of the syndesmosis.

Definition

When the sprain results in a complete rupture of the ligaments, a diastasis can occur with separation of the distal ends of the tibia and fibula. Diastasis refers to "any loosening in the attachment of the fibula to the tibia at the inferior tibiofibular joint, and is not confined to wide separation of the bones."[433] Although most cases of diastasis occur in conjunction with fractures of the tibia and/or fibula, this is not always the case.* When force on the syndesmosis is of sufficient magnitude to stretch one of the ligaments beyond the normal load zone for elastic deformation, then failure of the ligament ensues. This begins with failure of collagen bundles at the microscopic level and continues until gross disruption occurs. Therefore, it is possible to have a sprain of the syndesmosis without a fracture as well as without a diastasis.[435, 454] Furthermore, the configuration of the joint and the elasticity of the tissues make spontaneous reduction likely, and diastasis, when present, may be unapparent without some form of stress examination. Syndesmosis sprains encompass this entire continuum of injury from minor sprain to frank diastasis, and each grade of injury will be discussed under this heading.

Incidence

Although diastasis of the ankle without fracture has been discussed in only a small number of papers in the

---

**References 444, 445, 463, 464, 468, 474, 484.*

English literature, sprains to the syndesmosis have been estimated to occur in as many as 10% of all ankle sprains according to Cedel and Broström.[436, 438] In the closed population of cadets at the United States Military Academy, Hopkinson and coauthors reported 15 syndesmosis sprains among 1,344 ankle sprains—an incidence of 1%.[454] It has been suggested that many of these injuries go undiagnosed and may be the source of chronic ankle pain and arthrosis in some patients.[455] Calcification of the distal tibiofibular syndesmosis was found in 32% of professional football players attending training camp, thus suggesting a much higher incidence of this injury.[482] This is particularly likely in those athletes whose careers continue at a high level over a prolonged period of time. This was suggested in a more recent study of the Minnesota Vikings professional football team over a 6-year period.[435] There were 98 ankle sprains, 18 of which were classified as syndesmosis sprains (18%). Another report describes this injury in ten World Cup skiers during a 12-year period.[450] It is unclear exactly what percentage of syndesmosis sprains actually have instability since stress views are necessary for this determination and are not routinely performed. However, there are very few reports in the literature of diastasis without fracture, and one large trauma center documented only six cases of frank diastasis without fracture during a 5-year period.[445] The West Point study had only one case of frank diastasis.[454] We have had two cases of diastasis without fracture at Rice University during the past 25 years and see about one to two cases of syndesmosis sprain per year.

Anatomy

The tibia and fibula are connected throughout their length by fibrous structures. At the ankle these include three definable ligaments: (1) the anterior inferior tibiofibular (AITF) ligament, (2) the posterior inferior tibiofibular (PITF) ligament, and (3) the interosseous ligament[475] (Fig 27–38,A and B). Also contributing to the stability of the distal connection is the interosseous membrane through its lower fibers. The AITF ligament runs obliquely from the anterolateral tubercle of the tibia (Tillaux-Chaput tubercle) downward to the anterodistal fibular shaft at about a 45-degree angle to the plafond. It is approximately 20 mm wide and 20 to 30 mm long.[472] The ligament is often multifascicular, and its most inferior fascicle has been described as a separate structure—the accessory anterior tibiofibular ligament[429] (Fig 27–39). This ligament is distal to the main body of the AITF ligament but parallels its course across the anterolateral aspect of the ankle. The fibers can be seen during arthroscopy of the ankle and have been reported to be the source of pathologic impingement in certain cases.[429] The AITF ligament is the most commonly injured ligament in syndesmosis sprains and in frank diastasis.[433]

The PITF ligament has two components: (1) a deep portion also called the transverse tibiofibular ligament (classified as a distinct ligament by some authors[440, 442, 457] and (2) a superficial portion. The superficial PITF ligament originates on the posterior surface of the tibia at the posterolateral tubercle as well as from the periosteum of the posterodistal surface of the tibia.

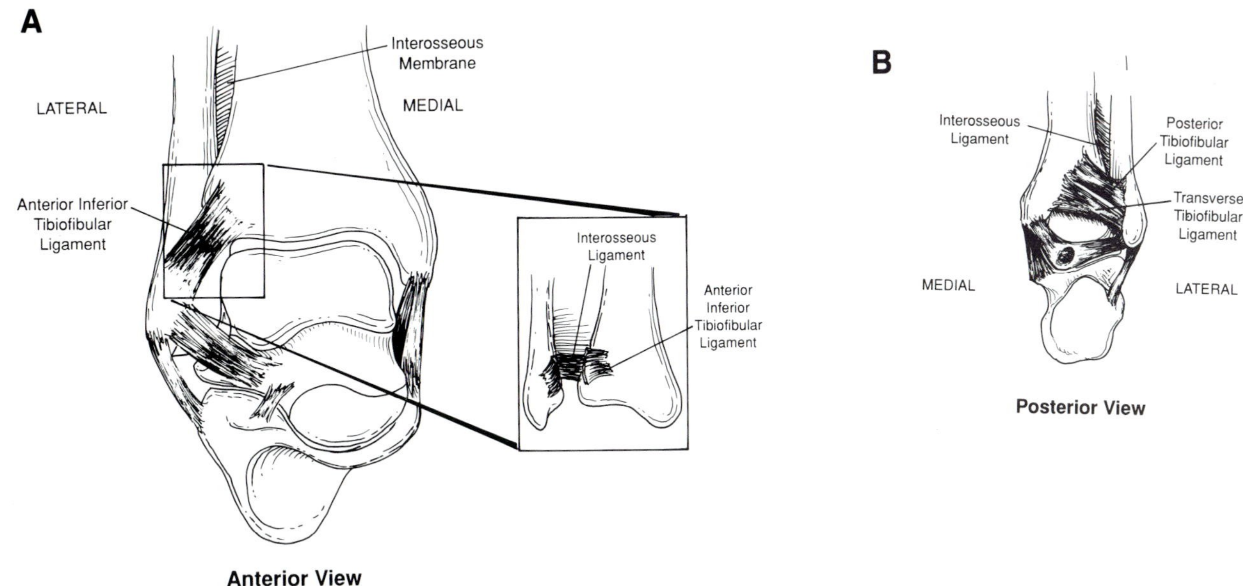

FIG 27–38.
Drawing of the anatomy of the tibiofibular articulation: **A,** anterior view; **B,** posterior view.

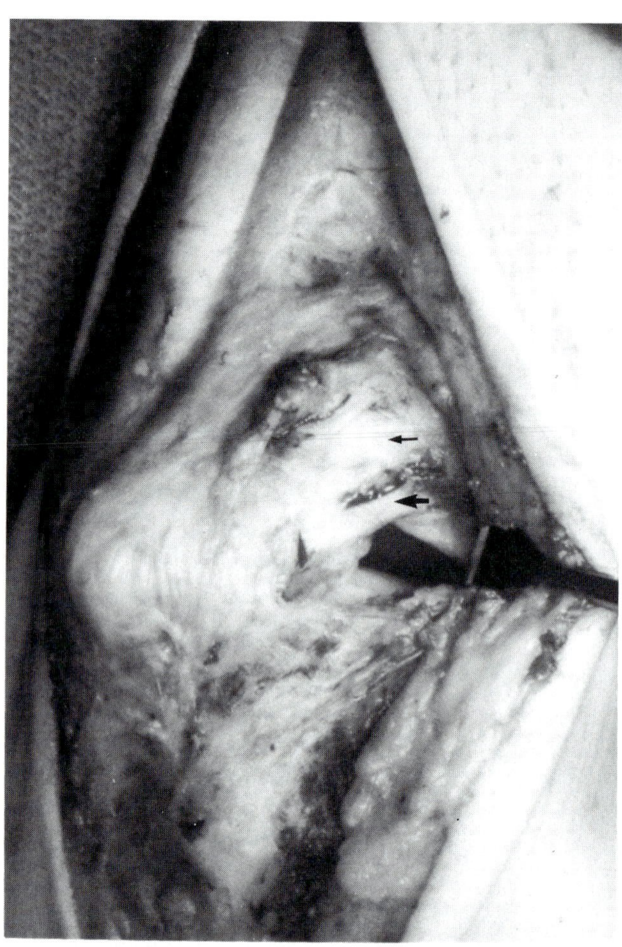

FIG 27–39.
Intraoperative photograph of the accessory anterior tibiofibular ligament *(large arrow)* of the anterior inferior tibiofibular ligament *(small arrow).*

It covers the back of the tibiotalar joint and runs obliquely down to the posterior aspect of the distal part of the fibula. It is approximately 20 mm wide, 30 mm long, and 5 mm thick.[472] The deep portion is anterior to the superficial part and forms the most distal aspect of tibial articulation with the talus, deepening the joint in a manner similar to a labrum. The fibers begin quite medially on the tibia and proceed transversely along the posterior aspect of the distal end of the tibia until they reach the lateral posterior surface of the tibia where they turn downward to insert on the posterior part of the fibula. This occurs at the upper edge of the fibular digital fossa very near its articular cartilage. Since the PITF ligament combines strength with elasticity, it is usually the last of the syndesmotic structures to tear.[457, 475]

The interosseus ligament interconnects the tibia and fibula approximately 0.5 to 2 cm above the plafond and surrounds the synovial recess, which extends upward from the tibiotalar joint approximately 1 cm. The interosseus ligament is the shortest of the interconnections and is considered the primary bond between the tibia and fibula.[442, 457, 469] Superiorly, the interosseus ligament is continuous with the interosseous membrane, which provides minimal additional strength to the stabilizing effect of the syndesmotic ligaments.

The bony anatomy of the distal ends of the tibia and fibula provides a variable degree of additional stability to their interconnection through containment of the distal portion of the fibula in the peroneal recess, a vertically oriented triangular groove with its apex superior and its base inferior. This concave groove in the lateral surface of the tibia is bounded anteriorly and posteriorly by tubercles of varying size. The size variance of the tubercles and the depth of the recess can make interpretation of diastasis by radiographic dimensions difficult.[433, 442] In fact, the study by Höcker and Pachucki indicates that the incisura fibularis is concave only 75% of the time and is convex in 16% of cases.[453] The remaining 8% were not characterized due to their irregularity.

Biomechanics

In the normal relationship between the distal ends of the tibia and fibula, a certain amount of motion is allowed in all three planes. As the ankle goes from full plantar flexion to full dorsiflexion, there is an increase in the intermalleolar distance that averages 1.5 mm.[442] Rotation of the ankle is also possible through the syndesmosis. During normal active or passive dorsiflexion or in walking, the tibia can rotate on the talus approximately 5 to 6 degrees.[442] McCullough and Burge noted up to 25 degrees of rotation in the horizontal plane in unloaded cadaveric ankles, with almost half this motion coming from the inferior tibiofibular joint.[465] Rasmussen and Tovberg-Jensen reported horizontal-plane motion averaging 7 degrees of internal rotation and 10 degrees of external rotation.[473] Finally, Scranton et al. have shown an average of 2.4 mm distal migration of the fibula during the stance phase of the gait cycle.[477]

The relative importance of the syndesmotic ligaments to ankle stability has been confirmed through experimental sectioning of the ligaments and evaluation of the change in mobility patterns for the ankle. Rupture of the AITF ligament produces up to 4 mm separation of the tibia and fibula according to Bonnin, and this can increase up to 1 cm with the additional rupture of the interosseous ligament.[433] Other authors have found this distance to be from 5 to 12 mm with sectioning of the AITF ligament.[428, 436, 439] Cutting this ligament has also been shown to increase external rotation of the fibula as well as forward-backward translation.[442, 472] Rasmussen's comprehensive study of the ankle ligaments showed only 1 to 2 degrees increase in external rotation of the fibula with isolated section of the AITF ligament.[472] There was no effect on frontal-plane motion. Including the interosseus ligament in the transection caused an additional 1.2 ± 0.45 degrees increase in external rotation. Adding the PITF ligament to the sectioning of the other ligaments produced a 2.78 ± 1.64 degrees increase in external rotation and a 2.44 ± 1.67 degrees increase in internal rotation. Section of the PITF ligament alone increased internal rotation by 0.75 ± 0.5 degrees without affecting external rotation. Adding the interosseus ligament to the PITF ligament transection increased internal rotation mobility only slightly to 1.25 ± 0.5 degrees. This work led Rasmussen to conclude that the ligaments of the syndesmosis play little role in the stability of the ankle as long as the other ligamentous structures are intact. It is of interest to note that no study has been able to produce a purely ligamentous injury to the syndesmosis through externally applied stress (usually external rotation and/or abduction).

Mechanism of Injury

Despite the inability of researchers to duplicate the lesions of a syndesmosis sprain or diastasis without fracture, most clinicians are in agreement that external rotation is the most significant force.[450, 454, 457, 472] It is possible to have a syndesmosis injury with abduction, but the deltoid ligament or medial malleolus must fail also. Persistence of the external rotation force can result in tearing of the interroseous ligament and interosseous membrane in addition to the AITF ligament. The PITF ligament is usually preserved in this mechanism. Greater amounts of external rotation force can lead to spiral fractures of the fibula at levels as high as the proximal end of the fibula (Maisonneuve fracture). O'Donoghue relates the syndesmosis sprain in athletes to hyperdorsiflexion of the ankle, and this mechanism is suggested in at least two other reports.[445, 454, 468]

Creation of a syndesmosis injury by external rotation in skiing has been well described by Fritschy.[450] In this unique situation the movement of the ankle is constrained by a rigid ski boot. When a slalom skier misses a gate by straddling it, the internal ski is forced into rapid external rotation. If the force is sufficiently violent, either the knee ligaments will fail, or a syndesmosis injury with or without concomitant fibula fracture will result. In the study of syndesmosis sprains by Hopkinson et al., injuries occurred in a variety of sports ranging from football to wrestling and with a variety of mechanisms.[454] Edwards and DeLee's study of diastasis injuries included no sports injuries but noted two twisting injuries, two slips, and two falls.[445] It has been our experience that athletes are often incapable of describing exactly what the mechanism of injury was at the time of injury, but they recognized that it was not that of a typical ankle sprain.

Diagnosis

Clinical Evaluation

Following an acute injury to the ankle, the patient will present with well-localized anterolateral ankle pain located over the anterior syndesmosis of the ankle. The patient's pain and swelling are usually more precisely localized than in cases of severe lateral ankle sprains of the traditional inversion type. This is particularly true if the athlete is seen soon after the injury. Careful palpation will reveal minimal if any tenderness over the anterior talofibular and calcaneofibular ligaments. There may be tenderness medially over the deltoid ligament, especially in cases where there has been an abduction component to the injury mechanism. It is crucial that the examiner palpate the malleoli and the entire length of the fibula including the proximal tibiofibular joint to rule out associated injury. Provocation of pain at the syndesmosis by squeezing the fibula at the midcalf can be helpful in focusing attention on possible injury to the syndesmotic ligaments (Fig 27–40). This test was popularized at West Point by Dr. Ed Pillings and was the basis for follow-up on eight patients with ten syndesmosis injuries in a recent study by Hopkinson et al.[454]

Anterior drawer and talar tilt testing are routinely performed and should have negative results. A feeling of side-to-side play may be appreciable in cases of diastasis. The most revealing test is external rotation of the foot while holding the leg stabilized with the knee flexed at 90 degrees (Fig 27–41). This reproduces pain at the syndesmosis. When this test is positive, one should presume that a syndesmosis injury exists until determined otherwise.

Realistically, it should be acknowledged that many of these injuries go undetected initially and are seen only later when it is evident that they are not following the pattern of healing of the "normal ankle sprain." This may make the diagnosis more obscure unless one is alert to the problem of syndesmosis sprains and diastasis. They typically produce more disability and longer missed playing time than do lateral sprains. Being alert to this problem in the initial evaluation of the athlete can save much time in answering questions and may provide an explanation when the coach wonders why the athlete is still not playing after 6 weeks.

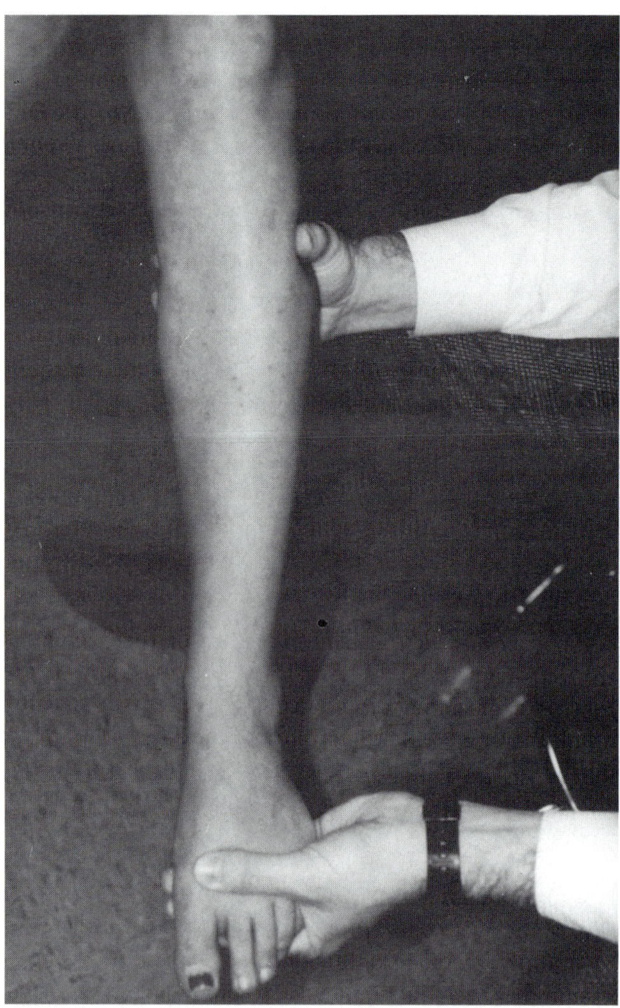

FIG 27–40.
The "squeeze test" can be used to diagnose sprains of the tibiofibular syndesmosis. (Modified from Hopkinson WJ, St. Pierre P, Ryan JB, et al: *Foot Ankle* 10:325–330, 1990.)

Radiographic Evaluation

Routine Radiographs.—The next step in the evaluation of the patient suspected of having a syndesmosis injury is routine radiography. This is essential since it has been shown that 10% to 50% of cases of syndesmosis injury will have a bony avulsion.[433, 435, 450] This can be seen as a variably sized fragment coming from the anterior tubercle or the posterior tubercle of the tibia, or much less commonly, the avulsion fragment comes from the fibula. Needless to say, x-ray films should be used to exclude more significant fractures of the tibia, fibula, and talus.

The evaluation of tibial and fibular relationships is as important as viewing the bony continuity. These relationships include (1) the medial clear space between the medial malleolus and the medial border of the talus, (2) the tibiofibular clear space at the incisura fibularis, and (3) the absolute amount and percentage of overlap of the tibia and fibula at the incisura (Fig 27–42). These relationships and the radiographic criteria for detection of widening of the syndesmosis have been thoroughly reviewed by Harper and Keller.[452] The most commonly cited measurements will be reviewed.

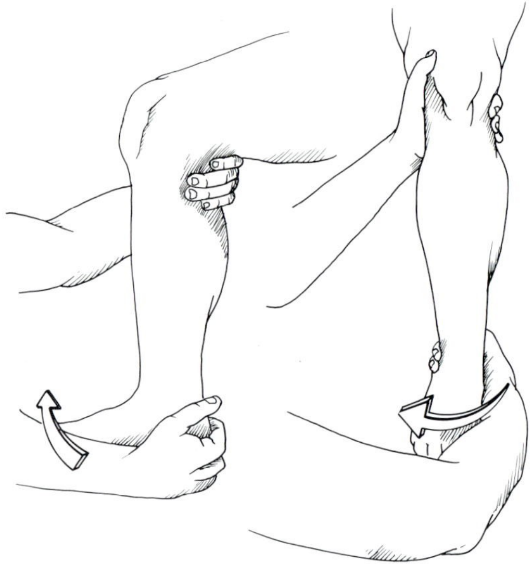

FIG 27–41.
The abduction/external rotation stress test produces extreme pain in syndesmosis sprains and is the method for eliciting latent diastasis by stress radiography.

The diagnosis of diastasis of the tibiofibular syndesmosis can be made by determining that the distance between the lateral aspect of the medial malleolus and the medial aspect of the talus (medial clear space) has increased (Fig 27–43). Normally this distance should be no more than 2 to 4 mm.[480] Noting the difference on a comparison view with the uninjured ankle is often recommended. However, Bonnin has delineated several reasons why this method of using the medial clear space is too variable to allow reliability in the diagnosis of diastasis.[433]

Various authors have recommended measurement of the overlapping shadow of the tibia and fibula and have given absolute millimeters for normal or as a percentage of the fibular width[433, 466, 470] (Fig 27–44). Quenu used 5 mm of overlap on the AP radiograph, and Pettrone used a figure of 1 mm of overlap or greater on the mortise view as the criterion of normal.[433, 470, 470a] McDade and Pettrone et al. both described normal by the width of the fibula on the AP x-ray film and stated that overlap of a third or greater of its width was normal.[466, 470] The inverse of this measurement was advocated by Ashhurst and Bromer, who measured from the lateral

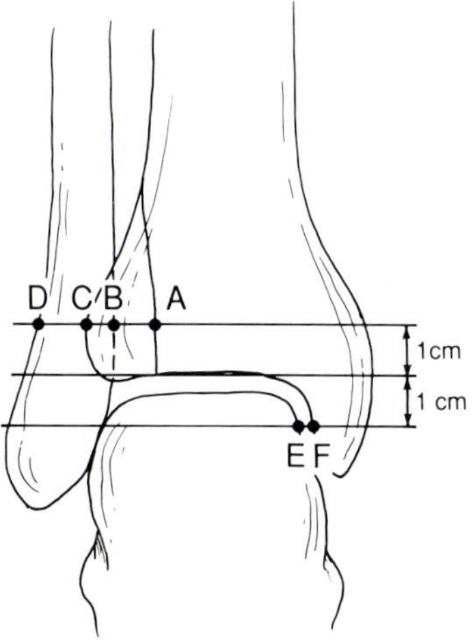

FIG 27–42.
Normal radiographic relationships important in the evaluation of the tibiofibular articulation. Clear spaces are *EF and AB.*

aspect of the fibula to the lateral edge of the anterior tubercle of the tibia.[428] They believed that a space of more than two thirds the width of the fibula was indicative of a diastasis.

The final method proposed for determining the presence of a diastasis radiographically is measurement of the tibiofibular clear space. The range of normal in various studies is from 3 to 6 mm as measured on the AP radiograph.[452, 460, 466, 469, 476] Leeds and Ehrlich measured the tibiofibular clear space 1 cm proximal to the tibial plafond on the mortise view of 34 ankles and found the average to be 3.84 mm (range, 2.5 to 5.0 mm).[460] Harper and Keller performed a radiographic evaluation of 12 fresh cadaver ankles to determine the reliability of the different measurements of the tibiofibular syndesmosis.[452] Based on their research, they recommended the following criteria to be consistent with a normal tibiofibular relationship at a 95% confidence level: (1) a tibiofibular clear space of less than 6 mm on the AP and mortise radiographs, (2) overlap of the tibia and fibula at the incisura fibularis of 6 mm or more (or ≥ 42% of the fibular width), and (3) overlap of the tibia and fibula of greater than 1 mm on the mortise view. They felt that the measurement of the tibiofibular clear space was the most accurate means of determining diastasis.[452]

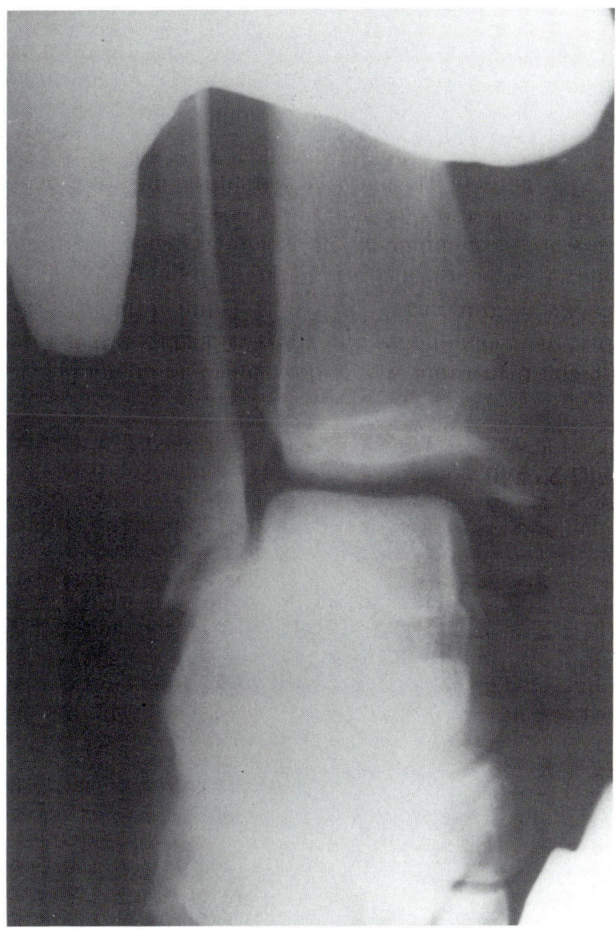

FIG 27–43.
Radiograph demonstrating widening of the medial clear space.

Stress Radiographs.—When routine x-ray findings are negative in the patient who is suspected of having a syndesmosis injury, stress radiographs with application of an external rotation and abduction force can expose an occult diastasis. Henning has recommended stress radiographs as standard practice for this injury.[435] Edwards and DeLee used the external rotation and abduction stress view to classify diastasis injuries into two varieties.[445] *Frank* diastasis is readily visible on routine radiographs, while *latent* diastasis is apparent only after stress. The authors used a difference of greater than 1 mm in the medial clear space when compared with the uninjured side as the determining figure. We prefer to use the same radiographic criteria as used on the unstressed radiograph as noted in the preceding paragraph. Because of the painful nature of this examina-

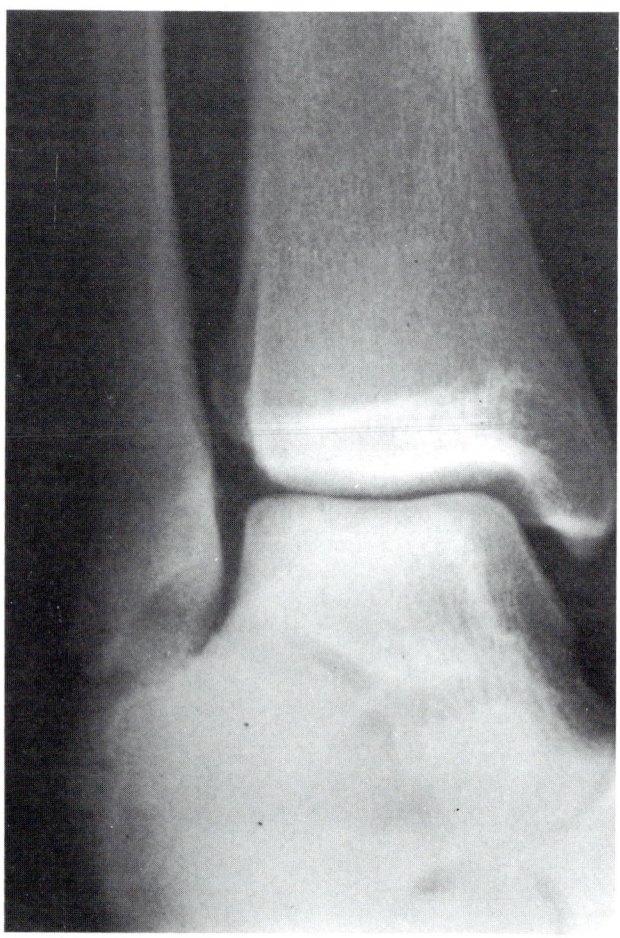

FIG 27–44.
Radiograph demonstrating widening of the tibiofibular clear space.

tion, it may be necessary to use some form of anesthesia such as a local or regional block.

Arthrography.—Up until the recent advances in diagnostic imaging, the most accurate study for visualizing injury to the syndesmosis has been arthrography of the ankle joint. The use of ankle arthrography to diagnose injury to the syndesmosis has been proved effective by several studies.[427, 431, 437, 455, 487] The method involves injection of radiographic contrast dye into the ankle joint away from the site of potential ligament injury. Routine x-ray studies are then performed to demonstrate leakage of dye superior to the plafond by greater than 1 cm at the syndesmosis. Berridge and Bonnin showed as early as 1944 that the use of this technique could disclose an isolated rupture of the tibiofibular ligaments at the syndesmosis.[431] Broström and coauthors reported on the use of arthrography to diagnose five such cases, which were all confirmed at surgery.[437] A sixth case confirmed at surgery had negative arthrography findings, but it was performed 8 days following the injury. This led the authors to conclude that the arthrogram would not be useful after a week from the date of injury. This time limitation has been refuted by Katznelson et al.[455] Although we have not used this method for diagnosing tibiofibular ligament injury, it has been used extensively in Europe and appears to be very sensitive.[427, 444, 449, 474, 487] One study of 2,020 arthrographies used for the diagnosis of acute diastasis without fracture found 114 positive arthrograms.[487] A comparison of arthrographic diagnoses with the intraoperative diagnoses revealed a sensitivity of 90% and a specificity of 67%.

Scintigraphy.—Ankle scintigraphy with ^{99m}Tc-pyrophosphate is another method for disclosing injury to the syndesmosis.[435, 454, 464] Trauma to these ligaments is reflected on the bone scan by localized uptake at the distal tibiofibular joint (Fig 27–45). Additional increased activity extends proximally along the lateral margin of the distal end of the tibia where the interosseous membrane attaches. In the only study of this technique, Marymont et al. compared ankle scintigraphy with stress radiographs in 27 athletes suspected of having ankle diastasis without fracture.[464] All 20 patients with positive stress test results were identified by positive bone scans as well. There were two cases of negative stress x-ray studies but positive scintigraphy. This study states that bone scintigraphy is 100% sensitive, 71% specific, and 93% accurate in the diagnosis of ankle diastasis without fracture. The advantages of scintigraphy are its noninvasive nature and freedom from pain. Disadvantages are the cost (although little different from that for an arthrogram) and the necessity for special equipment. Also, the reliability is unconfirmed and is probably sensitive to the familiarity of the diagnostician with the performance and interpretation of the study.

CAT Scan and MRI.—Recent advances in technology have improved the imaging techniques for bone and soft-tissue pathology. Their usefulness in the evaluation of foot and ankle pathology is still being defined.* The ability of these techniques to perform axial, sagittal, frontal, and three-dimensional imaging allows a more critical evaluation of the relationship between the tibia and the fibula at the ankle. Because of their expense and the requirement for specialized equipment and experienced interpretation, neither the CAT scan nor MRI are recommended as primary tests for the evaluation of diastasis. Nevertheless, both studies have been recommended for the diagnosis of diastasis without frac-

**References 443, 456, 458, 461, 481, 486.*

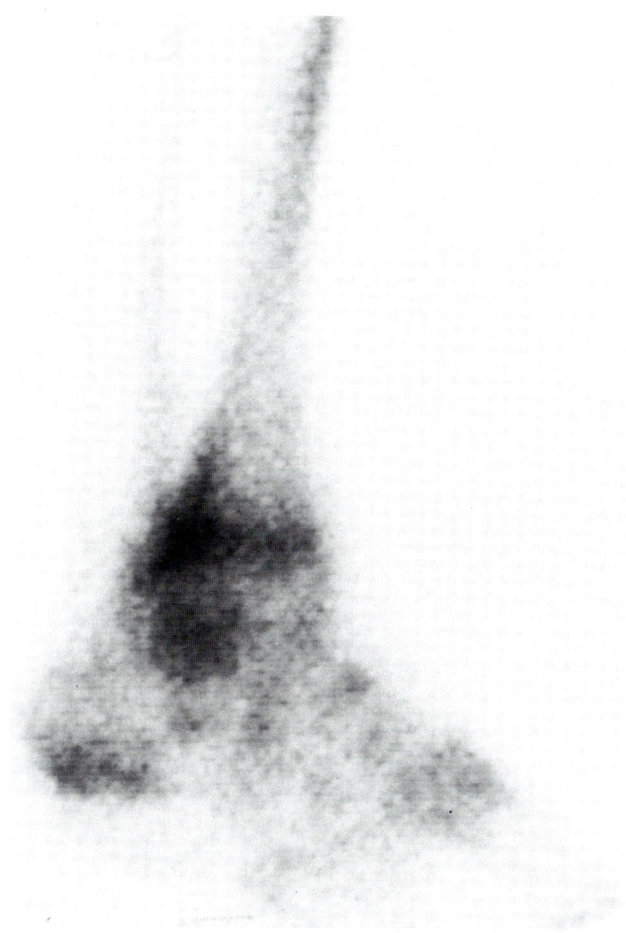

FIG 27–45.
Bone scintigraphy is useful in identifying occult injury to the syndesmosis. (Courtesy of John Marymont, M.D.)

ture.[443, 450] DenHartog and coworkers recently reported on the use of MRI in the evaluation of 44 patients with chronic ankle pain.[443] A widened syndesmosis was detected in 7%. The value of these techniques over other methods remains unclear pending further study.

Classification

Since several of the classification schemes depend upon radiologic evaluation, this seems the most appropriate place for discussing the classification of sprains and diastasis of the syndesmosis. First of all, it is necessary to classify the lesions as either acute or chronic since this has a bearing on treatment and the pathology to be encountered. It is also necessary to distinguish traumatic from congenital since the latter is an altogether different entity that presents in infancy in association with other skeletal abnormalities[434, 451, 478] Edwards and DeLee have classified diastasis without fracture into latent diastasis and frank diastasis.[445] The latent variety becomes obvious only after stress radiographs comparing injured and uninjured ankles following a normal routine radiograph of the injured ankle. Frank diastasis is apparent on the routine radiograph. They subdivide frank diastasis into four types based upon their experience and the cases in the literature (Table 27–6). Type I is frank diastasis with lateral subluxation of the fibula and no fibula fracture. Type II is similar, but close inspection of the x-ray film will disclose a plastic deformation in the fibula that prevents maintence of a reduction of the syndesmosis at surgery. Type III is a rare posterior rotary subluxation of the fibula where the fibula becomes displaced behind the tibia outside the incisura fibularis[459, 462, 485] (Fig 27–46). Type IV diastasis is equally rare, with superior dislocation of the talus wedging itself between the tibia and fibula without associated fibular fracture[467, 484] (Fig 27–47).

A classification system for the acute injury without frank diastasis or fracture was proposed by Marymont et al. based on the stress radiograph and scintigraphic results.[464] They classified patients with negative stress x-ray findings and negative scans as grade 0. Presumably these were patients with syndesmosis sprains on the basis of clinical examination but inappropriately diagnosed with diastasis by x-ray. Patients with positive scans but negative stress radiographs were classified as grade 1. Patients with positive scans and widening of the ankle mortise less than 1 mm in comparison to the uninjured ankle were considered grade 2, and widening

TABLE 27–6.
Classification of Syndesmosis Disorders*

- I. Congenital
- II. Acquired: Atraumatic (e.g., osteochondroma of the distal ends of the tibia or fibula near the syndesmosis)
- III. Acquired: Traumatic
  - A. Acute
    - 1. Sprain without diastasis
    - 2. Latent diastasis
    - 3. Frank diastasis
      - a. Lateral subluxation without fracture
      - b. Lateral subluxation with plastic deformation of the fibula
      - c. Posterior subluxation/dislocation of the fibula
      - d. Superior subluxation/dislocation of the talus into the mortise
  - B. Subacute (3 wk to 3 mo)
    - 1. Without tibiotalar arthritis
    - 2. With tibiotalar arthritis
  - C. Chronic (over 3 mo)
    - 1. Without tibiotalar arthritis
      - a. Without synostosis
      - b. With synostosis
    - 2. With tibiotalar arthritis

*Adapted from Edwards GS Jr, DeLee JC: *Foot Ankle* 4:305–312, 1984.

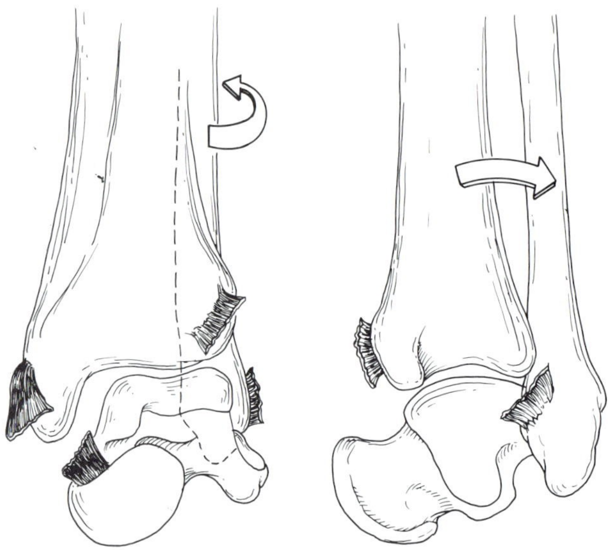

FIG 27–46.
Type III diastasis.

greater than 1 mm was grade 3. Since we do not believe that the technique used in stress radiographs allows accurate measurement down to a 1-mm difference and since treatment is identical for grade 1 and grade 2 injuries, we have eliminated the grade 2 category from our own classification scheme.

The authors' classification system is a modification of the above schemes. It is described in Table 27–6 and relates directly to treatment. Traumatic injuries are divided into those that present acutely, subacutely, and with a chronic condition. Acute injuries are divided into sprains without diastasis, sprains with latent diastasis, and sprains with frank diastasis on the basis of the clinical examination, routine radiographs, stress radiographs, and ankle scintigraphy. Traumatic injuries to the syndesmosis of greater than 3 weeks' duration are considered subacute disorders since the treatment and prognosis are altered. Finally, syndesmosis injuries present for 3 months or longer are considered chronic. The subacute and chronic categories are subdivided on the basis of arthritic changes in the tibiotalar joint, while chronic cases are further subdivided depending on the presence or absence of a synostosis.

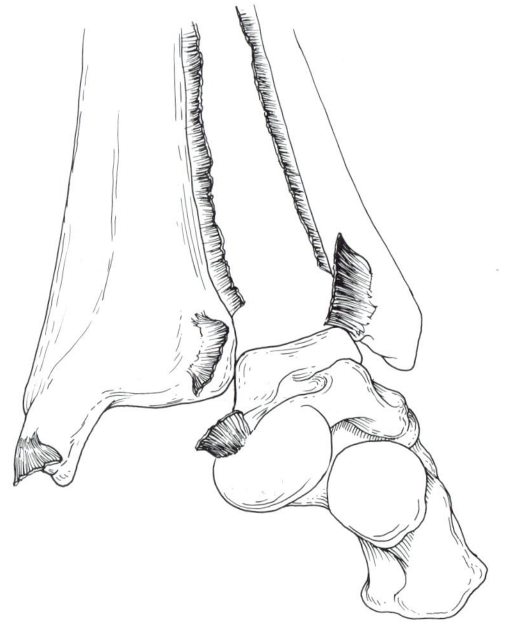

FIG 27–47.
Type IV diastasis.

Treatment

In the discussion to follow on the treatment of syndesmosis injuries, the reader is referred to Table 27–6, which describes the classification system utilized. Treatment will relate only to traumatic conditions, with congenital and acquired atraumatic problems receiving attention elsewhere. It should be kept in mind that there are few series dealing with the treatment of this entity, much less its separate subcategories.

Acute Injury

The ankle with an acute injury to the syndesmosis must be treated as quickly as possible while still arranging the necessary studies to allow proper diagnosis. The RICE formula of rest, ice, compression, and elevation is applied by using a splint, taping, and/or a brace, with crutch-walking during the immediate postinjury period.

Type 3.—If the clinical examination suggests a syndesmosis injury, routine radiographs are performed and analyzed by the criteria described previously. If frank diastasis without fracture is evident, the patient is taken to the operating room as soon as the soft-tissue condition allows (i.e., abrasions are allowed to heal before an open procedure is performed). Type 3c and 3d injuries have all been treated satisfactorily with closed reduction by longitudinal traction and cast immobilization according to the literature, except in a single report of an irreducible posterior dislocation of the fibula.[459, 462, 467, 484, 485] We would only suggest that postreduction radiographs be carefully analyzed and any persistent diastasis be treated by open reduction and internal fixation.

Type 3a and 3b injuries with frank diastasis and no apparent fracture of the fibula are both treated by surgical stabilization. This can be performed by any of the anesthetic methods with the patient in the supine position and a bolster under the ipsilateral hip.

Surgical Technique

1. The syndesmosis is approached through a straight longitudinal incision beginning directly over the midfibula approximately 3 cm above the tibial plafond. At the level of the plafond, the incision is curved slightly anteriorly.

2. The lateral branch of the superficial peroneal nerve often passes directly over the syndesmosis and must be sought out and protected during the exposure.

3. The distal tibiofibular joint is inspected after noting the tear in the AITF ligament. If there is an avulsion fragment from the anterior tubercle, it is evaluated to determine whether it is large enough to handle a screw without fragmenting. If so, a small cancellous screw with a soft-tissue washer is used to reattach the fragment.

4. Any ligamentous tissue or debris that is in the tibiofibular space is extracted, and a trial reduction is performed by pressing on the lateral aspect of the fibula.

5. If great force is necessary to achieve reduction or the reduction cannot be obtained, a medial incision is performed over the deltoid ligament to remove any interposed tissue blocking reduction. Sutures are placed but not tied.

6. A second attempt at reduction is then made. If the fibula can still not be reduced in the peroneal groove, the preoperative x-ray films are reevaluated to see whether a plastic deformation of the fibula might have been missed. When present, this deformation requires that an osteotomy of the fibula be performed prior to stabilization of the distal tibiofibular joint with a syndesmosis screw. Edwards and DeLee recommend that the osteotomy of the fibula be performed proximally due to instability of a distal osteotomy in the presence of damage to the interosseous membrane.[445]

7. Once anatomic reduction of the fibula in the groove is accomplished, a drill hole is made transversely from the posterolateral aspect of the fibula into the tibia with a slight anterior orientation. A fully threaded cortical screw is used to cross three cortices (Fig 27–48). A malleolar screw or fully threaded cancellous screw can be used as long as one is careful not to overtighten the screw through a lag effect. Fixation with the ankle in dorsiflexion helps to avoid this. Other fixation devices have been reported, but we have had no experience

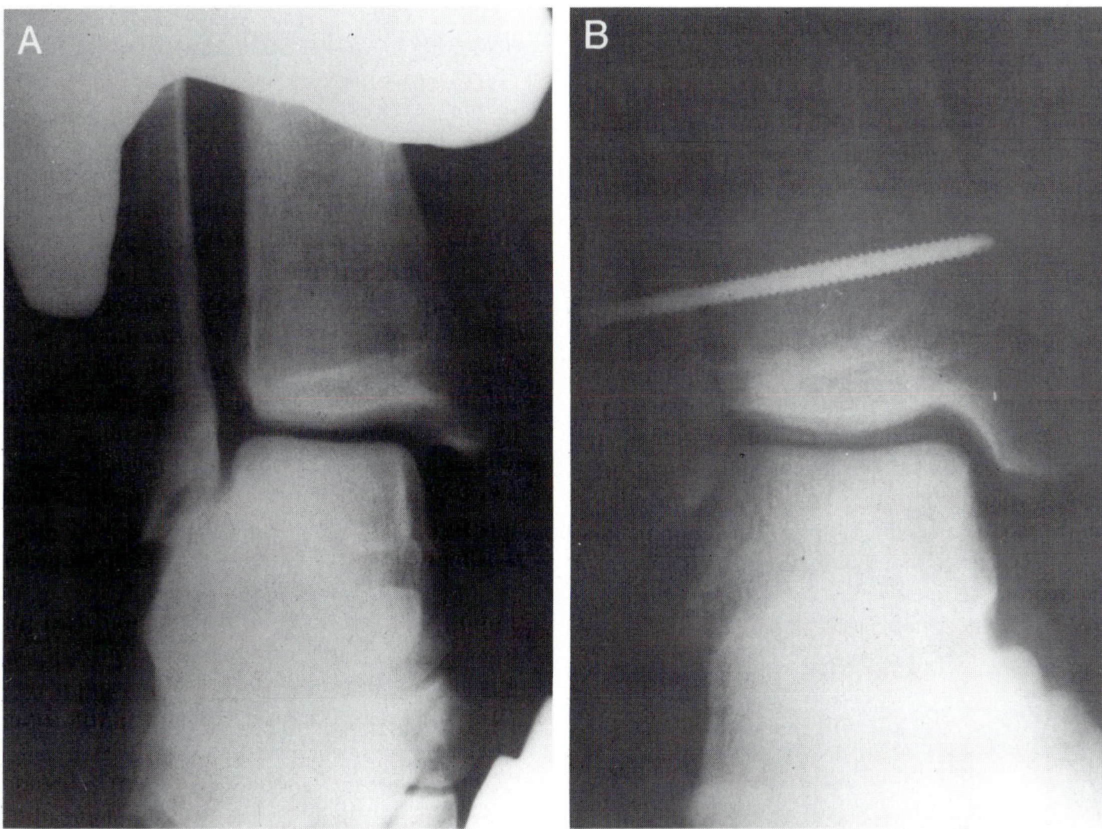

FIG 27–48.
Radiographs demonstrating treatment of a tibiofibular diastasis: **A,** preoperative; **B,** postoperative.

with their use.[426, 446, 447, 479] The transsyndesmotic screw works satisfactorily but does have certain disadvantages, such as the need for removal.[437]

8. Once the screw is in place, the previously placed deltoid sutures are tied (if a medial incision was necessary), and absorbable sutures are placed and tied in the AITF ligament.

9. The skin and subcutaneous tissues are closed in routine fashion, and a splint is applied.

Postoperative Care.—Postoperatively, the patient is kept non–weight bearing in a short-leg cast or walking boot for 4 weeks and started on partial weight bearing at that point. Full weight bearing is usually achieved by 6 weeks, and the screw is removed at 6 to 8 weeks. We have seen no difficulties from allowing this short period of full weight bearing with the screw in place. Immobilization is discontinued at 8 to 10 weeks, and the patient increases rehabilitation work in anticipation of returning to full activities, including sports, by 5 to 6 months postinjury.

Type 2.—Cases of type 2 syndesmosis injury with latent diastasis do not require surgery if the reduction of the fibula is anatomic in the incisura fibularis. Treatment is immobilization with a non–weight-bearing cast or brace for 4 weeks. A progressive increase in weight bearing is then allowed for an additional 2 to 4 weeks. Repeat weight-bearing x-ray films of the ankle should be taken at 2 to 3 weeks to confirm maintenance of the reduction.

Type 1.—Type 1 injuries are assumed to be stable. Treatment is symptomatic with weight bearing as tolerated. The importance of making the diagnosis of a syndesmosis sprain is as much informational as therapeutic. It allows proper counseling of the player and his coaches as to the expected length of disability and avoids unrealistic expectations as to a quick return to play. The West Point study reported a recovery time averaging 43 days for syndesmosis sprains without diastasis and barring reinjury (reinjury in 2 athletes increased the overall recovery time to 51 days).[454] It has also been our experience that syndesmosis injury almost doubles the time to return to play in comparison with a grade 3 lateral ankle sprain (Jackson's classification as noted in the previous section on lateral ankle sprains).

Subacute Injury

There is no guideline for the treatment of syndesmosis problems in the subacute period, although this is often the most perplexing presentation of this disorder. In the patient being evaluated for continued ankle pain following a "sprain," the examiner must always consider the possibility of a syndesmosis injury. Evaluation proceeds as noted previously. The presence of calcification in the interosseous membrane is indicative of a previous injury to the syndesmosis.[454]

If there is frank diastasis, then an assessment must be made of the degree of arthritic change in the tibiotalar joint. Since as little as 1 mm lateral displacement in the fibula has been shown to reduce the available tibiotalar contact area in weight bearing by 42%,[471] it is easy to understand why anatomic reduction is important and why a lack of anatomic reduction can lead to abnormal mechanics and resultant arthritis. If there is significant tibiotalar arthritis present, anything short of an ankle arthrodesis is of little benefit, so patients are treated nonoperatively until symptoms warrant arthrodesis.

If no arthritis is present, then the patient is treated surgically in an attempt to restore the normal relationship between the tibia and fibula. Exposure of both the medial portion of the ankle and the syndesmosis is usually required. The joints must be cleared of any interposed tissue blocking reduction. If the reduction can be achieved at this point with firm manual pressure on the tibia, then a syndesmosis screw is inserted as described previously and the remnants of the AITF ligament repaired.

If the ligaments are inadequate for late repair, a tendon graft can be taken from the plantaris or the extensor tendon to the third toe for creation of an anterior tibiofibular ligament. There is one report of using a Stryker Dacron ligament to reconstruct the syndesmotic ligaments in 11 patients. Results are reported as good with follow-up as long as 4 years.[430] The use of artificial ligaments in extra-articular locations has been successful in other locations and could be useful for this difficult reconstructive problem. The authors' personal preference is autogenous tissue.

If the reduction cannot be achieved with firm pressure and there is no evidence of plastic deformation of the fibula, then creation of an iatrogenic synostosis is a reasonable alternative.[455, 469] In this case, the adjacent surfaces of the tibia and fibula are roughened with an osteotome and/or a burr. A bone graft is taken from the medial portion of the tibia through a vertically oriented window, and the corticocancellous bone fragment is placed into a slot created between the tibia and fibula 1 cm above the plafond.[441] Cancellous bone is packed into the tibiofibular space above. While the tibiofibular synostosis can at times be symptomatic,[483] the symptoms are usually minimal, and the patient is improved from the preoperative condition.[455]

Chronic Injury

When diastasis has been present longer than 3 months, it is highly likely that significant arthritis has begun. In this case, arthrodesis of the tibiofibular joint may be necessary if symptoms are sufficiently severe. In those cases with diastasis but no significant arthritis of the tibiotalar joint, late reduction of the syndesmosis and reconstruction of the ligaments are advisable. If a synostosis is present and symptomatic, it can be taken down and an attempt made to reduce the diastasis prior to insertion of transfixing screws between the tibia and fibula. In this situation, two screws are usually warranted, and all four cortices are engaged. The screws are tightened with the ankle in full dorsiflexion to help avoid overtightening and loss of motion. Since the desired outcome is reduction of the diastasis, recurrence of a synostosis is not considered problematic as long as good reduction has been obtained. The presence of a partial or complete synostosis is compatible with high-level athletic performance.[483]

Results

Studies reporting the long-term results of treatment of acute or chronic diastasis of the ankle are notably few in number. The West Point series of patients with syndesmosis sprains, including one operatively treated diastasis, all returned to full duty without long-term problems and had full range of ankle motion.[454] The six cases of frank diastasis in Edward and DeLee's series had follow-up ranging from 4 months to 60 months.[445] There was one postoperative skin slough that healed uneventfully and one broken fixation device. Four patients had good results, and two patients with mild ankle pain and restriction in ankle motion had fair results. No results were given in the seven patients treated operatively in the series of Marymont et al.[464] In the ten patients with acute syndesmosis injury in Fritschy's report, three were treated surgically and seven with walking casts.[450] All returned to World Cup competition, but one patient had persistent pain and instability in the tibiofibular joint. Katznelson et al. reported on five patients with subacute or chronic syndesmosis injury.[455] All were treated by operative stabilization and a bone graft to the tibiofibular joint to create a synostosis. Fusion was achieved in all cases by 10 weeks, and there were no perioperative complications. One patient developed Sudeck's atrophy, which resolved after 6 months, but this patient continued to have mild loss of dorsiflexion. It appears that the properly selected patient has an excellent chance for good long-term function with appropriate treatment.

SUBTALAR SPRAINS

It is only in the past few years that considerable attention has been directed to the subtalar joint as an area of pathology in and of itself.[533] This is particularly the case for subtalar instability, which will be reviewed in this section. The matter of chronic lateral ligamentous instability of the ankle has been thoroughly described in the previous section. It was noted that some of the methods described for lateral reconstruction do not address subtalar instability. Since this is the case, it is important to recognize and direct specific treatment toward subtalar instability when it exists.

Historical Perspective

The clinical significance of subtalar instability was first suggested in 1962 by Rubin and Witten when they proposed a method for evaluation and diagnosis.[525] This radiographic method involved a stress tomogram of the subtalar joint from an AP projection whereby a tibiocalcaneal angle could be calculated. This method of evaluation was first used to actually diagnose subtalar instability in three patients by Brantigan et al. in 1977.[489] During this same time period, Laurin and coworkers proposed an alternative radiographic method of evaluation for subtalar instability and confirmed its legitimacy through cadaver ligament sectioning.[515] These studies provide the historical basis for evaluating subtalar instability, while the clinical study of Chrisman and Snook documented intraoperative subtalar instability in three of seven cases corrected by their tendon transfer procedure.[495] Clearly, in the patient presenting with symptoms of lateral ankle instability, it is difficult to distinguish from the history and physical examination alone where the underlying anatomic lesion is primarily located.

Anatomy

The section on lateral ligamentous instability has described the anatomy of this region in some detail. However, there are some specific anatomic features of the subtalar joint that are important in the understanding of subtalar sprains and instability. This is especially true since there has been some confusion over the soft-tissue anatomy of this region. The initial description of the ligamentous structures within the sinus tarsi and tarsal canal was provided by Wood Jones in 1944.[538] He used the terms "ligamentum frondiforme" for the tissue derived from the lateral stem of the inferior extensor retinaculum and "ligamentum cervicis" for the more medial ligament extending from the neck of the talus to the neck of the calcaneous. Other authors noted three ligamentous structures in this area, including a component derived from the retinacular tissues, the cervical ligament, and the more medial ligament of the tarsal canal.[494, 513, 529] More recently, Schmidt, Viladot et al., and Harper have contributed further to our understanding of the complicated anatomic features of this region.[505, 527, 536] Figure 27–49,A and B provide a visual representation of the most common anatomic pattern in this area, while Table 27–7 categorizes these tissues into superficial, intermediate, and deep layers.[505] Surgical reconstruction of the subtalar joint demands a thorough working knowledge of these features.

TABLE 27–7.
Lateral Ligamentous Support of the Subtalar Joint*

Superficial layer
Lateral root of the inferior extensor retinaculum
Lateral talocalcaneal ligament
Calcaneofibular ligament
Intermediate layer
Intermediate root of the inferior extensor retinaculum
Cervical ligament
Deep layer
Medial root of the inferior extensor retinaculum
Interosseous talocalcaneal ligament

*From Harper MC: *Foot Ankle* 11:354–358, 1991. Used by permission.

Diagnosis

Clinical Evaluation

Since the anatomic basis for subtalar instability has already been detailed in the preceding section, the patients' complaints and findings on physical examination will be described on that basis, as will the later section on reconstructive procedures. As mentioned, it is virtually impossible from the history alone to distinguish between tibiotalar and subtalar instability. Patients complain of frequent inversion mechanism sprains. The ankle "turns under" or "turns over" during the course of normal walking or running or during sports activities. The patients will often acknowledge that it is necessary to look at the surface when they are walking at night or that they are unable to walk comfortably on an irregular surface. Those runners who have this problem generally will not run at night. There may be lateral pain in the area of the sinus tarsi, and there appears to be some overlap of subtalar instability with sinus tarsi syndrome. When the instability problem becomes severe, it is not unusual to see patients develop a dependency on ankle supports, braces, or constant visual cueing.

The physical examination varies slightly from the patient with tibiotalar instability, and it must be recognized that the two conditions of tibiotalar and subtalar instability may coexist (Fig 27–50). Increased inversion and/or internal rotation of the subtalar joint is the prerequisite finding on physical examination, but it is extremely difficult to fully appreciate this at times, even in the hands of an experienced examiner. While the radiographic technique to be described assesses subtalar tilt or gapping between the posterior facets of the talus and the calcaneus, the finding at surgery is more one of excessive gliding of the calcaneus on the talus into a

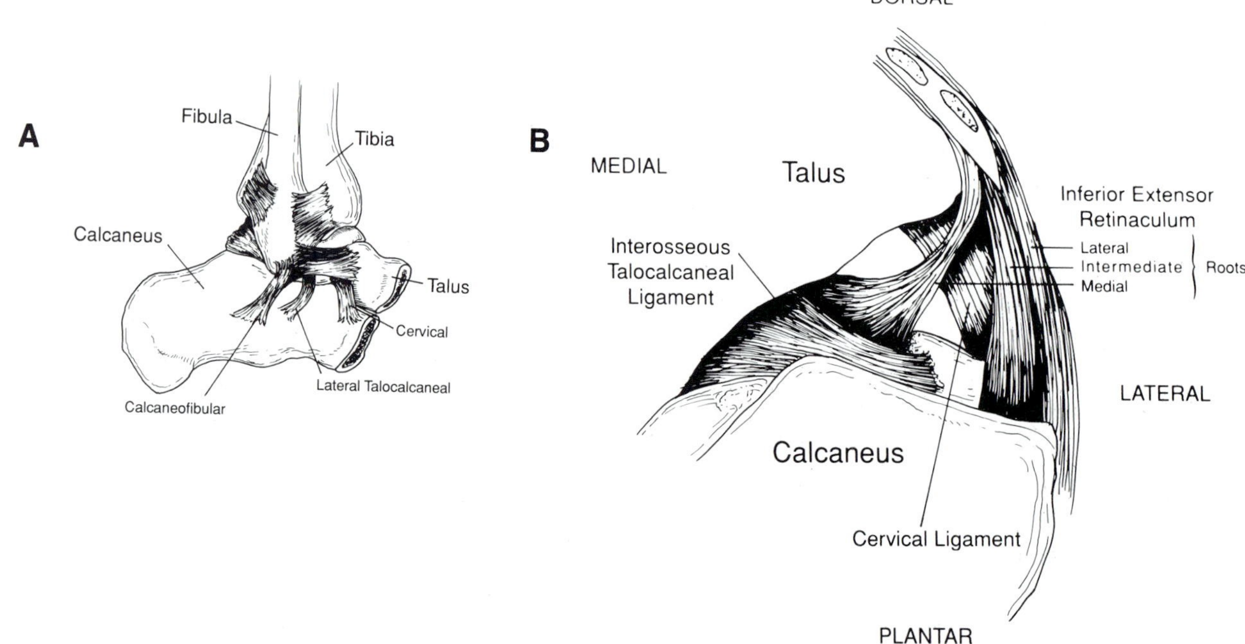

FIG 27–49.
A and **B**, drawings depicting the anatomy of the subtalar joint.

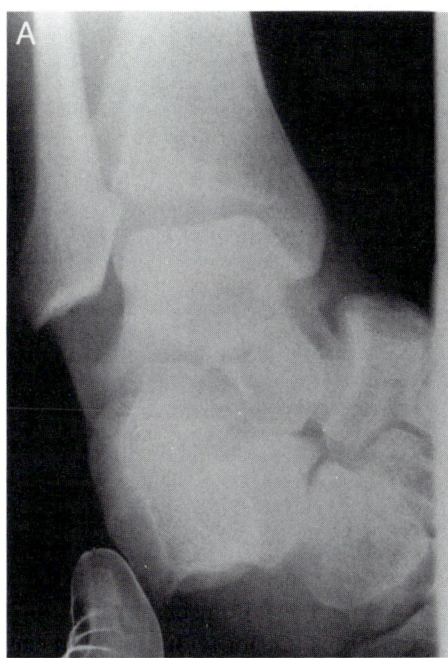

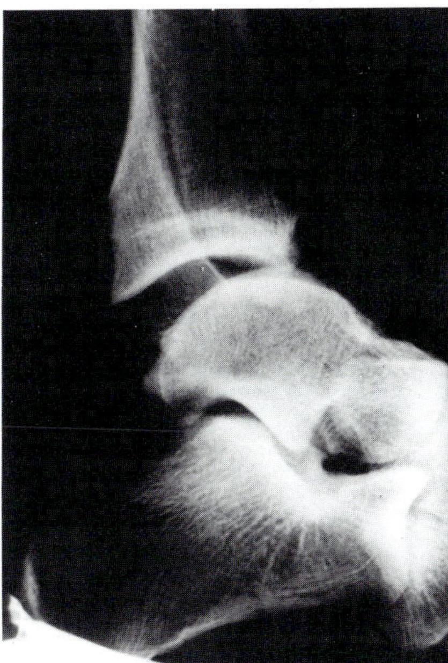

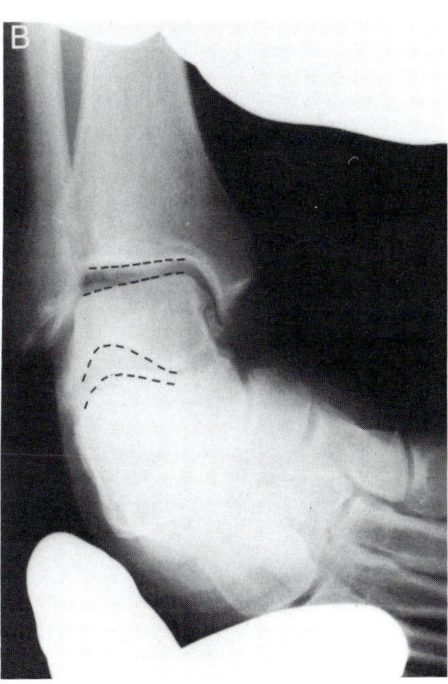

FIG 27–50.
Stress x-ray films demonstrating tibiotalar and subtalar instability. **A,** College athlete with combined instability: **1,** AP talar/subtalar stress radiograph; **2,** lateral anterior drawer stress radiograph. **B,** former athlete with chronic changes and combined instability. While the individual talar or subtalar tilt may not be impressively large, taken together they represent significant varus instability.

more distal and internally rotated position. A comparison with the normal side is efficacious, but must be done with the understanding that there may be excessive movement that is asymptomatic.

Radiographic Evaluation

Standard AP x-ray studies are always performed to rule out any underlying bony abnormality such as a loose body, osteochondrosis, or arthrosis. The patient with subtalar instability rarely has any significant findings on the routine radiographs.

Stress Radiographs.—Stress radiographs of the tibiotalar joint have been discussed under the topic of lateral ankle ligament instability and are performed as part of the evaluation of a patient with lateral ankle complex instability symptoms. If one is careful with hand placement or uses a holding device that is nonradiopaque, it is possible to visualize the talocalcaneal joint simultaneously with the tibiotalar joint.[497, 498] For the anterior drawer stress test, there is no need to alter the normal technique to allow good visualization of both joints. However, with the traditional AP stress test in order to look at the tibiotalar joint for divergence in the articular surface at the ankle, it is necessary to use additional technique in order to penetrate the dense bone of the hindfoot and allow adequate exposure of the posterior facets of the talocalcaneal joint. In the stable situation there is close congruity of the surfaces of the talus and calcaneus (Fig 27–51,A). In the unstable situation, there is a separation of these surfaces of 3 mm or more (Fig 27–51,B). The laterally viewed anterior drawer stress test can show translation of the calcaneus on the talus in addition to translation of the talus on the tibia. Figures 27–50,A and 27–52) demonstrate the normal and abnormal translation seen with subtalar instability.

In the situation where one is specifically looking for subtalar instability or documenting its existence radiographically, the best view is a combination of the method described by Laurin and colleagues and that of Brodén used in evaluating the degree of joint involvement in calcaneal fractures.[490, 515] This method, with minor modifications, has been used by several investigators to document subtalar instability.[496, 506, 507, 542]

The radiographic method that I employ is a 40-degree Brodén (projection I) view with inversion stress applied to to the calcaneus and fifth metatarsal head laterally while stabilizing the distal end of the tibia (Fig 27–53). This method directly visualizes the posterior facets of the subtalar joint, which are parallel in normal circumstances. Laurin et al. hypothesized that any loss of parallelism is diagnostic of subtalar instability[515] (Fig 27–54,A). Heilman and coworkers used a 5-mm separation between the talus and calcaneous as the diagnostic

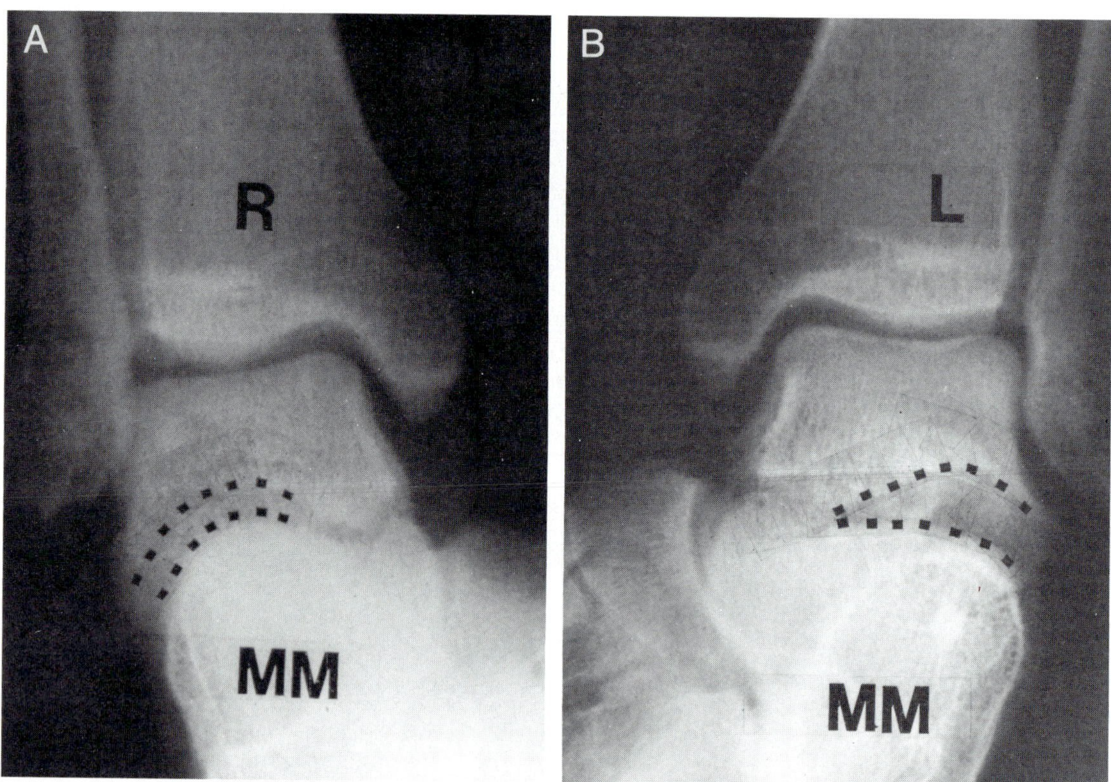

FIG 27–51.
A, stress radiograph demonstrating normal subtalar stability with parallelism of the posterior facets. **B,** stress radiograph demonstrating over 3 mm separation of the posterior facets in subtalar instability.

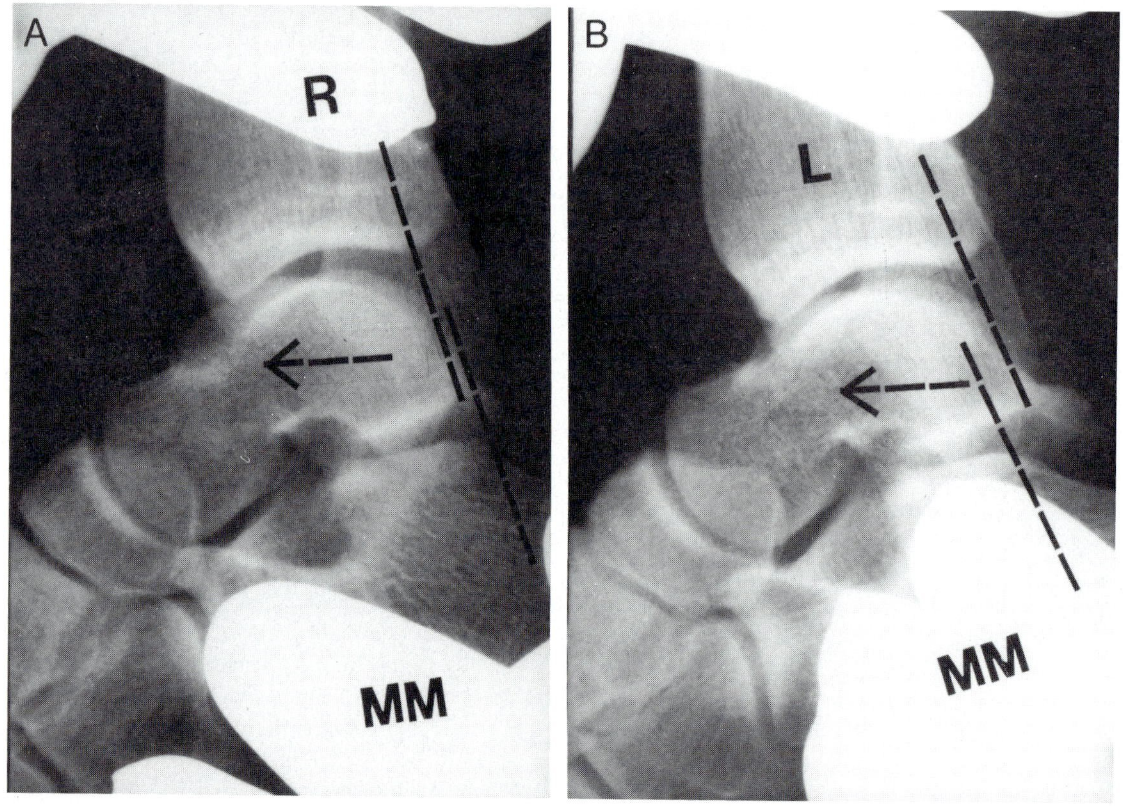

FIG 27–52.
Radiograph demonstrating the appearance of the subtalar joint with anterior drawer stress: **A,** normal; **B,** abnormal.

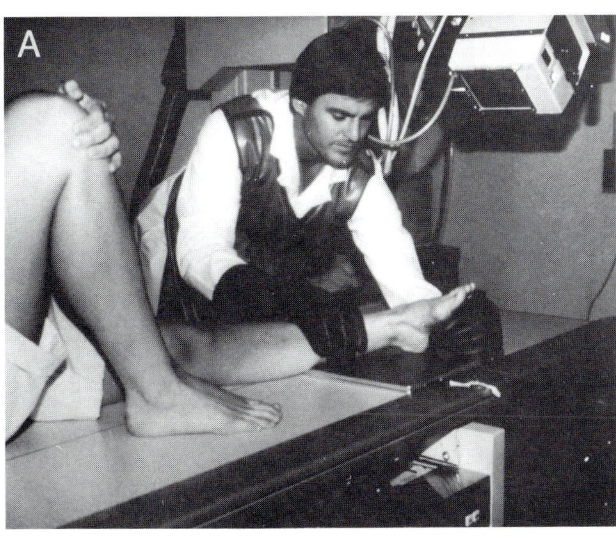
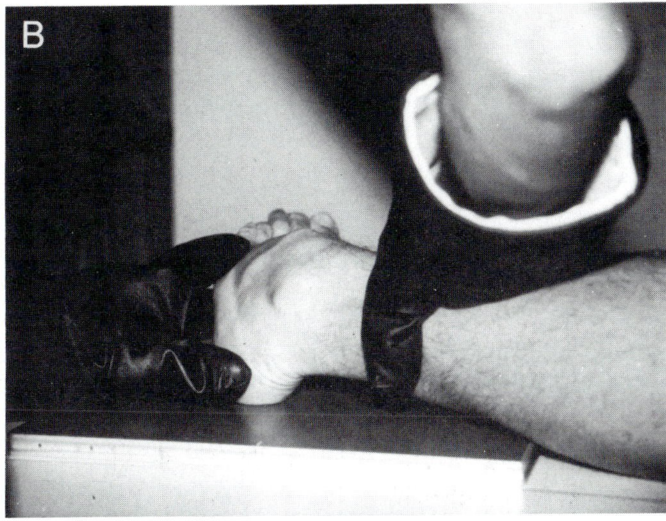

FIG 27–53.
Method of performing the stress Brodén view to visualize subtalar instability. **A,** the radiographic beam is tilted 40 degrees toward the head and directed at the sinus tarsi. **B,** method of applying varus stress to allow visualization of both the tibiotalar and subtalar joints (From Clayton TO: *Orthop Clin North Am* 20:583–592, 1989. Used by permission.)

cutoff.[507] My own experience is that parallelism is the norm, but I do not consider the stress Brodén view to be diagnostic of subtalar instability until the separation is over 3 degrees (Fig 27–54,B). While this is a very small angle, it is consistent with the small increments of increased movement noted in the experimental work of Kjaersgaard-Anderson and coworkers.[510, 512]

Stress Tomography.—The original method described for radiographic confirmation of subtalar instability was the tomographic technique of Rubin and Witten.[525] A special foot-holding device is required, and the patient must remain in this position while the tomograms are being completed. This can be somewhat time-consuming and uncomfortable—just two of the reasons why

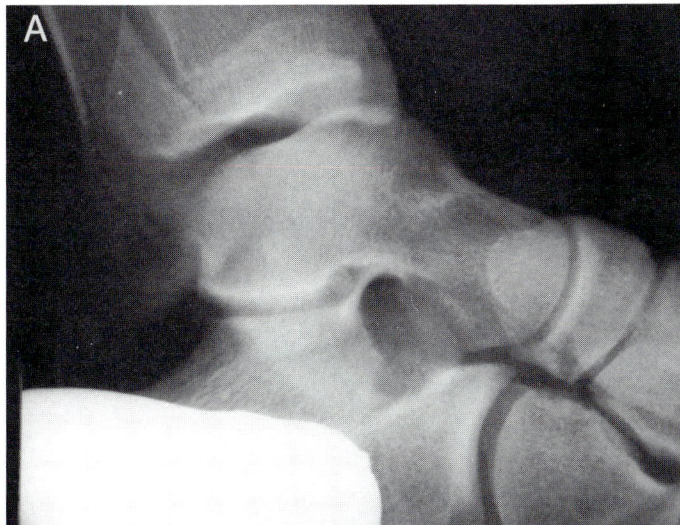
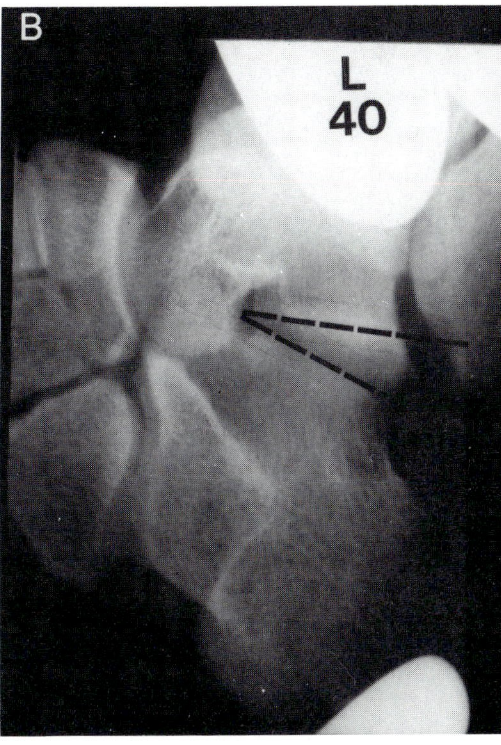

FIG 27–54.
Stress Brodén radiograph. **A,** the normal side shows parallelism of the posterior facets. **B,** the abnormal side shows varus tilt of the posterior facets.

we do not advocate this method. Nevertheless, it has been used by others with success[489, 540] (Fig 27–55). The original method called for calculation of a tibiocalcaneal angle, which was normally between 40 and 50 degrees.[525] Brantigan et al. used 38 ± 6 degrees as the norm.[489] Due to the difficulty of precisely defining the landmarks, this angle does not appear to be reproducible.

Other Evaluative Techniques.—Other techniques have been described for visualization of the subtalar joint and its pathology. These include fluoroscopy,[539] subtalar arthrography,[515, 520–522, 534] and a combination of the two with or without stress.[497] The arthrographic technique is fully described under the section on sinus tarsi syndrome, while the stress arthrogram with an image intensifier is shown in Figure 27–56.

Treatment

Historical Perspective

There has been very little written on the treatment of subtalar instability because it has been a poorly defined entity in the past. Although Rubin and Witten described the tomographic criteria for diagnosing this instability, they had no cases that they treated.[525] Brantigan et al. diagnosed three patients by the tomographic method but treated two by triple arthrodesis because of advanced arthritic changes.[489] It was Chrisman and Snook who noted satisfactory stabilization of subtalar instability in three of their seven patients with ankle instability treated by a modification of the Elmslie procedure.[495] This tendon transfer reconstructs both the anterior talofibular and calcaneofibular ligaments, effectively limiting subtalar motion. The Watson-Jones procedure has also been used for

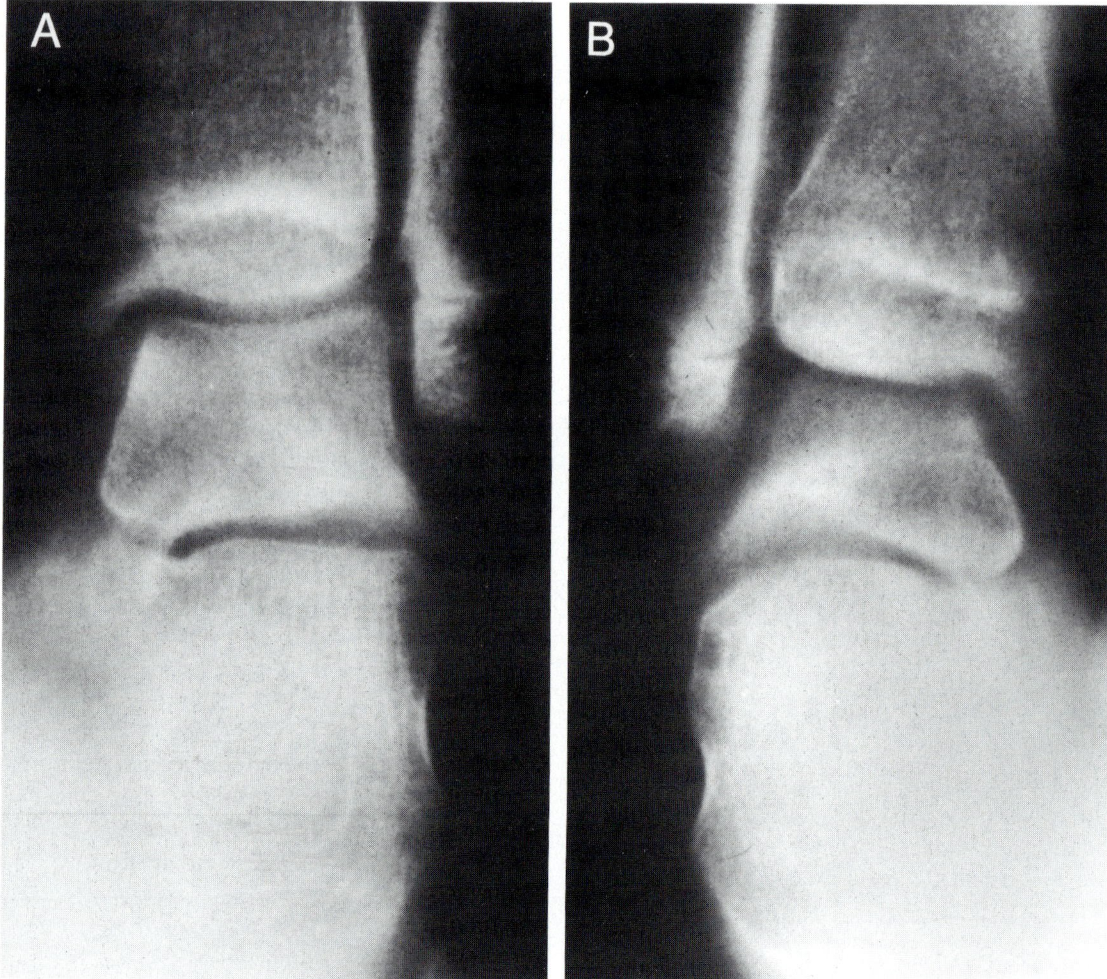

FIG 27–55.
Stress tomograms of the subtalar joint: **A,** normal side; **B,** abnormal side. (From Zollinger H, Meier CH, Waldis M: Diagnostik der Unteren Sprunggelenksinstabilitat Mittels Stress-Tomographie (Diagnosis of subtalar instability utilizing stress tomography). In *Hefte zur Unfallheilkunde,* Heft 165. Heidelberg, Springer-Verlag, 1983, pp 175–177. Used by permission.)

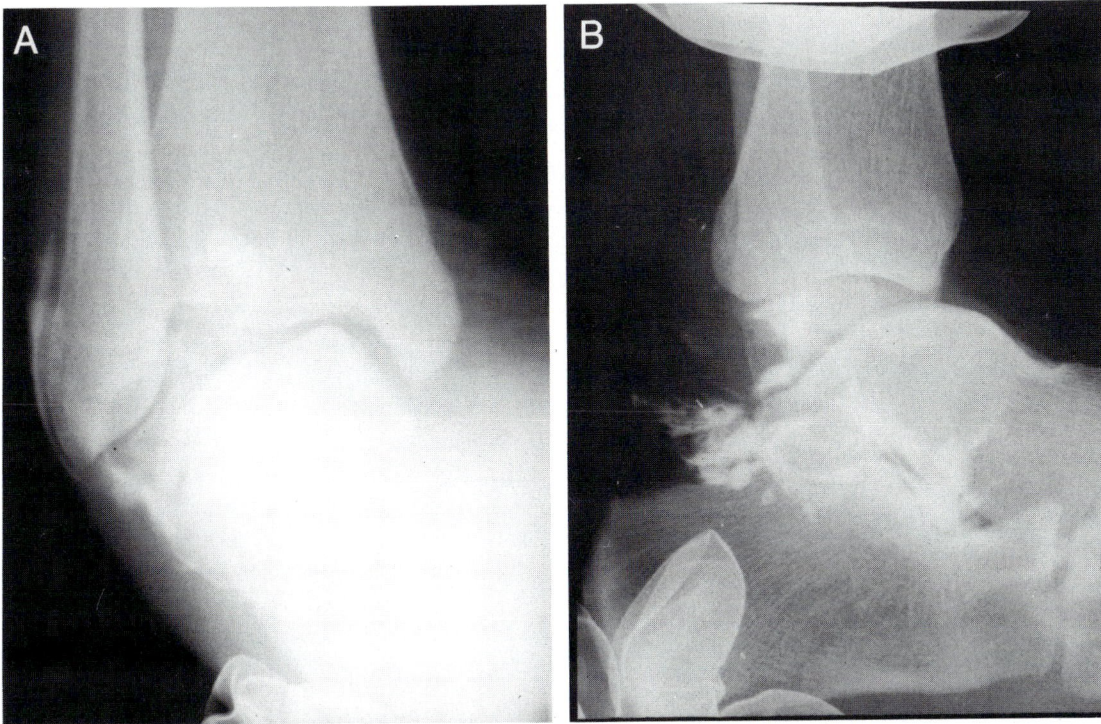

FIG 27–56.
Stress arthrogram in an acute injury to the anterior talofibular and calcaneofibular ligaments. Contrast dye injected into the subtalar joint communicates with the ankle joint and extravasates out the capsule. **A,** AP view; **B,** lateral view.

lateral ankle instability but does not correct subtalar instability.[537] Therefore, it is critical to understand the underlying pathology before proceeding with a reconstruction.

Acute vs. Chronic Treatment

In the discussion of treatment for subtalar instability it is important to differentiate between the acute and the chronic situation. An acute injury to the subtalar joint rarely warrants surgical intervention, while a chronic condition with instability often requires surgical stabilization. The only study dealing specifically with acute subtalar sprains and advocating surgical management is that of Meyer et al.[520, 521] They reported in 1988 on a group of 40 patients evaluated by talar tilt and anterior drawer stress x-ray films and subtalar arthrography following an acute inversion mechanism injury to the ankle. Leakage of contrast dye from subtalar arthrography in 32 of these patients led them to form two groups of patients with four injury patterns in the group with dye leakage. Although the pathology was confirmed surgically in only 12 patients, the study does support the relationship between inversion mechanism ankle sprains and subtalar instability. Furthermore, the study correlates well with the experimental work done on cadavers.[499, 515, 517]

While it is clear from this work that the supporting structures of the subtalar joint can be damaged through the same mechanism as the lateral ligaments of the ankle, it is seldom necessary to specifically treat the subtalar pathology in an acute situation. As previously discussed, there is still considerable controversy over the role of surgery in acute injury to the lateral ligaments of the ankle. It is obvious from the work of Drez et al. and Smith and Reischl that the majority of these patients respond well to immobilization with the ankle in dorsiflexion.[500, 530] By extrapolation from this, it can be assumed that their subtalar pathology is also addressed adequately by this method.

Nonoperative Treatment

Although the acute situation does not call for surgical intervention, the patient with chronic instability symptoms frequently requires surgical stabilization. Nevertheless, the treatment is initially nonoperative and is similar in many ways to the treatment for typical lateral ligamentous instability of the ankle, including peroneal strengthening, proprioceptive training, Achilles stretching, and use of a brace. All of these methods have an effect on inversion of the foot through the subtalar joint and are therefore just as effective for the subtalar joint sprain as for the more common ankle sprain. Interestingly, there has been little specific research of a basic science or clinical nature directed to the actual results obtained with therapeutic modalities such as these.

This paucity of supportive research is particularly true in the area of bracing of the ankle, where countless varieties of ankle braces exist, but there is little experimental work documenting their adequacy with regard to restricting motion of the ankle joint (much less the subtalar joint). We have had experience with most of these braces and found by personal experience that, of the braces that have been available for some time, the Aircast and its variations seem to provide the greatest degree of stability. Unfortunately, they are cumbersome for athletic participation (Fig 27–57). The canvass and lace braces (e.g., Swede-O) and the neoprene and nylon braces with Velcro straps (e.g., Kallassey) seem to provide less stability with correspondingly less inhibition of performance and a minimum of bulkiness (Fig 27–58). Without any supportive laboratory data to back it up, it is our opinion that the latter category of braces provides a similar order of stability as taping done by a skilled athletic trainer with a traditional method. A promising new brace for ankle and subtalar instability incorporates a heat-moldable heel cup and foot piece to allow it to hold the subtalar joint in a neutral position or one of slight heel valgus (Fig 27–59). Empirically one would think that this would provide a greater degree of control to the subtalar joint. In our limited experience with it, the brace has been effective but has required several adjustments before providing a comfortable fit.

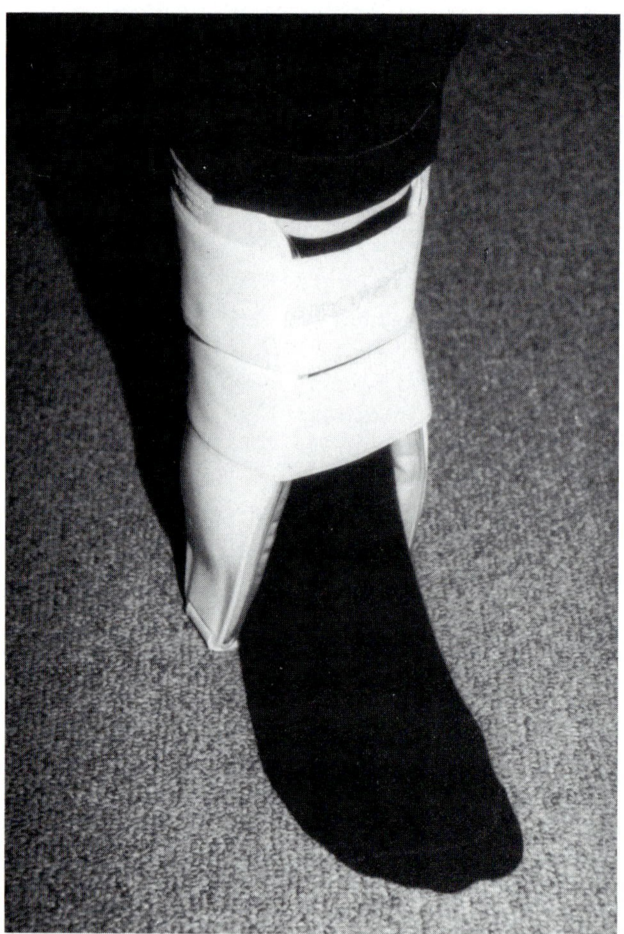

FIG 27–57.
Aircast ankle brace.

Surgical Treatment

If the patient fails to respond to nonoperative treatment or is intolerant of bracing, then operative treatment becomes the logical alternative. Since the reconstructive alternatives for lateral ankle instability have been discussed previously, this section will look specifically at reconstructions appropriate to the subtalar joint. Remember that the calcaneofibular ligament plays a crucial role in both the tibiotalar and talocalcaneal joints. Lesser degrees of instability result from isolated injury to the lateral talocalcaneal and/or the cervical ligaments. Most of the reconstructive procedures described include a reconstruction of the calcaneofibular ligament, e.g., Chrisman-Snook or Larsen procedures.[495, 514] An isolated reconstruction of the cervical ligament has been described without any documentation of results.[528] Our experience has been that the majority of individuals who present with subtalar instability requiring surgical treatment call for a procedure that addresses both the cervical and calcaneofibular ligaments.

Secondary Anatomic Repair.—Anatomic reconstruction of stabilizing structures has become the standard in both the shoulder for anterior instability and the knee for anterior cruciate ligament insufficiency. Anatomic reconstruction of the lateral ligaments of the ankle was described over 25 years ago by Broström and is a very simple and reliable method for treating chronic lateral ankle instability.[491, 502, 503, 508] The method is capable of correcting subtalar instability only if the calcaneofibular ligament is isolated and imbricated along with anterior talofibular ligament imbrication. In addition, it is efficacious to use the inferior extensor retinaculum through its connections into the subtalar joint to further tighten this joint and restrict inversion. The abundance of elastic fibers within the retinacular tissue and the variable location and degree of the pathology to the calcaneofibular ligament make this form of delayed primary reconstruction a less useful method when the stability problem is marked and particularly when it is isolated to the subtalar joint.

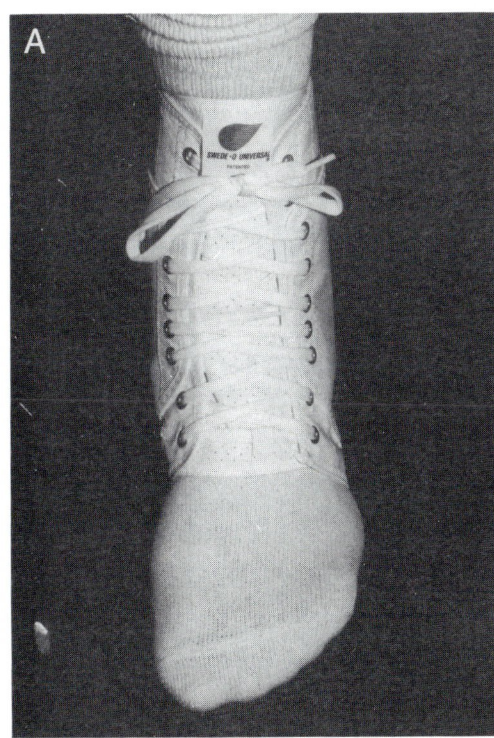

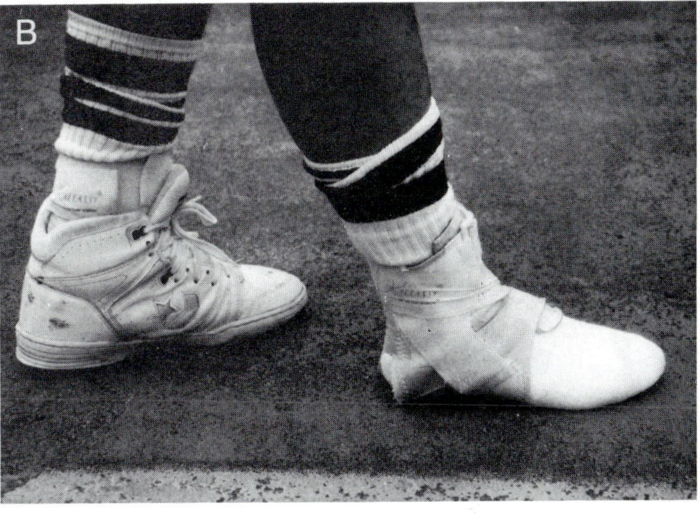

FIG 27–58.
Ankle braces: **A,** Swede-O; **B,** Kallassey.

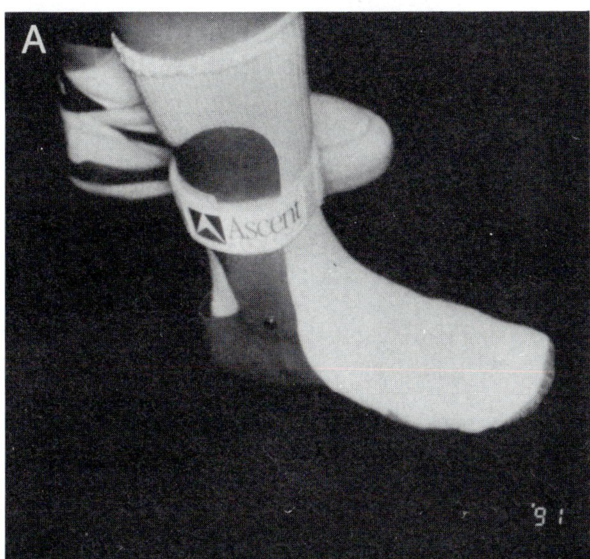

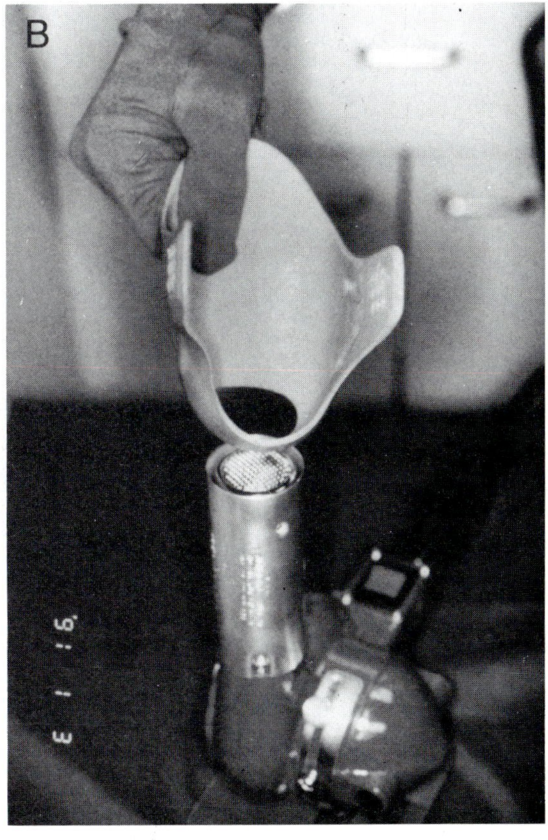

FIG 27–59.
A and **B,** ascent brace incorporating a thermomoldable heel cup.

Reconstructive Procedures.—The procedures that have the best history for stabilizing the subtalar joint are those that use a tendon graft or transfer to reconstruct the lateral ligaments. Elmslie's original procedure for the ankle joint described in 1934, used a strip of fascia lata placed through drill holes in the distal end of the fibula, talus, and calcaneus to recreate the calcaneofibular and anterior talofibular ligaments.[501] Most of the procedures subsequently described for instability of the subtalar joint or for the combination of subtalar and ankle joint instability have used a modification of the Elmslie procedure.[498, 528] Chrisman and Snook split the peroneus brevis and reconstructed the anterior talofibular and calcaneofibular ligaments with effective correction of subtalar instability in three of their seven patients who had this pattern of instability.[495] Others have described using half or all of the peroneus brevis, the plantaris tendon, or a portion of the Achilles tendon.*

There are certain technical points that are critical to the outcome of any of these procedures. These procedures are primarily designed to stabilize the lateral aspect of the ankle and subtalar joints against excessive inversion stress in the young, healthy athletic patient. It should be obvious that the procedure will not correct symptomatology that is derived from other sources such as anterior tibiotalar impingement, tears of the peroneal tendons (unless they are recognized and addressed simultaneously),[526] or significant arthrosis involving either the ankle, subtalar joint, or both. From a technical standpoint, it is helpful to place a bolster under the ipsilateral hip or to place the patient on his side to facilitate exposure of the lateral area of the ankle. Regardless of the reconstructive method, it is imperative to (1) handle the soft tissues delicately, (2) avoid injury to the sural nerve and the lateral branch of the superficial peroneal nerve, and (3) avoid overtensioning the graft or transfer and thereby "capturing" the subtalar joint, effectively eliminating all inversion. Symptoms arising from problems created by failures in any of these areas can negate any beneficial results from the reconstruction.

Authors' Surgical Technique.—The different forms of the modified Elmslie procedure are pictured in Figure 27–60. When correcting symptomatic subtalar instability, we prefer to use a modification of the Chrisman-Snook procedure that we have previously described as a triligamentous reconstruction.[528]:

*References 498, 514, 516, 528, 531, 532, 535, 541.

1. A lateral incision is made just posterior to the fibula beginning approximately 10 to 15 cm proximal to the tip of the fibula. (The incision parallels the course of the peroneal tendons and extends to just proximal and dorsal to the base of the fifth metatarsal).
2. The incision is carried sharply down to the tendon sheath, and flaps are created to allow exposure of the anterior lateral ankle joint and sinus tarsi region.
3. Care is taken to avoid the lateral branch of the superficial peroneal nerve at the anterolateral aspect of the ankle and the sural nerve as it crosses superficial to the peroneal tendons at the lateral hindfoot. (With appropriate incision placement, the sural nerve is kept protected in the inferior soft tissues on the plantar side of the incision).

The surgical procedure is similar to what has been described earlier, except that the dissection is carried more distally and the flexor digitorum brevis and inferior extensor retinaculum are reflected up out of the sinus tarsi.

4. Exposure must include the distal lateral calcaneus (where the first drill hole enters), the location of the cervical ligament insertion in the sinus tarsi (where the drill hole exits from the lateral calcaneus), the lateral ridge of the talus including the site of insertion of the anterior talofibular ligament on the talus (where the

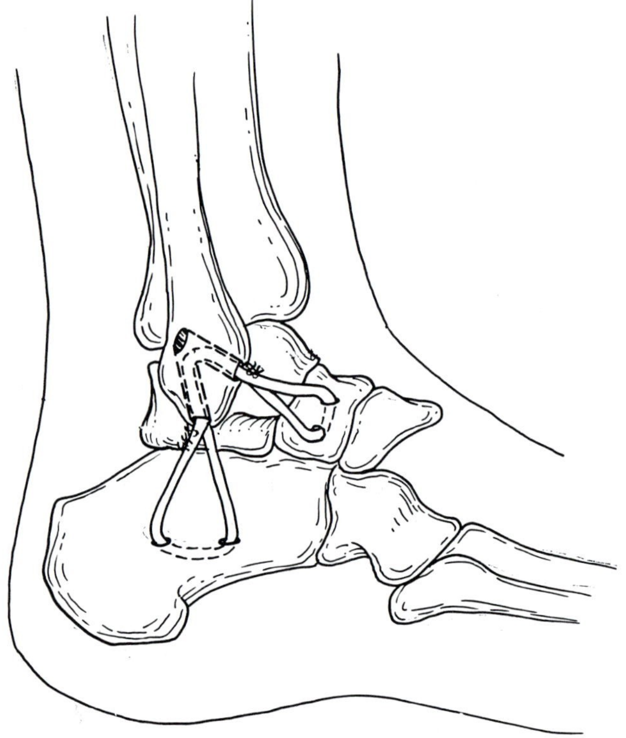

FIG 27–60.
Elmslie procedure and its modifications.

next drill hole is made to enter the sinus tarsi at the origin of the cervical ligament on the undersurface of the talar neck), the distal end of the fibula (where drill holes are made from the posterior portion of the fibula to the anterior attachment of the anterior talofibular ligament and from this same posterior hole to the tip of the fibula where the calcaneofibular ligament originates), and the lateral calcaneus under the peroneal tendons (where the calcaneofibular ligament inserts) (Figs 27–61 and 27–62).

5. The tendon transfer or graft may be anchored by one of several available methods. The sutures in the tendon can be passed through a bony tunnel in the calcaneus into which the tendon end is pulled and the sutures tied over a button-and-felt anchor on the skin of the plantar heel. (This is the least favorable method due to potential skin necrosis and the requirement for relatively rigid long-term immobilization.) If the tendon transfer or graft is of sufficient length, it can be passed through a bony tunnel in the lateral calcaneus and sutured back to itself at the entrance into the first tunnel.

6. Alternatively, the tendon can be sutured back on to itself at the calcaneal tunnel or into surrounding periosteum. Other methods are to anchor the tendon in a bony trough in the lateral calcaneus with a staple or to use a Mitek or Statak anchor.[498, 516, 528]

7. The basis for this procedure is an anatomic creation of ligamentous stability for the subtalar joint by using the tendon graft or transfer to rebuild the cervical ligament and the calcaneofibular ligament. Tensioning is done to allow some subtalar inversion (approximately 10 to 15 degrees).

Postoperative Care.—The patient is splinted in neutral dorsiflexion and neutral to slight subtalar eversion

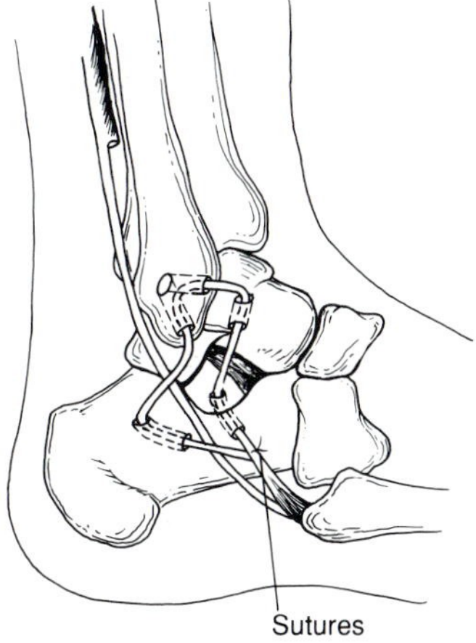

FIG 27–61.
Illustration of the technique for triligamentous reconstruction of subtalar instability.

postoperatively. When the splint is changed at 7 to 10 days, the patient is placed into a removable short-leg brace if he is relatively reliable, and limited dorsiflexion movement is started along with full weight bearing. At 3 weeks the patient begins active dorsiflexion and plantar flexion with limited inversion and eversion. At 6 weeks the patient is placed into an Aircast or similar brace, and strengthening exercises and functional activities are instituted. Patients return to sports at 3 to 6 months depending on their progression through this latter phase of therapy.

Other Considerations.—Kelikian, Mann, and Hanson as well as Brunner and Gaechter have all described the use of the plantaris tendon to anatomically reconstruct the lateral ankle ligaments as a preferred method in order to avoid sacrificing a peroneal tendon.[493, 504, 509, 518] We have previously described the use of this method for a triligamentous reconstruction of subtalar instability.[528] Those using this method must be prepared for the absence of this tendon (the case for approximately 7% of the population). Furthermore, it is critical to have a knowledge of the anatomy since it can be difficult to locate in the leg. Extra medial incisions are occasionally required if the tendon stripper meets obstacles. Excessive force with the stripper can rupture the tendon. At times the tendon is quite small and fragile, which makes it inadequate for this type of reconstruction. Several additional incisions are necessary for this method, thus making it a less cosmetic procedure—an important consideration for certain patients. It is difficult to harvest the plantaris tendon under ankle block anesthesia with a calf tourniquet. Despite these considerations, the plantaris tendon is useful since it does not sacrifice an important structure such as the peroneus brevis tendon, nor does it have the potential for compromising function to the degree that transferring this tendon might. Brunner and Gaechter reviewed 52 ankle ligament reconstructions performed with the plantaris tendon and found results that were quite favorable in comparison to the 128 peroneal tendon transfers that they reviewed simultaneously.[493] They mention the usefulness of the plantaris for subtalar instability symptoms, but their described technique reconstructs only the anterior talofibular and calcaneofibular ligaments.

Results

Since subtalar instability has been infrequently recognized except at the time of surgery for chronic lateral ligamentous instability of the ankle, there are limited reports of results, and most are commingled with results of lateral ankle instability procedures. Chrisman and Snook had three patients with subtalar as well as ankle instability treated by their method.[495] One case was a failed prior Watson-Jones procedure with persistent instability symptoms. The three cases of subtalar instability had 20-degree limitation of inversion in comparison to their normal side and no symptoms of instability at follow-up ranging from 2 years to 6 years from the date of surgery. Vidal used the modified Chrisman-Snook procedure on two patients with combined tibiotalar and subtalar instability and four patients with isolated subtalar instability and had satisfactory results in all six.[535] Zwipp and Krettek reported 17 patients with isolated subtalar instability who were successfully treated with a modified Chrisman-Snook technique.[541] Larsen used the entire peroneus brevis tendon to rebuild the lateral ligaments of the ankle in 73 patients (79 ankles).[514] There were 25 cases of combined subtalar instability. All patients resumed normal activity including sports, with only 9 complications in the 79 operations (11%). These complications included 2 patients with deep venous thrombosis who recovered uneventfully, 4 cases of fifth-toe hypesthesia, painful calcification at a lateral malleolar drill hole site in 1 patient (requiring reoperation for removal of the calcification), 1 superficial infection, and 1 dysesthetic scar. Zell and his coauthors reported a single case of combined ankle and subtalar instability treated with the Chrisman-Snook operation, with the patient capable of running and jumping and free of instability at the 2-year follow-up.[539]

Our own results have been equally as good in correcting this form of instability with the triligamentous reconstruction described in 1990.[497] It is a modification of the Chrisman-Snook procedure designed to address combined tibiotalar and subtalar instability. We have also found it to be the most reliable method for isolated subtalar instability. Among the 15 patients who were

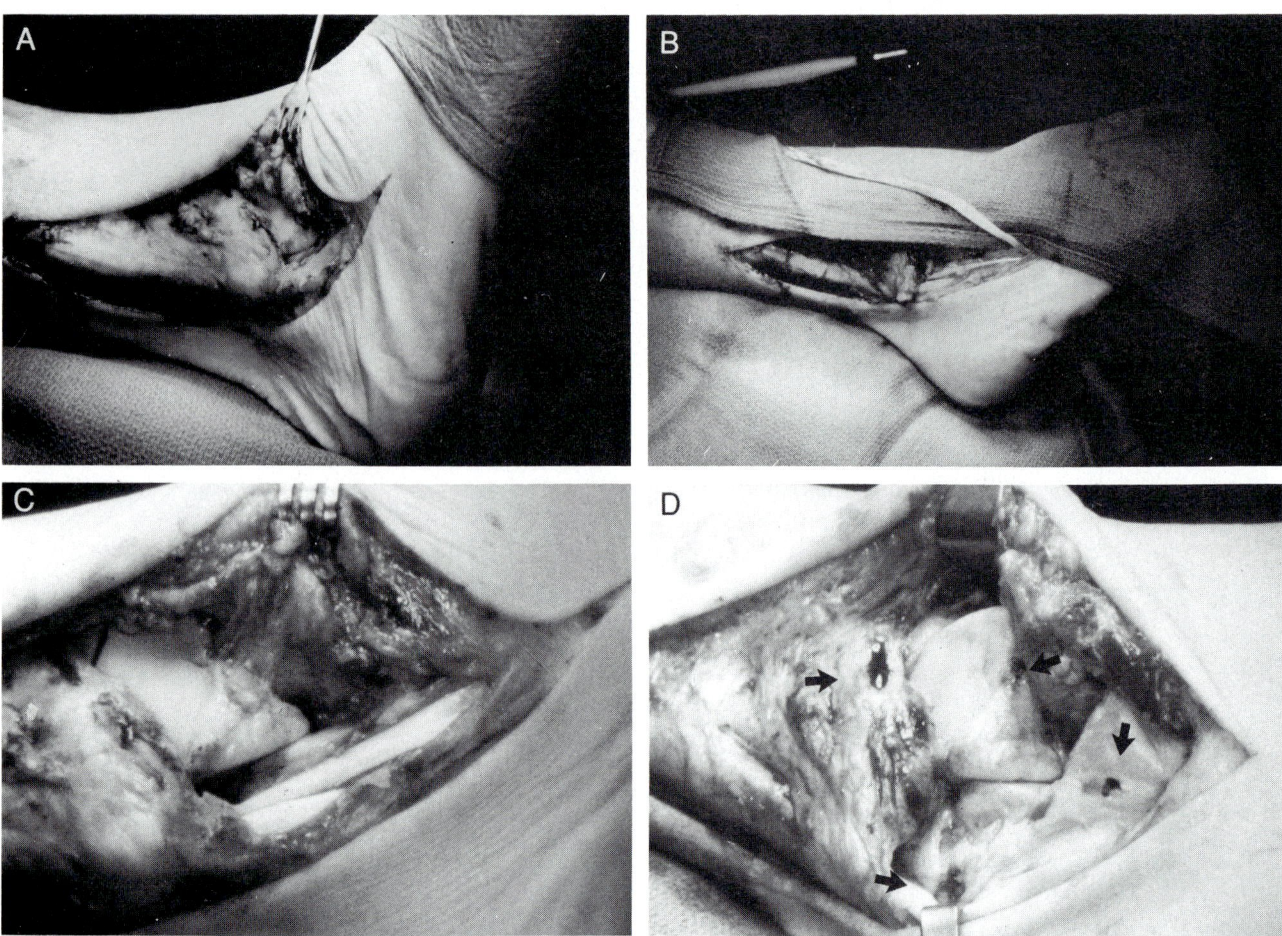

FIG 27–62.

Intraoperative photographs of triligamentous reconstruction of subtalar instability. **A,** surgical exposure. **B,** half of the peroneus brevis tendon harvested. **C,** exposure of the unstable subtalar joint. **D,** sites for bony tunnels. **E,** tendon graft passed through the sinus tarsi to reconstruct the cervical ligament. **F,** graft passed through the talus and into the fibula to recreate the anterior talofibular ligament. **G,** graft passed back through the fibula to the tip prior to insertion into the calcaneous to recreate the calcaneofibular ligament.

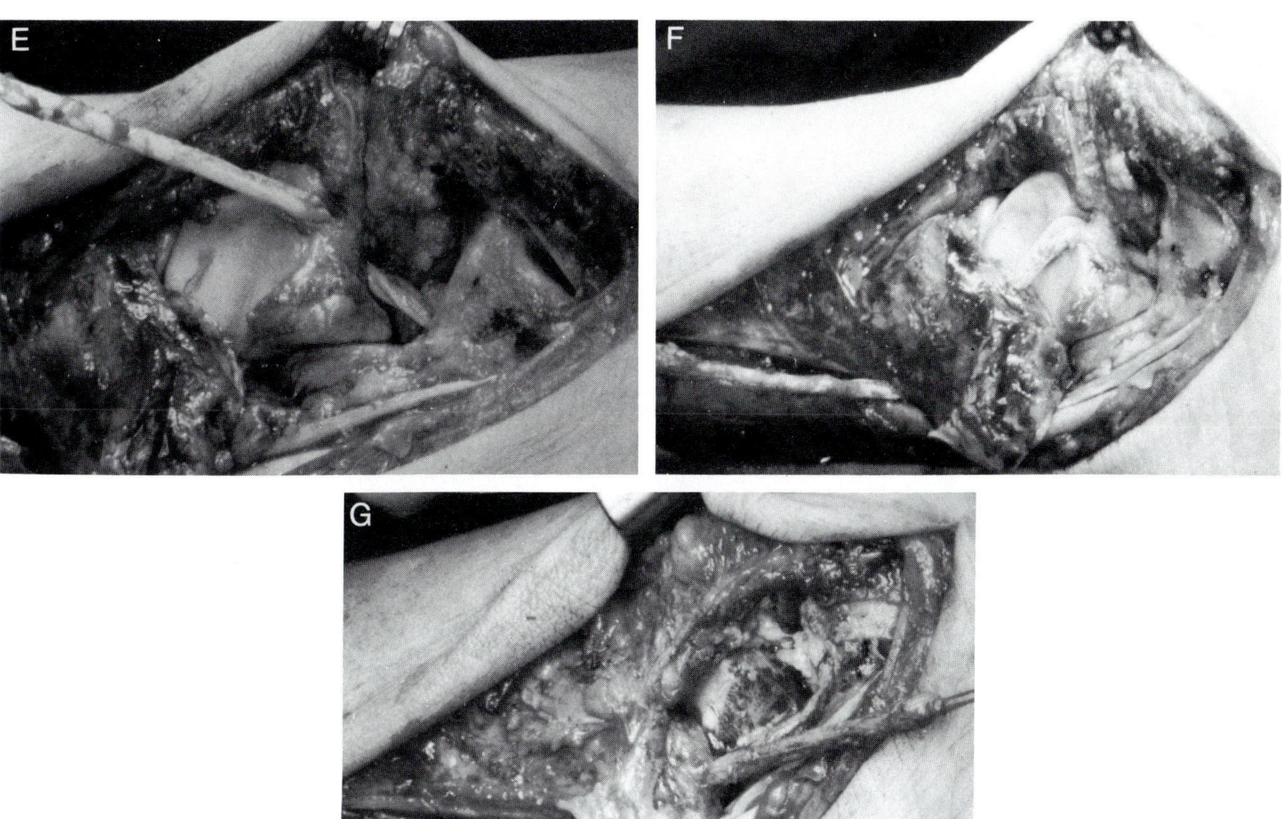

FIG 27–62 (cont.).

treated for subtalar instability, there was 1 complication of persistent lateral ankle pain that did not restrict activity and 1 case of decreased sensation in the sural nerve distribution. One patient with bilateral reconstructions has been able to resume sports from which she was previously restricted by her instability.

SINUS TARSI SYNDROME

Sinus tarsi syndrome is a related condition that may represent minor subtalar instability. With the use of the diagnostic tests described in the previous section, we feel that it is possible to distinguish between these two related subtalar problems—sinus tarsi syndrome and subtalar instability.

Historical Perspective

Initially described in 1958 by Denis O'Connor,[523] the sinus tarsi syndrome is a rather nebulous condition characterized by pain in the lateral region of the ankle and sinus tarsi. Very little has been written about the subject, and there are few objective diagnostic criteria. Furthermore, the pathologic anatomy associated with the condition is not clearly defined. As mentioned, some authorities have claimed that the condition is simply a subtle variation of subtalar instability.[522, 534, 535] The classic description of the pathoanatomy is scarring or degenerative changes to the soft-tissue elements of the sinus tarsi.[522–524, 535] Meyer and Lagier have demonstrated these changes histologically from surgically obtained biopsy specimens of the sinus tarsi.[522] The demonstration of nerve endings in the ligamentous tissue within the sinus and tarsal canals suggests the possibility that injury to the nerves and loss of their proprioceptive function could also be a factor in this condition. Baxter has proposed that there may be injury to the origin to the flexor digitorum brevis.[488] Whatever the etiology, it is certain that the changes are rather unimpressive at the time of surgical exploration in the majority of cases.

Diagnosis

Clinical Evaluation

Pain in the lateral part of the ankle and hindfoot over the sinus tarsi, often related to a prior inversion mechanism injury, is the primary complaint. Symptomatic instability is generally absent, and swelling is variable. Tenderness over the sinus tarsi is mandatory for this diagnosis. Other subjective and objective findings are absent or minimal.

Radiographic Evaluation

Objective documentation of the condition through radiographic means is difficult. Routine radiographs are negative, as are stress views. Meyer has popularized the use of the subtalar arthrogram for diagnosis of this condition.[519] The normal subtalar joint easily accepts 3 mL of contrast dye and demonstrates multiple microrecesses or interdigitations within the joint capsule. This is particularly true in the area of the interosseous and cervical ligaments. When these microrecesses are absent and

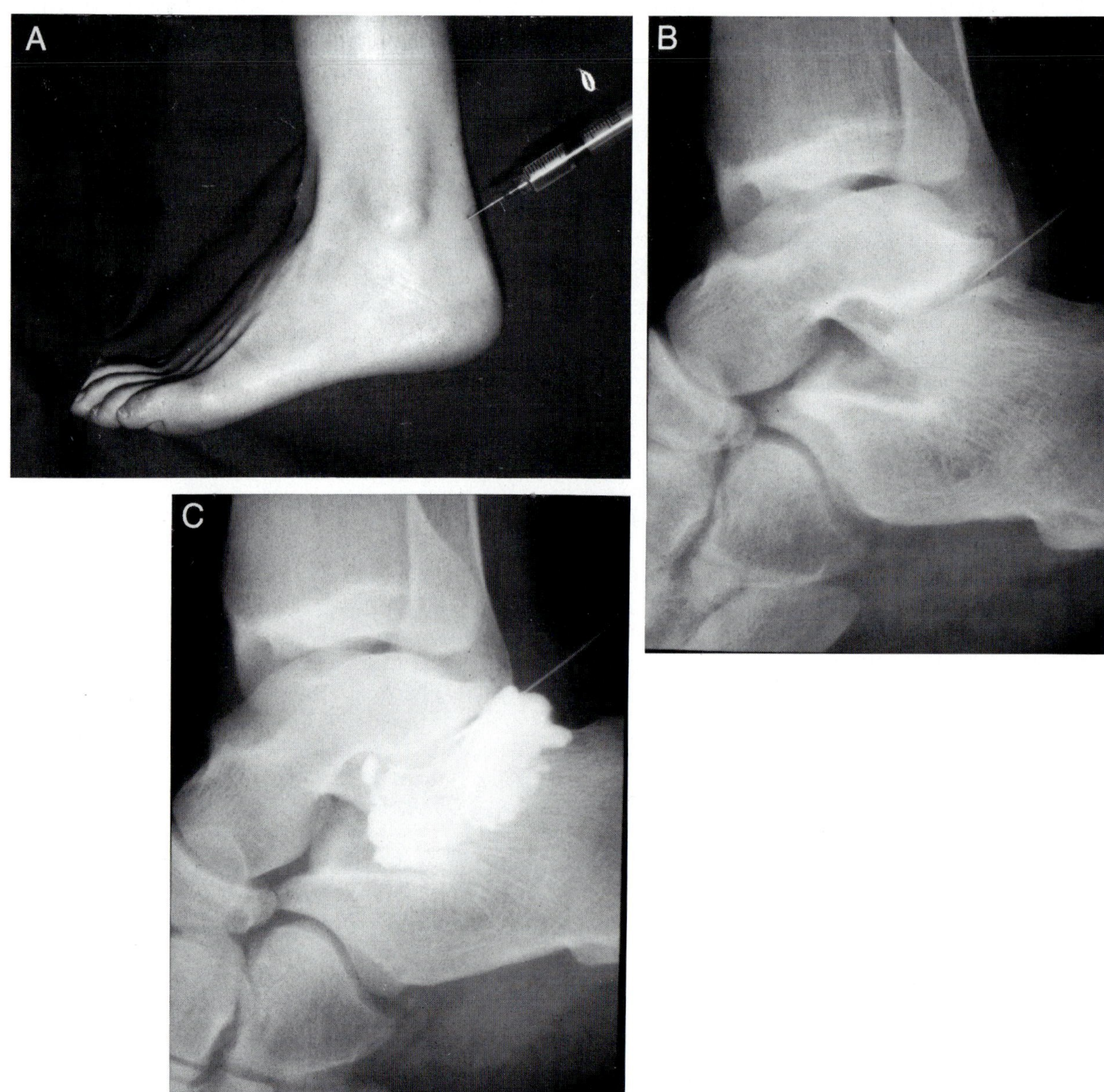

FIG 27–63.
Photographs of the method for performing subtalar arthrography. **A,** clinical photograph demonstrating posterior-to-anterior placement of the needle next to the Achilles tendon to inject dye into the posterior subtalar joint. **B,** radiograph demonstrating the needle in the posterior subtalar joint. **C,** radiograph demonstrating dye within the subtalar joint.

when the cutoff of dye at the interosseous ligament is abrupt, Taillard and Meyer hypothesized a relationship with sinus tarsi syndrome.[519, 522, 534]

The technique of performing subtalar arthrography is easily mastered. The patient is placed in the supine position on the table, and the skin is sterilely prepared. A 22-gauge needle is inserted just lateral to the Achilles tendon at the level of the ankle joint, which is palpated anteriorly. The needle is directed 20 to 30 degrees in the plantar direction until bone is encountered (Fig 27–63). A radiograph is taken to confirm the position at the posterior aspect of the posterior subtalar joint, and 3 mL of contrast dye is then injected prior to taking an additional film. Despite attempts to confirm the findings of Meyer and Taillard, we have been unable to do so conclusively.

Treatment

In the patient who fits this emerging picture of sinus tarsi syndrome, selection of a plan for treatment is necessary. An important aspect of both diagnosis and therapy has been the injection of an anesthetic agent and cortisone into the sinus tarsi. If this does not provide at least temporary relief, then the diagnosis must be questioned. In some patients one to three injections will provide permanent resolution of the symptoms. If significant pain recurs after temporary relief by injection, then surgical intervention is recommended.

It is unusual to find a patient who meets all the above considerations and arrives finally at the point of surgery. When this does occur one must carefully explain to the patient the exploratory nature of the procedure and the possibility of persistent symptoms. The surgical approach is a standard lateral oblique incision over the sinus tarsi that avoids the lateral branch of the superficial peroneal nerve. The extensor retinaculum is reflected distally along with the origin of the flexor digitorum brevis. The capsule of the subtalar joint is entered and the posterior talocalcaneal articulation inspected. Lateral talar osteophytes, if present, are removed to eliminate potential impingement (sinus impingement or abutment). The crux of the procedure as described by O'Connor was excision of the "fat pad in the sinus tarsi and resection of the superficial ligamentous floor."[523] Taillard et al. confined the excision to the tissue filling the lateral 1 to 1.5 cm of the sinus to avoid damage to the blood supply of the talus.[534] Regnauld has advised currettage of the fatty neurovascular tissue of the sinus with preservation of the interosseous ligament unless it is obviously damaged.[524] We prefer to preserve the interosseous talocalcaneal and cervical ligaments if possible and to resect the fibrofatty tissue and the extensions from the inferior extensor retinaculum. The extensor brevis is carefully reattached. Patients are treated with splint immobilization in the immediate postoperative period. This immobilization is then continued in a removable walking boot for a total of 4 weeks.

Results

Results of treatment in carefully selected surgical patients are quite acceptable. In O'Connor's original series of 45 patients, 14 were treated operatively, with 9 patients having complete relief of symptoms and improvement in the remaining 5.[523] Taillard and coworkers reviewed the cases found in the literature and added 15 of their own.[534] They had 11 excellent, 3 good, and 1 poor result. Summarizing the literature, there have been 96 surgically treated cases diagnosed as sinus tarsi syndrome with 66 excellent results (69%), 24 good results (25%), and 6 failures (6%).[492, 523, 524, 534]

PERONEAL TENDON SUBLUXATION AND DISLOCATION

Subluxation or dislocation of the peroneal tendons is an uncommon injury that is frequently misdiagnosed as a lateral ankle sprain in the acute setting (Fig 27–64). Although uncommon, peroneal tendon dislocation was considered "a well-recognized condition" as early as 1895.[621] Despite this, the acute injury still goes unrecognized. When the treatment is inadequate initially, recurrent dislocation is the usual consequence. In the chronic condition, the patient may be more aware of the actual pathology by having witnessed the movement of the tendon(s) around the lateral malleolus. Sports are the common setting for the acute injury, but the chronic condition may occur in a nonathletic situation.

Etiology

The majority of peroneal tendon dislocations can be traced directly to a traumatic event. Sports are involved in an overwhelming number of cases. Among 265 cases reported in the literature, 97% originated during an athletic activity, with 189 (71%) related to snow skiing and football coming in a distant second at 7%.* Running, basketball, soccer, and ice-skating were the most frequent of the remainder.

Chronic subluxation or dislocation has also been reported without a traumatic etiology. Frey and Shereff have divided subluxing peroneal tendons into two varieties: (1) traumatic and (2) habitual or voluntary.[564] In

---

**References 544, 548, 556, 558, 560, 561, 578, 580, 583, 587, 589, 606, 607, 612, 614.*

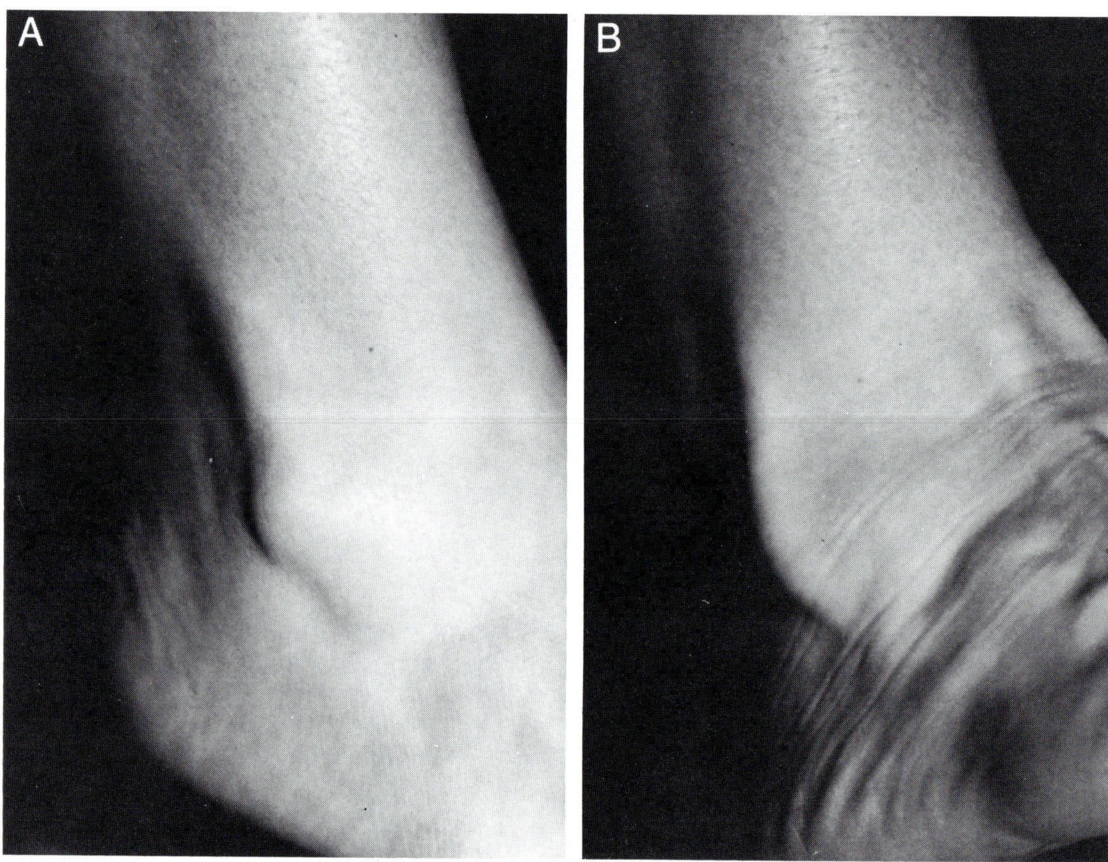

FIG 27–64.
Clinical photographs of an athlete with a dislocating peroneal tendon: **A**, reduced; **B**, dislocated.

the latter case, congenital deficiencies in the superior peroneal retinaculum and a shallow retrofibular groove have been ascribed the role of causative factors.[560, 569, 614] Congenital dislocation of the peroneal tendons was noted in 22 of 659 (3.3%) neonates and infants examined at one institution over a 15-month period.[573] Although these all went untreated and resolved spontaneously, it supports the possibility that these infants may carry a predisposition for subsequent dislocation of the tendons during adulthood. This form of congenitally related predisposition could account for some of the 31 patients with no history of trauma in Huber and Imhoff's series of 54 patients with dislocating peroneal tendons.[569]

Historical Perspective

The initial description of this condition has been attributed to Monteggia in 1803 when he described the problem in a ballet dancer.[586] The first papers dealing specifically with this subject and its treatment were by Blanulet in 1875 and Gutierrez in 1877.[550, 568] The anatomic relationships of the region were described by Tracey in 1909 and Edwards in 1928.[560, 618] Diagnosis of the injury radiologically from the presence of a posterior avulsion of bone at the distal end of the fibula was first mentioned by Moritz in 1959, although Dupuytren has been credited with first describing the avulsion fracture in this area.[580, 587] Since that time, the subject of peroneal tendon dislocation has received little attention in the English literature in comparison to what has been written in other languages. Stover and Bryan wrote an excellent review of the subject in 1962, and a further review was done by McLennan in 1980.[580, 614] The majority of papers deal with specific repair or reconstruction techniques for the chronic condition.

Anatomy

The peroneal tendons course from the lateral aspect of the leg to their insertion sites in the foot by passing around the lateral part of the ankle within a fibro-osseous tunnel.[547] This is formed by the fibula, a thickening of the tendon sheath enclosing the tendons, and the calcaneofibular and posterior talofibular ligaments (Fig 27–65). The tendons are positioned on the posterior as-

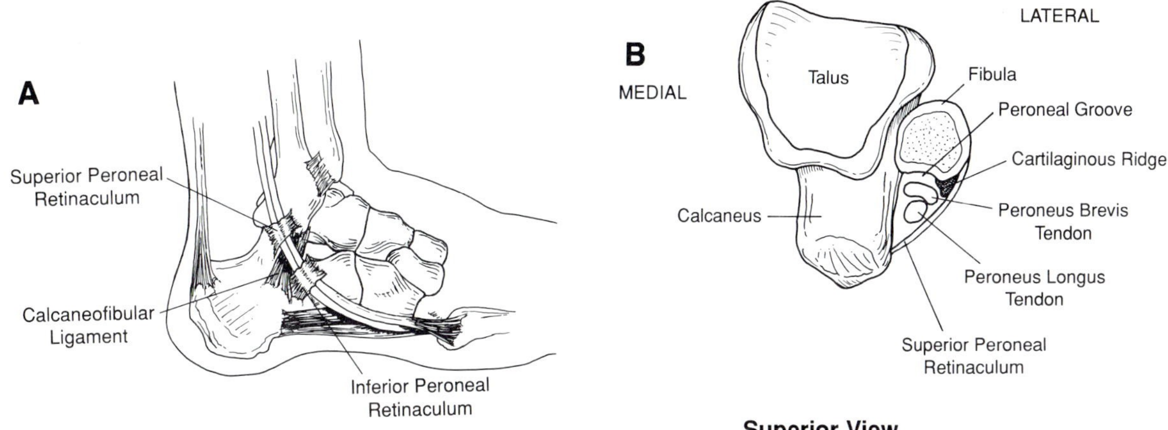

FIG 27–65.
Anatomic relationships of the ankle with the peroneal tendons held in position by the superior and inferior peroneal retinacula and the fibrous rim on the posterolateral aspect of the fibula. The calcaneofibular ligament lies below the peroneal tendons. **A,** lateral view; **B,** superior view.

pect of the distal end of the fibula in the retromalleolar sulcus. The depth of this sulcus is quite variable, however, even to the degree of being absent or convex in almost 20% of cases.[560] The width of the sulcus varies from 5 to 10 mm. The depth is often enhanced by a lateral bony ridge that is present in about 70% of cases, varies in height from 2 to 4 mm, and has an additional 1 to 2 mm of height contributed by cartilage. At times the entire ridge is formed by cartilage.[560, 605] Eckert and Davis examined this tissue microscopically and found it to be "a very dense aggregation of collagen fibers mixed with some elastin which is connected only loosely with the periosteum."[559]

The superior peroneal retinaculum is an important structure in maintaining the position of the peroneal tendons behind the fibula. However, despite this importance, it has been shown experimentally that division of the retinaculum alone is insufficient to cause dislocation of the peroneal tendons.[548] The superior peroneal retinaculum is formed as a condensation of the superficial fascia of the leg and the sheath of the peroneal tendons in the region of the posterior part of the fibula beginning approximately 2 cm proximal to the tip. The superior retinaculum is variable in its width, typically being well defined over a 1 to 2 cm area. It then tapers gradually into normal tendon sheath and fascia both proximally and distally. The origin of the retinaculum is the periosteum of the distal end of the fibula, and the insertion is the fascia surrounding the Achilles tendon and the periosteum of the lateral posterior calcaneus.[547, 559, 560, 605] The inferior peroneal retinaculum covers the tendons about 2 to 3 cm distal to the tip of the fibula. It is continuous with the inferior extensor retinaculum in the foot, originates near the sinus tarsi, and forms an arch over the peroneal tendons, with its superficial and deep layers inserting into the calcaneus near the peroneal, or posterolateral, tubercle.[605] This inferior retinacular structure apparently plays no significant role in the pathology of dislocating peroneal tendons.

The principal structure injured in the acute form of this problem is the superior peroneal retinaculum.[591] Although Jones and others have described the pathology as a rupture of this structure,[571, 580, 596] others have denied that such a lesion occurs.[547, 555, 559] Eckert and Davis explored 73 cases of acute injury and classified them into three gradations.[559] In *grade I* injuries the retinaculum with attached periosteum is stripped away from the posterolateral border of the distal end of the fibula (Fig 27–66,B). The tendons dislocate into this pocket and lie between the periosteum and the bare bone of the fibula. In *grade II* injuries the cartilaginous ridge is avulsed up with the periosteum off the distal portion of the fibula in a manner resembling a Bankart lesion of the shoulder (Fig 27–66,C). In a smaller number of cases, there is a *grade III* injury with bony avulsion of the posterolateral cortical rim of the fibula along with the cartilaginous rim and periosteum (Fig 27–60). In no case was an actual tear of the retinaculum discovered.

Mechanism of Injury

The most common mechanism of injury for dislocation of the peroneal tendons and/or injury to the superior peroneal retinaculum is a sudden dorsiflexion stress with a violent reflex contraction of the peroneal musculature.[547, 559, 561, 614, 625] Others have noted that the

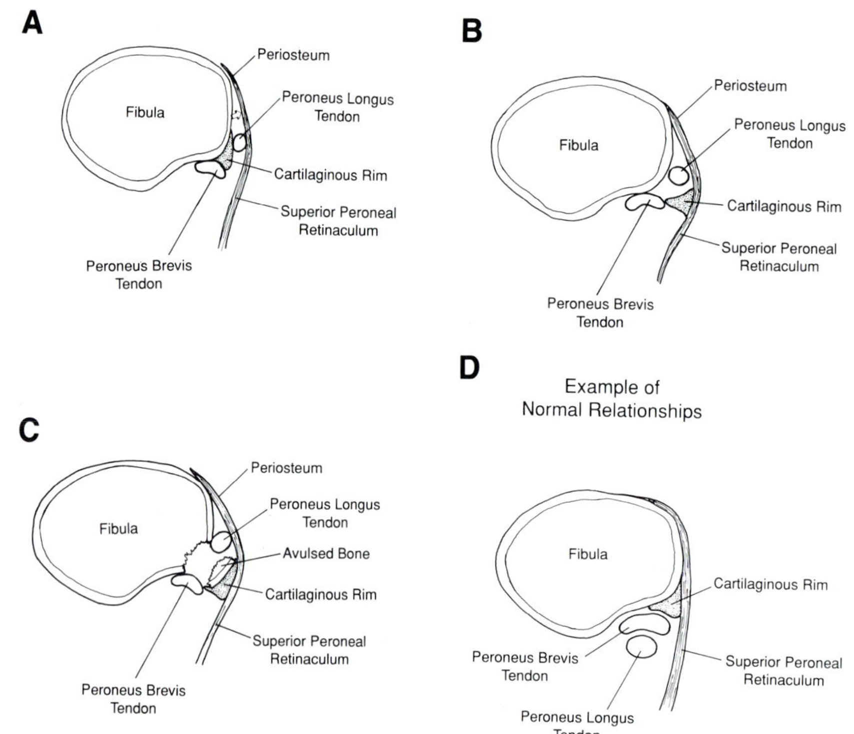

FIG 27–66.
Classification of pathology in peroneal tendon dislocations (Adapted from Eckert WR, Davis EA Jr: *J Bone Joint Surg [AM]* 58:670–673, 1976.) **A,** normal **B,** grade I: superior peroneal retinaculum stripped off the fibula. **C,** grade II: fibrous rim avused from the posterolateral aspect of the fibula along with the superior peroneal retinaculum. **D,** grade III: bony avulsion of the posterolateral part of the fibula by the superior peroneal retinaculum.

foot position could also be plantar flexion, slight eversion, or inversion, but all agree that there must be maximum tension in the peroneal muscles.[551, 579] When this is not the case, then a trimalleolar fracture is likely to occur.[592]

The frequent occurrence of this injury from skiing has been highlighted in several reports describing the mechanism of digging the ski tips into the snow to cause a sudden deceleration with ankle dorsiflexion followed by a forceful contraction of the peroneals.[589, 614] The rigid ski boot limits torque on the skeleton but allows force that is generated in the muscles to be concentrated on the soft-tissue constraints. Another mechanism attributed to skiing is the forced eversion used to edge the downhill ski while performing turns.[561] Eversion tenses the calcaneofibular ligament and narrows the fibro-osseous tunnel, thereby forcing the tendons against the retinaculum.[614, 618]

Diagnosis

Clinical Evaluation

In patients who present following an acute injury, it may be difficult to distinguish a tear of the superior peroneal retinaculum with or without peroneal tendon dislocation from an acute sprain of the lateral ankle ligaments unless the clinician has an awareness of this less common condition. Lateral swelling with tenderness and ecchymosis is present following an acute injury in an athletic setting. All these features point to the familiar ankle sprain. However, there are some distinguishing characteristics. First of all, the patient is often at a loss to explain exactly what happened, unlike the patient with a typical ankle sprain who generally recognizes that the foot has "turned under." Next, tenderness and swelling are maximum posterior to the fibula or along its posterior border. There is appreciably less tenderness anteriorly and in particular over the anterior talofibular ligament. The anterior drawer sign is negative. Extreme discomfort or apprehension during attempted eversion of the foot against resistance is a key feature of the acute injury. Rarely, the tendons will redislocate during this maneuver, which makes the diagnosis obvious.

The chronic condition of dislocating peroneal tendons presents a different diagnostic dilemma. In this setting, the patient relates a popping or snapping sensation around the lateral aspect of the ankle. This may or may not be associated with pain. Sometimes the patient complains more of an instability or a potential giving way of the ankle with little discomfort. This may suggest the presence of lateral ligamentous injury, but the anterior drawer and talar tilt tests are negative. (There is only one report of the two conditions of lateral ankle instability and peroneal tendon dislocation coexisting.[611]) The foot and ankle often appear entirely normal in the chronic case. There may be mild swelling or tenderness at the posterolateral aspect of the ankle. Testing the ankle by having the patient move the inverted and plantar-flexed foot through a range of motion to maximum dorsiflexion and eversion against resistance will normally reproduce the dislocation of the tendons or cause sufficient apprehension that the diagnosis is strongly suggested. The absence of demonstrable dislocation does not exclude the possibility of this being the etiology of the patient's complaint.

Radiographic Evaluation

Routine radiographs are essential since they can disclose the characteristic rim fracture of the distal portion of the fibula that is produced by avulsion of the superior peroneal retinaculum[598] (Fig 27–67). This can be present in 15% to 50% of cases.[553, 587] It is seen most clearly on the internally rotated oblique view. Unfortunately, in most series, the majority of cases have entirely normal radiographs. When this is the case and the diagnosis remains in question, one can consider the use of the other radiologic studies. According to McLennan,[580] the peroneal tenogram may show dye leakage anteriorly, but its primary usefulness is in distinguishing additional pathology within the peroneal tendons.[566, 599, 600] Due to the invasive nature of the tenogram and difficulty in its interpretation, other studies have been advocated. CAT scans allow precise definition of the anatomy of the retromalleolar sulcus as well as the position of the peroneal tendons.[601, 602, 615] More recently, MRI has been recommended for its ability to define the soft-tissue structures more exactly, including the superior and inferior peroneal retinaculum.[609, 624] In most circumstances we have found it unnecessary to utilize additional studies other than routine radiography.

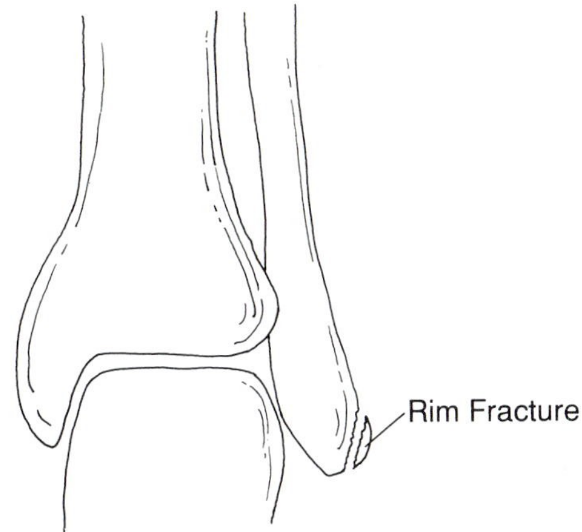

FIG 27–67.
Drawing of a characteristic rim fracture associated with dislocating peroneal tendons.

Treatment

Acute Treatment

Nonoperative Treatment.—When the diagnosis of dislocating peroneal tendons or rupture of the superior peroneal retinaculum is made immediately following an injury, two legitimate treatment options exist. Treatment with immobilization in a well-molded splint or cast with non–weight-bearing ambulation for 6 weeks is a safe approach that yields good results in over 50% of cases.[580, 614] Anything short of this results in a high rate of recurrence.[561] In fact, because of the potential for recurrence even with adequate conservative management, a number of authors recommend surgical treatment for the acute injury.[558, 559, 579, 590] The authors favor this approach for the majority of patients because this injury predominantly occurs in a young, athletic population who want to return to their active life-style as quickly as possible.

Authors' Operative Technique.—The operation can be performed with the patient in either the supine or the prone position. We favor the latter since it allows easy visualization of the retromalleolar sulcus and the tendons. The anesthetic method may vary from general anesthesia, to regional with a spinal or epidural, to local with direct infiltration or an ankle block.

1. The incision begins just posterior to the fibula over the peroneal tendons starting 5 cm above the tip of the lateral malleolus and follows the course of the tendons to just past the tip (Fig 27–68,A). Care is taken to protect the sural nerve in the posterior skin flap.
2. The superior retinaculum is identified as a thickening in the sheath, and the sheath is divided just proximal to the retinaculum. On inspection, there is typically a stripping of the retinaculum and periosteum off the posterolateral border of the distal end of the fibula as described by Eckert and Davis.[559] In some cases the fibrocartilaginous lateral ridge or bone has been avulsed.
3. Regardless of the pathology identified, the repair involves a direct repair of the retinaculum and periosteum back to bone through three or four drill holes in the posterolateral aspect of the fibula (Fig 27–68,B and C). Slowly absorbing suture of 0 or 00 size is utilized.

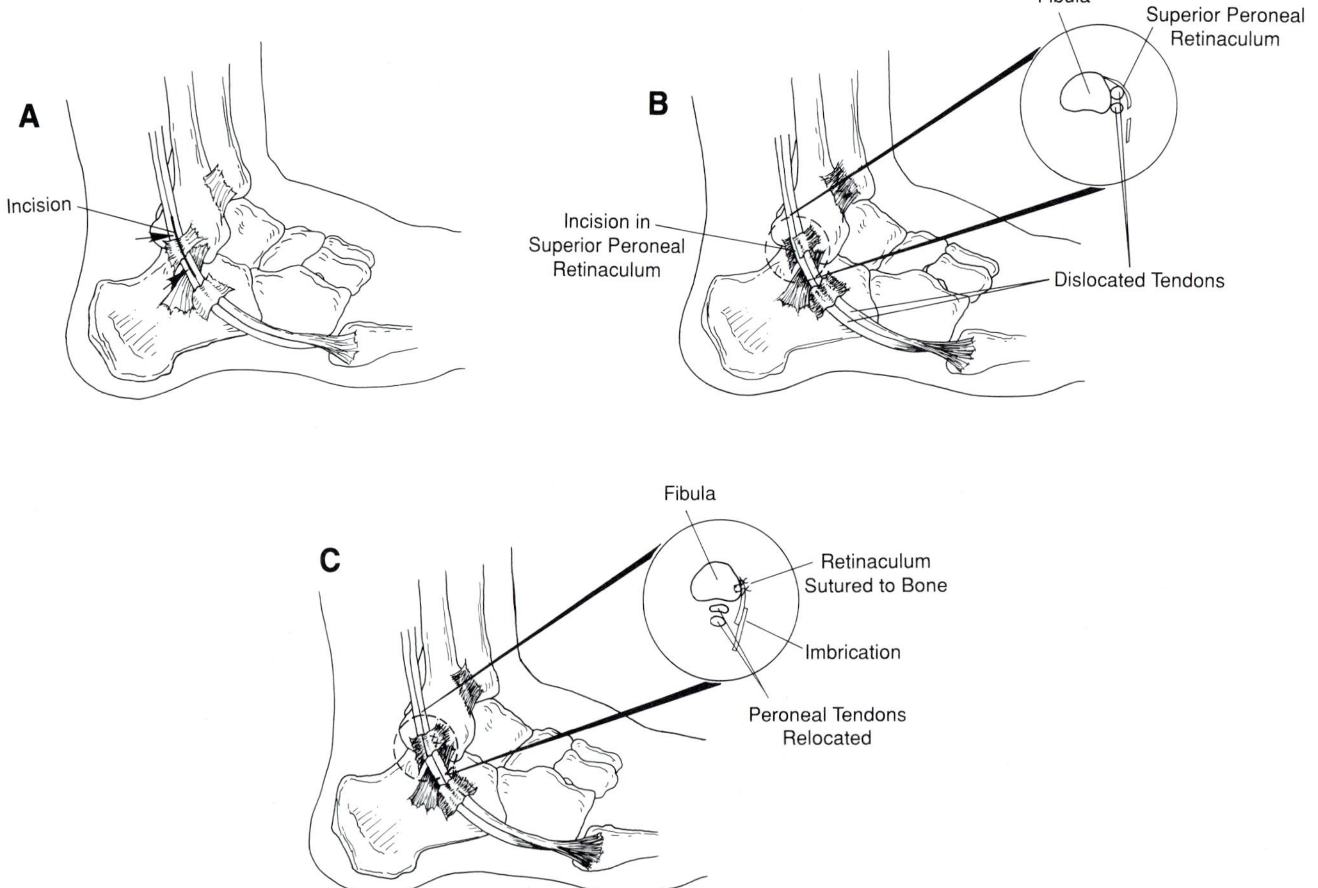

FIG 27–68.
Surgical repair of an acute peroneal tendon dislocation. **A,** surgical approach. **B,** pathologic anatomy. **C,** repair of the superior peroneal retinaculum by direct repair through drill holes in the posterolateral portion of the fibula.

4. Once the retinaculum is firmly reattached to the fibula, the incisions in the sheath and retinaculum are closed without undue imbrication. The skin is reapproximated with a running subcuticular closure, and a compressive dressing and splint are applied.

5. The foot and ankle are positioned in relaxed plantar flexion and slight eversion, which places the least tension on the repair.[618]

Postoperative Care.—Patients are kept non–weight bearing in their splint or cast for 6 to 10 days until their first postoperative visit, at which time they are placed in a short-leg walking cast or walking boot that is worn for an additional 4 weeks. Return to sports participation is allowed when the patient has regained full range of motion and strength. This has usually occurred by 3 to 4 months following the operation.

In the acute injury situation we have not found it necessary to address a shallow or convex fibular groove, although we are always prepared to do so if there is no other obvious pathology. This should be inspected in each case to ensure that it is not a contributing factor. If a shallow or convex groove is present with little apparent retinacular pathology, then a groove-deepening procedure as described below under treatment of the chronic disorder is advisable.

Chronic Treatment

In the more common situation where the patient appears with a chronic problem of recurrent dislocation of the peroneal tendons, the treatment is surgical. There is little to be gained from nonoperative management other than a temporary reduction in inflammatory symptoms, which tend to recur once treatment is discontinued. The most difficult decision is determining which of the over 20 different operations to utilize. The available procedures fall into five basic categories and several subcategories: (1) reattachment of the retinaculum and reinforcement with local tissue[544, 548, 549, 559, 620]; (2) bone block procedures;* (3) reinforcement of the superior peroneal retinaculum with transferred tissue—Achilles tendon,[561, 571, 606] periosteum,[567] peroneus brevis,[547, 612] peroneus quartus,[584, 610] or plantaris;[583] (4) rerouting procedures, i.e., under the calcaneofibular ligament[578, 596, 597, 604] or anterior transposition[577]; and (5) groove-deepening procedures.[547, 607, 625] Each method has advantages and disadvantages.

Anatomic Soft-tissue Reconstruction.—Chronic dislocation of the peroneal tendons has similarities to anterior dislocation of the shoulder where there is a pathologic pouch of tissue into which the dislocation occurs. Similarly, in dislocation of the peroneal tendons, the retinaculum and periosteum (occasionally accompanied by the fibrocartilaginous rim or bone) strip away from their bony attachment on the fibula. This lesion is similar to the Bankart lesion in the shoulder.[556] If this pathology has been created by a traumatic event, its direct reattachment should eliminate the problem, barring some underlying anatomic predisposing factor. Advantages to the direct repair method are its anatomic approach, lack of disturbance to other anatomy, small incision, and avoidance of osteotomy. A disadvantage is its failure to correct any predisposing anatomic feature such as an insufficient retinaculum or sulcus deformity. A review of the literature concerning this technique reveals a recurrence rate of 1 in 31 cases (3%).[544, 548, 549, 555]

Bone Block Procedures.—The bone block procedures have a long history of usage for this condition, and one of the methods was originally described in the first edition of this textbook[557] (Fig 27–69). The methods are all variations of the techniques described by Kelly in 1920[572] (Fig 27–70). The treatment principle is coverage and containment of the peroneal tendons with a bone block created from the fibula. Advantages are preservation of the fibro-osseous tunnel for smooth gliding of the tendons, creation of a physiologically deeper groove, and provision for bony rather than soft-tissue healing.[583] The disadvantages include the failure of the technique to address the underlying problem (i.e., the pouch into which the tendons dislocate), technical complexity, screw-related problems, and potential for worsening the patient's original condition (e.g., through graft nonunion, graft fracture, fibula fracture, or screw penetration into the ankle joint or retromalleolar sulcus). The redislocation/resubluxation rate after bone

*References 557, 572, 576, 579, 583, 590, 623.

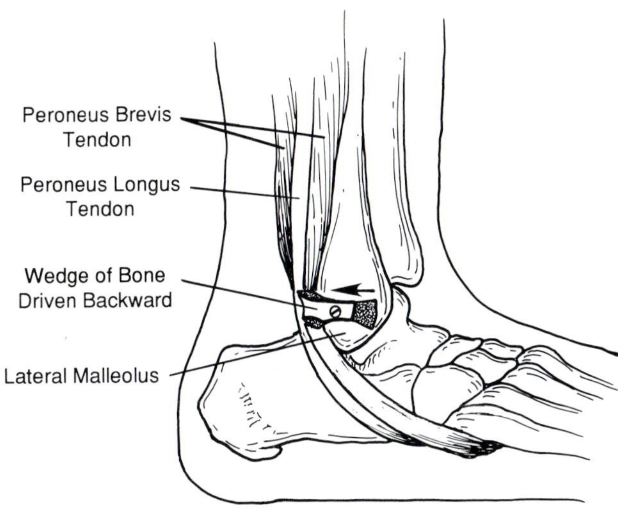

FIG 27–69.
DuVries procedure for dislocating peroneal tendons. (Adapted from DuVries HL: *Surgery of the foot,* St Louis, 1959, Mosby–Year Book, pp 253–255.)

block procedures is 7 in 89 cases (8%) with an overall complication rate of 30% (27 in 89 cases).*

Tissue Transfer Procedures.—Procedures that use periosteal flaps or transferred tissue to recreate or reinforce the superior peroneal retinaculum are designed to correct any incompetency in this structure and to prevent dislocation of the tendons by holding them behind the fibula. The most commonly recognized method is that described by Ellis Jones in 1932 using a strip of Achilles tendon[571] (Fig 27–71). Advantages are the

*References 572, 576, 579, 580, 583, 590.

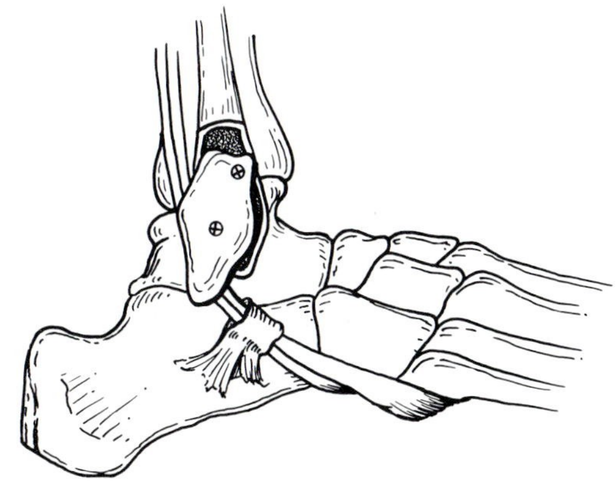

FIG 27–70.
Kelly bone block procedure (Adapted from Kelly RE: *Br J Surg* 7:502–504, 1920.)

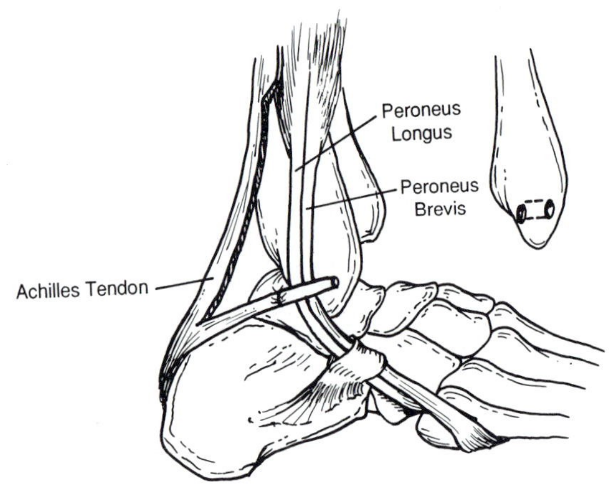

FIG 27–71.
Jones procedure utilizing a strip of Achilles tendon to reconstruct the superior peroneal retinaculum. The *inset* shows a drill hole in the fibula. (Adapted from Jones E: *J Bone Joint Surg* 14:574–576, 1932.)

nonreliance on potentially injured tissue, ability to correct the dislocation pocket, preservation of the fibro-osseous groove, avoidance of osteotomy, and the availability of several tissue options. Disadvantages include the small number of cases reported with some of the methods,† potential limitation of motion through a tenodesis effect, and weakening or alteration of function of normal tissue. Among 27 Jones procedures reported, there have been no redislocations, but 1 case of a sensation of instability and 4 cases with loss of ankle motion occurred for a complication rate of 19%.[561, 571, 606] Techniques other than the Jones procedure have only been used on one or two cases.‡

Rerouting Procedures.—The rerouting procedures primarily rely on use of the calcaneofibular ligament to constrain the peroneal tendons in order to prevent redislocation. There is one case report of rerouting the peroneal tendons by transferring them anterior to the lateral malleolus in a college football player.[577] Although he is said to have returned to play, there is no length of follow-up given. We can find nothing to advocate this method. On the contrary, the calcaneofibular ligament rerouting method maintains the tendons in their normal physiologic position behind the lateral malleolus. Advantages to this method are the lack of disturbance of the fibro-osseous groove and limited scarring around the tendons. The major disadvantage is the necessity for detachment or division of some normal structure. In the method of Platzgummer, the calcaneofibular ligament is divided and resutured over the tendons[595] (Fig 27–72). Sarmiento and Wolf modified this by dividing the peroneal tendons, passing the ends of the tendons under the calcaneofibular ligament, and resuturing the tendon ends[604] (Fig 27–73). Pozo and Jackson further developed the technique by taking the origin of the calcaneofibular ligament off with a fragment of predrilled distal fibula[597] (Fig 27–74). The tendons were replaced in their sulcus, and the ligament was then reattached with

†*References 547, 567, 571, 584, 585, 612.*

‡*References 547, 567, 571, 584, 585, 612.*

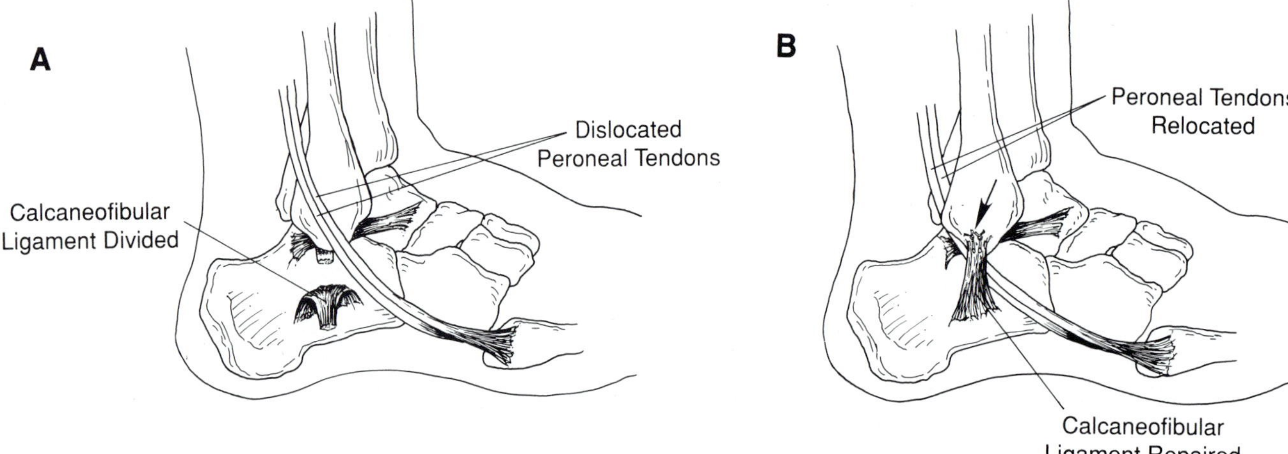

FIG 27–72.
Platzgummer method of reconstruction for dislocating peroneal tendons by rerouting the peroneal tendons underneath the calcaneofibular ligament. **A,** calcaneofibular ligament divided. **B,** peroneal tendons relocated under the repaired calcaneofibular ligament. (Adapted from Platzgummer H: *Arch Orthop Unfallchir* 61:144–150, 1967.)

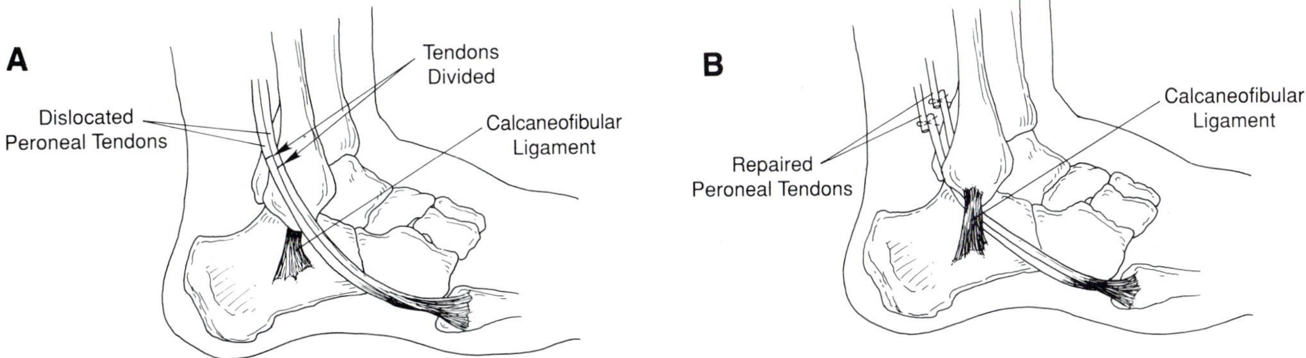

FIG 27–73.
Sarmiento and Wolf method of rerouting the peroneal tendons under the calcaneofibular ligament by dividing the tendons, placing the tendons under the ligament, and then resuturing the tendons. **A,** pathologic anatomy. **B,** Peroneal tendons relocated under the calcaneofibular ligament after division and repair. (Modified from Sarmiento A, Wolf M: *J Bone Joint Surg [AM]* 57:115–116, 1975.)

screw fixation. At the same time, Pöll and Duijfjes reported a similar method approached from the opposite direction by detaching the insertion of the calcaneofibular ligament on the calcaneus[596] (Fig 27–75). In the 23 cases reported there have been no recurrences. Fourteen "minor" complications have been noted, including 6 sensory abnormalities (2 specifically noted to be sural nerve injuries), 7 cases of minor discomfort and/or swelling, and 1 case of decreased motion in inversion.[578, 596, 597, 604]

Groove-deepening Procedures.—Groove deepening of the retromalleolar sulcus of the fibula for recurrent peroneal dislocation is derived from the study of Edwards.[560] She found that 19 of 178 fibulas (11%) had a flat posterior surface, and 13 of 178 fibulas (7%) had a convex posterior surface with no lateral or medial ridge. Jones and McLennan both mention earlier surgeons who have advocated deepening the retromalleolar groove, usually with a gouge.[571, 580] This has the obvious disadvantage of creating a rough bone surface to which the tendons would adhere. The modern method for accomplishing this deepening of the groove has been attributed to F.R. Thompson.[625] In this method, the posterior portion of the fibula is osteotomized on three sides and the medial side left hinged (Fig 27–76). With

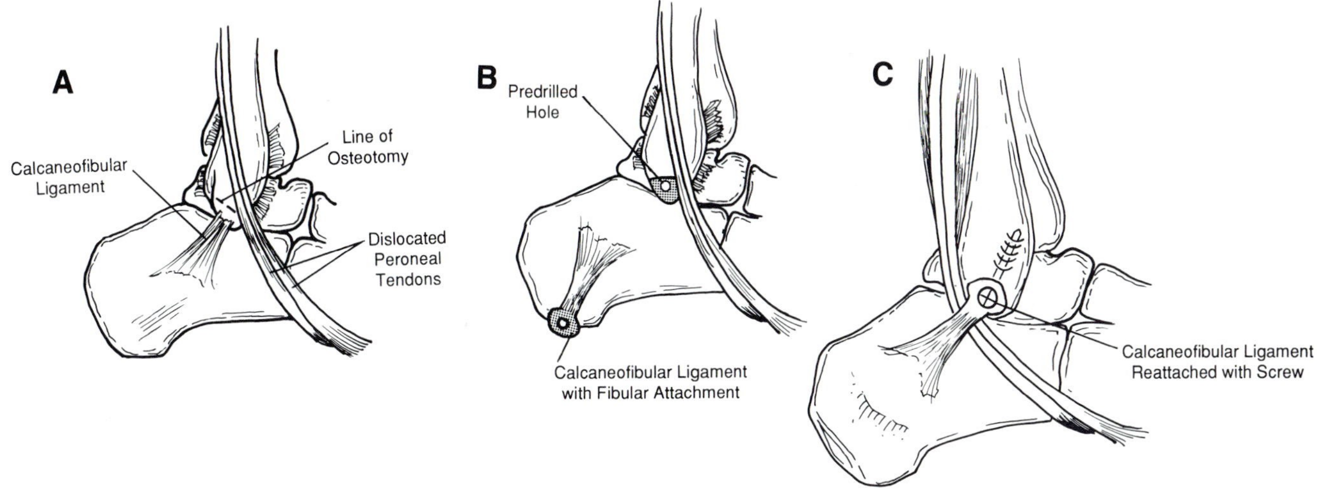

FIG 27–74.
Pozo and Jackson method of rerouting the peroneal tendons by removing a bone block from the fibula containing the origin of the calcaneofibular ligament. **A,** pathologic anatomy. **B,** calcaneofibular ligament with predrilled bone from the fibular attachment osteotomized. **C,** tendons and the calcaneofibular ligament relocated. (Adapted from Pozo JL, Jackson AM: *Foot Ankle* 5:42–44, 1984.)

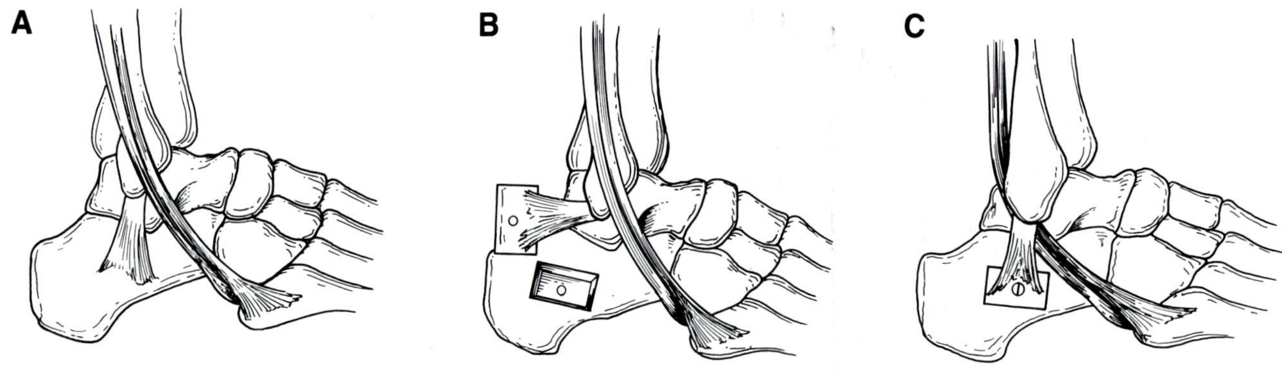

FIG 27–75.
Pöll and Duijfjes method of rerouting the peroneal tendons by removing a bone block from the part of the calcaneus containing the insertion of the calcaneofibular ligament. **A,** pathologic anatomy. **B,** calcaneofibular ligament detached from the bony insertion site, which has been predrilled. **C,** tendons relocated under the reattached calcaneofibular ligament. (Adapted from Pöll RG, Duijfjes F: *J Bone Joint Surg [Br]* 66:98–100, 1984.)

this flap of bone lifted up, the underlying cancellous bone of the fibula is curetted, and the flap is then reinserted in the deepened bed. Advantages include correction of any inherent groove deficiency and maintenance of the cartilaginous gliding layer. Disadvantages are the technique-sensitive nature of the procedure, possible irritation of the tendons on the bone edges created by the osteotomy, and failure to correct the dislocation pouch unless this is addressed simultaneously. In the 16 cases reported in the literature, there have been no cases of redislocation, resubluxation, or instability symptoms.[547, 607, 625] There have been no other complications reported with this method. Interestingly, in all 16 cases, the surgeons reinforced or repaired the superior retinaculum simultaneously with the groove-deepening osteotomy.[547, 607, 625]

Authors' Operative Technique.—As discussed above, there are a number of available methods for surgically treating the patient with chronically dislocating peroneal tendons. Time and space do not allow a complete discussion of all these methods, but the more classic techniques are illustrated in Figures 27–72 to 27–76. The authors' preferred technique includes addressing the dislocation pouch as detailed in the section on acute treatment and utilization of groove deepening as described by Zoellner and Clancy and by Slätis and coworkers.[607, 625] When the retinaculum is deficient, we employ the Achilles tendon transfer of Ellis Jones.[571]

1. The ankle is approached through a similar incision as described above for treatment of the acute condition, but it is lengthened by about 1 cm in both the proximal and distal directions.
2. The sural nerve is protected in the posterior flap.
3. The sheath and retinaculum are exposed and inspected prior to incising the sheath just posterior to the posterior border of the fibula.
4. This incision begins above the superior retinaculum and extends to just past the tip of the fibula.
5. The peroneal tendons are carefully inspected for evidence of attritional tears. This has been reported by Arrowsmith et al., and we have noted similar pathology in almost half our cases.[547]
6. If there is significant tenosynovitis, a tenosynovectomy is performed. Tears in the peroneal tendon(s) are addressed as described in the section on peroneal tendon tears.
7. Once the peroneal tendons have been inspected and any associated pathology corrected, the retromalleolar sulcus is exposed.
8. A micro-oscillating saw is used to create a 3-cm-long by 1-cm-wide trapdoor that is hinged medially (see Fig 27–76). A small osteotome is used to carefully lift this fragment up and expose the underlying cancellous bone of the fibula. A curette or burr is then used to remove 7 to 9 mm of cancellous bone before replacing the trapdoor.
9. With the tendons replaced in the groove, the trapdoor is held in place while the retinaculum and periosteum are reattached to the posterolateral border of the fibula by using suture placed through drill holes.
10. If the retinaculum appears to be inadequate to maintain the position of the tendons in the deepened groove, the Achilles tendon is exposed after lengthening the incision by several centimeters in the proximal direction.
11. A strip of Achilles tendon approximately 10 cm in length and 6 to 7 mm wide is harvested and left attached distally.
12. The sural nerve is at risk and must be avoided in the superficial tissue flap. Since the retromalleolar sul-

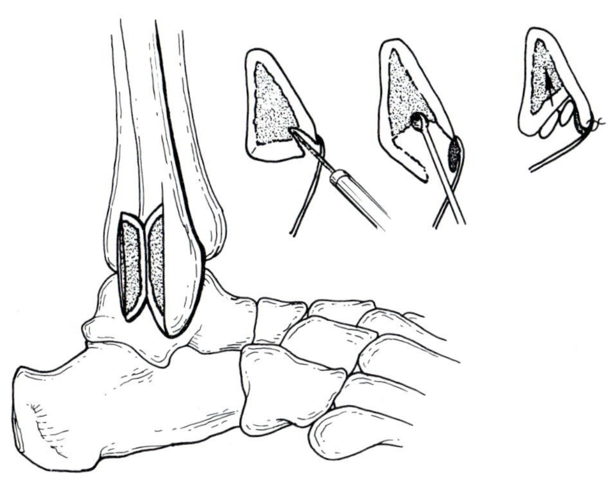

FIG 27–76.
Surgical reconstruction for peroneal tendon dislocation by deepening the peroneal groove. (Adapted from Slätis P, Santavirta S, Sandelin J: *Br J Sports Med* 22:16–18, 1988, and Zoellner G, Clancy W Jr: *J Bone Joint Surg [Am]* 61:292–294, 1979.)

cus has already been deepened by this point, a 2-mm drill hole is made from the anterolateral part of fibula at a location 1 cm above the tip. The hole is directed posteriorly to a point at the depth of the trough created in the retromalleolar sulcus. It is important to make the bone bridge in the fibula of sufficient width since the posterior part of the fibula has already been weakened by the previous osteotomy.

13. The hole in the fibula is carefully enlarged with a burr until the tendon graft can pass through the hole and be sutured back on itself. This should be done with the foot held in dorsiflexion and neutral inversion/eversion in order to prevent restriction in motion postoperatively.

14. The available retinaculum and periosteum are then sutured for reinforcement.

Postoperative Care.—The patient is splinted for 1 week, and a short-leg walking cast or walking boot is then applied for 4 to 6 weeks. After an adequate rehabilitation program, the patient can resume sports participation, usually at 4 to 6 months following the surgery.

Our own experience with this procedure reflects what is found in the literature: no redislocations and no significant complications. The patients have been able to resume sports participation without limitation. Two tennis players had more prolonged recovery periods with persistent swelling and aching during vigorous tennis play. Both had longitudinal tears of the peroneus brevis that were debrided and repaired. Their symptoms resolved after 8 and 12 months, respectively.

PERONEAL TENDINITIS AND RUPTURES

There are a variety of conditions that affect the peroneal tendons other than subluxation and dislocation. The most common affliction for the athlete is tenosynovitis or peritendinitis. This is defined as inflammation of the paratenon and/or the surrounding synovial lining where present. Some authors have described the pathology as stenosing tenosynovitis due to thickening of the tendon sheath and constriction of the underlying tendons.[545, 552, 593, 619, 622] When the inflammatory process involves the tendon itself, then the diagnosis of tendinitis is appropriate. Finally, *tendinosis* is a term that describes degenerative lesions of the tendon with no associated inflammatory response in the paratenon and no symptomotology present.[554]

A final condition, tendon rupture, can occur with or without pre-existing symptoms. The rarity of peroneal tendon rupture is reflected in the few cases reported in the literature on tendon ruptures plus a limited number of case reports.* In these cases of rupture, only two occurred in patients under 25 years of age[562, 574] and only four cases have been reported in athletes.[574, 575, 616] It is likely that the condition is more common than is traditionally recognized given the finding of Sobel and coworkers that 14 ankles among 124 autopsy specimens examined (11%) had varying degrees of attritional changes in the peroneus brevis tendon.[608] McMaster has shown that intratendinous rupture is much less common than failure of the musculotendinous unit at either the insertion to bone, within the muscle itself, or at the musculotendinous junction.[581] This suggests the presence of pre-existing disease within the tendons prior to their failure.

Etiologic Factors

Peroneal tenosynovitis is relatively rare as a source of significant symptoms for athletes. It is primarily related to repetitive movement, prolonged usage, increased training intensity, and/or direct trauma. In the athlete, the problem typically occurs from overuse. The problem may be either acute (less than 2 weeks of symptoms), subacute (2 to 6 weeks of symptoms), or chronic (greater than 6 weeks of symptoms).

Tendinitis may be classified identically, but it is more commonly associated with some identifiable trauma or anatomic factor rather than with overuse.[554] Only a small number of cases of peroneal tendon rup-

---

**References 543, 546, 562, 565, 570, 574, 575, 581, 588, 613, 616, 617.*

ture have been reported, and the majority of these have not been from an athletic setting. This suggests some primary degenerative process within the tendon. The role of altered vascularity has been discussed and may be a critical factor, particularly in cases with intratendinous degeneration.[608] Meyer proposed that abrasion on the tendon from the calcaneofibular ligament or the lateral cartilaginous ridge of the fibula was the initiating factor in the longitudinal tears seen in the peroneus brevis.[582] Others concur with the etiologic role of this ridge and the pressure of the peroneus longus tendon against the peroneus brevis.[608]

Diagnosis

Clinical Evaluation

Athletes with peroneal tenosynovitis or tendinitis are usually seen soon after the onset of symptoms, which include pain and swelling at the lateral portion of the ankle. Acutely, one can often appreciate some warmth and even some crepitus during movement of the tendon. Pain with eversion of the supinated foot against resistance from the examiner is helpful but not conclusive. In the acute setting, the possibility of a lateral compartment syndrome complicating a ruptured tendon must be considered.[555] Symptoms and signs may be almost identical in cases of tendinitis and rupture, with pain and swelling noted at the side of the ankle or foot. However, there is often a sensation of ankle instability or a history of recurrent lateral sprains with tears or ruptures of the peroneal tendons.[543, 574, 576, 603] Although the diagnosis is usually made from the history and physical examination, there are other studies that may be useful. Fitzgerald and Coventry recommended the injection of 1 to 2 mL of local anesthetic into the tendon sheath.[563]. Relief of pain strongly infers the diagnosis of peroneal tendinitis or tenosynovitis.

Radiographic Evaluation

Routine radiographs are necessary to exclude other sources of lateral pain and the occasional exostosis, osteochondroma, or hypertrophic peroneal tubercle of the calcaneus that might induce the tendon problem. Furthermore, it is sometimes possible to diagnose a rupture of the peroneus longus by noting proximal migration of the os peroneum, the sesamoid located within the tendon found near the calcaneocuboid joint in normal circumstances.[616, 617] Also, fracture of the os peroneum with rupture of the peroneus longus tendon has been reported.[594] Peroneal tenography has been used by several authors to diagnose peroneal tendon disorders.[566, 599, 600] Gilula et al. classified tenographic findings into four groups: (1) normal, (2) minimal marginal irregularity, (3) moderate or marked marginal irregularity, and (4) occluded tendon sheath.[566] Group 3 findings were diagnostic for synovitis, while group 4 findings were consistent with scarring or fibrosis. Fitzgerald and Coventry injected the sheath proximal to

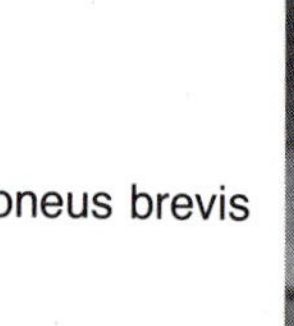

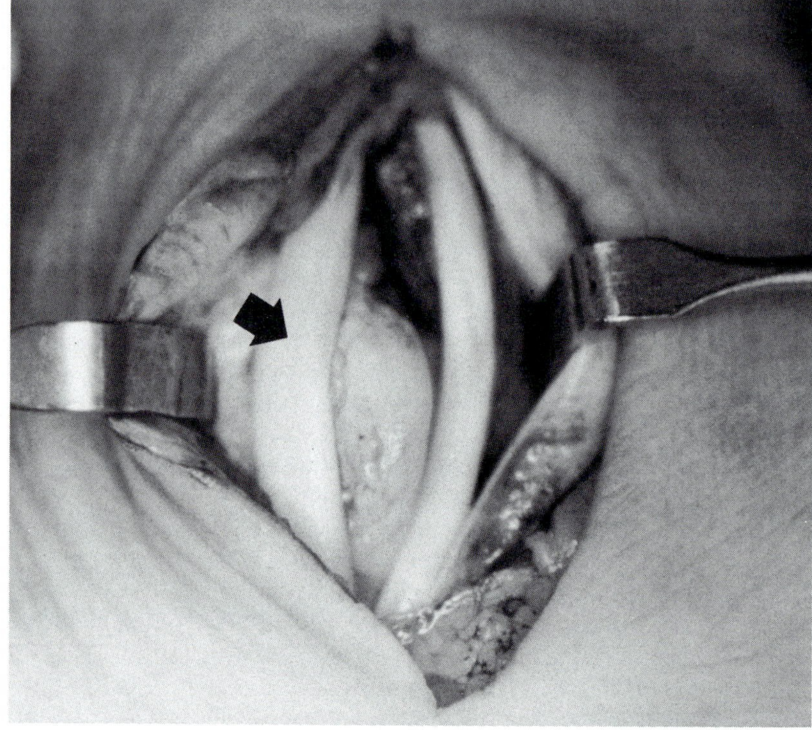

FIG 27–77.
Longitudinal tear of the peroneus brevis tendon.

the ankle in 12 patients suspected of having peroneal tendon pathology and discovered complete blockage or constriction of the sheath in all 12 cases.[563] More recently the CAT scan and MRI have been recommended for visualization of peroneal tendon abnormalities.[601, 602, 609, 624] In the patient who presents a difficult diagnostic dilemma or for whom objective documentation is necessary prior to surgery, one of these tests is often quite beneficial.

Treatment

Nonoperative Treatment

Treatment of athletic individuals with tendinitis or peritendinitis seen in the acute stage is RICE (rest, ice, compression, and elevation). When caught in the early stages, the problem usually resolves quickly with appropriate treatment. In the subacute phase, the response is slower, and some of these individuals require some form of immobilization (e.g., a brace, walking boot, or cast). Anti-inflammatory medication is a valuable adjunct. Once patients reach the chronic phase, the response to conservative measures is often disappointing. For these individuals, surgery is recommended only after they have failed an adequate program of conservative management. Athletes with chronic tendinitis often have not given the area sufficient rest to allow a proper healing response. Many runners, for example, will take 2 or 3 weeks off from their usual running program when faced with a painful tendinitis, but in the meantime they will try to run a shorter distance every few days just to "see how it's doing." Along this same line, they will take anti-inflammatory medication on a sporadic basis and then state that "it doesn't help me." For these reasons, it is imperative that athletes be educated concerning their condition and be brought to an understanding of what constitutes adequate medical management and rest. If the problem remains active or recurs immediately upon resumption of training, then surgery is offered as a treatment alternative.

Surgical Treatment

Surgery for the resistant case of tenosynovitis involves incising the tendon sheath and performing a tenosynovectomy. The superior and inferior retinaculum are preserved when possible and carefully repaired when their release is necessary. The tendons of the peroneus brevis and longus are carefully inspected for evidence of tears or degeneration. When there are tears of the tendons, they are generally longitudinal in nature (Fig 27–77). Depending on the chronicity, there may be significant fraying and fibrillation as well as fusiform enlargement and small masses of degenerative tendon (Fig 27–78). These areas are debrided and the tendon narrowed prior to repairing the tear with small absorbable suture. The tear is sewn in running fashion by using a method to invert the torn edge of the tendon. When the tendon is torn into two separate longitudinal sections, described by Don Jones as a bucket handle tear, the smaller or more severely damaged portion can be excised.[570] Five of six injuries treated in this fashion in young, active individuals did well with return to full activity. These cases of major longitudinal tears become less frequent as the diagnosis is made earlier, and this allows repair rather than excision of the tendon. When the peroneal tendons are ruptured with separation of the tendon ends, primary repair should be performed when possible. If primary repair is not achievable because of tendon retraction, then tenodesis of the proximal muscle-tendon remnant to the adjacent intact peroneal muscle and tendon is effective in maintaining function and relieving pain.[617]

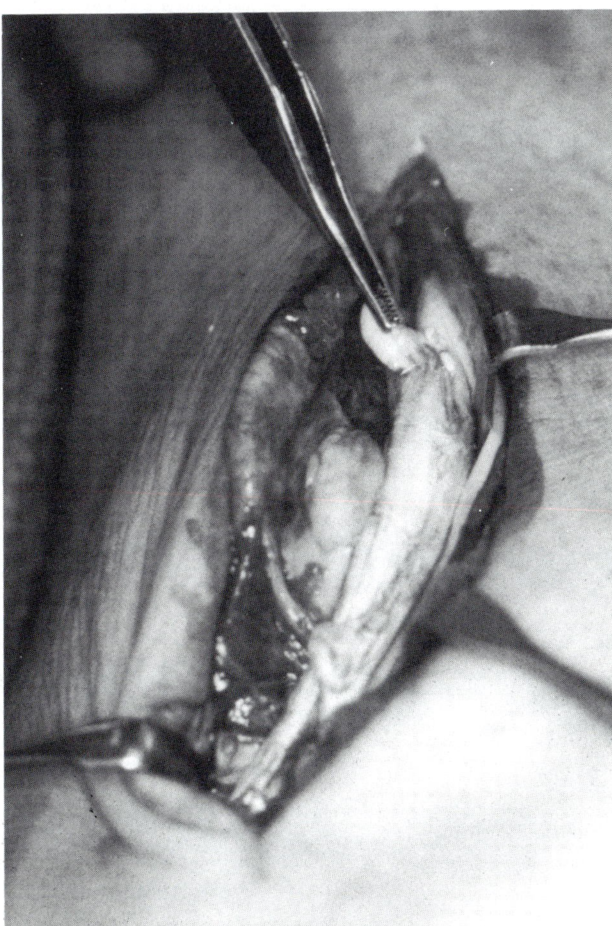

FIG 27–78.
Degenerative mass of a previously torn peroneus longus tendon.

POSTERIOR TIBIAL TENDINITIS AND TENDON RUPTURE

Other than overuse-related tenosynovitis, the vast majority of posterior tibial tendon problems, particularly ruptures, occur in middle-aged females.[629, 630, 634] Several studies of sports injuries mention tendinitis of the posterior tibial tendon among overuse problems.[626, 627, 632, 633] In the nonathletic population, rupture of the posterior tibial tendon has received considerable attention as a debilitating injury without a completely reliable solution, especially in the chronic condition.[629, 630, 634] For this reason it is critical to recognize its presentation and, preferably, institute treatment prior to rupture.

Incidence

A review of the literature on ruptures of the posterior tibial tendon reveals only four cases occurring in patients under the age of 30 years.[628, 631, 635, 636] Of these, only one case was in an athlete—a 20-year-old female runner with gradual onset of pain who had received several local steroid injections.[636] She was discovered to have a partial rupture near the navicular insertion. The only case of complete rupture in a young, healthy individual without prodromal symptoms occurred in a 26-year-old male who experienced sudden medial foot pain while stepping up into a bus.[631] At surgery he was found to have a complete rupture 1.5 cm from the navicular insertion. The only report to focus attention on

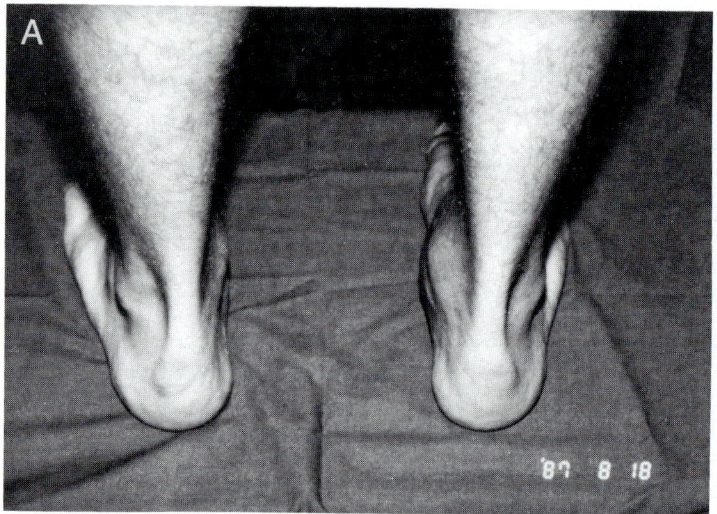

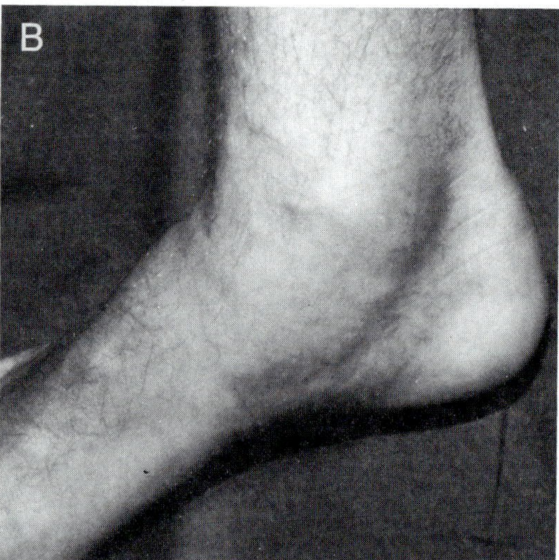

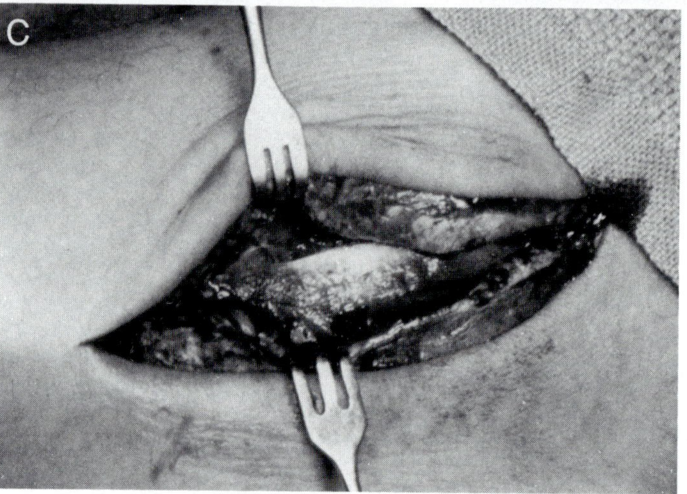

FIG 27–79.
Thirty-year-old athletic male with chronic posterior tibial tenosynovitis. **A,** posterior view showing thickening of the posterior tibial tendon sheath of the right ankle. **B,** medial view. **C,** intraoperative photograph demonstrating chronic posterior tibial tenosynovitis.

posterior tibial tendon ruptures in athletic individuals is that of Woods and Leach, who report six cases of complete or partial rupture.[636] They emphasize the importance of recognizing and treating this problem in the earlier stages.

Although tendon rupture does not appear to be a problem for athletes, tendinitis and tenosynovitis do occur with some frequency. Lysholm and Wiklander reported 2 cases in 55 injuries (3.6%) seen in 39 runners,[632] Macintyre and coauthors found a 2.3% incidence of posterior tibial tendinitis among 5,992 runners seen in their sports medicine clinic,[633] Clancy's study had 2 cases in 310 runners with injuries (0.6%),[627] and Cavanagh mentions a study of 974 injured runners with a 6% incidence of posterior tibial tendinitis. We see posterior tibial tendinitis, or more properly tenosynovitis, in a relatively small number of athletes (Fig 27–79,A and B). Most have sustained some injury to the foot or have an underlying anatomic reason for the problem. Examples of this include patients with an accessory navicular, a large navicular tuberosity, or a hyperpronated foot.

Treatment

Management of the athlete with posterior tibial tenosynovitis follows the generally prescribed regimen for other inflammatory conditions. If the patient does not respond, then cast or walking boot immobilization is recommended for a period of 4 to 6 weeks. If the problem persists longer than 4 to 6 months despite adequate conservative treatment, then surgery is recommended. This involves opening the tendon sheath and performing a tenosynovectomy (Fig 27–79). The tendon is carefully inspected for evidence of tear, and this is repaired if possible or debrided if badly frayed or hypertrophic. The patient is splinted postoperatively and use of a removable walking boot begun at 1 week. Progressive weight bearing begins, and the patient discontinues the use of crutches at 3 weeks. The walking boot is removed at 6 weeks. Athletic participation can usually begin around 4 months after the surgery.

ACHILLES TENDINITIS AND RUPTURES

The Achilles tendon has been a source of difficulty for both athletes and their physicians since antiquity. Whether the problem is peritendinitis, tendinitis, or rupture, the player's ability to continue or return to sports participation is jeopardized. Etiologically, most of these problems can be linked to overuse in the athletic environment.[644, 646, 657] While running is the most frequent sport involved, the Achilles tendon has proved vulnerable in most other sports as well.*

Epidemiology

Determining the incidence of Achilles tendon disorders in sports is difficult since most studies do not differentiate which tendon is involved in their "tendinitis" category or the studies do not separate Achilles tendinitis from Achilles ruptures in their reporting. In one of the original studies of running injuries, James et al. found Achilles tendinitis in 11% of their running clinic patients.[654] In other studies of runners, the percentage has ranged from 2.7 to 20.3.† In football, Zemper's study of 6,229 college football players noted Achilles tendon or heel problems in 0.8% of players, or 0.05 injuries per 1,000 athlete exposures.[674] In gymnastics, a study of injuries in 50 competitive gymnasts found a 5.4% incidence of injury to the heel or Achilles tendon.[639] Shaw's study of dance students at the University of Utah (an unpublished master's thesis quoted in Sohl and Bowling) reported a 4% incidence of Achilles tendon problems.[667] Rovere and coworkers found a 9% incidence of Achilles tendinitis in their study of 352 injuries to 185 theatrical dance students at the North Carolina School of the Arts.[664] A study of Danish championship tennis players reported a 4.3% incidence of injury to the Achilles tendon (2 in 89 players).[673] In ice skating, Achilles tendinitis from overuse was noted in 1 case among 49 injuries (2%).[666] This potpourri of studies provides good evidence of the pervasive nature of Achilles tendon problems in sports.

Among the epidemiologic studies, it is rare to see a report of an actual rupture of the Achilles tendon in competitive athletes. One volleyball participant ruptured her Achilles tendon, but she played in the women's senior division.[665] Rupture of the Achilles tendon is notably rare in dance forms from classical ballet to modern dance.[645] An 18-year-old dancer with a ruptured Achilles tendon is described in one report, but no statistical data are provided.[647] Likewise, a comprehensive study of dancers by Washington mentions three Achilles tendon ruptures without providing an incidence rate.[670] The best epidemiologic data come from the study by Józsa et al. of 292 Achilles ruptures.[655] They found 15 cases of rupture in the 20-year-old and under group, only 5 of which were sports related. Indeed, the most common age range for a sports-related rupture of

---

**References 639, 640, 644, 646, 654, 658, 660, 671, 674.*
†References 640, 641, 648, 653, 658, 659, 669, 671.

the Achilles tendon was 41 to 50 years of age. Overall, 173 (59%) of their 292 ruptures occurred in sports. Football, track and field, and basketball were the most common sports cited. This study also provides a table showing the distribution of Achilles tendon ruptures by sports from various studies in the literature (Table 27–8). In our experience at Rice University, there have been no cases of Achilles tendon rupture in an intercollegiate athlete during the past 25 years. It appears that the vast majority of Achilles tendon ruptures occur in the over-30 age group and in recreational athletes.

Etiology

When the problem is tendinitis or tenosynovitis, a detailed history will generally disclose a training-related problem.[642] James has referred to "accumulated impact loading," while others point out the problem of doing "too much, too soon."[648, 654, 669, 672] In running this may mean too much mileage early in the training schedule, while in ice skating it may be too many jumps prior to developing adequate leg strength. The young dancer trying to vigorously improve her pointe or relevé may irritate the Achilles tendon, or it may be the cyclist who is training hard and has the saddle positioned too low with the ankle kept in excessive dorsiflexion. Regardless, for the athlete under 25 years of age, there is almost always a discoverable mechanical source for the difficulty. Common etiologic factors other than overtraining include overpronation, poor gastrocnemius-soleus flexibility and strength, and faulty footwear.[642] After 25 years of age, there is a gradually increasing propensity for some intrinsic problem within the tendon to be the source. Many of these individuals have been relatively sedentary for a period of time before renewing an active athletic life-style. This is the setting in which the majority of Achilles tendon ruptures occur. This is particularly true when the 40-year-old former athlete tries to demonstrate his skill on the basketball or volleyball court once a year. In these instances where the tendon fails, histologic studies have confirmed pre-existing degenerative changes within the tendon.[637, 641, 649, 650, 663] These changes will often be silent in terms of producing symptomotology prior to actual failure of the tendon. In contrast, those athletes with symptoms of tenosynovitis rarely go on to a complete rupture of the tendon.[672]

Diagnosis and Treatment

Clinical Evaluation

Since the evaluation and treatment of Achilles tendon disorders have already been covered extensively in Chapter 19, the remaining discussion will be consider-

TABLE 27–8.

Distribution of Achilles Tendon Injuries by Sports From the Literature*

Sport	Holz[645] 1983 Germany	Frings[643] 1968 Germany	Schedl[662] 1983 Austria	Nillius et al.[655] 1976 Sweden	Kellam et al.[649] 1985 Canada	Zollinger[670] 1983 Switzerland	Cetti & Christensen[639] 1981 Denmark	Inglis[647] 1981 USA	Jozsa et al.[648] 1988 Hungary
Football	168	102	13	35	33	300	7	18	58
Handball	57	32		9			19	4	10
Volleyball	6		14		5			4	3
Basketball	6							29	23
Badminton		4		38			20		
Tennis	23	5	4	15					12
Table tennis		4		5				20	2
Other ball games		9				230		20	5
Gymnastics	47	43	7	19		110	5		12
Running	42	46	5	6					14
Jumping	18	31			17			5	14
Diving									
Climbing							1		
Rock climbing									3
Weight lifting									6
Trampoline							1		
Bicycling	39							1	3
Skiing	73	6	19		4	570		12	4
Dancing								10	7
Jogging								9	
Others		30	6	7		30			
Total	479	317	68	134	59	1,240	53	131	173

*From Jozsa L, Kvist M. Balint B, et al: *Am J Sports Med* 17:338–343, 1989. Used by permission.

ably abbreviated, and the reader is referred to the prior material. While Achilles tendon pain is not difficult to diagnose, it may present a challenge in differentiating peritendinitis from actual tendinitis. The "painful arc" sign may be useful in this case[672] (Fig 27–80). When the foot is moved from dorsiflexion to plantar flexion, the tenderness and swelling remain fixed in reference to the malleoli when the problem is in the tendon sheath, i.e., peritendinitis (Fig 27–80,A). When the lesion is in the tendon, the tenderness and swelling move with the tendon as the foot goes from dorsiflexion to plantar flexion (Fig 27–80,B). In combined lesions, one sees some movement of the physical signs and some fixation.

Nonoperative Treatment

The nonoperative treatment of Achilles tendinitis has produced variable results. When discovered early, it is almost always possible to alleviate the problem of acute tenosynovitis with rest and various physical therapy modalities.[642, 643] We have actually noticed a decreased prevalence of Achilles tendinitis over the past 10 years that we relate to improvements in shoe wear and the use of the ice-water whirlpool after workouts by our athletes. Others have noted this same reduction in Achilles tendinitis during this time period, with a corresponding increase in the incidence of knee and leg problems.[640, 659] Perhaps the protective value of the shoe and its modifications is merely transferring stress from one site and placing it on another.

Surgical Treatment

There are certain instances where conservative treatment of Achilles tendon lesions fails and one must proceed with surgery. We feel that the young athlete with a ruptured Achilles tendon falls into this category (Fig 27–81). There have been numerous studies detailing the advantages and disadvantages of operative and nonoperative treatment of Achilles tendon ruptures.* The consensus seems to be that the results are relatively the same other than a higher rerupture rate in the nonoperative group. This may be the case, but operative patients seem to regain function more quickly, and we are more confident in allowing their return to sports.

The other situation where we consider surgical intervention is the athlete with symptoms of tendinitis who has not responded to an adequate nonoperative treatment program of 4 months' duration, including a period of relative immobilization. This immobilization is provided by a walking boot rather than a cast in order to allow continued use of physical therapy modalities and gentle stretching exercises. When the individual remains significantly disabled from his normal life-style, the choice of surgery vs. continued avoidance of stressful sports is offered with the risks and benefits of each alternative. At surgery, the paratenon is exposed from the calcaneal insertion to the musculotendinous junction. The paratenon and any associated fibrosis are excised over approximately two thirds of the tendon's circumference. The tendon is inspected and palpated for any abnormality and is split longitudinally to visualize the underlying tendon substance. Necrotic tendon or areas of nodularity are excised, and the tendon is closed

---

**References 638, 649, 651, 652, 656, 661, 662, 668.*

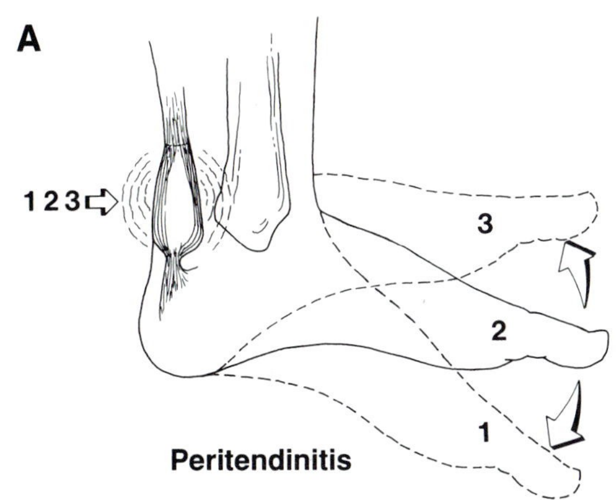

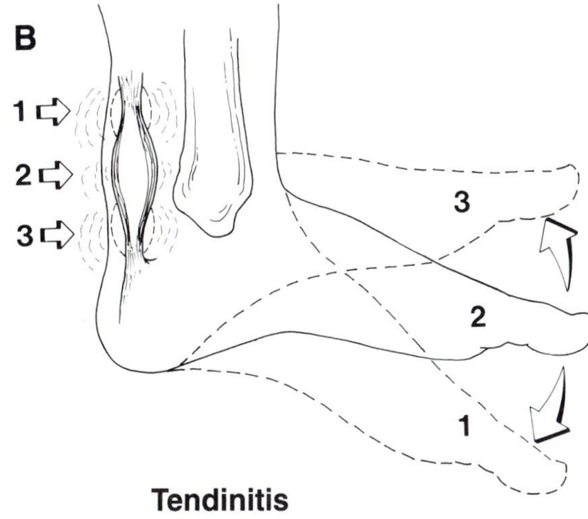

FIG 27–80.
Painful arc sign. **A,** in peritendinitis, the tenderness remains in one position despite moving the foot from dorsiflexion to plantar flexion. **B,** in the case of partial tendon rupture or tendinitis, the point of tenderness moves as the foot goes from dorsiflexion to plantar flexion. (From Williams JGP: *Sports Med* 3:114–135, 1986. Used by permission.)

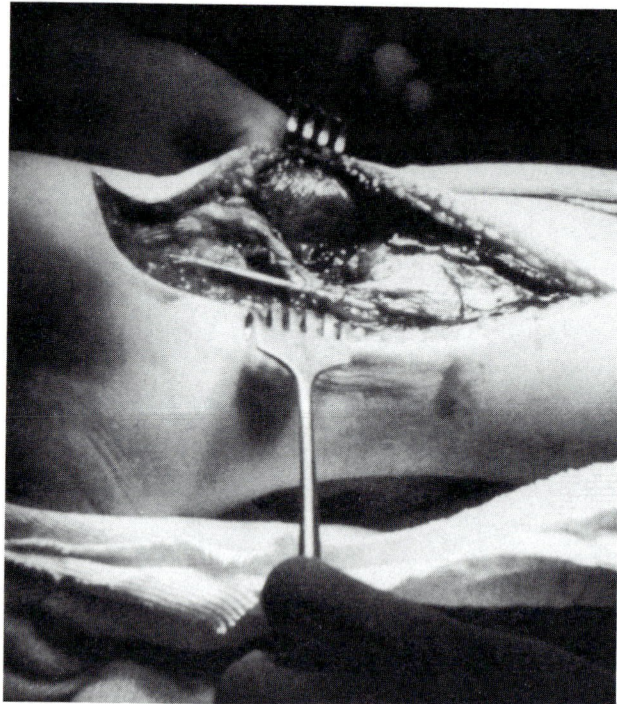

FIG 27–81.
Achilles tendon rupture in the young athlete is an indication for surgical repair.

with a small absorbable suture placed with a running technique using buried knots. Postoperative management allows motion in all cases where the tendon is not completely ruptured. The degree of movement and the amount of weight bearing are determined by the extent of the pathology. In complete ruptures, we apply a cast in slight plantar flexion to produce some tension on the repaired tendon. Weight bearing in a walking boot with a heel lift is allowed at 6 weeks. The athlete rarely returns to athletic activity prior to 6 months, and it is usually a year before full rehabilitation has been achieved.

MIDFOOT SPRAINS

Definition of Injury

Sprains involving the ligaments of the transverse tarsal (midtarsal), intertarsal, and tarsometatarsal joints are poorly defined injuries. On the other hand, much has been written concerning fractures and dislocations to these joints. As discussed in previous sections, there is a continuum of injury between sprains with stretching of the ligament (grade 1), sprains with partial ligamentous rupture (grade 2), and complete rupture of the ligaments (grade 3). Furthermore, the injury may cause no instability at the affected joint, or there may be subluxation or even dislocation as the degree of injury increases. The ligamentous injury can be an in-substance tear of the ligament or a failure at the attachment site by bony avulsion. The more severe stages of injury to the midfoot are covered thoroughly in the chapter on fractures and dislocations of the foot (Chapter 35) and will not be discussed here at length. However, the lesser grades of injury are occasionally seen in athletes and can become a persistent source of difficulty if not treated appropriately.

Incidence

The incidence of midfoot sprains in sports is impossible to determine from statistics found in the existing literature on individual sports or on sports in a collective sense. The primary problem is a lack of specificity in the reporting of injuries. Either the study categorizes injuries by type (e.g., contusion, fracture, strain, sprain, etc.) or by anatomic location in general (e.g., hand, arm, shoulder, hip, leg, knee, ankle, foot, etc.). As an example, Marti et al. have reported on the epidemiology of running injuries among 4,358 males and noted a 3.2% incidence of midfoot injuries.[690] Unfortunately, there are no data provided concerning the exact nature of these injuries. From studies such as these, one can only determine that some sports have very low rates of injury to the foot (e.g., swimming and skiing), while other sports have significant rates of foot-related problems (e.g., running and football). Some studies go further in their analysis of injury and give a categorization of the type of injury by anatomic site. In such reports "foot sprains" account for a very small percentage of the overall injuries in sports. This ranges from 0% to 6.7%.* The sports studies reporting the highest incidence of foot sprains were badminton and racquetball.[686, 700] In one of the few reports specifically devoted to foot and ankle injuries in a sport, Meyer reported 4 sprains and 1 dislocation of the foot among a total of 35 injuries to the foot occurring during a major league baseball season.[692] This degree of specificity is the best that is found in the available literature and provides little insight into the incidence of midfoot sprains, or any other specific diagnosis in the foot for that matter. In a retrospective review of records from 1971 to 1985 of 1,063 Rice University athletes, there were 188 foot injuries that required treatment.[675] Of these, the most common injury was a sprain of the metatarsophalangeal joint (63 injuries in 53 athletes). Upon a review

---

**References 676, 677, 679, 680, 686, 691, 694, 699, 700, 703.*

of injury records, it was found that the second leading category of foot injury was sprain of the midfoot, which accounted for 24 separate injuries, or 12.7% of all foot injuries in intercollegiate athletes at Rice.

Approaching the analysis of midfoot injuries from a different direction leads to a similar paucity of information. In the studies reporting injury to the tarsometatarsal joint, the majority of injuries are reported to occur from falls or jumps from a height, motor vehicle accidents, or crush injuries to the midfoot. There are only a few reports that mention sports-related causes.[681, 682, 687, 696] LaTourette and coauthors report one fracture-dislocation of the tarsometatarsal joint from sliding into a base in baseball.[687] Foster and Foster's series of tarsometatarsal fracture-dislocations includes one case of injury while playing handball.[682] The other reports do not specify the sport involved.[681, 696] Two papers addressing this subject have recently been presented at national orthopaedic meetings.[678, 693] Moyer et al. described 13 patients with traumatic diastasis of the proximal first and second metatarsal joints from a sports-related injury.[693] Four of these individuals were injured playing football. Curtis and coworkers reviewed 20 patients with tarsometatarsal injuries sustained during athletic activities ranging from baseball to sailboarding.[678] In their series, 7 were injured in basketball, 5 while running, 4 while sailboarding, and the rest in baseball, soccer, or gymnastics. It appears that there is an increasing awareness of this injury in sports, particularly for the minor grades of injury, which do not have such dramatic findings on clinical or radiographic evaluation.

Despite this growing awareness, there is still a lack of information on the sports-related incidence of injury to the transverse tarsal (midtarsal) joint and intertarsal joints. The classic article on this subject by Main and Jowett does not include a single athletic injury in 71 cases.[688] Hooper and McMaster have reported bilateral midtarsal subluxations occurring in a 19-year-old female who stumbled while running.[684] Zwipp and Krettek found instability in the midtarsal joints in three patients who ultimately required surgical stabilization.[704] A rather ill-defined problem that may have some relationship to midtarsal subluxation or instability is cuboid syndrome, a condition described by Newell and Woodle and discussed in the dance literature.[683, 689, 695] Newell and Woodle report a 4% incidence of this condition from their review of 3,600 athletes with foot injuries.[695] Among the other reports of this condition, there is no statistical information provided.[683, 689] (Further discussion of this entity can be found in the following section on injuries in dancers.) A discussion of joint subluxations in the midfoot is found in the chiropractic literature, but there is no objective test documenting these subluxations, and there are no epidemiologic data concerning their incidence or prevalence.[698] From both a review of the literature and personal experience, the authors believe that midtarsal joint sprains are quite uncommon as isolated injuries and are usually associated with significant fractures to the bones in this region. This diverts attention from the associated ligamentous injury. Whether these acute sprains or chronic overuse problems can develop into chronic instability patterns or subluxation of the transverse tarsal joint remains open to question.

Mechanism of Injury

The most common mechanism of injury to the midfoot in sports is twisting of the foot. This can be related to fixation of the foot in artificial grass as noted in three of the patients of Moyer et al.[693] Twisting the foot while sliding into a base has been a reported etiology and could probably be eliminated by usage of breakaway bases as suggested by Janda et al.[685] In football we have seen the injury from having the midfoot stepped on—a source of considerable load when it involves a 300-lb lineman. Curtis et al. noted that the mechanism of injury in their series of patients was combined forced plantar flexion and rotation, with or without abduction of the forefoot.[678] In sailboarding, the added factor of having the foot strapped onto the board slightly alters the mechanism. These individuals are injured in sudden backward falls that force the fixed forefoot into equinus and damage the dorsal stabilizers of the tarsometatarsal joints. The mechanism of injury for midtarsal joint and metatarsophalangeal injury is discussed more fully in the section devoted to these topics under fractures and dislocations of the foot.

Diagnosis

Anatomic Considerations

Proper clinical evaluation of these injuries requires a thorough understanding of the underlying anatomy, the biomechanics, and the mechanism of injury. There is an abundance of capsular and ligamentous tissue in this region, and the tendons of the peroneus longus and brevis, posterior tibialis, and anterior tibialis muscles attach here as well (Fig 27–82). Stability provided by the metatarsocuneiform ligament (Lisfranc's ligament) at the base of the second metatarsal is the key to preventing diastasis in this area (Fig 27–83).

Clinical Findings

When evaluating the patient with a midfoot injury, a thorough history will generally reveal the mechanism of

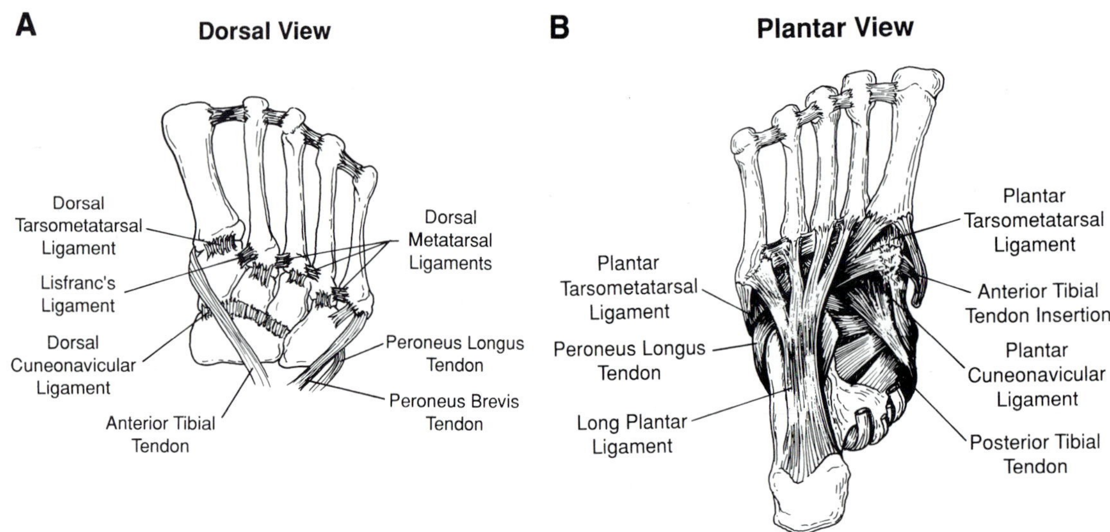

FIG 27–82.
Anatomic relationships of the ligaments and tendons at the midfoot: **A,** dorsal view; **B,** plantar view.

injury. Patients complain of pain in the midfoot region, but it can vary considerably in severity depending upon the degree of injury. Pain with weight bearing is a common feature, and there is an inability to run or jump on the involved foot. It is important to perform a careful examination of the foot to pinpoint the area of maximum tenderness if possible. Tenderness at the base of the first and second metatarsals is an important finding in subtle diastasis injuries. Tenderness over the articulation between the fourth and fifth metatarsals with the cuboid may be the only objective finding in the case of a lateral tarsometatarsal injury. In more severe injuries, palpation of specific locations may be precluded by pain and swelling. Testing the joints by manipulation can at times disclose excessive movement indicative of instability. In the patient suspected of having a severe injury to the midfoot who will not allow an adequate examination in the office or training room, examination under anesthesia including stress radiographs is warranted (Fig 27–84).

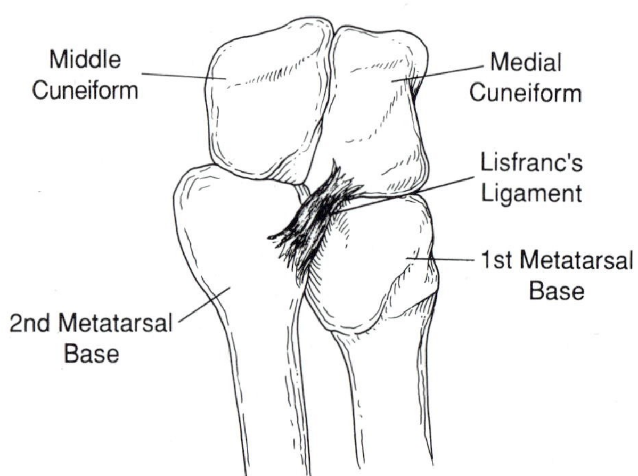

FIG 27–83.
Anatomic drawing of Lisfranc's ligament stabilizing the first and second tarsometatarsal joints.

Radiographic Evaluation

In the radiographic assessment of patients with midfoot injuries, close attention to bone alignment and detail is necessary to avoid overlooking subtle signs of significant injury (Fig 27–85). Diastasis of the proximal first and second metatarsal joints can easily be neglected if one is not cognizant of this problem. The average distance between the first and second metatarsal bases in uninjured feet measures 1.3 mm. When the measurement of this interval is 2 mm or more, a diastasis is considered to be present.[681] Further confirmation is demonstrated by an increase of 1 mm or more in this interval when a comparison is made with radiographs of the uninjured side. The use of a weight-bearing radiograph for these measurements is important (Fig 27–86). Faciszewski et al. have recently recommended the use of the weight-bearing lateral radiograph as an important prognosticating test for tarsometatarsal joint injuries.[681] They measure the distance from the plantar aspect of the fifth metatarsal to the plantar aspect of the medial cuneiform and compare it between the injured and uninjured feet (Fig 27–87). Normally, the medial cuneiform lies dorsal to the fifth metatarsal, which gives the measurement a positive value in the authors' system (Fig 27–87,A). The average measurement in normal feet was 1.5 mm (range, 0 to 4 mm). No normal feet

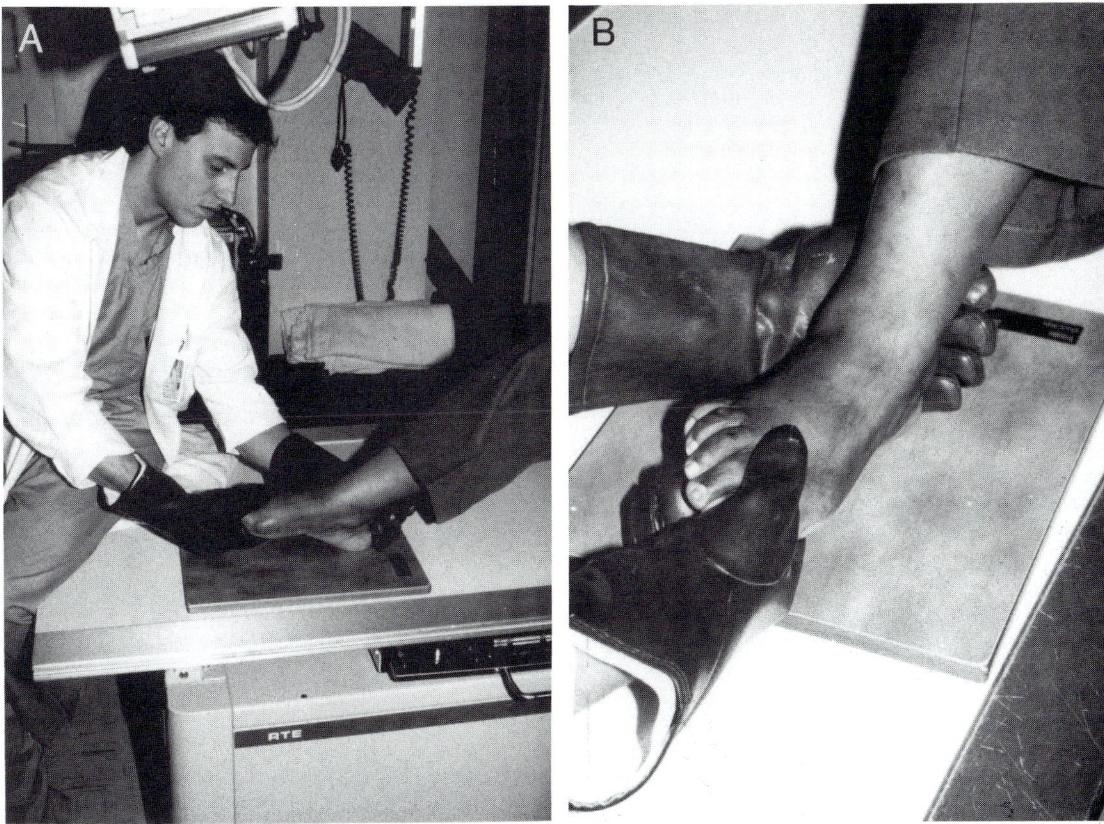

FIG 27–84.
Method for stress testing the midfoot by using pronation and abduction: **A,** overview; **B,** close-up.

had negative values (plantar border of the medial cuneiform lower than the plantar border of the fifth metatarsal base). The authors relate loss of the longitudinal arch to a negative value on this measurement and correlate it to poor results in their series of patients (Fig 27–87,B). They did not find a correlation between the amount of diastasis and the end result. We have been unable to confirm these conclusions in our own patients and disagree with their statement that "the extent of the diastasis does not correlate with the patient's functional result."[681]

In the evaluation of the initial radiographs, it is also important to search for small avulsion fractures since they can be indicative of serious ligamentous injury. As an example, fracture of the base of the second metatarsal or the medial cuneiform is not uncommon in the presence of a significant Lisfranc joint injury.[701, 702] Minor changes in the relationship of the metatarsal and tarsal bones reflect a major loss of capsular and ligament integrity. Stress radiographs with pronation-abduction and supination-adduction can assist in disclosing subtle grades of tarsometatarsal joint instability. Zwipp and Krettek have utilized a stress radiograph method to document transverse tarsal joint instability[704] (Fig 27–88). Because of the overlapping nature of the small bones in the midfoot and their varying joint congruity, the use of comparison radiographs can be helpful, and utilization of CAT scanning is frequently essential to properly define the bone injury and relationships. Only recently has the use of the MRI been suggested as a method for delineating soft-tissue trauma to the midfoot.

Treatment

Acute Injury

Treatment of injuries to the midfoot must be based on the extent of the injury and the degree of instability. Acute treatment begins with the RICE formula of rest, ice, compression, and elevation. If the patient has significant pain with weight bearing, the use of crutches with weight bearing as tolerated is allowed. Minor sprains are treated in this fashion, and athletes are returned to participation with supportive taping and a stiff-soled shoe or the use of a spring stainless steel–reinforced insole inside the shoe (Fig 27–89). This return to play can take as long as 4 to 6 weeks in

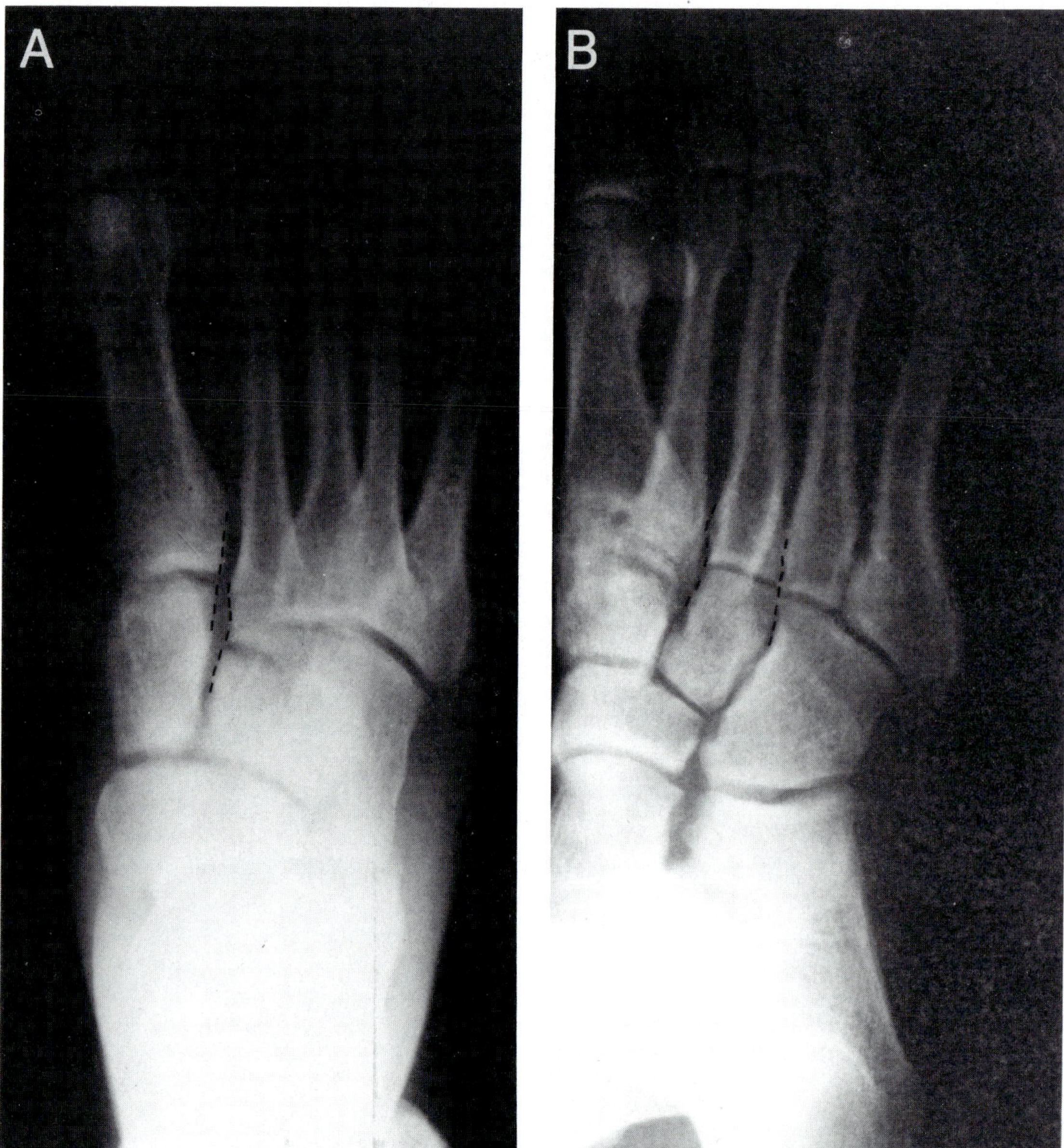

FIG 27–85.
Radiographic relationships at the midfoot in the uninjured foot. **A,** AP view showing the lateral base of the first metatarsal lining up with the lateral base of the medial cuneiform and the medial base of the second metatarsal lining up with the medial aspect of the middle cuneiform. **B,** oblique view showing the medial base of the third metatarsal lining up with the medial base of the lateral cuneiform and the medial base of the fourth metatarsal lining up with the medial aspect of the cuboid.

some of these "minor" sprains. If there is instability present by examination in any of the joints of the midfoot, a more thorough evaluation is undertaken. The presence of a diastasis is treated by surgical correction. If examination of the midfoot under anesthesia reveals instability (without displacement noted on the routine radiographs), consideration is given to stabilization of the joints by the insertion of percutaneous Kirschner wires under fluoroscopic control followed by application of a cast (Fig 27–90). Immobilization continues in a non–weight-bearing cast for 4 weeks followed by a walking cast or brace for an additional 4 weeks. The presence of any displacement is not tolerated well in this region, and therefore open reduction–internal fixa-

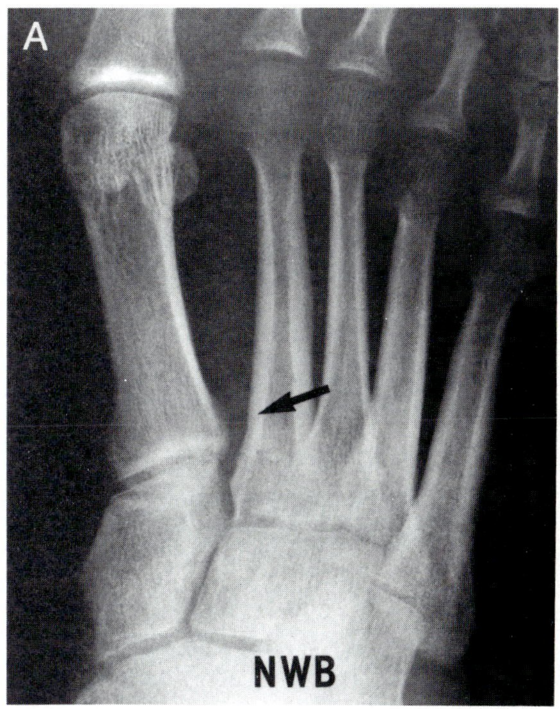

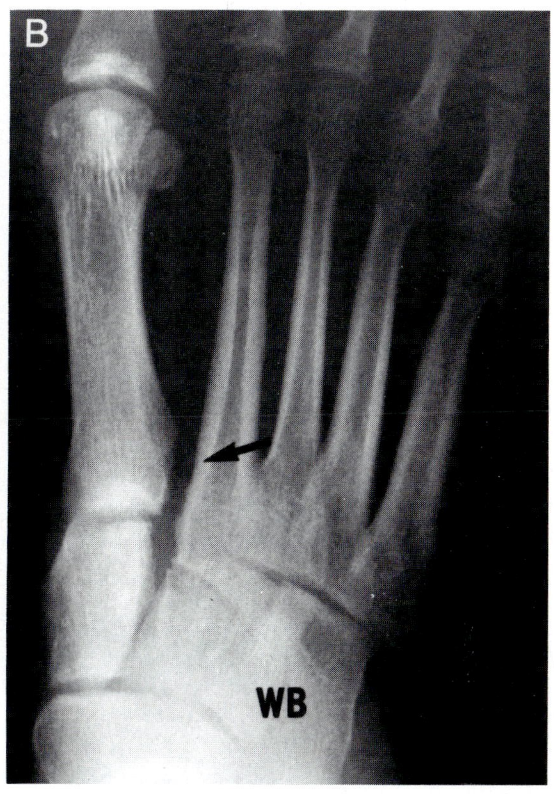

FIG 27–86.
Occult diastasis *(arrows)* of the first and second metatarsal bases may be missed on a non–weight-bearing radiograph. **A,** initial radiograph of the injured midfoot taken with the patient non–weight bearing *(NWB).* **B,** a weight-bearing *(WB)* radiograph of the same foot demonstrates significant diastasis.

tion is the procedure of choice when this is present (Fig 27–91).

Chronic Injury

Chronic instability in the joints of the midfoot does not permit athletic participation and has not been previously discussed as an entity seen among athletes. Surgical treatment of transverse tarsal joint instability has been reported in the German literature by Zwipp and Krettek, who used a modification of the Chrisman-Snook procedure.[704] Hooper and McMaster performed arthrodesis on the talonavicular and calcaneocuboid

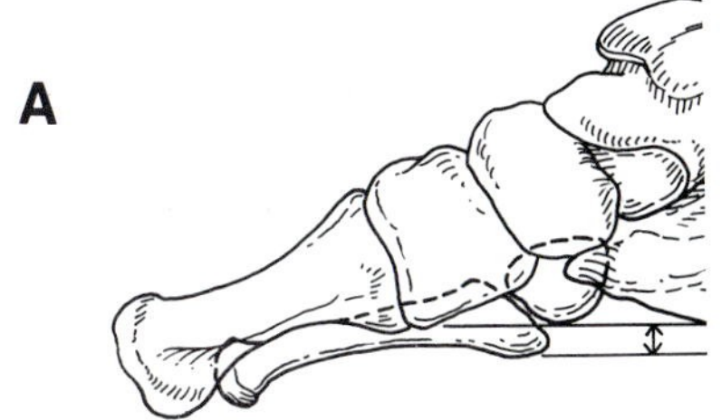

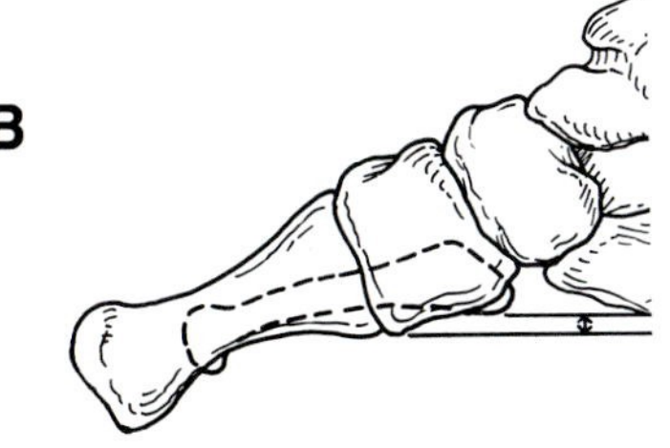

FIG 27–87.
Radiographic method for diagnosing significant injury to the tarsometatarsal joints. **A,** the normal relationship of the medial cuneiform and the base of the fifth metatarsal. It is considered a positive value when the inferior border of the medial cuneiform is dorsal to the inferior border of the fifth metatarsal base by some distance. **B,** with significant injury to the midfoot, there is flattening, with the medial cuneiform plantar to the fifth metatarsal base by some distance (a negative value). (From Faciszewski T, Burks RT, Manaster BJ: *J Bone Joint Surg [Am]* 72: 1519–1522, 1990. Used by permission.)

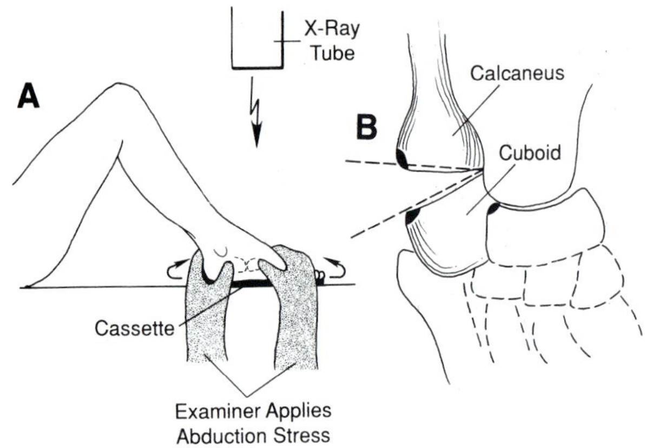

FIG 27–88.
Method for evaluating the transverse tarsal joint for instability. (Adapted from Zwipp H, Krettek C: *Orthopäde* 15:472–478, 1986.)

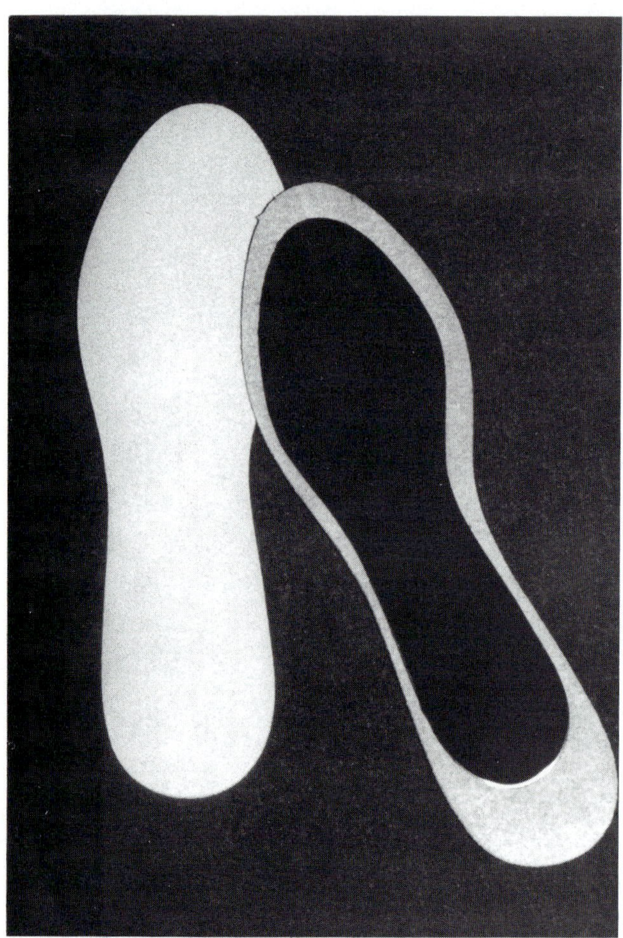

FIG 27–89.
A full-length reinforced insole can be used for protection of the athlete with a previous midfoot sprain. (Turf Toe Insert, Product no. 726, Scott Foot Care Products, Omaha, Neb.)

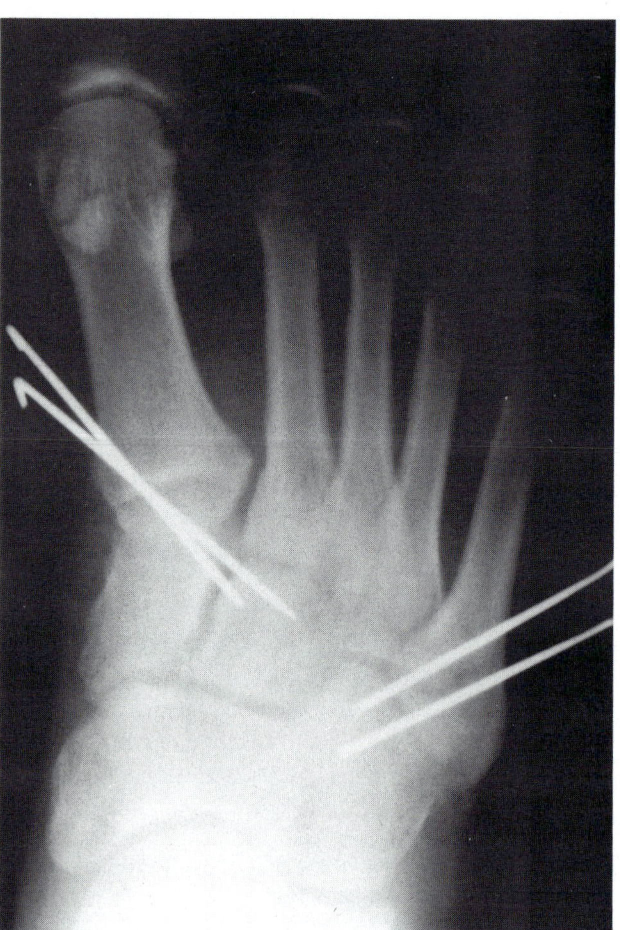

FIG 27–90.
In a potentially unstable but well-reduced tarsometatarsal joint injury, adequate treatment may be accomplished with the use of percutaneously inserted smooth Kirschner wires.

joints in their patient with bilateral midtarsal subluxation.[684] This seems to be the logical alternative in the nonathletic patient with significant instability, but it would certainly limit future athletic involvement for most individuals.

In conclusion, soft-tissue injuries to the midfoot, including both the tarsometatarsal joint and transverse tarsal joint, are seen in sports but often go unrecognized initially. The degree of injury may be masked initially, and proper diagnosis requires a thorough understanding of the anatomy of the area coupled with knowledge of the mechanism of injury. When this is applied along with a detailed physical examination and radiographic evaluation, one can avoid the difficulties that can arise from chronic unrecognized injury to this region. Early aggressive treatment, including the use of open reduction and internal fixation for displacement, produces the best results in these injuries.

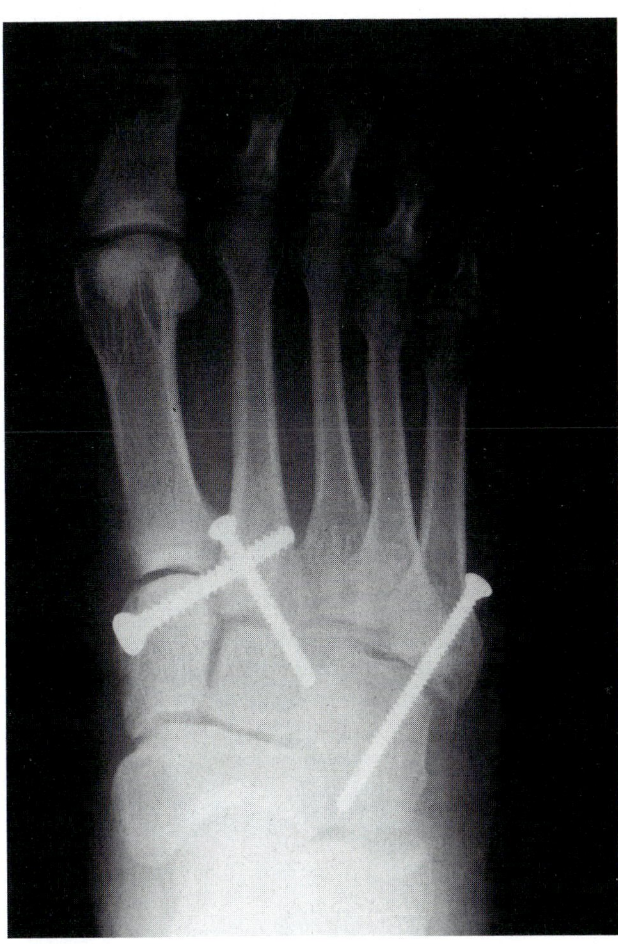

FIG 27–91.
An unstable tarsometatarsal joint injury with diastasis or joint displacement requires anatomic reduction and rigid fixation.

FOREFOOT SPRAINS

The athletic foot injury that has received the greatest notoriety recently is the sprain of the first metatarsophalangeal joint—commonly called "turf toe"[721] (Fig 27–92). This has apparently resulted from the importance that our society places on professional sports and the publicity that these athletes receive when they miss a game due to injury. Another factor is the controversy over the role of artificial playing surfaces in the production of injuries in professional sports.[737] As a result, one can now find information in major city newspapers listing the athletes injured on a particular team including those who have "turf toe." While other forefoot sprains certainly occur, none have received as much attention as this injury to the first metatarsophalangeal joint. Therefore, this section will primarily focus on sprains of the great toe.

Historical Perspective

Although sprains in the forefoot occurred in sports prior to the introduction of artificial grass in 1966, the injury was considered a minor problem. In 1975, during a roundtable discussion on the pros and cons of artificial turf, the relationship between sprains of the first metatarsophalangeal joint and artificial grass playing surfaces was first mentioned in the medical literature.[728] The term "turf toe" was later coined in the literature by Bowers and Martin in 1976 when they attributed the injury to the combination of the hard artificial playing surface and the use of flexible shoe wear.[709] The prevalence of this condition and its increasing recognition in college football was evident from the study by Coker et al. from the University of Arkansas in 1978.[713] They surveyed athletic trainers at 94 colleges and universities and found this sprain of the first metatarsophalangeal joint to be increasingly more common and a significant source of missed playing time.

Epidemiology

The true incidence of forefoot sprains in sports has never been accurately defined. At West Virginia University, 27 first metatarsophalangeal joint sprains were reported in a five-season period.[709] This is a 5.4 injury-per-season average in a population of approximately 500 players. Eighteen forefoot injuries occurring over three seasons were reported among University of Arkansas football players—a six injury-per-season average.[713] During a 14-year period at Rice University, Clanton et al. reported 63 metatarsophalangeal joint injuries in 53 athletes.[710] This report included all sports, and the average was 4.5 such injuries per year. Each year of their study had at least 1 injury, with a maximum of 9 reported injuries to the metatarsophalangeal joints in 1 year. Rodeo and coworkers found that 45% of 80 active professional football players had sustained a turf toe injury.[727] Only the study by Clanton et al. documents injury to the lesser metatarsophalangeal joints; they found 13 injuries in seven athletes.[710]

Severity of Injury

Having established the prevalence of forefoot sprains, the question now arises as to the severity of this injury. Comparing first metatarsophalangeal joint sprains with the more familiar lateral ankle sprain, Coker and coauthors found ankle sprains to be four times more common but accounted for less than double the number of missed practices.[713] In fact, there were more missed games from the great toe injuries (7) than from ankle sprains (6). In the study from Rice Univer-

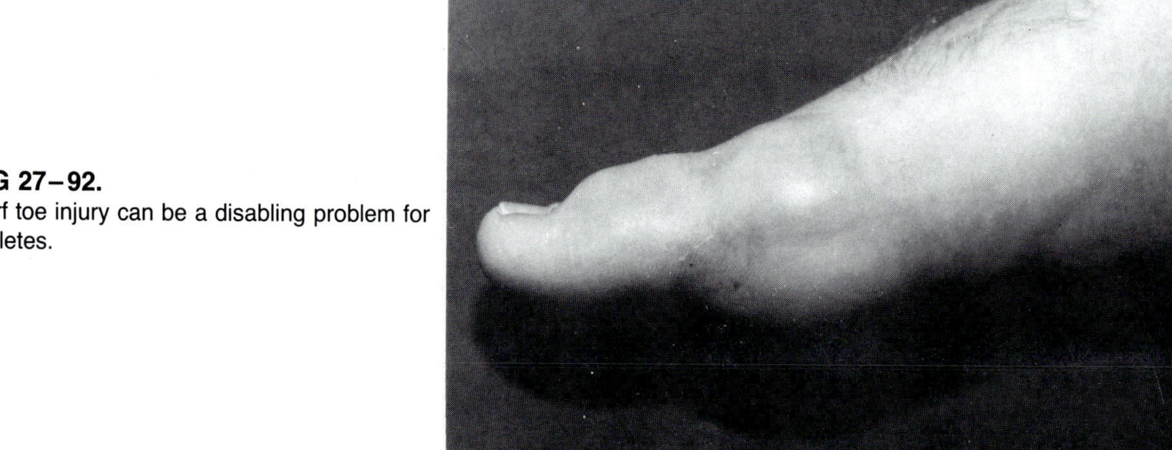

FIG 27–92.
Turf toe injury can be a disabling problem for athletes.

sity, players averaged missing 6 days of athletic participation.[710] From a study of the local newspaper during the football season, it is quite evident that professional players frequently miss games due to turf toe injury. It has even been implied that chronic pain from this entity has led to the retirement of certain professional footbal players.[737]

Mechanism of Injury

Since the original description of the problem, turf toe injuries have been known to occur primarily from the mechanism of hyperextension of the great toe metatarsophalangeal joint. Ryan et al. described this mechanism in football linemen driving off the foot from their stance.[728] Others have added various components to this mechanism, including having the forefoot fixed in the turf and having the heel raised.[709] A similar hyperextension force is seen when a player is in a pileup with his forefoot on the ground and the heel raised and another player lands on the back of his leg and forces the metatarsophalangeal joints into hyperextension[713] (Fig 27–93). Other less common mechanisms described are hyperflexion and valgus.[713] Hyperflexion can occur when a ball carrier is tackled from behind and the knee is forced forward; a plantar-flexed foot is pushed further in this direction, and the metatarsophalangeal joints are sprained at the same time. Valgus is often a variable in the hyperextension injury and is produced by the force of pushing off on the foot from stance. It is the mechanism responsible for symptoms of a more chronic nature according to Coker et al.[713] Depending on the mechanism of injury, different structures can be damaged.

Another mechanism of injury that is seldom seen in turf-related injuries of the metatarsophalangeal joint is varus stress. Mullis and Miller have reported one such injury in a basketball player who externally rotated on a fixed foot and sustained a tear of the adductor hallucis tendon from the base of the proximal phalanx along with a tear in the lateral capsule and collateral ligament.[722] No other similar case has been reported in sports or otherwise.

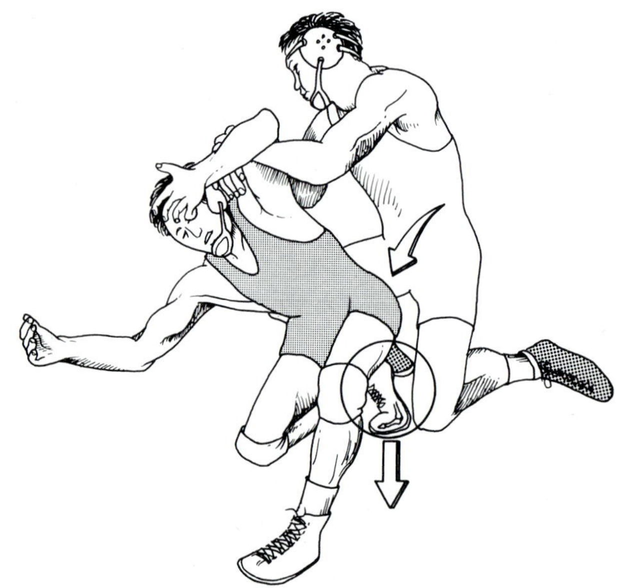

FIG 27–93.
Illustration of a common mechanism for turf toe injury with one player falling on the leg of another player whose foot is fixed on the turf. (From Rodeo SA, O'Brien S, Warren RF, et al: *Am J Sports Med* 18:280-285, 1990. Used by permission.)

Anatomy and Biomechanics

The capsuloligamentous complex of the metatarsophalangeal joint is the key factor contributing to its stability.[732] Relatively minor stability is provided by the shallow socket of the proximal phalangeal base articulating with the ball of the metatarsal head. The tendinous portions of the abductor and adductor hallucis provide some support to the medial and lateral capsule, respectively. The long flexor and extensor tendons contribute minimally to stability, while the short flexor and extensor tendons blend with the capsule and provide important stabilizing elements (Fig 27–94,A). The medial and lateral sides of the joint are supported by strong collateral ligaments that have two components (Fig 27–94,B). At the first metatarsophalangeal joint, these are the metatarsophalangeal and metatarsosesamoid ligaments. These ligaments have a narrow origin on the medial or lateral border of the metatarsal head and fan out to insert on the medial or lateral border of the proximal phalanx and the medial and lateral borders of the plantar plate. The plantar plate is a thickened fibrous portion of the capsule that blends with the sesamoids and the tendons of the short flexor for the great toe. The medial and lateral sesamoid bones are intrinsic to the stability provided by the capsuloligamentous complex (Fig 27–94,C). Sesamoids are much less common in the lesser metatarsophalangeal joints and occur in fewer than 10% of normal feet.[732] The plantar plate is firmly attached at its insertion to the base of the proximal phalanx, with a less firm attachment at its origin from the metatarsal neck via the capsule.[717] The nonuniform size of the metatarsal head creates a cam effect for the collateral ligaments that puts a different portion of the fibers under tension during different positions during the range of motion. When the metatarsophalangeal joint is forced into hyperextension, it has been shown that the plantar portion of the capsuloligamentous complex tears at the weaker area near its origin from the metatarsal head and neck.[717]

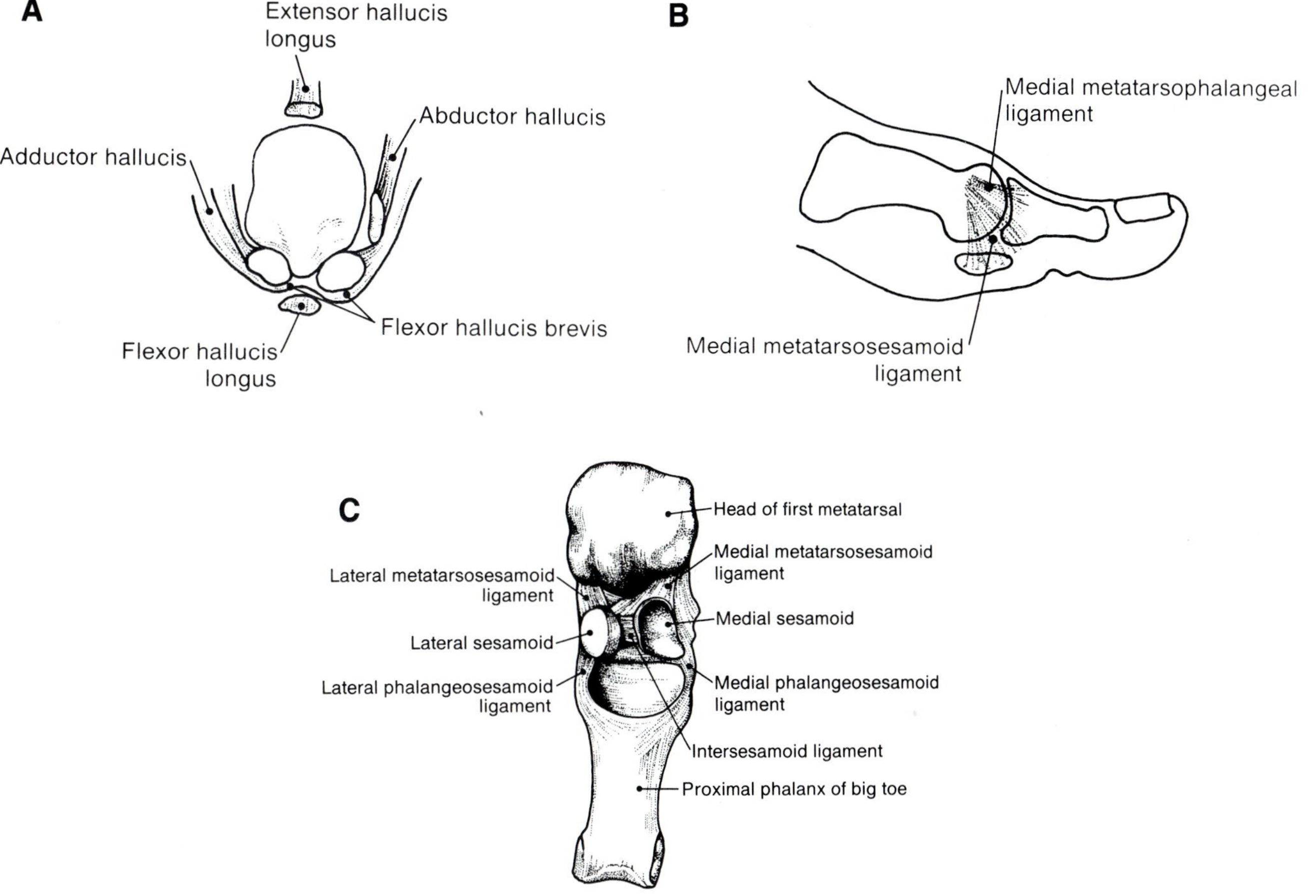

FIG 27–94.
Anatomic relationships of the first metatarsophalangeal joint: **A,** frontal-plane view; **B,** sagittal-plane view; **C,** cutaway view. (From Clanton TO, Butler JE, Eggert A: *Foot Ankle* 7:162–176, 1986. Used by permission.)

The biomechanics of the foot and ankle have been thoroughly reviewed in the opening chapter, and only pertinent aspects will be reiterated here. The importance of the first metatarsophalangeal joint to proper gait and to the normal weight-bearing function of the foot is self-evident. The great toe typically supports more than twice the load of the lesser toes, with maximum force reaching 40% to 60% of body weight in normal walking.[718, 730, 735] During more stressful activities such as running and jumping, these forces are increased proportionately.[725] When the first metatarsophalangeal joint is sprained, the athlete walks and runs with the foot in supination to unload the joint and to limit first metatarsophalangeal joint motion. This increases stress on the lesser metatarsals and can cause compensatory problems in this area.

The instant center of motion for the first metatarsophalangeal joint falls within the first metatarsal head[730] (Fig 27–95). This means that during range of motion of the metatarsophalangeal joint there is a gliding motion taking place at the joint surface. In full extension, this gliding motion is replaced by compression of the dorsal articular surfaces of the first metatarsal head and the base of the proximal phalanx. This fact has led to the postulate that the hyperextension injury mechanism in turf toe injuries can lead to compression fractures of the first metatarsal head.[710]

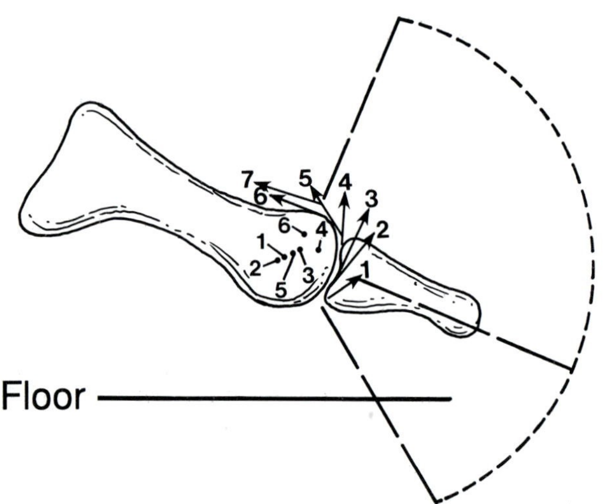

FIG 27–95.
The instant center of motion falls within the metatarsal head and creates a gliding motion of the joint surfaces except in dorsiflexion, where compression occurs. (From Sammarco GJ: Biomechanics of the foot. In Frankel VH, Nordin M, editors: *Biomechanics of the skeletal system,* Philadelphia, 1980, Lea & Febiger, pp 193–219. Used by permission.)

The range of motion of the metatarsophalangeal joints is important for understanding injuries in this location. Since motion in this area has been measured in two different ways, it is critical to understand the reference point when discussing metatarsophalangeal joint range of motion.[734] The line of the first metatarsal shaft is the reference line in most reports, although the natural inclination seems to be to use the sole of the foot as the reference. There is a great deal of variability in first metatarsophalangeal joint range of motion, and there is a tendency for motion to decrease with age. These points were brought out in the study by Joseph, who found the average total dorsiflexion to be 74 degrees when the line of the first metatarsal shaft was used as the neutral line.[720] In standing, the joint rests at 16 degrees of dorsiflexion on average, and active plantar flexion averages 23 degrees. Approximately 60 degrees of dorsiflexion is considered "normal" during barefoot walking on a flat surface.[708, 710, 718] A stiff-soled shoe can restrict first metatarsophalangeal joint motion to 25 or 30 degrees without changing an individual's gait appreciably.[708]

Etiologic Factors

Since these injuries were relatively uncommon in sports prior to the era of artificial playing surfaces, it is clear that some etiologic role must be present. Bowers and Martin theorized that the combination of the hard artificial playing surface together with flexible soccer-style shoes created a shoe-surface interface that potentiated first metatarsophalangeal joint sprains.[709] A poll of 66 athletic trainers found that 34% believed turf to be the responsible factor, 21% attributed the problem to the shoes, and 24% believed that the two factors were equally responsible.[713] (Sixteen percent rendered no opinion.) The change from the traditional grass shoe with seven cleats attached by posts into the sole of the shoe to more flexible varieties of soccer shoes and later to turf shoes seems to have been a major contributing factor in the natural history of the turf toe problem. The traditional shoe incorporated a steel plate in the sole that increased the shoe's stability but also increased its weight. As speed became an increasingly important factor in the game of football, more lightweight shoes were introduced, and stability was often sacrificed. Stress across the forefoot of the shoe was then applied more directly to the metatarsophalangeal joints, and an increasing incidence of sprains was the natural consequence. This is not to say that the surface plays no role in the injury, but we feel that it is secondary to the shoe. Also, sprains can occur in the traditional seven-cleated grass shoe, although this is relatively uncommon.[727]

The hardness of the artificial grass playing field has been accused of causing turf toe.[709] With aging the artificial playing surface loses resiliency and shock absorbency. In the older-generation turfs, the nylon ribbon wore away, and the foam underpad quickly packed down to leave a thin green carpet lying on top of an asphalt base.[719, 737] No doubt, this was a hard surface. Nevertheless, the study by Clanton et al. demonstrated no major time relationship with the aging of the Rice University artificial grass or with the introduction of new artificial grass during the time period of the study.[710] There were 13 turf toe injuries in the three seasons prior to the replacement of the artificial grass at Rice Stadium in 1980, and 12 turf toe injuries were recorded during the three seasons following replacement of the turf. This does not seem to support the hypothesis that harder turf from aging is a factor in the production of turf toe injury. Our impression is that the problem with the artificial grass surface is friction rather than hardness. Nigg and Segesser have demonstrated a generalized increase in the incidence of sports injuries related to enhanced surface friction.[726] This appears to hold true for turf toe injuries because the forefoot becomes fixed on the artificial grass and an externally applied force pushes the foot over the top of the toe and takes the first metatarsophalangeal joint through an abnormal range of dorsiflexion.

The stress of excessive dorsiflexion as a mechanism of injury has led to the hypothesis that athletes with a pre-existing loss of motion in the first metatarsophalangeal joint are at increased risk for turf toe injury.[710] By protecting athletes with 60 degrees or less of dorsiflexion, it was felt that the turf toe injury rate and severity could be reduced. Other studies have denied an association between range of motion and turf toe injury.[713, 727] A recent study has examined this in a prospective fashion by using matched controls and found that the range of motion prior to injury has no effect on the propensity for injury.[711] However, there is a significant reduction in motion following injury, even at late follow-up.

In analyzing metatarsophalangeal joint sprains, it is clear that the majority involve the great toe and the majority occur in football. Similar injuries have been reported in basketball and track.[710, 713] Surprisingly, there has been no mention of turf toe problems in the articles on soccer injuries, although this sport is similar to American football and is also played on artificial grass to some extent.[706, 716, 724] Nelson and associates have pointed out that there were no turf toe injuries in their study of injuries in another sport similar to football—lacrosse.[723] This occurred despite the fact that over half of the games and practices were played on artificial grass and shoes were similar to those worn in football. The high rate of turf toe injury in American football suggests that there are more complex factors involved in this injury other than artificial grass and shoewear.

Other etiologic factors in turf toe injury have been suggested. These include player position, age, years of participation, player weight, a flattened first metatarsal head, and range of ankle motion.[711, 713, 727] The report by Coker et al. suggested that running backs were at increased risk for injury,[713] and this was subsequently confirmed in the study by Rodeo and associates.[727] They concluded that offensive players were at higher risk for turf toe than defensive players, with running backs (including the quarterback), wide receivers (including tight ends), and linemen being most at risk. Their raw data suggest that defensive backs were just as vulnerable. The study by Clanton and coworkers does not show any statistical difference between positions, but offensive and defensive players were grouped by similar skills to increase numbers for the purpose of obtaining statistically valid numbers in each group.[711] The study of professional football players showed the mean age for the injured players to be 27.4 years vs. 24.7 years for controls, and the mean number of playing years was 5.2 for those injured vs. 3.0 for controls.[727] Player weight had no bearing on injury risk,[711] but mean range of ankle dorsiflexion was greater (13.3 degrees) when compared with ankle dorsiflexion for uninjured players (7.9 degrees).[727] There has been a suggestion of an increased propensity for turf toe injury in athletes with pes planus, but the results were not statistically significant.[727] A further predisposing factor that remains unconfirmed by subsequent reports is flattening of the first metatarsal head as noted by Coker and associates.[713]

Diagnosis

Clinical Evaluation

As mentioned previously, injury to the metatarsophalangeal joints can occur from a variety of mechanisms and produce an array of injuries including sprains, fractures (avulsions of ligaments, proximal phalanx, metatarsal, or sesamoid), dislocations, or some combination. Chronic sprain of the metatarsophalangeal joint and traumatic synovitis related to athletic participation have been reported.[733] The more severe grades of acute injury are usually obvious from the clinical or radiographic assessment. However, the player who presents with mild pain and swelling in the area of the metatarsophalangeal joint is frequently diagnosed as having a sprain and expected to perform. It is hoped that the preceding discussion has exposed this as a disabling problem often hindering athletic participation.

In the case of turf toe injuries, the initial pain and swelling may be relatively minor, but the swelling and pain tend to worsen over the course of 24 hours, and the player hobbles into the training room the following day. Three grades of injury have been described by clinical features.[710] Grade 1 sprains have a stretching injury to the capsuloligamentous complex about the first metatarsophalangeal joint and present with localized plantar or medial tenderness, minimal swelling, and no ecchymosis. The player is able to continue athletic participation but is uncomfortable. Grade 2 sprains have a partial tear of the capsuloligamentous complex and more severe symptoms and signs. The tenderness is more intense and diffuse with increased swelling and ecchymosis. There is usually some restriction in range of motion due to guarding. The player is unable to perform at his normal level. Grade 3 sprains present with severe pain along with marked swelling and ecchymosis. Tenderness is severe on both the plantar and dorsal surfaces. The pathology (in the hyperextension mechanism) involves tearing of the plantar plate from its origin on the metatarsal head-neck junction and impaction of the proximal phalanx into the metatarsal head dorsally. There may be a fracture of a sesamoid or separation of a bipartite sesamoid in this injury grade (Fig 27–96). Players are unable to bear weight on the medial portion of the forefoot and are clearly unable to play.

Sprains of the metatarsophalangeal joints also present in a more chronic form with generalized pain and pain with range of motion despite the absence of an acute injury event. In football, this is frequently the case for offensive and defensive linemen, who are constantly driving off their forefoot. This particular condition seems to be less common since the introduction of improved artificial turf shoe wear with reduced forefoot flexibility. This condition may be difficult to distinguish from metatarsophalangeal joint synovitis, although the patient population is different. In synovitis, the tenderness is directly over the joint, as is the swelling. Pain is usually present with passive motion of the joint, particularly into plantar flexion. Smith and Reischl have reported on this condition in 23 athletic individuals involved in sports, including running (6), walking (9), tennis (6), football (1), and aerobics (1).[733] They noted no major differences in this condition between their athletic and nonathletic patients, nor was there a difference in response to treatment. Therefore, interested readers are referred to the section devoted to synovitis of the metatarsophalangeal joint in the previous section of this textbook for a more complete discussion of its diagnosis and treatment.

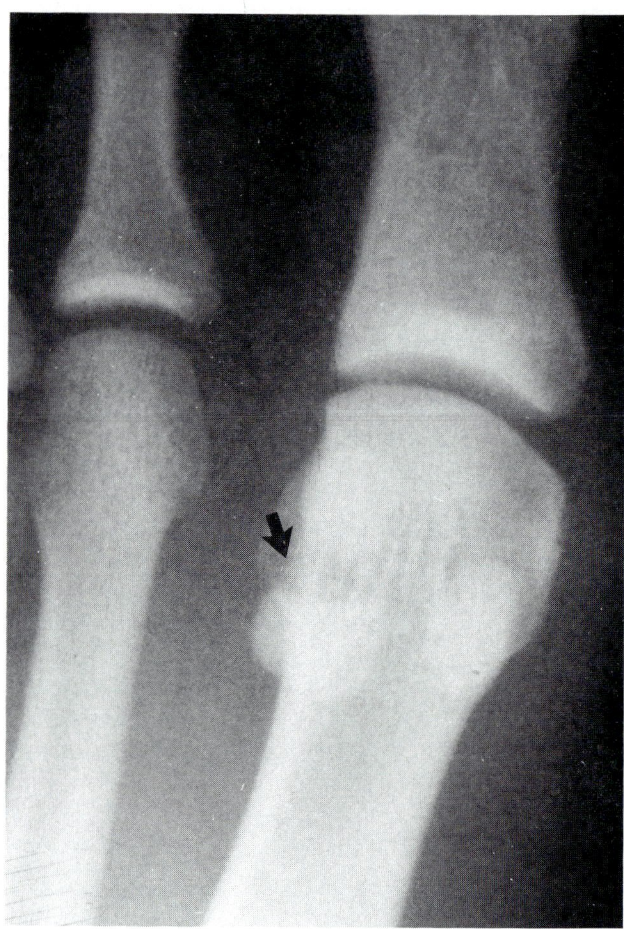

FIG 27–96.
Radiograph demonstrating separation of a bipartite sesamoid in a football player with a turf toe injury.

Radiographic Evaluation

Routine AP, oblique, and lateral radiographs are taken in some grade 2 and all grade 3 injuries to exclude underlying bony pathology. In the study by Coker and associates, several sesamoid, metatarsal, and proximal phalangeal fractures were noted in their football players with mechanisms of injury similar to that for turf toe injuries.[713] Another radiographic study of 17 patients (18 feet) in a study population of 53 athletes found the majority to have negative finding.[710] A few had small flecks of bone thought to represent ligament or capsular avulsions (Fig 27–97,A). There was one case with a cystlike change on the dorsal aspect of the first metatarsal head (Fig 27–97,B) and one case of a small divotlike area on the dorsomedial metatarsal head (Fig 27–97,C). The long-term significance of these findings is undetermined. In the radiologic assessment, it is important to recognize an associated sesamoid fracture since these can be a source of long-term symptomotology.[715]

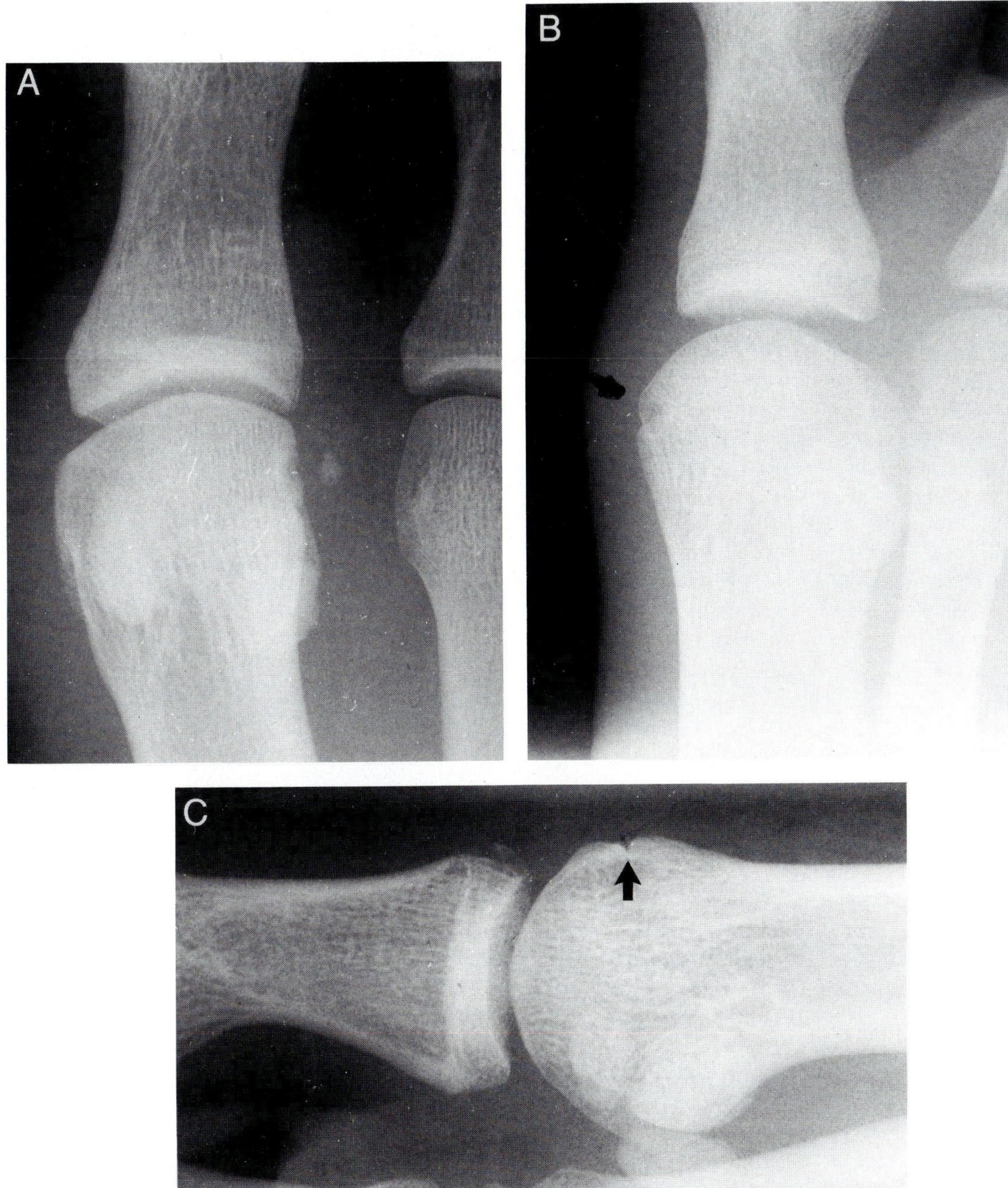

FIG 27–97.
Radiographic findings in athletes with turf toe injury. **A,** ligamentous avulsions can be seen in a turf toe injury. **B,** cystlike change on the first metatarsal head *(arrow)*. **C,** divot on the dorsal aspect of the first metarsal head *(arrow)*. (From Clanton TO, Butler JE, Eggert A: *Foot Ankle* 7:162–176, 1986 Used by permission.)

Other methods of evaluating sprains of the metatarsophalangeal joints have gained little acceptance. Stress radiographs were advocated by Mullis and Miller as a method to document instability of the first metatarsophalangeal joint.[722] Arthrography of the first metatarsophalangeal joint was mentioned by Coker and associates as an adjunct to establishing the definitive diagnosis in cases of capsular tears.[713] Bone scintigraphy might be useful in determining the degree of bony injury, and MRI would possibly define more precisely the extent of soft-tissue injury. However, the use of these methods does not seem warranted in a condition that almost always responds satisfactorily to nonoperative treatment methods.

Treatment

Nonoperative Treatment

The initial treatment of sprains of the metatarsophalangeal joint(s) proceeds along the same lines as discussed in the earlier sections on sprains of the ankle and midfoot. Rest, ice, compression, and elevation are the essential elements in the treatment protocol.[731] We have found that rest is the most important aspect of treatment and usually the most difficult to enforce. The coach and injured player both want an immediate cure or a treatment that will restore complete function spontaneously. It is sometimes difficult for them to understand that a "simple toe sprain" can affect performance so dramatically and cause such an extended downtime. Nevertheless, too early a return to competition almost always extends the period of impairment, occasionally in a dramatic fashion. Cryotherapy is best delivered by placing the foot in a bucket of ice water for 10 to 15 minutes. Compression is provided by taping the toe. Caution must be exercised in taping the toe following an acute injury since it is theoretically possible to restrict circulation as swelling continues.

Following a grade 1 injury, players are placed in more supportive shoe wear with an insole incorporating a stainless steel plate in the forefoot (Fig 27–98). For the athlete with a more chronic condition or difficulty adapting to the insole, it is possible to make a custom insole that conforms well to the foot and restricts motion just as adequately. Upon return to an athletic participation, the player has the toe taped to restrict dorsiflexion (in the hyperextension mechanism injury)[714] (Fig 27–99). Soreness is treated with mild analgesics.

The athlete with a grade 2 injury is usually unable to participate in sports for a few days to as long as a week or two. He is treated in a similar fashion to an athlete with a grade 1 injury, but enforcement of restricted activity and protection from reinjury is critical. The use of crutches for protected weight bearing is seldom necessary, whereas athletes with a grade 3 injury usually require crutches for a few days. Treatment is otherwise similar for the grade 3 injury except that loss of playing time is longer, often 3 to 6 weeks. We have found that it is usually those athletes who try to resume play too early who end up with the more prolonged disability. The majority of these injuries, if properly treated from the outset and protected for 3 to 4 weeks, will heal by the end of that period regardless of the severity of the sprain.

The use of cortisone and anesthetic injections is widespread in sports medicine circles to allow continued performance in the face of pain. When there is a significant ligamentous injury, this practice is obviously contraindicated (as it perhaps is in all situations). The deleterious effects of cortisone injections into joints or around ligaments and tendons is well established.[705, 707, 729, 736, 738] The complete loss of sensation in a toe produced by a nerve block can easily lead to much further damage. If an injection is to be used (and we are not advocating the practice), a long-acting anesthetic agent should be used and injected only in a very localized area and only when the joint is mobile and stable.

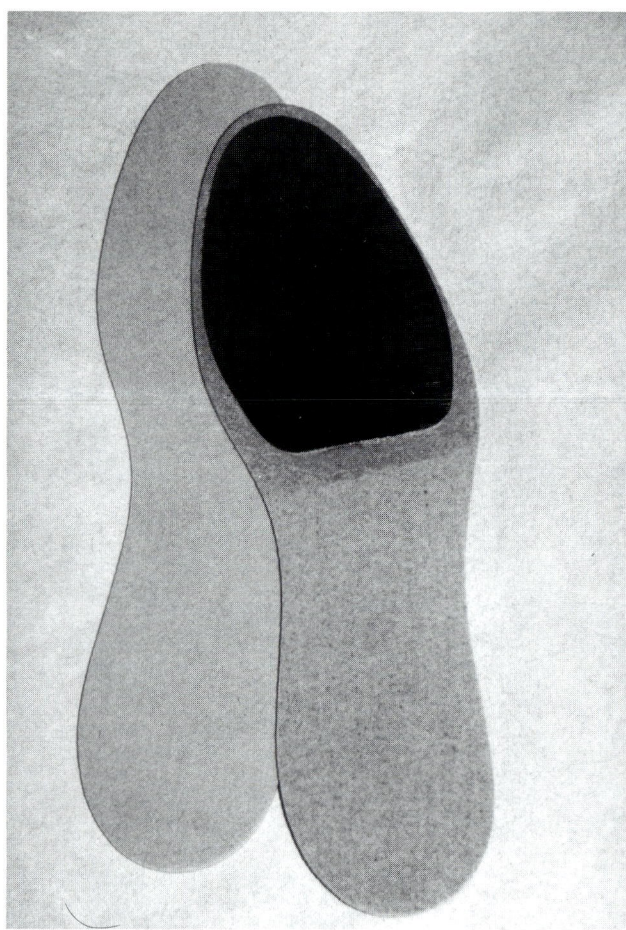

FIG 27–98.
A commercially available orthosis incorporating a stainless steel plate can provide protection for the athlete with a turf toe injury. (Turf Toe Insert, Product NO. 725, Scott Foot Care Products, Omaha, Neb.)

Surgical Treatment

Operative treatment of sprains of the metatarsophalangeal joints is seldom necessary. Coker et al. operated

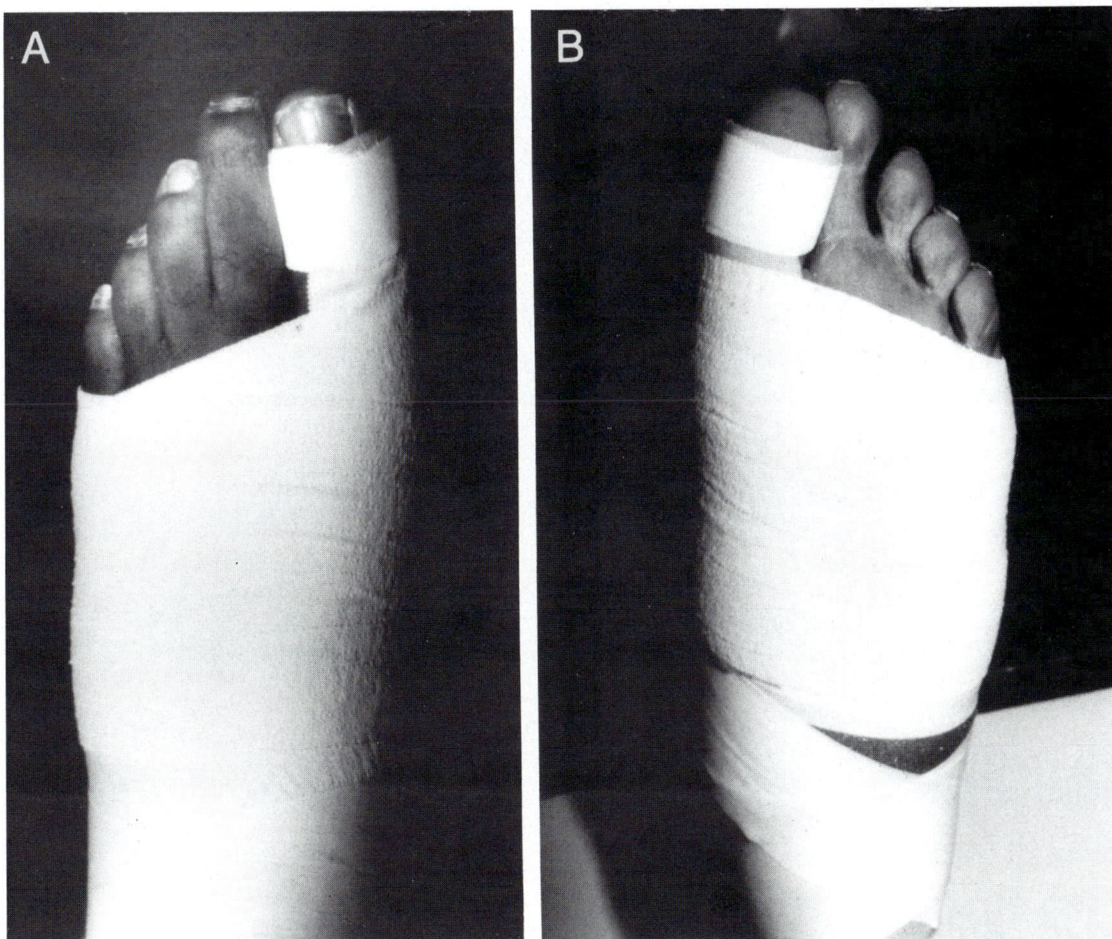

FIG 27–99.
Taping of the foot and great toe can restrict movement at the first metatarsophalangeal joint and provide protection for the athlete with a turf toe injury. **A,** dorsal view; **B,** plantar view.

on four patients including one with a sesamoid fracture.[713] No patients were operated on acutely. Among the three athletes with injury other than the sesamoid fracture, one patient had loose bodies within the first metatarsophalangeal joint, another had chondromalacia involving the first metatarsal head, and a third had calcification of the soft tissues over the first metatarsal head. There was evidence of prior capsular injury in all three of these patients. In the study by Clanton and associates, only one patient underwent delayed surgery for the removal of a symptomatic fragment of avulsed bone.[710] No other patients with metatarsophalangeal joint injury have undergone surgery at Rice University since that case. One patient with a turf toe injury separated a bipartite sesamoid but responded well to nonoperative management and resumed play. He still had mild discomfort at the 1-year follow-up.

The one exception to the rule that these sprains should be treated nonoperatively is the situation where there is obvious instability. These cases probably represent spontaneously reduced dislocations. Mullis and Miller reported one case of such an injury in a basketball player who tore the adductor tendon, lateral capsule, and lateral collateral ligament.[722] Persistent pain, swelling, and instability despite nonoperative treatment resulted in a delayed surgical repair that effectively eliminated the symptoms.

Results

Long-term sequelae from metatarsophalangeal joint injury, specifically turf toe, were first noted by Coker and associates.[713] Persistent pain with athletic activity and restricted motion were the remaining symptoms at follow-up among nine patients reported. *Sports Illustrated* has published several articles on the problems of artificial turf and suggested lasting consequences from turf toe injuries in professional football players.[719, 721, 737] Specific long-term consequences were re-

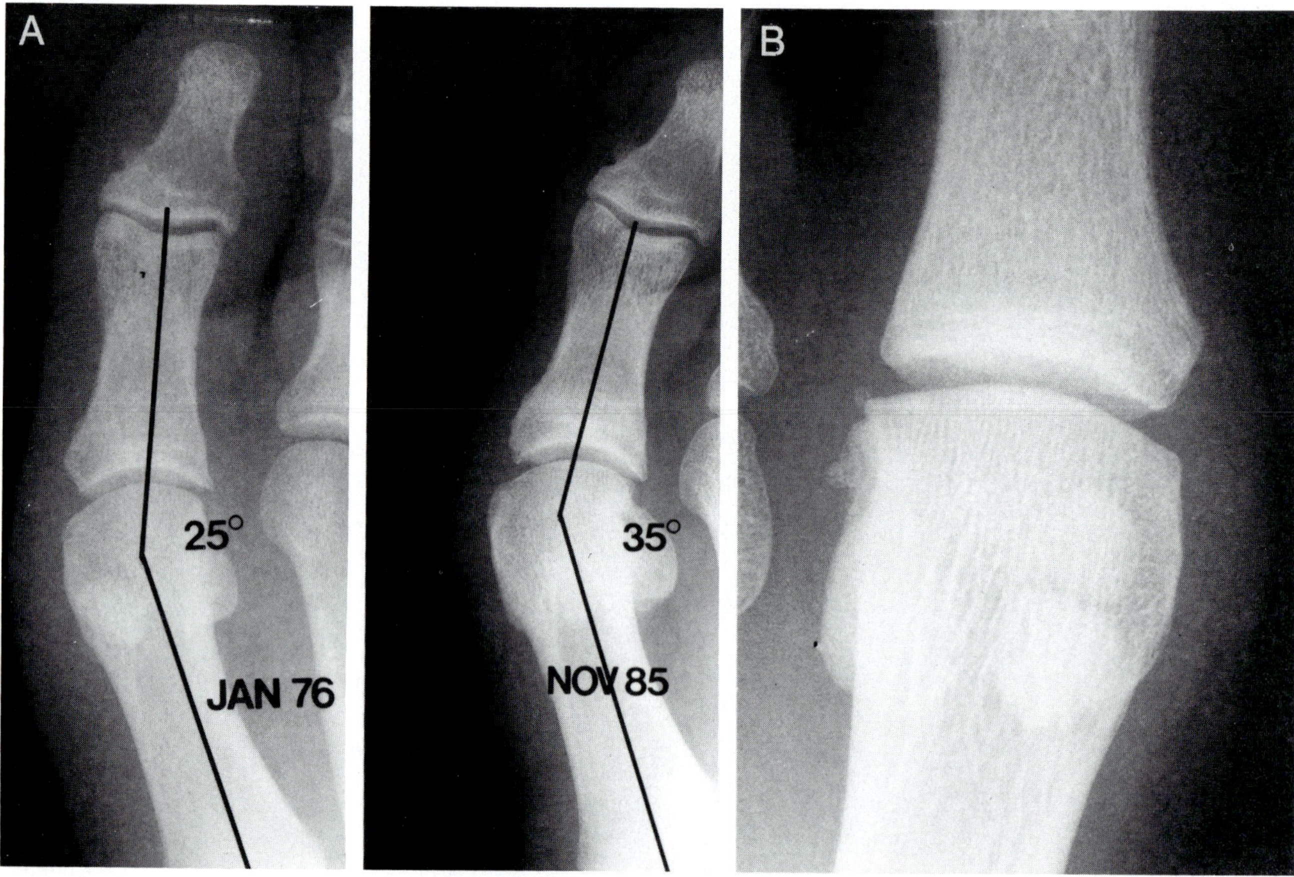

FIG 27–100.
Chronic problems can be seen in some cases of turf toe injury. **A,** hallux valgus developing in an athlete with prior turf toe injury; **1,** Rice football lineman 1 year following a severe turf toe injury with 25 degrees of valgus at the metatarsophalangeal joint; **2,** same player 10 years later with symptomatic hallux valgus and hallux rigidus and a 10-degree increase in his hallux valgus angle. **B,** early change of hallux rigidus in an athlete with prior turf toe injury. (From Clanton TO, Butler JE, Eggert A: *Foot Ankle* 7:162–176, 1986. Used by permission.)

ported by Clanton et al. and included hallux valgus and early hallux rigidus[710] (Fig 27–100). In an unpublished report, Clanton and Seifert have reviewed 20 athletes with prior turf toe injury at greater than 5-year follow-up and noted a 50% incidence of persistent symptoms.[712] It remains unclear whether these sprains will ultimately result in arthritic changes in the affected joint.

BUNIONS IN ATHLETES

Hallux valgus and hallux rigidus (dorsal bunion) have been discussed in detail in a previous section in this textbook. The majority of patients with these problems are middle-aged females and/or nonathletes. When a bunion problem occurs in an athlete, it can be a more complicated diagnostic and therapeutic dilemma. The present section will address this condition strictly from the point of view of its presence in the young athlete.

Etiology

A hallux valgus deformity in the athletic population may develop for several reasons. Acute injuries such as hyperextension of the first metatarsophalangeal joint may tear not only the plantar plate but also the medial capsule of the first metatarsophalangeal joint[741, 742](Fig 27–100,A). Acute subluxation and dislocations of the first metatarsophalangeal joint may also result in a posttraumatic hallux rigidus and/or hallux valgus.[744] More commonly, chronic repetitive injuries are responsible for the development of these deformities. Pronation in athletes who participate in running sports increases the lateral stress on the hallux during toe-off (Fig 27–101). Sports that require frequent "cutting" may increase val-

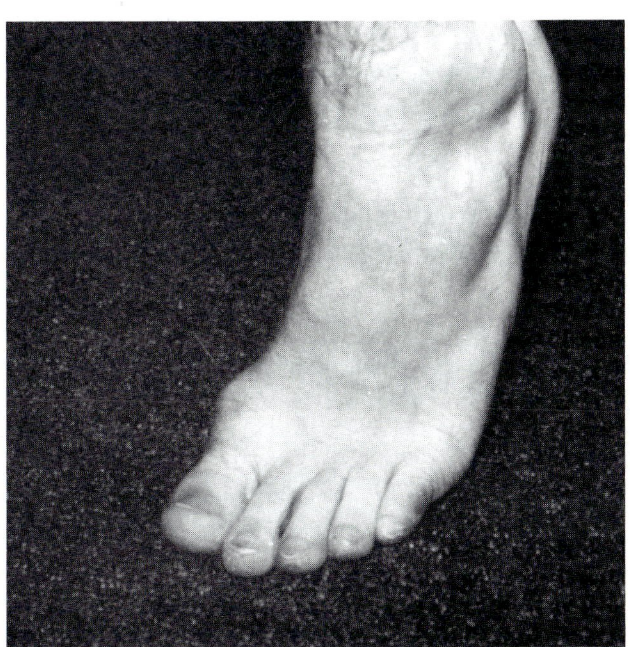

FIG 27–101.
Pronated feet in runners will increase valgus stresses on the hallux during toe-off.

gus stress on the first metatarsophalangeal joint. Athletes who squat, such as football linemen or catchers, increase the dorsally directed force on the first metatarsophalangeal joint. This is also observed in male dancers, who dorsiflex the first metatarsophalangeal joint in the demi-pointe position (Fig 27–102). In ballet, forcing a turnout or "rolling in" leads to pronation of the foot with abduction of the hallux (Fig 27–103). Furthermore, maintaining the pointe stance also involves foot abduction and increases the forces leading to the development of a bunion (Fig 27–104). Abduction stress on the first metatarsophalangeal joint are also high in the back foot in certain golfers, bowlers, and fencers. During the serve in tennis, the front of the forefoot is stressed in abduction and dorsiflexion, which may increase symptoms from a bunion or hallux rigidus (Fig 27–105).

Athletic footwear is often culpable in the pathogenesis of a symptomatic bunion. Shoes may fit improperly and/or provide inadequate protection. Improper fit occurs commonly when one foot is longer or larger (either width or volume) than the other foot. The athlete may unwittingly size the shoes by having the smaller or shorter foot measured. A smaller shoe will increase the squeezing of the forefoot and jamming of the toes, which will increase symptoms. Also, patients with narrow hindfeet and midfeet when associated with relatively broader forefeet may opt for a smaller shoe since a wider one may not fit the heel snugly. The development of more anatomic lasts for running shoes has, to some degree, decreased the incidence of these problems.

Certain shoes notoriously provide little protection to the forefoot. The change in shoe design that accompanied the conversion to synthetic turf was felt to be partially responsible for the increased incidence of turf toes. The flexible forefoot in the rubber-soled, multicleat soccer shoes provided inadequate protection against hyperdorsiflexion injuries (Fig 27–106).[740, 741] Dance shoes made of soft leather provide minimal support and do not adequately protect the dancer's forefoot (Fig 27–107). Toe shoes worn by ballerinas have a rigid toe box that increases the stress when performing on pointe (Fig 27–108). These above factors when com-

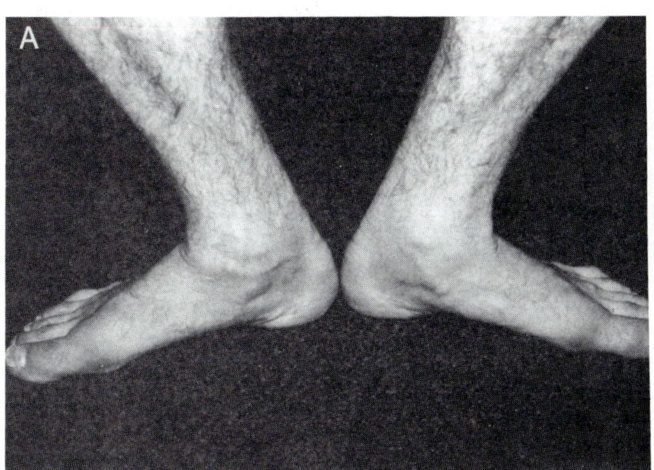

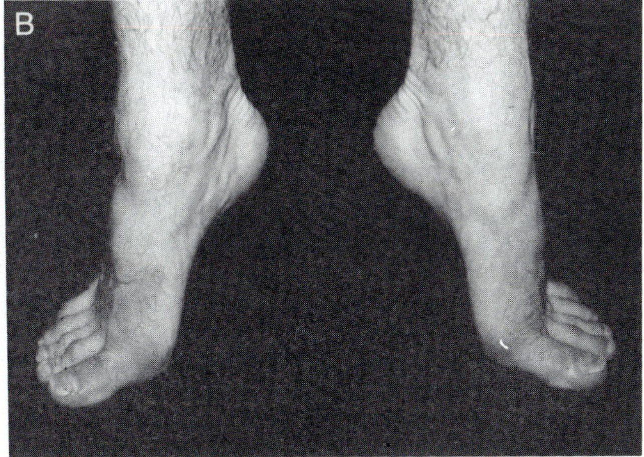

FIG 27–102.
Photograph of a male dancer with hallux valgus whose deformity increased in demi-pointe. **A,** male dancer standing in the first position. **B,** same dancer rising to demi-pointe.

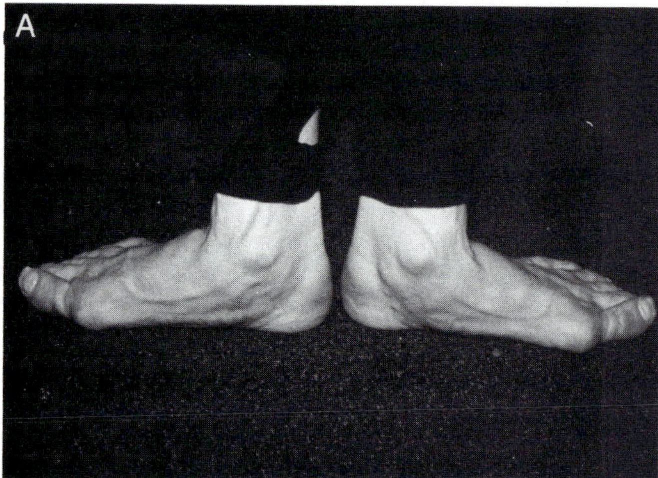

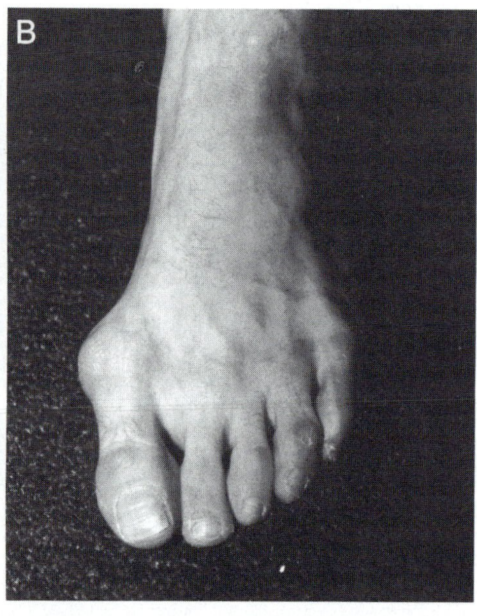

FIG 27–103.
"Rolling in" can lead to pronation of the foot with abduction of the hallux in ballet dancers. **A,** a female dancer in the first position demonstrates "rolling in" to achieve turnout. **B,** same dancer with a significant bunion and hallux valgus.

bined with hereditary predisposition, training/style errors, anatomic irregularities, generalized ligamentous laxity, and constricting work or pleasure shoes lead to the development of a hallux valgus deformity.

Diagnosis

Clinical Evaluation

Evaluation of the athlete with a bunion deformity includes a thorough history and physical examination pertaining to the feet, a limited general examination, radiographs, and rarely, other studies. The patient should be asked questions regarding the onset of the deformity and possible inciting events. The duration of pain, character of the symptoms, exacerbation, and relief of pain should be included. Any recent change in shoe wear, activity, or running surfaces must be elicited. Additional information regarding hereditary, metabolic, endocrine, and rheumatologic disorders should be sought.

Examination of the hallux and forefoot should proceed in systematic fashion, including inspection, palpation, and determination of range of motion. The foot should be inspected for the presence and severity of a hallux valgus, pronation deformity, prominence of the medial eminence, hallux valgus interphalangeus (valgus deformity occurring in the hallux interphalangeal joint), and medial and/or dorsal swelling and erythema. The physician should also note the presence of calluses and ingrown nails or other nail deformities. Perhaps the most critical part of the examination is identification of the point of maximum tenderness. Typically, a symptomatic bunion will be tender over the prominent medial eminence, but there may be tenderness dorsomedially or at the interphalangeal joint. Transfer lesions with callouses under the second metatarsal head may also be tender. The fibular and tibial sesamoids must also be palpated for tenderness. Tenderness of the medial or lateral hallucal nerves as well as the medial dor-

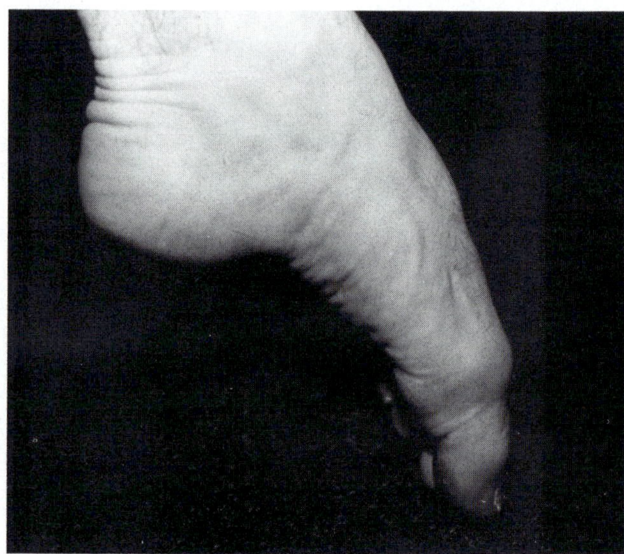

FIG 27–104.
Dancing on pointe increases abduction stresses on the first metatarsophalangeal joint.

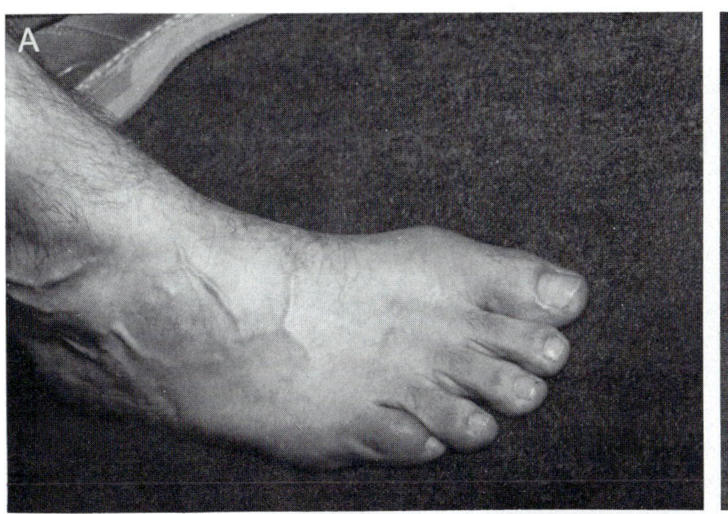

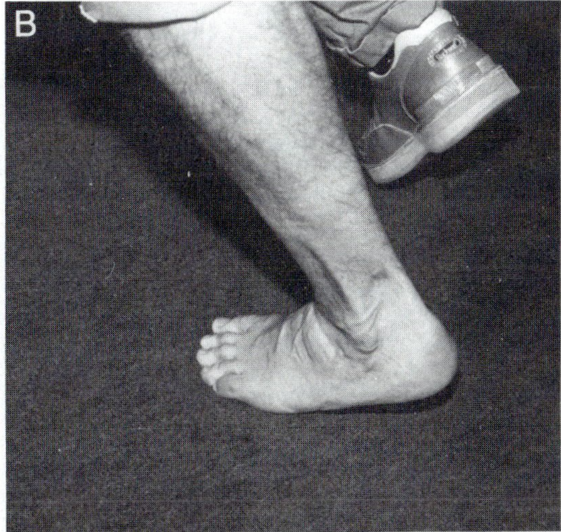

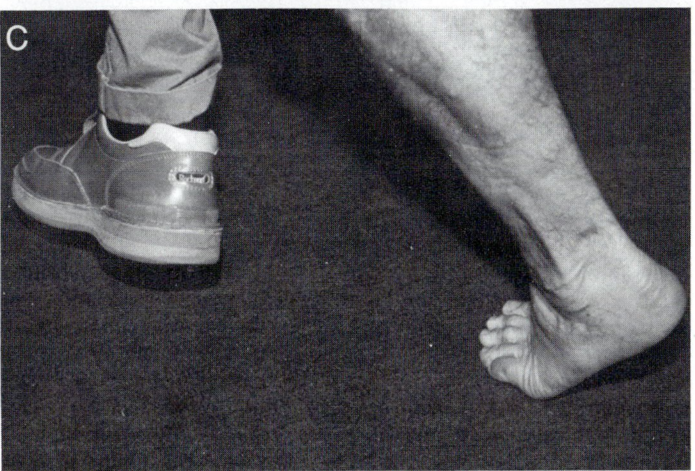

FIG 27–105.
During this patient's tennis serve, his bunion deformity became symptomatic. **A,** natural stance. **B,** rising onto toes at beginning of the tennis serve with increasing valgus stress. **C,** near completion of the serve with further valgus and dorsiflexion stress on the first metatarsophalangeal joint.

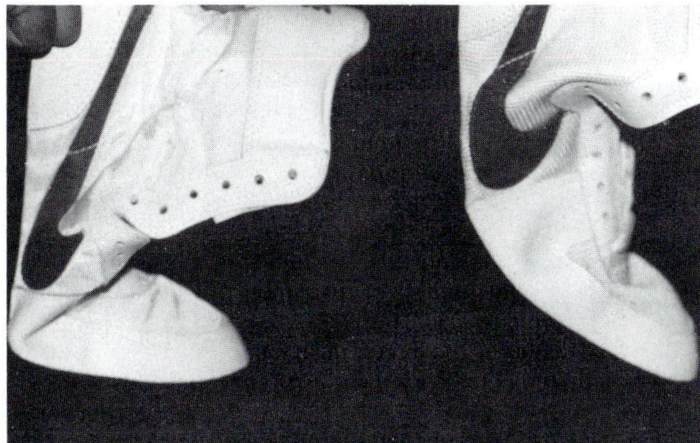

FIG 27–106.
Early models of football shoes had little support incorporated into the forefoot of the shoe as demonstrated by the shoe model on the *left,* which flexes markedly in the forefoot with minor compression load in comparison to the newer-model shoe on the *right* with improved forefoot support.

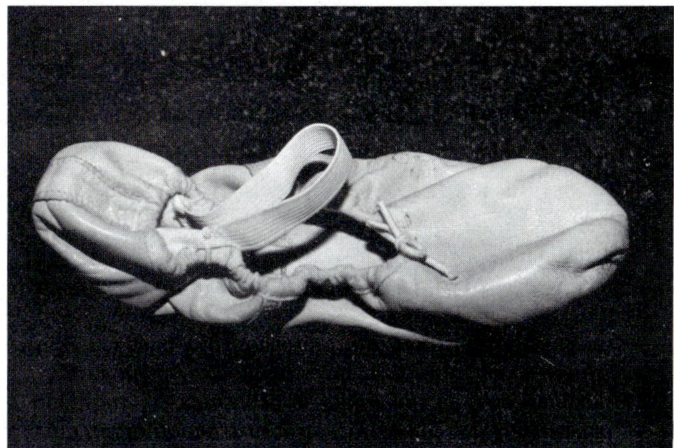

FIG 27–107.
Soft leather dance shoes provide minimal protection.

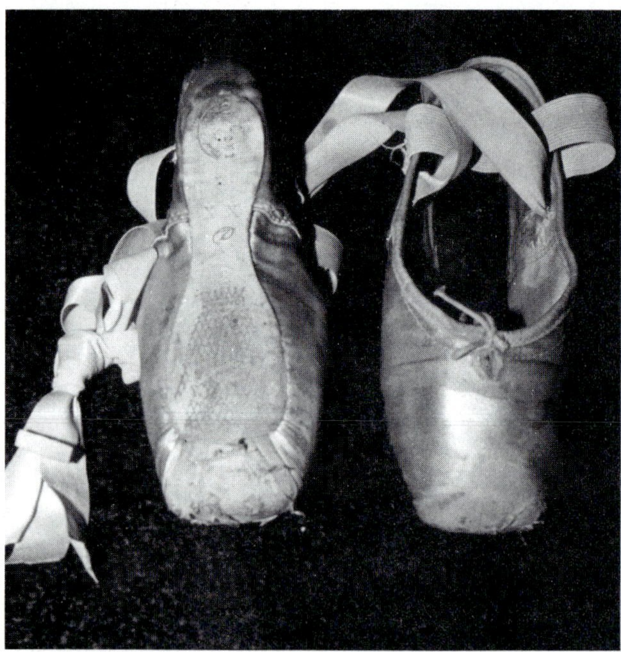

FIG 27–108.
Toe shoes have rigid toe boxes that squeeze the forefoot and increase symptoms from bunions.

sal cutaneous and deep peroneal nerves should also be noted. The specific evaluation of the hallux is completed by determining the range of motion of the first metatarsophalangeal joint. Although there is considerable variation from person to person, the normal arc of motion is approximately 100 degrees, with 70 degrees of dorsiflexion and 30 degrees of plantar flexion.[743, 745, 746]

A comparison with the contralateral side will aid considerably in evaluation. Dorsiflexion of less than 60 degrees may lead to problems depending on ankle flexibility, shoe wear, and activities.[741] Less than 30 degrees of dorsiflexion is usually symptomatic in any running or walking sport.

After examining the hallux, it is important to determine the mobility of the first metatarsocuneiform, midfoot, subtalar, and ankle joints. The physician should check for the presence of symptomatic clawtoes, subluxation or dislocation of the lesser metatarsophalangeal joints, medial or lateral deviation of toes, and painful callosities. Interdigital neuromas, athlete's foot, and metatarsal imbalance should be identified as well. The quality of the metatarsal fat pads should be assessed. General evaluation should also include an appreciation of the standing and non–weight-bearing alignment of the feet and lower extremities. The mobility of the lower-extremity joints and leg lengths should be measured. We have found it particularly useful to have the patient perform in the office the activity that causes the symptoms so that a more dynamic evaluation can be provided. (Fig 27–109).

Radiographic Evaluation

Routine radiographs should include AP, lateral, and oblique views of the feet. The AP view should be taken with the patient bearing weight. These views will permit an evaluation of hallux valgus, metatarsus primus varus, subluxation or abnormalities of the sesamoid, accessory ossicles, and osteophytes. Occasionally, a sesamoid view is helpful.

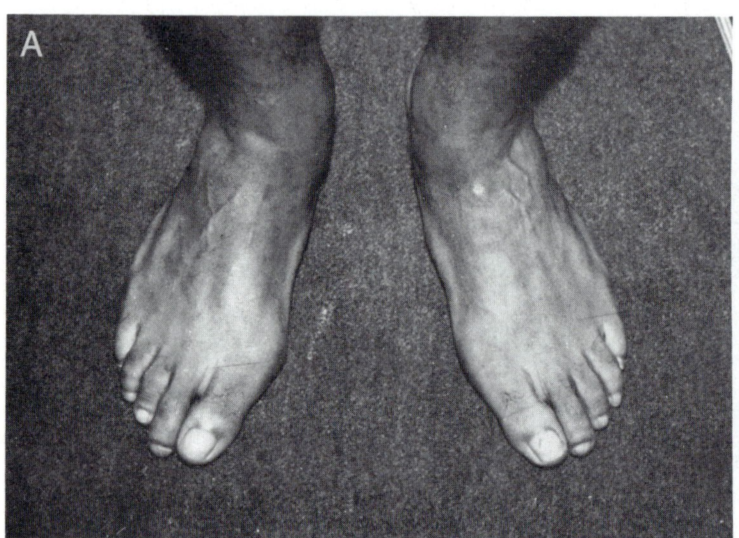

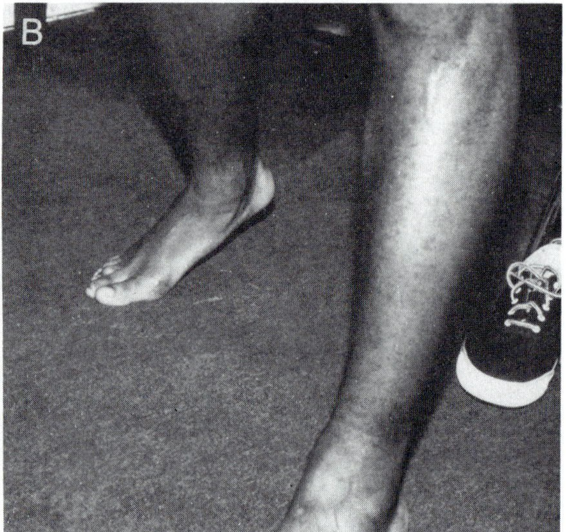

FIG 27–109.
Dynamic evaluation of a 20-year-old football running back with a chronic sprained medial first metatarsophalangeal joint capsule associated with a mild bunion. **A,** static examination. **B,** dynamic examination that exacerbates symptoms.

Stress fractures, avascular necrosis, arthritis, and sesamoid pathology may warrant ordering a bone scan. A CAT scan or MRI is rarely necessary, but they may be useful for evaluation of osteochondritis of the metatarsal head.

Differential Diagnosis

The differential diagnosis of a patient who presents with a painful forefoot in the presence of a bunion should include several conditions. Not uncommonly, there is coexistence of several problems. For example, a bunion may be present with or without bursitis (Fig 27–110), dorsal or dorsomedial osteophytes, or hallux rigidus. The main differential includes hallux rigidus, osteochondritis of the first metatarsal head, sesamoid osteochondritis, sesamoid avascular necrosis, sesamoid fracture (acute, chronic, or stress), posttraumatic capsular or ligamentous injury (i.e., turf toe), local neuritis, stress fracture, hallux valgus interphalangeus, or ingrown toenails.

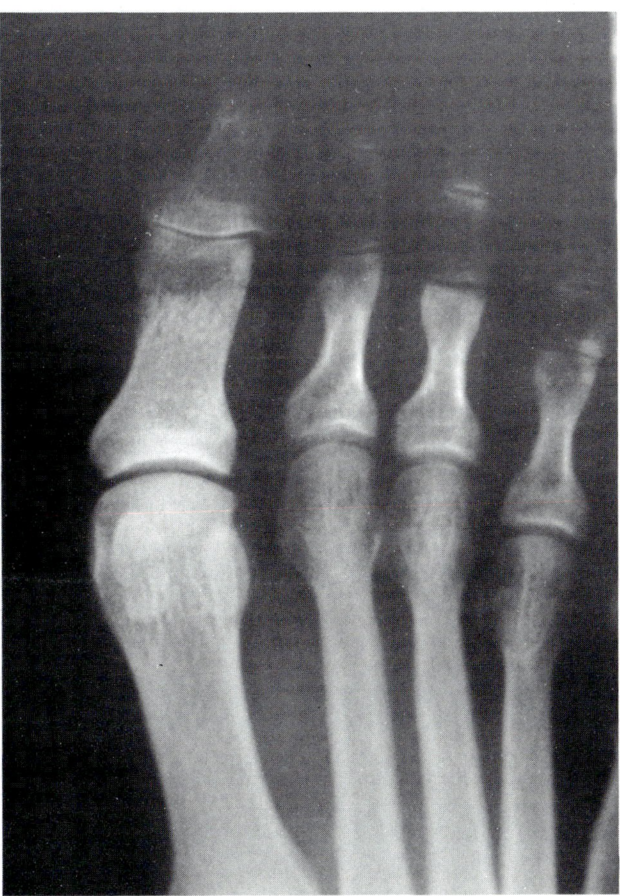

FIG 27–110.
AP radiograph of the forefoot of the tennis player pictured in Figure 27–105 demonstrates a moderately large bursa but minimal malalignment.

Treatment

Nonoperative Treatment

Conservative treatment remains the primary approach for all the above-mentioned conditions. Shoe modification can begin with larger or wider sizes or models with higher, wider toe boxes. Thicker and stiffer soles in the forefoot are especially useful for cases that involve reduced mobility of the first metatarsophalangeal joint. A metatarsal bar will decrease the stresses at the first metatarsophalangeal joint but is poorly tolerated by runners. A medial sole wedge may also be useful for patients who pronate. A spring steel plate incorporated into an orthosis may be inserted into the sole of the shoe to limit flexibility and decrease symptomatic dorsiflexion pain.

Orthotic devices made of lightweight flexible material have on rare occasions been helpful in alleviating a symptomatic bunion. This is especially true in patients who pronate or who have increased mobility of the first metatarsal cuneiform joint. Typically, we would recommend a medium- or high-density plastazote medial longitudinal arch support covered with a Spenco insole. Relief under the sesamoids can be provided by building up the orthosis proximal to the metatarsal heads. A Morton's extension for hypermobility of the first ray is sometimes useful.

Perhaps the simplest method of addressing the bunion deformity is to use a toe spreader made of rubber, foam, lamb's wool, or cotton to decrease pain from pressure between the first and second toes. A horseshoe pad can be individually fabricated to relieve localized nerve or sesamoid pain. Doughnut pads using mole skin or a foam material can be used for various symptomatic bony prominences. Hallux valgus taping or clawtoe taping may be useful for dynamic deformities. Other conservative modalities including massage, physical therapy, nonsteroidal anti-inflammatory medications, or trigger point injection may be tried in selected individuals.

Surgical Treatment

If the patient reaches the stage of considering surgical intervention, it is assumed that nonoperative treatment has been attempted and has failed. The athlete must be informed that the surgery has the potential to increase their pain and limit their ability to compete in sports. In general, we have found that sprinters and ballet dancers are poor candidates for bunion surgery since the high demands on their forefoot may exceed the functional results following any corrections. In considering operations for hallux valgus, the surgeon should address one specific disabling problem and not attempt to correct every associated deformity, ache, or pain.

The choice of procedure depends largely on the individual patient and the experience of the surgeon. Typically, a first metatarsophalangeal joint arthroplasty is required to treat hallux rigidus. Although a dorsal approach is standard, we have performed cheilectomies through medial and/or lateral incisions.[756] Occasionally, a proximal phalangeal dorsal closing wedge osteotomy is indicated in situations where sufficient dorsiflexion is not achieved following cheilectomy (see Chapter 14).

Various procedures for hallux valgus have been described, but simple bunionectomy (without a metatarsal osteotomy) combined with medial capsular reefing leads to a high incidence of recurrence and dissatisfaction.[739, 747] In a patient whose intermetatarsal angle is less than 12 degrees, a Chevron osteotomy may be the best alternative.[739] In cases with greater deviation between the first and second metatarsals, a proximal osteotomy is required. Obviously, fusion of the first metatarsophalangeal joint, interphalangeal joint, or metatarsal cuneiform joint should be avoided since these decrease mobility and lead to deficient stress transfer. Resection arthroplasty of the first metatarsophalangeal joint (Keller procedure) creates a floppy, mobile toe and transfer of stress to the second or third metatarsals. It should never be performed on an athletic individual. A similar statement can also be made for silicone implants.

Following surgery, it is important to start non–weight-bearing rehabilitation earlier and to splint the toes for a longer period of time than would be required for nonathletes. The typical rehabilitative protocol includes using an exercise bike at 1 to 2 weeks, instituting swimming at 3 to 4 weeks, walking at 6 weeks, and beginning full weight-bearing exercises at 8 weeks. The athletes may begin a full training program at about 3 months and resume competitive activity by 6 months. Individualization of the rehabilitation program depends on the patient, his activity, and the exact procedure performed.

Although mostly asymptomatic, bunion deformities do occur in athletes and are occasionally symptomatic. Biomechanical stresses inherent in various sport activities may contribute to the deformity and/or symptomatology. Evaluation of the athlete must include localized and general examination to determine the exact nature of the pathology. Even though conservative treatment is successful in the overwhelming majority of cases, a symptomatic hallux valgus deformity may occasionally require operative intervention. The choice of procedure is based on the patient's requirements and the specific underlying pathology as discussed in the earlier section on hallux valgus. When surgery becomes necessary, a bony procedure should generally be selected.

REFERENCES

Etiology of Injury in Sports

1. Abbot HG, Kress JB: Preconditioning in the prevention of knee injuries, *Arch Phys Med Rehabil* 50:326–333, 1969.
2. Agre JC: Hamstring injuries. Proposed aetiological factors, prevention, and treatment, *Sports Med* 2:21–33, 1985.
3. Anderson LJ: Ligamentous laxity and athletics, *JAMA* 256:527, 1986.
4. Andréasson G, Lindenberger U, Renström P, et al: Torque developed at simulated sliding between sport shoes and an artificial turf, *Am J Sports Med* 14:225–230, 1986.
5. Andréasson G, Olofsson B: Surface and shoe deformation in sport activities and injuries. In Nigg BM, Kerr BA, editors: *Biomechanical aspects of sport shoes and playing surfaces*, Calgary, 1983, The University of Calgary Press, pp 51–61.
6. Appen L, Duncan PW: Strength relationship of the knee musculature: effects of gravity and sport, *J Orthop Sports Phys Ther* 7:232–235, 1986.
7. Athletics. In *Encyclopaedia Britannica*, vol 1, Chicago, 1987, Encyclopaedia Britannica, pp 668–670.
8. Backous DD, Friedl KE, Smith NJ, et al: Soccer injuries and their relation to physical maturity, *Am J Dis Child* 142:839–842, 1988.
9. Bender JA, Pierson JK, Kaplan HM, et al: Factors affecting the occurrence of knee injuries, *J Assoc Phys Ment Rehabil* 18:130–134, 1964.
10. Bensel CK: *The effects of tropical and leather combat boots on lower extremity disorders among US marine corps recruits.* Clothing, equipment and materials engineering laboratory, US Army Natick Research and Development Command, Technical Report No 76-49-CEMEL, March 1976.
11. Berger-Vachon C, Gabard G, Moyen B: Soccer accidents in the French Rhone-Alps Soccer Association, *Sports Med* 3:69–77, 1986.
12. Bernhang AM, Winslett G: Equestrian injuries, *Physician Sports Med* 11:90–97, 1983.
13. Berson BL, Passoff TL, Nagelberg S, et al: Injury patterns in squash players, *Am J Sports Med* 6:323–325, 1978.
14. Biener K, Caluori P: Tennissportunfälle (Sports accidents in tennis players), *Med Klin* 72:754–757, 1977.
15. Bixby-Hammett DM: Youth accidents with horses, *Physician Sports Med* 13:105–117, 1985.
16. Blair SN, Kohl HW, Goodyear NN: Rates and risks for running and exercise injuries: studies in three populations, *Res Q* 58:221–228, 1987.
17. Blitzer CM, Johnson RJ, Ettlinger CF, et al: Downhill skiing injuries in children, *Am J Sports Med* 12:142–147, 1984.
18. Blyth CS, Mueller FO: Football injury survey: part 1. When and where players get hurt, *Physician Sports Med* 2:45–52, 1974.
19. Brody DM: Running injuries, *Clin Symp* 32:1–36, 1980.
20. Brody DM: Running injuries—prevention and management, *Clin Symp* 39:1–36, 1987.
21. Brown EW, McKeag DB: Training, experience, and

medical history of pairs skaters, *Physician Sports Med* 15:101–114, 1987.

22. Burkett LH: Causative factors in hamstring strains, *Med Sci Sports Exerc* 2:39–42, 1970.
23. Caine D, Cochrane B, Caine C, et al: An epidemiologic investigation of injuries affecting young competitive female gymnasts, *Am J Sports Med* 17:811–820, 1989.
24. Canale ST, Cantler ED, Sisk TD, et al: A chronicle of injuries of an American intercollegiate football team, *Am J Sports Med* 9:384–389, 1981.
25. Christensen CS, Wiseman DC: Strength, the common variable in hamstring strain, *Athletic Training* 7:36, 1971.
26. Clancy WG Jr: Tendinitis and plantar fasciitis in runners. In D'Ambrosia RD, Drez D Jr, editors: *Prevention and treatment of running injuries*, ed 2, Thorofare, NJ, 1989, Slack, Charles B, pp, 121–131.
27. Clanton TO: Etiology of injury to the foot and ankle. In Drez D Jr, DeLee JC, editors: *Orthopaedic sports medicine*, Philadelphia, 1992, WB, Saunders.
28. Clanton TO: Sport shoes, insoles and orthoses. In Drez D Jr, DeLee JC, editors: *Orthopaedic sports medicine*, Philadelphia, 1992, WB Saunders.
29. Clanton TO, Eggert KE, Pivarnik JM, et al: First metatarsophalangeal joint range of motion as a factor in turf toe injuries, *Am J Sports Med* 1992 (submitted for publication).
30. Culpepper MI, Niemann KMW: An investigation of the shoe-turf interface using different types of shoes on poly-turf and Astro-turf: torque and release coefficients, *Ala J Med Sci* 20:387–390, 1983.
31. Culpepper MI, Niemann KMW: High school football injuries in Birmingham, Alabama, *South Med J* 76:873–878, 1983.
32. Davis MW, Litman T, Crenshaw RW: Bicycling injuries, *Physician Sports Med* 8:88–96, 1980.
33. DeLee JC, Farney WC: Incidence of injury in Texas high school football. Unpublished study.
34. DeVan WT, Carlton DC: The march fracture persists. A report on 143 cases during a fifteen-month period at an infantry basic training center, *Am J Surg* 87:227–231, 1954.
35. Dowling PA: Prospective study of injuries in United States Ski Association freestyle skiing—1976–77 to 1979–80, *Am J Sports Med* 10:268–275, 1982.
36. Ekstrand J, Gillquist J: Soccer injuries and their mechanisms: a prospective study, *Med Sci Sports Exerc* 15:267–270, 1983.
37. Ekstrand J, Gillquist J: The avoidability of soccer injuries, *Int J Sports Med* 4:124–128, 1983.
38. Ekstrand J, Gillquist J: The frequency of muscle tightness and injuries in soccer players, *Am J Sports Med* 10:75–78, 1982.
39. Ekstrand J, Gillquist J, Liljedahl SO: Prevention of soccer injuries. Supervision by doctor and physiotherapist, *Am J Sports Med* 11:116–120, 1983.
40. Feriencik K: Trends in ice hockey injuries: 1965–1977, *Physician Sports Med* 7:81–84, 1979.
41. Ferkel RD, Mai LL, Ullis KC, et al: An analysis of roller skating injuries, *Am J Sports Med* 10:24–30, 1981.
42. Gardner L, Dziados JE, Jones BH, et al: Prevention of lower extremity stress fractures: a controlled trial of a shock absorbent insole, *Am J Public Health* 78:1563–1567, 1988.
43. Garfinkle D, Talbot AA, Clarizio M, et al: Medical problems on a professional baseball team, *Physician Sports Med* 9:85–93, 1981.
44. Garrick JG: Ballet injuries, *Med Probl Performing Arts* 1:123–127, 1986.
45. Garrick JG, Gillien DM, Whiteside P: The epidemiology of aerobic dance injuries, *Am J Sports Med* 14:67–72, 1986.
46. Garrick JG, Requa RK: Epidemiology of women's gymnastics injuries, *Am J Sports Med* 8:261–262, 1980.
47. Gilbert RS, Johnson HA: Stress fractures in military recruits—a review of twelve years' experience. *Milit Med* 131:716–721, 1966.
48. Gottlieb G, White JR: Responses of recreational runners to their injuries, *Physician Sports Med* 8:145–149, 1980.
49. Grace TG: Muscle imbalance and extremity injury. A perplexing relationship, *Sports Med* 2:77–82, 1985.
50. Grahame R: Joint hypermobility—clinical aspects, *Proc R Soc Med* 64:692–694, 1971.
51. Greaney RB, Gerber FH, Laughlin RL, et al: Distribution and natural history of stress fractures in U.S. Marine recruits. *Radiology* 146:339–346, 1983.
52. Greece. In *Encyclopaedia Britannica*, vol 20, Chicago, 1987, Encyclopaedia Britannica, p 375.
53. Haberl R, Prokop L: Physiological aspects of synthetic tracks. Foot motions during support phase of various running types on different track materials, *Biotelemetry* 1:171–178, 1974.
54. Hamilton WG: Foot and ankle injuries in dancers, *Clin Sports Med* 7:143–173, 1988.
55. Henry JH, Lareau B, Neigut D: The injury rate in professional basketball, *Am J Sports Med* 10:16–18, 1982.
56. Hoff GL, Martin TA: Outdoor and indoor soccer: injuries among youth players, *Am J Sports Med* 14:231–233, 1986.
57. *Holy Bible*, New International Version, International Bible Society, Grand Rapids, Michigan, 1984, Zondervan Bible Publishers, p. 36.
58. Horan FT, Beighton PH: Recessive inheritance of generalized joint hypermobility, *Rheum Rehabil* 12:47–49, 1973.
59. Howse J: Disorders of the great toe in dancers, *Clin Sports Med* 2:499–505, 1983.
60. Hummel G, Gainor BJ: Waterskiing-related injuries, *Am J Sports Med* 10:215–218, 1982.
61. James SL, Bates BT, Osternig LR: Injuries to runners. *Am J Sports Med* 6:40–50, 1978.
62. Janda DH, Wojtys EM, Hankin FM, et al: Softball sliding injuries. A prospective study comparing standard and modified bases, *JAMA* 259:1848–1850, 1988.
63. Janda DH, Wojtys EM, Hankin FM, et al: A three-phase analysis of the prevention of recreational softball injuries, *Am J Sports Med* 18:632–635, 1990.
64. Johnson RJ, Ettlinger CF, Campbell RJ, et al: Trends in skiing injuries. Analysis of a 6-year study (1972–1978), *Am J Sports Med* 8:106–113, 1980.
65. Jones BH, Harris JM, Vinh TN, et al: Exercise-induced stress fractures and stress reactions of bone:

epidemiology, etiology, and classification, *Exerc Sport Sci Rev* 17:379–422, 1989.
66. Kibler WB, Goldberg C, Chandler TJ: Functional biomechanical deficits in running athletes with plantar fasciitis, *Am J Sports Med* 19:66–71, 1991.
67. Kiburz D, Jacobs R, Reckling F, et al: Bicycle accidents and injuries among adult cyclists, *Am J Sports Med* 14:416–419, 1986.
68. Klemp P, Chalton D: Articular mobility in ballet dancers. A follow-up study after four years, *Am J Sports Med* 17:72–75, 1989.
69. Klemp P, Stevens JE, Isaacs S: A hypermobility study in ballet dancers, *J Rheumatol* 11:692–696, 1984.
70. Knapik JJ, Bauman CL, Jones BH, et al: Preseason strength and flexibility imbalances associated with athletic injuries in female collegiate athletes, *Am J Sports Med* 19:76–81, 1991.
71. Kulund DN, Dewey JB, Brubaker CE, et al: Olympic weight lifting injuries, *Physician Sports Med* 6:111–119, 1978.
72. Kwong PK, Kay D, Voner RT, et al: Plantar fasciitis. Mechanics and pathomechanics of treatment, *Clin Sports Med* 7:119–126, 1988.
73. Levy IM, Skovron ML, Agel J: Living with artificial grass: a knowledge update. Part 1: basic science, *Am J Sports Med* 18:406–412, 1990.
74. Lok V, Yuceturk G: Injuries of wrestling, *J Sports Med* 2:324–328, 1975.
75. Macera CA, Pate RR, Powell KE, et al: Predicting lower-extremity injuries among habitual runners, *Arch Intern Med* 149:2565–2568, 1989.
76. Mann RA, Baxter DE, Lutter LD: Running symposium, *Foot Ankle* 1:190–224, 1981.
77. Mann RA, Clanton TO: Hallux rigidus: treatment by cheilectomy, *J Bone Joint Surg [AM]* 70:400–406, 1988.
78. Mann RA, Coughlin MJ: Hallux valgus and complications of hallux valgus. In Mann RA, editor: *Surgery of the foot*, ed 5. St Louis, 1986, Mosby–Year Book, pp 70–71.
79. Marshall P: The rehabilitation of overuse foot injuries in athletes and dancers, *Clin Sports Med* 7:175–191, 1988.
80. Marti B, Vader JP, Minder CE, et al: On the epidemiology of running injuries. The 1984 Bern Grand-Prix study, *Am J Sports Med* 16:285–294, 1988.
81. McCarroll JR, Gioe TJ: Professional golfers and the price they pay, *Physician Sports Med* 10:64–70, 1982.
82. McCarroll JR, Rettig AC, Shelbourne KD: Injuries in the amateur golfer, *Physician Sports Med* 18:122–126, 1990.
83. McLennan JG, Ungersma J: Mountaineering accidents in the Sierra Nevada, *Am J Sports Med* 11:160–163, 1983.
84. McNeal AP, Watkins A, Clarkson PM, et al: Lower extremity alignment and injury in young, preprofessional, college and professional ballet dancers. Part II: dancer-reported injuries, *Med Probl Performing Arts* 5:83–88, 1990.
85. Meyers MC, Elledge JR, Sterling JC, et al: Injuries in interscholastic rodeo athletes, *Am J Sports Med* 18:87–91, 1990.
86. Micheli LJ, Riseborough EM: The incidence of injuries in rugby football, *J Sports Med* 2:93–98, 1974.
87. Milgrom C, Burr DB, Boyd RD, et al: The effect of a viscoelastic orthotic on the incidence of tibial stress fractures in an animal model, *Foot Ankle* 10:276–279, 1990.
88. Milgrom C, Giladi M, Kashtan H, et al: A prospective study of the effect of a shock-absorbing orthotic device on the incidence of stress fractures in military recruits, *Foot Ankle* 6:101–104, 1985.
89. Millar AP: An early stretching routine for calf muscle strains, *Med Sci Sports* 8:39–42, 1976.
90. Moretz A III, Grana WA: High school injuries, *Physician Sports Med* 6:92–95, 1978.
91. Mueller FO, Blyth CS: A survey of 1981 college lacrosse injuries, *Physician Sports Med* 10:87–93, 1982.
92. Mueller FO, Blyth CS: North Carolina high school football injury study: equipment and prevention, *Am J Sports Med* 2:1–10, 1974.
93. Nelson WE, DePalma B, Gieck JH, et al: Intercollegiate lacrosse injuries, *Physician Sports Med* 10:86–92, 1981.
94. Nichols C, Johnson RJ: Cruciate ligament injuries: nonoperative treatment. In Scott WN, editor: *Ligament and extensor mechanism injuries of the knee. Diagnosis and treatment*, St Louis, 1991, Mosby–Year Book, pp 227–238.
95. Nielson AB, Yde J: Epidemiology and traumatology of injuries in soccer, *Am J Sports Med* 17:803–807, 1989.
96. Nigg BM: Assessment of load effects in the reduction and treatment of injuries. In Skinner JS, Corbin CB, Landers DM, et al, editors: *Future directions in exercise and sport science research*, Champaign, Ill, 1989, Human Kinetics, pp 181–193.
97. Nigg BM: Biomechanical aspects of running. In Nigg BM, editor: *Biomechanics of running shoes*, Champaign, Ill, 1986, Human Kinetics, pp 1–25.
98. Nigg BM: The assessment of loads acting on the locomotor system in running and other sport activities, *Semin Orthop* 3:197–206, 1988.
99. Nigg BM, Denoth J, Kerr B, et al: Load sport shoes and playing surfaces. In Frederick EC, editor: *Sport shoes and playing surfaces. Biomechanical Properties*, Champaign, Ill, 1984, Human Kinetics, pp 1–23.
100. Olympic games. In *Encyclopedia Britannica*, vol 25, Chicago, 1987, Encyclopedia Britannica, pp 197–201.
101. Park RD, Castaldi CR: Injuries in junior ice hockey, *Physician Sports Med* 8:81–90, 1980.
102. Perlik PC, Kalvoda DD, Wellman AS, et al: Roller-skating injuries, *Physician Sports Med* 10:76–80, 1982.
103. Peterson TR: Blocking at the knee, dangerous and unnecessary, *Physician Sports Med* 1:46–50, 1973.
104. Peterson TR: Knee injuries due to blocking: a continuing problem, *Physician Sports Med* 7:99–104, 1979.
105. Peterson TR: The Cross-body block, the major cause of knee injuries, *JAMA* 211:449–452, 1970.
106. Petras AF, Hoffman EP: Roentgenographic skeletal injury patterns in parachute jumping, *Am J Sports Med* 11:325–328, 1983.
107. Physical tests. Sport research review. Beaverton, Ore, Nike Sport Research Laboratory, Jan/Feb, 1990.
108. Pino EC, Colville MR: Snowboard injuries, *Am J Sports Med* 17:778–781, 1989.
109. Powell KE, Kohl HW, Caspersen CJ, et al: An epidemiological perspective on the causes of running injuries, *Physician Sports Med* 14:100–114, 1986.

110. Requa R, Garrick JG: Injuries in interscholastic wrestling, *Physician Sports Med* 9:44–51, 1981.
111. Rheinstein DJ, Morehouse CA, Niebel BW: Effects on traction of outsole composition and hardnesses of basketball shoes and three types of playing surfaces, *Med Sci Sports Exerc* 10:282–288, 1978.
112. Rice SG: Epidemiology and mechanisms of sports injuries. In Teitz CC, editor: *Scientific foundations of sports medicine*, Philadelphia, 1989, BC Decker, pp 3–23.
113. Richie DH Jr, Delso SF, Bellucci PA: Aerobic dance injuries: a retrospective study of instructors and participants, *Physician Sports Med* 13:130–140, 1985.
114. Robbins SE, Gouw GJ: Athletic footwear and chronic overloading. A brief review, *Sports Med* 9:76–85, 1990.
115. Robbins SE, Gouw GJ: Athletic footwear: unsafe due to perceptual illusions, *Med Sci Sports Exerc* 23:217–224, 1991.
116. Robbins SE, Hanna AM: Running-related injury prevention through barefoot adaptations, *Med Sci Sports Exerc* 19:148–156, 1987.
117. Rodeo SA, O'Brien S, Warren RF, et al: Turf-toe: an analysis of metatarsophalangeal joint sprains in professional football players, *Am J Sports Med* 18:280–285, 1990.
118. Rothenberger LA, Chang JI, Cable TA: Prevalence and types of injuries in aerobic dancers, *Am J Sports Med* 16:403–407, 1988.
119. Rovere GD, Webb LX, Gristina AG, et al: Musculoskeletal injuries in theatrical dance students, *Am J Sports Med* 11:195–198, 1983.
120. Rowe ML: Varsity football. Knee and ankle injury, *N Y State J Med* 69:3000–3003, 1969.
121. Roy SP: Intercollegiate wrestling injuries, *Physician Sports Med* 7:83–91, 1979.
122. Schafle MD, Requa RK, Patton WL, et al: Injuries in the 1987 National Amateur Volleyball Tournament, *Am J Sports Med* 18:624–631, 1990.
123. Schlaepfer F, Unold E, Nigg BM: The frictional characteristics of tennis shoes. In Nigg BM, Kerr BA, editors: *Biomechanical aspects of sport shoes and playing surfaces*, Calgary, 1983, University of Calgary Press, pp 153–160.
124. Schwellnus MP, Jordaan G, Noakes TD: Prevention of common overuse injuries by the use of shock absorbing insoles. A prospective study, *Am J Sports Med* 18:636–641, 1990.
125. Silver RL, De La Garza J, Rang M: The myth of muscle balance, *J Bone Joint Surg [Br]* 67:432–437, 1985.
126. Sim FH, Simonet WT, Melton LJ, et al: Ice hockey injuries, *Am J Sports Med* 15:30–40, 1987.
127. Simkin A, Leichter I, Giladi M, et al: Combined effect of foot arch structure and an orthotic device on stress fractures, *Foot Ankle* 10:25–29, 1989.
128. Skovron ML, Levy IM, et al: Living with artificial grass: a knowledge update. Part 2: epidemiology, *Am J Sports Med* 18:510–513, 1990.
129. Smith AD, Micheli LJ: Injuries in competitive figure skaters, *Physician Sports Med* 10:36–47, 1982.
130. Snook GA: Injuries in intercollegiate wrestling; a five year study, *Am J Sports Med* 10:142–144, 1982.
131. Snook GA: The father of sports medicine, *Am J Sports Med* 6:128–131, 1978.
132. Snook GA: The history of sports medicine. Part I, *Am J Sports Med* 12:252–254, 1984.
133. Soderstrom CA, Doxanas MT: Raquetball. a game with preventable injuries, *Am J Sports Med* 10:180–183, 1982.
134. Sohl P, Bowling A: Injuries to dancers, *Sports Med* 9:317–322, 1990.
135. Solomon RL, Trepman E, Micheli LJ: Foot morphology and injury patterns in ballet and modern dancers, *Kinesiol Med Dance* 12:20–40, 1989.
136. Spiegl PV, Johnson KA: Heel pain syndrome: which treatments to choose? *J Musculoskel Med* 1:66–71, 1984.
137. Sports injuries. Accident facts. Report of the National Safety Council, 1990, p 88.
138. Stafford MG, Grana WA: Hamstring/quadriceps ratios in college football players: A high velocity evaluation, *Am J Sports Med* 12:209–211, 1984.
139. Steiner ME: Hypermobility and knee injuries, *Physician Sports Med* 15:159–165, 1987.
140. Sullivan JA: Outdoor and indoor soccer: injuries among youth players, *Am J Sports Med* 14:231–233, 1986.
141. Sutherland GW: Fire on ice, *Am J Sports Med* 4:264–269, 1976.
142. Temple C: Hazards of jogging and marathon running, *Br J Hosp Med* 29:237–239, 1983.
143. Tomczak RL, Wilshire WM, Lane JW, et al: Injury patterns in rock climbers, *J Osteopath Sports Med* 3:11–16, 1989.
144. Torg JS, Quedenfeld T: Effect of shoe type and cleat length on incidence and severity of knee injuries among high school football players, *Res Q* 42:203–211, 1971.
145. Torg JS, Quedenfeld T: Knee and ankle injuries traced to shoes and cleats, *Physician Sports Med* 1:39–43, 1973.
146. Torg JS, Quedenfeld TC, Landau S: Football shoes and playing surfaces: from safe to unsafe, *Physician Sports Med* 1:51–54, 1973.
147. Torg JS, Quedenfeld TC, Landau S: The shoe-surface interface and its relationship to football knee injuries, *Am J Sports Med* 2:261–269, 1974.
148. Van Gheluwe B, Deporte E, Hebbelinck M: Frictional forces and torques of soccer shoes on artificial turf. In Nigg BM, Kerr BA, editors: *Biomechanical aspects of sport shoes and playing surfaces*, Calgary, 1983, University of Calgary Press, pp 161–168.
149. Walsh WM, Blackburn T: Prevention of ankle sprains, *Am J Sports Med* 5:243–245, 1977.
150. Walter SD, Hart LE, McIntosh JM, et al: The Ontario cohort study of running-related injuries, *Arch Intern Med* 149:2561–2564, 1989.
151. Washington EL: Musculoskeletal injuries in theatrical dancers: site, frequency, and severity, *Am J Sports Med* 6:75–98, 1978.
152. Winge S, Jorgensen U, Nielsen AL: Epidemiology of injuries in Danish championship tennis, *Int J Sports Med* 10:368–371, 1989.
153. Wyatt MP, Edwards AM: Comparison of quadriceps and hamstring torque values during isokinetic exercise, *J Orthop Sports Phys Ther* 3:48–56, 1981.
154. Zelisko JA, Noble HB, Porter M: A comparison of men's and women's professional basketball injuries, *Am J Sports Med* 10:297–299, 1982.
155. Zemper ED: Injury rates in a national sample of college football teams: a 2-year prospective study, *Physician Sports Med* 17:100–113, 1989.

Chronic Leg Pain in Athletes

156. Allen JM, Barnes MR: Exercise pain in the lower leg, *J Bone Joint Surg [Br]* 68:818–823, 1986.
157. Almdahl SM, Samdal F: Fasciotomy for chronic compartment syndrome, *Acta Orthop Scand* 60:210–211, 1989.
158. Amendola A, Rorabeck, CH, Vellett D, et al: The use of magnetic resonance imaging in exertional compartment syndromes, *Am J Sports Med* 18:29–34, 1990.
159. Andrish JT, Bergfeld JA, Walheim J: A prospective study on the management of shin splints, *J Bone Joint Surg [Am]* 56:1697–1700, 1974.
160. Armstrong RB: Initial events in exercise-induced muscular injury, *Med Sci Sports Exerc* 22:429–435, 1990.
161. Armstrong RB: Mechanisms of exercise-induced delayed onset muscular soreness: a brief review, *Med Sci Sports Exerc* 16:529–538, 1984.
162. Arner O, Lindholm A: What is tennis leg? *Acta Chir Scand* 116:73–74, 1958.
163. Awbrey BJ, Sienkiewicz, PS, Mankin HJ: Chronic exercise-induced compartment pressure elevation measured with a miniaturized fluid pressure monitor. A laboratory and clinical study, *Am J Sports Med* 16:610–615, 1988.
164. Bell S: Intracompartmental pressures on exertion in a patient with a popliteal artery entrapment syndrome, *Am J Sports Med* 13:365–366, 1985.
165. Blank S: Transverse tibial stress fractures. A special problem, *Am J Sports Med* 15:597–602, 1987.
166. Bourne RB, Rorabeck CH: Compartment syndromes of the lower leg, *Clin Orthop* 240:97–104, 1989.
167. Burrows HJ: Fatigue infraction of the middle of the tibia in ballet dancers, *J Bone Joint Surg [Br]* 38:83–94, 1956.
168. Brody DM: Running injuries, *Clin Symp* 32:1–36, 1980.
169. Carter AE, Eban R: A case of bilateral developmental abnormality of the popliteal arteries and gastrocnemius muscles, *Br J Surg* 51:518–522, 1964.
170. Casscells SW, Fellows B, Axe MJ: Another young athlete with intermittent claudication. A case report, *Am J Sports Med* 11:180–182, 1983.
171. Chevalier J, Enon B, Walder J, et al: Endofibrosis of the external iliac artery in bicycle racers: an unrecognized pathological state, *Ann Vasc Surg* 1:297–303, 1986.
172. Clement DB: Tibial stress syndrome in athletes, *J Sports Med* 2:81–85, 1974.
173. Collins PS, McDonald PT, Lim RC: Popliteal artery entrapment: an evolving syndrome, *J Vasc Surg* 10:484–490, 1989.
174. D'Ambrosia RD, Zelis RF, Chuinard RG, et al: Interstitial pressure measurements in the anterior and posterior compartments in athletes with shin splints, *Am J Sports Med* 5:127–131, 1977.
175. Darling RS, Buckley CJ, Abbott WM, et al: Intermittent claudication in young athletes: popliteal artery entrapment syndrome, *J Trauma* 14:543–552, 1974.
176. Davey JR, Rorabeck CH, Fowler PJ: The tibialis posterior muscle compartment. An unrecognized cause of exertional compartment syndrome, *Am J Sports Med* 12:391–397, 1984.
177. Delaney TA, Gonzalez LL: Occlusion of popliteal artery due to muscular entrapment, *Surgery* 69:97–101, 1971.
178. Detmer DE: Chronic shin splints: classification and management of medial tibial stress syndrome, *Sports Med* 3:436–446, 1986.
179. Detmer DE, Sharpe K, Sufit RL, et al: Chronic compartment syndrome: diagnosis, management, and outcomes, *Am J Sports Med* 13:162–170, 1985.
180. Devas MB: Stress fractures of the tibia or "shin soreness," *J Bone Joint Surg [Br]* 40:227–239, 1958.
181. di Marzo L, Cavallaro A, Sciacca V, et al: Diagnosis of popliteal artery entrapment syndrome: the role of duplex scanning, *J Vasc Surg* 13:434–438, 1991.
182. di Marzo L, Cavallaro A, Sciacca V, et al: Surgical treatment of popliteal artery entrapment syndrome: a ten-year experience, *Eur J Vasc Surg* 5:59–64, 1991.
183. Duwelius PJ, Kelbel JM, Jardon OM, et al: Popliteal artery entrapment in a high school athlete. A case report, *Am J Sports Med* 15:371–373, 1987.
184. Ebbeling CB, Clarkson PM: Exercise-induced muscle damage and adaptation, *Sports Med* 7:207–234, 1989.
185. Fong H, Downs AR: Popliteal artery entrapment syndrome with distal embolization. A report of two cases, *J Cardiovasc Surg (Torino)* 30:85–88, 1989.
186. Friden J, Sfakianos PN, Hargens AR, et al: Residual muscular swelling after repetitive eccentric contractions, *J Orthop Res* 6:493–498, 1988.
187. Froimson A: Tennis leg, *JAMA* 209:415–416, 1969.
188. Garfin SR, Tipton CM, Mubarak SJ, et al: The role of fascia in the maintenance of muscle tension and pressure, *J Appl Physiol* 51:317–320, 1981.
189. Garrett JC: The lower leg. In Scott WN, Nisonson B, Nicholas JA, (editors): *Principles in sports medicine*, Baltimore, 1984, Williams & Wilkins, pp 342–347.
190. Garth WP Jr, Miller ST: Evaluation of claw toe deformity, weakness of the foot intrinsics, and posteromedial shin pain, *Am J Sports Med* 17:821–827, 1989.
191. Gorard DA: Effort thrombosis in an American football player, *Br J Sports Med* 24:15, 1990.
192. Green NE, Rogers RA, Lipscomb AB. Nonunions of stress fractures of the tibia, *Am J Sports Med* 13:171–176, 1985.
193. Greenwood LH, Yrizarry JM, Hallett JW Jr: Popliteal artery entrapment: importance of the stress runoff for diagnosis, *Cardiovasc Intervent Radiol* 9:93–99, 1986.
194. Gudas CJ: Patterns of lower extremity injury in 224 runners. *Compr Ther* 6:50–59, 1980.
195. Gyftokostas D, Koutsoumbelis C, Mattheou T, et al: Post stenotic aneurysm in popliteal artery entrapment syndrome, *J Cardiovasc Surg (Torino)* 32:350–352, 1991.
196. Haimovici H: Peroneal sensory neuropathy entrapment syndrome, *Arch Surg* 105:586–590, 1972.
197. Hamming JJ: Intermittent claudication at an early age, due to an anomalous course of the popliteal artery, *Angiology* 10:369–371, 1959.
198. Harvey JS Jr: Effort thrombosis in the lower extremity of a runner, *Am J Sports Med* 6:400–402, 1978.
199. Holder LE, Michael RH: The specific scintigraphic pattern of "shin splints in the lower leg," *J Nucl Med* 25:865–869, 1984.
200. Insua JA, Young JR, Humphries AW: Popliteal artery entrapment syndrome, *Arch Surg* 101:771–775, 1970.

201. Jackson DW, Bailey D: Shin splints in the young athlete: a non-specific diagnosis, *Physician Sports Med* 3:45–51, 1975.
202. Järvinnen M, Aho H, Niittymäki S: Results of the surgical treatment of the medial tibial syndrome in athletes, *Int J Sports Med* 10:55–57, 1989.
203. James SL, Bates BT, Osternig LR: Injuries to runners, *Am J Sports Med* 6:40–50, 1978.
204. Jones DC, James SL: Overuse injuries of the lower extremity: shin splints, iliotibial band friction syndrome and exertional compartment syndromes, *Clin Sports Med* 6:273–290, 1987.
205. Kirby NG: Exercise ischemia in the fascial compartment of the soleus, *J Bone Joint Surg [Br]* 52:738–740, 1970.
206. Leach RE: Editorial comment, *Am J Sports Med* 5:193, 1977.
207. Leach RE, Purnell MB, Saito A: Peroneal nerve entrapment in runners, *Am J Sports Med* 17:287–291, 1989.
208. Love JW, Whelan TJ: Popliteal artery entrapment syndrome, *Am J Surg* 109:620–624, 1965.
209. Lysens RJ, Renson LM, Ostyn MS, et al: Intermittent claudication in young athletes: popliteal artery entrapment syndrome, *Am J Sports Med* 11:177–179, 1983.
210. Mackey D, Colbert DS, Chater EH: Musculocutaneous nerve entrapment, *Irish J Med Sci* 146:100, 1977.
211. Martens MA, Backaert M, Vermaut G, et al: Chronic leg pain in athlete due to a recurrent compartment syndrome, *Am J Sports Med* 12:148–151, 1984.
212. Martens MA, Moeyersoons JP: Acute and recurrent effort-related compartment syndrome in sports, *Sports Med* 9:62–68, 1990.
213. Marti B, Vader JP, Minder CE, et al: On the epidemiology of running injuries: the Bern Gran-Prix Study, *Am J Sports Med* 16:285–294, 1988.
214. Martti V: Decompression for peroneal nerve entrapment, *Acta Orthop Scand* 57:551–554, 1986.
215. Massey EW, Pleet AB: Neuropathy in joggers, *Am J Sports Med* 6:209–211, 1978.
216. McAuliffe TB, Fiddian NJ, Browett JP: Entrapment neuropathy of the superficial peroneal nerve: a bilateral case, *J Bone Joint Surg [Br]* 67:62–63, 1985.
217. McDonald PT, Easterbrook JA, Rich NM, et al: Popliteal artery entrapment syndrome. Clinical, noninvasive and angiographic diagnosis, *Am J Surg* 139:318–325, 1980.
218. Mennen U: Letter to the editor, *J Bone Joint Surg [Am]* 65:1030, 1983.
219. Michael RH, Holder LE: The soleus syndrome. A cause of medial tibial stress (shin splints), *Am J Sports Med* 13:87–94, 1985.
220. Miles S, Roediger W, Cooke P, et al: Doppler ultrasound in the diagnosis of the popliteal artery entrapment syndrome, *Br J Surg* 64:883–884, 1977.
221. Millar AP: Strains of the posterior calf musculature ("tennis leg"), *Am J Sports Med* 7:172–174, 1979.
222. Miller WA: Rupture of the musculotendinous juncture of the medial head of the gastrocnemius muscle, *Am J Sports Med* 5:191–193, 1977.
223. Miniaci A, Rorabeck CH: Compartment syndrome as a complication of repair of the hernia of the tibialis anterior, *J Bone Joint Surg [Am]* 69:1444–1445, 1986.
224. Moller BN, Kadin S: Entrapment of the common peroneal nerve, *Am J Sports Med* 15:90–91, 1987.
225. Mozan LC, Keagy RD: Muscle relationship in function fascia, *Clin Orthop* 67:225–230, 1969.
226. Mozes M, Ouaknine G, Nathan H: Saphenous nerve entrapment simulating vascular disorder, *Surgery* 77:299–303, 1975.
227. Mubarak SJ: Exertional compartment syndromes. In Mubarak SJ, Hargens AR, editors: *Compartment syndromes and Volkmann's contracture*, Philadelphia, 1981, WB Saunders, pp 209–226.
228. Mubarak SJ, Gould RN, Lee YF, et al: The medial tibial stress syndrome. A cause of shin splints, *Am J Sports Med* 10:201–205, 1982.
229. Muller N, Morris DC, Nichols DM: Popliteal artery entrapment demonstrated by CT, *Radiology* 151:157–158, 1984.
230. Nussbaum AR, Treves ST, Micheli L: Bone stress lesions in ballet dancers: scintigraphic assessment, *AJR* 150:851–855, 1988.
231. O'Donoghue DH: Injuries of the leg. In *Treatment of injuries to athletes*, ed 4, Philadelphia, 1984, WB Saunders, pp 586–600.
232. Orava S, Puranen J: Athletes' leg pain, *Br J Sports Med* 13:92–97, 1979.
233. Pedowitz RA, Hargens AR, Mubarak SJ, et al: Modified criteria for the objective diagnosis of chronic compartment syndrome of the leg, *Am J Sports Med* 18:35–40, 1990.
234. Persky JM, Kempczinski RF, Fowl RJ: Entrapment of the popliteal artery, *Surg Gynecol Obstet* 173:84–90, 1991.
235. Prost WJ: Biomechanics of the foot, *Can Family Physician* 25:827–831, 1979.
236. Puranen J: The medial tibial syndrome. Exercise ischemia in the medial fascial compartment of the leg, *J Bone Joint Surg [Br]* 56:712–715, 1974.
237. Puranen J, Alavaikko A: Intracompartmental pressure increase on exertion in patients with chronic compartment syndrome in the leg, *J Bone Joint Surg [Am]* 63:1304–1309, 1981.
238. Reneman RS: The anterior and the lateral compartmental syndrome of the leg due to intensive use of muscles, *Clin Orthop* 113:69–80, 1975.
239. Rettig AC, Shelbourne KD, McCarroll JR, et al: The natural history and treatment of delayed union stress fractures of the anterior cortex of the tibia, *Am J Sports Med* 16:250–255, 1988.
240. Rorabeck CH: Exertional tibialis posterior compartment syndrome in athletes, *Clin Orthop* 208:61–64, 1986.
241. Rorabeck CH, Bourne RB, Fowler PJ: The surgical treatment of exertional compartment syndrome in athletes, *J Bone Joint Surg [Am]* 65:1245–1251, 1983.
242. Rorabeck CH, Bourne RB, Fowler PJ, et al: The role of tissue pressure measurement in diagnosing chronic anterior compartment syndrome, *Am J Sports Med* 16:143–146, 1988.
243. Rorabeck CH, Fowler PJ, Nott L: The results of fasciotomy in the management of chronic exertional compartment syndrome, *Am J Sports Med* 16:224–227, 1988.
244. Rudo ND, Noble HB, Conn J Jr, et al: Popliteal artery

entrapment syndrome in athletes, *Physician Sports Med* 10:105–114, 1982.
245. Schon LC, Baxter DE: Neuropathies of the foot and ankle in athletes, *Clin Sports Med* 9:489–509, 1990.
246. Sejersted OM, Hargens AR, Kardel KR, et al: Intramuscular fluid pressure during isometric contraction of human skeletal muscle, *J Appl Physiol* 56:287–295, 1984.
247. Severance HW, Bassett FH: Rupture of the plantaris—does it exist? *J Bone Joint Surg [Am]* 64:1387–1388, 1982.
248. Sidey JD: Weak ankles: a study of common peroneal entrapment neuropathy, *Br Med J* 3:623–626, 1969.
249. Slocum DB: The shin splint syndrome. Medical aspects and differential diagnosis, *Am J Surg* 114:875–881, 1967.
250. Snook GA: Intermittent claudication in athletes, *J Sports Med* 3:71–75, 1975.
251. Stuart TPA: Note on a variation in the course of the popliteal artery, *J Anat Physiol* 13:162, 1879.
252. Styf J: Chronic exercise-induced pain in the anterior aspect of the lower leg. An overview of diagnosis, *Sports Med* 7:331–339, 1989.
253. Styf J: Diagnosis of exercise-induced pain in the anterior aspect of the lower leg, *Am J Sports Med* 16:165–169, 1988.
254. Styf J: Entrapment of the superficial peroneal nerve. Diagnosis and results of decompression, *J Bone Joint Surg [Br]* 71:131–135, 1989.
255. Styf J, Korner L: Chronic anterior compartment syndrome of the lower leg: results of treatment with fasciotomy, *J Bone Joint Surg [Am]* 69:1338–1347, 1986.
256. Styf JR, Korner LM: Diagnosis of chronic anterior compartment syndrome in the lower leg, *Acta Orthop Scand* 58:139–144, 1987.
257. Taunton JE, Maxwell TM: Intermittent claudication in an athlete—popliteal artery entrapment: a case report, *Can J Appl Sport Sci* 7:161–163, 1982.
258. van Bockel JH, Biemans RG: Popliteal artery entrapment. Claudication during youth, *Arch Chir Neerl* 28:251–260, 1976.
259. Viitasalo JT, Kvist M: Some biomechanical aspects of the foot and ankle in athletes with and without shin splints, *Am J Sports Med* 11:125–130, 1983.
260. Wallensten R: Results of fasciotomy in patients with medial tibial syndrome or chronic anterior compartment syndrome, *J Bone Joint Surg [Am]* 65:1252–1255, 1983.
261. Wallensten R, Eriksson E: Intramuscular pressures in exercise induced lower leg pain, *Int J Sports Med* 5:31–35, 1984.
262. Williams LR, Flinn WR, McCarthy WJ, et al: Popliteal artery entrapment: diagnosis by computed tomography, *J Vasc Surg* 3:360–363, 1986.
263. Worth RM, Kettelkamp DB, Defalque RJ, et al: Saphenous nerve entrapment: a cause of medial knee pain, *Am J Sports Med* 12:80–81, 1984.
264. Zigun JR, Schneider SM: "Effort" thrombosis (Paget-Schroetter's syndrome) secondary to martial arts training, *Am J Sports Med* 16:189–190, 1988.

Lateral Ankle Sprain

265. Adler H: Therapie und prognose der frischen aussenknöchelbandläsion (Treatment and prognosis of fresh ankle ligament ruptures). *Unfallheilkunde* 79:101–104, 1976.
266. Anderson KJ, LeCocq JF, Clayton ML: Athletic injury to the fibular collateral ligament of the ankle, *Clin Orthop* 23:146–160, 1962.
267. Anderson ME: Reconstruction of the lateral ligaments of the ankle using the plantaris tendon, *J Bone Joint Surg [Am]* 67:930–934, 1985.
268. Attarian DE, McCrackin HJ, DeVito DP, et al: Biomechanical characteristics of human ankle ligaments, *Foot Ankle* 6:54–58, 1985.
269. Balduini FC, Tetzlaff J: Historical perspectives on injuries of the ligaments of the ankle, *Clin Sports Med* 1:3–12, 1982.
270. Balduini FC, Vegso JJ, Torg JS, et al: Management and rehabilitation of ligamentous injuries to the ankle, *Sports Med* 4:364–380, 1987.
271. Barbari SG, Brevig K, Egge T: Reconstruction of the lateral ligamentous structures of the ankle with a modified Watson-Jones procedure, *Foot Ankle* 7:362–368, 1987.
272. Baxter DE: Traumatic injuries to the soft tissues of the foot and ankle. Ligamentous injuries. In Mann RA, editor: *Surgery of the foot*, ed 5, St Louis, 1986, Mosby–Year Book, pp 456–472.
273. Berg EE: The symptomatic os subfibulare, *J Bone Joint Surg [Am]* 73:1251–1254, 1991.
274. Bergfeld JA, Cox JS, Drez D Jr, et al: Symposium: management of acute ankle sprains, *Contemp Orthop* 13:83–116, 1986.
275. Berridge FR, Bonnin JG: The radiographic examination of the ankle joint including arthrography, *Surg Gynecol Obstet* 79:383–389, 1944.
276. Björkenheim JM, Sandelin J, Santavirta S: Evans' procedure in the treatment of chronic instability of the ankle, *Injury* 19:70–72, 1988.
277. Black H: Roentgenographic considerations, *Am J Sports Med* 5:238–240, 1977.
278. Black HM, Brand RL, Eichelberger MR: An improved technique for the evaluation of ligamentous injury in severe ankle sprains, *Am J Sports Med* 6:276–282, 1978.
279. Bonnin JG: *Injuries to the ankle*, Darien, Conn, 1970, Hafner, pp 109–118.
280. Bonnin JG: Radiologic diagnosis of recent lesions of the lateral ligament of the ankle, *J Bone Joint Surg [Br]* 31:478, 1949. (Comment on paper by J. Roland Hughes by this title.)
281. Brand RL, Collins MDF: Operative management of ligamentous injuries to the ankle, *Clin Sports Med* 1:117–130, 1982.
282. Brand RL, Collins MDF, Templeton T: Surgical repair of ruptured lateral ankle ligaments, *Am J Sports Med* 9:40–44, 1981.
283. Brooks SC, Potter BT, Rainey JB: Treatment for partial tears of the lateral ligament of the ankle: a prospective trial, *Br Med J* 282:606–607, 1981.
284. Broström L: Sprained ankles. I. Anatomic lesions in recent sprains, *Acta Chir Scand* 128:483–495, 1964.
285. Broström L: Sprained ankles. V. Treatment and prognosis in recent ligament ruptures, *Acta Chir Scand* 132:537–550, 1966.
286. Broström L: Sprained ankles. VI. Surgical treatment of

"chronic" ligament ruptures, *Acta Chir Scand* 132:551–565, 1966.
287. Broström L, Liljedahl S, Lindvall N: Sprained ankles. II. Arthrographic diagnosis of recent ligament ruptures, *Acta Chir Scand* 129:485–499, 1965.
288. Cahill DR: The anatomy and function of the contents of the human tarsal sinus and canal, *Anat Rec* 153:1–18, 1965.
289. Cass JR, Morrey BF: Ankle instability: Current concepts, diagnosis, and treatment, *Mayo Clin Proc* 59:165–170, 1984.
290. Cass JR, Morrey BF, Katoh Y, et al: Ankle instability: comparison of primary repair and delayed reconstruction after long-term follow-up study. *Clin Orthop* 198:110–117, 1985.
291. Chapman MW: Part II. Sprains of the ankle, *Instr Course Lect* 24:294–308, 1975.
292. Chirls M: Inversion injuries of the ankle, *J Med Soc N J* 70:751–753, 1973.
293. Chrisman OD, Snook GA: Reconstruction of lateral ligament tears of the ankle. An experimental study and clinical evaluation of seven patients treated by a new modification of the Elmslie procedure, *J Bone Joint Surg [Am]* 51:904–912, 1969.
294. Clark BL, Derby AC, Power GRI: Injuries of the lateral ligament of the ankle. Conservative vs. operative repair, *Can J Surg* 8:358–363, 1965.
295. Colville MR, Marder RA, Boyle JJ et al: Strain measurement in lateral ankle ligaments, *Am J Sports Med* 18:196–200, 1990.
296. Cox JS, Hewes TF: "Normal" talar tilt angle, *Clin Orthop* 140:37–41, 1979.
297. Daseler EH, Anson BJ: The plantaris muscle. An anatomic study of 750 specimens, *J Bone Joint Surg* 25:822–827, 1943.
298. DenHartog B, Cardone BW, Johnson JE, et al: The role of magnetic resonance imaging in evaluating chronic ankle pain after sprain, American Orthopaedic Foot and Ankle Society Meeting, Boston, July 27, 1991.
299. Derscheid GL, Brown WC: Rehabilitation of the ankle, *Clin Sports Med* 4: 527–544, 1985.
300. Diamond JE: Rehabilitation of ankle sprains, *Clin Sports Med* 8:877–891, 1989.
301. Drez D Jr, Young JC, Waldman D, et al: Nonoperative treatment of double lateral ligament tears of the ankle, *Am J Sports Med* 10:197–200, 1982.
302. Ekstrand J, Tropp H: The incidence of ankle sprains in soccer, *Foot Ankle* 11:41–44, 1990.
303. Elmslie RC: Recurrent subluxation of the ankle-joint, *Ann Surg* 100:364–367, 1934.
304. Evans GA, Hardcastle P, Frenyo SD: Acute rupture of the lateral ligament of the ankle. To suture or not to suture? *J Bone Joint Surg [Br]* 66:209–212, 1984.
305. Flotterod K, Reichelt HG: Arthrography—expanded diagnosis in capsule-ligament injuries of the upper ankle joint, *Unfallchirurg* 13:207–217, 1987.
306. Francillon MR: Distorsio pedis with an isolated lesion of the ligamentum calcaneo-fibulare, *Acta Orthop Scand* 32:469–475, 1962.
307. Freeman MAR: Treatment of ruptures of the lateral ligament of the ankle, *J Bone Joint Surg [Br]* 47:661–668, 1965.
308. Garrick JG: The frequency of injury, mechanism of injury, and epidemiology of ankle sprains, *Am J Sports Med* 5:241–242, 1977.
309. Glasgow M, Jackson A, Jamieson AM: Instability of the ankle after injury to the lateral ligament, *J Bone Joint Surg [Br]* 62:196–200, 1980.
310. Glick JM, Gordon RB, Nishimoto D: The prevention and treatment of ankle injuries, *Am J Sports Med* 4:136–141, 1976.
311. Good CJ, Jones MA, Livingstone BN: Reconstruction of the lateral ligament of the ankle, *Injury* 7:63–65, 1975.
312. Gould N, Seligson D, Gassman J: Early and late repair of lateral ligament of the ankle, *Foot Ankle* 1:84–89, 1980.
313. Grønmark T, Johnsen O, Kogstad O: Rupture of the lateral ligaments of the ankle: a controlled clinical trial, *Injury* 11:215–218, 1980.
314. Hamilton WG: Foot and ankle injuries in dancers, *Clin Sports Med* 7:143–173, 1988.
315. Hamilton WG: Sprained ankles in ballet dancers, *Foot Ankle* 3:99–102, 1982.
316. Hansen H, Damholt V, Termansen NB: Clinical and social status following injury to the lateral ligaments of the ankle. Follow-up of 144 patients treated conservatively, *Acta Orthop Scand* 50:699–704, 1979.
317. Hardaker WT Jr, Margello S, Goldner JL: Foot and ankle injuries in theatrical dancers, *Foot Ankle* 6:59–69, 1985.
318. Harper MC: The lateral ligamentous support of the subtalar joint, *Foot Ankle* 11:354–358, 1991.
319. Harrington KD: Chronic ankle instability: what it is and what can be done for it, *J Musculoskeletal Med* 6:35–63, 1989.
320. Heilman AE, Braly WG, Bishop JO, et al: An anatomic study of subtalar instability, *Foot Ankle* 10:224–228, 1990.
321. Hendel D, Peer A, Halperin N: A simple operation for correction of chronic lateral instability of the ankle, *Injury* 15:115–116, 1983.
322. Henning CE, Egge LN: Cast brace treatment of acute unstable ankle sprain. A preliminary report, *Am J Sports Med* 5:252–255, 1977.
323. Horibe S, Shino K, Taga I, et al: Reconstruction of lateral ligaments of the ankle with allogeneic tendon grafts, *J Bone Joint Surg [Br]* 73: 802–805, 1991.
324. Horstman JK, Kantor GS, Samuelson KM: Investigation of lateral ankle ligament reconstruction, *Foot Ankle* 1:338–342, 1981.
325. Hughes JR: Sprains and subluxations of the ankle-joint, *Proc R Soc Med* 35:765–766, 1942.
326. Hyslop GH: Injuries to the deep and superficial peroneal nerves complicating ankle sprain, *Am J Surg* 51:436–438, 1941.
327. Jackson DW, Ashley RL, Powell JW: Ankle sprains in young athletes. Relation of severity and disability, *Clin Orthop* 101:201–215, 1974.
328. Jakob RP, Raemy H, Steffen R, et al: Zur funktionellen behandlung des frischen aussenbändrrisses mit der Aircast-schiene (Functional treatment of the fresh lateral ankle ligament ruptures by aircast brace). *Orthopäde* 15:434–440, 1986.
329. Jaskulka R, Fischer G, Schedl R: Injuries of the lateral

ligaments of the ankle joint. Operative treatment and long-term results, *Arch Orthop Trauma Surg* 107:217–221, 1988.

330. Javors JR, Violet JT: Correction of chronic lateral ligament instability of the ankle by use of the Broström procedure. A report of 15 cases, *Clin Orthop* 198:201–207, 1985.
331. Johannsen A: Radiological diagnosis of lateral ligament lesion of the ankle. A comparison between talar tilt and anterior drawer sign, *Acta Orthop Scand* 49:295–301, 1978.
332. Kannus P, Konradsen L, Holmer P, et al: Early mobilizing treatment for grade III ankle ligament injuries, *Foot Ankle* 12:69–73, 1991.
333. Kannus P, Renström P: Current concepts review. Treatment for acute tears of the lateral ligaments of the ankle. Operation, cast, or early controlled mobilization, *J Bone Joint Surg [Am]* 73:305–312, 1991.
334. Karlsson J, Bergsten T, Lansinger O, et al: Reconstruction of the lateral ligaments of the ankle for chronic lateral instability, *J Bone Joint Surg [Am]* 70:581–588, 1988.
335. Kelikian H, Kelikian A: *Disorders of the ankle*, Philadelphia, 1985, WB Saunders.
336. Kjaersgaard-Andersen P, Wethelund J, Helmig P, et al: Effect of the calcaneofibular ligament on hindfoot rotation in amputation specimens, *Acta Orthop Scand* 58:135–138, 1987.
337. Kjaersgaard-Andersen P, Wethelund J, Helmig P, et al: The stabilizing effect of the ligamentous structures in the sinus and canalis tarsi on movements in the hindfoot: an experimental study, *Am J Sports Med* 16:512–516, 1988.
338. Kjaersgaard-Andersen P, Wethelund J, Nielsen S: Lateral talocalcaneal instability following section of the calcaneofibular ligament: a kinesiologic study, *Foot Ankle* 7:355–361, 1987.
339. Klein J, Schreckenberger C, Röddecker K, et al: Operative oder konservative behandlung der frischen aussenbandruptur am oberen sprunggelenk. Randomisierte klinische studie (Operative or conservative treatment of recent rupture of the fibular ligament in the ankle. A randomized clinical trial). *Unfallchirurg* 91:154–160, 1988.
340. Konradsen L, Hølmer P, Søndergaard L: Early mobilizing treatment for grade III ankle ligament injuries, *Foot Ankle* 12:69–73, 1991.
341. Korkala O, Lauttamus L, Tanskanen P: Lateral ligament injuries of the ankle. Results of primary surgical treatment, *Ann Chir Gynaecol* 71:161–163, 1982.
342. Korkala O, Rusanen M, Jokipii P, et al: A prospective study of the treatment of severe tears of the lateral ligament of the ankle, *Int Orthop* 11:13–17, 1987.
343. Kristiansen B: Evans' repair of lateral instability of the ankle joint, *Acta Orthop Scand* 52:679–682, 1981.
344. Kristiansen B: Surgical treatment of ankle instability in athletes, *Br J Sports Med* 16:40–45, 1982.
345. Larsen E: Tendon transfer for lateral ankle and subtalar joint instability, *Acta Orthop Scand* 59:168–172, 1988.
346. Larsen E, Lund PM: Peroneal muscle function in chronically unstable ankles. A prospective preoperative and postoperative electromyographic study, *Clin Orthop* 272:219–226, 1991.
347. Lassiter TE Jr, Malone TR, Garrett WE, Jr: Injury to the lateral ligaments of the ankle, *Orthop Clin North Am* 20:629–640, 1989.
348. Laurin CA, Ouellet R, St-Jacques R: Talar and subtalar tilt: an experimental investigation, *Can J Surg* 11:270–279, 1968.
349. Leach RE, Namiki O, Paul GR, et al: Secondary reconstruction of the lateral ligaments of the ankle, *Clin Orthop* 160:201–211, 1981.
350. Leach RE, Schepsis AA: Acute injuries to ligaments of the ankle. In Evarts CM, editor: *Surgery of the musculoskeletal system*, vol 4, New York, 1990, Churchill Livingstone, pp 3887–3913.
351. Leonard MH: Injuries of the lateral ligaments of the ankle. A clinical and experimental study, *J Bone Joint Surg [Am]* 31:373–377, 1949.
352. Lightowler CDR: Injuries to the lateral ligament of the ankle, *Br Med J* 289:1247, 1984.
353. Lucht U, Vang PS, Termansen NB: Lateral ligament reconstruction of the ankle with a modified Watson-Jones operation, *Acta Orthop Scand* 52:363–366, 1981.
354. Maehlum S, Daljord OA: Acute sports injuries in Oslo: a one-year study, *Br J Sports Med* 18:181–185, 1984.
355. McCullough CJ, Burge PD: Rotatory stability of the load-bearing ankle. An experimental study, *J Bone Joint Surg [Br]* 62:460–464, 1980.
356. McCulloch PG, Holden P, Robson DJ, et al: The value of mobilisation and non-steroidal anti-inflammatory analgesia in the management of inversion injuries of the ankle, *Br J Clin Pract* 2:69–72, 1985.
357. McMaster PE: Treatment of ankle sprain. Observations in more than five hundred cases, *JAMA* 122:659–660, 1943.
358. Meals RA: Peroneal-nerve palsy complicating ankle sprain. Report of two cases and review of the literature, *J Bone Joint Surg [Am]* 59:966–968, 1977.
359. Meyer JM, Hoffmeyer P, Savoy X: High resolution computed tomography in the chronically painful ankle sprain, *Foot Ankle* 8:291–296, 1988.
360. Milachowski KA, Wirth C: The results of reconstruction of the lateral ligaments of the ankle, *Int Orthop* 12:51–55, 1988.
361. Møller-Larsen F, Wethelund JO, Jurik AG, et al: Comparison of three different treatments for ruptured lateral ankle ligaments, *Acta Orthop Scand* 59:564–566, 1988.
362. Niedermann B, Andersen A, Andersen SB, et al: Rupture of the lateral ligaments of the ankle: operation or plaster cast? A prospective study, *Acta Orthop Scand* 52:579–587, 1981.
363. Niethard FU: Die stabilitat des sprunggelenkes nach ruptur des lateralen bandapparates (The mechanical stability of the ankle joint after rupture of the lateral ligament). *Arch Orthop Unfallchirurg* 80:53–61, 1974.
364. Nitz AJ, Dobner JJ, Kersey D: Nerve injury and grades II and III ankle sprains, *Am J Sports Med* 13:177–182, 1985.
365. Orava S, Jaroma H, Weitz H, et al: Radiographic instability of the ankle joint after Evans' repair, *Acta Orthop Scand* 54:734–738, 1983.
366. Petrov O, Blocher K, Bradbury RL, et al: Footwear and ankle stability in the basketball player, *Clin Podiatr Med Surg* 5:275–290, 1988.
367. Prins JG: Diagnosis and treatment of injury to the lat-

eral ligament of the ankle. A comparative clinical study, *Acta Chir Scand Suppl* 486:1–152, 1978.
368. Rasmussen O: Stability of the ankle joint. Analysis of the function and traumatology of the ankle ligaments, *Acta Orthop Scand Suppl* 211:1–75, 1985.
369. Redler I, Brown GG Jr, Williams JT: Operative treatment of the acutely ruptured lateral ligament of the ankle, *South Med J* 70:1168–1171, 1977.
370. Reichen A, Marti R: Die frische fibulare bandruptur—diagnose, therapie, resultate (rupture of the fibular collateral ligaments—diagnosis, surgical treatment, results), *Arch Orthop Unfallchirurg* 80:211–222, 1974.
371. Riegler HF: Reconstruction for lateral instability of the ankle, *J Bone Joint Surg [Am]* 66:336–339, 1984.
372. Rubin G, Witten M: The talar-tilt angle and the fibular collateral ligaments. A method for the determination of talar tilt, *J Bone Joint Surg [Am]* 42:311–326, 1960.
373. Ruth CJ: The surgical treatment of injuries of the fibular collateral ligaments of the ankle, *J Bone Joint Surg [Am]* 43:229–239, 1961.
374. Sandelin J: Acute sports injuries. A clinical and epidemiological study (dissertation), University of Helsinki, 1988, pp 1–66.
375. Sarrafian SK: *Anatomy of the foot and ankle: descriptive, topographic, functional*, Philadelphia, 1983, JB Lippincott.
376. Savastano AA, Lowe EB Jr: Ankle sprains: surgical treatment for recurrent sprains. Report of 10 patients treated with the Chrisman-Snook modification of the Elmslie procedure, *Am J Sports Med* 8:208–211, 1980.
377. Schaap GR, de Keizer G, Marti K: Inversion trauma of the ankle, *Arch Orthop Trauma Surg* 108:273–275, 1989.
378. Schmidt HM: Gestalt und befestigung der bandsysteme im binus und canalis tarsi des menschen (Shape and fixation of band systems in human sinus and canalis tarsi), *Acta Anat* 102:184–194, 1978.
379. Schon LC, Baxter DE: Neuropathies of the foot and ankle in athletes, *Clin Sports Med* 9:489–509, 1990.
380. Schon LC, Clanton TO, Baxter DE: Reconstruction for subtalar instability: a review, *Foot Ankle* 11:319–325, 1991.
381. Schon LC, Hansen ST Jr: Anatomic reconstruction of the lateral ligaments of the ankle using the plantaris tendon: the modified Kelikian procedure, American Academy of Orthopaedic Surgeons Comprehensive Foot and Ankle Course, Chicago, Nov 1988.
382. Schrøder HM, Lind T, Andersen K, et al: The Ottosson repair in lateral instability of the ankle, *Arch Orthop Trauma Surg* 107:280–282, 1988.
383. Sedlin ED: A device for stress inversion or eversion roentgenograms of the ankle, *J Bone Joint Surg [Am]* 42:1184–1190, 1960.
384. Sefton GK, George J, Fitton JM, et al: Reconstruction of the anterior talofibular ligament for the treatment of the unstable ankle, *J Bone Joint Surg [Br]* 61:352–354, 1979.
385. Siegler S, Block J, Schneck CD: The mechanical characteristics of the collateral ligaments of the human ankle joint, *Foot Ankle* 8:234–242, 1988.
386. Smith JW: The ligamentous structures in the canalis and sinus tarsi, *J Anat* 92:616–620, 1958.
387. Smith RW, Reischl S: The influence of dorsiflexion in the treatment of severe ankle sprains: an anatomical study, *Foot Ankle* 9:28–33, 1988.
388. Smith RW, Reischl SF: Treatment of ankle sprains in young athletes, *Am J Sports Med* 14:465–471, 1986.
389. Snook GA, Chrisman OD, Wilson TC: Long-term results of the Chrisman-Snook operation for reconstruction of the lateral ligaments of the ankle, *J Bone Joint Surg [Am]* 67:1–7, 1985.
390. Solheim LF, Denstad TF, Roaas A: Chronic lateral instability of the ankle. A method of reconstruction using the Achilles tendon, *Acta Orthop Scand* 51:193–196, 1980.
391. Sommer HM, Arza D: Functional treatment of recent ruptures of the fibular ligament of the ankle, *Int Orthop* 13:157–160, 1989.
392. St. Pierre R, Allman F Jr, Bassett FH III, et al: A review of lateral ankle ligamentous reconstructions, *Foot Ankle* 3:114–123, 1982.
393. St. Pierre RK, Andrews L, Allman F Jr, et al: The Cybex II evaluation of lateral ankle ligamentous reconstructions, *Am J Sports Med* 12: 52–56, 1984.
394. Standard nomenclature of athletic injuries. Report of the Committee on the Medical Aspects of Sports, Chicago, American Medical Association, 1966.
395. Staples OS: Ruptures of the fibular collateral ligaments of the ankle. Result study of immediate surgical treatment, *J Bone Joint Surg [Am]* 57:101–107, 1975.
396. Stewart MJ, Hutchins WC: Repair of the lateral ligaments of the ankle, *Am J Sports Med* 6:272–275, 1978.
397. Stormont DM, Morrey BF, An K, et al: Stability of the loaded ankle. Relation between articular restraint and primary and secondary static restraints, *Am J Sports Med* 13: 295–300, 1985.
398. Van Moppens FI, Van Den Hoogenband CR: Diagnostic and therapeutic aspects of inversion trauma of the ankle joint (Thesis), University of Maastricht, The Netherlands, 1982.
399. Verhaven EFC, Shahabpour M, Handelberg FWJ, et al: The accuracy of three-dimensional magnetic resonance imaging in the diagnosis of ruptures of the lateral ligaments of the ankle, *Am J Sports Med* 19:583–587, 1991.
400. Viladot A, Lorenzo JC, Salazar J, et al: The subtalar joint: embryology and morphology, *Foot Ankle* 5:54–66, 1984.
401. Williams JGP: Plication of the anterolateral capsule of the ankle with extensor digitorum brevis transfer for chronic lateral ligament instability, *Injury* 19:65–69, 1988.
402. Younes C, Fowles JV, Fallaha M, et al: Long-term results of surgical reconstruction for chronic lateral instability of the ankle: comparison of Watson-Jones and Evans techniques, *J Trauma* 28:1330–1334, 1988.
403. Zenni EJ Jr, Grefer M, Krieg JK, et al: Lateral ligamentous instability of the ankle: a method of surgical reconstruction by a modified Watson-Jones technique, *Am J Sports Med* 5:78–83, 1977.

Medial Ankle Sprain

404. Attarian DE, McCrackin HJ, DeVito DP, et al: Biomechanical characteristics of human ankle ligaments, *Foot Ankle* 6:54–58, 1985.
405. Bonnin JG: Injury to the ligaments of the ankle, *J Bone Joint Surg [Br]* 47:609–611, 1965.
406. Bruns J, Dahmen G: Involvement of the inner malleo-

lus and deltoid ligament in supination trauma of the ankle joint, *Aktuel Traumatol* 17:209–213, 1987.
407. Cedell C: Supination-outward rotation injuries of the ankle. A clinical and roentgenological study with special reference to the operative treatment, *Acta Orthop Scand Suppl* 110:1–148, 1967.
408. Close JR: Some applications of the functional anatomy of the ankle joint, *J Bone Joint Surg [Am]* 38:761–781, 1956.
409. Duriau F, Tondeur G: Faut-il reparer chirurgialement les lesion du ligament lateral interne de la cheville? *Acta Orthop Belg* 40:96–103, 1974.
410. DuVries HL: Reconstruction of the medial collateral (deltoid) ligament. In Inman VT, editor: *DuVries' surgery of the foot*, St Louis, 1973, Mosby–Year Book, pp 477–478.
411. Grath G: Widening of the ankle mortise. A clinical and experimental study, *Acta Chir Scand Suppl* 263:1–88, 1960.
412. Harper MC: An anatomic study of the short oblique fracture of the distal fibula and ankle stability, *Foot Ankle* 4:23–29, 1983.
413. Harper MC: Deltoid ligament: an anatomical evaluation of function, *Foot Ankle* 8:19–22, 1987.
414. Harper MC: The Deltoid ligament: an evaluation of function and need for surgical repair, *Clin Orthop* 226:156–168, 1988.
415. Jackson R, Wills RE, Jackson R: Rupture of the deltoid ligament without involvement of the lateral ligament, *Am J Sports Med* 16:541–543, 1988.
416. Kelikian H, Kelikian A: Disruptions of the deltoid ligament. In Kelikian H, Kelikian A, editors: *Disorders of the ankle*, Philadelphia, 1985, WB Saunders, pp 339–370.
417. Lauge-Hansen N: "Ligamentous" ankle fractures: diagnosis and treatment, *Acta Chir Scand* 97:544–550, 1949.
418. Leach RE, Schepsis AA: Acute injuries to ligaments of the ankle. In Evarts CM, editor: *Surgery of the Musculoskeletal System*, vol 4, New York, 1990, Churchill Livingstone, pp 3887–3913.
419. Monk CJE: Injuries to the tibio-fibular ligaments, *J Bone Joint Surg [Br]* 51:330–337, 1969.
420. Pankovich AM, Shivaram MS: Anatomic basis of variability in injuries of the medial malleolus and the deltoid ligament. I. Anatomical studies, *Acta Orthop Scand* 50:217–223, 1979.
421. Pankovich AM, Shivaram MS: Anatomical basis of variability in injuries of the medial malleolus and the deltoid ligament. II. Clinical studies, *Acta Orthop Scand* 50:225–236, 1979.
422. Rasmussen O: Stability of the ankle joint. Analysis of the function and the traumatology of the ankle ligaments, *Acta Orthop Scand Suppl* 211:1–75, 1985.
423. Sarrafian SK: *Anatomy of the foot and ankle*, Philadelphia, 1983, JB Lippincott.
424. Staples OS: Injuries to the medial ligaments of the ankle, *J Bone Joint Surg [Am]* 42:1287–1307, 1960.
425. Wiltberger BR, Mallory TM: A new method for the reconstruction of the deltoid ligament of the ankle. *Orthop Rev* 1:37–41, 1972.

Syndesmosis Sprains of the Ankle

426. Abdrakhmanov AZ, Baimagambetow SA, Grishin AN, et al: Biomechanical substantiation of osteosynthesis of distal intertibial syndesmosis with wire, *Ortop Travmatol Protez* 5:40–43, 1990.
427. Arlinghaus E, Mayer F: Die Isolierte Ruptur der Vorderen Distalen Syndesmose. Ein Diagnostisches Problem (Isolated rupture of the anterior distal syndesmosis. A diagnostic problem), *Aktuel Traumatol* 20:184–187, 1990.
428. Ashhurst APC, Bromer RS: Classification and mechanism of fractures of the leg bones involving the ankle, *Arch Surg* 4:51–129, 1922.
429. Bassett FH III, Gates HS III, Billys JB, et al: Talar impingment by the anteroinferior tibiofibular ligament. A cause of chronic pain in the ankle after inversion sprain, *J Bone Joint Surg [Am]* 72:55–59, 1990.
430. Becker D: Funktionsgerechte Rekonstrucktion Veralteter Syndesmosensprengungen durch Implantation von Dacron Ligament (Function-related reconstruction of chronic syndesmosis ruptures by implantation of a Dacron ligament). *Beitr Orthop Traumatol* 37:551–561, 1990.
431. Berridge FR, Bonnin JG: The radiographic examination of the ankle joint including arthrography, *Surg Gynecol Obstet* 79:383–389, 1944.
432. Boden SD, Labropoulos PA, McCowin P, et al: Mechanical considerations for the syndesmosis screw. A cadaver study, *J Bone Joint Surg [Am]* 71:1548–1555, 1989.
433. Bonnin JG: *Injuries to the ankle*, Darien, Conn, 1970, Hafner, pp 147–185.
434. Bose K: Congenital diastasis of the inferior tibiofibular joint. Report of a case, *J Bone Joint Surg [Am]* 58:886–887, 1976.
435. Boytim MJ, Fischer DA, Neumann L: Syndesmotic ankle sprains, *Am J Sports Med* 19:294–298, 1991.
436. Broström L: Sprained ankles. III. Clinical observations in recent ligament ruptures, *Acta Chir Scand* 130:560–569, 1965.
437. Broström L, Liljedahl S, Lindvall N: Sprained ankles. II. Arthrographic diagnosis of recent ligament ruptures, *Acta Chir Scand* 129:485–499, 1965.
438. Cedell C: Ankle lesions, *Acta Orthop Scand* 46:425–445, 1975.
439. Cedell C: Supination–outward rotation injuries of the ankle. A clinical and roentgenological study with special reference to the operative treatment, *Acta Orthop Scand Suppl* 110:1–148, 1967.
440. Chapman MW: Part II. Sprains of the ankle, *Instr Course Lect* 24:294–308, 1975.
441. Clanton TO, Clain MR, Baxter DE: Distal tibial bone graft: Operative technique, *Foot Ankle* 1992 (in press).
442. Close JR: Some applications of the functional anatomy of the ankle joint, *J Bone Joint Surg [Am]* 38:761–781, 1956.
443. DenHartog B, Cardone BW, Johnson JE, et al: The role of magnetic resonance imaging in evaluating chronic ankle pain after sprain, American Orthopaedic Foot and Ankle Society Meeting, Boston, July 27, 1991.
444. Dittmer H, Huf R: Die Sprengung der Distalen Tibiofibularen Syndesmose ohne Knöchelfraktur (Rupture of the distal tibiofibular syndesmosis without ankle fracture). *Aktuel Traumatol* 17:179–181, 1987.
445. Edwards GS Jr, DeLee JC: Ankle diastasis without fracture, *Foot Ankle* 4:305–312, 1984.

446. Engelbrecht E: Die Versorgung Tibio-fibularer Syndesmosensprengungen mit dem Syndesmosen-Haken [The treatment of tibiofibular diastasis with the syndesmosis hook], *Chirurg* 42:92–94, 1971.
447. Engelbrecht E, Engelbrecht H, Huynh PL: Erfahrungen mit dem Syndesmosenhaken bei der Tibiofibularen Bandverletzung (Experiences with the syndesmosis hook in tibiofibular ligament injuries), *Chirurg* 55:749–755, 1984.
448. Farhan MJ, Smith TWD: Fixation of diastasis of the inferior tibiofibular joint using the syndesmosis hook, *Injury* 16:309–311, 1985.
449. Frick H: Diagnostik, Therapie und Ergebnisse der Akuten Instabilität der Syndesmose des Oberen Sprunggelenkes (Isolierte Vordere Syndesmosenruptur) (Diagnosis, therapy, and results of acute instability of the syndesmosis of the upper ankle joint [isolated anterior rupture of the syndesmosis]), *Orthopade* 15:423–426, 1986.
450. Fritschy D: An unusual ankle injury in top skiers, *Am J Sports Med* 17:282–286, 1989.
451. Gabarino JL, Clancy M, Harcke T, et al: Congenital diastasis of the inferior tibiofibular joint: A review of the literature and report of two cases, *J Pediatr Orthop* 5:225–228, 1985.
452. Harper MC, Keller TS: A radiographic evaluation of the tibiofibular syndesmosis, *Foot Ankle* 10:156–160, 1989.
453. Höcker K, Pachucki A: Die Incisura Fibularis Tibiae. Die Stellung der Fibula in der distalen Syndesmose am Querschnitt (The fibular incisure of the tibia. The cross-sectional position of the fibula in the distal syndesmosis). *Unfallchirurg* 92:401–406, 1989.
454. Hopkinson WJ, St. Pierre P, Ryan JB, et al: Syndesmosis sprains of the ankle, *Foot Ankle* 10:325–330, 1990.
455. Katznelson A, Lin E, Militiano J: Ruptures of the ligaments about the tibio-fibular syndesmosis, *Injury* 15:170–172, 1984.
456. Kaye RA: Stabilization of ankle syndesmosis injuries with a syndesmosis screw, *Foot Ankle* 9:290–293, 1989.
457. Kelikian H, Kelikian AS: *Disorders of the ankle*, Philadelphia, 1985, WB Saunders.
458. Kingston S: Magnetic resonance imaging of the ankle and foot, *Clin Sports Med* 7:15–28, 1988.
459. Kirschenmann JJ: Rotated fibula, *N Y State J Med* 37:1731–1732, 1937.
460. Leeds HC, Ehrlich MG: Instability of the distal tibiofibular syndesmosis after bimalleolar and trimalleolar ankle fractures, *J Bone Joint Surg [Am]* 66:490–503, 1984.
461. Lindsjö U, Hemmingsson A, Sahlstedt B, et al: Computed tomography of the ankle, *Acta Orthop Scand* 50:797–801, 1979.
462. Lovell ES: An unusual rotatory injury of the ankle, *J Bone Joint Surg [Am]* 50:163–165, 1968.
463. Manderson EL: The uncommon sprain. Ligamentous diastasis of the ankle without fracture or bony deformity, *Orthop Rev* 15:664–668, 1986.
464. Marymont JV, Lynch MA, Henning CE: Acute ligamentous diastasis without fracture. Evaluation by radionuclide imaging, *Am J Sports Med* 14:407–409, 1986.
465. McCullough CJ, Burge PD: Rotatory stability of the load-bearing ankle. An experimental study, *J Bone Joint Surg [Br]* 62:460–464, 1980.
466. McDade WC: Diagnosis and treatment of ankle fractures, *Instr Course Lect* Mosby Company, 24:251–293, 1975.
467. Milliken SM: Complete dislocation of ankle without fracture of leg bone, *Ann Surg* 69:650–651, 1919.
468. O'Donoghue DH: *Treatment of injuries to athletes*, ed 2, Philadelphia, 1970, WB Saunders.
469. Outland T: Sprains and separations of inferior tibiofibular joint without important fracture, *Am J Surg* 59:320–329, 1943.
470. Pettrone FA, Gail M, Pee D, et al: Quantitative criteria for prediction of the results after displaced fracture of the ankle, *J Bone Joint Surg [Am]* 65:667–677, 1983.
470a. Quénu E: Du diastasis de l'articulation tibio-péronier, *Rev Chir* 45:416–438, 1912.
471. Ramsey PL, Hamilton W: Changes in tibiotalar area of contact caused by lateral talar shift, *J Bone Joint Surg [Am]* 58:356–357, 1976.
472. Rasmussen O: Stability of the ankle joint. Analysis of the function and traumatology of the ankle ligaments, *Acta Orthop Scand Suppl* 211:1–75, 1985.
473. Rasmussen O, Tovberg-Jensen I: Mobility of the ankle joint. Recording of rotatory movements in the talocrural joint in vitro with and without the lateral collateral ligaments of the ankle, *Acta Orthop Scand* 53:155–160, 1982.
474. Ruf W, Friedl P, Frobenius H: Die Ruptur der Tibiofibularen Syndesmose ohne Knöcherne Fibulaverletzung (Rupture of the tibiofibular syndesmosis without osseous fibular injury). *Aktuel Traumatol* 17:153–156, 1987.
475. Sarrafian SK: *Anatomy of the foot and ankle. Descriptive, topographic, functional*, Philadelphia, 1983, JB Lippincott.
476. Sclafani SJA: Ligamentous injury of the lower tibiofibular syndesmosis: Radiographic evidence. *Radiology* 156:21–27, 1985.
477. Scranton PE, McMaster JH, Kelly E: Dynamic fibular function, *Clin Orthop* 118:76–81, 1976.
478. Sedgwick WG, Schoenecker PL: Congenital diastasis of the ankle joint. Case report of a patient treated and followed to maturity, *J Bone Joint Surg [Am]* 64:450–453, 1982.
479. Seitz WH Jr, Bachner EJ, Abram LJ, et al: Repair of the tibiofibular syndesmosis with a flexible implant, *J Orthop Trauma* 5:78–82, 1991.
480. Shereff MJ: Radiographic analysis of the foot and ankle. In Jahss MH, editor: *Disorders of the foot and ankle*, ed 2, Philadelphia, 1991, WB Saunders.
481. Solomon MA, Gilula LA, Oloff LM, et al: CT scanning of the foot and ankle: 2. Clinical applications and review of the literature, *AJR* 146:1204–1214, 1986.
482. Vincelette P, Laurin CA, Lévesque HP: The footballer's ankle and foot, *Can Med Assoc J* 107:872–875, 1972.
483. Whiteside LA, Reynolds FC, Ellsasser JC: Tibiofibular synostosis and recurrent ankle sprains in high performance athletes, *Am J Sports Med* 6:204–305, 1978.
484. Wilson MJ, Michele AA, Jacobson EW: Ankle dislocations without fracture, *J Bone Joint Surg* 21:198–204, 1939.

485. Woods RS: Irreducible dislocation of the ankle-joint, *Br J Surg* 29:359–360, 1942.
486. Woolson ST, Dev P, Fellingham LL, et al: Three-dimensional imaging of the ankle joint from computerized tomography, *Foot Ankle* 6:2–6, 1985.
487. Wrazidlo VW, Karl E, Koch K: Die Arthrographische Diagnostik der Vorderen Syndesmosenruptur am Oberen Sprunggelenk (Arthrographic diagnosis of rupture of the anterior syndesmosis of the upper ankle joint), *ROFO* 148:492–497, 1988.

Subtalar Sprains and Sinus Tarsi Syndrome

488. Baxter DE: Personal communication.
489. Brantigan JW, Pedegana LR, Lippert FG: Instability of the subtalar joint: Diagnosis by stress tomography in three cases, *J Bone Joint Surg [Am]* 59:321–324, 1977.
490. Brodén B: Roentgen examination of the subtaloid joint in fractures of the calcaneus, *Acta Radiol* 31:85–91, 1949.
491. Broström L: Sprained ankles. VI. Surgical treatment of "chronic" ligament ruptures, *Acta Chir Scand* 132:551–565, 1966.
492. Brown JE: The sinus tarsi syndrome, *Clin Orthop* 18:231–233, 1960.
493. Brunner R, Gaechter A: Repair of fibular ligaments: comparison of reconstructive techniques using plantaris and peroneal tendons, *Foot Ankle* 11:359–367, 1991.
494. Cahill DR: The anatomy and function of the contents of the human tarsal sinus and canal. *Anat Rec* 153:1–17, 1965.
495. Chrisman OD, Snook GA: Reconstruction of lateral ligament tears of the ankle: an experimental study and clinical evaluation of seven patients treated by a new modification of the Elmslie procedure, *J Bone Joint Surg [Am]* 51:904–912, 1969.
496. Clanton TO: Assessment and classification of subtalar instability, Foot and Ankle Society annual meeting, St Paul, Minn, July 24, 1988.
497. Clanton TO: Instability of the subtalar joint, *Orthop Clin North Am* 20:583–592, 1989.
498. Clanton TO, Schon LC, Baxter DE: An overview of subtalar instability and its treatment, *Perspect Orthop Surg* 1:103–113, 1990.
499. Dias LS: The lateral ankle sprain: an experimental study. *J Trauma* 19:266–269, 1979.
500. Drez D, Young JC, Waldman D, et al: Nonoperative treatment of double lateral ligament tears of the ankle, *Am J Sports Med* 10:197–200, 1982.
501. Elmslie RC: Recurrent subluxation of the ankle-joint, *Ann Surg* 100:364–367, 1934.
502. Gould N, Selligson D, Gassman J: Early and late repair of lateral ligament of the ankle. *Foot Ankle* 1:84–89, 1980.
503. Hamilton WG, Thompson FM: The Brostrum-Gould procedure for lateral ankle instability, American Orthopaedic Foot and Ankle Society meeting, Sun Valley, Idaho, Aug 6, 1989.
504. Hansen ST Jr: Personal communication.
505. Harper MC: The lateral ligamentous support of the subtalar joint, *Foot Ankle* 11:354–358, 1991.
506. Heilman A, Bishop J, Braly WG, et al: Anatomic study of subtalar instability, American Orthopaedic Foot and Ankle Society annual meeting, St Paul, Minn, July 24, 1988.
507. Heilman AE, Braly WG, Bishop JO, et al: An anatomic study of subtalar instability, *Foot Ankle* 10:224–228, 1990.
508. Karlsson J, Bergsten T, Lansinger O, et al: Surgical treatment of chronic lateral instability of the ankle joint. A new procedure, *Am J Sports Med* 17:268–274, 1989.
509. Kelikian H: Personal communication. As quoted in Mann RA, editor: *Surgery of the foot*, St Louis, 1986, Mosby–Year Book, p 308.
510. Kjaersgaard-Andersen P, Wethelund J, Helmig P, et al: Effect of the calcaneofibular ligament on hindfoot rotation in amputation specimens, *Acta Orthop Scand* 58:135–138, 1987.
511. Kjaersgaard-Andersen P, Wethelund J, Helmig P, et al: The stabilizing effect of the ligamentous structures in the sinus and canalis tarsi on movements in the hindfoot: an experimental study, *Am J Sports Med* 16:512–516, 1988.
512. Kjaersgaard-Andersen P, Wethelund J, Nielsen S: Lateral talocalcaneal instability following section of the calcaneofibular ligament: a kinesiologic study, *Foot Ankle* 7:355–361, 1987.
513. Last RJ: Specimens from the Hunterian collections. 7. The subtalar joint (specimens S 100 1 and S 100 2), *J Bone Joint Surg [Br]* 34:116–119, 1952.
514. Larsen E: Tendon transfer for lateral ankle and subtalar joint instability, *Acta Orthop Scand* 59:168–172, 1988.
515. Laurin CA, Ouellet R, St-Jacques R: Talar and subtalar tilt: An experimental investigation, *Can J Surg* 11:270–279, 1968.
516. Leach RE, Namiki O, Paul GR, et al: Secondary reconstruction of the lateral ligaments of the ankle, *Clin Orthop* 160:201–211, 1981.
517. Leonard MH: Injuries of the lateral ligaments of the ankle: a clinical and experimental study, *J Bone Joint Surg [Am]* 31:373–377, 1949.
518. Mann RA: Major surgical procedures for disorders of the ankle, tarsus, and midtarsus. In Mann RA, editor: *Surgery of the foot*, St Louis, 1986, Mosby–Year Book, pp 284–308.
519. Meyer JM: L'arthrographie de l'articulation sousastragalienne posterieure et de l'articulation de Chopart (Arthrography of the subtalar joint and Chopart's joint). *These Med Geneve* no. 3318, 1973.
520. Meyer JM, Garcia J, Hoffmeyer P: Subtalar sprain: a radiological study, American Orthopaedic Foot and Ankle Society annual meeting, Atlanta, Feb 7, 1988.
521. Meyer JM, Garcia J, Hoffmeyer P, et al: The subtalar sprain. A roentgenographic study, *Clin Orthop* 226:169–173, 1988.
522. Meyer JM, Lagier R: Post-traumatic sinus tarsi syndrome: an anatomical and radiological study, *Acta Orthop Scand* 48:121–128, 1977.
523. O'Connor D: Sinus tarsi syndrome. A clinical entity, *J Bone Joint Surg [Am]* 40:720, 1958.
524. Regnauld B: Sinus tarsi syndrome. In *The foot. Pathology, etiology, semiology, clinical investigation and therapy*, New York, 1986, Springer-Verlag, pp 498–500.
525. Rubin G, Witten M: The subtalar joint and the symptom of turning over on the ankle: a new method of eval-

uation utilizing tomography, *Am J Orthop* 4:16–19, 1962.

526. Sammarco GJ, DiRaimondo CV: Surgical treatment of lateral ankle instability syndrome, *Am J Sports Med* 16:501–511, 1988.
527. Schmidt H: Gestalt und Befestigung der Bandsysteme im Sinus und Canalis Tarsi des Menschen (Shape and fixation of band systems in human sinus and canalis tarsi), *Acta Anat* 102:184–194, 1978.
528. Schon LS, Clanton TO, Baxter D: Reconstruction of subtalar instability: a review, *Foot Ankle* 11:319–325, 1991.
529. Smith JW: The ligamentous structures in the canalis and sinus tarsi, *J Anat* 92:616–620, 1958.
530. Smith RW, Reischl SF: Treatment of ankle sprains in young athletes, *Am J Sports Med* 14:465–471, 1986.
531. Solheim LF, Denstad TF, Roaas A: Chronic lateral instability of the ankle. A method of reconstruction using the achilles tendon, *Acta Orthop Scand* 51:193–196, 1980.
532. Stören H: A new method for operative treatment of insufficiency of the lateral ligaments of the ankle joint, *Acta Chir Scand* 117:501–509, 1959.
533. Symposium on subtalar instability, American Orthopaedic Foot and Ankle Society annual meeting, St Paul, Minn, July 24, 1988.
534. Taillard W, Meyer JM, Garcia J, et al: The sinus tarsi syndrome, *Int Orthop* 5:117–130, 1981.
535. Vidal J, Fassio B, Buscayret C, et al: Instabilité externe de la cheville. Importance de l'articulation sour-astragalienne: nouvelle technique de Réparation (Lateral ankle instability. The importance of the subtalar joint: new technique of repair), *Rev Chir Orthop* 60:635–642, 1974.
536. Viladot A, Lorenzo JC, Salazar J, et al: The subtalar joint: embryology and morphology, *Foot Ankle* 5:54–66, 1984.
537. Watson-Jones R: *Fractures and joint injuries*, ed 4, vol 2, Baltimore, 1962, Williams & Wilkins, pp 821–823.
538. Wood Jones F: The talocalcaneal articulation, *Lancet* 24:241–242, 1944.
539. Zell BK, Shereff MJ, Greenspan A, et al: Combined ankle and subtalar instability, *Bull Hosp J Dis Orthop Inst* 46:37–46, 1986.
540. Zollinger H, Meier CH, Waldis M: Diagnostik der Unteren Sprunggelenksinstabilitat Mittels Stress-Tomographie (Diagnosis of subtalar instability utilizing stress tomography) In *Hefte zur Unfallheilkunde* Heft 165, Heidelberg, 1983, Springer-Verlag, pp 175–177.
541. Zwipp H, Krettek C: Diagnostik und Therapie der Akuten und Chronischen Bandinstabilität des Unteren Sprunggelenkes (Diagnosis and therapy of acute and chronic ligament instability of the transverse tarsal joint), *Orthopäde* 15:472–478, 1986.
542. Zwipp H, Tscherne H: Die radiologische diagnostik der rotationsinstabilität im hinteren unteren sprunggelenk (Radiological diagnosis of instability of the subtalar joint), *Unfallheilkunde* 85:494–498, 1982.

Peroneal Tendon Dislocation and Tendinitis

543. Abraham E, Stirnaman JE: Neglected rupture of the peroneal tendons causing recurrent sprains of the ankle. Case report, *J Bone Joint Surg [Am]* 61:1247–1248, 1979.
544. Alm A, Lamke LO, Liljedahl SO: Surgical treatment of dislocation of the peroneal tendons, *Injury* 7:14–19, 1975.
545. Andersen E: Stenosing peroneal tenosynovitis symptomatically simulating ankle instability, *Am J Sports Med* 15:258–259, 1987.
546. Anzel SH, Covey KW, Weiner AD, et al: Disruption of muscles and tendons. An analysis of 1,014 cases, *Surgery* 45:406–414, 1959.
547. Arrowsmith SR, Fleming LL, Allman FL: Traumatic dislocations of the peroneal tendons, *Am J Sports Med* 11:142–146, 1983.
548. Beck E: Operative treatment of recurrent dislocation of the peroneal tendons, *Arch Orthop Trauma Surg* 98:247–250, 1981.
549. Behfar AS: Peronealsehnenluxation (Dislocation of the peroneal tendons), *Sportverletz Sportschaden* 1:223–228, 1987.
550. Blanulet C: De la luxation des tendons des muscles peroniers lateraux (On the dislocation of the tendons of the lateral peroneal muscles), These 242, Paris, 1875.
551. Bonnin JG: *Injuries to the ankle*, Darien, Conn, 1970, Hafner, p 302.
552. Burman M: Stenosing tendovaginitis of the foot and ankle. Studies with special reference to the stenosing tendovaginitis of the peroneal tendons at the peroneal tubercle, *Arch Surg* 67:686–698, 1953.
553. Church CC: Radiographic diagnosis of acute peroneal tendon dislocation. *AJR* 129:1065–1068, 1977.
554. Clancy WG Jr: Tendinitis and plantar fasciitis in runners. In D'Ambrosia RD, Drez D Jr, editors: *Prevention and treatment of running injuries*, ed 2, Thorofare, NJ, 1989, Slack, Charles B, pp 121–131.
555. Das De S, Balasubramaniam P: A repair operation for recurrent dislocation of peroneal tendons, *J Bone Joint Surg [Br]* 67:585–587, 1985.
556. Davies JAK: Peroneal compartment syndrome secondary to rupture of the peroneus longus. A case report, *J Bone Joint Surg [Am]* 61:783–784, 1979.
557. DuVries HL: *Surgery of the foot*, St Louis, 1959, Mosby–Year Book, pp 253–255.
558. Earle AS, Moritz JR, Tapper EM: Dislocation of the peroneal tendons at the ankle: An analysis of 25 ski injuries, *Northwest Med* 71:108–110, 1972.
559. Eckert WR, Davis EA Jr: Acute rupture of the peroneal retinaculum, *J Bone Joint Surg [Am]* 58:670–673, 1976.
560. Edwards ME: The relations of the peroneal tendons to the fibula, calcaneus, and cuboideum, *Am J Anat* 42:213–253, 1928.
561. Escalas F, Figueras JM, Merino JA: Dislocation of the peroneal tendons. Long-term results of surgical treatment, *J Bone Joint Surg [Am]* 62:451–453, 1980.
562. Evans JD: Subcutaneous rupture of the tendon of peroneus longus. Report of a case. *J Bone Joint Surg [Br]* 48:507–509, 1966.
563. Fitzgerald RH, Coventry MB: Post-traumatic peroneal tendinitis. In Bateman JE, Trott AW, editors: *The Foot and ankle*, A selection of papers from the American Orthopaedic Foot Society Meetings, New York, 1980, Brian C Decker, pp 103–109.

564. Frey CC, Shereff MJ: Tendon injuries about the ankle in athletes, *Clin Sport Med* 7:103–118, 1988.
565. Gilcreest EL: Ruptures and tears of muscles and tendons of the lower extremity. Report of fifteen cases, *JAMA* 100: 153–160, 1933.
566. Gilula LA, Oloff L, Caputi R, et al: Ankle tenography: A key to unexplained symptomotology. Part II: Diagnosis of chronic tendon disabilities. *Radiology* 151:581–587, 1984.
567. Gould N: Technique tips: footings. Repair of dislocating peroneal tendons, *Foot Ankle* 6:208–213, 1986.
568. Gutierrez I: De la luxation des tendons, des muscles peronier laterauz (On the dislocation of the tendons of the lateral peroneal muscles), These 356, Paris, 1877.
569. Huber H, Imhoff A: Habituelle Peronealsehnenluxation (Habitual peroneal tendon dislocation), *Z Orthop* 126:609–612, 1988.
570. Jones DC: Bucket handle tears of the peroneus brevis. American Orthopaedic Foot and Ankle Society meeting, Santa Fe, NM, July 17, 1987.
571. Jones E: Operative treatment of chronic dislocation of the peroneal tendons, *J Bone Joint Surg* 14:574–576, 1932.
572. Kelly RE: An operation for the chronic dislocation of the peroneal tendons, *Br J Surg* 7:502–504, 1920.
573. Kojima Y, Kataoka Y, Suzuki S, et al: Dislocation of the peroneal tendons in neonates and infants, *Clin Orthop* 266:180–184, 1991.
574. Konradsen L, Sommer H: Ankle instability caused by peroneal tendon rupture. A case report, *Acta Orthop Scand* 60:723–724, 1989.
575. Larsen E: Longitudinal rupture of the peroneus brevis tendon, *J Bone Joint Surg [Br]* 69:340–341, 1987.
576. Larsen E, Flink-Olsen M, Seerup K: Surgery for recurrent dislocation of the peroneal tendons, *Acta Orthop Scand* 55:554–555, 1984.
577. LeNoir JL: A new surgical treatment of peroneal subluxation-dislocation. A case report with a 27-year follow up, *Orthopedics* 9:1689–1691, 1986.
578. Martens MA, Noyez JF, Mulier JC: Recurrent dislocation of the peroneal tendons. Results of rerouting the tendons under the calcaneofibular ligament, *Am J Sports Med* 14:148–150, 1986.
579. Marti R: Dislocation of the peroneal tendons, *Am J Sports Med* 5:19–22, 1977.
580. McLennan JG: Treatment of acute and chronic luxations of the peroneal tendons, *Am J Sports Med* 8:432–436, 1980.
581. McMaster PE: Tendon and muscle ruptures. Clinical and experimental studies on the causes and location of subcutaneous ruptures, *J Bone Joint Surg* 15:705–722, 1933.
582. Meyer AW: Further evidences of attrition in the human body, *Am J Anat* 34:241–267, 1924.
583. Micheli LJ, Waters PM, Sanders DP: Sliding fibular graft repair for chronic dislocation of the peroneal tendons, *Am J Sports Med* 17:68–71, 1989.
584. Mick CA, Lynch F: Reconstruction of the peroneal retinaculum using the peroneus quartus. A case report, *J Bone Joint Surg [Am]* 69:296–297, 1987.
585. Miller JW: Dislocation of peroneal tendons—a new operative procedure. A case report, *Am J Orthop* 9:136–137, 1967.
586. Monteggia GB: *Instituzini chirurgiche, parte secondu*, Milan, Italy, 1803, pp 336–341.
587. Moritz JR: Ski injuries, *Am J Surg* 98:493–505, 1959.
588. Munk RL, Davis PH: Longitudinal rupture of the peroneus brevis tendon, *J Trauma* 16:803–806, 1976.
589. Murr S: Dislocation of the peroneal tendons with marginal fracture of the lateral malleolus, *J Bone Joint Surg [Br]* 43:563–565, 1961.
590. Orthner E, Polcik J, Schabus R: Die Luxation der Peroneussehnen (Dislocation of peroneal tendons), *Unfallchirurg* 92:589–594, 1989.
591. Orthner E, Wagner M: Die Peroneussehnenluxation (Dislocation of the peroneal tendon), *Sportverletz Sportschaden* 3:112–115, 1989.
592. Orthner E, Weinstabl R, Schabus R: Experimentelle Untersuchung zur Klärung des Pathomechanismus der Traumatischen Peroneussehnenluxation (Experimental study for clarification of the pathogenic mechanism in traumatic peroneal tendon dislocation), *Unfallchirurg* 92:547–553, 1989.
593. Parvin RW, Ford LT: Stenosing tenosynovitis of the common peroneal tendon sheath. Report of two cases, *J Bone Joint Surg [Am]* 38:1352–1357, 1956.
594. Peacock KC, Resnick EJ, Thoder JJ: Fracture of the os peroneum with rupture of the peroneus longus tendon. A case report and review of the literature, *Clin Orthop* 202:223–226, 1986.
595. Platzgummer H: Uber ein einfaches Verfahren zur operativen Behandlung der habituellen Peronaeussehnenluxation (on a simple procedure for the operative therapy of habitual peroneal tendon luxation), *Arch Orthop Unfallchir* 61:144–150, 1967.
596. Pöll RG, Duijfjes F: The treatment of recurrent dislocation of the peroneal tendons, *J Bone Joint Surg [Br]* 66:98–100, 1984.
597. Pozo JL, Jackson AM: A rerouting operation for dislocation of peroneal tendons: operative technique and case report, *Foot Ankle* 5:42–44, 1984.
598. Rask MR, Steinberg LH: The pathognostic sign of tendoperoneal subluxation: report of a case treated conservatively, *Orthop Rev* 8:65–68, 1979.
599. Reinus WR, Gilula LA, Lesiak LF, et al: Tenography in unresolved ankle tenosynovitis, *Orthopedics* 10:497–504, 1987.
600. Resnick D, Goergen TG: Peroneal tenography in previous calcaneal fractures, *Radiology* 115:211–213, 1975.
601. Rosenberg ZS, Feldman F, Singson RD: Peroneal tendon injuries: CT analysis, *Radiology* 161:743–748, 1986.
602. Rosenberg ZS, Feldman F, Singson RD, et al: Peroneal tendon injury associated with calcaneal fractures: CT findings, *AJR* 149:125–129, 1987.
603. Sammarco GJ, DiRaimondo CV: Chronic peroneus brevis tendon lesions, *Foot Ankle* 9:163–170, 1989.
604. Sarmiento A, Wolf M: Subluxation of peroneal tendons. Case treated by rerouting tendons under calcaneofibular ligament, *J Bone Joint Surg [Am]* 57:115–116, 1975.
605. Sarrafian SK: *Anatomy of the foot and ankle. Descriptive, topographic, functional*, Philadelphia, 1983, JB Lippincott.
606. Savastano AA: Recurrent dislocation of the peroneal tendons. In Bateman JE, Trott AW, editors: *The Foot and Ankle. A selection of papers from the American ortho-*

paedic foot society meetings, New York, 1980, Brian C Decker, pp 110–115.
607. Slätis P, Santavirta S, Sandelin J: Surgical treatment of chronic dislocation of the peroneal tendons, *Br J Sports Med* 22:16–18, 1988.
608. Sobel M, Bohne WHO, Levy ME: Longitudinal attrition of the peroneus brevis tendon in the fibular groove: an anatomic study, *Foot Ankle* 11:124–128, 1990.
609. Sobel M, Bohne WHO, Markisz JA: Cadaver correlation of peroneal tendon changes with magnetic resonance imaging, *Foot Ankle* 11:384–388, 1991.
610. Sobel M, Levy ME, Bohne WHO: Congenital variations of the peroneus quartus muscle: an anatomic study, *Foot Ankle* 11:81–89, 1990.
611. Sobel M, Warren RF, Brourman S: Lateral ankle instability associated with dislocation of the peroneal tendons treated by the Chrisman-Snook procedure. A case report and literature review, *Am J Sports Med* 18:539–543, 1990.
612. Stein RE: Reconstruction of the superior peroneal retinaculum using a portion of the peroneus brevis tendon. A case report, *J Bone Joint Surg [Am]* 69:298–299, 1987.
613. Stiehl JB: Concomitant rupture of the peroneus brevis tendon and bimalleolar fracture: A case report, *J Bone Joint Surg [Am]* 70:936–937, 1988.
614. Stover CN, Bryan DR: Traumatic dislocation of the peroneal tendons, *Am J Surg* 103:180–186, 1962.
615. Szczukowski M Jr, St. Pierre RK, Fleming LL, et al: Computerized tomography in the evaluation of peroneal tendon dislocation. A report of two cases, *Am J Sports Med* 11:444–447, 1983.
616. Tehranzadeh J, Stoll DA, Gabriele OM: Case report 271. Diagnosis: posterior migration of the os peroneum of the left foot, indicating a tear of the peroneal tendon, *Skeletal Radiol* 12:44–47, 1984.
617. Thompson FM, Patterson AH: Rupture of the peroneus longus tendon. Report of three cases, *J Bone Joint Surg [Am]* 71:293–295, 1989.
618. Tracy EA: The calcaneo-fibular ligament and its neighborhood, based on dissections, *Boston Med Surg J* 160:369–371, 1909.
619. Trevino S, Gould N, Korson R: Surgical treatment of stenosing tenosynovitis at the ankle, *Foot Ankle* 2:37–45, 1981.
620. Viernstein K, Rosemeyer B: Ein Operationsverfahren zur Behanlung der Rezidivierenden Peronaealschnenluxation beim Leistungssportler (A method of operative treatment of recurrent displacement of peroneal tendons), *Arch Orthop Unfallchir* 74:175–181, 1972.
621. Walsham WJ: On the treatment of dislocation of the peroneus longus tendon, *Br Med J* 2:1086, 1895.
622. Webster FS: Peroneal tenosynovitis with pseudotumor, *J Bone Joint Surg [Am]* 50:153–157, 1968.
623. Wirth CJ: Eine Modifizierte Operationstechnik nach Viernstein und Kelly zur Behebung der Chronischrezidivierenden Peronealsehnenluxation (A modified Viernstein and Kelly surgical technique for correction of chronic recurrent peroneal tendon dislocation), *Z Orthop* 128:170–173, 1990.
624. Zeiss J, Saddemi SR, Ebraheim NA: MR imaging of the peroneal tunnel, *J Comput Assist Tomogr* 13:840–844, 1989.
625. Zoellner G, Clancy W Jr: Recurrent dislocation of the peroneal tendon, *J Bone Joint Surg [Am]* 61:292–294, 1979.

Posterior Tibial Tendinitis and Tendon Rupture

626. Cavanagh PR: *The running shoe book*, Mountain View, Calif, 1980, Anderson World, p 270.
627. Clancy WG Jr: Lower extremity injuries in the jogger and distance runner, *Physician Sports Med* 2:46–50, 1974.
628. Henceroth WD II, Deyerle WM: The acquired unilateral flatfoot in the adult: some causative factors, *Foot Ankle* 2:304–308, 1982.
629. Holmes GB Jr, Cracchiolo A III, Goldner JL, et al: Symposium. Current practices in the management of posterior tibial tendon rupture, *Contemp Orthop* 20:79–108, 1990.
630. Johnson KA: Tibialis posterior tendon rupture, *Clin Orthop* 177:140–147, 1983.
631. Kettelkamp DB, Alexander HH: Spontaneous rupture of the posterior tibial tendon, *J Bone Joint Surg [Am]* 51:759–764, 1969.
632. Lysholm J, Wiklander J: Injuries in runners, *Am J Sports Med* 15:168–171, 1987.
633. Macintyre JG, Taunton JE, Clement DB, et al: Running injuries: a clinical study of 4,173 cases, *Clin Sports Med* 1:81–87, 1991.
634. Mann RA, Thompson FM: Rupture of the posterior tibial tendon causing flat foot, *J Bone Joint Surg [Am]* 67:556–561, 1985.
635. Trevino S, Gould N, Korson R: Surgical treatment of stenosing tenosynovitis at the ankle, *Foot Ankle* 2:37–45, 1981.
636. Woods L, Leach RE: Posterior tibial tendon rupture in athletic people, *Am J Sports Med* 19:495–498, 1991.

Achilles Tendinitis and Ruptures

637. Arner O, Lindholm A: Subcutaneous rupture of the Achilles tendon. A study of 92 cases, *Acta Chir Scand Suppl* 239:1–51, 1959.
638. Beskin JL, Sanders RA, Hunter SC, et al: Surgical repair of Achilles tendon ruptures, *Am J Sports Med* 15:1–8, 1987.
639. Caine D, Cochrane B, Caine C, et al: An epidemiologic investigation of injuries affecting young competitive female gymnasts, *Am J Sports Med* 17:811–820, 1989.
640. Cavanagh PR: *The running shoe book*, Mountain View, Calif, 1980, Anderson World, pp 261–276.
641. Clancy WG Jr, Neidhart D, Brand RL: Achilles tendonitis in runners: a report of five cases, *Am J Sports Med* 4:46–57, 1976.
642. Clement DB, Taunton JE, Smart GW: Achilles tendinitis and peritendinitis: etiology and treatment, *Am J Sports Med* 12:179–184, 1984.
643. Drez D Jr: *Therapeutic modalities for sports injuries*, St Louis, 1989, Mosby–Year Book.
644. Ekstrand J, Gillquist J: Soccer injuries and their mechanisms: a prospective study, *Med Sci Sports Exerc* 15:267–270, 1983.
645. Ende LS, Wickstrom J: Ballet injuries, *Physician Sports Med* 10:101–118, 1982.
646. Garrick JG: Ballet injuries, *Med Probl Perform Arts* 1:123–127, 1976.
647. Gelabert R: Preventing dancers' injuries, *Physician Sports Med* 8:69–76, 1980.

648. Gottlieb G, White JR: Responses of recreational runners to their injuries, *Physician Sports Med* 8:145–149, 1980.
649. Hattrup SJ, Johnson KA: A review of ruptures of the Achilles tendon, *Foot Ankle* 6:34–38, 1985.
650. Holmes GB Jr, Mann RA, Wells L: Epidemiologic factors associated with rupture of the Achilles tendon, *Contemp Orthop* 23:327–331, 1991.
651. Inglis AE, Scott WN, Sculco TP, et al: Ruptures of the tendo Achillis. An objective assessment of surgical and non-surgical treatment, *J Bone Joint Surg [Am]* 58:990–993, 1978.
652. Jacobs D, Martens M, Van Audekercke R, et al: Comparison of conservative and operative treatment of Achilles tendon rupture, *Am J Sports Med* 6:107–111, 1978.
653. Jacobs SJ, Berson BL: Injuries to runners: a study of entrants to a 10,000 meter race, *Am J Sports Med* 14:151–155, 1986.
654. James SL, Bates BT, Osternig LR: Injuries to runners, *Am J Sports Med* 6:40–50, 1978.
655. Józsa L, Kvist M, Bálint BJ, et al: The role of recreational sport activity in Achilles tendon rupture. A clinical, pathoanatomical, and sociological study of 292 cases, *Am J Sports Med* 17:338–343, 1989.
656. Kvist H, Kvist M: The operative treatment of chronic calcaneal paratenonitis, *J Bone Joint Surg [Br]* 62:353–357, 1980.
657. Leach RE, James S, Wasilewski S: Achilles tendinitis, *Am J Sports Med* 9:93–98, 1981.
658. Lysholm J, Wiklander J: Injuries in runners, *Am J Sports Med* 15:168–171, 1987.
659. Macintyre JG, Taunton JE, Clement DB, et al: Running injuries: a clinical study of 4,173 cases, *Clin Sports Med* 1:81–87, 1991.
660. Mellion MB: Common cycling injuries. Management and prevention, *Sports Med* 11:52–70, 1991.
661. Nistor L: Surgical and non-surgical treatment of Achilles tendon rupture. A prospective randomized study, *J Bone Joint Surg [Am]* 63:394–399, 1981.
662. Percy EC, Conochie LB: The surgical treatment of ruptured tendo Achillis, *Am J Sports Med* 6:132–136, 1978.
663. Puddu G, Ippolito E, Postacchini F: A classification of Achilles tendon disease, *Am J Sports Med* 4:145–150, 1976.
664. Rovere GD, Webb LX, Gristina AG, et al: Musculoskeletal injuries in theatrical dance students, *Am J Sports Med* 11:195–198, 1983.
665. Schafle MD, Requa RK, Patton WL, et al: Injuries in the 1987 National Amateur Volleyball Tournament, *Am J Sports Med* 18:624–631, 1990.
666. Smith AD, Ludington R: Injuries in elite pair skaters and ice dancers, *Am J Sports Med* 17:482–488, 1989.
667. Sohl P, Bowling A: Injuries to dancers. Prevalence, treatment and prevention, *Sports Med* 9:317–322, 1990.
668. Stein SR, Luekens CA: Methods and rationale for closed treatment of Achilles tendon ruptures, *Am J Sports Med* 4:162–169, 1976.
669. Temple C: Sports injuries. Hazards of jogging and marathon running, *Br J Hosp Med* 37:237–239, 1983.
670. Washington EL: Musculoskeletal injuries in theatrical dancers: site, frequency, and severity, *Am J Sports Med* 6:75–98, 1978.
671. Watson MD, DiMartino PP: Incidence of injuries in high school track and field athletes and its relation to performance ability, *Am J Sports Med* 15:251–254, 1987.
672. Williams JGP: Achilles tendon lesions in sport, *Sports Med* 3:114–135, 1986.
673. Winge S, Jørgensen U, Lassen Nielsen A: Epidemiology of injuries in Danish championship tennis, *Int J Sports Med* 10:368–371, 1989.
674. Zemper ED: Injury rates in a national sample of college football teams: a 2-year prospective study, *Physician Sports Med* 17:100–113, 1989.

Midfoot Sprain

675. Clanton TO, Butler JE, Eggert A: Injuries to the metatarsophalangeal joints in athletes, *Foot Ankle* 7:162–176, 1986.
676. Clarke KS, Buckley WE: Women's injuries in collegiate sports. A preliminary comparative overview of three seasons, *Am J Sports Med* 8:187–191, 1980.
677. Collins RK: Injury patterns in women's intramural flag football, *Am J Sports Med* 15:238–242, 1987.
678. Curtis M, Myerson MS, Szura B: Tarsometatarsal joint injuries in the athlete. American Orthopaedic Foot and Ankle Society meeting, Boston, July 28, 1991.
679. DeHaven KE, Lintner DM: Athletic injuries: comparison by age, sport, and gender. *Am J Sports Med* 14:218–224, 1986.
680. Estwanik JJ, Bergfeld J, Canty T: Report of injuries sustained during the United States olympic wrestling trials, *Am J Sports Med* 6:335–340, 1978.
681. Faciszewski T, Burks RT, Manaster BJ: Subtle injuries of the Lisfranc joint, *J Bone Joint Surg [Am]* 72:1519–1522, 1990.
682. Foster SC, Foster RR: Lisfranc's tarsometatarsal fracture-dislocation, *Radiology* 120:79–83, 1976.
683. Hamilton WG: Foot and ankle injuries in dancers, *Clin Sports Med* 7:143–173, 1988.
684. Hooper G, McMaster MJ: Recurrent bilateral midtarsal subluxations. A case report, *J Bone Joint Surg [Am]* 61:617–619, 1979.
685. Janda DH, Wojtys EM, Hankin FM, et al: Softball sliding injuries. A prospective study comparing standard and modified bases, *JAMA* 259:1848–1850, 1988.
686. Jørgensen U, Winge S: Injuries in badminton, *Sports Med* 10:59–64, 1990.
687. LaTourette G, Perry J, Patzakis MJ, et al: Fractures and dislocations of the tarsometatarsal joint. In Bateman JE, Trott AW, editors: *The foot and ankle. A selection of papers from the American orthopaedic foot society meetings,* New York, 1980, Brian C Decker, pp 40–51.
688. Main BJ, Jowett RL: Injuries of the midtarsal joint, *J Bone Joint Surg [Br]* 57:89–97, 1975.
689. Marshall P: The rehabilitation of overuse foot injuries in athletes and dancers, *Clin Sports Med* 7:175–191, 1988.
690. Marti B, Vader JP, Minder CE, et al: On the epidemiology of running injuries. The 1984 Bern Grand-Prix Study, *Am J Sports Med* 16:285–294, 1988.
691. McNeal AP, Watkins A, Clarkson PM, et al: Lower extremity alignment and injury in young, preprofessional, college and professional ballet dancers. Part II: dancer-reported injuries, *Med Probl Perform Arts* 5:83–88, 1990.

692. Meyer PW: Problems of the foot and ankle in professional baseball players. In Kiene RH, Johnson KA, editors: *American Academy of Orthopaedic Surgeons symposium on the foot and ankle,* St Louis, 1983, Mosby–Year Book, pp 27–33.
693. Moyer RA, Betz RR, Clements DB: Diastasis of the first and second tarsometatarsal joints, American Orthopaedic Foot and Ankle Society meeting, Las Vegas, 1985.
694. Mueller FO, Blyth CS: A survey of 1981 college lacrosse injuries, *Physician Sports Med* 10:87–93, 1982.
695. Newell SG, Woodle A: Cuboid syndrome, *Physician Sports Med* 9:71–76, 1981.
696. Resch S, Stenström A: The treatment of tarsometatarsal injuries, *Foot Ankle* 11:117–123, 1990.
697. Roy SP: Intercollegiate wrestling injuries, *Physician Sports Med* 7:83–91, 1979.
698. Schaffer RC: *Chiropractic management of sports and recreational injuries,* Baltimore, 1986, Williams & Wilkins, pp 526–529.
699. Shively RA, Grana WA, Ellis D: High school sports injuries, *Physician Sports Med* 9:46–50, 1981.
700. Soderstrom C, Doxanas MT: Racquetball. A game with preventable injuries, *Am J Sports Med* 10:180–183, 1982.
701. Turco VJ: Injuries to the ankle and foot in athletics, *Orthop Clin North Am* 8:669–682, 1977.
702. Wiley JJ: The mechanism of tarso-metatarsal joint injuries, *J Bone Joint Surg [Br]* 53:474–482, 1971.
703. Yde J, Nielsen AB: Sports injuries in adolescents' ball games: soccer, handball and basketball, *Br J Sports Med* 24:51–54, 1990.
704. Zwipp H, Krettek C: Diagnostik und Therapie der Akuten und Chronischen Bandinstabilität des Unteren Sprunggelenkes (Diagnosis and therapy of acute and chronic ligament instability of the transverse tarsal joint, *Orthopade* 15:472–478, 1986.

Forefoot Sprain

705. Bentley G, Goodfellow JW: Disorganization of the knees following intra-articular hydrocortisone injections, *J Bone Joint Surg [Br]* 51:498–502, 1969.
706. Berger-Vachon C, Gabard G, Moyen B: Soccer accidents in the French Rhone-Alpes Soccer Association, *Sports Med* 3:69–77, 1986.
707. Berkin CR: Effects of cortisone on the healing of tendons in rabbits, *Proc R Soc Med* 48:610–613, 1955.
708. Bojsen-Møller F, Lamoreux L: Significance of free dorsiflexion of the toes in walking, *Acta Orthop Scand* 50:471–479, 1979.
709. Bowers KD Jr, Martin RB: Turf-toe: a shoe-surface related football injury, *Med Sci Sports Exerc* 8:81–83, 1976.
710. Clanton TO, Butler JE, Eggert A: Injuries to the metatarsophalangeal joints in athletes, *Foot Ankle* 7:162–176, 1986.
711. Clanton TO, Eggert KE, Pivarnik JM, et al: First metatarsophalangeal joint range of motion as a factor in turf toe injuries, *Am J Sports Med* 1992 (in press).
712. Clanton TO, Seifert S: Long-term sequelae of turf toe injury. Unpublished observations; study in progress.
713. Coker TP, Arnold JA, Weber DL: Traumatic lesions of the metatarsophalangeal joint of the great toe in athletes, *Am J Sports Med* 6:326–334, 1978.
714. Cooper DL, Fair J: Turf toe, *Physician Sports Med* 6:139, 1978.
715. Coughlin MJ: Sesamoid pain: causes and surgical treatment, *Instr Course Lect* 39:23–35, 1990.
716. Ekstrand J, Nigg BM: Surface-related injuries in soccer, *Sports Med* 8:56–62, 1989.
717. Giannikas AC, Papachristou N, Papavasiliou N, et al: Dorsal dislocation of the first metatarso-phalangeal joint, *J Bone Joint Surg [Br]* 57:384–386, 1975.
718. Johnson KA, Buck PG: Total replacement of the first metatarsophalangeal joint, *Foot Ankle* 1:307–314, 1981.
719. Johnson WO: The tyranny of phony fields, 63:34–47, 1985.
720. Joseph J: Range of movement of the great toe in men, *J Bone Joint Surg [Br]* 36:450–457, 1954.
721. Lieber J: Turf toe: the NFL's most pesky agony of da feet. *Sports Illus* 69:401–402, 1988.
722. Mullis DL, Miller WE: A disabling sports injury of the great toe, *Foot Ankle* 1:22–25, 1980.
723. Nelson WE, DePalma B, Gieck JH, et al: Intercollegiate lacrosse injuries, *Physician Sports Med* 9:86–92, 1981.
724. Nielsen AB, Yde J: Epidemiology and traumatology of injuries in soccer, *Am J Sports Med* 17:803–807, 1989.
725. Nigg BM: Biomechanical aspects of running. In Nigg BM, editor: *Biomechanics of running shoes,* Champaign, Ill, 1986, Human Kinetics, pp 1–25.
726. Nigg BM, Segesser B: The influence of playing surfaces on the load on the locomotor system and on football and tennis injuries, *Sports Med* 5:375–385, 1988.
727. Rodeo SA, O'Brien S, Warren RF, et al: Turf-toe: an analysis of metatarsophalangeal joint sprains in professional football players, *Am J Sports Med* 18:280–285, 1990.
728. Ryan AJ, Behling F, Garrick JG, et al: Round table. Artificial turf: pros and cons, *Physician Sports Med* 3:41–50, 1975.
729. Salter RB, Gross A, Hall JH: Hydrocortisone arthropathy. An experimental investigation, *Can Med Assoc J* 97:374–377, 1967.
730. Sammarco GJ: Biomechanics of the foot. In Frankel VH, Nordin M, editors: *Biomechanics of the skeletal system,* Philadelphia, 1980, Lea & Febiger, pp 193–219.
731. Sammarco GJ: How I manage turf toe, *Physician Sports Med* 16:113–118, 1988.
732. Sarrafian SK: *Anatomy of the foot and ankle. Descriptive, topographic, functional,* Philadelphia, 1983, JB Lippincott.
733. Smith RW, Reischl SF: Metatarsophalangeal joint synovitis in athletes, *Clin Sports Med* 7:75–88, 1988.
734. Smith RW, Reynolds JC, Stewart MJ: Hallux valgus assessment: report of the research committee of the American Orthopaedic Foot and Ankle Society, *Foot Ankle* 5:92–103, 1984.
735. Stokes IAF, Hutton WC, Stott JRR, Forces under the hallux valgus foot before and after surgery, *Clin Orthop* 142:64–72, 1979.
736. Sweetnam R: Editorials and annotations. Corticosteroid arthropathy and tendon rupture, *J Bone Joint Surg [Br]* 51:397–398, 1969.
737. Underwood J: Just an awful toll, *Sports Illus* 63:48–62, 1985.
738. Wrenn RN, Goldner JL, Markee JL: An experimental study of the effect of cortisone on the healing process

and tensile strength of tendons, *J Bone Joint Surg [Am]* 36:588–601, 1954.

Bunions in Athletes

739. Baxter DE, Lillich JS: Bunionectomies and related surgery in the elite female middle distance and marathon runner. *Am J Sports Med* 14:491–493, 1976.
740. Bowers KD Jr, Martin RB: Turf-toe: a shoe-surface related football injury, *Med Sci Sports Exerc* 8:81–83, 1976.
741. Clanton TO, Butler JE, Eggert A: Injuries to the metatarsophalangeal joints in athletes, *Foot Ankle* 7:162–176, 1986.
742. Fahey T: *Athletic training: principles and practice*, Palo Alto, Calif, 1986, Mayfield, p 410.
743. Kelikian H: *The functional anatomy of the forefoot in hallux valgus, allied deformities of the forefoot and metatarsalgia*, Philadelphia, 1965, WB Saunders, pp 31–33.
744. Jahss MH: Traumatic dislocations of the first metatarsophalangeal joint, *Foot Ankle* 1:15–21, 1980.
745. Joseph J: Range of movement of the great toe in men, *J Bone Joint Surg [Br]* 36:450–457, 1954.
746. Mann RA, Clanton TO: Hallux rigidus: treatment by cheilectomy, *J Bone Joint Surg [Am]* 70:400–406, 1988.
747. Sammarco GJ, Drez D Jr, Elkus RA, et al: Symposium: overuse syndromes of the leg, foot, and ankle in athletes, *Contemp Orthop* 12:67–93, 1986.

CHAPTER

28

The Foot in Running

Donald E. Baxter, M.D.*

History
Physical examination
Standing
Sitting
Supine
Prone
Diagnostic studies
Primary and secondary injuries
Surface injuries
Torsional joint injuries
Short-leg syndrome
Stress fractures
Leg pain
Heel pain
Tendinitis
Impingement syndromes
Forefoot disorders
Orthoses and complications of rigid orthoses
Shoes
Rehabilitation of the injured runner

The population of today is very active, with 59% of adults participating in some form of exercise. Eleven percent of those surveyed were joggers, with 25% running at least 2 miles a day.[21] With the impact forces during running ranging from three to eight times body weight and an average of 800 footstrikes occurring per mile,[37] one can expect injuries secondary to the tremendous demands placed on the joints and supporting structures of the foot and ankle. Indeed, in one study of running athletes followed for 1 year, two thirds experienced at least one injury.[31] Therefore, in order to provide optimal care for the population of today, a physician should have an understanding of injuries that occur in the running athlete.

Injuries sustained by the running athlete are usually a result of training errors, anatomic factors, or are secondary to problems with shoes or the running surface.[15] Sixty percent of the injuries are felt to be secondary to training errors such as a rapid increase in mileage. Mild anatomic abnormalities, which may not cause symptoms under normal activities, can lead to significant disability when running. This chapter is written so as to provide a rational approach to the diagnosis of running injuries with an emphasis on determining the primary underlying cause. Only by understanding the primary predisposing factor can a physician institute training alterations, prescribe appropriate orthotic devices, and suggest surgical interventions that will allow the patient to return to running.

HISTORY

Forms may be used in taking a history, thus allowing the runner to make an outline of his complaints while seated in the waiting room. A suggested format follows:

1. Chief complaint. The most severe problem should be listed first, with the duration and nature of the onset of the symptom. Lesser problems should then be listed in order of their significance.

The author would like to thank Roy S. Benedetti, M.D., for his assistance in preparing this chapter.

2. Occurrence of pain during runs or after runs.
3. Type of previous treatment the patient has undergone.
4. Nature of the patient's training program. Is the runner a beginner, recreational noncompetitive jogger, or a competitive runner? Has there been a recent increase in the training mileage? Has there been increased speed associated with the workouts?
5. Any recent change in shoe wear. Are the shoes rotated among two or three types to avoid similar stresses? Does the patient note a specific abnormal wear pattern?
6. Use of orthotic devices. If used, have the devices been rigid or flexible orthoses, and what symptoms were changed by their use?
7. Type of surface the training is carried out on. Is it hard or soft, circular or slanted?
8. Related exercises used, such as stretching and strengthening exercises. Is a systematic stretching or yoga program used? Are weights used to build up strength in a balanced manner?
9. Nutritional aspects of the runner. Are supplemental vitamins or minerals used? Is sufficient water consumed with increased training, racing, and weather conditions?

PHYSICAL EXAMINATION

The physical examination must encompass the entire lower extremity and back. This should be carried out with the patient in the standing position first and then allowing him to walk and run if possible. The examination should then be continued with the patient sitting, followed by an examination with the patient in the prone and supine positions.

Standing

With the patient in the standing position, the back is observed for evidence of scoliosis, which would result in malalignment of the spine. An increase in the lumbar lordosis associated with weakened abdominal musculature should be carefully observed. The level of the iliac wings gives one a good idea as to leg length. The patient is asked to touch the floor with his hands to give the examiner some idea as to flexibility of the hamstrings and Achilles tendons. The overall alignment of the knee is important to determine whether there is any abnormality involving the patella as well as whether genu varum and valgum are present. Next, the overall alignment of the foot is observed to see whether both feet are in approximately the same amount of external rotation. The heel alignment gives indication not only of symmetry of the forefoot but also of increased varus or valgus configuration of the heel during running. The patient should be asked to stand on his toes to be sure that the proper subtalar joint mechanism is functioning. The general configuration of the forefoot is observed next. The configuration of the arch is noted, and the toes are observed for possible dynamic clawing or possibly a single hammer toe. The patient is now asked to walk, and the overall alignment of the lower extremity is carefully observed. Specific observations are made of the patella to determine whether there is any evidence of femoral anteversion with increased internal rotation of the patella. Symmetry of the transverse rotation of the foot and ankle should likewise be carefully noted. External tibial torsion combined with rotation with pronation of the foot results in a high risk for shin splints or possibly medial knee problems. It is useful to have the individual jog, if space permits, and to look for any gross biomechanical asymmetries, particularly in the transverse rotation of the lower extremities and angle of foot placement (Fig 28–1).

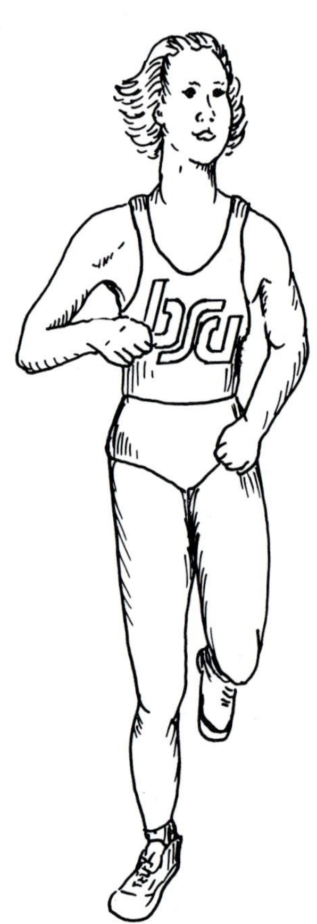

FIG 28–1.
A runner exhibiting external rotation and pronation.

Sitting

With the patient in the sitting position, the leg lengths are again observed by having the runner place his back flat against the wall or chair back and extending the knees. By examining the patient in this manner, the possibility of pelvic obliquity is eliminated. While the leg lengths are noted, the tightness of the hamstrings and the sciatic nerve is tested. Next the patient's knee ligaments are tested, and the patella is palpated while the knee is actively extended to look for possible chondromalacia. The degree of malleolar torsion is noted as to symmetry. The ankle joint is examined for dorsiflexion and plantar flexion and the subtalar joint for eversion and inversion. The total range as well as the symmetry of motion is recorded. The hindfoot is placed in the neutral position, and the alignment of the forefoot is observed to see whether it is in the neutral, varus, or valgus position. Hypermobility of the first metatarso-cuneiform joint is checked. The pattern of callus configuration on the plantar aspect of the foot is observed. The toes are carefully examined for any fixed or dynamic contractures.

Supine

With the patient in the supine position the range of motion of the hips and knees is once again checked. Any further examination of the knee can be carried out with the patient in this position. The sciatic nerve can be evaluated by elevating the extended lower extremity.

Prone

The examination of the patient in the prone position is important for evaluation of the Achilles tendon area. With the knee flexed to 90 degrees, the heel-leg alignment is observed along with the configuration of the longitudinal arch.

DIAGNOSTIC STUDIES

To complete the patient's workup, one or more diagnostic studies may be indicated. Routine x-ray films of the involved area should be the initial study. Disorders such as osteoarthritis, infection, osteochondritis, and tendon and ligament avulsions as well as the presence of extra ossicles (e.g., accessory navicular, os trigonum) can be diagnosed. A stress fracture, if over 3- to 4-weeks-old, may be discovered by callus formation or periosteal reaction. Weight-bearing views can add information with respect to foot alignment. In those cases with suspected ligamentous instability of the ankle or Lisfranc's joint, stress views can be quite helpful. This is especially true when a Lisfranc type of injury is suspected and plain x-ray films reveal no abnormalities. Subtalar stress views are less predictable, and subtalar instability may need to be determined by excluding other diagnoses.

When symptoms are vague and the physical findings difficult to interpret, a bone scan may be helpful. The bone scan is extremely helpful in the early diagnosis of stress fractures where plain x-ray films are still normal. A computed tomographic (CT) scan can assist in the evaluation of osteoarthritis of the ankle and subtalar joint, as well as the smaller joints of the midfoot. Osteochondral lesions of the talus are well visualized with a CT scan, which can be instrumental in preoperative planning.

Magnetic resonance imaging (MRI) is becoming increasingly useful in the evaluation of foot and ankle disorders. MRI provides excellent contrast between bone marrow, tendons, cartilage, ligaments, cortical bone, muscles, and allows clear visualization of these structures.[17] T1 images are very sensitive to changes in bone marrow quality and can aid in the diagnosis of an occult fracture or early avascular necrosis. T2 images enhance areas with fluid collection such as occur with effusions and tendinitis. Tendon ruptures and areas of degenerative changes within tendons can be visualized. MRI can also allow an assessment of articular cartilage and the presence of soft-tissue masses. Ligament injuries of the foot and ankle can sometimes be confirmed by using MRI. As our interpretive skills improve, MRI will become even more useful as a diagnostic tool.

PRIMARY AND SECONDARY INJURIES

In assessing running injuries it is important to determine which is the primary problem and what secondary problem the primary problem has caused.[25] Often, if one leg is injured, the opposite leg will develop an injury by overcompensating for the weaker leg. For instance, if one hamstring muscle is pulled, a stress fracture may occur in the opposite leg. If hyperpronation of the foot is present, patellar subluxation may occur secondarily. For such a problem, placing a longitudinal arch support in the running shoe and diminishing hyperpronation of the foot will result in correction of the knee pain or secondary problem.[15] Sciatica will develop at times because of underdevelopment of the abdominal muscles and overdevelopment of the back muscles. By treating the primarily weak muscles with a regimen of sit-ups, the secondary sciatica diminishes. Peroneal muscular spasm along the lateral aspect of the calf can develop as a result of a hypermobile or short first metatarsal. This is caused by inadequate support of the medial aspect of the foot so that the peroneus longus overpulls and causes a peroneal spasm to develop. Again, by inserting a longitudinal arch support with a Morton extension under the first metatarsal head the peroneal spasm can be corrected (Fig 28–2).

Needless to say, there are numerous problems that develop in runners. It is important for the physician to analyze the problems carefully and always ask himself during the examination whether the problem presented is primary or secondary.

Often, the etiology of running injuries can be traced to a change, or faults in the training schedule, the shoe type, or the running surface. Running diaries can be maintained to record how much training was done, the shoes that were worn, and the surface that was run on. Also, rapid weight changes may result in a musculoskeletal injury from a nutritional deficiency. Not all biomechanical imbalances need to be corrected. For instance, leg length inequality that has never been treated and has not caused secondary problems may not need treatment. Mild pronational deformity that causes minimal problems may not require treatment. One runner with forefoot varus had several secondary problems, including stress fractures of the fibula, compartment syndrome necessitating fascial releases, and recurrent Achilles tendinitis from pronation during toe-off. Possibly, by correcting the primary problem of forefoot varus by inserting a slight wedge into the midsole on the medial aspect of her running shoe, some of these problems might have been prevented.

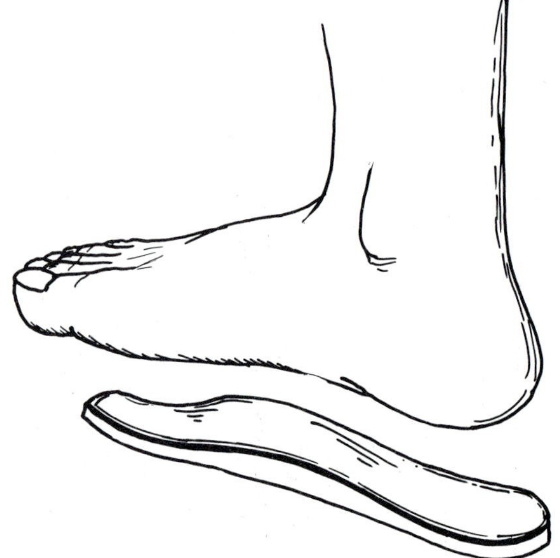

FIG 28–2.
An orthotic device with a Morton extension.

SURFACE INJURIES

Synthetic surfaces, which have replaced cinders and grass in the past 20 years, have brought a great number of athletic records. However, these synthetic tracks are also causing injuries as technically aided performances push the body toward and beyond the breaking point. Synthetic carpets are faster, longer lasting, and weatherproof, but muscles and bones, it appears, are suffering from their use. By eliminating the skid phase of running that is seen with imperfect surfaces such as grass and cinders, there is a more powerful push-off and more efficient running, but more stressful forces in the joints as well. Synthetic surfaces cause "shock vibration" to an extent not known on conventional cinder tracks. This leads to jarring, which in turn leads to damage of the ankle, lower portion of the thigh, knee, leg, and even the spine. Jarring, a well-known hazard of road racing, can be lessened if the surface elasticity is modified during its production. Another factor with synthetic surfaces is the increased torque in various joints. With cinders and grass, the foot can slide and pivot during running. This eliminates some of the torquing forces transmitted to the ankle, knee, and hip. With synthetic surfaces, the foot does not slide, which causes a greater shearing force on the foot and more torque on the ankle, knee, and hip. Shoe manufacturers are attempting to develop shoes that will cushion heel strike and lessen shear forces. Some torque can be decreased by changing sole design, but this does not equate to grass or cinders as a forgiving surface. Thus training should usually be done on grass and cinders and running on synthetic surfaces limited to racing and periodic training sessions.

TORSIONAL JOINT INJURIES

In training and giving advice to runners, coaches, trainers, and physicians have stressed linear stretching of the hamstrings, gastrocnemius-soleus, and lower part of the back. Minimal emphasis, except in yoga, has been given to rotational stretching of the hip, pelvic, and back rotators. If there is limited hip, pelvic, or back rotation, more torque is placed on the knee, leg, and ankle during running, especially during the foot-plant phase of running. For instance, if there is an external rotational deformity of the hip, more torque is placed on the knee during running as the speed is increased and the lower extremity attempts to rotate inwardly. By doing internal rotational stretching of the hip and having the runner run with the foot slightly externally rotated, knee pain can often be eliminated. Other rotational deformities that can cause similar torquing problems exist. Congenital femoral retroversion and external tibial torsion often cause knee pain in running as the runner attempts to rotate the leg internally during normal swing phase and foot plant. Rarely does femoral anteversion or internal tibial torsion cause problems since these are more anatomic positions for running.

SHORT-LEG SYNDROME

When a runner is evaluated, care should be taken to examine the leg lengths. This has been described previously. If there is a leg length inequality, there often is a history of repeat injuries to the short leg. These may include stress fractures, medial knee strain from genu valgus, hyperpronation with resultant plantar fasciitis or patellar subluxation, iliotibial band tendinitis, and lateral knee joint impingement.[13] Quadriceps strain from weakness of the shorter leg or external rotation of the shorter leg may also be observed. A short leg develops from a congenitally short tibia or femus or a fixed pelvic obliquity from scoliosis. A functional short-leg syndrome occurs by running on the same tilt of the road or in the same direction on a circular track. It can also occur from a flexion contracture in the knee or ankle. If a short leg is present, it is corrected by adding a lift to the inner lining of the shoe. The insole of the running shoe is built up gradually in ⅛- to ¼-in. increments. The inside of the running shoe can be elevated approximately ½-in. if necessary. Should more elevation be needed, it must be made to the midsole of the shoe.

Occasionally problems develop in the long leg. These problems include lateral hip pain as the iliotibial band rubs over the greater trochanter on the longer leg. Occasionally, iliotibial band problems develop distally in the longer leg. By placement of a lift in the shorter leg, the iliotibial band problem may be lessened.

STRESS FRACTURES

A stress fracture occurs because of the failure of normal bone reparative processes to keep pace with microdamage. Normally, physiologic bone remodeling occurs at sites of fatigue microdamage and leads to increased strength of bone at the site of increased stress. However, under conditions that cause sudden changes in stress concentration or excessively high stresses, the rate of bone fatigue fractures can overwhelm the reparative process, and bone weakening occurs. If the imbalance of fatigue microdamage to repair continues, a stress fracture may occur.

In the runner, stress fractures can occur secondary to sudden increases in loading. One situation that can cause this is an injury to the opposite limb. This would lead to increased forces on the normal side. Muscle fatigue also has been shown to cause sudden increases in loading. Normally functioning muscle has a protective effect on bone by providing even stress distribution along its insertion onto bone.[11] However, with muscle fatigue, the runner's gait becomes altered and causes increased shock absorption and increased impact loads. Also, the protective effect of muscle on bone is diminished with fatigue. This combination of increased impact loads and impaired stress distribution may lead to a stress fracture.

Biomechanical imbalances may also lead to stress fractures in the running athlete. Runners who run on hard surfaces, wear poorly cushioned shoes, and have a heavy heel strike experience especially high impact loads. Runners with rigid cavus feet will have decreased shock absorption of the midfoot during the loading response phase of gait that will lead to increased metatarsal stresses. Runners with hyperpronation may transfer increased stresses along the medial aspect of the tibia or, if the pronation is severe enough, may actually cause fibular stress fractures by transmitting forces into the distal end of the fibula. A hypermobile first metatarsal or a long second metatarsal will cause increased forces on the second metatarsal and lead to a possible stress fracture.

The diagnosis of stress fractures may be quite difficult secondary to the vague symptoms and insidious onset. Physical examination may reveal little or no swelling but will usually show focal tenderness upon palpation at the site of the fracture. X-ray findings are often normal until 3 to 4 weeks postinjury. Suspicion alone may be adequate to initiate treatment, but if a more definite early diagnosis is desired, a bone scan is usually quite sensitive.

The treatment of stress fractures in the running athlete must involve not only treatment of the fracture but also correction of the underlying cause. Common locations of stress fractures in runners include the tibial diaphysis, fibula, metatarsals, hallucal sesamoids, tarsal navicular, and rarely the medial malleolus.[41, 46] Most stress fractures can be treated by limiting running mileage to the level of comfort. If pain persists, running is stopped, and non-gravity exercises such as swimming and bicycling are initiated. Casting is usually not required and should be avoided since the muscle atrophy and joint stiffness may cause significant disability in the competitive runner. Healing of the fracture can be expected in 4 to 15 weeks. An exception to the above treatment is when a stress fracture of the hip or femur is suspected. In these cases, cessation of activity is enforced until all pain resolves. This will prevent displacement of the fracture, which would require operative intervention.

Most biomechanical imbalances can be corrected with shoe modifications. If the stress fracture is secondary to running on hard surfaces or a heavy heel strike, a well-cushioned shoe may be all that is necessary. A rigid cavus foot should be treated with a flexible arch support in a highly cushioned shoe. The runner with hyperpronation or with a hypermobile first metatarsal can be given a soft medial arch support. For the runner with a long second metatarsal, a metatarsal pad just proximal to the second metatarsal head will provide necessary unloading.

In the patient with no significant biomechanical imbalances who does not respond to normal treatment modalities, one must consider an underlying metabolic disorder. Hormonal imbalances as well as nutritional or anemic disorders may contribute to bone breakdown. Routine laboratory studies such as calcium and phosphate levels and a complete blood count should be obtained as an initial screen.

LEG PAIN

There can be multiple causes of leg pain in the running athlete. Shinsplints have been used to describe a variety of exercise-induced leg pains.[16, 42] Current thought is that the term "shinsplints" describes the symptoms resulting from numerous causes such as soft-tissue injuries, periostitis, compartment syndrome, and stress fractures. As such, a more definitive diagnosis should be sought.

Medial tibial stress syndrome is a term used to describe pain at the posterior medial aspect of the distal end of the tibia that is associated with exercise.[9, 33] This area is tender to palpation, and a local injection of lidocaine relieves the symptoms. Compartment pressures have been found to be normal with this entity.[8] Theories as to the etiology of this syndrome include periostitis and soleus insertional fasciitis (Fig 28–3). The bone scan can be of assistance in the diagnosis by demonstrating a characteristic appearance: the uptake area involves the posterior cortex of the tibia, is longitudinally oriented, and involves one third or more of the length of the bone with varying intensity.[29] Initial treatment consists of rest, well-cushioned shoes, and isometric exercises. When symptoms resolve, a gradual return to running can begin. This disorder has been shown to be more common in the runner with increased subtalar excursion and increased pronation during the loading

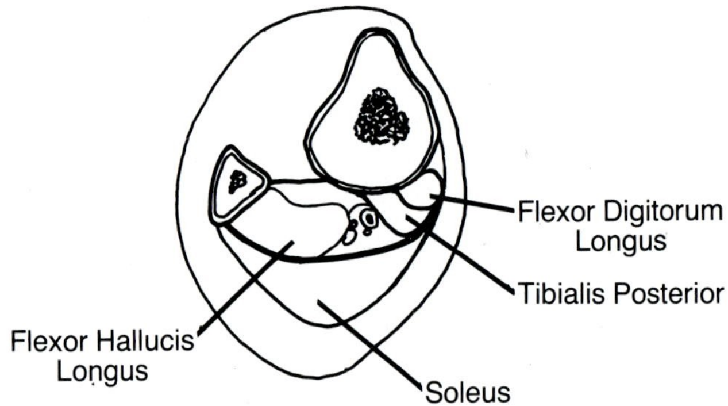

FIG 28–3.
This diagram illustrates the location of the inflammation associated with medial tibial stress syndrome.

response.[48] Therefore, a soft longitudinal medial arch support that would limit pronation may also be helpful. If conservative treatment fails, a fasciotomy of the posteromedial insertion of the soleus has been performed with success.[30]

Stress fractures of the tibia or fibula may be another cause of leg pain in the runner. The patient may give a history of running on hard surfaces or a recent rapid increase in mileage. There may be an underlying hyperpronation of the foot that could lead to increased fibular stress. Although the symptoms may be vague, physical examination usually reveals point tenderness over the tibia or lateral aspect of the fibula at the site of the stress fracture. As previously mentioned, X-ray findings are usually normal for the first 3 to 4 weeks, and if a specific diagnosis is desired, a bone scan can be obtained. The symptoms usually resolve in time with decreased activity and correction of the underlying biomechanical imbalance.

A compartment syndrome may be another cause of leg pain.[10, 27, 31, 34, 35] A complete discussion of the etiology, diagnosis, and treatment of this disorder is included in Chapter 27, and therefore, only a brief discussion is included. The runner typically presents with pain in the involved compartment that occurs after running several miles. With time, the symptoms become more consistent and limit the patient's activities. Paresthesias of the superficial peroneal nerve are quite common in runners with chronic anterior compartment syndrome. In the patient with chronic posterior compartment syndrome, pain and paresthesias in the posterior tibial nerve distribution (i.e., the planter aspect of the foot) may be described.

Initial treatment should consist of decreased activity, a change in shoe wear, and anti-inflammatory medication. If symptoms persist, a fasciotomy of the involved compartment may be performed. The results of anterior fasciotomies for chronic anterior compartment syndromes are quite good, with 92% to 100% percent of patients returning to previous activity levels.[12, 38, 39] The success of fasciotomy for posterior compartment syndromes is not as high. Consequently, if a fasciotomy of the deep posterior compartment is indicated, current recommendations are to include a formal release of the tibialis posterior muscle.[39]

HEEL PAIN

The most common causes of heel pain in the runner include fat pad trauma, plantar fasciitis, and compression of the first branch of the lateral plantar nerve. Fortunately, most cases resolve with conservative treatment, although it is common for symptoms to persist 10 to 12 months. Fat pad trauma is caused by repetitive compression and shear stresses upon the heel that occur during running. This type of heel pain has been termed fat pad inflammation,[14] fat pad shear syndrome,[25] and achillodynia[20] by other authors. It is characterized by diffuse tenderness that is limited to the fat pad of the heel. Treatment consists of a semirigid heel cup and limitation of activity.

Plantar fasciitis refers to heel pain produced by microtears of the plantar fascia and chronic inflammation at the medial tubercle of the calcaneus where the plantar fascia attaches. Patients give a history of severe pain in the morning upon arising that decreases as they begin to walk. The pain is exacerbated by running, especially with hill climbing and sprinting. Tenderness is elicited at the medial tubercle of the calcaneus and occasionally over the fascia itself. The discomfort may be increased with forced toe dorsiflexion or by having the patient stand on his toes. Important in the examination is to rule out tarsal tunnel syndrome as a cause of the heel pain. Tarsal tunnel syndrome is characterized by tenderness not only at the medial tubercle of the calcaneus but also along the course of the posterior tibial nerve. The neurogenic pain secondary to tarsal tunnel syndrome is also more typically described as burning in nature. Treatment of plantar fasciitis consists of decreased activity, heel cord stretching, contrast baths, and anti-inflammatory medication. If symptoms persist over 6 months but preferably 12 months, surgery may be considered. The procedure recommended is a partial plantar fascial release with removal of all the inflamed necrotic fascia as well as the calcaneal spur if present. This provides an environment most conducive to healing of the plantar fascial attachment. In one study of 13 runners, 12 were able to return to full activity after surgical treatment of their plantar fasciitis.[20]

Another cause of heel pain in the runner is compression of the first branch of the lateral plantar nerve[2, 3] (Fig 28–4). This nerve corresponds to the motor branch to the abductor digiti minimi muscle and is the third nerve branch from the posterior tibial nerve (Fig 28–5). This nerve courses deep to the deep fascia of the abductor hallucis muscle and then passes transversely superficial to the quadratus plantae and innervates the abductor digiti minimi (Fig 28–6). In the runner, there is significant hypertrophy of the abductor hallucis muscle, and this may lead to compression of the nerve as it passes deep to this muscle. Another site of compression is as the nerve passes over the medial edge of the quadratus plantae to assume a horizontal course. The last site of possible compression is where the nerve passes distal to the medial calcaneal tuberosity. It is at this location that chronic inflammation, thickening of the plantar fascia, and the presence of a calcaneal spur may lead to nerve compression.

The symptoms of compression of the first branch of the lateral plantar nerve may be similar to those of plantar fasciitis, although the pain may be described as having a more burning quality. Often the patient will complain of proximal radiation of the pain up the leg. The diagnostic physical finding is tenderness along the

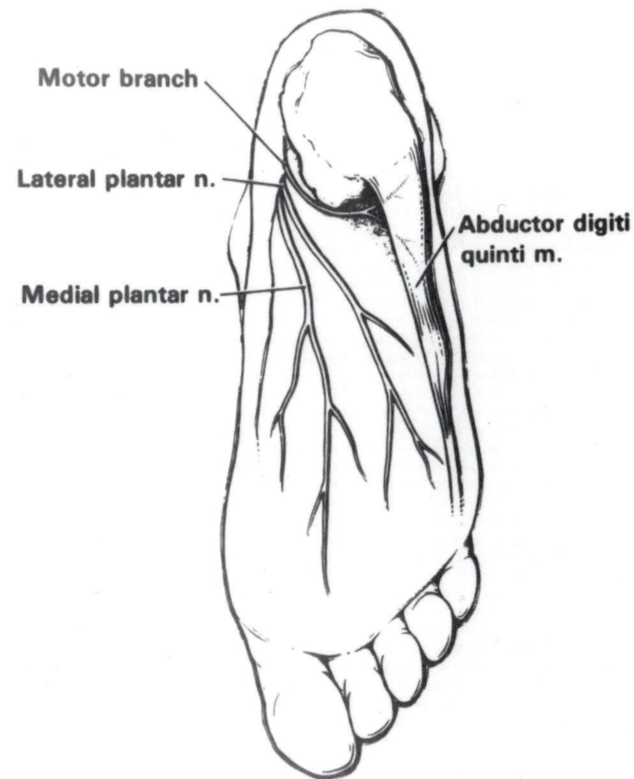

FIG 28–4.
Motor branch to the abductor digiti quinti muscle. (From Baxter D, Thigpen M: *Foot Ankle* 5:16, 1984. Used by permission.)

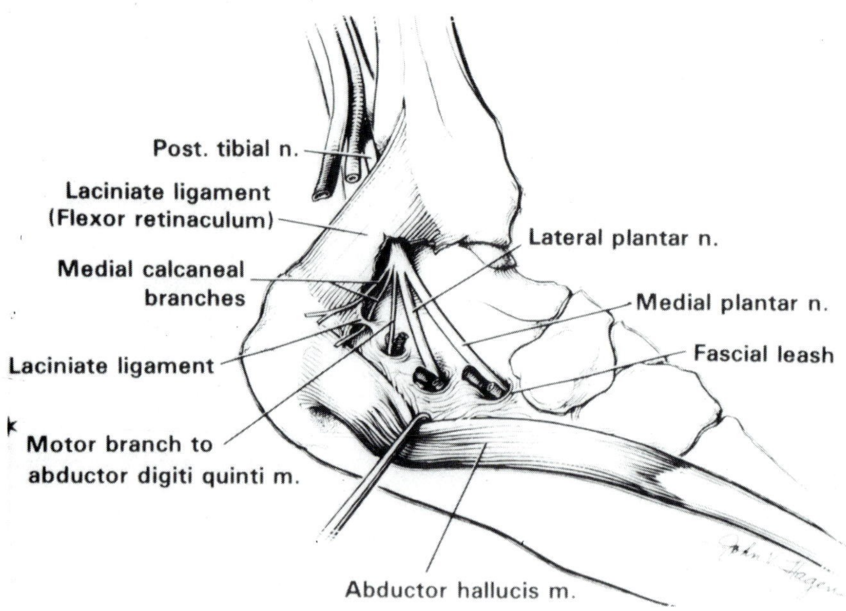

FIG 28–5.
Nerve to the abductor digiti quinti muscle as it migrates into the deep fascia of the abductor hallucis muscle. Deeper than more superficial calcaneal nerves, this nerve is the third branch of posterior tibial nerve or, on occasion, a branch of the lateral plantar nerve. (From Baxter D, Thigpen M: *Foot Ankle* 5:16, 1984. Used by permission.)

course of the nerve and maximal tenderness in the medial plantar surface just anterior to the medial tubercle of the calcaneus. In some patients, pressure at the point of maximal tenderness leads to paresthesias along the course of the nerve. Conservative treatment consists of rest, heel cord stretching, contrast baths, anti-inflammatory medication, and steroid injections. A heel pad may be helpful, and a medial arch support should be prescribed for the runner with hyperpronation. If conservative measures are not effective after 6 months, sur-

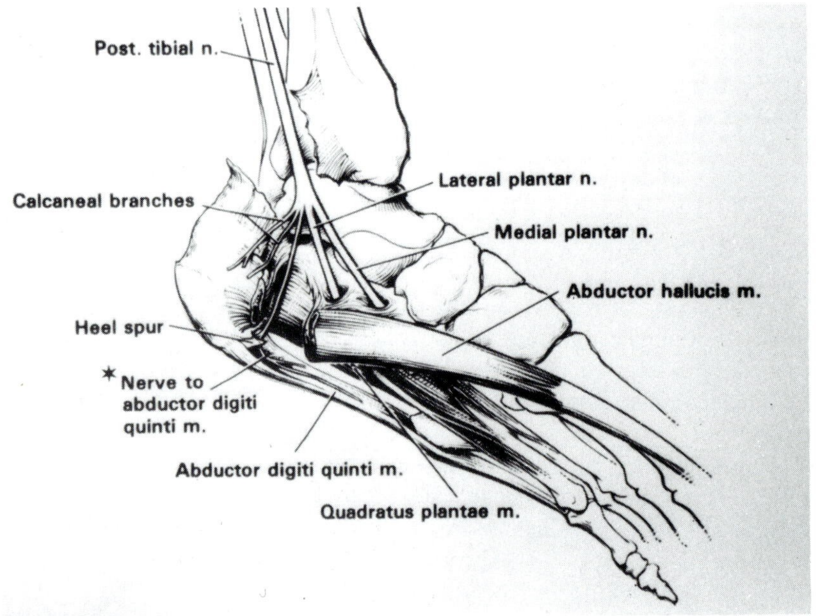

FIG 28–6.
The deep fascia of the abductor hallucis muscle has been incised to expose the nerve to the abductor digit quinti. This nerve can be compressed by the abductor hallucis muscle, medial tuberosity of the calcaneus, or on occasion, a heel spur or the plantar fascia. (From Baxter D, Thigpen M: *Foot Ankle* 5:16, 1984. Used by permission.)

gical decompression may be considered. The nerve decompression can be performed through either an oblique medial incision or a plantar incision. A small portion of the medial plantar fascia is removed to provide adequate visualization, and the deep fascia of the abductor hallucis is then incised and any calcaneal spur removed. The most recent follow-up of 69 cases treated surgically had 89% good or excellent results.[1]

TENDINITIS

Running places tremendous functional demands on the tendons of the foot and ankle and often leads to complaints of tendinitis.[43] Although the Achilles tendon is the most commonly affected, the posterior tibial and peroneal tendons may also be involved. Since the treatment of chronic tendinitis and tendinosis can be very challenging and ultimately lead to cessation of running, prevention of chronic tendinitis should be the goal. Frequent stretching and variation of training patterns should be emphasized and will often prevent the occurrence of tendinitis.

Achilles tendinitis is very common in the running athlete, with an incidence ranging from 6.5% to 18%.[7, 18] It also can be quite disabling. In one study of competitive track athletes with chronic Achilles tendinitis, 16% were forced to abandon their sport permanently, while 54% competed with significant discomfort.[49] Achilles tendinitis represents a continuum of disease presenting initially as an inflammation of the peritendinous structures and bursae and progressing to involvement of the tendon itself. In an article by Puddu et al.[32] the pathology of Achilles tendinitis is divided into three stages: peritendinitis, peritendinitis with tendinosis, and tendinosis. In the peritendinitis stage, it is the structures surrounding the tendon including the peritendinous sheath and bursae that become inflamed. The tendon itself is not involved. With the last two stages, there is a degree of tendinosis that implies damage to the tendon itself in the form of tears of the tendon, necrosis, or calcification within the tendon.

Achilles tendinitis can occur in two forms: insertional and noninsertional. Insertional Achilles tendinitis implies that the pathology is located near its insertion at the calcaneal tuberosity. These patients often have an associated Haglund deformity, i.e., a posterosuperior prominence of the calcaneal tuberosity. This bony prominence causes inflammation of the retrocalcaneal and superficial calcaneal bursae and leads to tendinitis (Fig 28–7). Often, runners with pronation will have more tenderness medially, and those with supination will have more symptoms laterally. A cavus foot brings the bony prominence closer to the anterior edge of the distal part of the Achilles tendon, thus increasing the risk of this disorder developing. Symptoms include pain at the posterior aspect of the heel, especially when running uphill. The patient is tender at the Achilles insertion and may have crepitance with dorsiflexion and plantar flexion. There is often an associated tight heel cord and a palpable bony prominence posteriorly. X-ray films may reveal calcification within the Achilles tendon near or at its insertion (Fig 28–8). Conservative treatment includes rest, intermittent ice massage, Achilles stretching, anti-inflammatory medication, and a heel lift to be used in all shoes including running shoes. If the patient has a pronated foot with symptoms medially, a medial sole and heel wedge may be helpful. Similarly, if there is supination of the foot with lateral pain, a lateral sole and heel wedge are indicated. For the runner with a Haglund deformity and a cavus foot, a heel lift will increase the distance between the anterior edge of the Achilles tendon and the posterosuperior bony prominence. Steroid injections are not recommended

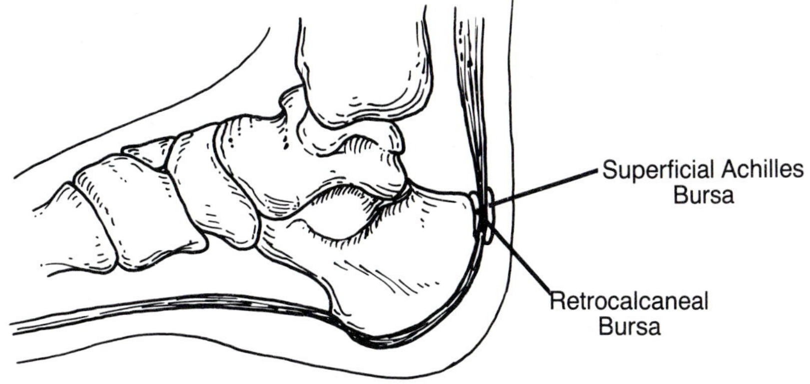

FIG 28–7.
The superficial Achilles bursa and the retrocalcaneal bursa are often involved in insertional Achilles tendinitis.

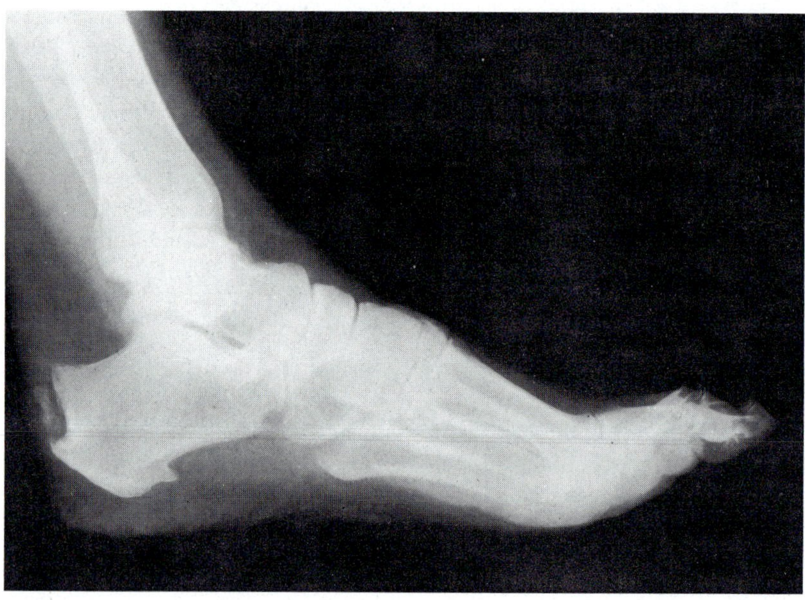

FIG 28–8.
Radiograph illustrating severe calcific insertional Achilles tendinosis associated with a Haglund deformity. There also is a calcaneal spur.

for Achilles tendonitis because of a risk of tendon rupture.

If conservative measures are not effective after 1 year, surgery may be considered. The suggested procedure by this author is to remove the Haglund deformity and debride the Achilles tendon of necrotic debris and calcification. This should be performed through longitudinal incisions medially and/or laterally depending on the area of greatest involvement. One should make longitudinal incisions into the tendon to remove the calcifications so that as much of the Achilles tendon insertion can be left intact as possible. If significant disruption of the tendon occurs, a tendon transfer may be required to provide additional strength in the Achilles tendon. Several tendons are appropriate for the transfer, and they include the peroneus brevis, the flexor digitorum longus, or the flexor hallucis longus.[26, 45, 47] Postoperatively, the patient is treated with immobilization and cast braces for 6 to 10 weeks depending upon the amount of disruption of the Achilles tendon insertion and whether a tendon transfer was performed. The runner usually can return to full activities within approximately 6 months.

Noninsertional Achilles tendinitis is characterized by pain and tenderness approximately 2 to 6 cm above the insertion. It has been shown that this region corresponds to the area of the most tenuous blood supply to the Achilles tendon.[19] With the exception of the location of symptoms, the patient's complaints are similar to those with the insertional form. Conservative treatment is identical to that for insertional tendinitis with the exception that an injection of bupivacaine (Marcaine) into the tendon sheath, which may disrupt adhesions, may provide relief. Surgical intervention may be considered if symptoms persist for 1 year in spite of conservative measures. The tendon and peritenon should be debrided, and if significant tendon weakening is evident, a tendon transfer or reinforcement with the plantaris tendon may be performed. Post operative care is similar to that of insertional tendinitis. Overall, the surgical results for insertional Achilles tendinitis have been less satisfactory than for noninsertional tendinitis.[40]

Posterior tibial tendinitis may present with acute symptoms that occur from a sudden pronation of the foot or may develop more gradually. The insertional form of posterior tibial tendinitis is usually associated with an accessory navicular and will have symptoms near its insertion at the medial aspect of the navicular. The noninsertional form may be tender throughout the course of the tendon or mainly posterior to the medial malleolus. The runner with hyperpronation is especially at risk to develop this disorder. Conservative treatment is similar to Achilles tendinitis and consists of rest, intermittent ice massage, anti-inflammatory medication, and stretching of the Achilles tendon as well as the posterior tibial tendon. A medial heel and sole wedge should be used, especially in the patient with hyperpronation. If symptoms persist, an injection of

Marcaine in the tendon sheath may disrupt adhesions and provide relief. Casting may be necessary in order to allow the inflammation to subside.

If conservative treatment is not successful after a prolonged period of time, surgery may be considered. For insertional tendinitis, excision of the accessory navicular may be performed. To gain access to the accessory ossicle, one should make longitudinal dorsal incisions in the tendon, which can be repaired. If significant tendon disruption occurs, a tendon transfer using the flexor digitorum longus or the flexor hallucis longus with attachment through a drill hole in the navicular may be added. In chronic noninsertional posterior tibial tendinitis, a release of the tendon sheath with debridement may lead to the resolution of symptoms.

Tendinitis of the peroneal tendons occasionally occurs in the runner. It is usually seen in the runner with either a cavovarus deformity or a hypermobile first metatarsal cuneiform joint. In both cases, increased stresses are placed on the peroneal tendons. Symptoms may occur posterior to the distal end of the fibula or at the point where the tendons are separated by the peroneal tubercle along the lateral border of the calcaneus. The symptoms may radiate up the lateral aspect of the leg and will be increased by forced supination of the foot. Peroneal subluxation during the toe-off phase of gait may be a predisposing factor. Conservative treatment consists of rest, intermittent ice massage, anti-inflammatory medication, and peroneal stretching. If the patient has a hypermobile first metatarsal-cuneiform joint, a medial arch support with a Morton extension may be helpful. For the runner with a cavovarus deformity, an orthotic device that keeps the foot in neutral position should be ordered. Conservative measures are usually effective. In recalcitrant cases, release of the peroneal sheath may be indicated.

IMPINGEMENT SYNDROMES

There are three sites in which an impingement syndrome may occur. One common area is the first metatarsophalangeal joint, in which impingement occurs as the runner increases his speed and the great toe is placed in more dorsiflexion. Initially the pain is vague, but it becomes more severe as hallux rigidus develops. When this syndrome begins to develop, a metatarsal pad or a metatarsal bar should be placed on the shoe to eliminate excessive dorsiflexion of the joint. Another area of impingement is in the anterior aspect of the ankle. The impingement occurs on the neck of the talus as it contacts the anterior part of the tibia. A synovitis develops in the area of the transcruciate ligament. The deep peroneal nerve passes underneath the transcruciate ligament at this level and can be irritated by this impingement. Initial treatment includes rest, anti-inflammatory medications, and a heel lift in the shoe. Another site of impingement is in the side of the ankle in runners who excessively pronate. The impingement occurs at the lateral subtalar joint or in the fibulotalar joint. Treatment of this problem is to support the medial aspect of the foot with a longitudinal arch support.

FOREFOOT DISORDERS

Forefoot disorders in the runner can be quite disabling, and their treatment requires a thorough understanding of gait biomechanics. The forefoot is subjected to a combination of linear, rotational, and shear stresses throughout its multiple joints. The impact forces of running can be three to eight times body weight[37] and will cause the stresses within the forefoot to be very high. Mild anatomic abnormalities, which may otherwise go unnoticed, may cause significant problems for the runner.

Metatarsalgia can have many underlying causes. A tight Achilles tendon or an anterior ankle impingement can lead to increased metatarsal impact by limiting ankle dorsiflexion. This limited dorsiflexion can subsequently cause clawtoes from the overactive pull of the extensor digitorum longus. Clawtoes in themselves increase the likelihood of metatarsalgia by displacing the plantar pad distally from under the metatarsal heads. Treatment consists of heel cord stretching exercises or an ankle arthroplasty to increase ankle dorsiflexion. If the clawtoes are the underlying cause, a metatarsal lift should be tried initially. If this is not successful, correction of the clawtoes can be considered.

A hypermobile first metatarsal-cuneiform joint or long second metatarsal can lead to metatarsalgia under the second or third metatarsals. Treatment can be the placement of a pad just proximal to the symptomatic metatarsal to decrease the pressure, or a medial longitudinal arch support with a Morton extension can be used to increase the weight-bearing contribution of the first metatarsal. If conservative treatment is not effective, a metatarsophalangeal joint arthroplasty with removal of a small amount of the plantar condyle is recommended. Metatarsal osteotomies are more unpredictable and may lead to a transferred metatarsalgia. It is important in refractory cases of metatarsalgia to not overlook nerve entrapment between the second and third metatarsals as a cause of pain. This usually accompanies clawtoe deformities and can be treated by a metatarsal pad or, if necessary, by nerve resection.

Sesamoid injuries are often secondary to overuse in the runner. Predisposing factors include a cavus foot secondary to a plantar-flexed first metatarsal, hyperpronation, and limitation of dorsiflexion at the first metatarsophalangeal joint. The cause of the pain can usually be classified as sesamoiditis, osteochondritis, or fracture of one or both sesamoids, with the tibial sesamoid being the most commonly affected. The patient will usually complain of a several-week history of pain at the first metatarsophalangeal joint. There will usually be no swelling, but the injured sesamoid will be locally tender, and the pain will be increased with passive dorsiflexion of the great toe. Initial x-ray studies should include anteroposterior (AP), lateral, and oblique views of the foot with an axial view (Lewis view) of the sesamoids. If no abnormalities are seen, a bone scan may be helpful in localizing the pathology to the sesamoids. If the x-ray findings are normal, a diagnosis of sesamoiditis is made and conservative treatment begun. This includes a reduction in activity and the use of an orthotic device incorporating a Morton extension and a U-shaped pad to unload the symptomatic sesamoid. Runners who hyperpronate should also have a soft medial longitudinal arch incorporated in their orthotic device. Sesamoid osteochondritis is diagnosed by mottling of the sesamoid on radiographs; however, treatment should be the same as with sesamoiditis. As symptoms resolve, activity can increase. The orthotic device, however, should be used for a minimum of 6 months. If the sesamoid disorder was secondary to a plantar-flexed first metatarsal, a proximal dorsal closing wedge osteotomy of the first metatarsal may be effective in unloading the sesamoids and preventing recurrence.

Fracture of a sesamoid can be treated similarly or with casting. A recent study has found conservative treatment ineffective for sesamoid fracture or severe osteochondritis.[36] Sesamoid excision is recommended for the following conditions: displaced fracture of a sesamoid, nondisplaced sesamoid fracture that has failed conservative treatment for 12 weeks, and sesamoiditis or osteochondritis if symptoms persist for 6 months in spite of treatment. An alternative to sesamoid excision that may be considered is bone grafting of the sesamoid.[28] Sesamoidectomy should be done with caution because it can lead to angular deformities of the hallux and decreased push-off strength of the great toe.[23]

Occasionally, a runner presents with complaints suggestive of a sesamoid disorder but will not be tender over the sesamoids. In this instance, a proximal nerve entrapment may be present. The location of the entrapment may be at the tarsal tunnel with involvement of the posterior tibial nerve or at the distal end of the abductor hallucis where the medial plantar nerve exits. The patient is commonly a hyperpronator, and palpation over the site of compression will usually reproduce the symptoms. Treatment consists of preventing hyperpronation, if present, along with decreased activity. If symptoms persist, decompression of the nerve or, rarely, excision of the nerve may be considered.

Hallux rigidus occurs in the runner and causes limited and painful motion of the first metatarsophalangeal joint. The runner commonly complains of pain upon squatting or starting from a stance. X-ray films are usually diagnostic and reveal degenerative changes of the first metatarsophalangeal joint with medial, lateral, and dorsal osteophytes. Conservative treatment consists of a metatarsal bar and a rigid-soled shoe. If symptoms persist, a cheilectomy-arthroplasty of the first metatarsophalangeal joint can be effective. It is usually necessary to remove the medial and lateral as well as the dorsal osteophytes of the first metatarsal head and any osteophytes on the dorsum of the proximal phalanx. Occasionally, only the dorsal or fibular osteophyte should be removed, especially in the elite athlete with only local symptoms. The goal is to achieve 60 degrees of dorsiflexion at the first metatarsophalangeal joint. If after removal of the osteophytes dorsiflexion is less than 60 degrees or if significant articular erosion is present at the dorsal aspect of the first metatarsal head, a dorsal closing wedge osteotomy of the proximal phalanx can be included to decompress the first metatarsophalangeal joint. We recommend a dorsolateral incision with the addition of a medial incision, if necessary. Care is taken to protect the sheath of the extensor hallucis longus in order to limit postoperative morbidity. A Silastic implant for treatment of this disorder in the running athlete is not recommended because of the high loads experienced by the first metatarsophalangeal joint. An arthrodesis of the first metatarsophalangeal joint can be used as a salvage procedure if the recommended arthroplasty fails.

Pain in the forefoot may develop secondary to a hallux valgus deformity. A hallux valgus deformity may lead to pain at the medial imminence initially but may eventually lead to secondary disorders such as metatarsalgia, clawtoes, and neuromas. As the hallux valgus worsens, the first metatarsal drifts into more varus and causes increased weight to be transferred to the second and third metatarsals. This may lead to metatarsalgia. Clawtoe deformities of the lesser toes and subluxation of the second metatarsophalangeal joint may also occur. Neuromas may develop secondary to traction as a result of the worsening clawtoes. Thus, a hallux valgus deformity can present with a variety of symptoms and findings.

In treating the hallux valgus deformity, one must remain aware of the high stresses placed on the forefoot during running. Also, during running, the range of motion of the joints of the foot may increase 50%. Treatment of hallux valgus must attempt to provide stable and durable correction as well as maintain adequate range of motion of the first metatarsophalangeal joint. Conservative treatment consists of training alterations and shoe modifications. A shoe with a wide toe box and well-padded forefoot may be helpful. Orthotic devices such as a metatarsal lift may improve symptoms secondary to metatarsalgia as well as secondary to clawtoes and neuromas. A lightweight medial arch support may relieve the valgus stress on the first metatarsophalangeal joint in the runner with hyperpronation. If pain persists and surgery is considered, it is recommended by the author that a bunionectomy with a distal osteotomy of the first metatarsal be performed. This has led to good results in middle-distance and marathon runners.[22] The postoperative regimen includes non-gravity exercises 1 to 2 weeks postoperatively and a return to running at 8 weeks.

For the runner with evidence of an interdigital neuroma, initial treatment should consist of a metatarsal bar placed behind the metatarsal head in an attempt to decrease the traction on the nerve. If this is not successful, an injection of steroid can be attempted. For resistant cases, nerve excision through a dorsal incision with release of the distal half of the intermetatarsal ligament may be indicated.

Callosities are frequently seen in running athletes and can be classified into three types.[4] A hard callus is secondary to external pressure of a bony prominence. A large diffuse callus is produced by shearing forces. A soft corn is located between the toes and is secondary to pressure between bony prominences of adjacent toes in a moist environment. Hard callosities can be treated by removing the external pressure through shoe modifications and padding. If these measures are not successful, removal of the bony prominence may be performed. Diffuse callosities are treated by reducing shear forces through the use of orthotic devices and shoe modifications and running on surfaces with less traction. Soft corns are initially treated with pads between the toes, and if persistent, excision of bony prominences can be considered.

Running athletes can develop toenail disorders secondary to repetitive trauma. The trauma is commonly secondary to toe hyperextension causing the toenails to be in contact with the dorsum of the shoe. Poorly fitting shoes can be another cause. A shoe that is too small will not allow enough space for the toes. A shoe that is too wide in the midfoot will allow the foot to slide forward within the shoe and cause the toes to strike the distal end of the shoe. The resulting nail deformity may be a simple thickening of the nail, subungual hematoma, or an ingrown toenail of the great toe. Treatment consists of metatarsal pads for toe hyperextension and properly fitting shoes with a snug midfoot and adequate toe box.

Blisters occur because of excessive shear. They are more likely when running in conditions of increased traction that cause high shear stresses on the plantar skin. This situation occurs with runners using spikes and running on artificial surfaces. Treatment consists of shear-reducing measures such as double socks, skin lubrication, and training on low-traction surfaces without spikes. Acutely, blisters should be treated by drainage of fluid with a sterile needle and covering the blister with an adhesive pad.

ORTHOSES AND COMPLICATIONS OF RIGID ORTHOSES

In some runners an overuse syndrome can occur as a result of the repetitive stress of running. These people tend to have a more pronated foot than the average population, but a few may also have a cavus-type foot. There are other malalignment problems such as genu varus and valgum and toeing in and toeing out that also lead to clinical problems secondary to the stress of running. Various types of orthotic devices have been used by runners, and the question always arises: what if anything does an orthosis do from a biomechanical point of view? An orthosis primarily prevents hyperpronation. Cavanaugh et al. selectively placed increasing thicknesses of felt along the medial border of the foot, to the eventual equivalent of 9.5 mm, and demonstrated a decrease in the degree of pronation and a decrease in the angular velocity of pronation.[5] They further studied subjects by using a force plate, and the only significant change was in the medial and lateral shear; the medial shear was decreased considerably in the subjects using the medial support. It appears that an orthosis providing a medial arch support does play a role in control of the foot by decreasing the degree as well as the rate of pronation of the foot. According to Stipe,[44] orthoses actually cause more energy consumption. It was felt that if orthoses helped correct problems with a runner's gait, it could be assumed that the runner would experience an improvement in running economy as a result of wearing running orthoses. A study comparing the energy demands of running with and without orthoses was made between the responses of the subjects to running in the controlled condition (the shoes with no orthosis) and the two orthotic conditions (shoes with soft orthoses and shoes with semirigid orthoses).

The study was carried out by collecting expired air during the final 2 minutes of each run and analyzing it to determine the volume of oxygen consumed per kilogram of body weight per minute (VO_2). The study demonstrated that athletes running without orthoses required less oxygen than did the athletes running with orthoses. While this situation was present at most running speeds, it was most significant during running at a pace of 7 min/mile or faster. The added weight of the orthoses alone could not account for the increased oxygen consumption, and it was hypothesized that the orthosis diminished the cushioning effects of the running shoe. This meant that the athlete had to do more work to absorb the vertical impact of each stride.

This research suggests that an athlete does not gain running economy when he runs with orthoses in his shoes. Instead, it appears that runners who wear orthoses actually encounter an increase in the aerobic demands of running. This should not be construed as a recommendation not to wear orthoses while running a race. A decision should be made for medical reasons independent of the energetic consequences of wearing orthoses.

There are three groups of orthoses. The soft type is generally inexpensive and can be made in the office or obtained ready-made. These are the type that many runners make themselves. They use orthopaedic felt, semiflexible cork, or leather. Many of the orthopaedic supply houses have a large selection of precut orthoses that can be used as either a temporary orthosis or a long-term orthosis to be changed intermittently.

The second type of orthosis is semiflexible. These may be made in the office but need to be fabricated by someone who understands the biomechanics of the foot and understands what function is being altered. One type may be made out of Orthoplast or Plastizote. These are heat-sensitive, semiflexible materials that become quite pliable when warm. Orthoplast is heated with warm water and Plastizote in a baking oven. Once the material is pliable, it is molded onto the foot or the cast of the foot while an attempt is made to hold the foot in a neutral position. Additional height of the longitudinal arch can be fabricated in layers. Once this orthosis cools, it is finished by smoothing the edges.

The third type of orthosis is a rigid orthosis that is fabricated from a positive plaster mold. A negative mold is made from the individual's foot with the foot held in the appropriate position. Once this has been done, a positive plaster cast is poured. Acrylic is poured over the positive plaster cast, and posting "bars and wedges" are added to finish the orthosis.

Indications for any orthosis are to relieve pressure from an area of the foot, to transfer pressure to a specific area, or to prevent specific motion. The main indication is in the prevention of pronation in the individual with a hypermobile foot or pes planus. The use of a rigid orthosis for a high-arched, rigid, cavovarus foot is less effective because it attempts to push the rigid foot into a different position. Selection of the orthosis is dependent on the amount of control that is needed and whether the foot is hypermobile or rigid. Rigid orthotic devices should be avoided if possible. Complications that occur with rigid orthoses include neuromas and sesamoiditis just distal to the edge of the rigid orthosis. Other problems include stress fractures of the leg as a result of inflexibility and decreased shock absorption in the foot. Cost configuration is something that must be brought into consideration. The soft orthoses are obviously the least expensive. The ideal orthosis has several characteristics. It is durable, controls motion, transfers pressure points, and is inexpensive and easy to fabricate.

SHOES

There are a multitude of shoes on the market today. More and more sophisticated shoes are being designed for training, for racing, for the heavy runner, or for the runner with a narrow foot. Good racing shoes are lightweight and should not be worn over prolonged mileage for fear of developing overuse syndromes and strains of the foot. Good training shoes have adequate compressability of the heel to cushion heel strike. They have adequate medial support to prevent hyperpronation, and they are adequately flexible to eliminate stress on the Achilles tendon from a rigid lever arm. In advising runners on buying shoes, quality control should be evaluated. Evaluation of the shoes should be carried out to ensure that the sole layers are securely fastened to each other and to the upper portion of the shoe. The inner aspect of the shoes should be evaluated for protrusions and indentations. In fitting the shoe, the shoes should be fitted to the longer foot. A minimum of ¼ to ⅜ of an inch in front of the long toe should be left when measuring the length of the shoe. The calcaneus should not slip or rub excessively in the rear of the shoe. The lacing and tongue must feel comfortable on the instep to avoid irritating the superficial nerves and bony prominences.

REHABILITATION OF THE INJURED RUNNER

It is important for the athlete to stay physically fit while undergoing treatment for a specific injury. This will allow a quicker return to the previous activity level and prevent recurrent injuries. If the injury is minor and relatively acute, merely a decrease in mileage or a change of surface may be necessary. In this case, minimal rehabilitation is necessary. If the symptoms are more severe such that a cessation of running is required, alternate activities must be suggested to maintain fitness.

Cross-training is a very effective method to maintain a runner's conditioning during injury. Cross-training substitutes one activity for another in order to maintain cardiovascular conditioning and to exercise similar muscle groups while allowing the injured area to heal. For the running athlete with a foot disorder, bicycling, swimming, roller-skating, or cross-country skiing are recommended cross-training activities.[6] In those with stress fractures, running in a pool to minimize impact loads may be suggested as another form of cross-training.

Running can usually begin when the injured area is asymptomatic. It is essential that a gradual increase in mileage be initiated. A reasonable approach is to start running every other day for half the normal preinjury mileage. Cross-training can be done on alternate days. If after 2 weeks no symptoms return, a gradual increase in mileage and frequency can begin with a return to preinjury levels by 6 to 8 weeks. Interval activities and hill climbing (especially with plantar fasciitis and Achilles tendinitis) should be avoided in the first 6 to 8 weeks. It is essential that the runner avoid the pitfalls of his previous training regimen in order to avoid recurrence. If orthotic devices have been prescribed, they should be used at all times while running. If symptoms return, cross-training exercises should resume as well as treatment for the specific injury.

REFERENCES

1. Baxter DE, Pfeffer GB: Treatment of chronic heel pain by surgical release of the first branch of the lateral plantar nerve (submitted for publication).
2. Baxter DE, Pfeffer GB, Thigpen M: Chronic heel pain treatment rationale, *Orthop Clin North Am* 20(4):563–570, 1989.
3. Baxter DE, Thigpen M: Heel pain—operative results, *Foot Ankle* 5:16–25, 1984.
4. Bordelon RL: Management of disorders of the forefoot and toenails associated with running, *Clin Sports Med* 4:717–724, 1985.
5. Cavanaugh PR, Clarke T, Williams K, et al: An evaluation of the effect of orthotics on force distribution and rearfoot movement during running, American Society for Sports Medicine meeting, Lake Placid, NY, June 1978.
6. Clancy WG Jr: Specific rehabilitation for the injured recreational runner, *Instr Course Lect* 38:483–486, 1989.
7. Clement DB, Tauton JE, Smart GW: A survey of overuse running injuries, *Physician Sports Med* 9:47–58, 1981.
8. D'Ambrosia RD, Zelis RF, et al: Interstitial pressure measurements in the anterior and posterior compartments in athletes with shin splints, *Am J Sports Med* 5:127–131, 1977.
9. Detmer DE: Chronic shin splints: classification and management of medial tibial stress syndrome, *Sports Med* 3:436–446, 1986.
10. Detmer DE, Sharpe K, et al: Chronic compartment syndrome: diagnosis, management, and outcomes, *Am J Sports Med* 13:162–170, 1985.
11. Frankel VH: Fatigue fractures: biomechanical considerations, *J Bone Joint Surg [Am] 54:1345, 1972.*
12. Fronek J, Mubarek SJ, Hargens AR, et al: Management of chronic exertional anterior compartment syndrome of the lower extremity, *Clin Orthop* 220:217–227, 1987.
13. Green WT: *Discrepancy in leg length of lower extremities,* American Academy of Orthopaedic Surgery Instructional Course Lecture, Ann Arbor, Mich, 1951, JW Edwards.
14. Jahss MH: *Disorders of the foot and ankle,* ed 2, Philadephia, 1991, WB Saunders.
15. James SL, Bates BT, Ostering LR: Injuries to runners, *Am J Sports Med* 6:40–50, 1978.
16. Jones DC, James SL: Overuse injuries of the lower extremity: shin splints, iliotibial band friction syndrome, and exertional compartment syndromes, *Clin Sports Med* 6:273–290, 1987.
17. Kingston S: Magnetic resonance imaging of the ankle and foot, *Clin Sports Med* 7:15–28, 1988.
18. Krissoff WB, Ferris WD: Running injuries, *Physician Sports Med* 7:64, 1978.
19. Lagergren C, Lindholm A: Vascular distribution in the Achilles tendon, *Acta Chir Scand* 116:491–495, 1958.
20. Leach RE, Seavey MS, Salter DK: Results of surgery in athletes with plantar fasciitis, *Foot Ankle* 7:156–161, 1986.
21. Lehman WL: Over-use syndromes in runners, *Am Fam Physician* 29:157–164, 1984.
22. Lillich J, Baxter DE: Bunionectomies and related surgery in the elite female middle-distance and marathon runner, *Am J Sports Med* 14:491–493, 1986.
23. Lillich JS, Baxter DE: Common forefoot problems in runners, *Foot Ankle* 7:145–151, 1986.
24. Lysholm J, Wiklander J: Injuries in runners, *Am J Sports Med* 15:168–171, 1987.
25. Mann RA, Baxter DE, Lutter LD: Running symposium, *Foot Ankle* 1:190–224, 1981.
26. Mann RA, Holmes GB Jr, et al: Chronic rupture of the Achilles tendon: a new technique of repair, *J Bone Joint Surg [Am]* 73:214–219, 1991.
27. Martens MA, Backaert M, Verant G, et al: Chronic leg pain in athletes due to a recurrent compartment syndrome, *Am J Sports Med* 12:148–151, 1984.
28. McBryde AM Jr, Anderson RB: Sesamoid foot problems in the athlete, *Clin Sports Med* 7:51–60, 1988.
29. Michael RH, Holder LE: The soleus syndrome: a cause of medial tibial stress (shin splints), *Am J Sports Med* 13:87–94, 1985.
30. Mubarek SJ, Gould RN, Fon Lee Y, et al: The medial tibial stress syndrome. A cause of shin splints, *Am J Sports Med* 10:201–205, 1982.
31. Mubarek SJ, Hargens AR: Exertional compartment syn-

dromes. In *Symposium on the foot and leg in running sports*, St Louis, 1982, Mosby–Year Book.
32. Puddu G, Ippolito E, Postacchini F: A classification of Achilles tendon disease, *Am J Sports Med* 4:145–150, 1976.
33. Puranen J: The medial tibial syndrome, *J Bone Joint Surg [Br]* 56:712–715, 1974.
34. Reneman RS: *The anterior and lateral compartment syndrome of the leg*, The Hague, 1968, Mouton.
35. Reneman RS: The anterior and lateral compartment syndrome of the leg due to intensive use of muscles, *Clin Orthop* 113:69–80, 1975.
36. Richardson EG: Injuries to the hallucal sesamoids in the athlete, *Foot Ankle* 7:229–244, 1987.
37. Riegler HE: Orthotic devices for the foot, *Orthop Rev* 16:27–37, 1987.
38. Rorabeck CH, Bourne RB, Fowler PJ: The surgical treatment of exertional compartment syndrome in athletes, *J Bone Joint Surg [Am]* 65:1245–1255, 1983.
39. Rorabeck CH, Fowler PJ, Nott L: The results of fasciotomy in the management of chronic exertional compartment syndrome, *Am J Sports Med* 16:224–227, 1988.
40. Schepsis AA, Leach RE: Surgical management of Achilles tendinitis, *Am J Sports Med* 15:308–315, 1987.
41. Shelbourne KD, Fisher DA, Rettig AC, et al: Stress fractures of the medial malleolus, *Am J Sports Med* 16:60–63, 1988.
42. Slocum DB: The shin splint syndrome: medical aspects and differential diagnosis, *Am J Surg* 114:875–881, 1967.
43. Stanish WD, Curwin S, Rubinovich M: Tendinitis: the analysis and treatment for running. *Clin Sports Med* 4:593–609, 1985.
44. Stipe P: The effects of orthotics on rearfoot movement in running, *Nike Res Newsl* 2, No 3, 1983.
45. Teuffer AP: Traumatic rupture of the Achilles tendon: reconstruction by transplant and graft using the lateral peroneus brevis, *Orthop Clin North Am* 5:89–93, 1974.
46. Ting A, King W, et al: Stress fractures of the tarsal navicular in long-distance runners, *Clin Sports Med* 7:89–101, 1988.
47. Turco VJ, Spinella AJ: Achilles tendon ruptures—peroneus brevis transfer, *Foot Ankle* 7:253–259, 1987.
48. Viitasalo JT, Kvist M: Some biomechanical aspects of the foot and ankle in athletes with and without shin splints, *Am J Sports Med* 11:125–130, 1983.
49. Welsh RP, Clodman J: Clinical survey of Achilles tendinitis in athletes, *Can Med Assoc J* 122:193–196, 1980.

CHAPTER

29

Foot and Ankle Injuries in Dancers*

William G. Hamilton, M.D.

Toes

Corns
Calluses
Blisters
Fracturers and dislocations
  Toe fractures
Chronically unstable fifth proximal interphalangeal joint
Mallet toes
The "proud" fourth toe
Subungual hematomas
Subungual exostoses
Painful fifth toenails

The interphalangeal joint of the hallux

The subhallux sesamoid
Dorsal impingement

The metatarsophalangeal joint of the hallux

Bunions
Lateral instability
Hallux rigidus
  Grade I
  Grade II
  Grade III
Sesamoid injuries
  Differential diagnosis of sesamoid pain

The lesser metatarsophalangeal joints

Freiberg's disease
Acute dislocation
Metatarsophalangeal instability
Idiopathic synovitis

The metatarsals

"Pseudotumor" of the first web space
Metatarsal stress fractures
  Base of the second metatarsal
  Dancer's-view radiograph of the foot
  Treatment
Third and fourth metatarsals
Fifth metatarsal
Fracture of the proximal tubercle of the fifth metatarsal
Bunionettes

The midtarsal area

Painful accessory navicular
Stress fracture of the tarsal navicular
Degeneration in the tarsometatarsal joints
Lisfranc's dislocation
Sprains at the base of the fourth and fifth metatarsals

The medial ankle

Posterior tibial tendonitis
Medial sprains of the ankle

The anterior ankle

Impingement syndrome
Tendonitis

The lateral ankle

Classification of ankle sprains
Treatment
  Conservative treatment
  Surgical treatment
  Postoperative care
  The sprained ankle that will not heal

The posterior ankle

Posterior impingement syndrome
  Treatment
  Tendonitis of the flexor hallucis longus tendon

The Achilles tendon

Achilles tendonitis
Rupture of the Achilles tendon
Accessory soleus muscle, the pseudotumor of the calf

Heel pain

Heel spur syndrome
Plantar fasciitis
Rupture of the plantar fascia
Stress or hairline fracture
Plantar calcaneal bursitis
Entrapment of Baxter's nerve
Bone cysts and tumors

Leg pain

Stress fractures of the distal isthmus of the fibula
Shinsplints
Stress fractures of the tibia

Dancers, whether they are ballet, modern, "Broadway," "show," tap, folk, ethnic, etc., all have unique requirements for their particular art form and, at the professional level, are the result of a Darwinesque selection process that has usually weeded out the ones unsuited for that profession. The dancer's feet are the equivalent of the musicians' hands—they earn their living with them; they are their "instrument." This foot is a unique structure, the result of years of endless training, classes, and "barres." It tends to be slightly cavus (at least the dancer wishes it were, even if it is not), with a rounded arch, thickened metatarsals to support body weight when dancing on the ball of the foot ("demi-pointe"), and calluses on appropriate areas where the skin also needs to be tough. Indeed, this toughness of skin and bone is necessary for its normal function, and blisters and metatarsal stress fractures occur when the necessary toughness is not present.

Normally, a dancer's foot is also quite strong, i.e., it is intrinsic plus. Intrinsic minus feet are characterized by splaying of the metatarsals and clawing of the toes,[12] whereas the opposite, the intrinsic plus foot, has narrowing of the metatarsals and straightening of the toes. The dancer's foot may be unsightly due to callus formation, but a claw-toe in a dancer is hardly ever seen.

In addition to strength, the dancer's foot and ankle need to have an extreme range of motion.[7, 8, 14] Most dancers have 10 to 15 degrees of recurvatum at the knee and, in order for the ankle to be in a vertical position on relevé, there ideally should be 90 to 100 degrees of plantar flexion in the foot-ankle complex. If the ankle is vertical, the dancer needs 90 to 100 degrees of dorsiflexion in the first metatarsophalangeal (MTP) joint in order to relevé onto demi-pointe (Fig 29–1). Few people are born with this much motion, and in order to get it, most female dancers have to begin their training early so that the immature skeleton can be molded as it grows.[5]

There are several different foot types found in dancers.

The *"Grecian" or Morton's foot* with foreshortening of the first and fifth rays is the most common. Difficulties are sometimes encountered in the relatively long second, third, and fourth rays, but problems found in the general population, such as transfer metatarsalgia and loosening of the second MTP ligaments with instability are surprisingly rare.

The *"Egyptian" foot* with its long hallux is the oppo-

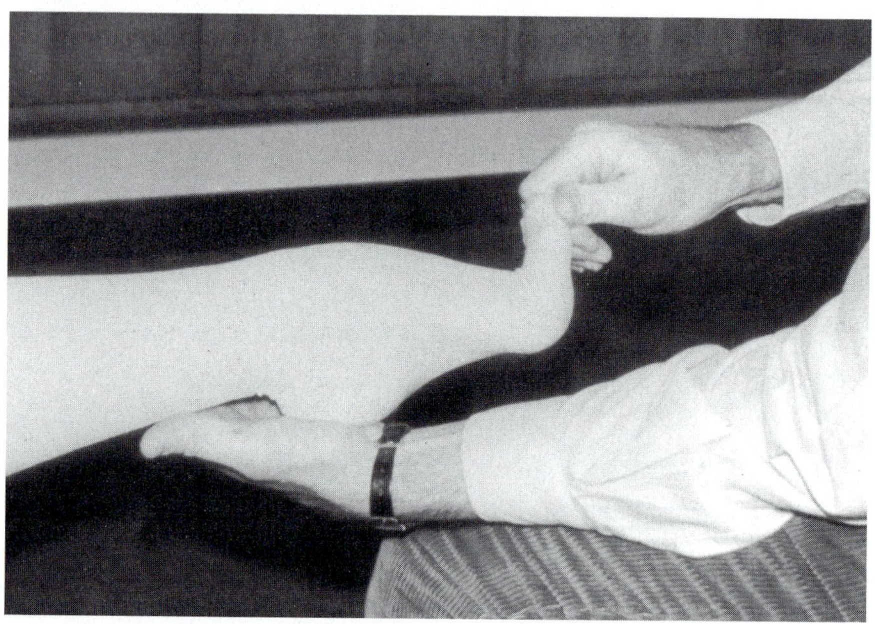

FIG 29–1.
The 90 degrees of dorsiflexion needed in the dancer's first MTP joint.

site of the Grecian foot and is predisposed to difficulties with the first MTP joint: degenerative joint disease (DJD), osteophyte formation, and hallux rigidus. This is probably due to the increased lever arm of the long hallux acting on the joint through an extreme range of motion.

The *"model's" foot* is narrow and pleasing to look at, with an exaggerated taper in metatarsal length from the first to the fifth rays, but it bears weight unevenly on demi-pointe and tends to be hypersensitive. It is a poor foot for a dancer.

The *"simian" foot* with its metatarsus primus varus is the bunion-prone foot. As the first metatarsal migrates into varus, it becomes hypermobile, does not bear weight well, and leads to transfer metatarsalgia, which can be a problem. Bunion surgery, however, should be avoided in a professional dancer because it is impossible to operate on the bunion and leave the dancer with the 90 degrees of dorsiflexion in the first MTP joint that she needs in her profession.

The *"peasant's foot"* is a broad, square foot with uniform metatarsal length providing stability and an equal distribution of forces among the metatarsals. It is the ideal foot for the dancer.

TOES

Dancers have a remarkable ability to tolerate pain in their feet and toes and often have developed elaborate systems to control the discomfort so that they can continue to dance.

Corns

Corns are a necessity for the ballet dancer so that she may bear weight on her toes in the toe shoe. When they become hypertrophied, they may need to be trimmed, preferably with a pumice stone, but most dancers know all about these things—they deal with them every day. Ballet dancers usually use lamb's wood or paper towels in their toe shoes to redistribute the forces within the toe box. They become experts at this, and it is usually best to let them do this on their own because they can do it better than you can; they have been doing it since they were 12 years old! If the toe box is made too tough, however, it takes away their proprioception and "feel of the floor," and they cannot dance in it. Minor complications can occur with a corn, such as bleeding or infection beneath it. In these cases it may be best to drain or unroof the corn and use antibiotics. Repeated infections may be a sign of undiagnosed early diabetes. (We have had such a case in the New York City Ballet.)

Soft corns in the fourth web space are a common problem in dancers who have a shortened fifth metatarsal. Ideally, the proximal interphalangeal (PIP) joint of the fifth toe should lie in the concavity of the diaphysis of the adjacent phalanx of the fourth toe. When the fifth ray is foreshortened, the PIP joint comes to rest against the head of the fourth metatarsal, and a soft corn forms. Usually, these can be managed nonsurgically by trimming the corn and placing lamb's wool or a foam rubber spacer between the fourth and fifth toes to hold them apart. Dancers with this problem may need to be instructed in management and hygiene because these soft corns can develop local infections and, on occasion, a deep sinus into the fourth web space. When surgery is necessary, there are several choices. In Europe they excise the skin and web the fourth and fifth toes together (this is not popular in North America). Usually it will be necessary to perform some combination of excision of the medial condyle, excision of all of the distal portion of the proximal fifth phalanx, and/or excision of the lateral portion of the fourth metatarsal head (see soft corn surgery in Chapter 8). An x-ray film with a radiopaque marker on the soft corn will help determine which resections are necessary. Not infrequently, there is also a painful corn with a small osteophyte beneath it on the lateral condyle of the PIP joint of the fifth toe. In this situation the distal portion of the proximal phalanx should be removed with both the medial and lateral condyles. Care should be taken in making incisions on the fifth toe because numbness or incisional neuromas here can be a real problem in the dancer.

Calluses

Calluses, like corns, are essential for toughness. The dancer will usually develop areas on the ball of the foot that resemble intractable plantar keratoses (IPKs). Usually they are not true IPKs because they are not painful; they are simply areas of concentrated weight bearing. Occasionally they may need trimming, but the dancers know how to do this. When these normal calluses are painful, it may be a sign that something else is going on. Usually it is either a plantar wart or an invaginated callus ("seed corn"). A *plantar wart* will usually not be found on a weight-bearing surface of the sole of the foot, and black spicules and capillary bleeding will be found when the wart is pared down. Treatment consists of trimming the excess callus and treatment with one of the salicylic acid products such as "Wart-Off." Surgical excision is rarely if ever indicated. When a *seed corn* is present, trimming will reveal a white nidus. It will sometimes penetrate deeply into the callus. This nidus must be entirely removed, even if multiple trimming sessions are required. Dramatic relief of pain usually follows removal of this nidus. Care should be taken to avoid causing bleeding, and sterility of the instruments used in these trimming procedures is essential to prevent possible human immunodeficiency (HIV) contamination. In my office we use disposable, sterile scalpels on a "one-use-only" basis.

Very thick calluses are needed by the modern dancer to dance barefoot on the stage. They may occasionally become hypertrophic and need to be trimmed, but dancers live with these corns and calluses throughout their whole career and usually know how to deal with them. Hygiene is difficult when dancing barefooted all day in a dirty studio. These modern dancers occasionally develop a massive callus under the ball of the foot, and this callus tends to tear at its margins and leave little crevices that contain breaks in the skin. These raw creases can become infected, usually with a local cellulitis that can be managed with local hygiene, soaks, and oral antibiotics. On occasion, however, this can lead to a major foot infection requiring hospitalization, appropriate intravenous antibiotics, and open drainage via marginal incisions *off the weight-bearing surface of the foot.* (Fasting blood sugar levels, a glucose tolerance test, and HIV testing in these cases are also needed.) The author has seen several of these infections, and it is important to be able to recognize this situation when it occurs.

Orthoses are frequently prescribed for dancers, but I have never known a professional dancer who could wear an orthosis when she performed. Certainly they can be worn in street shoes and sometimes in the rehearsal shoes, but they cannot be used when seriously dancing, so it is a mistake to prescribe them for this use.

Blisters

Blisters are part of the everyday life of a dancer. They are a necessary part of the toughening process leading to the calluses that allow weight bearing on the toes. The dancers usually know how to manage these from past experience and "dancer's folklore." For example, they favor unroofing a blister and using "Benzodent" as a local anesthetic so that they can continue dancing with the pain. (If the physical therapist treating a dancer has a cold red laser available, it can be used to aid healing of these blisters remarkably fast.) Occasionally, a blister can form underneath a corn. This blister may contain blood and may need to be drained or unroofed. These may also be accompanied by local cellulitis requiring oral antibiotics and soaks with Epsom Salts (1 heaping tbsp of Epsom Salts in a quart of warm water, with soaking twice daily for 20 to 30 minutes).

Fractures and Dislocations

Dancers wear many different kinds of shoes when performing:

The *toe shoe* is worn by the female ballet dancer when dancing on full pointe on the tips of the toes. It contains a hardened cardboard toe box in which the toes are "rosebudded." The forces are dissipated both axially and circumferentially within this box. It dates from the early 19th century and separates ballet dancing from all other forms of dancing.

The *ballet slipper* is a soft glovelike shoe with a small sole that is worn by male and female dancers when they are dancing on demi-pointe only (i.e., not on the toes, but on the ball of the foot). The toe shoe and the ballet slipper are made on a straight last. There is no "right" or "left" shoe.

The *character shoe* is a special shoe or boot worn for a specific role in a ballet. It may be flat, or it may have a heel. It is also used by Spanish dancers.

The *jazz shoe* is a soft, laced shoe with a sole and small heel. Older teachers often wear this shoe when teaching class (Fig 29–2).

All of these shoes protect the toes to some degree. It is virtually impossible to fracture a toe while wearing a toe shoe. In the ballet slipper that male dancers wear, the toes are less protected, and toe injuries usually occur either when wearing this shoe or when dancing barefooted. A common cause of PIP dislocations occurs when the male dancer is exiting the stage and accidentally kicks one of the lead weights used to hold down the scenery (Fig 29–3). These dislocations are usually "complex," i.e., they are not reducible by closed means because the plantar plate is subluxed into the joint or

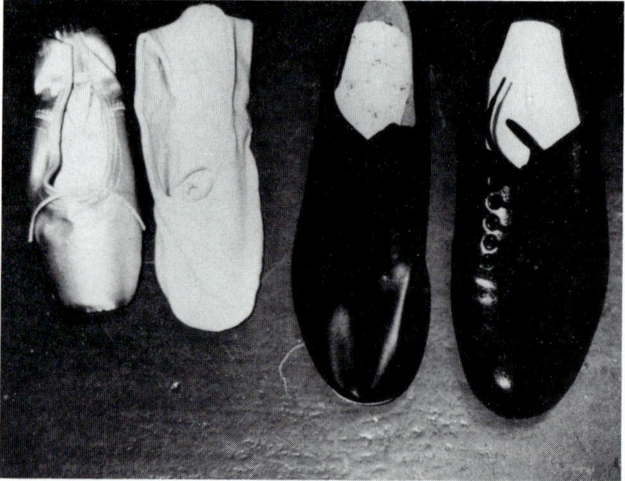

FIG 29–2.
The toe shoe, ballet slipper, and jazz shoe.

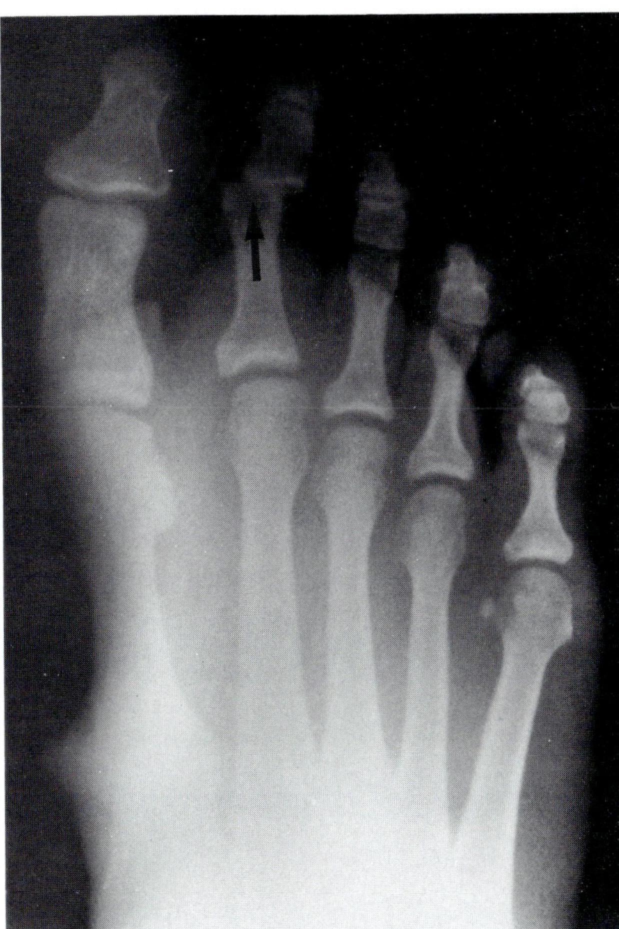

FIG 29–3.
Acute dislocation of the second PIP joint.

dorsal to the head of the proximal phalanx and prevents reduction. Open release of the collateral ligaments under a digital block will usually allow an easy reduction. An intramedullary Kirschner wire across the PIP joint (not crossing the MTP joint) for stability is used for 3 weeks. Phalangeal fractures and dislocations are more common in modern dancers who dance barefooted and unprotected than in other dancers who wear shoes.

Toe Fractures

Toe fractures in dancers are common, but they usually occur like everyone else, at home, in the middle of the night, barefooted. These fractures most frequently occur in the diaphysis of the phalanx and rarely involve the joint. I usually treat them by taping them to the adjacent toe for 3 to 4 weeks while they heal: the "buddy system." I have never performed an open reduction of a phalangeal fracture. If they should cause trouble later, a PIP or distal interphalangeal (DIP) resection can be performed as a salvage procedure with a high degree of success.

Chronically Unstable Fifth Proximal Interphalangeal Joint

The chronically unstable fifth PIP joint can be a problem. It usually follows an untreated lateral dislocation of the fifth PIP joint with complete rupture of the medial collateral ligament of the joint. Often it is difficult to recognize because the patient does not know exactly what is wrong with the toe, only that it hurts. The x-ray findings will be normal. It is easy to detect on physical examination if you remember to look for it. A valgus force will cause the toe to dislocate, and the patient will usually say "that's what happens when it hurts" (Fig 29–4). Surgery will usually be necessary for this condition. A PIP resection corrects the problem nicely by removing the fulcrum on which the distal phalanges dislocate and allows the joint to scar down.

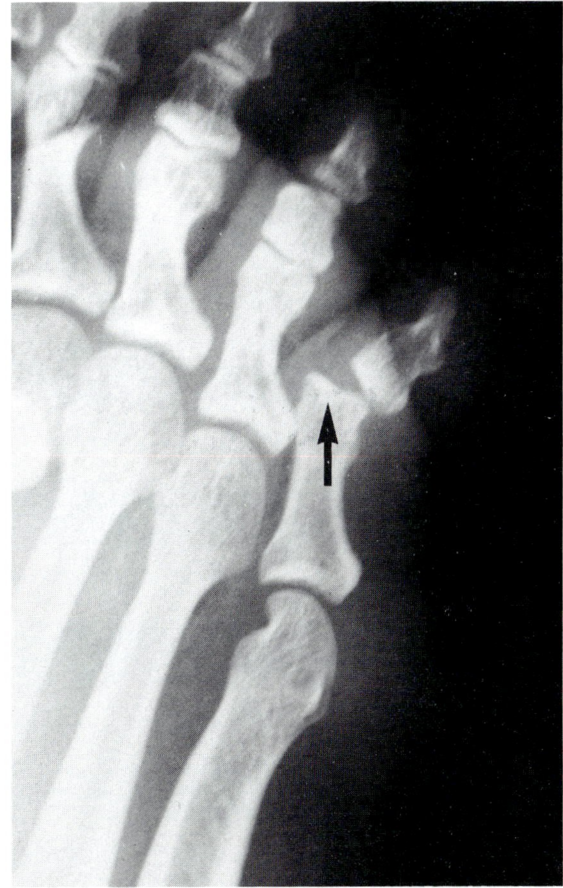

FIG 29–4.
Recurrent dislocation of the fifth PIP joint.

Mallet Toes

Mallet toes do not usually need treatment. If surgery is needed, a DIP resection with an intramedullary toe wire will correct the problem. It is usually not necessary to tenotomize the long flexor tendon (see mallet toes in Chapter 8).

The "Proud" Fourth Toe

In some dancers the fourth toe is too long in relation to its adjacent toes. The toe reacts by either curling under the third toe to form a mallet toe or a hammer toe. If surgery is warranted, the condition can be corrected by a DIP or PIP resection, depending upon the location of the deformity (see hammer toes in Chapter 8). The toe should be shortened so that the tip of the resected fourth toe lines up with the base of the nail of the third toe. The patient should be warned that the toe will be "fat" for 6 months to a year following the operation.

Subungual Hematomas

Subungual hematomas are quite common in ballet dancers, particularly in the first and second toes. In the acute phase, symptoms may warrant drilling a hole in the nail to relieve the pressure (Fig 29–5). Later, it is best to tell the dancer to keep the old toenail on as long as possible to protect the sensitive new nail beneath it. In the late stages it may be necessary to save the old nail after it has fallen off and tape it over the new nail when wearing toe shoes.

Subungual Exostoses

Subungual exostoses are occasionally seen and, at times, may be large. They seem to be more common in ballet dancers; perhaps the toe shoe irritates the periosteum of the distal phalanx and gives rise to this tumorlike growth (Fig 29–6). Removal is usually curative (see subungual exostoses in Chapter 25).

Painful Fifth Toenails

Some female dancers have fifth toes that are rotated toward the fourth toes so that in the toe shoe they are bearing weight directly on the fifth toenails. This condition can be very uncomfortable and may warrant permanent removal of the nails. For this situation, I prefer the Thompson-Terwilliger operation in which the nails,

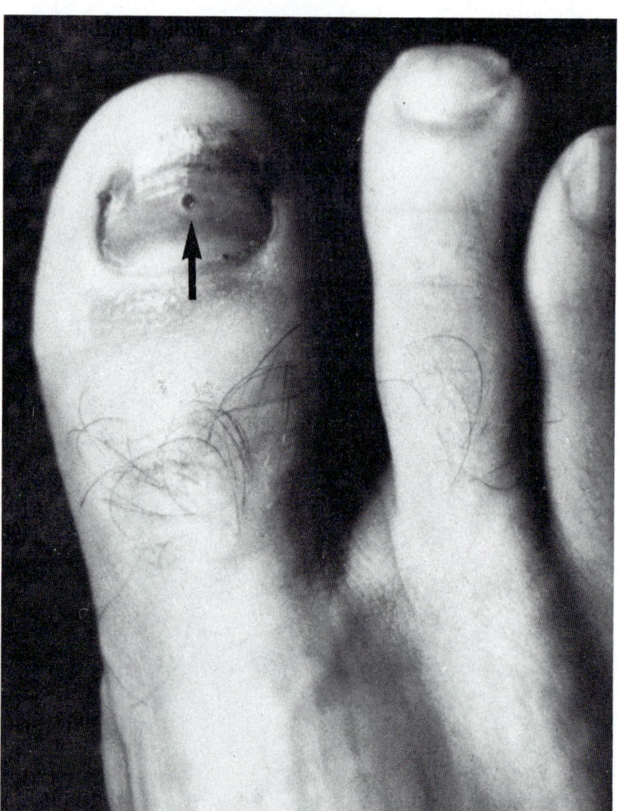

FIG 29–5.
A subungual hematoma. Note the drainage hole.

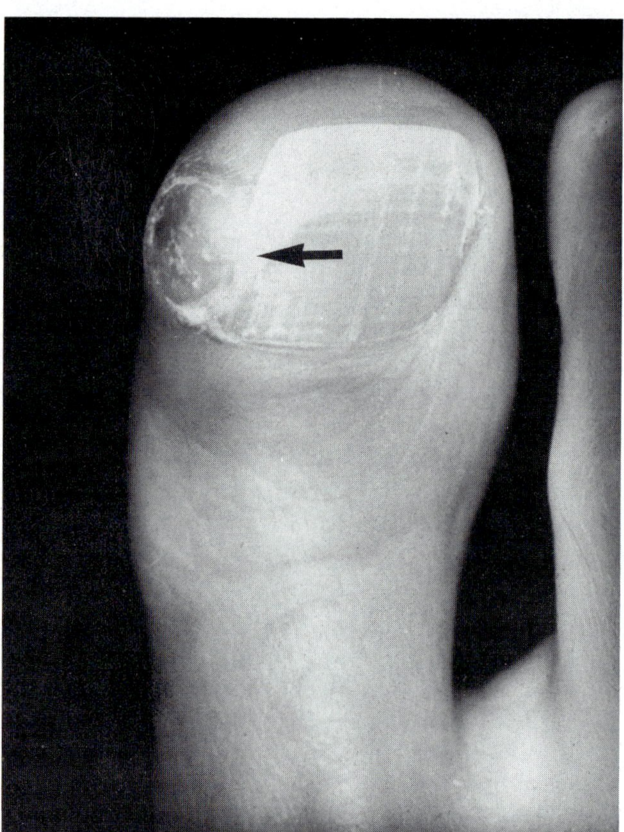

FIG 29–6.
A subungual exostosis growing out through the skin.

nail beds, and terminal portion of the distal phalanx are removed to allow a Syme-type primary closure of the wound (see Chapter 25 for this procedure). This has worked well for me. The dancer should be warned that she will need at least 2 months to recover, perhaps 3 months to get into a pair of toe shoes, and will not be totally free of pain for 6 to 9 months. Care should be taken when performing this simple operation because incisional neuromas or incomplete removal of the nail bed can leave you with a very unhappy patient.

THE INTERPHALANGEAL JOINT OF THE HALLUX

Similar to the first MTP joint, a remarkable variation in the formation of this joint can be found. Frequently, dorsiflexion at the interphalangeal (IP) joint will compensate for a lack of motion in the MTP joint, especially if the first ray is foreshortened (the Grecian foot). I once saw a dancer who had a congenital fibrous ankylosis of both first MTP joints with no dorsiflexion in these joints at all. She had short first rays and had developed 90 degrees of dorsiflexion in the IP joints of both great toes, which allowed her to dance normally.

The Subhallux Sesamoid

The IP joint of the hallux will occasionally have a sesamoid on the plantar aspect of the joint that causes a fullness. (This sesamoid is *not* in the insertion of the flexor hallucis longus (FHL) tendon; it is in the plantar plate dorsal to the tendon.) The prominence caused by the sesamoid is best left alone. If symptoms warrant, a small pad can be worn beneath the proximal phalanx to flex the IP joint slightly. This will usually alleviate the discomfort and callus that forms under the joint.

Dorsal Impingement

If the first MTP joint motion is poor, either from an early hallux rigidus or from congenital stiffness, the IP joint will be forced into dorsiflexion to compensate for the lack of motion in the other joint. Osteophytes, DJD, and even some mild dorsal and lateral instability can occur secondary to these forces. On several occasions I have performed a cheilectomy, similar to the operation performed on the first MTP joint, for dorsal osteophyte formation. The surgeon should keep in mind, however, that this is a "forgiving" joint and that one must base one's decisions regarding surgery on the patient's symptoms and disability and not on the x-ray findings. I have seen some very shoddy IP joints that were hardly symptomatic.

THE METATARSOPHALANGEAL JOINT OF THE HALLUX

Bunions

There is a general feeling that dancing causes bunions. It is my clinical impression that bunions are no more common in dancers than in any other group of females. Dancers, like everyone else, are born with "bunion-proof" and "bunion-prone" feet that run in their families. If you take a bunion-prone foot and put it in a toe shoe, it will rapidly form a bunion, but it is the foot that causes the bunion, not the dancing. The bunion-proof foot will form calluses over the bunion area, but like other calluses, they are a necessary part of dancing. The foot surgeon should keep in mind that the dancer needs 90 to 100 degrees of dorsiflexion in the first MTP joint. Anything (such as bunion surgery) that takes away that motion will adversely affect the dancer's career. *I strongly feel that all bunion surgery in a serious dancer should be deferred until their professional career is over.* Hobby dancers or dance teachers may be able to function after bunion surgery if their bunions are moderate and if the surgery is performed carefully. (Obviously, they should be warned in advance that they will loose motion in the joint and will, in all likelihood, have to "sickle" when they relevé.) Unfortunately, I see all too many young dancers who claim that their budding careers in dancing were ended by well-meaning bunion surgeons.

Even severe bunions can usually be managed conservatively with toe spacers to hold the toe in alignment (Fig 29–7) and "horseshoe" pads to relieve the pressure over the medial eminence.

Lateral Instability of the First Metatarsophalangeal Joint

I have seen several cases of rupture of the medial collateral ligament of the first MTP joint. All have gone unrecognized at the time of the acute injury, and all have had difficulties later. Based on this experience, I recommend that when this injury occurs, it is best to open the medial ligament complex and repair the torn ligaments (analogous to third-degree ankle sprains). I have performed late repair by using local tissues on two occasions, both of which were successful. (One was associated with recurrent dislocation of the sesamoid mechanism into the first web space. See under the section on sesamoid injuries.)

Hallux Rigidus

This condition can be a major disability in the dancer. As previously noted, loss of the 90 degrees of

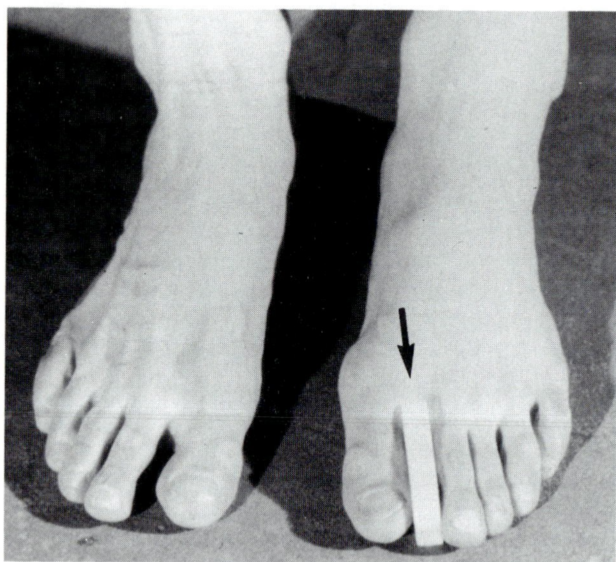

FIG 29–7.
Spacer in the first web spaces for conservative management of hallux valgus.

dorsiflexion normally present in this joint prevents a proper relevé onto demi-pointe and forces the dancer to roll onto the lateral rays of the foot. (The dancers call this "sickling.") I like to think of hallux rigidus as a spectrum presenting in three types:

Grade I

The joint is essentially normal, and the osteophytes are located marginally around the dorsum of the joint. This is the simplest type because generous removal of the spurs is usually curative. Unfortunately, this type of hallux rigidus is uncommon.

Grade II

There is both osteophyte formation and some degree of degeneration within the joint. Some early narrowing of the cartilage space is seen on the x-ray film. This type is amenable to a "radical cheilectomy," but the dancer should be warned of the following:

1. The result will not be perfect, only "better."
2. Even though the procedure is relatively simple, it often takes an unexpectedly long time to recover—at least 3 to 6 months.
3. The underlying degeneration may progress to osteoarthritis in spite of the surgery, and further surgery may be needed later if this should occur.

The procedure is done under an ankle block as an outpatient. A midmedial incision is made. The dorsal and plantar flaps are mobilized with care taken to avoid damage to the adjacent digital nerves, the FHL, and the extensor hallucis longus (EHL). The head of the metatarsal is exposed and inspected. Usually the damage to the articular cartilage is on the dorsolateral portion of the head. The dorsal half of the metatarsal head is then removed with an osteotome or thin oscillating saw. The dorsal portion of the base of the proximal phalanx is then exposed, with care taken not to injure the EHL. The dorsal third of the articular portion of the phalanx is then osteotomized and removed. Ideally, the bone removed will excise the most damaged portion of the joint. The sesamoids are then mobilized by blunt dissection until 90 to 100 degrees of dorsiflexion is obtained. If the patient is not allergic to bees, the raw surfaces are covered with a thin layer of bone wax. There is a tendency to not remove a dorsolateral osteophyte, but it is important to do so. The surgeon can expect to obtain about 60% of what is obtained at the time of surgery, so every effort should be made to obtain as much motion as possible. A layered closure with chromic catgut is performed. The patient is encouraged to bear weight as soon as possible following the surgery, and early active and passive motion is begun as soon as the wound is healed.

Grade III

The dorsal osteophytes are secondary to obvious DJD within the joint. This presents a dilemma for the surgeon and the dancer. The results with cheilectomy are not reliable, although a "radical cheilectomy" will sometimes maintain some MP motion. A first MP fusion will eliminate all motion in the joint, which is usually incompatible with dancing.

If the patient has 1st and 2nd metatarsals that are relatively the same length, and needs to preserve MP motion, then I have performed a capsular arthroplasty. The patient needs to be warned that this may not work, and, if it does, it may not hold up over time. If it fails then an MP fusion can be done for salvage. The operation is basically a resection arthroplasty but the thick dorsal capsule of the joint is pulled down between the metatarsal head and the base of the proximal phalanx and sutured to the stumps of the flexor brevi, distal to the sesamoids. One must be careful not to remove too much of the proximal phalanx, 25% to 30% at the most. If the EHL tendon is tight, it should be lengthened to prevent the hallux from riding upward. I perform a tenotomy of the extensor hallucis brevis proximally so that the whole dorsal sleeve of the MP joint, including EHB insertion, can be pulled down into the gap between the bones. I have had mixed results with this procedure, sometimes surprisingly good and sometimes disappointing. If the first ray is foreshortened, this operation will not work as well, because the patient will almost certainly get a transfer lesion on the 2nd metatarsal head.

Silastic implants have been abandoned in active patients by all reputable foot surgeons, because the long-term results have been so poor. They simply cannot hold up under the demands of the active dancers and athletes:

Sesamoid Injuries

In view of the forces that are placed on the sesamoids by the dancer, it is a wonder that they do not have more problems with them than they do. Over the 20-year period that I have been seeing injured dancers, I have developed a great respect for the sesamoids to heal themselves. On many occasions I have seen older dancers whose sesamoids appeared as though they had been smashed with a hammer. Upon questioning, the dancers invariably stated that they had had a year or so of pain in the area, but it eventually went away, and most of the time they had been unaware of what the problem was and had just continued dancing with the pain until it resolved. Careful physical examination and an accurate diagnosis are essential in this area, for all pain around the plantar aspect of the first MTP joint is not always "sesamoiditis."

Differential Diagnosis of Sesamoid Pain

Sesamoiditis.—True sesamoiditis can be due to the following:

1. Stress or hairline fracture (positive bone scan).
2. Sprain or avulsion fracture of the proximal pole.
3. Sprain of a bipartite sesamoid. X-ray films will show widening of the space between the two fragments.
4. Sprain of the distal pole. This is a very rare injury and usually accompanies a strong dorsiflexion force, similar to a "turf toe" in football.
5. Osteonecrosis that is not yet apparent on the x-ray film. The symptoms may precede the x-ray changes by as much as 6 months. A bone scan is indicated when the diagnosis is not clear.
6. DJD in the sesamoid-metatarsal articulation.

Sesamoid Bursitis.—There is a bursa beneath the sesamoids that can become swollen and inflamed. This sesamoid bursitis is frequently misdiagnosed as sesamoiditis. It can be recognized on physical examination if it is kept in mind. The diagnosis can be confirmed by injecting a local anesthetic into the bursa. Treatment consists of a small amount of corticosteroid injected into the bursa and a pad to unweight the area so that the inflammation can subside. Unfortunately, the condition heals slowly, and it can leave bands of fibrous tissue within the bursa that can be painful later, especially if these bands lie directly underneath the sesamoid where they are rolled upon when the dancer relevés. If the condition fails to heal, a bursectomy via a plantar-medial incision can be performed, similar to chronic olecranon bursitis. The plantar proper digital nerve in this area must be identified and protected.

Sesamoid Instability.—On rare occasions, rupture of the medial collateral ligament of the tibial sesamoid can lead to sesamoid instability. I have seen two cases of recurrent lateral dislocation of the sesamoid mechanism into the first web space. The dancers presented with a complaint that their great toe was "dislocating" when they relevéd. When the dancer is examined barefooted, the dislocation is rather dramatic. A sudden "clunk" occurs when the sesamoids slip laterally. This condition requires surgery to correct the instability. On two occasions I have performed a lateral sesamoid release and reconstructed the medial ligament of the tibial sesamoid with local tissues. One must keep in mind the anatomy of the medial ligament structures so that the reconstruction can be performed at the isometric center of motion and the all-important MTP join motion maintained. (On both occasions the operation worked, but two cases hardly make a series.)

Neural Entrapment Around the Sesamoids.

Joplin's Neuroma.—Caused by entrapment of the proper digital nerve adjacent to the medial sesamoid, this condition will have a positive Tinel sign, whereas sesamoiditis will not. Dancers who "roll in" (pronate) are prone to this problem. Chronic cases may need surgical neurolysis and transposition of the nerve away from the sesamoid.

Entrapment of the Lateral Proper Digital Nerve.—This rare condition is difficult to diagnose. It presents as a neuralgic-type pain radiating into the hallux from the lateral side. It is not possible to elicit a Tinel sign due to the location of the nerve. The diagnosis must be confirmed by injecting a small amount of local anesthetic into the area of the nerve just as it exits from beneath the deep transverse metatarsal ligament insertion into the lateral sesamoid. The symptoms are not usually disabling enough to warrant surgery. When they are, the deep transverse metatarsal ligament can be divided and the trapped nerve released, similar to the median nerve release for carpal tunnel syndrome. The nerve will lie directly beneath the ligament and is usually found to be flattened by the pressure of the ligament.

THE LESSER METATARSOPHALANGEAL JOINTS

Freiberg's Disease

Freiberg's disease[29] is no more common in dancers than in the general population. It can be symptomatic for as long as 6 months before it appears on the x-ray film. A bone scan will usually make the diagnosis early. Freiberg's infraction comes in four variations:

In *type I*, the head of the metatarsal dies and then heals by "creeping substitution." In this type it heals completely, with little or no collapse, and leaves the articular surface intact and almost as good as it was before the event occurred.

In *type II*, the head collapses during revascularization, the articular surface remains intact, but osteophytes form along the dorsal margin of the joint and limit dorsiflexion. This type is amenable to a dorsal clean-out, which should leave the joint intact and restore dorsiflexion. The surgeon should remember to remove more bone than he thinks is necessary when this operation is performed.

In *type III*, the head collapses, and the articular surface loosens and falls into the joint to leave the joint totally destroyed. Obviously, simply removing the osteophytes will not suffice in this case—arthroplasty is required. All the necrotic bone must be excised from the metatarsal head, and all the dorsal osteophytes must be removed. Usually the plantar portion of the head is left when this has been done. Again, the surgeon should be generous in the excision in order to have full dorsiflexion later.

In *type IV*, there are multiple heads involved in the process (Fig 29–8). This type is very rare and may actually be a form of epiphyseal dysplasia. Each metatarsal head must be evaluated and treated individually.

Acute Dislocation of the Lesser Metatarsophalangeal Joints

This injury is more common in males than females because their feet are less protected by the shoes they wear when dancing. Unfortunately, for some reason it often goes unrecognized. Perhaps this is due to the swelling that accompanies the injury in the metatarsal region. Obviously, the dislocation must be reduced and immobilized so that it can heal. If the joint has been dislocated for a long time, i.e., a month or more, it may not be possible to reduce it and maintain vascularity. In this case it is usually necessary to perform either a resection or a Du Vries type of arthroplasty in order to allow reduction without stretching the neurovascular bundles. If this is done, it should be remembered that the dancer will need excessive dorsiflexion postoperatively, so the pin placed across the joint at the time of surgery should be removed earlier than usual (no later than 2 weeks) to allow early motion. (In spite of this the joint will occasionally end up with limited motion. In these cases one can perform a manipulation under anesthesia in the office with a local anesthetic block.) An al-

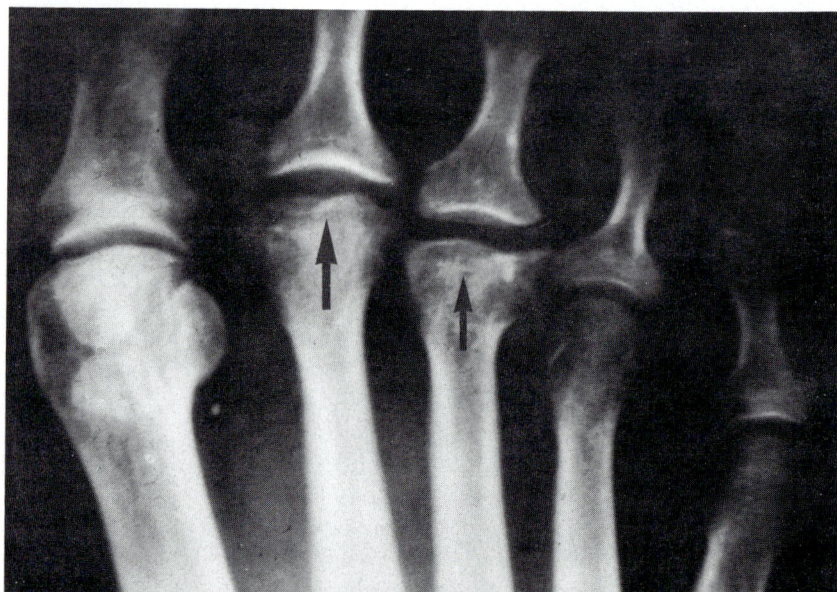

FIG 29–8.
Freiberg's disease in two MTP joints.

ternative would be to perform a Keller-type arthroplasty, especially if the joint involved is the fourth MTP joint. If this is done, one should not remove too much of the proximal phalanx (no more than a fourth to a third at the most), but should remove the plantar condyles of the metatarsal head. This is necessary because some laxity in the joint will likely be present later, with metatarsalgia.

Metatarsophalangeal Instability

Metatarsalgia is not common in this young healthy population. When it is encountered, one should suspect either early Freiberg's disease or MTP instability. This subtle problem often goes unrecognized because the x-ray and bone scan findings will be normal. The patient presents with isolated metatarsalgia. There is plantar tenderness under the metatarsal head and dorsal tenderness where the phalanx subluxes on top of the head when the patient relevés. The subluxed phalanx pushes the head of the metatarsal downward to produce the metatarsalgia. It is easily recognized on physical examination if one remembers to look for it. The "Lachman test" of the MTP joint will be positive.[29] The base of the proximal phalanx is grasped in the fingers, and an anteroposterior force is applied. The instability is easily recognized when the phalanx dislocates on top of the metatarsal head (Fig 29–9). Conservative treatment consists of padding to unweight the painful metatarsal head and taping or wearing a toe retainer to try to control the instability. It is often a frustrating situation for dancers because they do not want to undergo surgery, but once the ligaments and plantar plate are stretched out, they can be tightened again only by surgery. The surgical options for this problem in a dancer are tricky. The usual operations for this condition (stabilizing procedures such as the Girdlestone-Taylor operation) may stabilize the joint, but they will also limit dorsiflexion—an unacceptable solution. I have had success, in a limited number of dancers, with a resection arthroplasty, especially in the fourth MTP joint—a joint that seems especially prone to this problem. As noted above, one should not remove too much of the proximal phalanx (a quarter to a third at most), but should remove the plantar condyles of the metatarsal head, use a toe wire, and remove it early (2 weeks).

Idiopathic Synovitis

This condition[29] is characterized by MTP swelling, the so-called sausage toe. Its cause is controversial (it is not usually associated with systemic inflammatory diseases, but of course, these need to be ruled out). It is usually associated with laxity of the joint and MTP instability. Whether the looseness irritates the joint and leads to chronic synovitis or vice versa is not known. My own feeling is that this condition is related to the former sequence of events because I have seen several cases where eventual surgical exploration of the joint revealed chondral fractures and joint damage. Conservative therapy involves reduced activities and anti-inflammatories followed by one or two (at most!) intra-articular injections of steroids. If this fails, exploration and appropriate surgery are indicated (see above).

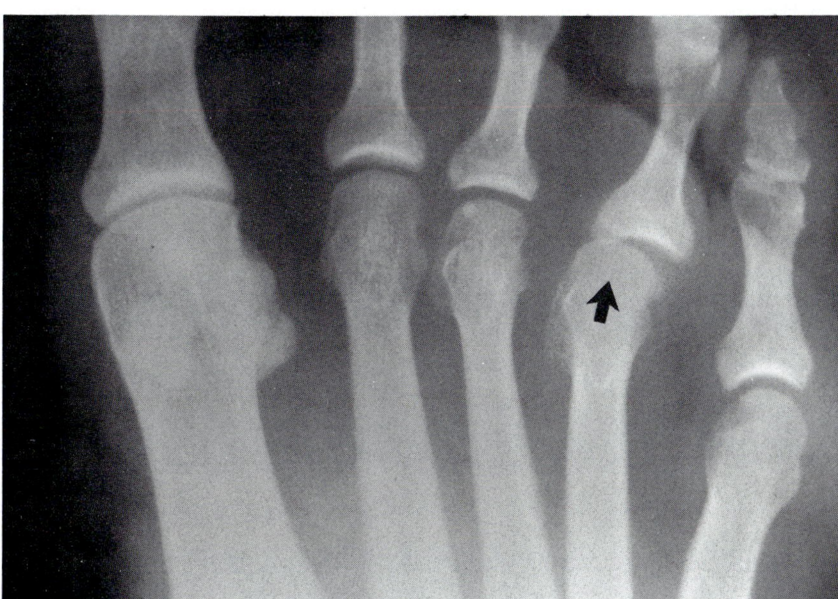

FIG 29–9.
An unstable fourth MTP joint.

THE METATARSALS

"Pseudotumor" of the First Web Space

A slowly enlarging mass in the first web space of the foot that does not aspirate fluid (is not a ganglion) will usually turn out to be muscle fibers of the extensor hallucis brevis. In these cases, the muscle fibers extend down the tendon, almost to the MTP joint, and can resemble a tumor.

Metatarsal Stress Fractures

A radiogram of a dancer's foot shows a characteristic thickening of the lateral cortex of the first metatarsal and the shafts of the second and third metatarsals (Fig 29–10). This hypertrophy is due to "Wolff's law" i.e., bone will respond to the stresses placed upon it. Most dancers are selected for a mild cavus foot, and this foot is rigid. It absorbs energy poorly. Normally, by starting dancing early, there is time for the metatarsals to hypertrophy as body weight increases so that the loads placed upon the foot as an adult will not fracture the bones. Metatarsal stress fractures do occur, especially at the base of the second metatarsal. Some predisposing factors include the following:

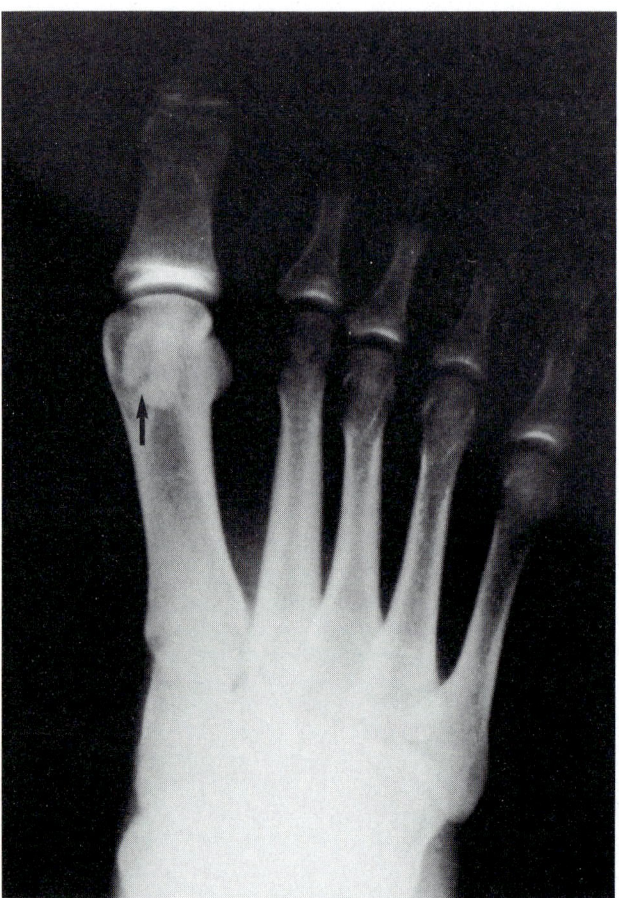

FIG 29–10.
Metatarsal thickening of the lateral cortex of the first metatarsal and shafts of the second and third. Note the fracture of the tibial sesamoid.

1. The dancer's cavus foot, as noted above.
2. A long second metatarsal (the "Grecian" foot).
3. Dancers who start dancing late and try to catch up with their peers before they have developed the necessary hypertrophy in their metatarsals.
4. Amenorrhea.[5, 31]

The Base of the Second Metatarsal

The medial, middle, and lateral cuneiforms are wedged shaped and sit together like the stones of a Roman arch. The middle cuneiform is the keystone in this arch. This middle cuneiform is recessed to accept the base of the second metatarsal, which adds rigidity to the second ray. This anatomy creates a stress riser at the proximal metaphysis of the second metatarsal, and it is at this location that the metatarsal tends to fracture. These factors result in the characteristic stress fracture that dancers get at the base of the second metatarsal. *Pain and tenderness at the base of the first web space or on the proximal portion of the second metatarsal is a stress fracture until proved otherwise.* It is by far the most common location of stress fractures in the dancer's foot. It may or may not be seen on the x-ray film depending upon how long it has been present.

On rare occasions, the fracture may occur at the very base of this bone, and these fractures may enter the cuneiform-metatarsal joint. This fracture will usually heal by bony or asymptomatic fibrous union.

The "Dancer's-View" Radiograph of the Foot

Because of the cavus foot present in the dancer, the normal x-ray of the forefoot taken in an anteroposterior projection will usually yield a very poor visualization of this area. An x-ray taken "upside down" with the dorsum of the forefoot against the cassette will give a much better view of the proximal metatarsals (Fig 29–11). A bone scan will confirm the diagnosis if necessary; however, the physical findings are so characteristic of the problem that I often do not bother to get a scan.

Treatment

If the fracture is *acute*, immobilization in a short-leg walking cast or a removable walking boot for 4 to 6

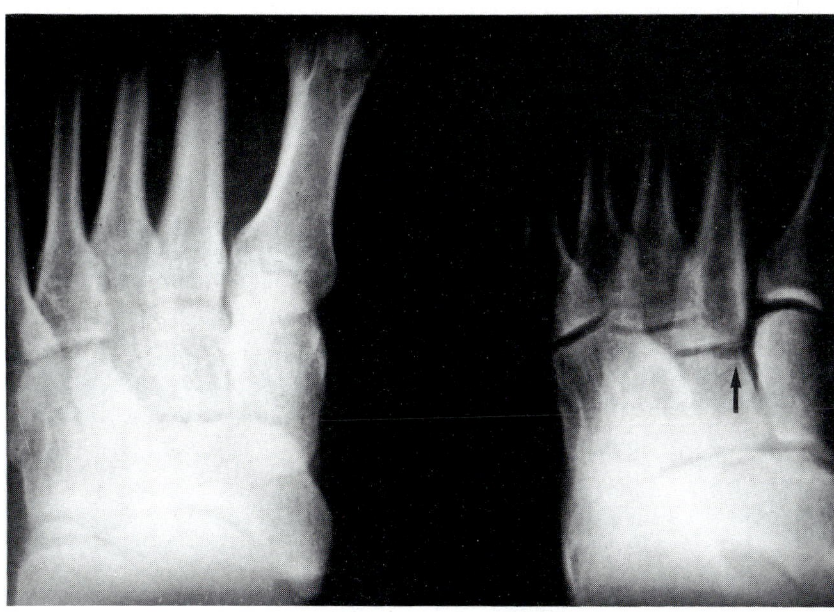

FIG 29–11.
The AP normal view *(left)* vs. the PA "Dancers view" *(right)*. Note the chip fracture of the second tarsometatarsal joint.

weeks is the safest thing to do. (The removable boot allows the dancer to take it off for sleeping and swimming to maintain conditioning.) A *chronic stress fracture* is usually treated by modified activities, i.e., the dancer should not do what hurts until it does not hurt to do it anymore. The healing time will be 4 to 6 weeks or, if they have been ignoring the pain and dancing with it, longer, i.e., 6 to 8 weeks. Healing is usually judged by the disappearance of pain rather than by the x-ray findings.

The Third and Fourth Metatarsals

Injuries and stress fractures in the third and fourth metatarsals are not common. Pain and tenderness in these bones can be due to an *osteoid osteoma* or to a *"stress reaction"* (forces on the bones leading eventually to a stress fracture but prior to the actual fracture of the bone).

The Fifth Metatarsal

A spiral fracture of the distal shaft of the fifth metatarsal is the most common acute fracture in the dancer (Fig 29–12). It is often called *"the dancer's fracture."*[7] It usually happens when the dancer loses balance while dancing on demi-pointe and rolls over on the outer border of the foot.

The *Jones fracture*, or a fracture of the proximal diaphysis of the fifth metatarsal shaft, is a dangerous fracture if it is not recognized for what it is (Fig 29–13). It can occur acutely or chronically, or the symptoms can build up gradually, and then the bone can fracture acutely. It is more common in "show" and modern dancers, who dance plantigrade, than in ballet dancers, who dance mostly on the ball of the foot (demi-pointe). It occurs in a portion of the bone that has a meager blood supply, so it often heals poorly and has a propensity to go to nonunion. This fracture should be treated in a short-leg, *non–weight-bearing* cast until it heals, and this can be 6 to 12 weeks or longer. I have never had one of these fractures go to nonunion when treated in this manner. The nonunions that I have seen have been treated with weight-bearing casts, or the seriousness of the injury was not recognized, and it was mistaken for the benign fractures that occur at either end of this bone. Some orthopaedists recommend primary percutaneous intramedullary fixation in high-level or professional athletes. In cases with established nonunion, the bone should be internally fixed and bone-grafted.

Fracture of the Proximal Tubercle of the Fifth Metatarsal

This common, benign fracture usually happens on the way to the theater rather than when the dancer is dancing. It is really an avulsion fracture of the insertion

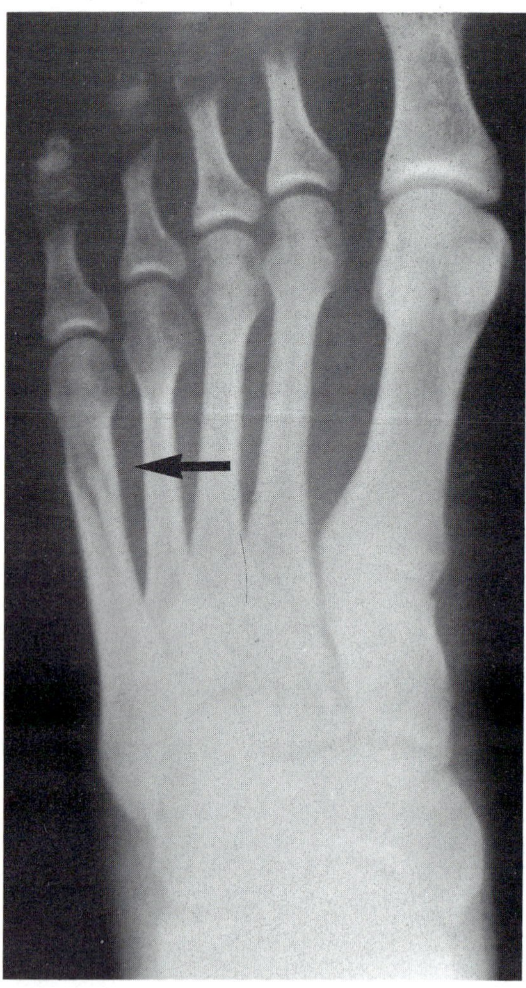

FIG 29–12.
The "dancer's fracture" of the fifth metatarsal.

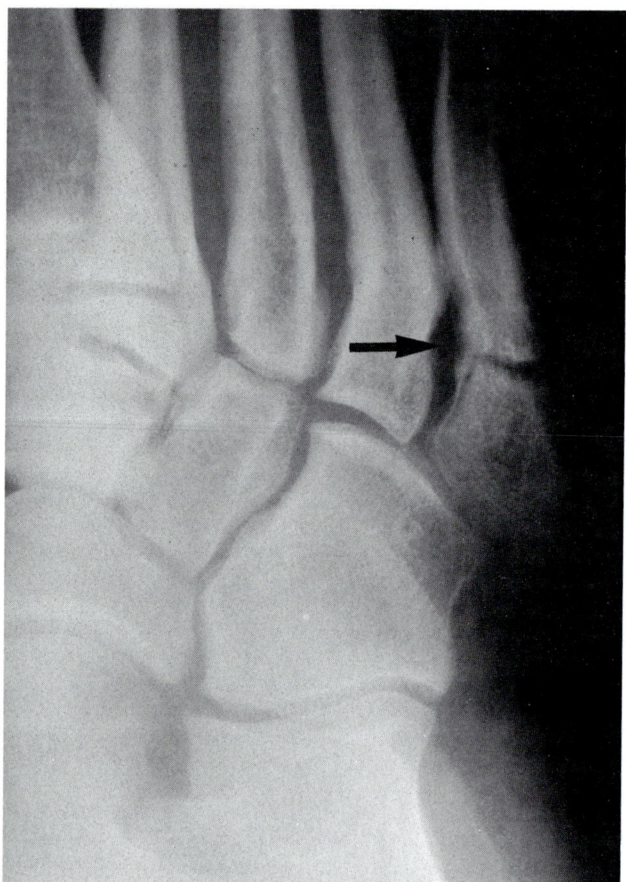

FIG 29–13.
The Jones' fracture of the fifth metatarsal.

of the peroneus brevis. It is usually safe to treat this injury in a loose shoe or removable cast. A great deal of displacement can be accepted here. It rarely needs to be operated upon because fibrous unions at this location are usually pain free. It is important to recognize the difference between this fracture and the Jones fracture of the proximal diaphysis (see above).

Bunionettes

Bunionettes frequently accompany bunions. They can be removed if they are symptomatic, but usually they do not need to be. The dancer should be warned that it can take an extraordinarily long time for the tenderness to subside following these procedures so that they can get into a toe shoe comfortably. For this reason, I usually try to postpone this surgery in professionals until retirement.

THE MIDTARSAL AREA

The Painful Accessory Navicular

Fortunately, for some reason this condition is not common in young dancers. It can become symptomatic following contusion (I have had one case of a fracture of an accessory navicular and one case of a partial avulsion.) When the symptoms warrant, I have had success with simply shelling out the bone rather than the Kidner procedure. Cast immobilization following the procedure is very important. The recovery is often longer than one would expect.

Stress Fracture of the Tarsal Navicular

Stress fracture of the tarsal navicular is rare in dancers. It must be kept in mind, however, and is best diagnosed with a bone scan.

Degeneration in the Tarsometatarsal Joints

Older female dancers routinely develop degeneration of the first and, to a lesser degree, the second tarsometatarsal joints. The appearance of these joints on the x-ray film can be quite dramatic. It is amazing how few symptoms the dancers have from this problem. Decisions regarding debridement of tarsometatarsal fusions must be carefully made on the basis of the clinical disability.

Lisfranc's Dislocation

Lisfranc's dislocation is rare in dancers. It can happen, and when it does, it is usually a pure valgus injury, with disruption of the medial ligaments of the naviculocuneiform or cuneiform-metatarsal joints. This injury can be very subtle, and a careful physical examination, x-ray studies (including a valgus forefoot stress film with a local anesthetic if necessary), and bone scan are advisable. Lisfranc's injury in dancers, as in anyone else, demands anatomic reduction either by closed or open means, usually with internal fixation and non–weight-bearing immobilization.

Sprains at the Base of the Fourth and Fifth Metatarsals

In this area of the foot, the plantar tarsometatarsal ligaments are thick and the dorsal tarsometatarsal capsules are thin. If the dancer falls over the dorsolateral foot in plantar flexion, the tarsometatarsal joints that are normally subjected only to a dorsal force are forced into extreme plantar flexion. This often tears the dorsal capsules at the base of the fourth and fifth tarsometatarsal joints. On several occasions I have seen these capsules trapped in sprained joints producing symptoms. On two occasions, I have had to explore this area for intractable pain. At surgery the invaginated tissue was removed from the joint, and the symptoms were relieved.

THE MEDIAL ANKLE

Posterior Tibial Tendonitis

Posterior tibial tendonitis, so commonly seen in athletes, is a rare occurrence in dancers—an example of altered kinesiology producing changes in the patterns of injury normally found. Working primarily in the equinus position produces stress on the FHL tendon, "the Achilles tendon of the foot," as it passes through its pully behind the medial malleolus. In this position, the posterior tibial tendon is relatively shortened, and the subtalar joint is in inversion. In addition, dancers are selected for, and usually have cavus feet, and these seem less prone to posterior tibial tendonitis. Indeed, more often than not, a dancer diagnosed as having posterior tibial tendonitis will, on careful examination, be found to have FHL tendonitis instead—"dancer's tendonitis."[6, 7, 11, 13]

Medial Sprains of the Ankle

Medial sprains of the ankle are rare because the medial structures are strong and rigid in comparison to the lateral ones. Persistent symptoms on the medial side may be due to an unrecognized stress fracture of the sustentaculum tali that can be picked up on a bone scan or a localized posteromedial fibrous tarsal coalition. Sprains of the medial aspect of the ankle do occur, usually from landing off balance with sudden pronation, but this will be more likely to produce a sprain of the deltoid ligament than a strain of the posterior tibial tendon. The sprain will usually affect the portion of the ligament under tension when the force was applied: the anterior deltoid if the foot was in equinus, the middle deltoid if it was plantargrade, and the posterior portion if the foot was in dorsiflexion (very rare). If a significant injury to the deltoid ligament is found, one must always look for damage to the lateral structures, especially the syndesmosis and proximal end of the fibula. Isolated injuries to the lateral portion of the ankle are common, but isolated injuries to the medial side are rare. An accessory bone, the os subtibiale, may be present in the deep layer of the deltoid (see section on Accessory Bones of the Foot, Chapter 10), and this bone can be involved in the sprain and become symptomatic when it had not been before. An x-ray study should be performed to rule out bone, syndesmosis, or epiphyseal injury. Recovery is usually uneventful. Occasionally, trigger points can form in the deltoid, usually around a chip fracture or accessory ossicle. These may require a corticosteroid injection if they do not respond to conservative therapy. Nodules may form on the flexor digitorum longus or posterior tibial tendons following medial strains, but these are usually not symptomatic.

In the differential diagnosis of medial ankle pain one must keep in mind the possibility of *osteochondritis dissecans* of the talus (Table 29–1). This condition usually occurs in the *posterior* portion of the medial talar dome and the *anterior* portion of the lateral dome. It can cause

TABLE 29–1.
Differential Diagnosis of Medial Ankle Pain in the Dancer

Occurrence	Anatomic Location
Most common	Flexor hallucis longus tendonitis
Less common	Deltoid ligament sprain
Rare	Posterior tibial tendonitis
Very rare	Flexor digitorum longus tendonitis
	The soleus syndrome[22]

vague pains that are hard to localize, and symptoms can be present before the lesion appears on regular x-ray films. If it is suspected, a bone scan, computed tomography (CT), or magnetic resonance imaging (MRI) may be indicated.

In dancers, a common cause of pain around the medial malleolus comes from "rolling in" (pronating) to obtain proper turnout (Fig 29–14). This produces a chronic strain of the deltoid ligament and is one of many overuse syndromes seen in dancers.

Contusion of the medial prominence of the tarsal navicular can occur. This usually happens when one foot is brought forward past the other and, as they pass, the navicular strikes the medial malleolus of the other ankle. These contusions usually heal with symptomatic treatment. On rare occasions a fracture of the medial tubercle or disruption of an accessory navicular can occur. If the symptoms warrant, it should be treated in a short-leg walking cast or ankle-foot orthosis (AFO) for 4 to 6 weeks to prevent the injury from becoming chronic.

Sprains of the spring ligament and/or the plantar fascia can be mistaken for medial ankle pain, but a careful physical examination should make the diagnosis apparent.

Another cause of medial pain just above the medial malleolus is the *soleus syndrome*.[22] This presents as chronic pain resembling a shinsplint but too far distal on the posteromedial tibial metaphysis to be a true shinsplint. It is caused by an abnormal slip in the origin of the soleus muscle, usually 3 to 6 cm above the medial malleolus. Normally, the tibial origin of the soleus ends at the junction of the middle and distal thirds of the tibia. In this syndrome, the origin continues down the tibia to just above the medial malleolus. This condition, similar to a compartment syndrome, is much more common in athletes who engage in sustained muscular activity than in dancers, whose efforts are usually intermittent. It will usually respond to conservative therapy. On rare occasions, subcutaneous release of the tight band may be necessary.

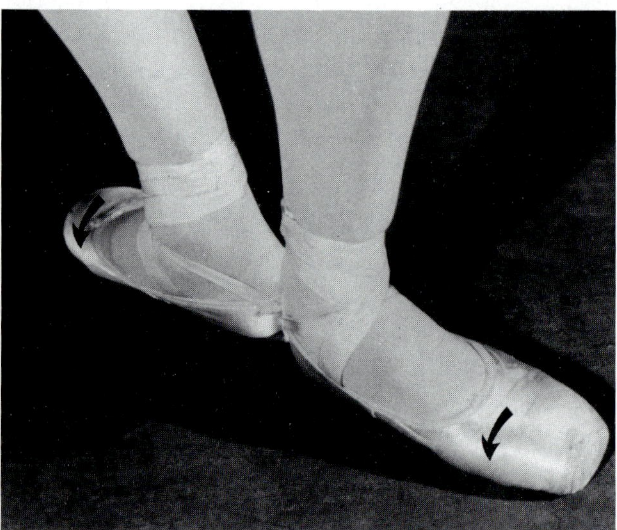

FIG 29–14.
"Rolling in" (pronating) to gain additional turnout.

THE ANTERIOR ANKLE

Impingement Syndromes

Dancers are selected for an extreme range of motion in their joints and for cavus feet to give them maximum plantar flexion of the foot and ankle. In spite of this extreme motion they will constantly take the joints of the lower extremity to the limits of their motion. The cavus foot has increased plantar flexion but decreased dorsiflexion. For this reason impingement syndromes of the ankle are very common. They occur anteromedially and posterolaterally. When motion in the ankle is limited by impingement, dancers and sometimes dance teachers will blame the Achilles tendon for the lack of dorsiflexion and will spend hours trying to stretch the posterior structures of the calf to obtain a better plié when, in reality, there is no more dorsiflexion possible in the talocrural joint. (It would not increase, even if the Achilles were severed.) This fact must often be explained to the dancer, i.e., that the lack of dorsiflexion is not due to tightness in the Achilles.

The most common cause of anterior ankle pain in the dancer is the *anterior impingement syndrome*.[7, 19, 20, 24] It is typically seen in the older male dancer with cavus feet who has spent his career dancing the "bravura" technique, i.e., high jumps and deep pliés. The impingement of the bones, one on the other, stimulates the cambium layer of the periosteum to form exostoses, like stalactites in a cave. When they form, they limit dorsiflexion, facilitate further impingement, result in more periosteal stimulation, etc., thus setting up a repetitive cycle. As the spurs build up, they can break off and become loose bodies.

Diagnosis is made on the basis of the history, physical examination and x-ray studies. On physical examination the following signs are usually present:

1. Anterior tenderness and thickening of the synovium, often with an effusion.
2. Palpable osteophytes.
3. Limited dorsiflexion when compared with the opposite ankle.
4. A positive "dorsiflexion sign" i.e., pain with forced dorsiflexion of the ankle with the knee flexed.

A standard lateral x-ray film of the ankle will usually show the spurs. If further information is needed, a weight-bearing lateral view in maximum dorsiflexion can be taken (Fig 29–15).

Conservative treatment consists of making the dancer aware of the problem and having him not "hit bottom" in his plié. Heel lifts will help open up the front of the ankle and relieve the symptoms, but dancers often find these difficult to dance in. "Show dancers" (Broadway or Las Vegas–type dancers) who dance in "character shoes" will often tolerate heel lifts and orthoses much better than ballet dancers do.

Dancers with loose ankles secondary to repeated ankle sprains also tend to form these impingement spurs. In this situation, consideration should be given to tightening the ankle ligaments at the time of the anterior cleanout—preferably by the Brostrom-Gould procedure, q.v.

If symptoms are disabling, an anterior debridement either through a small anteromedial incision or through the arthroscope may be indicated. The anterior impingement syndrome of the ankle usually occurs in one of three types depending upon the location of the exostoses:

1. Primarily on the anterior lip of the tibia.
2. Primarily on the neck of the talus.
3. A combination of both.

The first type can be easily removed with the arthroscope. In my opinion, the second and third types are best treated with a small arthrotomy behind the anterior tibial tendon. The open method in these cases is faster and more thorough than arthroscopy. When ankle arthroscopy became popular, I performed many arthroscopic anterior debridements in the hope of facilitating an earlier return to dancing. I found that it took 3 months to return to full dancing with either technique and the arthroscopic cases were taking 1 to 1½ hours vs. 20 to 30 minutes with the open technique. I presently do them open except for the type that involves only the anterior lip of the tibia, which I do arthroscopically.

One should always look for an impingement exostosis on the medial shoulder of the talus that impinges against the anterior portion of the medial malleolus. This spur can be hard to visualize on an x-ray film but can contribute considerably to the symptoms. Dancers undergoing this operation should be warned that although the cleanout is a relatively minor procedure with minimal risk, it may take 3 to 4 months before they will get back all of their plié.

There are several conditions that can mimic the anterior impingement syndrome:

1. Osteochondritis dissecans of the talus.
2. An acute or chronic "high" ankle sprain involving the anterior tibiofibular (ATF) ligament.
3. "Bassett's ligament," an aberrant distal insertion of the ATF ligament that can cause persistent symptoms[1] (Fig 29–16)
4. DJD of the tibiotalar or talonavicular joints, especially in the early phases when the x-ray findings are subtle.
5. An osteoid osteoma in the tarsal navicular (Fig 29–17).

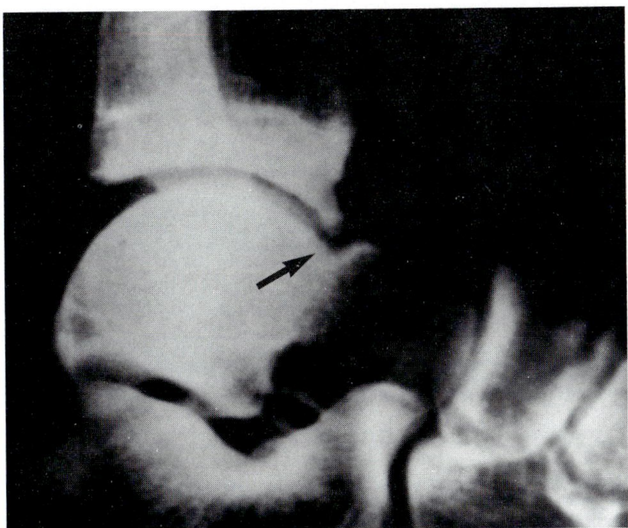

FIG 29–15.
Anterior impingement of the ankle.

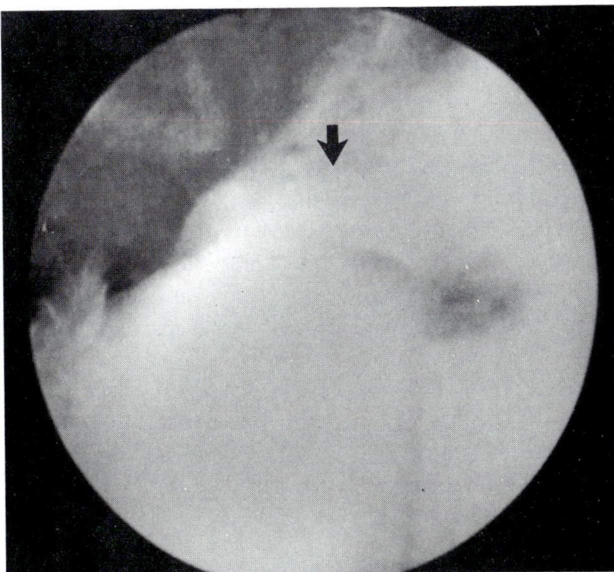

FIG 29–16.
"Bassett's" ligament: arthroscopic view of the right ankle seen through the anteromedial portal.

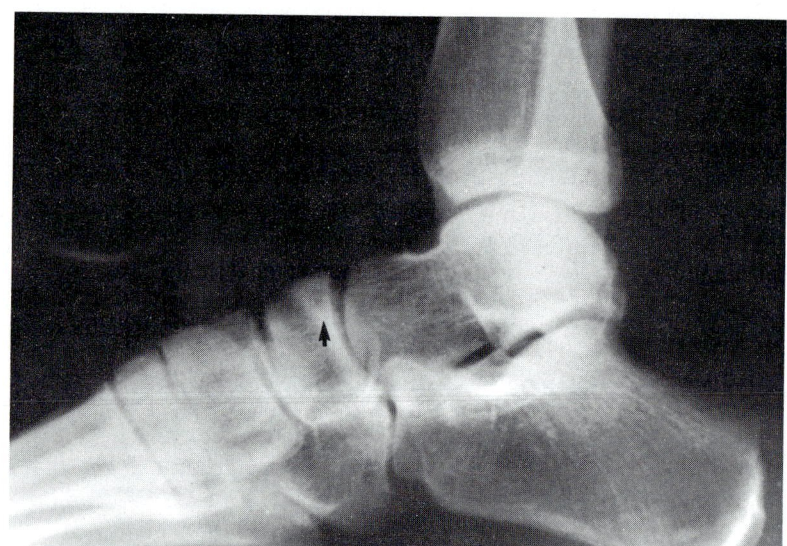

FIG 29–17.
An osteoid osteoma in the tarsal navicular.

These conditions will usually give a characteristic picture on either the radiograph or the bone scan.

Tendonitis

Anterior tibial, EHL, and extensor digitorum longus tendonitis, like posterior tibial tendonitis, is very rare in dancers. Symptoms in this area are almost always due to ankle impingement. Irritation of the extensor tendons in the anterior extensor retinaculum can occur. This is often due to either a ganglion in the region or to tightness in an elastic strap passing over this area. This strap is sewn into the shoe by the dancer to hold the shoe on. The position of the strap on the dance shoe should be adjusted so that it does not press against the extensor retinaculum if there are symptoms in that area.

Irritation of the EHL can occur in the region of the medial cuneiform–first metatarsal joint. A bossing, or exostosis, is often found on the dorsum of this joint in older dancers, exactly where the EHL tendon and the deep branch of the peroneal nerve pass over it. Any tight shoe or strap in this area will press the tendon down against the underlying bone and cause pain and irritation. It is rarely necessary to remove this exostosis surgically; instead, the dancer should simply avoid direct pressure on the tendon in the region of the exostosis. Recurrent or recalcitrant symptoms may be an indication for surgery. The surgeon should be extremely careful when operating in this area—incisional neuromas are very common here!

THE LATERAL ANKLE

The most common acute injury in dance is an inversion sprain of the ankle.[10, 20] (Remember, ligaments "sprain," and tendons and muscles "strain.") Sprains may occur in any ligament in the foot or ankle, but the most common ones involve the lateral ligament complex of the ankle (the ATF, the calcaneofibular (CF), and the posterior talofibular ligaments); the ATF ligament; the lateral talocalcaneal ligament; and occasionally, the medial (deltoid) ligament. The posterior talofibular ligament is rarely if ever injured.

Other conditions, however, can closely resemble the classic lateral ankle sprain. The exact mechanism of injury may not always be apparent, especially in dancers who may have been in the pointe position when the injury occurred. In this position, many possible combinations of forces may have taken place. Some of these injuries even occur in a helical or corkscrew manner whereby both inversion and eversion forces are placed on the ankle in the same injury. The physician is well advised to examine the patient carefully for the following conditions that can simulate or accompany a simple sprain:

1. A complete tear of the lateral collateral structures (in actuality, a medial dislocation of the talus that has spontaneously reduced, or the ultimate grade III sprain).
2. An injury to the anterior inferior tibiofibular ligament, the "high" ankle sprain (more common in pronation/external rotation injuries than in inversions).
3. A complete tear of both the distal anterior and posterior tibiofibular ligaments (the syndesmosis) and the interosseous membrane without fracture of the malleoli but with diastasis of the ankle mortise and, frequently, fracture of the proximal isthmus of the fibula—the "Maisonneuve fracture."
4. A sprain of the subtalar joint with disruption of the CF ligament and the lateral talocalcaneal ligament.
5. A fracture of the base of the fifth metatarsal.

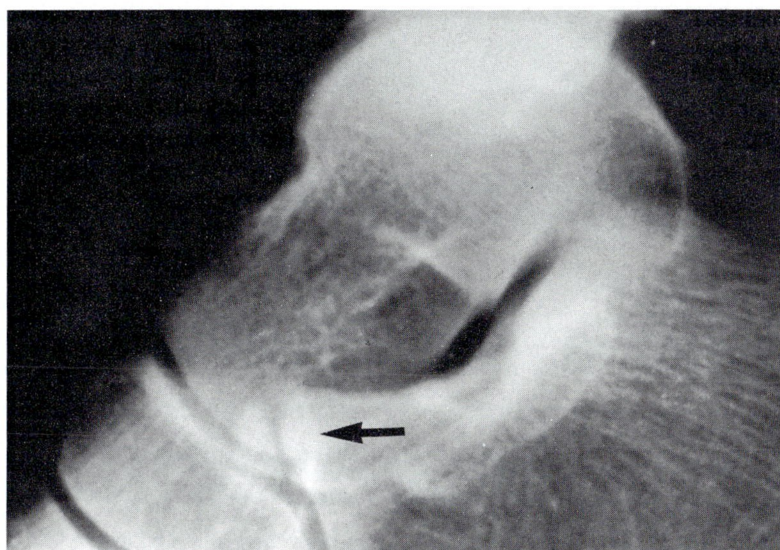

FIG 29–18.
An anterior process fracture of the os calcis.

6. An undisplaced fracture of the lateral malleolus or, in a young dancer, the malleolar epiphysis.
7. A fracture of the lateral process of the talus.[17]
8. A fracture of the anterior process of the os calcis in the sinus tarsi[16] (Fig 29–18).
9. Subluxation of the cuboid.[21, 23]
10. A fracture of the posterior lip of the distal end of the tibia or fracture of a trigonal process behind the talus (shepherd's fracture).[27] (See section on Accessory Bones of the Foot, Chapter 10.)
11. A lateral sprain of the tarsometatarsal (Lisfranc's) joints.
12. Rupture of the Achilles tendon.

Classification of Ankle Sprains

Ankle sprains are usually graded as I, II, or III depending upon the extent of the injury[10] (Table 29–2).

Grade I sprains are partial tears, usually of the ATF ligament or occasionally the ATF ligament with little or no resultant instability. On physical examination the drawer sign and the stress films are normal. After the initial 48 hours of "RICE" (rest, ice, compression, elevation), the patient should begin early active use of the limb with a compression bandage, taping, or an "Aircast."

Grade II sprains are complete tears, usually of the ATF ligament, with minimal damage to the CF ligament. They produce a moderately positive drawer sign but a normal or minimal talar tilt on the stress film. They often result in some residual instability, although this can usually be controlled by good peroneal strength. Treatment consists of some type of support, either taping, Aircast, or a walking plaster cast for 3 to 6 weeks followed by aggressive peroneal rehabilitation.

The Grade II sprain is the type of ankle sprain most commonly seen in dancers. It usually occurs when they are on demi-pointe (up on the ball of the foot). In this position, the ATF ligament is almost vertical—in the position normally taken by the CF ligament when the foot is plantargrade, and it is easily torn when an adduction-inversion force is applied. In this position, the CF ligament is almost parallel to the floor; it is out of harm's way and is rarely injured.

TABLE 29–2.
Working Classification of Acute Ankle Sprains*

Grade	Anatomic Injury†	Physical Examination (Drawer Sign)	X-ray Findings
I	Partial tear; ATF or CF	Negative or 1+ drawer sign	Neg. drawer sign Neg. talar tilt
II	Torn ATF, intact CF	2+ Drawer sign	Pos. drawer sign Neg. talar tilt
III	Torn ATF, torn CF	3+ Drawer sign	Pos. drawer sign Pos. talar tilt

*Adapted from Hamilton WG: "Dancer's tendonitis" of the FHL tendon, American Orthopedic Society for Sports Medicine, Durango, Colo, July, 1976.
†ATF = anterior talofibular; CF = calcaneofibular.

The *grade III sprain* is fortunately a rare injury. It consists of complete rupture of the lateral ligament complex (i.e., the ATF and the CF ligaments—I have never seen a tear of the posterior talofibular ligament and doubt that such a thing exists). This injury results in gross instability. It is actually a spontaneously reduced medial dislocation of the talus. The drawer sign and stress films are grossly positive on physical examination and x-ray studies. The healing time is long and uncertain, 3 to 4 months, and the likelihood of persistent laxity of the ligaments is significant. Dancers with residual laxity of the lateral ankle ligaments from this injury usually complain more of *rotatory instability* than of varus instability, i.e., they develop anterolateral rotatory instability of the ankle analogous to ligament injuries of the knee. For this reason, many orthopaedists, including myself, feel that grade III lateral ankle sprains in **professional** athletes and dancers should be surgically repaired primarily (within 7 to 10 days of the injury if possible). The repair itself is a simple procedure done under regional anesthesia with a small incision over the distal portion of the fibula (see the Brostrom-Gould procedure described below). The ligaments are easily identified, as they are within the capsule, similar to the anterior capsule of the shoulder. They are usually avulsed from the fibula rather than torn in their midsubstance, which makes them easy to reattach. Occasionally, the CF ligament is avulsed from the calcaneus rather than the fibula, thus making the repair somewhat more difficult. Postoperative immobilization in a short-leg walking cast for 4 weeks is followed by protection in an Aircast and early rehabilitation. Recreational dancers should be treated in a short-leg walking cast or analogous removable splint for a month.

Stress films can be performed in the office with a local anesthetic if necessary. I have found, along with other authors, that the drawer sign is a better sign of the extent of the injury as well as a better predictor of later dysfunction than is the stress x-ray film.[7, 15]

Treatment

Conservative Treatment

Regardless of the method of treatment, adequate physical therapy and proper rehabilitation are necessary to restore normal use following injury. Restoration of full peroneal strength is essential. Unrecognized peroneal weakness is a common condition in dancers[9, 10] and can be the cause of a myriad of obscure symptoms such as unexplained swelling and discomfort or poor timing with "beats." Any dancer complaining of these symptoms should be checked for weak peroneals. This is done by having the dancer place her foot in full plantar flexion and neutral abduction/adduction (the "tendu" position) and asking her to hold this position against varus and then valgus stress (Fig 29–19). A well-conditioned dancer should be able to resist as much force as one can manually apply to the foot in this position. The uninjured side can be checked for comparison if necessary. Often, they have either not been adequately rehabilitated, or they have been exercising in the neutral position rather than full plantar flexion. (Cybex and other exercise machines are not very good for ankle rehabilitation because they cannot be placed in full plantar flexion.) I use a home exercise program over the end of a sofa or couch with the dancer on her side using a weight bag in *full plantar flexion* (Fig 29–20). Abduction exercises are performed with the ankle supported so that it can only move upward in valgus and the patient can re-

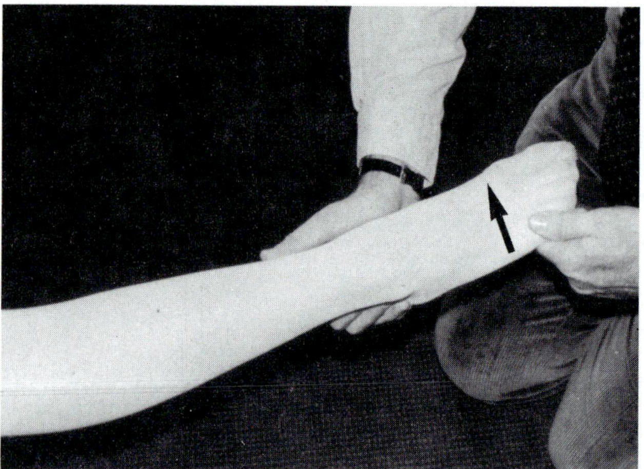

FIG 29–19.
Testing peroneal strength; the dancer should be able to resist full manual pressure.

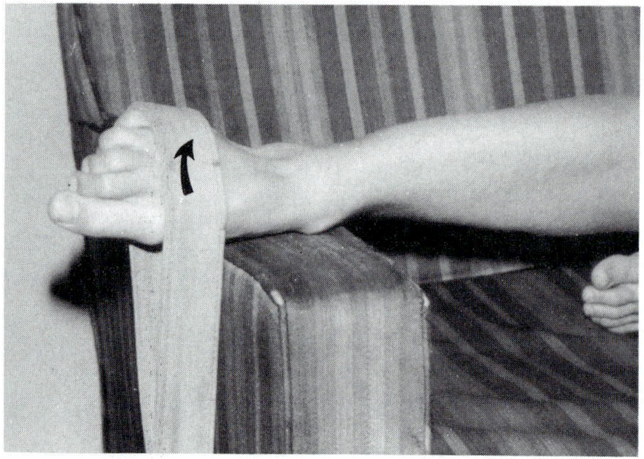

FIG 29–20.
Peroneal exercises done in full plantar flexion.

lax the ankle between lifts. They lift 3 lb, 25 times slowly, morning and evening, and increase the weight in the bag by 3 lb each week to a total of 15 lb. When they can lift 15 lb slowly 25 times they are adequately rehabilitated. I have never seen this method fail to restore normal peroneal strength. The symptoms do not always disappear, and if they do not you have to look elsewhere for the problem (when in doubt, get a bone scan).

Surgical Treatment

Secondary or delayed ankle ligament reconstruction is occasionally necessary in a dancer, but it should only be considered after full peroneal strength has been obtained (see above) and the dancer is still unable to dance. Often, as previously mentioned, the problem is rotatory instability rather than varus instability. It must be emphasized that reconstruction should be done only for *functional* difficulties and not simply on the basis of a drawer sign or a positive stress x-ray finding. There are many professional dancers dancing quite well with loose ankles that are not symptomatic enough to warrant surgical repair.

I feel strongly that the peroneus brevis tendon should not be used for ankle reconstruction in a professional dancer for two reasons. First, the peroneus brevis is too important as a support tendon for dancing on full pointe to be sacrificed. Second, it is not necessary to use it—I have had excellent results with the Brostrom repair as described by Gould et al.[3] The procedure is simply a reefing of the ATF and CF ligaments with reattachment to their anatomic locations on the fibula and then sewing the lateral extensor retinaculum over the tip of the fibula in a "pants-over-vest" manner to limit inversion. The patient is placed in a short-leg walking cast for 1 month, and then the leg is taken out for rehabilitation and swimming and protected in a removable Aircast for another 2 to 3 weeks. In 20 professional dancers, this technique has not failed to give an excellent result with full range of motion and normal strength. A 10-year follow-up of my first case has not revealed any stretching out of the repaired ligaments in spite of another sprain in the same ankle.[15]

Technique for the Modified Brostrom Repair for Acute and Chronic Lateral Ankle Instability

1. The operation is performed with the patient in the lateral decubitus position. A thigh tourniquet is used over cast padding, so general, spinal, or epidural anesthesia is needed.
2. A curvilinear incision is made along the anterior border of the distal portion of the fibula and stops at the peroneal tendons (Fig 29–21,A). (The sural nerve is just below this area, lying directly upon the peroneal tendons.) The lesser saphenous vein usually crosses the distal end of the fibula at this level and will have to be divided.
3. The dissection is carried down to the joint capsule along the anterior border of the lateral malleolus.
4. The lateral portion of the extensor retinaculum is then identified (Fig 29–21,B). It is dissected off the capsule and mobilized so that it can be pulled over the repair at the end of the procedure. Care should be taken when working anterior to the malleolus because the lateral branch of the superficial peroneal nerve often lies in this area and can be damaged by dissection or a sharp retractor.
5. The capsule is then divided along the anterior border of the fibula down to the peroneal tendons and a 2- to 3-mm cuff left. The ATF ligament lies within this capsule, similar to the anterior glenohumeral ligaments of the shoulder. It can frequently be identified as a thickening in the capsule.
6. The CF ligament must now be identified. It lies deep to the peroneal tendons and runs obliquely downward and posterior to the calcaneus. It will often be stretched out and attenuated, or it may be dislodged so that it lies *outside* the peroneals. If it is in continuity, it is divided and a cuff left at its insertion in the fibula. By leaving a cuff of tissue at the insertion of the ligaments, the surgeon will be able to repair the ligaments in their anatomic locations, thus preserving isometry and supplying an unrestricted range of motion.
7. The ligaments must now be shortened and repaired. The ankle should be placed in the fully reduced position in neutral dorsiflexion and slight eversion. The stumps of the ligaments are pulled up, and the redundancy is trimmed (Fig 29–21,C).
8. The ligaments are then sutured to their anatomic locations with 2–0 nonabsorbable sutures, starting with the CF ligament (because it is the most difficult to visualize) and then proceeding to the ATF ligament (Fig 29–21,D). This repair can be done by end-to-end suture, "pants over vest," or into drill holes.
9. At this point the ankle should be examined for stability and range of motion.
10. The previously identified lateral extensor mechanism is then pulled over the repair and sutured to the tip of the fibula with 2–0 chronic catgut (Fig 29–21,E). This accomplishes three things:
    a. It reinforces the repair.
    b. It limits inversion (the position of injury).
    c. It helps correct the *subtalar component* of the in-

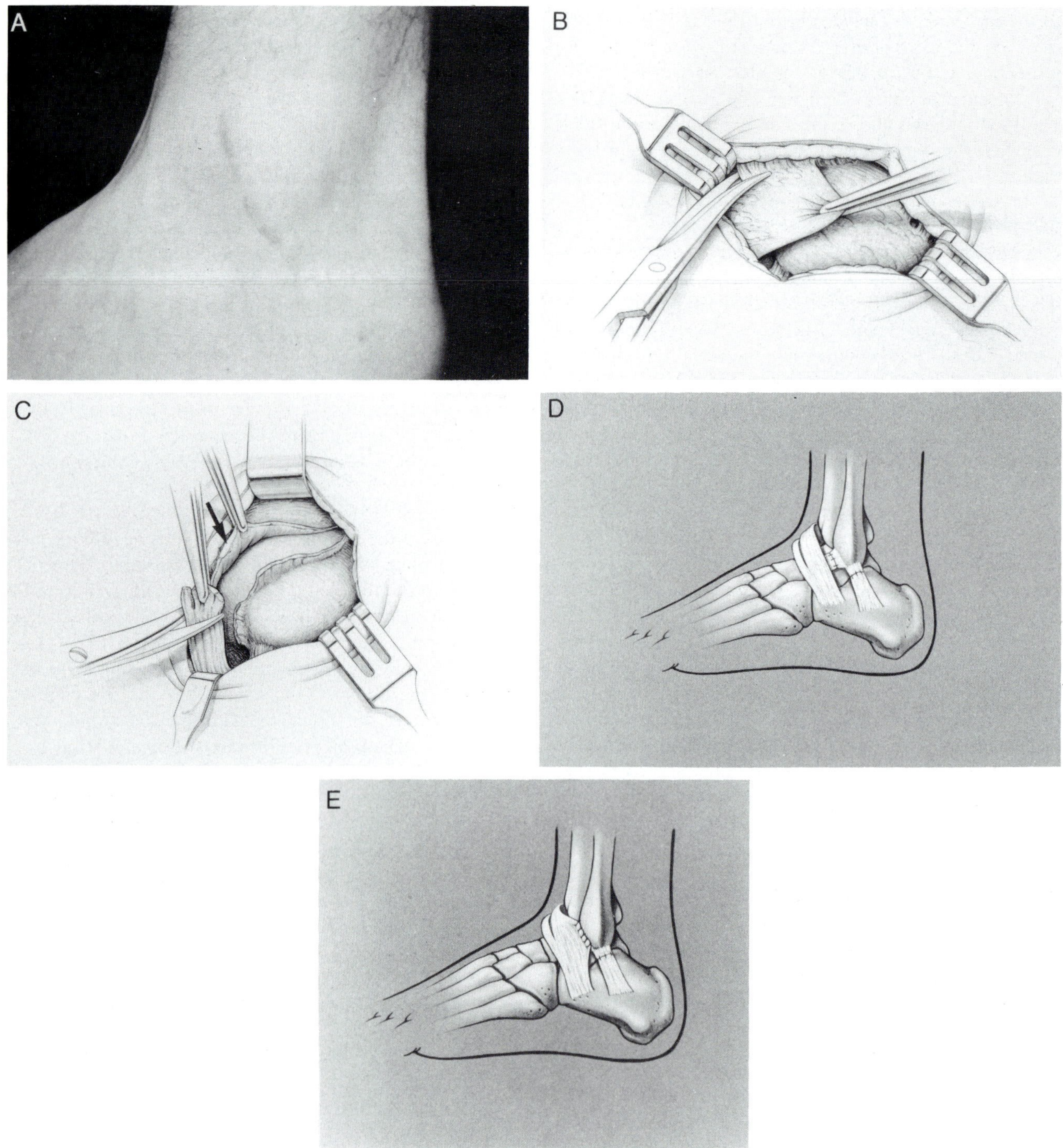

FIG 29–21.

A, the skin incision. **B,** the lateral external retinaulum is identified and mobilized (left ankle). **C,** the capsular incision. The calcaneofibular ligament is being trimmed. The anterior talofibular ligament is seen as a thickening in the capsule. **D,** capsular repair after the anterior talofibular and calcaneofibular ligaments have been shortened. **E,** the extensor retinaculum is sutured over the capsular repair. (From Westwood WB: *Strategies Orthop Surg* 9:1, 1990. Used by permission.)

stability. (If the CF ligament is attenuated, there will have to be some degree of subtalar instability—the CF ligament is one of the stabilizing ligaments of the subtalar joint.[7, 20]

11. The ankle is once again checked for stability and taken through a full range of motion. A layered closure is then performed with an absorbable subcutaneous suture and steri-strips. The patient is placed in anteroposterior plaster splints and discharged non-weight bearing with crutches.

Postoperative Care.—When the swelling has subsided, in 5 to 7 days, a short-leg walking cast is applied for 3 to 4 weeks. The cast is then removed and the ankle protected with an air splint. Swimming, range-of-motion, and isometric peroneal exercises are begun. Unrestricted activities are allowed at 10 to 12 weeks *if full peroneal strength is present.*

The Sprained Ankle That Will Not Heal

Miscellaneous problems following ankle sprains are not uncommon.

A trigonal process may be fractured (shepherd's fracture) at the time of the injury and may continue to be symptomatic after the sprain heals. (A bone scan is recommended.)

Dancers will often develop an FHL tendonitis and/or posterior impingement following an ankle sprain, occasionally involving an os trigonum that had previously been asymptomatic.[7, 10] These complications are not always related to the severity of the sprain.

A unique type of posterior impingement may follow grade III sprains with residual ligamentous laxity. In this condition, the loose ATF ligament cannot hold the talus under the tibial plafond in the full relevé position, and the talus slips forward and allows the posterior lip of the tibia to settle down upon the os calcis (Fig 29–22).

If there is looseness in the ankle, an anterior impingement may follow with osteophyte formation in the anterior tibiotalar joint secondary to rotatory instability, often opposite the tip of the medial malleolus.

An osteochondral fracture or osteochondritis dissecans may be present.

Problems around the tip of the fibula may persist after the sprain heals:

1. Soft-tissue entrapment (the "meniscoid" of the ankle).[32]
2. An avulsion fracture of the tip of the fibula.
3. A previously asymptomatic accessory ossicle (the os subfibulare).
4. An unrecognized fracture of the anterior process of the os calcis. This fracture is an avulsion fracture of the extensor digitorum brevis origin[16] (see Fig 29–18).
5. Damage to the peroneal tendons found following sprains. Often the peroneus brevis has longitudinal tears, and the tendon becomes enlarged and flattened. This condition can usually be diagnosed by a peroneal tenogram or with an MRI study.[26]
6. Peroneus longus tendonitis around the os peroneum.
7. A fracture of an os peroneum.
8. A lateral process fracture of the talus.[17]
9. The sinus tarsi syndrome.[28]
10. Subluxation of the cuboid.[21, 23]

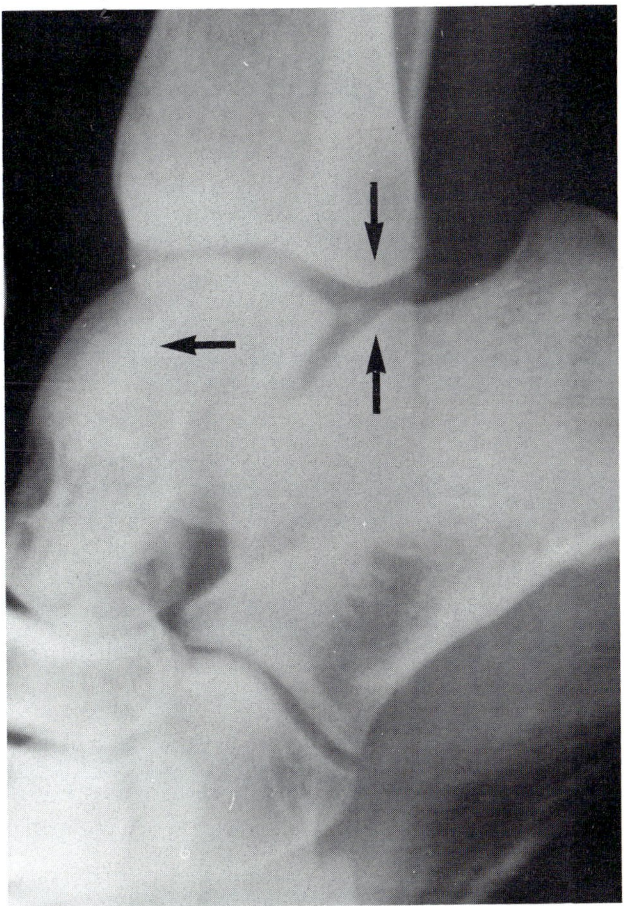

FIG 29–22.
Posterior impingement of the ankle secondary to loose lateral ligaments.

The *"high" ankle sprain* of the distal tibiofibular syndesmosis should be recognized as a different entity from the common sprained ankle seen at the lateral malleolus. This injury represents a partial tear of the anterior tibiofibular ligament in the syndesmosis, usually by pronation/external rotation. It can take an extraordinary long time to heal and may be associated with an avulsion fracture at the tibial or fibular origin of the ligament—the "fracture of Tillaux." Treatment of this injury should be aggressively conservative, and the dancer should be warned at the beginning that it can be symptomatic for as long as 3 to 6 months. There have been cases that remained symptomatic in spite of time and conservative therapy. Surgical exploration of these ankles has revealed the following states:

1. A rent in the ligament with a synovial hernia.
2. Entrapment of tissue in the syndesmosis.
3. A Tillaux fragment too small to see on the x-ray film.
4. "Bassett's ligament," a slip of the anterior inferior tibiotalar ligament that inserts so far down on the fibula that it causes irritation of the shoulder of the talus.[1]
5. "Ferkel's phenomenon," scar tissue in the anterolateral gutter, similar to Bassett's ligament.[2]

Acute peroneal dislocation is usually obvious, but chronic peroneal subluxation in dancers can sometimes be difficult to diagnose. This condition should be kept in mind in any dancer with vague but persistent symptoms such as "giving way" in the peroneal area. Repair of *recurrent dislocating peroneal tendons* is done similar to the Brostrom-Gould procedure, i.e., by taking down the retinaculum, shortening it to its proper length, and reattaching it to its anatomic location on the posterior border of the distal end of the fibula. The patient must be kept in a short-leg walking cast for 6 weeks. As usual, postoperative rehabilitation is essential.

THE POSTERIOR ANKLE

Two things separate ballet from other forms of dancing; the 180 degrees of turnout at the hips and the ballerina dancing on full pointe in a toe shoe. Thus, the full equinus position is essential for proper ballet technique, especially in females. Not only should there be at least 90 degrees of plantar flexion in the foot-ankle complex, but preferably 10 to 15 degrees more than that to compensate for the recurvatum usually present in the knee above.

The shape of the dome of the talus can vary considerably from one individual to another. Some are round like an oil drum and have excellent motion, both in plantar flexion and dorsiflexion. Others are congenitally flattened and have very limited motion. It is possible that these tali can be molded and improved to some degree by beginning training at an early age while the bones are growing, but a stiff flatfoot and flat, domed talus will never achieve the desired amount of motion, and this dancer is far better off choosing a career in some other form of dancing than ballet.

A considerable amount of this dorsiflexion and plantar flexion comes from the subtalar joint and from the basic turned-out position assumed by the dancer. This position of mild forefoot pronation and abduction loosens the subtalar joint and allows maximum motion. This can be seen by comparing a lateral x-ray film in the plantargrade position with one on relevé. The subtalar space will usually open considerably when the dancer goes on pointe (Fig 29–23). Dancers with a tarsal coalition are usually "weeded out" of ballet early because this condition limits motion in the foot-ankle complex and produces a poor relevé—often before the onset of pain and discomfort. Lack of subtalar motion can be very subtle, for tarsal coalitions can exist in a spectrum from solid and bony to cartilaginous or fibrous with moderate loss of motion. These subtle coalitions are usually located posteriorly (often in association with an os trigonum) (see section on Accessory Bones of the

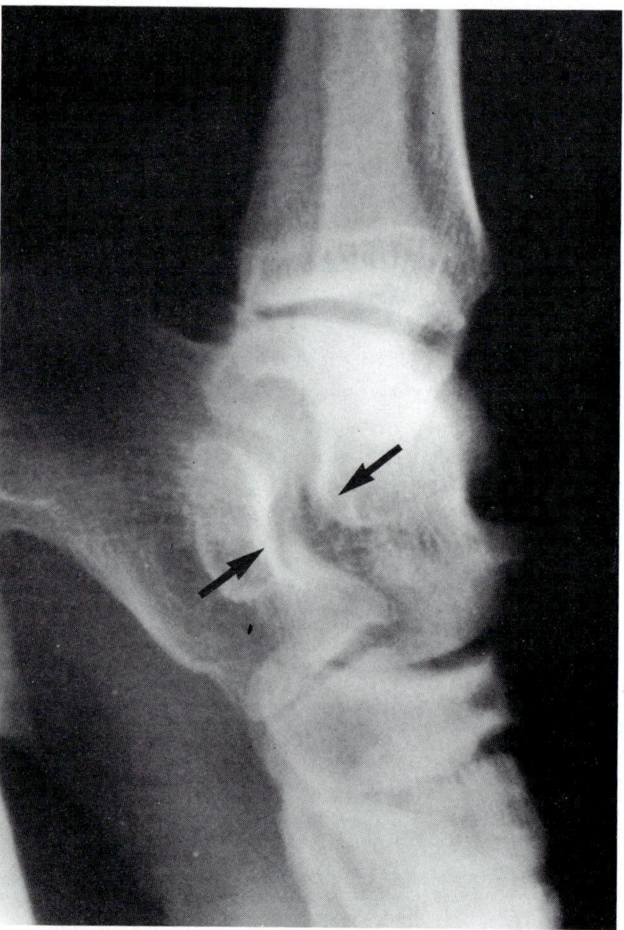

FIG 29–23.
Opening of the subtalar joint in relevé.

Foot, Chapter 10) and are caused by marked fibrosis and thickening of the posterior talocalcaneal ligament complex surrounding the os trigonum or posterior lateral tubercle of the talus.

Early training usually produces a notch in the neck of the talus to accept the anterior lip of the tibia and allow a deep plié (Fig 29–24). Conversely, some posterior molding may be necessary, especially if there is an os trigonum or trigonal process present. In the younger age group (13 to 16 years), posterior ankle pain frequently occurs when an os trigonum is present and full plantar flexion is limited, especially if the other ankle is normal. The symptoms in this situation are usually due to the machinations that the young dancer is going through to force the "bad" ankle to go down as far as the "good" one. These include hooking the toes underneath the piano and levering the forefoot into equinus, sitting on the heels with the foot in full plantar flexion or having one of their friends do this, etc. The diagnosis should be made and the problem explained to the dancer and her family. The symptoms will usually subside when she stops forcing the ankle and understands that the lack of motion is due to a bony block and that the ankle cannot go any further down, no matter how hard she pushes it.

Posterior Impingement Syndrome

The posterior impingement syndrome of the ankle, or "talar compression syndrome"[11, 18, 25] (Fig 29–25), is the natural result of full weight bearing in maximum plantar flexion of the ankle in the demi-pointe or full pointe position, especially if an os trigonum or trigonal process is present. It presents as posterior lateral pain (see Table 29–3) in the back of the ankle when the posterior lip of the tibia closes against the superior border of the os calcis as in the tendu, frappé, relevé, or leaving the ground in a jump. It can be confirmed on physical examination by tenderness behind the peroneal tendons in back of the lateral malleolus (it is often mistaken for peroneal tendonitis) and by pain with forced passive plantar flexion of the ankle—the "plantar flexion sign."[7] The syndrome is often but not always associated with an os trigonum or trigonal process in the back of the ankle. On occasion the syndrome can be caused by soft-tissue entrapment between the posterior lip of the talus and the os calcis. It also can be found in association with lateral ligament laxity. It is often mistaken for heel pain, Achilles' tendonitis, or peroneal tendonitis and is a common problem in ballet dancers.

The posterior aspect of the talus normally has two tubercles, the medial tubercle and the lateral tubercle.

TABLE 29–3.
Posterior Ankle Pain Syndromes in Dancers

Posteromedial	Posterolateral
Flexor hallucis longus tendonitis	Posterior impingement (os trigonum syndrome)
Soleus syndrome	Fracture of the trigonal process (shepherd's fracture)
Posterior tibial tendonitis	Peroneal tendonitis
Posteromedial fibrous tarsal coalition	Pseudomeniscus syndrome

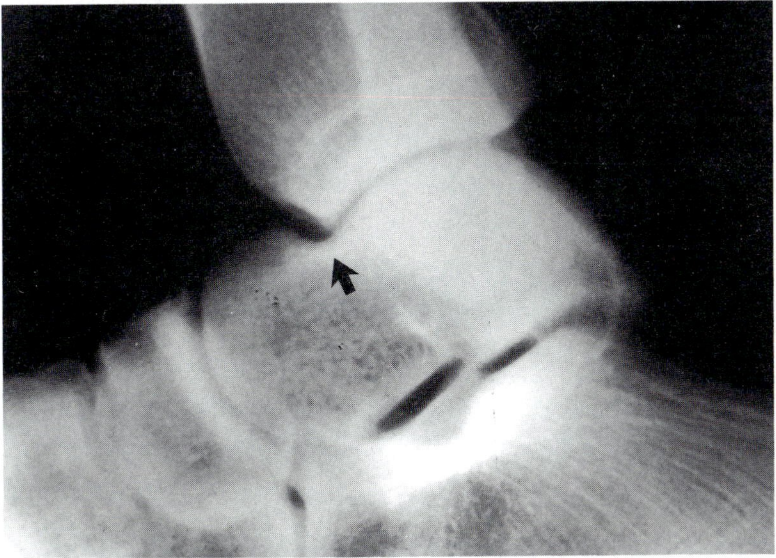

FIG 29–24.
The notch in the neck of the talus that allows a deep plié.

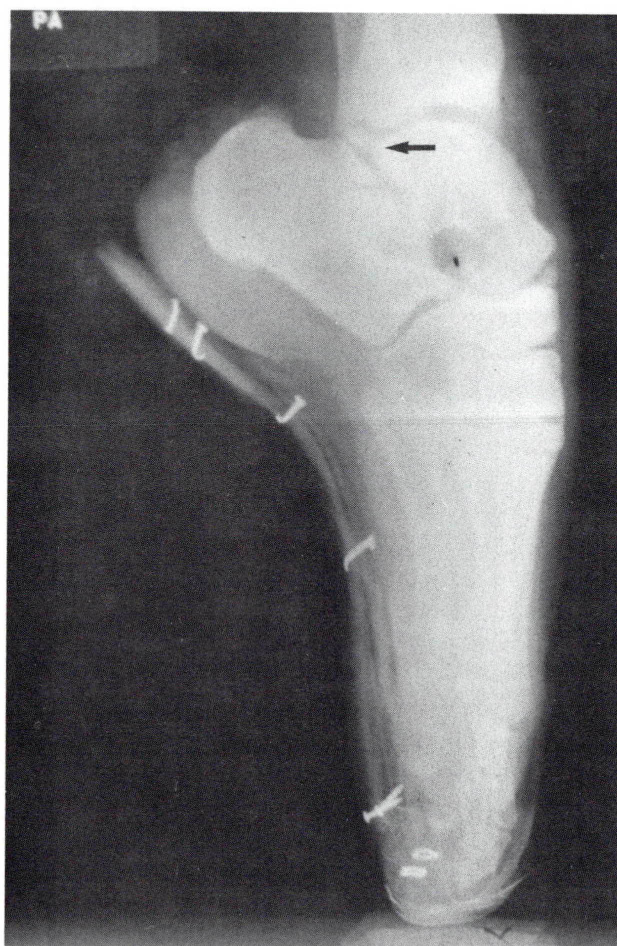

FIG 29–25.
Posterior impingement against an os trigonum.

Between the two tubercles lies the fibro-osseous tunnel of the FHL tendon. The os trigonum is the ununited lateral tubercle on the posterior aspect of the talus. It is present in 7% to 10% of people and has a 50% incidence of bilaterality.[4] Most people who have an os trigonum are not aware of its presence, and the posterior impingement syndrome is rare in athletes. In dancers, it may or may not be symptomatic, and the degree of symptomatology is not always related to the size of the os trigonum. Large ones can be minimally symptomatic, and small ones can sometimes be disabling. Usually the symptoms are mild, and on the whole, the os trigonum is more often asymptomatic than symptomatic. Many world-famous ballerinas have asymptomatic os trigona, and they work with them without any trouble. It is important to stress this fact to the patient and her mother when discussing the problem because the condition is frequently overdiagnosed and surgery may be recommended unnecessarily—perhaps due to the dramatic appearance of the bone on the x-ray film. It is best seen on a lateral view of the ankle on pointe or in full plantar flexion. Tomograms, bone scans, and CT may be helpful, but the diagnosis can usually be made by injecting ½ to ¾ cc of lidocaine (Xylocaine) into the posterior soft tissues behind the peroneal tendons. If the pain that was present is relieved by this small injection, the diagnosis is almost certain. If the patient is not pain free, then another diagnosis should be considered (see Tables 29–3 and 29–4). The differential diagnosis includes the following:

1. Posterior process fracture: hairline or stress.
2. FHL tendonitis ("dancer's tendonitis").
3. Peroneal tendonitis.
4. Posteromedial localized talocalcaneal coalition.
5. Osteoid osteoma.

Treatment

Treatment of the posterior impingement syndrome should follow an orderly sequence. The first approach, similar to that with tendonitis, is modification of activities ("Don't do what hurts."), nonsteroidal anti-inflammatory drugs (NSAIDs) if the dancer is over 16 years of age, and physical therapy. As noted above, if the patient is forcing the foot into equinus to achieve further plantar flexion, she must be instructed to not do this. Patients should be told that it will take a few weeks for the pain to subside—usually as long as they have been dancing with the condition before they begin treatment (e.g., if they have been working with the pain for a month, then it will often take a month of treatment and reduced activities before they can resume normal activities without discomfort). In cases where this approach has failed or the symptoms recur and the patient is 16 years or older, an injection of ½ to ¾ cc of a mixture of a long- and short-acting corticosteroid can often give dramatic and permanent relief of symptoms. Before injecting the steroid preparation the diagnosis should be confirmed with Xylocaine. If the Xylocaine does not relieve the symptoms, there is no point in injecting the

TABLE 29–4.
Flexor Hallucis Longus Tendonitis vs. Posterior Impingement of the Ankle

FHL Tendonitis	Posterior Impingement
Posteromedial	Posterolateral
Tenderness over the FHL tendon	Tenderness behind the fibula
Pain or triggering with motion of the hallux	Pain with plantar flexion of the ankle
Tomasen's sign[30]	Plantar flexion sign
Mistaken for posterior tibial tendonitis	Mistaken for peroneal tendonitis

steroids. It should be stressed that the os trigonum is not usually a surgical problem and that *most dancers with an os trigonum do not need to have it removed surgically.*

Occasionally, it does cause enough disability to warrant surgical excision, but as with most elective surgery, it is only indicated after the failure of conservative therapy in a serious dancer at least 16 years of age or older. If the problem is an isolated os trigonum with no medial symptoms, then it can be approached posterolaterally between the FHL and the peroneals (protect the sural nerve). Not infrequently, there is a combined problem of FHL tendonitis and the os trigonum syndrome. In these patients, the posteriormedial approach is used so that the neurovascular bundle can be isolated and protected. A tenolysis of the FHL and removal of the adjacent os trigonum can then be performed safely.

Other causes of posterior impingement include the following:

1. A previously asymptomatic os trigonum that becomes persistently symptomatic following an ankle sprain due to disruption of its ligamentous connections and a subtle shift in position.
2. Posterior impingement following an ankle sprain that stretches out the lateral ligaments that hold the talus under the tibia in relevé.[7] As the talus slips forward, the posterior lip of the tibia comes to rest upon the os calcis (see Fig 29–22). The treatment for this type of posterior impingement is to tighten the lateral ankle ligaments (preferably by the Brostrom-Gould technique). If the drawer sign can be corrected, the posterior impingement will usually disappear.
3. A posterior pseudomeniscus or plica in the posterior of the ankle, with or without an os trigonum.[7] It can cause the posterior impingement syndrome in the absence of an os trigonum or loose ligaments. Bucket handle tears in this structure have been seen to cause locking and other mechanical symptoms more often in the knee than the ankle.

Conservative Treatment.—Acute fracture of the posterior process of the talus if undisplaced should be treated with a short-leg walking cast. In the chronic condition, physical therapy modalities (cortisone phonophoresis), low-heeled shoes, and modified activities should be utilized.

If the pain is well relieved by a small injection of lidocaine (Xylocaine), the injection of 3/4 cc of cortisone acetate may give dramatic relief.

Operative Treatment.—Operative treatment is indicated when conservative therapy has failed and the diagnosis has been confirmed with Xylocaine. The posterior "cleanout" can be done from either the medial or lateral side of the Achilles tendon. The lateral approach should be used if the dancer has an isolated posterior impingement without a history of FHL tendonitis or medial difficulties. A medial incision is indicated if there is a combined problem of FHL tendonitis and posterior impingement or if the problem is primarily FHL tendonitis with an incidental os trigonum that you wish to remove along with a FHL tenolysis. The medial incision is safer and more utilitarian because the lateral side can be worked on safely from the medial but it is dangerous to work medially from the lateral side because the neurovascular bundle cannot be isolated and protected from that side.

Technique for Tenolysis of the Flexor Hallucis Longus and Excision of the Os Trigonum From the Medial Side.—This procedure can be performed with the patient supine because dancers usually have increased external rotation of the hip that will allow visualization of the posterior aspect of the ankle from the medial side. A bloodless field is desirable, so I use a tourniquet on the distal aspect of the thigh over cast padding. For this reason, the procedure cannot be done under local anesthesia or an ankle block.

1. A curvilinear incision is made over the neurovascular bundle behind the medial malleolus beginning just above the superior border of the os calcis and continuing to a line just posterior to the tip of the medial malleolus. This incision should be made carefully (Fig 29–26,A). The deep fascia and laciniate ligament in this area are often quite thin. If the incision is made too enthusiastically, the surgeon may find himself in the midst of the neurovascular bundle before he has planned to be there.
2. The deep fascia is then divided carefully and damage to the artery and nerve beneath it avoided (Fig 29–26,B). At this point it must be decided whether to go in front of the bundle or behind it. The posterior approach can involve the variable branches of the nerves to the os calcis. It is safer to pass anterior to the bundle. All branches of the tibial nerve at this level go posteriorly, so the safe plane is between the posterior aspect of the medial malleolus and the neurovascular bundle.
3. The bundle is taken down off the malleolus by blunt dissection (Fig 29–26,C). Several small vessels crossing the field may need to be ligated, but once the bundle is mobilized, it can be held with a blunt retractor such as a loop or Army-Navy retractor—never with a sharp rake. The posterior tibial nerve is larger than one expects, usually about the size of a pencil (Fig 29–26,D). The surgeon should examine the neurovascular bundle carefully. There are frequent anatomic variations within the tarsal tunnel. Both the nerve and

the artery divide into medial and lateral plantar branches as they leave the tarsal canal. It is not unusual for one or both of them to divide above this area and lead to reduplication within the tunnel. There may also be reduplication of the tendons—the flexor hallucis accessorius.

4. With the neurovascular bundle retracted posteriorly, the FHL tendon is easily identified by moving the hallux. The thin fascia is opened proximally, and a tenolysis is performed by opening the sheath proximally to distally (Fig 29–26,E). Usually it is stenotic and tough, and frequently the FHL can enter at an acute angle. Care should be taken distally because the FHL tunnel and the nerve are quite close together at this location. As the tenolysis approaches the area of the sustentaculum, the tunnel thins out so that there no longer seems to be anything more to divide.

5. The tendon should then be retracted with a blunt retractor and inspected for nodules and partial or longitudinal tears. If present, these should be debrided carefully or repaired.

6. At this point the FHL tendon can be retracted posteriorly with the neurovascular bundle. The os trigonum or trigonal process will be found just on the lateral side of the FHL tunnel. If the posterior aspect of the talus cannot be visualized, a capsulotomy should be performed. If there is difficulty in visualizing the os trigonum, it helps to identify the superior border of the os calcis and the subtalar joint (by moving the os calcis into adduction and abduction).

7. The subtalar joint is then dissected medially to laterally to get underneath the os trigonum. Once identified, it can be removed by circumferential dissection. Care should be taken to stay on the bone when per-

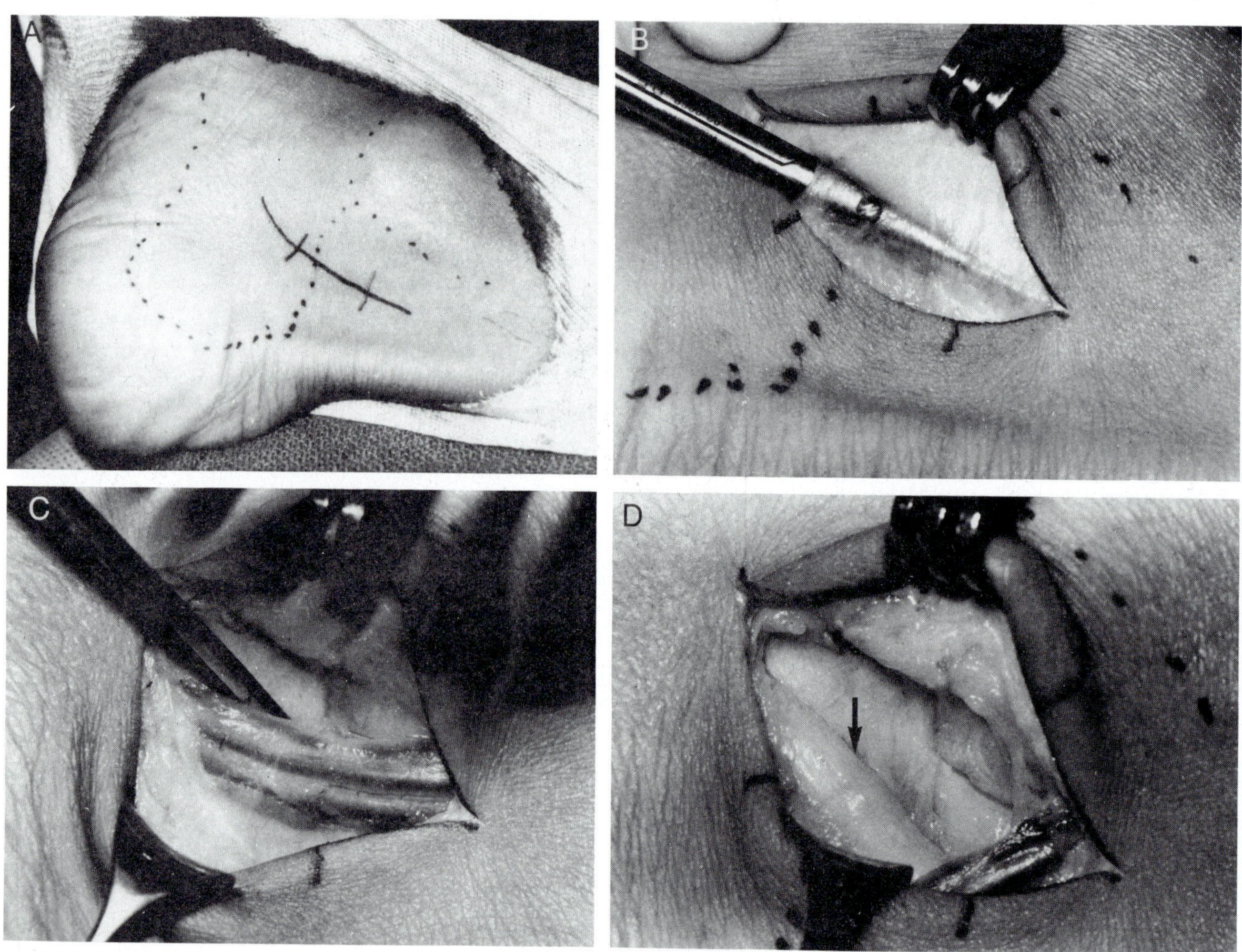

FIG 29–26.

A, the posteromedial incision. Tenolysis of flexor hallucis longus and excision of os trigonum. **B,** division of the laciniate ligament. **C,** taking down the neurovascular bundle. **D,** the posterior tibial nerve beneath the neurovascular bundle. **E,** tenolysis of the FHL. **F,** removal of the trigonal process. **G,** closure of the wound in neutral dorsiflexion.

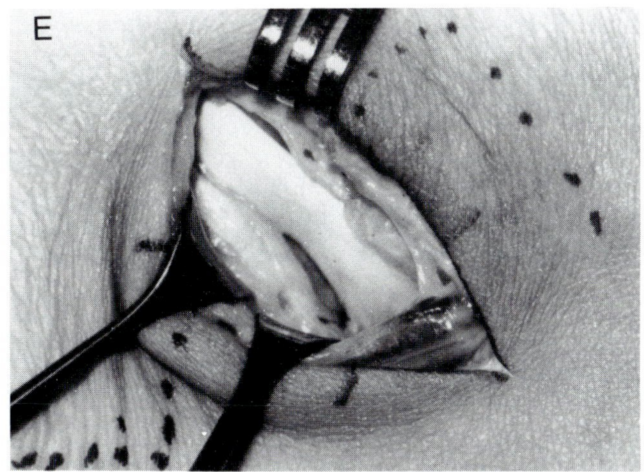

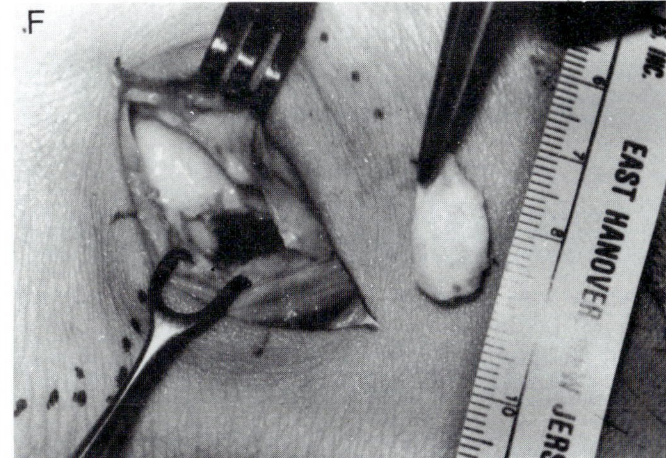

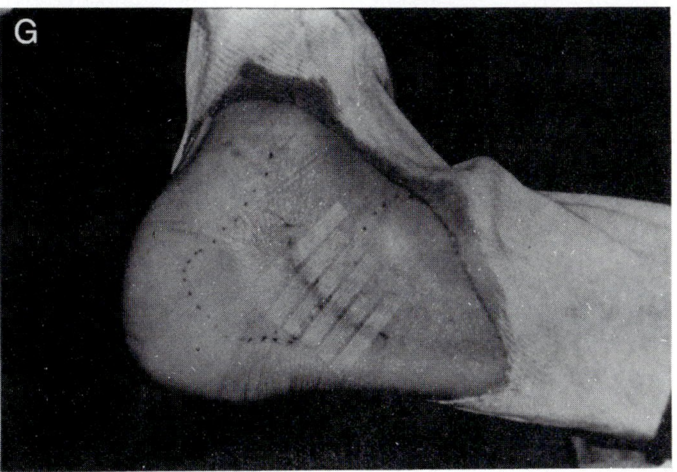

FIG 29–26 (cont.).

forming this part of the procedure. This can sometimes be somewhat difficult, especially if the os trigonum is quite large. Once it is removed, the posterior ankle joint should be inspected for remnants, bone fragments or loose bodies, soft-tissue entrapment, or a large articular facet on the upper surface of the os calcis that articulates with the os trigonum. If this is present, it may need to be removed with a thin osteotome (Fig 29–26,F).

8. The wound is then irrigated and checked for any residual impingement by putting the foot in maximum plantar flexion, the closing in the layers with plain catgut, and holding the ankle in the neutral position (Fig 29–26,G). (The FHL tunnel is *not* closed.)

Postoperative Care.—The patient is discharged with crutches and bears weight as tolerated; swimming and physical therapy are begun when the wound is healed. Early motion is encouraged to prevent adhesions. If the tenolysis is performed without excision of the os trigonum, the recovery period is usually 6 to 8 weeks. If the os trigonum is removed along with tenolysis, the recovery time is 8 to 12 weeks. If there is a large os trigonum, it is necessary to warn the dancer that once it is removed, the ankle does not just drop down into maximum plantar flexion. The dancer must realize that the bone has been there since birth and removing it does not result in immediate motion. The increase in plantar flexion is obtained slowly and can be accompanied by many strange symptoms, both anteriorly and posteriorly as the soft tissues adjust to the new range of motion.

Technique for Excision of the Os Trigonum by Using the Lateral Approach.—Under anesthesia, the patient is placed in the lateral decubitus position with a pneumatic tourniquet on the leg or thigh over cast padding. (Because dancers have increased external rotation of the hip, it is extremely difficult to perform this operation with the patient in the supine position.)

1. A curvilinear incision is made at the level of the posterior ankle mortise. There is a tendency to

make this incision a little too distal. Exposure will be easier if the approach is slightly proximal. The sural nerve is identified and protected in the subcutaneous tissues.
2. The dissection is carried down in the interval between the peroneal tendons laterally and the muscle belly of the FHL medially.
3. A posterior capsular incision is then made with the ankle in neutral or slight dorsiflexion. The os trigonum or trigonal process (Stieda's process) can be found on the superior surface of the posterior talus just on the lateral side of the FHL tendon. It has attachments on all its sides:
   a. Superior: the posterior capsule of the talocrural joint.
   b. Inferior: the posterior talocalcaneal ligament, at times quite thick and fibrous.
   c. Medial: the FHL tunnel with its sheath.
   d. Lateral: the origin of the posterior talofibular ligament.
4. The bone is removed by circumferential dissection. One should be careful not to stray too far medially because the posterior tibial nerve rests upon the FHL tunnel. The proximal entrance to this FHL tunnel can be opened if there are muscle fibers attached distally to the FHL tendon that crowd into the tunnel entrance when the hallux is brought into dorsiflexion (Tomasen's sign).[30] *Do not dissect medially without adequate visualization!* There are sometimes terminal branches of the posterior interosseus artery in the field that must be avoided or controlled. Check for loose bodies; I have found small ones in the FHL tunnel.
5. The foot should be brought into maximum plantar flexion to look for any residual impingement. At times it is necessary to remove more of the remnants of the posterior lateral tubercle. Frequently there is a facet on the cephalad portion of the os calcis that articulates with the os trigonum, and this can be large enough to impinge against the posterior lip of the tibia after the os trigonum has been removed. I often drain the wound with a small Hemovac because a postoperative hematoma will delay recovery and can make early motion difficult for the patient.
6. A layered closure is then performed with catgut sutures. I usually close the wound with a running absorbable suture.

Postoperative Care.—Weight bearing with crutches is begun as tolerated. The dancer is encouraged to swim and progress to barre exercises when the wound is healed. The average return to full dancing is 2 to 3 months.

Tendonitis of the Flexor Hallucis Longus Tendon

Tendonitis of the FHL tendon behind the medial malleolus of the ankle is so common that it is known as "dancer's tendonitis." It is often misdiagnosed as posterior tibial or Achilles tendonitis, but careful examination will usually reveal the true diagnosis. The FHL is the "Achilles tendon of the foot" for the dancer. It passes through a fibro-osseus tunnel from the posterior aspect of the talus to the level of the sustentaculum tali, like a rope through a pulley. As it passes through this pulley, it can be strained. When strained, rather than moving smoothly in the pulley, it begins to bind. This binding causes irritation and swelling, which in turn causes further binding, irritation, and swelling—setting up the familiar cycle: because it is swollen and irritated, it binds, and because it binds, it is swollen and irritated, etc. If a nodule or partial tear is present, triggering of the big toe may occur—"*hallux saltans*"[12] (Fig 29–27), or the tendon may become completely frozen in the sheath and cause a *pseudo–hallux rigidus*. This tendonitis typically responds to the usual conservative

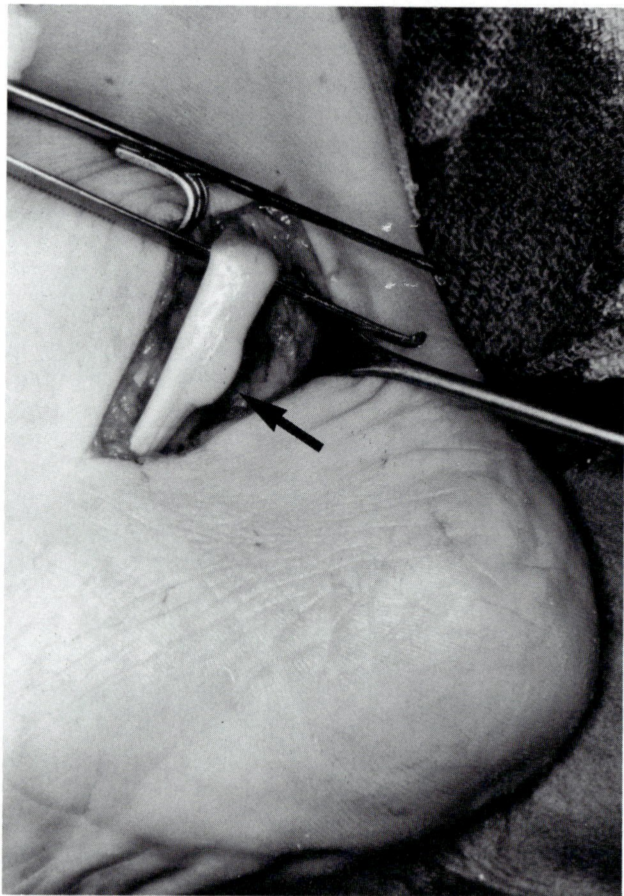

FIG 29–27.
A nodule on the FHL causing triggering of the hallux.

measures. Rest is an important component of the therapy so that the chronic cycle described above can be broken. NSAIDs can help, but they should only be used as part of an overall treatment program and not as medicine to kill the pain so that the dancer can continue dancing and ignore the symptoms. As with other tendon problems, steroid injections should be avoided. On some occasions, in professional or high-level amateur dancers, FHL tendonitis may be recurrent and disabling. In these cases operative tenolysis may be indicated (but only after the failure of conservative therapy). The situation is similar to De Quervain's stenosing tenosynovitis in the wrist.

FHL tendonitis will usually occur behind the medial malleolus, but it can occasionally be found at Henry's knot under the base of the first metatarsal where the flexor digitorum longus crosses over the FHL and under the head of the first metatarsal where it passes between the sesamoids. A *fibrous subtalar coalition* may be present in the posteromedial aspect of the ankle and mimic FHL tendonitis or the tarsal tunnel syndrome. This condition should be suspected when there is less-than-normal subtalar motion on physical examination.

THE ACHILLES TENDON

The tendo Achilles is the largest tendon in the body. It connects the triceps surae (medial and lateral gastrocnemius plus soleus muscles) to the os calcis and transmits the forces necessary to propel the body in walking, running, and jumping. These forces range from two to three times body weight in walking to four to six times body weight in running and jumping.[12] Their magnitude makes the Achilles tendon a common site for tendonitis secondary to repetitive overload or faults in technique in dancers and athletes, such as "rolling in" (pronation) and landing hard upon the heels.

Achilles Tendonitis

Achilles tendonitis, similar to other forms of tendonitis, is an inflammatory response surrounding the tendon that is triggered by microscopic tearing of the collagen fibers secondary to overload. The tearing may be on the surface or in the substance of the tendon (interstitial); thus clinically there are types and gradations of severity. The simplest type results in pain, tenderness, swelling, and thickening of the pseudosheath surrounding the tendon, usually at its isthmus or narrowest point. There may also be crepitus present on active motion. If the condition is chronic, nodules usually form around the tendon or on its surface. These may result in adhesions between the tendon and its sheath. A more severe strain results in a localized, fusiform swelling of the tendon itself, "like a snake that has swallowed a pig." This latter injury is slow to heal and has a guarded prognosis.

Certain factors can contribute to the development of Achilles tendonitis:

1. *Heel cord tightness,* the most common cause of Achilles strain in the recreational athlete and dancer.
2. A *"ribbon burn,"* from dancing with the toe shoe ribbons tied too tightly around the lower part of the leg. Dancers with this problem should sew elastics in their ribbons where they cross the Achilles (Fig 29–28).
3. *Congenitally small or thin Achilles tendons.* The size of the tendon varies considerably from person to person and from one side to the other and is not always related to body size. People with small tendons are prone to strains and overloads.
4. *Pronation* in runners, which is called "rolling in" in dancers.
5. A *cavus foot* with prominence of the posterosuperior os calcis, often a cause of *chronic retrocalcaneal bursitis* (Haglund's disease, or "pump bumps") and tendonitis of the Achilles overlying the bursa. Occasionally this con-

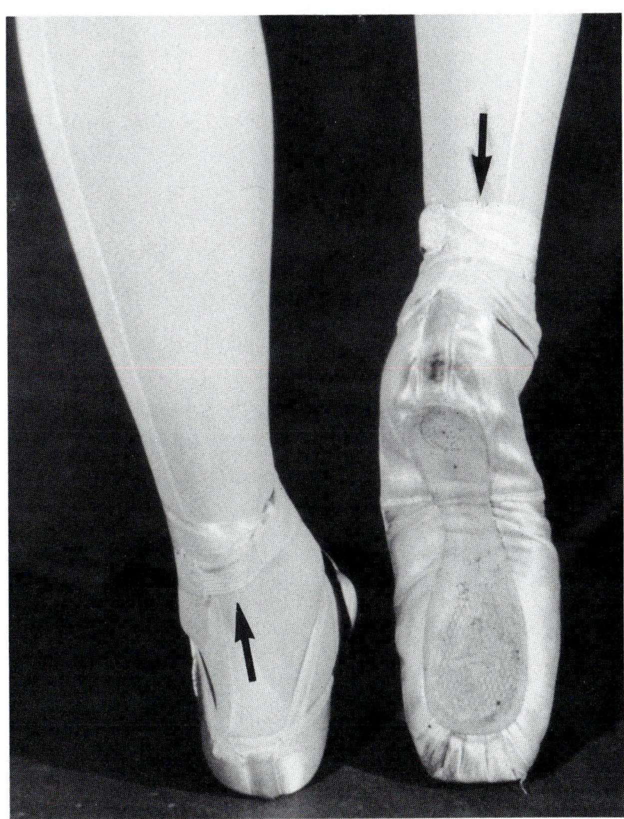

FIG 29–28.
Elastics sewn in the toe ribbons for tendonitis.

dition can result in a *partial tear of the Achilles tendon* just above its insertion and cause chronic pain and swelling. This condition is not uncommon in dancers since they are selected for having cavus feet. Exploration, debridement of the bursa, partial excision of the os calcis, and repair of the tendon may be necessary if the condition does not respond to conservative therapy. *Care should be taken when injecting steroids in the retrocalcaneal bursa. Repeated injections can weaken the Achilles insertion and may cause the tendon to pull loose. I have seen this happen in several professional dancers.*

Treatment of Achilles tendonitis, like so many other sports-related injuries, should be two-phased: first, the injured tendon must be allowed to heal. Rest, anti-inflammatory medicines, and physical therapy modalities such as ice, contrast baths, and ultrasound will promote healing. Second, rehabilitation is prescribed to restore strength and flexibility, along with correction of any predisposing factors to prevent recurrence prior to resumption of full activities. An injured athlete should not try to play himself back into shape but should get into shape and then play.

NSAIDs are helpful in the treatment of tendonitis. However, they should always be used as part of an overall treatment plan and not used simply to kill the pain so that the dancer can continue to do what caused the tendonitis in the first place.

In the New York City Ballet and the American Ballet Theater we have reduced the incidence of Achilles tendonitis considerably by the use of the "stretch box" (Fig 29–29), a wedge-shaped box that is kept in the wings during the season so that the dancers can stand on it to stretch their Achilles tendons while they are waiting backstage during performances and rehearsals. (Note: Steroids should NOT be injected into or around the Achilles tendon or into its insertion in the os calcis. They can weaken the tendon and lead to rupture!

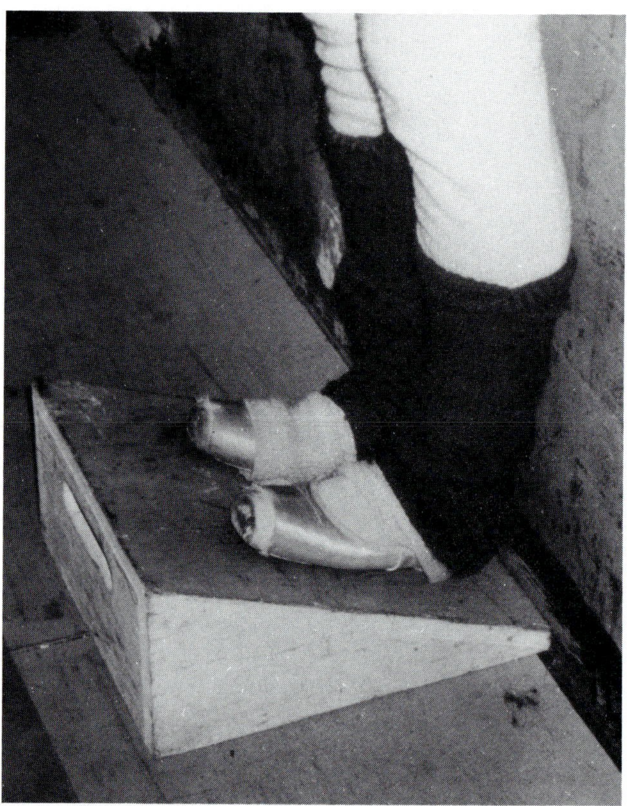

FIG 29–29.
The stretch box.

Rupture of the Achilles Tendon

This injury can occur without warning but is usually preceded by tendonitis or degeneration. A normal Achilles tendon can be lacerated but cannot be torn. Rupture usually occurs in male athletes and ballet dancers over 30 years of age and in the general male population in midlife. It is rare in females. Typically, the patient feels as if he has been "kicked in the back of the leg" and thereafter is unable to walk on his toes. The hematoma that forms may disguise the injury and lead to a missed diagnosis. The injury is often confused with the following:

1. An acute strain of the medial head of the gastrocnemius muscle.
2. A rupture of the plantaris tendon (this injury probably does not exist—one has never been documented).
3. An inversion sprain of the ankle.
4. A "partial tear" of the Achilles (it is almost always completely torn).

A ruptured Achilles tendon is easy to identify if it is suspected; the patient cannot walk on his toes, there is a palpable defect in the tendon, and the Thompson test is positive. (With the patient in the prone position, squeezing the calf muscles will normally produce noticeable plantar flexion in the foot and ankle. If the Achilles is torn, the foot will not move or will move very little when the calf is squeezed).

There are four methods of treating a ruptured Achilles tendon:

1. The *no-treatment method* is treatment by "judicious neglect." If the patient is too old, too inactive, or too sick, the situation is best left alone. The tendon will heal by the "law of the unsatisfied tendon," but it will heal elongated, and the patient will walk with a calcaneal gait.
2. *Cast immobilization* in the gravity-equinus position will produce a tendon with about 75% to 85% normal

function. This is usually quite satisfactory for the recreational athlete and dancer but has a rerupture rate of 25% to 30%.

3. A *percutaneous suture* will often obtain the correct length without open surgery. Incisional neuromas can be a problem with this procedure.

4. *Operative repair* will approximate normal function if the physiologic length of the tendon can be restored and if postoperative complications are avoided. It is the method of choice in serious or professional athletes and dancers.

It used to be said that a ruptured Achilles tendon was automatically the end of a professional athlete or dancer's career. This need not be the case. If the tendon can be restored to its original length and if the dancers are willing to devote the time and effort (1 full year) necessary for the postoperative rehabilitation, they can dance again or return to their sport. The type of repair used is not as important as the concept of the *restoration of physiologic length.* My preferred method is to use the plantaris tendon, if present, as an autogenous "figure-of-8"[11] suture to approximate the ends of the tendon under proper tension (Fig 29–30). This tension is best determined by having the uninjured leg prepared in the field so that the resting length of the contralateral Achilles is available when the tension is set in the repair. By sighting across both ankles the tension can be adjusted to place the injured and uninjured ankles in the same resting position relative to one another. An incision placed on the medial rather than the posterior aspect of the leg will minimize postoperative skin problems, and splitting the Achilles' sheath anteriorly prior to the repair will allow a layered closure of the wound at the end of the procedure. Postoperatively the patient is placed in a short-leg walking cast in slight equinus for 6 to 8 weeks depending upon the security of the repair and is then instructed to wear "clogs" or cowboy boots and to begin swimming and gentle stretching. Physical therapy is begun at 12 weeks and is continued until full strength is achieved.

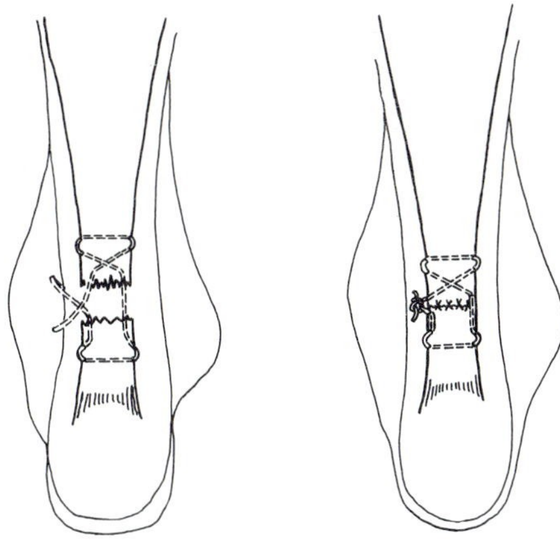

FIG 29–30.
A figure-of-8 Achilles tendon repair using the plantaris tendon.

Accessory Soleus Muscle, the Pseudo-Tumor of the Calf

A pseudotumor of the calf presents in teen-age dancers as a slowly enlarging mass in the distal third of the calf, usually on the medial side. It is painless, or only mildly uncomfortable, with a feeling of fullness or tightness. Obviously, it does not contain fluid, so aspiration will be negative. Division of the sheath will usually relieve the mild symptoms seen in this condition.

HEEL PAIN

Heel pain is not as common in dancers as one might expect. An accurate diagnosis here is important because there are many different types of heel pain.

Heel Spur Syndrome

Current opinion suggests that the heel spur often found on x-ray films is *not* usually the true source of the calcaneal pain in this syndrome. (The spur lies in the origin of the flexor digitorum brevis, not in the insertion of the plantar fascia.)

Plantar Fasciitis

Plantar fasciitis is the classic and most common type of heel pain. Tenderness is at the medial plantar insertion of the fascia.

Rupture of the Plantar Fascia

This is usually an acute injury, and the tenderness is in the midportion of the arch, not at the calcaneus. The tear may be partial or complete. If it is complete, a palpable defect can usually be found in the fascia when the toes and ankle are dorsiflexed (Fig 29–31).

Stress or Hairline Fracture

In this situation, the tenderness is usually on the *sides* of the os calcis rather than on the plantar surface. A bone scan will confirm the diagnosis.

Plantar Calcaneal Bursitis

There is a bursa directly beneath the calcaneus, and this bursa can become chronically inflamed. A careful

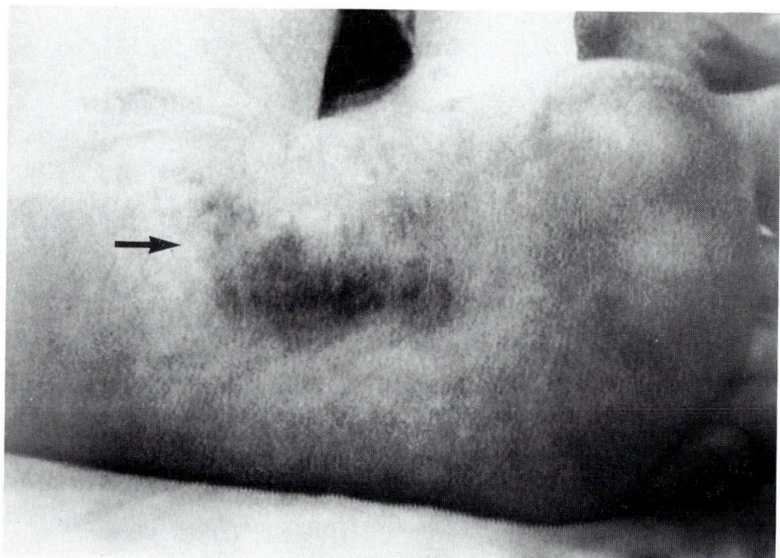

FIG 29–31.
An acute tear of the plantar fascia (left foot).

examination will sometimes reveal palpable fullness and thickened bands of inflamed synovial tissue within this bursa.

Entrapment of Baxter's Nerve

The motor branch to the abductor digiti quinti (FBLPN, or first branch lateral plantar nerve) can be trapped under the deep fascia of the abductor hallucis muscle as the nerve enters the sole of the foot near the medial calcaneal tuberosity (and the "spur," if present). This obscure condition can be the source of intractable heel pain. It is exacerbated by pronation ("rolling in") and is difficult to diagnose. The tenderness in this condition is usually directly over the nerve on the *medial* side of the calcaneus. A small injection of a local anesthetic may help make the diagnosis.

Bone Cysts and Tumors

Bone cysts and tumors are not that rare in this bone.

LEG PAIN

There are many causes of leg pain in the dancer. The usual differential diagnosis is between shinsplints, compartment syndromes, and stress fractures, although other more obscure conditions such as the osteoid osteoma must be kept in mind. Generally speaking, compartment syndromes are relatively rare in dancers. Dancing is an episodic rather than a sustained activity.

Stress Fracture of the Distal Isthmus of the Fibula

There is an isthmus in the proximal and distal portions of the fibula. Stress fractures are found in these locations. The distal narrowing is at the level where the toe shoe ribbons are wrapped tightly around the ankle, and this tightness, along with other factors such as pronation and external rotation, contributes to the condition. It is easy to diagnose because of the extent and precise location of the tenderness. The fracture itself can rarely be seen on the x-ray film, but a bone scan will be positive. Treatment is by modified activities until the pain is gone. When the lesion is healed and the dancer is ready to resume dancing, elastics should be sewn in the ribbons to decompress the fibula and Achilles tendon (see Fig 29–28). Many professional dancers routinely use these elastics in their toe shoe ribbons.

Shinsplints

Shinsplints, due to traction periostitis, can be found along the anterior or posterior borders of the tibia. They can usually be differentiated from stress fractures by the fact that the tenderness is usually spread out over a three-finger breadth area along the tibia. The tenderness associated with a stress fracture, however, is very localized and can be found with the tip of one finger. They also tend to occur at the beginning of the season, after a summer layoff, when the dancers are getting back into shape. Stress fractures, on the other hand, are usually seen in midseason or later, when the pounding and jumping are beginning to take their toll.

1. The *posterior* shinsplint is the most common in dancers. It is usually mistakenly identified as the origin of the posterior tibial muscle. It is, in fact, the origin of the flexor digitorum longus. (The posterior tibial muscle origin is on the proximal portion of the interosseus membrane between the tibia and the fibula.) Physical therapists who work with dancers feel that posterior

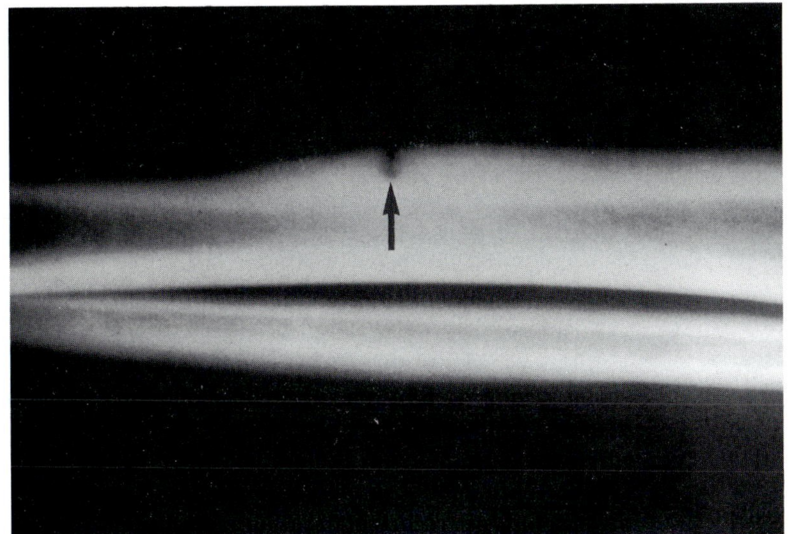

FIG 29–32.
The "dreaded black line" (anterior tibial stress fracture).

shinsplints are more common in dancers who "grab the floor" with their toes when they dance, and they should be taught not to do this.

2. The *anterior* shinsplint usually occurs in the origin of the anterior tibial muscle. Weakness and/or tightness is felt to be a predisposing factor.

The *soleus syndrome*[22] produces shinsplint-like pain just above and posterior to the medial malleolus. It is caused by tension on an abnormal slip of the origin of the soleus muscle that runs further down the posteromedial aspect of the tibia than is normal. Surgical release, similar to that done with compartment syndromes, is hardly ever necessary.

Stress Fractures of the Tibia

Predisposing factors to stress fractures include the following:

1. Dancers with an *anterior bow* in their tibia.
2. The *"Bravura" technique*. This style of choreography is danced in the 19th century classics. It is characterized by dramatic leaps that often land in a "balance," or pose, and produce large deceleration forces on the tibia. (In New York City there are two major ballet companies, the New York City Ballet and the American Ballet Theater. The American Ballet Theater uses the bravura technique in its productions of *Swan Lake* and *Giselle*, etc. Stress fractures of the tibia are relatively common in this company. The New York City Ballet, on the other hand, dances the "Balanchine" technique, which is known for its fluidity and rapid movements that rarely have a dancer decelerate. Stress fractures of the tibia in this company are extremely rare—only two or three in almost 20 years).
3. *Amenorrhea*, commonly found in female dancers, is associated with stress fractures of the metatarsals.[31] Whether it predisposes them to stress fractures of the tibia is probable, but this has not been proved.

An unrecognized or untreated anterior tibial stress fractures often progresses to the *"dreaded black line"*[7] (Fig 29–32). It is analogous to nonunion of a fracture (the tissue in the black line is granulation tissue). Once the black line appears, conservative treatment will often take an extremely long time to heal the fracture, 6 months to a year. It is difficult for a professional to be "out" for this length of time. Drilling these lesions can accelerate the healing process. The procedure is done with a small drill, as an outpatient, under anesthesia, with the image intensifier. (This technique is called "ferrage," after the French). The patient is put on crutches for a month following the procedure and kept away from jumps and grand pliés until healing is seen on the radiograph. In eight patients over the past 10 years, all have healed in 6 to 12 weeks.

REFERENCES

1. Bassett FH, Gates HS, Billys JB, et al: Talar impingement by the anteriorinferior tibiofibular ligament, *J Bone Joint Surg [Am]* 72:55–59, 1990.
2. Ferkel RD, Karzel RP, Del Pizzo W, et al: Arthroscopic treatment of anteriorlateral impingement of the ankle, *Am J Sports Med* 19:440–446, 1991.
3. Gould N, Seligson D, Gassman J: Early and late repair of the lateral ligament of the ankle, *Foot Ankle* 1:84–89, 1980.
4. Grant JCB: *A method of anatomy*, Baltimore, 1958, Williams & Wilkins.
5. Hamilton WG: Ballet. In Reider B, editor: *The school-age athlete*, Philadelphia, 1991, WB Saunders.

6. Hamilton WG: "Dancer's tendonitis" of the FHL tendon, American Orthopedic Society for Sports Medicine, Durango, Colo, July 1976.
7. Hamilton WG: Foot and ankle injuries in dancers. In Yokum L, editor: *Sports Clinics of North America*, Philadelphia, 1988, Williams & Wilkins.
8. Hamilton WG: Physical prerequisites for ballet dancers, *J Musculoskeletal Med* 13:61–66, 1986.
9. Hamilton WG: Post traumatic peroneal tendon weakness in classical ballet dancers, American Orthopaedic Society for Sports Medicine, Lake Placid, NY, July 1978.
10. Hamilton WG: Sprained ankles in ballet dancers, *Foot Ankle* 3:99–102, 1982.
11. Hamilton WG: Stenosing tenosynovitis of the flexor hallucis longus tendon and posterior impingement upon the os trigonum in ballet dancers. *Foot Ankle* 3:74–80, 1982.
12. Hamilton WG: Surgical anatomy of the foot and ankle, *CIBA Clin Symp* 37, 1985.
13. Hamilton WG: Tendonitis about the ankle joint in classical ballet dancers; "dancer's tendonitis," *J Sports Med* 5:84, 1977.
14. Hamilton WG, Hamilton LH, Marshall P, et al: A physical profile of the musculoskeletal characteristics of elite professional ballet dancers, *Am J Sports Med* 20:267-273, 1992.
15. Hamilton WG, Thompson FM: The Brostrom/Gould repair for lateral ankle instability, *Foot Ankle* (in press).
16. Harburn T, Ross H: Avulsion fracture of the anterior calcaneal process, *Physician Sports Med* 15:73–80, 1987.
17. Hawkins LG: Fractures of the lateral process of the talus, *J Bone Joint Surg [Am]* 52:991, 1970.
18. Howse AJG: Posterior block of the ankle joint in dancers, *Foot Ankle* 3:81–84, 1982.
19. Kleiger B: Anterior tibiotalar impingement syndromes in dancers, *Foot Ankle* 3:69–73, 1982.
20. Kleiger B: Mechanisms of ankle injury, *Orthop Clin North Am* 5:127, 1974.
21. Marshall PM, Hamilton WG: Subluxation of the cuboid in professional ballet dancers, *Am J Sports Med* 20:169–175, 1992.
22. Michael RH, Holder LE: The soleus syndrome, *Am J Sports Med* 13:87–94, 1985.
23. Newell S, Woodie A: Cuboid syndrome, *Physician Sports Med* 9:71–76, 1981.
24. Parkes JC, Hamilton WG, Patterson AH, et al: The anterior impingement syndrome of the ankle, *J Trauma* 20:895–898, 1980.
25. Quirk R: The talar compression syndrome in dancers, *Foot Ankle* 3:65–68, 1982.
26. Sammarco JG, DiRaimondo CV: Chronic peroneus brevis tendon lesions, *Foot Ankle* 9:163–170, 1989.
27. Shepherd FJ: A hitherto undescribed fracture of the astragalus, *J Anat Physiol* 17:79–81, 1882.
28. Taillard W, Meyer J, Garcia J, et al: The sinus tarsi syndrome, *Int Orthop* 5:117–130, 1981.
29. Thompson FM, Hamilton WG: Problems of the second metatarsophalangeal joint, *Orthopedics* 10:83–89, 1987.
30. Tomasen E: *Diseases and injuries of ballet dancers*, Denmark, Universitetsforlaget I, 1982, Arhus.
31. Warren M, Brooks-Gunn J, Hamilton L, et al: Scoliosis and fractures in young ballet dancers: relationship to delayed menarcheal age and amenorrhea, *N Engl J Med* 314:1338–1353, 1986.
32. Wolin I, Glassman F, Sideman S, et al: Internal derangement of the talofibular component of the ankle, *Surg Gynecol Obstet* 91:193–200, 1950.

C H A P T E R

30

Arthroscopy of the Ankle and Foot

Richard D. Ferkel, M.D.*

History

Advantages and disadvantages

Indications and contraindications

Ankle arthroscopy

Arthroscopic portals
  Anterior portals
  Posterior portals
Normal ankle arthroscopic anatomy
  Fifteen-point examination of the ankle
  Eight-point anterior ankle examination
  Seven-point posterior ankle examination
Equipment and setup
  Arthroscope
  Instruments
  Ankle distractors
  Leg holder
  Arthroscopy pumps
Author's preferred technique
  Patient positioning
  External anatomic landmark
  Ankle distractor
  Anterior portal establishment
  Posterior portals
Soft-tissue lesions
Congenital plicae
Trauma
  Nonspecific generalized synovitis
  Nonspecific localized synovitis
  Anterior soft-tissue impingement
  Posterior soft-tissue impingement
  Syndesmotic impingement
Technique of ankle synovectomy
Arthroscopic treatment of osteochondral lesions of the talus
  Terminology
  Incidence
  Diagnosis
  Surgical treatment
  Operative techniques
  Specific lesions
  Postoperative care
  Conclusion
Arthroscopic treatment of chondral and osteochondral lesions of the ankle
  Loose bodies
  Osteophytes
  Chondral lesions
  Traumatic and degenerative arthritis
Arthroscopic treatment of chronic ankle fractures
Arthroscopic treatment of lateral ankle instability
  Diagnostic evaluation
  Technique of arthroscopic stabilization of the ankle
Arthroscopic ankle arthrodesis
  Surgical technique
  Postoperative care
  Results
  Discussion

Arthroscopy of the subtalar joint

Anatomy of the subtalar joint
Indications and contraindications
Portals
Instrumentation
Surgical technique
  Author's preferred technique
Diagnostic examination
Pathology

Great toe arthroscopy

Anatomy of the great toe
Indications and contraindictions
Portals
Instrumentation
Surgical technique

The author would like to thank Hank C.K. Whu, M.D., for his assistance in preparing this chapter.

Arthroscopic normal examination
Postoperative care

Complications of ankle arthroscopy

How to avoid complications

Future of ankle arthroscopy

HISTORY

Arthroscopy was first performed in 1918 by Takagi in Tokyo when he inspected a cadaver knee with a cystoscope.[71] This eventually led to the development of a 7.3-mm arthroscope in 1920 and a 3.5-mm arthroscope in 1931. Kreuscher[60] became the first American to report the use of an arthroscope in the knee joint in 1925. In 1931, Burman[17] reported his experience of arthroscopic examination of multiple joints in a cadaver. At that time, the ankle was not believed suitable for arthroscopic examination because the joint space was too narrow. In 1939, Takagi[90] developed a standard method of arthroscopic examination of the ankle that was published in the *Journal of the Japanese Orthopedic Association*. In 1972, Watanabe[97] reported on 28 ankle arthroscopies performed with the newly developed fiber-optic arthroscope. In this report, the anteromedial, anterolateral, and posterior approaches to the ankle during arthroscopic examination were described in detail. In 1976, Chen[22] reported his experience with ankle arthroscopy in 67 clinical and 17 cadaver cases. In this report, Chen offered an extensive description and discussion of the compartments within the ankle and their surgical anatomy. More recently, Drez, Guhl, Andrews, Parisien, and Ferkel* have described their techniques and approaches for arthroscopy of the ankle joint.

Within the last 10 years, clinical experience with ankle arthroscopy has significantly increased. It is expected that ankle arthroscopy will continue to advance as an important diagnostic and therapeutic technique for the documentation and treatment of disorders of the ankle and foot. Techniques of arthroscopy have continued to advance with the development of small-joint arthroscopes and instrumentation that have allowed improved visualization and surgical access to the foot and ankle.

ADVANTAGES AND DISADVANTAGES

Arthroscopy of the ankle and foot allows direct visualization of all intra-articular structures without the need for an extensive surgical approach, arthrotomy, or malleolar osteotomy. Direct inspection of the ankle provides the best assessment of articular surface changes and damages. In addition, ligamentous structures may be observed directly by using the arthroscopic approach. Intraoperative stress testing maneuvers may be performed to determine the specific sites of laxity or incompetency of the ligamentous structures. A plethora of surgical procedures may be performed by using arthroscopic techniques, including biopsy, debridement, synovectomy, loose body removal, and "plasty" procedures. Postoperatively, advantages of the arthroscopic approach include decreased patient discomfort, decreased morbidity, a faster rate of rehabilitation, and an earlier return to daily and athletic activities.

Cartilage and soft-tissue injuries of the ankle may be associated with recurrent effusion, nonspecific tenderness, restricted range of motion, popping, or a feeling of instability. All these physical findings may present a diagnostic challenge for the orthopaedic surgeon. Arthroscopic examination of the ankle and foot allows one the opportunity to directly visualize and evaluate articular cartilage and soft-tissue pathology.

Disadvantages of ankle and foot arthroscopy are similar to those for arthroscopy of other joints. These include the potential for numerous complications (discussed later in the chapter), the need for special equipment and operating team, a propensity for equipment failure, and expense.

INDICATIONS AND CONTRAINDICATIONS

There are numerous indications for arthroscopy of the ankle and foot. The diagnostic indications include unexplained pain, swelling, stiffness, instability, hemarthrosis, locking, and popping. The therapeutic indications for ankle and foot arthroscopy include articular injury, soft-tissue injury, bony impingement,[32, 33, 79] arthrofibrosis, fracture, synovitis, loose bodies,[65] osteophytes, and osteochondral defects.[6, 76, 82] Depending on the patient and the specific condition involved, arthroscopy may also be indicated in ankle stabilization[54] and arthrodesis.[69]

The relative contraindications for ankle and foot arthroscopy include moderate degenerative joint disease with restricted range of motion, a significantly reduced joint space, severe edema, and tenuous vascular status.

The absolute contraindications for ankle and foot arthroscopy include localized soft-tissue infection and severe degenerative joint disease. In severe degenerative joint disease, it is difficult to achieve successful distrac-

---

**References 4, 25, 26, 29, 34, 43, 44, 51, 58, 76, 77–79.*

tion and adequate range of motion for visualization of the joint. A localized soft-tissue infection is an absolute contraindication to ankle arthroscopy. The potential for dissemination of localized infection intra-articularly and thus for septic arthritis must be avoided. However, if septic arthritis is present, ankle and foot arthroscopy is indicated since it is a useful tool for drainage and debridement of the joints.

ANKLE ARTHROSCOPY

Arthroscopic Portals

A thorough understanding of the extra-articular anatomy of the ankle is of paramount importance in placing the arthroscopic portals. The greatest concern is injury to the neurovascular structures. However, one must also be aware of potential injury to the tendons traversing the ankle joint.[30]

Anterior Portals

The three most commonly used anterior portals are shown in Figure 30–1. The anteromedial portal is placed just medial to the anterior tibial tendon at the joint line. Care must be taken to not injure the saphenous vein and nerve traversing the ankle joint along the anterior edge of the medial malleolus. The anterolateral portal is placed just lateral to the tendon of the peroneus tertius. This is at a level at or slightly proximal to the joint line. The superficial peroneal nerve divides 6.5 cm proximal to the tip of the fibula into the intermediate and medial dorsal cutaneous branches.[1] The intermediate dorsal cutaneous nerve passes over the inferior extensor retinaculum, crosses the common extensor tendons of the fourth and fifth digits, and then runs in the direction of the third metatarsal space prior to dividing into dorsal digital branches. The medial terminal branch of the superficial peroneal nerve, the medial dorsal cutaneous nerve, passes over the anterior aspect of the ankle overlying the common extensor tendons. It runs parallel to the extensor hallucis longus (EHL) tendon and divides distal to the inferior extensor retinaculum into the three dorsal digital branches. These nerve branches must be avoided during portal placement.

Between these portals, an anterocentral portal may be established between the tendons of the extensor digitorum communis (EDC). This is done to avoid possible injury to the neurovascular structures including the dorsalis pedis artery and the deep branch of the peroneal nerve. The dorsalis pedis artery and the deep branch of the peroneal nerve lie deep in the interval between the EHL and the medial border of the EDC tendons. Medial branches of the superficial peroneal nerve must also be avoided when using this portal. The use of this portal is strongly discouraged due to the increased potential for complications.

Posterior Portals

Posterior portals are also useful during arthroscopy of the ankle, as illustrated in Figure 30–2. These portals are commonly placed directly medial to, lateral to, or traversing the Achilles tendon just distal to or at the joint line. The posterolateral portal is established just lateral to the Achilles tendon, 2.5 cm above the tip of the fibula. Branches of the sural nerve and the small sa-

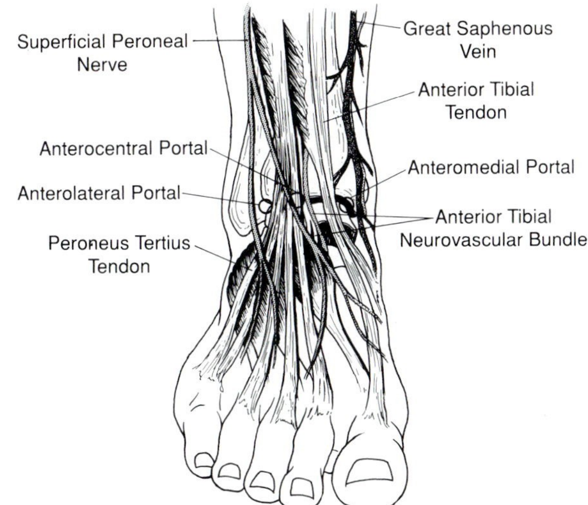

FIG 30–1.
The three anterior portals used for ankle arthroscopy are illustrated. The anterocentral portal is rarely used.

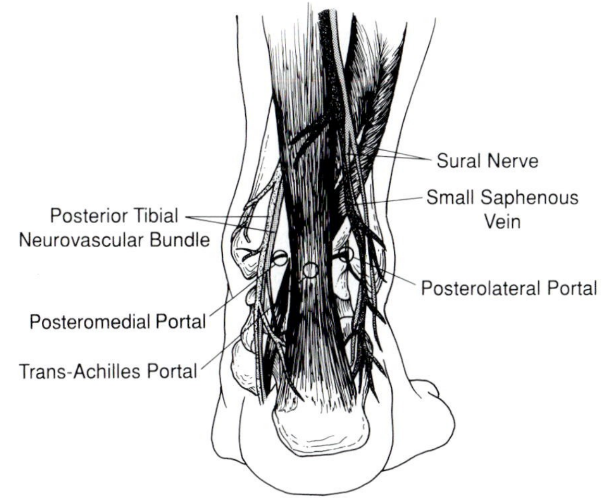

FIG 30–2.
The three posterior portals are diagrammatically represented. The posterolateral portal is the most commonly used portal.

phenous vein must be avoided with the posterolateral approach. The trans-Achilles portal is established at the same level as the posterolateral, but through the center of the Achilles tendon. The posteromedial portal is made just medial to the Achilles tendon at the joint line. With the posteromedial portal, the posterior tibial artery and the tibial nerve must be avoided. In addition, the tendons of the flexor hallucis longus and flexor digitorum longus must also be protected. The calcaneal nerve and its branches may separate from the tibial nerve proximal to the ankle joint and traverse in an interval between the tibial nerve and the medial border of the Achilles tendon.[66] Because of the potential for serious complications, the posteromedial portal is contraindicated in most instances.

During surgery, the anterolateral, anteromedial, and posterolateral portals are routinely established. Occasionally, transmalleolar portals[30] may be used for operative techniques, particularly for drilling of Kirschner wires under fluoroscopic and endoscopic control through either the tibia or fibula into the talar dome for the purpose of establishing new vascularity into an osteochondral lesion.

Normal Ankle Arthroscopic Anatomy

The intra-articular anatomy of the ankle during arthroscopic examination has been described extensively by Chen.[22] In addition, Drez et al.[26] have divided the ankle joint into an anterior and a posterior cavity, each of which are subdivided further into three compartments for a methodical inspection of the joint. More recently, a 15-point arthroscopic examination of the ankle has been developed.[30, 34]

Fifteen-Point Examination of the Ankle

As in the shoulder and the knee, it is imperative to use a methodical, systematic approach during arthroscopic examination of the ankle. This allows one to document in a reproducible fashion the arthroscopic findings, to accurately diagnose any potential intra-articular pathology, and to improve the quality of future clinical studies of the ankle arthroscopy patient population.

The author has devised a 15-point systematic examination of the anterior and posterior ankle joint that increases accuracy and reproducibility of the arthroscopic examination.

Eight-Point Anterior Ankle Examination

The eight-point anterior examination is shown diagrammatically in Figure 30–3 and includes the deltoid ligament, medial gutter, medial talus, central talus, lateral talus, talofibular articulation, lateral gutter, and the anterior gutter.

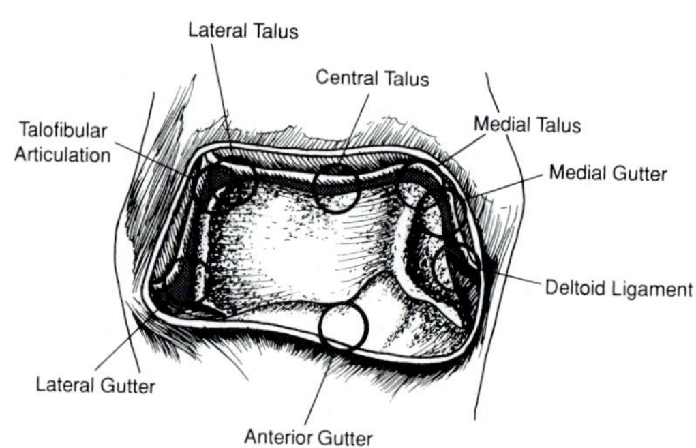

FIG 30–3.
The eight-point anterior examination of the ankle through the arthroscope.

Seven-Point Posterior Ankle Examination

The seven point posterior examination is shown diagrammatically in Figure 30–4 and includes the medial gutter, medial talus, central talus, lateral talus, talofibular articulation, lateral gutter, and the posterior gutter.

Generally, the combination of the anteromedial, anterolateral, and posterolateral portals allows excellent visualization of the entire joint. However, if an area is not well seen, the other described portals may be occasionally used to improve visualization and access.

Equipment and Setup

Arthroscope

Both the 4.0-mm and 2.7-mm arthroscopes are used for ankle arthroscopy. In general, the 4.0-mm arthroscope provides a large, clear picture and is more resistant to bending or breakage. This is the arthroscope normally used in the knee and shoulder joints. The 2.7-mm short arthroscope is somewhat more delicate, but it also provides an excellent picture and a wide angle field of vision. It is excellent for visualization throughout the ankle, but particularly in the tighter spots in the medial and lateral gutters and posterior aspect of the ankle. Both the 4.0 and 2.7-mm arthroscopes

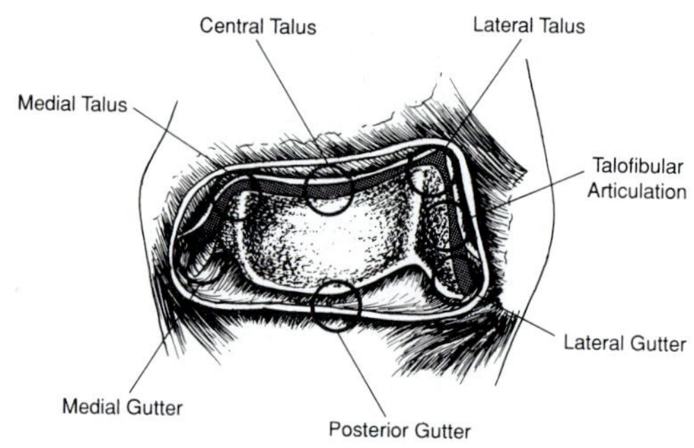

FIG 30–4.
The seven-point posterior examination of the ankle joint through the arthroscope.

have a 30-degree obliquity for improved field of vision. In addition, a 70-degree arthroscope is also available and is particularly helpful in seeing over the medial or lateral domes of the talus and looking into the gutters, as well as evaluating certain osteochondral lesions of the talus. Because the 2.7-mm 30-degree arthroscope is short and smaller, less instrument crowding and inadvertent chondral damage occurs. It is also important to have an interchangeable cannula system that allows the arthroscope to be switched from portal to portal without constant reinstrumentation of the portals with possible nerve and wound damage (Fig 30–5).

Instruments

Although standard-size instruments can be used for ankle arthroscopy, small-joint instruments are preferred. These instruments are easier to maneuver within the tight joint spaces and are much more efficient in their use than larger ones. Instruments typically used include 2.9-mm shavers and burrs, 3.5-mm ring curettes, 1.5-mm probes, 2.9-mm grasper and baskets, and small banana blades (Table 30–1 and Fig 30–6).

Ankle Distractors

Visualization of the ankle can be significantly improved by the use of an ankle distractor[49] to increase the space between the tibia and the talus. Without the distractor, certain areas of the ankle, such as the central tibial plafond and talar dome, the posterior talofibular ligament, and the calcaneofibular ligament, are poorly seen (Figure 30–7,A).

Distraction methods applied to the ankle may be either noninvasive or invasive. Noninvasive techniques include manual distraction and gravity distraction, which are "uncontrolled" methods. Other types of noninvasive methods such as the modified clove-hitch knot around the ankle can be termed "semicontrolled." Several new devices allow the ankle to be distracted noninvasively while also permitting the amount of pressure and force to be monitored and maintained mechanically. These are termed "controlled" devices (Fig 30–7,B). A variety of invasive distractors are also available that use pins in the tibia and talus or calcaneus to provide mechanical distraction. Most of these devices

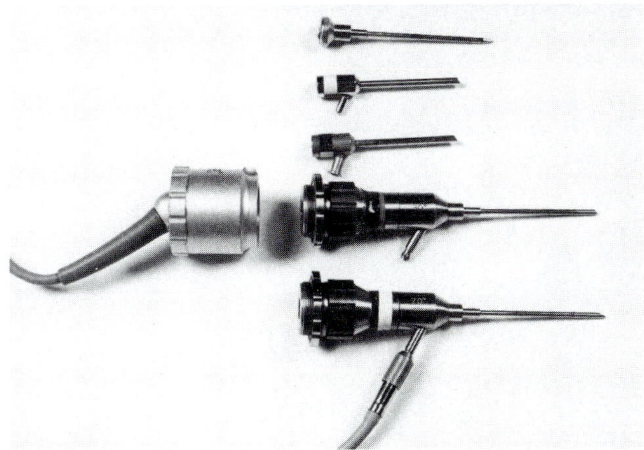

FIG 30–5.
Small-joint arthroscopes. The 30-degree 2.7-mm arthroscope is shown above, and the 70-degree arthroscope is shown below with their corresponding interchangeable cannulae.

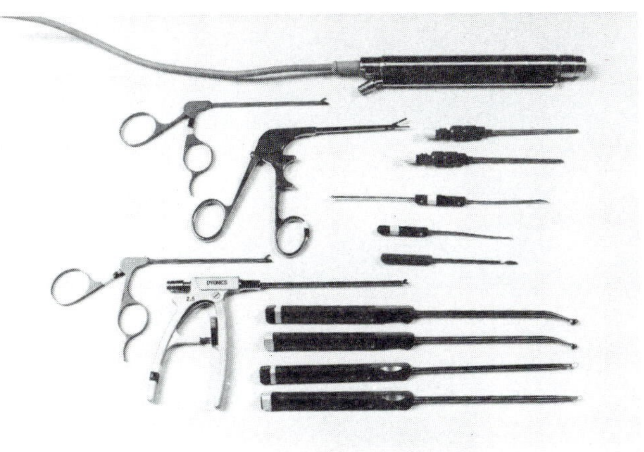

FIG 30–6.
Small-joint instrumentation, including a 2.9 shaver and burr, 3.5 and 4.5 ring curettes, probe, grasper, basket, and small banana blades.

TABLE 30–1.
Instruments for Ankle and Foot Arthroscopy

CHP camera with an adapter to a light source
Compatible light source
Small- and large-joint shaver system
TV monitor
Ankle and thigh holder
Power reamer with a Jacobs chuck and key
Ankle distractor—both invasive and soft tissue
3/16 in. threaded "trochar-tipped" Steinmann pins
4.0-mm, 30 degree standard scope and 2.7-mm, 30 degree short scope with corresponding cannulae
No.11 scalpel and mosquito clamp
22-gauge, 1½-in. needle with an 18-gauge spinal needle
10-cc syringe with IV extension tubing
2, 50-cc syringes
Small ring curettes and pituitary rongeurs
Minidriver with K-wire attachment and K-wires
Miniprobes, graspers and bites, including a 2.7-mm grasper and suction basket
Drill guide
3.5-, 2.9-, 2.0-mm shavers and burrs
Shoulder holder and toe trap for toe arthroscopy
2.7-mm, 70-degree arthroscope (optional)

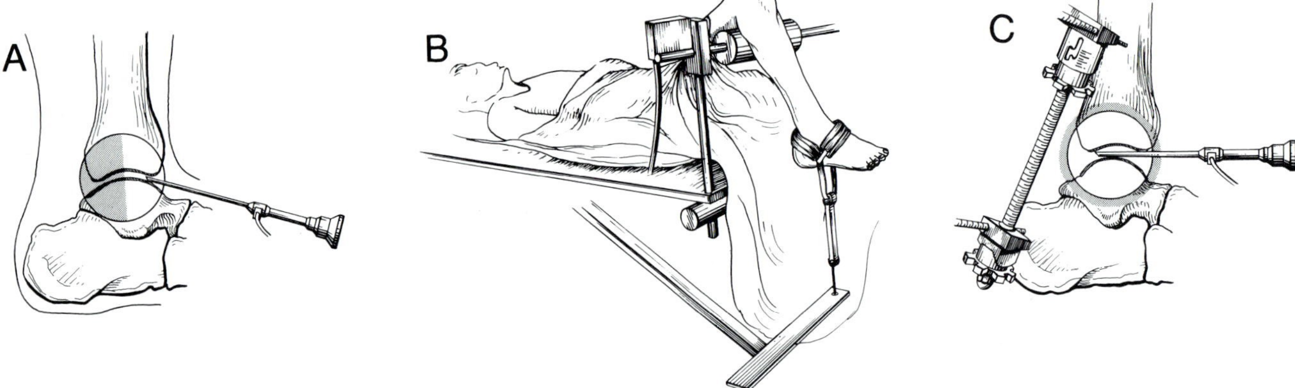

FIG 30–7.
A, lateral view of the ankle during arthroscopic examination without distraction. **B,** lateral view of the ankle during arthroscopic examination with a controlled noninvasive distraction device. **C,** lateral view of the ankle during arthroscopic examination with an invasive distraction device.

have a strain gauge to measure the amount of force and permit some degree of freedom within the ankle joint (Figure 30–7,C). More recently, a "multimode" distraction system has been developed by Guhl to allow both invasive and noninvasive distraction in the same device. Contraindications for invasive distraction include reflex sympathetic dystrophy, open epiphysis, pyarthrosis, chronic infection, and high-performance athletes who need to return to their sport quickly.[47]

Leg Holder

The thigh is usually supported by a nonsterile leg holder that is positioned underneath the tourniquet. This is set in such a way as to flex the hip proximally 45 to 50 degrees and keep the popliteal fossa free from pressure. An alternative method is to use a urology leg holder positioned in the popliteal fossa, but one must be very careful to keep the pressure in this area to a minimum. Since the thigh support is nonsterile, it should be applied preoperatively. Following preparation and draping of the patient, a sterile foot holder with a sterile clamp is applied to the side of the table to support the foot and ankle if the arthroscopy is done with the patient in a supine position (Fig 30–8).

Another way to do ankle arthroscopy is to use a thigh holder commonly utilized with knee arthroscopy and flex the knee 90 degrees over the end of the table.

Arthroscopy Pumps

In ankle arthroscopy, it is critical to have a high inflow and outflow system. Generally, this can be accomplished with gravity drainage into the posterolateral portal of the ankle. However, in situations where a posterior portal is difficult to obtain or maintain or higher fluid pressure is desired, an arthroscopy pump can be used. It provides a high flow volume and maintenance of pressure around the ankle. It is also helpful in obtaining hemostasis, permits improved visualization, and can be adjusted through the operative procedure. *Caution:* Arthroscopy pumps can be very dangerous in the foot and ankle if not monitored carefully and a good outflow system is not maintained. The fluid can extravasate into the foot or up into the anterolateral compartment, and the potential for increased compartmental pressure can be significant. In addition, some systems require special cannulas that are difficult to use, depending on the arthroscope.

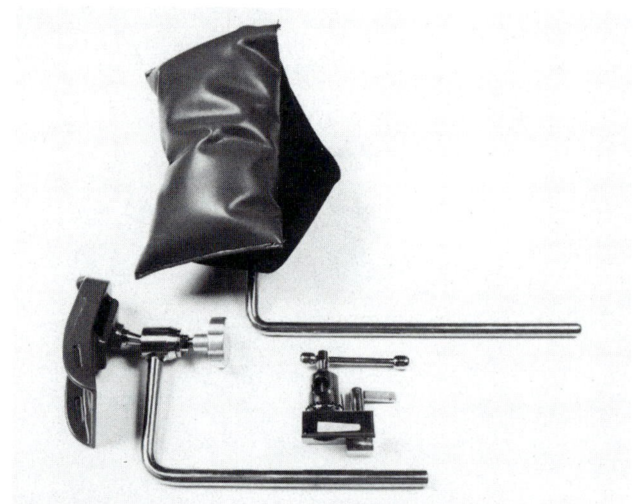

FIG 30–8.
Thigh and ankle holder used during arthroscopic examination in the supine position. Normally, the ankle holder is sterile as is the clamp that attaches to the table.

Authors' Preferred Technique

Patient Positioning

1. The position of the patient is a matter of the surgeon's preference. The author prefers the patient to be in the supine position, with the thigh secured by an unsterile thigh holder supporting the proximal aspect of the thigh, superior to the popliteal fossa. This area is well padded to avoid injury to the sciatic nerve.

2. The thigh is positioned with the hip flexed 45 to 50 degrees.

3. A sterile foot holder is utilized to support the foot and ankle in the desired position. It is secured to the table with a sterile clamp that goes over the drapes on the side of the table.

4. With this set up, the surgeon is able to sit or stand during sùrgery, and both the anterior and posterior portions of the ankle are easily accessible without further manipulation of the patient's extremity (Fig 30–9,A and B).

5. Other authors have described techniques with the knee flexed over the end of the table[4] or the patient in an oblique, decubitus position.[79]

6. A tourniquet is routinely placed around the patient's thigh, and the thigh is secured by using a thigh-holding device.

7. Special care should be taken to pad all the areas of bony prominence to prevent potential neurovascular compromise secondary to pressure.

8. The patient is then prepared and draped in the standard fashion.

External Anatomic Landmark

1. The dorsalis pedis should be carefully palpated, and its position should be marked.

2. Likewise, the saphenous vein and the anterior tibial and peroneus tertius tendons are outlined over the surface of the ankle.

3. Marking the superficial peroneal nerve branches is particularly important since it is the structure most at risk for injury when the anterolateral portal is created. Its identification is facilitated by holding the foot in plantar flexion and inversion. The nerve should be palpated along its course anterior and inferior to the lateral malleolus.[95] The joint line is then identified anteriorly by palpation with dorsiflexion and plantar flexion of the ankle.

Ankle Distractor

Various joint distraction techniques have been described above to improve visualization and ease of access for operative instrumentation. Both noninvasive soft-tissue distraction setups as well as invasive mechan-

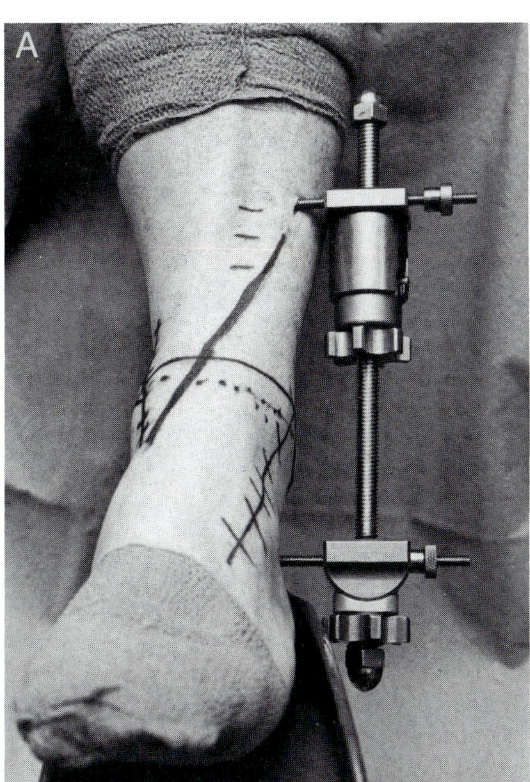

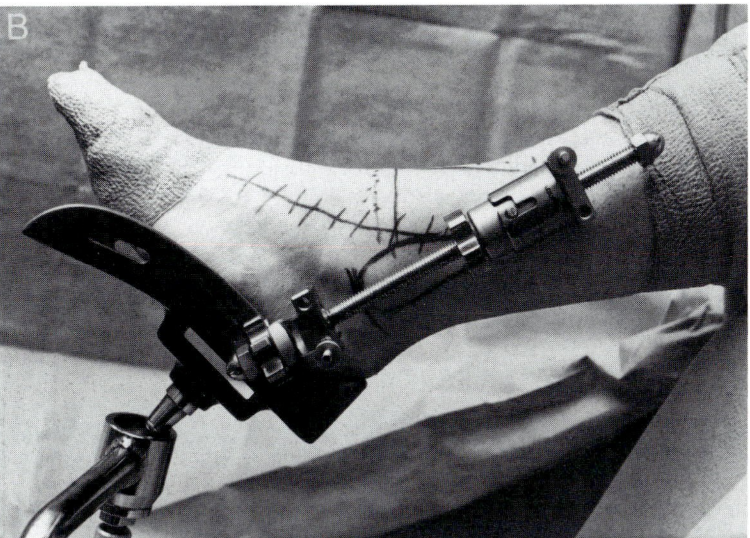

FIG 30–9.
Ankle arthroscopy setup with the ankle holder and distraction device in place. **A** anterior view; **B** lateral view.

ical distractors using tibial and calcaneal pins may be used.[28, 48, 50] The decision to use a noninvasive or invasive distractor is made at the time of surgery and depends upon the tightness of the ankle joint and location of the pathology. The technique for invasive distraction has been described by Guhl[49] (see Fig 30–7,C).

1. Two threaded trochar-tipped Steinmann pins measuring 4.5 in. long and 3⁄16 in. in diameter are used. Both pins are drilled laterally to medially. The tibial pin should be placed 6.5 to 7.5 cm (2½ to 3 in.) above the joint line. The calcaneal pin should be placed 2.5 cm (1 in.) anterior and 2.5 cm (1 in.) superior to the posteroinferior calcaneal margin at a 30 degree angle from the coronal plane toward the head.
2. A stab incision is made in the skin 6.5 to 7.5 cm above the tibiotalar joint and a thumb's breadth below the anterior tibial crest.
3. A soft-tissue trochar with attached cannula is used to tunnel through the subcutaneous tissue anterior to the tibialis anterior tendon.
4. A Steinmann pin is then drilled across the lateral cortex to but not through the medial cortex (Fig 30–10).
5. The distal calcaneal pin is placed so as to avoid the peroneal tendons and the subtalar joint.
6. The skin stab incision in the calcaneus is performed by using a technique similar to that for tibial pin placement. However, a 20-degree caudal inclination is used to direct the pins.
7. The pins should be drilled through the lateral cortex up to but not through the medial cortex. Care should be taken during placement of the tibial pin to avoid violating the tibialis anterior during insertion.
8. Once a nick is made in the skin, a cannula should be used to protect the soft tissues around the pin while drilling. Both pins should be unicortical and should not penetrate the medial cortex.
9. The joint is slowly distracted about 4 to 5 mm. Additional distraction is applied as relaxation of the capsular tissues takes place. Distraction should not exceed more than 7 or 8 mm, which usually corresponds to a reading of 50 lb on the distractor.
10. Care should be taken to minimize bending of the pins. Distraction should be limited to 50 lb of force for 60 minutes' or less duration.
11. If a soft-tissue distractor is used, I prefer a device that grips around the inferior aspect of the ankle and foot and is attached to a strain gauge. However, care must be taken to make sure that the device does not exert excessive pressure over the anterior tibial neurovascular bundle, so periodic relaxation of this device aids in preventing complications.

Invasive Distraction

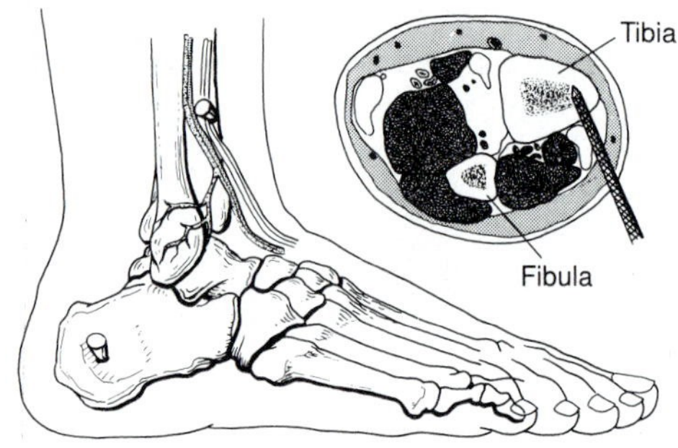

FIG 30–10.
Invasive distraction. Note that the tibial pin is inserted subcutaneously anterior to the anterior tibial tendon to avoid injury to the neurovascular bundle.

Anterior Portal Establishment

1. Sterile lactated Ringer's solution is infused into the ankle joint with an 18-gauge needle to establish the position of the anteromedial portal.
2. A no. 11 scalpel is then used to make a vertical skin incision while palpating the anterior tibial tendon.
3. Blunt dissection using a mosquito clamp is then performed through the subcutaneous tissue to the capsule.
4. A blunt trochar with attached arthroscopic cannula is then carefully placed into the ankle joint.
5. Additional lactated Ringer's solution is then infused into the joint through the arthroscope, and the joint is visualized from the anteromedial portal.
6. An 18-gauge spinal needle is then inserted into the ankle joint to locate, under direct vision, the position for the anterolateral portal.
7. By using a similar technique, the skin is incised and bluntly dissected with a mosquito clamp followed by insertion of an inflow cannula into the ankle joint.
8. Sequential examination of the anterior ankle joint and its structures is now performed by using the eight-point anterior examination system.
9. If an anterocentral portal is necessary, blunt dissection down to the joint capsule is absolutely necessary to protect the deeper neurovascular structures.

Posterior Portals

1. Commonly, the posterolateral portal is used for inflow or visualization. The key to establishing the posterior portal is good joint distension with constant distraction. The posterolateral portal is established under

direct visualization, if possible, by using an 18-gauge spinal needle.

2. The cannula should penetrate the posterior capsule medial to the posterior inferior tibiofibular and transverse tibiofibular ligaments.

3. When the posterolateral portal is used, distraction will often need to be increased for adequate visualization.

4. The cannula should be inserted with care to avoid injury to the branches of the sural nerve and the short saphenous vein.

5. The posterolateral portal is initially used as the primary inflow portal and may be subsequently used for visualization or instrumentation by means of an interchangeable system of cannulas.

TABLE 30–2.
Sources of Synovial Irritation

Congenital	Plica
	Congenital bands within the ankle
Traumatic	Sprains
	Fractures
	Previous surgeries
Rheumatic	Rheumatoid arthritis
	Pigmented villonodular synovitis
	Crystal synovitis
	Hemophilia
	Synovial chondromatosis
Infectious	Bacterial
	Fungal
Degenerative	Primary
	Secondary
Neuropathic	Charcot joints
Miscellaneous	Ganglions
	Arthrofibrosis

Soft-Tissue Lesions

Soft-tissue lesions account for approximately 30% to 50% of pathology in the ankle joint. It has traditionally been a diagnostic challenge to the orthopaedic surgeon since the definitive pathology is frequently not apparent by history, physical examination, or radiographic examination. Since the advent of ankle arthroscopy, the ability to diagnose and treat soft-tissue lesions around the ankle has increased significantly. Generally, soft-tissue lesions of the ankle involve the synovium. However, the capsule and the ligamentous tissues of the ankle may also be affected. The sources of synovial irritation are summarized in Table 30–2 and may include congenital, traumatic, rheumatic, infectious, degenerative, neuropathic, and miscellaneous causes.

Congenital Plicae

Congenital plicae have been well described in the knee.[80] However, little is known about the plicae in the ankle, but they appear to be more congenital than traumatic in origin.

Trauma

Nonspecific Generalized Synovitis

Following a traumatic injury to the ankle joint, a generalized or localized synovitis may occur. The patient with generalized nonspecific synovitis will usually complain of swelling, aching, and soreness. The history of trauma may be significant or trivial. Sometimes, no specific inciting event can be recalled. If the patient fails to respond to prolonged conservative treatment following an adequate workup, ankle arthroscopy is indicated.

Ankle sprains and fractures are the most common causes of nonspecific generalized synovitis. The author has performed arthroscopic debridement with lysis of adhesions and partial synovectomy in 25 patients after fracture. Ankle arthroscopy under this setting may be technically challenging. The key to success is a high–flow volume system using a posterolateral inflow cannula. The distractor may be very helpful in these cases to improve visualization and access to the joints.

Systematic evaluation of the entire ankle with the 15-point examination system should be performed. The ankle should be evaluated through both the anterior and posterior portals. The entire joint should be debrided and freed from scar, fibrotic material, and synovitis. Debridement of associated chondromalacia and removal of loose bodies may be performed after improvement in visualization. It is important to note that in patients with rheumatoid arthritis or other synovial diseases, the capsule may be quite thin and friable. One should use a whisker shaver tip when debriding anteriorly under the neurovascular structures to avoid injury to these structures.

The portals should be sutured postoperatively. A compressive dressing with a short-leg stocking should be applied. The postoperative regimen should include early range of motion and weight bearing as tolerated.

Nonspecific Localized Synovitis

Following trauma, some patients will develop a localized synovitis in the medial or lateral malleolar joints. X-ray examinations are generally negative or may show small ossicles consistent with previous trauma. Magnetic resonance imaging (MRI) may signal a change in the area of pain with or without fluid. Arthroscopic examination will reveal mild or localized synovitis, papillary formation, and fibrosis. Excision of this localized synovitis will often produce excellent results if a patient has failed conservative management.

Anterior Soft-Tissue Impingement

Chronic ankle pain after an ankle "sprain" is a well-documented problem and is seen in 20% to 40% of cases. This pain is usually located anterolaterally, rarely anteromedially. The borders of the lateral gutter of the ankle include the talus medially, fibula laterally, and tibia superiorly bordered by the anterior inferior tibiofibular (AITF) ligament (Fig 30–11). The anteroinferior section of the lateral gutter is bordered by the anterior talofibular, calcaneofibular, and anterior talocalcaneal ligaments (Fig 30–12).[35] The posteroinferior borders are composed of the posterior talofibular, calcaneofibular, and posterior talocalcaneal ligaments (Fig 30–13).

The classic sequence of events associated with inversion injuries of the ankle is as follows:

Torn anterior talofibular ligament
↓ ↘
Torn calcaneofibular ligament — Torn anterior inferior tibiofibular ligament
↓
Torn posterior talofibular ligament

Wolin et al,[98] was the first to describe a "meniscoid" band between the fibula and the talus. This mass was thought to be hyalinized connective tissue from the talofibular joint capsule. It was felt that repeated pinching (or impingement) of this meniscoid tissue led to pain and swelling in the ankle. Waller in 1982[96] described the anterolateral corner compression syndrome. The pain in this syndrome was noted to be along the anteroinferior border of the fibula and the anterolateral talus, and the pain was thought to be a result of repetitive inversion injuries.

The differential diagnosis for chronic sprain pain secondary to ankle sprain includes osteochondral lesions of the talus, calcific ossicles, peroneal subluxation or dislocation, tarsal coalition, subtalar joint dysfunction, degenerative joint disease, and "soft-tissue impingement."

There are three primary sites where anterolateral impingement of the ankle occurs. The first site is the superior portion of the AITF ligament. The second site is the distal portion of the AITF ligament, which may involve a separate fascicle. The third site is along the anterior talofibular ligament and lateral gutter near the area of the lateral talar dome (Fig 30–14).

Over the last 7 years, the author has treated over 75 patients with pain in the anterolateral gutter of the ankle following an inversion stress injury. The results

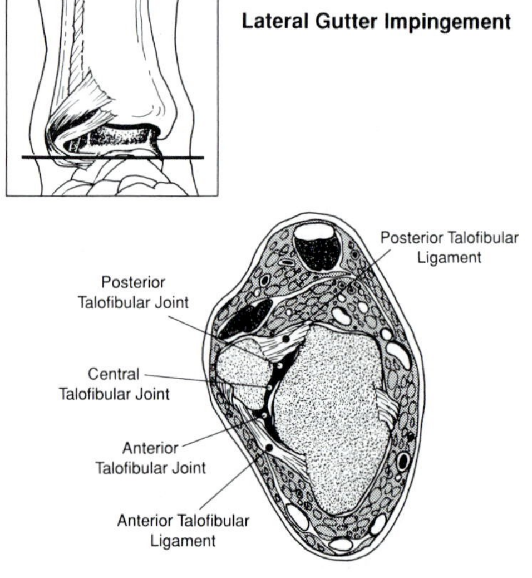

FIG 30–11.
Cross section through the talus to demonstrate the lateral gutter anatomy.

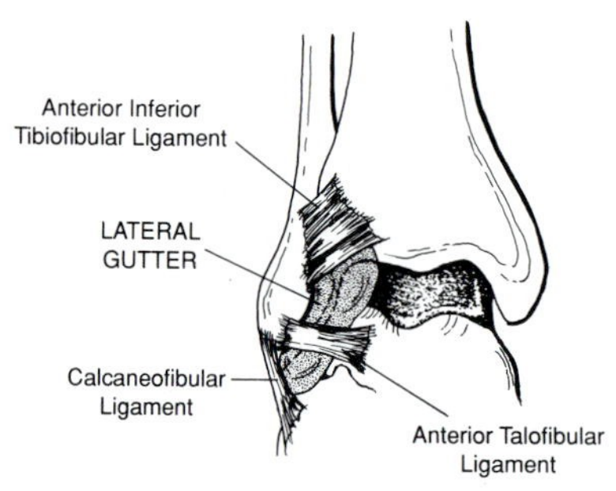

FIG 30–12.
Anterior anatomy of the lateral gutter. The space is bordered by the bone and capsular and ligamentous structures.

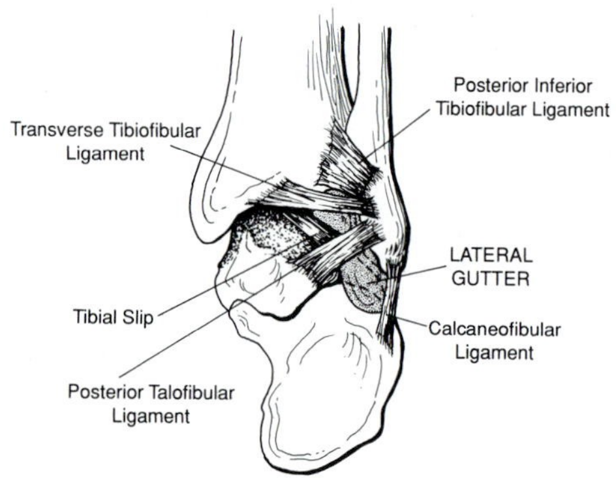

FIG 30–13.
Posterior anatomy of the lateral gutter. Note that the tibial slip runs between the transverse tibiofibular ligament and the posterior talofibular ligament.

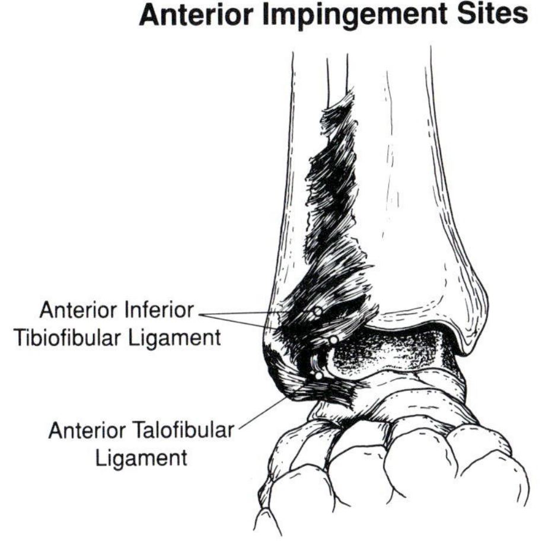

FIG 30–14.
Anterior impingement sites. Note that the anterior inferior tibiofibular ligament may have a separate fascicle that can impinge against the lateral dome of the talus.

were analyzed in a smaller group with longer follow-up.[31, 36] The average patient age was 34 years, with an average follow-up of 34 months. All patients had tenderness over the anterolateral corner of the talar dome and the lateral gutter. All patients had a history of previous sprain, with an average interval from injury to surgery of 24 months. In every case, the patients had failed a complete course of conservative management, including nonsteroidal anti-inflammatories (100%), physical therapy (100%), bracing (75%), casting (50%), and steroid injection (62%). X-ray findings were normal in 50% of the patients; others had mild spurs, calcification, and joint space narrowing. Stress x-ray films were done on all patients and showed no evidence of chronic ligamentous instability. MRI revealed synovial thickening consistent with impingement in the anterolateral gutter (Fig 30–15).

At the time of surgery, all patients had synovitis and fibrosis of the anterolateral gutter, with some patients showing chondromalacia of the talus and fibula (Fig 30–16,A). In some patients, a thick band of tissue could be identified and excised, which probably corresponded to the meniscoid lesion Wolin described.

At the time of surgery, debridement of the anterolateral gutter was performed with complete removal of the inflamed synovium. The chronic synovial impingement lesion may be removed by using baskets, rongeurs, or motorized shaver equipment. It is necessary to remove not only the synovium but also any inflamed capsular or ligamentous tissue. However, care must be taken to not excise any of the functional remnants of the anterior talofibular ligament (Fig 30–16,B).

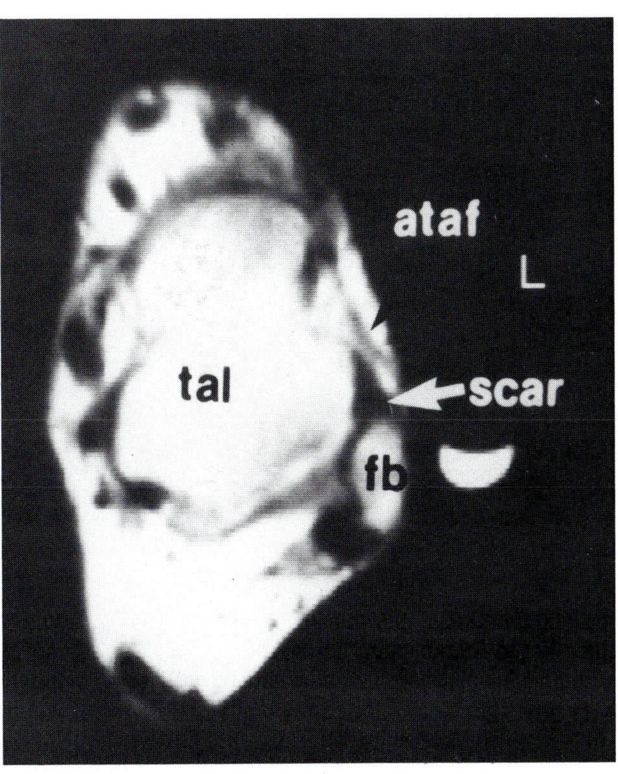

FIG 30–15.
T1-weighted axial view of the ankle with anterolateral impingment. Scar tissue appears as a decreased single intensity between the talus and the fibula.

Postoperatively, patients use crutches for support and ambulate weight bearing as tolerated. The support is discarded at 1 week, at which point rehabilitation is started. Sports activities are reserved for 4 to 6 weeks.

Moderate synovial hyperplasia with subsynovial capsular proliferation was seen histologically in all patients. Postoperative assessment found 84% of the patients rated good to excellent. Based upon these results, the current sequence of events leading to chronic ankle pain is described in Figure 30–17.

The author feels that the term "chronic ankle sprain" should be replaced by "anterolateral impingement of the ankle" as a more accurate description of this chronic condition around the ankle joint. The term "meniscoid" is misleading and should be omitted in the future.

Posterior Soft-Tissue Impingement

In addition to anterolateral impingement, posterolateral impingement of the ankle may also be seen clinically. Posterolateral impingement may occur in combination with anterolateral impingement problems. Diagnostic testing is generally nonrevealing for a posterolateral impingement lesion. It is generally difficult to evaluate and visualize these lesions without the use of

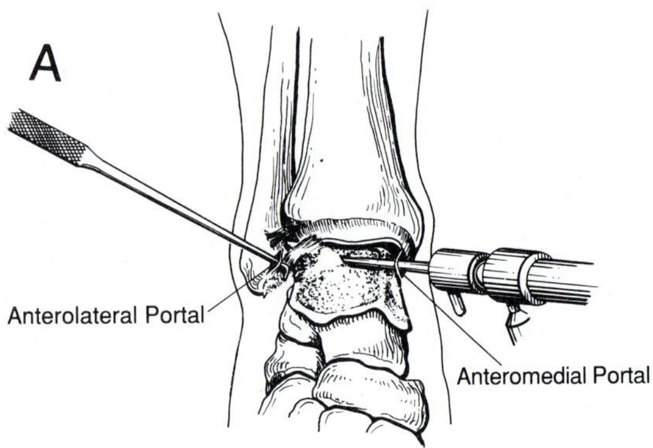

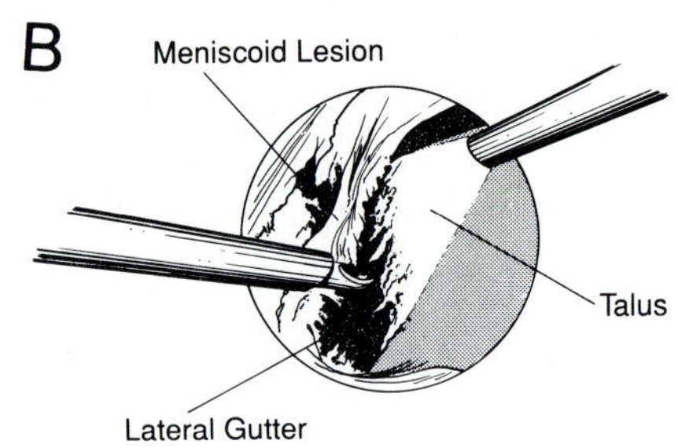

FIG 30–16.
A, anterolateral soft-tissue impingement. The probe is palpating the synovitis and fibrosis of the anterolateral gutter. **B,** synovectomy and debridement of the lateral gutter with a 2.9-mm full-radius shaver.

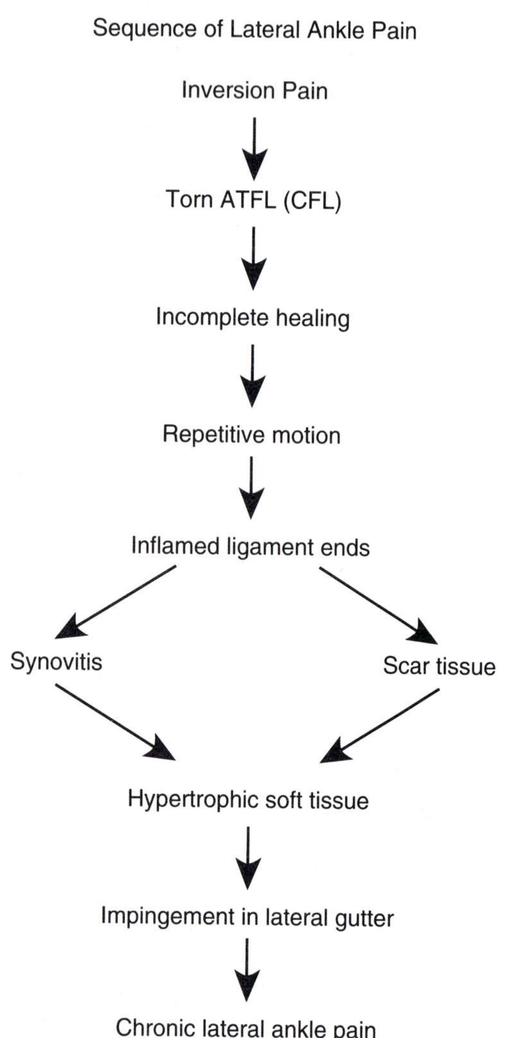

FIG 30–17.
Sequence of lateral ankle pain. *ATFL* = anterior talofibular ligament; *CFL* = calcaneofibular ligament.

a distractor. In addition, generalized posterolateral impingement may also occur with fibrosis, capsulitis, and synovial swelling. It is important to note that both localized and generalized posterolateral impingement may be missed during ankle arthroscopy if visualization from the posterolateral portal is not performed. Furthermore, it is routinely difficult to see synovial pathology in the posterolateral aspect of the ankle without the use of a distraction device.

Posterior impingement can also be caused by hypertrophy or a tear in the posterior inferior tibiofibular ligament, transverse tibiofibular ligament, tibial slip, or pathologic labrum on the posterior ankle joint (Fig 30–18). The transverse tibiofibular ligament can become hypertrophied and pathologic in certain instances. The ligament may be associated with a specific tibial slip; however, this is a rare occurrence. When both ligaments are seen together, there is a higher incidence of

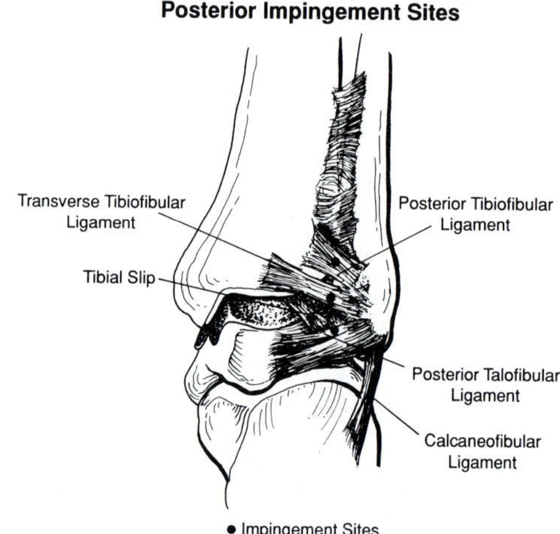

FIG 30–18.
Posterior impingement sites. Note the direction and orientation of the tibial slip.

impingement-type problems. Although excision of this hypertrophied ligament may lead to significant pain relief, great caution must be used in the diagnosis and treatment of this lesion.[21]

The tibial slip can also hypertrophy and be a cause of posterior soft-tissue impingement. The tibial slip runs between the posterior inferior tibiofibular ligament and the transverse ligament.[5] This ligament can develop fibrosis following trauma to the ankle with subsequent pain and swelling.

In addition, Hamilton[47] has also described a tibial labrum on the posterior lip of the tibia. This may become pathologic just like the superior labrum in the shoulder. This is a relatively rare finding for which the author has little clinical experience.

Syndesmotic Impingement

Injuries to the syndesmosis are among the most serious that occur to the ankle. Unfortunately, the incidence of these injuries has been underestimated in the past, particularly after an inversion mechanism. During an acute ankle sprain, if the talus inverts and the tibia rotates, stress is placed across the syndesmosis, and a tear of the syndesmosis occurs. The injury usually affects the AITF ligament and occasionally the interosseous membrane and posterior inferior tibiofibular ligament (Fig 30–19).

After injury, synovitis and scarring can occur in the area of the AITF ligament and corresponding joint. Soft-tissue impingement can develop with increased activity around the area of the ligament and the undersurface of the joint. Often at surgery, reddened synovium

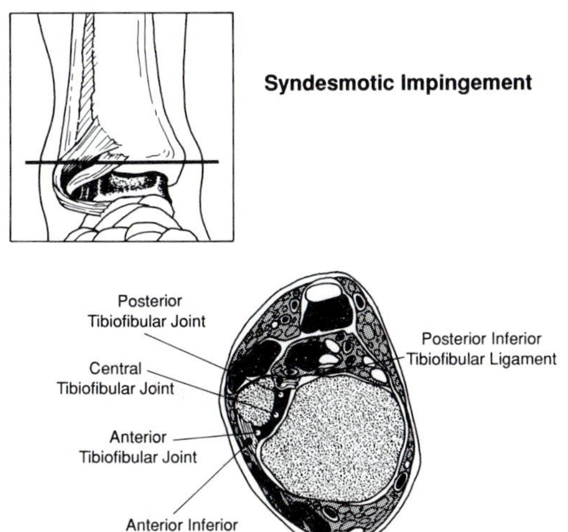

FIG 30–19.
Syndesmotic impingement. Note the cross-sectional anatomy through the syndesmosis demonstrating the confines of the lateral gutter at this level.

is seen surrounding the AITF and extruding into the distal tibiofibular joint. Sometimes the synovitis can extend through the joint all the way to the posterior articulation.

Bassett et al. reported impingement from a separate fascicle of the AITF ligament.[10] They did an anatomic study and found the fascicle to be present in 10 out of 11 cadavers. They suggested that with a tear of the anterior talofibular ligament, the patient can develop increased laxity, and the talar dome may extrude anteriorly in dorsiflexion and cause soft-tissue impingement. I have also seen a fascicle of the AITF ligament cause impingement and feel that this is traumatically induced rather than a normal variant (see Fig 30–14).

Treatment for syndesmotic soft-tissue impingement includes debriding the AITF ligament and tibiofibular joint. In addition, if a separate fascicle is seen, it should be removed. It appears from anatomic studies that approximately 20% of the syndesmotic ligament is intra-articular. On rare occasions, we have excised this portion of the ligament without any untoward effects to the patient at long-term follow-up.

Technique of Ankle Synovectomy

Several technical aspects of arthroscopic ankle synovectomy are important to emphasize. The authors prefer to have patients in the supine position with the use of thigh and ankle holders. This allows the foot to be secured in place and permits easy simultaneous access to the anteromedial, anterolateral, posterolateral, and the trans-Achilles portals. For localized anterior synovitis, distraction is not always necessary. However, distraction is helpful to permit complete visualization, especially in cases of generalized synovitis. I prefer to use the 2.9- or 3.5-mm full-radius blade for ankle synovectomy (Fig 30–20,A). In addition, I generally use a 2.7-mm, 30-degree oblique scope with a wide-angle lens and a large-screen picture.

An important key to a "successful" synovectomy is the maintenance of a high fluid flow system into the ankle and suction outward. This is best accomplished by using a separate inflow cannula placed through the posterolateral portal. The two anterior portals are used for the arthroscope and instruments including shavers, baskets, burrs, etc. In addition, it is important to have an interchangeable cannula system that allows the scope, baskets, shavers, and inflow to be switched easily without losing the portal sights. A systematic 15-point examination of the entire ankle should be routinely carried out. Synovectomy and debridement should be performed sequentially and thoroughly.

Caution: patients with rheumatoid arthritis have friable synovium. When debriding posteromedially or an-

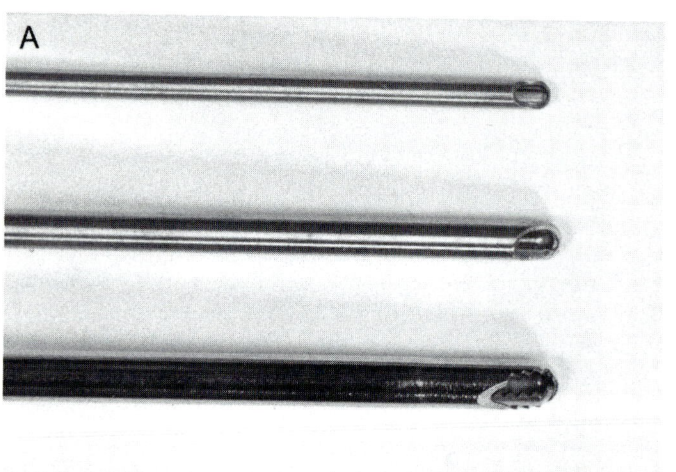

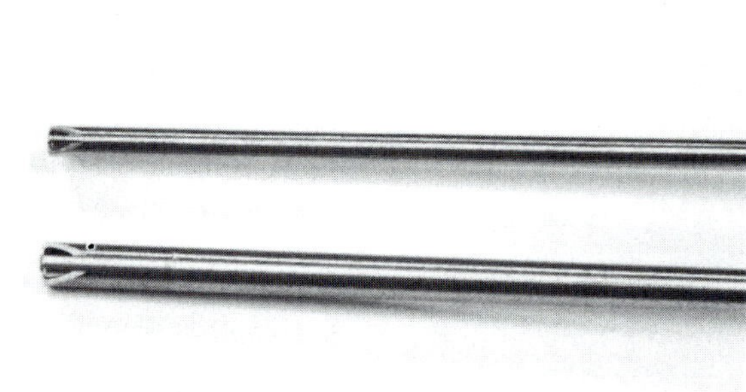

FIG 30–20.
Small-joint shavers. **A,** shaver blade tips utilized for small-joint arthroscopy. The 2.9-mm blade is above, and the 3.5-mm full-radius blade is below. **B,** "whisker" blades. Note that the blades are protected so that only a small amount of tissue is excised with each revolution.

terodorsally, extreme caution should be exercised so as not to injure the neurovascular structures. The full-radius blade should not be used for these areas. Instead the "whisker" is utilized to prevent injury to the neurovascular structures (Fig 30–20,B). Following complete synovectomy, the tourniquet should be released and drains inserted if extensive bleeding is noted. The portals should be closed with a nonabsorbable suture and a compression dressing applied. Splinting the ankle for a short period of time (5 to 7 days) may be performed, and then early range of motion is strongly encouraged.

Osteochondral Lesions of the Talus

Recent advances in operative ankle arthroscopy have resulted in the development of improved techniques, advanced arthroscopic instrumentation, and adequate visualization of the talar dome through the arthroscope. As a result, arthroscopic management of osteochondral lesions of the talus is becoming an increasingly attractive alternative.* More importantly, arthroscopic management of osteochondral lesions of the talus may reduce the morbidity associated with an extensive surgical approach, ankle arthrotomy, and malleolar osteotomy.

Terminology

Numerous terms have been used to describe osteochondral lesions of the talar dome, including transchondral fracture, osteochondral fracture, osteochondritis dissecans, talar dome fracture, and flaked fracture. The controversy in the lack of uniform terminology is, in part, the result of a lack of a clearly defined, universally accepted mechanism of injury. In 1922, Kappis first applied the term "osteochondritis dissecans" to the ankle joint. This term was accepted and remained in use until Berndt and Harty's classic treatise in 1959.[8, 12, 21] In this treatise, the term "transchondral fractures of the talus" was proposed, and trauma was established as the principle etiologic factor. In 1966, Campbell and Ranawat concluded that osteochondritis is a disease process resulting in pathologic fracture through necrotic bone as a result of ischemia.[18] The argument in support of idiopathic osteonecrosis as the underlying pathology is supported by the fact that trauma is not documented in all cases of osteochondral lesions of the talus. However, the authors feel that a traumatic etiology plays an important role in the pathogenesis of osteochondral lesions of the talus. The lesion likely represents the chronic phase of a compressed or avulsed talar dome fracture. Isolated incidents of macrotrauma or repeated cumulative microtrauma may contribute to initiation of the lesion in an individual predisposed to talar dome ischemia. An osteonecrotic process resulting in subchondral fracture and bony collapse may exist. The author advocates the use of the term *osteochondral lesions of the talus* (OLT) to describe these lesions. The presence of subchondral cysts with overlying chondromalacia and osteochondral fragments and loose bodies may all represent stages in the progression of this disease entity.

Incidence

The incidence of OLT has been reported as ranging from 0.09% of all talar fractures based on a series report

**References 5, 6, 40, 41, 50, 76, 82, 93.*

during World War II[24] to 6.5% of 133 ankle sprains reported by Bosien et al.[15] OLT is reported to occur in 4% of all cases of osteochondritis dissecans.[50] However, the actual incidence of OLT may be much higher than previously reported. The incidence of misdiagnosis or delayed diagnosis of OLT in a group of patients with unexplained chronic ankle pain has been reported to be as high as 81%.[37] Several series indicate that the incidence of bilateral lesions ranges around 10%.[12, 14, 46] Medial lesions are more common than lateral lesions.* In general, medial lesions tend to be more posterior, and lateral lesions tend to be more anterior[12, 13] (Fig 30–21,A). In addition, medial lesions tend to be deeper and cup shaped and are usually nondisplaced. On the other hand, lateral lesions are usually shallow, wafer shaped, and frequently displaced (Fig 30–21,B).

Diagnosis

Indications of OLT may be immediate following an acute ankle injury. More frequently, however, it is associated with chronic ankle pain, particularly following associated trauma such as an inversion injury to the lateral ligamentous complex. The history of chronic lateral ankle pain or chronic ankle sprain pain is frequently noted. In addition, a history of associated injuries such as ankle or lower-extremity fractures or falls from a height may be elicited. Other presenting symptoms may include recurrent ankle swelling, stiffness, weakness, or giving way. In certain patients, no specific mechanism of injury or associated causes may be documented. In this group of patients, an idiopathic osteonecrotic process or accumulative microtrauma may be the proposed etiology.

The differential diagnosis should include ankle soft-tissue impingement syndrome, reflex sympathetic dystrophy, degenerative arthrosis, occult fractures, lateral ankle instability, infection, tarsal coalition, peroneal subluxation or tendinitis, and subtalar dysfunction. A high index of suspicion must be maintained when patients with chronic ankle pain are evaluated. Periodic follow-up, examination, and selective lidocaine injections may be useful in making the correct diagnosis.

Following the history and physical examination, the diagnosis of OLT has traditionally been made by using plain roentgenograms. In 1959, a staging system was described by Berndt and Harty.[12] With advancements in technology such as computed tomography (CT) and MRI, our diagnostic capability is significantly improved. As a result, the author has proposed a new staging system modified from the Berndt and Harty classification that is based on his experience with high-resolution CT scanning of OLT (Fig. 30–22,A–C and Table 30–3). In addition, multiplanar tomography may be indicated in cases in which high-resolution CT scan may not be available.

Surgical Treatment

Surgical treatment of OLT has traditionally involved extensive ankle arthrotomy for excision of loose bodies, joint debridement, and drilling or abrasion at the site of the lesion. Numerous studies have reported the results of open techniques.* In addition, a number of methods

**References 6, 11, 18, 37, 40, 50, 64, 76, 93.*

**References 2, 12, 20, 39, 68, 70, 73, 81, 100.*

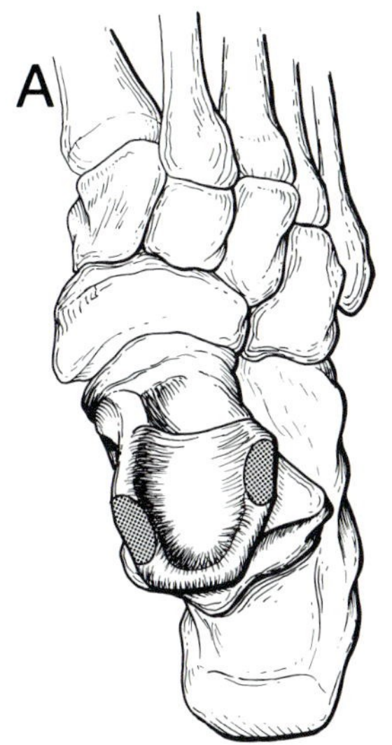

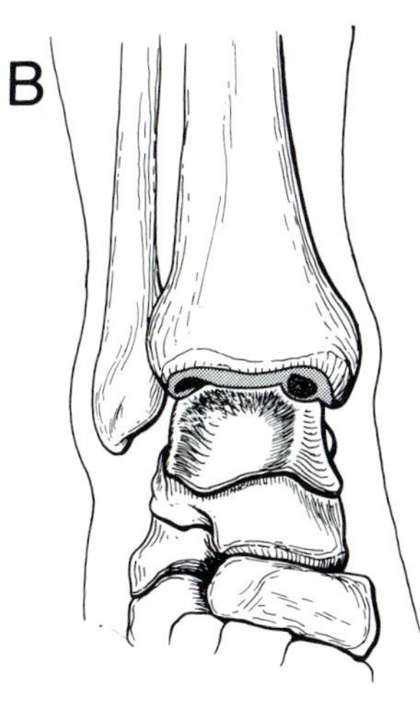

FIG 30–21.
Osteochondral lesions of the talus. **A,** the location of medial lesions tends to be more posterior, and the lateral lesions tend to be more anterior. **B,** the shape of the lateral lesions is usually shallow and waferlike and frequently displaced; the medial lesions tend to be deeper, cup shaped and usually nondisplaced.

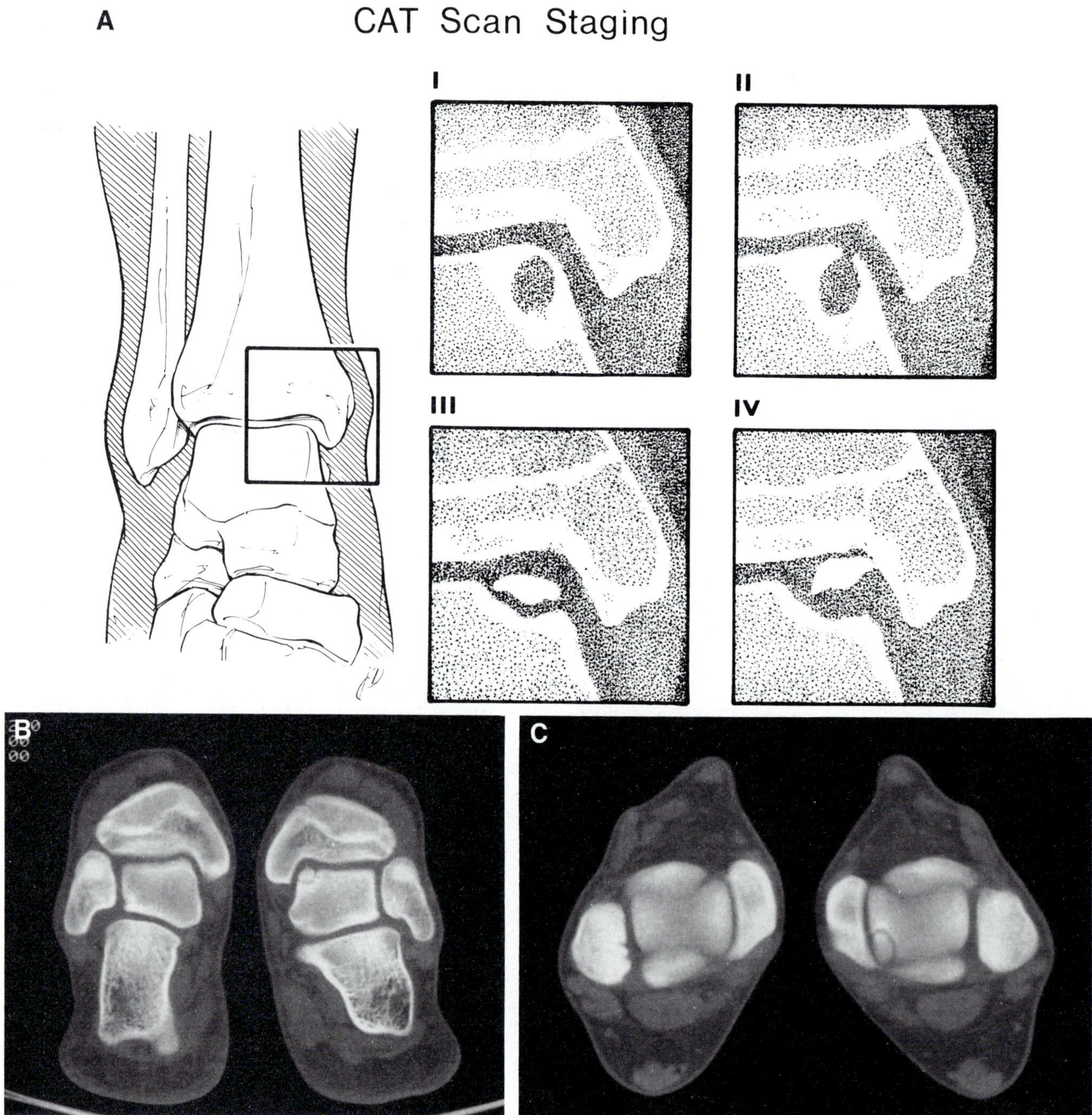

FIG 30–22.
Computerized axial tomography (CAT) staging. **A,** classification of stages. **B,** stage 3 CAT scan, coronal view. **C,** stage 3 CAT scan, axial view.

have been reported for the treatment of posterior lesions, particularly those involving the posteromedial aspect of the talar dome, including the use of extensive arthrotomy,[92] distal tibial articular surface grooving,[39, 45] medial and lateral malleolar osteotomies,[2, 12, 20, 64, 73, 74] and percutaneous fluoroscopic drilling.[41] These approaches require significant tissue trauma and may be associated with nonunion or malunion of the malleoli, postoperative joint stiffness, prolonged rehabilitation time, suboptimal cosmetic appearance, and inadequate posterior visualization of the talar dome lesion. With the development of improved instrumentation and technology, ankle arthroscopy has evolved to become a useful tool for both the diagnosis and treatment of osteochondral lesions of the talus. Ankle arthroscopy provides an alternative approach to open procedures and may pro-

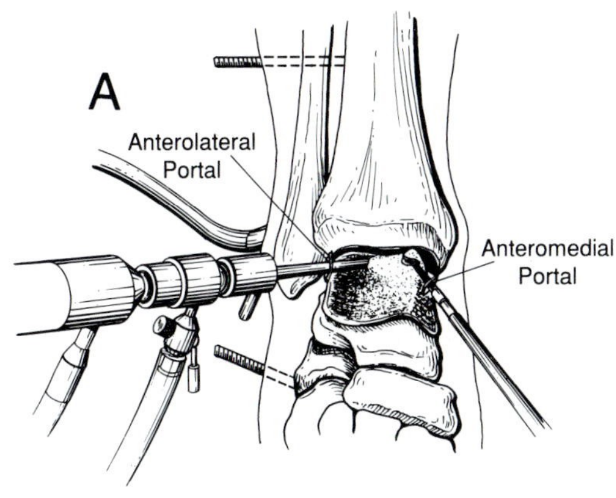

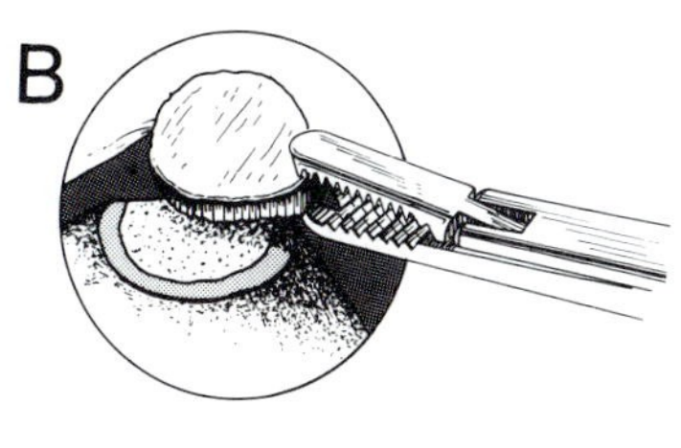

FIG 30–23.
Excision of osteochondral lesions of the talus. Note the inflow is through the posterolateral portal. **A,** the lesion is removed while visualizing through the anterolateral portal and inserting a banana knife anteromedially. **B,** once the lesion has been freed, it can be extracted with a grasper.

vide superior visualization of the talar dome and improved access to the lesion without an extensive surgical approach. This may serve to reduce the morbidity associated with ankle arthrotomy or malleolar osteotomy.

Operative Techniques

1. The design and use of small-joint arthroscopic instruments have greatly facilitated operative techniques for OLTs. Inspection, identification, and staging of all lesions in articular surfaces is performed intraoperatively.
2. Any loose bodies and osteochondral fragments are excised and extracted.
3. Palpation of the talar articular surface is essential for an appreciation of the extent of the overlying cartilaginous softening and blistering and to adequately stage the lesion.
4. Various instruments are used, including the 2.9-mm-diameter full-radius shaver, 2.9-mm-diameter high-speed burr, mini–suction punch, 3.5- and 4.5-mm ring curettes, mini–pituitary grasper, and arthroscopic scalpels.
5. Following debridement, a scalpel may be used to excise loose chondral fragments and areas of surface blistering (Figure 30–23,A).
6. A grasper is then utilized to remove the chondral pieces (Fig 30–23,B). However, caution must be exercised, and this technique should be limited to debridement of significant chondral flaps. The authors do not advocate removing softened but intact cartilage.
7. Transmalleolar drilling is performed from a percutaneous stab incision at a supermalleolar level. A mini–drill guide (MicroVector) has been developed to improve triangulation and facilitate precise positioning of the drill pin (Fig 30–24).
8. Occasionally, fluoroscopy may be used to assist with drilling. This is not frequently required since the advent of mechanical distraction techniques.
9. Distraction of the ankle allows dorsiflexion and plantar flexion of the ankle so that drilling may be performed throughout the entire lesion to eliminate passage of the drill through the tibial plafond.
10. Drilling is performed with 0.062-in. Kirschner wires to create osseous vascular channels. All lesions, particularly those involving subchondral bone, are drilled at 3- to 5-mm intervals to a depth of 10 mm.

TABLE 30–3.
Radiographic Staging of Osteochondral Lesions of the Talus

Stage	Berndt and Harty System[12]	CT System[37]
I	Compressed	Cystic lesion with an intact roof
II	Disrupted	Lesion extending to the surface
III	Partially displaced	Open lesion with fragments
IV	Displaced	Open lesion with displaced fragments

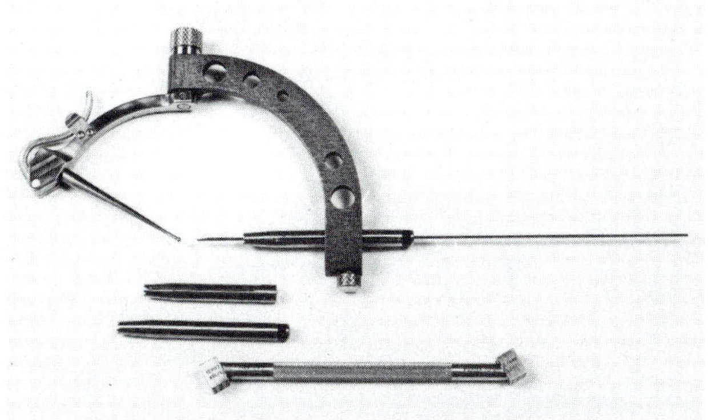

FIG 30–24.
MicroVector drill guide with a retractable tip and offset guide.

Drilling may be performed through the three basic arthroscopic portals from inferior to superior or through a transmalleolar technique in a superior-to-inferior fashion (Fig 30–25, A and B).

11. Lateral lesions, especially anterior ones, may be more amenable to pinning than medial ones. The advent of absorbable pins has allowed accurate fixation with early motion and has avoided additional surgery for pin removal (Fig 30–26A to C).

Specific Lesions

Anterolateral Lesions.—The anterolateral or central lesions of the talar dome may best be approached through the anteromedial and anterolateral portals. Drilling or pinning using the mini–drill guide may be performed through the anterolateral portal while visualizing through the anteromedial portal. The posterolateral portal is used for fluid inflow.

Anteromedial Lesions.—The anteromedial lesions are less common and may be instrumented and drilled through an anteromedial portal, with visualization through an anterolateral portal. The posterolateral portal is used for fluid inflow.

Posterolateral Lesions.—Posterolateral lesions are also relatively rare and may be instrumented through the posterolateral portal or through the tibia while visualization is performed through the posterolateral and anterolateral portals. The anteromedial portals may be used for fluid inflow.

Posteromedial Lesions.—Posteromedial or posterocentral lesions are best approached by visualization through the posterolateral portal and drilling performed transmalleolarly with the drill guide. Instruments such as the shaver, curette, and extractors may be inserted through the anteromedial portal. The instrument cannula may be exchanged with the inflow cannula anteriorly, and an accessory posterolateral portal may be established to facilitate instrumentation as needed. This is particularly useful with more posteriorly situated lesions (Fig 30–27).

Postoperative Care

Following drilling, the tourniquet is deflated and the fluid flow turned off. This allows one to visualize the area of pathology and to evaluate whether adequate vascular access was created over the site of pathology. It continues to remain controversial whether drilling or abrasion of the subchondral surfaces remains the treatment of choice. At the present time, the author advocates drilling intact symptomatic lesions. If the lesion is loose, it should be removed. Abrasion of smaller lesions is recommended, but larger lesions (greater than 1 cm) should be treated by drilling.

Following irrigation of the joint, the distractors and pins are removed and all portals and incisions sutured with monofilament nylon suture material. The ankle is wrapped with a bulky compression dressing and a posterior plaster splint applied in the neutral position for 5 to 7 days. Following this, patients are started on early range-of-motion and strengthening exercises. All patients are generally kept non–weight bearing for a period of 6 to 8 weeks.

Conclusion

The evolution of smaller instrumentation and improved technology has made ankle arthroscopy an effective alternative for the diagnosis and treatment of osteochondral lesions of the talus. The arthroscopic approach has provided good to excellent results in 84% of the patients in the author's series of 65 patients. The advan-

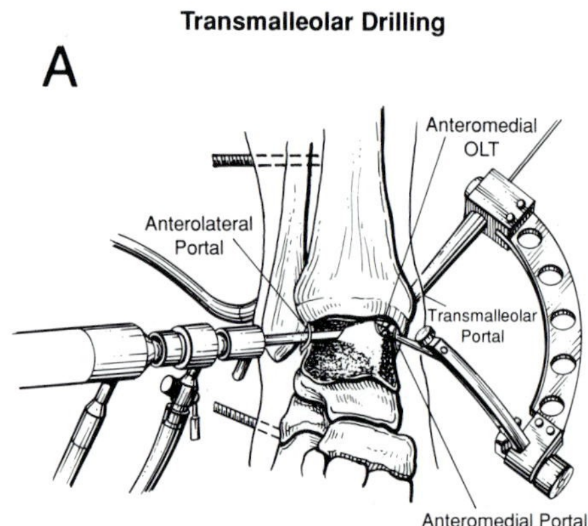

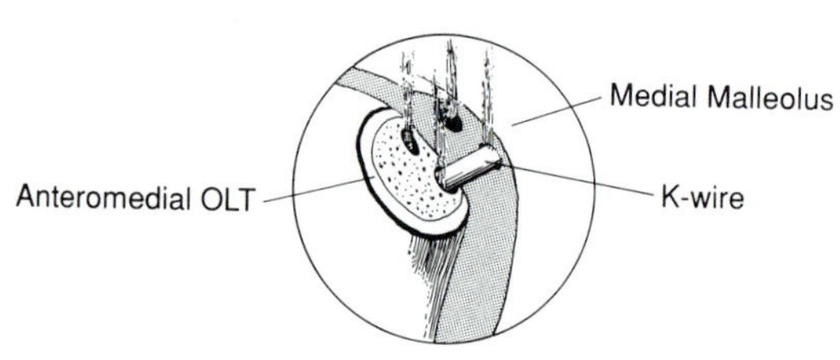

FIG 30–25.
A, transmalleolar drilling of an osteochondral lesion of the medial dome of the talus using the MicroVector. Note visualization is through the anterolateral portal and the inflow is placed through the posterolateral portal. **B**, the drill holes are established through the medial malleolus into the talus down to areas of bleeding bone.

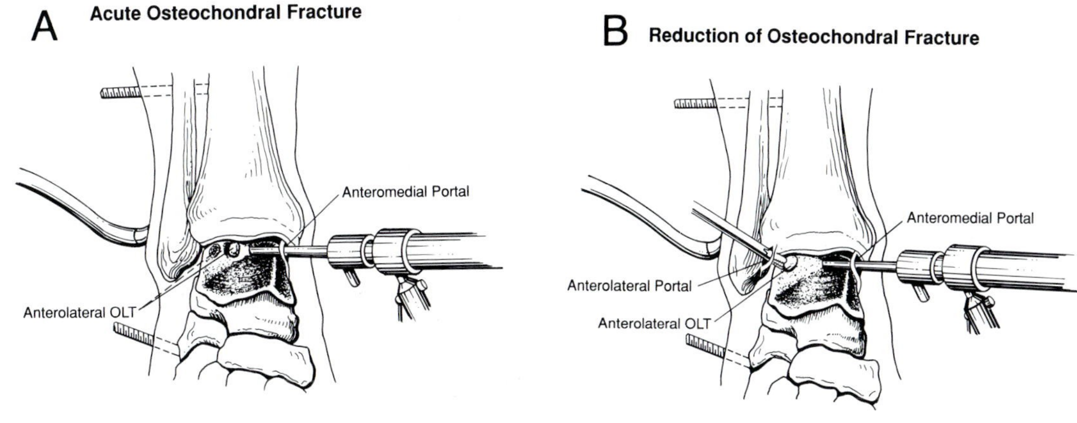

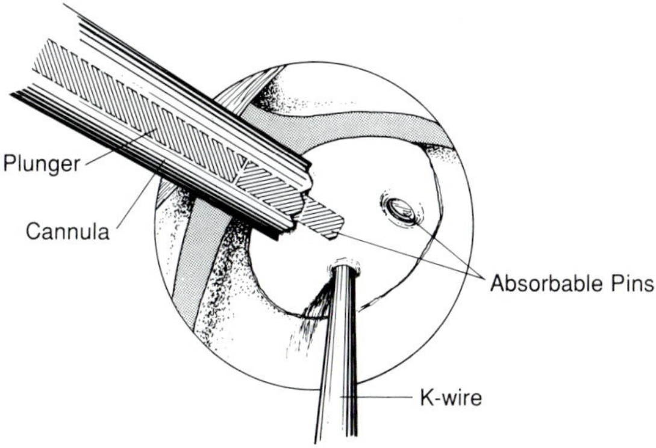

FIG 30–26.
Internal fixation of an osteochondral lesion of the lateral dome of the talus. **A**, osteochondral fracture visualized from the anteromedial portal with inflow posterior and anterolateral portal used for probing and instrumentation. **B**, insertion of the clamp or other device to reduce the acute fracture to its fracture bed on the lateral talar dome. **C**, internal fixation of the acute osteochondral fracture with absorbable pin fixation.

tages of arthroscopy include decreased morbidity, shortened hospitalization, early range of motion, and return of strength. An extensive surgical approach in ankle arthrotomy or a malleolar osteotomy is not required. Visualization is superior, and access to difficult-to-reach lesions is achievable with the use of distraction devices. High-resolution CT scanning of the ankle preoperatively has been found to be helpful in staging and operative preplanning.

Arthroscopic Treatment of Chondral and Osteochondral Lesions of the Ankle

The following section discusses the arthroscopic management of chondral and osteochondral lesions of the ankle joint, excluding osteochondral lesions of the talus (osteochondritis dissecans).

Osteochondral lesions of the ankle joint may include osteophytes, chondral and osteochondral loose bodies, protuberances secondary to fracture and trauma, chondral lesions involving the tibia and talus, degenerative and posttraumatic arthritic changes, and cystic lesions. A spectrum of symptoms may result from chondral and osteochondral lesions of the ankle, including the symptoms of pain, swelling, popping, locking, and limited range of motion. These lesions have frequently been a diagnostic challenge to orthopaedic surgeons, particularly for those lesions that are chondral or soft tissue in nature. Advancement in arthroscopy of the ankle has allowed the orthopaedic surgeon to directly visualize the ankle joint for evaluation of such pathology and enables arthroscopic management of these lesions without an extensive surgical approach and ankle arthrotomy.

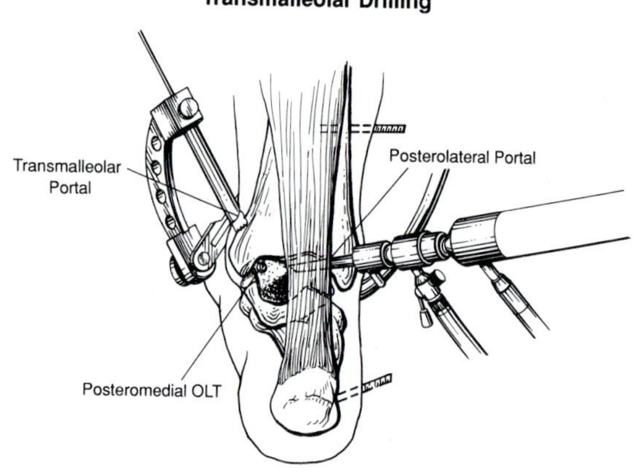

FIG 30–27.
Posteromedial osteochondral lesion of the talus. Note that the arthroscope is through the posterolateral portal to visualize the lesion while the instruments are brought in through the anteromedial portal and inflow is done through the anterolateral portal.

Loose Bodies

Etiology.—Loose bodies may be either chondral or osteochondral in origin. The causes of loose bodies are many, and they range from a minor ankle sprain to major ankle trauma. In addition, multiple loose bodies may form in synovial chondromatosis or synovial osteochondromatosis. The former is difficult to diagnose with radiography, CT, or MRI. This is due to the fact that cartilaginous lesions are, in general, radiolucent. Although this disorder is more common in the larger joints, it may certainly involve the ankle joint.

Signs and Symptoms.—Loose bodies in the ankle joint may cause symptoms of catching and locking with resultant pain, swelling, and limitation of range of motion. Symptoms may be intermittent due to the fact that a loose body may become fixed in the synovial lining, therefore becoming asymptomatic until it is loosened and enters the ankle joint. The physical examination is generally unrevealing. Frequently, it is difficult to detect a specific area of tenderness. Rarely is a loose body palpable.

Diagnostic Evaluation.—Although plain radiographs will generally reveal the presence of an osseous loose body, chondral loose bodies are not visible on plain x-ray examination (Fig 30–28,A and B). The arthrogram, however, will effectively reveal the presence of chondral loose bodies, particularly in the presence of synovial chondromatosis. Bone scans are rarely informative. MRI holds greater promise for revealing chondral lesions not otherwise visible on plain radiographs; however, its role has not been clearly established in the detection of chondral loose bodies. Therefore, a combination of diagnostic tests, including radiographs, arthrograms, CT scans, or MRI scans, should be effectively utilized to diagnose the presence and origin of the loose bodies preoperatively.

It is of critical importance to determine the general

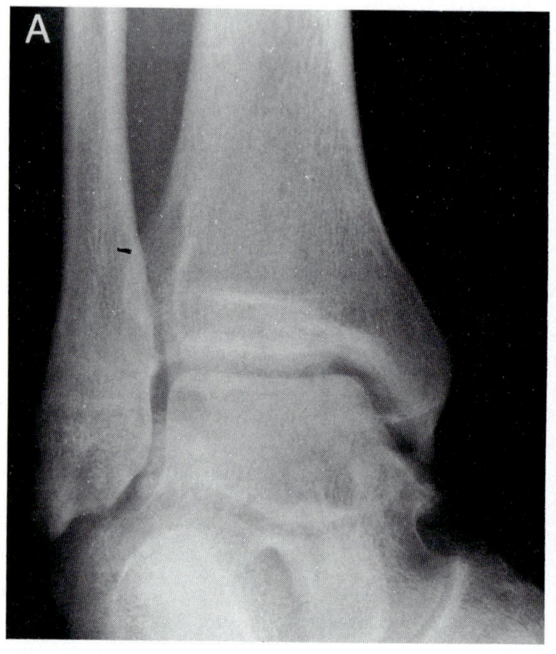

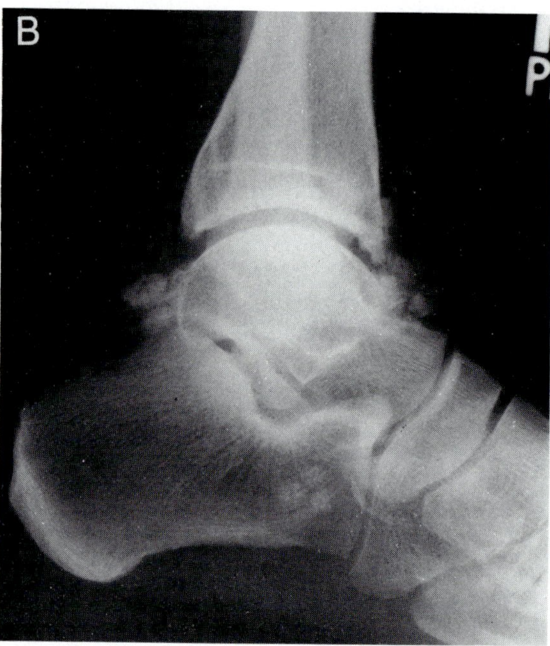

FIG 30–28.
Synovial chondromatosis of the ankle. **A,** anteroposterior view; **B,** lateral view.

location of the loose body, whether it is intra-articular, intracapsular, or extra-articular, as part of the preoperative planning.

Treatment.—Treatment of loose bodies should entail the standard ankle arthroscopic technique. It is critical to employ the 15-point ankle examination protocol in order to systematically evaluate the entire ankle, including both anterior and posterior compartments. Distraction of the ankle joint may be particularly helpful, both in visualization of the loose body as well as surgical access to the loose body in difficult-to-reach areas.

Portals.—A loose body in the anterior compartment may usually be removed from the anterior portals. However, it may be necessary to place the arthroscope in the posterolateral portal and utilize the anteromedial or anterolateral portals for removal of the loose body. A loose body in the posterior compartment of the ankle may be best removed with the arthroscope placed in either of the anterior portals and accomplishing removal of the loose body through instrumentation placed in the posterolateral portal or by pushing the loose body into the anterior compartment.

Following loose body removal, a repeat examination of the entire ankle joint surfaces should be performed to detect any residual loose body and determine the origin of the lesion. If a substantial chondral or osteochondral defect is detected, debridement, burring, and possibly drilling should be performed. If a significant osteophyte was responsible for the loose body, the osteophyte should be aggressively debrided with an arthroscopic burr.

Postoperative Care.—Postoperatively, a bulky compressive dressing with a posterior splint is applied. The patient is started on range-of-motion exercises at 5 to 7 days postoperatively. The exercise routine is then gradually advanced to include strengthening and increased range of motion. The clinical results of loose body removal are dependent upon the underlying cause of the loose body and the presence of degenerative or posttraumatic arthritis in the ankle joint. In the presence of significant degenerative or posttraumatic arthritis, the results tend to be less predictable.[62]

Osteophytes

Osteophytes in the ankle joint are most commonly seen at the anterior lip of the tibia. They usually present as a beaklike prominence and are associated with a corresponding area over the neck of the talus. Talar lesions may be either a defect or an opposing "kissing" lesion osteophyte. This lesion may be the result of direct trauma following forced dorsiflexion injuries to the ankle or may be the result of forced plantar flexion causing capsular avulsion injury. Anterior impingement secondary to osteophyte formation is quite common following athletic injuries with a 45% incidence reported in football players and a 59.3% incidence in dancers.[72, 89]

These osteophytes may cause impingement resulting in limited range of motion, pain, catching, and joint swelling.[53] Normally the angle between the distal end of the tibia and the talus is greater than 60 degrees (Fig 30–29). However, with osteophytic formation on the distal part of the tibia and/or talar neck, this angle diminishes to under 60 degrees (Fig 30–30). Occasionally, exostosis may occur anterolaterally between the talus and the lateral malleolus. This may be a source of symptomatic complaint and disability in the athlete.[85] In addition, osteophytes have also been noted on the anterior aspect of the medial malleolus and may be a source of symptoms when they impinge upon the talus. Posterior ankle joint osteophytes may also form and cause clinical symptoms with plantar flexion of the ankle.

It is important during preoperative evaluation to determine the relative medial and lateral extent of the osteophytes. The anatomic location of the osteophytes should be determined to the extent possible preoperatively. Surgical localization may be difficult.

Signs and Symptoms.—Clinically, a patient may have evidence of anterior ankle pain exacerbated by walking up stairs, squatting, or running. Tenderness may be localized over the bony prominence of the anterior ankle joint and exacerbated by passive ankle dorsiflexion. Range of motion may be limited, particularly in dorsiflexion. Plain x-ray studies will frequently demonstrate

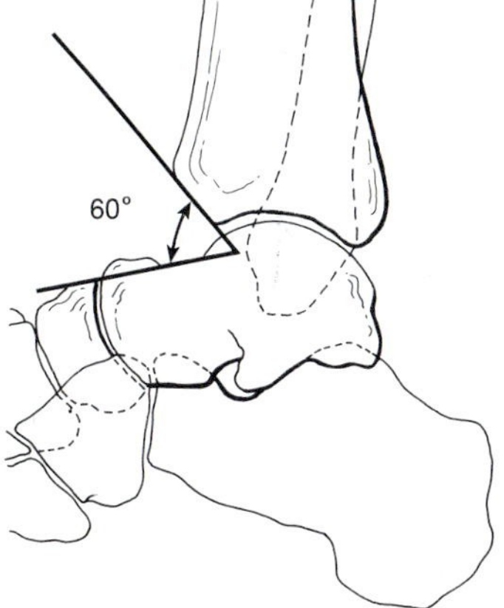

FIG 30–29.
The normal angle between the distal tibia and talus is 60 degrees or greater.

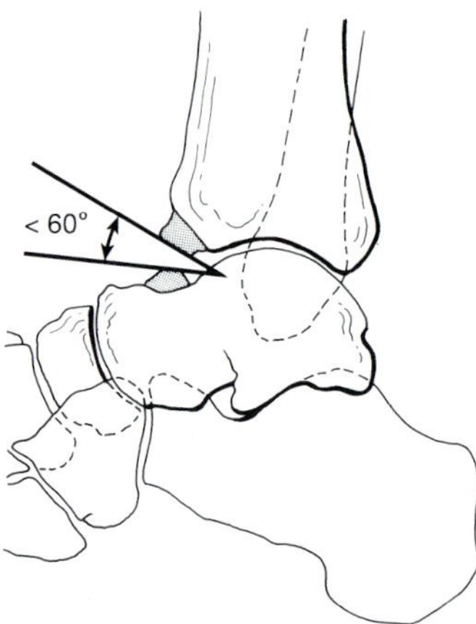

FIG 30–30.
Osteophytic formation on the distal tibia and/or talar neck with the angle diminished to under 60 degrees.

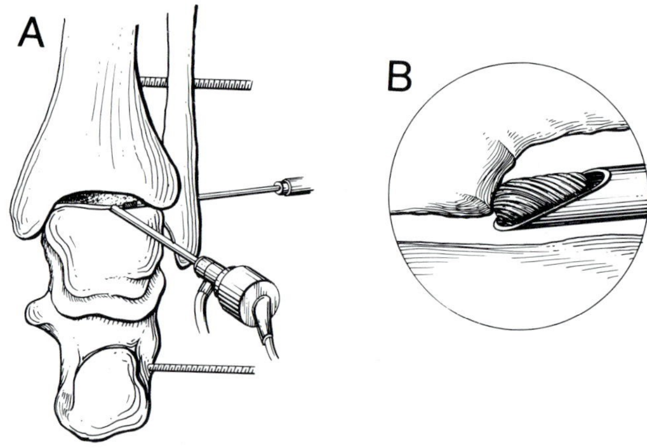

FIG 30–31.
Excision of the anterior osteophyte through posterolateral visualization. **A**, note the anterior overhang of the osteophyte well seen visualizing through the posterolateral portal. **B**, excision of the osteophyte can be done with a motorized burr or osteotome.

the anterior osteophyte, and lateral stress radiographs performed in maximum dorsiflexion may demonstrate impingement of the two osteophytes anteriorly. A bone scan would show evidence of an increased uptake in the area of the osteophytes in symptomatic lesions. A CAT scan in the coronal and axial planes may also be helpful in localizing the size and extent as well as the location of osteophytes.

Treatment.—Arthroscopic resection of ankle osteophytes may be performed in patients with progressive symptoms, pain well localized to the anterior aspect of the palpable bony prominence, and limitation of range of motion. Anterior osteophytes are usually accessible to arthroscopic technique for resection. Anterior osteophytes may generally be visualized without the use of distraction. However, distraction is often necessary to "get around" the osteophytes during resection. Most osteophytes can be excised by utilizing the anteromedial and anterolateral portals with a burr, osteotome, or rongeur. Occasionally, it is necessary to place the arthroscope through the posterolateral portal to remove these osteophytes. Mechanical distraction of the ankle is frequently necessary in order to visualize the anterior osteophytes through the posterior portals (Fig 30–31). Systematic evaluation of the entire ankle joint should be performed to evaluate the coexistence of other intra-articular pathology or the presence of loose bodies. If significant synovitis is present as part of the inflammatory reaction to the presence of an osteophyte, synovectomy may be performed to improve visualization.

Postoperative Care.—Postoperatively, patients are managed with a heavy, bulky dressing and a posterior splint. Range of motion is started 5 to 7 days postoperatively, with increased strengthening and range-of-motion exercises.

Chondral Lesions

Etiology.—Chondral lesions of the articular surface of the talus or tibia may result following acute or accumulative trauma to the ankle joint. The spectrum of injury to the joint surface ranges from softening or fibrillation of the cartilage surface to gross separation and detachment of the articular cartilage from the underlying subchondral bone. The most common etiology for chondral injuries is acute trauma such as an ankle sprain. The talar dome is more frequently injured than the tibial plafond.

Diagnostic Evaluation.—Pure chondral lesions of the ankle may be difficult to detect with plain radiographs. Bone scans will show abnormalities only if the chondral injury is associated with injury to or a reaction of the underlying subchondral bone. Plain CT is unlikely to reveal the underlying lesion. However, a CT arthrogram or an arthrographic tomogram may be able to pick up a defect in the chondral surface. In addition, as MRI techniques continue to advance, there is great promise to be able assess areas of chondral injuries previously difficult to diagnose. Clinical symptoms of a chondral lesion may include pain, swelling, catching, and limited range of motion. This is frequently a diagnostic challenge for the orthopaedic surgeon, and ankle arthroscopy is an excellent tool in the direct diagnosis of chondral lesions in patients who are symptomatic with a nonrevealing radiographic examination.

Treatment.—A systematic 15-point examination of the ankle should be performed to evaluate the entire joint surface and to document all associated pathology. Distraction of the ankle with the ankle distractor is frequently helpful in improving visualization and access to all parts of the ankle joint. Both the anterior and posterior compartments of the ankle should be carefully evaluated. In particular, the posteromedial talar dome should be evaluated because chondral and osteochondral lesions are frequently found in this area.

In addition to visualization, the entire articular surface of the talus and tibia should be gently probed to detect changes in surface texture and consistency. Fibrinous cartilage should be gently debrided to stable and adherent cartilage. If subchondral bone is exposed secondary to the lesion or debridement, drilling is generally recommended to establish vascular channels in the subchondral bone with eventual formation of fibrocartilage surface.[23]

If the chondral lesion is posteromedial, transmalleolar drilling may be performed. This may be best accomplished by using a triplaned vector guide designed by Ferkel to localize the specific area of the lesion. Transmalleolar drilling may then be performed with sequential dorsiflexion and planter flexion of the ankle. Multiple drill holes are placed in the lesion. The tourniquet is then let down and the flow pressure decreased in order to visualize and establish the vascular channels within the lesion. Postoperatively, the ankle is mobilized with bulky dressing and a posterior splint for 5 to 7 days. Active motion is then begun. Weight bearing is delayed for 6 to 8 weeks to optimize fibrocartilaginous healing of the lesion.

Traumatic and Degenerative Arthritis

Specific indications must be selected in order for arthroscopy of the ankle to be effective in the presence of degenerative changes. Arthritic ankle joints with advanced joint destruction, marked joint line narrowing, extensive fibrosis, and a significant degree of instability or deformity, should be excluded from ankle arthroscopy. Candidates for ankle arthroscopy include those patients with ankles having only limited motion secondary to capsulitis; a minimal to moderate degree of fibroarthrosis, osteophytes, chondral defects, or loose bodies; and only a minimal degree of instability. Patients' symptoms, length of conservative treatment, and expectations are important and realistic concerns in the selection of candidates for ankle arthroscopy.

During ankle arthroscopy, a variety of pathology may be encountered, so each lesion must be dealt with separately. Loose bodies should be removed; osteophytes may be debrided; synovial impingement lesions, whether local or generalized, should be resected; and chondral and osteochondral defects over joint surfaces should be debrided. Abrasion of exposed subchondral bone with reestablishment of vascular channels and fibrocartilage formation may be advantageous. Postoperatively, early range of motion must be established. Progressive strengthening, stretching, and range-of-motion exercises should be performed.

Arthroscopic Treatment of Chronic Ankle Fractures

Ankle arthroscopy may be a useful diagnostic and therapeutic tool in the management of patients following chronic ankle fractures. Use of the ankle distractor is generally recommended since in many of these patients the ankle joint is contracted and motion is limited secondary to arthrofibrosis. Therefore, visualization is initially quite difficult without the use of ankle distraction. A cannula should always be inserted in the posterolateral portal, and a high inflow portal should be established.

Fifteen-point examination of the anterior and posterior compartments of the ankle should be performed in a systematic fashion. Proliferative synovitis and arthrofibrosis should be carefully debrided so that visualization of the entire joint is possible. All loose bodies should be removed. The entire joint should be debrided free of scar, fibrotic tissues, and synovitis. The presence of any cartilaginous or osteochondral lesions should be identified and treated. In view of a contracted joint capsule and significant scarring, care must be taken to avoid injury to the dorsal neurovascular structures at all times.

Arthroscopic Treatment of Lateral Ankle Instability

Lateral ankle sprains due to forced inversion are one of the most common ankle injuries seen by the orthopaedic surgeon.[41] Treatment for lateral ankle sprains has traditionally been conservative. However, recurrent lateral ankle sprains may result in chronic instability that may not respond favorably to conservative management.[56] Surgical repair may be necessary to correct chronic lateral ankle instability.[84, 86] Over recent years, techniques of ankle arthroscopy have advanced, and it may now be a viable tool for both the diagnosis and treatment of chronic lateral ankle instability.

Diagnostic Evaluation

The major complaint in patients with lateral ankle instability is pain and swelling following each episode of injury. This is followed by a sense of instability and giving way. Other complaints may include weakness, stiffness, tenderness, a sense of looseness, and sensitivity to damp or cold weather.

Thorough preoperative evaluation is necessary before a diagnosis of chronic lateral instability can be made. Ankle arthroscopy is an excellent diagnostic tool in confirming the diagnosis of lateral instability with its direct visualization of the ligamentous structures around the ankle joint.

Technique of Arthroscopic Stabilization of the Ankle

The technique for arthroscopic stabilization of the ankle for lateral instability will not be discussed in detail in this section since the author does not utilize this technique. Hawkins has lectured and written extensively about this technique.[52] Initially, a staple was utilized to secure the soft tissues to the bone after the talus had been abraded. Because of problems with the staples, more recently a suture anchor technique using Mitek anchor sutures has been developed. These are placed percutaneously through the lateral portal and planted parallel to the tibiotalar joint. Postoperative management includes a weight-bearing cast for 6 weeks and then subsequent rehabilitation.

Arthroscopic Ankle Arthrodesis

Arthrodesis of the ankle joint is an excellent procedure for the treatment of end-stage degenerative joint disease of the ankle. Patients have been able to return to work, including heavy labor. The efficacy of a variety of techniques of ankle fusion has been established by numerous authors.[7, 19, 55, 59, 61, 63, 91] More than 30 distinct techniques for ankle arthrodesis have been described. Techniques differ in terms of surgical approach, mode of fixation, type of bone grafting, and clinical success.* Many potential complications exist in ankle fusion, and the incidence has been reported to be as high as 60%.[57] Potential complications of ankle fusion may include nonunion, delayed union, wound infection, pain, tibial fracture, hardware failure, and unsightly scars. The reported incidence of pseudarthrosis in the literature is as high as 23%.[3, 7, 16, 27, 83, 87] Open ankle arthrodesis typically requires an extensive surgical approach and significant tissue dissection. It may be partly responsible for devascularization of the bony tissue and potential high incidence of infection.

The goal of arthroscopic ankle arthrodesis is to allow preparation of the joint surfaces for successful arthrodesis without extensive arthrotomy, soft-tissue dissection, devascularization of the bony tissue, and unsightly scars.

Arthroscopic ankle arthrodesis, similar to open ankle arthrodesis, involves three basic principles: first, debridement and removal of all hyaline cartilage and underlying avascular subchondral bone; second, reduction in the appropriate position for fusion of the ankle; and third, rigid and stable internal fixation in the reduced position.

Surgical Technique

1. Position the patient supine on the operating table with a fluoroscopic attachment. The operative leg should be placed so that the ankle is easily accessible to fluoroscopy and use of the image intensifier.
2. Ankle distraction should be performed intraoperatively for maximum visualization and access to the entire ankle joint.
3. The standard arthroscopic portals are used: anterolateral, anteromedial, and posterolateral. The arthroscope is first inserted in the anterolateral portal to assess the amount of distraction. Once adequate visualization is achieved, the posterolateral portal is established for fluid flow and eventual instrumentation to the posterior compartment.
4. The entire articular surface of the tibial plafond, talar dome, and the medial and lateral talomalleolar surfaces should be systematically abraded by using a motorized abrader placed through the anteromedial portal.
5. All remaining hyaline cartilage and sclerotic subchondral bone should be removed. Debridement should be carried out until underlying viable cancellous bone is exposed.
6. Care should be taken to maintain the anatomic bony contour of the talar dome and the tibial plafond.
7. Previously existing varus/valgus deformity may be corrected at this time, although advanced deformities should be treated by open techniques. One must be careful to avoid resecting too much bone or squaring off the surfaces to prevent the creation of a varus/valgus deformity that may result in a delayed union or malunion (Fig 30–32,A and B).
8. In general, the posterior compartment may be

**References 7, 19, 55, 59, 61, 63, 88, 91, 94.*

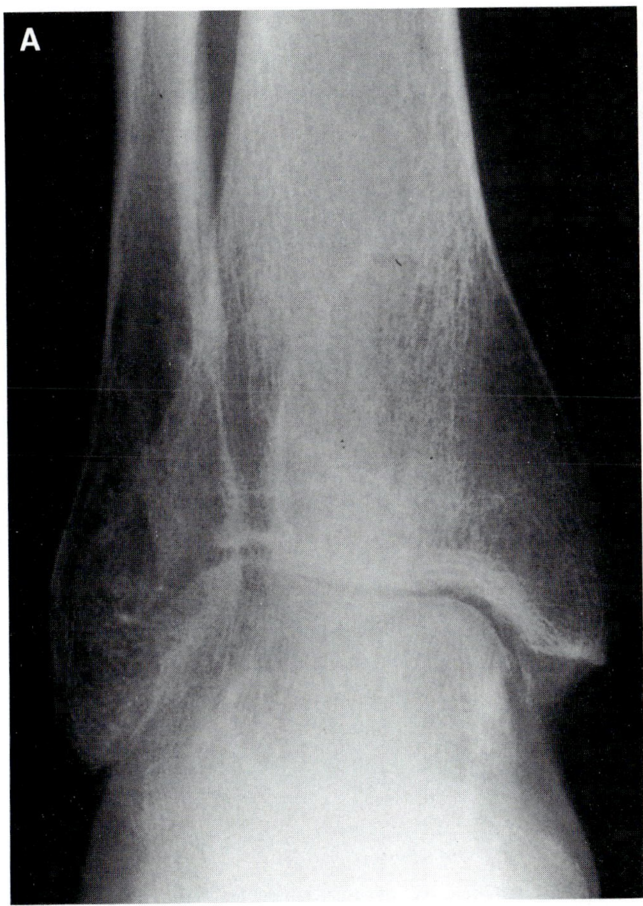

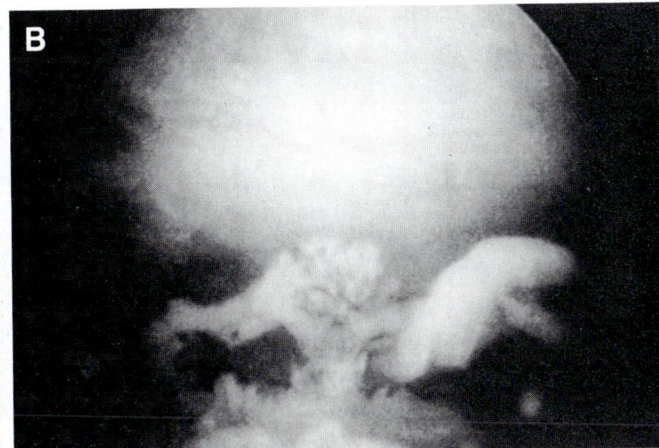

FIG 30–32.
Arthroscopic fusion of the ankle. **A,** preoperative radiograph. **B,** arthroscopic view.

abraded from the anterior portals. If the motorized burr does not reach adequately into the posterior compartment, a 15-degree angle curette may be used.

9. In addition, it is occasionally easier to reach the posterior compartment by abrading through the posterolateral portal while viewing through the anterolateral portal.

10. In general, the medial portion of the debridement process is performed with the arthroscope placed anterolaterally and the abrader placed anteromedially.

11. Conversely, the lateral half of the debridement process is generally accomplished with the arthroscope placed anteromedially and the abrader placed anterolaterally.

12. An anterior lip osteophyte should be removed so that it does not block reduction of the talar dome convexity into the tibial plafond cavity. This may be achieved by abrading and viewing through the anterior portals.

13. If the anterior capsule is adherent to the anterior osteophyte, visualization through the posterolateral portal will make it possible to assess the amount of bone required to be removed.

14. A small osteotome may be placed through a ½-in. incision made directly over the osteophyte to facilitate its rapid removal.

15. Once cancellous bone with viable vascularity is established over the entire fusion area, two guidepins may be drilled percutaneously into the tibial plafond and lateral malleolus under direct vision.

16. The first pin is drilled from the proximal part of the medial malleolus just above the joint line. The second pin is drilled laterally through the lateral malleolus and the posterior aspect of the joint line. The medial pin is directed slightly posteriorly, and the lateral pin is directed anteriorly.

17. The tips of the pins should penetrate the tibial plafond and lateral malleolus and may be viewed directly by using the arthroscope.

18. The pins are then advanced into the talus under direct vision with the arthroscope to confirm their correct position.

19. These pins are then backed out so that the tips are level with the denuded surfaces of the tibial plafond and the lateral malleolus.

20. The distraction should then be released and the arthroscopic instruments removed. The ankle surfaces are then compressed.

21. Fluoroscopy should be used at this time to confirm satisfactory positioning of the ankle position of fusion. The fusion surfaces should be in intimate contact, and the foot should be in the desired position.

22. While maintaining this position, the guidepins should be advanced back into the talus. The depth of the pins may be determined by using the image intensifier.

23. Small stab skin incisions should be made around both the medial and lateral guidepins.

24. The length of the cannulated screws to be used may be established by using a second guidepin of equal length.

25. A 7.0-mm cannulated screw is then placed over the guidepin and advanced through the malleoli and into the talus.

26. The position of the fusion is confirmed throughout insertion of the hardware.

27. The final position of the ankle should be confirmed by using fluoroscopy following placement of the screw under direct image intensification.

Postoperative Care

Postoperatively, the ankle is immobilized by using a fracture boot with the hinges locked, or the patient is placed in a posterior splint to reduce swelling. Weight bearing is allowed at 1 week in the fracture boot or cast and weight bearing gradually increased.

Results

Early clinical functional results with arthroscopically assisted ankle arthrodeses were good to excellent in 92%.[67] Complications have included dorsalis pedis artery aneurysm secondary to nicking the artery during instrument placement. There was one case of a nonunion, a broken drill bit in the tibia during pin distraction, and a disabling equinus position of the ankle that required revision of the fusion (Fig 30–33,A and B).

Discussion

Arthroscopically assisted ankle arthrodesis minimizes the amount of devascularization, soft-tissue dissection, and surgical arthrotomy necessary during ankle arthrodesis. It allows for removal of the minimal amount of subchondral bone and maintenance of the shape of the talus and tibial surfaces.

Arthroscopically assisted ankle arthrodesis allows rapid postoperative mobilization. This is particularly appealing for elderly patients and patients with inflammatory arthritis who cannot easily tolerate prolonged non–weight-bearing postoperative periods. It is hoped that the limited soft-tissue dissection and devasculariza-

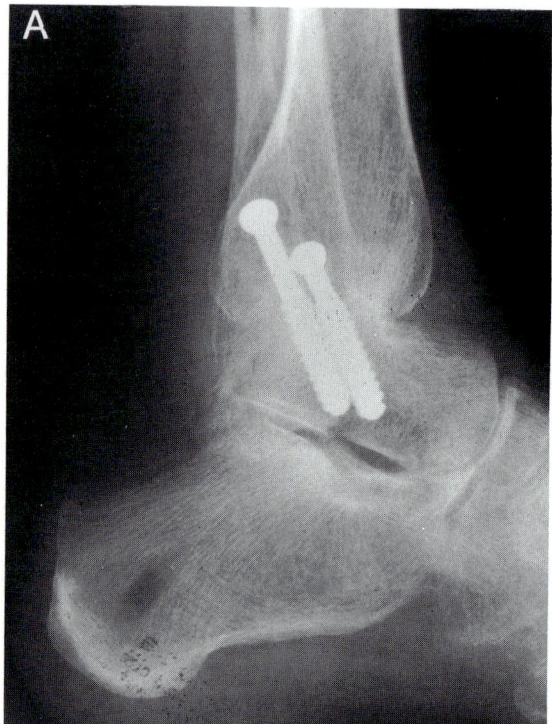

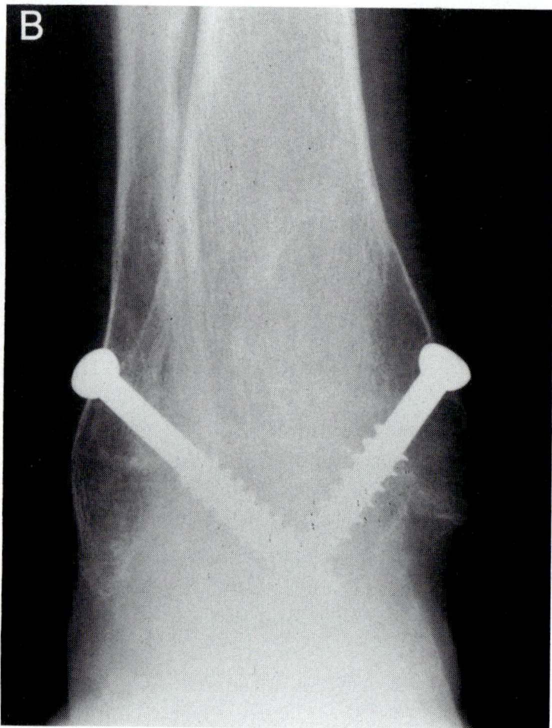

FIG 30–33.
Healed ankle fusion via the arthroscope. **A,** anteroposterior view. **B,** lateral view.

tion will increase the fusion rate and decrease the incidence of infection. Although we are still early in the learning stages, arthroscopically assisted ankle arthrodesis offers a viable alternative to traditional methods of the open approach for ankle fusion. While arthrodesis techniques are the preferred method at this time, with further experience we hope to define the role and indications for arthroscopic ankle fusion.

This section of the chapter has been included to inform the reader of the latest in technological advances. In time, with further experience by the more highly trained arthroscopists, the clinical efficacy of these procedures will be better defined. These are not procedures that should be undertaken by the occasional arthroscopist.

ARTHROSCOPY OF THE SUBTALAR JOINT

Arthroscopy of the subtalar joint was described by J.S. Parisien in 1986.[75] Since that time, there have only been a few other reports on the subject. Currently, techniques for arthroscopy of the subtalar joint are still evolving, and improvements have been made. Although subtalar arthroscopy may not be utilized as frequently as arthroscopy of other joints, I have found it to be useful in the diagnosis and treatment of pathology of the hindfoot. At the present time subtalar arthroscopy is still considered somewhat experimental and is in its infancy from a technical standpoint. For this reason, this procedure should not be carried out except by the very experienced arthroscopist.

Anatomy of the Subtalar Joint

The subtalar joint is divided into anterior (talocalcaneonavicular joint) and posterior (talocalcaneal joint) joints (refer to previous chapters). The anterior and posterior joints are separated by the tarsal canal and sinus tarsi. The bony configurations of the anterior subtalar joint are composed of the talus, posterior surface of the tarsal navicular, anterior surface of the calcaneus, plantar calcaneonavicular or spring ligament, and posterior portion of the capsule that forms the anterior part of the interosseous talocalcaneal ligament. The posterior subtalar joint is composed of synovium-lined articulation and includes a posterior calcaneal facet and posterior talar facet. There is a convex orientation of the subtalar joint that is directed upward. In the subtalar joint the cervical ligament limits inversion and eversion and is well seen on arthroscopy. The talocalcaneal interosseous ligament is hard to see. The posterior subtalar joint has a lateral gutter where reflection of the calcaneofibular and lateral talocalcaneal ligaments is seen. The posterior space is larger than the anterior space.

Indications and Contraindications

Diagnosing problems in the subtalar joint can be somewhat difficult. Although various scans are available to three-dimensionally analyze the subtalar joint, even these modalities are sometimes limited, and the only way to make the correct diagnosis is by direct visualization. The diagnostic indications for subtalar arthroscopy include pain, swelling, stiffness, and locking. Therapeutic indications include treatment of chondromalacia, osteophytes, arthrofibrosis, synovitis, loose bodies, osteochondritis dissecans, excision of a painful os trigonum, and arthrodesis.

Absolute contraindications include localized soft-tissue infection and advanced degenerative joint disease. Relative contraindications include severe edema and poor vascular status.

Portals

Two primary portals and two accessory portals are utilized for subtalar arthroscopy. The anterolateral portal is located approximately 2 cm anterior and 1 cm distal to the tip of the lateral malleolus (Fig 30–34). The posterolateral portal is located approximately 1 cm proximal to the tip of the fibula and closer to the fibula than to the Achilles. Accessory anterior and posterior portals can also be made and are sometimes quite useful when removing loose bodies or shaving anteriorly or posteriorly in the posterior subtalar region.

Instrumentation

Because of the small size and convex nature of the posterior subtalar joint, small instrumentation is critical; 1.9-

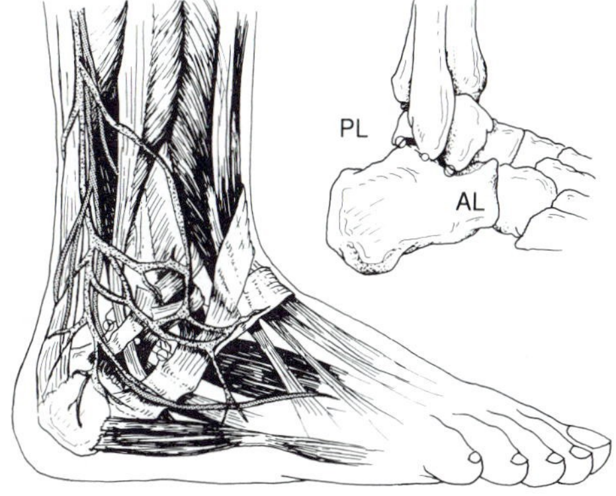

FIG 30–34.
Subtalar arthroscopic portals. Note the position of the anterolateral and posterolateral incisions. Care should be taken to avoid injury to the small saphenous vein and sural nerve.

and 2.7-mm, 30-degree short oblique scopes are utilized. Also used is a small chip camera attached to the scope (video scope); a similar light source and shaver system are utilized as described for the ankle. However, in the subtalar joint, the small-joint shaver blades, as well as whiskers and burrs, are between 1.9 and 2.9 mm. Smaller graspers and baskets are also utilized, as are small curettes, freers, and probes.

Surgical Technique

Subtalar arthroscopy can be performed with the patient supine in a foot holder, in the lateral decubitus position, or with the knee bent over the table 90 degrees. My preferred technique is with thigh and ankle holders and the patient in the supine position. Anesthesia can be general, spinal, epidural, or local. A noninvasive or invasive distractor can be applied to the joint, particularly if operative arthroscopy is necessary.

Author's Preferred Technique

1. The patient is placed in the supine position with a thigh and sterile ankle and foot holder.
2. Distraction can initially be tried by using a noninvasive semicontrolled device; if this is not successful, an invasive distractor can be applied to the distal end of the tibia and calcaneus to facilitate opening the joint space, as previously described.
3. The posterior portal is located and the subtalar joint distended with a 19-gauge needle and a 30-cc syringe. It is important to avoid injury to the sural nerve and the small saphenous vein as well as the peroneal tendons. If the needle is inserted too proximally, the ankle joint instead of the subtalar joint will be distended.
4. After the subtalar joint is distended, a 19-gauge needle is used to establish the location and direction of the anterolateral portal.
5. The arthroscope is then inserted anteriorly (Fig 30–35). A larger inflow cannula can be inserted posteriorly. In addition, the inflow can be placed on the arthroscope and a probe inserted via the other portal (Fig 30–36).

Diagnostic Examination

1. The anterior portion of the posterior subtalar joint is visualized initially. The cervical ligament is generally well seen, as is a portion of the interosseous talocalcaneal ligament.
2. The articular surfaces of the talus and calcaneus are carefully evaluated for integrity (Fig 30–37).
3. As the arthroscope is inserted into the lateral recess and lateral gutter, the reflection of the calcaneofibular and lateral talocalcaneal ligaments are seen.
4. From the anterolateral portal, occasionally the arthroscope can be inserted all the way into the posterior recess and the posterior aspect of the joint. However, sometimes the arthroscope needs to be switched through the posterolateral portal to facilitate visualization.
5. With the arthroscope through the posterolateral portal, the medial posterior subtalar joint can be well visualized.
6. All of the articulation of the ankle with the talus can be ascertained and inversion and eversion stress performed to determine the integrity of the subtalar joint itself.
7. The lateral gutter with its ligamentous reflections is also well noted from this approach, and occasionally, the arthroscope can be maneuvered into the anterior portal for complete visualization as well.

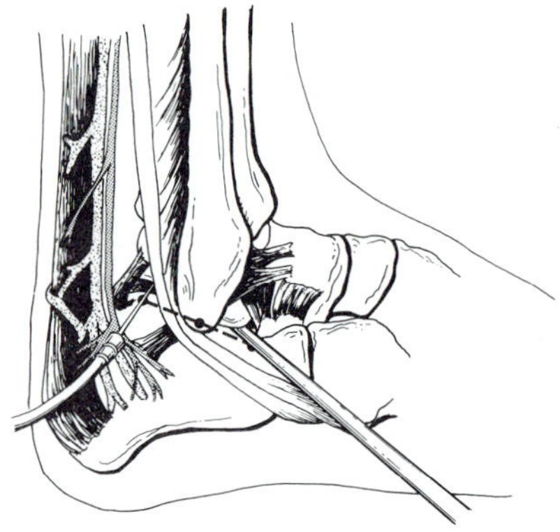

FIG 30–35.
After distending the subtalar joint through the posterolateral portal, the arthroscope can be inserted through the anterolateral portal.

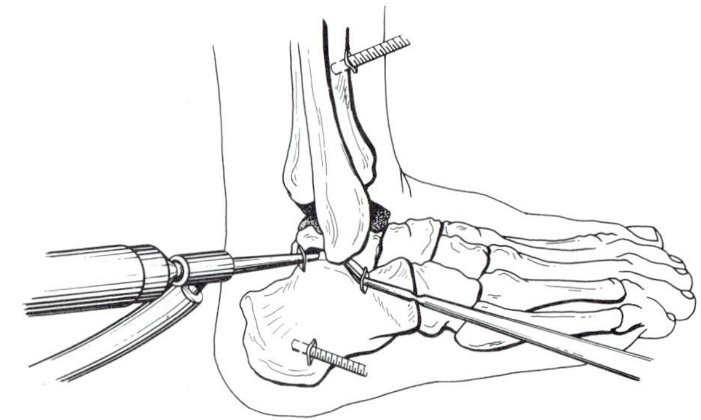

FIG 30–36.
Subtalar arthroscopy with visualization through the posterolateral portal and palpation through the anterolateral portal. Invasive distraction can be utilized in cases where the subtalar joint is quite tight, to improve visualization.

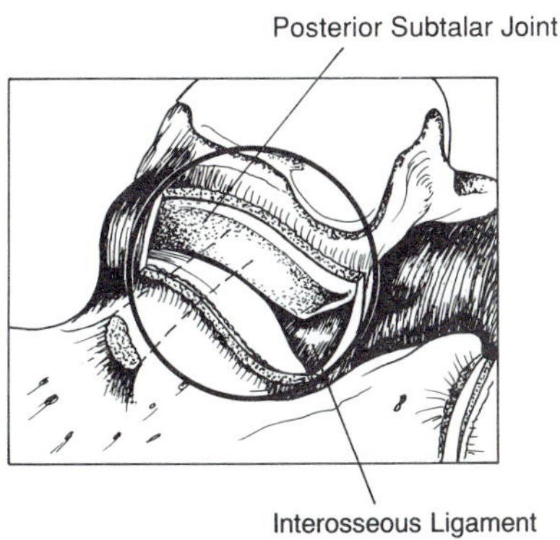

FIG 30–37.
Normal anatomy of the posterior subtalar joint. The posterior joint is separated from the anterior by the interosseous and cervical ligament.

8. By using interchangeable cannulas, the arthroscope can be inserted into the posterior portal and inflow through the anterior portal and the remaining portion of the subtalar joint is well visualized.

9. For surgical procedures, either a two- three- or four-portal system is utilized to facilitate the insertion of small-joint probes, shavers, baskets, and other instrumentation.

10. The key to success is maintaining a high inflow system with good outflow. It is important to do a systematic examination each time so that the entire joint is inspected carefully.

Pathology

With complete examination of the posterior subtalar joint, the articular surfaces are well seen for the presence of chondromalacia and degenerative joint disease as well as loose bodies. From the posterolateral portal, the os trigonum and lateral process are well visualized and can be removed if pathologic or abnormal. However, it is important to remember that the flexor hallucis longus and associated neurovascular bundle are very near the area of excision and that damage can occur if careful attention to detail is not maintained. Surgery is done by utilizing as many portals as necessary, but usually the anteromedial, anterolateral, and posterolateral portals are the primary ones used (Fig 30–38).

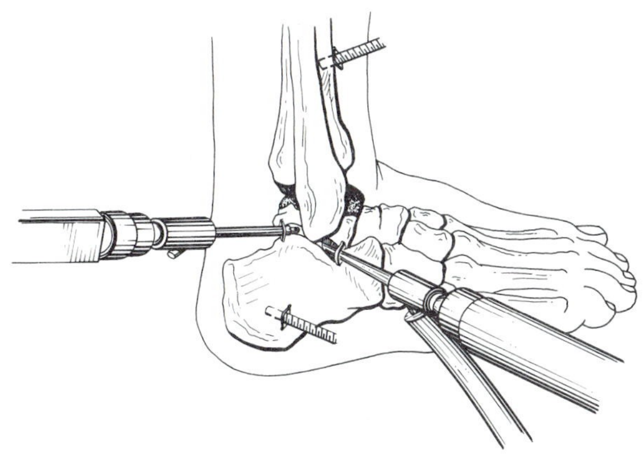

FIG 30–38.
Debridement of the subtalar joint with the arthroscope through the anterolateral portal and the shaver through the posterolateral portal.

GREAT TOE ARTHROSCOPY

Arthroscopic examination of the great toe metatarsophalangeal (MTP) joint was first described by Watanabe.[97] In 1986, Yovich reviewed the use of the arthroscope for the purpose of debridement of osteochondral fractures and MTP joint forces.[99] In 1987, Lundeen reported on 11 great toe arthroscopies in the podiatric literature. There were no specific clinical results reviewed.[21] Bartlett was the first to describe successful arthroscopic debridement of an osteochondritis dissecans lesion in the first metatarsal head.[49] Recently, Ferkel and Van Buecken have described the technique of great toe arthroscopy and reported on the results.[38] Although arthroscopic evaluation of the first metatarsophalangeal joint is described, it is still in its infancy and should not be undertaken except by the most highly trained arthroscopist.

Anatomy of the Great Toe

The anatomy of the great toe MTP joint has been previously elaborated upon in detail. No further statement about anatomy will be made except to remind the reader that it is critical that the surgeon know and understand the anatomy of the great MTP joint prior to initiating arthroscopy.

Indications and Contraindications

The diagnostic indications for great toe arthroscopy include persistent pain, swelling, stiffness, and locking, just as in the subtalar joint. Therapeutic indications include the treatment of chondromalacia, osteophytes (particularly dorsal ones), arthrofibrosis, synovitis, loose bodies, osteochondritis dissecans, and perhaps in the future, arthrodesis.

Absolute contraindications include localized soft-tissue infection, severe narrowing, and degenerative joint disease of the great MTP joint. Relative contraindications include severe edema of the foot, particularly the forefoot, and poor vascular status.

Portals

There are three portals most commonly used in arthroscopy of the great toe. The dorsomedial portal is placed just medial to the extensor hallucis longus tendon at the joint line. The dorsolateral portal is placed just lateral to the extensor hallucis longus tendon at the joint line (Fig 30–39). The straight medial portal is placed through the medial capsule midway between the dorsal and plantar aspects of the joint and usually made under direct vision (Fig 30–40).

Instrumentation

Instrumentation for the great toe is similar to the subtalar joint. The primary difference is that traction is applied in a different manner. For the great toe, traction is applied with a modified finger trap device suspended with weights. The arthroscopes utilized are the 2.7- or 1.9-mm, 30-degree oblique scopes with wide-angle lenses. A small chip camera is essential so that a light lever arm will be produced. Otherwise, the possibility of breakage of the equipment, particularly the arthroscopes, can be alarmingly high. The small-joint shaver with the 2.9- or 1.9-mm, full-radius blades, burrs, and whiskers is also used.

Surgical Technique

1. The patient is placed in the supine position, and general, spinal, epidural, or local anesthesia is provided.
2. The foot pad is removed from the end of the bed to allow the foot to sink down into this area while traction is applied.
3. A sterile finger trap suspension is used to maintain distraction while the procedure is performed. Enough weight is used to lift the foot off the operative table in a balanced position.
4. The dorsolateral portal is established with a 19-gauge needle, and 5 cc of sterile Ringer's lactate is injected. Flow is verified under direct vision.
5. A no. 11 blade is used to make skin incisions, and a small clamp is used to spread the incision down to the capsule to avoid injuring the neurovascular structures.
6. Once the arthroscope is inserted through the dorsolateral portal, the dorsomedial and medial portals can be established with the needle under direct vision.
7. The arthroscope and the instruments are rotated through the various portals by using interchangeable cannulas to allow optimal visualization of the entire joint and management of the intra-articular pathology (Fig 30–41). As in the rest of the ankle, the key to success is maintaining a high inflow system with constant distension of the joint.

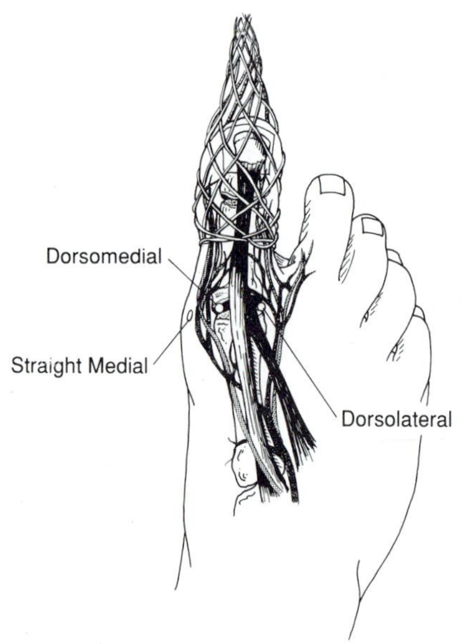

FIG 30–39.
Great toe arthroscopy portals. Note the position of the dorsmedial and dorsolateral incisions.

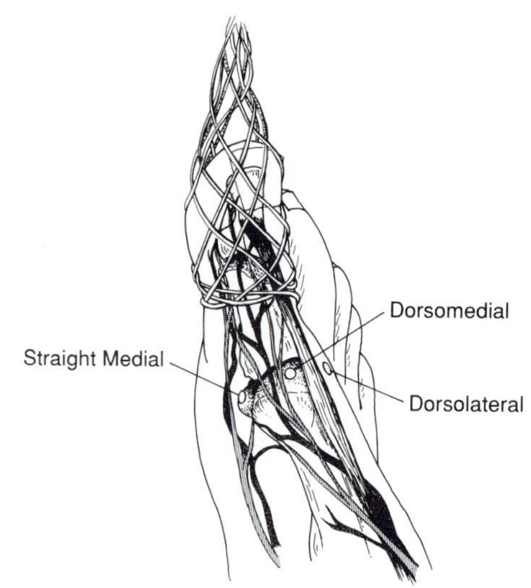

FIG 30–40.
Oblique view of the great toe arthroscopic portals. Note the position of the straight medial portal.

Arthroscopic Normal Examination

The entire MTP joint is inspected by starting through the lateral recess and progressing along the medial articulation, across the MTP first joint, and into the lateral gutter. The rest of the articular surface is well visualized through the use of multiple portals. The medial portal in particular allows inspection of the dorsal aspect of the proximal phalanx and metatarsal head as well as visualization of the medial and lateral sesamoids.

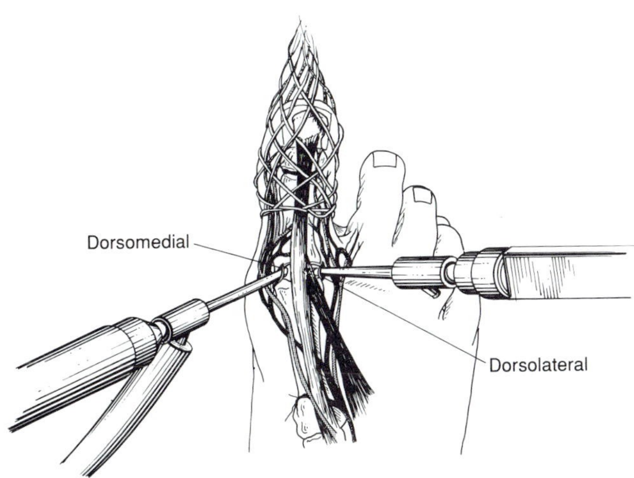

FIG 30–41.
Debridement of the great toe through the dorsolateral portal while visualization is done through the dorsomedial portal. Note the proximity to the neurovascular structures.

As with arthroscopic examination in any other joint, a systematic approach is essential for the MTP joint. A ten-point examination has been developed by the author. The ten-point arthroscopic examination of the MTP joint has been performed through the dorsolateral portal and includes the following: (1) lateral gutter, (2) lateral corner of the metatarsal head, (3) central portion of the metatarsal head, (4) medial corner of the metatarsal head, (5) medial gutter, (6) medial portion of the proximal phalanx, (7) central portion of the proximal phalanx, (8) lateral portion of the proximal phalanx, (9) medial sesamoid, and (10) lateral sesamoid. In addition, the dorsal medial and straight medial portals may be used to better visualize certain portions of the joint.

Postoperative Care

Postoperatively, all wounds are sutured with nylon, and a bulky compression dressing is applied for the first 4 to 7 days. The stitches are then removed and the patient started on active range of motion and strengthening activities as soon as the swelling and pain subside. Postoperatively a wooden shoe is used for several weeks until the swelling and pain have been eliminated.

COMPLICATIONS OF ANKLE ARTHROSCOPY

Arthroscopy has many potential complications, whether it is done in the knee, shoulder, ankle, or other joints. Although ankle arthroscopy has been done since 1939, no accurate assessment of the complication rate has previously been available in a large number of patients. In a series of 518 cases presented by Ferkel et al.,[35] the overall complication rate was 9.8%, or 51 complications in the group. The most common complication was neurologic (25/51 or 49%), primarily involving the superficial peroneal nerve 56% of the time; the saphenous nerve 24%; the sural nerve 20%. Other complications included superficial infection (6), adhesions (3), fractures (3), deep infection (2), instrument failure (2), ligament injury (2), and incisional pain (2), with several other complications seen in only 1 patient each. An invasive distractor was utilized in 317 of the 518 cases. Distraction pins were associated with some transient pin tract pain that resolved in all situations. No ligament injuries occurred in the ankle, but two stress fractures of the tibia occurred early in the series when the pins were placed either too anteriorly or too posteriorly in the tibia. One stress fracture occurred when the pin was placed in the fibula. The overall complication rate was not affected by the use of an invasive distractor, however. Superficial wound infection appeared to be related to the closeness of portal placement, the type of cannula used, and early mobilization. The deep wound infections correlated with the lack of preoperative antibiotics. Experience of the arthroscopist was associated with a lower complication rate.

Since this was a series involving primarily two experienced arthroscopists, it emphasizes the extreme caution that must be undertaken when ankle arthroscopy is performed.

How to Avoid Complications

Adherence to surgical protocol and to meticulous technique is important for all aspects of orthopaedic surgery. Care must be taken in portal selection. It is important to have a clear understanding of surface anatomy as well as the intra-articular anatomy prior to portal selection. Superficial surface anatomy should be well delineated preoperatively, prior to portal selection. The superficial peroneal nerve is the most at risk during the anterolateral portal entry, followed by the saphenous and sural nerves. By incising only the skin with the scalpel blade in a vertical orientation and by careful spreading of the subcutaneous tissue with a mosquito clamp, neurovascular injury may be significantly minimized. In addition, avoiding the anterocentral and posteromedial portals would also decrease the likelihood of neurovascular injury. The use of arthroscopic cannulas will diminish repetitive trauma to soft tissue around the portal site. Suturing of the portal and care during instrument insertion and removal would also serve to protect the soft tissue and minimize wound problems. In addition, it is important to avoid multiple portals in close proximity. Care must be taken when distraction pins are placed to avoid potential neurovascular compromise, tendinous injury, or bony fractures. The use of 3/16-in. pins eliminates the likelihood of pin slippage and provides additional safety by allowing the inherent bending in the pin. Both the tibial and calcaneal pins should be unicortical to minimize the establishment of stress risers, which may potentially lead to future fractures.

Although the vast majority of complications reported with ankle arthroscopy have been minor and transient, the potential for serious complications does exist. Therefore, attention to details and meticulous surgical technique must be followed. Care must be taken in portal selection, portal entry technique, as well as the placement of ankle distractors.

FUTURE OF ANKLE ARTHROSCOPY

The future of ankle arthroscopy is bright because better equipment and more innovative ideas are being developed. The use of the endoscopic carpal tunnel system to release the plantar fascia is currently being investigated, and it has some promise. However, problems with injuries to the medial nerves provide potential complications. Furthermore, many patients with heel pain require neurolysis of the nerves in the deep abductor hallucis fascia, which is not routinely done via this endoscopic method.

Arthroscopic Achilles tendon repairs have been performed in both Japan and the United States, with good results for acute injuries that have not retracted or become further necrotic. Moreover, the small-joint arthroscope can be used for removing spurs off the calcaneus that go into the undersurface of the Achilles tendon.

Although lasers first became operational in the 1960s, they have since occupied a permanent place in the surgical armamentarium. The word "laser" is an acronym for "light amplified by stimulated emission of radiation." There is still much debate as to which laser is the most appropriate one to use arthroscopically, with the least amount of tissue damage. The advantages of the laser arthroscopically are that it allows complete and rapid removal of articular surface debris. With increasing interest in use of the laser, various new lasers will be available in the near future.

REFERENCES

1. Adkinson DP, Bosse MJ, et al: Anatomic variations in the course of superficial peroneal nerve, *J Bone Joint Surg* 73(A):112–114, 1991.
2. Alexander AH, Lichtman DM: Surgical treatment of transchondral talar-dome fractures (osteochondritis dissecans), *J Bone Joint Surg [Am]* 62:646, 1980.
3. Anderson R: Concentric arthrodesis of the ankle joint: A trans-malleolar approach, *J Bone Joint Surg [Am]* 27:37, 1945.
4. Andrews JR, Previte WJ, Carson WG: Arthroscopy of the ankle: Technique and normal anatomy, *Foot Ankle* 6:29, 1985.
5. Axe MJ, Casscells SW: Arthroscopic assistance in osteochondritis dissecans of the talus, *Orthop Consultation* 4:1, 1983.
6. Baker CL, Andrews JR, Ryan JB: Arthroscopic treatment of transchondral talar dome fractures, *Arthroscopy* 2:82, 1986.
7. Barr JS, Record EE: Arthrodesis of the ankle joint: indications, operative technique, and clinical experience, *N Engl J Med* 248:53, 1953.
8. Barth A: Die Enstehung and das Wachstum der freien Gelen Kkorper, *Arch Klin Chir* 56:507, 1988.
9. Bartlett DH: Arthroscopic management of osteochondritis dissecans of the first metatarsal head. *Arthroscopy* 4:51, 1988.
10. Bassett FH III, Gates HS III, Billys JB: Talar impingement by anteroinferior tibiofibular ligament. *J Bone Joint Surg* 72A:55, 1990.
11. Bauer M, Jonsson K, Linden B: Osteochondritis dissecans of the ankle; a 20-year follow-up study, *J Bone Joint Surg [Br]* 69:93, 1987.
12. Berndt AL, Harty M: Transchondral fractures (osteochondritis dissecans) of the talus, *J Bone Joint Surg [Am]* 41:988, 1959.
13. Bessen J, Wellinger C: L'osteochondrite dissequante de l'astragale a propos def 12 observations, *Rev Rhum* 34:552, 1967.
14. Blom JM, Strijk SP: Lesions of the trochlea tali, *Radiol Clin* 44:387, 1975.
15. Bosien WR, Staples OS, Russell SW: Residual disability following acute ankle sprains, *J Bone Joint Surg [Am]* 37:1237, 1955.
16. Brittain HA: *Architectural principles in arthrodesis*, ed 2, Edinburgh, 1952, Livingstone, p 8.
17. Burman MS: Arthroscopy of direct visualization of joints: An experimental cadaver study, *J Bone Joint Surg* 13:669, 1931.
18. Campbell CJ, Ranawat CS: Osteochondritis dissecans: The question of etiology, *J Trauma* 6:201, 1966.
19. Campbell CJ, Rinehart WT, Kalenek A: Arthrodesis of the ankle. Deep autogenous inlaid grafts with maximum cancellous bone apposition, *J Bone Joint Surg [Am]* 56:63, 1974.
20. Canale ST, Belding RH: Osteochondral lesions of the talus, *J Bone Joint Surg [Am]* 62:97, 1980.
21. Chen Y: Arthroscopy of the ankle joint. In Watanabe M, editor: *Arthroscopy of small joints*. New York, 1985, Igaku-Shoin.
22. Chen YC: Clinical and cadaver studies on the ankle joint arthroscopy, *J Jpn Orthop Assoc* 50:631, 1976.
23. Cheung HS, Cottrell WH, Stephenson K, et al: In vitro collagen biosynthesis in healing and normal rabbit articular cartilage, *J Bone Joint Surg [Am]* 60:1076, 1978.
24. Coltart WD: Aviator's astragalus, *J Bone Joint Surg [Br]* 34:545, 1952.
25. Drez D, Guhl JF, Gollehon DL: Ankle arthroscopy: Technique and indications, *Clin Sports Med* 1:35, 1982.
26. Drez D, Guhl JF, Gollehon DL: Ankle arthroscopy: Technique and indications, *Foot Ankle* 2:138, 1981.

27. Eggers GWN, Shindler TO, Pomeret CM: The influence of the contact-compression factor of osteogenesis in surgical factors, *J Bone Joint Surg [Am]* 31:693, 1949.
28. Ewing JW: Ankle arthroscopy, Arthroscopy Surgery Update, 1989, Scottsdale, Ariz.
29. Ferkel RD: *Arthroscopy of the foot and ankle*, New York, JB Lippincott (in press).
30. Ferkel RD: *An illustrated guide to small joint arthroscopy*, Andover, Maryland, 1989, Dyonics, Inc.
31. Ferkel RD: Soft tissue pathology of the ankle. In McGinty JB, editor: *Operative arthroscopy*, New York, 1991, Raven, pp 713–725.
32. Ferkel RD: Treatment of chronic ankle sprain, American Orthopaedic Foot and Ankle Society meeting, San Francisco, January 27, 1987.
33. Ferkel RD, Del Pizzo W, Friedman MJ, et al: Arthroscopic treatment of anterolateral impingement of the ankle, Western Orthopaedic Association meeting, Coronado, Calif, April 28, 1987.
34. Ferkel RD, Fischer SP: Progress in ankle arthroscopy, *Clin Orthop* 240:210–220, 1989.
35. Ferkel RD, Guhl J, et al: Complications in 518 ankle arthroscopies, American Academy of Orthopaedic Surgeons annual meeting, Washington, DC, February 1992.
36. Ferkel RD, Karzel RP, Del Pizzo W, et al: Arthroscopic treatment of anterolateral impingement of the ankle. *Am J Sports Med* 19:440, 1991.
37. Ferkel RD, Sgaglione NA: Arthroscopic treatment of osteochondral lesions of the talus, 1991 (in press).
38. Ferkel RD, Van Buecken KP: Great toe arthroscopy: Indications, technique and results. Arthroscopy Association of North America meeting, San Diego, April 1991.
39. Flick AB, Gould N: Osteochondritis dissecans of the talus (transchondral fractures of the talus): Review of the literature and new surgical approach for medial dome lesions, *Foot Ankle* 5:165, 1985.
40. Frank A, Cohen P, Beaufils P, et al: Arthroscopic treatment of osteochondral lesions of the talar dome, *Arthroscopy* 5:57, 1989.
41. Gebstein R, Conforty B, Weiss RE, et al: Closed percutaneous drilling for osteochondritis dissecans of the talus, *Clin Orthop* 213:197, 1986.
42. Glasgow M, Jackson A, Jamieson AM: Instability of the ankle after injury to the lateral ligament, *J Bone Joint Surg [Br]* 62:296, 1980.
43. Gollehon DL, Drez D: Ankle arthroscopy approaches and technique, *Orthopedics* 6:1150, 1983.
44. Gollehon DL, Drez D: Arthroscopy of the ankle. In McGinty J, editor: *Arthroscopic surgery update*, Rockville, Md, 1985, Aspen, pp 161–173.
45. Gould N: Technique tips, *Foot Ankle* 3:184, 1982.
46. Guhl JF: Ankle arthroscopy, International Arthroscopy Association biennial meeting, Rome, 1989.
47. Guhl JF, editor: *Ankle arthroscopy: pathology and surgical techniques*, Thorofare, NJ, 1988, Charles B Slack.
48. Guhl JF: New concepts (distraction) in ankle arthroscopy, *Arthroscopy* 4:160, 1988.
49. Guhl JF: New techniques for arthroscopic surgery of the ankle: preliminary report, *Orthopedics* 9:261, 1986.
50. Guhl JF: Osteochondritis dissecans, In Guhl JF, editor: *Ankle arthroscopy*, Thorofare, NJ, 1988, Charles B Slack, pp 95–106.
51. Harrington KD: Degenerative arthritis of the ankle secondary to long-standing lateral ligament instability, *J Bone Joint Surg [Am]* 61:354, 1979.
52. Hawkins RB: Ankle instability surgery from an arthroscopist's perspective. In McGinty JB, editor: *Operative arthroscopy*, New York, 1991, Raven Press, pp 747–752.
53. Hawkins RB: Arthroscopic treatment of sports related anterior osteophytes in the ankle, *Foot Ankle* 9:87, 1988.
54. Hawkins RB: Arthroscopic reconstruction for chronic lateral instability of the ankle, In McGinty JB, editor: *Arthroscopic surgery update*, Rockville, Md, 1985, Aspen, pp 175–181.
55. Heinig CF, Dupuy DN: Anterior dowel fusion of the ankle. In Bateman JE, editor: *Foot science*, Philadelphia, 1976, WB Saunders, pp 150–155.
56. Johnson EE, Markolf KL: The contribution of the anterior talofibular ligament to ankle laxity, *J Bone Joint Surg [Am]* 65:81, 1983.
57. Johnson EW Jr, Boseker EH: Arthrodesis of the ankle, *Arch Surg* 97:766, 1968.
58. Johnson LL: *Diagnostic and surgical arthroscopy*, ed 2, St Louis, 1981, Mosby–Year Book, pp 412–419.
59. Kennedy JC: Arthrodesis of the ankle with particular reference to the Gallie procedure: a review of 50 cases, *J Bone Joint Surg [Am]* 42:1308, 1960.
60. Kreuscher PH: Semilunar cartilage diseases. A plea for early recognition by means of the arthroscope and early treatment of this condition. *Ir Med J* 47:290, 1925.
61. Marcus RE, Balourdas GM, Heiple KG: Ankle arthrodesis by chevron fusion with internal fixation and bone graft, *J Bone Joint Surg [Am]* 65:833, 1983.
62. Martin DF, et al: Operative ankle arthroscopy, long term followup, *Am J Sports Med* 17:16, 1989.
63. Mazur JM, Schwartz E, Simon SR: Ankle arthrodesis: Long term followup with gait analysis, *J Bone Joint Surg [Am]* 61:964, 1979.
64. McCullough CJ, Venugopal V: Osteochondritis dissecans of the talus, the natural history, *Clin Orthop* 144:264, 1979.
65. McGinty JB: Arthroscopic removal of loose bodies, *Orthop Clin North Am* 13:313, 1982.
66. McMinn RMH, Hutchings RT, Logann BM: *Color atlas of foot and ankle anatomy*, New York, 1982, Appleton-Century-Crofts.
67. Morgan CP: Arthroscopic tibiotalar arthrodesis. In McGinty JB, editor: *Operative arthroscopy*, New York, 1991, Raven Press, pp 695–701.
68. Mukherjee SK, Young AB: Dome fractures of the talus. A report of ten cases, *J Bone Joint Surg [Br]* 55:319, 1973.
69. Myerson MS, Allon SM: Arthroscopic ankle arthrodesis. *Contemp Orthop* 19:21, 1989.
70. Naumetz VA, Schweigel JF: Osteocartilaginous lesions of the talar dome, *J Trauma* 20:924, 1980.
71. O'Connor RL: *Arthroscopy*, Kalamazoo, Mich, 1977, Upjohn, pp 12–16.
72. O'Donoghue DH: Chondral and osteochondral fractures, *J Trauma* 6:469, 1966.
73. O'Farrell TA, Costello BG: Osteochondritis dissecans of the talus. The late results of surgical treatment, *J Bone Joint Surg [Br]* 64:494, 1982.
74. Ove PN, Bosse MJ, Reinert CM: Excision of posterolateral talar dome lesions through a medial transmalleolar approach, *Foot Ankle* 9:171, 1989.
75. Parisien JS: Arthroscopic treatment of osteochondral lesions of the talus, *Am J Sports Med* 14:211, 1986.

76. Parisien JS: Arthroscopy of the posterior subtalar joint: a preliminary report. *Foot Ankle* 6:219, 1986.
77. Parisien JS: Arthroscopy of the ankle: state of the art, *Contemp Orthop* 5:21, 1982.
78. Parisien JS, Shereff MJ: The role of arthroscopy in the diagnosis and treatment of disorders of the ankle, *Foot Ankle* 2:144, 1981.
79. Parisien JS, Vangsness T: Operative arthroscopy of the ankle: three years' experience, *Clin Orthop* 199:46, 1985.
80. Patel D: Arthroscopy of the plicae—synovial folds and their significance, *Am J Sports Med* 6:217–225, 1978.
81. Pettine KA, Morrey BF: Osteochondral fractures of the talus, a long term follow-up, *J Bone Joint Surg [Br]* 69:89, 1987.
82. Pritsch M, Horoshovski H, Farine I: Arthroscopic treatment of osteochondral lesions of the talus, *J Bone Joint Surg [Am]* 68:862, 1986.
83. Ratliff AHC: Compression arthrodesis of the ankle and subtalar joint, *J Bone Joint Surg [Am]* 38:50, 1956.
84. Ruth CJ: The surgical treatment of the fibular collateral ligaments of the ankle, *J Bone Joint Surg [Am]* 43:229, 1961.
85. St. Pierre RK, et al: Impingement exostosis of the talus and fibula secondary to an inversion sprain, a case report, *Foot Ankle* 3:282, 1983.
86. Sefton GK, George J, Fitton GM, et al: Reconstruction of the anterior talofibular ligament for the treatment of the unstable ankle, *J Bone Joint Surg [Br]* 61:352, 1979.
87. Soren A: Safe inlay of bone graft in arthrodesis, *Clin Orthop* 58:147, 1968.
88. Staples OS: Posterior arthrodesis of the ankle and subtalar joints, *J Bone Joint Surg [Am]* 38:50, 1956.
89. Stoller SM: A comparative study of the frequency of anterior impingement exostosis of the ankle in dancer and non-dancer, *Foot Ankle* 4:201, 1984.
90. Takagi K: The arthroscope, *J Jpn Orthop Assoc* 14:359, 1939.
91. Thomas FB: Arthrodesis of the ankle, *J Bone Joint Surg [Br]* 51:53, 1969.
92. Thompson JP, Loomer RL: Osteochondral lesions of the talus in a sports medicine clinic, *Am J Sports Med* 12:460, 1984.
93. Van Buecken KP, Barrack MD, Alexander AH, et al: Arthroscopic treatment of transchondral talar dome fractures, *Am J Sports Med* 17:350, 1989.
94. Verhelst MP, Mulier JC, Hoogmartens MJ, et al: Arthrodesis of the ankle joint with complete removal of the distal part of the fibula: Experience with a trans-fibular approach in three different types of fixation, *Clin Orthop* 118:93, 1976.
95. Voto SJ, Ewing JW, Fleissner PR Jr, et al: Ankle arthroscopy: neurovascular and arthroscopic anatomy of standard and trans-Achilles tendon portal placement, *Arthroscopy* 5:41, 1989.
96. Waller JF: Hindfoot and midfoot problems of the runner in symposium on the foot and leg. In Mack RP, editor: *Running Sports*, St Louis, 1982, Mosby–Year Book, pp 64–71.
97. Watanabe M: Selfoc-Arthroscope (Watanabe No. 24 Arthroscope) (Monograph), Tokyo, Teishin Hospital, 1972.
98. Wolin I, Glassman F, Sideman F, et al: Internal derangement of the talofibular component of the ankle, *Surg Gynecol Obstet* 91:193–200, 1950.
99. Yovich JV, McIlwraith CW: Arthroscopic surgery for osteochondral fractures of the proximal phalanx, the metacarpophalangeal and metatarsophalangeal joints in horses. *J Am Veterinary Med Assoc* 188:273, 1986.
100. Zinman C, Reis ND: High resolution CT scan in osteochondritis dissecans of the talus, *Acta Orthop Scand* 53:697, 1982.

SECTION

VIII

PEDIATRICS

CHAPTER

31

Congenital Foot Deformities

Walter W. Huurman, M.D.

Embryology
Growth and development
Genetics in the foot
Talipes deformities
Clubfoot (talipes equinovarus)
  Incidence
  Pathologic anatomy
  Etiology
  Radiographic evaluation
  Treatment
  Uncorrected or residual clubfoot in the older child
Metatarsus adductus and metatarsus varus
  Anatomy
  Etiology
  Treatment of metatarsus adductus
  Treatment of resistant metatarsus varus in the older child
Talipes calcaneovalgus
Flatfoot
Flexible pes planus
  Treatment
  Accessory navicular (prehallux)
Rigid flatfoot
  Peroneal spastic flatfoot (tarsal coalition)
  Congenital convex pes valgus (congenital vertical talus)
Arthrogryposis multiplex congenita
Talectomy
Abnormalities of toes
Abnormalities of the great toe
  Congenital hallux varus
  Congenital hallux rigidus
Abnormalities of the lesser toes
  Polydactyly
  Syndactyly
  Macrodactyly
  Congenital hammer toe
  Overlapping toes
  Congenital underlapping toes
Torsional deformities of the lower extremities
Physical examination and normal parameters
Treatment
  Toeing out
  Toeing in as a result of foot abnormalities
Tibial torsion
  Technique of supramalleolar tibial derotational osteotomy
Femoral anteversion
  Technique of supracondylar femoral derotational osteotomy

Congenital deformities, those present at or before birth, may result from inherited (genetic) or extrinsic (environmental) influences. To understand the pathophysiology of congenital foot disorders, one must have a working knowledge of prenatal growth and foot development. Only with this background can the treatment of these disorders be systematically and competently approached.

EMBRYOLOGY

The skeletal elements of the foot are blastemic by the fifth gestational week; all are present and begin to chondrify between 5 and 6½ weeks. The cartilage anlage of each individual bone begins to ossify at a particular time in development; the pattern of ossification is quite regular. The metatarsals and distal phalanges demonstrate a periosteal collar of bone at 9 weeks, the calcaneus develops a lateral perichondral area of ossification at 13 weeks, and the talus shows an enchondral center after 8 months. The tarsonavicular does not ossify until the third to fourth postnatal year.

Joints are formed with the appearance of homogeneous interzones—intermediate cell masses—beginning at the sixth gestational week. The interzones then become fissured (9½ weeks), followed by synovial tissue invasion at 11 weeks.

Differentiation of tendons begins as early as the sixth week, and by the eighth week most ligaments of the foot and ankle are differentiated as cellular condensations.[1]

Hence we see that differentiation of the blastemas into elements arranged like those of the adult occurs between 5 and 7 weeks after conception. Individual elements of the limb appear generally in a proximal-distal sequence, and the specific time of differentiation has been determined with reasonable accuracy.[4] Knowing the time of blastemic insult in the case of a specific skeletal abnormality may guide one to search for less obvious congenital malformations in organs differentiating at precisely the same time.[3]

GROWTH AND DEVELOPMENT

Maturation begins during the fetal period and continues postnatally through adolescence. Extrinsic and intrinsic influences that are separate from the genetic code can affect growth and development of the foot at any time during these years. Because of the unique properties of the growing foot, maturation may adversely affect the developing limb by enhancing an existing pathologic condition.

Conversely, the same phenomenon, growth, can be turned to advantage by the knowledgeable clinician to lessen or eliminate functional disability secondary to an abnormal condition. In turn, the physician must not forget that the continuing effect of growth and development may cause a reappearance of the deformity or development of a compensating iatrogenic deformity after treatment.

GENETICS IN THE FOOT

Congenital anomalies of the foot may be seen as part of a genetic disorder adhering to the Mendelian rules of inheritance. As such, the foot abnormality frequently appears in association with other obvious anomalies or, on occasion, may be the only phenotypic indication of a generalized syndrome. Heritable anomalies follow either the dominant or recessive mode of transmission and may result from the influence of an autosome or the sex chromosome.[2]

Zimbler and Craig have presented a large series of birth defect syndromes and identified the specific disorder via abnormalities seen in the foot.[6] Excluded from this list were foot disorders unassociated with other defects. McKusick lists several such isolated anomalies (relative length of the first and second metatarsals, rotational deformity of the fifth toe, number of phalanges contained in the fifth toe) that demonstrate a dominant mode of inheritance.[5]

A review of Zimbler and Craig's compilation has facilitated classification of most disorders according to an appropriate mode of inheritance (see Table 31–1). Some (e.g., Silver's syndrome) have yet to show a clear genetic code but quite possibly will be classified in the future. For problems more specifically dealt with in the text, genetics are discussed under the individual disorder.

TALIPES DEFORMITIES

Talipes, derived from the Latin words *talus* ("ankle bone") and *pes* ("foot"), is a term used to describe any congenital foot anomaly. Congenital hindfoot deformities are correctly designated *talipes* followed by a descriptive term for the morbid anatomy. A plantar-flexed hindfoot is therefore talipes equinus; if dorsiflexed, talipes calcaneus; if inverted, talipes varus; and if everted, talipes valgus.

Currently the simple contraction *talipes* is commonly used in reference to the classic clubfoot deformity. Clinically the true clubfoot present with a triad of (1) midfoot and forefoot adductus, (2) hindfoot varus, and (3) heel equinus. Anatomically, then, *talipes equinovarus* is the appropriate descriptive term, and the use of simple *talipes* should probably be avoided.

Clubfoot (talipes equinovarus)

A relatively common malformation and certainly the continuing subject of heated discussion among experts, clubfoot remains an unsolved and enigmatic congenital foot deformity. The orthopaedic literature continues to abound with articles espousing methods of treatment nearly as numerous as the number of their authors. Despite this vast experience, the etiology remains obscure, and a single best form of treatment is elusive.*

As Lloyd-Roberts (1964) knowingly stated: "This is an undeniably disheartening state of affairs which is in no way redeemed by the knowledge that little or no improvement has occurred since Brockman's review was published 35 years ago."

TABLE 31–1.
Foot Deformities Associated With Other Primary Problems*

PLANOVALGUS	**CAVUS**
Achondrogenesis (type 1)	Mucopolysaccharidosis
Chromosome 18 trisomy	Homocystinuria
Chromosome 13 trisomy	Carpal tarsal osteolysis and chronic progressive glomerulopathy
Dysplasia epiphysealis hemimelica	Phytamic acid storage disease
Larsen syndrome	Urticaria, deafness, and amyloidosis
Marfan syndrome	**POLYDACTYLY**
Mucopolysaccharidosis IV	Chondroectodermal dysplasia
Multiple exostoses	Chromosome 13 trisomy
Popliteal pterygium syndrome	Cleft lip without cleft palate
Ehlers-Danlos syndrome	Cleft tongue
Bird-headed dwarfism	Cyclopia
Chromosome 5P syndrome	Focal dermal hypoplasia
Diaphyseal dysplasia	Orofaciodigital syndrome II
METATARSUS ADDUCTUS	Polysyndactyly
Acrocephalosyndactyly	Retinal dysplasia
Smith-Lemli-Opitz syndrome	Stippled epiphyses
Carpenter syndrome	**SYNDACTYLY**
Cerebrohepatorenal syndrome	Acrocephalosyndactyly
Clasped thumbs	Aglossia-adactyly
EQUINOVARUS	Ankyloblepharon
Arthrogryposis multiplex congenita	Chromosome 18P syndrome
Bird-headed dwarfism	Oligophrenia
Chromosome 18Q syndrome	Familial static ophthalmoplegia
Chromosome 13 trisomy	Focal dermal hypoplasia
Craniocarpotarsal dystrophy	Holoprosencephalus
Diastrophic dwarfism	Hypertelorism
Ehler-Danlos syndrome	Laryngeal web or atresia
Larsen syndrome	Lissencephaly
Oculoauriculovertebral dysplasia	Meckel syndrome
Radioulnar synostosis	Monosomy G syndrome, type II
Situs inversus viscerum	Oculomandibulofacial syndrome
Stippled epiphyses	Orocraniodigital syndrome
VARUS	Orofaciodigital syndrome, I and II
Carpenter syndrome (acrocephalopolysyndactyly, type II)	Popliteal web syndrome
Hypochondroplasia	Retinal dysplasia
Laryngeal web or atresia	Silver syndrome
CALCANEUS	Smith-Lemli-Opitz syndrome
Chromosome 18 trisomy	Stippled epiphyses
Chromosome 13 trisomy	

*From Zimbler S, Craig C: *Orthop Clin North Am* 7:331, 1976. Used by permission.

Incidence

The commonly accepted incidence in the general population is approximately 1 per 1,000 births. Wynne-Davies notes the incidence as 1.24 per 1,000; when broken down by sex, the male incidence is 1.62 per 1,000, and that for females is 0.8 per 1000.[32] This represents a distinct 2.17 to 1 predominance of male over female incidence. There are strong hereditary factors, and if one child in a family has the deformity, the incidence among siblings rises to 2.9 per 100, or 1 in every 35 births. If the index patient is female, the incidence among male siblings rises to 1 in 16; however, if the index patient is male, there appears to be no significant increase in the 1 per 35 sibling incidence.[32] Although there may be a genetic factor involved, the specific Mendelian characteristics with regard to sex linkage, dominance or recessiveness, etc., have not been worked out. It can, however, be stated with some certainty that penetrance does appear to be variable. As Cowell has pointed out, clubfeet associated with other clearly Mendelian-based syndromes (e.g., diastrophic dwarfism, Freeman-Sheldon syndrome) should not be included in genetic studies of talipes equinovarus. Currently, a multifactorial mode of inheritance seems most plausible. Nongenetic, extrinsic factors that may result in clubfoot deformity include arthrogryposis multiplex congenita, amniotic band (Streeter's) syndrome, and certain drugs taken during pregnancy (aminopterin).

Pathologic Anatomy

Despite the fact that clubfoot has been recognized as a handicapping deformity since ancient times, relatively few anatomic studies have been published. A careful review of most writing reveals that dissections were usually performed on a fetus or infant who also had other significant congenital malformations.

The anatomic findings in the deformed foot of a stillborn anencephalic, myelodysplastic, or fetus with other congenital malformations potentially affecting foot development should not be used as the anatomic basis for a discussion of idiopathic clubfoot. Before the excellent studies of Irani and Sherman, no satisfactory series of dissections on the isolated idiopathic deformity had been reported.[20] Although Settle confirmed the findings of Irani and Sherman later the same year,[27] 14 of his 16 specimens had other significant deformities. Waisbrod contributed the study of eight additional idiopathic clubfeet occurring without any other significant congenital anomaly.[30] Ippolito and Ponsetti reported their findings in five fetuses with clubfeet that were aborted between 15 and 20 weeks' gestation.[19] At the present time these studies provide the basis for our knowledge of the pathologic anatomy.

The reason for this rather sparse information seems clear: isolated clubfoot deformity is not a cause of fetal or infant mortality, and therefore specimens are not readily available for study. Nonetheless, the idiopathic clubfeet that have been studied have demonstrated rather constant findings. A primary deformity seems to be present in the head and neck of the talus: the neck is foreshortened to absent and medially deviated, the articular surface of the head is inclined plantarward. Other bony and soft-tissue anomalies that may be present seem to be adaptive to this primary talar deformity (Fig 31–1).

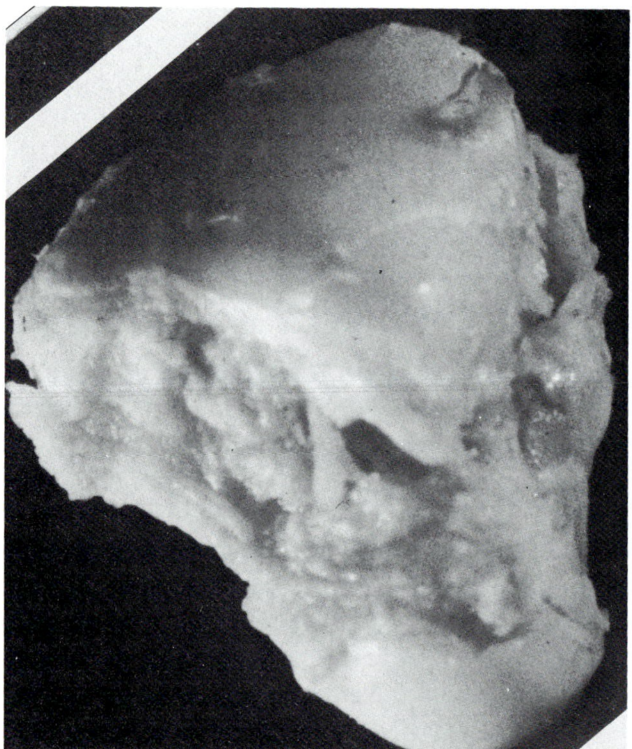

FIG 31–1.
Dorsomedial view of the left talus of an idiopathic clubfoot in a 5-year-old child. Note the shortening of the neck and medial and plantar deviation of the navicular articular surface.

The normal talar neck has an angle of incidence with its body of 150 to 155 degrees.[17, 25] Irani and Sherman found in their dissected specimens an angle varying between 115 and 135 degrees.[20] Other than adaptive changes resulting from this primary deformity, the muscles, tendons, neurovascular and other osseous structures of the foot and leg seemed to be basically normal.

Because of the plantarward declination of the talar neck, the talar body lies more anterior in the ankle mortise than in the normal foot. The hindfoot therefore declines into equinus, and developmental contracture of both the ankle and subtalar joint capsules is accompanied by atrophy and contracture of the triceps surae muscle group.[31] Adaptive changes are present in the osseous structure of the talus itself. The articulations of the subtalar joint are noticeably deformed, the medial- and plantar-deviated head of the talus articulating with the anteromedial portion of the calcaneus. The posterior calcaneus is rotated laterally and held in close proximity to the fibular malleolus by a thick, strong, deformity-inducing fibulocalcaneal ligament. Settle noted in his directions that the subtalar joints were slanted medially with a single articular facet.[27] This combination of rotation and varus of the calcaneus widens the sinus tarsi and brings the Achilles tendon insertion medial to the calcaneal midline axis. This medial displacement of the Achilles tendon causes its line of pull to promote further hindfoot varus[16] (Fig 31–2).

The midfoot likewise adapts to changes in the head and neck of the talus. The navicular is smaller than normal and medially "dislocated."[9, 26] This medial dislocation, however, is only apparent insofar as the navicular articulates rather properly with the medially deviated talar head and covers its articular surface.[27, 30] It is true that the navicular is deviated medially relative to the longitudinal axis of the talar body, but this is because the anterior talus is inclined medially and plantarward. On occasion, depending on the angle of incidence of the talar neck, the navicular may be so far swung around that its medial margin articulates with the medial malle-

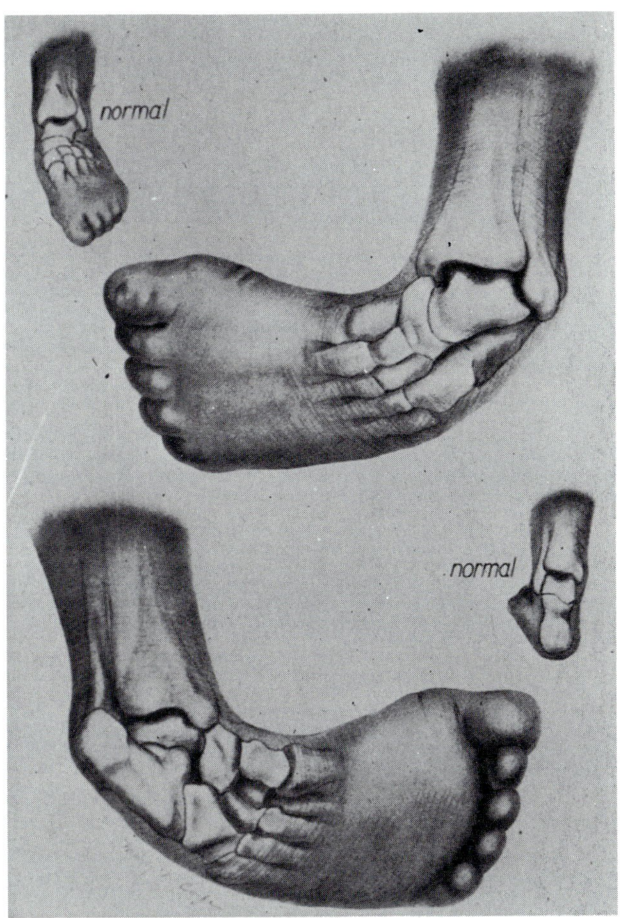

FIG 31–2.
Pathologic anatomy of the clubfoot. A medially and plantar-deviated talar neck is the primary deformity; medial deviation of the navicular and hindfoot varus and equinus are adaptive. (From Settle GW: *J Bone Joint Surg [Am]* 45:1341, 1963. Used by permission.)

olus. The remainder of the midfoot seems to follow the talar neck and the rotated calcaneus: the cuboid is actually displaced beneath the third cuneiform and rotated toward the medial side of its normal articulation with the calcaneus. The forefoot follows the varus and adducted contour of the midfoot to complete the clinical equinovarus appearance.

If the talar deformity is severe, all adaptive changes are accentuated. The medial border of the calcaneus may be concave, the lateral column of the foot elongated, and the medial column foreshortened. With the foot swung around into equinovarus, during development the ligamentous and capsular structures on the posterior and medial side of the foot eventually become foreshortened, thickened, and quite rigid. This includes capsules of the ankle, subtalar, talonavicular, and naviculocuneiform joints. Furthermore, the deltoid and talocalcaneal interosseous ligaments become contracted and thickened. The tendinous structures (tibialis posterior, tibialis anterior, Achilles tendon), if allowed to come into opposition with deformed osseous structures, may adhere to them. This apparent abnormality of tendon insertion is adaptive and secondary to the distorted hindfoot and midfoot. On dissection, normal insertion of these tendinous structures is always present.

When treating the idiopathic clubfoot, the physician must constantly keep in mind the pathologic anatomy and dynamics of the growing foot. Successful treatment relies primarily on the ability of growing osseous structures to adapt and alter their shape in response to the influence of extrinsic force.

Etiology

Because the literature contains no report of an idiopathic clubfoot dissection in a fetus under 7 weeks' gestation, it has not been established whether the deformity is blastemic in origin or arises during the embryonic period. However, the presence of significantly fewer vessels in the talar neck of a fetal clubfoot, with marked disorganization of these vessels, seems to indicate that the deformity originates during the blastemic period.[30]

Bohm described four stages of normal fetal foot positioning, proceeding from a stance of equinovarus immediately after the embryonic period and progressing through gradual supination, ankle dorsiflexion, and finally by the fourth month, pronation.[8] A partial arrest of development during the blastemic or early embryonic stage may well be the insult that causes the deformity recognized at birth.

Radiographic Evaluation

Because the osseous structures of the infant foot are small, it is nearly impossible to ascertain their true anatomic relationship by simple clinical examination. Indeed, the rather abundant heel fat pad can easily hide a great deal of hindfoot equinus. Likewise, the absence of soft-tissue definition can make even a moderate amount of hindfoot varus clinically difficult to appreciate. For this reason, radiographic evaluation performed initially and intermittently during the course of treatment is necessary to adequately assess correction.

Standard radiographic views should be obtained in the anteroposterior (AP) and lateral projections. The AP view is obtained with the plantar surface flat on the film cassette in a pseudostanding position. The ankle should be slightly plantar-flexed and the x-ray tube caudally directed 30 degrees. This positioning will permit visualization of the hindfoot and allow accurate measurement of the talocalcaneal (Kite's) angle[23] (Fig 31–3).

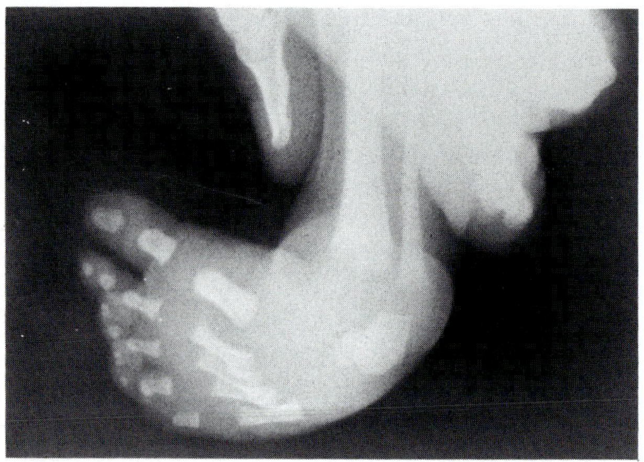

FIG 31–3.
AP view of a clubfoot in a neonate. Note the reduction in Kite's angle; the talus is nearly parallel with the calcaneus. Neither hindfoot structure aligns with the forefoot.

The lateral view should likewise be obtained in a pseudostanding position with the ankle as neutral as possible. If the film cassette is aligned parallel with the lateral border of the foot, an oblique view of the hindfoot will result, and the talus will spuriously appear to be flat topped with the fibula displaced posteriorly.[29] An accurate lateral view is obtained when the hindfoot is parallel with the cassette, and in the true projection the talus is recognized as having a normal dorsally convex but anteriorly displaced articular surface.

In the AP view the longitudinal axis of the normal talus aligns well with a similar axis of the first metatarsal, and the longitudinal axis of the calcaneus aligns with the fifth metatarsal. These two axes converge posteriorly to form Kite's angle (normally 20 to 40 degrees). With hindfoot varus the calcaneus is rotated beneath the talus, plantar-flexed, and if the deformity is severe, medially bowed. This causes a decrease in Kite's angle, occasionally to 0 degrees (Fig 31–4). With correction of hindfoot varus, the abnormal talocalcaneal relationship reverses, the anterior calcaneus rotates laterally and the

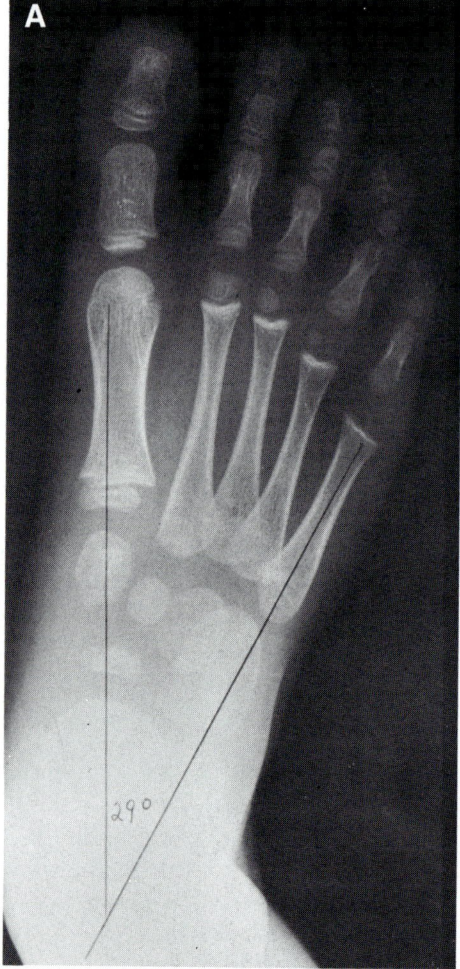

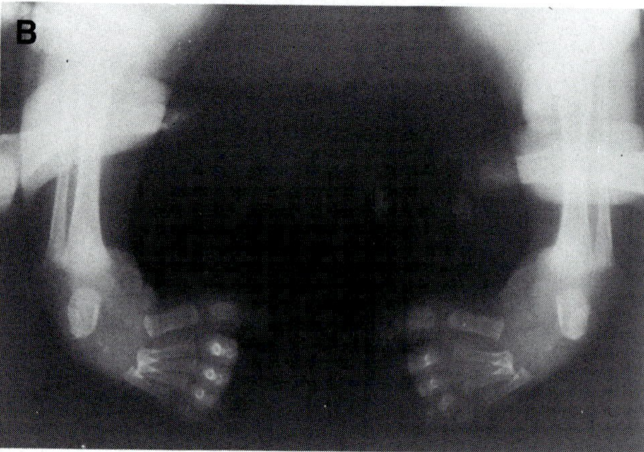

FIG 31–4.
A, normal talocalcaneal (Kite's) angle. **B,** bilateral clubfoot in a newborn; note that neither the midfoot nor the forefoot align with the longitudinal axes of the talus and calcaneus.

posterior calcaneal tuberosity medially, and the entire structure everts. Without a normal talocalcaneal angle in the AP projection, the hindfoot varus has not been fully corrected.

In the lateral view the talocalcaneal angle is derived from a line drawn through the midlongitudinal axis of the ossific nucleus and a second converging line drawn along the plantar surface of the calcaneus. This angle is not static and in the normal foot will decrease with plantar flexion and increase with dorsiflexion. In the normal standing lateral projection the talocalcaneal angle measures between 35 and 50 degrees.[21] A distinct overlap of the anterosuperior margin of the calcaneus on the anteroinferior margin of the talus is normally present. With clubfoot deformity and hindfoot varus, the normal lateral talocalcaneal angle is reduced, and the two structures are parallel. Furthermore, relatively little change in the angle occurs with dorsiflexion and plantar flexion. (Fig 31–5).

Careful evaluation of the calcaneotibial relationship will demonstrate hindfoot equinus uncorrected with forced dorsiflexion. The ossific nucleus of the talus is displaced anteriorly because of the equinus deformity, and when severe, the posterior calcaneus nearly approximates the posterior malleolus.

Forefoot deformity is seen on both AP and lateral projections. On the AP view, both adduction and inversion with shortening of the medial column and lengthening of the lateral column are present. Viewed laterally, possible foreshortening of the plantar soft-tissue structures may cause forefoot equinus and result in a cavus deformity (Fig 31–6).

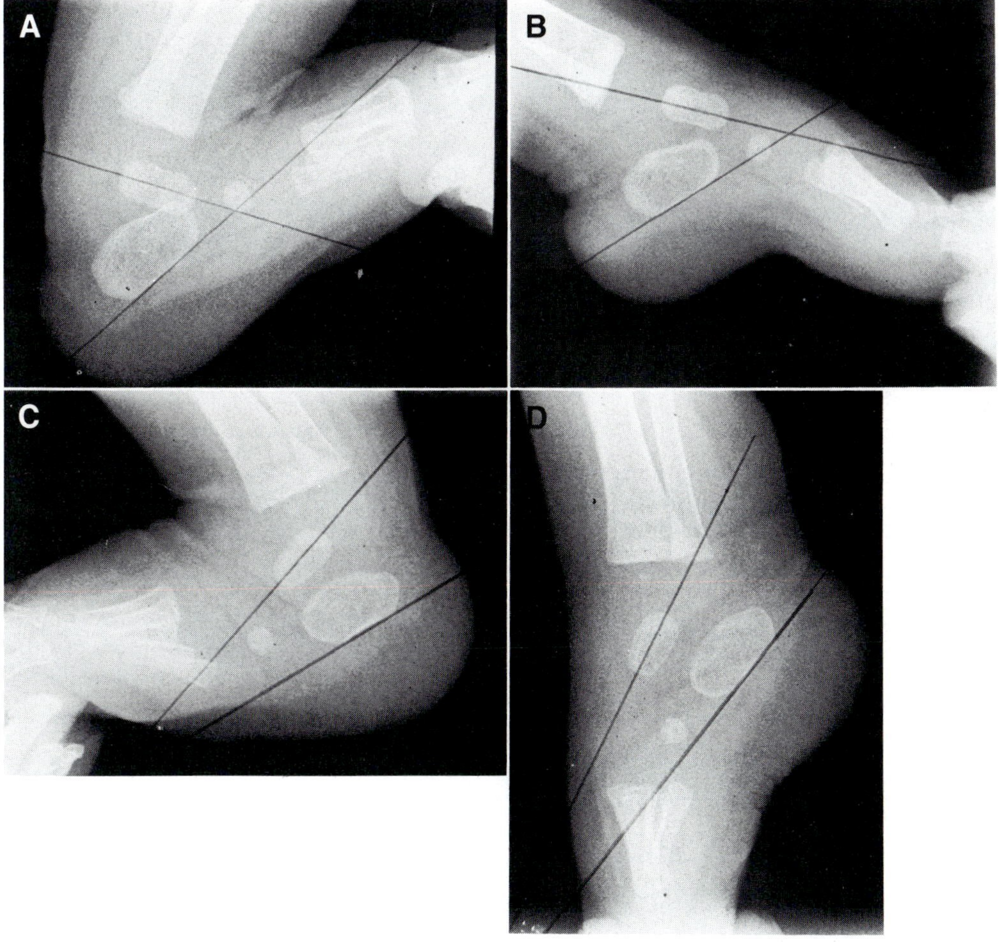

FIG 31–5.
Clubfoot in a 3-month-old child. **A** and **B,** stress dorsiflexion—plantar flexion views of the normal foot. On stress dorsiflexion, the lateral talocalcaneal angle measures 45 degrees; on stress plantar flexion, it is 58 degrees. Note the overlap of the anteroinferior talus and anterosuperior calcaneus on dorsiflexion. **C** and **D,** stress dorsiflexion—plantar flexion lateral views of the opposite clubfoot. Despite stress, the talocalcaneal angle is not reduced and remains unchanged at 17 degrees. On dorsiflexion, the calcaneus remains in equinus, and the talus does not overlap the anterior process of the os calcis.

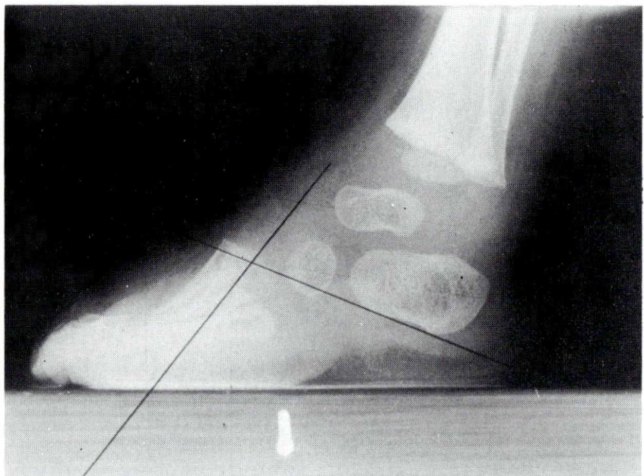

FIG 31–6.
Cavus deformity in a clubfoot with foreshortened plantar soft tissues.

Until all the radiographic alterations have returned to normal, one cannot be satisfied that the clubfoot deformity has been corrected. Active treatment should continue until talocalcaneal parallelism is reversed in both the AP and lateral views and until the stress plantar flexion–dorsiflexion radiographs demonstrate unlocking of the subtalar articulation with adequate dorsiflexion of the hindfoot. The standing lateral radiograph should present a normal plantigrade appearance with no hindfoot equinus, cavus deformity, or break of the midfoot.

Treatment

As each color has many shades and hues, so are there many degrees of clubfoot deformity. Treatment necessary to bring the foot to a plantigrade, longitudinally aligned posture depends on the degree of deformity present. Each foot must be carefully examined both clinically and radiographically, and the treatment program must be designed to meet the demands of the deformity present.

Waisbrod, in studying his eight specimens,[30] found that the response to manual manipulation was dependent on the degree of deformity in the talar neck. In his series he was able to passively correct three feet and found, on dissection, the talar neck in each of these to have an angle in excess of 150 degrees with the body. It is quite likely that the apparent clubfoot that responds rapidly and readily to manipulation and casting has, in fact, little deformity in the talar neck; the initial clinical presentation may be more a postural problem. This is not to ignore these feet or to downgrade the importance of early active treatment, for the postural deformity, if persistent, can result in secondary structural change. A rather large number of clubfeet belong in the postural deformity category, and if they are treated early (from the day of birth), secondary resistant changes do not have an opportunity to develop. The longer one waits before initiating treatment, the more significant and resistant are the secondary structural changes. Active treatment should begin as soon after birth as possible.

If plantar and medial inclination of the foreshortened distal talus exists to any degree, the osseous structures must be placed in an aligned position and held there during the formative years of growth and development for the foot to anatomically permit normal ambulation and normal footwear. To align the foot with the rest of the extremity may require dividing secondarily shortened, thickened capsules and ligaments as well as lengthening secondarily abbreviated muscle-tendon units.[24] One must always remember that the primary talar neck deformity with secondary structural change in other osseous components persists but may be altered over time by use of Wolff's law. Holding the foot in a corrected position during growth and development will create adaptive changes in the distal talus,[11] distal calcaneus, and subtalar joint and cause them to revert to near normal. However, the talus will continue to have a short neck with a somewhat flattened head, the navicular and talar body may continue to be smaller than normal, and indeed, the entire foot and calf will probably never match the opposite member in size. If, after alignment of the foot is obtained by either serial casting or soft-tissue release, the foot is not held in the corrected position for a significant period of growth and development, the neck of the talus will continue to deviate medially, the navicular and calcaneus will gradually realign with their previous articulations about the talar neck, and the hindfoot will drift back into varus and equinus and the forefoot into cavus and adduction.

It would therefore seem reasonable that once alignment is obtained and reasonably stable, the foot should be held in the corrected position day and night for a moderate period of time and subsequently at night alone through at least the second period of accelerated growth and development (7 to 8 years of age). Anything less may lead to a reappearance of the deformity.

Treatment at Birth.—The foot of a neonate with talipes equinovarus deformity is often no larger than the thumb of the treating physician. This small structure, on careful examination, is frequently quite supple.

Longitudinal traction applied at the distal first through third metatarsals with the heel plantar-flexed will result in the gradual formation of a dimple over the superolateral aspect of the midfoot. This represents progressive lateral subluxation of the navicular on the medially deviated talar head as the medial column elongates with traction. The dimple or void develops at the lateral junction of the talar neck with the talar body (Fig 31–7). Lateral subluxation of the midfoot produces normal forefoot alignment with the tibia and, if held in this position, will allow soft-tissue structures of the medial column to elongate and stretch. With traction on the forefoot, the physician stretches the tightened deltoid and talocalcaneal interosseous ligaments and is able to push the posterior calcaneus into eversion and medial rotation with the thumb and forefinger of the opposite hand. Forceful attempts at dorsiflexing the ankle against tightened posterior ligaments will result in a nutcracker effect,[12, 22] with the contracted posterior structures acting as a hinge and the talar body within the mortise like a fulcrum. To prevent a longitudinal midfoot break with development of a rocker-bottom deformity, the physician should not attempt forceful ankle dorsiflexion.

After manipulation, the foot can be held in its realigned position by application of a corrective cast or, as is my preference, adhesive strapping. The taping technique, a modification of the Jones method, is preferred because of the difficulty encountered in attempting to apply a corrective cast with appropriately placed pressure points on the extremely small foot of a neonate. Furthermore, taping of the newborn foot permits dynamic and passive stretching exercises during the entire time of treatment, thereby avoiding progressive joint stiffness and further muscle atrophy (Fig 31–8).

Tape Application.

1. After manipulation and reduction of the clubfoot deformity and with traction applied to the distal first through third metatarsals by an assistant, apply tincture of benzoin to the foot, leg, and distal portion of the thigh in the areas to be covered by tape.
2. Place a piece of ⅛-in. orthopaedic felt about 1¼ inches wide over the distal aspect of the thigh with the knee flexed 90 degrees and the free ends extending 1½ in. down the medial and lateral aspects of the leg.
3. Wrap a piece of felt of similar width about the forefoot, the free ends meeting on the lateral border of the foot.
4. At this point, or earlier, it is most helpful to follow Kite's suggestion: give the baby a bottle in an attempt to promote muscle relaxation.[23] A parent may play an active role in the treatment by assisting with this task.
5. Apply the first strip of tape, a long one, over the felt surrounding the forefoot. Begin at the lateral plantar margin, course medially over the dorsum of the foot, make the turn around the medial border, continue laterally on the plantar surface, and complete the circle about the foot. At all times be sure that the assistant continues longitudinal traction on the forefoot while maintaining the corrected position. Continue the strip up the lateral border of the leg (it tends to bowstring a bit at the ankle) over the felt draped on the distal portion of the thigh (the knee must be flexed 90 degrees)

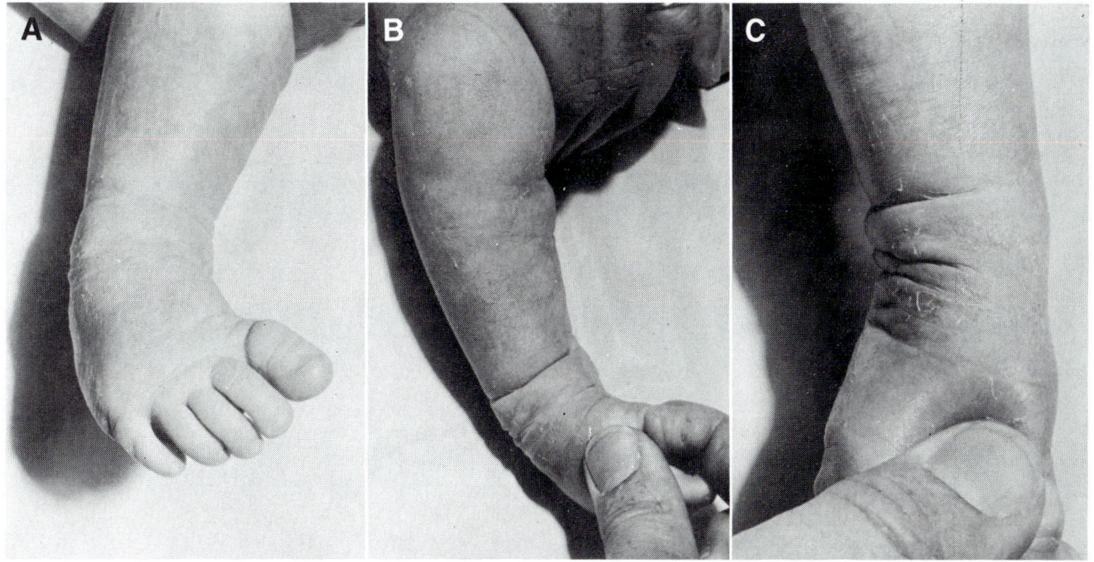

FIG 31–7.
Neonatal clubfoot deformity. **A,** moderate equinovarus deformity. **B,** this responds to traction on the medial metatarsal heads. **C,** by developing a recess at the lateral border of the talar neck, the navicular and forefoot are brought into alignment with the tibia. It represents lateral subluxation of the midfoot on the medially deviated head of the talus.

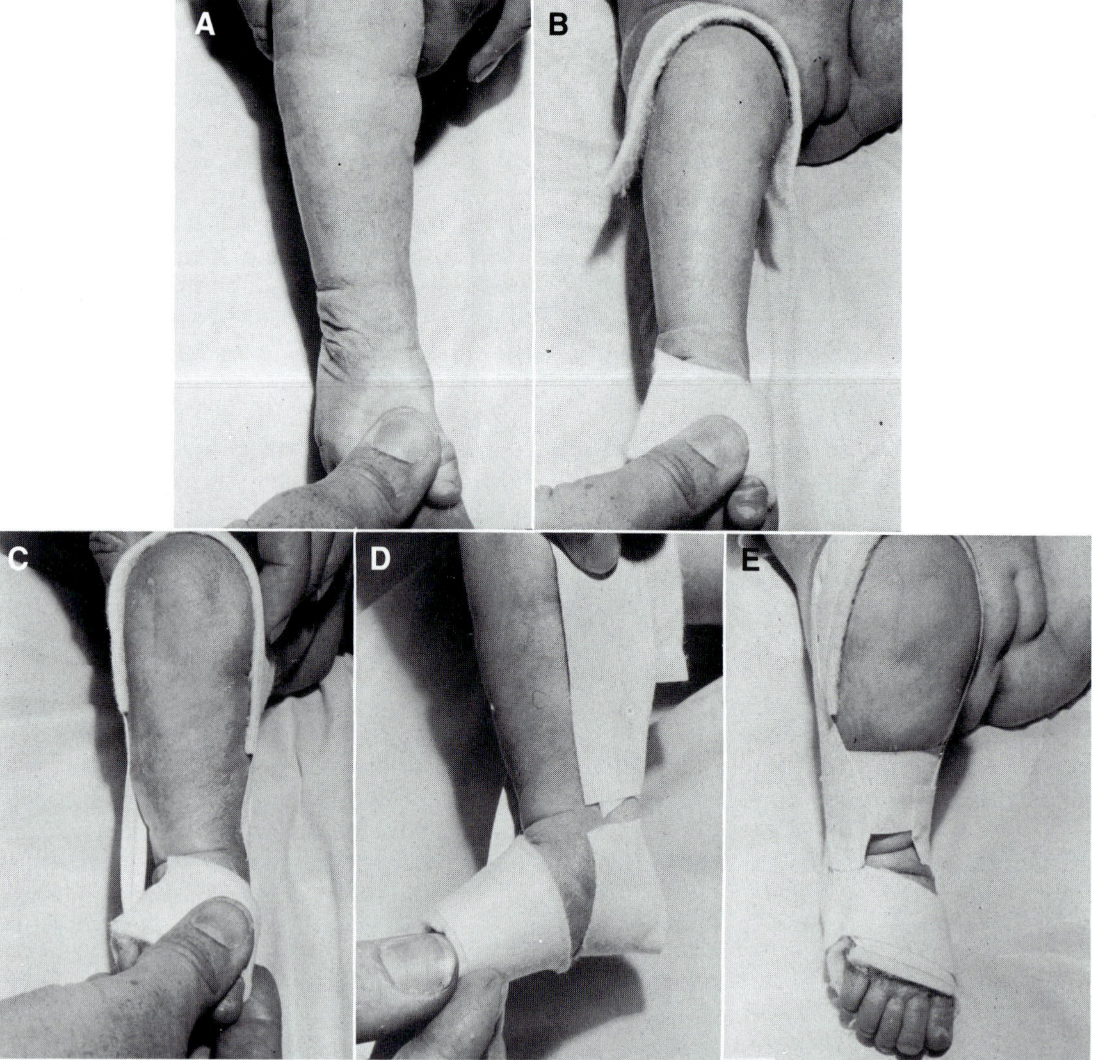

FIG 31–8.
Adhesive strapping of the neonatal clubfoot depicted in Figure 31–7. **A,** gentle traction for several minutes applied to the medial metatarsal heads aligns the foot with the leg. Note the recess at the lateral margin of the talar neck. **B,** the areas to be covered by tape are painted with tincture of benzoin. A 1¼-in.-wide strip of orthopaedic felt covers the distal portion of the thigh, and a second strip surrounds the forefoot. **C,** a long strip of 1-in. adhesive tape encircles the foot and courses up the lateral aspect of the leg over the distal part of the thigh (knee flexed) and three fourths of the way down the medial portion of the leg. **D,** the second long strip of tape beginning just at the medial malleolus runs under the calcaneus, up the lateral aspect of the leg, over the distal part of the thigh, and down the medial portion of the leg (overlying the initial tape). **E,** two short anchoring strips encircle the distal part of the leg and foot. The foot is held in the corrected position. Active and passive stretching exercises are still possible.

and halfway down the medial side of the leg. As the tape crosses over the thigh, allow its upper margin to contact ½ in. of thigh skin proximal to the felt. This initial strip serves to align the forefoot and correct the adductus and supination.

6. Use a second long strip of tape to correct heel varus and equinus. Begin just below the medial malleolus (do not overlap or connect with the end of the first strip), course beneath the heel medially to laterally, and push the calcaneus out of varus. Make sure that this strip is no further distal than the cuboid. Continue up the lateral portion of the leg, overlying for the most part the first applied strip, over the distal thigh felt, and again down the medial aspect of the leg. The final corrected position now has been accomplished.

7. The last two strips of tape, 4 to 6 in. in length, are used to anchor the long pieces. With the first, circle the distal part of the leg above the malleoli. This will

tend to contain (but not eliminate) the bowstringing. Encircle the foot with the second strip by overlapping the felt and previously applied adductus-correcting tape. If necessary (it usually is), apply a third smaller strip in horseshoe fashion over the thigh just proximal to the felt and leg tapes. With this strip connecting the skin of the distal portion of the thigh to the previously applied tape, the latter is prevented from slipping distally off the knee as it is actively extended.

During the immediate postnatal period the strapping is changed daily. Nurses and parents are encouraged to exercise and stretch the foot frequently during the day, and after leaving the hospital, the parent is instructed to perform stretching exercises with each diaper change. After discharge, usually the third or fourth day after delivery, the tape is changed in the physician's office at least twice weekly for the first 3 to 4 weeks. During this period of rapid growth and development, plantigrade alignment and progressive correction are encouraged by the corrective taping and stretching. If the plantar deviation of the talar neck is not too severe, the foot can be nearly or completely corrected by adhesive strapping alone for a period of 2 to 3 months. By 8 weeks of age, the foot is usually large enough to allow application of a corrective cast with discretely applied pressure points (Fig 31–9). Fiberglass or other synthetic casting materials do not permit the accurate molding and contouring necessary for correction and hence are not an adequate substitute for plaster. If radiographs demonstrate adequate dorsiflexion of the hindfoot with unlocking of the subtalar joint and a normal Kite's angle, the foot may be merely held in the corrected position by plaster until it is large enough to be fitted with a shoe.

Despite the fact that separate centers of ossification may appear on radiographic examination to have normal relationships, it must be remembered that the unossified anterior talus is still directed medially and plantarward and, unless the foot is held in a corrected position, the forefoot will realign itself with the maldirected anterior talus and calcaneus. All three components of the deformity—hindfoot equinus, inversion, and forefoot adduction-supination—will recur. For this reason, once radiographic evidence of full correction has been obtained, the foot must be held in the corrected position with either plaster or a well- fitting brace. The device is worn day and night until walking age has been reached (10 to 12 months). As long as the radiograph continues to show adequate correction of the deformity, the child may then wear the brace at night only.

With single-foot involvement a Phelps brace with a medial upright, lateral valgus–inducing T-strap and 90-degree downstop is recommended. A plastic window at the counter of the shoe will allow the mother to visualize the heel of the child as it is placed in the shoe, thus ensuring proper heel seating. It is a good practice to obtain lateral radiographs of the foot in the brace to be sure that the hindfoot has not persisted in equinus. If both feet are under treatment, bilateral Phelps braces maybe joined by a Denis-Browne bar bent into some valgus.

Surgical Treatment.—When treatment is begun at birth, the foot is usually supple enough to obtain at

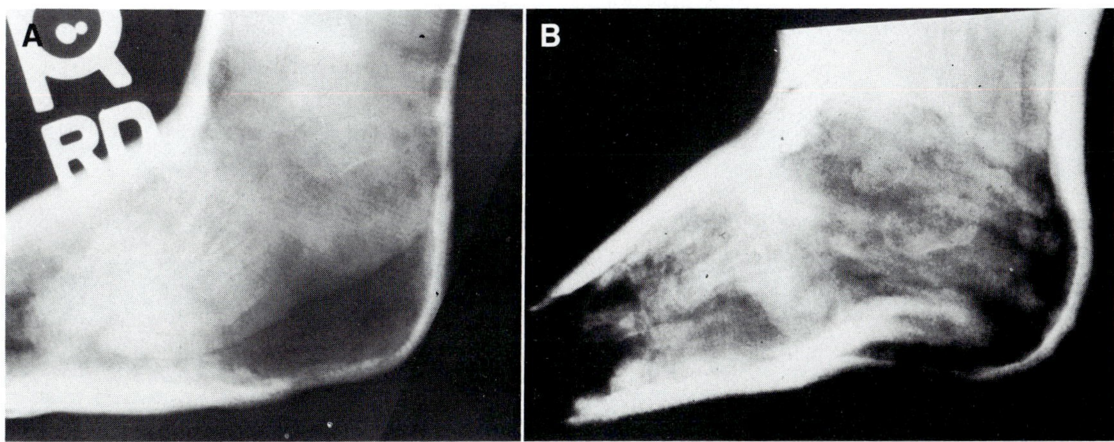

FIG 31–9.
A, poorly molded cast. Externally it gives the impression of clubfoot correction; however, a radiograph demonstrates a loose fit and persistent hindfoot equinus and varus. Note the absence of molding beneath the calcaneocuboid joint and behind the Achilles tendon. **B,** with better molding, the foot is locked in position and will not slide up into the cast. The calcaneocuboid joint is further posterior than would be clinically suspected. An occasional radiographic check to verify appropriate placement of the molded contours is advisable.

least some correction of the secondary deformity with strapping and casting. Depending on the severity of the primary osseous deformity, a time usually arises at about 3 to 4 months of age when further correction is no longer attainable by nonoperative means.

Surgery on an infant's foot is technically demanding because of the small structures. Violation of articular cartilage during an operative procedure can and frequently does result in permanent stiffness and deformity. A demonstration of the singular importance of the posterior tibial artery to blood supply of the entire clubfoot further points out the care and expertise required for successful surgical intervention. Surgery should be delayed until it can safely be performed without damaging articular cartilage and tendons, nerves, and vascular structures can be readily identified. Even at 3 to 4 months of age, the foot is so small that the use of operating telescopes or magnifying loupes during the procedure is recommended.

The most frequent deformities remaining after conservative treatment are hindfoot varus and equinus. Taping, stretching, and casting may frequently correct the forefoot adduction-supination. Surgical release of posterior and posteromedial soft-tissue structures will often allow completion of the correction in the less rigid clubfoot (Fig 31–10). The surgeon must be able, however, to make an accurate assessment of the completeness of soft-tissue release intraoperatively and be prepared to extend the procedure to the degree required by the residual deformity. Advances in surgical technique over the past decade have removed clubfoot surgery from the armamentarium of the occasional foot surgeon.

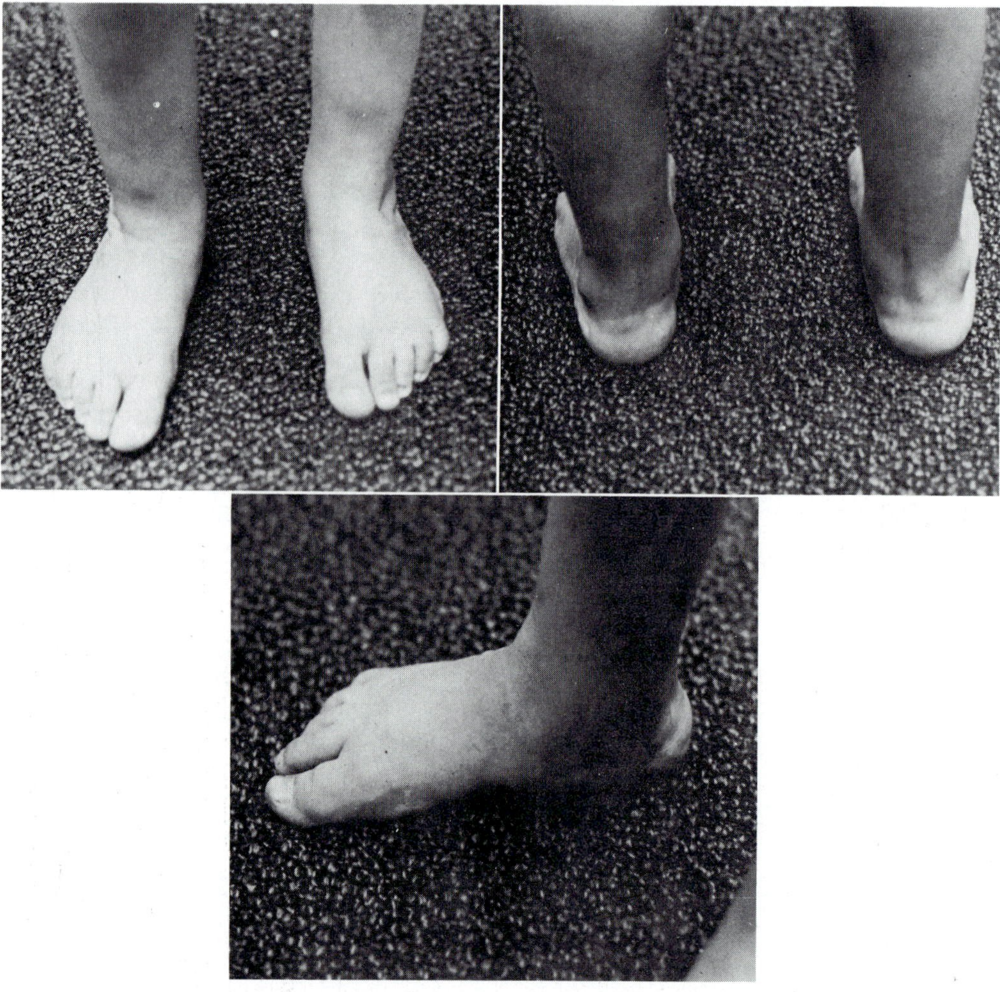

FIG 31–10.

Appearance of bilateral clubfeet at 3½ years of age. The child was treated by adhesive strapping until 3 months of age, corrective casts until 6 months, and then posteromedial release was performed. Casts were continued until 11 months of age and followed with night braces.

Before undertaking the task, the surgeon must have an in-depth understanding of the pathologic anatomy and broad experience in clubfoot surgery.

Although the Achilles tendon may appear to be the primary impediment to equinus correction, this is rarely the case. In a true clubfoot, the entire posterior capsule and posterior ligamentous structures are contracted and thickened.[28] Therefore subcutaneous tenotomy of the Achilles tendon should be performed only as a preliminary procedure to formal division of the remaining resistant posterior soft tissues.

Surgical Release.

1. The Cincinnati incision as described by Crawford et al.[10] has been my choice for a surgical approach to most problems of the foot that include the hindfoot. The versatility of the incision allows one to perform total circumtalar clubfoot release, and it serves admirably in whole or part for all other hindfoot problems.

Begin the incision on the medial aspect of the foot, just distal to the first metatarsocuneiform joint. Course posteriorly in a somewhat curvilinear fashion to a point one-half finger breadth distal to the medial malleolus. Continue around the posterior portion of the ankle, and cross the Achilles tendon just proximal to the flexion skin crease. Continue laterally and somewhat distally to a point 0.5 cm distal to the lateral malleolus and then anteriorly, crossing the peroneal tendons; swing somewhat medially over the sinus tarsi toward the lateral talonavicular joint (Fig 31–11).

2. Divide and spread the soft tissues sharply and bluntly while taking care to preserve the sural nerve, which crosses the wound midway between the lateral margin of the Achilles tendon and lateral malleolus.

3. Longitudinally open the sheath, and divide the Achilles tendon by bisecting it in the sagittal plane. It will be necessary to strongly retract the skin and subcutaneous tissue of the calf proximal to the incision to obtain a sufficient length of tendon for reapproximation after dorsiflexion has been restored. Complete the tenotomy by freeing its lateral half proximally at the musculotendinous junction and its medial half distally at the insertion into the calcaneal tuberosity. When repaired, this will decrease the tendency for the triceps to invert the heel on plantar flexion.

4. A critical evaluation of dorsiflexion will usually demonstrate little change in equinus after heel cord tenotomy. Identify the flexor hallucis longus tendon deep and slightly medial to the Achilles tendon. Place the foot in plantar flexion, and medially identify and retract the flexor digitorum longus, posterior tibial tendon, and neurovascular bundle to expose the posterior surface of the tibia.

5. Make a small longitudinal incision in the posterior retinaculum and dense ankle capsule. This allows identification of the tibiotalar joint without injury to the distal tibial epiphysis. With care and by using small scissors, divide the entire posterior capsule transversely. The division should be carried laterally to the sheath of the peroneal tendons. A rather dense structure, the calcaneofibular ligament, will be encountered as it courses

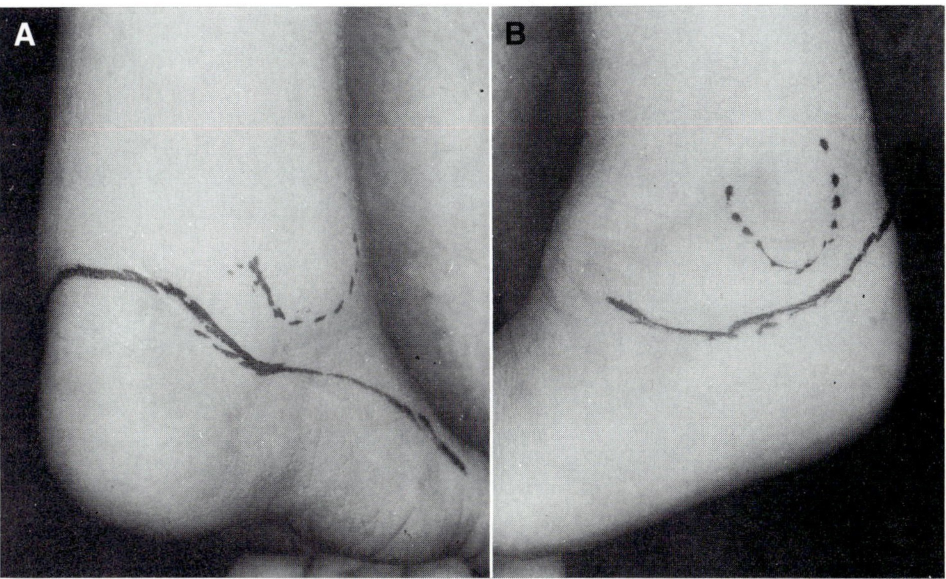

FIG 31–11.
Preoperative skin marking delineating the course of the Cincinnati incision. **A,** posteromedial view. **B,** posterolateral view.

from the tip and posterior aspect of the lateral malleolus to the calcaneous; a division of this structure is critical and facilitated by the Cincinnati incision.

6. Continue the release medially, and include the most posterior fibers of the deep deltoid ligament; take care to not transect the midsubstance of the deep deltoid ligament, and protect the neurovascular contents of the tarsal tunnel.

7. Dorsiflex the foot to bring the articular surface of the talar dome into view. Divide the posterior inferior tibiofibular ligament.

8. Identify the subtalar joint in the same manner as the ankle (posteriorly it will lie only a few millimeters distal to the ankle joint). Begin with a longitudinal incision, and after the joint space is visualized, divide its posterior capsule from the tip of the lateral malleolus to the midportion of the medial malleolus while protecting the flexor hallucis longus.

9. Carefully examine the foot under stress, and assess the correction of equinus, hindfoot varus, and forefoot adductus. In a small number of cases, this degree of release will be sufficient to effect correction. If deformity persists, one must be prepared to proceed with extreme caution and continue the complete release.

10. Identify the course of the tibialis posterior tendon by passing a probe through its sheath beginning proximally above the malleolus to its insertion into the inferior-medial navicular distally. Open the sheath along its course, and preserve only a small pulley at the medial malleolus. Use of the probe in this fashion allows one to identify the navicular with ease.

11. Lengthen, in Z fashion, the tibialis posterior tendon proximal to the medial malleolus. Pull the distal portion of the tendon through the sheath, and retract distally. This will allow identification of the navicular; very often it nearly approximates the medial malleolus.

12. Open the entire talonavicular joint (the identification of this may be a very demanding task). The medial most portion of the joint may actually parallel the longitudinal axis of the foot due to the medial orientation of the talar head. Open the talonavicular joint medially and dorsally (protecting the dorsal neurovascular structures and extensor tendons by retraction). Avoid dissection along the dorsal aspect of the talar neck because so doing may interrupt the critical blood supply to the talus. Similarly, the inferior capsule of the talonavicular joint should be divided as far laterally as can be safely reached.

13. While in the depths of the wound medially, attempt to visualize the calcaneonavicular (spring) and Y ligaments. Divide these in similar fashion to the talonavicular joint.

At the medial malleolus, identify the sheath of the flexor digitorum communis tendon. Divide this into the plantar surface of the foot by pushing open scissors along its course. A thickening in the sheath beneath the navicular will identify the master knot of Henry; at this point, the flexor hallucis longus crosses the flexor digitorum communis. Divide the master knot, and free both tendons.

14. Bluntly divide the fibers of the abductor hallucis muscle as it arises from the medial calcaneus. Take care to avoid interruption of the medial plantar nerve, which penetrates its substance.

15. Plantar retraction of the divided abductor hallucis muscle opens the deep plantar structures to visualization. One should be able to identify the flexor hallucis longus tendon crossing to the medial side of the flexor digitorum communis tendon. If it is not clearly seen, Henry's knot is still intact and should be incised.

16. Retract the deeper plantar structures plantarward so as to visualize the medial portion of the calcaneocuboid capsule. Open this joint dorsally, medially, and on its plantar surface. I prefer small scissors or an elevator to accomplish this task safely.

17. Complete the division of the subtalar joint capsule medially by dividing the entire superficial deltoid ligament. At the anterior margin of the posterior facet, the talocalcaneal interosseous ligament may be visualized.

18. The medial release having been completed, examine the foot once more for any residual equinus, forefoot adductus, or hindfoot varus. Be very critical at this point, and proceed to the posterolateral portion of the wound if any evidence of hindfoot deformity persists.

19. Identify the peroneal tendons, and ensure that the capsule and ligaments of the subtalar joint are divided posteriorly and laterally. Completion of the calcaneal fibular ligament incision will allow the posterior calcaneus to rotate medially and unlock the subtalar joint.

20. Dorsiflex the foot to bring the talar dome well into view posteriorly. Examination of the posterior talus will reveal a flattened posterolateral surface that had articulated with the medial surface of the fibular malleolus. With talar dorsiflexion and fibula-talar ligamentous division, the posterior talus rotates toward the medial malleolus and exposes this facet.

21. Distract the posterior calcaneus into dorsiflexion. The subtalar joint will open, and the talocalcaneal interosseous ligament can be seen traversing the joint medially to laterally. A blunt nerve hook slipped anterior to the ligament will facilitate its division with a thin scalpel blade.

22. In the anterolateral portion of the wound, enter the sinus tarsi. This allows visualization and complete

division of the most lateral part of the talonavicular capsule. In addition, any remainder of the interosseous talocalcaneal ligament will be evident and may be sectioned, if necessary, to allow full visualization of the subtalar joint laterally.

23. Divide the lateralmost calcaneal cuboid capsule.

24. It should now be possible to place the foot into a fully corrected position. With the talonavicular joint held in a reduced position, pass a smooth Kirschner wire through the posterolateral portion of the talus, anteromedially through the navicular and out the dorsum of the foot. Be careful not to overreduce the navicular laterally because this will create a Z-foot deformity. From where it exits the dorsum of the foot, withdraw the Kirschner wire until it is flush with the posterior articular surface of the talus.

25. Insert a smooth Kirschner wire transversely through the posterior calcaneus medially to laterally. I avoid placing a wire vertically through the subtalar joint to eliminate the possibility of articular surface disruption.

The flexor hallucis longus is often tight on dorsiflexion of the foot. This will usually stretch out over a few weeks without lengthening. If extremely tight, division of the intramuscular portion of this tendon and that of the flexor digitorum cammunis is helpful.[8a]

26. Repair the lengthened Achilles tendon and tibialis posterior with the foot in a corrected position. Close the skin with interrupted subcuticular stitches and plastic strip bandages. Apply a long-leg cast with the pins incorporated; do not attempt maximum manipulative correction until the first cast change, 10 days to 2 weeks later.

27. Two weeks later, change the case with the patient under anesthesia, and by using the transverse calcaneal pin, obtain maximum correction of hindfoot equinus and varus. Leave the second cast on for 6 weeks; remove the transfixion pins 8 weeks postoperatively.

This approach toward the clubfoot allows the physician to correct both moderate and severe clubfoot deformity. The use of magnification and iris scissors combined with a thorough knowledge of both normal and abnormal anatomy allows the experienced surgeon to accomplish a total release without damage to articular cartilage. One should not attempt surgery of this magnitude until the child is at least 6 months of age, when osseous structures have reached a size that makes identification of the small joints more certain. Postoperative casting for a total of 2 to 3 months should be followed by bracing full-time until the child nears walking age. Normal shoe wear during the day is appropriate after the child begins independent ambulation. If the child is older when complete release is first performed, postoperative casting with intermittent free periods to foster ankle and subtalar joint motion should be continued for at least 4 to 6 months. Night bracing is routinely recommended until the individual has passed through the second growth spurt (usually 7 to 8 years of age).

Uncorrected or Residual Clubfoot in the Older Child

After the age of 2 years, clubfoot correction by soft-tissue release alone becomes more difficult. By the time the child is 4, some form of bony reconstruction is usually necessary. The goal in these late cases is not to create a normal foot but rather to convert the existing deformity to one that is plantigrade and allows normal shoe wear.

Many procedures have been described, including metatarsal osteotomy, lateral wedge resection of the tarsus, excochleation of the cuboid,[21] fusion of the calcaneocuboid joint (the Dilwyn-Evans procedure).[7, 14] calcaneal osteotomy after the method of Dwyer,[13, 15] and ultimately triple arthrodesis. Each of these procedures has its place in the armamentarium of reconstructive clubfoot surgery, and each case must be individually evaluated to select the appropriate form of treatment.

Metatarsus Adductus and Metatarsus Varus

Much confusion surrounds the terminology of the metatarsus adductus and varus deformities. Many authors use the words *adductus* and *varus* interchangeably; to additionally confuse the issue, metatarsus adductus varus has been further delineated as a separate entity.[43] As noted in earlier editions of this book, the distinction may be academic and the difference merely a matter of degree.

Assuming that the entities metatarsus adductus and metatarsus varus are merely variations in degree of the same deformity, metatarsus varus is the more involved of the two.[39] Metatarsus adductus varus is perhaps the most severe grade of the deformity. The most important thing to recognize is that the hindfoot is in neither equinus nor varus.[45] In the mildest form of the problem, metatarsus adductus, little or no supination persists with weight bearing. Just after the turn of the century the problem was not widely recognized—only 4 cases were noted among 5,000 patients in Hoffa's clinic. Today it appears at least ten times as frequently as clubfoot deformity,[59] is quite supple, and can be corrected easily with passive stretching and corrective immobilization (Fig 31–12).

As the degree of deformity progresses, metatarsus

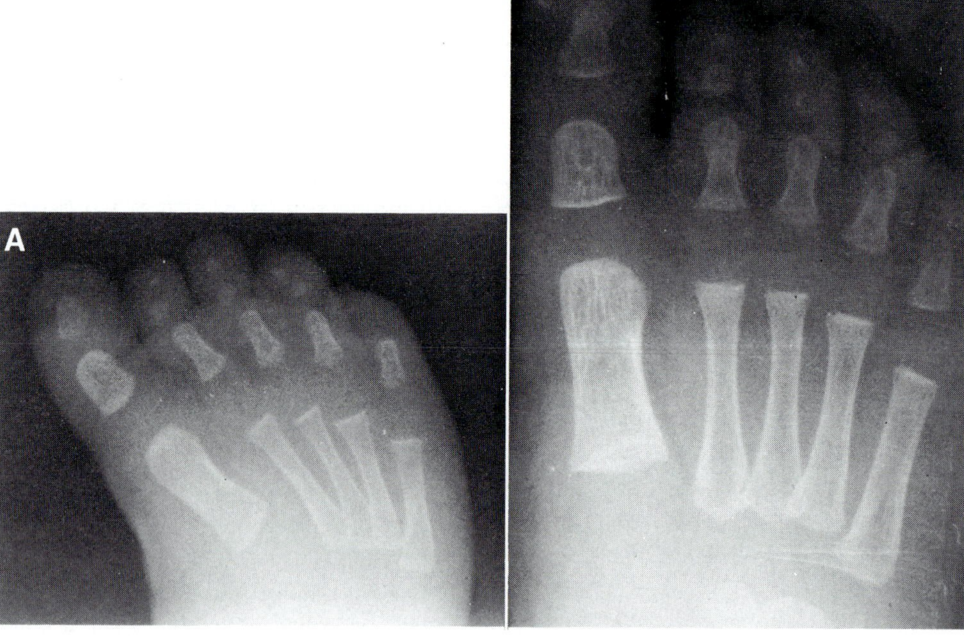

FIG 31–12.
Metatarsus adductus. **A,** at 7 months of age there is convexity of the lateral border of the foot. The lateral three metatarsals have a slight medial bow, with actual inturning (adductus) greatest in the first metatarsal and least in the fifth. **B,** standing radiograph at the age of 18 months. Treatment was serial casting for 8 weeks beginning at 3 months of age.

varus occurs, and in this case the forefoot demonstrates supination as well as adduction with weight bearing. Metatarsus varus tends to be hereditary,[40] is a more resistant problem, and more frequently requires surgical intervention.

Anatomy

In metatarsus adductus or varus the head of the talus is directed inward but not plantarward as in clubfoot deformity. No hindfoot equinus is present, but the hallmark of the problem, incurving of the lateral border of the foot, is noted. The metatarsal shafts are deviated medially, the deviation increasing laterally to medially. Actual incurving of the lateral metatarsal diaphyses may occur as the child grows. The first metatarsal is straight, but at the metatarsal base the first cuneiform articulates with its medial aspect. Generally the cuneiforms are rotated into varus, each, however, remaining lateral to the navicular. The heel is never in varus, either remaining neutral or deviating into valgus. With weight bearing the lateral border of the foot is in contact with the ground, and the medial border is elevated.

In the absence of hindfoot varus or equinus, Kite termed the deformity *one third of a clubfoot.*[40] The probable interrelationship of these deformities is noted in the common finding of talar neck medial deviation. Bleck's[34] explanation and description of persistent medial deviation of the talar neck as a cause for childhood toe-in may point out the clinical presentation of the same deformity of an even lesser degree.

McCormick and Blount coined the term *skewfoot* to describe the condition when forefoot and midfoot varus is very severe and combined with cavus and hindfoot valgus.[44] Lloyd-Roberts and Clark have termed the deformity *metatarsus adductus varus* when fixed adduction and supination of the forefoot are accompanied by valgus deformity of the heel.[43] It would appear that these authors were using different terminology to describe the same problem.

Etiology

As yet no microscopic studies have been reported that investigate the possibility that a developmental defect in the fetal talar neck can, if mild, lead to metatarsus adductus or metatarsus varus.

Kite felt that muscle imbalance with overpull of the tibialis anterior and tibialis posterior might be the cause.[40] Abnormal insertion of the tibialis anterior into the base of the first metatarsal, with slips of tendon extending to the neck of the first metatarsal and without insertional fibers into the first cuneiform, has also been implicated as a cause of forefoot imbalance leading to metatarsus adductus.

Like clubfoot, an increased familial incidence has

been noted. Hip dysplasia has also been associated with metatarsus adductus; hence careful evaluation of the hips should accompany an assessment for this problem.[37] Any suggestion of hip pathology demands a pelvic radiograph.

Treatment of Metatarsus Adductus

In general, milder cases of metatarsus adductus recognized in early infancy respond promptly to conservative management.[46] Often, the early deformity is merely dynamic and caused by overpull of the anterior tibial or posterior tibial tendon. If a dynamic deformity is allowed to persist, however, a more fixed adductus will develop.[47] Hence, early intervention is preferred because treatment is simplified.

The small foot of a neonate is quite supple, and because of its small size a well-molded cast with appropriately placed pressure points is difficult to apply. Passive stretching of the forefoot by the mother at each diaper change combined with frequent stroking of the lateral border during the day to stimulate active forefoot eversion may be enough to reverse the inturning. In North America, infants are placed in the prone position for sleeping. The resultant reflex posture of hip and knee flexion, combined with internal rotation of the foot, promotes structural change in supple metatarsus adductus. Since very young infants are not capable of rolling over, the inturned foot remains in this position so long as the baby is left prone. The adverse effect of such posturing can be reversed by poking two holes in the heels of soft infant shoes. When a shoelace, woven through the four holes, is tied tightly and the shoes placed upon the infant's feet, the baby will then lie with the feet externally rotated, even when prone. Worn when in bed, this may reverse, over 2 or 3 months, the tendency for progression of dynamic metatarsus adductus to a structural deformity (Fig 31–13).

If the child is over 3 months of age and the deformity persists, no matter to what degree, it is best to initiate treatment. The ideal goal in treating metatarsus deformity is to limit active intervention to nonsurgical methods and complete treatment before walking age. Therefore as soon as the foot is large enough and if any degree of deformity persists, one should proceed directly to serial casting or corrective bracing.[48] In the absence of equinus, a well-molded below-knee cast is adequate. Since in the first few months of life the child is growing quite rapidly, osseous structures and articular surfaces remodel readily; hence permanent correction can be achieved. The cast should be changed weekly, with progressive correction obtained until the lateral border of the foot is either straight or slightly concave. It is probably best to continue casting until slight overcorrection is noted; a final holding cast should be applied for 2 weeks after overcorrection has been achieved.

Serial casting, despite its effectiveness, has distinct disadvantages. Time, finances, and convenience are all consumed to a significant degree. Recently multiadjustable footwear has been introduced which permits variable positioning of the foot's components. The shoe may be progressively adjusted into forefoot abduction as required for gradual correction of the deformity. It is important to avoid midfoot and forefoot pronation during adjustments. The shoe/brace should be worn at all times, with the exception of time spent bathing; the duration of treatment in my hands has been no longer (or shorter) than when serial casting is used.

Despite the fact that the soft bones of the infant's foot should remodel and achieve a permanent correction, it has been my practice, after casting or bracing for metatarsus adductus, to place the child's foot in either straight-last shoes or tennis shoes with a straight lateral border. Reversing normal shoes, right for left, is inadvisable since this may tend to promote heel valgus. The location of the longitudinal arch along the medial portion of the midfoot of the shoe creates a pronating force when the shoe is placed on the opposite foot and the medial arch mold is placed under the lateral midfoot. When the child reaches walking age, he or she should be able to proceed directly to normal footwear.

The approach toward more resistant metatarsus varus deformity is essentially the same as that used for metatarsus adductus. More time may be required for correction, and unless full correction with slight overcorrection is achieved, recurrence is common. Again, aiming for completion of treatment before walking age is important. After the child reaches 1 year of age, growth of the foot slows considerably, and therefore remodeling takes much longer. Cast treatment of a child over 1 year of age tends to be measured in months rather than weeks as in the infant. However, plaster treatment can be effective.

Application of the Cast.—The basic steps in applying a cast are as follows:

1. A knowledgeable assistant stands at the outer side of the leg and grasps the foot with index and long fingers between the heads of the first and second metatarsals. With the other hand the thigh is held to stabilize the extremity with the knee flexed 90 degrees.
2. Place a 3-in. length of 2-in. stockinette on the upper part of the calf to serve as a cuff for the proximal end of the cast.
3. Wrap the extremity from the tip of the toes to just below the knee with a single layer of Webril. Place ex-

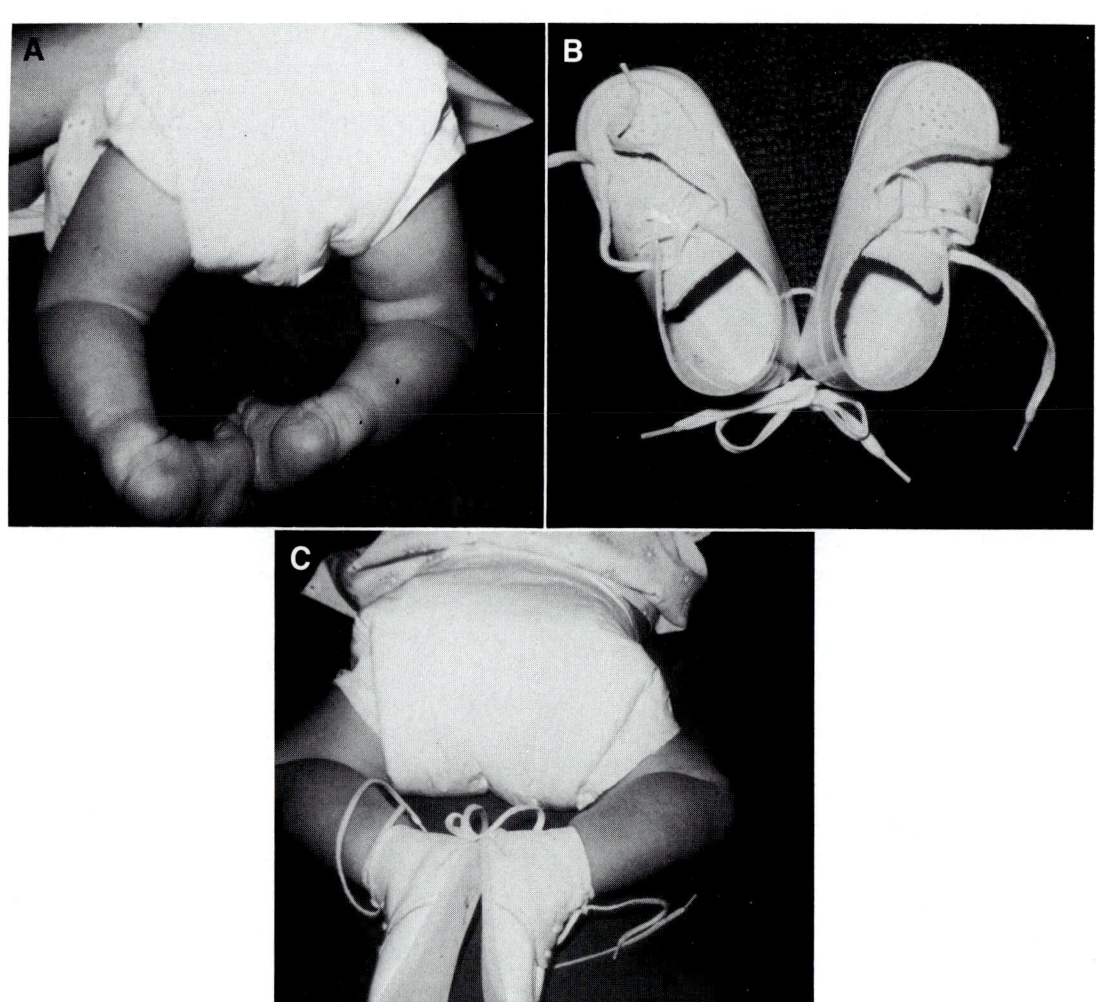

FIG 31–13.
A, sleeping posture contributing to the persistence of forefoot adductus deformity. **B,** soft shoes tied together at the heel and worn **(C)** at nap and bedtime to keep the feet externally rotated.

tra padding under the heel, over the lateral border of the cuboid, and medial to the first metatarsal head.

4. With 2-in.-wide extra-fast–setting plaster, wrap circumferentially, coursing medially to laterally when crossing the plantar surface of the forefoot. The cast may be applied in one stage; incorporate a small splint covering the plantar surface of the foot and posterior part of the calf as reinforcement. When the final 2 in. of bandage is reached, fashion a small tag to initiate removal if the parents are to soak the cast off just before recasting.

5. Apply molding pressures by stabilizing the hindfoot with your outer hand (right hand for the left foot, left hand for the right foot). The calcaneus is held in a neutral position and the heel cradled so that the thenar eminence of the individual applying the cast falls at the infant's calcaneocuboid joint. There it will serve as a fulcrum over which the forefoot can be laterally displaced. The ankle should be maintained at neutral or in slight equinus, the index finger of the outer hand creating an impression over the distal portion of the Achilles tendon. This prevents the foot from sliding proximally and/or the child from kicking the cast off.

6. With the inner hand, apply forefoot abduction pressure to push the head of the first metatarsal laterally. The pressure should never be applied distal to the first metatarsophalangeal joint (creating a hallux valgus). Also resist the tendency to force the forefoot into pronation.

7. After the cast has dried, the stockinette may be turned down over the proximal margin and held in place with a single strip of plaster. The lateral margin of the cast at the small toe should be split and turned back to allow visualization of the sides of all toes.

In the small infant I prefer to soak the cast off rather than remove it with a cast saw. The noise of the saw is frightening and causes the child to cry and the foot to go tense. A good cast can be applied only over a relaxed foot; the child should be given a bottle or pacifier during cast application.

Operative Treatment.—By the time the child reaches 2 years of age, growth has slowed considerably, and cast treatment, although occasionally effective, must be unduly prolonged. In this age group, soft-tissue procedures are effective in gaining permanent correction.

In some feet with metatarsus adductus deformity, the abductor hallucis tendon is the primary deforming force.[41] When attempts at passive correction of the adducted forefoot lead to bowstringing of the abductor hallucis, lengthening this tendon can result in permanent correction (Fig 31–14). The procedure is simple and is carried out through a small longitudinal incision over the distal medial first metatarsal. The abductor tendon is identified and divided obliquely or in Z fashion. This allows the tendon to lengthen; reattachment is not necessary. The skin is then closed and a corrective cast applied for 6 weeks. Overcorrection of forefoot adduction can result, but if the tendon is lengthened rather than excised, overcorrection is unlikely to occur (Fig 31–15).

After 3 years of age, Heyman et al recommend mobilization of the tarsometatarsal and intermetatarsal joint for correction of resistant forefoot adduction.[36] Transfer of the anterior tibial tendon laterally into the cuboid has been recommended but runs a significant risk of creating a pes valgus deformity.[49] Splitting the tibialis anterior longitudinally and moving the lateral portion of the tendon into the third cuneiform have been recommended as an alternative to avoid iatrogenic creation of the opposite deformity. I have found this approach very helpful.

Split Anterior Tibial Transfer.

1. Make a longitudinal incision over the dorsal aspect of the first cuneiform at the insertion of the tibialis anterior tendon.

2. Make a second linear incision about 1½ in. long on the lateral side of the tibial crest at the junction of its middle and lower thirds.

3. Separate the lateral half of the tendon from its dis-

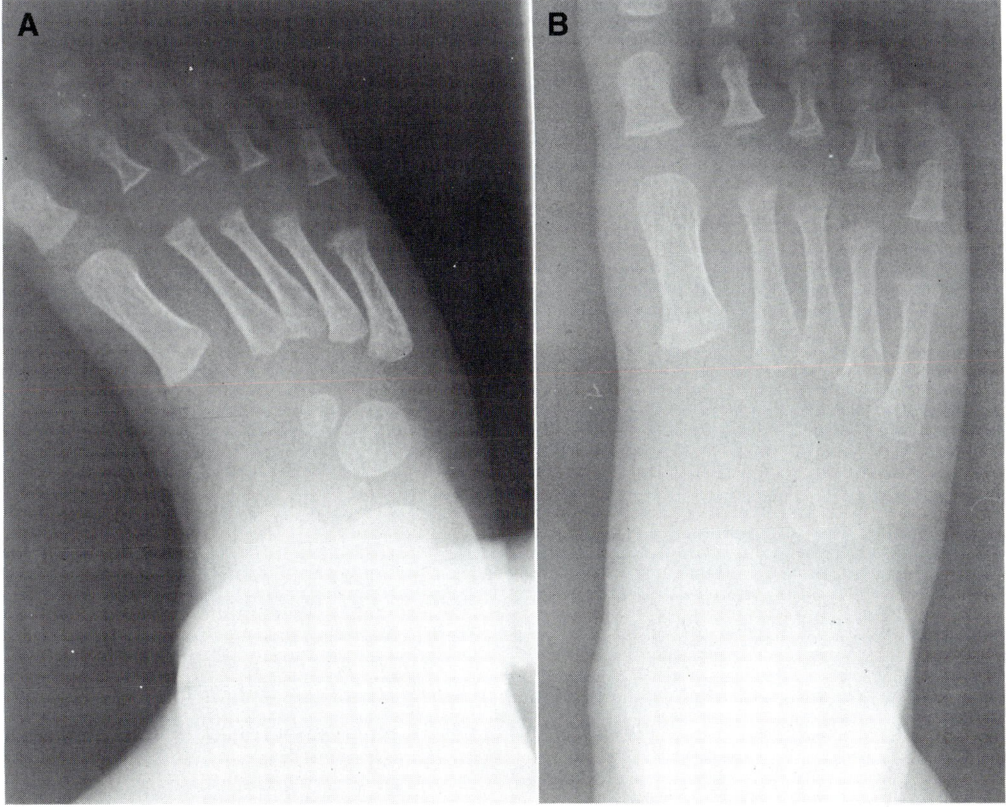

FIG 31–14.
A, metatarsus adductus in a child 1 year and 8 months old. **B,** at the age of 1 year and 10 months, after lengthening of the abductor hallucis tendon.

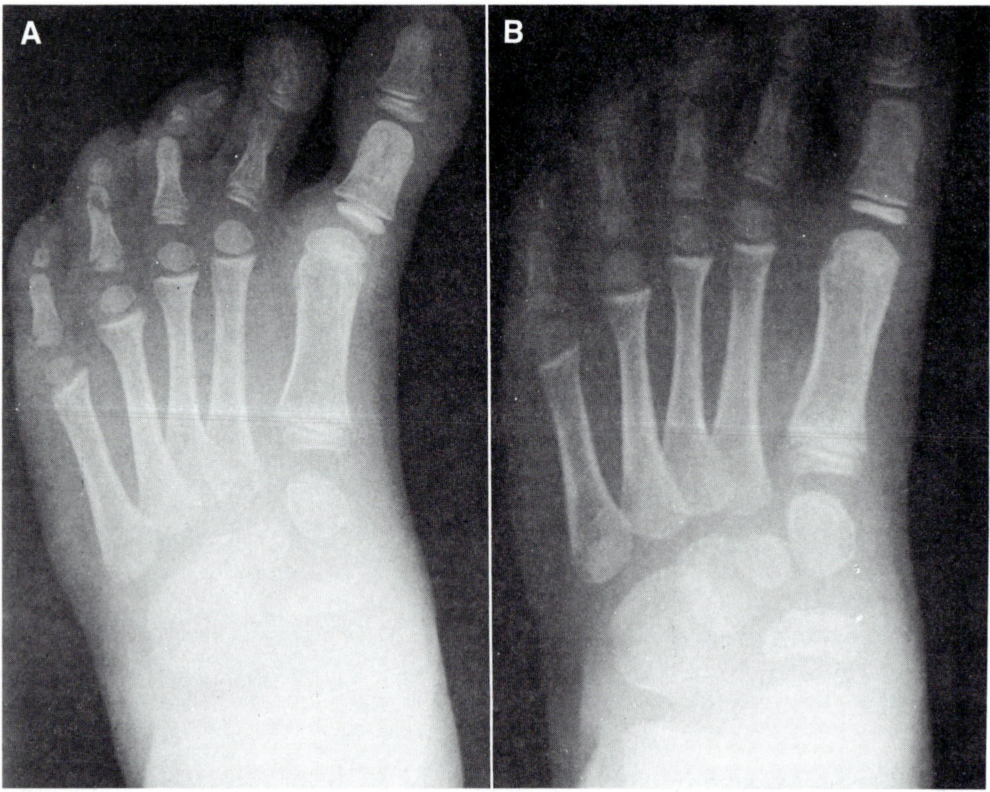

FIG 31–15.
A, persistent metatarsus adductus in a 5-year-old boy who was casted for clubfoot from birth to 11 months of age. Note the continuing medial deviation of the talar head. **B,** 6-months after lengthening of the abductor hallucis, hallux valgus has not occurred.

talmost insertion and begin a longitudinal incision in the tendon substance that bisects it and courses proximally, thereby creating a free lateral slip of tendon.

4. Insert a tendon passer into the sheath of the anterior tibialis at the proximal incision; guide it under the extensor retinaculum, and pass it into the distal portion of the wound.

5. Attach a silk whip suture to the free lateral portion of the tendon, grasp the suture ends with the tendon passer, and withdraw them into the proximal part of the wound. Traction on the suture will then draw the lateral half of the tibialis anterior into the proximal part of the wound and split the distal aspect of the tendon into two segments. When initially applying traction on the suture, guide the free end of tendon back on itself and completely within the tendon sheath distally. If the tendon passer has not remained within the sheath or the distal slip becomes entrapped on filaments of sheath, the lateral slip will not glide and separate from the medial half of tendon; the suture will pull out of its anchor.

6. Make a short longitudinal incision over the third cuneiform. Insert the tendon passer into the third incision and guide it subcutaneously under the transverse retinacular ligament and out the proximal segment of the wound.

7. Pull the tendon through the subcutaneous tunnel, under the transverse retinacular ligament, and into the incision over the third cuneiform.

8. Weave a stainless steel wire through the distal inch of the withdrawn tibialis anterior tendon after the method of Bunnell, and insert a pullout wire through its most proximal loop.

9. Drill a vertical hole through the tarsus in the region of the third cuneiform, and pass the two ends of wire through the bone and plantar skin with straight needles. Pass the pullout loop through skin on the dorsum of the foot.

10. Anchor the tendon in bone by passing the free ends of wire through a foam sponge or ½-in. orthopaedic felt, and tie them over a button.

11. Close all incisions while making certain that the foot is held in dorsiflexion and mild eversion at all times by an assistant.

12. Apply a plaster cast from the toes to the groin with the knee flexed. The cast and pullout wires may be

removed after 8 weeks. Correction of forefoot varus should be permanent.

Mobilization of Tarsometatarsal Joints.—Releasing soft tissues and aligning the forefoot to correct adductus are effective so long as sufficient growth remains to allow for remodeling of deformed articular surfaces[38] (Fig 31–16). Capsulotomies and soft-tissue release should therefore be limited to the child under 7 years of age with persistent adduction deformity. Since treatment with this method relies on the remodeling potential of bone, the foot must be held in the corrected position until such remodeling can occur.

1. The approach can be made via a distally curved incision across the dorsum of the midfoot. Begin medially at the first tarsometatarsal joint and extend laterally to the base of the fifth metatarsal. Alternatively, two longitudinal incisions may avoid the occasional complication of skin slough and transection of longitudinal neurovascular structures. Visualization, however, is better with a transverse incision. When longitudinal incisions are used, they should be made between the first and second metatarsals and between the fourth and fifth. Capsulotomies proceed similarly by either approach.
2. Retract the skin flap to expose the deep fascia covering the tarsal articulation at the base of the first metatarsal. Identify the tibialis anterior tendon, and protect its insertion.
3. Make a longitudinal incision in the deep fascia overlying the interosseous space between the first and second metatarsals. Divide the interosseous ligaments, beginning distally and proceeding proximally. This permits accurate identification of the first metatarsocuneiform joint. Avoid damage to the physeal plate of the first metatarsal or the dorsalis pedis vessels.
4. Incise the entire dorsal and medial capsule of the first tarsometatarsal joint; flex and apply distal traction to the metatarsal to expose and carefully divide the entire medial two thirds of the plantar capsule. Leave the lateralmost margin of the plantar capsule intact.
5. The second tarsometatarsal articulation is proximal to the others. Because of this variation, osteotomy of the second metatarsal alone at the level of the other tarsometatarsal joints more readily permits adductus

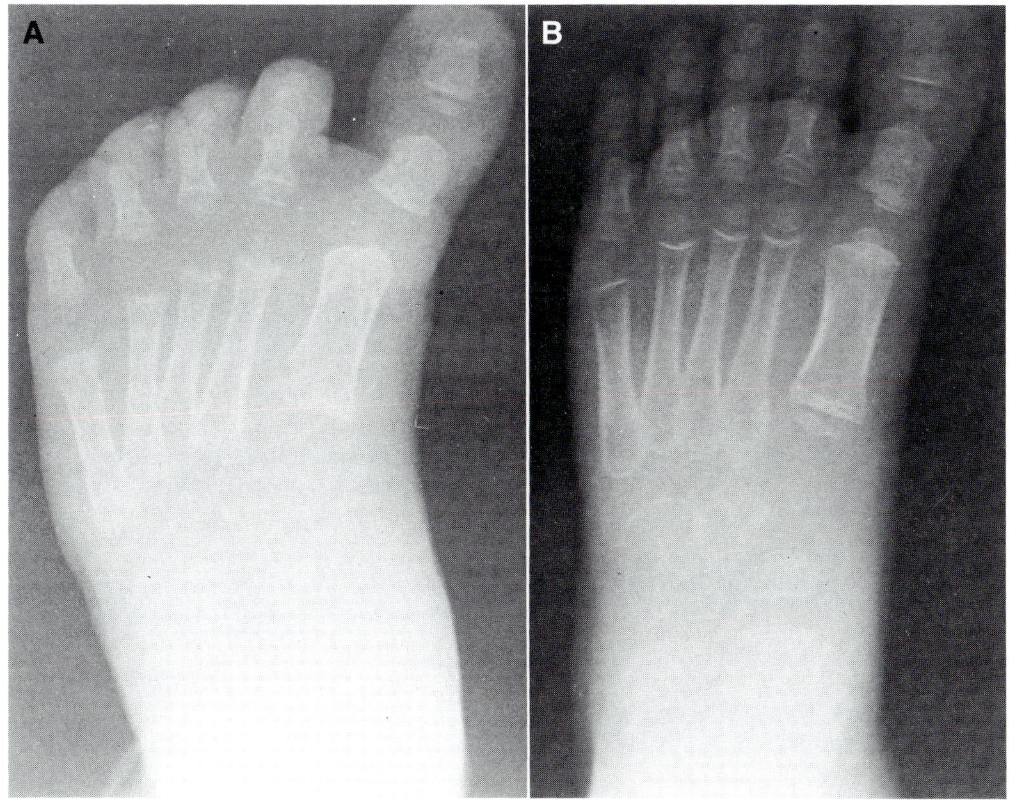

FIG 31–16.
A, persistent metatarsus adductus at the age of 2 years and 11 months. **B,** at 3 years and 10 months, correction after tarsometatarsal and intermetatarsal capsulotomies. The second metatarsal was not osteotomized.

correction than does capsulotomy; a transverse osteotomy done subperiosteally is sufficient. During exposure of the second metatarsal, carefully protect the extensor tendons and longitudinally oriented neurovascular structures.

6. Proceed laterally, and completely divide all interosseous ligaments and then the capsules at each tarsometatarsal articulation medially and dorsally; on the plantar aspect divide only the medial two thirds of each capsule.

7. After the intermetatarsal ligaments and tarsometatarsal capsules have been thoroughly divided, the forepart of the foot will swing laterally at the tarsometatarsal joints. One must be careful to avoid subluxation of the metatarsal bases, either dorsally or plantarward. I have not found it necessary to transfix the joints with pins. Close the skin, and apply a well-molded short-leg corrective cast to hold the forefoot in as much abduction as possible; however, avoid excessive forefoot pronation or hindfoot valgus.

8. Remove the cast with the patient under anesthesia after 2 weeks to examine the wound and gain further correction if necessary. The casting program should continue for an extended time to allow articular surface remodeling at the tarsometatarsal joints. Depending on the age of the child (longer in the older child), ambulatory immobilization should continue for 3 to 5 months.

Treatment of Resistant Metatarsus Varus in the Older Child

In children over the age of 8 years soft-tissue release is insufficient to effect adequate correction of significant metatarsus varus.[38, 42] Correction of the deformity is ensured only by osteotomizing and realigning the bony structures of the forefoot. If the primary deformity is metatarsus adductus with little forefoot supination, metatarsal osteotomy will correct the deformity.

Metatarsal osteotomy can be performed through the same approach used for tarsometatarsal capsulotomies.[36] Either a curving transverse or two longitudinal incisions may be used. Berman and Gartland have recommended using a hollow drill and making dome-shaped, apex-proximal osteotomies in each of the metatarsals.[33] Special care and occasionally even radiographic localization must be used to avoid damaging the epiphyseal plate at the proximal end of the first metatarsal (Fig 31–17). Carrying out the osteotomy subperiosteally tends to promote union and avoid displacement of the fragments.

After osteotomies it is safest to hold the foot in a corrected position with longitudinal pins through the first and fifth metatarsals. A cast to maintain the foot in the corrected position is applied at surgery and left intact until the pins are removed at 6 weeks. Because the child will inevitably walk on a short-leg cast and bend the pins, a long-leg cast with the knee flexed 90 degrees is necessary. Concerns for knee stiffness and convenience encountered when dealing with adults are not problems in children. If union at this point is radiographically limited, further short-leg casting for an additional 3 to 4 weeks may be necessary. However, bony union is usually rapid, and recurrence after successful osteotomy is rare.

If significant forefoot supination or cavovarus is present, plantar release accompanied by abductor hallucis tenotomy may be combined with metatarsal osteotomy or open wedge osteotomy of the tarsal bones to correct the deformity.[35, 42] In older children, shortening the lateral column of the foot by excising a wedge of tarsus based laterally may likewise be indicated. A thorough neurologic evaluation should be carried out when dealing with a progressive adductus or cavovarus deformity. Complex deformities are often the result of space-occupying lumbar canal lesions or neuromuscular pathology, and such diagnoses must be ruled out prior to surgery.

Talipes Calcaneovalgus

Reported to be the most common congenital foot malformation,[52] talipes calcaneovalgus may exist to some degree in up to 50% of all births.[51] Its most striking feature is marked dorsiflexion of the foot, the dorsal aspect of the metatarsals approximating the anterior portion of the tibia. There is a significant increase in hindfoot valgus with occasional contracture of the anterior dorsiflexion musculature. There seems to be abnormal mobility in pronation and frequently a significant decrease in active or passive plantar flexion.

The differential diagnosis is most important. The appearance of the foot with calcaneovalgus deformity can simulate that of congenital convex pes valgus. The basic anatomic difference between the two abnormalities is the position of the calcaneus: in congenital convex pes valgus the calcaneus is fixed in plantar flexion with contracture of the Achilles tendon and dislocation of the navicular onto the dorsal neck of the talus; in talipes calcaneovalgus the calcaneus is dorsiflexed and somewhat in valgus, and most importantly, the relationships between all osseous structures are normal. There are no luxations and therefore no adaptive bony changes.

Active treatment of the deformity has generally been recommended; however, a follow-up of 110 calcaneovalgus feet by Larsen et al. indicated no significant differ-

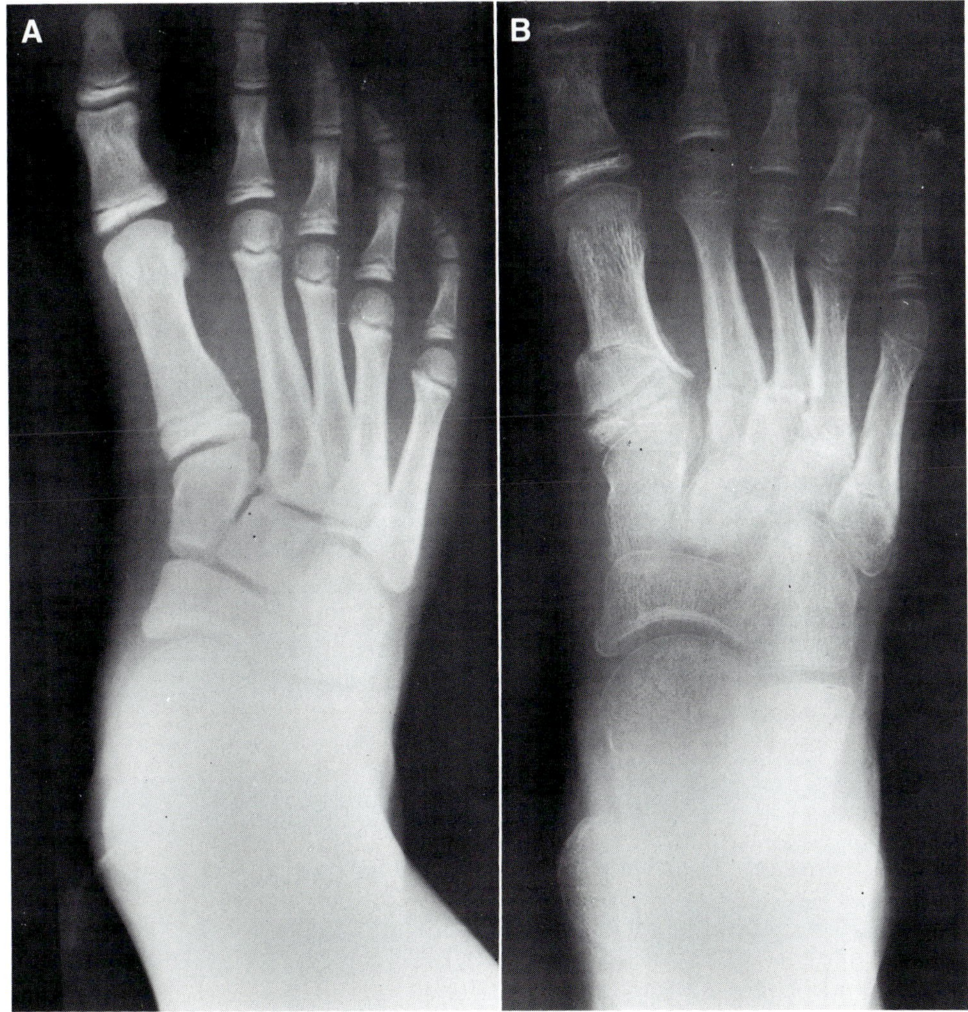

FIG 31–17.
A, persistent metatarsus adductus as part of a flexible skewfoot deformity in a 10-year-old. **B,** after metatarsal osteotomy, the entire foot alignment, although not normal, improved.

ence was later found between patients treated actively and those allowed to go untreated.[51] The experience of these authors would indicate that even in the presence of dorsiflexor contracture, the ultimate result is excellent, with or without treatment.

The only residual seen after congenital talipes calcaneovalgus is persistent hindfoot valgus and slight depression of the medial arch. Neither of these problems is often symptomatic, and the occasional symptomatic case may respond to orthotic support.

In my experience, this deformity is frequently over treated with serial casting, and I would echo the sentiments of Larsen et al, who espoused stretching and observation.[51]

In my practice the parents are taught to manipulate and massage the foot into plantar flexion. Since no abnormal bony relationship exists and secondary adaptive changes do not occur, maintenance of the corrected position in plaster is not necessary. If plantar flexion is limited to less than a neutral ankle position, I have sometimes undertaken a short period of adhesive strapping (taping into plantar flexion) to accelerate correction.

FLATFOOT

Two of the more common reasons a child is brought to a physician with lower extremity complaints are flat feet and toeing in. An analytic, scientific approach to either of these problems paves the way to successful treatment.

Pes planus may be congenital in nature if the normal anatomy is distorted at birth. As in other congenital anomalies, the degree of deformity varies from patient to patient. Treatment depends on the degree of deformity and resistance to passive correction. Pes planus may also exist in the absence of congenital bony anomalies and is then caused by an abnormality of soft-tissue structures: loose ligaments, a contracted Achilles tendon, etc. Indeed, the vast majority of flat feet in children are flexible, correct passively, and display a longitudinal arch with non–weight bearing.

The common finding on examination of either a flexible or rigid flatfoot is depression or loss of the longitudinal arch on weight bearing. The head of the talus or medial aspect of the navicular may be prominent at the normal midarch position. The forefoot is abducted, and the calcaneus may be in valgus (Fig 31-18). Sometimes the normal longitudinal arch can be restored by external rotation of the tibia with the foot fixed in a weight-bearing position.[67] Excessive internal tibial torsion, genovalgum, or simple ligamentous laxity are the common causes when such a response is noted.

Weight-bearing radiographs should be obtained before initiation of treatment. The lateral view must include the entire foot and ankle; the AP view is taken with the x-ray tube angled 30 degrees toward the heel to better visualize the talocalcaneal angle (Fig 31–19).

Flexible Pes Planus

Although most flat feet are flexible and passively correct early in life, persistence of the deformity can result in structural change as the foot grows and develops.[65] The deformity disappears with non–weight bearing and frequently with external rotation of the leg on a fixed foot. Often the patient is capable of actively correcting the deformity by contracting the tibialis anterior.

Heel alignment is normal when 0 to 5 degrees of valgus is present and the forefoot is straight.[53] In children up to 2 or 3 years of age, the normal arch is obscured by an overabundance of fat tissue on the plantar aspect of the heel; hence one cannot use the clinical appearance of the toddler's foot to diagnose flat feet. Radiographs must be obtained.

Normal weight-bearing radiographs show a divergence of the talus and calcaneus in the AP projection of

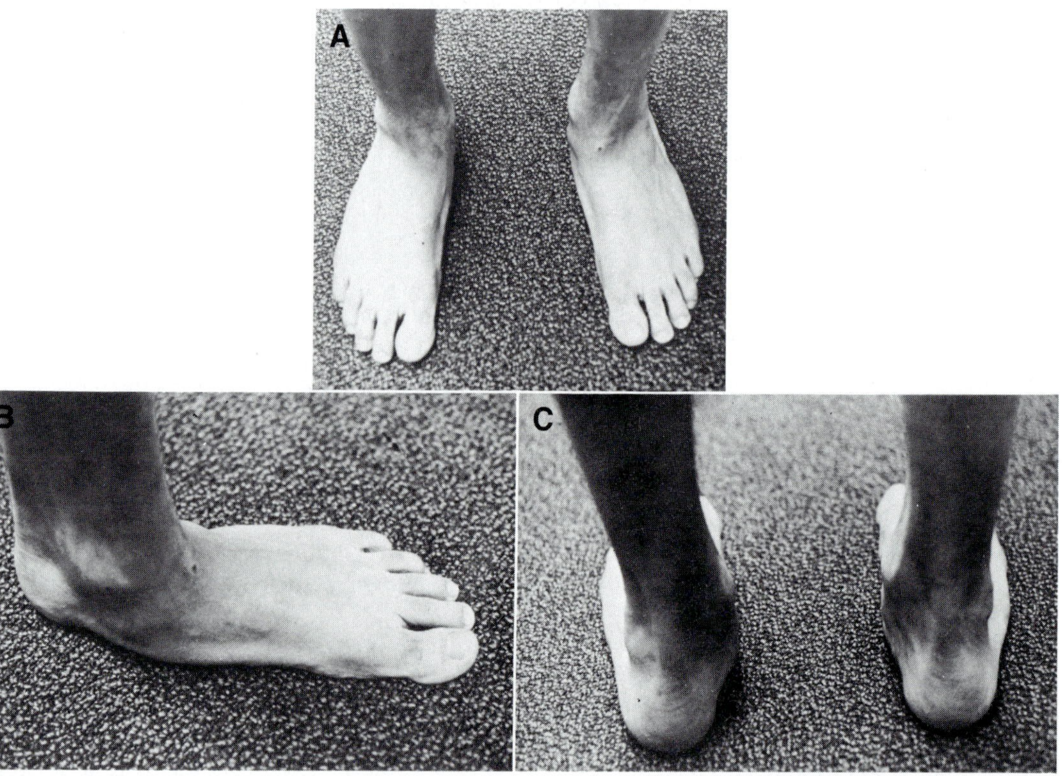

FIG 31–18.
A, symptomatic flatfoot in a 16-year-old boy. **B,** the medial arch is depressed, and the head of the talus is prominent on the plantar aspect of the arch. **C,** slight hindfoot valgus is evident when viewed from behind.

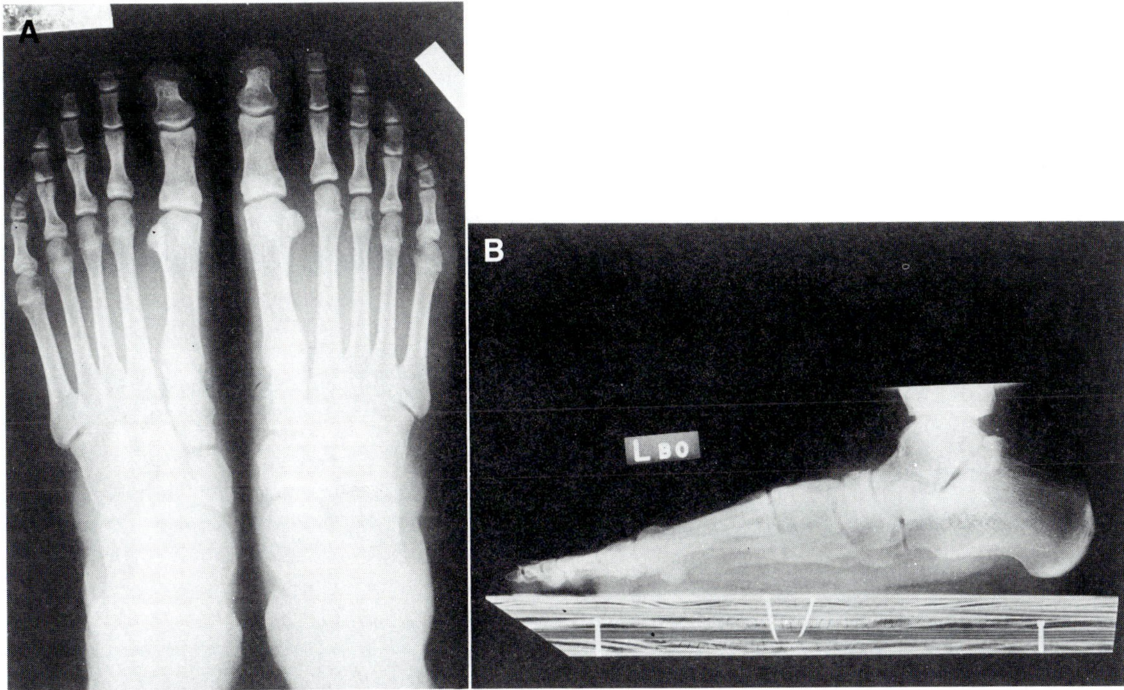

FIG 31–19.
Radiograph of the feet of the boy in Figure 31–18. **A,** AP view. Note the medial deviation of the talar neck. The longitudinal axis of the talus falls medially, away from the axis of the first metatarsal. **B,** lateral view. The talus is plantar-flexed, and the navicular sags but is not displaced on the neck of the talus. The normal dorsiflexion angle of a weight-bearing calcaneus is lost.

approximately 20 degrees (18 ± 5 degrees). In the lateral view a line bisecting the body of the talus is inclined in plantar flexion approximately 25 degrees from the horizontal; a line drawn along the inferior border of the calcaneus shows a similar 20 to 25 degrees of dorsiflexion.[54] With a flexible flatfoot the talocalcaneal angle in the AP projection is increased because of divergence of the talus and calcaneus, and on lateral views an interruption in the longitudinal arch is noted. Normally a line through the body and neck of the talus parallels the first metatarsal; with loss of the longitudinal arch the talar neck is depressed to some degree, and this line lies at an angle and inferior to the shaft of the first metatarsal[71] (Fig 31–20). Sagging of the talonavicular and/or naviculocuneiform joint is often noted. In a mild flat foot, the radiographic talar–first metatarsal angle measures between 1 and 15 degrees; in severe pes planus it is over 15 degrees.[55]

Treatment

Symptoms are rarely present during childhood. However, the stresses of weight bearing, shoe wear, and hard surfaces may result in fatigue-type discomfort during the teenage years.

Few truly scientific reports documenting the lasting value of corrective devices are present in the literature. Bleck and Berzins[54] and Bordelon[55] have shown that passive correction with an orthotic device in early childhood may result in permanent and significant restoration of the longitudinal arch.

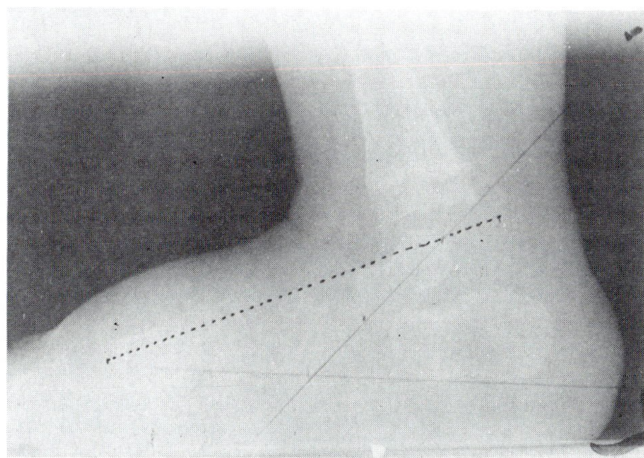

FIG 31–20.
Flexible flatfoot in a toddler. The lateral talocalcaneal angle is 50 degrees, and the longitudinal axis of the talus falls at a significant angle below the axis of the first metatarsal *(dotted line).* There is no fixed hindfoot (calcaneal) equinus.

As in other congenital abnormalities, growth and development can be effectively used to gain permanent correction so long as the orthotic device is worn faithfully and for a prolonged period of time. If the talar plantar flexion angle exceeds 45 degrees the University of California Biomechanics Laboratory (UCBL) insert has achieved improvement in up to 74% of cases.[54, 60] For less severe deformity, with the talus plantar-flexed 34 to 45 degrees, the Helfet heel seat is reportedly effective in 85% of cases.[59] Bordelon prefers a custom-molded insert fabricated from a plaster mold fashioned with the foot in relaxed plantar flexion.[55] As might be expected, the longer the corrective device is used, the greater will be the improvement; correction can be attained at the rate of 5 degrees per year if worn in a supportive shoe for several years.

An occasional cause of flatfoot, one often overlooked when the patient presents for examination and treatment, is contracture of the Achilles tendon (Fig 31–21). When evaluating potential Achilles tendon contracture by assessing hindfoot dorsiflexion, one must take particular care to invert the subtalar joint and forefoot before applying dorsiflexion stress. Doing so locks the calcaneus under the talus, thus ensuring that observed motion occurs only at the ankle joint and that spurious dorsiflexion does not occur at the midfoot. If flatfoot is found in conjunction with a tight Achilles tendon, heel cord stretching exercises or serial casting may restore the longitudinal arch.[58, 59, 65] Surgical Achilles tendon lengthening may occasionally be required to prevent progressive deformity.

Unless osseous abnormalities are evident, a flexible flatfoot in childhood rarely requires surgery. The operations of Miller[66] and Hoke[61] involve arthrodesis of the midfoot joints and hence are inappropriate for the very young, growing foot. Even in the adolescent, I find that symptoms significant enough to require surgical intervention are extremely rare. In a 5-year postoperative review of 46 naviculocuneiform fusions performed for mobile flatfoot, Jack reported 82% good or excellent results among adolescents.[62] Longer follow-up of the same group at 16 years postoperatively revealed a deterioration to unsatisfactory in 50%; this was caused primarily by stress-induced degenerative change in other joints.[69] When the Achilles tendon is contracted and depression of the longitudinal arch in the young adolescent is symptomatic, the technique of Young remains, in my hands, the treatment of choice.[72] Miller[65] has recently reported excellent or good results with Chamber's procedure in 95% of 81 feet.[56] I have no experience with Silastic interposition arthroereisis as reported by Smith and Millar but would hesitate to place this type of foreign implant in the foot of a child for this relatively benign condition.[70] I have used the arthroereisis procedure with a staple in the sinus tarsi as described by Crawford for the reducible flatfoot encountered in neurologically compromised children (cerebral palsy, myelodysplasia) and have found it to be satisfactory.[57] Ongoing postoperative use of an orthotic is necessary. This procedure may also have a place in the treatment of supple pes planus without a neuromuscular etiology. However, use of these procedures should be restricted to the very rare maximally symptomatic flatfoot.

Accessory Navicular (Prehallux)

On occasion, a patient will seek treatment for flat feet and complain of tenderness over a palpable prominence at the medial aspect of the depressed longitudinal arch.[63] Radiographs demonstrating the presence of an accessory ossicle adjacent to the proximal medial aspect of the navicular confirm the diagnosis of prehallux. The navicular is described as cornuate when the ossicle has fused with the main body of the bone (Fig 31–22). Because of this osseous overgrowth, a painful bursa aggravated by footwear frequently forms directly over the prominence.

Normally the tibialis posterior swings under the medial aspect of the navicular to insert into the plantar aspect of the first and second cuneiforms as well as the base of the second and fourth metatarsals. With either a cornuate or an accessory navicular, the major insertion of the tibialis posterior has been reported to be into the abnormal projection of bone.[73] This insertional abnormality arguably interferes with the dynamic support of the longitudinal arch that is provided by the tibialis posterior. Surgical treatment of the condition according to the method of Kidner[63] relieves the local discomfort secondary to the bursa and elevates the longitudinal arch by redirecting the tendon of the tibialis posterior (see Chapter 16). Recent studies dispute the abnormal tendinuous insertion[72] and others report equally satisfactory surgical results with or without rerouting the tendon.[50a, 64]

Rigid Flatfoot

The flatfoot whose abnormal appearance is not corrected with non–weight bearing requires more attention and often a more aggressive approach.

Rigid flat feet, as opposed to the flexible type, tend to have a greater incidence of symptoms and cause more disability. Physical examination reveals a prominence of the talar head or navicular along the medial border of the longitudinal arch as well as a loss or limitation of subtalar motion, persistent hindfoot equinus, and pain-

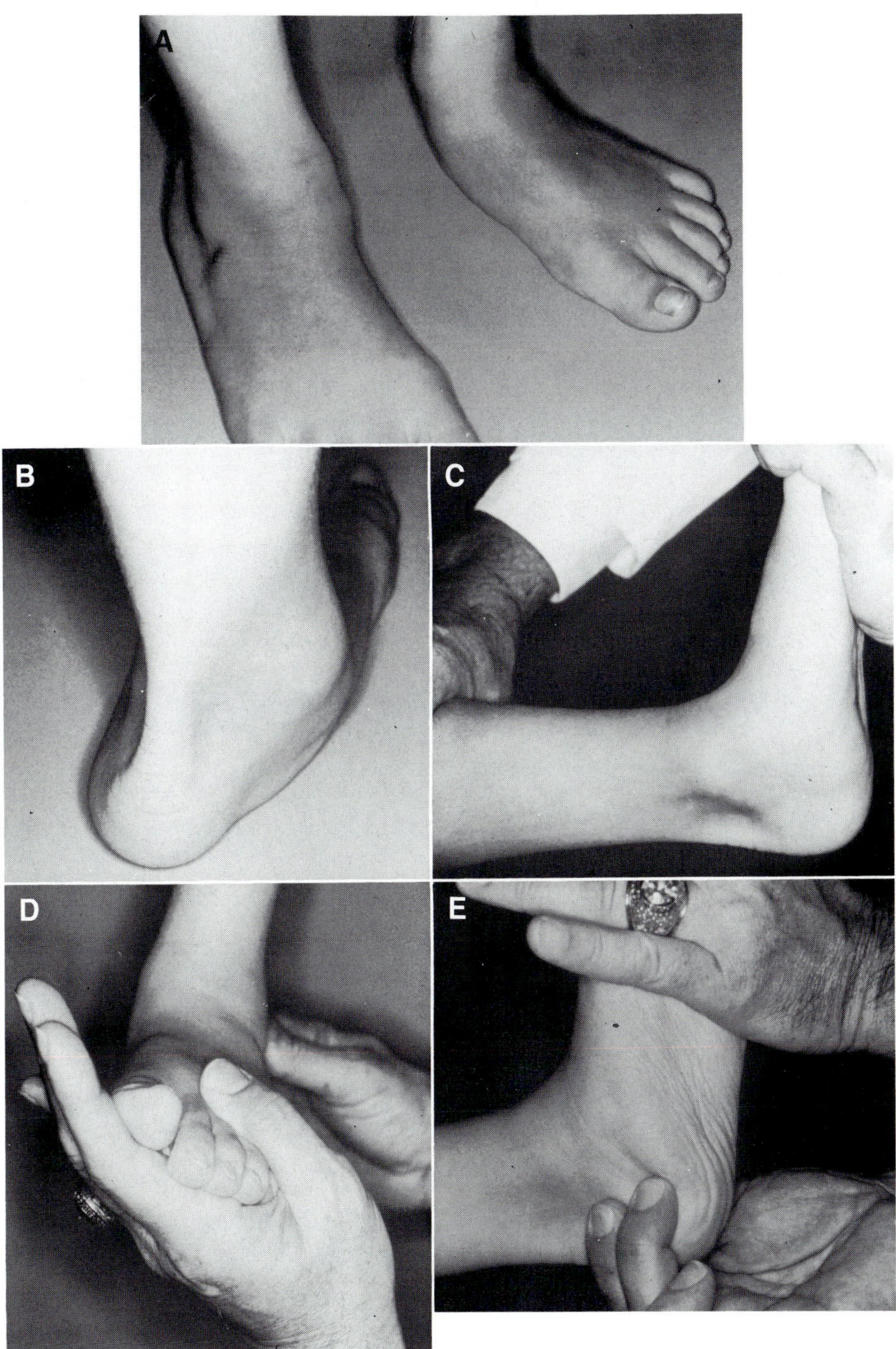

FIG 31–21.
A and **B,** flatfoot as the result of Achilles tendon contracture. **C,** incorrect method of assessing heel cord contracture or performing stretching exercises. Note the passive inversion (**D** and **E**) of the forefoot and hindfoot to lock the subtalar joint and prevent midfoot break when correctly assessing dorsiflexion. The hindfoot does not reach neutral on maximum dorsiflexion.

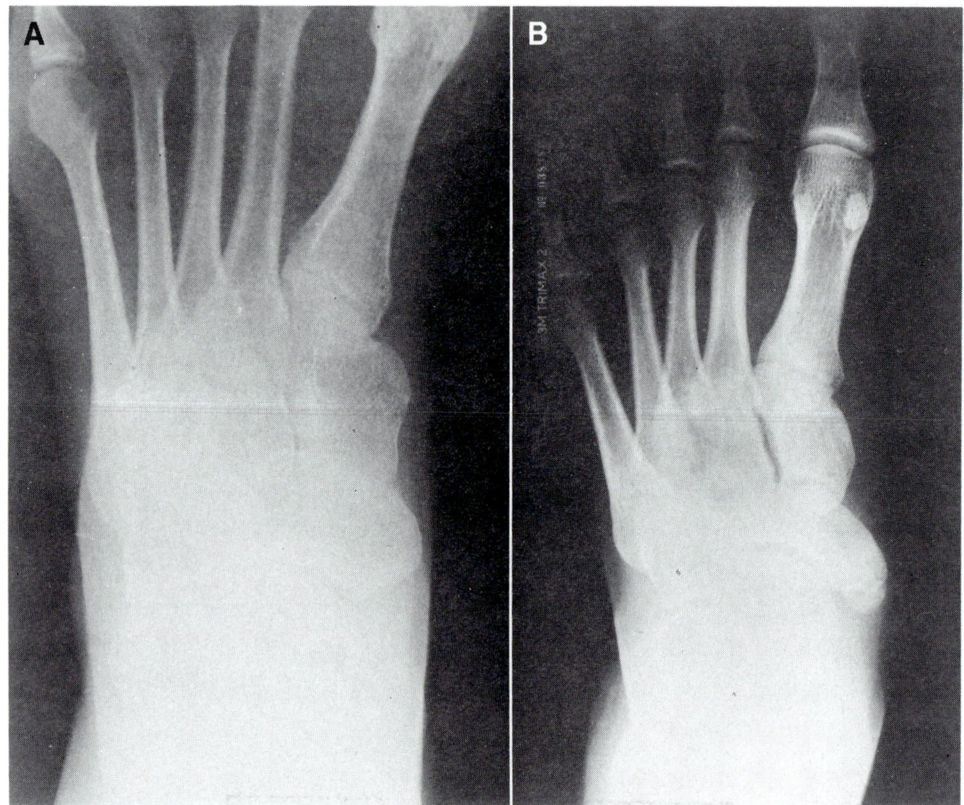

FIG 31–22.
A, cornuate navicular causing pain and discomfort in a 15-year-old girl. After the Kidner procedure, the symptoms resolved. **B,** unfused prehallux requiring treatment because of symptoms.

ful callosities signifying abnormal mechanics. Radiographs often demonstrate osseous abnormalities, and more frequently surgical intervention is required.

Several types of rigid flatfoot exist. These are grouped according to etiology in the discussions that follow.

Peroneal Spastic Flatfoot (Tarsal Coalition)

Various abnormalities in the development of normal articulations between the tarsal bones have long been recognized. Unions between the talus and navicular, the calcaneus and talus, the calcaneus and navicular, and the calcaneus and cuboid have been noted. This union can take the form of a fibrous connection (syndesmosis), a cartilaginous bond (synchondrosis), or a bony bridge (synostosis). These are grouped together into a common category termed *tarsal coalition*.

Slomann was the first to recognize the association of peroneal tendon spasm resulting in a rigid flat foot with coalition of the tarsal bones.[87] Badgley described the anatomy of a coalition uniting the navicular calcaneus.[74] He also observed that certain severe cases of rigid flatfoot seemed to be associated with a calcaneonavicular coalition.

Tarsal coalition is an autosomal dominant condition, the talocalcaneal type being most common in some studies[90] and the calcaneonavicular in others.[89] There does not appear to be any association between fusion of the tarsal bones and fusion of the carpus. Leonard, in a review of 31 patients with calcaneonavicular or talocalcaneal coalitions, found similar deformities in 50% of first-degree relatives.[82]

Conway and Cowell[75] postulated that the congenital deformity does not begin as a failure of segmentation but rather is seen in early childhood as a syndesmosis. Although the union remains fibrous, motion appears to be normal, and no symptoms are noted. Hence identification of the problem in infancy or early childhood is rare. As time passes, the syndesmosis becomes a cartilaginous bar, and motion is progressively restricted. By the time early adolescence is reached, the cartilaginous bar becomes ossified, and significant restriction in hindfoot motion occurs.

This restriction places an abnormal stress on the tarsus. Abnormal stress in the region results in pain and discomfort, occasionally leading to protective spasm of the peroneal muscles. As motion is progressively restricted and the peroneal muscles become tightened, the midfoot is forced into more pronation, and a rigid type of flatfoot eventually develops. Symptoms often appear before the development of a spastic flatfoot, frequently following a rather minor wrenching-type injury to the foot after the bridge has become cartilaginous or osseous. Actual fracture of the coalition has been noted, and healing of such a fracture can occur.

An individual complaining of discomfort and demonstrating a rigid-type flatfoot must be carefully examined, including appropriate radiographic views. Physical findings include significant loss of subtalar motion, which may be demonstrated with the foot at 90 degrees to the leg and the hand of the examiner firmly grasping the calcaneus. In this position the talus is well locked in the ankle mortise, and passive inversion and eversion of the calcaneus create motion only in the subtalar joint. In the presence of tarsal coalition, such motion is markedly reduced or absent. When the coalition has been present a long time, hindfoot valgus results in shortening of the peroneal muscle-tendon unit. Attempts at inverting the midfoot cause the peroneal tendon to stand out as if in spasm. In an instance such as this, only the peroneal spasm is apparent. However, when ligamentous strain in the hindfoot has occurred because of loss of flexibility, the peroneal spasm can be real and painful.[79]

Peroneal spasm may also be caused by degenerative arthritis or inflammatory processes within the midfoot or hindfoot. In such instances, unless marked gross deformity has occurred, subtalar motion is less limited.[77, 84] In addition, not all instances of tarsal coalition develop peroneal spasm. To use the term *peroneal spastic flatfoot* synonymously with tarsal coalition is therefore inappropriate.

Standing AP and lateral radiographs should be taken and in addition an oblique view should be obtained at approximately 45 degrees to delineate a potential calcaneonavicular coalition[81] (Fig 31–23). An axial view of

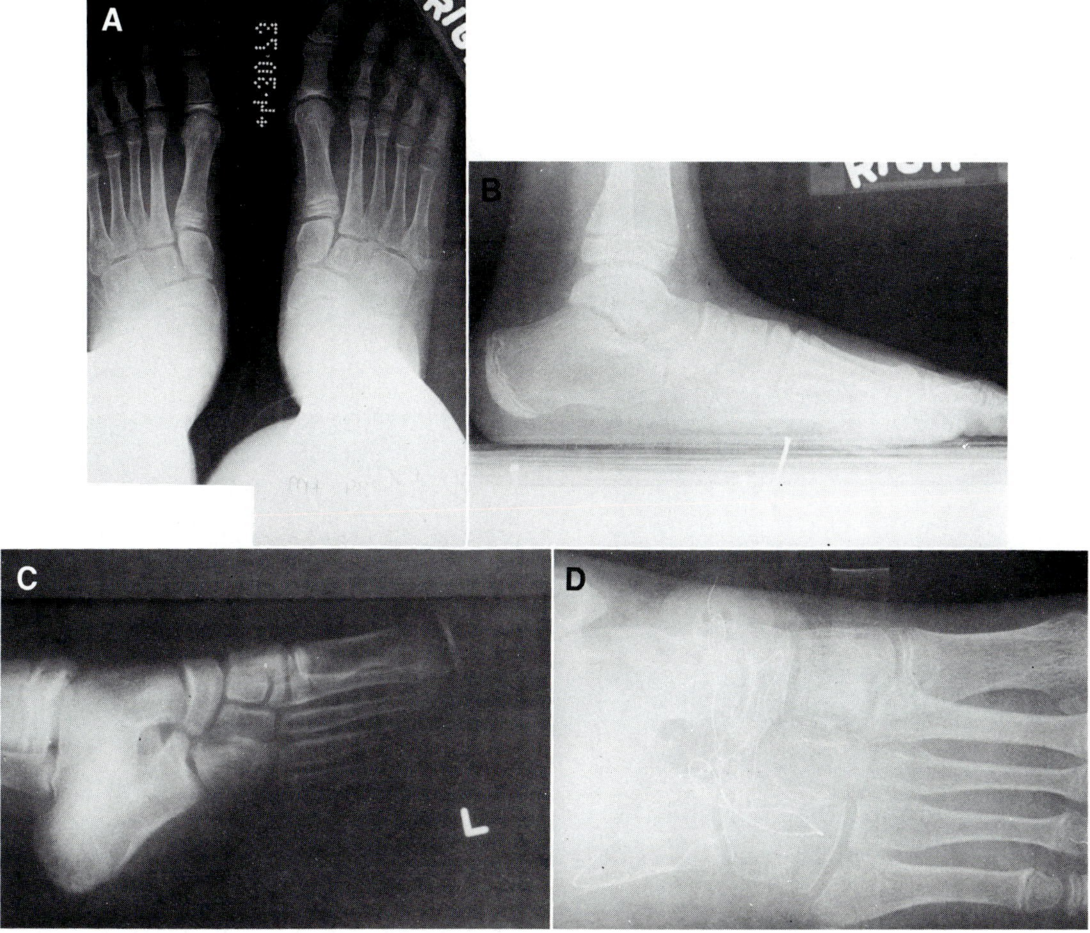

FIG 31–23.
Calcaneonavicular coalition. **A** to **C,** not easily appreciated on routine lateral or AP views. The oblique view however, obtained at 45 degrees, clearly shows a bar. **D,** after resection of the bar and interposition of the extensor brevis origin. The wire is a pullout suture tied over a button holding the muscle in place immediately after the operation.

the hindfoot acquired at a 45-degree angle will normally demonstrate the joints of the posterior facet and sustentaculum tali, the middle facet. If a bony coalition is present, the facet joint is obliterated on this tangential view. Occasionally the x-ray beam does not pass directly through the joint when tilted 45 degrees; if the joint on such a film appears abnormal, the lateral standing radiograph should be examined to determine the actual angle of the joint. If it varies significantly from 45 degrees a film with the tube tilted appropriately so that the beam passes through the subtalar joint should be obtained.

It has been pointed out that a synostosis or synchondrosis of the middle facet is present if the facet joint appears oblique rather than horizontal on the tangential view (Fig 31–24). Only if the union is osseous does complete obliteration of the joint occur, and if cartilaginous or fibrous, the coalition may be difficult to appreciate. A radiographic finding of facet obliquity and/or irregularity, however, is strong evidence that a coalition is probably present.[80]

The most difficult area to examine radiographically for a coalition is the anterior facet between the calcaneus and talus. Conway and Cowell recommend tomography in the lateral projection to demonstrate this joint.[75] Computed tomography (CT)[77a, 88] has added to our ability to delineate less obvious coalitions and is now a part of routine evaluation for the disorder (Fig 31–25).

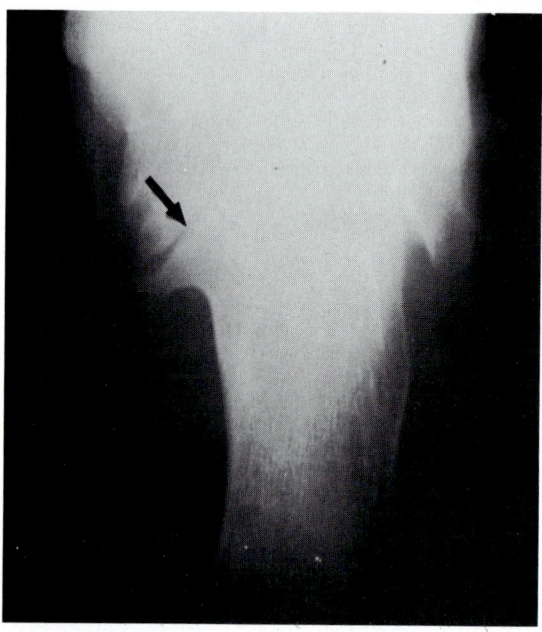

FIG 31–24.
Synchondrosis of the middle facet (talocalcaneal coalition). Note the obliquity of the joint *(arrow)*. Resection is not usually successful; if the condition is symptomatic, resection and talocalcaneal fusion are necessary. Degenerative changes in the talonavicular joint may additionally necessitate fusion there.

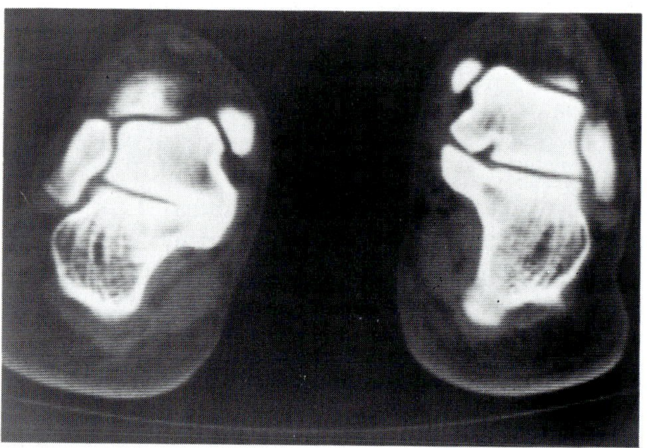

FIG 31–25.
CT view of middle facet coalition on the left.

In addition to the primary radiographic findings of coalition, secondary changes at radiography are also noted. The most significant of these is the "talar beak" (Fig 31–26). Lipping of the superoanterior surface of the talar head at the talonavicular joint is secondary to abnormal motion of the tarsal complex. Talar beaking is not present early in life but, as time passes, develops as a remodeling process. Other secondary changes include narrowing of the talocalcaneal joint as seen on lateral views.[79]

Treatment.—As previously mentioned, symptoms do not usually occur until early adolescence. Talonavicular

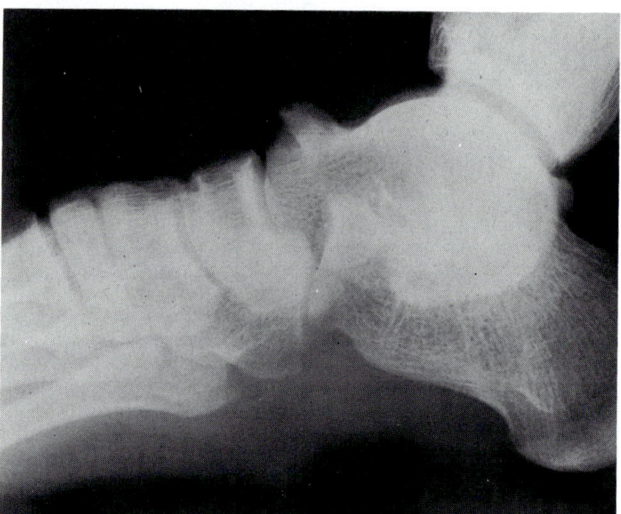

FIG 31–26.
Talar beaking—osteophyte formation caused by abnormal stress on the talonavicular joint secondary to middle facet talocalcaneal coalition.

coalition is rarely the cause of symptoms and is usually an incidental radiographic finding.

When an individual first notices symptoms secondary to calcaneonavicular or talocalcaneal coalition, 6 weeks of immobilization in a short-leg walking cast often results in resolution of this discomfort. If it is not completely resolved or recurs shortly after treatment, a second period in plaster may be necessary. Further treatment is dependent on the age of the patient and the presence or absence of degenerative changes in other joints.

If coalition has occurred between the calcaneus and navicular and the patient is less than 12 years of age, resection of the bar may be carried out at this early age. Structural changes are unlikely to have developed in other joints, and normal, pain-free motion may be surgically restored. Through a standard lateral approach to the sinus tarsi, a rectangular portion of the bar is removed with interposition of the extensor digitorum brevis[77] (Fig 31–23,D). If the patient is beyond early adolescent years or the coalition is between the talus and calcaneus, successful resection is not routinely possible. In the absence of radiographic evidence for early degenerative disease in nearby joints, it is not unreasonable to attempt resection of the bridge and interposition of fat or bone wax in an effort to prevent reformation.[83a] If the effort fails and symptoms recur, a second procedure may be necessary.[83, 85, 86] In such instances arthrodesis of the talonavicular, calcaneocuboid, and subtalar joints is necessary. For middle facet coalition, Harris recommends a medial approach with resection of the bar followed by talonavicular and subtalar fusion.[78] Arthrodesis of this type should be delayed until the individual is 11 or 12 years of age and the foot has obtained nearly full growth. Symptomatic talocalcaneal coalition of the anterior facet that is unresponsive to a period of cast immobilization should be treated similarly at an appropriate age with triple arthrodesis.

Congenital Convex Pes Valgus (Congenital Vertical Talus)

Rigid flatfoot, other than that seen with peroneal spasm, is also noted with this deformity. The imprecise term *congenital vertical talus* should probably be abandoned since the talus is vertically inclined to a varying degree with any significant degree of flatfoot, both flexible and rigid. The term *congenital convex pes valgus* is preferable; it is more appropriate and most descriptive.

The essential difference between the flexible flatfoot and congenital convex pes valgus is dorsal dislocation of the navicular onto the neck of the talus in the latter. In flexible flatfoot the navicular may sag plantarward but articulates more normally with the head of the talus (Fig 31–19,*B*). Other salient findings are additional hallmarks of congenital convex pes valgus: fixed equinus deformity of the calcaneus, lateral rotation of the anterior calcaneus, dorsiflexion and supination of the forefoot, and a typical rocker-bottom appearance. The talar head is prominent on the medial plantar aspect of the midfoot.

Concerning the differential diagnosis, other entities may present a similar superficial appearance. With congenital calcaneal valgus, hindfoot equinus is absent; this is therefore a different problem. Unlike flexible flatfoot and tarsal coalition, congenital convex pes valgus can usually be recognized at birth.[103] If it remains untreated, the initial problems concern footwear. The gait is awkward because of the shape of the foot, and shoe wear, particularly along the medial border, is excessive. As the child approaches adolescence, callosities form over the medial aspect of the tarsus, ligamentous structures are strained, and the foot becomes painful.

Herndon and Heyman believe that the abnormality is caused by an insult during the first trimester of pregnancy and may well be related to clubfoot deformity.[99] To date, however, no absolute proof exists that either congenital convex pes valgus or clubfoot is caused by changes during the embryonic period. Congenital convex pes valgus is frequently seen in association with other neurologic abnormalities such as myelodysplasia, neurofibromatosis, or arthrogryposis. Because of the association of congenital convex pes valgus with congenital neurologic abnormalities, a careful search for such problems should be carried out when the deformity is encountered.[95, 101, 102] As with clubfoot, very little specimen dissection has been reported.

Patterson et al. described the anatomic findings at dissection of a 6-week-old infant with congenital convex pes valgus who died of congenital heart disease; the spinal cord of the specimen was not examined. Findings in their study indicated that not until the shortened extensor tendons—including the tibialis anterior, extensor hallucis longus, extensor digitorum longus, and peronei—were serially lengthened was reduction of the talonavicular subluxation possible. Correction of hindfoot equinus was possible only after heel cord lengthening. Section of the talonavicular, subtalar, and posterior ankle capsules was carried out before tendon division but did not reduce the navicular or the talus. Moderate abnormalities in the talus and calcaneus were felt to be secondary changes and not the primary cause of the deformity.[104] Therefore these authors contended that the primary abnormality was shortening of the muscle-tendon unit.

Drennan and Sharrard pointed out the marked association of congenital convex pex valgus with central nervous system abnormalities and presented their dissection of this deformity in a myelodysplastic child. They too felt that the deformity was secondary to shortening or overpull of the dorsiflexors and everters of the foot unopposed by a weakened invertor—the tibialis posterior.[95]

Physical Findings.—The problem as it presents clinically is a rigid foot with the heel in equinus and a convex sole with the head of the talus prominent on the plantar medial aspect of the tarsus. The forefoot is dorsiflexed and everted; passive correction of the deformity is not possible.

Radiographic Findings.—AP radiographs of the foot with the patient in a standing position demonstrate increased divergence of the talus and calcaneus. On lateral views the calcaneus is noted to be in equinus, the talus vertical, and if ossified, the navicular dislocated onto the dorsal neck of the talus. If plantar flexion, non–weight-bearing stress projections are obtained, unlike the flexible flatfoot, the abnormal relationship between the talus and the forefoot persists (Fig 31–27). Jayakumar and Ramsey point out the essential difference between radiographic findings of the oblique or plantar-flexed talus seen in association with a flexible flatfoot and the vertical talus of congenital convex pes valgus.[100]

Treatment.—Conservative treatment, although usually unsuccessful, should be initiated as soon as possible after the patient is first seen.[91] Efforts should be made at stretching the contracted anterior structures by maximally plantar-flexing and inverting the forefoot, pressing the talar head dorsally, and attempting to push the navicular into a more normal relationship with the ta-

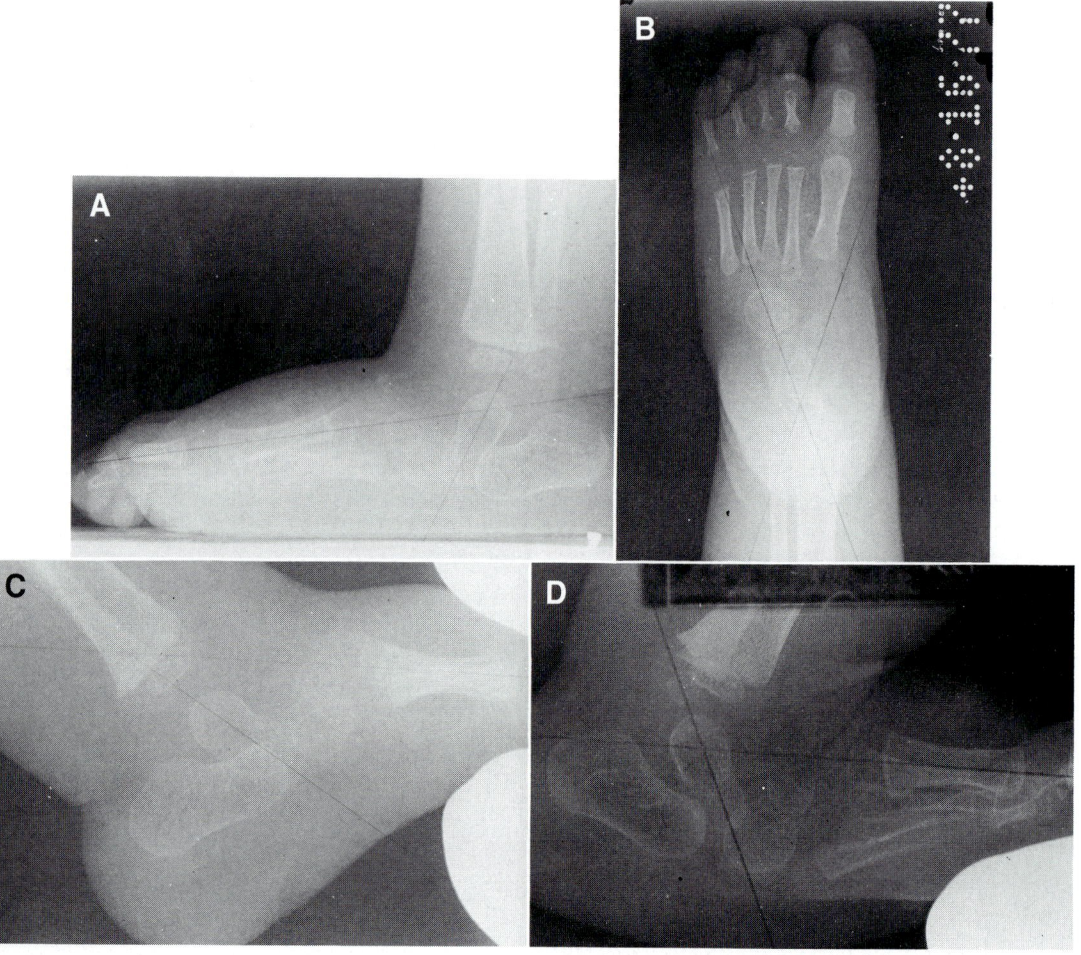

FIG 31–27.
Congenital convex pes valgus in an 18-month-old child. **A** and **B,** the talar axis falls at an angle medial and plantar to that of first metatarsal. **C,** plantarflexion stress fails to align the talus and first metatarsal. **D,** dorsiflexion stress demonstrates the persistence of hindfoot equinus. An unossified navicular is dislocated on the talar neck.

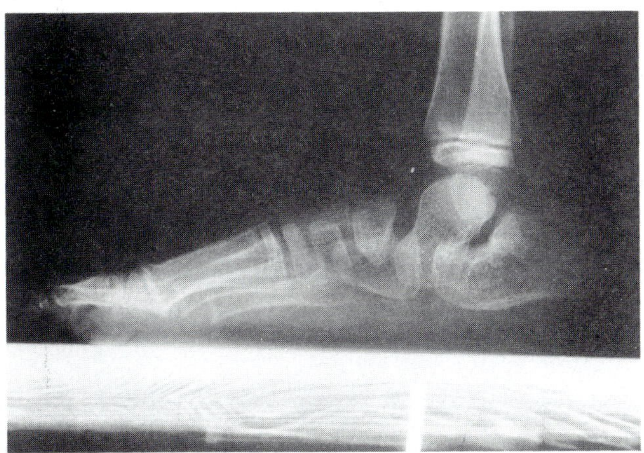

FIG 31–28.
Foot of 9-year-old whose vertical talus was treated at the age of 2 years with closed reduction and percutaneous pinning. Despite 3 months of casting, anatomic pathology recurred.

lus. Although it is not likely, serial casting after these maneuvers may result in correction of the deformity (Fig 31–28); more likely, casting will assist in making surgical correction more successful by stretching contracted dorsal soft-tissue structures.[92]

Operative treatment as advocated by Lamy and Weissman combines partial or total talectomy with lengthening of peroneal and extensor tendons as necessary.[101] Colton has recommended peritalar release with navicular excision as described by Stone (Fig 31–29).[94, 105] Most authors agree that soft-tissue procedures necessary to effect reduction include capsulotomies of the talonavicular, subtalar, and ankle joints and routine lengthening of the Achilles tendon.[92, 98] The peroneal, anterior tibial, extensor digitorum communis, extensor hallucis longus, and posterior tibial tendons may be lengthened as necessary[97] (Fig 31–30). In addition, Eyre-Brook excised a dorsally based wedge from the navicular and placed it beneath the neck of the talus for support. He also shortened the spring ligament. Because he believed that the calcaneus was not in equinus, he did not recommend posterior release.[96] Jayakumar and Ramsey have recommended transplantation of the anterior tibial tendon into the talar neck after reduction has been obtained, thus providing dynamic support to the reduction.[100]

I would generally recommend preoperative stretching of the anterior tendons by serial casting followed by soft-tissue release of tightened talonavicular, subtalar, calcaneocuboid, and posterior ankle capsules through a Cincinnati incision (see page 31-15). The Achilles tendon should be lengthened and reduction of the deformity attempted by plantar-flexing the forefoot; if it is tight, dorsal tendons should be lengthened as necessary. Reduction, once obtained, should be maintained by Kirschner-wire fixation through the first metatarsal and navicular into the neck and body of the talus. Reduction of the deformity is possible only by acutely plantar-flexing the forefoot and bringing the navicular into a normal relationship with the talar head. If reduction following complete capsular and extensor tendon division is still impossible, navicular excision should be carried out. A second Kirschner wire transversely placed through the tuberosity of the calcaneus but avoiding the apophysis is incorporated in plaster and serves as a lever to gradually bring the hindfoot out of equinus. Correction should be maintained in long-leg casts for 4 to 6 months; the Kirschner wires may be removed at 3 months.

If the patient is an adolescent or older, reduction of the deformity by soft-tissue release and navicular excision is unlikely to be successful. By this time, foot strain and abnormal mechanics have altered other

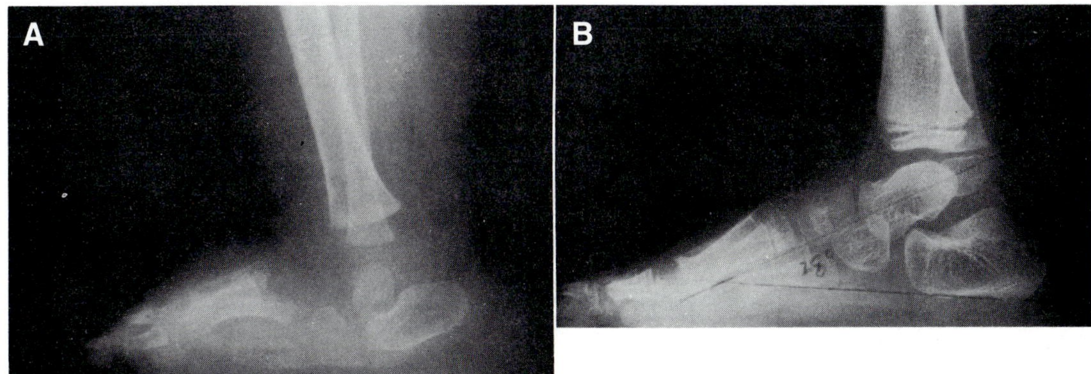

FIG 31–29.
A, preoperative view of a 14-month-old with vertical talus. **B,** 4 years after open reduction, soft-tissue release, and naviculectomy, the foot is supple, plantigrade, and painfree.

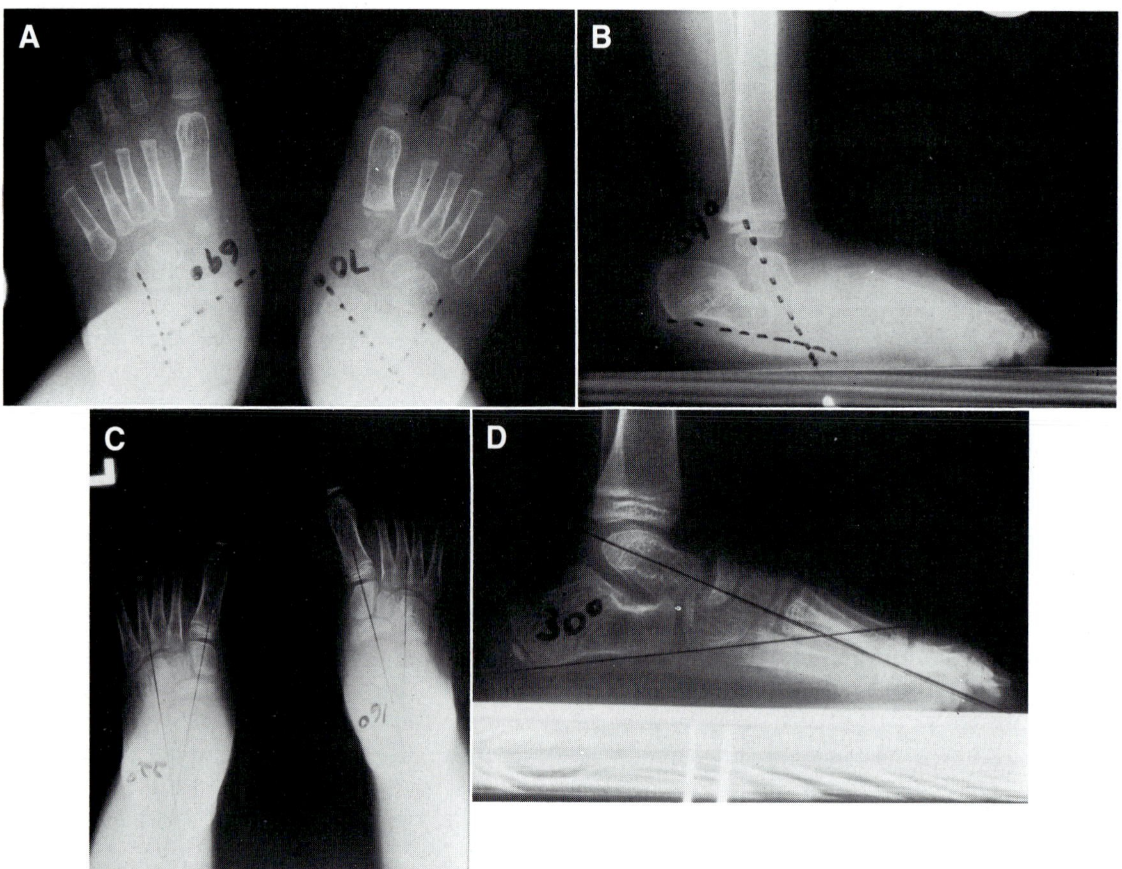

FIG 31–30.
A and **B,** standing AP and lateral views of a vertical talus in a 3-year-old girl. **C,** and **D,** 4 years after open reduction accomplished by posterior capsulotomy with Achilles tendon lengthening, talonavicular capsulotomy, and peroneal and extensor tendon lengthenings followed by 4 months of casting in a reduced position.

joints, and triple arthrodesis with resection of enough bone to create a plantigrade foot is the only solution. Heel cord lengthening and posterior capsulotomy may be required along with the triple arthrodesis to bring the calcaneus out of equinus.

ARTHROGRYPOSIS MULTIPLEX CONGENITA

Arthrogryposis multiplex congenita is an affliction in which multiple rigid joint deformities are evident at birth.[116] The severity of both deformity and rigidity may vary from patient to patient and joint to joint. It is currently felt that the broad term *arthrogryposis* encompasses any disorder that presents with a congenital, nonprogressive limitation of movement due to soft-tissue contracture, not bony malformation, in two or more joints. More commonly involved regions of the skeleton include the fingers, wrists, elbows, and shoulders as well as hips, knees, and feet. Not infrequently the spine is involved with a congenital-type scoliosis. Normally, the skin is smooth, muscle bulk is diminished, and the fingers are rather long and slender.[119a, 120] In even the mildest cases the presence of long tapered fingers may be a tip-off to the diagnosis of arthrogryposis.

Two types exist, neuropathic and myopathic forms.[106] In many circles it is felt that the myopathic form is a type of muscular dystrophy and should be classified with the myodystrophies.[107, 118] The etiology of arthrogryposis is generally unknown. Because many of the deformities appear to be teratologic in nature, the problem must arise sometime during the prenatal period.[110] Several causes have been proposed: intrauterine disturbances (decreased amniotic fluid, increased intrauterine pressure, mechanical compression of the fetus), inflammatory processes (rubella, viral infections, central nervous system infections),[109] and environmental damage (teratogenic agents). Several attempts to work out the genetics have been made, but published series tend to be too small for any definite conclusions to be reached. At present most authorities believe that heredity does not play a significant role.

Microscopic studies of arthrogrypotic specimens have shown major abnormalities in both muscle and nerve tissue. Involved muscles tend to be small, pale, and pink; some muscles are simply not present. In other areas muscle fibers may be extensively replaced by fat and connective tissue. Nervous tissue involvement includes abnormalities of the spinal cord (i.e., a decrease or absence of anterior horn cells in the thoracic and lumbar regions). In addition, the anterior roots have few fibers. The posterior roots and posterior horn cells appear to be normal.[106, 112]

In arthrogryposis the foot tends to manifest the most severe and most resistant of all deformities. Equinovarus is the most common foot deformity and varies from quite mild to quite severe.[113] The most resistant and the most difficult to treat clubfeet are seen in arthrogryposis (Fig 31–31). Although principles of management follow those for idiopathic clubfoot, conservative treatment often fails, and the surgical approach must be extensive and radical.[111, 119a]

As with the idiopathic clubfoot, treatment should begin as soon as possible after birth. Adhesive strapping in the nursery with frequent passive manipulation by nurses and parents should begin promptly. The deformity will generally not be corrected with longitudinal traction at the head of the first and second metatarsals, and its rigidity can be appreciated immediately.

After some foot growth and with the assumption that correction, although slow, is progressing, serial casting should begin as soon as the foot is large enough. Unlike other congenital problems, arthrogryposis does not tend to be progressive; however, suspension of treatment commonly results in a relapse to the initial deformity.[119] Since the basic problem is abnormal or absent muscles and abnormal nerve structures, the goal of treatment in the arthrogrypotic clubfoot differs from that in the idiopathic condition. In arthrogryposis the goal of treatment is to change a stiff, rigid, deformed foot to one that is stiff, rigid, and plantigrade.[115] To date, no form of treatment has been successful in obtaining or restoring any significant degree of increased mobility.

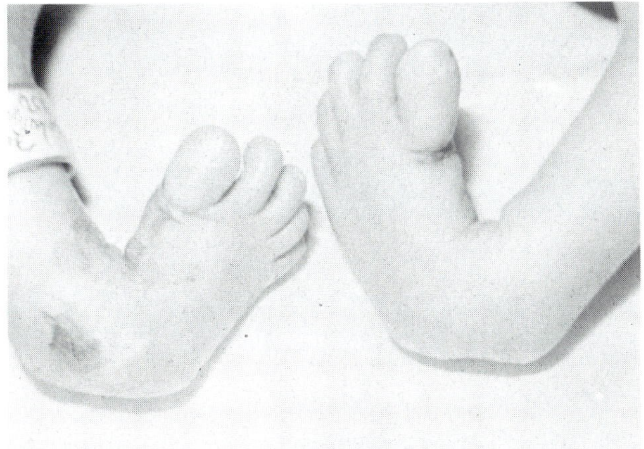

FIG 31–31.
Rigid, severe clubfoot in a newborn arthrogrypotic.

If after a period of conservative treatment it becomes obvious that full correction has not been obtained (and this is usually the case), operative intervention should proceed directly. Correction of the hindfoot is of prime importance, and if the equinus and varus can be neutralized, any residual forefoot deformity is unlikely to interfere with function. If the deformity is mild or moderate, posterior release with capsulotomy of the ankle and subtalar joints combined with segmental excision (not lengthening) of the Achilles tendon and posterior tibial tendon, accompanied by division of the posterior talofibular and deltoid ligaments, may result in a plantigrade foot. Under such circumstances the foot should be maintained in plaster in the corrected position 3 or 4 months postoperatively. It is then advisable to continue maintenance of correction in an appropriate day-night brace.

Often a moderate deformity will require a formal medial as well as posterior release. In addition to those structures released via the posterior approach, the capsules of the talonavicular, subtalar, and naviculocuneiform joints must be excised. Postoperative treatment is the same as for posterior release alone.[7, 112] When the foot deformity is severe, soft-tissue release can effect correction only by opening joints widely on the medial side of the foot. The situation has been likened to the opening of a suitcase; often there is insufficient skin and subcutaneous tissue for adequate wound closure. With such severe deformity, the "suitcase" simply closes again after removal of cast immobilization, and the deformity can be obtained recurs. In this instance correction of the deformity can be obtained only by shortening skeletal elements.[117]

In a young child, arthrodesis of the growing foot is inappropriate. Excision of the talus is an effective method of gaining alignment and allows skin closure without tension.[114] In an immature, severely involved foot, talectomy results are best when the patient is between the ages of 1 and 5 years; the procedure can result in a plantigrade functional foot. The procedure is a

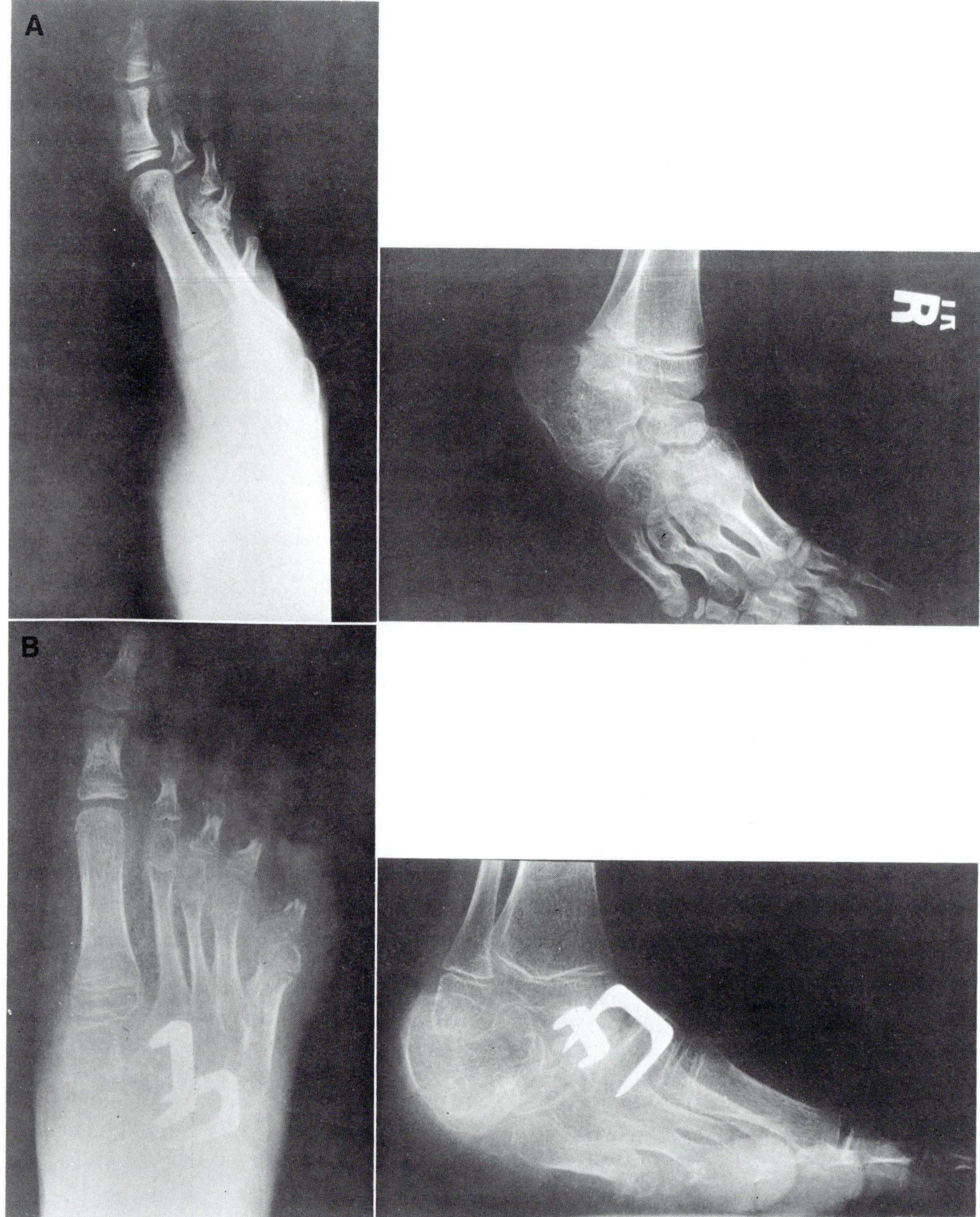

FIG 31–32.
A, AP and lateral views of 12-year-old arthrogrypotic foot that underwent talectomy at 15 months. **B,** result after midtarsal dorsolateral wedge resection. The residual equinus could be corrected, if necessary, by supramalleolar osteotomy to provide a better weight-bearing surface.

demanding one, and attention to detail is of prime importance.

Talectomy

A lateral curved incision following the line of the subtalar and talonavicular joints provides adequate exposure. Subcutaneous tissues should be protected and the incision carried directly to the capsule of these joints. The joints should be entered and the capsule excised; to prevent damage to the articular cartilage, iris scissors and loupe magnification should be used. As the dissection proceeds, the hindfoot can be manipulated into equinovarus to permit division of the posterior and posteromedial ligaments. The entire talus must be excised; any remnants left behind can grow and produce a recurrent progressive deformity. After excision of the talus, a portion of the Achilles tendon should be excised. The calcaneus may then be placed in the ankle mortise; if it does not fit well, partial excision of the tip of the lateral malleolus and division of the anterior tibiofibular ligament may be necessary. The calcaneus is usually fairly stable within the ankle mortise, but it is a good practice to hold the reduction with a Kirschner wire or small Steinmann pin placed up through the heel into the tibia. If excision of the talus is inadequate and the deformity is not fully corrected, the navicular may also be excised to provide further correction. One must, however, avoid excising any portion of the calcaneus because this will have an adverse effect on the size of the foot. Postoperatively, the foot should be maintained in plaster for 3 months; the Kirschner wire can be removed at 3 to 4 weeks.

Follow-up of talectomy for arthrogryposis has generally demonstrated good results, with a plantigrade functional foot, so long as the appropriate indications for surgery were present.[121] The procedure is indicated for badly deformed rigid equinovarus feet when additional musculoskeletal abnormalities make prolonged standing and extended ambulation unlikely. When the surgical resection is incomplete or postoperative care is inadequate, deformity will certainly recur (Fig 31–32,*A*).

For the older child, triple arthrodesis is the procedure of choice. Adequate shortening of the skeletal elements to effect correction and closure of the skin without tension can be carried out during the procedure. If the triple arthrodesis does not effect complete correction, fusion of the ankle joint with appropriate resection of bone from the distal end of the tibia may be necessary in the severely involved arthrogrypotic foot.[108] Triple arthrodesis should probably not be performed when significant foot growth remains (i.e., in children under the age of 12 years).

Midtarsal wedge resection is effective in correcting cavus or forefoot equinus deformity (Fig 31–32,*B*). Supramalleolar osteotomy can be used to correct hindfoot equinus in the older child, although Drummond et al. believe that this should be the last line of defense.[112]

ABNORMALITIES OF TOES

Congenital abnormalities of the toes include polydactyly, syndactyly, macrodactyly, congenital hammer toe, and overlapping and underlapping toes. Congenital abnormalities of the great toe include hallux rigidus, hallux varus, and interphalangeal valgus. More than any other group of foot abnormalities, congenital toe deformities tend to be hereditary. Furthermore, some toe abnormalities are found in concert with generalized syndromes as noted in the compilation by Zimbler and Craig[141] (see Table 31–1).

Abnormalities of the Great Toe

Congenital Hallux Varus

Congenital hallux varus is a rare deformity and differs from that seen as an adducted first toe accompanying metatarsus primus varus. There is no hereditary tendency for this deformity, and it is often associated with supernumerary phalanges or metatarsals; on occasion, the first metatarsal is duplicated and fused.

Clinically the deformity presents as an adduction deviation of the great toe, occasionally as much as 90 degrees to the long axis of the foot (Fig 31–33). Most often the deformity occurs at the metatarsophalangeal joint; however, it is sometimes seen at the interphalangeal joint. McElvenny described hallux varus in association with (1) a short thick metatarsal, (2) accessory bones or toes, (3) varus deformity of one or more of the lateral four metatarsals, and (4) a firm fibrous band along the medial aspects of the foot.[131] This firm band, interpreted as being the abductor hallucis, has been implicated as a causative factor.[140]

Surgery for the condition must be tailored to meet the needs of the individual deformity. In general, sufficient skin must be retained by fashioning appropriate flaps to provide cover for the inner border of the foot. Farmer described a skin-fat flap that he uses to lengthen the short medial side of the foot after adapting the technique to the demands of the deformity.[123] To obtain reduction, all structures along the medial side, including the metatarsophalangeal joint capsule, must be transected. To obtain correction and prevent recurrence of the deformity, the abductor hallucis must be divided. If the deformity is limited to the distal phallanx or the interphalangeal joint, symptoms may develop in adoles-

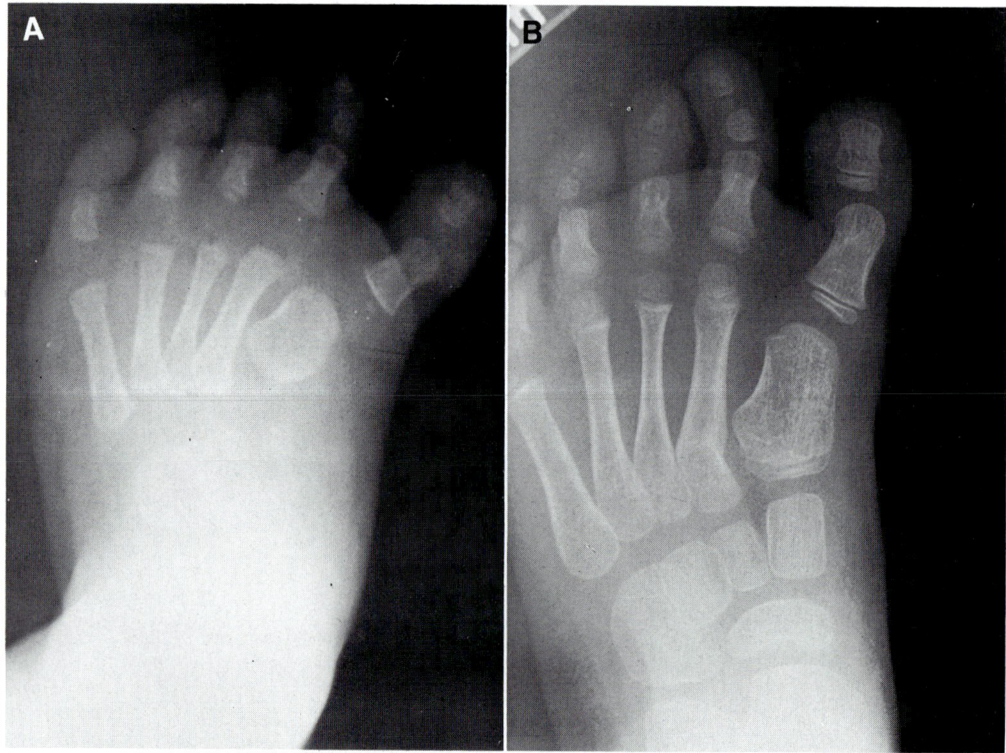

FIG 31–33.
Congenital hallux varus (atavistic first toe). **A,** at 10 months of age, there is shortening of the first metatarsal accompanied by medial subluxation of the metatarsophalangeal joint. **B,** at 2 years and 7 months, early release of the abductor hallucis has resulted in better cosmesis and alignment.

cence and require surgical intervention. Angular deformity of the distal or proximal phalanx (*hallux* interphalangeus), either varus or valgus, can be corrected by appropriate osteotomy. The surgeon must be aware of and protect the physis of the digital bone; hence intraoperative use of image intensification fluoroscopy is recommended.

Existence of a hemicircumferential medial epiphysis on the first metatarsal as described by Jones and more recently by Mubarak can lead to a hallux varus deformity.[132a] When the great toe deformity is accompanied by a short (atavistic) first metatarsal, a CT scan may outline the C-shaped or 'bracket' epiphysis. Treatment in such a case involves meticulous resection of the juxta-diaphyseal portion of the epiphysis. The ideal age for this procedure is between 12 and 24 months.

Congenital Hallux Rigidus

Congenital hallux rigidus is extremely rare. Its presence has been ascribed to an abnormality of the first metatarsal: elevation, excessive length, or hypermobility. More commonly the deformity appears secondary to trauma, with involvement of the first metatarsophalangeal joint or development of osteochondritis dissecans of the first metatarsal head.[127] Anomalies of the first metatarsal head that cause abnormal joint surfaces can have the same effect as trauma and lead to abnormal stress and degenerative joint disease. Treatment of symptomatic congenital hallux rigidus is the same as for the acquired type. Since symptoms are not usually present before adolescence, interference with future growth of the toe is not necessarily a consideration.

Abnormalities of Lesser Toes

Polydactyly

Often inherited as an autosomal dominant,[128] polydactyly is frequently part of a generalized syndrome and may be accompanied by supernumerary fingers. If the extra digit occurs on the tibial side of the foot, it is termed *preaxial;* on the fibular side, it is called *postaxial.*[133] The literature contains many references to polydactyly, but for the most part these references are made only in passing when describing the clinical characteristics of a generalized syndrome.

Recognition of the deformity in biblical times is found in 2 Samuel 21:20: "And there was again war at

Goth, where there was a man of great stature who had six fingers on each hand and six toes on each foot, 24 in number; and he also was descended from the giants." Frazier noted a 12-fold increase in polydactyly among the southern black population as compared with southern whites. He described an incidence of 3.6 per 1,000 live births among black children born in Baltimore with an overall incidence of 1.7 per 1,000.[124]

Supernumerary toes are a clinical problem since they interfere with footwear. For this reason surgical excision is often indicated, but one must adhere to a few basic principles. Because polydactyly frequently interferes with shoe wear, excision at walking age is appropriate. At 1 year the foot and its individual structures are usually large enough to identify easily and deal with safely. Unlike the hand, treatment of the foot does not necessitate making a decision as to which is the most rudimentary of the digits and then excising that particular one. More appropriately, the contour of the entire foot should be considered and for the most part, the peripheral extra digit excised.[139] This is irrespective of whether it appears to be the more major digit. On the medial side of the foot, the toe closest to the tibia is usually excised; and on the lateral side, that closest to the fibula is removal. If an abnormality of the metatarsals (bifurcation, duplication) is demonstrated radiographically, appropriate excision to obtain a normal contour of the entire foot must be considered (Fig 31–34).

Surgical technique should be tailored to the individual case. In usual circumstances, disarticulation is carried out via a racquet-shaped incision with division and repair of ligaments and tendons as needed to prevent progressive deformity. Damage to remaining growth plates and articular cartilage must be avoided.

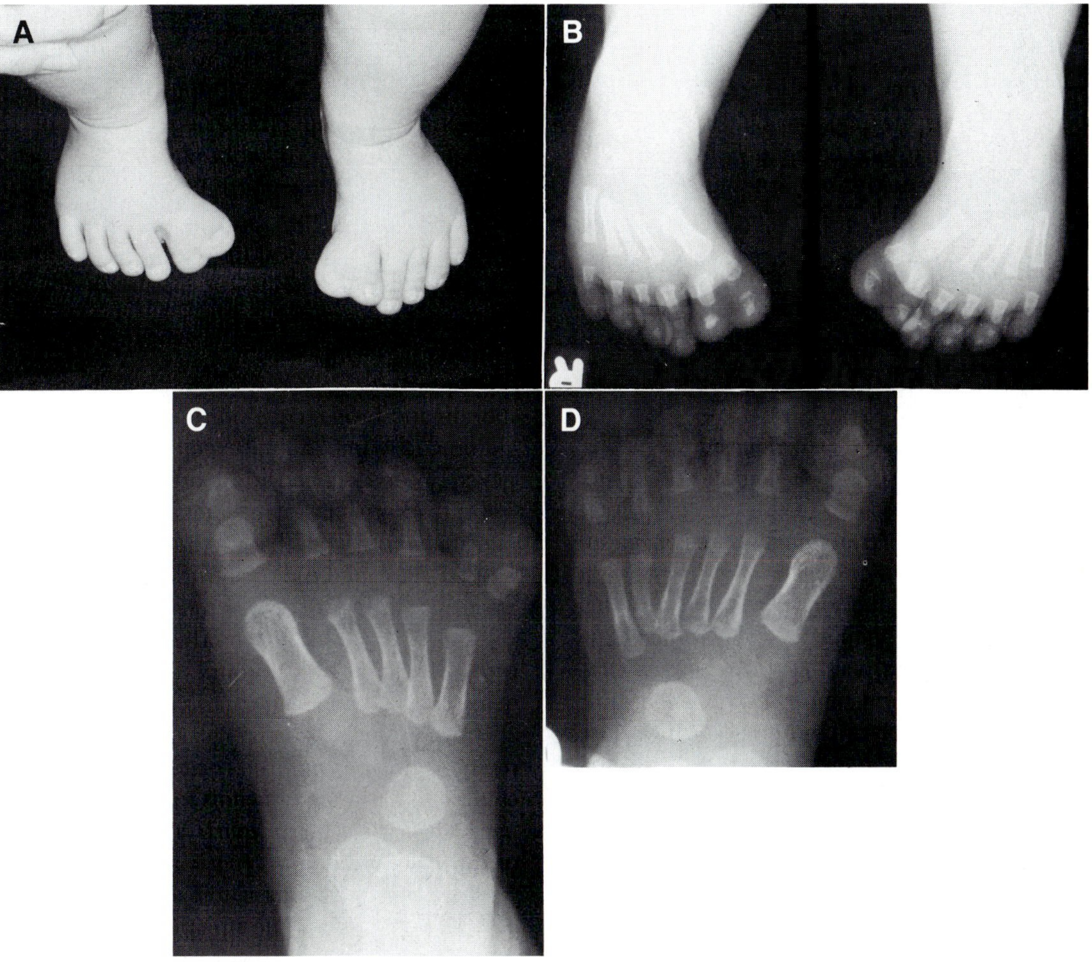

FIG 31–34.
A, bilateral duplication and syndactyly of the hallux. The tibialmost toe should be removed and the abductor hallucis reattached to the remaining proximal phalanx. If the abductor hallucis is lenthened, the metatarsus adductus will resolve. **B,** radiograph of the same feet. **C,** duplication of the fifth toe; the fibularmost (lateral) digit should be removed. **D,** polydactyly with six fully developed metatarsals. If surgery is required, ray resection as well as toe amputation is necessary.

Muscle attachment is a more significant consideration with an accessory hallux than with other accessory toes. In a review of 16 hallux duplications, Phelps et al. found that 14 had a residual varus deformity at long-term (15.1 years) follow-up.[134] The tibialmost hallux had been excised but no effort to balance soft-tissue structures carried out. If the tibial hallux is excised, the abductor hallucis must be reinserted into the remaining proximal phalanx to avoid a hallux valgus deformity. Similarly, if the fibular hallux is grossly deformed and is to be excised, the adductor hallucis must be resutured into the proximal phalanx of the remaining hallux to avoid a hallux varus deformity secondary to overpull of the abductor hallucis.

If a block metatarsal is present, the proximal phalanx should be centralized onto the head of the metatarsal and held in place with a longitudinal pin and cast for 6 to 8 weeks.

When the duplication of the great toe involves only the distal phalanx, excision of the tibialmost phalanx or portion thereof with longitudinal removal of the nail, its bed, and the underlying epiphysis is recommended. Meticulous closure of the eponychium and again, temporary pin centralization of the remaining phalanx are important.[135]

Syndactyly

Like polydactyly, syndactyly is also seen in association with other congenital anomalies and syndromes. McKusick[132] described five types of syndactyly, all transmitted as autosomal dominant traits. In the feet three types are seen:

1. Type I (zygodactyly): partial or complete webbing of the second and third toes; the hands are also involved at times.
2. Type II (synpolydactyly): syndactyly of the lateral two toes and polydactyly of the fifth toe in the syndactyly web.
3. Type III: syndactyly associated with metatarsal and metacarpal fusion.

Surgical intervention for simple syndactyly of the foot is rarely indicated. The deformity is functionally insignificant and rarely becomes symptomatic. When surgery for cosmetic reasons is necessary, techniques of syndactyly release for the fingers apply as well to the toes.

The basic surgical technique involves outlining dorsal and volar skin flaps, based proximally. Flaps are incised, and this skin is used to close the cleft and reconstruct the web by suturing the flaps side to side. Opposing surfaces of the toes are then covered with free split-thickness skin grafts as required. Attempts to close flaps without using skin grafts lead to inevitable contracture and deformity.

Macrodactyly

Usually seen as a manifestation of a generalized problem (neurofibromatosis, arteriovenous fistula, hemangioma), gigantism of a toe can result in significant functional as well as cosmetic problems (Fig 31–35). Both gait abnormalities and difficulty with foot wear occur and make surgery necessary. The toe may be reduced in length by a partial or total proximal or middle phalangectomy. The circumference of a toe can be reduced by staged defatting procedures. If the third or fourth toe is involved, amputation may be acceptable. However, amputation of a gigantic second toe can result in progressive hallux valgus deformity. Tachdjian has recommended syndactyly of the second to the fourth toes if a gigantic third toe is amputated.[139] Overgrowth of the metatarsal may be managed by epiphysiodesis at an appropriate time.

Congenital Hammer Toe

A rare congenital deformity, hammer toe is recognized as a flexion contracture of the proximal interphalangeal joint with or without fixed deformity of the distal interphalangeal joint. With ambulation and footwear the metatarsophalangeal joint eventually becomes hyperextended. Like syndactyly and polydactyly, hammer toe is frequently a familial problem, most often involving the middle toes. With shoe wear, callus formation over the dorsal aspect of the proximal interphalangeal joint can result in symptoms.

Because the deformity usually eventually becomes symptomatic, early treatment is indicated. In infancy, adhesive strapping combined with stretching of the contracted volar capsule of the proximal interphalangeal joint is often effective. Early surgical treatment is usually not necessary since the deformity does not become symptomatic until adolescence. After the foot has reached an appropriate size, correction can easily be obtained surgically by partial phalangectomy and interphalangeal fusion. If contracture of the dorsal metatarsophalangeal joint capsule has occurred, capsulotomy must also be carried out. Specifics of surgical treatment are described in Chapter 8.

Overlapping Toes

Often familial, overriding is most commonly seen as the fifth toe overlapping the fourth. There is dorsiflexion of the metatarsophalangeal joint with adduction and external rotation of the digit. The condition is usually bilateral and, in about 50% of the cases, causes dis-

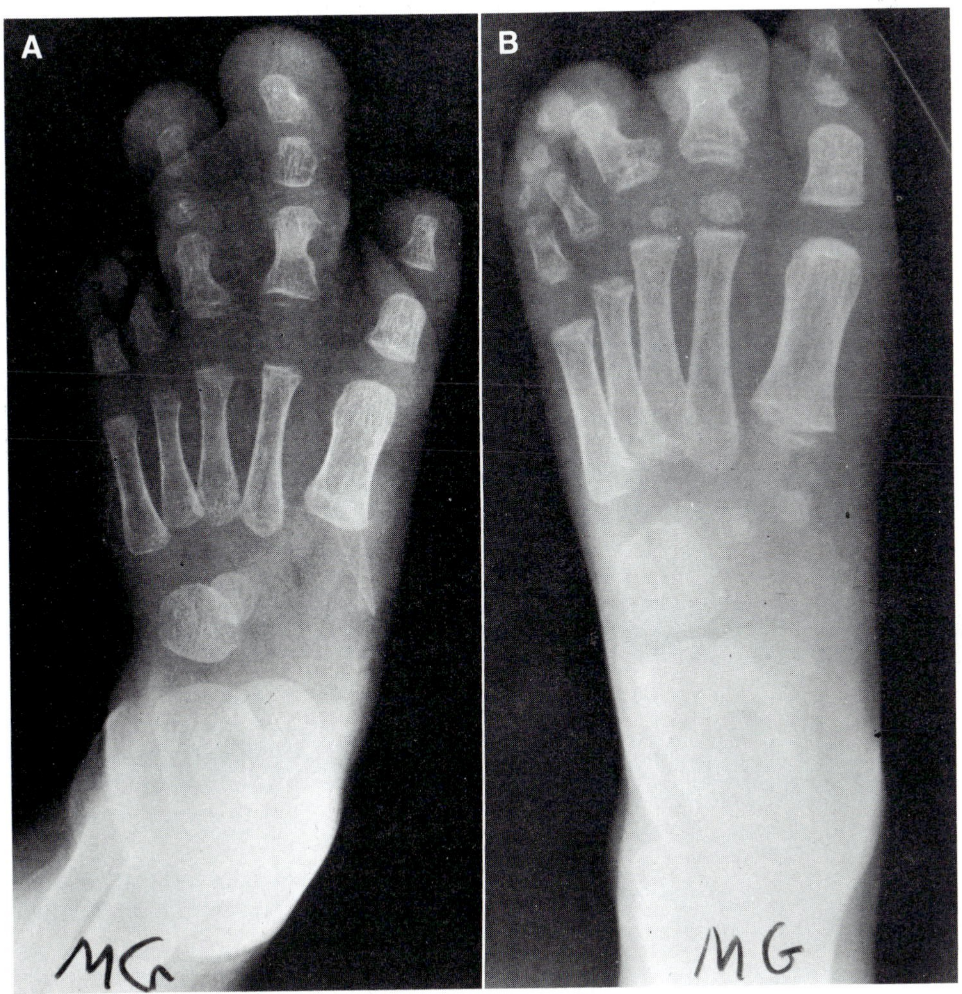

FIG 31–35.
A, macrodactyly involving the second and third toes. The digits are adult sized at 2 years of age. **B,** the initial procedure included epiphyseodeisis and soft-tissue resection. Three years later interphalangeal resection and fusion with further soft-tissue removal resulted in better cosmesis and shoe fit. (Courtesy of Dr. Semour Zimbler, Boston.)

abling symptoms.[122] Discomfort is aggravated by shoe wear and accompanying callus formation over the dorsal aspect of the proximal interphalangeal joint.

Because, as in hammer toe and congenital curly toe, symptoms are likely to develop later in life, early treatment may be of some benefit. In infancy, stretching the medial collateral ligament structure and dorsal medial capsule with adhesive taping into the correct position may be of some benefit. In most cases, surgical correction can be carried out without bone resection or interference with growth; therefore treatment in early childhood is possible.

Treatment.—Most procedures described involve tenotomy of the extensor digitorum communis to the fifth toe as well as capsulotomy of the dorsal medial metatarsophalangeal joint.

Lapidus did the extensor tenotomy at the midtarsal level, rerouted the distal tendon stump plantarward around the medial side of the small toe and inserted the stump into the abductor digiti minimi.[129]

I have been particularly pleased with Butler's operation.[122] In this procedure the entire toe is freed via a racquet incision at its base with proximal extensions dorsally and at the plantar lateral margin. After extensor tenotomy and dorsal capsulotomy the plantar capsule, if adherent, is freed from the metatarsal head. Closure of the skin is then completed with the toe in the corrected position; no postoperative cast is necessary.[122]

Syndactylization of the fifth to the fourth toe is advocated by Scrase[136] and Kelikian et al.[126] A double-U incision between the fourth and fifth toes with excision of the intervening skin permits the syndactyly. Correction via capsulotomy and extensor digitorum tenotomy can be accompanied by removal of enough proximal phalanx to correct the deformity.[130]

Amputation for an overlapping fifth toe generally results in pain and pressure at the head of the fifth metatarsal and is therefore not recommended. If the deformity is too severe, attempted correction without bony resection can result in vascular compromise. For this reason procedures restricted to soft tissues tend to be more applicable to children and adolescents than to adults, although satisfactory results may also be seen in the adult population (see Chapter 8).

Congenital Underlapping Toes (Congenital Curly Toe)

Congenital underlapping toes is a common familial deformity most often seen in the lateral three toes. It presents as a combination of flexion, adduction, and internal rotation primarily at the distal interphalangeal joint (Fig 31–36). In severe cases the proximal interphalangeal joint is also rotated and the toenail pointed laterally.

Unlike congenital overlapping toes, the congenital curly toe rarely becomes symptomatic. Early conservative treatment does not seem to be of benefit in correcting curly toe deformity.

Sweetman evaluated the long-term results of 50 cases, 21 patients treated and 29 untreated. In no patient, either treated or untreated, did the deformity progress; 25% improved whether treated or not. Even though the deformity persisted in many cases, most patients had forgotten that it was present.[138]

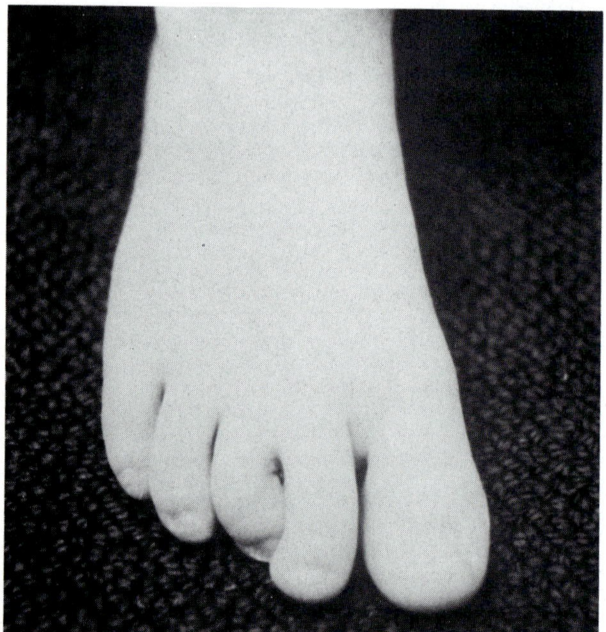

FIG 31–36.
Congenital curly toes. The lateral deviation of the second toe is secondary to an underlapping third digit.

If surgery is required because of symptoms, syndactylization of the curly toe to its neighbor may be performed.[125] Correction may be obtained by excising an appropriate wedge from the superolateral aspect of the distal interphalangeal joint. Sharrard recommended transfer of the extensor digitorum longus of the affected toe to the dorsolateral aspect of the extensor hood. He found that this was of benefit, particularly if the deformity was not too severe.[137] In my hands, tenotomy of the flexor digitorum longus through an oblique incision underlying the middle phalanx, when performed in early childhood, has been curative. One must take care to not cross the joint flexor crease with the incision. Postoperatively a soft dressing is sufficient.

TORSIONAL DEFORMITIES OF THE LOWER EXTREMITIES

In the daily practice of a primary-care physician, perhaps the most common orthopaedic problem noted among skeletally immature patients seen in the office is some form of rotational malalignment of the lower extremities. Rarely does the problem present as a complaint of the individual but rather the result of concern on the part of parents, grandparents, or other well-meaning individuals. Diagnosis can sometimes be elusive, speculative, or unrecognized. Perhaps millions of dollars annually are spent for orthotics, braces, or other devices that are reputedly therapeutic but in fact offer no scientifically proven benefit.

The rotational deformity may obviously be either internal or external and is most often referred to as in-toeing or out-toeing. If the treating physician is able to make a specific diagnosis by physical examination, then appropriate treatment or advice can be advanced on a judicious basis. The anatomic site responsible for toeing in or toeing out can be located anywhere between the toes and the pelvis. Torsional malalignment of the foot, ankle, leg, thigh, or pelvis will result in a clinical picture most obvious at the foot. Therefore, a complete appreciation of the various diagnostic possibilities, their anatomic location, and associated physical findings allows one to treat appropriately, avoiding overtreatment and unnecessary expense.

Physical Examination and Normal Parameters

With lower-extremity rotational problems, physical assessment should begin with an evaluation of the individual's coordination and gait if he/she is ambulatory. The angle of gait or foot progression angle is that angle subtended by the foot relative to the line of progression as it strikes the floor. Under normal circumstances, the angle of gait ranges between 5 and 15 degrees external (Fig 31–37). While observing the individual ambulate, the examiner should note the position of the knee as related to the line of progression; this should be observed from both the front and the back. The relationship of the foot to the knee is important in delineating the source of rotational malalignment, either above or below the knee joint.

After observing the gait pattern, sequential examination of the lower limbs should be carried out. The feet should be the first specific structure examined. Starting distally allows the examiner to remain outside the patient's "*space*" and thereby puts the child at ease; one may then usually carry out this and the remainder of an examination with enhanced patient cooperation. I prefer to begin the examination with the child on a parent's lap; this allows excellent visualization of the foot's plantar surface. With the child supine, the plantar surface of the foot should be observed, with careful attention paid to the contour of its outer border as well as the alignment of the great toes in relation to the longitudinal axis of the first metatarsal. The outer border of the foot should normally be straight; the great toe should continue on the long axis of the first metatarsal. The tendon of the abductor hallucis muscle should not be particularly prominent when the great toe is passively deviated toward the midline.

With the patient moving to a sitting position on the edge of the examining table, the transmalleolar axis should next be evaluated. Clinically this can be accomplished by placing your index finger of the hand opposite that of the leg being examined on the lateral malleolus with the thumb on the medial malleolus. With the index finger of the other hand resting on the tibial tubercle and by using this as a guide, sight down the leg from above and determine the relationship of the transmalleolar axis to the horizontal (Fig 31–38,*A* and *B*). Normally, the medial malleolus should be anterior to the lateral malleolus by approximately 5 degrees at birth and progress to 20 degrees in adulthood.[142]

While the child remains in the sitting position, one may then assess the axis of the femoral neck and its relationship to the transcondylar axis of the femur. Since the femoral neck is in a direct line with the greater trochanter (Fig 31–39,A and B), rotating the extremity until the greater trochanter is palpably most lateral will allow one to determine the longitudinal axis of the neck (Fig 31–40). The degree of femoral anteversion (relationship of the femoral neck axis to the transcondylar axis) is represented in the angle subtended by the longitudinal axis of the leg and the vertical.

Final assessment on physical examination is carried out with the patient prone. In this position, with the hip extended, the knee flexed 90 degrees, and the ankle in a plantigrade position, one may determine the thigh-foot axis. With the patient prone, the longitudinal axis of the foot as compared with the longitudinal axis of the thigh is normally between 0 and 10 degrees external (Fig 31–41). A deviation from this indicates the presence of a torsional malalignment below the knee. If the lateral border of the foot is straight, the deformity is further isolated to the area between ankle and knee.

Rotational motion of the hip in extention is also assessed in this position. Total normal rotation is approximately 90 degrees. This should consist of nearly equal internal and external rotation; in the normal individual there may be slightly more external rotation available than internal.[147]

By using these procedures as a means of physical assessment, the examiner is able to delineate the anatomic site responsible for the rotational malalignment and approach treatment on a more scientific basis.

Treatment

Toeing Out

External rotational posturing of the lower extremities is most often physiologic. Two pathologic entities that may result in this picture include a vertical talus or a neurologic disorder. If both careful neurologic assessment and examination for the presence of a vertical talus are negative, the parents may be assured that the external rotational posture of the extremity is physiologic and does not require treatment. One occasionally finds that internal rotation of the hip is limited in the infant by tight external hip rotators, perhaps because of heavy diapering or large thighs that keep the infant's hip flexed and externally rotated. External rotator stretch-

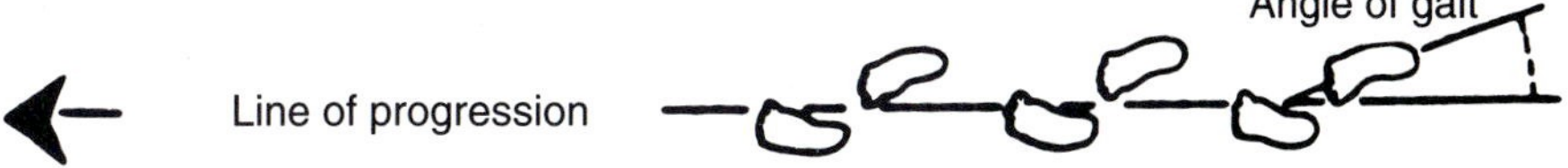

FIG 31–37.
Angle of gait in the presence of intoeing.

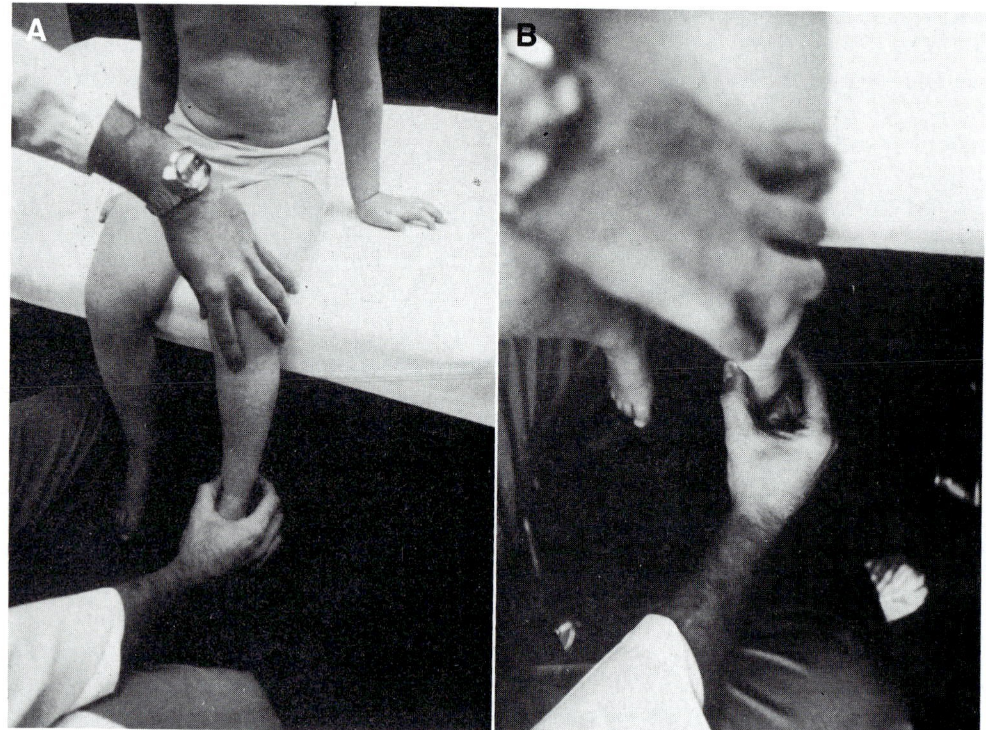

FIG 31–38.
A, placement of the hand for clinical measurement of the tibial torsional angle. **B,** as viewed from above, the normal medial malleolus is anterior to the lateral malleolus by 15 degrees.

ing at the time of diaper change by internally rotating the thigh and using the flexed knee as a handle may be of some benefit. However, it is most probable that the tight muscular and capsular structures will normally elongate as the child grows.

In the ambulatory child, external rotational posturing of the lower extremity is common before the age of 2 years. This may appear with initial ambulation as an effort on the part of the individual to provide stability in standing. This, too, normally resolves by 24 months of age without specific treatment.[144]

Toeing in as Result of Foot Abnormalities

The entities of the foot responsible for internal malalignment of the foot are addressed elsewhere in this chapter (Metatarsus Adductus, atavistic first toe, abductor hallucis tightness). Treatment of the specific foot anomaly should follow the guidelines recommended.

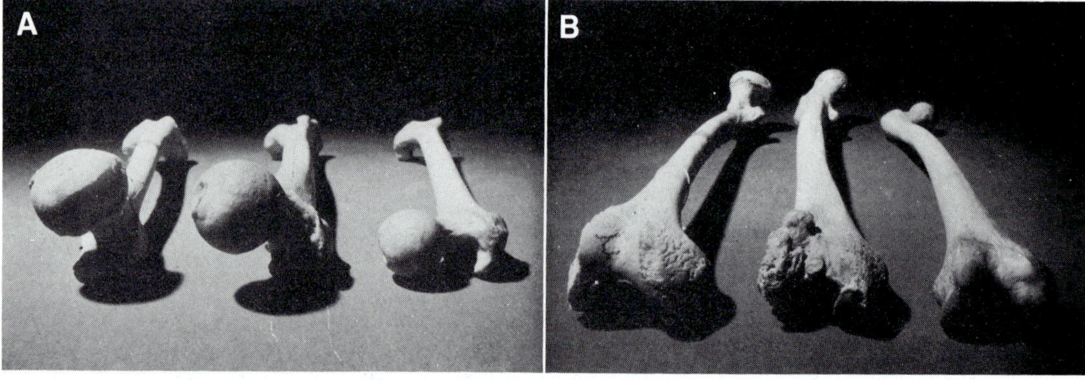

FIG 31–39.
Adult femora with varying angles of anteversion. **A,** view from above. Note the position of the greater trochanter in relation to the femoral neck. **B,** view from below. The femoral condyles are in identical positions; these femoral necks vary from 80 to 0 degrees of anteversion. (Courtesy of Shands Bone Museum. A.I. duPont Institute.)

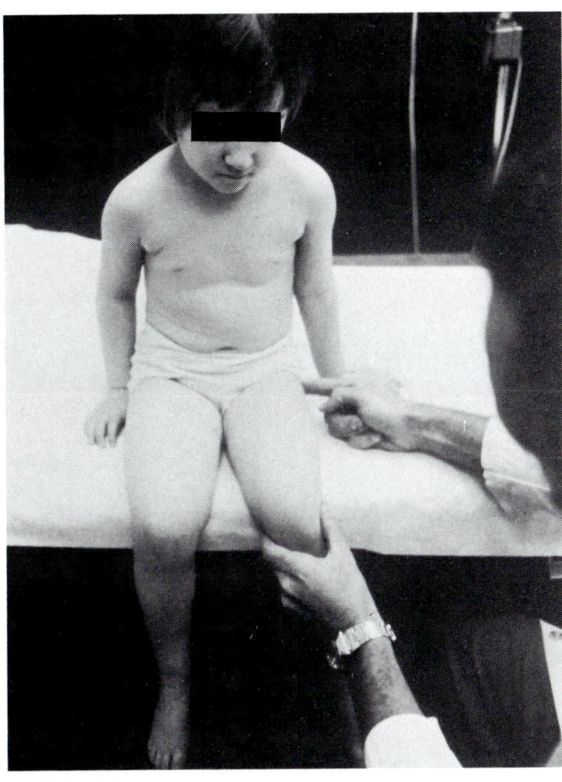

FIG 31–40.
Determination of the anteversion angle by palpation of the greater trochanter. The angle subtended by the tibia as compared with a vertical line is equal to the angle of the femoral neck with the transcondylar axis.

Tibial Torsion

Torsional malalignment of the leg, either external or more commonly internal, is determined by the transmalleolar axis as described under "Physical Examination." At birth the transmalleolar axis may be neutral and progress to its normal 15 degrees external by 2 to 3 years of age. The child who is seen between 6 months and 2 years of age with a complaint of toeing in has, most commonly, persistent internal tibial torsion. It is generally felt that as growth and development proceed, a normal transmalleolar axis will develop with ambulation, and active treatment is rarely indicated. Occasionally, persistent internal torsion or deformities with a negative transmalleolar angle are of enough concern to warrant active intervention. If one is to treat a perceived problem that is potentially a phase of normal development, the induction of secondary iatrogenic problems must be avoided. A Denis-Browne bar no longer than the width of the individual's pelvis with the feet externally rotated no more than 45 degrees may be applied (Fig 31–42). More elaborate devices such as the Blount derotation brace have been used to keep the knee flexed and thereby concentrate torsional force to

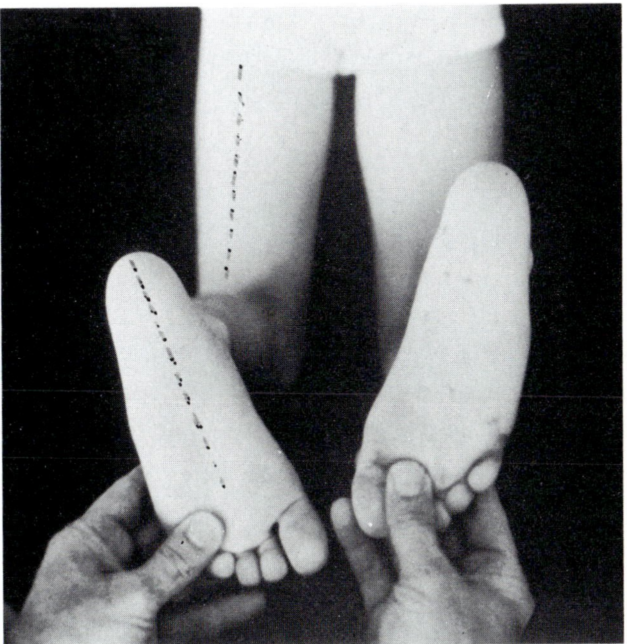

FIG 31–41.
Abnormal thigh-foot axis bilaterally, worse on the left than the right.

the ankle and leg. A bar wider than the pelvis or external rotation beyond 45 degrees can result in secondary ligamentous laxity at the ankle or valgus deformity of the knee. Tolerance to motion-inhibiting devices is limited in the ambulatory child, and newer night splints have been designed that allow some motion, induce correction, and minimize the potential for iatrogenic deformity.

It is advisable to avoid initiation of brace treatment until the child has reached 18 to 24 months of age and failure of improvement has been documented by serial accurate thigh-foot angle and transmalleolar axis mea-

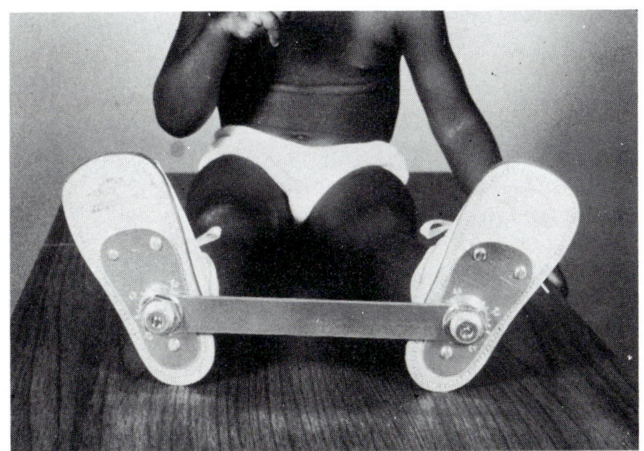

FIG 31–42.
Appropriately measured and configured Denis-Browne bar.

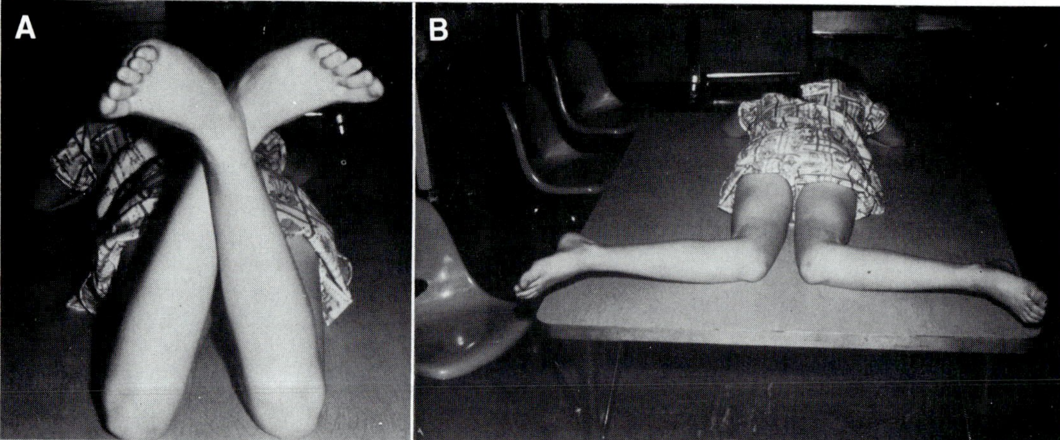

FIG 31–43.
Degree of external hip rotation available **(A)** and internal rotation possible **(B)** in the presence of femoral anteversion clinically measuring 70 degrees.

surements performed over a 6-month period. Brace wear at night and nap time may then be justified, and improvement should be complete in 6 months.

Significant external torsional deformities of the tibia are less commonly encountered. When seen, they are most frequently secondary to internal torsional deformities of the femur or malalignment of the foot as a result of neuromuscular problems. Consequently, isolated treatment of external torsional malrotation of the leg is rarely indicated.

Because of the benign nature of the problem and its probable physiologic basis, a surgical approach to torsional deformities of the tibia should be performed only under rare circumstances and following a great deal of thoughtful consideration. Rotational osteotomies performed subperiosteally through a small incision in the supramalleolar area may be performed without internal fixation, thus avoiding the problems associated with pins, plates, screws, etc. Maintaining corrected alignment in a long-leg cast with the knee bent 90 degrees for 6 weeks carries the least risk of complication from nonunion, infection, failure of correction, etc.

Technique of Supramalleolar Tibial Derotational Osteotomy

The goal of the procedure is to create a normal transmalleolar axis relative to the femoral transcondylar axis.

1. With the patient supine and a tourniquet about the upper portion of the thigh, the entire limb is draped free. A 4-cm longitudinal incision slightly lateral to the tibial crest just proximal to the tibial physis allows one to divide the deeper tissues along the crest and expose the tibial subperisoteally. I prefer to use the image intensifier to ensure avoidance of the physis and a perfectly transverse osteotomy.

2. A second incision along the distal shaft of the fibula is necessary if the rotation is to be corrected more than 20 degrees. This helps to prevent reoccurrence of the torsional malalignment. Subperiosteal fibular osteotomy should precede the tibial osteotomy.

3. Divide the fibula 4 to 5 cm proximal to the level of the tibial osteotomy. Incise the periosteum longitudinally, elevate it with sharp and blunt elevators, and complete the cut by using an appropriately sized osteotome after drilling the cortex in two or three sites.

4. In similar fashion, elevate the tibial periosteum; drill the cortex medially, laterally, and posteriorly; and then complete the osteotomy with an osteotome.

5. I avoid the use of internal fixation because the periosteal sleeve provides sufficient stability. Rotate the foot so as to align the tibial tubercle with the first to second metatarsal interspace; close the wounds.

6. Place the limb in a long-leg cast with the knee flexed 90 degrees and the foot held in proper rotational alignment. After 6 weeks the cast may be removed and motion and protected weight bearing begun.

Femoral Anteversion

Those individuals over 2 $\frac{1}{2}$ years of age with persistent or recently noticed toeing in most frequently have a torsional abnormality in the proximal shaft of the femur. At birth, the longitudinal axis of the femoral neck subtends an angle of approximately 40 degrees when compared with the transcondylar axis of the femur. During the first 2 years of life, this angle declines to 20 degrees; a further decrease to slightly over 10 degrees in the adult occurs during the latter years of growth.[145] Anterior inclination of the neck is referred to clinically as femoral anteversion. Excessive anteversion results from incomplete derotation of the upper portion of the femur as it assumes a position of extension, adduction, and internal rotation from its initial early position in the fetal limb bud. When weight bearing, unless the acetabulum is abnormally inclined so as to receive the head of the excessively anteverted femoral neck, the extremity must internally rotate to avoid anterior subluxation. The stresses of weight bearing, influence of growth, and capsular pressures will induce remodeling and decrease the anteversion angle. Longitudinal anteversion studies have demonstrated that an individual retains the potential for remodeling until approximately 8 years of age. In children who persistently alter their gait pattern or sit in the reversed tailor position, the stresses that induce the remodeling processes are decreased. In such cases, excessive anteversion persists.

On physical examination, a significant increase in internal rotation at the hip is noted. External rotation, on the other hand, is limited to only a few degrees (Fig 31–43,*A* and *B*).

It has been suggested in the past and noted in studies by Fabray and MacEwen[143] that bracing has little or no effect on the anteversion angle. Treatment with a Denis-Browne bar, twister cables, etc., has never shown a decrease in anteversion angle that withstood scientific scrutiny. Therefore, beyond recommending appropriate sitting habits (e.g., avoiding the reversed tailor position), the child under 8 years of age with persistent femoral anteversion and toeing in should not be actively treated. There is no place in the treatment of this entity for prescription footwear; similarly bracing has no effect.

If, after 8 to 9 years of age, a significant cosmetic or functional deformity is present, surgical intervention may be required. Functional impairment is commonly seen in individuals who have no more than 10 degrees of passive external rotation at the hip. It has been our policy to do a supracondylar subperiosteal derotational osteotomy without internal or external fixation. When performed as described, the risk of asymmetric or excessive derotation is minimal. Again, the complications associated with pins, plates, screws, etc., are avoided.

Technique of Supracondylar Femoral Derotational Osteotomy

Before surgery, the total amount of femoral anteversion is evaluated fluoroscopically. With the patient prone on the x-ray table, the knees are bent and the hip internally rotated until the longest image of the femoral neck is present on the screen. At that point, the neck is parallel to the x-ray table; determination of the anteversion angle is possible by measuring the angle subtended by the leg against the vertical. At surgery, this degree of derotation is carried out.

1. With the patient supine on the fracture table and the legs abducted 45 degrees, the extremity is prepared and draped so as to allow for a medial approach to the distal portion of the femur. With use of an image intensifier, the supracondylar region of the femur is identified 2.5 cm above the distal femoral physis.
2. A 4-cm longitudinal skin incision is made just anterior to the intramuscular septum, beginning just distal to the growth plate and coursing proximally. Dissection through the subcutaneous tissue is carried out, the fascia lata divided, and the vastus medialis retracted anteriorly.
3. The posteromedial aspect of the femoral shaft is identified, and epiphyseal vessels crossing the field are protected. A 2.5-cm longitudinal incision in the posteromedial periosteum is made, and with care the periosteum elevated circumferentially from the femoral metaphysis at this point.
4. The femur may be divided either by predrilling the osteotomy site with a small drill bit followed by osteotomes or with a power saw. Of great importance is maintenance of the osteotomy in a line absolutely perpendicular to the longitudinal axis of the femoral shaft.
5. Following completion of the osteotomy, the foot plate of the fracture table is externally rotated, thus derotating the extremity distal to the osteotomy site. The intact periosteal sleeve provides sufficient stability and limits the amount of derotation possible. Further external rotation of the foot will result in rotation at the hip, not at the osteotomy site. A 4-cm circumferential periosteal stripping will permit approximately 40 degrees of derotation. It has been unnecessary to place drains within the wound or add internal fixation devices.
6. After manipulative derotation and wound closure the extremity is placed in a long-leg bilateral hip spica cast with the foot (or feet) externally rotated 90 degrees.

Postoperatively, the patient is kept nonambulatory in the cast for a period of 6 weeks. On cast removal, hospitalization for vigorous physical therapy over a period of 4 to 6 days is necessary to regain 60 degrees of knee motion. The patient is kept on crutch-assisted weight bearing until 90 degrees of knee motion has been realized.

Results of applying this approach to the well-selected patient in my hands have been universally excellent. The use of a small medial incision avoids cosmetic problems of a readily visable surgical scar. Complications of nonunion, infection, loss of position, entry into the suprapatellar pouch of the knee, or less than complete patient satisfaction have been avoided.

REFERENCES

Embryology and Genetics

1. Blechschmidt E: *The stages of human development before birth*, Philadelphia, 1961, WB Saunders.
2. Cowell HR, Wein BK: Current concepts review: genetic aspects of club foot, *J Bone Joint Surg [Am]* 62:1381–1384, 1980.
3. Fuller DJ, Duthie RB: The timed appearance of some congenital malformations and orthopaedic abnormalities, *Instr Course Lect* 23:53–71, 1974.
4. Gardner E, Gray DJ, O'Rahilly R: The prenatal development of the skeleton and joints of the human foot, *J Bone Joint Surg [Am]* 41:847, 1959.
5. McKusick VA: *Mendelian inheritance in man*, ed 4, Baltimore, 1975, Johns Hopkins.
6. Zimbler S, Craig C: Foot deformities, *Orthop Clin North Am* 7:331, 1976.

Clubfoot (Talipes Equinovarus)

7. Abrams RC: Relapsed clubfoot: the early results of an evaluation of the Dillwyn Evans operation, *J Bone Joint Surg [Am]* 51:270, 1969.

8a. Atar D, Lehman WB, Grant AD, et al: Fractional lengthening of the flexor tendons in clubfoot surgery, *Orthop Clin North Am* 264:267, 1991.

8. Bohm M: The embryologic origin of clubfoot, *J Bone Joint Surg* 11:229, 1929.
9. Brockman EP: *Congenital clubfoot*, London, 1930, John Wright & Sons.
10. Crawford AH, Marxen JL, Osterfeld DL: The Cincinnati incision: a comprehensive approach for surgical procedures of the foot and ankle in childhood, *J Bone Joint Surg [Am]* 64:1355–1358, 1982.
11. Denham PA: Congenital talipes equinovarus, *J Bone Joint Surg [Br]* 49:583, 1967.
12. Dunn HK, Samuelson KM: Flat topped talus: a long term report of 20 clubfeet, *J Bone Joint Surg [Am]* 56:57, 1974.
13. Dwyer FC: The treatment of relapsed clubfoot by insertion of a wedge into the calcaneum, *J Bone Joint Surg [Br]* 45:67, 1963.
14. Evans D: Relapsed clubfoot, *J Bone Joint Surg [Br]* 43:722, 1961.
15. Fisher RL, Shaffer SR: An evaluation of calcaneal osteotomy in congenital clubfoot and other disorders, *Clin Orthop* 70:141, 1970.
16. Fried A: Recurrent congenital clubfoot, *J Bone Joint Surg [Am]* 41:424, 1959.
17. Gardner E: Osteogenesis in the human embryo and foetus. In Bourne G, editor, *Biochemistry and physiology of bone*, New York, 1956, Academic Press.
18. Heywood AWB: The mechanics of the hindfoot in clubfoot as demonstrated radiographically, *J Bone Joint Surg [Br]* 46:105, 1964.
19. Ippolito E, Ponseti IV: Congenital clubfoot in the human fetus: a histological study, *J Bone Joint Surg [Am]* 62:8–22, 1980.
20. Irani RN, Sherman MS: The pathological anatomy of clubfoot, *J Bone Joint Surg [Am]* 45:45, 1963.
21. Johanning K: Exocochleatio ossis cuboidei in the treatment of pes equino varus, *Acta Orthop Scand* 27:310, 1958.
22. Keim HA, Ritchie GW: Nutcracker treatment of clubfoot, *JAMA* 189:613, 1964.
23. Kite JH: The non-operative treatment of congenital clubfoot, *South Med J* 23:337, 1930.
24. Lowe LW, Hannon MA: Residual adduction of the forefoot in treated congenital club foot, *J Bone Joint Surg [Br]* 55:809, 1973.
25. Paturet G: *Traite d'anatomie humaine*, vol 2, Paris, 1951, Masson.
26. Ponseti IV, Smoley EN: Congenital clubfoot: the results of treatment, *J Bone Joint Surg [Am]* 45:261, 1963.
27. Settle GW: The anatomy of congenital clubfoot talipes equinovarus: sixteen dissected specimens, *J Bone Joint Surg [Am]* 45:1341, 1963.
28. Smith WA, Campbell P, Bonnett C: Early posterior ankle release in treatment of congenital clubfoot, *Orthop Clin North Am* 7:889, 1976.
29. Swann M, Lloyd-Roberts GC, Catterall A: The anatomy of uncorrected club feet, *J Bone Joint Surg [Br]* 51:263, 1969.
30. Waisbrod H: Congenital clubfoot: an anatomical study, *J Bone Joint Surg [Br]* 55:796, 1973.
31. Wiley AM: Club foot: an anatomical and experimental study of muscle growth, *J Bone Joint Surg [Br]* 41:821, 1959.
32. Wynne-Davies R: Family studies and the cause of congenital club foot, *J Bone Joint Surg [Br]* 46:445, 1964.

Metatarsus Adductus and Metatarsus Varus

33. Berman A, Gartland JJ: Metatarsal osteotomy for the correction of adduction of the fore part of the foot in children, *J Bone Joint Surg [Am]* 53:498, 1971.
34. Bleck EE, Minaire P: Persistent medial deviation of the talar neck: a common cause of intoeing in children, American Academy of Orthopaedic Surgeons annual meeting, New Orleans, 1976.
35. Fowler B, Brooks AL, Parrish TF: The cavo-varus foot, *J Bone Joint Surg [Am]* 41:757, 1959.
36. Heyman CH, Herndon CH, Strong JM: Mobilization of the tarsometatarsal and intermetatarsal joints for the correction of resistant adduction of the fore part of the foot in congenital clubfoot and congenital metatarsus varus, *J Bone Joint Surg [Am]* 40:299, 1958.
37. Jacobs JE: Metatarsus varus and hip dysplasia, *Clin Orthop* 16:203–213, 1960.
38. Kendrick RE, Sharma NK, Hassler WE, et al: Tarsometatarsal mobilization for resistant adduction deformity of the fore part of the foot: a follow-up study, *J Bone Joint Surg [Am]* 52:61, 1970.
39. Kite JH: Congenital metatarsal varus, *J Bone Joint Surg [Am]* 32:500, 1950.
40. Kite JH: Congenital metatarsal varus, *J Bone Joint Surg [Am]* 49:388, 1967.
41. Lichtblau S: Section of the abductor hallucis tendon for correction of metatarsus varus deformity, *Clin Orthop* 110:227, 1975.

42. Lincoln CR, Wood KE, Bugg EI: Metatarsus varus corrected by open wedge osteotomy of the first cuneiform bone, *Orthop Clin North Am* 7:795, 1976.
43. Lloyd-Roberts GC, Clark CR: Ball and socket joint in metatarsus adductus varus, *J Bone Joint Surg [Br]* 55:193, 1973.
44. McCormick DW, Blount WP: Metatarsus adductovarus—"skewfoot," *JAMA* 141:449, 1949.
45. Peabody CW, Muro F: Congenital metatarsus varus, *J Bone Joint Surg* 15:171, 1933.
46. Ponseti IV, Becker JR: Congenital metatarsus adductus: the results of treatment, *J Bone Joint Surg [Am]* 48:702, 1966.
47. Reimann I: Congenital metatarsus varus: on the advantages of early treatment, *Acta Orthop Scand* 46:857, 1975.
48. Reimann I, Werner HH: Congenital metatarsus varus, *Clin Orthop* 110:223, 1975.
49. Specht EE: Major congenital deformities and anomalies of the foot. In Inman VT, editor: *DuVries' surgery of the foot*, ed 3, St Louis, 1973, Mosby–Year Book.
50. Wynne-Davies R: Family studies and the cause of congenital clubfoot: talipes equinovarus, talipes calcaneovalgus and metatarsus varus, *J Bone Joint Surg [Br]* 46:445, 1964.

Talipes Calcaneovalgus

50a. Bennett GL, Weiner DS, Heighler B, et al: Surgical treatment of symptomatic accessory tarsal navicular, *J Ped Orthop* 10:445, 1990.
51. Larsen B, Reimann I, Becker-Anderson H: Congenital calcaneovalgus with special reference to its treatment and its relation to other foot deformities, *Acta Orthop Scand* 45:145, 1974.
52. Wetzenstein H: Prognosis of pes calcaneovalgus congenita, *Acta Orthop Scand* 41:122, 1970.

Flatfoot

53. Bleck EE: The shoeing of children—sham or science? *Dev Med Child Neurol* 13:188, 1971.
54. Bleck EE, Berzins UE: Conservative management of pes valgus with plantar flexed talus, flexible, *Clin Orthop* 122:85, 1977.
55. Bordelon RL: Hypermobile flatfoot in children, *Clin Orthop* 181:7, 1983.
56. Chambers EFS: An operation for the correction of flexible flatfoot of adolescents, *Surg Gynecol Obstet* 54:77, 1946.
57. Crawford AH, Kucharzyk D, Roy DR, et al: Subtalar stabilization of the planovalgus foot by staple arthroereisis in young children who have neuromuscular problems, *J Bone Joint Surg [Am]* 72A:840–845, 1990.
58. Harris RI, Beath T: Hypermobile flatfoot with short tendo Achillis, *J Bone Joint Surg [Am]* 30:116, 1948.
59. Helfet AJ: A new way of treating flat feet in children, *Lancet* 1:262, 1956.
60. Henderson WH, Campbell JW: *UCBL shoe insert: casting and fabrication*, Technical Report 53, 1967, University of California, Berkeley, Biomechanics Laboratory.
61. Hoke M: An operation for the correction of extremely relaxed flat feet, *J Bone Joint Surg* 13:773, 1931.
62. Jack EA: Naviculo-cuneiform fusion in the treatment of flatfoot, *Am J Roentgenol* 35:75, 1953.
63. Kidner FC: The prehallux (accessory scaphoid) in its relation to flatfoot, *J Bone Joint Surg* 11:831, 1929.
64. Manicol JF, Voutsinas S: Surgical treatment of the symptomatic accessory navicular, *J Bone Joint Surg [Br]* 66:218–226, 1984.
65. Miller GR: Hypermobile flatfeet in children. *Clin Orthop* 122:95, 1977.
66. Miller OL: A plastic foot operation, *J Bone Joint Surg* 9:84, 1927.
67. Rose GK: Correction of the pronated foot, *J Bone Joint Surg [Br]* 44:642, 1962.
68. Sella EJ, Lawson JP, Ogden JA: The accessory navicular synchondrosis, *Clin Orthop* 209:280–285, 1986.
69. Semour N: The late results of naviculo-cuneiform fusion. *J Bone Joint Surg [Br]* 49:558, 1967.
70. Smith SD, Millar EA: Arthrorisis by means of a subtalar polyethylene peg implant for correction of hindfoot pronation in children, *Clin Orthop* 181:15, 1983.
70a. Sullivan JA, Miller WA: The relationship of the accessory navicular to the development of the flatfoot, *Clin Orthop* 144:233, 1979.
71. Templeton AW, McAlister WH, Zim ID: Standardization of terminology and evaluation of osseous relationships in congenitally abnormal feet, *Am J Roentgenol* 93:374, 1965.
72. Young CS: Operative treatment of pes planus, *Surg Gynecol Obstet* 68:1099, 1939.
73. Zadek I: The accessory tarsal scaphoid, *J Bone Joint Surg [Am]* 30:957, 1948.

Peroneal Spastic Flatfoot (Tarsal Coalition)

74. Badgley CE: Coalition of the calcaneus and navicular, *Arch Surg* 15:75, 1927.
75. Conway JJ, Cowell HR: Tarsal coalition: clinical significance and roentgenographic demonstration, *Radiology* 92:799, 1969.
76. Cowell HR: Diagnosis and management of peroneal spastic flatfoot, *Instr Course Lect* 24:94, 1975.
77. Cowell HR: Talocalcaneal coalition and new causes of peroneal spastic flatfoot, *Clin Orthop* 85:16, 1972.
77a. Deutsch AL, Resnick D, Campbell G: Computed tomography and bone scintigraphy in the evaluation of tarsal coalition, *Radiology* 144:137, 1982.
78. Harris RI: Rigid valgus foot due to talocalcaneal bridge, *J Bone Joint Surg [Am]* 37:169, 1955.
79. Harris RI, Beath T: Etiology of peroneal spastic flatfoot, *J Bone Joint Surg [Br]* 30:624, 1948.
80. Jayakumar S, Cowell HR: Rigid flatfoot, *Clin Orthop* 122:77, 1977.
81. Korvin H: Coalitio talocalcanea, *Z Orthop Chir* 60:105, 1934.
82. Leonard M: The inheritance of tarsal fusion and the relationship to spastic flatfoot, British Orthopaedic Research Society meeting, 1972.
83. Mosier K, Asher M: Tarsal coalitions and peroneal spastic flat foot—a review. *J Bone Joint Surg [Am]* 66:976, 1984.
83a. Olney BW, Asher MA: Excision of symptomatic coalition of the middle facet of the talonavicular joint, *J Bone Joint Surg* 69A:539, 1987.
84. Outland T, Murphy ID: The pathomechanics of peroneal spastic flat foot, *Clin Orthop* 16:64, 1960.
85. Pineda C, Resnick D, Greenway G: Diagnosis of tarsal coalition with computed tomography, *Clin Orthop* 208:282, 1986.

86. Scranton PE: Treatment of symptomatic talo-calcaneal coalitions, *J Bone Joint Surg [Am]* 69:533, 1987.
87. Slomann HC: On coalitio calcaneo-navicularis, *J Orthop Surg* 3:586, 1921.
88. Smith RW, Staple TW: Computerized tomography (CT) scanning technique for the hindfoot, *Clin Orthop* 177:34–38, 1983.
89. Stormont DM, Peterson HA: The relative incidence of tarsal coalition, *Clin Orthop* 181:28, 1983.
90. Wray JB, Herndon CH: Hereditary transmission of congenital coalition of the calcaneus to the navicular, *J Bone Joint Surg [Am]* 45:365, 1963.

Congenital Convex Pes Valgus (Congenital Vertical Talus)

91. Becker-Anderson H, Reimann I: Congenital vertical talus, *Acta Orthop Scand* 45:130, 1974.
92. Coleman SS, Jarrett J: Congenital vertical talus: pathomechanics and treatment, *J Bone Joint Surg [Am]* 48:1026, 1966.
93. Coleman SS, Stelling FH, Jarrett J: Pathomechanics and treatment of congenital vertical talus, *Clin Orthop* 70:62, 1970.
94. Colton CL: The surgical management of congenital vertical talus, *J Bone Joint Surg [Br]* 55:566, 1973.
95. Drennan JC, Sharrard WJ: The pathological anatomy of convex pes valgus. "Persian slipper foot," *J Bone Joint Surg [Br]* 53:455, 1971.
96. Eyre-Brook AL: Congenital vertical talus, *J Bone Joint Surg [Br]* 49:618, 1967.
97. Fitton JM, Nevelös AB: The treatment of congenital vertical talus, *J Bone Joint Surg [Br]* 61:481, 1979.
98. Hark FW: Rocker bottom foot due to congenital subluxation of the talus, *J Bone Joint Surg [Am]* 32:344, 1950.
99. Herndon CH, Heyman CH: Problems in the recognition and treatment of congenital convex pes valgus, *J Bone Joint Surg [Am]* 45:413, 1963.
100. Jayakumar S, Ramsey P: Vertical and oblique talus: a diagnostic dilemma, Scientific exhibit at the annual meeting of the American Academy of Orthopaedic Surgeons, Las Vegas, 1977.
101. Lamy L, Weissman L: Congenital convex pes valgus, *J Bone Joint Surg* 21:79, 1939.
102. Lloyd-Roberts GC, Spence AJ: Congenital vertical talus, *J Bone Joint Surg [Br]* 40:33, 1958.
103. Osmond-Clarke H: Congenital vertical talus in infancy, *J Bone Joint Surg [Br]* 48:578, 1966.
104. Patterson WR, Fritz DA, Smith WS: The pathologic anatomy of congenital convex pes valgus, *J Bone Joint Surg [Am]* 50:458, 1968.
105. Stone KH (for Lloyd-Robert GC): Congenital vertical talus: a new operation, *Proc R Soc Med* 56:12, 1963.

Arthrogryposis Multiplex Congenita

106. Adams RC, Denny-Brown D, Pearson CM: *Diseases of muscle: a study in pathology*, ed 2, New York, 1953, Harper & Brothers, 1953.
107. Banker BQ, Victor M, Adams RD: Arthrogryposis multiplex congenita due to congenital muscular dystrophy, *Brain* 80:319, 1957.
108. Carmack JC, Hallock H: Tibiotarsal arthrodesis after astragalectomy: a report of eight cases, *J Bone Joint Surg* 29:476, 1947.
109. Drachman DB, Banker BQ: Arthrogryposis multiplex congenita, *Arch Neurol* 5:77, 1961.
110. Drachman DB, Coulombre AJ: Experimental clubfoot and arthrogryposis multiplex congenita, *Lancet* 2:523, 1962.
111. Drummond DS, Cruess RL: The management of the foot and ankle in arthrogryposis multiplex congenita, *J Bone Joint Surg* [Br] 60:96, 1978.
112. Drummond D, Siller TN, Cruess RL: Management of arthrogryposis multiplex congenita, *Course Lect* 23:79, 1974.
113. Gibson DA, Urs NDK: Arthrogryposis multiplex congenita, *J Bone Joint Surg* [Br] 52:483, 1970.
114. Green A, Fixsen J, Lloyd-Roberts GC: Talectomy for arthrogryposis multiplex congenita, *J Bone Joint Surg* [Br] 66:697, 1984.
115. Lloyd-Roberts GC, Lettin AWF: Arthrogryposis multiplex congenita, *J Bone Joint Surg* [Br] 52:494, 1970.
116. Mead NL, Lithgow WC, Sweeney HJ: Arthrogryposis multiplex congenita, *J Bone Joint Surg* [Am] 40:1285, 1958.
117. Menelaus MB: Talectomy for equinovarus deformity in arthrogryposis and spina bifida, *J Bone Joint Surg* [Br] 53:468, 1971.
118. Middleton DE: Studies on prenatal lesions of skeletal muscle as a cause of congenital deformity. I. Congenital tibial kyphosis. II. Congenital high shoulder. III. Myodystrophia foetalis, *Edinburgh Med* 41:401, 1934.
119. Oh WH: Arthrogryposis multiplex congenita of the lower extremities: report of two siblings, *Orthop Clin North Am* 7:511, 1976.
119a. Sarwark JF, Macewen GD, Scott CI: Amyoplasia (a common form of arthrogryposis, *J Bone Joint Surg* 72A: 465, 1990.
120. Sheldon W: Amyoplasia congenita, *Arch Dis Child* 7:117, 1932.
121. Tompkins SF, Miller RJ, O'Donoghue DH: An evaluation of astragalectomy, *South Med J* 49:1128, 1956.

Abnormalities of Toes

122. Cockin J: Butler's operation for an overriding fifth toe, *J Bone Joint Surg* [Br] 50:78, 1968.
123. Farmer AW: Congenital hallux varus, *Am J Surg* 95:274, 1958.
124. Frazier TM: A note on race specific congenital malformation rates, *Am J Obstet Gynecol* 84:184, 1960.
125. Kelikian H: *Hallux valgus, allied deformities of the forefoot and metatarsalgia*, Philadelphia, 1965, WB Saunders, p 330.
126. Kelikian H, Clayton L, Loseff H: Surgical syndactylia of the toes, *Clin Orthop* 19:208, 1961.
127. Kessel L, Bonney G: Hallux rigidus in the adolescent, *J Bone Joint Surg* [Br] 40:668, 1958.
128. Kirtland LR, Russell RO: Polydactyly: report of a large kindred, *South Med J* 69:436, 1976.
129. Lapidus PW: Transplantation of the extensor tendon for correction of the overlapping fifth toe, *J Bone Joint Surg* 24:555, 1942.
130. Leonard MH, Rising EH: Syndactylization to maintain correction of overlapping 5th toe, *Clin Orthop* 43:241, 1965.
131. McElvenny RT: Hallux varus, *Q Bull Northwest Univ Med Sch* 15:277, 1941.

132. McKusick VA: *Mendelian inheritance in man: catalogues of autosomal dominant, autosomal recessive, and X-linked phenotypes,* ed 2, Baltimore, 1968, Johns Hopkins.
132a. Mubarak SJ, O'Brien TJ, Davids JR, et al: Metatarsal epiphyseal bracket; treatment by central epiphysiolysis, presented at the Pediatric Orthopedic Society of North America, May, 1992.
133. Nathan PA, Keniston RC: Crossed polydactyly: case report and review of the literature, *J Bone Joint Surg [Am]* 57:847, 1975.
134. Phelps OA, Grogan DP: Polydactyly of the foot, *J Pediatr Orthop* 5:446, 1985.
135. Robertson WW: The bifid great toe: a surgical approach, *J Pediatr Orthop* 7:25, 1987.
136. Scrase WH: The treatment of dorsal adduction deformities of the fifth toe, *J Bone Joint Surg [Br]* 36:146, 1954.
137. Sharrard WJW: The surgery of deformed toes in children, *Br J Clin Pract* 17:263, 1963.
138. Sweetman R: Congenital curley toe: an investigation into the value of treatment, *Lancet* 2:398, 1958.
139. Tachdjian MO: *Pediatric orthopaedics,* Philadelphia, 1972, WB Saunders.
140. Thompson SA: Hallux varus and metatarsus varus, *Clin Orthop* 16:109, 1960.
141. Zimbler S, Craig C, Oh WH, et al: Exhibit presented at the annual meeting of the American Academy of Orthopaedic Surgeons, Las Vegas, 1977.

Torsional Deformities of Lower Extremity

142. Engel GM, Staheli LT: The natural history of torsion and other factors influencing gait in childhood: a study of the angle of gait, tibial torsion, knee angle, hip rotation and development of the arch in normal children, *Clin Orthop* 99:12–17, 1974.
143. Fabray G, MacEwen GD, Shands AR Jr: Torsion of the femur, *J Bone Joint Surg [Am]* 55:1726, 1973.
144. Hensinger RF: Rotational problems of the lower extremity, *Postgrad Med* 60:161, 1976.
145. MacEwen GD: Anteversion of the femur, *Postgrad Med* 60:154, 1976.
146. Staheli L: Rotational problems of the lower extremities, *Orthop Clin North [Am]* 18:563, 1987.
147. Staheli L, Corbett M, Wyss C, et al: Lower extremity rotational problems in children, normal values to guide management, *J Bone Joint Surg [Am]* 67:39, 1985.

ADDITIONAL READINGS

Clubfoot

Cowell HR, Wein BK: Current concepts review: genetic aspects of club foot, *J Bone Joint Surg [Am]* 62:1381–1384, 1980.

Grider TD, Siff SJ, Gerson P, et al: Arteriography in clubfoot, *J Bone Joint Surg [Am]* 64:837–840, 1982.

Lloyd-Roberts GC: Congenital clubfoot, *J Bone Joint Surg [Br]* 46:369, 1964.

Turco VJ: Resistant congenital clubfoot, *Instr Course Lect* 24:104, 1975.

Turco VJ: Surgical correction of the resistant clubfoot, *J Bone Joint Surg [Am]* 53:477, 1971.

Metatarsus Varus

Helbing C: Ueber den Metatarsus varus, *Dtsch Med Wochenschr* 21:1312, 1905.

Flatfeet

Bordelon RL: Correction of hypermobile flatfoot in children by inserts, *Foot Ankle* 1:143, 1980.

Lusted LB, Keats TE: *Atlas of roentgenographic measurements,* ed 2, St Louis, 1967, Mosby–Year Book.

SECTION

IX

TRAUMA

CHAPTER

32

Soft-Tissue Trauma—Acute and Chronic Management

Mark Myerson, M.D.

General principles in the initial evaluation and determination of salvageability

Initial treatment

Zone of injury

Acute compartment syndrome

Specific requirement of foot and ankle coverage

Primary closure with or without skeletal shortening: Coverage of hallux and digital amputations
Skin grafting
Split-thickness skin excision
Transpositional and island pedicle flaps
Free tissue flaps
Cross-leg flaps

Chronic compartment syndromes of the foot

This chapter will cover many aspects of trauma to the foot and ankle but will focus more specifically on injury to the soft tissues. This will encompass both open and closed injuries, crush injuries, and compartment syndromes and will provide guidelines for determining salvageability of the foot. The evaluation and treatment of chronic foot pain and the sequelae of untreated compartment syndromes and nerve injury are also discussed. The chapter has been divided for convenience and ease of reference into the following sections:

1. General principles in initial evaluation and guidelines for salvage
2. The zone of injury
3. Acute compartment syndromes
4. Options for soft-tissue coverage
   a. Skeletal shortening and primary closure
   b. Split-thickness skin grafting
   c. Split-thickness skin excision
   d. Local rotation flaps
   e. Free tissue transfer
   f. Cross-leg flaps
5. Coverage of hallux and digital amputations
6. Chronic compartment syndromes

GENERAL PRINCIPLES IN THE INITIAL EVALUATION AND DETERMINATION OF SALVAGEABILITY

It is essential to obtain a thorough history of the circumstances of the injury and to perform a consistent and complete initial examination of the foot since both have significant implications for subsequent treatment. The history should include the mechanism of injury, duration of potential ischemia, and any known environmental pathogens, particularly since these may be associated with subsequent infection. Agricultural, immersion, industrial, and household injuries are associated with different organisms, and appropriate and timely antibiotic prophylaxis should be instituted.[12] Crush injuries of the foot occur under many different circumstances, and it is often helpful to know the type or mechanism of the force involved. Generally, the amount of force or energy expended on injury to the foot is determined by the mass and acceleration of the vehicle, both of which have a bearing on the magnitude and outcome of injury and treatment. All injuries associated with an element of crushing should be carefully examined for a compartment syndrome.[36, 37] The duration of elapsed time since the injury and the patient's age, activity level, occupation, and expectations regarding the outcome of treatment are all relevant. Pertinent medical information, including diabetes and cardiovascular disease, also have a bearing on the initial treatment and subsequent decision making, particularly in the case of attempted salvage of the foot in severe trauma.

The wound should be carefully inspected for the approximate extent of tissue loss and any exposed tendons, nerves, vessels, bones, and joints identified.[40,47,48] Any manipulation of the foot at this stage is extremely painful for the patient, and the goal of examination here is to determine in general what the treatment alternatives are. If articular surfaces, bone, or tendon is exposed, this may limit the options available for simpler forms of coverage. This initial assessment is therefore directed toward the immediate operative course to be taken, with particular emphasis on salvageability. This decision is best made early, if possible, in the emergency department. The emergency department is, however, not the ideal setting to carefully examine the foot. The lighting is often inadequate, contaminated wounds appear far worse prior to definitive irrigation and debridement, and decision making is often influenced by the overall apprehension of the patient. One may there-

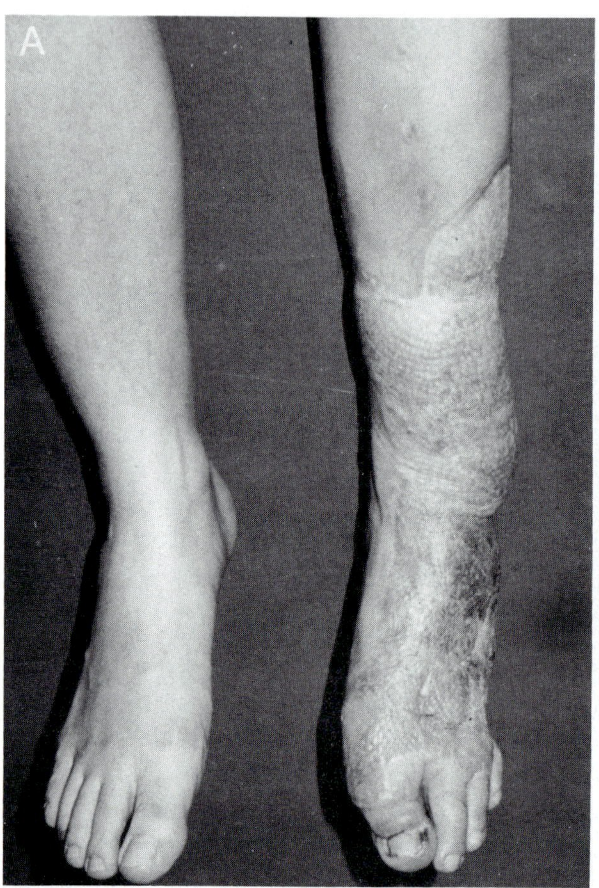

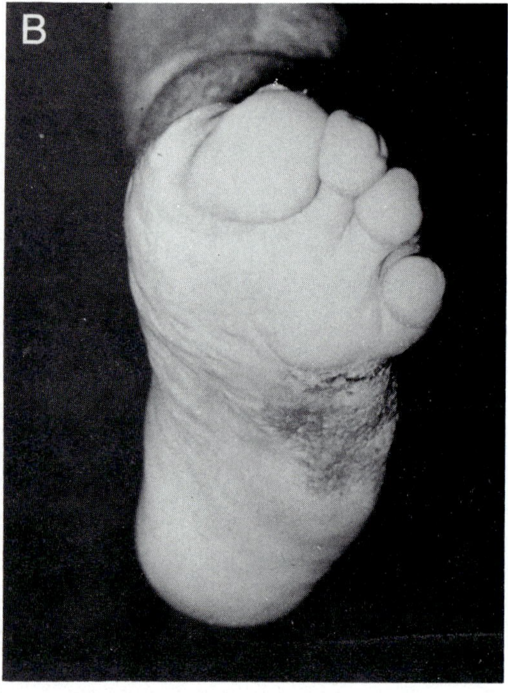

FIG 32–1.
This patient sustained a severe crush injury to her foot and ankle, predominantly involving the dorsal and lateral aspects. Soft-tissue coverage was achieved with extensive free tissue transference for split-thickness skin grafting **(A).** She has a painful deformed foot that is stiffened in equinovarus. Partial plantar tissue loss is present **(B).** After 2 years of repeated salvage attempts aimed at achieving a plantigrade foot, this patient acknowledged that she would have been better off with an amputation at the time of her injury.

fore misinterpret the severity of the injury initially, and where possible, it is best to defer decision making regarding salvage until the initial evaluation has been thoroughly completed in the operating room. Despite this, it is probably best to communicate all concerns to the patient and family immediately. We have experienced problems with the patient who has expectations regarding the outcome of treatment that are nurtured by unrealistic attempts at salvage.[14, 15] While one cannot reliably predict the outcome following initial treatment, it is useful to use sound judgment to determine the likelihood of success of salvage or the need for amputation. This should be determined before the patient becomes attached to the foot (no pun intended). It becomes increasingly difficult for both the physician and the patient to accept the necessity of an amputation following repeated early operative procedures. We are unfortunately all too familiar with the patient who years following salvage of severe extremity trauma requests an amputation that should have been done during the initial course of treatment.

Having said this, it is becoming increasingly difficult to determine which wounds are beyond the scope of salvage. With increasing experience in microvascular repair and free tissue transfer there are few severe wounds of the foot and ankle that cannot be covered.[8, 31, 45] There are, however, certain patterns of injury that are better off with a primary amputation. Injuries associated with neurovascular deficit should be very carefully assessed, particularly if the plantar weight-bearing surfaces of the foot are involved.[33] While it is possible to cover all plantar deficits, tissue loss rarely occurs without injury to the skeletal structures. One should appreciate the overall injury to the joints and bones, particularly of the hindfoot and ankle. If one can anticipate the potential need for immediate or delayed arthrodesis of the hindfoot or ankle, salvage of plantar deficits may not be advisable. The more rigid the foot, the less able the patient is to compensate for any structural alterations on the weight-bearing surface of the foot. Following multiple reconstructive procedures each followed by prolonged immobilization, the foot is often markedly stiff. This is poorly tolerated under normal circumstances, but made far worse in the presence of inadequate plantar soft tissues, particularly if insensate. Loss of motion may of course be present even without arthrodesis, and if the foot is structurally altered or deformed, tissue breakdown will occur regardless of the method of coverage (Fig 32–1). Even if sensate, deformity is not well tolerated if it involves the weight-bearing surfaces, and if this is associated with significant plantar soft-tissue loss, an amputation may be prudent. Extensive dorsal soft-tissue loss is well tolerated and rarely necessitates amputation (Fig 32–2). A lack of plantar sensation is reasonably tolerated, particularly if this does not involve major portions of the weight-bearing sur-

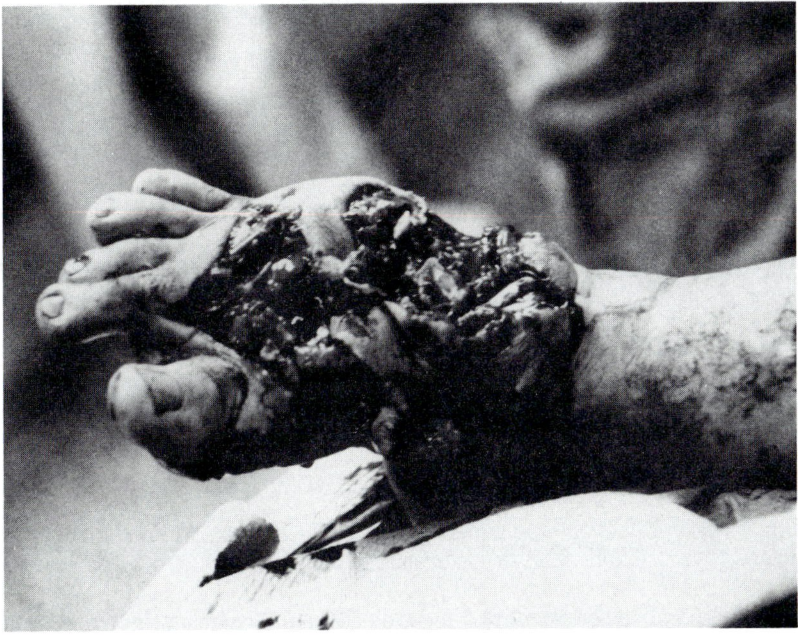

FIG 32–2.
This patient sustained a crush injury of the foot when run over by a tractor trailer. Despite the mangled appearance, crushing and soft-tissue loss were limited to the dorsal aspect of the foot. Following rigid internal fixation of the fracture dislocation, dorsal soft-tissue coverage was attained with a free tissue transfer using a fasciocutaneous flap.

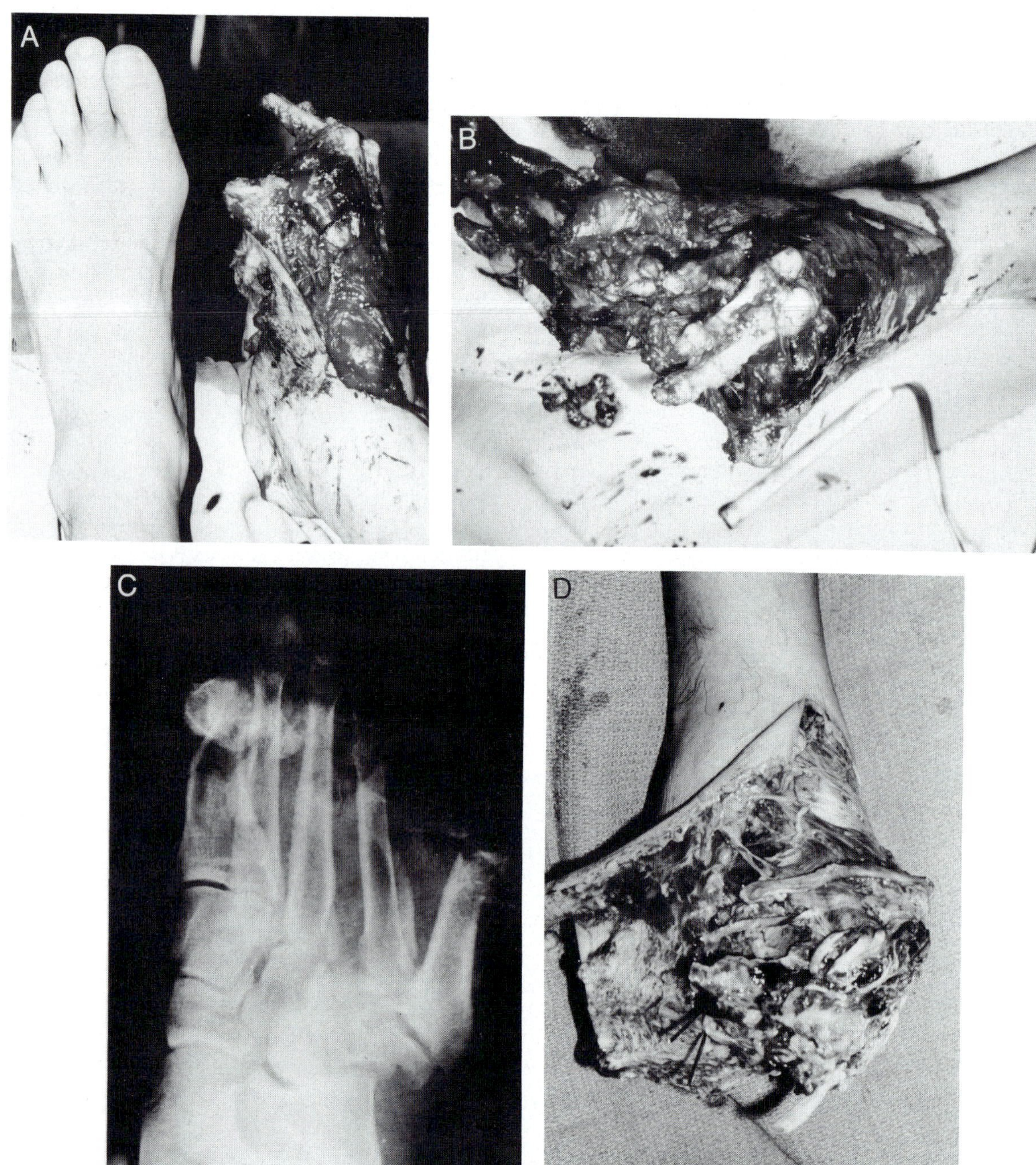

FIG 32–3.
This patient sustained a crush injury to the foot in a railway accident. Severe degloving of the dorsal and plantar surfaces **(A** and **B)** was further associated with a Lisfranc fracture dislocation **(C).** This was treated with debridement; skeletal shortening to a short transmetatarsal amputation; open reduction and rigid internal fixation of the dislocation; local rotation flaps using the abductor hallucis, flexor brevis, and abductor digiti quinti muscles **(D);** and immediate coverage using the technique of split-thickness skin excision **(E).** The capillary bleeding indicates the viable margin of the skin flap. Complete coverage was performed in one operative procedure **(F).**

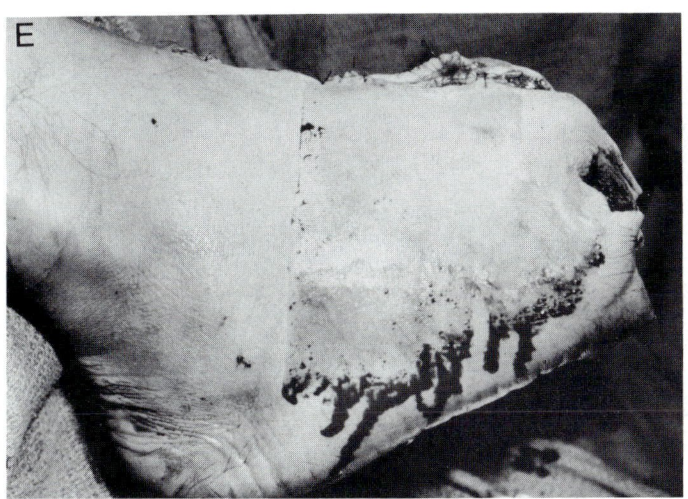

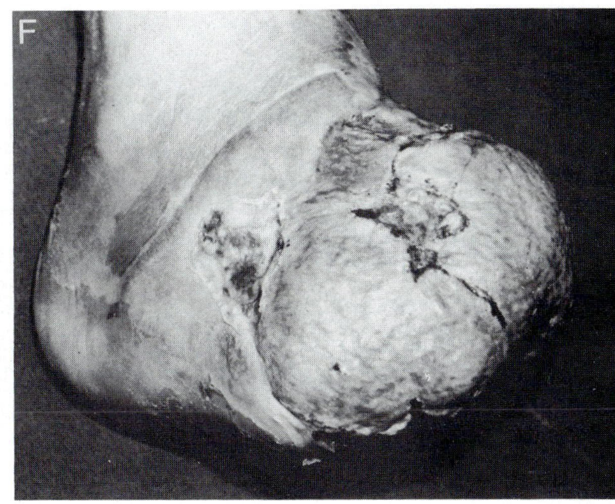

FIG 32–3 *(cont.)*.

face.[7, 32, 38, 44] However, if this insensitivity is associated with deformity of either the forefoot or hindfoot, recurrent ulceration and infection are likely. The same concerns apply to severe avulsion injuries associated with bone and joint injury. If the foot is mobile and the range of motion, particularly in the hindfoot and ankle, is relatively normal, then salvage may be worth the effort. This is well demonstrated in the patient in Figure 32–3,A and B, who sustained a crush injury of the foot between the couplings of a train. On initial evaluation, significant dorsal soft-tissue loss extending up to the ankle was present. Plantar skin was partially present but not viable. A severe fracture dislocation of the tarsometatarsal joint was present (Fig 32–3,C). Options for treatment would have included skeletal shortening and a hindfoot amputation, free tissue transfer to preserve the length of the foot, or the use of local rotation flaps to cover the distal weight-bearing surface of the foot. Since the remainder of the hindfoot and ankle was normal, maximum preservation of tissue and length of the foot was attempted by using a combination of local rotation muscle flaps and the technique of split-thickness skin excision (STSE) (see below) (Fig 32–3,D). Despite the application of a split-thickness skin graft over the distal plantar weight-bearing surface of the foot, no breakdown has occurred over the past 4 years, probably due to the mobility of the ankle and hindfoot. The same principles that apply to salvage of foot injury with soft-tissue coverage procedures have relevance to replantation and revascularization of the foot. Replantation efforts in the foot have lagged behind those of the upper extremity, perhaps due to the ready availability of satisfactory partial-foot and below-knee prostheses. There have been numerous isolated reports of replantation of the foot, but these are insufficient to make strong recommendations for salvage.[19, 21–23, 30, 39] We have had limited experience with replantation and, despite a few successes, have much to learn regarding the ideal candidate for replantation. Our philosophy is that all amputated parts[26] may potentially be salvaged with replantation. This enhances our understanding of these injuries, and with increasing experience we hope to refine this further. Salvage efforts should be coordinated and readily available and require the combined expertise of microvascular and orthopaedic services. It has been our experience that children are more suitable candidates for revascularization, and to this end we are prepared to salvage most amputation injuries in the child provided that considerable crushing and avulsion has not occurred. Unfortunately, nerve injuries are usually complex and difficult to repair since most are associated with tearing and not simple laceration. Insensibility is, however, less of a consideration provided that the foot is well perfused since adequate coverage can be provided with free tissue transfer. The insensate foot that lacks adequate perfusion should probably not be salvaged. Severe degloving or avulsion injuries of the plantar weight-bearing surface of the foot are difficult to salvage (Fig 32–4). Soft-tissue loss of limited portions of the plantar surfaces can be successfully covered, but not if the deficit includes both the heel and metatarsal weight-bearing surfaces. Avulsion of the heel pad may be successfully restored with revascularization provided that this is an isolated injury and marked crushing has not occurred. Consideration for primary amputation must also be made in the context of the severity of injury and individual patient needs.

Before embarking on complex coverage techniques one should therefore clearly define the intended goals, which must be individualized for each patient. In addi-

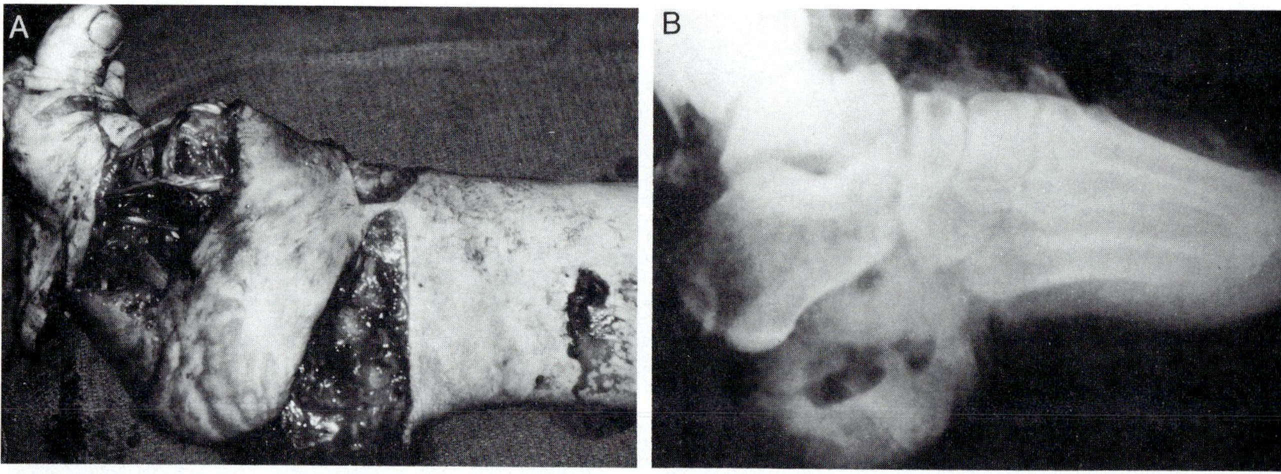

FIG 32–4.
This degloving injury of the foot occurred in an industrial accident (**A** and **B**). In addition to the heel pad avulsion, significant crushing and avulsion of the plantar and dorsal surfaces of the foot are present. This should not be salvaged.

tion to plantar sensation, the duration of ischemia associated with vascular insufficiency and the potential for repair must be determined. The patient's age, occupation, and expectations must be considered prior to initiating a course of treatment often associated with multiple surgical procedures and a prolonged recovery extending over several years. One should always consider amputation positively in an effort to minimize overall morbidity and not as a failure of treatment.

INITIAL TREATMENT

Once it has been decided to proceed with reconstruction, it should be performed with the goal of maximizing function in the absence of infection. Additional considerations include limited scarring, cosmesis, and the ability to wear normal footwear. Treatment should be commenced immediately, with wound cultures, prophylactic wound-specific broad-spectrum antibiotics, followed by definitive and repeated surgical debridement as needed.[1,3,5] For minor open injuries of the foot, we use a second-generation cephalosporin antibiotic for 2 days postoperatively or until coverage is obtained. For significantly contaminated wounds, agricultural accidents, and those where deep soft-tissue planes are involved with potential contaminants and debris that are not identified, we use a combination of penicillin, clindamycin, and gentamicin for 3 days or until the wound is covered.[24,25,27,28,41] It is useful to have a standardized protocol for treating these injuries. In the emergency department only one member of the orthopaedic team should evaluate the injury. A common problem that occurs in this setting is the curiosity of various staff members to inspect these severe, sometimes "sensational" wounds. Repeated dressing changes are extremely painful for the patient and are associated with an increased incidence of contamination and subsequent infection. Following a thorough evaluation along the lines mentioned above and a careful neurovascular examination, cultures are obtained and a regional ankle block administered. We use a mixture of 10 cc of 1% lidocaine and 10 cc of ½% bupivicaine, both without epinephrine, and block the tibial, superficial and deep peroneal, and if necessary, the sural nerves. This is extremely effective in alleviating pain and allaying anxiety and in many circumstances allows us to perform a more complete examination immediately. Minor open wounds of the toes and forefoot can be treated immediately in the emergency department following the administration of an adequate ankle block. Most patients are not adequately prepared for emergency surgery under general anesthesia, and since a delay in performing the initial debridement is associated with an increased incidence of infection, immediate treatment is a distinct advantage. This works particularly well with the cooperation of the staff in the emergency department since debridement with thorough and copious irrigation is the mainstay of treatment for these wounds.[2, 3, 11, 12, 13, 29, 43] This, however, tends to create quite a mess unless an adequate catchment is available to contain this irrigation. We manage this by suspending the foot over the edge of the stretcher and irrigate directly into a large trash bin.

THE ZONE OF INJURY

The injury to the foot is often far worse than what is immediately and grossly apparent. There is always an extended area of pathologic involvement involving soft tissue and bone beyond the point of impact on the foot. This we refer to as the zone of injury. This has significant implications for treatment since the extent of the zone of injury is often underestimated. Although this extended area at risk is a common problem associated with crushing, it is present with almost all injuries to the soft-tissue envelope as well as bone, regardless of the mechanism of injury.[35]

Since we are accustomed to debriding only what is obviously nonviable, there is a tendency to underestimate and possibly inadequately treat these injuries.[16] The absolute extent of this extended zone of injury is never apparent macroscopically and, as such, forms the basis for serial debridement of soft tissue and bone. This is integral to successful management of the wound since all nonviable tissue has to be removed prior to definitive wound closure or coverage. It is frequently advocated that one let the wound settle down over a few days until the true extent of the injury becomes apparent. In this manner, the nonviable areas become demarcated, and final debridement is more easily accomplished. This problem of gradual demarcation of the wound is well illustrated in the patient in Figure 32–5, a 54-year-old male whose foot was crushed between the couplings of a train. Although the overall appearance of the foot is relatively benign and the only fracture was a small avulsion off the base of the first metatarsal, the extended zone of injury is clearly evident. The patient refused to undergo a more aggressive form of treatment, which may have included free tissue transfer, and we awaited demarcation of the nonviable tissue. However, over the ensuing 10 days he developed a severe infection of the plantar fascial spaces that significantly compromised any form of delayed coverage. This was finally achieved 5 weeks later with split-thickness skin grafts. This "wait-and-see" approach is not ideal, and under most circumstances, the earlier definitive coverage is obtained, the less the likelihood of wound compromise, infection, and failure. I believe that we are by nature either "debriders or keepers," some of us being more inclined to let things be and others treating nonvitalized areas of bone and soft tissue more aggressively. One should certainly be loathe to remove potentially viable tissue, particularly if these are vital structures or integral constituents of form and function.[69] Yet, one does not want to face an ever-expanding area of necrosis due to inadequate debridement. This occurs due to an expanding zone of cellular necrosis associated with edema and finally followed by increased focal fibrosis and stiffness.

Certain exposed tissues such as cortical bone, articular cartilage, and tendon devoid of peritenon do not survive if exposed. One is therefore faced with the dilemma of covering these wounds as soon as possible to protect the underlying structures but recognizing the increased potential for infection where the recipient bed is marginal. In fact, as is discussed below, the risk of infection is actually less following immediate coverage. As an alternative to early coverage, one can attempt to keep these vital structures viable with moist or wet dressing changes performed every 6 to 8 hours (Fig 32–6). The goal of this form of treatment is the formation of granulation tissue that would support a simpler form of coverage such as a split-thickness skin graft. Unfortunately, we have found that these tissues invariably desiccate despite wet dressings, and one is faced with an extending margin of necrosis. In these patients, one may end up sacrificing tissue, perhaps vital structures that may have been preserved by earlier coverage. This is well illustrated in a patient whom we treated for salvage of a crush injury of his foot and ankle that was sustained in an industrial accident. The wound was apparently initially clean, but the anterior tibial tendon was exposed. During the ensuing 4 days, the tendon and the articular surface of the ankle desiccated. Although a free flap had been planned all along, the tendon had to be sacrificed, and an ankle fusion was performed. The flap failed, however, and the recipient bed was ultimately covered with a split-thickness skin graft. This patient presented to us for treatment 6 months later with a very stiff foot positioned in equinovarus. This was eventually salvaged with a triple arthrodesis and extensive releases of fixed-toe deformities. This postoperative course was also complicated, perhaps not unexpectedly, by a minor dorsomedial wound slough and a nonunion of the talonavicular joint, which was treated by repeat arthrodesis with a bone graft and split-thickness skin grafting for a second wound slough. This patient is currently ambulatory and, despite intermittent aching and complaints of stiffness, functions reasonably well. This scenario is unfortunately not uncommon and could potentially have been avoided with earlier coverage. Even had the anterior tibial tendon been lost, the best alternative for treatment would have been an early free flap followed by a tendon graft or transfer to maintain dorsiflexion at a later stage.

There are clearly significant advantages to a more aggressive approach to debridement and definitive earlier coverage. It has been our bitter experience that the longer we wait before final coverage, the greater the incidence of wound contamination, bacterial colonization, and infection.[16, 17, 18, 42, 49, 62] On occasion this is determined by the condition of the wound, but also due to patient problems and physician prevarication. Perhaps the milestone in the treatment of these complex open extremity injuries came out of Yugoslavia approxi-

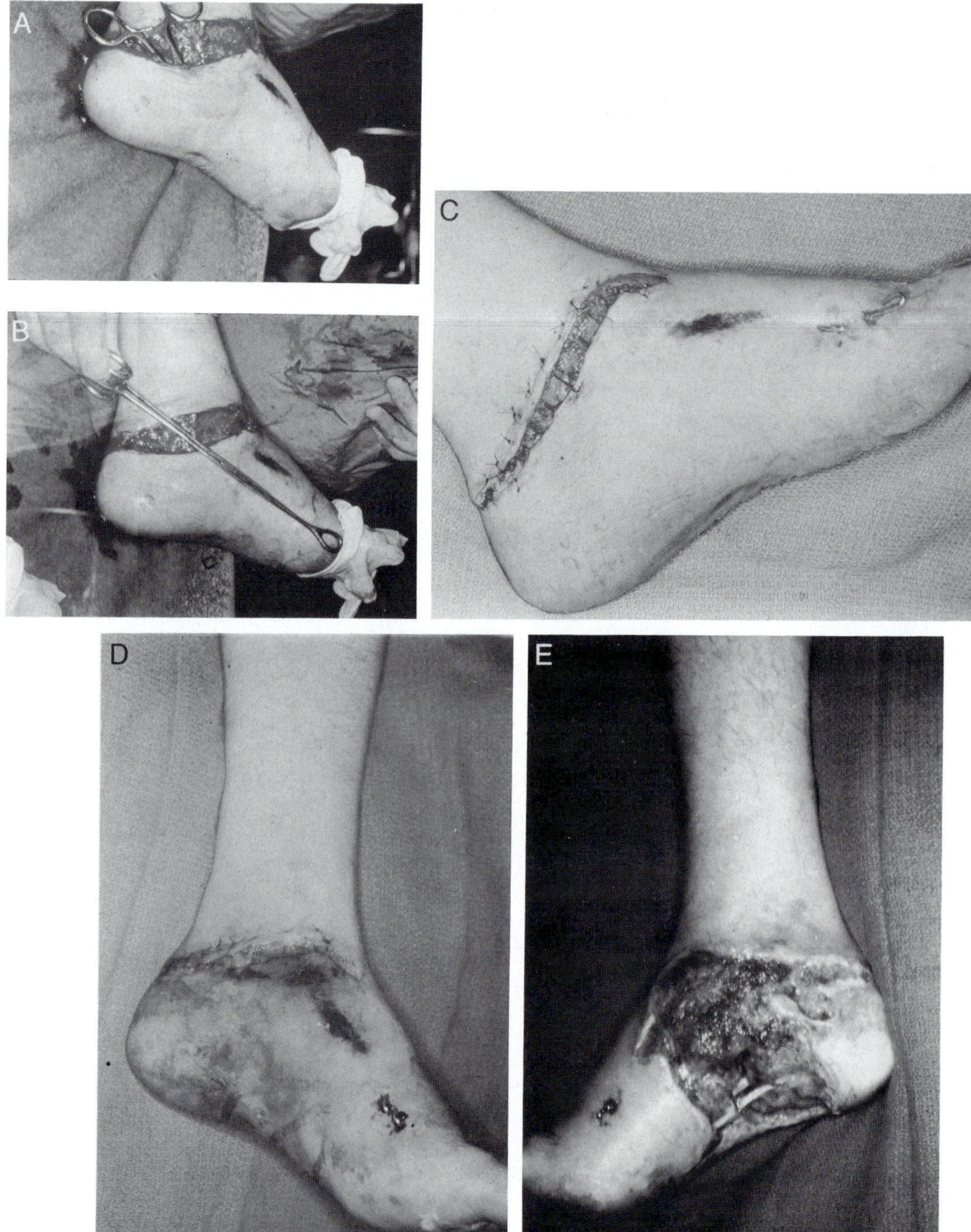

FIG 32–5.
This patient sustained a crush injury to the foot and ankle in a railway accident. On presentation, significant degloving of the subcutaneous tissue was evident **(A** and **B)**. This patient refused a more aggressive treatment approach to the wound, which was sutured with minimal tension **(C)**. Not unexpectedly, most of the skin flap was nonviable and underwent necrosis **(D)**. This was followed by severe infection **(E** and **F)** and finally covered with a split-thickness skin graft **(G)**, with ultimate healing.

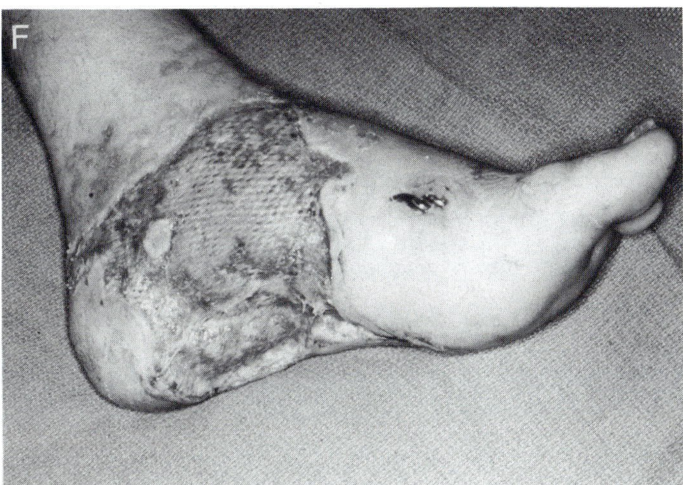

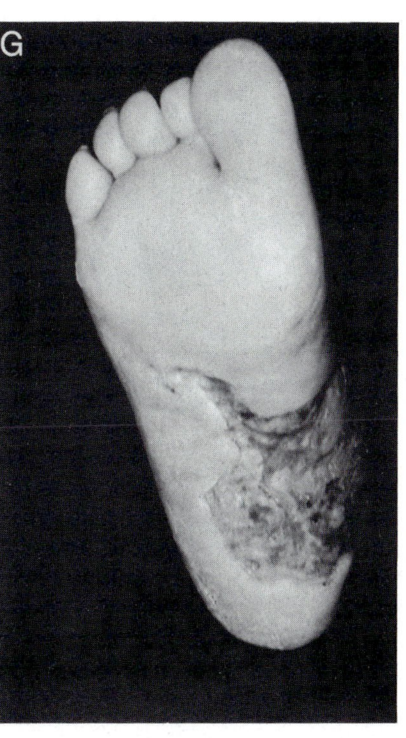

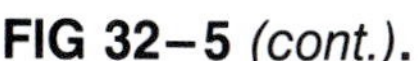

FIG 32–5 *(cont.).*

mately 6 years ago. In a series of 532 patients undergoing microsurgical reconstruction following extremity trauma, Godina demonstrated far better results if closure was performed within the initial 72 hours following injury. Early coverage provided an overall lower failure rate, decreased infection rate, fewer overall operations, an increased rate of bone union, and a decreased hospital stay.[52] Godina demonstrated failure rates of 0.75% for early (less than 72 hours) microsurgical procedures as compared with 12% when performed between 72 hours and 3 months and 9% if later than 3 months. These results were attributed to increased fibrosis in the wounds that were treated in the delayed and later groups. It was found that this fibrosis extended up to 10 cm from the wound into all tissues, including tendons, muscles, and neurovascular structures. The infection rate in this series was highest in the delayed reconstructions (17.5%) as compared with 6% in the late reconstructions and 1.5% in the early group. These concepts have since been verified repeatedly, and the current treatment recommended to maximize fracture union rate and decrease infection is with early soft-tissue coverage.

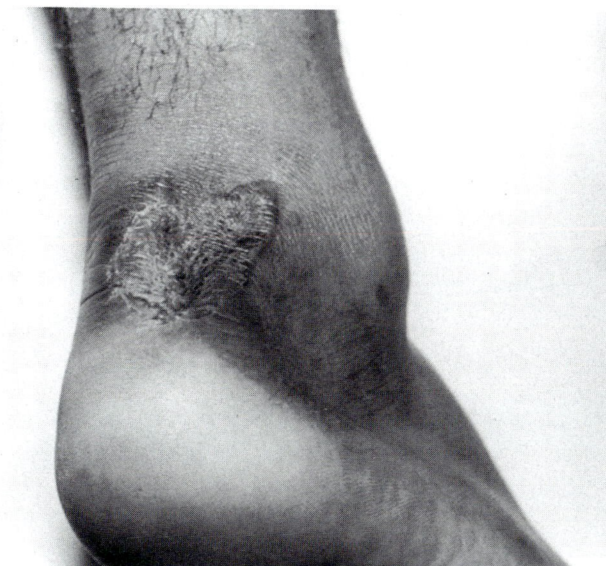

FIG 32–6.
This patient lost most of the lateral soft-tissue support in the retrocalcaneal space, and the lateral half of the Achilles tendon was exposed and found to be devoid of peritenon. This was treated with wet to dry dressings, followed by the application of a split-thickness skin graft.

Whatever the choice and form of soft-tissue coverage, we too have found that a more aggressive approach to obtaining earlier coverage has led to our most optimal results. A delay in coverage is associated with an increasing zone of injury and a progression of the level of unusable recipient vessels. We treat approximately 30 to 40 patients every season with lawn mower injuries to the foot and have found that delayed coverage of these wounds was also associated with an increased incidence of infection and failure of coverage.[10, 20] Significant contamination and devitalization of tissue is present in these wounds, and it is tempting to return the patient to the operating room every 48 hours for serial debridement.[9, 56, 63, 68] However, it is this remaining necrotic tissue that is the cause of infection and an extended zone of tissue loss and fibrosis. We have found that there is no substitute for meticulous debridement with loupe magnification. Following initial debridement and pulsatile lavage, no matter how thorough we have been, more debris and contaminants are found, and the process is laboriously continued and repeated until completely clean. This is particularly true for lawn mower injuries but also for any injuries that involve high energy, crushing, and contamination. Soil, grass, and other debris are embedded in multiple tissue planes and are difficult to remove even with lavage. (Fig 32–7). Lawn mower blades revolve at speeds of 2,000 to 3,000 rpm and with a kinetic energy greater than a low-velocity bullet.[55, 68] It is therefore important to carefully inspect between muscle and soft-tissue planes to look for more debris that can only be removed manually. A similar problem is encountered with a "road burn," where the dirt and gravel are extremely difficult to remove without mechanical abrasion. In addition to vigorous cleansing of the skin and exposed subcutaneous tissue with a sterile scrubbing brush, these tissues have to be sharply excised, often leaving large areas exposed that require skin grafting. When performing this debridement it is important to identify the branches of the superficial peroneal and sural nerves. It is preferable to preserve these nerves unless they are avulsed or crushed, in which case they should be sharply divided and buried in the nearest available muscle. On the dorsal surface of the foot, the nerve is usually buried in the

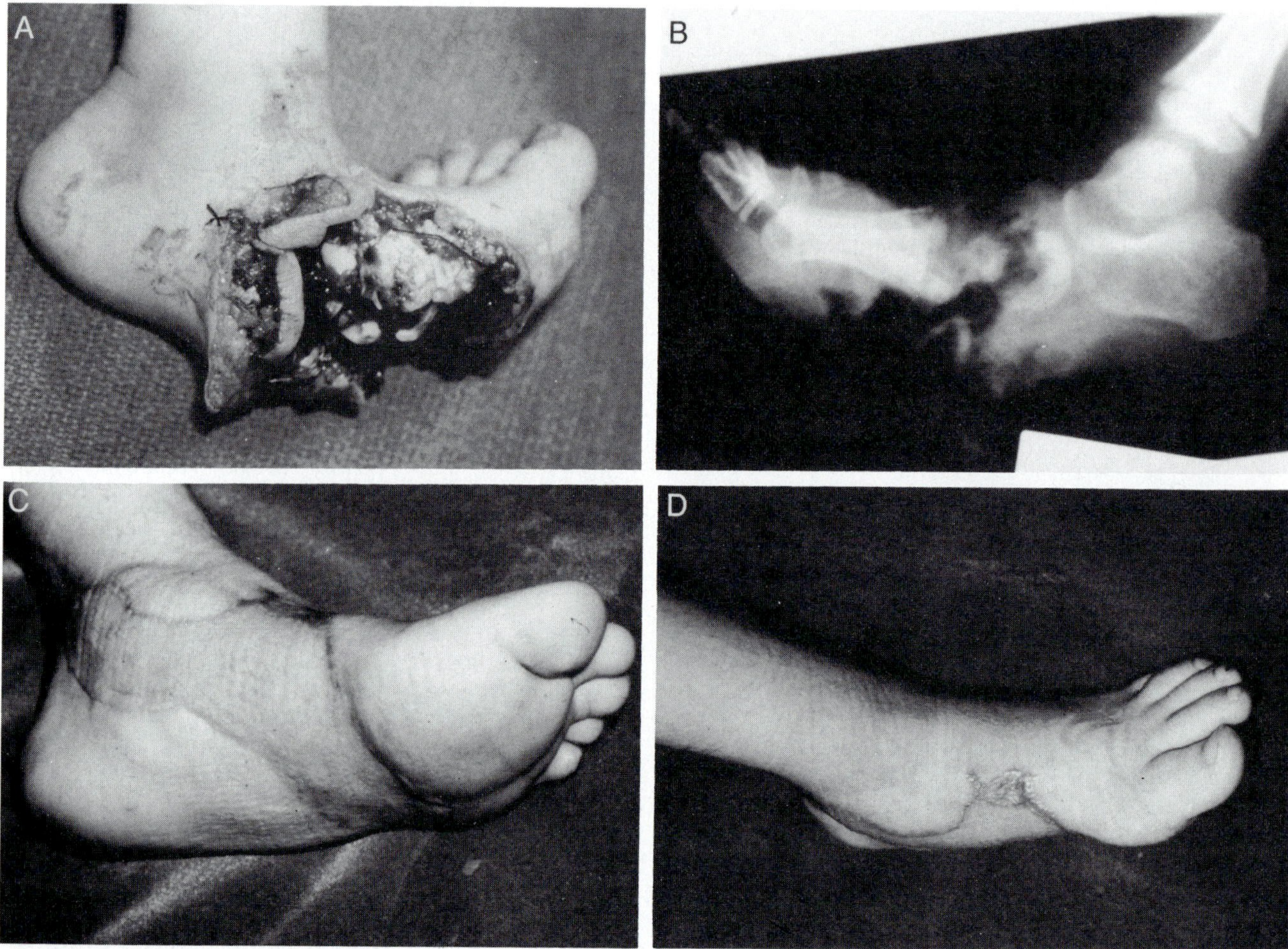

FIG 32–7.
A and **B,** this 4-year-old child sustained a partial foot amputation in a lawn mower accident. Following revascularization, meticulous debridement was performed. Despite the use of copious Parsiton lavage, glass and debris were still identified in the deeper muscle and soft-tissue planes. The debridement lasted approximately 2 hours and was followed around 24 hours later by further debridement and lavage and the application of a free gracilis flap. **C** and **D,** the final functional and cosmetic results 2 years later are excellent.

extensor brevis muscle by imbricating the muscle over the nerve with a buried absorbable 4–0 or 5–0 suture. With these avulsion shear-type injuries one should also try to preserve any peritenon over exposed tendons. The peritenon is often lacerated or avulsed and can be gently reapproximated and sutured with an absorbable 5–0 or 6–0 suture. A split-thickness skin graft will "take" over peritenon but not exposed tendon, and it is important to identify and preserve the peritenon. While this may not be significant for the intrinsic extensors, it is particularly relevant if the anterior or posterior tibial or peroneal tendons are involved. Another difficult wound to cleanse and debride is one contaminated with oil or grease. Degreasing agents can be purchased at the hardware or grocery store and are more effective than some of the more abrasive solvents that are commercially available. This requires frequent applications followed by pulsatile lavage.

It is important to recognize the zone of injury as early as possible and identify contused, crushed, and devitalized tissue in a reproducible, easy, and reliable manner. The conventional parameters used to determine tissue viability include color, bleeding, contractility, and consistency of muscle. These are unfortunately often inconclusive and do not allow a clear differentiation of viable from nonviable tissue. The differentiation of viable from nonviable tissue should ideally be performed in a bloodless field. In addition to thorough debridement of obviously necrotic muscle and contaminated tendon and bone, non essential vessels are ligated. We prefer not to excise any skin at this stage even if obviously nonviable since these contused skin flaps may be used as a donor site for a skin graft. Although debridement of grossly contaminated tissue is obvious, several more accurate methods are available to determine tissue viability and include fluorescein labeling, cutaneous capillary circulation using laser Doppler flowmetry, and STSE.

Fluorescein is a phenolphthalein dye that in the presence of an intact capillary circulation fluoresces when exposed to ultraviolet light.[54, 60, 61, 64] Fluorescence is a type of luminescence where light energy is absorbed without the dissipation of any energy.[64, 65, 66] Ultraviolet light affects the fluorescein molecule by raising an electron to a higher energy level and releasing a photon as the electron returns to its prior energy level, with resultant green fluorescence. The intensity of the fluorescence depends on the extracellular concentration of fluorescein in the skin rather than the absolute amount of blood flow or intravascular concentration. Fluorescein is quite nontoxic in the usual dose range of 10 to 15 mg/kg, and an allergic reaction is rare. I would recommend giving 1 cc intravenously as a test dose and the balance over a period of 5 minutes. Fluorescence is checked 15 minutes later when the peak extracellular concentration is reached. Fluorescein is rapidly excreted by the kidneys, and the intense yellow discoloration of the skin that occurs usually dissipates after 24 hours. I have used fluorescein testing frequently and have found it to be quite useful to delineate the extent of muscle and skin necrosis (Fig 32–8). We occasionally find it difficult to interpret the true extent of skin viability with fluorescein, partly due to bleeding from adjacent healthy tissue onto nonviable areas. In these and other patients we have used the technique of STSE to determine viability and have added it to our armamentarium for managing crush injuries of the foot associated with shearing and degloving of skin and subcutaneous tissue.[67, 71]

ACUTE COMPARTMENT SYNDROMES OF THE FOOT

A compartment syndrome develops as a result of an elevation of tissue fluid pressure within a closed space. The foot has numerous separate spaces or compartments rigidly bound by various osseous and fascial structures. Following injury, bleeding into these closed spaces elevates the local tissue fluid pressure. The compartment syndrome complex develops as the local tissue interstitial fluid pressure increases and capillary perfusion drops below what is required to maintain tissue viability. Due to the inelastic surrounding osseofascial structures, the elevated tissue pressure is not dissipated and, unless reduced, will eventually cause vascular occlusion and myoneural ischemia.

Many theories have been proposed to account for the sequence of events leading from tissue injury to myoneural ischemia. Experimental studies have demonstrated that tissue perfusion will progressively decrease as tissue compression increases and that blood flow in the microcirculation will stop when local tissue pressure equals the diastolic blood pressure.[72, 74] Blood ceases at levels below the mean arterial pressure secondary to passive capillary collapse when local tissue pressure increases above intracapillary pressure.[79] A currently accepted theory for the pathogenesis of compartmental ischemia involves local venous hypertension. Under normal circumstances, intravenous pressure must exceed the surrounding tissue pressure for the veins to remain patent. Local increases in venous pressure will reduce the arteriovenous gradient and will therefore reduce capillary blood flow.[73] When pressures are below diastolic levels, blood flow can then no longer sustain local metabolic demands. This is important since myoneural ischemia can therefore occur in the presence of arterial flow. This obviously has implications regarding evaluation and treatment of myoneural ischemia where pulses are still palpable in patients with actual or potential compartment syndromes. We have demonstrated that the pulses are not palpable in over 80% of these injuries, predominantly due to swelling, but that the pulse is almost always audible with Doppler ultrasound evaluation.[82] This concept has particular relevance in patients who have systemic hypotension inasmuch as they do not tolerate these lower pressures well and may require fasciotomy at a level lower than what is currently considered to be pathologic. Similarly, patients who are hypertensive will theoretically tolerate much higher levels of interstitial fluid pressure. Once established, the compartment syndrome complex will lead to vascular occlusion and myoneural ischemia, and if this ischemic process continues, irreparable damage occurs with myoneural necrosis and fibrosis.

The osseofascial spaces subdivide the foot into well-demarcated areas. For the purposes of understanding compartment syndromes, the foot is best viewed in coronal section (Fig 32–9). The medial compartment, which contains the abductor hallucis and flexor hallucis brevis muscles, is bounded medially and inferiorly by the extension of the plantar aponeurosis, laterally by an intermuscular septum, and dorsally by the first metatarsal. The central compartment contains (from plantar to dorsal) the flexor digitorum brevis, the lumbricales, the quadratus plantae, and the adductor hallucis muscles; its boundaries are the thick plantar aponeurosis inferiorly, the osseofascial tarsometatarsal structures dorsally, and the intermuscular septae medially and laterally. The lateral compartment contains the flexor, abductor, and opponens muscles of the fifth toe; its boundaries are the fifth metatarsal dorsally, the plantar aponeurosis inferiorly and laterally, and an intermuscular septum medially. The interosseous compartment contains the seven interossei and is bounded by the interosseous fascia and the metatarsal.[81, 85] Manoli has identified additional compartments, including a deep central compartment that contains the quadratus plantae muscle.[75] This we believe has particular relevance to calcaneus fractures. There are many other anatomic compartments of the foot that can be identified with appropriate dye or gelatin injection studies, but they have little clinical relevance. For practical purposes, although these osseofascial spaces provide the anatomic setting for a compartment syndrome, communication between them may occur during trauma due to disruption of the limiting fascial membranes. We have also noted experimentally that leakage of dye from one space into another occurs with high pressures.[34, 81] Under normal physiologic pressures, however, there is no communication or direct extension between the fascial spaces of the foot or the leg. We have delineated the experimental basis for fasciotomy in managing these injuries and concluded that alternative approaches to fasciotomy are available and equally effective in resolving the raised interstitial pressure. It was found that although the medial fasciotomy incision more rapidly decompressed the compartments than did fasciotomy through two dorsal incisions, either approach satisfactorily decompressed the measured compartments.[81]

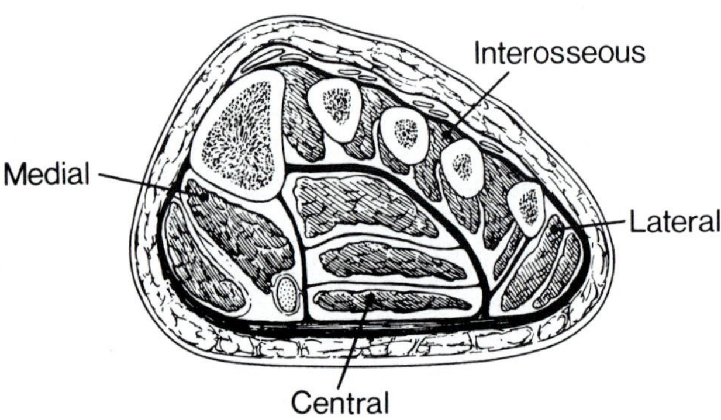

FIG 32–9.
On coronal section, many compartments of the foot may be identified. Each interosseous muscle is probably contained in a separate compartment but for practical purposes may be regarded as one. The medial, central, lateral, and interosseus compartments are illustrated in coronal section through the base of the metatarsals.

The foot is in an extremely vulnerable location and is particularly prone to isolated injury. Most of the devastating injuries of the feet associated with compartment syndromes that we treat are caused by various crushing forces (Fig 32–10). These patients typically present with massive swelling, and under these circumstances, the diagnosis is relatively obvious provided that one is aware of the potential for compartment syndromes. Most crushing-type injuries are associated with fractures and dislocations of the midfoot, yet the presence of an open fracture does not automatically decompress the fascial spaces of the foot. We have found that compartment syndromes may occur in open fractures of the foot with the same frequency as they occur with other open extremity fractures. The spectrum of injury causing compartment syndromes is varied. Although we associate compartment syndromes with crushing injury, they occur following almost any injury regardless of the mechanism or forces involved. One form of crush injury we commonly see is where the crushing force comes into contact with the foot over a gradual or slow period of time. This results in bursting of tissue, typically on the plantar aspect of the foot, and is akin to the wringer injury in the upper extremity. Despite the be-

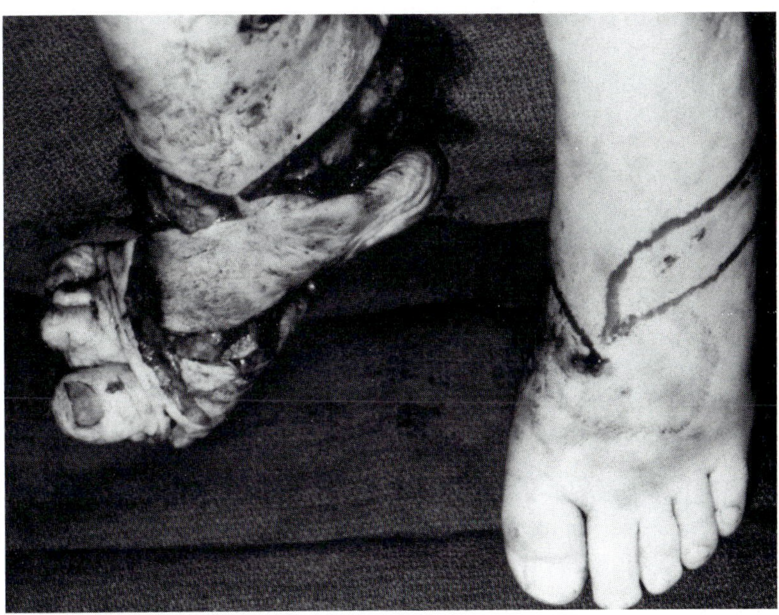

FIG 32–10.
This patient sustained bilateral crush injuries to the feet when they were struck by a 2-ton steel beam, with massive swelling in the left foot associated with an open fracture dislocation of the tarsometatarsal joint and a compartment syndrome. The right foot was not salvaged, and a below-knee amputation was performed.

nign appearance of the wound, significant degloving of the plantar subcutaneous tissue is present, and the skin envelope is often avulsed off the deeper fascial structures (Fig 32–11). Suffice it to say that compartment syndromes may occur in the setting of a variety of injuries to the foot, even calcaneus fractures. Over the years we have treated numerous patients with chronic sequelae following calcaneus fractures, some of whom manifested symptoms and signs of chronic myoneural ischemia. This prompted us to look more closely at the

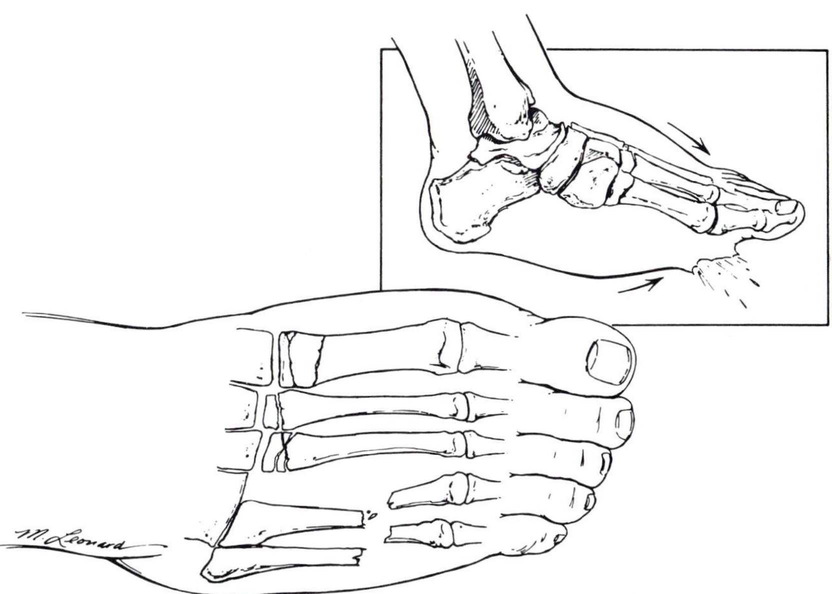

FIG 32–11.
If the crushing force comes into contact with the foot gradually, bursting of tissues on the plantar aspect of the foot may occur. Despite the open wound, these crush injuries are often associated with compartment syndromes.

potential for compartment syndromes associated with calcaneus fractures, regardless of the clinical findings, which may at times be quite misleading. We all recognize that profound pain and considerable swelling occur with calcaneus fractures, far more so than with other devastating fractures of the foot and ankle. This is probably related to the large bleeding cancellous bone surfaces and the limited osseofascial compartments into which this hematoma may be dissipated. While marked swelling may be suggestive of the possibility of a compartment syndrome, it is not diagnostic. The swelling associated with calcaneus fractures is usually significant but depends more on the duration from the time of injury and the intervening treatment prior to examination. The calcaneal compartment is small and contains only the quadratus muscle and the posterior tibial neurovascular bundle and branches. Interestingly, magnetic resonance imaging (MRI) can delineate the hematoma of a compartment syndrome, and although this is of academic interest only, it confirms the clinical findings by demonstrating the location of the hematoma. MRI should never be used to determine treatment since any delay may be associated with myoneural ischemia. The overall incidence of compartment syndromes associated with calcaneus fractures at our institution is approximately 10%, although this probably depends to some extent on the circumstances of the injury.

As demonstrated with compartment syndromes of the foot in other settings, the only reliable method of diagnosis is by clinical suspicion and measurement of raised intracompartmental pressures. The diagnosis is based on the history of the injury and the findings of signs and symptoms compatible with myoneural ischemia. Fortunately, functional losses precede myoneural necrosis by a few hours, which allows us some latitude for earlier diagnosis of ischemia and prevention of tissue necrosis.[76–78] The earliest clinical finding of muscle and nerve ischemia is pain. However, all severely injured feet associated with multiple fractures are painful, and it may be difficult to distinguish the pain of injury from that of a developing compartment syndrome. The pain secondary to compartment syndrome or ischemia does not, however, abate with adequate immobilization of the foot and is usually quite out of proportion to the injury. We have found that this pain can be markedly exacerbated by gentle, passive dorsiflexion of the toes that stretches the intrinsic muscles of the foot. Lack of sensation is generally accepted as an important sign of nerve ischemia, but we have not found this to be reliable in the foot. A diminution in sensation over time may be more helpful. In the foot, two-point discrimination and light touch over the plantar aspect of the foot and toes is more reliable than a loss of pinprick sensation. Pain is present in all patients, but it is difficult to distinguish the pain of the injury from that of an impending compartment syndrome. The presence or absence of a dorsalis pedis or posterior tibial pulse is notoriously unreliable in diagnosing an early compartment syndrome. We have repeatedly documented the presence of both the pulses and normal capillary refill time in a foot with compartmental ischemia. The pathogenesis of the compartment syndrome clearly underscores the potential for misdiagnosis when based on the presence or absence of pulses. Nevertheless, a thorough vascular evaluation, including a routine Doppler examination, should be an integral part of managing these injuries because it can assist one in preoperative planning.

During the initial evaluation, all dressings should be removed. No circumferential dressings, particularly splints or casts, should be used in the management of these injuries where the potential for compartmental ischemia exists. In equivocal cases, high-risk patients should be checked frequently since compartment syndromes are usually progressive. The foot should not be maximally elevated but placed at heart level to ensure venous drainage without compromising local arteriolar pressures any further. In some patients who present late in the course of events, irreversible myoneural necrosis may have occurred by the time the ischemia is diagnosed.[80, 82–84] The diagnosis of compartment syndrome cannot be made clinically in patients with head, cord, or peripheral nerve injuries, although it seldom represents a problem for the isolated foot injury. Nevertheless, for patients with multisystem trauma, as well as in patients in whom the diagnosis is equivocal, the only objective and accurate test is by invasive catheterization of the involved compartments. These pressure-measuring devices should be liberally used, with the understanding that changes in compartment pressures often precede the clinical signs of an incipient compartment syndrome.

The method we prefer is utilization of a small, digital, hand-held monitor based on the slit-catheter system (Stryker Co., Kalamazoo, Mich). An 18-gauge needle is inserted first into the central and then the interosseous compartment. To measure the pressure in the central compartment, the surface landmark is the base of the first metatarsal, and the needle is passed between the metatarsal and the abductor hallucis muscle. The needle is advanced 1.5 in., with care taken to obtain the reading when the needle can be felt to be in soft tissue and not up against bone or tendon. The central compartment can also be monitored from a dorsal approach by measuring the interosseous compartment pressure when passing through it. The interosseous compartment pressure should be measured in two positions by introducing the needle through the intermetatarsal space. The second and fourth web spaces are preferable because these avoid inadvertent puncture of the dorsalis pedis and its branches. Although either pressure recording is probably sufficient, we have found that pressures in the central and interosseous compartments may differ by as much as 12 mm Hg. The calcaneal or quadratus compartment is measured by inserting the needle 5 cm distal and 2 cm inferior to the medial malleolus and advancing it through the abductor muscle.

Treatment should be based on a combination of clinical findings and pressure measurements, particularly in the presence of an upward trend in pressures. On the basis of the preceding symptoms, history, physical examination, and measurement of compartment pressures, one should treat the patient expeditiously with decompressive fasciotomy. Some clinicians advocate fasciotomy when the pressure is greater than 45 mm Hg;[77] however, most clinical and animal studies have demonstrated the need for fasciotomy when pressures greater than 30 mm Hg persist for more than 8 hours.[78, 81, 86] Controversy exists, however, as to what is the critical threshold pressure above which irreversible ischemic changes occur. We cannot know exactly when the pressures begin to elevate unless they are measured continuously, and I would recommend performing fasciotomy for an acute injury associated with pressure greater than 40 mm Hg. There is evidence that an individual's tolerance for increased tissue pressure varies and that the same degree of pressure may cause neuromuscular deficit in some patients but not in others.[76] Fasciotomy is also recommended when the compartment pressure is within 30 mm Hg of the patient's diastolic blood pressure.[86]

There are several fasciotomy techniques that one may use. The dorsal approach for fasciotomy utilizes two longitudinal incisions based over the second and fourth metatarsals. These should be placed slightly medial to the second metatarsal and lateral to the fourth metatarsal to ensure as wide a bridge of skin as possible (Fig 32–12). When the foot is swollen, the skin and subcutaneous tissues are also stretched and expanded. Following fasciotomy, the skin resumes a more normal

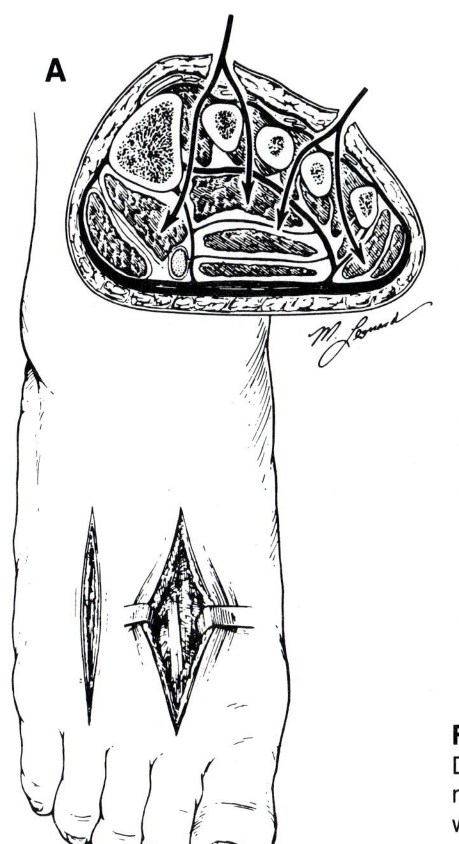

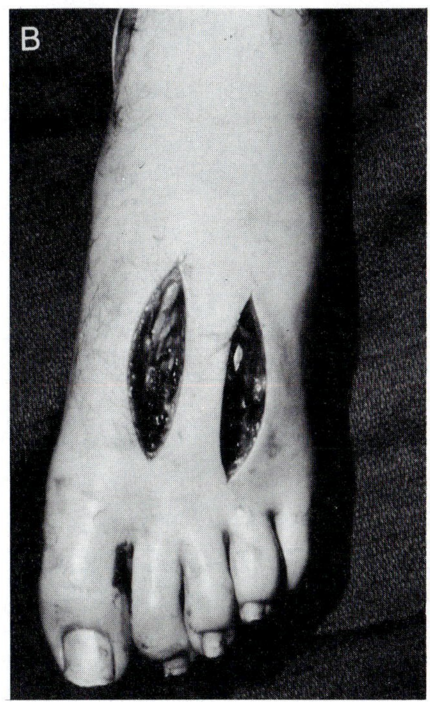

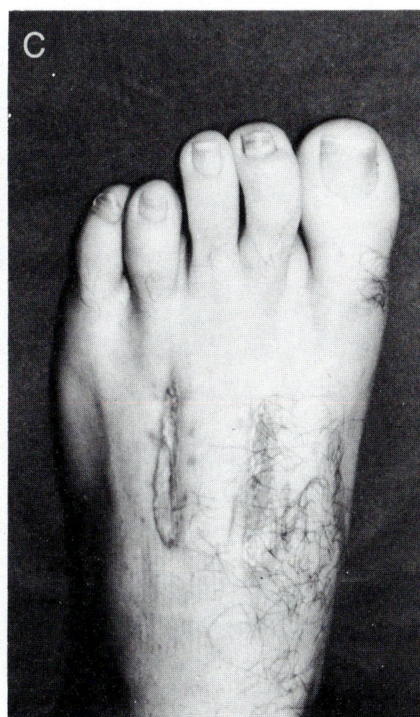

FIG 32–12.
Dorsal fasciotomy incisions are performed on the medial aspect of the second metatarsal and the lateral aspect of the fourth metatarsal so as to ensure as wide a skin bridge as possible **(A** and **B).** Provided that no horizontal plane dissection is performed, the skin bridge rarely undergoes slough. This was treated at 5 days with leg closure using a small split-thickness skin graft **(C).**

turgor, and the intervening skin bridge narrows. Although this bridge of skin is narrow, it seldom undergoes necrosis. Once the skin incision for fasciotomy is made, it is deepened to the bone by using a small hemostat to spread the tissue longitudinally. No subcutaneous dissection is performed in order to avoid compromise of already tenuous dorsal skin. When the bone is reached with the hemostat, further longitudinal dissection is performed in each interosseous space. From these dorsal incisions, reaching the medial and lateral compartments requires precise dissection and may not always be possible despite the use of a curved hemostat clamp. The medial approach follows the length of the inferior surface of the first metatarsal, enters the medial compartment between the metatarsal and the abductor hallucis muscle, and provides direct access into the other compartments. Once the abductor hallucis muscle is retracted inferiorly, we prefer to use blunt finger dissection and gentle longitudinal tissue spreading with a hemostat (Fig 32–13). To avoid injuring the neurovascular bundle when cutting across the central compartment, scissors or sharp instruments are not used. The skin incision can be extended more proximally to decompress the entire posterior tibial neurovascular bundle.

The same principles that apply to fasciotomy elsewhere in the extremities apply to fasciotomy in the foot: no tourniquet is used, generous incisions are made, and subcutaneous fasciotomy is not advised. No debridement of muscle at the time of fasciotomy is performed because it is difficult to determine muscle contractility in the foot and, once decompressed, the muscle may recover postoperatively. The decision to perform the fasciotomy dorsally or medially is based on the presence or absence of fractures amenable to open reduction and internal fixation. Many crushing injuries are associated with midfoot fractures and dislocations, and it is preferable to treat these injuries after fasciotomy with open reduction and internal fixation. Under these circumstances, the double–dorsal incision approach is utilized for fasciotomy because it provides simultaneous access for fracture reduction and fixation. When a compartment syndrome is associated with a fracture pattern unsuitable for internal fixation or when crushing occurs without fracture-dislocation, then the medial incision is preferable. Needless to say, once the fasciotomy has been completed, the pressures should be checked and additional incisions made as needed. We have found that a medial fasciotomy incision has to be performed following adequate dorsal incisions approximately 5% to 10% of the time. Skeletal stabilization, whether by external or internal fixation or a combination of the two, facilitates wound healing. Rigid skeletal stability enhances the environment for soft-tissue healing, decreases pain, and allows more rapid mobilization of the extremity. Early return of full function following fractures and the avoidance of "fracture disease" can be achieved only by anatomic reduction of fractures with resumption of early range of motion and partial loading. These prerequisites are only possible in the presence of stable fixation. With inadequate methods of fixation, full return of function is rarely achieved, and then only after prolonged and arduous rehabilitation.

These fasciotomy incisions are left open, and the

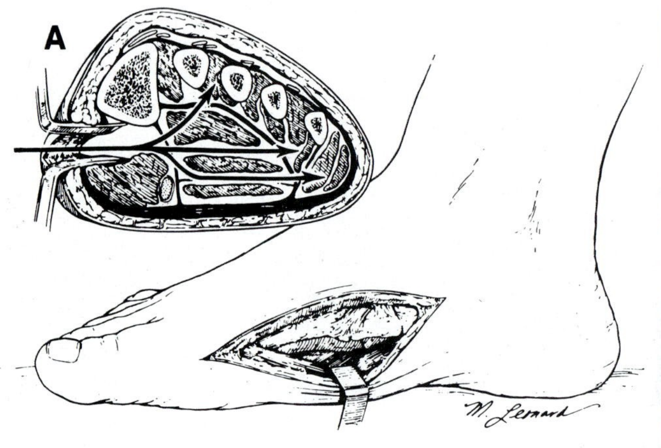

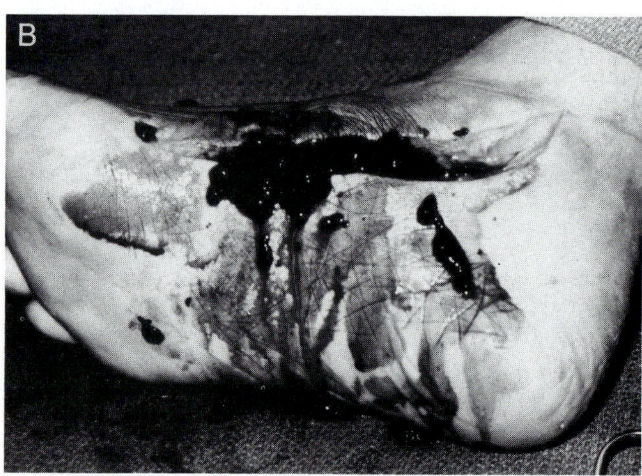

FIG 32–13.
The skin marking for the medial fasciotomy incision is just below the inferior aspect of the first metatarsal **(A** and **B)**. The medial compartment is opened, the abductor hallucis muscle retracted inferiorly, and the central compartment entered. The hematoma in this patient is characteristic.

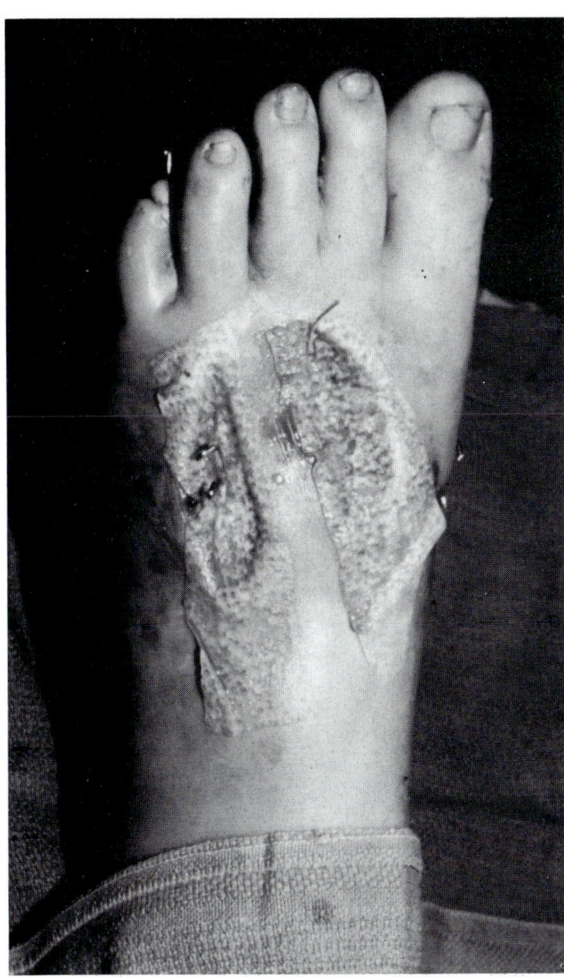

FIG 32–14.
Following a fasciotomy, this wound was covered temporarily with a porcine allograft, which provides a biologic covering for the wound, prevents desiccation, and when removed at 48 hours gives a good indication as to the potential contamination of the underlying wound.

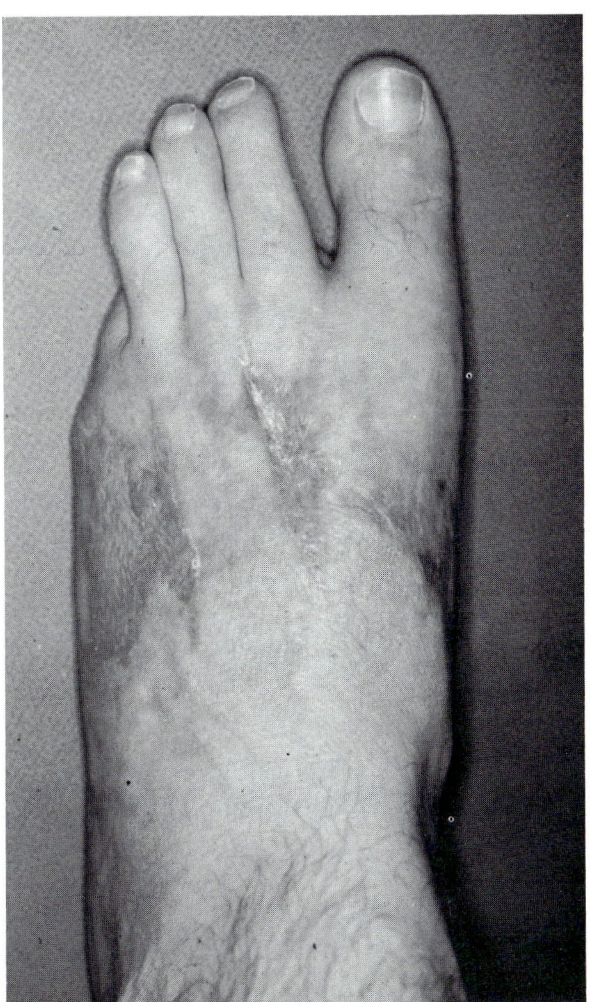

FIG 32–15.
This crush injury was associated with compartment syndrome and soft-tissue loss dorsolaterally. Following fasciotomy, closure was performed with split-thickness skin grafting, with a satisfactory functional result.

wounds should not be closed before the fifth day. We frequently use porcine allograft to provide temporary coverage of the fasciotomy incisions, and these are changed at the bedside every 48 to 72 hours (Fig 32–14). The dorsal skin may still be tenuous, and if so, the wounds are preferably closed with split-thickness skin grafts. These contract during healing to provide a satisfactory cosmetic appearance to the foot (Fig 32–15). Closure of the dorsal incisions by suturing is possible but should be performed judiciously since the skin edges may be tenuous and can undergo necrosis. Medial fasciotomy incisions approximate more easily with delayed primary closure than do dorsal incisions, but split-thickness grafts can be used as well in this location.

SPECIFIC REQUIREMENTS OF FOOT AND ANKLE COVERAGE

The soft tissues covering the foot and ankle perform specific functions connected with locomotion. The dorsal soft-tissue covering is a distal extension of the leg that provides support and protection to the underlying neurovascular structures, extensor tendons, and bones. The plantar surface consists of highly specialized tissue well adapted to meeting the unique demands imposed by weight bearing.[53] The surfaces under the heel and metatarsal heads are thick with an abundant subcutaneous layer divided by multiple fibrous septae anchored to the underlying fascia.[91, 96] This provides highly durable shock absorption as well as resistance to the shear stresses necessary during weight bearing.[97] Cutaneous ligaments link the skin with the more rigid deeper structures in the forefoot and limit skin motion over the metatarsal heads and plantar aspect of the toes. Proprioception and protective sensation are also dependent upon adequate support and function of these weight-bearing surfaces, which are unfortunately not possible to duplicate. The choice of substitute coverage is determined by the final defect size, composition, and specific requirements of tissues lost, as well as the condition of the remaining adjacent tissues. Since the closest match is produced by "like tissues," it is preferable to use local tissue when appropriate provided that they are available and expendable. However, coverage of defects of the foot and ankle is frequently quite challenging due to the relative scarcity of tissue available for local transfer.[93, 94] When selecting from a plethora of coverage options, one should consider simpler solutions before embarking on a complex reconstruction that is associated with increased complications and morbidity. The spectrum of treatment options is extensive and includes the following:

1. Skeletal shortening and primary closure
2. Split-thickness skin grafting
3. Split-thickness skin excision
4. Local rotational (transpositional) flaps
5. Free flaps
6. Cross-leg flaps

Primary Closure With or Without Skeletal Shortening: Coverage of the Hallux and Digital Amputations

The simplest solution to some wounds of the forefoot is skeletal shortening followed by primary closure. This should, however, not be resorted to when an alternative form of coverage is possible that would better preserve function. This is particularly true when a more sophisticated method of coverage would preserve the length of the foot. When considering skeletal shortening as an option, the final function of the foot should be considered, particularly since any ablative procedure is irreversible. Nevertheless a correctly performed amputation may provide better function than a partially sensate foot that

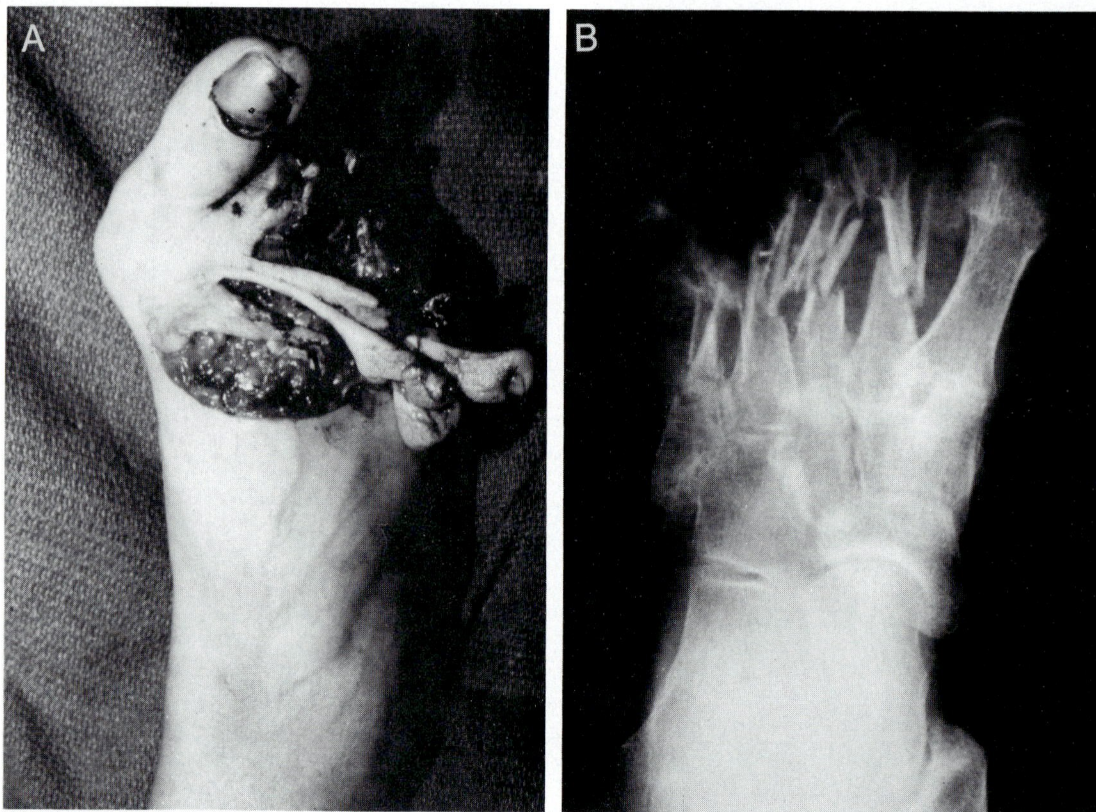

FIG 32–16.
A and **B,** this 74-year-old patient sustained crushing of tissue and severely comminuted fractures of the metatarsals in a lawn mower accident. Following debridement, a transmetatarsal amputation was performed successfully.

is not balanced or plantigrade.[89] This is well illustrated in the 74-year-old patient in Figure 32–16 who sustained a severe lawn mower injury to her foot. In addition to significant contamination and devastating bone injury, she had fairly significant pre-existing hallux valgus. Although the first metatarsal could have been preserved and covered with a local rotation flap, it was felt that the final function of her foot would be compromised and probably no better than that of a functional amputation. This was performed 2 weeks later following serial wound debridement for a wound infection with a short transmetatarsal amputation. It has been our experience that the longer the foot, the more functional ambulation is. This applies to not only the foot as a whole but also the digits, particularly the hallux. This has encouraged us to perform nonstandard amputations when the plantigrade position of the foot is maintained and the range of motion in the remaining parts of the foot and ankle preserved. This function is best attained with the judicious use of tendon transfers, particularly in midfoot and hindfoot amputations. A Lisfranc or short transmetatarsal amputation will function extremely well provided that equinus or varus contracture is avoided by careful assessment of the foot and reattachment of the extensor tendons with or without lateral transfer of the anterior tibial tendon. Wherever possible, we attempt to preserve the length of the digits and foot with local tissue, and if such is not available, then consider coverage from a distant source.

Preservation of digits and parts of the forefoot may, however, not be in the patient's best interests if the appendage left has no function and involves complex reconstructive procedures to achieve salvage. Amputation of one or more lesser toes does not generally result in any significant loss of function. If the second toe is involved, it is preferable to preserve length albeit with a short segment of the base of the proximal phalanx. If a short stump of the proximal phalanx is present, valgus drift of the hallux is less likely to occur. It has always been felt that the loss of the hallux impairs function, and we have recently confirmed this with clinical and pedobarographic analysis.[88] Amputation of the hallux is followed by retraction of the sesamoids, dysfunction in toe-off, lesser toe metatarsalgia, and a sense of imbalance with rapid walking. The windlass mechanism depends on an intact plantar aponeurosis through its attachment to the hallux via the flexor brevis and sesamoids. During the stance phase of gait, this windlass mechanism helps to stabilize and elevate the medial longitudinal arch and invert the heel.[87] We were able to ascertain that the flexor mechanism of the hallux remains intact provided that at least 8 mm of the base of the proximal phalanx is preserved. We were unable to differentiate this group of patients in whom the base of the proximal phalanx was maintained from patients with a normal hallux. We concluded from this study that amputation of the hallux at the metatarsophalangeal joint or proximal to the bulk of the insertion of the aponeurosis leads to instability of the first ray, loss of intrinsic strength, and a lateral shift of forefoot pressure toward the lesser rays.

There are numerous options for closure of the skin following digital or hallux amputation. Traditionally, a long plantar flap is created and closure made by rotating the flap dorsally. These closures are associated with the formation of "dog-ear" deformities that do not always shrink over time and can be a persistent problem (Fig 32–17). Even when these edges gradually retract, they are still bulbous, and the medial edge rubs against the shoe or the lateral prominence against the second toe (Fig 32–18). To close the hallux amputation with a

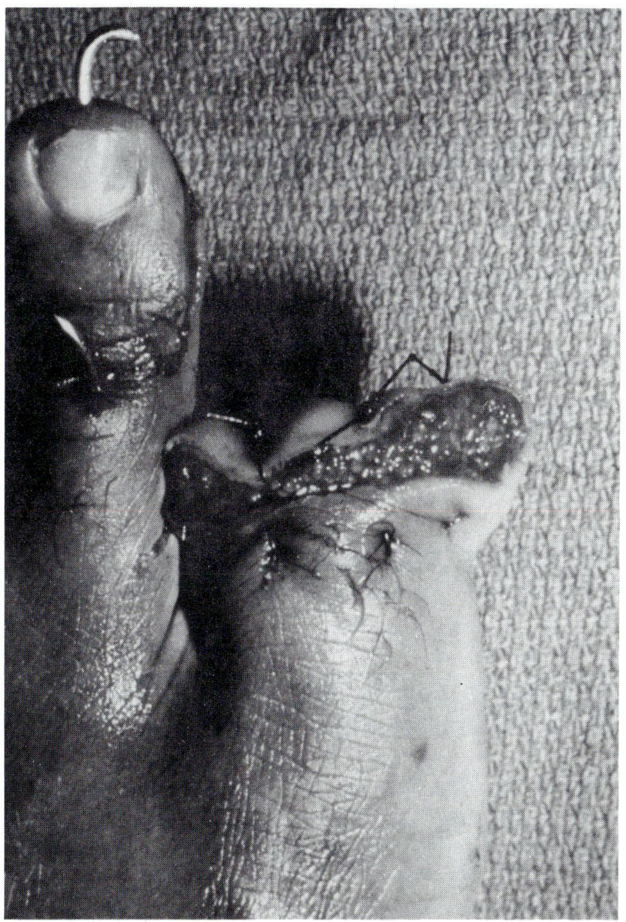

FIG 32–17.
Closure of this hallux amputation was performed with a plantar dorsal skin closure creating large medial and lateral dog-ears.

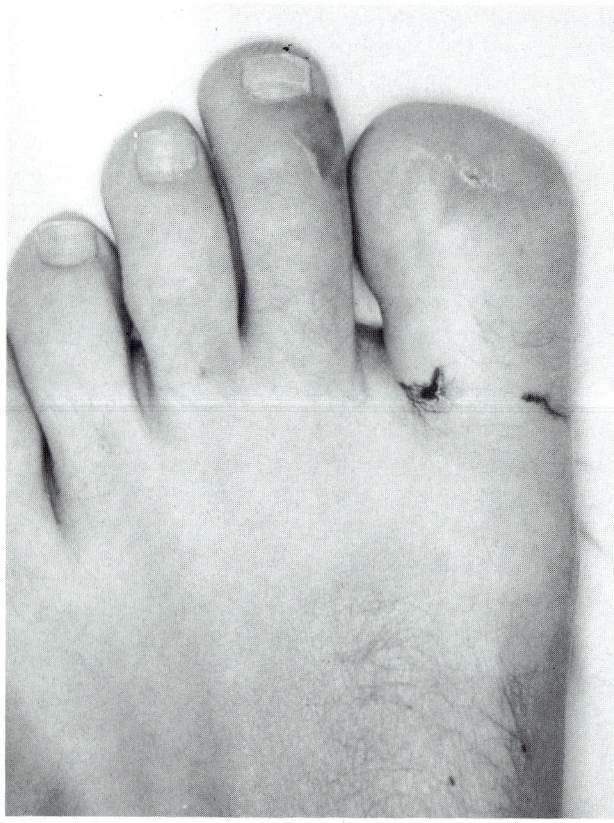

FIG 32–18.
This patient had persistent discomfort from the closure of the hallux amputation where the bulbous lateral edge rubbed against the second toe. This was the result of a large dog-ear formation that did not shrink or atrophy with time.

plantar-to-dorsal flap requires significantly more bone shortening. The subcutaneous tissue is much thicker, and the volar plates of both the metatarsophalangeal and interphalangeal joints add bulk to the flap and limit closure. For these reasons, wherever possible I prefer to create medial and/or lateral skin flaps with side-to-side rather than plantar-to-dorsal closure. Not only does this preserve the length of the hallux and toes since less bone has to be resected, but the final cosmetic appearance is also more acceptable, again due to the increased length obtained (Fig 32–19).

The type of flap used depends to a large extent on the available soft tissues and the obliquity of the laceration or partial amputation present. This is particularly relevant in closing partial amputation following lawn mower injury. A side-to-side closure is ideal for an oblique shear partial amputation or when the tip of the digit is crushed and intact plantar skin left proximally. Where the injury to the hallux is shearing and the plane of the partial amputation is long and oblique, tubing or side-to-side closure does not work well unless more bone and distal skin is resected. For these long shearing injuries of the hallux, I prefer to create a local rotation flap designed according to the plane of the injury and the tissue available (Fig 32–20). This is essentially a skin flap that is rotated either from distal lateral to dorsal proximal and medial directions or from the distal medial to dorsal lateral areas (Fig 32–21). In addition to preserving the length of the hallux, it is important to establish and maintain flexor strength. If the amputation is distal to the insertion of the flexor brevis, then sufficient flexor strength is maintained, but I also attempt to preserve the flexor hallucis and extensor hallucis longus attachments if possible, even if the amputation is proximal to the interphalangeal joint. These tendons can be retrieved with a tendon-grabbing forceps and either sutured to each other or sutured separately to the surrounding soft tissues. The flexor hallucis longus tendon is the more important of the two, and if no available tissue is present to secure the tendon, it can be reattached through drill holes in the proximal phalanx. Generally injuries about the hallux and digits can be closed with available local tissue.

There are certain patterns of injury of the hallux where a small split-thickness skin graft is the easiest method of coverage. This is harvested under local anesthesia and preserves maximal length and function of the hallux. (Figs 32–22 and 32–23). This coverage is used when minimal plantar tissue is present and cancellous bone is exposed. Split-thickness skin grafts may even be used to cover the hallux when articular cartilage is exposed. This is well illustrated in the patient in Figure 32–24 who sustained a crushing injury of the hallux with partial amputation and intra-articular fractures of the hallux metatarsophalangeal joint. Following meticulous debridement, open reduction and screw fixation of the articular fracture were performed and a local rotation flap used to cover the flexor tendon repair. The articular surface was covered with a small split-thickness skin graft, with an excellent functional and cosmetic result. Following these digital injuries, patients are kept non–weight bearing for 2 weeks, until the tissue flap has matured, and then walk in a hard surgical shoe until comfortable.

Skin Grafting

Skin grafting of soft-tissue defects of the foot is a simple and frequently very effective technique of coverage. These grafts are typically applied to the dorsal surface of the foot over a healthy recipient bed.[95] Split-thickness grafts may also be applied to the plantar aspect of the foot, particularly to the non–weight-

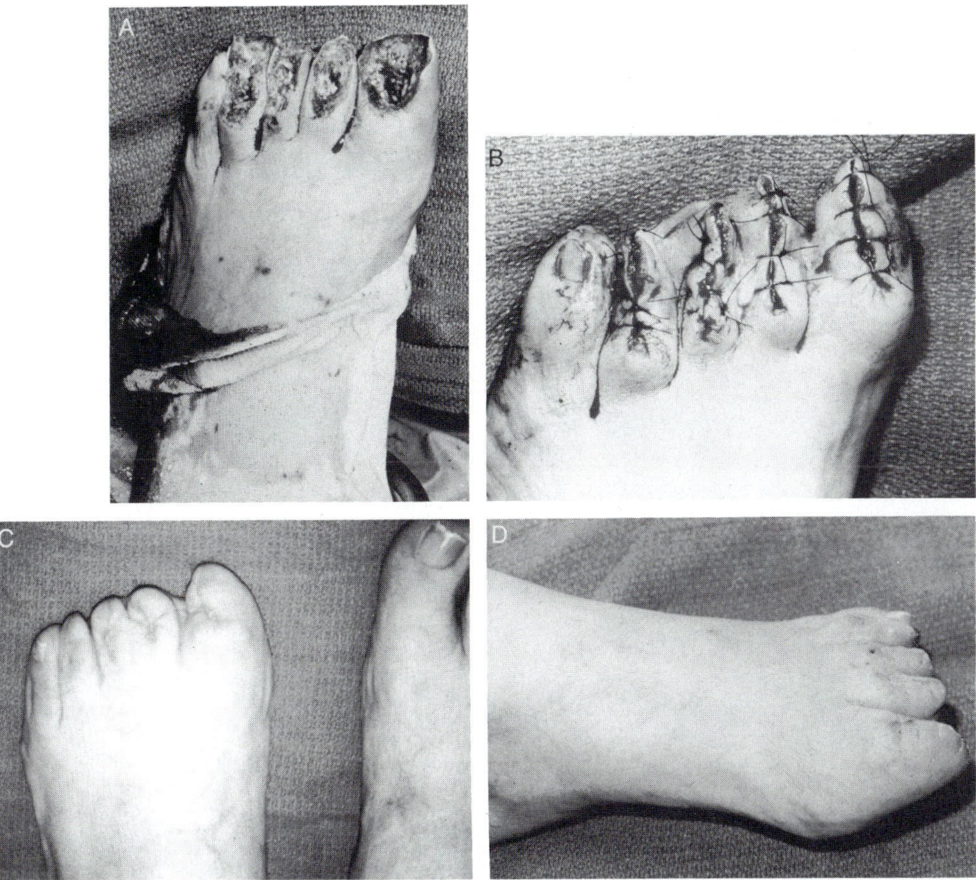

FIG 32–19.
A–D, these digital amputations were sustained in a lawn mower injury. The oblique plane of the amputation necessitated either bone shortening and closure with a plantar dorsal flap or, as was performed here, a side-to-side, medial-to-lateral skin closure. The final cosmetic result is acceptable and in fact is preferred by many patients since the apparent length of the digits is preserved.

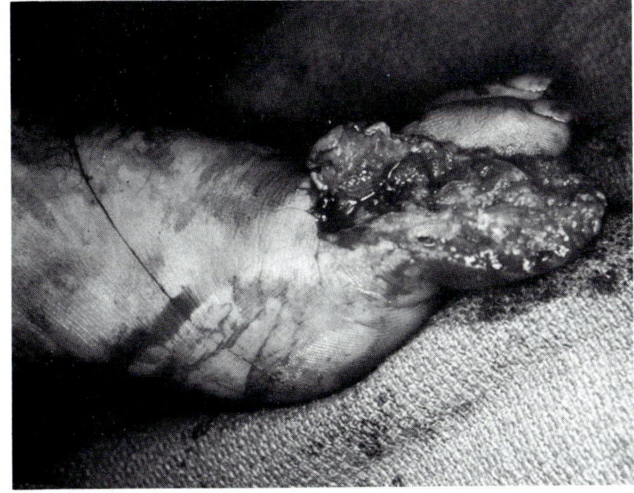

FIG 32–20.
This long shear oblique amputation of the hallux was sustained in a lawn mower injury. This could not be closed with tubing, i.e., medial-to-lateral closure, and a plantar-to-dorsal closure would have created unacceptable large medial and lateral dog-ears.

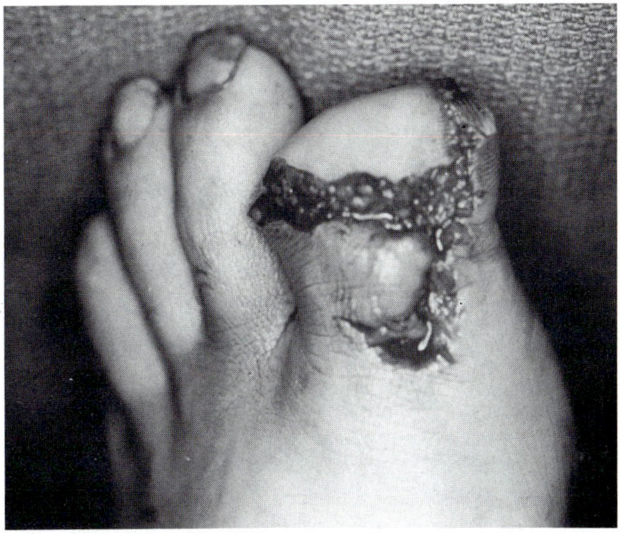

FIG 32–21.
Local rotation skin flaps were created for a long oblique shear amputation of the hallux from a plantar lateral flap that was fashioned and rotated over the dorsum of the phalanx.

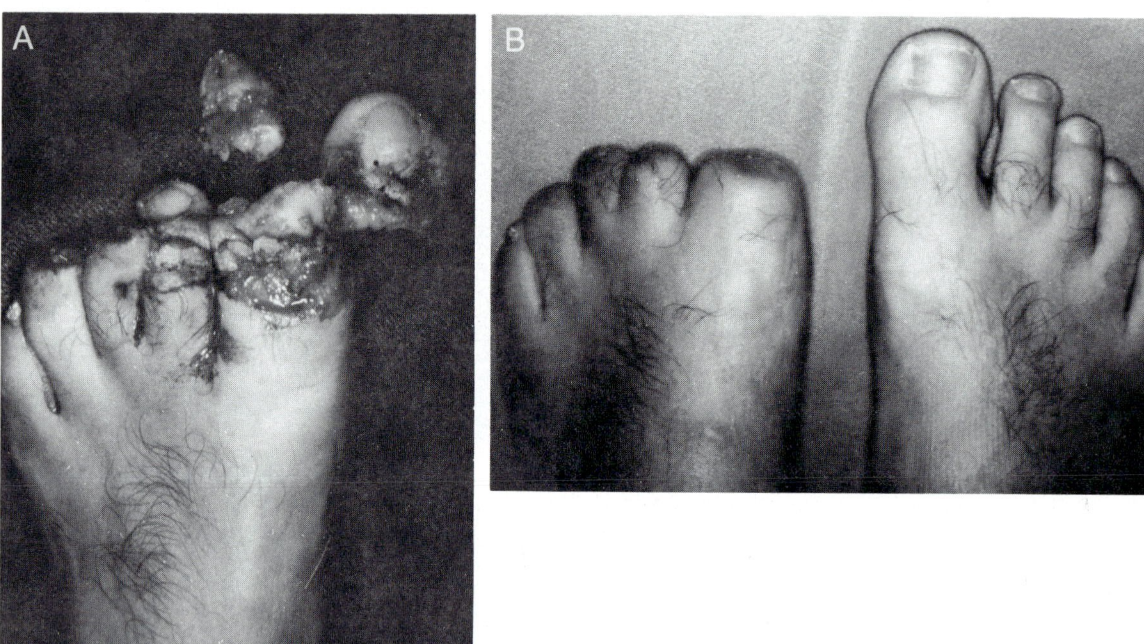

FIG 32–22.
This crush injury of the forefoot resulted in digital crushing and loss. This pattern of amputation is easy to close with skeletal shortening and side-to-side skin closure. Alternatively, if adequate soft tissue is available, a small split-thickness graft can usually be harvested off the amputated toes and applied directly to the open wound as illustrated here.

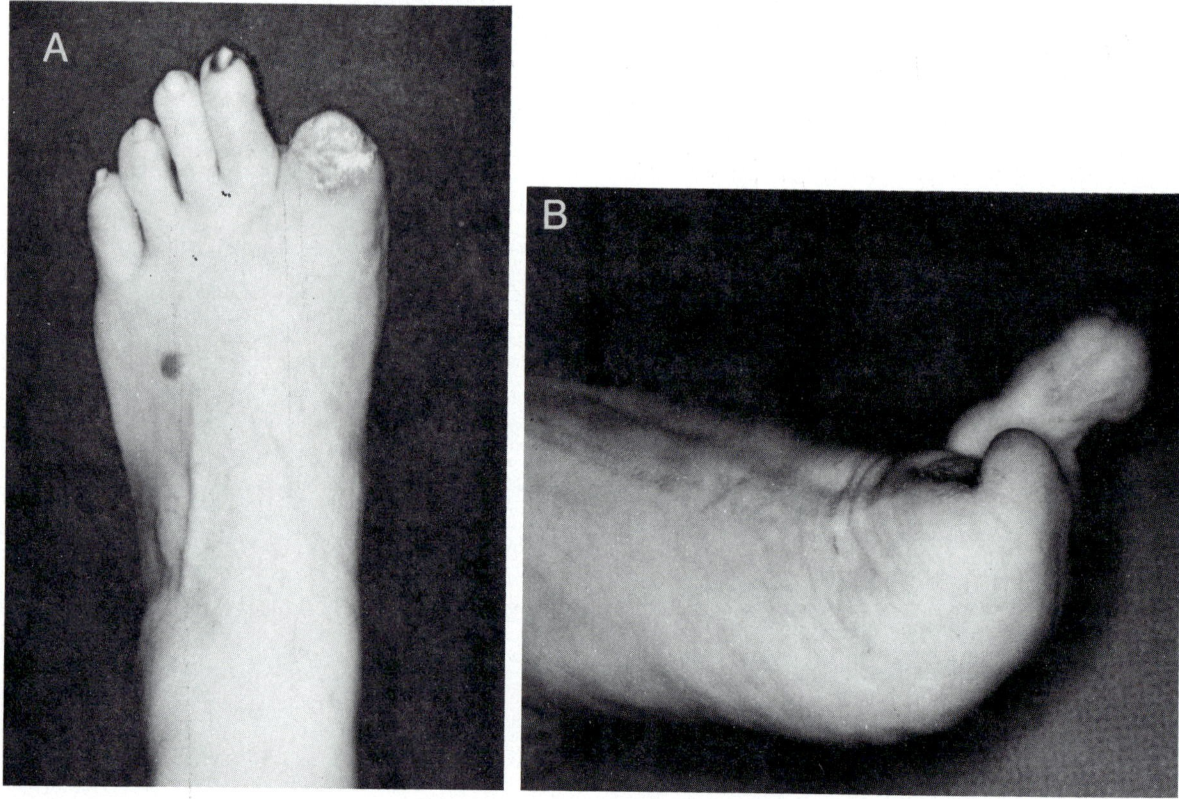

FIG 32–23.
A and **B,** this crushing amputation of the hallux was treated with reattachment of the intrinsic flexor and extensor tendons, with maintenance of active dorsiflexion and plantar flexion. Coverage of the defect was performed with a small split-thickness skin graft harvested off the amputated hallux.

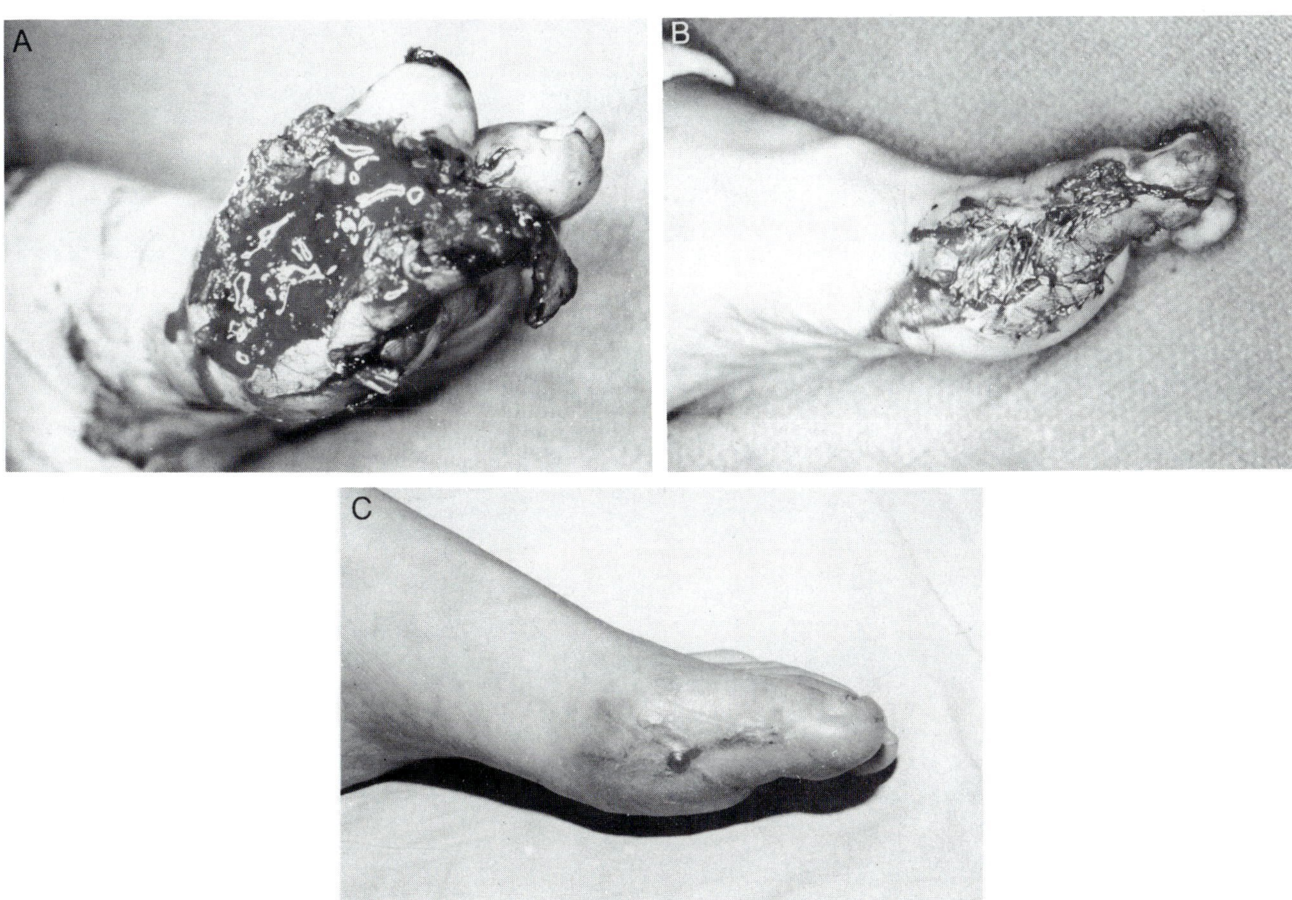

FIG 32–24.
A–C, this patient sustained a crush injury of the hallux associated with partial amputation, laceration of the flexor tendons, and an intra-articular fracture of the metatarsophalangeal joint. Following debridement, a local rotation flap was used to cover the flexor tendon repair, and the exposed articular surface was successfully covered with split-thickness grafts. The final cosmetic result is excellent.

bearing surfaces (Fig 32–25).[90] Although split-thickness grafts may be applied to portions of the weight-bearing surface of the foot, this often fails unless the rest of the foot is by and large normal with range of motion preserved. The best results are obtained when a well-vascularized granulating bed is present without exposed bone, cartilage, or tendon devoid of peritenon. This rule does not apply to children, in whom split-thickness graft will adhere to just about any bed, including cortical bone or tendon, and bridge small defects over articular cartilage. Skin grafts may in fact be applied directly onto cancellous bone surfaces even in adults, and in children grafts will adhere to cortical bone with an intact periosteum (Figs 32–26 and 32–27). This is useful over the dorsum of a foot associated with shear, avulsion, or crushing injuries. In these patients, the entire length of the foot can be maintained without resorting to more sophisticated forms of coverage or skeletal shortening. If the distal extensor tendons are exposed and the peritenon is missing, it is unlikely that a split-thickness graft will adhere, and a decision should be made whether to sacrifice the tendons or perform tissue transfer from a distant source. Generally, we have not performed free tissue transfers unless large areas of the dorsal skin including bone are missing. If the defect involves only limited areas of soft tissue, then it is prudent to remove some or all of the extensor tendons to facilitate application of a split-thickness graft. It is not advisable to leave tendon exposed since rapid desiccation occurs and may be followed by infection. We have tried to preserve the function of the extensor tendons with wet dressings but have found that they desiccate rapidly. One method of preventing a torn or lacerated tendon from desiccation is to tag it with a nonabsorb-

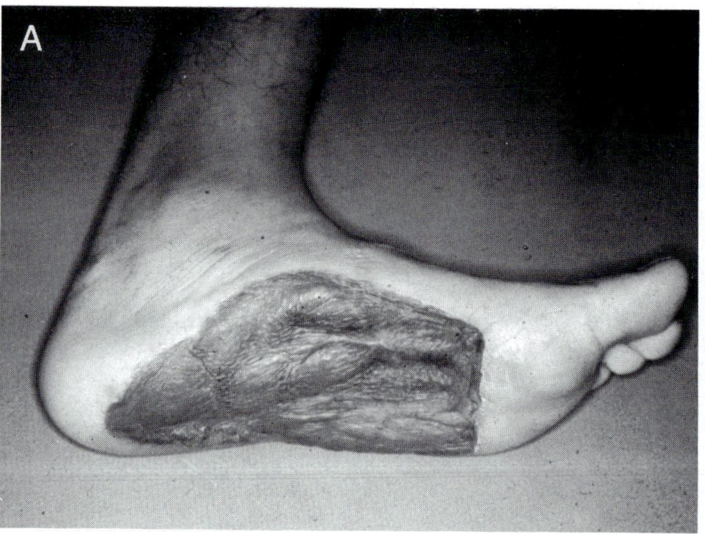

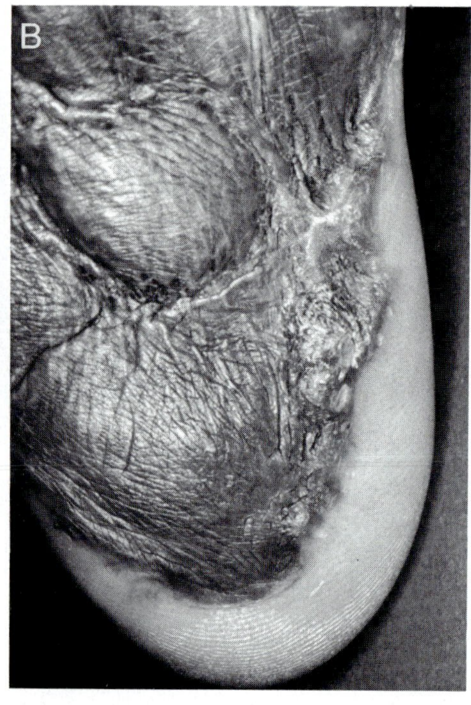

FIG 32–25.
A and **B,** a split-thickness skin graft was applied to the plantar aspect of the foot in this patient. The graft extends from the non–weight-bearing portion of the plantar forefoot distally and includes part of the weight-bearing surface of the heel approximately. Note the junctional keratosis between the normal skin and the split-thickness skin graft.

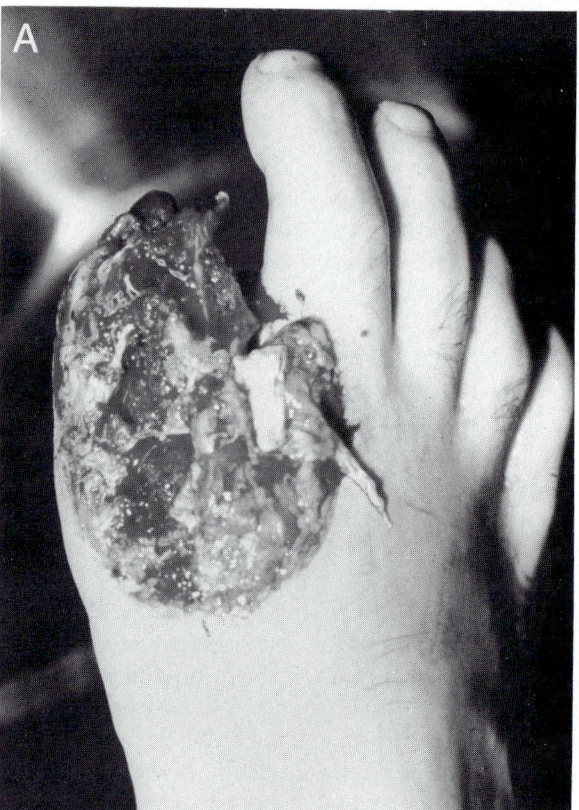

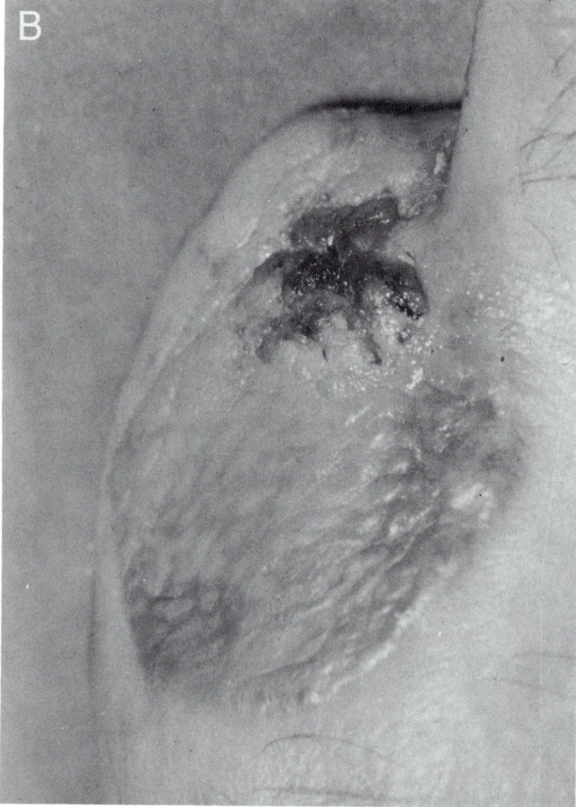

FIG 32–26.
A and **B,**this amputation was covered with a split-thickness skin graft directly onto the exposed cancellous bone of the distal first metatarsal and the base of the proximal phalanx.

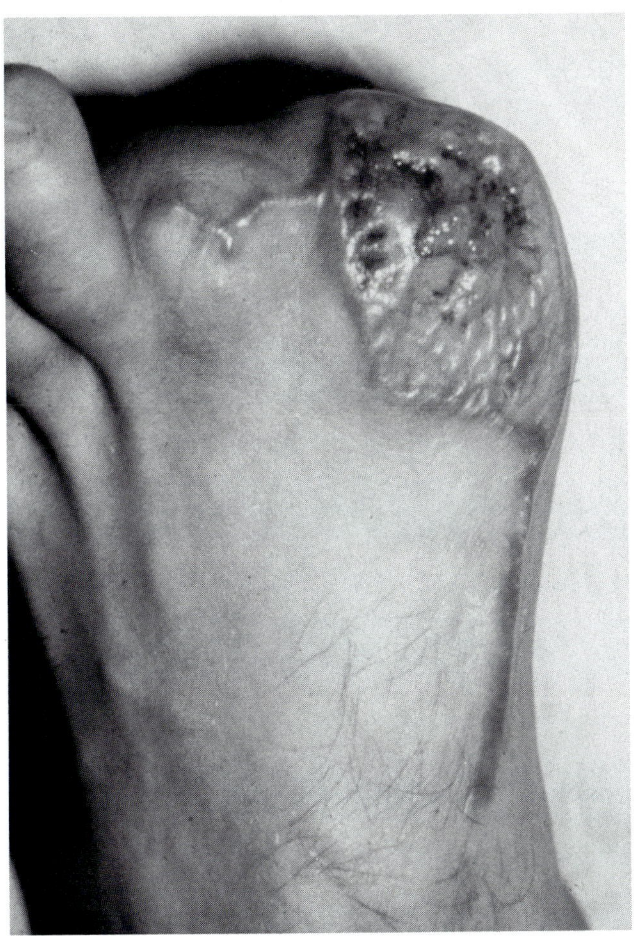

FIG 32–27.
Hyperkeratosis, common following the application of a split-thickness graft directly to bone, is illustrated in this patient.

able suture and bury it under viable tissue for later retrieval. Digital extensor tendons may have to be sacrificed to obtain early and simple coverage. Following crush and mangling injuries, the foot is often quite stiff, and I prefer to obtain early coverage even if it means sacrificing a few nonessential distal extensor tendons. Although this is not ideal, the alternate form of coverage would be free tissue transfer, and this extensive procedure may not be worth the effort to preserve digital extensor tendon function.

We have extended the indications for using split-thickness skin grafts on both the dorsal and plantar surfaces. As stated above, the ideal recipient bed is well vascularized, with no exposed cortical bone or tendon devoid of peritenon. Although this is generally correct, we have successfully applied skin grafts to the plantar aspect of the foot, including the weight-bearing surface, and used them in situations where free tissue transfer is the only other alternative. There are, however, circumstances where skin grafts may be quite feasible but are not the preferred method of coverage. This occurs if the deficit is very large or where later reconstruction of deeper tissues is anticipated. For example, if the deficit extends across the dorsum of the midfoot or hindfoot and injury to the ankle and or transtarsal joints has occurred, one must anticipate the possibility of an ankle arthrodesis in the future; in these patients, a split-thickness graft is not the ideal bed to work with since sloughing of the graft may occur. This principle holds true when there is a possibility of future major tendon repair or tendon transfer. In many patients, both split-thickness grafts or free tissue transfer are equally effective, and one obviously has to choose between the two depending on the size of the defect and the potential morbidity associated with each. This is well illustrated in the 63-year-old male in Figure 32–28 who sustained an injury to his foot in a lawn mower accident. The entire medial aspect of the foot was exposed from the hallux metatarsophalangeal joint proximally to the talonavicular joint. The hallux was crushed and nonviable, a large skin flap over the dorsal and medial aspects of the foot was avulsed, and the intrinsic muscles were partly lacerated and contused. The articular cartilage of the metatarsophalangeal, metatarsocuneiform, and talonavicular joints were exposed. In addition to these injuries described, significant contamination of the wound in the form of deeply ingrained dirt and fragments of grass was present. The options for treating this wound include free tissue transfer or local rotation flaps to cover the joint surfaces followed by skin grafts. These can be performed early or following serial debridement once the wound has stabilized and is free of infection. As I have outlined above, the longer we wait for coverage under these circumstances, the higher the incidence of failure. Although there is a risk of infection with immediate coverage, the contaminants present can most definitely be removed. Interestingly enough, the incidence of infection in these wounds at our institution is lowest with early or even immediate coverage. I have found that when some egress for drainage is present, coverage may be performed immediately. It is difficult to predict which form of coverage will maximize this patient's ultimate function. Free tissue transfer adds bulk to the foot, provides form, and possibly prevents delayed problems with shoe fitting. More importantly, free tissue transfer prevents the potential problems with tendon and joint exposure. Alternatively, immediate closure with local rotation flaps has merit in that the coverage uses like tissue to minimize the morbidity from a lengthy operation with its own incidence of failure and therefore was selected for this patient. After meticulous debridement followed by pulsatile lavage

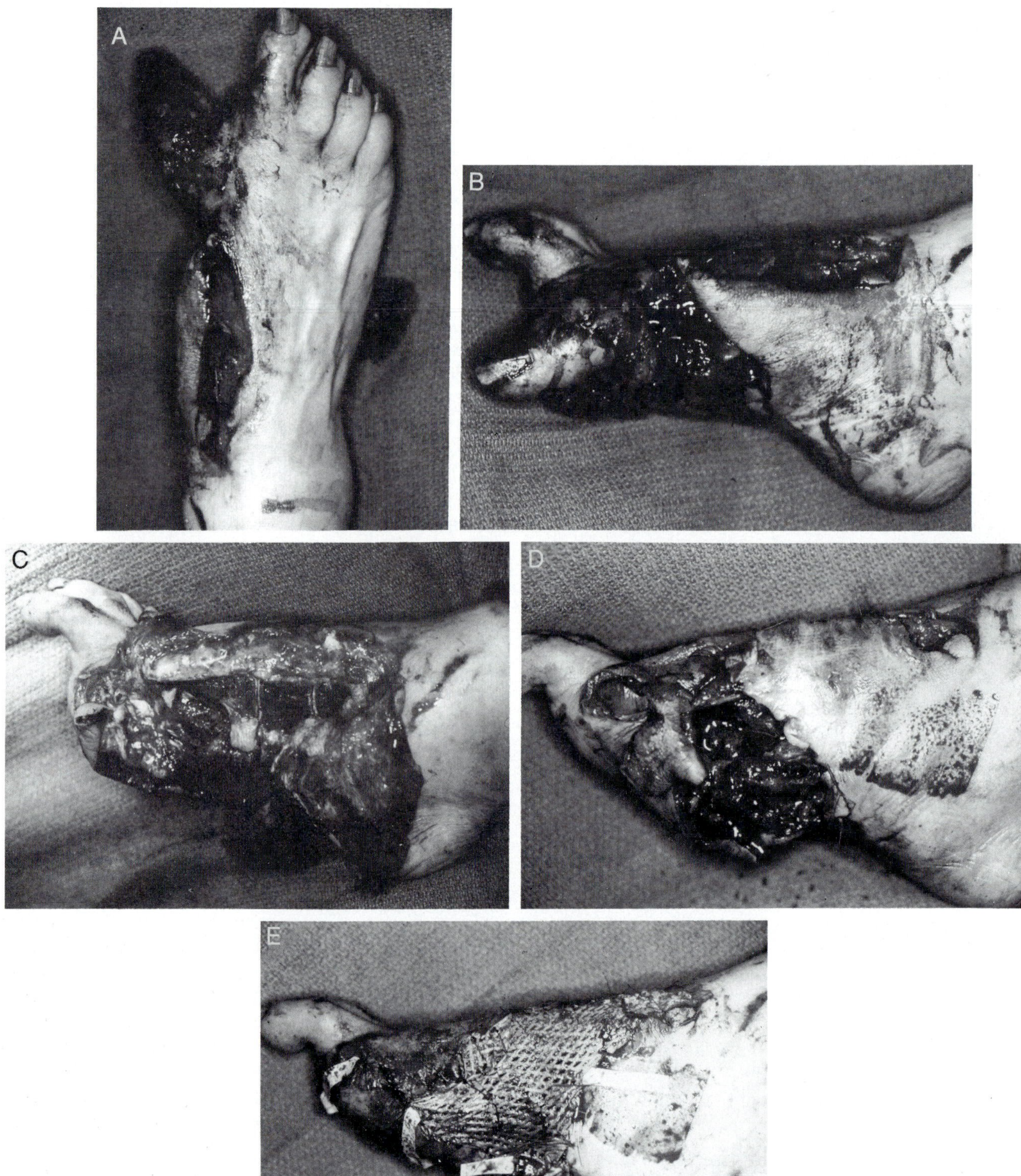
A
B
C
D
E

and manual removal of contaminants, the intrinsic muscles were found to be viable and suitable for use in local rotation flaps. The large dorsomedial skin flap was reattached and a split-thickness skin graft harvested by using the technique of STSE (see below). The nonviable skin was excised, the abductor hallucis and flexor digitorum brevis muscles mobilized and used as rotation flaps to cover the articular surfaces, and the entire wound covered by using the harvested split-thickness skin graft. The patient recovered rapidly without complication. Antibiotic prophylaxis was continued for 3 days with a combination of a clindamycin, gentamicin, and penicillin, which is our recommended treatment for significantly contaminated wounds. A similar problem with decision making in wound closure follows gunshot injuries to the foot. These often appear quite extensive at first, but following adequate debridement of soft tissue and bone where necessary, the defect often granulates in and can be covered with split-thickness skin.

Harvested skin may be full or split thickness, autologous or heterologous. The choice of the donor site depends on regional requirements of the defects being covered. Skin graft coverage of plantar foot defects is probably best performed with full-thickness skin devoid of hair follicles or sebaceous glands, which are frequently present on the dorsum of the foot. Hair-bearing donor skin (i.e., from the groin crease) placed on the weight-bearing surface of the foot will frequently undergo hyperpigmentation. Hyperkeratosis occurs frequently at the junction of the normal skin with the skin graft on the plantar surface. This junctional or marginal keratosis (see Fig 32–25,B) can be quite uncomfortable and requires frequent paring and soft Plastizote orthotic support. Although we attempt to provide a more durable surface other than split-thickness skin to the plantar weight-bearing surfaces, this is not always feasible. This applies particularly to amputations of the midfoot and forefoot where a free flap is an alternative but may not be necessary. The other option is skeletal shortening and primary closure, one that I rarely recommend. Depending on the overall pattern of the amputation, we are often able to preserve the length of the foot with skin grafts. These have been quite successful, even in children provided that there is a plantigrade weight-bearing surface for ambulation without an equinus contracture (Figs 32–29 and 32–30). In the child, growth of the foot may cause pressure necrosis of the distal aspect of the graft, but this too has not proved to be a problem, and we have treated this with periodic ostectomy if needed. In these patients skin grafts hold up well provided that the range of motion of the remaining portion of the foot is normal. I would not recommend skin grafting for a weight-bearing surface whether plantar or distal if an arthrodesis is planned or if tendon function is not normal.

If one is uncertain about the status of a wound or the advisability of coverage, then a better alternative than wet dressings is to use homograft, porcine allograft, or semisynthetic skin substitute (Epigard, Ormed, Santa Barbara, CA).[92] This temporary skin coverage is an excellent alternative to immediate coverage since it minimizes postoperative wound edema and simultaneously supplies a bacteriostatic coverage for the foot (Fig 32–31). The porcine xenograft covering is changed every 48 to 72 hours and the synthetic covering every 24 hours. The temporary coverage provides a barrier to bacterial invasion, protects underlying vital structures, decreases pain by covering exposed sensory nerve endings, and promotes epithelial proliferation beneath the graft.[92] When these dressings are changed, one is able to ascertain the overall viability of the wound as well as the extent of bacterial colonization. If the allograft adheres to the wound, a more favorable milieu is present for definitive coverage or closure. This contrasts with situations where the graft does not adhere to the wound or literally "floats" off when the dressing is removed. Under these circumstances, more aggressive wound care with debridement and frequent dressing changes is performed until a more favorable milieu is present for closure. Xenograft skin was initially popularized in burn care, and porcine allograft is now commercially available.

Split-Thickness Skin Excision

The technique of STSE was initially developed by Ziv and associates for the management of severe degloving injuries of the extremities.[70, 107, 108] We have applied these principles to its use in the foot and have since expanded its indications to include crushing, degloving, and partial amputation injuries.[57, 58, 59, 103, 106] The goal of STSE is to carefully delineate the margin of

←FIG 32–28.
This partial foot amputation was sustained in a lawn mower accident **(A and B).** Following debridement, the tarsometatarsal, navicular cuneiform, and cuneonavicular joints were exposed. These were covered with local rotation flaps by using the abductor hallucis and flexor brevis muscles, and final coverage was performed by using the technique of split-thickness skin excision. Note the capillary bleeding at the proximal extent of the skin flap that denotes viable skin **(C–E).**

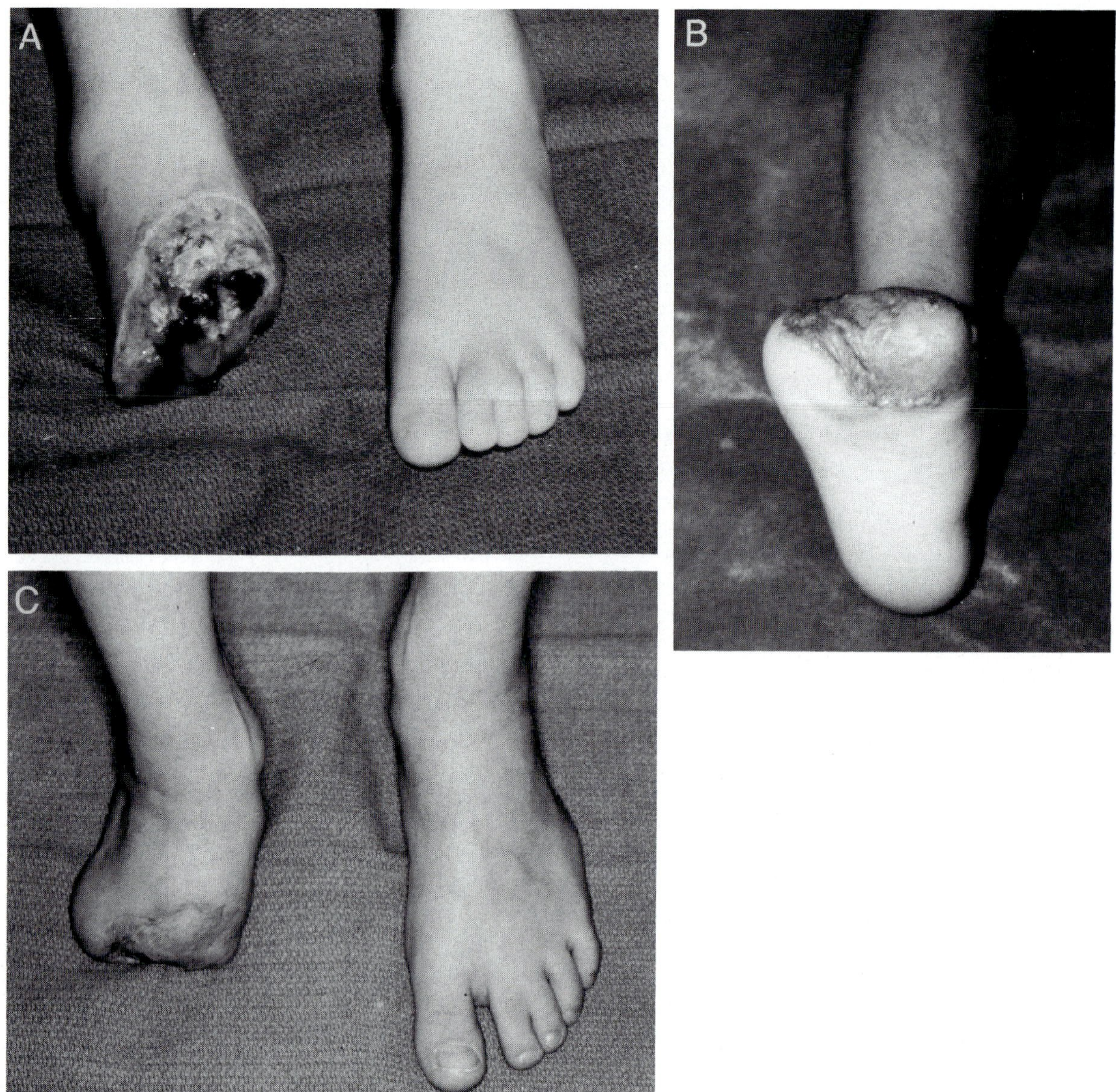

FIG 32–29.
A–C, this 5-year-old child sustained a midfoot amputation. Replantation was attempted, but due to severe crushing, this was abandoned. In order to maintain the length of the foot, a split-thickness skin graft was applied directly to the wound with the intention of performing a free flap sometime in the future if this failed. Three years later, with growth of the foot, no bone protrusion has occurred, and function is preserved.

necrosis of any devitalized skin flap and simultaneously provide a split-thickness skin graft for immediate use and primary coverage of the wound. The technique of STSE commences by suturing the avulsed or sheared flap of skin temporarily down to its original bed.[107] A split-thickness skin graft 0.010 to 0.015 in. thick is then harvested from the potentially nonviable skin flap as well as the adjacent normal skin. Since it is unclear as to the extent of the skin viability, one can estimate the amount of skin graft that will be required and remove more potentially "normal" skin. If a closed crush injury is present with devitalized skin, the STSE technique works as well, and the skin graft is harvested similarly. Although the contour of the dorsal surface of the foot is irregular, the smaller electric dermatomes work well enough to harvest the graft. Since the areas that are nonviable do not bleed, dermal capillary bleeding is used as an indicator of skin viability (see Fig 32–3,E).

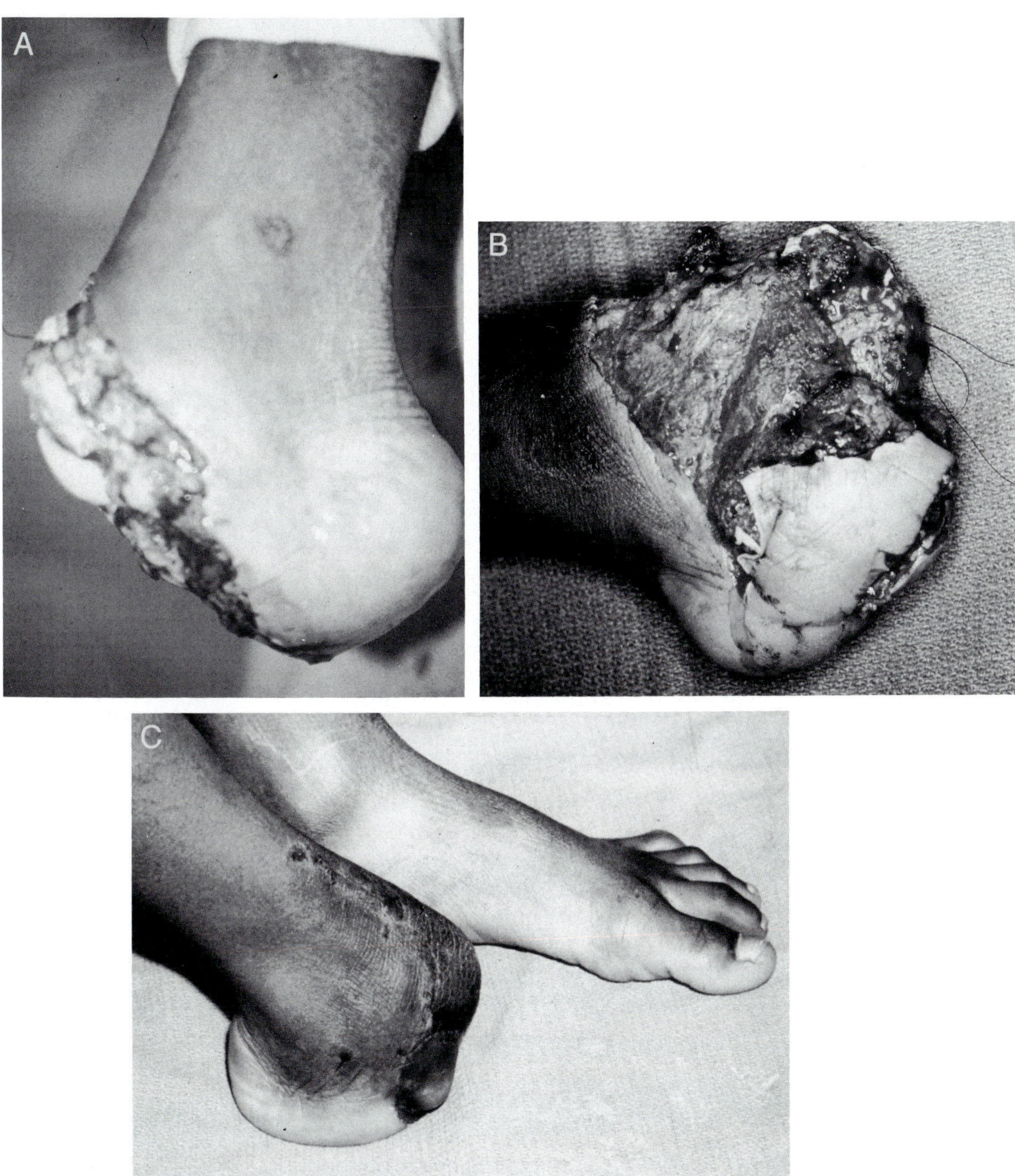

FIG 32–30.
A–C, a traumatic Chopart amputation was sustained by this 5-year-old child in a railway accident. The length of the foot was preserved, and coverage options included a free tissue transfer or split-thickness sking grafting, the latter of which was chosen. Two years later, with growth of the foot, a minor exostectomy was performed for bone overgrowth. Function of the foot has been preserved since the anterior tibial tendon was reattached.

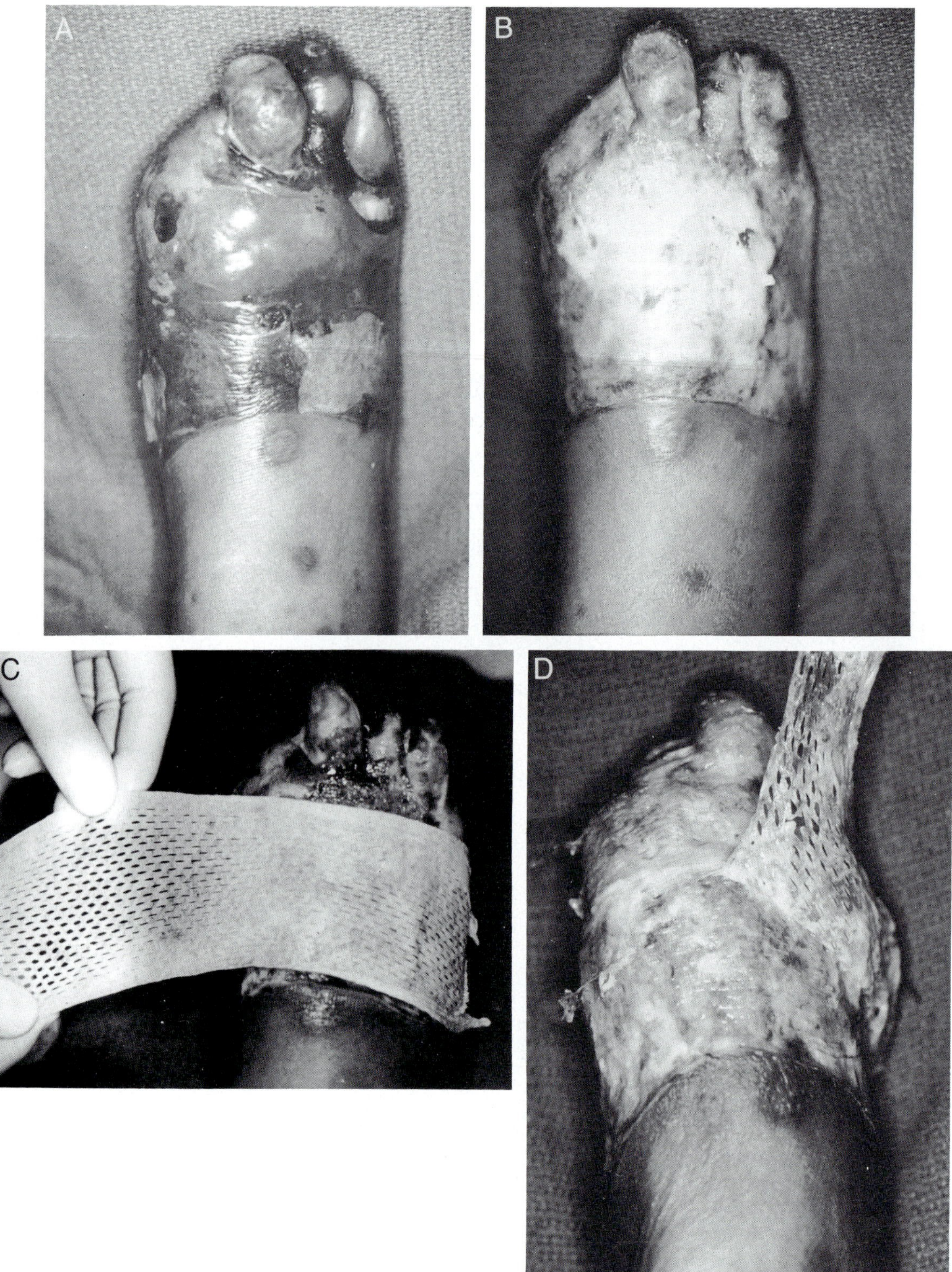

FIG 32–31.
A–D, this diabetic patient sustained a full-thickness burn to the forefoot. She presented late, with blistering and cellulitis. Debridement was staged, and following tangential excision of the full-thickness skin loss, a porcine allograft was applied. This adhered well to the underlying bed, as demonstrated here.

The nonviable skin flap that is clearly demarcated by the zone of capillary bleeding is then excised. The skin that was harvested across both the normal and nonviable skin may be used and is then meshed 1:1.5 and reapplied to the denuded area. We have used this form of coverage extensively in many crushing and mangling injuries of the foot. The technique is ideally suited to definitive management immediately following injury since cellular necrosis occurs after 24 to 48 hours and the epidermal layers would probably no longer be suitable. Although the skin harvested from the nonviable portions of the flap would not be suitable under these circumstances, the STSE technique can nevertheless still be used to delineate the margin of viability.

The utilization of skin from a potentially nonviable flap for immediate use on a degloved extremity is not new.[50, 98–101] Both split- and full-thickness grafts used during the initial surgical procedure have been shown to be superior to techniques in which salvage of the flap is attempted. Immediate reapplication of the flap and fixation with compression dressings usually fail, with necrosis of at least part of the flap likely.[102] Delayed coverage of the wound is of course an alterative and may be achieved with grafting 7 to 10 days after injury. This procedure has the potential for secondary infection of the wound compounded by the delayed treatment and prolonged hospitalization. Primary wound coverage currently appears to be the treatment of choice in shear avulsion injuries of the extremities. These concepts, however, are controversial, and primary coverage is not universally accepted as the treatment of choice. One may argue that primary closure of certain crush injuries will increase the potential for infection. I would certainly exercise caution in closing any farm injury primarily as well as those where potentially necrotic muscle is present. However, we have not experienced any deep wound infections following the application of STSE. This is probably due to aggressive intraoperative wound care, thorough irrigation and debridement, as well as appropriate selection of suitable wounds for the STSE coverage. In fact, the wound is not completely closed since free drainage may occur following meshing of the grafts. The ideal setting for the STSE technique is with shear avulsion injuries. These typically occur in association with motor vehicle injuries where the foot is run over at lower speeds and the dorsal skin surface sheared off its deeper fascial planes and bone.[106] Large skin flaps are created, often with questionable viability. In these shear injuries (Fig 32–32), the STSE technique accurately determines the extent of viability of the flap as well as provides additional skin for immediate coverage. We have extended the indication for the use of the STSE technique to many injuries associated with degloving and crushing of skin. The technique may also be used in crush-amputation injuries, where the amputated part is temporarily reat-

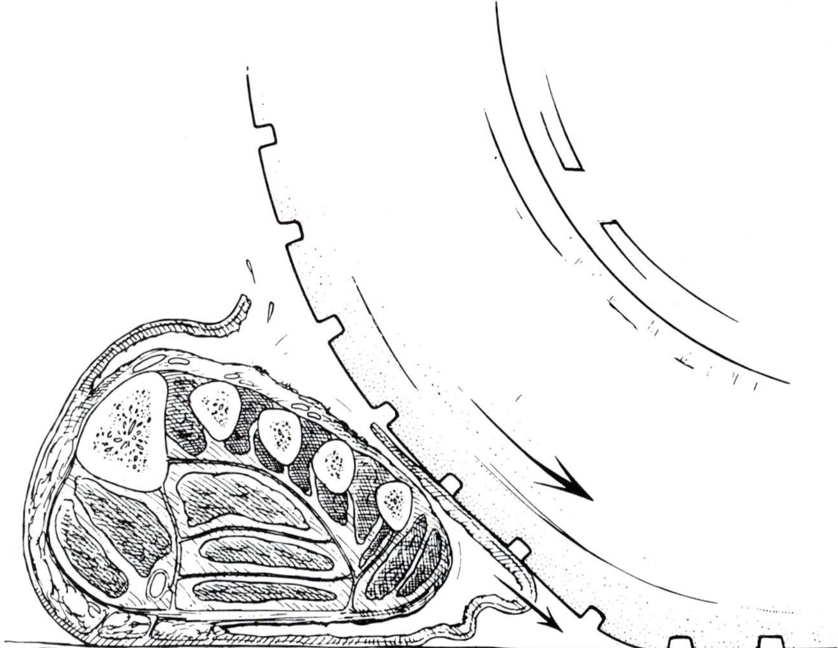

FIG 32–32.
A shear avulsion injury typically occurs when the foot is run over by a car at low speed. The injury sustained is not as much as a result of crushing as shearing of superficial layers from the deeper fascial planes and bones.

tached, the graft harvested, and following appropriate debridement and bone trimming, the graft applied as a one-stage procedure (Fig 32–33). The common surgical goal in managing these complex crush injuries of the foot is to provide optimum skin coverage with minimum morbidity. Alternative methods for attaining these goals are clearly available but have increasing complexity and morbidity. We have applied these techniques of STSE to harvesting the graft in both open and closed injuries, as well as those where the foot is clearly nonviable and amputated. For example, the technique of STSE may be used in a partial or complete amputation. The amputated part is secured or sutured back to its original bed and a graft harvested from it. We frequently use the amputated or crushed digits to harvest small pinch grafts. Although it is difficult to secure the digit firmly while the graft is being harvested, it can be performed with an assistant and small pinch grafts then removed from the dorsal, medial, and lateral surfaces.

The results of primary wound coverage depend on thorough debridement of the devascularized flap and wound bed, an observation in keeping with current philosophy that a fresh wound is a suitable site for donor tissue. The success of this procedure also depends on careful delineation of the viable and nonviable portions of the flap, particularly when dealing with crushing injuries of the foot involving shearing or avulsion of tissue. In these circumstances, the subcutaneous segmental vessels are disrupted, the dermal circulation is compromised, and accurate assessment of the flap becomes critical.

Techniques such as STSE and fluorescein testing, which enhance identification of tissue viability and predict flap survival, are integral to aggressive primary wound care.[104, 105] Other methods such as visual inspection of the flap and "clinical judgment" are satisfactory but clearly lack accuracy. We have found that fluorescein testing is a useful modality but that, on occasion, it has proved to be unreliable in predicting flap viability, perhaps as a result of altered perfusion of the dermal plexus in the flap due to arteriovenous shunting. We now use the STSE technique as both a diagnostic (delineation of the flap margins) and a thera-

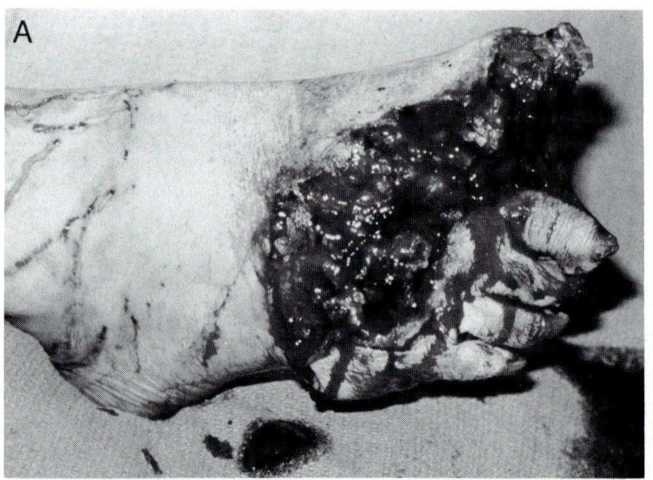

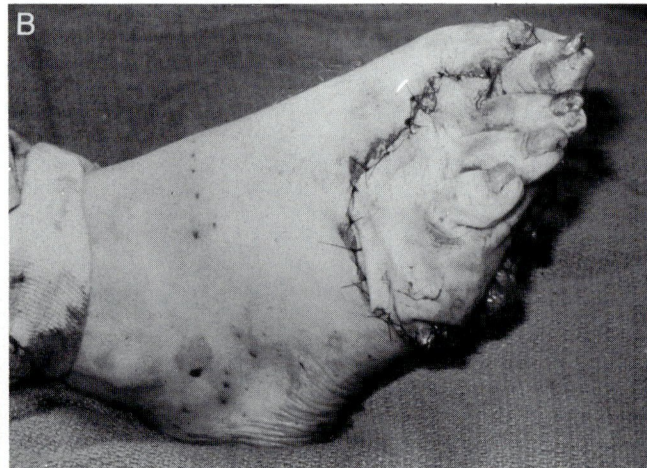

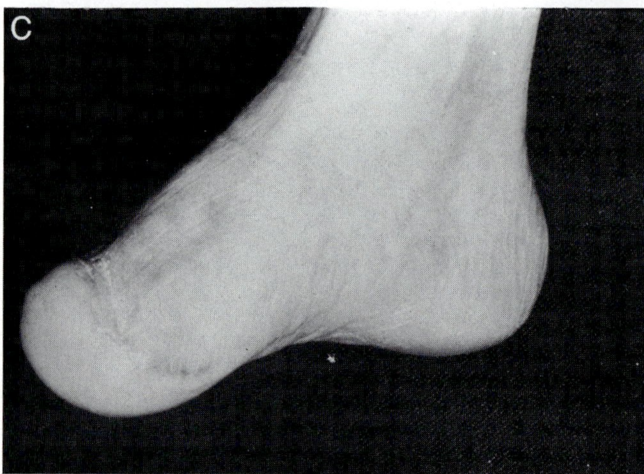

FIG 32–33.
This patient sustained a crush of the forefoot resulting in partial amputation **(A).** The amputated part was reattached **(B),** a split-thickness skin graft harvested from the dorsal surface of the foot was placed directly over the amputated part and more proximally, and the split-thickness skin graft was covered via the technique of split-thickness skin excision. This one-stage procedure healed uneventfully, and a functional forefoot amputation was present **(C).**

peutic (application of available skin graft) modality. The STSE technique cannot, however, be optimally utilized in all crushing injuries of the foot. In farm injuries or others where significant contamination is present, immediate coverage may be injudicious. There are other situations when the bed is not suitable for application of a split-thickness graft of any nature, e.g., where bare bone is exposed or where the deeper tissues are nonviable. Such injuries may be better suited to application of a free flap.

Transpositional and Island Pedicle Flaps

When sufficient and available, local tissue is optimal for coverage of many defects. The use of a like tissue donor provides the closest substitution for lost tissue. A variety of such local flaps can be effectively employed for coverage of relatively small defects.[109, 111–114] Their use is generally limited by defect size, with election of specific flap type based on deficit location.[115, 119, 122, 123] In addition, consideration must be given to the effect of distal vascular supply when axial-type flaps based on a major vessel are used (i.e., medial or lateral plantar arteries). Proper utilization of local tissue flaps requires an intricate knowledge of the regional neurovascular anatomy.[122, 125–127]

Cutaneous flaps based on the proximal plantar subcutaneous plexus (PPSP) can provide excellent coverage for defects up to 6 cm in diameter that involve the proximal plantar area. The PPSP is an extensive superficial vascular plexus receiving contributions primarily from branches of the dorsalis pedis and lateral plantar arteries and to a lesser extent from the medial plantar artery.[133, 137, 139, 141, 142, 146] It is this rich vascular network that allows cutaneous flaps to be raised superficial to the plantar fascia in the region extending from the most proximal plantar heel area to midway between the heel and the metatarsal heads. This essentially results in a random pattern–type flap.

The instep or medial plantar flap has proved effective in the coverage of limited defects overlying both the weight-bearing and the posterior non–weight-bearing heel area as well as the medial malleolus.[112, 123, 133, 139, 142, 143] When taken as a fasciocutaneous flap, excellent skin quality with adequate sensibility can be provided to cover defects up to 5 cm in diameter without resulting in an unacceptable donor site deficit. Vascularity of this flap is based on the medial plantar artery, and the flap is innervated by cutaneous branches of the medial plantar nerve. This neurovascular bundle passes between the abductor hallucis and quadratus plantae muscles and terminates in branches to the first and second toes. This neurovascular bundle with its accompanying fasciocutaneous flap can be passed subcutaneously to cover proximal defects. Mobility can be maximized by maintaining a narrow pedicle. Vascularity of distal plantar tissues is dependent on intact flow to the plantar arch via the deep branch of the dorsalis pedis artery and is therefore a prerequisite to flaps based either on the medial or lateral plantar arteries.

Similar to the medial plantar flap, an axial-pattern flap may be based on the lateral plantar artery. This may be a fasciocutaneous, myocutaneous, or an arterial skin flap.[113, 114, 120, 146] Local pedicle-type flaps may also be based on the lateral calcaneal artery (terminal branch of the peroneal artery). This flap may be used to cover small defects over the posterior of the heel and the Achilles tendon. In addition to the lateral calcaneal artery, the flap usually incorporates the lesser saphenous vein and the sural nerve. The intrinsic muscles of the foot can all be used to cover small soft-tissue defects about the foot and ankle. These may be muscle and covered with split-thickness skin grafts or myocutaneous flaps. The abductor hallucis can best be employed to cover small proximal deep defects distal to the medial malleolus. Likewise, the abductor digiti minimi can be used for similar defects below the lateral malleolus. The flexor digitorum brevis muscle is ideal for small defects over the posterior non–weight-bearing area of the heel. Numerous authors have described use of the extensor digitorum brevis or extensor hallucis brevis flap to cover small defects below as well as directly over the malleoli.

When the above local transposition flaps are inadequate or unavailable, the dorsalis pedis island pedicle flap may provide a good alternative to distant flaps for coverage of small defects.[121, 131, 132] Defects up to 5 cm in diameter overlying the distal end of the tibia, malleoli, and heel can be addressed. Intact plantar vessels are a necessary prerequisite before mobilizing this flap based on the dorsalis pedis artery. Potential problems with the donor site may occur fairly frequently, however, and include hyperkeratosis as well as delayed healing. The reverse pedicled–anterior tibial flap is a distally based flap that can be used to cover small deficits of the lower part of the leg and foot. Adequate plantar circulation is a prerequisite since blood supply is dependent on retrograde flow through anastomoses between the dorsalis pedis and anterior tibial vessels with branches of the posterior tibial and peroneal arteries. This flap is quite versatile and can reach the distal aspect of the plantar surface of the foot. The donor defect produced lacks significant morbidity.

Although there are numerous options for local coverage, these local flaps work extremely well, and one should be familiar with the basic anatomy and possibilities for their use. I would recommend the abductor hallucis flap on the medial aspect of the foot and the extensor brevis flap to cover small defects on the dorsal and lateral surfaces.

Free Tissue Flaps

Free tissue transfer provides well-vascularized composite tissues with primary closure of donor and recipient sites in a single procedure and relatively rapid recovery time.[110, 116–119, 129, 145] This technique, however, can be technically demanding and requires meticulous attention to detail as well as microsurgical skills. The presence of adequate recipient vessels is an essential requirement of free tissue transfer and, due to the frequently encountered extended zone of injury, is often the limiting factor. The selection of donor site is based on the size and specific requirements of the missing tissue and often personal preference. Other factors such as durability, sensibility, as well as structural bulk and contour are less important.

The radial forearm fasciocutaneous flap is a reliable durable procedure capable of covering a wide variety of foot and ankle defects. It is a thin flap and, I think, is particularly useful for covering defects over the dorsum of the foot and ankle. Hallock has referred to this flap as the "workhorse for coverage of acute defects of all foot regions."[122] The flap is based on the radial artery and incorporates the nonhirsute volar skin. The lateral antebrachial cutaneous nerve may be included to provide increased sensibility, but we rarely resort to this. The advantage of this flap is its large size and lack of bulk. Unfortunately donor site closure generally requires skin grafting resulting in suboptimal cosmesis and a focal area of sensory loss. This may be treated in time with tissue volume expanders, excision of the skin graft, and closure of the wound, which is far more cosmetically acceptable. We used this flap in a patient who sustained a severe crush avulsion of his foot at the level of the midfoot, not unlike the patient illustrated in Figure 32–30,C. Following debridement, it was apparent that a more proximal amputation would have to be performed to obtain a plantigrade foot. The long lateral soft-tissue flap could not be used to cover the distal exposed areas due to the bulk of the thick plantar subcutaneous tissue. An alternative for closure in this patient was a split-thickness skin graft directly over the distal part of the foot and ankle; since the plantar surface was intact, this was an appealing alternative. However, to support a functional Chopart amputation, it is imperative to provide optimal dorsiflexion of the foot and avoid an equinus contracture, which is otherwise quite common. This can only be accomplished by reattachment of the anterior tibial tendon into the neck of the talus with lengthening of the Achilles tendon. In this patient, the anterior tibial tendon was completely exposed and the peritenon avulsed, thus indicating that simple coverage with a skin graft would fail. The tendon was tagged with a suture and buried under the viable distal skin flap for later use, and coverage was obtained with a radial forearm fasciocutaneous flap.

A variety of free muscle flaps are available that when covered with a split-thickness skin graft represent an excellent coverage solution for many foot and ankle defects. We have found the latissimus dorsi flap based on the thoracodorsal artery to be reliable and quite versatile. Very large flaps can be harvested and easily contoured and, when covered with a skin graft, still remain less bulky than a myocutaneous flap.[118, 134] The latissimus offers minimal donor site morbidity and has a long pedicle that makes it useful when the recipient vessel is farther away from the defect. For smaller defects, a gracilis flap is very useful, but can also cover larger defects if required. The disadvantage of the gracilis flap is a relatively shorter pedicle that occasionally requires more dissection into the groin to obtain the maximum length. These muscle flaps have proved quite durable even when subjected to weight-bearing stresses (Fig 32–34). Resistance to weight-bearing shear stresses has been explained in part by May by the formation of fibrous shear planes between both the skin graft and muscle as well as between the muscle and bone.[116, 134, 140, 145] These shear planes are shown to dissipate weight-bearing shear forces. These muscle flaps covered with a split-thickness graft are our treatment of choice for defects involving the heel and plantar foot surface.

We have occasionally used a fasciocutaneous scapular flap for coverage of large dorsal wounds where shearing of the tissues with weight-bearing is not a factor.[145] The flap is harvested with the patient prone and is based on the circumflex scapular artery, a branch of the subscapular artery. It is relatively thin and can cover large defects, and where needed the flap can include bone by using a segment of the spine of the scapula. Primary closure of the donor site results in minimal cosmetic deformity and essentially no functional loss. Although it is not our preferred source for coverage, it is occasionally useful as illustrated in the patient in Figure 32–35, a 4-year-old who fell under a tractor and had the dorsomedial aspect of his forefoot sheared off, including the distal aspect of the first metatarsal and proximal phalanx. The plantar tissues were healthy, and we wanted to fill the dorsal defect and simultaneously reconstitute the weight-bearing surface under the first metatarsal head. The length of the hallux was temporarily maintained with a mini–external fixator and the defect closed by using a scapular flap. The flap was raised at 4

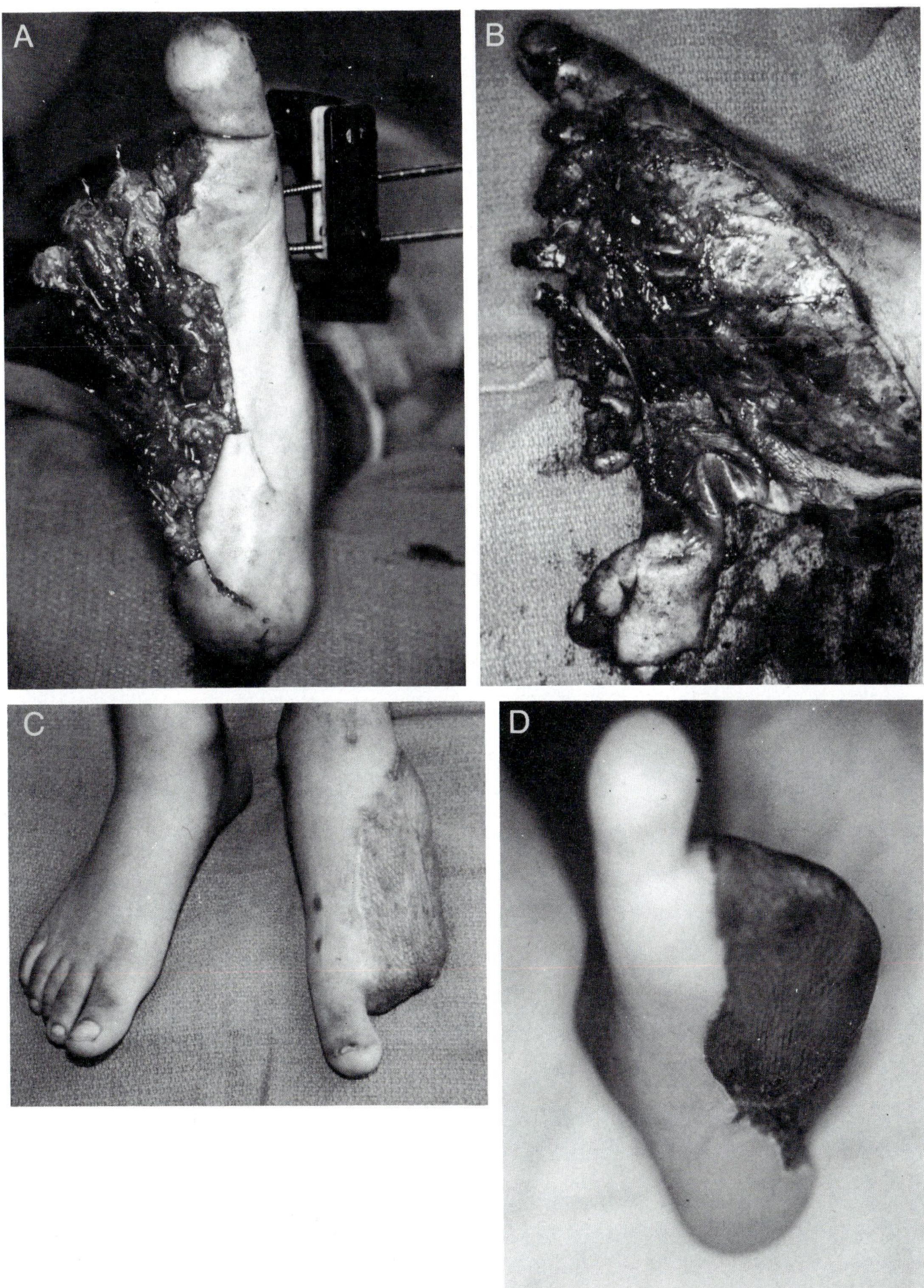

FIG 32–34.
This 11-year-old child sustained a crush amputation of his foot **(A** and **B)** in a railway accident. Note the marked avulsion of tissue both on the dorsal and plantar surfaces. The external fixator is used to immobilize the foot in neutral and facilitate suspension postoperatively. This was treated with immediate latissimus dorsi flap coverage. One year following his accident, he has a functional plantigrade foot with no tendency to break down **(C** and **D).**

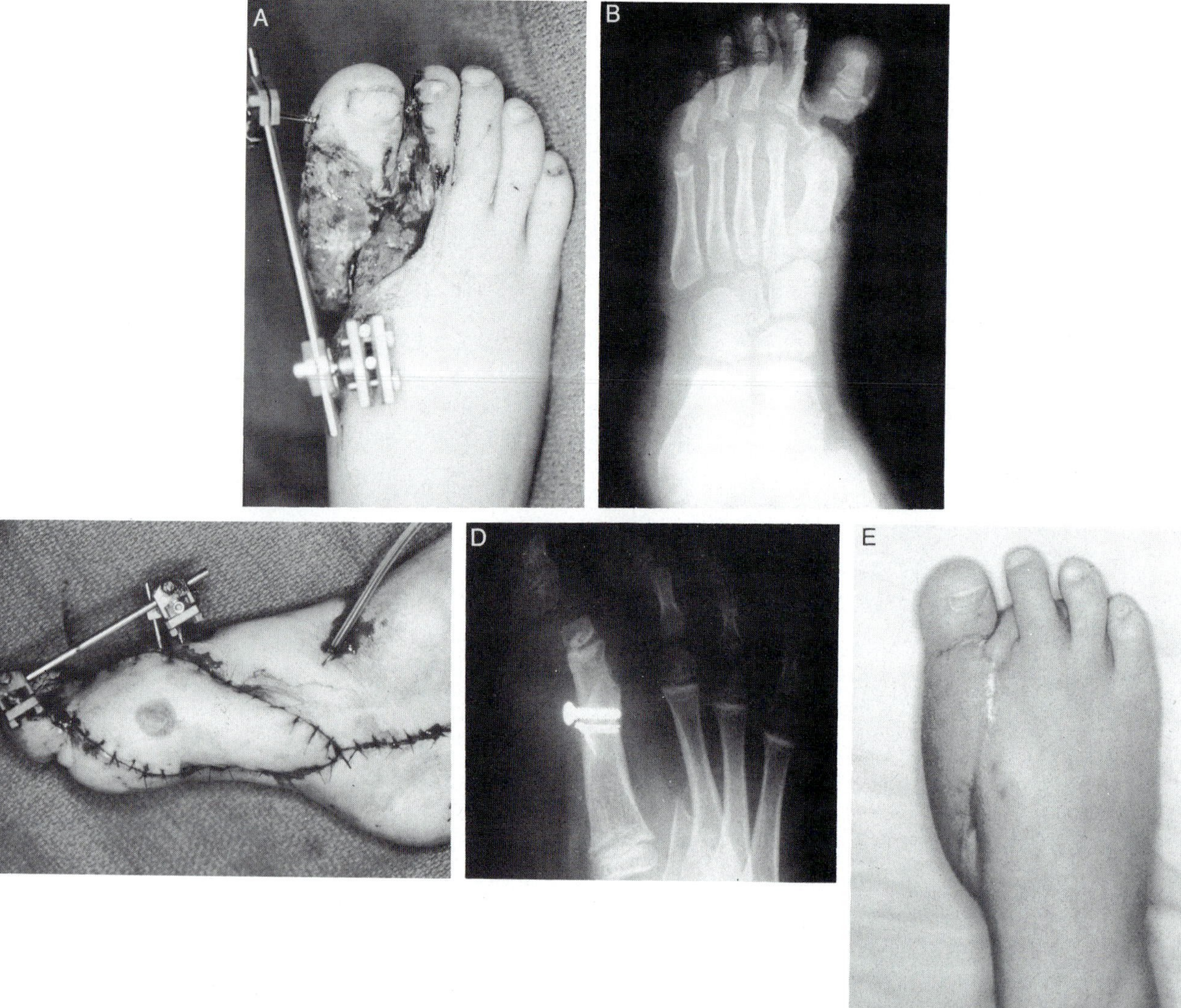

FIG 32–35.
A–E, this child sustained a mangling injury to the hallux with dorsal soft-tissue loss and maintenance of the plantar tissue including the flexor hallucis. Coverage was obtained with a scapular flap and staged amputation of the nonviable second toe with transposition of the second metatarsal including its physis. This vascularized transfer has continued to function and grow over the past 2 years.

weeks to bone-graft the first metatarsal head. Alternatives for grafting would include a free nonvascularized iliac crest graft or a vascularized fibular graft. Since the fibular graft was not felt to be adequate in terms of size, shape, and potential for future growth, it was not selected initially. Since the second toe was not viable and had been ablated in a prior procedure, a second ray resection was performed. The distal second metatarsal was used to substitute for the deficient first in the hope that a vascularized transfer could be performed with potential for growth through the physis. An oblique osteotomy was performed through the distal second metatarsal, and it was medially transposed while attached to its intrinsic muscles as a vascularized transfer (see Fig 32–35).

The importance of flap sensibility on the plantar weight-bearing surfaces of the foot is no longer controversial.[116, 126] It had always been thought that good flap sensibility was essential for protective sensation. However noninnervated heel flaps have proved to be quite viable since almost all retain deep pressure sensation, which is all that appears to be required to maintain durability. We have found that although intermittent ulceration occurs, this is easy to address and does not imply flap failure. Most patients, even children, adjust to the demands of flap care and the routine of daily inspection of their feet (Fig 32–36). Several authors have even stated that sensibility has no significant effect on long-term flap success.

Cross-Leg Flaps

Cross-leg flaps were popular before the successes of free tissue transfer made the latter form of soft-tissue coverage the treatment of choice for covering large defects that were out of the scope of split-thickness skin grafts or local fasciocutaneous flaps.[148–152] However, there are still certain indications for this flap, particularly when free tissue transfer is not available or is not a viable alternative. This occurs in the presence of severe crushing or vascular injuries in which the survival of a free flap may be compromised or a free flap has failed and to repeat a free tissue transfer is not acceptable. The cross-leg flap certainly has a place in the treatment

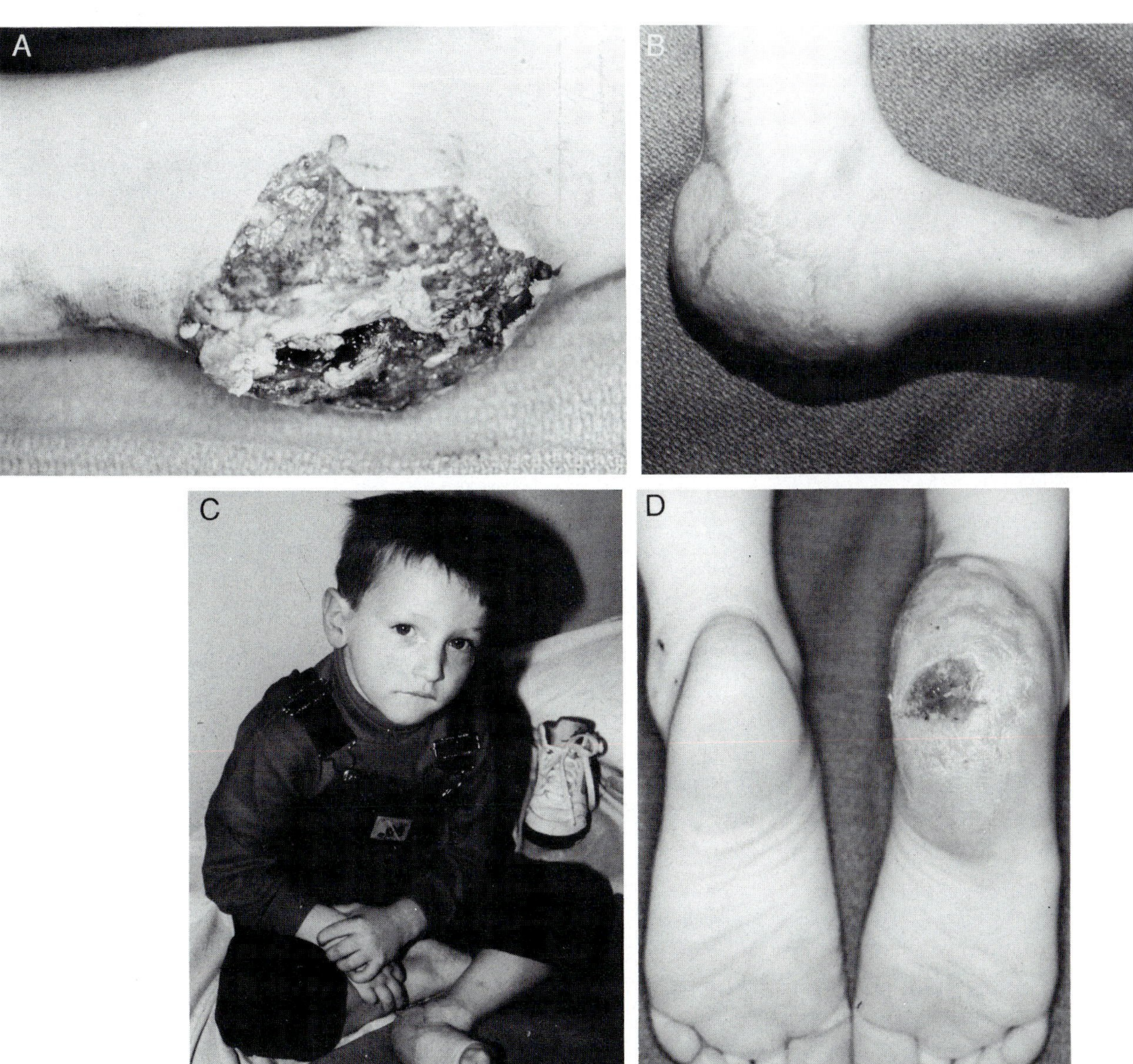

FIG 32–36.
This 3-year-old child sustained an amputation of his heel in a lawn mower accident, which was treated successfully with a latissimus dorsi free flap **(A** and **B).** Over the ensuing year, minor recurrent ulceration occurred that was eventually controlled with the appropriate shoe inserts and parental education **(C** and **D).**

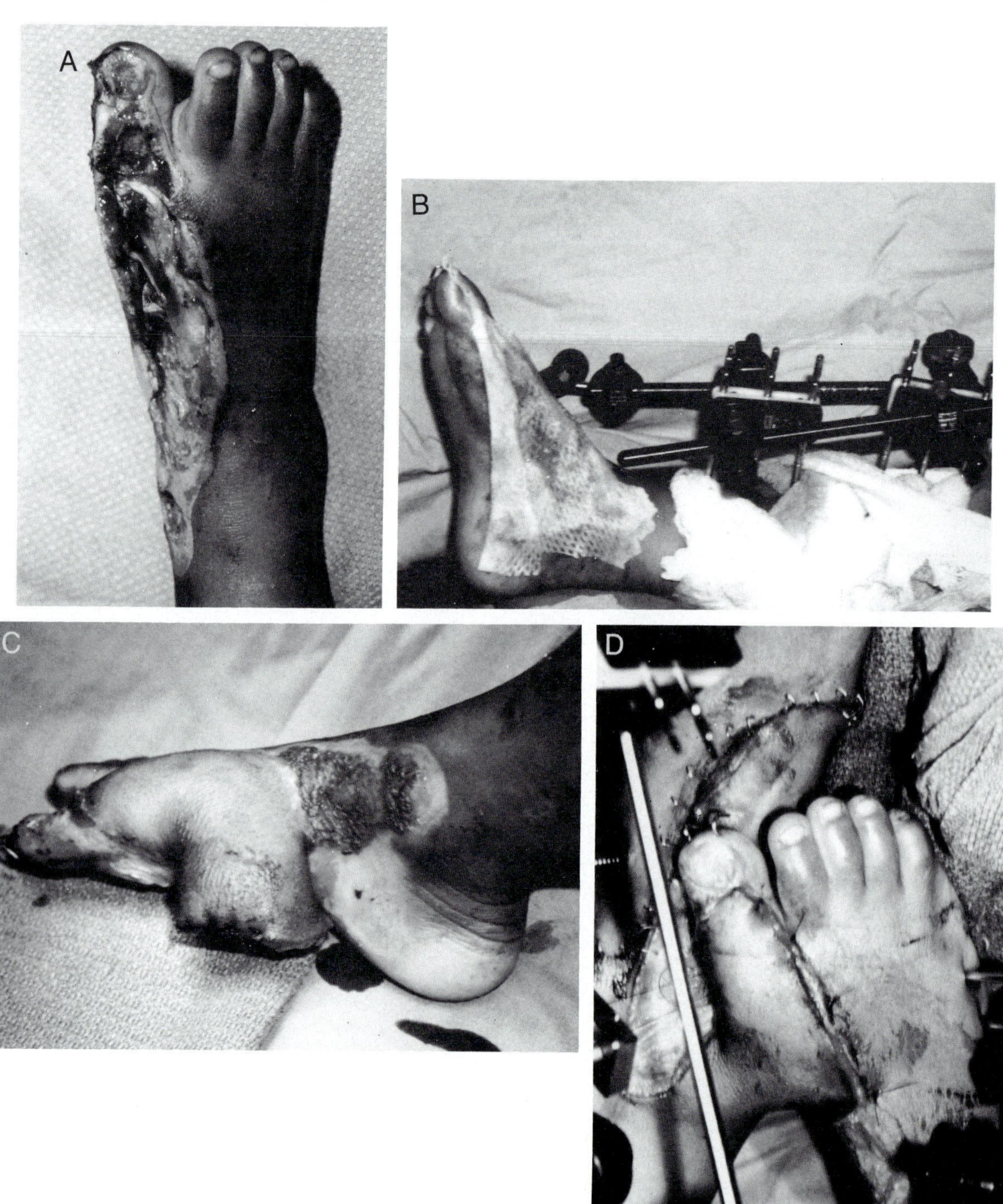

FIG 32–37.
A–D, this 4-year-old child sustained a crush injury to the foot and leg in a motor vehicle accident. In addition to the dorsomedial soft-tissue loss noted here, an ipsilateral tibia fracture associated with a compartment syndrome was present. This was treated with fasciotomy and the limb immobilized with external fixation. Although a free flap would have been our preferred method of coverage, due to the profound ischemia and potential for vessel spasm a cross-leg flap was utilized, as demonstrated here. The flap was mobilized at 14 days and staged reapplication to the foot performed. Although the final functional result is good, the cosmetic result of the cross-leg flap is far from satisfactory.

of soft-tissue loss of the foot and is well reported in the literature.[147, 151, 156] Due to the prolonged immobilization of both limbs during healing, this flap has limited applicability in the adult.[153, 154] Children tolerate the contorted position required to hold the opposite leg to the foot, which may be accomplished with casting but is just as easily tolerated with bilateral external fixation devices, particularly where external fixation is required for treating the injured limb or foot.[152, 155] A simple unilateral external pin construction may be designed to enhance immobilization and facilitate elevation of the limb. This is illustrated in the child in Figure 32–37 who sustained a severe crush injury to her foot and leg in association with a compartment syndrome of the leg and profound ischemia. Due to the ischemia and an extended zone of injury, it was felt that a free flap, which would otherwise be the choice for coverage, would be risky due to potential vessel spasm. A cross-leg flap was selected. The final cosmetic result is fair but unfortunately associated with significant donor site morbidity from the extensive scarring present.

The cross-leg flap depends on neovascularization, which occurs either through the recipient bed or through the three sides of the normal adjacent healthy skin. The former is less likely in view of the poor perfusion of the bone or tendon that the flap is intended to cover. The cross-leg flap becomes a bipedicled flap once perfusion occurs with the adjacent normal tissue. Once this occurs, the flap may be detached from the donor leg, usually between 2 and 3 weeks. The viability of the flap may be ascertained with fluorescein prior to division by occluding the circulation in the donor leg and determining the viability of the flap by the presence of fluorescence. An interesting modification of the cross-leg flap has been described by Uhm et al., who recommend horizontal division of the flap at 10 days. The attached flap is split horizontally in the subcutaneous layer and leaves behind a subcutaneous fat-fascia flap and a skin-subcutaneous flap. The fat-fascia flap pedicle is divided and covered with a split-thickness skin graft. The skin-fat flap can be repositioned on the donor leg over its original site, thereby minizing the marked donor site scarring otherwise present.[156]

CHRONIC COMPARTMENT SYNDROMES OF THE FOOT

Despite an increased awareness of the spectrum of these injuries, the signs and symptoms of increased intracompartmental pressures within the foot are often overlooked. The consequences of untreated compartment syndromes of the feet are serious since these patients have profound sensory and motor disturbances. Chronic pain, stiffness, contracture, intrinsic atrophy, fixed clawing of the toes, soft-tissue dystrophy, and disuse atrophy with osteopenia are some of the delayed sequelae of an untreated compartment syndrome of the foot. In many patients these problems are compounded by chronic immobilization necessitated by the injury, further adding to the dystrophic changes in the juxta-articular structures.

The end result of an untreated compartment syndrome of the foot is a dysfunctional, painful extremity. If the intrinsic muscles of the foot atrophy, particularly the interossei and lumbricales, the critical balance between the intrinsic and extrinsic flexion of the toes is lost. The long extensor tendons then hyperextend the metatarsophalangeal joints, while the long flexor tendons flex both the proximal and distal interphalangeal joints. These deformities eventually become fixed and lead to further dysfunction (Fig 32–38). The remaining intrinsic muscles may also atrophy, and as the foot loses its contour and bulk, and patients complain of discomfort from pressure around bony prominences. The foot is stiff, frequently from unresolved problems dating to the original injury. This ischemic process may also involve sensory deficits, a source of considerable additional debility. We have identified two basic types of forefoot deformity associated with chronic compartment syndromes: one where the toes are clawed and the other where they are stiff and hyperflexed. In some patients, diffuse clawtoe deformities develop by hyperextension of the metatarsophalangeal joints and flexion of the proximal and distal interphalangeal joints. Intrinsic atrophy is noted by wasting of the interossei, the abduc-

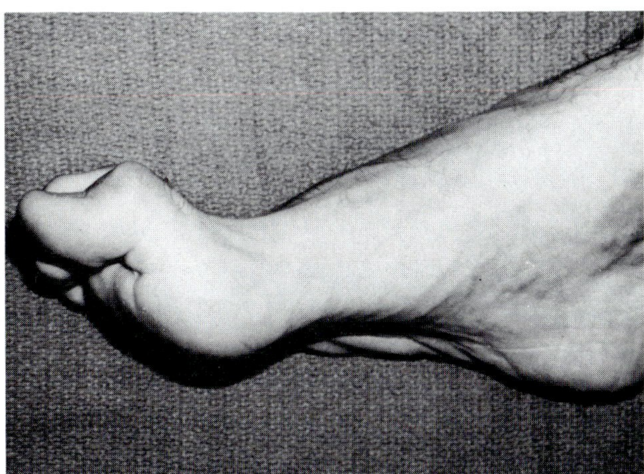

FIG 32–38.
This patient sustained a crush injury of the foot not associated with fracture or dislocation. Following immobilization, he developed fixed clawtoe deformities as illustrated here. Note also the intrinsic atrophy typical of chronic myoneural ischemia.

tor hallucis, and occasionally the extensor brevis muscles. This gives rise to a typical intrinsic minus deformity. The interosseous muscle that attaches to the plantar base of the proximal phalanx is the strongest flexor of the metatarsophalangeal joint, and when it undergoes atrophy, the extensor digitorum longus tendon extends the metatarsophalangeal joint. The delicate balance between the intrinsic and extrinsic musculotendinous units at the metatarsophalangeal joint is lost, and this leads to further extension at the joint. The interosseous tendon subluxes dorsal to the axis of the metatarsal head and fixes the joint in extension, further perpetuating this imbalance. In the alternative deformity, the toes are all acutely flexed at the metatarsophalangeal and interphalangeal joints. These joints are extremely stiff, and little active dorsiflexion of the digits is possible. It is my belief that these two very different forms of contracture of the digits both occur as a result of acute myoneural ischemia. In the first group, the intrinsic minus deformity is due to atrophy of the involved muscles, probably as a result of neural ischemia. This is the same deformity identified in the upper extremity and hand that gives rise to an intrinsic minus deformity of the hand. The fixed flexion deformities in the second group are due to intrinsic muscle fibrosis, including the interossei, lumbricales, and the flexor digitorum brevis. This sequence follows muscle edema, necrosis, and ultimate fibrosis after ischemia.

In some patients, a combination of unrecognized myoneural ischemia in both the foot and the deep posterior compartment of the leg occurs (Fig 32–39). In these patients, in addition to the forefoot deformities as described above, additional contracture occurs in the extrinsic flexors, including the posterior tibial, flexor hallucis, and flexor digitorum longus tendons. The entire foot is extremely stiff, the toes immobile, and equinovarus contracture present. We have treated these deformities with excision of the involved musculotendinous units in the deep compartments. Although tendon lengthening may occasionally work, it is preferable to excise not only the tendon but also the fibrotic muscle to prevent recurrence. The muscles no longer function, and full correction of the deformity is difficult to achieve without excision. Whether or not this should include the entire compartment or be limited to the contracted tendons in the foot and ankle is unclear. We have achieved satisfactory correction of the deformity by complete excision of the posterior tibial, flexor hallucis, and flexor digitorum longus tendons through a posteromedial incision, which can be extended to include a lengthening of the Achilles tendon as needed. Although the incision is longer than a simple tenotomy, which may be performed percutaneously, excision is the mainstay of treatment.

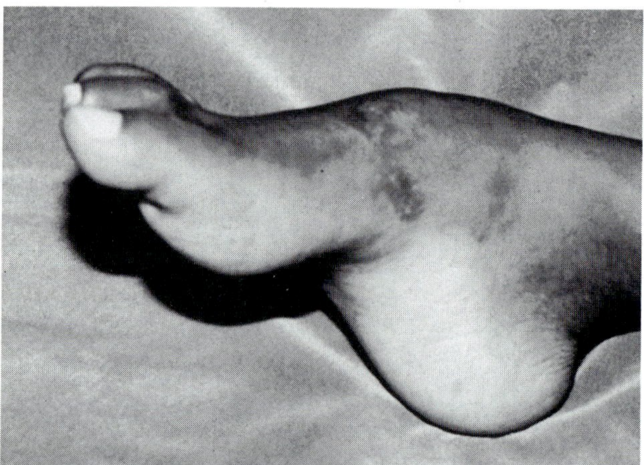

FIG 32–39.
This patient sustained a crush injury of the leg and foot followed by myoneural ischemia that was untreated. The resulting fixed equinovarus deformity is characteristic, but also noted here are fixed clawtoe deformities associated with atrophy of all the intrinsic foot muscles.

Correction of the toe deformities is difficult, and satisfactory function is never regained. Unfortunately, most of these feet are extremely stiff, and the goal in treating these patients is to maximize function and relieve pain. Arthrodesis of the proximal interphalangeal joints is perhaps the best form of treatment when combined with appropriate tendon lengthening or tenotomy. The soft-tissue releases will depend on which type of intrinsic deformity is present. For the fixed flexion contracture, I prefer to lengthen both the short and long flexors with a percutaneous tenotomy through the proximal flexion crease. Passive dorsiflexion returns, and provided that the extrinsic extensor tendons are still functioning, some active dorsiflexion is regained. In the presence of intrinsic atrophy and fixed hyperextension at the metatarsophalangeal joint, proximal interphalangeal arthrodesis is combined with appropriate soft-tissue releases at the metatarsophalangeal joint. If functioning, the long flexor tendons will function to flex the metatarsophalangeal joint. Needless to say, these deformities are best treated by prevention.

To summarize a chapter of this nature is difficult. My approach to treating these severe injuries is constantly evolving. Clearly, the soft-tissue envelope is of paramount importance in managing trauma to the foot and ankle. Through an aggressive multidisciplinary approach, we have managed these wounds by successfully maximizing the ultimate function of the foot. In many if not most facilities where foot trauma is treated, there is and will continue to be a dichotomy of treatment between orthopaedic and plastic reconstructive services.

This, I believe, is wrong and does not enhance the outcome of treatment. There should be close cooperation between these two services from the outset. All too often, we treat patients from other facilities who, following excellent microsurgical reconstructive coverage, have a foot that is still deformed and contracted and requires further orthopaedic treatment. Achilles tendon contracture, toe deformities, and general dysfunction of the foot due to stiffness can all be avoided by careful planning between the orthopaedic and plastic reconstructive teams from the outset. The patient should be evaluated by both teams and a decision made how to proceed with salvage. If soft-tissue coverage by the microsurgeon takes precedence initially, the orthopaedic team should be involved with the treatment at that stage. We frequently use simple uniaxial external fixation to support the foot, which facilitates elevation postoperatively and prevents contracture. The external fixator can be placed on either the medial or lateral side of the foot depending on the wound, the need for dressing changes, and the microsurgical approach to be used. One should also anticipate the timing for major orthopaedic procedures following soft-tissue coverage. I do not recommend that these be performed simultaneously with the free flap since swelling and bleeding may jeopardize the outcome of soft-tissue coverage. An ankle or hindfoot arthrodesis should be deferred until adequate coverage has been obtained and the flap can be safely raised at its edges without fear of compromising its survival. One should also be aware that these severely traumatized feet require constant supervision, monitoring and modification of shoes, and protective orthoses. While it is beyond the scope of this chapter to deal with rehabilitation of these injuries, it is important to recognize that these patients experience problems that change and evolve with time. Plastic and bone revision, patient education for the insensate foot, and periodic supervision all enhance the likelihood of ultimate success.

REFERENCES

General Principles, Salvageability

1. Altemeier WA, Gibbs EW: Bacterial flora of fresh accidental wounds, *Surg Gynecol Obstet* 78:164, 1944.
2. Brown LL, Shelton HT, Bornside GH, et al: Evaluation of wound irrigation by pulsatile jet and conventional methods, *Ann Surg* 187:170–173, 1978.
3. Brown PW: The prevention of infection in open wounds, *Clin Orthop* 96:42, 1973.
4. Burkhalter WE, Butler G, Metz W, et al: Experience with delayed primary closure of war wounds of the hand in Vietnam, *J Bone Joint Surg [Am]* 50:945, 1968.
5. Custer J, Edlich RF, Prusak M, et al: Studies in the management of the contaminated wound, *Am J Surg* 121:522, 1971.
6. Etter C, Burri C, Claes L, et al: Treatment by external fixation of open fractures associated with severe soft tissue damage of the leg. Biomechanical principles and clinical experience, *Clin Orthop* 178: 80–88, 1983.
7. Gidumal R, Carl A: Functional evaluation of nonsensate free flaps to the sole of the foot, *Foot Ankle* 7:118–129, 1986.
8. Gould J: Reconstruction of soft tissue injuries of the foot and ankle with microsurgical techniques, *Orthopaedics* 10:151, 1987.
9. Graham WP, Miller SH, DeMuth WE, et al: Injuries from rotary power lawnmowers, *Am Fam Physician* 13:75, 1976.
10. Grosfeld JL, Morse TS, Eyring EJ: Lawn mower injuries in children, *Arch Surg* 100:582, 1970.
11. Gross A, Cutright ED, Bhaskar SN: Effectiveness of pulsating water jet lavage in treatment of contaminated crushed wounds, *Am J Surg* 124:373, 1972.
12. Gustilo RB, Mendoza RM, Williams DN: Problems in the management of type III (severe) open fractures: a new classification of type III open fractures, *J Bone Joint Surg [Am]* 58:453–458, 1976.
13. Hamer ML, Robson MC, Krizek TJ, et al: Quantitative bacterial analysis of comparative wound irrigations, *Ann Surg* 181:819, 1975.
14. Hansen S: Overview of the severely traumatized lower limb: Reconstruction versus amputation, *Clin Orthop* 243:17, 1989.
15. Hansen ST: The type III tibial fracture. Salvage or amputation, *J Bone Joint Surg [Am]* 69:799–805, 1987.
16. Haury G, Rodeheaver G, Benski J, et al: Debridement: an essential component of traumatic wound care, *Am J Surg* 135:238–242, 1978.
17. Heckman J, Champine M: New techniques in the management of foot trauma, *Clin Orthop* 240:105, 1989.
18. Heggers JP, Robson MC, Doran ET: The quantitative assessment of bacterial contamination of open wounds by a slide technique, *Trans R Soc Trop Med Hyg* 63:532, 1969.
19. Hoehn JG, Jacobs RL, Karmody A: Replantation of a severed foot. *In* Batement J, Trorr A, editors: *The foot and ankle*, New York, 1979, Thieme-Stratton.
20. Horowitz JH, Nichter LS, Kenney JG, et al: Lawnmower injuries in children: lower extremity reconstruction, *J Trauma* 25:1138, 1985.
21. Huany CT, Li PH, Kong GI: Successful restoration of a traumatic amputated leg, *Chin Med J* 84:641, 1965.
22. Jupiter J, Tsai T-M, Kleinert JE: Salvage replantation in lower limb amputations, *Plast Reconstr Surg* 69:1, 1982.
23. Kleinert HE, Jablon M, Tsai TM: An overview of replantation and results of 347 replants in 245 patients, *J Trauma* 20:390, 1980.
24. Kovaric JJ, Matsumoto T, Dobek AS, et al: Bacterial flora of one hundred and twelve combat wounds, *Milit Med* 133:662, 1968.
25. Krizek TJ, Robson MC: Evolution of quantitative bacteriology in wound management, *Am J Surg* 130:579–584, 1975.
26. Lesavoy MD: Successful replantation of lower leg and foot, with good sensibility and function, *Plast Reconst Surg* 64:760, 1979.
27. Levine NS, Lindberg RB, Mason AD, et al: The quantitative swab culture and smear: a quick, simple method

for determining the number of viable aerobic bacteria in open wounds, *J Trauma* 16:89–94, 1976.
28. Lindsey D: Quantitative bacteriological study of tissues, fluids, and exudates, *J Lab Clin Med* 53:299–307, 1959.
29. Madden J, Edlich RF, Schaverhamer R, et al: Application of principles of fluid dynamics to surgical wound irrigation, *Curr Top Surg Res* 3:85, 1971.
30. Magee HR, Parker WR: Replantation of the foot: results after two years, *Med J Aust* 1:751, 1972.
31. May J, Halls M, Simon S: Free microvascular muscle flaps with skin graft reconstruction of extensive defects of the foot: a clinical and gait analysis study, *Plast Reconstr Surg* 75:627, 1985.
32. May JW, Rohrich R: Foot reconstruction using free neurovascular muscle flaps with skin grafts, *Clin Plast Surg* 13:681–689, 1986.
33. McAndrew M, Lantz B: Initial care of massively traumatized lower extremities, *Clin Orthop* 243:20, 1989.
34. Myerson M: Experimental decompression of the fascial compartments of the foot—the basis for fasciotomy in acute compartment syndromes, *Foot Ankle* 8:308, 1988.
35. Myerson MS: Crush injuries of the foot. In Jahss MH, editor: *Disorders of the foot*, Philadelphia, 1991, WB Saunders.
36. Myerson MS: The diagnosis and treatment of compartment syndromes of the foot, *Orthopedics* 13:711–717, 1990.
37. Myerson MS, Burgess AR: The initial evaluation of the acutely traumatized foot and ankle. *In Jahss MH, editor: Disorders of the foot*, Philadelphia, 1991, WB Saunders.
38. Noever G, Bruser P, Kohler L: Reconstruction of heel and sole defects by free flaps, *Plast Reconstr Surg* 78:345, 1986.
39. O'Brien B: Replantation surgery, *Clin Plast Surg* 1:405–426, 1974.
40. Omer G, Pomerantz G: Initial management of severe open injuries and traumatic amputations of the foot, *Arch Surg* 105:696, 1972.
41. Patzakis M, Wilkins J: Factors influencing infection rate in open fracture wounds, *Clin Orthop* 243:36, 1989.
42. Robson MC, Duke WF, Krizek TJ: Rapid bacterial screening in the treatment of civilian wounds, *J Surg Res* 14:426, 1973.
43. Rodeheaver GT, Pettry D, Thacker JG, et al: Wound cleansing by high-pressure irrigation, *Surg Gynecol Obstet* 141:357–362, 1975.
44. Roth J, Urbaniak J, Koman A, et al: Free flap coverage of deep tissue defects of the foot, *Foot Ankle* 3:150, 1982.
45. Sommerlad BC, McGrouther DA: Resurfacing the sole: long-term follow-up and comparison of techniques, *Br J Plast Surg* 31:107, 1978.
46. Trueta J: *The treatment of war wounds and fractures*, New York, 1940, Paul B Hoeber.
47. Trueta J, Barnes JM: The rationale of complete immobilization in treatment of infected wounds, *Br Med J* 2:46, 1940.

The Zone of Injury

48. Bragdon RW: Delayed excision in the severely injured hand, *Orthop Trans* 3:70, 1979.
49. Brown PW: The prevention of infection in open wounds, *Clin Orthop* 96:42, 1973.
50. Corps BVM, Littlewood M: Full-thickness skin replacement after traumatic avulsion, *Br J Plast Surg* 19:229, 1966.
51. Entin MA: Roller and wringer injuries: clinical and experimental studies, *Plast Reconstr Surg* 15:290–312, 1955.
52. Godina M: Early microsurgical reconstruction of complex trauma of the extremities, *Plast Reconstr Surg* 78:285, 1986.
53. Gould J: Management of soft-tissue loss on the plantar aspect of the foot, *AAOS Instr Course Lect* 39:121–136, 1990.
54. Graham WP, Miller SH, DeMuth WE, et al: Injuries from rotary power lawnmowers, *Am Fam Physician* 13:75, 1976.
55. Grosfeld JL, Morse TS, Eyring EJ: Lawn mower injuries in children, *Arch Surg* 100:582, 1970.
56. Hulme JR, Askew AR: Rotary lawn mower injuries, *Injury* 5:217, 1974.
57. Innes CO: Treatment of skin avulsion injuries of the extremities, *Br J Plast Surg* 10:122–136, 1957.
58. Kalisman M, Wexler MR, Yeschua R, et al: Treatment of extensive avulsions of skin and subcutaneous tissues, *J Dermatol Surg Oncol* 4:322–327, 1978.
59. Kudsk KA, Sheldon GF, Walton RL: Degloving injuries of the extremities and torso, *J Trauma* 21:835–839, 1981.
60. Lange K: The use of fluorescent dyes as tracers in biology and medicine, *J Electrochem Soc* 95:131, 1949.
61. Lange K, Boyd LJ: The use of fluorescein to determine the adequacy of circulation, *Med Clin North Am* 26:943, 1942.
62. Levine NS, Lindberg RB, Mason AD, et al: The quantitative swab culture and smear: a quick, simple method for determining the number of viable aerobic bacteria in open wounds, *J Trauma* 16:89–94, 1976.
63. Madigan RR, McMahan CJ: Power lawn mower injuries, *J Tenn Med Assoc* 72:653, 1979.
64. McCraw JB: The value of fluorescein in predicting the viability of arterialized flaps, *Plast Reconst Surg* 60:710, 1977.
65. McGrouther DA, Sully L: Degloving injuries of the limbs: long-term review and management based on whole-body fluorescence, *Br J Plast Surg* 33:9–24, 1980.
66. Myers MB: Prediction of skin slough at the time of operation with the use of fluorescein dye, *Surgery* 51:158–162, 1962.
67. Myerson MS: Split-thickness skin excision: Its use for immediate wound care in crush injuries of the foot, *Foot Ankle* 10:54–60, 1989.
68. Park WH, DeMuth WE: Wounding capacity of rotary lawnmowers, *J Trauma* 15:36, 1975.
69. Tophoj K, Madsen E: Delayed primary operation for open injuries of the extremities, especially the hand (two-stage treatment), *Injury* 2:51–54, 1970.
70. Zeligowski AA, Ziv I: How to harvest skin graft from the avulsed flap in degloving injuries, *Ann Plast Surg* 19:89–90, 1987.
71. Ziv L, Zeligowski AA, Mosheiff R, et al: Split-thickness skin excision in severe open fractures, *J Bone Joint Surg [Br]* 70:23–26, 1988.

Acute Compartment Syndromes

72. Ashton H: Critical closure in human limbs, *Br Med Bull* 19:149, 1963.

73. Ashton H: The effect of increased tissue pressure on blood flow, *Clin Orthop* 113:15–26, 1975.
74. Jennings AMC: Some observations of cortical dosing pressures in the peripheral circulation of anesthetized patients, *Br J Anaesth* 36:683, 1964.
75. Manoli A: Compartment syndromes of the foot: current concepts, *Foot Ankle* 10:340-344, 1990.
76. Matsen FA III: Compartmental syndrome. A unified concept, *Clin Orthop* 113:8–14, 1975.
77. Matsen FA III, Krugmire RB Jr: Compartmental syndromes, *Surg Gynecol Obstet* 147:943–949, 1978.
78. Mubarak S, Owen CA: Compartmental syndrome and its relation to the crush syndrome: a spectrum of disease. A review of 11 cases of prolonged limb compression, *Clin Orthop* 113:81–89, 1975.
79. Mubarak SJ, Hargens AR: *Compartment syndromes and Volkmann's contracture*, Philadelphia, 1981, WB Saunders.
80. Myerson MS: Acute compartment syndromes of the foot, *Orthopedics* 13:711–717, 1990.
81. Myerson MS: Experimental decompression of the fascial compartments of the foot—the basis for fasciotomy in acute compartment syndromes, *Foot Ankle* 8:308–314, 1988.
82. Myerson MS: The diagnosis and treatment of compartment syndromes of the foot, *Orthopedics* 13:711–717, 1990.
83. Rorabeck CH, Caastle TS, Hardie R, et al: Compartment pressure measurements. An experimental investigation using the slit catheter, *J Trauma* 21:446–449, 1981.
84. Rorabeck CH, Macnab I: Anterior tibial–compartment syndrome complicating fractures of the shaft of the tibia, *J Bone Joint Surg [Am]* 58:549–550, 1976.
85. Sarraffian SK: *Anatomy of the foot and ankle*, Philadelphia, 1983, JB Lippincott.
86. Whitesides TE Jr, Haney TC, Morimoto K, et al: Tissue pressure measurements as a determinant for the need of fasciotomy, *Clin Orthop* 113:43–51, 1975.

Skeletal Shortening

87. Hicks JH: The mechanics of the foot. The plantar aponeurosis and the arch, *J Anat* 88:25–30, 1954.
88. Quill GE, Myerson MS, Schwartz LW: Clinical, radiographic and pedobarographic analysis of the involved and contralateral foot after hallux amputation, American Academy of Orthopedic Surgeons annual meeting, Anaheim, Calif, 1991.
89. Roach JJ, McFarlane DS: Midfoot amputations. Application of pioneer procedures in a new age, *Contemp Orthop* 18:577–584, 1989.

Skin Grafting

90. Avellan L, Johanson B: Full thickness skin graft from the dorsum of the foot to its weight-bearing areas, *Acta Chir Scand* 126:497, 1963.
91. Bennett J, Kahn R: Surgical management of soft tissue defects of the ankle-heel region, *J Trauma* 12:696, 1972.
92. Elliott RA, Hoehn JG: Use of commercial porcine skin for wound dressings, *Plast Reconstr Surg* 53:401–405, 1973.
93. Hallock G: Cutaneous coverage for the difficult wound of the foot, *Contemp Orthop* 16:19, 1988.
94. Hidalgo D, Shaw W: Reconstruction of foot injuries, *Clin Plast Surg* 13:663, 1986.
95. Liedberg NCF, Reiss E, Artz CP: Effects of bacteria on take of split-thickness skin grafts in rabbits, *Ann Surg* 142:92, 1955.
96. Sommerlad BC, McGrouther DA: Resurfacing the sole: long-term follow-up and comparison of techniques, *Br J Plast Surg* 31:107, 1978.
97. Southers S: Skin grafts from the sole of the foot: case report and literature review, *J Trauma* 20:163, 1980.

Split-Thickness Skin Excision

98. Corps BVM, Littlewood M: Full-thickness skin replacement after traumatic avulsion, *Br J Plast Surg* 19:229, 1966.
99. Entin MA: Roller and wringer injuries: clinical and experimental studies, *Plast Reconstr Surg* 15:290–312, 1955.
100. Innes CO: Treatment of skin avulsion injuries of the extremities, *Br J Plast Surg* 10:122–136, 1957.
101. Kalisman M, Wexler MR, Yeschua R, et al: Treatment of extensive avulsions of skin and subcutaneous tissues, *J Dermatol Surg Oncol* 4:322–327, 1978.
102. Kudsk KA, Sheldon GF, Walton RL: Degloving injuries of the extremities and torso, *J Trauma* 21:835–839, 1981.
103. Mandel MA: The management of lower extremity degloving injuries, *Ann Plast Surg* 6:1, 1981.
104. McGrouther DA, Sully L: Degloving injuries of the limbs: long-term review and management based on whole-body fluorescence, *Br J Plast Surg* 33:9–24, 1980.
105. Myers MB: Prediction of skin slough at the time of operation with the use of fluorescein dye, *Surgery* 51:158–162, 1962.
106. Myerson MS: Split-thickness skin excision: its use for immediate wound care in crush injuries of the foot, *Foot Ankle* 10:54–60, 1989.
107. Zeligowski AA, Ziv I: How to harvest skin graft from the avulsed flap in degloving injuries, *Ann Plast Surg* 19:89–90, 1987.
108. Ziv I, Zeligowski AA, Mosheiff R, et al: Split-thickness skin excision in severe open fractures, *J Bone Joint Surg [Br]* 70:23–26, 1988.

Free Tissue Transfer

109. Angelats J, Albert LT: Sural nerve neurocutaneous cross-foot flap, *Ann Plast Surg* 13:239, 1984.
110. Barwick W, Goodkind D, Serafin D: The free scapular flap, *Plast Reconstr Surg* 69:779, 1982.
111. Bennett J, Kahn R: Surgical management of soft tissue defects of the ankle-heel region, *J Trauma* 12:696, 1972.
112. Bostwick J: Reconstruction of the heel pad by muscles transposition and split skin graft, *Surg Gynecol Obstet* 143:973, 1976.
113. Colen LB, Buncke HJ: Neurovascular island flaps from the plantar vessels and nerves for foot reconstruction, *Ann Plast Surg* 12:327, 1984.
114. Crocker A, Moss A: The extensor hallucis brevis muscle flap, *J Bone Joint Surg [Br]* 71:532, 1989.
115. Duncan MJ, Zuker RM, Manktelow RT: Re-surfacing weight-bearing surfaces of the heel. The role of the dorsalis pedis innervated free tissue transfer, *J Reconstr Microsurg* 1:201, 1985.
116. Gidumal R, Carl A: Functional evaluation of nonsensate free flaps to the sole of the foot, *Foot Ankle* 7:118–129, 1986.
117. Godina M: Early microsurgical reconstruction of com-

plex trauma of the extremities, *Plast Reconstr Surg* 78:285, 1986.
118. Gordon L, Buncke HJ, Alpert BS: Free latissimus dorsi muscle flap with split-thickness skin graft cover: a report of 16 cases, *Plast Reconstr Surg* 70:173, 1982.
119. Gould J: Reconstruction of soft tissue injuries of the foot and ankle with microsurgical techniques, *Orthopaedics* 10:151, 1987.
120. Grabb W, Argenta L: The lateral calcaneal artery skin flap (the lateral calcaneal artery, lesser saphenous vein, and surak nerve skin flap), *Plast Reconstr Surg* 68:723, 1981.
121. Gulyas G, Mate F, Kartik I: A neurovascular island flap from the first web space of the foot to repair a defect over the heel: case report, *Br J Plast Surg* 37:398, 1984.
122. Hallock G: Cutaneous coverage for the difficult wound of the foot, *Contemp Orthop* 16:19, 1988.
123. Harrison DH, Morgan DGB: The instep island flap to resurface plantar defects, *Br J Plast Surg* 34:315, 1981.
124. Hartrampf CR, Scheflan M, Bostwick J: The flexor digitorum brevis muscle island pedicle flap: a new dimension in heel reconstruction, *Plast Reconstr Surg* 66:264, 1980.
125. Hidalgo D, Shaw W: Anatomic basis of plantar flap design, *Plast Reconstr Surg* 78:627, 1986.
126. Hidalgo D, Shaw W: Reconstruction of foot injuries, *Clin Plast Surg* 13:663, 1986.
127. Hidalgo DA: Lower extremity avulsion injuries. *Clin Plast Surg* 13:701, 1986.
128. Holmes J, Rayner C: Lateral calcaneal artery island flaps, *Br J Plast Surg* 37:402, 1984.
129. Iwaya T, Hari K, Yamada A: Microvascular free flaps for the treatment of avulsion injuries of the feet in children, *J Trauma* 22:15, 1982.
130. Lai MF: Degloved sole and heel, *Med J Aust* 1:598, 1979.
131. Land A, Soragni O, Monteleone M: The extensor digitorum brevis muscle island flap for soft-tissue loss around the ankle: case report, *Plast Reconstr Surg* 75:892, 1985.
132. Leitner D, Gordon L, Buncke H: The extensor digitorum brevis as a muscle island flap: case report. *Plast Reconstr Surg* 76:777, 1985.
133. Leung P, Hung Leung K: Use of the medial plantar flap in soft tissue replacement around the heel region, *Foot Ankle* 8:327, 1988.
134. May J, Halls M, Simon S: Free microvascular muscle flaps with skin graft reconstruction of extensive defects of the foot: a clinical and gait analysis study, *Plast Reconstr Surg* 75:627, 1985.
135. May JW, Rohrich R: Foot reconstruction using free neurovascular muscle flaps with skin grafts, *Clin Plast Surg* 13:681–689, 1986.
136. May JW Jr, Gallico GG III, Lukash FN: Microvascular transfer of free tissue for closure of bony wounds of the distal lower extremity, *N Engl J Med* 306:253, 1982.
137. McCabe WP, Kelly AP Jr, Behan FC: Reconstruction of the plantar pad after degloving injuries of the foot, *Surg Gynecol Obstet* 137:971, 1973.
138. Noever G, Bruser P, Kohler L: Reconstruction of heel and sole defects by free flaps, *Plast Reconstr Surg* 78:345, 1986.
139. Reiffel R, McCarthy J: Coverage of heel and sole defects: A new subfascial arterialized flap, *Plast Reconstr Surg* 66:250, 1980.
140. Roth J, Urbaniak J, Koman A, et al: Free flap coverage of deep tissue defects of the foot, *Foot Ankle* 3:150, 1982.
141. Serafin D, Georgiade N, Smith D: Comparison of free flaps with pedicled flaps for coverage of defects of the leg or foot, *Plast Reconstr Surg* 59:492, 1977.
142. Shanahan RE, Gingrass RP: Medial plantar sensory flap for coverage of heel defects, *Plast Reconstr Surg* 64:295, 1979.
143. Snyder GB, Edgerton MT: The principle of island neurovascular flap in the management of ulcerated aesthetic weight-bearing areas of the lower extremity, *Plast Reconstr Surg* 36:518, 1965.
144. Sommerlad BC, McGrouther DA: Resurfacing the sole: long-term follow-up and comparison of techniques, *Br J Plast Surg* 31:107, 1978.
145. Urbaniak J, Koman A, Goldner R, et al: The vascularized cutaneous scapular flap, *Plast Recontr Surg* 69:772, 1982.
146. Yana A, Park S, Iwao T, et al: Reconstruction of a skin defect of the posterior heel by a lateral calcaneal flap, *Plast Reconstr Surg* 75:642, 1985.

Cross-Leg Flaps

147. Barclay TL, Cardoso E, Sharpe DT, et al: Repair of lower leg injuries with fasciocutaneous flaps, *Br J Plast Surg* 35:127–131, 1982.
148. Barclay TL, Sharpe DT, Chisholm EM: Cross-leg fasciocutaneous flaps, *Plast Reconstr Surg* 72:843–849, 1983.
149. Cormack GC, Lamberty BGH: A classification of fasciocutaneous flaps according to their patterns of vascularization, *Br J Plast Surg* 37:80–86, 1984.
150. Millard DR: The Crane principle for the transport of subcutaneous tissue, *Plast Reconstr Surg* 43:451–462, 1969.
151. Ponten B: The fasciocutaneous flap: Its use in soft tissue defects of the lower leg, *Br J Plast Surg* 34:215–221, 1981.
152. Stark RB: The cross-leg flap procedure, *Plast Reconstr Surg* 9:173–182, 1952.
153. Thatte RL: De-epithelialized turn-over flaps for "salvage" operations, *Br J Plast Surg* 36:178–182, 1983.
154. Thatte RL, Laud N: The use of the fascia of the lower leg as a roll-over flap: its possible clinical application in reconstructive surgery, *Br J Plast Surg* 37:88–96, 1984.
155. Tolhurst DE, Haeseker B, Zeeman RT: The development of the fasciocutaneous flap and its clinical applications, *Plast Reconstr Surg* 71:597–602, 1983.
156. Uhm KI, Shin KS, Lew JD: Crane principle of the cross-leg fasciocutaneous flap: aesthetically pleasing technique for damaged dorsum of foot, *Ann Plast Surg* 15:257–261, 1985.

CHAPTER

33

Miscellaneous Soft-Tissue Injuries

G. James Sammarco, M.D.

Reflex sympathetic dystrophy syndrome — the orphan disease

Anatomy and physiology
Etiology
Classification
Stages of reflex sympathetic dystrophy
Clinical symptoms
Diagnosis
Treatment
  First level of treatment
  Second level of treatment
  Surgical treatment
  Discussion

Heat and cold injuries

Frostbite
  Treatment
Immersion and trench foot
  Treatment
Chilblain
  Treatment
Burns
  Classification of burns
  Treatment

Foreign bodies

The earliest description of causalgia, a type of reflex sympathetic dystrophy syndrome (RSDS), is credited to Weir Mitchell.[17] He gave a clear description of the severe, unrelenting, burning pain experienced by soldiers who had sustained penetrating wounds to a major nerve trunk in the Civil War.[20] Through the years many reports of more syndromes and case reports of neurovascular dysfunction related to the sympathetic nervous system have appeared in the medical literature. In most cases the symptoms and signs of the syndrome were similar except for certain factors. Patients with reflex sympathetic dystrophy had differing etiologies, presenting symptoms, and response to treatment.[31] Recently the term *reflex sympathetic dystrophy syndrome* has been used to characterize this group of disorders resulting from dysfunction of the sympathetic nervous system.[30]

Anatomy and Physiology

A study of the normally functioning sympathetic nervous system reveals the great number of interconnections in the spinal cord and central nervous system (CNS). The dysfunctional sympathetic nervous system may present a wide variety of symptoms from mild to severe involvement. The success of treatment requires a thorough understanding of these factors.

The sympathetic nervous system is the thoracolumbar division of the autonomic nervous system, and the parasympathetic nervous system is the craniosacral division (Fig 33–1). These divisions of the autonomic nervous system, along with the endocrine system, regulate the internal human environment and are not under voluntary control.[1]

The afferent sympathetic neuron cell bodies are lo-

**The author wishes to thank Sandra Adams Eisele, M.D., for her contributions to the section on "Reflex Sympathetic Dystrophy Syndrome" in this chapter.*

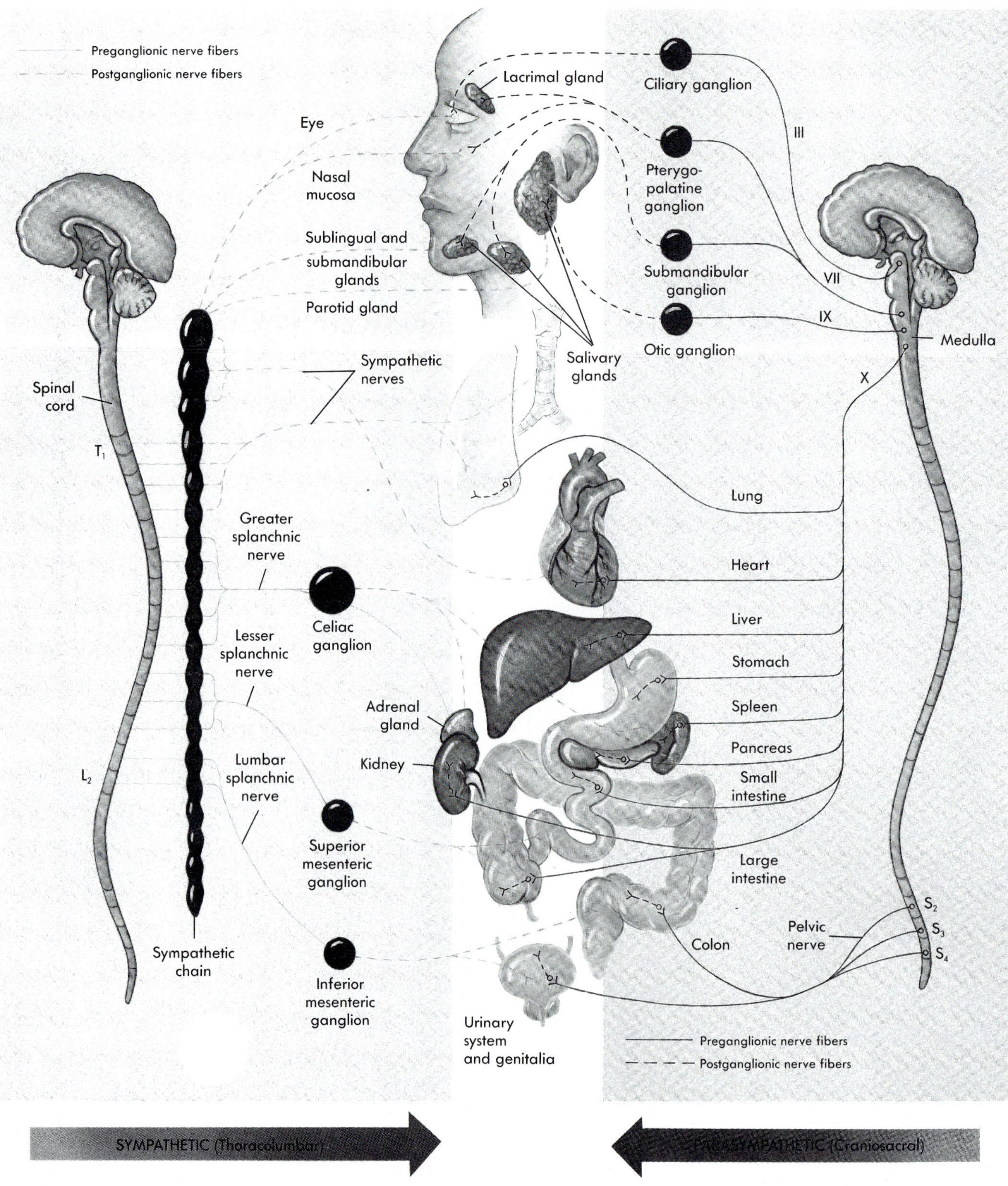

FIG 33–1.
In the sympathetic division of the autonomic nervous system, preganglionic fibers begin in the spinal cord (intermediolateral nucleus) and pass to peripheral autonomic ganglia. The postganglionic fibers pass from the peripheral ganglia to effector organs. In the parasympathetic division of the autonomic nervous system, preganglionic fibers begin in the brainstem and presacral segments and pass to peripheral ganglia. Postganglionic fibers pass from the ganglia to the effector organs. The hypothalamus helps regulate the system as does the supranuclear regulatory apparatus of the CNS. Preganglionic fibers are indicated by *solid lines,* and postganglionic fibers are indicated by *broken lines.* (From Seeley RR, Stephens TD, Tate R: *Anatomy and physiology,* St Louis, 1989 Times Mirror/Mosby College Publishing. Used by permission.)

cated in the lateral horns of the spinal cord gray matter from the first thoracic to the third lumbar level. The axons may pass up or down several levels before entering the paravertebral chain of ganglia via the white ramus communicans (Fig 33–2). They then travel up or down several levels before synapsing with the postganglionic neuron. They may also synapse with many postganglionic neurons, and each postganglionic neuron receives input from many preganglionic neurons. Some preganglionic neurons pass through the paravertebral chain to synapse in the prevertebral ganglia, the celiac, superior, or inferior mesenteric ganglia. The sympathetic supply to the cranium arises from the eighth cervical and first two thoracic ganglia, and the arm receives its sympathetic supply from the upper thoracic ganglia via the stellate ganglia. The lower three lumbar and first sacral ganglia supply only the legs, with no visceral connections.

In the sympathetic system the afferent sympathetic fibers carry information into the spinal cord and then synapse in the gray matter of the cord (see Fig 33–2). The preganglionic neuron then travels out the spinal nerve to the paravertebral ganglia. Here additional synapses occur. The postganglionic neuron now travels back to the spinal nerve via the gray ramus communicans and out the spinal nerve to the skin with vasomotor, sudodomotor, and pilomotor impulses. There are multiple connections at several levels for the sympathetic neurons. All this is under "automatic" control.

In the extremities, the most common sympathetic regulatory functions are vasomotor, i.e., control of constriction and dilation of the blood vessels; sudomotor, i.e., regulation of sweating; and piloerection, i.e., control of hair movement. The most common neurotransmitter for the sympathetic system is norepinephrine and for the parasympathetic system, acetylcholine. How-

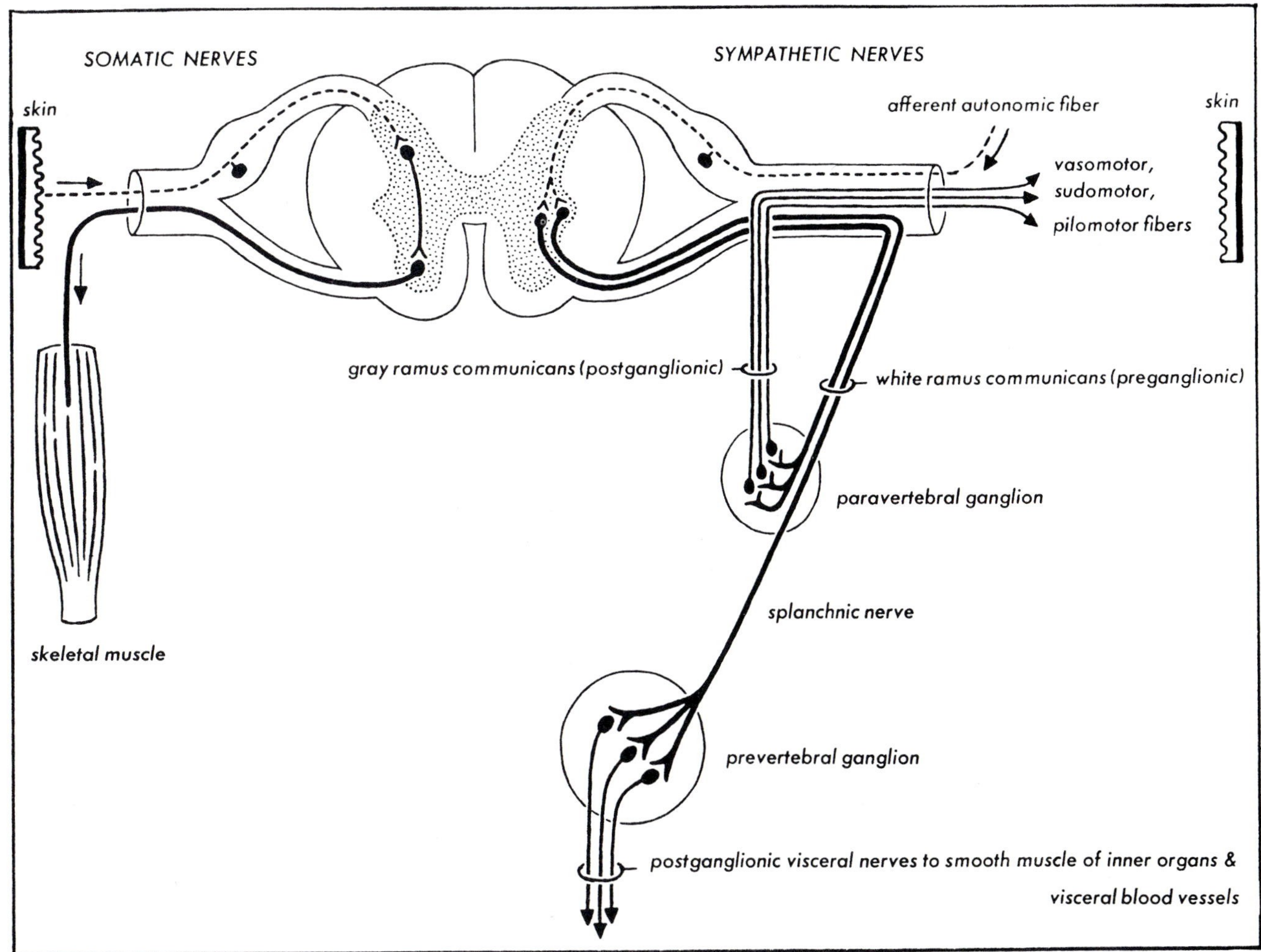

FIG 33–2.
Sympathetic outflow from the spinal cord and the course of sympathetic fibers. *Heavy lines* are preganglionic fibers. *Thin lines* are postganglionic fibers. (Adapted from Pick S: *The autonomic nervous system,* Philadelphia, 1970, JB Lippincott.)

ever, there are exceptions. The blood vessels, piloerector muscles, and sweat glands receive only sympathetic innervation, yet the sweat glands respond only to acetylcholine.

In the periphery, the sympathetic nervous system has both excitatory and inhibitory effects, depending on the type of receptors, either alpha, which are generally excitatory, or beta, which are generally inhibitory and are found in bronchial muscles and the sinoatrial node of the heart.

Drugs that interfere with neurotransmitters at the nerve endings can cause a blockade of nerve function. Local anesthetic agents cause a sympathetic blockade when used to block the lumbar paravertebral sympathetic chain for lower-extremity blockade. In a pure sympathetic blockade, somatic sensation and motor function remain intact. If incomplete relief of dysfunctional sympathetic symptoms occurs, then a complete blockade of somatic and sympathetic systems is required. This can be accomplished with local anesthetic agents such as lidocaine or bupivacaine (Marcaine), intravenous regional anesthesia for the upper extremity, and an epidural block in the lower extremity.

Etiology

There are several theories that attempt to explain the hyperactivity of the sympathetic nervous system which occurs after injury and occasionally in patients without a history of injury. Yet, the cause and mechanisms of RSDS remain unclear. Early theories were based on probability. More recently basic and clinical research has added to the growing information required to substantiate these theories.

Livingston[24] proposed a "vicious cycle of reflexes" that starts with chronic irritation of a peripheral nerve from trauma or some other cause resulting in increased afferent input to the spinal cord. This not only causes pain but also excites the "internuncial pool" of neurons in the lateral and anterior horns, which, in turn, increases sympathetic and efferent motor activity and causes the syndrome.

Melzak[20] expanded on the theory and proposed that the substantia gelatinosa in the spinal cord modulates afferent impulses before they reach effector neurons. Afferent impulses are carried by the small (C) and large (A) neural fibers to the substantia gelatinosa. Preferential stimulation of the small (C) fibers would suppress the substantia gelatinosa and "open the gate" to allow more afferent impulses into the spinal cord. If the large (A) fibers were preferentially stimulated, the substantia gelatinosa would have an enhanced inhibitory tone, and the "gate would close" and block afferent impulses. Selective prolonged stimulation of small (C) fibers would allow unrestrained afferent impulses to the spinal cord and to other interconnecting paths.

Schott[28, 29] reviewed the mechanisms for the etiology of RSDS and concluded that the CNS plays an important role for five reasons: (1) causalgia occurs in diseases confined to the CNS and in phantom limb pain; (2) an unusual pain distribution sometimes occurs, i.e., a stocking- or glove-like distribution in an injured limb or even in the contralateral limb; (3) a paradoxical widespread pain distribution can occur after sympathetic nervous system injury; (4) peripheral sympathetic blockade is effective even when the cause is in the CNS; and (5) the central interactions cause motor, sensory, and psychological phenomena.

A hypothesis proposed by Janig[36] considers RSDS to be caused by central lesions, peripheral nerve lesions, and "chronic excitation of visceral and deep somatic afferents." These include (1) a change in the processing of information in the spinal cord and supraspinal centers; (2) coupling between sympathetic postganglionic axons and afferent axons in the periphery with the establishment of a vicious circle; (3) coupling causing orthodromic impulse activity to the spinal cord and also antidromic afferent activity to the periphery, with the possible development of an "axon response" in the peripheral tissues; (4) with degeneration of their innervation, the development of supersensitivity to circulating catecholamines or other substances in blood vessels and other autonomic effector organs; and (5) central lesions and stimulation of visceral afferents such as angina pectoris, with production of the symptoms of RSDS.

A hypothesis proposed by Roberts and Stanton-Hicks et al.[25, 36] is based on the premise that spinal sensory neurons called wide-dynamic-range neurons receive excitatory input from low-threshold mechanoreceptors, which are influenced by trauma. These neurons are sensitized by this stimulation and become hyperexcitable. Subsequent sympathetic activation of the low-threshold mechanoreceptors causes excessive firing of the hyperexcitable neurons and spontaneous pain; further firing of the low-threshold mechanoreceptors results in excessive firing of those neurons and characteristic allodynia, i.e., painful sensation to touch.

Classification

The term *reflex sympathetic dystrophy* has been used to refer to a great number of different conditions, some of which apparently have several names themselves. All these conditions have in common the primary condition of sympathetically maintained pain. Weir Mitchell in 1864 coined the term *causalgia*. The injury involved an incompletely damaged nerve. Pain would usually start within 1 week of injury and was difficult to treat. The median, ulnar, and sciatic nerves were the most commonly damaged. Often the burning pain spread beyond the limits of the specific damaged nerve to include the entire extremity or even the contralateral extremity.[29]

Sudeck's atrophy,[28] described in 1900, included primarily bony resorption in the involved extremity. Swelling and redness of the extremity were also present (Fig 33–3).

Homans in 1940 used the term "minor causalgia" to refer to patients with this syndrome but no nerve injury and "major causalgia" for those with nerve damage as described by Mitchell. Since the symptoms are often equally severe and the disability the same, regardless of the etiology, these terms have not been practical in classifying patients.[20]

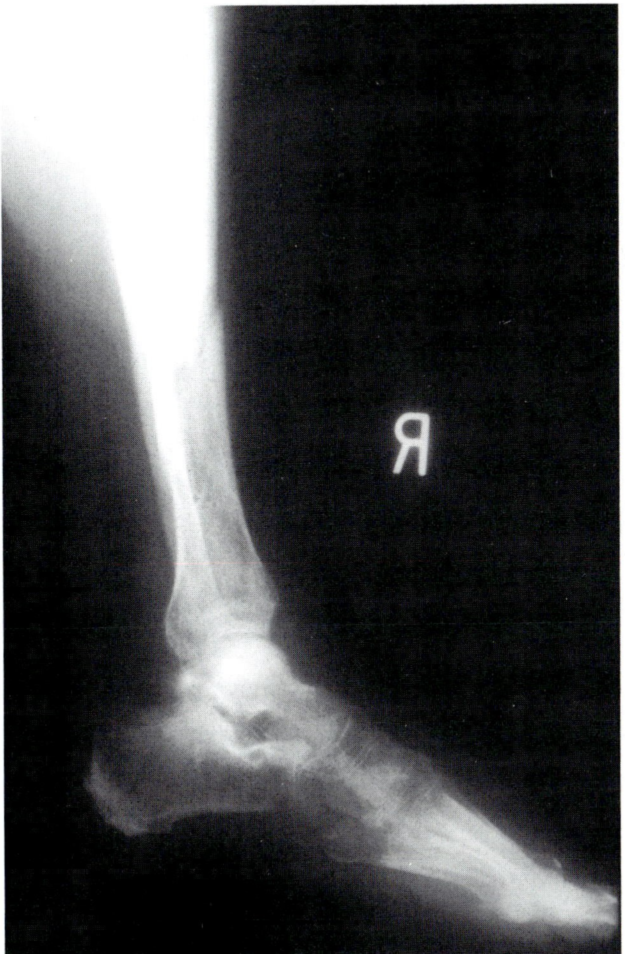

FIG 33–3.
Lateral radiograph of the foot and ankle in a 54-year-old male with RSDS. The disease has been present for more than 1 year. Note the healed fracture of the tibia. Gross osteoporosis is present, so-called Sudeck's atrophy.

Many other terms have been used. A partial list includes the following[11]: posttraumatic pain syndrome, posttraumatic osteoporosis, posttraumatic dystrophy of the extremities, reflex sympathetic dystrophy, sympathetic dystrophy, mimocausalgia, algoneurodystrophy, shoulder-hand syndrome, algodystrophy, reflex sympathetic imbalance, as well as reflex sympathetic dystrophy syndrome. RSDS is the most inclusive of all the varieties and manifestations of the abnormal functioning of the sympathetic nervous system and is the most commonly used term today.

Stages of Reflex Sympathetic Dystrophy Syndrome

It is generally held that there are three distinct stages of RSDS.[34, 36] Determining what stage a patient is in at the time of diagnosis will help in planning treatment and determining the prognosis. The first, or acute, phase lasts from the time of onset to 3 months and is thought to result from denervation of the sympathetic nervous system. The findings include burning pain, hyperpathia, i.e., prolonged painful sensation to touch, increased blood flow to the extremity resulting in higher temperature, dependent rubor, localized edema, accelerated hair and nail growth, and joint stiffness with reduced active and passive range of motion. The second stage is the dystrophic phase. Symptoms are more likely to be related to hyperactivity of the sympathetic nervous system and include persistent hyperpathia and burning pain, decreased blood flow to the extremity and lower-than-normal skin temperature, decreased hair growth and brittle nails, spreading brawny edema, pale cyanotic color, muscle stiffness along with muscle atrophy, localized osteoporosis, and personality or psychological changes associated with continued severe disability. This phase also lasts up to 3 months. The third and final phase is that of severe atrophy and is characterized by less hyperpathia and burning pain, more normal blood flow with a tendency to normalization of local temperature, coarse hair and rigid nails, smooth, glossy drawn skin with subcutaneous atrophy, atrophic muscles with severe weakness, arthrofibrosis of joints with tendon and muscle contractures, localized osteoporosis, and a chronic pain syndrome personality (Fig 33–4).

Clinical Symptoms

As much information as possible should be obtained from the patient concerning the circumstances surrounding the onset of RSDS. There are certain symptoms frequently seen in these patients.[26, 36] All patients have pain in the affected area, and most have some amount of tenderness. Some have hyperpathia and oth-

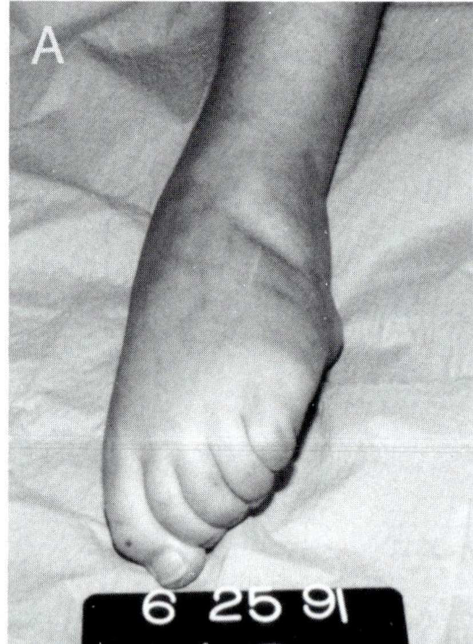

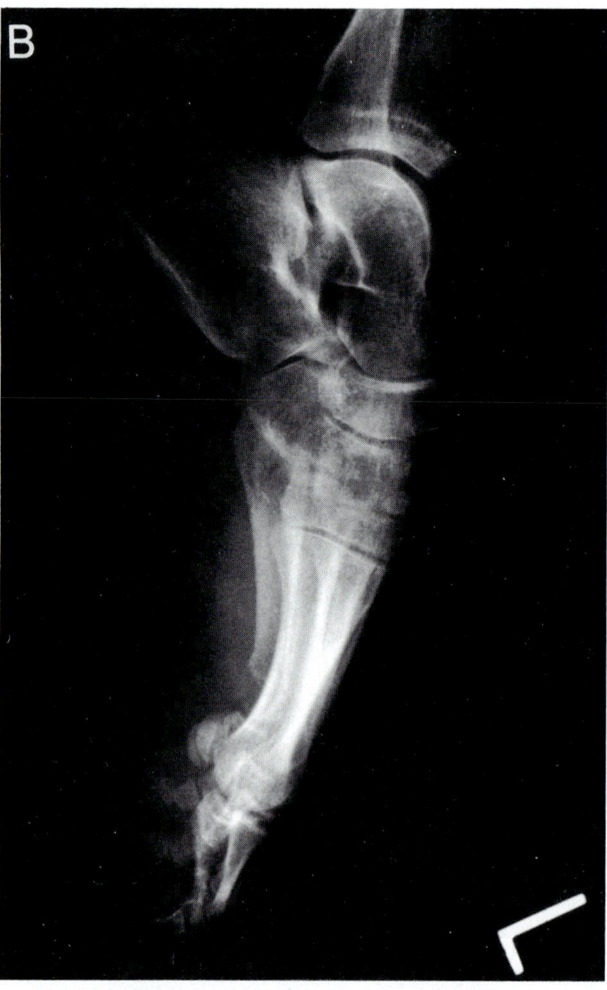

FIG 33–4.
A, photograph of a 23-year-old female with RSDS that developed immediately following arthroscopy. Eighteen months later she was unable to bear weight and had extensive flexion contractures of the knee, ankle, foot, and toes. **B,** lateral radiograph of the same patient showing bone atrophy and severe equinus of the ankle with clawing of all toes. The patient dragged her foot on the ground and was unable to wear even a soft sock for protection.

ers, allodynia. Pain is out of proportion to the injury and is often described as "burning" in nature, i.e., hyperalgesia. The leg may be swollen and will often have increased or decreased vasomotor reactions and sudomotor abnormalities with sweating or dryness of the skin. Medical diseases also known to cause RSDS include myocardial infarction, angina pectoris, arthritis, and herpes zoster after effects. Diseases of the CNS such as brain tumors, head injury, cervical fractures, and subarachnoid hemorrhage can also cause RSDS. Orthopaedic considerations include injuries as mild as an ankle sprain. But fractures, amputations, and surgical procedures during which nerves are manipulated or otherwise traumatized may trigger it. Its onset may occur quite early in the postoperative period and has been reported as beginning in the recovery room. RSDS has been reported to occur after intramuscular injections near the sciatic or lateral femoral cutaneous nerves.[15] RSDS has also been reported to occur with diabetic neuropathy.[27]

Typically, the patient complains of persistent postoperative or posttraumatic pain that gradually grows to become the primary complaint. The surgeon may be misled into thinking that the pain is due to unusual patient sensitivity or a mechanical problem, but symptoms rapidly increase beyond those of physical findings. Pain at rest, pain with active and passive motion, and pain at night are characteristic symptoms. Burning pain is common and often involves the extremity from just above the site of injury or surgery distally in a so-called stocking distribution. The burning and pain may also be localized without having the distribution of a single peripheral nerve or dermatome. At night limb sensitivity may be so exaggerated that the patient is unable to tolerate even the weight of a sheet on the foot. Symptoms may include the entire extremity as well as the bowel and bladder and may be so disabling as to prevent any voluntary motion of the leg without triggering continued muscle spasms of the entire extremity. Crutches are required. Chronic spasm may lead to fixed joint contracture including ankle equinus and toe flexion (see Fig 33–4). The patient may be so miserable that he may demand an amputation. In chronic severe cases, the patient is unable to work, and this may lead to social problems that complicate the treatment and prognosis.[36]

Demographically, RSDS is seen in males and females equally in adults of all ages. In children it is most common in adolescent girls.[13] Adolescents and children often have a spontaneous onset without a history of injury. However, the clinical course of the condition in children seems to be shorter. They may be treated with simple noninvasive modalities usually with good results.[10, 35]

Diagnosis

When a patient presents with a characteristic history and symptoms following injury, physical examination and radiographs should be obtained. Localized osteoporosis will often be seen as early as 3 to 4 weeks following the onset. Soft-tissue swelling and subperiosteal bone resorption are often present also, although this may occur later in the course of the disease, in the second or third phase. These findings are not specific for RSDS and may also be seen in hyperparathyroidism, thyrotoxicosis, and other conditions with high bone turnover.

The three-phase technetium bone scan has been used in recent years to aid in making this diagnosis.[36] The most common abnormality seen in adults is due to increased blood flow into the affected leg causing increased bone metabolism. Therefore, the early perfusion and blood pool activity may be increased, and the delayed images may also show increased periarticular activity in bone, especially if symptoms have been present for more than 6 weeks.[6, 16] Children, however, may have the opposite finding, with decreased uptake most of the time in all three phases.[11] The reason for this is as yet undetermined.

A lumbar sympathetic block using 5 cc of 0.25% bupivacaine (Marcaine) injected through a spinal needle directed into the paravertebral sympathetic plexus is a good test. An image intensifier is often used to ensure that the needle tip is at the correct anatomic site. This greatly increases the accuracy of the needle position and hence the validity of the test. When performed correctly, a warm flush is felt by the patient in the skin of the extremity. The characteristic burning pain may be relieved for more than 2 hours. The test may not necessarily relieve the pain, even when performed correctly, but this does not necessarily rule out RSDS.[36]

Another diagnostic test is the sympathetic block described by Schwartzman and McLellan.[31] An epidural spinal block is performed at 10-minute intervals with the following solutions in order of sequence: (1) 5 cc normal saline (placebo), (2) 5 cc of 0.2% procaine hydrochloride (critical sympathetic concentration), and (3) 5 cc of 0.5% procaine hydrochloride (critical motor concentration). The lowest level of procaine that relieves pain indicates whether the pain is sympathetically maintained, peripheral somatic, or central in origin.

Treatment

The rationale for treating RSDS is based on the need to alleviate symptoms while eliminating suspected or obvious causes. This is difficult to accomplish since the specific cause of the syndrome is not fully understood. The syndrome has been nicknamed "the orphan disease" because the symptoms are often so overwhelming and the treatment response so limited that the physician "refers the patient" to another specialist. Treatment is directed not only at interrupting the abnormal sympathetic input and the peripheral and central mechanisms that support this, but also directly at the targets of the disease, that is, the joints, bones, and muscles.[36]

First Level of Treatment

The first line of therapy is composed of anti-inflammatory medication and physical therapy. Physical therapy is prescribed on a daily basis. Modalities including active motion, flexibility exercises, a tilt board, progressive ambulation, ultrasound, contrast baths, and hydrotherapy are all utilized with concentration on the modalities that are the most successful in reducing pain and increasing function. The patient is not forced beyond his tolerance, but supervised therapy is recommended throughout the course, sometimes for as long as a year or more. Putting patients through painful physical therapy sessions may perpetuate the pain process. The best approach is to let patients progress through a program of active therapy at their own rate and allow them some control over their own pain symptoms. In addition to anti-inflammatory medication i.e., nonsteroidal anti-inflammatory drugs (NSAIDs), a tricyclic antidepressant such as amitriptyline, 25 mg for sleep, is prescribed. The dose may be increased to 50 mg for sleep if the symptoms do not abate and the patient is able to tolerate it.

Desipramine has also been used in like manner. Tricyclics are used primarily to reduce hypersensitivity in the affected area and secondarily to treat depression. Phenoxybenzamine causes a chemical sympathectomy with oral treatment and has been utilized with some improvement in symptoms. Hypotension episodes are a common side effect, and therefore this drug may be contraindicated in some patients.[31] Other medications such as propranolol, calcium channel blockers, prazosin nifedipine (Procardia), phenytoin, and calcitonin have been used, but their true efficacy is unknown.[31, 34, 36]

Transcutaneous nerve stimulation (TENS) has been used to treat RSDS.[36] Its mechanism of action is unknown, but Melzak notes that it produces stimulation of both large and small fibers, with large A fibers "closing the gate" to cyclic activity and small C fibers enhancing inhibitory areas of the brain stem and blocking pain transmission. The TENS unit can be used early in treatment to enhance the results of physical therapy.

The use of corticosteroids is controversial. They have been used both orally as well as in intravenous regional blocks along with lidocaine. Corticosteroids do not treat the sympathetic system itself but seem to affect the peripheral tissue effects of RSDS by stabilizing basement membranes, decreasing capillary permeability, and reducing perivascular inflammation.

There is no place for the use of narcotic medications in the treatment of RSDS. Such medication does not affect sympathetically maintained pain and leads to dependency with no relief of pain.[2]

Second Level of Treatment

If the previously described treatment modalities are ineffective in the first 4 to 8 weeks after the diagnosis of acute RSDS, additional treatment is indicated.

Lumbar sympathetic blocks used in diagnosis are often the first step in treatment as well and occasionally result in dramatic relief of pain. The sympathetic blocks may be repeated, with the patient requiring up to ten blocks over several weeks. The blocks should be repeated as soon as the symptomatic improvement begins to deteriorate, initially every few days and later on a weekly basis. As long as they provide pain relief adequate to allow physical therapy on the involved area, the sympathetic blocks are indicated. If there is not enough pain relief with the sympathetic block alone, a complete epidural spinal anesthetic may be effective.[4] This is performed as either an inpatient or outpatient procedure. If an indwelling catheter is inserted, intermittent injections may be performed for up to 1 week.[5, 19]

For advanced cases of RSDS unresponsive to sympathetic blocks, dorsal column stimulations can be implanted and significant pain relief expected in about 50% of patients; if all treatments fail, a morphine pump can be implanted. A daily dose of 30 mg of intrathecal morphine usually gives pain relief (Fig 33–5).

Intravenous regional blockade with guanethidine[14] and reserpine[36] has been used chiefly in cases involving the upper extremity.[8] Guanethidine is a false transmitter: it acts only in the periphery, displaces norepinephrine from its storage vesicles, and prevents its reuptake. It affects the adrenergically mediated aspects of the sympathetic nervous system by causing increased blood flow in the treated area. It does not affect the cholinergically mediated sudomotor aspect of the sympathetic system. This block is performed in a similar manner as a Bier block, with guanethidine and a local anesthetic. The resulting relief of pain may last from days to weeks. Reserpine has also been used like guanethidine in the intravenous regional method for sympathetic blockade. Reserpine blocks the reuptake of norepinephrine into storage vesicles in the periphery and eventually depletes the vesicles in the sympathetic nerve endings. Reserpine used by the intravenous regional method has been shown to not be as effective as guanethidine. Intravenous phentolamine blocks have been tried with variable success.

Surgical Treatment

If sympathetic blocks provide good but short-lived relief of pain, the patient may benefit from a surgical sympathectomy. Long-term results are good in carefully selected patients.[17, 23, 36] Often, by the time a patient is a candidate for lumbar sympathectomy, most other treatment modalities have been exhausted.

An important consideration in the treatment of RSDS is related to prior trauma or surgery since mechanical problems may be part of the cause, i.e., nerve scarring or entrapment, retained internal fixation, or malunion or nonunion.[30] There is a difference of opinion concerning whether surgical intervention to remove the suspected offending cause is indicated. Broken or misplaced plates and screws in malunion or nonunion with obvious deformity should be corrected early in the course of the disease.[2] This may be difficult since the patient may not be able to tolerate cast immobilization. Alternatively, surgical intervention for RSDS has been known to worsen symptoms. The decision for surgical intervention must therefore be based on all factors and the patient advised of the potential benefits and risks of surgery.

Fibrous ankylosis, joint deformity, and muscle contracture are the result of chronic disease. It is important

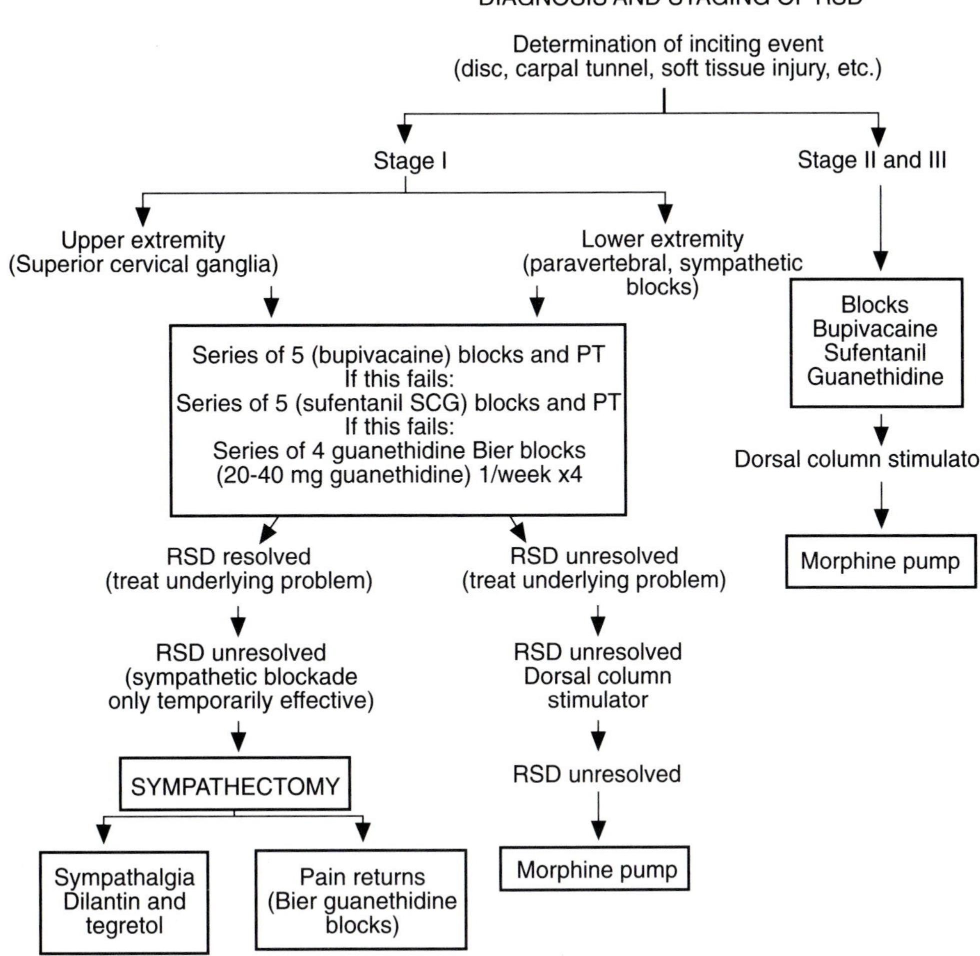

FIG 33–5.
An approach to the management of RSDS. *PT* = physical therapy; *SCG* = superior cervical ganglia. (Adapted from Schwartzman RJ: *Reflex sympathetic dystrophy in current therapy in neurologic disease,* ed 3, Philadelphia, 1990, BC Decker, p 68.)

to recognize that surgery under these circumstances will have a limited objective: making the foot plantigrade and aligning the ankle in neutral position. Indeed, although the deformity may be corrected, symptoms of RSDS may not be completely relieved.

Discussion

There is certainly a psychological component to any chronic pain syndrome. Although there is no evidence that RSDS is caused by psychological factors, as the condition progresses, patients develop characteristics of dependency, depression, insomnia, and personality changes.[36] Successful treatment not only of the painful disorder but of the patient as a whole will require appropriate attention to this aspect of the syndrome.[20] This often involves psychiatric therapy as well as social service consultation and rehabilitation counseling.

Because of the chronic nature of RSDS a patient support organization has formed:

Reflex Sympathetic Dystrophy Association
P.O. Box 821
Haddenfield, NJ 08083

Another organization specializing in RSDS and other rare disorders is NORD:

NORD (The National Organization for Rare Diseases)
P.O. Box 8923
New Fairfield, CT 06812

One persistent theme in reports of RSDS is that the results of treatment are best if the diagnosis is made early and appropriate therapy instituted before the dystrophic and atrophic stages of the disease develop.[5, 36] At that point, even if pain relief is achieved, permanent changes such as arthrofibrosis and weakness preclude a return to normal function.

HEAT AND COLD INJURIES

Cold injury to the foot is common. It occurs in mountainous areas, in arctic climates, and during warfare. Many injuries occur in temperate climates with the victims unaware of or unprepared for the weather. Skin temperature in cool weather ranges from 90 to 93°F (32 to 34°C) but can be as low as 70 to 73°F (21 to 23°C) before the body core starts cooling. The body generates and conserves heat to maintain itself in equilibrium with the environment (Tables 33–1 and 33–2). Heat is transferred to and from the feet in five ways (Table 33–3). The body's response to cold is variable, and therefore the extent of injury is unpredictable. There are two types of freezing injuries, those caused by wet and those caused by cold.[61] Any form of wetness, either from rain or perspiration, decreases the insulating properties of socks and shoes. Heat loss is five to six times faster when clothing is wet than when it is dry. If the feet are immersed in cold water, they can lose heat up to 25 times faster than if placed in cold air at the same temperature. Frostbite is caused by freezing cold. Immersion foot is caused by wet and cold. Freezing injuries have been classified, as have burns, by the degree of severity (Table 33–4).[48]

Temperature regulation of the extremities is an important factor in regulating the temperature of the body. Fifty percent of the body's surface lies on the extremities. The vasculature is arranged to be an effective heat exchanger so that the hands and feet are kept at the best working temperature. Normally there is a high blood flow to the toes. This is ensured by numerous arteriovenous shunts that pass warm arterial blood from arteries to superficial veins. From there the blood flows centrally. During this passage heat is exchanged from the blood to the surrounding tissue, which then ensures a higher temperature to the deeper structures such as the supporting tissues and nerves. Even in a very cold environment a person with a positive heat balance exhibits temperatures in the toes higher than those found proximally in the same extremity. When the temperature of the body core is threatened, these distal anastomoses are closed to minimize heat loss. This reduction in blood flow is so rapid that local temperatures in the toes fall at a rate similar to that seen with arterial occlusion under the same environmental conditions.[102] Local cooling above the level of freezing can cause local vasoconstriction. This does not cause injury if the patient is in positive heat balance. After some minutes a reactive vasodilation occurs and gives the sensation of prickling heat, the so-called Lewis hunting reaction.[76] If cold prevents the normal body temperature from being maintained, the arteriovenous anastomoses close and lead to irreversible changes.

It is impossible to produce boots that will prevent a freezing injury. The insulation of a boot only determines the rate of fall of temperature in the foot, not the final result. When the local temperature drops to 50°F (10°C), sensory nerves are inhibited from making the victim aware of ensuing frostbite. At 28.4°F (−2°C) tissue freezes. Some of the extracellular water is trans-

TABLE 33–1.
Generation of Body Heat*

Basal heat production: heat produced by oxidation of food at a fixed metabolic rate; maintains life processes under resting conditions; can be altered very little and is ineffective in preventing body cooling during exposure to cold environments
Muscular thermoregulatory heat: heat produced by shivering; increases heat production some three to five times the basal rate; consumes tremendous amounts of energy reserves and tends to reduce coordination and useful movement
High-intensity exercise-induced heat: heat produced by muscular activity during vigorous walking or running; can elevate heat production up to ten times the basal rate during very strenuous exercise; can be maintained for only a few minutes at a time owing to exhaustion of energy stores
Mild- to moderate-intensity exercise-induced heat: mechanism the same as high intensity; can elevate to five times the basal rate; can be maintained for much longer periods of time

*From Fritz RL, Perrin DH: *Clin Sports Med* 8:111–126, 1989. Used by permission.

TABLE 33–2.
Conservation of Body Heat*

Superficial vasoconstriction: body heat conserved by constriction of superficial blood vessels in the skin, especially over the extremities. Shunts blood away from the body surface, where it will lose heat to a cooler environment, to supply more blood flow to the brain, heart, lungs, and other internal organs
Body insulation: insulation against heat loss by layering of subcutaneous fat and, to a smaller measure, by growing body hair
External heat sources: insulation against heat loss through the use of proper clothing and by acquiring more heat by external means such as fire, sun exposure, hot food and drink, and contact with another body

*From Fritz RL, Perrin DH: *Clin Sports Med* 8:111–126, 1989. Used by permission.

TABLE 33–3.
Heat Transfer Mechanisms

Conduction: direct contact with a cold object
Convection: movement of air or water adjacent to skin
Radiation: energy emission to a colder object
Evaporation: loss of body heat by the conversion of water to gas (vapor)
Respiration: loss of heated air from the lungs by exhalation

TABLE 33–4.
Classification of Cold Injury According to Severity*

Severity	Symptoms
Superficial	
First degree: partial skin freezing	
Erythema, edema, hyperemia	Transient stinging and burning
No blisters or necrosis	Throbbing and aching possible
Occasional skin desquamation (5–10 days later)	May have hyperhidrosis
Second degree: full-thickness skin freezing	Numbness; vasomotor disturbances in severe cases
Erythema, substantial edema	
Vesicles with clear fluid	
Blisters that desquamate and form blackened eschar	
Deep	
Third degree: full-thickness skin and subcutaneous tissue freezing	Initially no sensation
	Involved tissue feels like a "block of wood"
Violaceous/hemorrhagic blisters	Later, shooting pains, burning, throbbing, aching
Skin necrosis	
Blue-gray discoloration	
Fourth degree: full-thickness skin, subcutaneous tissue, muscle, tendon, and bone freezing	Possible joint discomfort
Little edema	
Initially mottled, deep red, or cyanotic	
Eventually dry, black, mummified	

*From Delano Britt DL, Dascomebe WH, Rodriguez A: *Contemp Probl Trauma Surg* 71:345–370, 1991.

formed into ice, thereby increasing the hypertonicity of the remaining fluids and thus dehydrating cells in the toes. The longer the period of increasing dehydration, the more severe the injury. Rapid cooling tends to decrease the amount of this damage.

There are several factors that predispose an individual to cold injury. Hippocrates first observed that dark-skinned persons were more susceptible than those fair skinned to develop such conditions.[95] During the Korean War frostbite was noted to occur more frequently in black troops than white.[79] There are several other predisposing factors (Table 33–5).[54, 95, 100]

Frostbite

Frostbite is a specific type of cold injury that occurs between the actual freezing of all tissue and an immersion foot.[41, 44] Blair reported that of 100 cases of frostbite seen during the Korean War, 89 occurred in the foot and 11 in the hand.[42] The most common form of of frostbite is superficial (see Table 33–4). A white patch of frozen skin is all that may be visible, and in fact, this heals within a few days without tissue damage. Frostbite of the foot is considered a serious injury since there is only a small margin between the superficial and the deep type (Fig 33–6). When deep frostbite occurs, those portions of the foot become stiff and brittle. Symptoms and signs may be similar to those of a burn. Radiographic changes in bone resulting from frostbite have also been noted.[102] Pathologic evaluation includes tissue necrosis. Edwards and Leeper[51] analyzed 71 cases and noted that the extent of necrosis was in direct relation to the duration of freezing following the onset of symptoms. Heggers et al. illustrated the changes that occur during freezing injury (Fig 33–7).[59] Simeone noted a proliferation of adventitial cells in the capillaries of smaller vessels, clotting of the vascular tree with fibrin-poor clots typically seen in stagnant blood, and

TABLE 33–5.
Persons at Risk of Frostbite

Altered mental status
Psychiatric disorders
Alcohol abuse
Head injury
Military personnel exposed to cold, wet climates
Outdoor sporting enthusiasts
Skiers
Runners
Mountain climbers
Snowmobilers
Homeless, elderly, and malnourished persons
Laborers and industrial workers in cold environments
Oil and gas workers
Trucking, warehousing, protective services

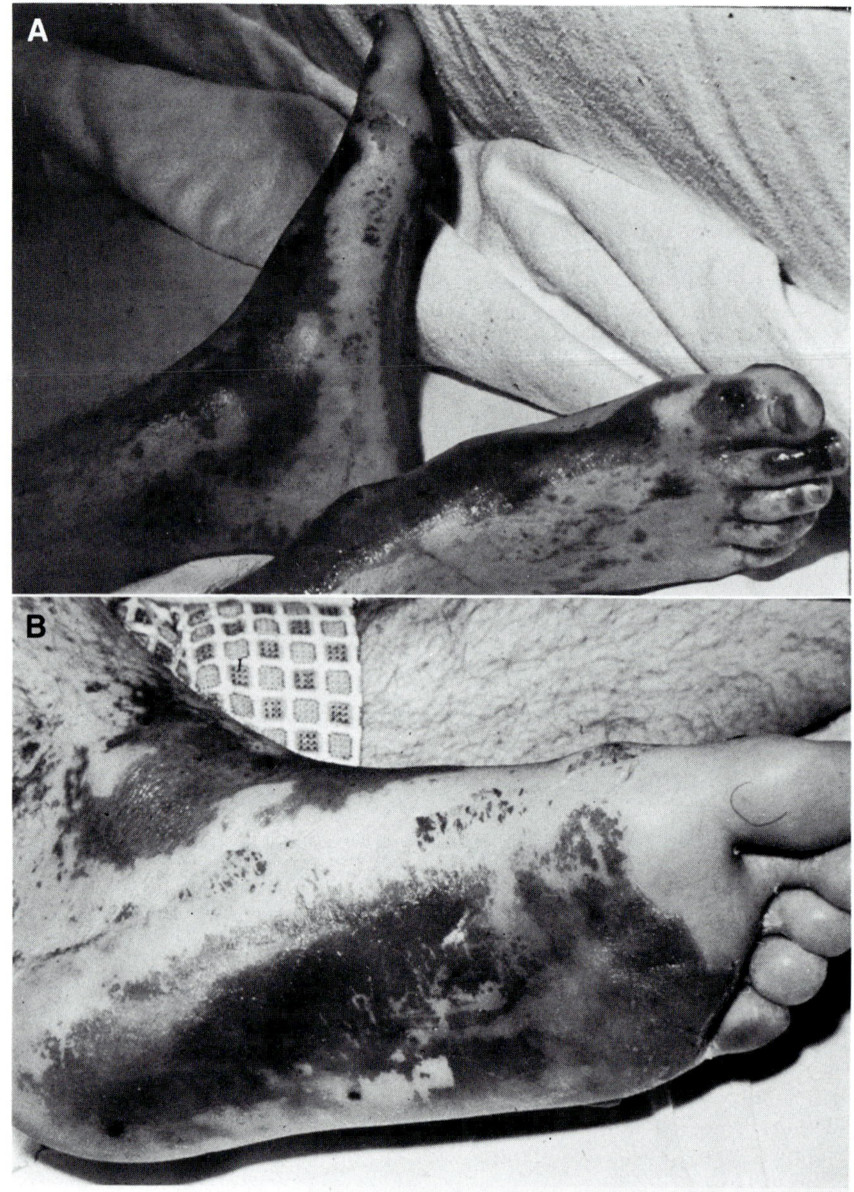

FIG 33–6.
A, severe frostbite of the feet. **B,** plantar aspect of the foot. Surgical debridement was withheld until clear demarcation of necrotic tissue developed. (Courtesy of Dr. J. Cranley.)

mural hemorrhage in the vessel walls.[96] He noted that most changes were thought to be a result of vascular occlusion.

Residual symptoms caused by severe freezing include cold and numbness in the feet, pain, hyperhidrosis, deformed toenails, scarring, and mutilation of the terminal phalanges.[43, 76]

Treatment includes the principle of rewarming of the foot and local care to maintain the surviving tissue. There are accounts of treatment of cold injury as early as biblical times:

> "Now King David was old and stricken in years; and they covered him with clothes, but he gat no heat. Wherefore his servants said unto him, 'Let there be sought for my lord the king a young virgin and let her stand before the king, and let her cherish him, and let her lie in thy bosom, that my lord the king may get heat.' " (*The Holy Bible*, I Kings 1:1–2.)

Treatment

Initial treatment includes warming the entire body and should be initiated prior to transporting the victim

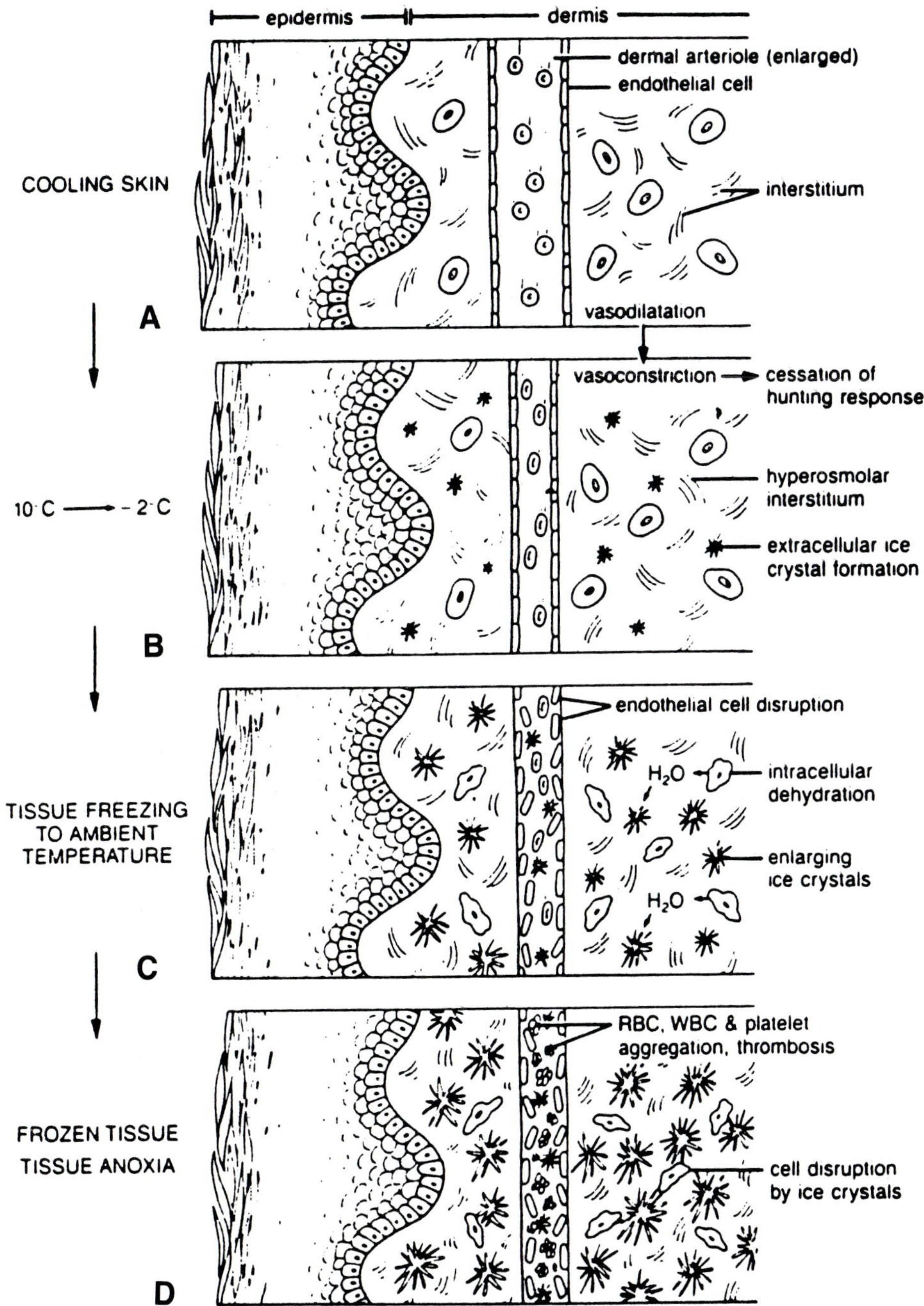

FIG 33–7.
Stages in cooling. **A,** the skin is exposed to a cool environment. **B,** as temperature declines, the hunting response ceases. Early ice crystal formation begins. **C,** freezing disrupts endothelial cell integrity. Water exits cells to contribute to growing extracellular ice crystals. **D,** circulatory stasis secondary to thrombosis and cell sludging results in tissue anoxia. (Adapted from Heggers JP, Robson MC, Manavalen K, et al: *Ann Emerg Med* 16:1056, 1987.)

to the hospital (Table 33–6). Rapid warming is recommended. A frozen foot should be placed in a water bath between 104 and 108°F (40 and 42°C).[69, 87, 103] The frostbite treatment protocol provides that the patient be admitted to the hospital (Table 33–7). As tissue thaws, additional pathologic changes occur (Fig 33–8). When general hypothermia is present, the normal body temperature should be restored before thawing the frozen foot. Analgesics may be necessary during the rewarming period. Strict cleanliness and asepsis of the feet are maintained during the first 7 to 10 days following the rewarming. The foot is splinted in neutral position, but

TABLE 33–6.

Care of the Frostbite Patient Prior to Admission to a Medical Facility*

1. Prevent further heat loss by avoiding the wind, protecting the area better, and drying all gear over exposed skin, especially wet gloves, socks, and boot liners
2. Protect the victim from further freezing by making an emergency camp and leaving him to get help only after a fire is started and ample firewood obtained
3. If there is any chance of a rescue search party, stay with the victim
4. If rapid rewarming by water immersion is possible, remember that this can be very painful and that shock is a possibility both from pain and the sudden reentry of lactic acid and other metabolic wastes into the circulation
5. Once thawed, a frozen foot or hand should be considered functionless during evacuation
6. A thawed and rewarmed foot swells rapidly and cannot be reinserted into the normal boot
7. Once frozen, progressive tissue damage is minimal; if immediate evacuation is not possible, it is preferable to leave a foot frozen
8. A frozen body part is unlikely to be further damaged by use
9. A thawed and rewarmed body part is very susceptible to further injury; avoid any pressure, normal function, or chance of refreezing
10. With rewarming of extremities, rapid and sometimes severe swelling may occur; watch for compartment syndromes
11. Once evacuated, all frostbite injuries should be examined in a medical facility or hospital

*From Fritz RL, Perrin DH: *Clin Sports Med* 8:111–126, 1989. Used by permission.

a flexibility program with active range of motion is encouraged even if gangrene is present. Intravenous low–molecular-weight dextran has been used in an attempt to reverse the tendency to intravascular sludging at low flow rates.[68, 104] Hyperbaric oxygen has been reported to be beneficial,[86, 103] but some have found no benefit.[55, 92] Following thawing of the injured foot, observation is important. McCauley et al. found that applying topical aloe vera while giving oral ibuprofen and intramuscular penicillin yielded less tissue loss with a lower amputation rate.[79] To aid tissue debridement, patients are also prescribed whirlpool baths at 38°C with povidone-iodine added followed by water rinsing twice daily. The affected foot area is air-dried and sterilely dressed to prevent skin maceration. After demarcation of necrosis has been established 2 weeks later, debridement of tissue is performed. Immediate amputation should not be performed, however, as long as there is motion and a chance for revitalization of the foot and toes.[64] The old dictum "frostbite in January, amputate in July," although exaggerated, indicates the need to be conservative early in the course of treatment since superficial injuries may only need debridement and skin grafting. Only uncontrolled infection requires early debridement. Mummified tissue should be debrided 1 to 3 months later when the level of gangrene is clearly demonstrated.[71]

TABLE 33–7.

Treatment Protocol for Frostbite*

Patients with frostbite injuries are admitted to the hospital

On admission, the affected area(s) are rewarmed rapidly in circulating warm water (104°–108°F) for 15–30 min. Patients presenting 24 hr after injury are not rewarmed

On completion of rewarming, the affected parts are treated as follows:

- All blisters are debrided, and topical treatment with aloe vera (Dermaide Aloe) every 6 hours is instituted
- Elevation of the affected part(s) with splinting as indicated
- Tetanus prophylaxis
- Analgesia, IV or IM morphine or meperidine as indicated
- Unless contraindicated by the medical history, ibuprofen, 12 mg/kg/day p.
- Penicillin: 500,000 units every 6 hr IM until edema resolves
- Daily hydrotherapy

*Data from Heggers JP, Robson MC, Manavalen K, et al: *Ann Emerg Med* 16:1056, 1987; and McCauley RL, Hing DN, Robson MC, et al: *J Trauma* 23:143, 1983.

Injuries in which deep frostbite has been thawed and refrozen behave like a deep burn. It is suggested that only 3 weeks of observation be made before definitive debridement and reconstructive surgery so that muscle wasting is held to a minimum and rehabilitation is not delayed. Early motion is encouraged. Spontaneous arthrodesis has not been found following frostbite. The bones of the foot show signs of demineralization, probably as a result of immobilization. This appears to be transient and reverses as the patient becomes active.[98]

Immersion and Trench Foot

Prolonged contact of the foot with subfreezing temperatures while activity is limited causes cold injury. Trench foot often affects the entire lower extremity, whereas chilblain more commonly affects the hands,

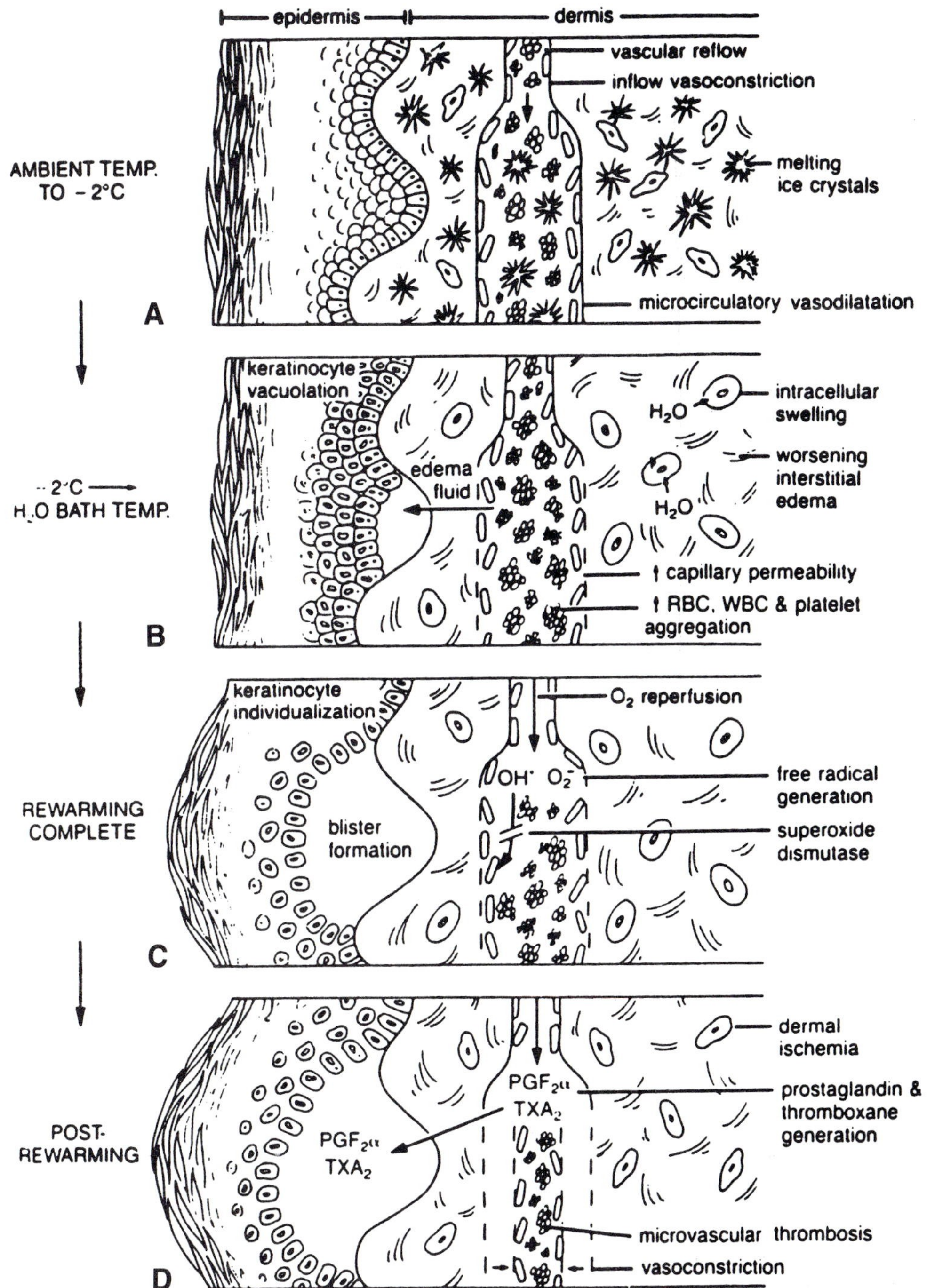

FIG 33–8.

Stages in thawing-rewarming. **A,** tissue rewarming begins. **B,** extracellular ice crystals melt. Freeze-induced endothelial cell disruption promotes the development of edema. **C,** continued endothelial cell injury occurs from free radicals, whose toxic effect is blocked by superoxide dismutase. Epidermal blisters may develop. **D,** prostaglandin- and thromboxane-induced microcirculatory vasoconstriction and platelet aggregation result in worsening dermal ischemia. (Adapted from Heggers JP, Robson MC, Manavalen K, et al: *Ann Emerg Med* 16:1056, 1987.)

feet, and face. If the feet are not removed from boots and stockings and allowed to dry and warm with regular intervals of massaging along with a change into dry clothes, a change in the metabolism at the cellular level begins to occur.[78] Metabolic changes present for long periods lead to irreversible damage. This condition was observed in survivors from sinking ships or aircraft downed over water. Webster et al.[105] and Fausel and Hamphill[52] studied large numbers of cases that also occurred in soldiers during combat. Symptoms tend to increase when boots are removed and the feet are dried and warmed. A dusky cyanosis with blanching is first observed followed by a rapid swelling. The feet then become hyperemic and red.[54] The temperature of the feet becomes markedly elevated, but there is no evidence of sweating. Tibial pulses are palpable. Subsequently, cyanosis with blebs, ecchymosis, and an obvious vasodilation develops. Paresthesias, burning, and numbness are usually present. This is most dramatic over the medial aspect of the foot along the hallux and the medial portion of the longitudinal arch. If the foot has been immersed in water for a long time, such as with survivors of a sinking ship, there is greater maceration of skin than seen in trench foot. This is associated with greater edema of the foot and leg.

Treatment

The principles involved in treating immersion foot include preservation of living tissue and supportive measures to prevent further injury by infection or trauma (see Table 33–7). Rewarming should be at temperatures between 104 and 108°F (40 and 42°C). This is the maximum allowable temperature without causing injury from heat, which is a serious possibility when rewarming the foot. Additional treatment includes bed rest and active motion of the feet with elevation. Massage and walking are not recommended.[99] The use of heparin is not helpful. Pathologic studies of blood clots within blood vessels indicate that these appear to be caused by stasis with little fibrin present. Low–molecular-weight dextran administered intravenously with hydration of the patient may be of benefit. Surgical debridement of the areas that appear necrotic is not recommended for several weeks following treatment. Areas of skin and deep tissue that initially appear dead often become revitalized, particularly in younger individuals. Debridement and amputation are reserved for areas that have become necrotic and clearly demarcated after several weeks. Sympathectomy is reserved for those patients who have clear evidence of increased sympathetic tone. This usually becomes clear several weeks after injury and is seen more frequently in patients with immersion foot or trench foot rather than other types of cold injury.[50] As with all cold-related injuries, areas of blistering and gangrene may reappear during reexposure to cold weather.

Chilblain

Chilblain (lupus pernio) is a neurocirculatory disturbance of the dorsum of the feet.[74] It also occurs on the face, anterior tibial surface, or dorsum of the hands.[45] It occurs in subfreezing weather from often-repeated exposure to cold in a wet or dry environment. Symptoms include dermatitis and occasionally ulceration of the skin. Microscopic examination of the tissues reveals a perivascular infiltration and intimal proliferation of vessels. Often subcutaneous tissue and skin show a chronic inflammatory reaction, and there may even be fat necrosis.[81] Chilblain has often been considered the same as a milder form of frostbite. Hauser notes that it occurs where the circulation is poorest, such as on the dorsal aspect of the toes, the heads of the first and fifth metatarsals, and the posterior surface of the heel.[58] Lake noted that chilblain tends to be more common in children than adults.[72] If exposure to cold is repeated and prolonged, the fibrotic changes around the blood vessels and in tissues sensitize the foot to future exposure to cold. Chilblain tends to appear in cold weather and disappear in dry summer months. In some patients, however, symptoms may persist year round. Excessively tight footwear aggravates symptoms.

Treatment

Treatment includes avoiding tight-fitting shoes, wearing comfortable socks that are appropriately thick for cold weather, and avoiding remaining in wet footwear for a long period. Workers in cold environments including meat cutters, frozen food handlers, and workmen whose occupations require them to be outside for a long time during the winter are particularly prone to this condition.

Burns

Thermal injury to the foot is common. A conservative estimate is that 2.5 million people obtain medical treatment for burns each year with more than 100,000 persons hospitalized and more than 12,000 victims dying of their injuries.[49] Burns can be caused by heat, chemicals, radiation, and electricity. It is important to properly diagnose the injury, institute immediate measures to prevent further injury, begin definitive care as early as possible, and rehabilitate the patient on a regular schedule so that total disability is kept to a minimum.

The survival rate of burn patients has steadily improved over the last several decades. Prior to 1940 the 50% mortality rate was below 30% burn of the total body surface area. The mean burn size for a 50% mortality rate today ranges from 65% to 75% of the body surface area. Fortunately, the vast majority of burn victims have less than 20% of the body surface involved, which is not life-threatening.[53, 62]

Burns to the foot caused by fire and contact with hot objects are less common because the foot is usually covered. They are seen more often in patients with severe burns on other parts of their body.[38, 39] Injury to the foot from electric burns is related to the duration and force of the insult. Alternating current injuries tend to produce tissue necrosis deep to the skin, much more than is visible on observation.[70] Early observation is important, and treatment may require long skin incisions to thoroughly debride dead deep tissue.

Isolated burns of the feet produced by hot liquids are common and often occur from spills. Most burns of the feet are caused by domestic accidents rather than work (Fig 33–9).[77] Burns from heating pads are also common causes of minor thermal injury.

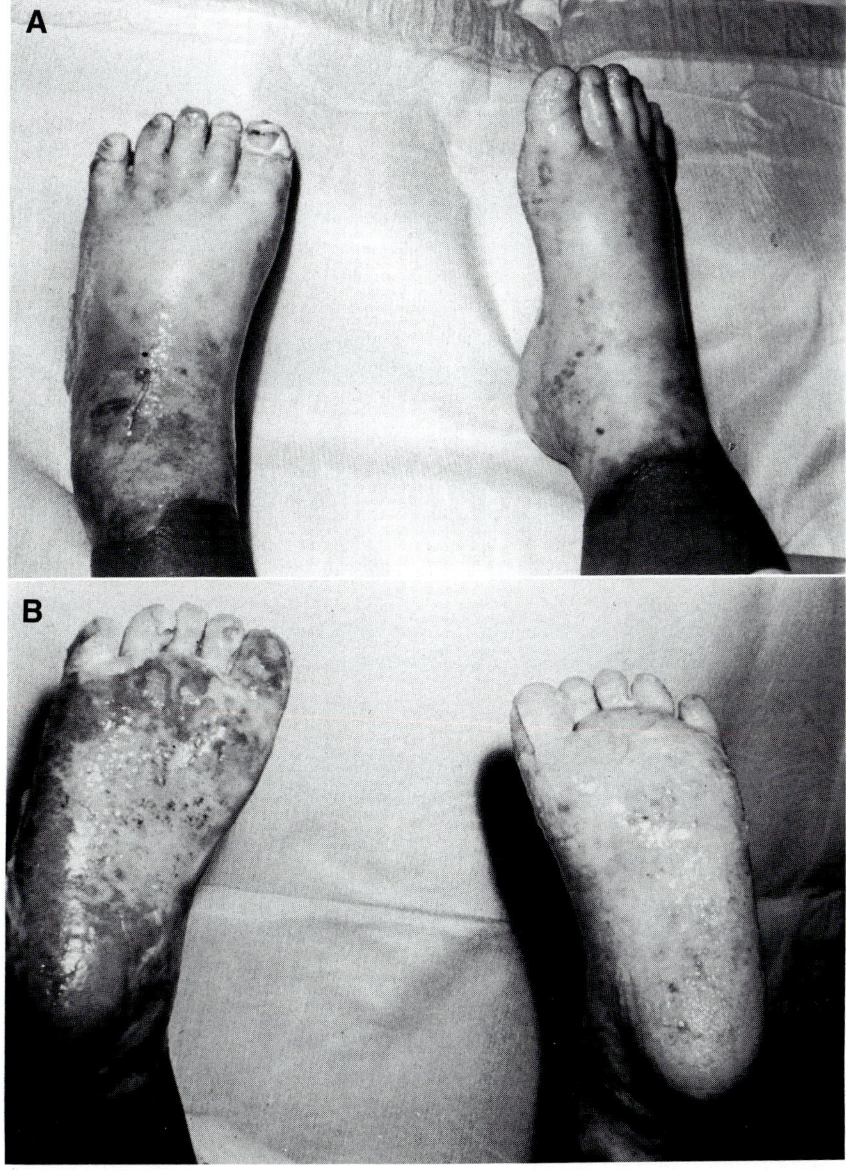

FIG 33–9.
Hot water burn to the feet of a 3-year-old boy. He was placed in a bathtub. Investigation revealed no evidence of child abuse. **A,** dorsal view. **B,** plantar view. (Courtesy of Dr. B. MacMillan.)

Symmetric scalds in a child should be viewed with the suspicion of child abuse. In determining the nature of lower-extremity burns in children it should be determined whether the burn or scald is *accidental*, that is, a lapse in the usual protection given to the child. *Neglected* children can be burned due to inadequate parenting such as a failure to protect the child. In *abused* children, scalds and burns are deliberately inflicted. Burns from child abuse are sadistic and associated with sexual and violent arousal in the adult. They may also be inflicted as punishment to evoke fear.[63] An adequate history must be taken. If abuse is suspected, appropriate investigative personnel must be contacted. Social service departments in hospitals often provide such a service, as do law enforcement agencies.

Classification of Burns

It is important to note three important facts concerning burns and their evaluation. First, tissues are overheated for periods longer than the burning agent is in contact with the skin. Following the removal of the burning agent, heat continues to penetrate deep into the tissue. Second, cooling the burned area shortens the period of overheating; therefore it is important to note that a burn injury progresses following removal of the heat source.[60, 65] Third, it is necessary to wait until the burn is well demarcated before attempting reconstructive surgery.

The peripheral area of a burn is hyperemic, blanches with pressure, and is epithelialized in about 7 days. A second area, closer to the central area of the burn, tends to be red and blanches on pressure immediately following the burn. However, capillary stasis occurs within the first 24 hours, after which blanching no longer occurs. Within the next 4 days it begins to appear as a central area that is coagulated and white and eventually becomes necrotic. The causes for continued ischemia and tissue death following a burn have been investigated by Robson et al.[90] and Sawacki[94] but are still unclear.

In evaluating burns it is important to determine whether the injury is of partial or full thickness. Since a partial-thickness injury extends through the epidermis and part of the dermis, damage is considerably less than a full-thickness injury, which includes destruction of the epidermis, the entire dermis, and the skin appendages. Burns are classified into first, second, and third degree.[39]

A *first-degree burn* is characterized by erythema and dryness of the skin (Table 33–8). A sunburn is a typical example. Usually blistering does not occur. *Second-degree burns* are often caused by hot liquid or a flash burn and appear as mottled redness of the skin with blistering, edema, and moistness and characteristically show decreased sensation. Partial-thickness burns are differentiated from *third-degree burns*, which involve epidermis, dermis, and the skin appendages and loss of sensation (Fig 33–10).

TABLE 33–8.
Classification of Burns

1. First degree: erythema without blistering
2. Second degree: erythema with blistering
3. Third degree: destruction of full thickness of skin and often deeper tissues

On initial examination it may be difficult to determine the nature and extent of a burn. Several methods have been reported, including the use of fluorescein[40] and thermography.[84, 88] Ultrasound has also been suggested to determine the nature of deep thermal burns.[56] There may be difficulty in determining the extent of a burn because following removal of the injury source, damage continues to progress from the burn tissue itself.[91]

Treatment

Treatment of burns of the foot includes determining how the burn occurred, what caused the injury, and when it occurred (Table 33–9). Associated injuries must be evaluated properly. Inspecting the wound and testing for sensation by pinprick provide most of the information needed to assess the depth of injury. The general health of the patient is important. Older patients with peripheral vascular disease and venous insufficiency will require greater care and a longer period for healing. Continuing care of the burn includes (1) prevention of progression of injury, (2) prevention and treatment of infection that may accompany the open wounds, and (3) development of an environment that promotes healing as rapidly as possible.

Emergency treatment includes the use of cool water at a temperature of 77°F (25°C) applied for periods of 30 minutes. In treating the burn patient it is important to note that the most important threat to life after initial treatment of the patient is infection, with burn sepsis and pneumonia being the leading causes.[47] Blisters should be left intact by covering the wound with gauze impregnated with petrolatum antiseptic in petroleum (Xeroform) or Adaptic dressings. Second- and third-degree burns of the foot usually require hospitalization. Circumferential wounds of the foot, lower part of the leg, and full-thickness burns may have an eschar that is constricting and causing vascular occlusion. In such cases escharotomy and, if necessary, fasciotomy must be performed to restore circulation. Topical antimicro-

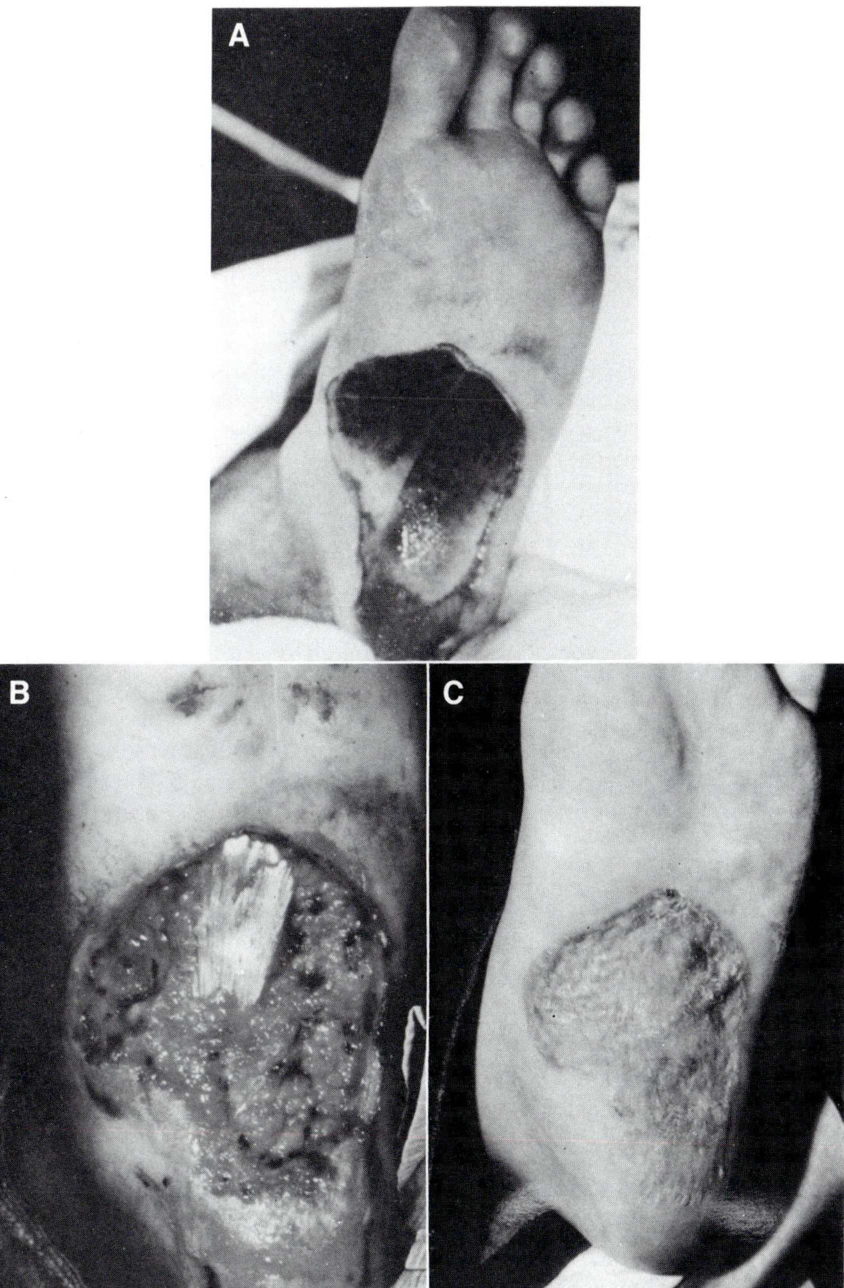

FIG 33–10.
Third-degree burn of the sole of the foot. **A,** burn before debridement. **B,** after debridement exposed plantar fascia can be seen. **C,** healed following a full-thickness graft. (Courtesy of Dr. John W. Brogan.)

bial agents are also important in addition to local wound care. The escharotomy may be performed at the margins of unburned skin. Since the eschar is asensory, no anesthetic is necessary. The use of Doppler ultrasound is a helpful adjunct to determine whether treatment has been effective. The edema accompanying the open burn along with poor circulation and damaged tissue predisposes the injury to infection. Elevation of the foot will help to control edema. Antibiotics are an important adjunct to therapy. Proper immunization is administered also.

Early treatment of wounds with skin grafts such as xenografts or homografts may slow the progression of dermal ischemia and provide early protection of the wound to aid in healing.[83] To control infection, debridement of infected tissue is recommended with wound

TABLE 33–9.
Outline for Care of the Burn Patient*

Evaluation
- Examine for evidence of respiratory distress or smoke-inhalation injury
- Evaluate cardiovascular status
- Determine the percentage of the body burned
- Determine the depth of burns
- Assess for other injuries

Systemic therapy†
- Intubate if respiratory distress is present or likely
- Start supplemental oxygen
- Perform volume resuscitation with Ringer's lactate solution based on the Parkland formula (4 mL/kg of body weight per percentage of body surface area burned); administer half of the calculated fluid needs during the first 8 hr after the injury
- Insert a nasogastric tube for gastric decompression
- Insert a Foley catheter to monitor urinary output

Wound care
- Clean burns and gently remove all devitalized tissue with aseptic technique
- Apply topical antimicrobial agent to all second-degree and third-degree burns
- Cover burns with closed dressing
- Keep the patient warm
- If there are circumferential third-degree burns of the extremities, assess the need for decompressive escharotomies
- Do not apply ice or cold dressings because of the risk of hypothermia

*From Deitch EA: *N Engl J Med* 323:1249–1253, 1990. Used by permission.
†Intravenous fluid resuscitation and the insertion of a nasogastric tube or a Foley catheter are generally not required in otherwise healthy patients with burns of less than 15% of their total body surface area.

closure when possible. Some authors contend that immediate debridement should be withheld except for relieving immediate circulatory compromise of the extremity.[39] Others[85] believe that even small burns that do not show evidence of healing with 8 to 10 days should be debrided and grafted. Wound cultures should be taken 2 days before surgery and appropriate intervenous antibiotics administered if infection exists. The conditions necessary for successful use of an autograft include absolute hemostasis, adequate debridement, and a quantitative bacterial count of the wound less than 10^5 bacteria per gram of tissue. Burns may be excised to fascia and covered with widely meshed skin grafts. If the burn is extensive, available donor sites may be limited. If it is determined that an autograft cannot be applied, the freshly debrided wound is protected from drying so as to protect the tissue from developing a new layer of necrotic tissue. Xenograft heterografts (pig skin) may be used as a biologic dressing but must be changed every 2 days until the wound is ready for autogenous grafts. Following skin grafting, the foot should be splinted in the position of function. Grafts should be protected with Adaptic gauze and wrapped with a light compression dressing using Kling bandage. A well-padded, molded splint should be used to protect the graft from motion. Non–weight-bearing ambulation is permitted in 10 days.

Contractures and scars following burns of the foot will necessitate reconstructive procedures and bracing to achieve a plantigrade foot (Fig 33–11). Of the several bony changes that occur following burns, one of the most common is bone demineralization. As many as 70% of burn victims show such changes. Seventeen percent develop reflex dystrophy. Bone necrosis from heat and from thrombosis of nutrient vessels also occurs. Inflammatory changes can cause lacelike periostitis and osteolysis with sequestration and sclerosis as healing occurs. Joint effusion is less common (3%), as is extensive myositis ossificans.[70]

Electrical burns of the foot occur if the victim steps on a live wire or is grounded through the foot. A number of bony and soft-tissue findings may be present (Table 33–10). Chemical burns of the skin coagulate protein through oxydation/reduction, corrosion, desiccation, and other metabolic methods.[67] Additional injury can occur as a result of the heat of reaction. If the chemical reaction is exothermic, the duration of contact, volume of chemical, mode of reaction, and pH of the chemical solution all influence the severity of the burn.

Emergency treatment includes removal of shoes, socks, and any particulate matter. Most chemical burns can be treated immediately with a continuous, copious supply of running tap water. This is usually available. It dilutes and debrides the chemical, reduces the rate of reaction, and restores the pH of the wound to normal. The exception to this rule includes treatment with 2% copper sulfate solution for injuries caused by white phosphorus and treatment with sodium bicarbonate (boric acid wash) for hydrofluoric acid burns. The copper sulfate solution will identify the phosphorus particles, which must then be debrided manually.[93] Following this, the care regimen is similar to that for other thermal wounds. It is important to note that chemical material may delay healing and that repeat debridement may be required if all particulate matter is not removed initially. Stiffness and joint pain may occur as sequelae.

Radiation burns are caused by α-particles, β-particles, x-ray examinations, or γ-rays. The burn may be acute or chronic. Ionizing radiation has a direct effect through biochemical changes at the cellular level and an indirect effect through damage to bones and joints. The orthopaedic effects on bone are induced by obliterative radiation-induced vascular disease. The extent of damage is determined by the type of radiation and the period of exposure of the victim. An acute burn may be mild in appearance and subside completely. However,

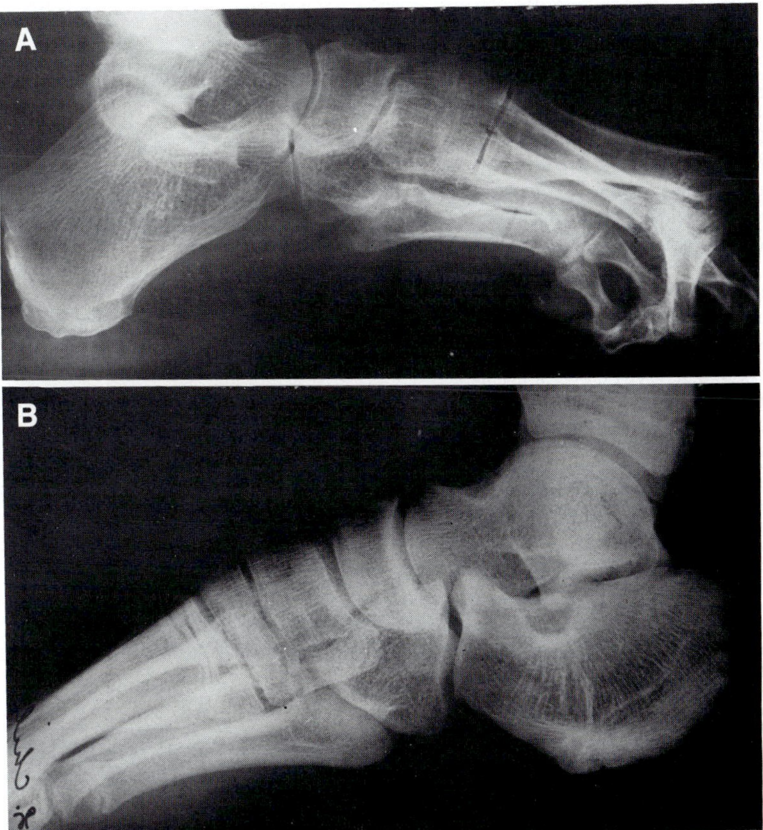

FIG 33–11.
A, severe plantar contracture of the toes resulting from a third-degree burn. **B,** destruction of the calcaneal tuberosity by a third-degree burn.

later affects can occur 6 months to 1 year later. The treatment of verrucae plantares with radiotherapy is a common cause of plantar radiation burn. Chronic effects include microscopic changes, endarteritis obliterans, excessive tissue fibrosis, and changes within the cell that affect cellular replication. Radiation from external sources can cause bone damage (Table 33–11).

Treatment of chronic ulceration depends on the severity of the radiodermatitis. Superficial necrosis may be treated with skin grafts if a well-vascularized wound bed is present. Deep injuries to skin and bone may require distant flaps or the use of a musculocutaneous free

TABLE 33–10.
Bone and Soft-Tissue Changes Associated With Electrical Burns

1. Skin and subcutaneous damage, which may be apparent on radiographs.
2. Fractures as a result of muscular cramps, mainly in the midthoracic vertebral bodies and humeral, femoral, and scapular neck. Longitudinal fractures, often following a zigzag contour, so-called osteoschisis, may result from a direct mechanical splitting effect of the passing current.
3. Melting of bone due to intense heat may result in small rounded osseous fragments resembling drips of wax, so-called bone pearls lying along the surface of bone.
4. Osteonecrosis may occur and result in osteolytic medullary, lucent cystic areas in both the diaphysis and metaphysis. Cortical sequestration, collapse of subchondral bone, epiphyseal collapse, and fragmentation have all been described.
5. Growth disturbances as a result of premature fusion of the epiphysis in children.
6. Laceration of the skin may allow access of microorganisms with resulting osteomyelitis and suppurative arthritis. The latter may result in joint ankylosis.
7. Scars and contractures of soft tissues and periarticular calcification and ossification may cause limitation of joint movement.

TABLE 33–11.
Radiation Burns*

1. *Grade I* is clinically silent with demineralization, mainly of trabecular bone but sometimes also of the inner surface of cortical bone. Repair of bone is not apparent.
2. *Grade II* changes include hypertrophic bone atrophy with spongiosclerosis. Pathologic fractures may occur, especially at predisposed sites such as the femoral neck, pubic bones, ribs, and mandible. These fractures are usually associated with pain and loss of function and may heal. However, complete normalization of bone never occurs.
3. *Grade III* is the stage of osteoradionecrosis that is often accompanied by fracture and/or infection. The latter may present clinically with the features of osteomyelitis. It is important that the clinician appreciate that the degree of underlying bone damage often does not correlate with the overlying skin changes. Surgical intervention may be necessary to remove necrotic bone and to drain the bone of infected material. Death is not an infrequent outcome, and chronic sinus drainage is also a common complication.
4. *Grade IV* consists of radiation-induced malignancy, usually osteogenic sarcoma or fibrosarcoma. There is usually a latent period between the time of exposure and the development of neoplasm, most often 10 years. The radiation dose is of the order of 20 Gy or more. The clinical and radiologic appearances of the tumors do not differ from those occurring spontaneously, and the prognosis is very poor.

*From Kohler J: *Baillieres Clin Rheumatol* 3:99–109, 1989. (Used by permission.)

flap.[46, 58, 82] Neoplasm following radiation of the foot is also well known.[57]

Treatment of these bony sequelae is both symptomatic and curative as each case dictates.

FOREIGN BODIES

Foreign bodies in the foot may be caused by a penetrating wound including wartime injuries from exploding bombs with metallic debris and from explosions wherein wood, glass, and other nonradiopaque objects penetrate the skin (Fig 33–12). The most common metallic foreign body is a needle or pin that penetrates the plantar aspect of the foot (Fig 33–13). Because such objects are on the ground and may have penetrated the shoe, the small puncture wound is contaminated. The patient may feel pain and recognize the problem immediately, or he may be unaware of the injury and not seek treatment until symptoms of pain or abscess become evident. On occasion such a foreign body may remain asymptomatic and becomes noticeable only when the foot is undergoing radiographic examination for some other reason (Fig 33–14). The most common infecting organism associated with foreign bodies in the soft tissues of the foot is *Staphylococcus aureus*, although gram-negative or anaerobic infections are occurring with increasing frequency. If the foreign body has penetrated bone and has remained undetected for a time the infection is often multibacterial in etiology, with *Pseudomonas* being the most commonly present.

A small foreign body present for a long time need not be removed unless it becomes symptomatic. Preoperative radiographs of the foot taken in the true anteroposterior and lateral planes as well as an oblique view are important to determine the exact position of the

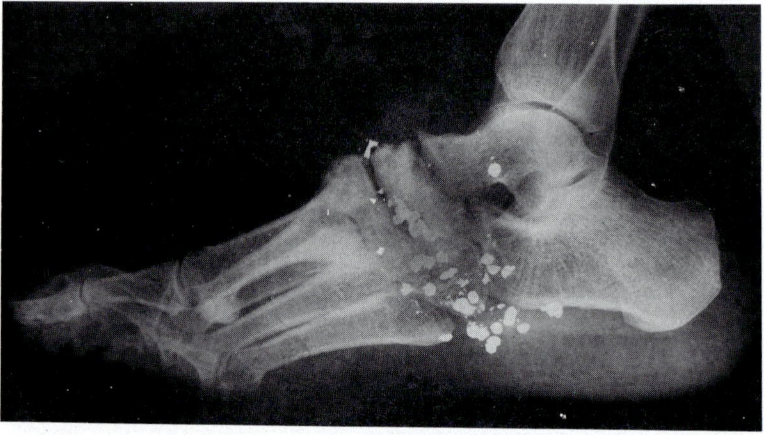

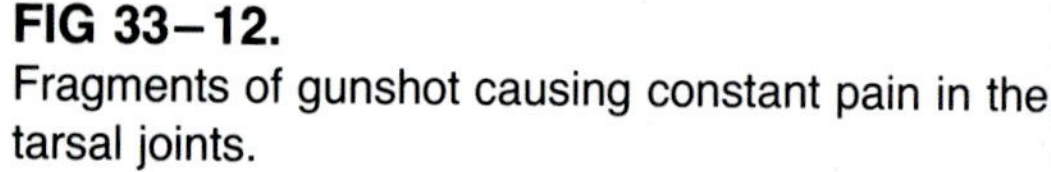

FIG 33–12.
Fragments of gunshot causing constant pain in the tarsal joints.

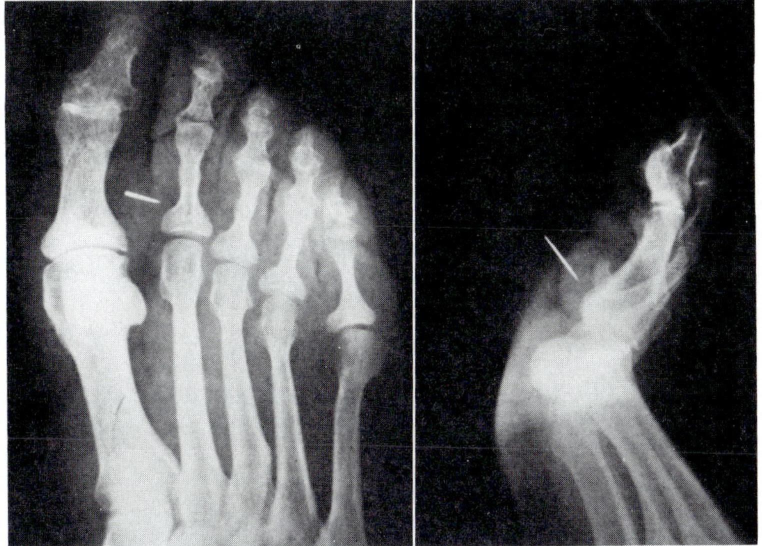

FIG 33–13.
Part of a needle in the foot. Acute symptoms occurred immediately after entrance.

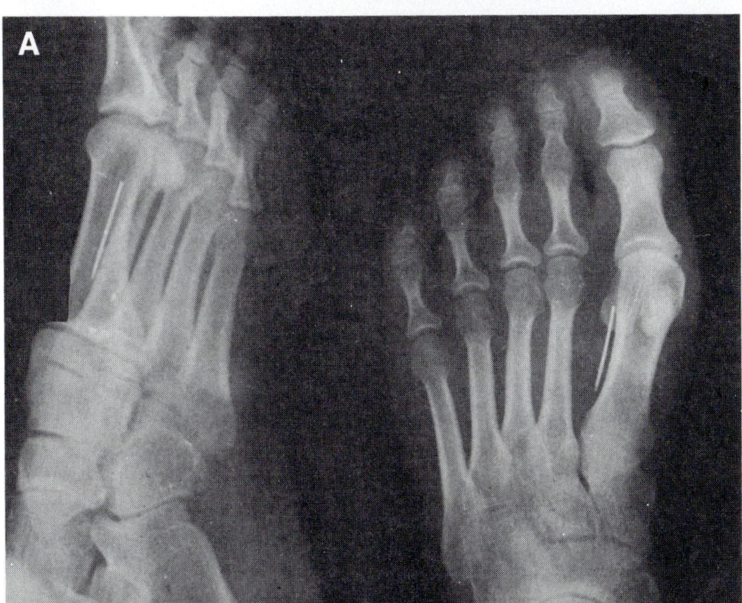

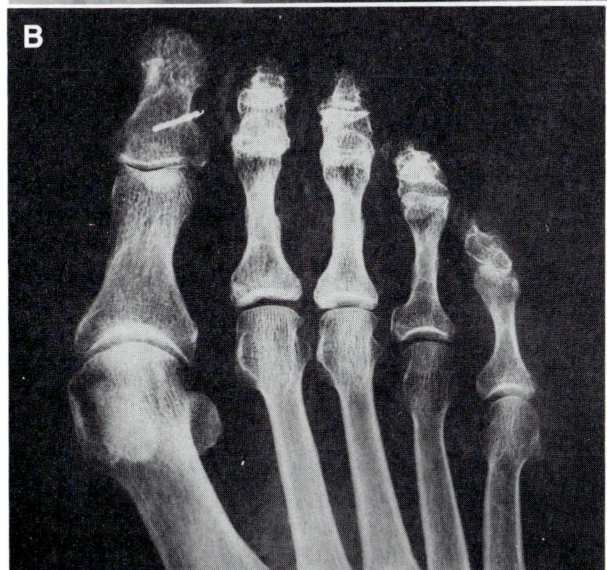

FIG 33–14.
A, radiographs taken for other purposes disclosed a needle—asymptomatic. **B,** part of the needle in the great toe. This foreign body, dormant for a long time, suddenly became symptomatic.

metal object (Fig 33–15). Since finding a needle may be difficult unless gross reaction, rust formation, or abscess is present, an x-ray image intensifier is helpful intraoperatively. Two needles or hemostats passed in the direction of the foreign body localize it by triangulation, that is, by determining the relationship of the foreign body to the tips of the metal instruments. The x-ray "mini C-arm" is convenient since the surgeon may operate the instrument alone without the need for cumbersome equipment in a small operating field. Shrapnel and gunshot particles, likewise, may remain dormant for a considerable period, several months or years, before developing a granulomatous reaction. Because they may be easily seen on radiographs, the same methods used for locating metal objects are used to find them.

The most common nonradiopaque foreign object in the sole is a splinter. Often the patient is unaware that he has stepped on a splinter until an abscess forms. Maceration then permits an abscess to form, in the center of which may be the splinter. Removal is often done by the patient. If the splinter is embedded and broken off deep into the dermis, local anesthesia may be neces-

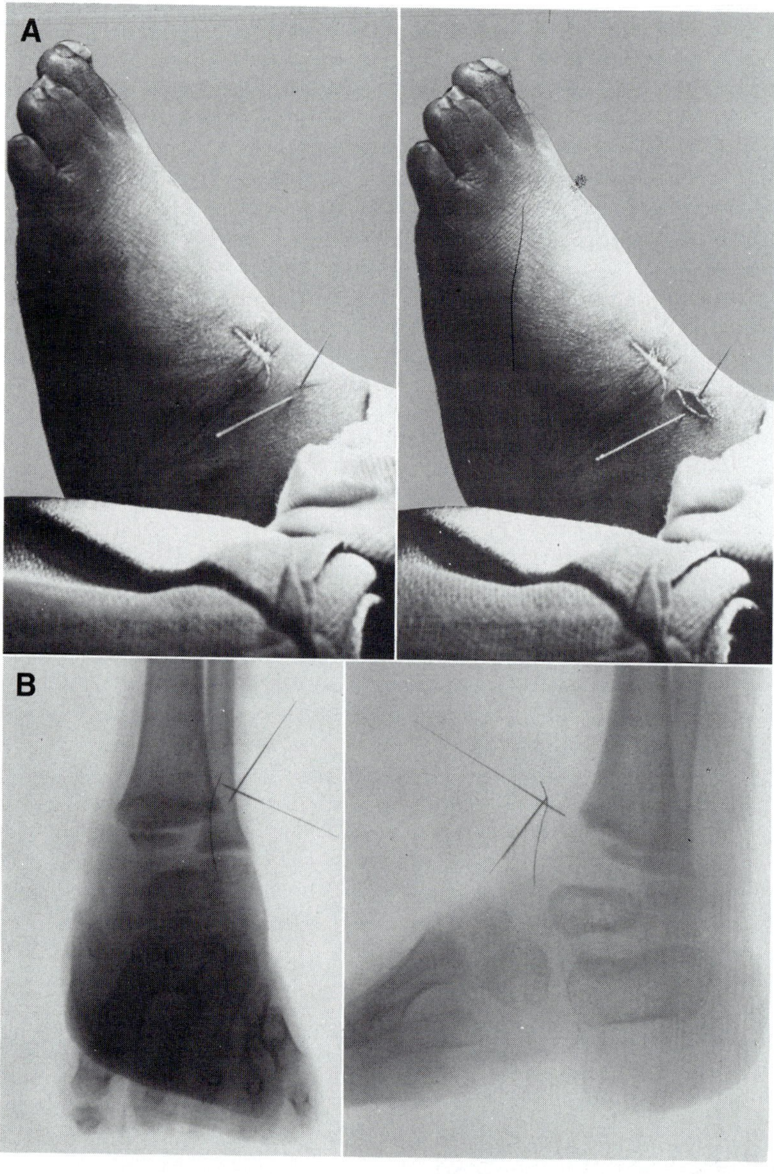

FIG 33–15.
Localization of a foreign body. **A,** two needles at right angles to each other in the region of the foreign body. An incision was made between the two needles. **B,** biplane radiographs show the needles localizing the foreign body.

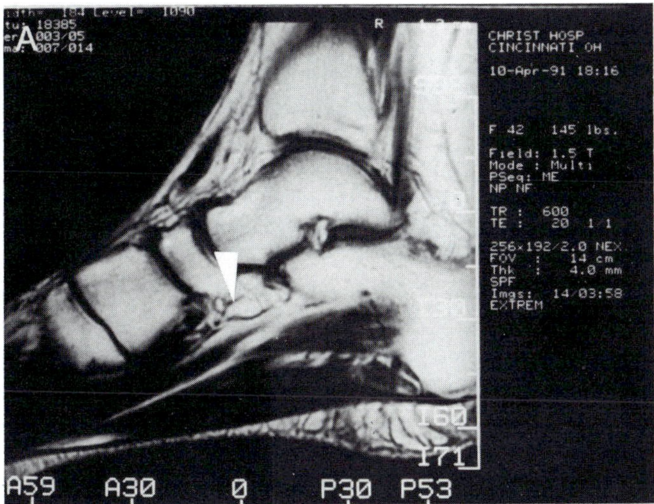

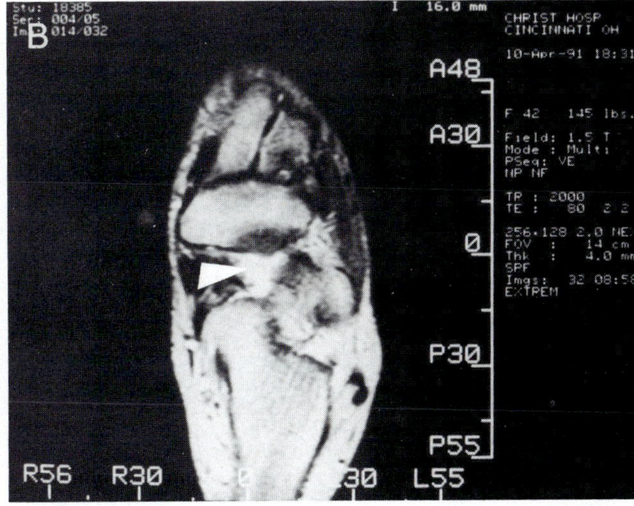

FIG 33–16.
A, MRI saggittal cut showing an abscess (white) from a toothpick fragment *(arrow)*. The patient had stepped on a toothpick 15 years previously and had undergone eight surgeries to debride and repair "arthritis." **B,** MRI transverse view of the same foot showing the abscess *(arrow)*.

sary to reduce pain so that it may be removed. The skin is simply pared down to the area of the tip of the splinter, and a thin forceps is used to grasp and withdraw it. It is important to note that nonradiopaque objects may be present for decades and slowly work themselves toward the skin, where they may then be spontaneously extruded. A useful diagnostic aid in determining the presence in the foot of nonradiopaque foreign objects is magnetic resonance imaging (MRI). Not only can the object be located through various cuts at differing "spins," but the presence and location of an associated abscess can also be determined (Fig 33–16,A and B).

Even a hair embedded in the epidermis of the sole that remains invisible may set up an inflammatory process later and require removal. Often it is not seen until a small abscess is incised and drained.

Glass made of nonradiopaque, soda lime silicate such as is used in glass bottles and windows does not appear on standard x-ray examinations and may be difficult to find.[89] It is important for the physician to recognize the inflammatory reaction and have the cooperation of the patient. Glass containing various amounts of barium or lead is not uncommon (Fig 33–17). Expensive lead crystal is no longer commonplace, but fluoroscopic screens

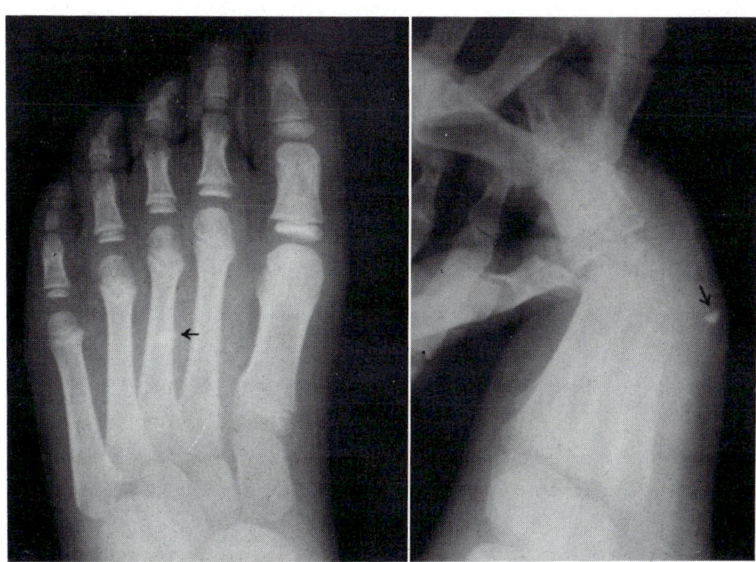

FIG 33–17.
Small piece of glass *(arrow)* embedded in the subcutaneous tissue of the plantar surface—painful.

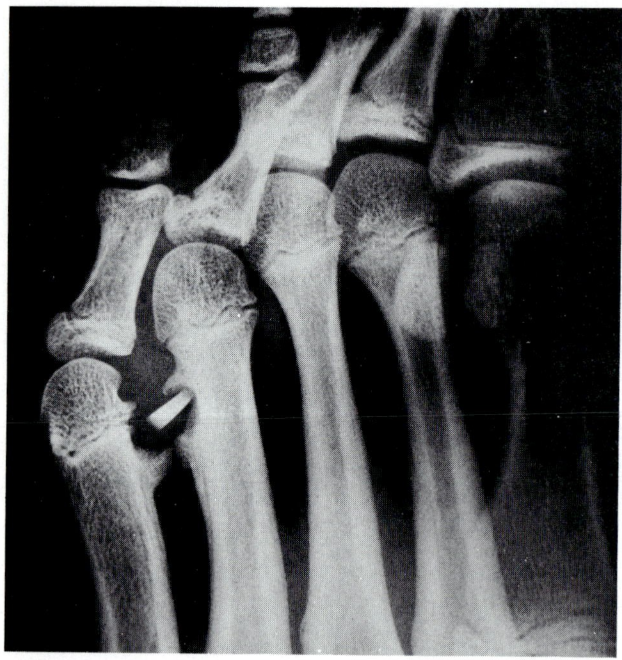

FIG 33–18.
A sharp piece of glass embedded between the fourth and fifth metatarsal heads caused extensive osseous proliferation.

and the base of light bulbs that contain barium are frequently found in wounds. Lead is highly visible (Fig 33–18). MRI is quite useful in locating such objects. Cultures should be taken of any wound, and an appropriate history of tetanus immunization should be obtained to ensure proper antitetanus therapy.

REFERENCES

Reflex Sympathetic Dystrophy Syndrome

1. Adams RD, Victor M: *Principles of neurology*, New York, 1977 McGraw-Hill.
2. Amadio PC: Pain dysfunction syndromes, *J Bone Joint Surg [Am]* 70:944–949, 1988.
3. Beresford HR: Iatrogenic causalgia. Legal implications, *Arch Neurol* 41:819–820, 1984.
4. Cicala RS, Jones JW, Westbrook LL: Causalgic pain responding to epidural but not to sympathetic nerve blockade, *Anesth Analg* 70:218–219, 1990.
5. Cooper DE, DeLee JC, Ramamurthy S: Reflex sympathetic dystrophy of the knee, *J Bone Joint Surg [Am]* 71:365–369, 1989.
6. Davidoff G, Morey K, Amann M, et al: Pain measurement in reflex sympathetic dystrophy syndrome, *Pain* 32:27–34, 1988.
7. Davidoff G, Werner R, Cremer S, et al: Predictive value of the three-phase technetium bone scan in diagnosis of reflex sympathetic dystrophy syndrome, *Arch Phys Med Rehabil* 70:135–137, 1989.
8. Davies JAH, Beswick T, Dickson G: Ketanserin and guanethidine in the treatment of causalgia, *Anesth Analg* 66:575–576, 1987.
9. Demangeat J, Constantinesco A, Brunot B, et al: Three-phase bone scanning in reflex sympathetic dystrophy of the hand, *J Nucl Med* 29:26–32, 1988.
10. Dietz F, Mathews KD, Montgomery WJ: Reflex sympathetic dystrophy in children, *Clin Orthop* 285:225–231, 1990.
11. Doury P: Algodystrophy. Reflex sympathetic dystrophy syndrome, *Clin Rheumatol* 7:173–180, 1988.
12. Escobar PL: Reflex sympathetic dystrophy, *Orthop Rev* 15:646–651, 1986.
13. Goldsmith DP, Vivino FB, Eichenfield AH, et al: Nuclear imaging and clinical features of childhood reflex neurovascular dystrophy: comparison with adults, *Arthritis Rheum* 32:480–485, 1989.
14. Holland JT: The causalgia syndrome treated with regional intravenous guanethidine, *Clin Exp Neurol* 15:166–173, 1978.
15. Horowitz SH: Iatrogenic causalgia, *Arch Neurol* 41:821–824, 1984.
16. Intenzo C, Jim S, Millin J, et al: Scintigraphic patterns of the reflex sympathetic dystrophy syndrome of the lower extremities, *Clin Nucl Med* 14:657–661, 1989.
17. Jebara VA, Saade B: Causalgia: a wartime experience—report of twenty treated cases, *J Trauma* 27:519–524, 1987.
18. Kesler RW, Saulsbury FT, Miller LT, et al: Reflex sympathetic dystrophy in children: treatment with transcutaneous nerve stimulation, *Pediatrics* 82:728–732, 1988.
19. Ladd AL, DeHaven KE, Thanik J, et al: Reflex sympathetic imbalance. Response to epidural blockade, *Am J Sports Med* 17:660–668, 1989.
20. Malkin LH: Reflex sympathetic dystrophy syndrome following trauma to the foot, *Orthopaedics* 13:851–858, 1990.
21. Mandel S, Rothrock RW: Sympathetic dystrophies, *Postgrad Med* 87:213–218, 1990.
22. McKain CW, Urban BJ, Goldner JL: The effects of intravenous regional guanethidine and reserpine, *J Bone Joint Surg [Am]* 65:808–811, 1983.
23. Mockus MB, Rutherford RB, Rosales C, et al: Sympathectomy for causalgia, *Arch Surg* 122:668–672, 1987.
24. Procacci P, Maresca M: Reflex sympathetic dystrophies and algodystrophies: historical and pathogenic considerations, *Pain* 31:137–146, 1987.
25. Roberts WJ: A hypothesis on the physiological basis for causalgia and related pains, *Pain* 24:297–311, 1986.
26. Rowlingson JC: The sympathetic dystrophies, *Int Anesthesiol Clin* 24:117–129, 1983.
27. Schapira D, Barron SA, Nahir M, et al: Reflex sympathetic dystrophy syndrome coincident with acute diabetic neuropathy, *J Rheumatol* 15:120–122, 1988.
28. Schott G: Clinical features of algodystrophy: is the sympathetic nervous system involved? *Funct Neurol* 4:131–134, 1989.
29. Schott G: Mechanisms of causalgia and related clinical conditions, *Brain* 109:717–738, 1986.
30. Schutzer SF, Gossling HR: The treatment of reflex sympathetic dystrophy syndrome, *J Bone Joint Surg [Am]* 66:625–629, 1984.
31. Schwartzman JR, McLellan TL: Reflex sympathetic dystrophy, *Arch Neurol* 44:555–561, 1987.

32. Schwartzman RJ, Kerrigan J: The movement disorder of reflex sympathetic dystrophy, *Neurology* 40:57–61, 1990.
33. Seale KS: Reflex sympathetic dystrophy of the lower extremity. *Clin Orthop* 243:80–85, 1989.
34. Shelton RM, Lewis CW: Reflex sympathetic dystrophy: A review, *Dermatology* 22:513–520, 1990.
35. Silber TJ, Majd M: Reflex sympathetic dystrophy syndrome in children and adolescents, *Am J Dis Child* 142:1325–1330, 1988.
36. Stanton-Hicks M, Janig W, Boas RA: *Reflex sympathetic dystrophy*, Workshop held in Kelkheim, West Germany, Oct 15–17, 1988, Boston, 1990, Kluwer.
37. Tahmoush AJ, Malley J, Jennings JR: Skin conductance, temperature and blood flow in causalgia, *Neurology* 33:1483–1486, 1983.

Heat and Cold Injuries and Foreign Bodies

38. Artz CP, Moncrief JA: *The treatment of burns*, ed 2, Philadelphia, 1969, WB Saunders.
39. Artz CP, Reiss E: *The treatment of burns*, Philadelphia, 1957, WB Saunders.
40. Becktold F, Lipin RJ: Differentiation of full thickness and partial thickness burn with the aid of fluorescein, *Am J Surg* 119:436, 1965.
41. Bigelow WG: The modern conception and treatment of frostbite, *Can Med Assoc J* 47:529, 1942.
42. Blair JR: *Proceedings of symposium on arctic medicine and biology*, vol 4, *Frostbite*, Ft Wainwright, Alaska, 1964, Arctic Aero Medical Laboratory.
43. Blair JR, Schatzki R, Orr KD: Sequelae to cold injury in one hundred patients, *JAMA* 163:1203, 1957.
44. Brownrigg GM: Frostbite in shipwrecked mariners, *Am J Surg* 59:232, 1943.
45. Christensen C, Steward C: Frostbite, *Am Fam Physician* 30:111, 1984.
46. Dabb, Conklin, 1981.
47. Deitch EA: The management of burns, *N Engl J Med* 323:1249–1253, 1990.
48. Delano Britt DL, Dascombe WH, Rodriguez A: New horizons in management of hypothermia and frostbite injury, *Contemp Probl Trauma Surg* 71:345–370, 1991.
49. Department of Health and Welfare: *Reports of the epidemiology and surveillance of injuries*, Atlanta, 1982, Centers for Disease Control, DHEW Publication No. (HSW) 73-10001.
50. Dinep M: Cold injury: A review of current theories and their application to treatment, *Conn Med* 39:8, 1975.
51. Edwards EA, Leeper RW: Frostbite: an analysis of seventy-one cases, *JAMA* 149:1199, 1952.
52. Fausel EG, Hamphill JA: Study of the late symptoms of cases of immersion foot, *Surg Gynecol Obstet* 81:500, 1945.
53. Feller I, Tholen D, Cornell RG: Improvements in burn care 1965 to 1979, *JAMA* 244:2074–2078, 1980.
54. Fritz RL, Perrin DH: Cold exposure injuries: Prevention and treatment, *Clin Sports Med* 8:111–126, 1989.
55. Gage AA, Ishikawa H, Winter PM: Experimental frostbite and hyperbaric oxygenation, *Surgery* 66:1044, 1969.
56. Goans RE: Ultrasonic pulse echo determination of thermal injury in deep dermal burns, *Ed Phys* 4:259, 1977.
57. Hartwell SW, Huger W Jr, Pickrell K: Radiation dermatitis and radiogenic neoplasms of the hand, *Ann Surg* 169:828, 1964.
58. Hauser EDW: *Diseases of the foot*, Philadelphia, 1939, WB Saunders.
59. Heggers JP, Robson MC, Manavalen K, et al: Experimental and clinical observations on frostbite, *Ann Emerg Med* 16:1056, 1987.
60. Henshaw RJ: Early changes in the depth of burn, *Ann NY Acad Sci* 150:548, 1978.
61. Hermann G, Schechter DC, Owens JC, et al: The problem of frostbite in civilian medical practice, *Surg Clin North Am* 43:519, 1963.
62. Herndon DN, Curreri PW, Abston S, et al: Treatment of burns. *Curr Probl Surg* 24:341–397, 1987.
63. Hobbs CJ: ABC's of child abuse burns and scalds, *Br Med J* 13:298, 1989.
64. Holm PCA, Vanggard L: Frostbite, *Plast Reconstr Surg* 54:544, 1974.
65. Jackson DM: The diagnosis of depth of burning, *Br J Surg* 40:588, 1953.
66. Jackson DM: Second thoughts on burn wound, *J Trauma* 9:839, 1969.
67. Jelenko C III: Chemicals that burn, *J Trauma* 14:65, 1974.
68. Knize DM, Weatherly-White RCA, Paton BC: Use of antisludging agents in experimental cold injuries, *Surg Gynecol Obstet* 129:1019–1026, 1969.
69. Knize DM, Weatherly-White RCA, Paton BC, et al: Prognostic factors in the management of frostbite, *J Trauma* 9:749, 1969.
70. Kolar J: Locomotor consequences of electrical and radiation injuries, burns and freezings, *Baillieres Clin Rheumatol* 3:99–109, 1989.
71. Kyosola K: Clinical experience in the management of cold injuries, *J Trauma* 14:32–36, 1974.
72. Lake MC: *The foot*, Baltimore, 1938, Wm Wood.
73. Larkin JM, Moylan JA: Tetanus following a minor burn, *J Trauma* 15:546, 1975.
74. Lewin P: *The foot and ankle*, Philadelphia, 1941, Lea & Febiger.
75. Lewis T: Observations on some normal and injurious effects of cold upon the skin and underlying tissues: frostbite, *Br Med J* 2:869, 1941.
76. Lewis T: Observations upon the reactions of the vessels in the human skin to cold, *J Heart* 15:177, 1930.
77. London PS: The burnt foot, *Br J Surg* 40:293, 1953.
78. Lyons JM: Phase transitions and control of cellular metabolism at low temperatures, *Cryobiology* 9:341, 1972.
79. McCauley RL, Hing DN, Robson MC, et al: Frostbite injuries: a rational approach based on pathophysiology, *J Trauma* 23:143, 1983.
80. Meehan JP: Individual and racial variations in a vascular response to cold stimulus, *Milit Med* 116:330–337, 1955.
81. Mennell JM: *Foot pain*, Boston, 1969, Little Brown.
82. Metaizeau JP, Gayet O, Prevot J: The use of free full thickness skin grafts in treatment of complications of burns, *Prog Pediatr Surg* 14:209, 1981.
83. Miller TA, Switzer WE, Foley WD, et al: Early homografting of second degree burns, *Plast Reconstr Surg* 40:117, 1967.
84. Mladick R, Georgiade H, Thorne F: Clinical evaluation of thermography in determining degree of injury, *Plast Reconstr Surg* 38:512, 1966.
85. Norris JEC: Burns of the foot. In Jahss M, editor: *Disorders of the foot*, Philadephia, 1982, WB Saunders.

86. Okuboye JA, Ferguson CC: The use of hyperbaric oxygen in the treatment of experimental frostbite, *Can J Surg* 11:78, 1968.
87. Owens JC: Treatment of cold injuries, *Postgrad Med* 48:160, 1970.
88. Randolph et al, 1969.
89. Roberts WC: Radiographic characteristics of glass, *Arch Indust Health* 18:470, 1958.
90. Robson MC, Kucan JO, Piak KI, et al: Prevention of derma ischemia after thermal trauma, *Arch Surg* 113:621, 1978.
91. Rudowski W: *Burn therapy and research*, Baltimore, 1976, John Hopkins University.
92. Salimi Z, Wolverson MK, Herbold DR, et al: Treatment of frostbite with IV streptokinase, *AJR* 149:773, 1987.
93. Salisbury RE, Pruitt BA: *Burns of the upper extremity*, vol 9. In *Major problems in clinical surgery*, Philadelphia, 1976, WB Saunders.
94. Sawacki BE: Reversal of capillary stasis and prevention of necrosis in burns, *Ann Surg* 180:98, 1974.
95. Schecter DC, Sarot IA: Historical accounts of injuries due to cold, *Surgery* 63:527–535, 1968.
96. Simeone FA: Cold injury, *Arch Surg* 80:396, 1960.
97. Starzl TE: The problem of frostbite in civilian medical practice, *Surg Clin North Am* 43:519, 1963.
98. Tishler JM: The soft tissue and bone changes in frostbite injuries, *Radiology* 102:511, 1972.
99. Ungley CC: Treatment of immersion foot by dry cooling, *Lancet* 1:681, 1943.
100. Urschel JD: Frostbite predisposing factors and predictors of poor outcome, *J Trauma* 30:340–342, 1990.
101. Vanggaard L: Arterial venous anastomosis in temperature regulation (abstract). *Acta Physiol Scand* 76:13, 1969.
102. Vinson HA, Schatzki R: Roentgenologic bone changes encountered in frostbite: Korea 1950–51, *Radiology* 63:685, 1954.
103. Washburn B: Frostbite, *N Engl J Med* 266:974, 1962.
104. Weatherly-White RCA, Paton BC, Sjostrom B: Observations on the treatment of frostbite, *Plast Reconstr Surg* 36:10, 1965.
105. Webster DR, Woolhouse FM, Johnston JL: Immersion foot, *J Bone Joint Surg [Am]* 24:785, 1942.

CHAPTER

34

Fractures and Fracture-Dislocations of the Ankle

Michael W. Chapman, M.D.

Criteria for treatment
Fracture classification
Vertical compression fractures
Diagnosis and emergency treatment
History
Physical diagnosis
Radiographic findings
Emergency treatment
Treatment
Soft-tissue considerations
Closed vs. open treatment
Surgical technique
Medial malleolus
Lateral malleolus
Posterior malleolus
Syndesmosis separations
Tibial pilon (plafond) fractures
Postoperative care
Epiphyseal injuries of the ankle in children
Fibula
Tibia
Tillaux fracture
Triplane fracture
Compartment syndrome

CRITERIA FOR TREATMENT

For best functional results in the treatment of ankle fractures, particularly those involving joints, four criteria must be filled:

1. *Dislocations and fractures should be reduced as soon as possible.* Fractures are most easily reduced early. Reduction is easier to obtain before swelling occurs and before the fracture hematoma between the fragments organizes. Furthermore, gross displacement—particularly in the ankle, subtalar, and midfoot joints—results in considerable distortion of the soft tissues and can lead to impairment of peripheral circulation, neuropraxis, and loss of skin. Early reduction minimizes these complications.

2. *All joint surfaces must be precisely reconstituted.* Nonanatomic reduction may lead to joint instability and/or joint surface incongruity, which predisposes to arthritis.

3. *Reduction of the fracture must be maintained during the period of healing.* Once anatomic reduction has been achieved, it must be held until healing of bone and ligaments sufficient to provide stability has occurred. This can be accomplished by external immobilization with a plaster cast or splints, by external fixation, or by internal fixation. External immobilization of injured joints has definite deleterious effects. The extent of these undesirable effects is largely dependent on the age of the patient: the older the patient, the more adverse the effects of long-term immobilization. In addition, holding ankle fractures anatomically by external means is difficult, and late loss of reduction in plaster is all too common.

An appreciation of the problems associated with external immobilization has prompted many surgeons, in spite of the possible risk of infection, to employ open reduction, internal fixation, and early mobilization as the treatment of choice.

4. *Motion of joints should be instituted as early as possible.* To maintain itself in a state of health, any organ or organ system must be used. Suppression of the normal functioning of the musculoskeletal system by immobilization of any of its parts is attended by numerous undesirable sequelae, including muscular atrophy, myostatic contracture, decreased joint motion, proliferation of the connective tissue in the capsular structures, internal synovial adhesions, cartilaginous degeneration, and bone atrophy. Furthermore, vascular changes occur during the period of immobilization, and these often result in edema after the external support is removed. Early mobilization obviates or decreases the possible occurrence of these abnormal processes.

The most ardent protagonist for early motion after the reduction of fractures was Lucas-Championnière,[23] who based his beliefs on clinical experience. Since that time, experimental evidence has gradually appeared in the medical literature to support his contentions.[32, 37]

FRACTURE CLASSIFICATION

Many classification systems for fractures and fracture-dislocations about the ankle joint exist and are based, for the most part, on the mechanism of injury.[1, 3, 18–22, 27] Knowledge of a classification system enables the surgeon to offer better treatment through the understanding it provides of the interrelationship between the mechanism of injury and the pathologic anatomy. Occult ligamentous injury will be detected, and the optimal position of the limb in a closed reduction can be determined.

Lauge-Hansen[19–22] has provided the most useful and comprehensive classification of ankle injuries; in spite of the complex variety of ankle fractures, 98% to 99% can be fit into his system. Most importantly he emphasizes the role of the ligaments in these injuries. Students of ankle injuries are strongly advised to read the articles of Lauge-Hansen cited in the reference section.

Table 34–1 briefly summarizes the Lauge-Hansen classification. The Lauge-Hansen system is quite complex, so from a practical point of view one can look at ankle fractures in a more simplified way—as advocated by Jergesen.[17]

When assessing fractures about the ankle within a

TABLE 34–1.
Lauge-Hansen Classification of Ankle Fractures

Type of Injury (Foot Position—Direction of Force)	Stage	Pathology
Supination—adduction	I	Transverse fracture of the lateral malleolus or Torn lateral collateral ligaments
	II	Stage I plus Fracture of the medial malleolus
Supination—eversion	I	Rupture (or avulsion fracture) of the anterior inferior tibiofibular ligament
	II	Stage I plus Spiral or oblique fracture of the lateral malleolus
	III	Stage II plus Fracture of the posterior lip of the tibia
	IV	Stage III plus Fracture of the medial malleolus or tear of the deltoid ligament
Pronation—abduction	I	Fracture of the medial malleolus or tear of the deltoid ligament
	II	Stage I plus Rupture of the anterior and posterior ligaments of the syndesmosis and fracture of the posterior lip of the tibia
	III	Stage II plus Oblique fracture of the fibula above the ankle mortise
Pronation—eversion	I	Fracture of the medial malleolus or tear of the deltoid ligament
	II	Stage I plus Tear of the anterior inferior tibiofibular and interosseous ligaments
	III	Stage II plus Tear of the interosseous membrane and spiral fracture of the fibula 5–6 cm above the plafond of the tibia
	IV	Stage III plus Avulsion fracture of the posterior lip of the tibia

functional framework, the practitioner should consider two concepts: (1) anatomic reduction is desirable because the restoration of normal anatomy to a weight-bearing joint is of primary importance, and (2) stability of the ankle is related to the integrity of the malleolar and syndesmosis ligaments.

The foot is securely bound to the leg by two osseous ligamentous shrouds consisting of (on the one side) the medial malleolus and the corresponding medial collateral ligament and (on the other side) the lateral malleolus and the lateral collateral ligaments. In addition, the intermalleolar space is maintained by the tibiofibular syndesmosis ligaments (Fig 34–1). Any number of fracture and ligamentous disruption combinations can occur that may destroy the normal stability of the ankle. If we speak of the foot in relation to the leg, the basic mechanisms of injury can be thought of as (1) external rotation–eversion or abduction, (2) internal rotation–inversion or adduction, and (3) vertical loading.

Ankle injuries result from abnormal motion of the talus within the ankle mortise. Fractures of the malleoli can result from the impact of the talus on the malleoli. Fractures can also occur in tension, and the malleoli can be avulsed because of the pull exerted by the intact collateral ligaments attached to the talus.

Impact fractures tend to be spiral or oblique. Avulsion fractures tend to be at right angles to the line of pull of the ligament. Ligament failure rather than fracture may occur, so instability in any given injury can be due to a combination of fracture and ligament rupture. Figure 34–2 illustrates the difference between these two mechanisms.

Figure 34–3 contains four radiographs showing some of the combinations of injuries seen in external rotation–eversion and abduction-type fractures. The possible varieties of injury include the following:

1. External rotation–eversion and abduction injuries
   a. Medial side
      (1) Transverse avulsion fracture of the medial malleolus
      (2) Ruptured deltoid ligament

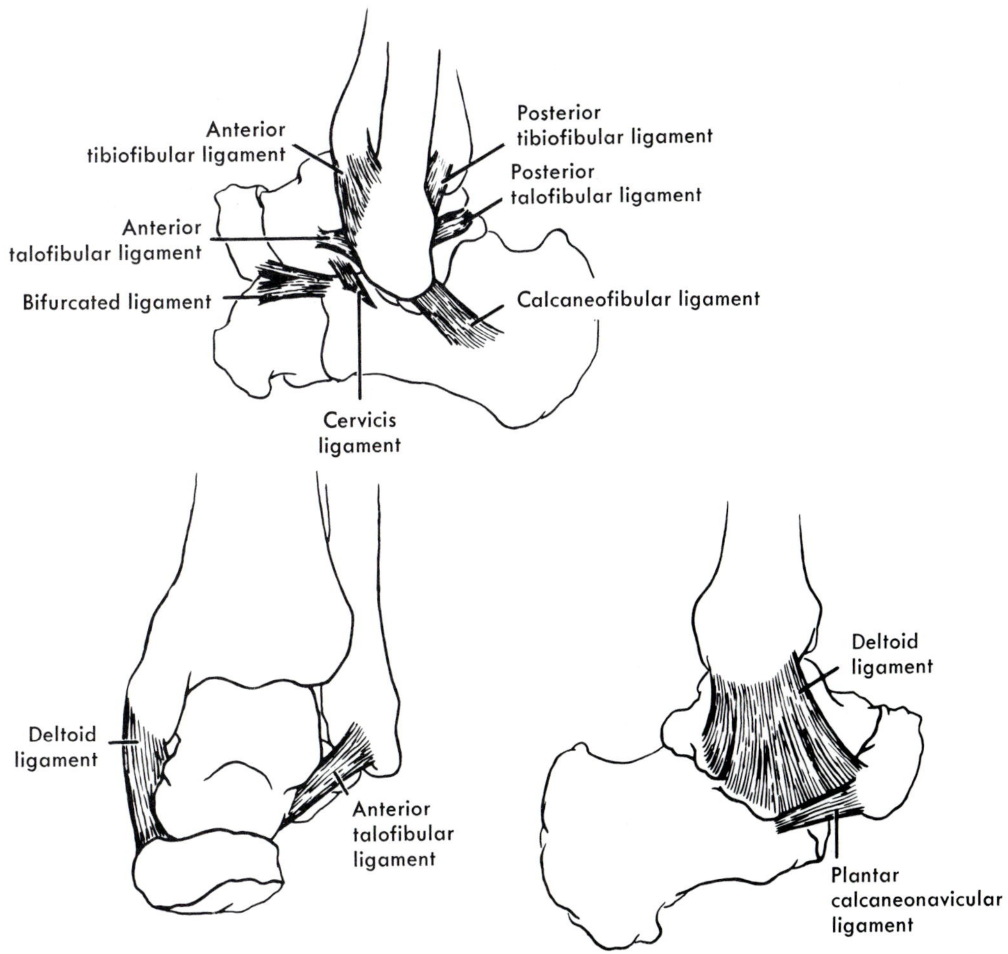

FIG 34–1.
Anatomy of the ankle. (From Chapman MW: Sprains of the ankle, *Instr Course Lect* 24:294, 1975. Used by permission.)

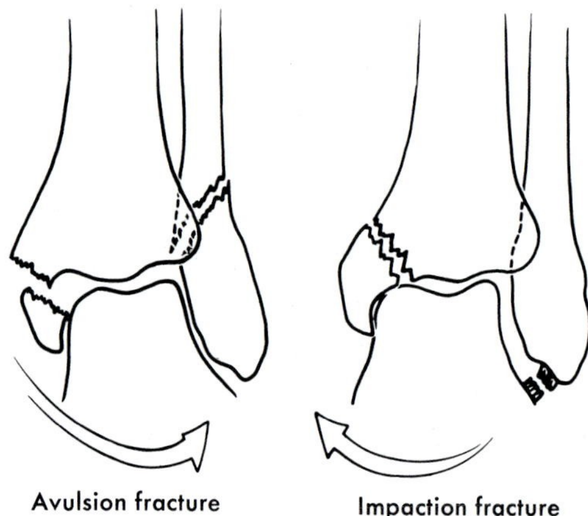

FIG 34–2.
Mechanism of injury.

b. Lateral side
   (1) Spiral fracture of the lateral malleolus with the fracture line proceeding from the distal anterior to the proximal posterior aspects (external rotation)
   (2) Spiral fracture of the shaft of the fibula above the syndesmosis, usually associated with disruption of the syndesmosis (external rotation)
   (3) Short oblique fracture of the fibula in the mediolateral plane below or above the syndesmosis, often with a small lateral butterfly fragment at the fracture (abduction)
c. Syndesmosis
   (1) Torn anterior tibiofibular ligament (external rotation) through a complete syndesmosis rupture (more common abduction mechanism)
   (2) Avulsion fracture of the posterior malleolus (external rotation)

Figure 34–4 is a radiograph of an adduction-inversion injury. The possible varieties of such an injury include the following:

2. Adduction-inversion injuries (Fig 34–4)
   a. Medial side
      (1) Oblique fracture of the medial malleolus extending from the corner of ankle mortise proximally and medially
   b. Lateral side
      (1) Transverse avulsion of the lateral malleolus below the syndesmosis
      (2) Rupture of the lateral collateral ligaments
   c. Syndesmosis
      (1) As part of a fibular fracture (torn inferior fibers rare in adduction injuries)
   d. Posterior malleolus
      (1) With posterior medial dislocation (occasional fracture of the posterior and medial malleoli)

When internal fixation is being considered, the Arbeitsgemeinschaft für Osteosynthese (A-O) system for classification of ankle fractures is very helpful.[33] The A-O system is based on the level of the fibula fracture. The higher the fracture of the fibula, the more extensive the damage to the syndesmosis ligaments and the more likely that the ankle mortise will be unstable. I will use this system when discussing operative treatment. The three types of fractures are as follows:

Type A	
Fibula	Transverse avulsion fracture below or at the level of the plafond (or ligament tear)
Medial malleolus	Intact or sheared with fracture angulating upward from the corner of the mortise
Posterior tibia	Usually intact, but a medial posterior fracture fragment may be present
Syndesmosis	Intact
Lauge-Hansen equivalent	Supination-adduction
Type B	
Fibula	Spiral fracture beginning at the level of the plafond and extending proximally
Medial malleolus	Intact or transverse avulsion fracture or rupture of the deltoid ligament
Posterior tibia	Intact or avulsion fracture
Syndesmosis	Interosseous ligament intact; anterior and posterior inferior tibiofibular ligaments torn depending on the level of the fracture and the severity of injury
Lauge-Hansen equivalent	Supination-eversion
Type C	
Fibula	Fractured above the syndesmosis
Medial malleolus	Transverse avulsion fracture or a deltoid ligament tear
Posterior tibia	Avulsion fracture can occur
Syndesmosis	Always torn
Lauge-Hansen equivalent	Pronation-eversion

See Figure 34–5 for an illustration of types A, B, and C.

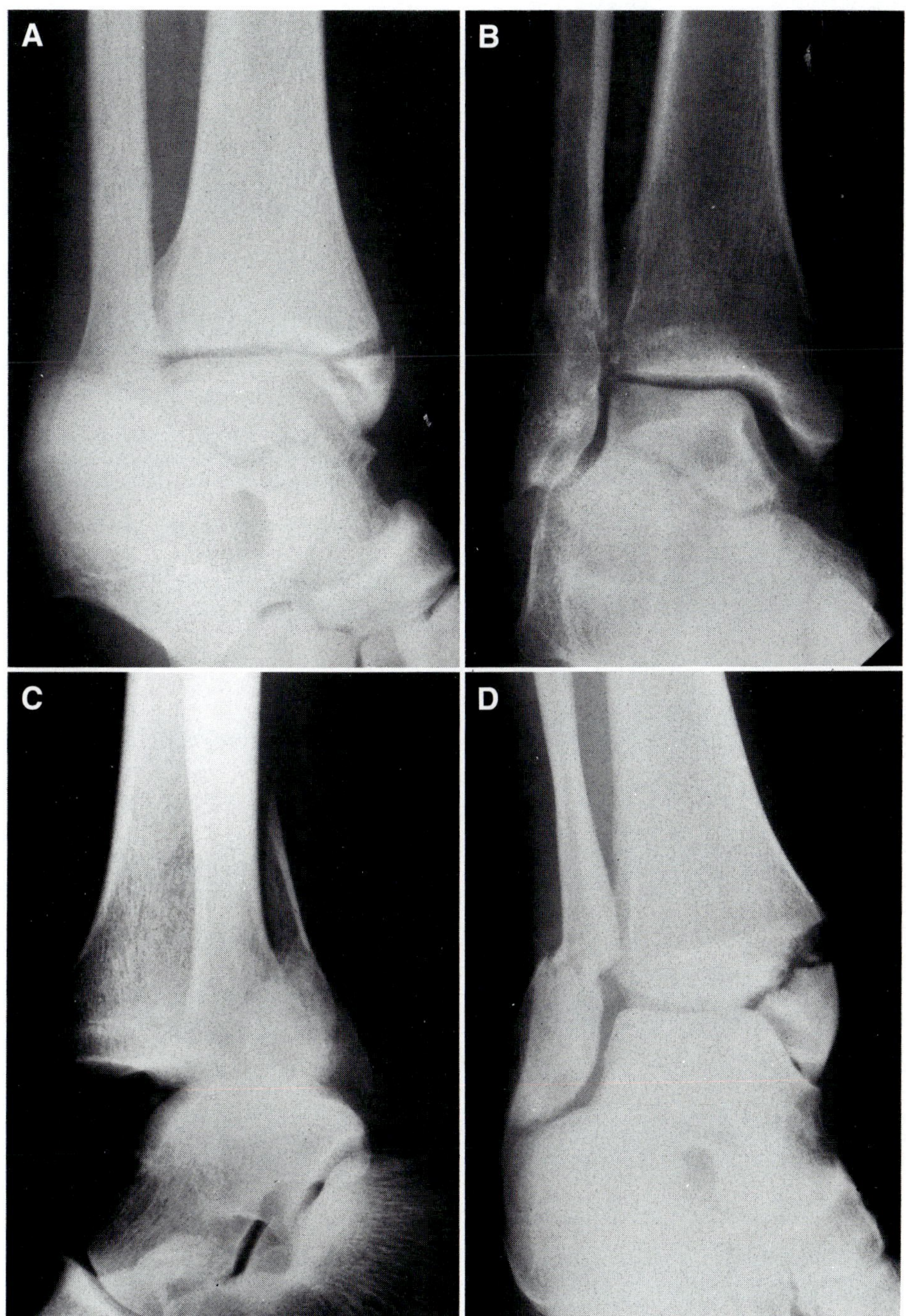

FIG 34–3.
External rotation–eversion and abduction injuries. **A,** external rotation–eversion with a transverse avulsion fracture of the medial malleolus. Look for associated syndesmosis ligament ruptures and/or a high proximal fracture of the fibula. **B,** external rotation–eversion with a short spiral-oblique fracture of the lateral malleolus and a deltoid ligament rupture. **C,** external rotation–eversion with a spiral fracture of the lateral malleolus and an avulsion fracture of the posterior malleolus. **D,** abduction. A transverse comminuted fracture of the fibula is fairly typical. An avulsion fracture of the medial malleolus is usually more transverse.

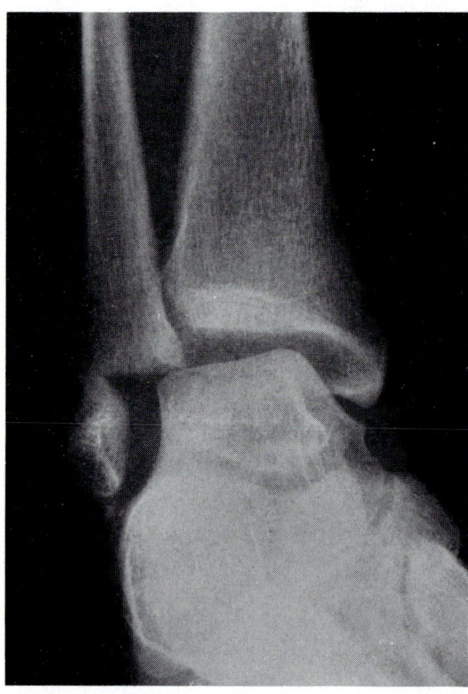

FIG 34–4.
Adduction-inversion injury showing a transverse avulsion fracture of the lateral malleolus below the level of the syndesmosis. The talus is hinging on an intact deltoid ligament.

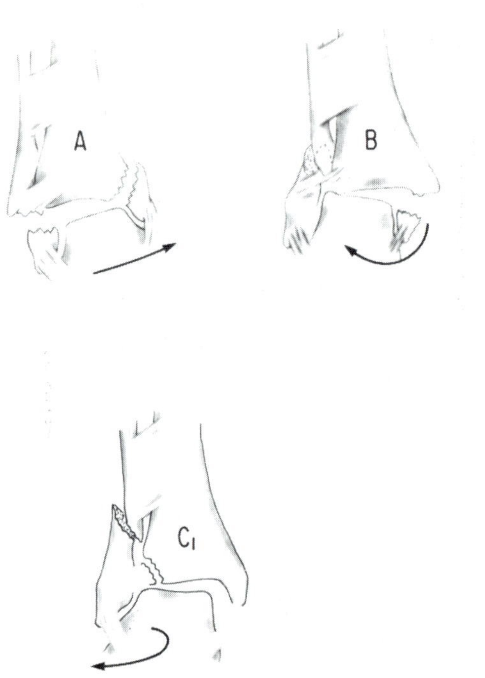

FIG 34–5.
Diagram of the A-O system for classifying ankle fractures based on the level of fibular fracture. See the text for details.

Historically, certain ankle fractures have come to be named after the surgeon who originally described them. Before the invention of x-rays, Sir Percivall Pott[35] described an ankle injury secondary to leaping or jumping that was a transverse fracture of the fibula 2 to 3 in. above the distal end and associated with a tear of the deltoid ligament and lateral subluxation of the talus.

In 1819, a Frenchman named Dupuytren described a fracture similar to Pott's: a fracture of the fibula about 2½ in. proximal to its tip accompanied by a rupture of the syndesmosis and either a fracture of the medial malleolus or a tear of the deltoid ligament. This fracture is a Lauge-Hansen pronation-eversion stage III.[12]

In 1840 Maisonneuve emphasized the importance of external rotation in the etiology of ankle injuries, and his name is associated with a spiral fracture of the fibula that occurs as high as the proximal third.[25]

An avulsion fracture of the tibial origin of the anterior inferior tibiofibular ligament, caused by abduction and external rotation, was described by Tillaux in 1872. An avulsion fracture of the fibular side can also occur.

VERTICAL COMPRESSION FRACTURES

Vertical compression fractures are typically caused by falls from a height or deceleration motor vehicle injuries. The configuration of these fractures is quite variable. The usual fracture is accompanied by hyperdorsiflexion of the ankle that produces a vertical shear fracture of the anterior tibial plafond. This injury is usually accompanied by upward impaction of the tibial plafond compressing the metaphyseal cancellous bone. With severe compression, an explosion-type fracture occurs in which the malleoli are displaced outward as the talus drives into the central plafond of the tibia (Fig 34–6).

Lauge-Hansen pointed out that these fractures occur in stages, with the sequence of fractures and ligament ruptures depending on the position of the foot at the time of injury.[19–22] These are also known as tibial plafond (French for "ceiling") fractures. When the fracture involves the metaphysis and distal shaft, it is known as a pilon (French for "rammer" or "hammer") fracture.

The A-O group classifies these into types I, II, and III, according to their severity. Type I fractures are undisplaced, type II have joint incongruity, and type III are comminuted with articular displacement and crushing of the cancellous bone of the metaphysis (Fig 34–7).

Osteochondral fractures of the talus are common and must be searched for diligently in all ankle injuries. These will be discussed in Chapter 35.

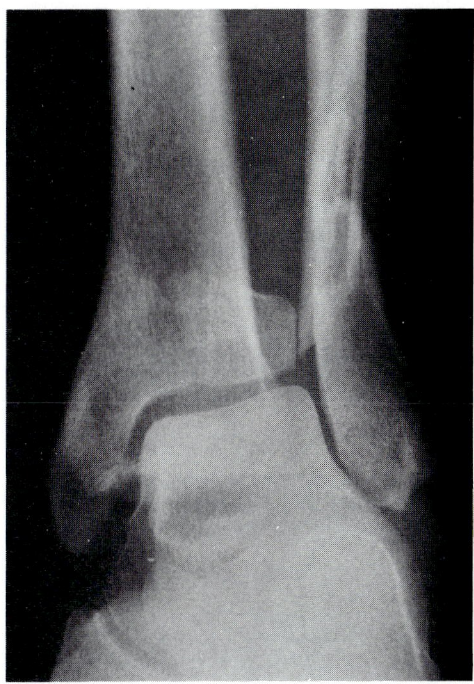

FIG 34–6.
Vertical loading type of fracture of the ankle. The fibular shaft is comminuted. The tibial plafond is driven proximally and has resulted in a crush fracture of the cancellous bone of the distal end of the tibia.

Diagnosis and Emergency Treatment

History

Most patients are unable to relate the exact mechanism of injury beyond the type of force involved. With a fall from a height or following a motor vehicle deceleration injury, the surgeon should look for occult impaction of the tibial plafond. The patient may describe complete dislocation of the foot on the leg with spontaneous relocation. This history, of course, would indicate a grossly unstable ankle with probable severe associated soft-tissue injuries. Pedestrians hit by motor vehicles frequently have unstable adduction or abduction fractures. Weight-bearing twisting injuries are usually of the external rotation–eversion type, which makes up about 60% of all ankle fractures.[1] Knee pain over the head of the fibula may suggest an unstable ankle with a high fibula fracture.[25]

Physical Diagnosis

Physical diagnosis is important in determining the degree of soft-tissue injury, in ascertaining the presence of ligamentous injuries not evident on radiographic examination by assessing joint stability, and in determining the neurovascular status of the foot. Radiographs will usually reveal the extent of bony injury. Careful systematic palpation to identify areas of tenderness and swelling will help localize disruptions in the structures about the ankle and the interosseous area; the full length of the fibula should also be examined.

The location of findings, plus crepitus, will usually indicate a fracture. In minor, seemingly stable injuries, such as an isolated undisplaced fracture of the lateral malleolus, one should look carefully for evidence of deltoid and syndesmosis ligament injury. Stability of the ankle should be gently tested in varus, valgus, and particularly external rotation. Premedication and local anesthetics may be necessary. Anterior instability of the talus in the mortise is helpful in detecting unstable ligament injuries. Peroneal muscle spasm may hide lateral instability. If there is a question in the examiner's mind, examination with stress radiographs under anesthesia may be indicated. The neurovascular status of the foot should be carefully assessed. In particular, one should look for partial or complete common peroneal nerve paralysis.

Radiographic Findings

Anteroposterior, lateral, and mortise views (the last, an oblique view with the foot internally rotated 15 to 20 degrees) should be obtained. Fractures involving the plafond may require multiple oblique projections and biplane tomograms for full delineation. After correlation of the physical examination findings with the initial radiographic findings, further assessment of the fracture with evaluation of the integrity of the ankle mortise and the tibiofibular syndesmosis is of paramount importance.

The integrity of the syndesmosis is best assessed on the anteroposterior projection, as is well described by McDade (based on Bonnin, 1970),[3, 28] since complete disruption, if undisplaced, will appear normal. The external rotatory malalignment that occurs when only the anterior inferior tibiofibular ligament is torn is subtle; the syndesmosis clear space, which represents the posterior tibiofibular joint, does not change as the fibula rotates outward. One must look instead at the extent of overlap of the fibula by the anterior tibial tubercle. Comparison views are often necessary because there is considerable anatomic variation (Fig 34–8).

On a good mortise view the superior articular surface of the talus should be fully congruous with the tibial plafond. The medial and lateral joint spaces should be equal and comparable to the superior joint space. A line extending distally from the posterior syndesmosis of the tibia should pass along the lateral aspect of the talus (*d-d* in Fig 34–9). On lateral views the talar dome should be concentric with the tibial plafond (*b-b*).

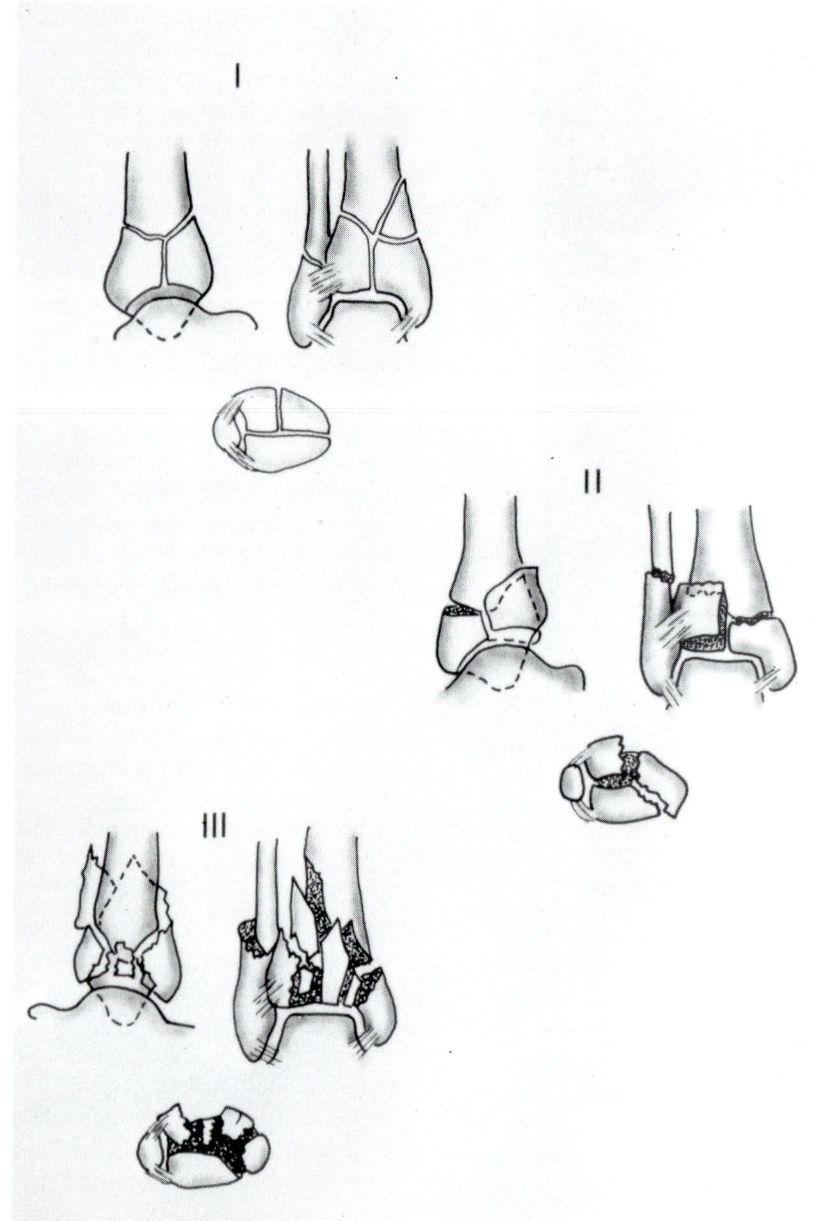

FIG 34–7.
Classification of tibial plafond fractures: **I,** undisplaced; **II,** joint incongruity; **III,** comminuted with articular displacement and crushing of cancellous bone.

Emergency Treatment

Excessive swelling can so compromise the treatment of even minor ankle sprains that patients should all have their lower extremities elevated higher than their heart while undergoing initial evaluation and treatment. This usually requires that they be placed on a gurney.

Wounds and abrasions should be cleansed and dressed. A soft compression dressing and radiolucent long-leg splint should be applied before radiographic examination.

Grossly distorted ankles with severe skin distortion should be reduced immediately in the emergency room to avoid skin necrosis and also eliminate tension on the neurovascular structures.

Treatment

Soft-tissue Considerations

Whether treatment of these fractures is by closed or open reduction, ultimate success depends on proper as-

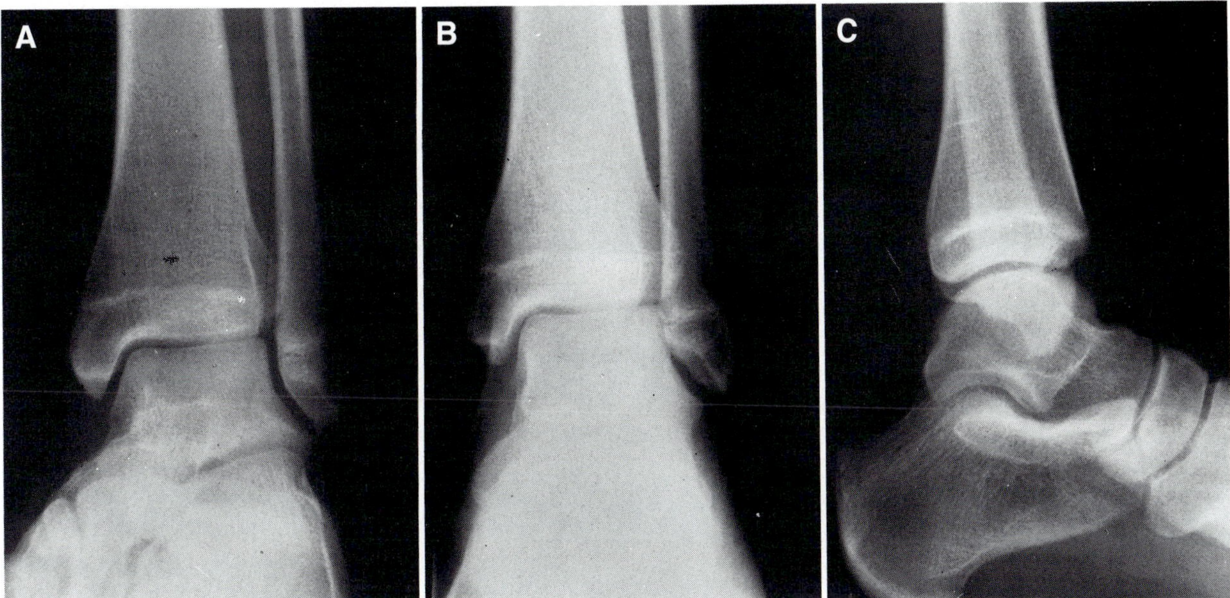

FIG 34–8.
Normal ankle in a young adult. **A,** mortise view (15 to 20 degrees of internal rotation). **B,** standard anteroposterior view. **C,** lateral view.

sessment and management of the associated soft-tissue trauma.

Abrasions should be carefully cleansed and sterily dressed. Abrasions into the dermis quickly become colonized by skin bacteria; therefore any surgery planned should be done within a few hours. After 12 to 24 hours, depending on how dirty it is, a deep abrasion may contraindicate surgery for 3 weeks or more. Neglected abrasions can lead to local cellulitis with possible infection of the fracture hematoma.

Early closed reduction and elevation with a good compression dressing and splints or a cast are important in preventing edema. Ankle and foot edema can be severe and cause fracture blisters. Gross edema may contraindicate surgery and lead to loss of the initial closed reduction. Surgeons should avoid early surgery on the tensely swollen shiny-skinned "watermelon" ankle since skin closure may be impossible and marginal wound necrosis can occur.

One should always be alert for a compartment syndrome in the leg and foot. The physical findings that should alert the clinician are tenseness in the calf, leg pain with passive stretch of the muscles, and paresis of the deep peroneal nerve.

Closed vs. Open Treatment

Undisplaced fractures without disruption of the ankle mortise are treated with cast immobilization. Treatment of undisplaced stable fractures of the lateral malleolus and distal medial malleolus can begin with immediate weight-bearing in a short-leg walking cast, which should be left in place for 6 weeks. Other stable injuries should be placed in a long-leg cast with the knee flexed 15 degrees. The cast must be molded to ensure the maintenance of position. Weekly radiographs for at least 4 weeks are usually necessary to ensure that these fractures do not become displaced. Depending on the surgeon's judgment about the stability of the ankle, weight bearing can begin in either a short- or a long-leg cast at 4 or 6 weeks. Any fracture, whether treated in a closed or open manner, will, if treated in a non–weight-bearing cast, rehabilitate more quickly and easily if given 2 weeks in a short-leg walking cast before complete cast removal.

Displaced fractures or fracture-dislocations may be treated by closed reduction and cast immobilization or by open reduction and internal fixation. Open reduction and internal fixation are almost always indicated if anatomic reduction cannot be achieved. If anatomic reduction is achieved by closed technique, it is often impossible to maintain, and late displacement is frequent.

In deciding whether to accept any displacement in an ankle fracture it is important to appreciate the effects of minor displacements on the congruity of the ankle mortise. Ramsey and Hamilton[36] showed that a 1-mm lateral shift of the talus in the mortise reduces the contact area of the ankle joint 42%. Yablon et al.[41] showed that the talus faithfully follows the lateral malleolus.

On the other hand, in a study of 150 patients with displaced fractures of the ankle caused by external rota-

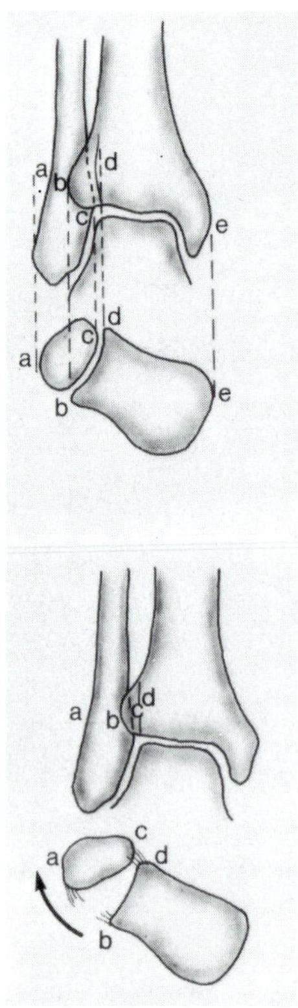

FIG 34–9.
Diagram of the anteroposterior projection of an ankle joint: *a,* lateral border of the lateral malleolus; *b,* lateral border of the anterior aspect of the tibia; *c,* medial border of the fibula; *d,* lateral border of the posterior aspect of the tibia. Rupture of the anterior syndesmosis with external rotation of the fibula does not affect the apparent width of the syndesmosis *(c-d)* or the intermalleolar distance *(a-e).* However, the amount of overlap of the anterior portion of the tibia on the fibula, distance *a-b* and distance *b-c,* change. Distance *a–b* increases and *b-c* decreases. In most ankles, distance *b-c* is over 50% of *a-c* on anteroposterior projections. Comparison radiographs of the normal ankle are very helpful.

tion-abduction forces that were treated by open reduction and rigid internal fixation and had an average follow-up of 3 1/2 years, De Souza, et al.[10] found that 90% satisfactory results could be obtained even if up to 2 mm of residual lateral displacement of the lateral and medial malleoli was present. Similar displacement of the talus was also compatible with a satisfactory result provided that there was anatomic restoration of the lateral side. I interpret these papers as indicating that somewhat more latitude is possible than that suggested by the studies of Ramsey and Hamilton.[36] There is no reason not to strive for anatomic alignment. The accuracy of alignment is much more important on the lateral side as compared with the medial. When faced with the decision whether to operate or not operate, it seems that up to 2 mm of displacement of the malleoli and 1 to 2 degrees of talar tilt are compatible with a satisfactory result. In the high-performance athlete, one might consider surgery if greater than 1-mm displacement is present, whereas in the more sedentary, elderly individual, 2 mm is acceptable.

In closed treatment interposition of the periosteum or other soft tissues, particularly when the medial malleolus is fractured, can prevent good fracture apposition and thereby lead to nonunion or fibrous union.

Open reduction and internal fixation are generally indicated if ankle fractures are displaced, particularly if the talus is subluxated in the ankle mortise. Closed treatment of displaced fractures may be indicated when (1) the condition of the soft tissues contraindicates surgery, (2) the patient is nonambulatory (paraplegic), (3) the patient is elderly and sedentary, and (4) the patient has sustained multiple trauma and surgery is contraindicated.

Closed Reduction.

External Rotation–Eversion and Abduction.—The mechanisms of these injuries are accompanied by posterolateral subluxation or dislocation of the foot on the leg; the foot is usually externally rotated with reference to the leg. For reduction to be achieved, the foot must be brought anteriorly and medially and internally rotated on the tibia.

The malleoli are attached to the foot by the collateral ligaments; the "distal fragment" is, in reality, the foot with the attached malleoli. Hence reduction entails regaining the proper relationship of the foot to the tibia. If the deltoid ligament rather than the medial malleolus is disrupted or if the medial malleolar fragment is small, a shoulder or buttress exists medially against which the foot (talus) can be reduced. If the medial malleolar fragment is large, internal fixation of the medial malleolus may be necessary to achieve stability of the joint.

A convenient way to carry out manipulative reduction, if an assistant is available, is to flex the patient's hip and knee approximately 30 degrees to allow the extremity to rotate externally approximately 30 degrees. The assistant holds the limb in this position by supporting the thigh with one hand and holding the first two toes with the other hand, thereby maintaining the foot in a vertical plane. Gravity produces medial and anterior replacement of the foot, and with the foot held in a vertical position, an attitude of internal rotation of the foot relative to the leg is achieved. A cast employing the principles of three-point molding can then be applied. The knee should be flexed only 15 degrees in the cast. Rotational control is gained through molding rather than knee flexion. These principles are embodied in the cast shown in Figure 34–10.

Adduction-Inversion Mechanisms.—In adduction-inversion injuries the reverse of the maneuvers described for the abduction–external rotation injury is required. There is less often a lateral buttress against which to reduce the joint, and the medial malleolar fracture line frequently runs proximally from the level of the joint.

Anterior Lip Fractures.—It is difficult to avoid anterior subluxation in this injury when the patient is recumbent with his limb supported in the usual fashion at the foot and knee. Again, the force of gravity can be used to assist the surgeon in reducing the fracture.

Suspend the leg over the end of the treatment table where an assistant can carry out a posterior thrust of the foot against the leg. Or, more simply, have the patient lie prone on the table with his knee on the injured side flexed approximately 60 degrees. An assistant supports the foot in this position, which permits the weight of the leg against the supported foot to reduce the subluxation. Reduction is maintained in this position while the surgeon applies the cast.

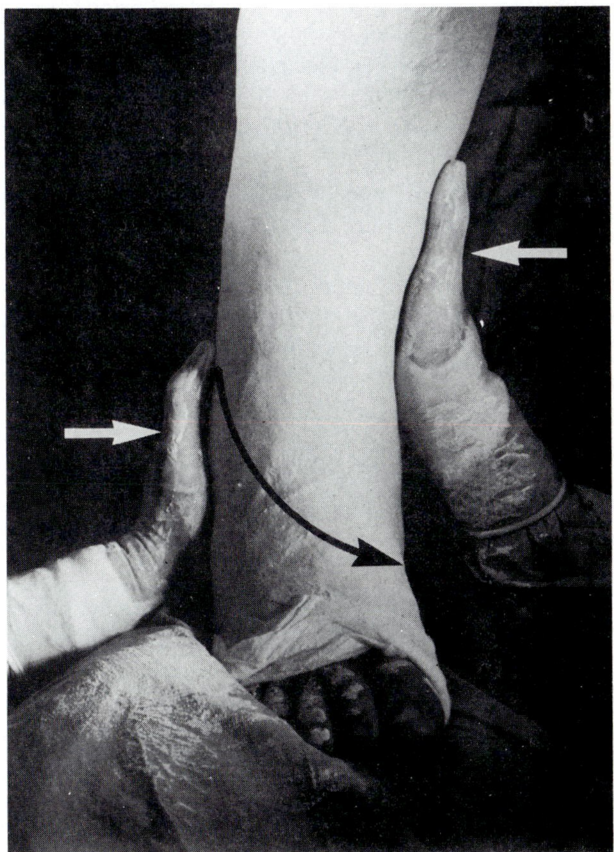

FIG 34–10.
Molding of a cast to reduce an external rotation–eversion type of injury.

Vertical Compression Fractures.—In stable impacted fractures with minimal displacement, immobilization in a neutral position with careful molding of the cast about the malleoli usually suffices. Unstable comminuted fractures present unique problems (see page 34–21).

Open Reduction With Internal Fixation – Indications and Philosophy.

Fracture of One Malleolus.—A fracture of one malleolus without involvement of its ligamentous component or the opposite malleolus permits using the uninjured side as a buttress to immobilize the part until healing takes place (see Fig 34–2). If only the malleolar tip is injured, simple protection from forced inversion (in the case of a lateral malleolus) or eversion (in the case of a medial malleolus) suffices. These are actually third-degree sprains with a small bone chip attached to the fragment.

Radiographic evidence of a fracture of just one malleolus does not guarantee stability; therefore clinical evaluation of the ligamentous structures at the distal tibiofibular junction and on the opposite side of the ankle is necessary to assess the stability of the injury.

Except for an avulsion fracture of the lateral malleolar tip, the most common isolated fracture of the lateral malleolus is a spiral fracture in the distal portion. Controversy exists over the indications for open reduction of these fractures. If the patient is young or middle-aged, the inability to achieve and hold an anatomic reduction is an indication for surgery.

What is a satisfactory reduction? Since the talus follows the lateral malleolus even in the presence of an intact deltoid ligament, small persistent displacement of the fracture can lead to talotibial incongruity. For this reason, assuming that the talus is anatomically reduced in the ankle mortise, I would accept 0.5 mm or less of shortening or widening. One millimeter or more of displacement is an indication for open reduction if the patient's age, activity level, etc., justify surgery.

Isolated fractures of the lateral malleolus per se are seldom associated with nonunion, although small avulsed fragments frequently do not unite.

Fractures of the medial malleolus, particularly those occurring below the level of the superior surface of the talus, may be asymptomatic even though they heal with fibrous union. Portis and Mendelsohn[34] and Aufranc[2] found little evidence to suggest that the isolated malleolar fracture, if not displaced, requires internal fixation. Fractures of the medial malleolus at the level of the plafond, however, result in complete functional loss of internal support provided by the medial collateral ligament. This fracture must be accurately reduced and internally fixed for the ankle to regain stability.

***Bimalleolar Fractures and Fracture-Dislocations.*—** The terms *bimalleolar fracture* and *fracture-dislocation* are used to describe fractures of both malleoli, fractures of one malleolus plus complete disruption of the ligament on the opposite side, or a fracture of the medial malleolus and rupture of the tibiofibular ligaments[14] in association with a fracture in the shaft of the fibula proximal to the tibiofibular ligament (see Fig 34–3).

A fibular fracture can occur at the proximal end of the fibula. If such a fracture is accompanied by ankle injury, one can assume that some disruption of the interosseous membrane has occurred anywhere from the distal tibiofibular syndesmosis to the level of the fibular fracture and that division of the distal tibiofibular ligaments has also taken place. Occasionally the injury will be manifested as a rupture of the deltoid ligament, with the line of dehiscence passing across the ankle capsule and continuing upward through the distal tibiofibular ligaments and interosseous membrane to the level of the proximal neck of the fibula. This particular combination is easy for the unwary examiner to miss since the ankle may be relocated when the technician positions it for radiographic examination. No fracture will be seen unless a full-length radiograph of the leg, including the upper end of the fibula, is taken.

Traditional teaching in English and American orthopaedics has held that with bimalleolar fractures, the majority of which are external rotation injuries, the key to reduction and stability of the ankle mortise is the medial malleolus. Fixation of the lateral side was not believed necessary because of the intact periosteal hinge.[7] This is now known to be not wholly true. McDade[28] and Yablon et al.[41] have emphasized the key role of the lateral malleolus in determining the position of the talus in the mortise. With an intact medial osseous ligamentous bridge, subluxation of the talus in the presence of an external rotation fracture of the lateral malleolus can occur. Because the talus faithfully follows the lateral malleolus, anatomic reduction of the lateral malleolus is a must in bimalleolar fractures. Yablon et al.[41] found that degenerative arthritis following displaced bimalleolar fractures is usually caused by incomplete reduction of the lateral malleolus with residual talar tilt.

Reduction of the lateral malleolus can be difficult. Fixation of the medial side first may lock the distal lateral malleolar fragment behind the shaft and prevent reduction. It is best to open both sides simultaneously, inspect and cleanse the joint space and fracture site(s) of debris, and reduce and then fix either the lateral side first or the medial side.

***Trimalleolar Fractures and Fracture-Dislocations.*—** Trimalleolar fractures and fracture-dislocations include all the combinations described for bimalleolar types of fracture and dislocation plus fractures of the posterior lip of the tibia.

The fragment may vary in size and may communicate with the medial malleolar fragment, or if it is laterally placed, it may carry the posterior tibiofibular ligament with it. If the fragment carries one fourth or more of the articular surface of the tibia with it, a high risk of posterior subluxation of the talus exists unless the fracture is internally fixed (see Fig 34–3).

Fortunately, most posterior lip fragments are small and do not, in themselves, compromise the stability of the ankle.[2] It has been generally accepted that in ankles with a posterior fragment involving more than 25% of the articular surface, open treatment is associated with better results than closed treatment.[29] This has been recently reinforced by the laboratory study of Macko et al.[24] They pointed out that the standard, lateral radiograph of a posterior malleolar fracture may underestimate the size of the fragment and therefore the joint surface area affected. If the lateral roentgenogram suggests 25% involvement of the articular surface, the odds are high that it may be much more. With a quarter of the articular surface involved, they found that with the ankle joint in a neutral position the average loss of contact area was approximately 12%; for a third of the surface involved, 20%; and for half involved, 35%. These represent substantial losses. On the other hand, Harper and Hardin[16] showed no statistical difference between posterior malleolar fractures that were fixed and those that were not. They studied 38 patients in whom the posterior malleolus fractures occupied 25% or more of the articular surface on the lateral radiograph and followed them for an average of 44 months. Fifteen patients had fixation of the posterior malleolus, and 23 did not. In the majority of cases, however, satisfactory reduction was obtained by closed methods. Ninety-one percent of the fragments that were treated without internal fixation reduced to within 2 mm of the articular surface, with reduction of the other components of the fracture. In their study, the key factor seems to be the quality of reduction of the medial and lateral malleoli.

In general, strive for anatomic reduction. In fragments involving 25% or less of the articular surface on the lateral view, the results do not seem to be influenced by the position of the posterior malleolus as long as the ankle joint is congruous. With larger fragments, strive for anatomic reduction because the fracture may involve a larger portion of the ankle articular surface than is apparent by radiographs. (This can be confirmed by computed tomography [CT]). Anatomic reduction and internal fixation are indicated if any element of incongruity, subluxation, or residual instability of the ankle is present.

Fractures of the Anterior Lip of the Distal Tibia.—Fracture of the anterior lip of the distal end of the tibia may accompany a malleolar fracture as a mirror image of the posterior trimalleolar fracture-dislocation; occasionally it occurs as an isolated injury.

It is generally the result of a vertical loading injury and therefore is not usually associated with fracture of the fibular shaft or disruption of the distal tibiofibular ligaments. The anterior lip of the tibia is more often comminuted than is the posterior lip; thus internal fixation techniques may be compromised.

Open reduction and fixation are indicated when the fracture is large enough to cause talar instability (25% to 35% of the articular surface) in association with talar subluxation or when the fracture is a component of a comminuted fracture that is amenable to open reduction.

Occasionally a rupture of the anterior inferior tibiofibular ligament manifests itself as an avulsion fracture from the fibula or tibia. The avulsion fracture from the tibia is most common and is known as a Tillaux fracture (see C1 fracture in Fig 34–4). If displaced this fracture should be internally fixed with a 4.0-mm cancellous bone screw to stabilize the mortise.

Fractures With Severe Comminution and Instability.—It may not be possible to reduce and internally fix severely comminuted fractures of the ankle. Such injuries can be managed with skeletal traction through the calcaneus or application of an external fixator from the tibia to the foot.

Early motion in these fractures is important to preserve ankle function and help mold the fracture surfaces. This can be achieved by performing a closed reduction with a Steinmann traction pin in the os calcis and then applying a bulky dressing or Delbet cast and placing the limb in traction on a Böhler-Braun frame. The traction will help maintain the reduction, and ankle motion can begin.

Occasionally both comminution and a complex-compound wound about the ankle create a situation in which it is impossible to employ the usual methods of malleolar fixation; yet to ensure the survival of the foot and permit management of the surrounding soft tissue, stability must be achieved. In this situation the technique of driving a vertical Steinmann pin through the calcaneus and the talus into the distal end of the tibia (Fig 34–11) can be used to preserve the foot.[8, 11] Because the Steinmann pin transgresses normal articular surfaces, I prefer to immobilize these fractures with an external fixator. The fixator is more versatile in that the position can be adjusted, better fixation is obtained, and conversion to a system that permits early motion is possible. A triangular frame is used with two pins in the tibia, one in the calcaneus, and one in the first and fifth metatarsals, respectively. This maintains a plantigrade foot (see Fig 34–12).

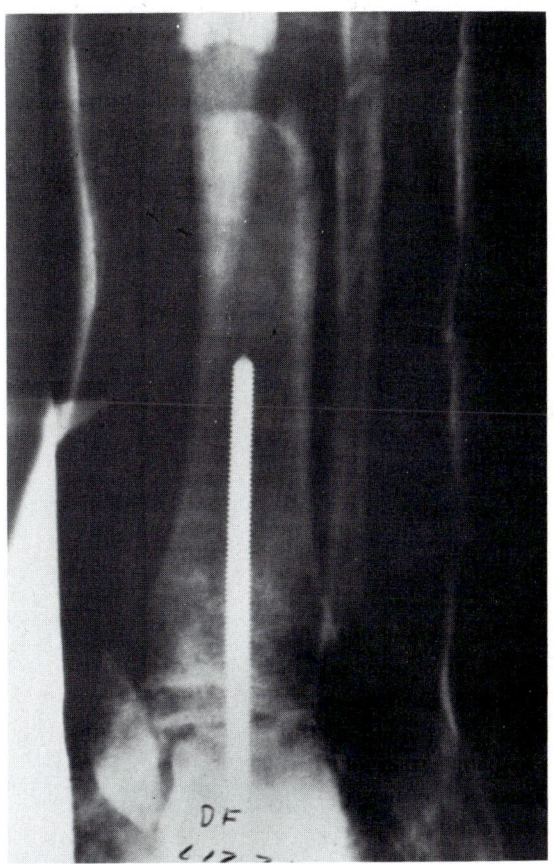

FIG 34–11.
Vertical Steinmann pin.

Fractures of the Lateral Malleolus With Posterior Displacement of the Proximal Fibular Fragment.—Bosworth,[4] Fleming and Smith,[13] and Meyers[31] all described bimalleolar types of fracture accompanied by displacement of the proximal portion of the fibula at the fracture site posteriorly on the tibia in a position that usually makes reduction by closed manipulation impossible. The ligamentous support of the syndesmosis apparently remains intact and holds the fibula in its dislocated position. In these types of fractures, open reduction is necessary, and a posterolateral approach is appropriate (Figs 34–13 and 34–14).

Open Fractures and Fracture-Dislocations of the Ankle.—The same principles of meticulous debridement, copious irrigation, and the use of systemic and lo-

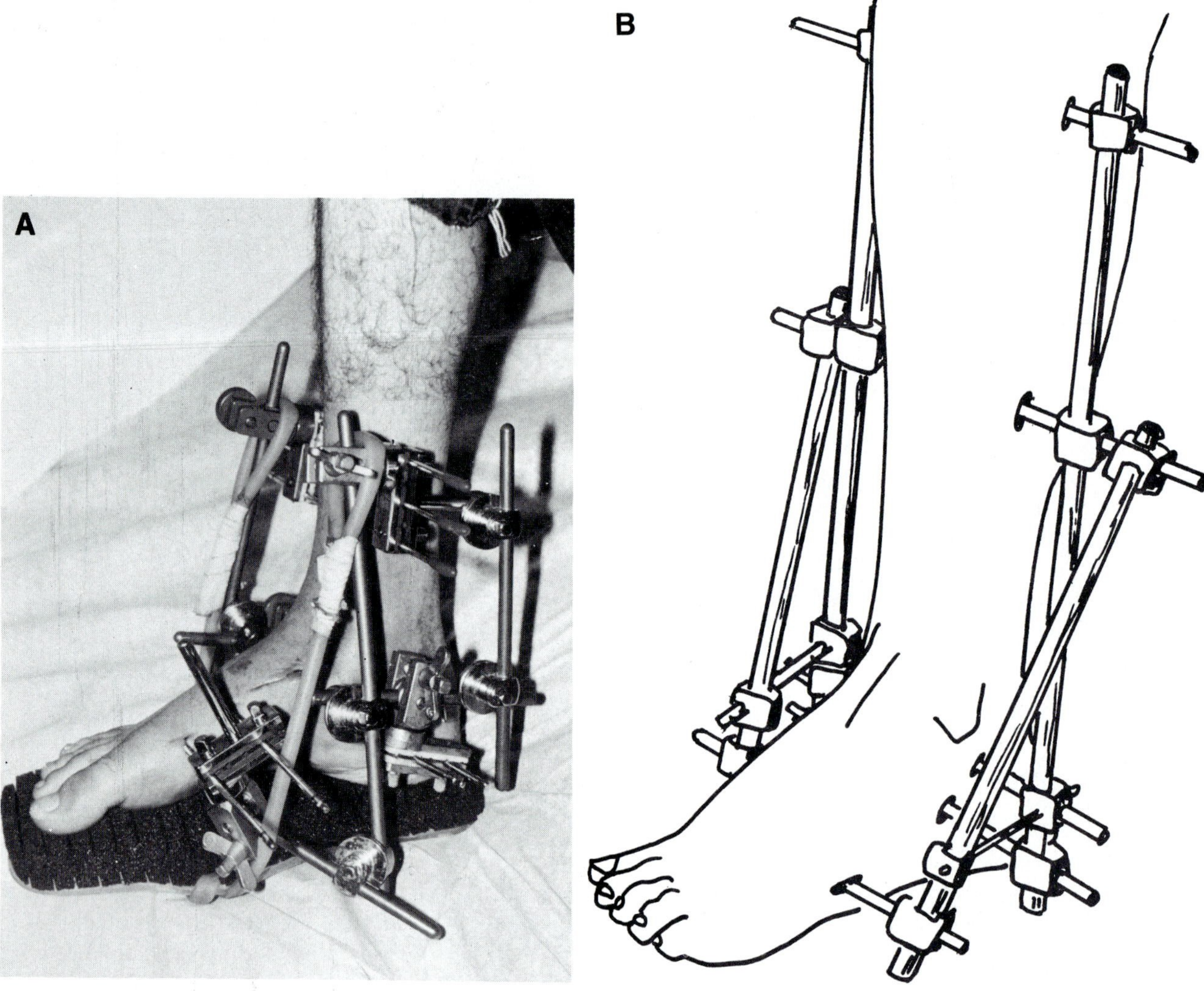

FIG 34–12.
A, immobilization of a severely comminuted fracture by using an external fixator. **B,** rather than the older Hoffman external fixator illustrated in **A,** I now prefer an external fixator with single, universal clamps and carbon fiber rods as illustrated in **B.** For the application of this fixator, first place a through-and-through threaded fixation pin in the shaft of the tibia at an appropriate distance proximal to the ankle joint and at right angles to the longitudinal axis of the tibia on the anterior view. Place a similar bicortical pin through the calcaneus in alignment with the tibial pin. Apply a carbon fiber bar, and use this preliminary external fixator to pull the fracture out to length and restore good alignment in the anterior, posterior, and lateral views. Once satisfactory alignment is obtained, lock the fixator by placing a second pin transversely through the tibia below the first. If the bone quality in the calcaneus is poor, two pins can be used. In addition, a pin can be placed in the talus. Generally, I avoid using talus pins because they are technically much more difficult to place. Next, place a half-pin into the proximal shaft—metaphyseal junction of the first and fifth metatarsals. Connect a carbon bar from the main frame bar to the metatarsal pins. Then cross-connect the carbon bar at the foot to form a triangle with the steel cross-connecting pins. This forms a lightweight, versatile, easy to adjust fixator that is radiolucent. This is superior to the Hoffman frame illustrated in **A,** through which it is almost impossible to see the ankle joint on a lateral view.

cal bactericidal antibiotics apply to open fractures of the ankle as apply to open fractures and injuries elsewhere in the body.

Wounds in this area almost always communicate with the ankle joint. The ankle joint must be explored. Although not essential, the ankle joint capsule is usually closed primarily; if this is done, a suction tube should be left in place to permit drainage. Joint closure, as either a primary or a delayed primary procedure, is essential.[17] The skin wound can be closed by primary clo-

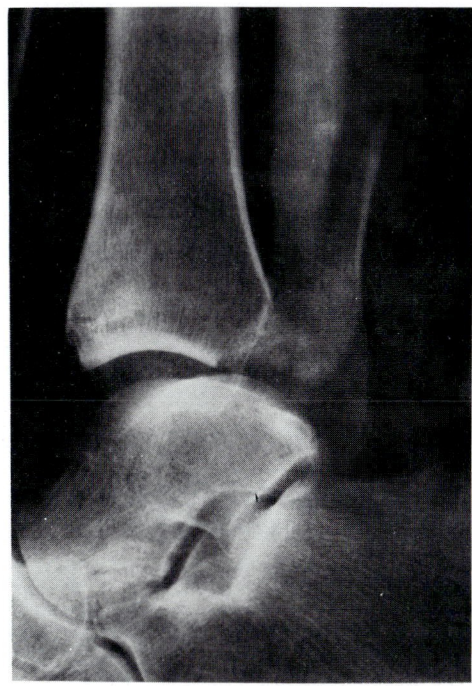

FIG 34–13.
Bosworth fracture with characteristic posterior displacement of the proximal aspect of the fibula.

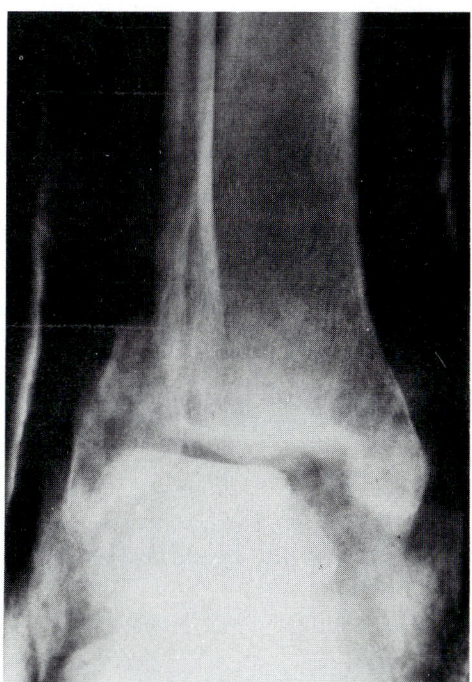

FIG 34–14.
This anteroposterior view of the ankle mortise in Figure 34–13 shows lateral subluxation of the talus.

sure, delayed primary closure, or secondary closure—depending on the degree of soft-tissue damage and contamination and on the amount of elapsed time since occurrence of the injury. The safest procedure, however, is to leave the wound above the joint capsule open and carry out a delayed primary closure.

Infection is the major complication to be avoided and can be related directly to the type of wound. Gustilo and Anderson[15] classified wounds as type I, II, or III, with type I being a wound less than 1 cm long and clean and type III having extensive soft-tissue damage. In their review of open fractures Chapman and Mahoney[6] noted that 60% of open ankle injuries had type I wounds and only 10% had type III wounds. In their series of open fractures in which immediate fixation was achieved, the infection rate in type I wounds was 2%; in type II wounds, 8%; and in type III wounds, 29%. This is significant insofar as it means that immediate internal fixation of ankles with type I wounds can be performed without an infection rate greater than that seen in closed fractures.

The risk of infection is much higher in type II and, in particular, type III open fractures, especially when high-energy fractures such as pilon fractures are present. Wiss et al.[40] in 76 open ankle fractures treated by immediate internal fixation had only a 5% deep infection rate. Twenty-eight of their 76 fractures had grade III wounds. Deep infection was a poor prognostic factor and always led to a poor result. Their series indicates that primary internal fixation of ankle fractures can be carried out with acceptable risks.

In the most commonly seen open fracture-dislocation about the ankle, a transverse wound occurs at the level of the medial malleolus centered on the medial side of the leg. The foot is dislocated posterolaterally; frequently the proximal surface of the avulsed medial malleolus and the articular surface of the tibia appear in the wound. In these injuries the wound is so close to the surface of the fracture and to the joint that rigid internal fixation is necessary to protect the overlying soft tissues from pressure and recurrent tension. Since the open wound lies directly over the medial malleolus, internal fixation of the medial malleolar side can usually be accomplished with one or two screws; little if any additional dissection is necessary after the wound has been debrided and irrigated and the dislocation has been reduced.

It is unlikely that the minimal surgery required to place medial malleolar screws will increase the risk of infection, and in fact, the opposite may be true since the stability achieved allows optimal treatment of the soft tissues. Again, by way of emphasis, the wounds should be closed by delayed primary closure (Fig 34–15).

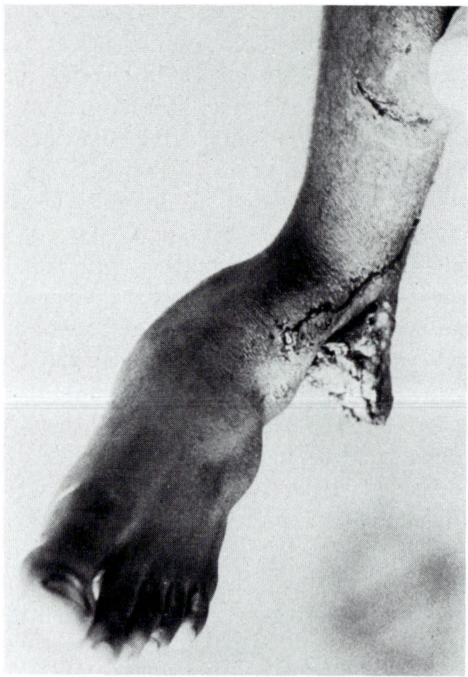

FIG 34–15.
Typical open fracture of the ankle.

Repair of Ligament Ruptures.—Ligamentous injuries associated with fractures are the subject of controversy in the literature and are discussed in more detail in Chapters 27 and 29.

The primary indication for repair is ligament interposition in the joint space, where exploration is necessary to achieve anatomic reduction.[9] Ruptured lateral collateral ligaments accompanying a fracture are almost always repaired. The ligaments of the tibiofibular syndesmosis usually require stabilization. Direct repair is rarely possible. Stabilization of the lateral malleolus is often sufficient; if not, a syndesmosis screw is used. Deltoid ligament ruptures accompanying lateral fractures do not have to be repaired if joint congruity is achieved. If early mobilization, free of plaster, is planned, repair may be necessary to achieve adequate stability.

Often repair of the ligaments will be done incidental to exploration of the ankle joint on the nonfractured side to effect debridement and to look for osteochondral fractures of the talus.

Surgical Technique

Early surgery is usually best for optimal results. It is best carried out on the day of injury, before edema occurs. Open reduction within 7 days of injury is little different from that achieved on the day of injury. Between 7 and 14 days, the hematoma organizes, and extensive debriding of the fracture fragments is necessary to achieve reduction; anatomic reduction can usually be achieved, however. Between 14 and 21 days, callus formation, soft-tissue scarring, resorption, and osteoporosis of the fractured bone ends create technical problems that compromise reduction. After 21 days, anatomic reduction is frequently impossible to achieve, and closed treatment may be indicated.

Bivalving of the cast and surgical preparation of the skin the evening before surgery are unwise, for an accidental nick of the skin may necessitate postponement of surgery.

Unless contraindicated, a tourniquet should be employed. Unexpected comminution is often encountered, so the surgeon should have a full armamentarium of bone instruments and fixation devices available. In addition to screws, Kirschner wires, small fragment screws, small plates, malleable wire, Steinmann pins, Rush rods, or Knowles pins may be useful. One should be prepared to take an iliac bone graft in vertical compression fractures.

Medial Malleolus

The skin incision should be vertical, parallel with the long axis of the tibia, and directly over the malleolus. Dissection is carried sharply to bone, and any undermining necessary should take place just above the periosteum. The incision must be long enough to offer good exposure without excessive retraction. It has the advantages of being extensile, being optimally located for the insertion of a screw, and avoiding significant undermining or flaps. I have never had a patient complain of a tender scar in this location. The J-shaped incision posterior or anterior and distal to the malleolus has the disadvantage of not being easily extended distally, therefore frequently compromising the exposure needed for screw insertion and requiring undermining (which leads to an increased incidence of marginal wound slough).

1. Elevate the periosteum from the edges of the fracture line for a distance of 2 to 3 mm with a no. 15 scalpel blade used edge on. The full anterior and posterior extents of the fracture must be seen to ensure accurate reduction.
2. Lightly curette and irrigate the fracture surfaces to remove all organized hematoma.
3. Explore the joint through the fracture site to detect occult chondral and osteochondral fractures of the talus and to debride and irrigate the joint as needed.
4. Anatomically reduce the fracture by grasping the malleolus transversely in a towel clip and guiding it into place with a periosteal elevator in the other hand. The

reduction should be securely maintained by mechanical means while the internal fixation is inserted. The best method I have found is to use two A-O towel clip–type bone clamps or two towel clips across the fracture at its anterior and posterior borders. The towel clips are held with 4 × 8s tied through their handles (Fig 34–16). A Bishop clamp can also be used, but I find them heavy, and they often interfere with hardware placement. The towel clip method does not interfere with hardware placement, and the clamps prevent slippage of the fracture.

5. The best fixation is obtained with two, 4-mm cancellous bone screws. A pointed drill guide is used to place two, 2-mm Kirschner wires from the tip of the malleolus at right angles to the plane of the fracture and as vertically as possible (Fig 34–17,*A*). Each Kirschner wire is then removed and replaced with a 4-mm cancellous bone screw (Fig 34–17,*B*) or cannulated screws can be used.

Note that in high vertical fractures caused by adduction injuries, placing the screws at right angles to the fracture line will result in the screws being parallel to the plafond of the ankle mortice.

Alternative fixation can be obtained with a 4.5-mm malleolar screw. The screw should enter the distal tip of the malleolus; otherwise, comminution may occur, and the screw head will be too prominent. The malleolar screws provided in the A-O equipment are ideal, although lag technique can be used with a standard bone screw (Fig 34–18). Small or comminuted fragments not amenable to screw fixation are best fixed with two or more Kirschner wires (Fig 34–19). I have had no experience with the Zuelzer hook plate.[42] Vertical adduction–type fractures tend to slip with a single screw. Fixation with two Kirschner wires as illustrated in Figure 34–19 before insertion of the screw will prevent displacement.

Very small fragments may be excised, and a repair of the deltoid ligament to a drill hole in the malleolus can be affected.

Lateral Malleolus

The same principles of incision and exposure described for the medial malleolus are applicable to the lateral malleolus. If syndesmosis repair is anticipated, the incision should be somewhat anterior, and if fixation of the posterior malleolus through the same incision is planned, the incision should be placed somewhat posterior.

The configuration of the fracture determines the type of fixation to be employed. Ideal fixation provides interfragmentary compression and rotational control. Oblique and spiral fractures whose lengths are greater than 1½ times the diameter of the bone at the level of the fracture are best fixed with interfragmentary lag screws.

Neutralization of the forces across the fracture should always be accomplished. A one-third tubular plate applied to the lateral border of the fibula is suffi-

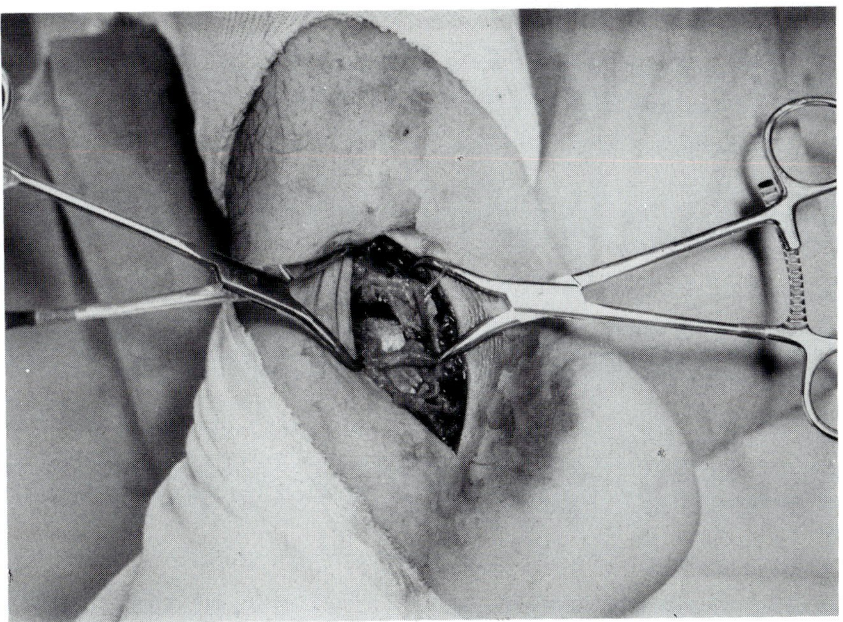

FIG 34–16.
Use of A-O bone forceps to stabilize the fracture site.

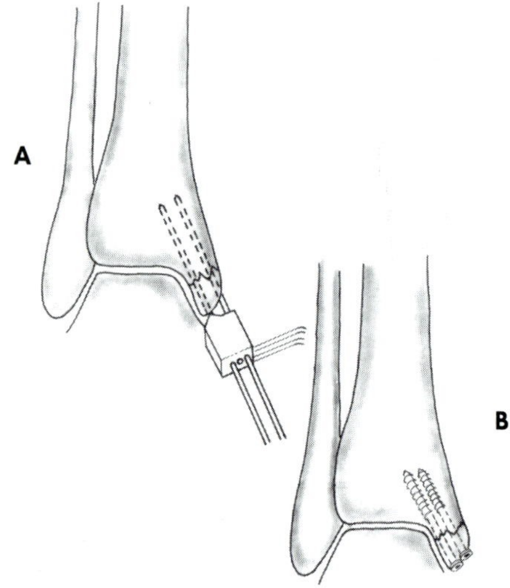

FIG 34–17.
A, double fixation with two, 2-mm Kirschner wires. These can be placed in the vertical or horizontal plane, depending on the configuration of the fracture. Pointed drill guides ensure parallelism of the wires. **B,** replacement of the Kirschner wires with two, 4-mm cancellous screws.

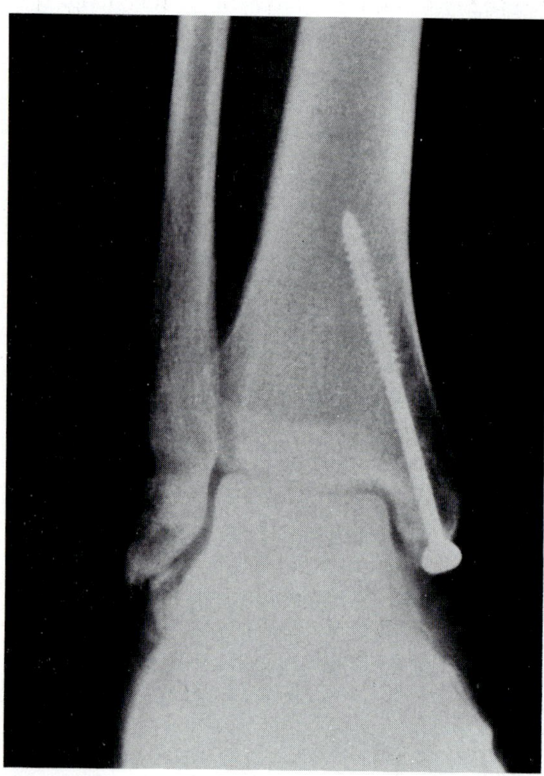

FIG 34–18.
A-O malleolar screw fixing a fracture of the medial malleolus by employing the principle of lag fixation.

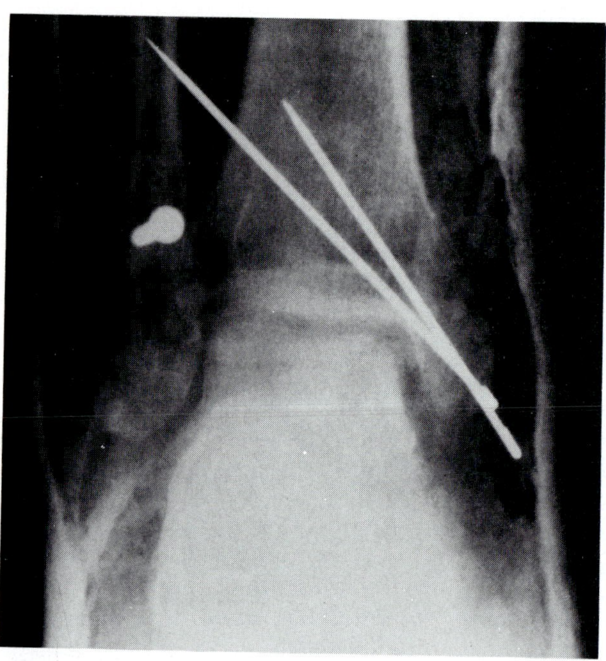

FIG 34–19.
Kirschner wire fixation of a comminuted medial malleolar fracture. Note that one wire was left excessively long.

cient. Ideally, five cortices of fixation above and below the fracture should be obtained. If a lateral plate is used and the fracture is at the syndesmosis, only unicortical screws will be possible in the distal fragment, and the plate will serve as a buttress.

This configuration of an anteroposterior interfragmentary screw and lateral plate provides biplanar fixation. The plate can be placed anteriorly or posteriorly, and the interfragmentary lag screw can then be placed through the plate. This is technically more difficult, however. Often the interfragmentary lag screw must be placed through a separate anterior stab wound.

For the interfragmentary screw, I prefer to use a 3.5-mm cortical screw with overdrilling of the near cortex. If comminution is a problem, then a 4.0-mm cancellous screw can be used. The best plate is a one-third tubular which is bent to fit the malleolus and fixed with 3.5- or 4.0-mm screws. Figure 34–20 shows a suggested configuration of fixation for various fractures of the lateral malleolus and fibula. Figure 34–21 is a radiograph of similar fixation for a fracture of the shaft of the fibula. The empty screw holes were not filled because of comminution.

I no longer use fixation with Rush rods or Steinmann pins because they offer poor rotational control and in oblique fractures shortening may occur.

The A-O tension-band wire technique is useful for

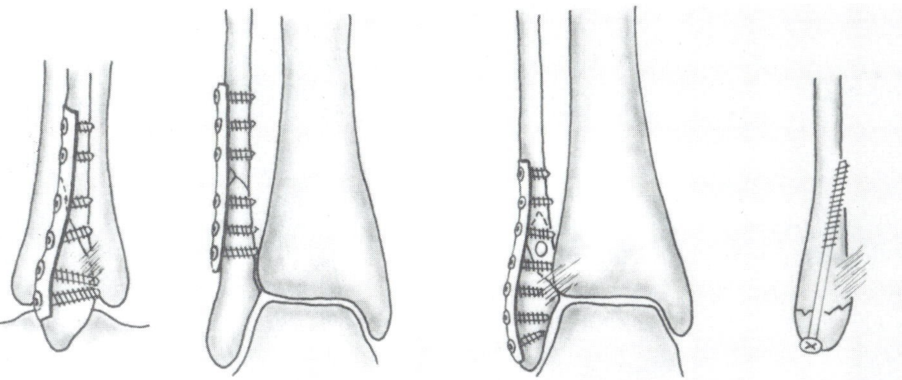

FIG 34–20.
A, lateral views showing a posterior plate applied to a fracture just above the syndesmosis. Note the interfragmentary lag screw through the plate. **B,** lateral plate for a fracture of the fibular shaft. **C,** lateral plate used a buttress plus an anteroposterior lag screw for fixation of an oblique fracture at the syndesmosis. **D,** single malleolar screw used to fix a transverse avulsion–type fracture below the syndesmosis.

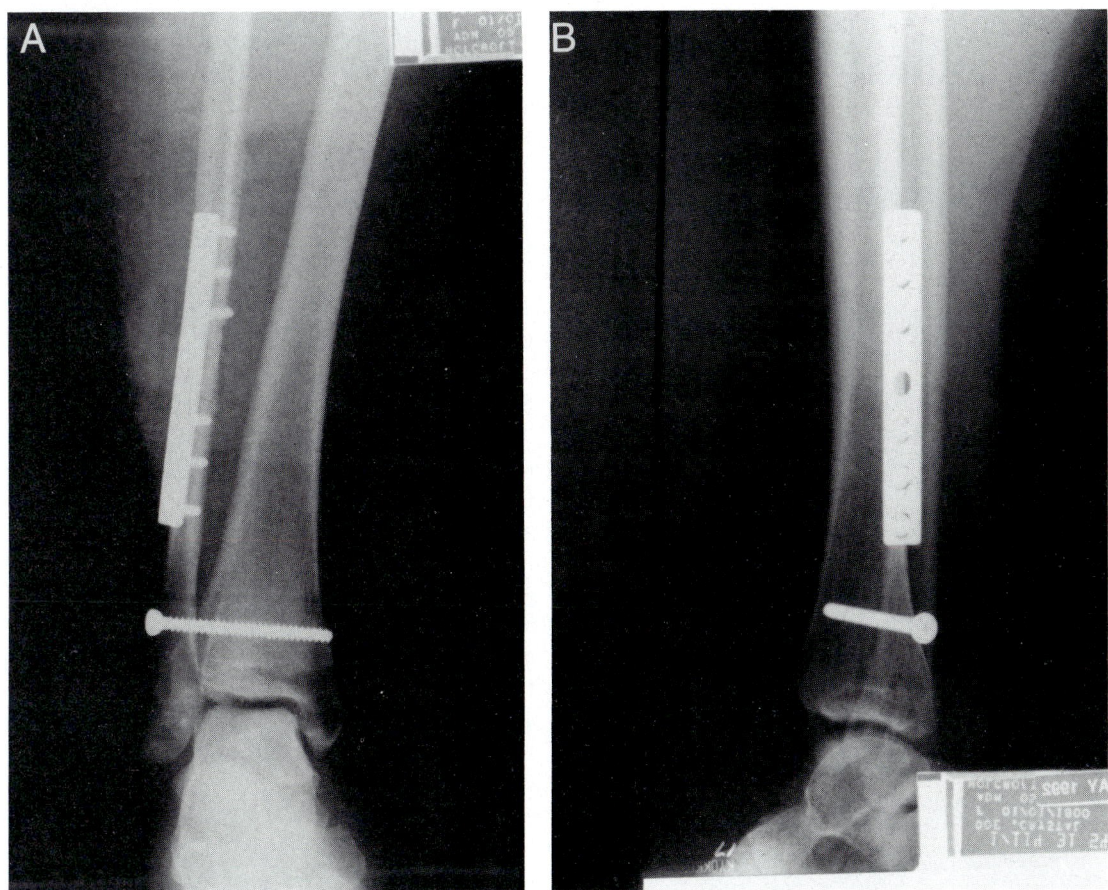

FIG 34–21.
Plate fixation of fracture of the fibula. Syndesmosis is stabilized with a transverse screw.

transverse fractures at or below the syndesmosis which have small fragments or are comminuted (Fig 34–22).

Posterior Malleolus

Injuries to the posterior malleolus are usually posterolateral and are best fixed through a posterolateral approach with the patient prone. The lateral and medial malleoli can easily be repaired with the patient prone. Preoperative radiographs should be carefully assessed. Occasionally a posterior malleolar fracture is an extension of a medial malleolar fracture and should be approached medially.

Because of limited exposure, posterior malleolar fractures can be difficult to internally fix. Since the intra-articular component of the fracture cannot be seen when reduced, the entire extra-articular portion of the fracture should be visualized to ensure the accuracy of reduction. Fixation with two Kirschner wires while the malleolus is held in place ensures that reduction will not be lost during screw placement. To guarantee optimal closure of the intra-articular component, the screw should be at right angles to the fracture and just above the tibial plafond.

If the screw cannot be easily placed from posterior to anterior, it can be placed from anterior to posterior through a small stab wound (Fig 34–23). Since preliminary K-wire fixation has been performed, cannulated screws are quite useful and are now available in both small and large fragment sizes.

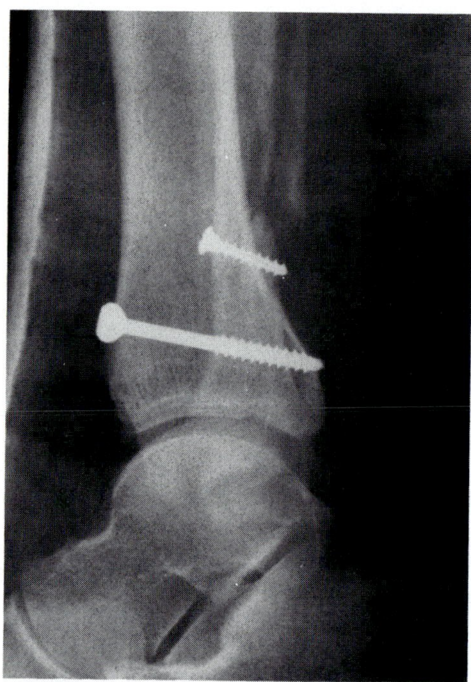

FIG 34–23.
Fracture of posterior malleolus fixed with interfragmentary malleolar screw placed through anterior stab wound. Before comminution there is a small defect in articular surface of tibial plafond.

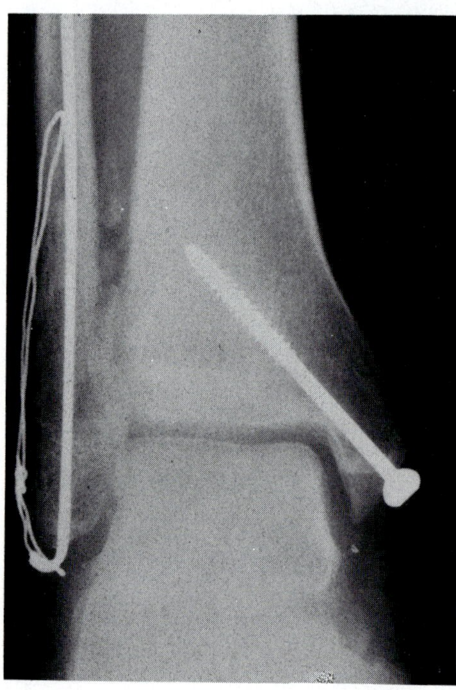

FIG 34–22.
Intramedullary Kirschner wires and tension-band figure-of-8 wire used to fix a fracture of the lateral malleolus.

Syndesmosis Separations

Syndesmosis separations that are unstable should be stabilized. Occasionally stabilization of an associated fibular fracture provides adequate stability, and fixation across the syndesmosis can be avoided. With fibular fractures above a syndesmosis separation, some surgeons elect to treat only the syndesmosis separation. This is acceptable, but great care must be exercised to avoid residual external rotational deformity of the distal fragment and avoid overtightening the syndesmosis screw, which can produce a valgus malposition of the lateral malleolus. Proximal migration of the lateral malleolus should be avoided by making certain that shortening at the fracture site has not occurred. It is usually best to stabilize the fibula first and then the syndesmosis. I always plate the fibula.

When transfixing the syndesmosis, the surgeon should take care to ensure that the fibula is reduced posteriorly into the tibial sulcus. Fixation is obtained with a screw (Fig 34–24). Fully threaded, 4.5-mm cortical screws are best because they avoid overreduction of the syndesmosis. Insert the screw through all four cortices.

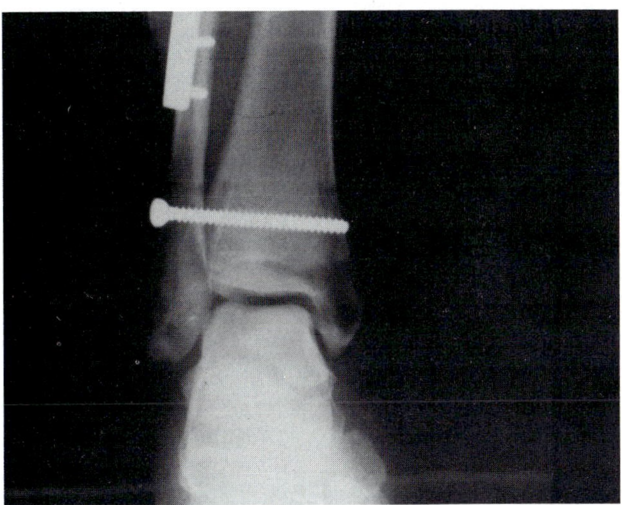

FIG 34–24.
Syndesmosis rupture stabilized with a fully threaded screw engaging four cortices.

The syndesmosis must be properly reduced when the screws are inserted, however. A malleolar screw can also be used, but with the lag effect possible, one must avoid overtightening the syndesmosis. The screw is best inserted at right angles to the distal tibiofibular joint so as to pass from the posterolateral border of the fibula anteromedially into the tibia.

Screws across the syndesmosis will generally not loosen or break if dorsiflexion of the ankle beyond neutral is not allowed. On this basis, these patients can be allowed to begin weight bearing in a short-leg cast or in a cam walker by 6 weeks after injury. Because of the dynamic function of the fibula,[30, 38] a small number of patients do require significant motion through the syndesmosis to achieve dorsiflexion of the ankle. In these cases, persistent motion of the ankle with the syndesmosis screw in place will result in a fracture of the screw or loosening of the screw in bone. Because it is impossible to guess which patient needs this motion, for the most part, routine removal of the syndesmosis screw by 8 to 12 weeks after injury is generally indicated.

Tibial Pilon (Plafond) Fractures

A comminuted fracture of the ankle is usually caused by vertical loading that produces compression of the cancellous bone above the tibial plafond. An unstable fracture of the distal shafts of the tibia and fibula may be associated (see Fig 34–7). Because the degree of comminution and the poor condition of the soft tissues make internal fixation impossible, closed treatment may be indicated. The surgeon must weigh the goals of surgery against such risks as increased soft-tissue trauma from multiple incisions and the ill effects of prolonged surgery. Some advocate restoration of the joint surfaces and treatment of the remainder of the fracture with a cast. This is the worst of all possible choices, however, inasmuch as one has taken the risk of surgery, not achieved sufficient stability for early motion, and subjected an intra-articular fracture to surgery and prolonged immobilization.

In this fracture the best results will be achieved with restoration of the normal anatomy, stabilization, and early motion to restore joint physiology.

Müller et al.[33] advocate total reconstruction of comminuted fractures with multiple fixation devices, including large buttress plates, to stabilize the shaft component and permit early mobilization in the absence of external fixation. The procedures are difficult and should be undertaken only by surgeons who are intimately familiar with the method and do more than an occasional fracture of this type. To avoid the complications of wound sloughing and infection, the surgeon's soft-tissue technique must be atraumatic and meticulous.

The preferable skin incisions are depicted in Figure 34–25. The anterior incision exploits the interval between the anterior tibial tendon and extensor hallucis longus. Flaps are developed at the level of the periosteum. The periosteum must be left attached to the anterior fragment, which can easily be opened like a book to reveal the central comminution of posterior fragments. Avoid entering the sheath of the anterior tibial tendon. If a wound complication develops and the wound must be left open, exposure of this tendon will result in desiccation and death of the tendon. If very extensive exposure is required, carry the incision distally to the talonavicular joint and lift medial and lateral flaps at the level of bone. This will give very adequate exposure for even the most difficult pilon fracture. Although not as versatile as the direct anterior approach, the transfibular approach can be used when the fibula is fractured and the syndesmosis ruptured.[39] A bone graft is usually required, and most commonly I remove it through a small window in the proximal portion of the tibia. Iliac crest bone can also be used.

The steps in reconstructing a comminuted pilon fracture of the tibia with an associated fracture of the fibula are as follows.

1. The fibula is brought out to length and internally fixed with a plate and screws. This restores normal length to the tibia fracture and reveals the extent of communication and crush of cancellous bone (Fig 34–26,*B*).
2. The tibia fracture is exposed and reduced. Typi-

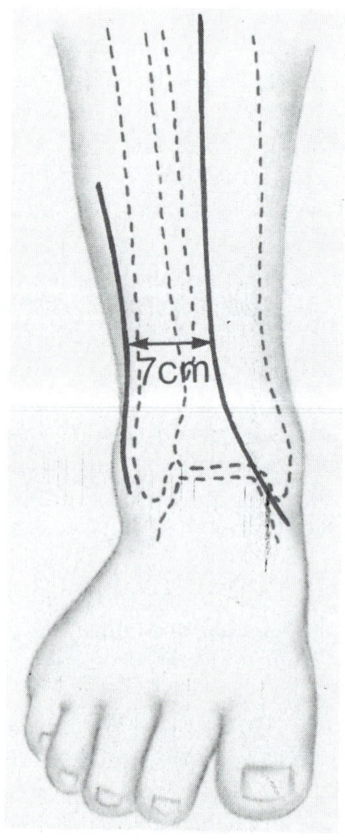

FIG 34–25.
Preferred incisions for operating on comminuted fractures of the distal ends of the tibia and fibula. A lateral incision is over the midlateral border of the fibula. Avoid injury to the superficial peroneal nerve. The tibia is approached anteriorly. The incision swings medially as one proceeds distally. Seven centimeters should separate the two incisions.

cally the plafond is in four pieces with some central comminution, as depicted in Figure 34–26,*A*. Because of interlocking, often all four major fragments must be reduced and temporarily fixed with Kirschner wires or screws (Fig 34–26,*C*). The goal is to reassemble the fracture into a main distal and proximal fragment, which can then be brought together. The talus can be used as a template against which the tibia is reconstructed. Before the plate and screws are applied, defects are filled with bone graft.

3. The Kirschner wires are then replaced with screws and a buttress plate. In Figure 34–26,*D*, the use of an anterior spoon plate is depicted. A T-plate or medial cloverleaf plate can also be used, depending on the configuration of the fracture. An example of the complex reconstruction often required is shown in Figure 34–27.

4. The wounds are then closed. Tension must be avoided. If necessary, a deep layer can be closed, the skin left open, and a delayed closure carried out.

Postoperative Care

In the immediate postoperative period the most frequent problem is swelling, which can be controlled by bed rest and elevation. I do not use casts postoperatively because the fractures are stable after fixation. In the vast majority of cases, a short-leg Robert Jones dressing with splints can be used. If a cast is used, it should be routinely univalved anteriorly and spread.

Fractures that are unstable after fixation usually require a long-leg non–weight-bearing cast for 6 weeks followed by 2 weeks in a short-leg walking cast. Signif-

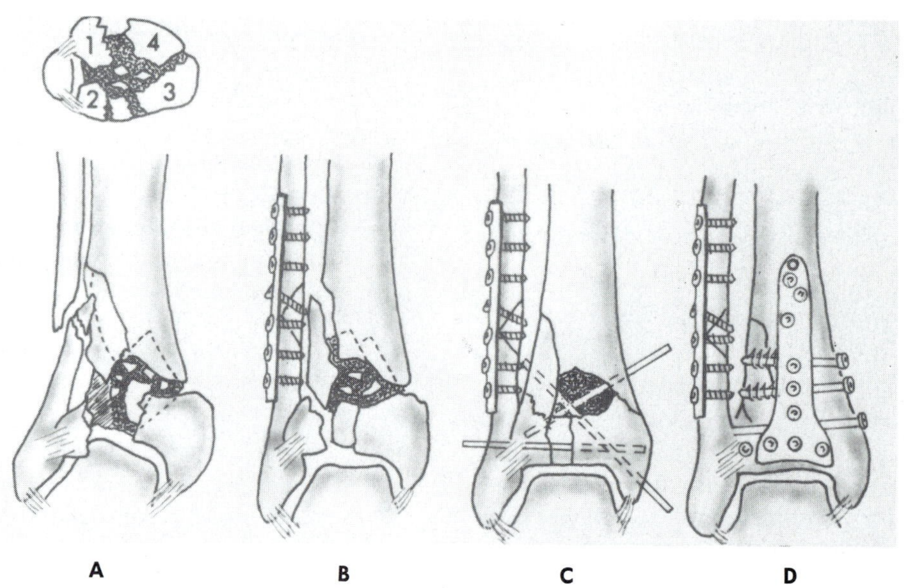

FIG 34–26.
Steps in the reconstruction of a typical pilon fracture.

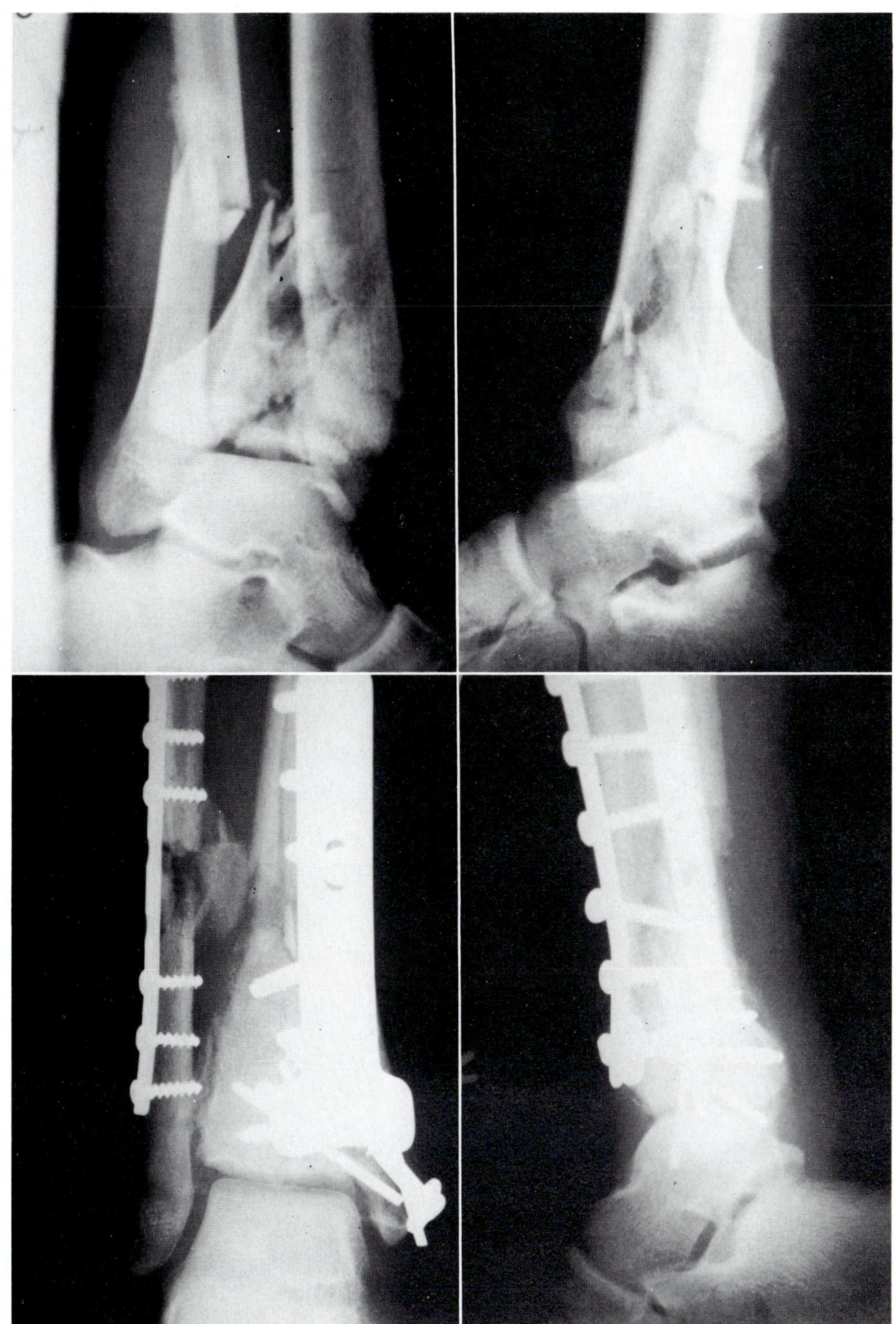

FIG 34–27.
Anteroposterior and lateral radiographs of fixation of a comminuted pilon fracture.

icant accompanying diaphyseal fractures may require prolonged non-weight bearing.

Stable fractures can be treated according to the need for early joint mobilization and the surgeon's confidence in the repair.

In their series of patients in whom a stable situation was produced at the time of internal fixation, Burwell and Charnley[5] described a minor modification of the usual postoperative care for internal fixation of ankle fractures. In the early postoperative period, the injured limb was removed from the protective plaster cast for active non–weight-bearing exercise, and a long-leg cast was replaced by a short-leg plaster cast. The authors reported an early recovery of maximum range of motion in patients thus treated.

In most cases I keep the Robert Jones dressing in place for 1 week. I then apply a brace or bivalved short-leg cast and begin supervised dorsiflexion and plantar flexion exercises. To avoid an equinus contracture, a splint must be in place when the patient is not exercising. This can be removed when the patient can actively dorsiflex within 5 degrees of the normal side. Unprotected weight bearing is delayed until 8 weeks, and in pilon fractures, until 12 weeks or longer if required for union.

EPIPHYSEAL INJURIES OF THE ANKLE IN CHILDREN

Ankle fractures are less common in children than adults. The ligaments are stronger than the physeal plates, so ligament tears are uncommon, and epiphyseal injuries are more common. The physeal plates are zones of weakness that produce fracture patterns different from those seen in adults. Growth disturbances from fractures about the ankle are common, and there is a tendency to underestimate the severity of the injury.

Diagnosis requires a high degree of suspicion. Radiographs are essential, and comparison views are very helpful. Stress radiography may be necessary to reveal an occult epiphyseal slip.

Fibula

A Salter-Harris (S-H) type I slip of the lateral malleolus is the most common injury. Reduction is rarely necessary because most of these are avulsion injuries that are minimally displaced. Treatment with a short-leg walking cast for 3 to 4 weeks suffices.

Tibia

Eversion–external rotation injuries tend to produce S-H type II displaced fractures of the tibial epiphysis with a greenstick fracture of the fibula above the syndesmosis. The ankle mortise is undisturbed. Closed reduction and cast immobilization for 3 to 6 weeks are adequate treatment. Because the perichondral ring is disrupted, weight bearing is not advisable. Damage to the lateral side of the tibial epiphysis can occur with these injuries. Follow-up yearly radiographs until maturity are advisable. Type I injuries of this epiphysis can occur but are rare. Treatment is as just outlined.

Fractures of the medial malleolus are usually S-H type III or IV injuries. Growth disturbance caused by these injuries is common. Open reduction and Kirschner wire fixation parallel to the physeal line are usually advisable.

TILLAUX FRACTURE

In early adolescence, the medial portion of the tibial epiphysis begins to close. An external rotation force may avulse the anterior lateral portion of the epiphysis and produce an S-H type III injury. The ankle is usually rotationally unstable. Although these can often be treated with closed reduction and a long-leg cast, open reduction and Kirschner wire fixation is indicated if anatomic position cannot be achieved by closed reduction.

TRIPLANE FRACTURE

Triplane fracture is a complex fracture of the distal tibial epiphysis that resembles an S-H type IV injury in the coronal plane medially, an S-H type II injury in the coronal plane laterally, and an S-H type III injury in the sagittal plane laterally (Fig 34–28). Diagnosis is often difficult. Tomograms and CT scans are often helpful. Anatomic reduction is essential. This can usually

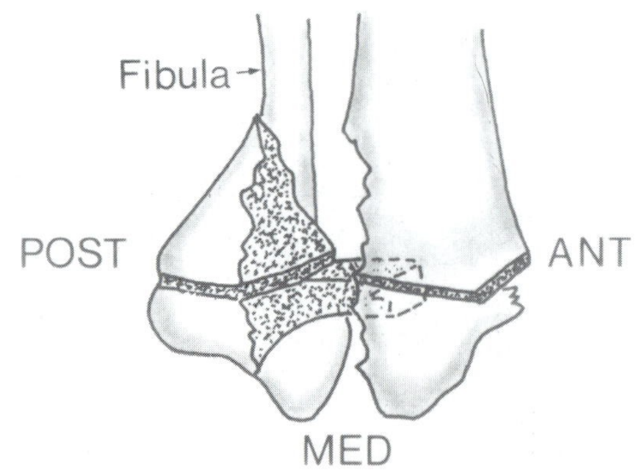

FIG 34–28.
Triplane fracture.

be achieved in a closed fashion, but open reduction may be required.

COMPARTMENT SYNDROME

Compartment syndrome of the leg or foot occurs where increased pressure within the fascial compartments compromises the circulation and function of the nerves and muscles in the compartment(s). The most common causes in the foot and leg are increased compartment content (from bleeding and/or edema) and externally applied pressure (from a tight cast). Decreased compartment volume (from closure of the fascia too tightly or from traction) can also be causal. Foot surgeons must be aware of this problem because the leg is the most common site of compartment syndrome.

The symptoms and signs of compartment syndrome are as follows:

1. Pain out of proportion to the clinical situation
2. Pain with passive stretch of the muscles in the involved compartment
3. Tenseness of the compartment
4. Hypesthesia and decreased sensation

Adjunctive diagnostic techniques are tissue pressure measurements and nerve function tests. Depending on the patient and the measuring technique used, normal is usually less than 10 mm Hg. Over 30 mm Hg is definitely abnormal (fasciotomy may be indicated), and fasciotomy is nearly always indicated if the pressure is over 50 mm Hg.

In the leg, all four compartments usually require decompression. This can be accomplished by the single-incision parafibular technique described by Matsen.[26]

In the foot, decompression of all compartments can be achieved through a single incision on the non–weight-bearing surface of the medial arch.

For further discussion of the compartment syndromes see Chapters 32 and 35.

REFERENCES

1. Ashhurst APC, Bromer RS: Classification and mechanism of fracture of the leg bones involving the ankle. Based on a study of three hundred cases from the Episcopal Hospital, *Arch Surg* 4:51, 1922.
2. Aufranc OE: Trimalleolar tracture dislocation, *JAMA*. 174:2221, 1960.
3. Bonnin JG: *Injuries to the ankle*, Darien, Conn, 1970, Hafner.
4. Bosworth DM: Fracture-dislocation of the ankle with fixed displacement of the fibula behind the tibia, *J Bone Joint Surg* 29:130, 1947.
5. Burwell HN, Charnley AD: The treatment of displaced fractures at the ankle by rigid internal fixation and early joint movement, *J Bone Joint Surg [Br]* 47:634, 1965.
6. Chapman MW, Mahoney M: The place of immediate internal fixation in the management of open fracture, *Abbott Soc Bull* 8:85, 1976.
7. Charnley J: *The closed treatment of common fractures*, Baltimore, 1963, Williams & Wilkins.
8. Childress HM: Vertical transarticular-pin fixation for unstable ankle fractures, *J Bone Joint Surg [Am]* 47:1323, 1965.
9. Coonrad RW, Bugg EI: Trapping of the posterior tibial tendon and interposition of soft tissue in severe fractures about the ankle joint, *J Bone Joint Surg [Am]* 36:744, 1954.
10. DeSouza LJ, Gustilo RB, Meyer TJ: Results of operative treatment of displaced external rotation-abduction fractures of the ankle, *J Bone Joint Surg [Am]* 67:1066–1074, 1985.
11. Dieterlé J: The use of Kirschner wire in maintaining reduction of fracture-dislocations of the ankle joint: a report of two cases, *J Bone Joint Surg* 17:990, 1935.
12. Dupuytren G: Of fractures of the lower extremity and luxations of the foot, *Med Classics* 4:151–172, 1939.
13. Fleming JL, Smith HO: Fracture-dislocation of the ankle with the fibula fixed behind the tibia, *J Bone Joint Surg [Am]* 36:556, 1954.
14. Glick BW: The ankle fracture with inferior tibiofibular joint disruption, *Surg Gynecol Obstet* 118:549, 1964.
15. Gustilo RB, Anderson JT: Prevention of infection in the treatment of one thousand and twenty-five open fractures of long bones, *J Bone Joint Surg [Am]* 58:453, 1976.
16. Harper MC, Hardin G: Posterior malleolar fractures of the ankle associated with external rotation-abduction injuries, *J Bone Joint Surg [Am]* 70:1348–1356, 1988.
17. Jergesen F: Open reduction of fractures and dislocations of the ankle, *Am J Surg* 98:136, 1959.
18. Kleiger B: The mechanism of ankle injuries, *J Bone Joint Surg [Am]* 38:59, 1956.
19. Lauge-Hansen N: Fractures of the ankle: analytic historic survey as the basis of new experimental, roentgenologic and clinical investigations, *Arch Surg* 56:259, 1948.
20. Lauge-Hansen N: Fractures of the ankle. II. Combined experimental-surgical and experimental-roentgenologic investigations, *Arch Surg* 60:957, 1950.
21. Lauge-Hansen N: Fractures of the ankle. III. Genetic roentgenologic diagnosis of fracture of the ankle, *Am J Roentgenol* 71:456, 1954.
22. Lauge-Hansen N: Fractures of the ankle. IV. Clinical use of genetic roentgen diagnosis and genetic reduction, *Arch Surg* 64:488, 1952.
23. Lucas-Championnère J: *Précis du traitement des fractures par le massage et la mobilisation*, Paris, 1910, G Steinheil.
24. Macko VW, Matthews LS, Zwirkoski P, et al: The joint-contact area of the ankle. The contribution of the posterior malleolus, *J Bone Joint Surg [Am]* 73:347–351, 1991.
25. Maisonneuve JG: Recherches sur la fracture du perone, *Arch Gen Med.* 7:165, 433, 1840.
26. Matsen FA, III: *Compartmental syndromes*, New York, 1980, Grune & Stratton.
27. Mayer V, Pohlidal S: Ankle mortise injuries, *Surg Gynecol Obstet* 96:99, 1953.

28. McDade WC: Treatment of ankle fractures, *Instr Course Lect* 24:251, 1975.
29. McDaniel WJ, Wilson FC: Trimalleolar fractures of the ankle. An end result study, *Clin Orthop* 122:37, 1977.
30. McMaster JH, Scranton PE: Tibiofibular synostosis: a cause of ankle disability, *Clin Orthop* 111:172, 1975.
31. Meyers MH: Fracture about the ankle joint with fixed displacement of the proximal fragment of the fibula behind the tibia, *J Bone Joint Surg [Am]* 39:441, 1957.
32. Mitchell N, Shepard N: Healing of articular cartilage in intra-articular fractures in rabbits, *J Bone Joint Surg [Am]* 62:628–634, 1980.
33. Müller ME, Allgower M, Willenegger H: *Manual external fixation*, New York, 1979, Springer-Verlag.
34. Portis RB, Mendelsohn HA: Conservative management of fractures of the ankle involving the medial malleolus, *JAMA* 151:102, 1953.
35. Pott P: *Some few general remarks on fractures and dislocations*, London, 1768, Hawes, Clarke, Collins.
36. Ramsey PL, Hamilton W: Changes in tibiotalar area of contact caused by lateral talar shift, *J Bone Joint Surg [Am]* 58:356–357, 1976.
37. Salter RB, Semmonds DF, Malcolm BW, et al: The biological effect of continuous passive motion on the healing of full-thickness defects in articular cartilage, *J Bone Joint Surg [Am]* 62:1232–1251, 1980.
38. Scranton PE, McMaster JH, Kelly E: Dynamic fibular function, a new concept, *Clin Orthop* 118:76, 1976.
39. Wiggins HE: Pronation-dorsiflexion fractures with involvement of distal tibial metaphysis—case studies, *Instr Course Lect* 24:309, 1975.
40. Wiss DA, Gilbert P, Merritt PO, et al: Immediate internal fixation of open ankle fractures, *J Orthop Trauma* 2:265–271, 1989.
41. Yablon IG, Heller FG, Shouse L: The key role of the lateral malleolus in displaced fractures of the ankle, *J Bone Joint Surg [Am]* 59:169, 1977.
42. Zuelzer WA: Use of hookplate for fixation of ununited medial tibial malleolus, *JAMA* 167:828, 1958.

ADDITIONAL READINGS

Akeson WH: An experimental study of joint stiffness, *J Bone Joint Surg [Am]* 43:1022, 1961.

Clark DD, and Weckesser EC: The influence of triamcinolone acetonide on joint stiffness in the rat, *J Bone Joint Surg [Am]* 53:1409, 1971.

Collins DH, McElligott TF: Sulphate ($^{35}SO_4$) uptake by chondrocytes in relation to histological changes in osteoarthritic human articular cartilage, *Ann Rheum Dis* 19:318, 1960.

Cooperman DR, Seigel PG, Laros GS: Tibial fractures involving the ankle in children, *J Bone Joint Surg [Am]* 60:140–146, 1978.

Davenport HK, Ranson SW: Contraction resulting from tenotomy, *Arch Surg* 21:995, 1930.

Dziewiatkowski DD, Benesch RE, Benesch R: On the possible utilization of sulfate sulfur by the suckling rat for the synthesis of chondroitin sulfate as indicated by the use of radioactive sulfur, *J Biol Chem* 178:931, 1949.

Ely LW, Mensor MC: Studies on the immobilization of the normal joints, *Surg Gynecol Obstet* 57:212, 1933.

Evans EB, Eggers GWN, Butler JK, et al: Experimental immobilization and remobilization of rat knee joints, *J Bone Joint Surg [Am]* 42:737, 1960.

Frankshteyn SI: Experimental studies on mechanism of development of contractures due to immobilization in casts, *Khirurgiia* 8:44, 1944.

Frugone JE, Thomsen P, Luco JV: Changes in weight of muscles of arthritic and immobilized arthritic joints, *Proc Soc Exp Biol Med* 61:31, 1946.

Gasser HS: Contractures of skeletal muscle, *Physiol Rev* 10:35, 1930.

Hall MC: Cartilage changes after experimental immobilization of the knee joint of the young rat, *J Bone Joint Surg [Am]* 45:36, 1963.

Harrison MHM, Schajowicz F, Trueta J: Osteoarthritis of the hip: a study of the nature and evolution of the disease, *J Bone Joint Surg [Br]* 35:598, 1953.

Mast JW, Spiegel PG, Pappas JN: Fractures of the tibial plateau, *Clin Orthop* 230:68–82, 1988.

McLean FC, Urist MR: *Bone: an introduction to the physiology of skeletal tissue*, Chicago, 1955, University of Chicago Press.

Menzel A: Ueber die Erkrankung der Gelenke bei dauernder Ruhe derselben: eine experimentelle Studie, *Arch Klin Chir* 12:990, 1871.

Müller W: Experimentelle Untersuchungenüber die Wirkung langdauernder Immobilisierung auf die Gelenke, *Z Orthop Chir* 44:478, 1924.

Peacock EE Jr: Some biochemical and biophysical aspects of joint stiffness: role of collagen synthesis as opposed to altered molecular bonding, *Ann Surg* 164:1, 1966.

Ranson SW, Sams CF: A study of muscle in contracture: the permanent shortening of muscles caused by tenotomy and tetanus toxin, *J Neurol Psychopathol* 8:304, 1923.

Salter RB, Field P: The effects of continuous compression on living articular cartilage: an experimental investigation, *J Bone Joint Surg [Am]* 42:31, 1960.

Salter RB, Harris WR: Injuries involving the epiphyseal plate, *J Bone Joint Surg [Am]* 45:587, 1963.

Scaglietti O, Casuccio C: Studio sperimentale degli effetti della immobilizzazione su articolazioni normali, *Chir Organi Mov* 20:469, 1936.

Sokoloff L, Jay GE Jr: Natural history of degenerative joint disease in the small laboratory animals. 4. Degenerative joint disease in the laboratory rat, *Arch Pathol* 62:140, 1956.

Solandt DY, Magladery JW: A comparison of effects of upper and lower motor neuron lesions on skeletal muscle, *J Neurophysiol* 5:373, 1942.

Thaxter TH, Mann RA, Anderson CE: Degeneration of immobilized knee joints in rats: Histological and autoradiographic study, *J Bone Joint Surg [Am]* 47:567, 1965.

Trias A: Effect of persistent pressure on the articular cartilage, *J Bone Joint Surg [Br]* 43:376, 1961.

Thomsen P, Luco JV: Changes of weight and neuromuscular transmission in muscles of immobilized joints, *J. Neurophysiol* 7:245, 1944.

Tschmarke G: Experimentelle Untersuchungenüber die Rolle des Muskeltonus in der Gelenkchirurgie. 3. Mitteilung: Fixationskontrakturen und die Beeinflussung ihrer Entwicklung, *Arch Klin Chir* 164:785, 1931.

CHAPTER

35

Fractures and Dislocations of the Foot*†

Jesse C. DeLee, M.D.

Clinical diagnosis
Radiographic diagnosis
Treatment
Compartment syndromes of the foot
Anatomy
Clinical presentation
Surgical decompression
Author's preferred method of treatment
Fractures of the calcaneus
Anatomy
Superior surface
Inferior surface
Lateral surface
Medial surface
Posterior surface
Anterior surface
The tuberosity joint angle
Crucial angle of Gissane
Classification
Mechanism of injury
Radiographic diagnosis
Standard radiographic views
Radiographic evaluation of the subtalar joint
Conventional tomography and computerized axial tomography

†The author would like to thank Kerry Donegan, M.D., for his assistance in preparing this chapter.

Treatment
Extra-articular fractures
Fractures of the anterior process of the calcaneus
Tuberosity fracture: beak and avulsion fractures
Fractures of the medial or lateral process of the calcaneus
Fractures of the body of the calcaneus not involving the subtalar joint
Intra-articular fractures
Fractures of the sustentaculum tali
Tongue, joint depression, and comminuted fractures of the os calcis
Stress fractures of the calcaneus
Dislocation of the calcaneus
Fracture and fracture-dislocations of the talus
Vascular anatomy
Extraosseous arterial supply
Intraosseous arterial supply
Intraosseous anastomoses
Skeletal anatomy
The head
The neck
The body
Open fractures of the talus
Author's preferred method of treatment
Fractures of the head of the talus
Mechanism of injury
Clinical diagnosis
Radiographic diagnosis
Treatment
Fractures of the neck of the talus
Anatomy
Mechanism of injury
Clinical diagnosis

Radiographic diagnosis
Treatment
Prognosis and complications
Fractures of the body of the talus
Group I: osteochondral fractures of the talar body
Groups II and V: shearing and comminuted fractures of the body of the talus
Group III: fractures of the posterior process of the talus
Group IV: fractures of the lateral process of the talus

Fractures of the midpart of the foot

Fractures of the tarsal navicular
Anatomy
Radiographic diagnosis
Fractures of the dorsal lip of the navicular
Clinical diagnosis
Treatment
Fractures of the navicular tuberosity
Clinical diagnosis
Treatment
Fractures of the body of the navicular
Clinical diagnosis
Treatment
Results
Stress fractures of the tarsal navicular
Clinical diagnosis
Radiographic diagnosis
Treatment
Author's preferred method of treatment
Dorsal chip fractures of the navicular
Fractures of the navicular tuberosity
Fractures of the body of the navicular
Stress fractures of the navicular

Fractures of the cuboid and cuneiform bones

Fractures of the cuboid
Clinical diagnosis
Radiographic diagnosis
Treatment
Author's preferred method of treatment
Cuneiform fractures
Clinical diagnosis
Radiographic diagnosis
Treatment
Author's preferred method of treatment

Fractures of the metatarsals

Anatomy
Mechanism of injury
Clinical diagnosis
Radiographic diagnosis
Treatment
Open fractures
Closed fractures
Metatarsal neck fractures
Metatarsal head fractures
Author's preferred method of treatment
Fractures of the base of the fifth metatarsal
Anatomy
Mechanism of injury
Clinical diagnosis
Radiographic diagnosis
Treatment
Author's preferred method of treatment
Stress fractures of the metatarsal diaphysis
Predisposing conditions and activities
Clinical diagnosis
Radiographic diagnosis
Treatment
Author's preferred method of treatment

Fractures of the phalanges

Mechanism of injury
Clinical diagnosis
Radiographic diagnosis
Treatment
Hallux phalangeal fractures
Lesser toe phalangeal fractures
Author's preferred method of treatment
Fractures of the hallux phalanges
Fractures of the lesser toe phalanges

Fractures of the sesamoid

Anatomy
Mechanism of injury
Clinical diagnosis
Radiographic diagnosis
Treatment
Nonoperative treatment
Surgical treatment
Author's preferred method of treatment
Stress fractures of the sesamoids
Author's preferred method of treatment
Dislocation of the sesamoids

Dislocations about the talus

Subtalar dislocations
Anatomy
Mechanism of injury
Clinical diagnosis
Radiographic diagnosis
Treatment
Results
Author's preferred method of treatment
Total dislocation of the talus
Mechanism of injury
Clinical diagnosis
Radiographic diagnosis
Treatment
Complications
Author's preferred method of treatment

Injuries to the midtarsal joint

Anatomy
Mechanism of injury
Clinical diagnosis
Radiographic diagnosis
Treatment
Complications
Author's preferred method of treatment
Medial injuries
Longitudinal injuries
Lateral injuries
Plantar injuries
Crushing injuries

Tarsometatarsal dislocations

Anatomy
Mechanism of injury
Clinical diagnosis
Radiographic diagnosis
Treatment
Results
Author's preferred method of treatment

Isolated talonavicular dislocations

Dislocations of the cuneiforms and cuboid

Dislocations of the cuneiforms
Isolated dislocations of the cuboid
Clinical diagnosis
Radiographic diagnosis

Treatment
Author's preferred method of treatment

Dislocations of the metatarsophalangeal joints

Anatomy
Hallux metatarsophalangeal joint
Lesser toe (II to V) metatarsophalangeal joints
Classification
Mechanism of injury
Hallux metatarsophalangeal dislocations
Lesser toe (II to V) metatarsophalangeal dislocations
Clinical diagnosis
Radiographic diagnosis
Hallux metatarsophalangeal dislocations
Lesser toe metatarsophalangeal dislocations
Treatment
Hallux metatarsophalangeal dislocations
Lesser toe (II to V) metatarsophalangeal dislocations
Results
Author's preferred method of treatment
Hallux metatarsophalangeal dislocations
Lesser toe metatarsophalangeal dislocations

Dislocations of the interphalangeal joints

Author's preferred method of treatment

Fractures and dislocations of the foot are among the most common injuries in the musculoskeletal system. Historically these injuries have been considered minor and their treatment often relegated to a secondary position. Hillegass[7] reports that of every 300 men working in heavy industry, 15 working days per month are lost as the result of foot problems, 65% of which are the result of trauma. The disability resulting from these injuries and their frequency warrant closer attention in their diagnosis and management.[8] The following general comments on the diagnosis and management of fractures and dislocations of the foot are meant to establish the basic principles. More detailed remarks are presented for each particular injury.

CLINICAL DIAGNOSIS

In evaluating patients with trauma to the foot, it is essential to obtain a thorough history. One must determine the general state of health with regard to such diseases as gout, diabetes, and circulatory problems before the initiation of treatment.[4] A detailed history of the mechanism by which the injury occurred will direct the examiner in his physical and radiographic examination.[4] In addition, it will provide a clue to the degree of soft-tissue injury associated with the fracture.

Once the history is taken, the physical examination must be carried out systematically. Klenerman[9] emphasizes that while forefoot injuries are easily diagnosed, midfoot and hindfoot injuries oftentimes go undetected. Because of the high incidence of multiple fractures in the injured foot,[4] careful palpation for points of tenderness is performed to detect any area of occult injury.[3, 14] The importance of evaluating the circulatory status of the foot cannot be overemphasized. It is important to compare the arterial pulsations of the involved foot with the normal foot, particularly in the elderly patient in whom absent pulsations may not be secondary to the fracture but to pre-existing vascular disease.

In displaced fractures and dislocations, evaluation of the overlying skin for signs of ischemia is important so that early reduction can be performed to prevent skin sloughing. Evaluation of the range of motion of the ankle, subtalar, midtarsal, and metatarsophalangeal joints is carried out within the limits of pain as part of a routine examination. A careful motor examination of intrinsic and extrinsic muscles is recorded both before and after treatment. The sensory examination is essential to detect loss secondary to the injury and such pre-existing conditions as diabetic neuropathy, which could produce a Charcot joint in the injured foot.

RADIOGRAPHIC DIAGNOSIS

Only after a careful history and physical examination are radiographs considered. The standard views used in evaluating the foot are the anteroposterior, lateral, and oblique views. The lateral view of the foot is helpful in evaluating fractures of the calcaneus and neck and body of the talus in addition to evaluating the midtarsal bones. Metatarsal overlap limits the usefulness of the lateral view in evaluation of the metatarsals and phalanges. The oblique view is particularly useful in evaluating the calcaneocuboid joint and in overcoming metatarsal overlap noted on the lateral view. Additional radiographs such as the anteroposterior view of the ankle are useful in evaluating the articular surface of the talus and the lateral aspect of the calcaneus. Axial views of the heel, special views of the subtalar joint, polytomography, and arthrography are also indicated in certain instances. The use of computed tomography (CT) in evaluating fractures and dislocations in the foot will be extended as experience with its use increases.

TREATMENT

The prime objectives in the treatment of fractures and dislocations of the foot are (1) avoiding stiffness and loss of mobility; (2) preventing bony prominences, which may result in pressure phenomena from the use of a shoe; and (3) restoring the articular surfaces. The goal of treatment of fractures and dislocations of the foot is a flexible plantigrade foot with good bony alignment.

Once the diagnosis is certain, dislocations and fractures of the foot should be reduced as soon as possible. The reduction is easier to achieve before swelling occurs and before hematoma forms between the fracture fragments. Additionally, gross displacement of dislocations and fractures of the foot can result in localized pressure on the skin with vascular compromise and skin loss. Immediate reduction of the displacement can limit these complications.

It is important to remember that a perfect anatomic result does *not* necessarily ensure that mobility will be maintained. In fact, McKeever[12] emphasizes that all too often a perfect radiograph is seen but the foot is so stiff that the patient cannot walk without pain. However, Klenerman[9] emphasizes the importance of restoring the foot to its normal shape even in cases in which joint mobility cannot be achieved. He stresses the importance of maintaining the relative lengths of the medial (talonaviculocuneiform) and lateral (calcaneocuboid) columns of the foot and avoiding any abnormal prominence on the plantar aspect of the foot.

Chapman[1] emphasizes the importance of anatomic restoration of joint surfaces within the foot and advocates open reduction and internal fixation where applicable in order to restore joint continuity. In addition, Klenerman[9] stresses that mobility of joints of the foot, so essential in normal function, is not likely to be regained if joint surfaces remain notably incongruous. He also emphasizes that although a period of immobilization may be beneficial to soft-tissue healing, it can lead to stiffness of joints, even those that are not involved in the injury, because of hemorrhage and extravasation about the adjacent joints.

Because of the close relationship of subtalar with midtarsal motion, limitation of motion of either of these joint complexes will secondarily limit motion in the other.[2, 10] Therefore, isolated injuries to midtarsal or subtalar joints must be actively mobilized to prevent secondary limitation of the linked joint.[2, 10]

Giannestras and Sammarco[5] emphasize that since the foot is a weight-bearing structure, the preservation of soft tissue is as important as the reduction of the fracture. They note that patients experience a great deal of difficulty when attempting to walk on scarred soft tissue, even if the bones of the foot are anatomically reduced.[5] Heck[6] also stresses the concept that fractures and dislocations of the foot are not solved simply by restoration of the continuity of a bone or joint complex, but rather by the simultaneous treatment and rehabilitation of the soft tissues. He emphasizes that the response to treatment of injuries to soft parts of the foot adjacent to a fracture is dependent on their early recognition and proper management. If for any reason one does not obtain supple soft tissues about the fracture, the final result will be impaired function of the foot and toes.

Lapidus and Guidotti[11] strongly emphasize the need for early mobilization in injuries of the foot. They note that the only two indications for immobilization of a fracture or dislocation are (1) to maintain reduction of the fragments and (2) to eliminate motion between fragments to prevent nonunion. They note that immobilization of a badly injured foot 6 weeks or longer (the time usually required for bony union) will almost invariably produce fibrous ankylosis of the small joints of the foot, with resultant muscular atrophy and limitation of joint motion.

Chapman[1] stresses that if immobilization can be accomplished by internal fixation, earlier institution of joint motion is possible and should be encouraged. However, if cast immobilization is required, leaving the toes free so that motion at the metatarsophalangeal joints can be encouraged will help decrease edema and stimulate muscle function in the calf and foot. In addition, I have found that by leaving the toes exposed in a cast and using them to pick up small objects, swelling can be decreased and earlier mobility stimulated.

In cases in which stability of the fracture or dislocation allows early weight bearing, Hillegass[7] reports that such early weight bearing decreases the period of disability following injury. He believes that it prevents the development of osteoporosis, decreases swelling by early muscle contraction, and permits slight motion in the small joints of the foot (even in a cast), which helps to prevent stiffness. Mullen and Gamber[13] also noted the importance of early mobilization and weight bearing to prevent long-term disability. Chapman[1] emphasizes that immobilization of the foot in a non–weight-bearing mode is accompanied by muscular atrophy, myostatic contracture, decreased joint motion, proliferation of connective tissue and capsular structures, internal synovial adhesions, and cartilaginous degeneration. Early mobilization obviates or decreases the possible occurrence of these abnormal processes.[1] In situations in which postoperative immobilization is indicated *without* weight bearing, consideration can be given to bivalving the short-leg cast and instituting early motion *without* weight bearing. Once motion is restored, immobilization can be continued until union occurs. The stability of the fracture or dislocation must be considered before this method is recommended. If weight bearing needs to be delayed, Omer and Pomerantz[14] suggest using a patellar tendon–bearing plaster cast or brace to relieve weight bearing but allow mobilization. Evaluation of stability, determined at the time of reduction, and cast immobilization will help decide whether early weight bearing, with its known benefits, can be instituted.

Following the period of fracture immobilization, an intensive rehabilitation program specialized for the foot should be instituted to ensure restoration of joint function and muscle strength. I have found that an Unna boot or Gelocast to gently support the foot and yet allow progressive motion of the joints for the first week after cast removal helps to prevent swelling. Exercises with the foot, including bunching a towel with the toes (Fig 35–1,A) and picking up small objects with the toes (Fig 35–1,B), help to institute muscle contraction and range of motion in the foot and ankle. McKeever[12] points out that many injuries to the foot result in crushing, stretching, or tearing of the soft tissues in addition to the fractures. This produces hemorrhage, which extravasates through the soft tissue and infiltrates the tissue interstices. The result is dense intra-articular and extra-articular adhesions and fibrosis, all of which severely limit the normal flexibility of the foot. In addition, this can be accompanied by demineralization of bone and can result in Sudeck's atrophy or reflex sympathetic dystrophy in the limb. It is McKeever's opinion[12] that prolonged immobilization of a foot distended with blood is a common precursor to this disabling syndrome. A discussion of the diagnosis and treatment of reflex sympathetic dystrophy is beyond the scope of this chapter; however, by early motion, elevation, and early weight bearing, it can often be prevented.[12]

Lapidus and Guidotti[11] recommend early mobilization combined with swimming pool walking exercises to treat fractures of the ankle or tarsal bones. These swimming pool walking exercises are performed on a daily basis. Walking is started in the deepest part of the pool so that the buoyancy of the patient's body in the water results in a weightless state. The patient is instructed to walk as though he were walking on normal ground. Although Lapidus and Guidotti recommend that some fractures of the foot be *initially* treated in this manner, if the fractures are unstable and require immobilization, I

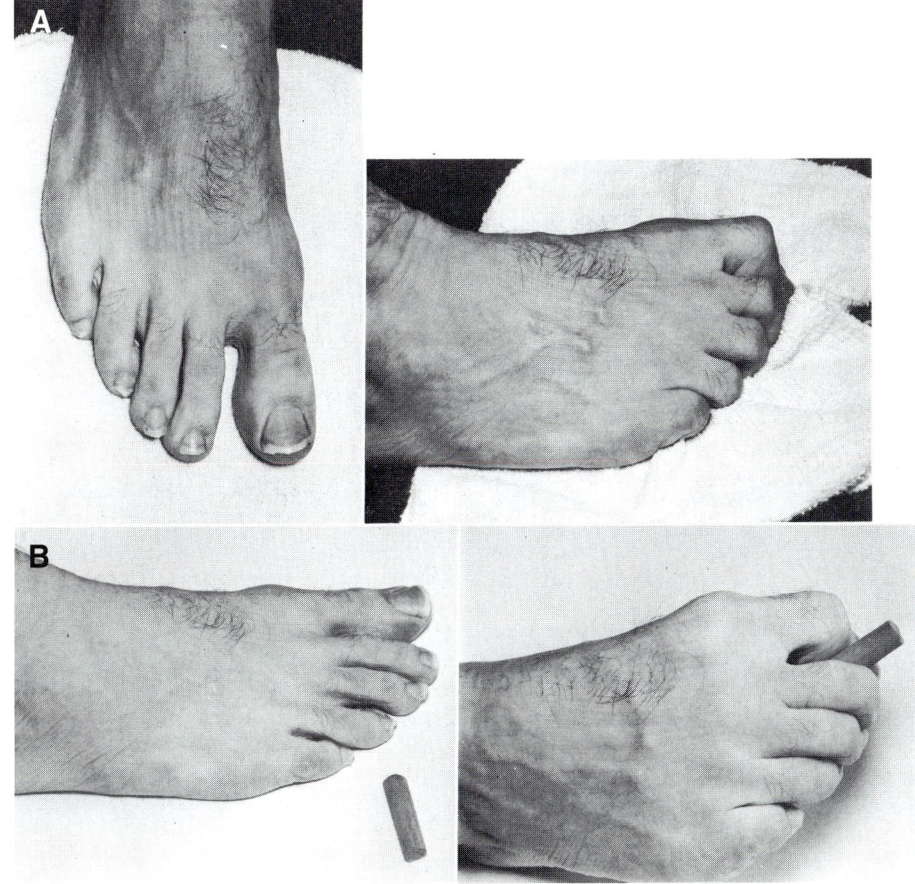

FIG 35–1.
Foot exercises used to institute early muscle contraction and range of motion. **A,** using the toes to bunch up a towel. Exercise can also be done in a cast if the toes are left free. **B,** picking up small objects with the toes helps to stimulate intrinsic muscle function.

have found this method very useful following a period of immobilization. Although a whirlpool used for soaking before instituting range-of-motion exercises is helpful in improving range of motion, it does not allow actual weight bearing with support of the water as swimming pool walking does.

I have found the use of an elastic bandage for gentle resisted dorsiflexion–plantar flexion, inversion-eversion, and abduction-adduction to be helpful early in restoring both joint motion and muscle power (Fig 35–2). Later, strengthening exercises including resisted ankle plantar flexion–dorsiflexion and inversion-eversion are added as pain permits. Proprioceptive exercises are instituted when strength allows painless ambulation. A simple means of proprioceptive training is the use of a board placed on a cylinder ("bongo board"), which helps in

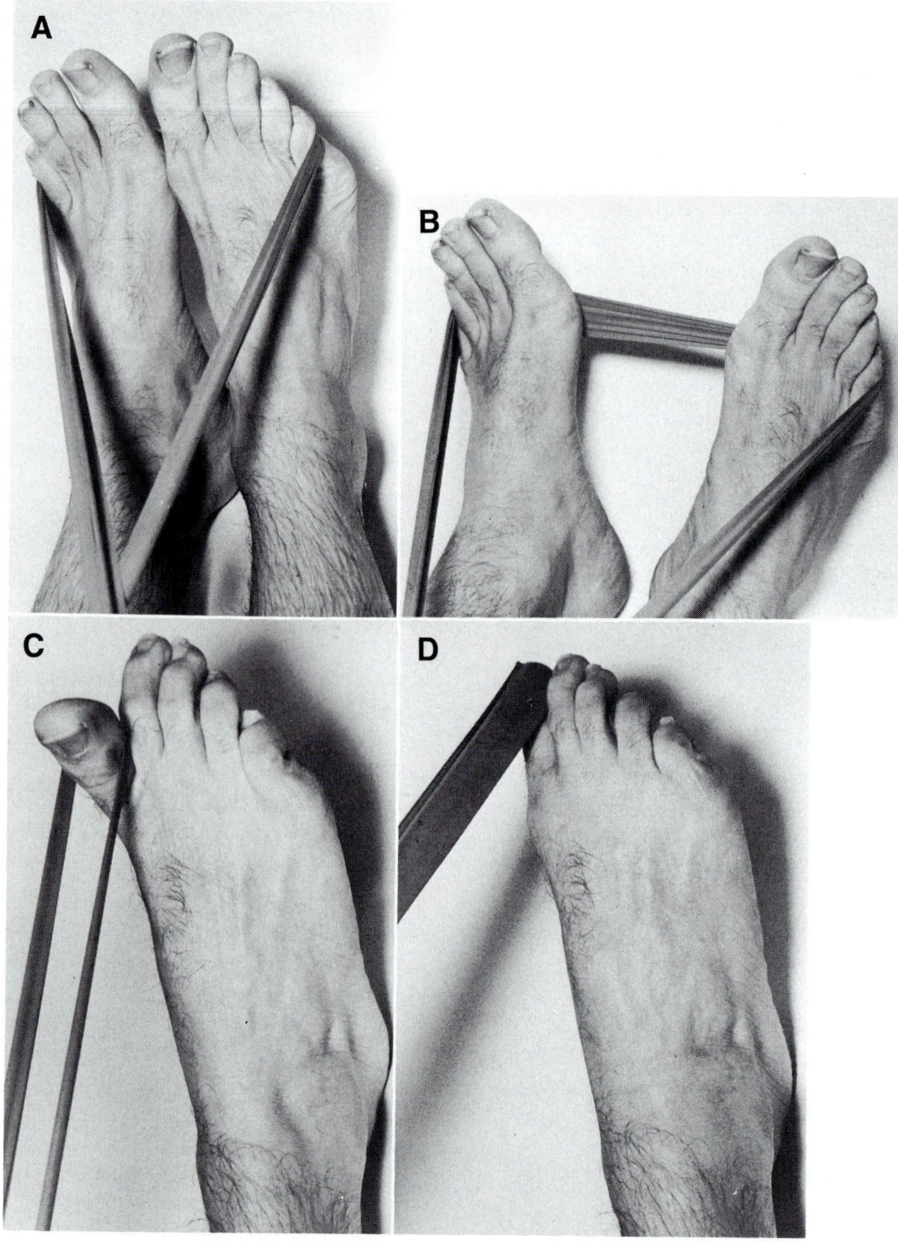

FIG 35–2.
An elastic bandage can be used to supply gentle resistance for early strengthening and motion exercises. This can be used for ankle dorsiflexion–plantar flexion **(A),** inversion-eversion **(B),** and metatarsophalangeal motion (even in a cast) of the foot **(C** and **D**).

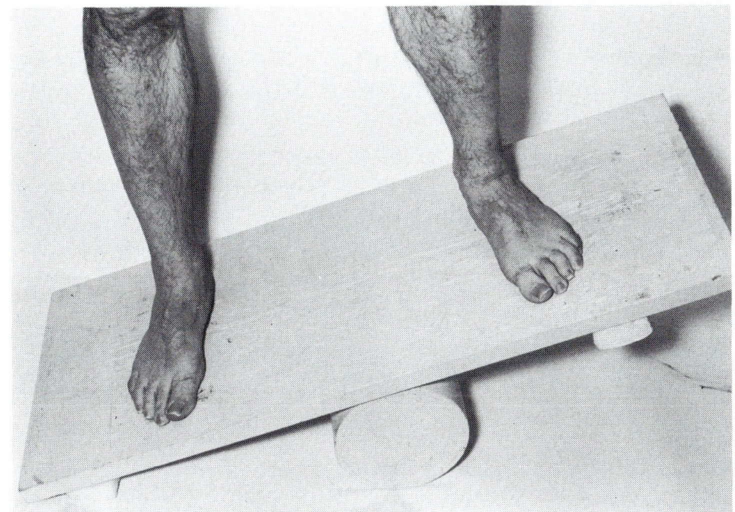

FIG 35–3.
Use of a "bongo board" to help retrain the foot in proprioception. Balancing on a board by using cylinders of increasing diameter facilitates the progression of proprioceptive development.

two-dimensional retraining (Fig 35–3). Eventually placing the board on a round ball will introduce three-dimensional tilt for proprioception education.

Stretching exercises for the Achilles tendon and gentle stretching of the subtalar, midtarsal, and metatarsophalangeal joints is also indicated. The metatarsophalangeal joints can be actively assisted in their range of motion, again, by using an elastic bandage (see Fig 35–2,C and D). If swelling occurs during this period of rehabilitation, consideration is given to a compression dressing such as a Jobst compression stocking or Ace wrap. Contrast baths with alternating heat and cold are used later if recurrent swelling becomes a permanent problem.

After rehabilitation is complete, the use of a longitudinal arch support, particularly for midtarsal injuries, and a protective liner in the shoe made of a material such as Plastizote to relieve the plantar aspect of the foot helps to restore the weight-bearing function of the foot. Special shoe alterations and appliances are mentioned later under each specific injury.

REFERENCES

General

1. Chapman MW: Fractures and dislocations of the ankle and foot. In Mann RA, (editor:) *DuVries surgery of the foot*, ed 4, St Louis, 1978, Mosby–Year Book.
2. Close JR, Inman VT, Poor PM, et al: The function of the subtalar joint, *Clin Orthop* 50:159–179, 1967.
3. Coker TP, Jr, Arnold JA: Sports injuries to the foot and ankle. In Jahss MH, editor: *Disorders of the foot*, vol 2, Philadelphia, 1982, WB Saunders.
4. Garcia A, Parkes JC: Fractures of the foot. In Giannestras NJ, editor: *Foot disorders: medical and surgical management*, ed 2, Philadelphia, 1973, Lea & Febiger.
5. Giannestras NJ, Sammarco GJ: Fractures and dislocations in the foot. In Rockwood CA Jr, Green DP, editors: *Fractures*, vol 2, Philadelphia, 1975, JB Lippincott.
6. Heck CV: Fractures of the bones of the foot (except the talus), *Surg Clin North Am* 45:103–117, 1965.
7. Hillegass RC: Injuries to the midfoot: A major cause of industrial morbidity. In Bateman JE, editor: *Foot science*, Philadelphia, 1976, WB Saunders.
8. Johnson VS: Treatment of fractures of the forefoot in industry. In Bateman JE, editor: *Foot science*, Philadelphia, 1976, WB Saunders.
9. Klenerman L: *The foot and its disorders*, ed 2, Boston, 1982, Blackwell.
10. Lapidus P: Mechanical anatomy of the tarsal joints, *Clin Orthop* 30:20, 1963.
11. Lapidus PW, Guidotti FP: Immediate mobilization and swimming pool exercises in some fractures of foot and ankle bones, *Clin Orthop* 56:197–206, 1968.
12. McKeever FM: Fractures of the tarsal and metatarsal bones, *Surg Gynecol Obstet* 90:735–745, 1950.
13. Mullen JP, Gamber HH: Management of severe open foot injuries, *J Bone Joint Surg [Am]* 54:1574, 1972.
14. Omer GE, Pomerantz GM: Principles of management of acute injuries of the foot, *J Bone Joint Surg [Am]* 51:813–814, 1969.

COMPARTMENT SYNDROMES OF THE FOOT

The significance of compartment syndromes in the forearm and lower portion of the leg have been appreciated for many years.[10, 11] Early management by fasciotomy of the acute muscle ischemia due to compartment syndromes is the mainstay of prevention of myonecrosis.[10, 17] Myerson has recently discussed the diagnosis and treatment of compartment syndromes of the foot.[12, 13] He emphasized that bleeding and edema fluid can produce ischemic necrosis of the muscles in four compartments of the foot just as it does in the forearm and lower part of the leg.[12, 13] In the foot, the end result of this ischemic process is a clawfoot deformity with permanent loss of function due to contracture, weakness, and sensory disturbance.[1, 3, 4, 7, 16, 18]

Anatomy

A compartment syndrome is a symptom complex that results from elevated tissue pressure in a closed osteofascial space. As the tissue pressure increases, it reduces capillary blood profusion below what is required for tissue viability. The inelastic nature of the structures compromising the osteofascial compartments of the involved limbs prevent dissipation of this tissue pressure. This eventually causes vascular occlusion and myoneural ischemia.

The osteofascial compartments of the foot have been recently reemphasized.[12 13, 15] Kamel and Sakla[8] divided the foot into four compartments: medial, central, lateral, and interosseous (Fig 35–4). The medial compartment consists of the abductor hallucis and flexor hallucis brevis muscles as well as the flexor hallucis longus, peroneus longus, and posterior tibial tendons. The medial compartment is bounded dorsally by the inferior surface of the first metatarsal shaft, medially by an extension of the plantar aponeurosis, and laterally by a flimsy intermuscular septum. The central compartment is bounded on the inferior surface by the thick plantar aponeurosis, medially and laterally by intermuscular septae and dorsally by the osseous tarsometatarsal structures, the interosseous ligaments, and fascial expansions. From plantar to dorsal, the central compartment contains the flexor digitorum brevis muscle, the flexor digitorum longus tendons and the lumbricales, the quadratus plantae muscle, the adductor hallucis muscle, and peroneus longus and posterior tibial tendons. The lateral compartment is bounded dorsally by the fifth metatarsal shaft, medially by an intermuscular septum, and laterally by the end of the plantar aponeurosis. It contains the abductor, short flexor, and opponens muscles of the fifth toe. Finally, the interosseous compartment is bounded by the interosseous fascia and metatarsals and contains the interosseous muscles.

Three methods have been described to decompress these four compartments of the foot. Mubarak and Hargens[11] described double longitudinal dorsal incisions with dissection extending between all metatarsal shafts to allow full decompression of the plantar spaces (Fig 35–5). Myerson[12, 13] and Bonuti and Bell[2] recommend a long medial longitudinal incision along the first metatarsal shaft through which one can access all the compartments of the foot (Fig 35–6). Grodinski,[5] Loeffler and Ballard,[9] and Heckman and Champine[6] utilize a plantar incision extending from the second metatarsal head proximally to the arch of the foot (Fig 35–7). If necessary, this can be extended posteriorly to the medial malleolus to decompress the tarsal tunnel.

Clinical Presentation

Compartment syndromes of the foot are often associated with crushing injuries, injuries in which there are multiple metatarsal fractures, and fractures and/or dislocations of the tarsometatarsal joints.[5, 10, 11] The diagnosis of a compartment syndrome is a clinical one and is based upon the signs of nerve and muscle ischemia.[5, 11]

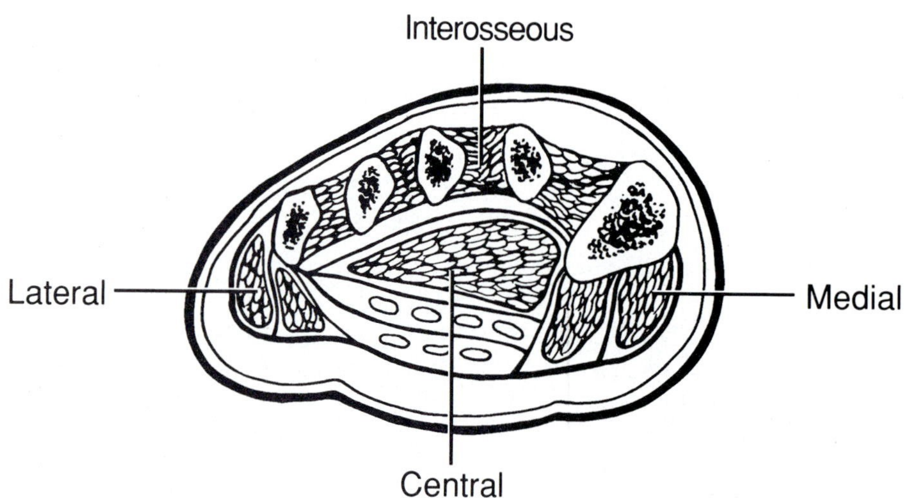

FIG 35–4.
The four osteofascial compartments of the foot: medial, central, lateral, and interosseous.

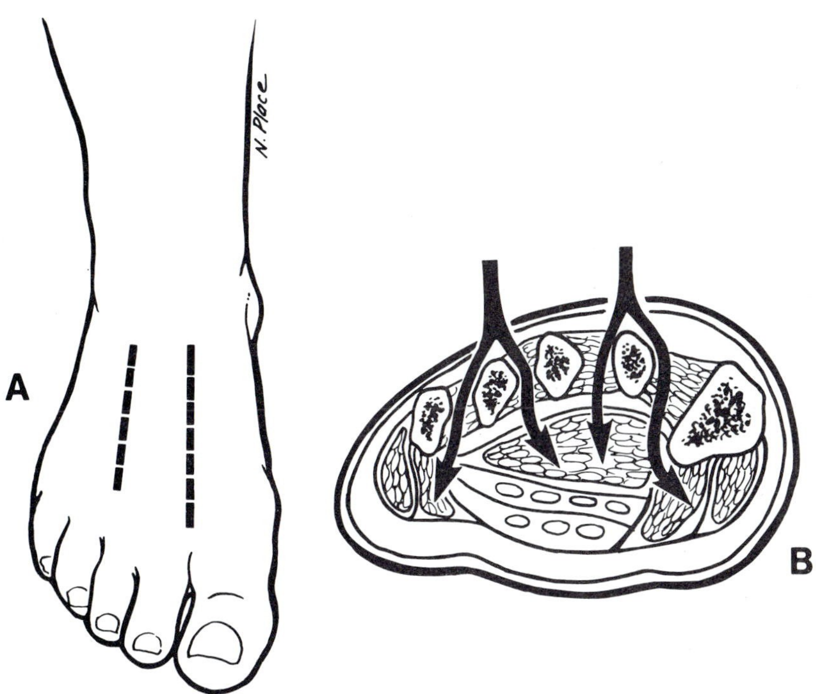

FIG 35–5.
The technique of Mubarak and Hargens[11] uses double dorsal longitudinal incisions **(A)** to decompress all four compartments **(B).**

Clinical and laboratory data suggest that in patients with an impending compartment syndrome, functional losses precede actual myoneural necrosis by several hours.[5, 10, 11] Recognizing these early clinical findings provides the basis for early diagnosis and prevention of tissue necrosis. Clinically, it is not possible to separate the different compartments of the foot to assess individual toe muscle function.

The suspicion of a compartment syndrome should be present in all patients with foot injuries in which there is any element of crushing. The majority of these injuries are closed injuries and are associated with multiple midfoot and forefoot fractures and dislocations. These patients usually present with a tense, swollen foot. It is also important to recognize that a crushed foot associated with large open injuries can also result in a compartment syndrome. Hence, one should not assume that the osteofascial spaces have been automatically decompressed by any associated open injury.

The hallmark of muscle and nerve ischemia of a compartment syndrome of the foot is pain. In the presence of multiple fractures of the foot, it may be difficult to determine whether a patient's pain is due to the fractures and soft-tissue injury or is due to an underlying compartment syndrome.[6, 14, 19] The presence of severe, unrelenting pain that does not respond to immobilization strongly suggests the presence of a compartment syndrome. Passive stretching of the involved ischemic muscles is also a reliable diagnostic test in the assessment of compartment syndrome. Dorsiflexion and plantar flexion of the toes involved in a foot with a compartment syndrome will always elicit discomfort. Decreased sensation is an important, early sign of nerve ischemia, particularly if there is a change in the pattern of sensation over time. Two-point discrimination and light touch over the plantar aspect of the toes are more sensitive than loss of pinprick sensation.[12, 13] It is important to recognize that the absence of peripheral pulses is an *unreliable* sign and plays no role in the early diagnosis of compartment syndrome. The associated presence of marked tenderness and tenseness in the foot is also a sign of a compartment syndrome. The foot needs to be repeatedly examined if the diagnosis of compartment syndrome is suspected. Myerson suggests that no circumferential dressings be used when a compartment syndrome is suspected.[12, 13] He also suggests that the foot not be elevated maximally under these circumstances, but instead placed at heart level to ensure venous drainage without compromising arterial pressure.[12, 13]

Due to the fact that a compartment syndrome is a progressive phenomenon, a patient suspected of having a compartment syndrome must be frequently monitored. A history of relentless pain, clinical proof of sen-

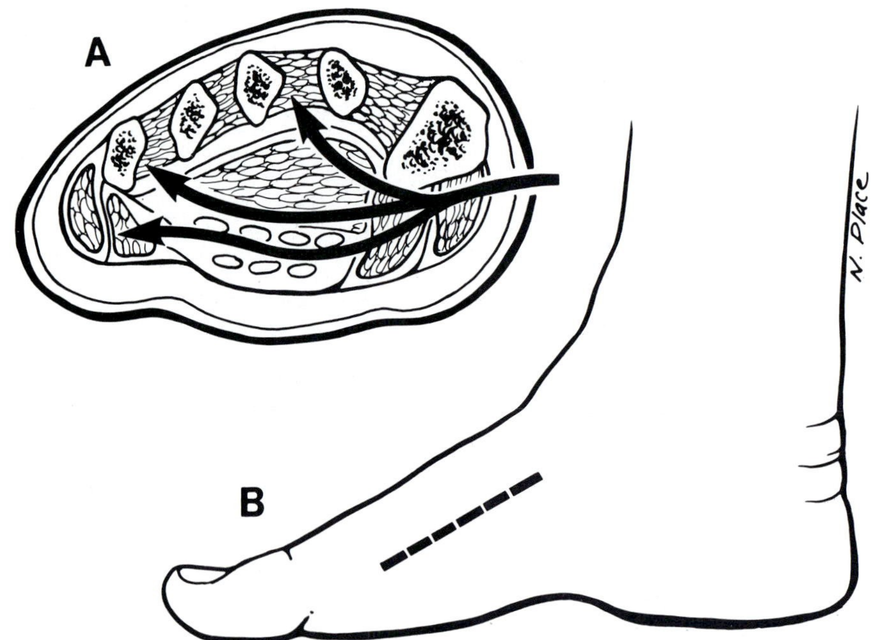

FIG 35–6.
The technique of Myerson[12, 13] uses a long medial incision **(B)** to decompress all four compartments **(A).**

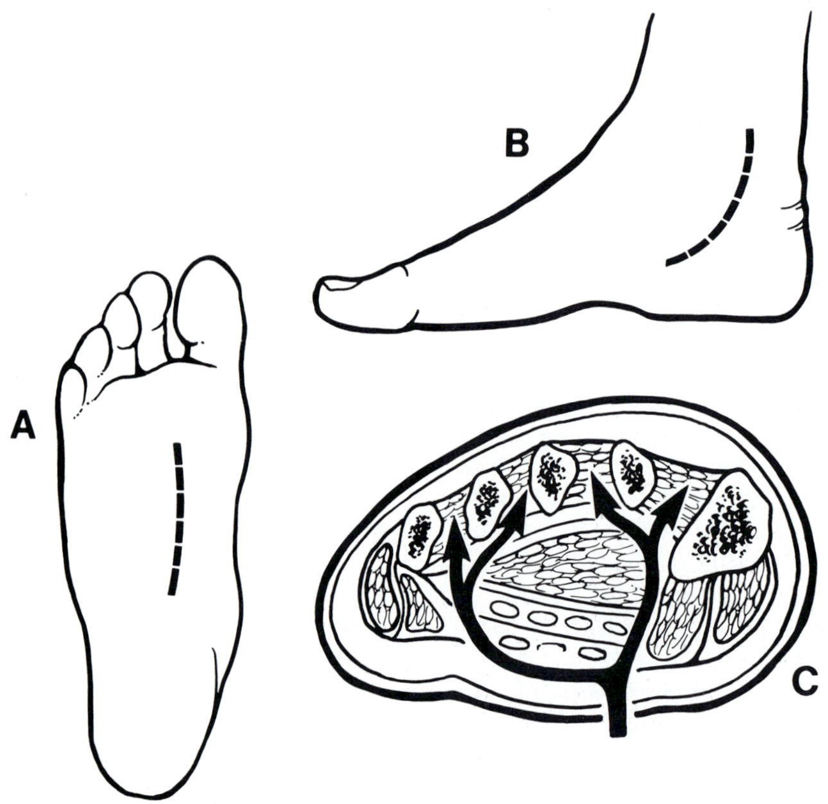

FIG 35–7.
The technique described by Grodinski[5] utilizes a plantar incision from the second metatarsal to the arch of the foot **(A)** to decompress all four compartments **(C).** If necessary, a second incision can decompress the tarsal tunnel **(B).**

sory deficit, or pain with passive stretch of the involved muscle indicate the necessity for fasciotomy.

The clinical signs of a compartment syndrome will not be present in a patient who is comatose or who has had spinal cord or peripheral nerve injury. Because of this, more objective tests have been introduced for measuring compartment pressure. Matsen,[10] Mubarak and Hargens,[11] Rorabeck et al.[14] and Whitesides et al.[17] have introduced different techniques for measuring compartmental pressure. While all of these techniques have potential pitfalls with their use, they are helpful in the diagnosis of compartment syndrome in patients who cannot cooperate with a physical evaluation. However, the diagnosis and decision to perform a fasciotomy on a foot with a suspected compartment syndrome is based upon the clinical evaluation. Myerson[12] states that it is his practice to decompress any acute injury associated with a measured pressure of 30 mm, particularly when the pressure is accompanied by other positive clinical findings. If clinical suspicions are high, however, I believe that a fasciotomy should be performed.

Surgical Decompression

Surgical decompression of an acutely traumatized foot with a compartment syndrome is the only method of preventing the ischemic complications of a clawfoot. Mubarak and Hargens[11] suggested the use of two longitudinal dorsal incisions located over the metatarsals. This approach was based on a similar experience with compartment syndromes of the hand.[11] The dorsal approach consists of two longitudinal incisions along the length of the second and fourth metatarsals. These incisions are carried down directly to bone without any subcutaneous dissection. Once the metatarsals are reached, longitudinal dissection is performed in each interosseous space until the interosseous fascia that separates the central and interosseous compartments is incised (see Fig 35–5). Myerson[12, 13] induced compartment syndromes in fresh cadaver feet and then decompressed them either through dorsal incisions or a long medial incision. He found that both approaches gave excellent access to the involved compartments for surgical decompression but that it took considerably longer for tissue pressures to normalize when the dorsal approach was used. He therefore recommends the use of a medial approach for fasciotomies in cases of crush injuries unassociated with midfoot or forefoot fractures. The medial approach utilizes an incision that follows the length of the inferior surface of the first metatarsal. Entry into the medial compartment is made just above the abductor hallucis muscle. From this point, access to the central, lateral, and interosseous compartments is easy (see Fig 35–6).

Myerson prefers the dorsal approach, however, for compartment syndromes associated with fractures of the metatarsals or tarsometatarsal joints. This is based upon the fact that it provides better access to fractures for rigid internal fixation, which is the treatment of choice for these injuries. Grodinski,[5] Loeffler and Ballard,[9] and Bonuti and Bell[2] prefer the use of a long plantar utilitarian incision from the second metatarsal head to the proximal arch of the foot for decompression of the foot. This incision can be extended posteriorly to the medial malleolus to decompress the tarsal tunnel (see Fig 35–7).

The same surgical principles utilized in fasciotomies of the upper and lower extremities apply to fasciotomies of the foot. The incisions should be adequate in length. It is important to recognize that the skin may become a limiting factor and can actually produce a compartment syndrome as a result of postischemic swelling after fasciotomy if it is not released adequately.[10, 11] Although it is often difficult to determine the viability of muscle in the foot, debridement of all necrotic tissue should be performed at the time of fasciotomy. Myerson[12, 13] emphasizes the importance of stabilizing all fractures in massively injured feet as rigidly as possible with a combination of internal and external fixation where appropriate. He emphasizes that rigid skeletal stability enhances soft-tissue healing.

All fasciotomy incisions are left open and covered with a dressing. The wound is debrided again in 24 to 48 hours. Irrigation with pulsating lavage is recommended. The wound is covered with either a dressing or allograft.[11] Myerson recommends that no efforts be made to close these incisions until the fifth or sixth day. He also states that the dorsal incisions do not close well, and because of this, he recommends the use of split-thickness skin grafts.

Ziv et al.[19] have introduced the concept of immediate one-stage management of crush injuries of the foot associated with a compartment syndrome. The authors describe their experience with a method that involves removal of a split-thickness skin graft from avulsed flaps at the time of the original injury, debridement of the injured area, decompression of the compartments of the foot including the tarsal tunnel, fixation of bony injuries, and finally coverage with the meshed skin graft. The authors also emphasize the importance of releasing the tarsal tunnel in association with a standard foot compartment syndrome release. The authors reported using this one-stage technique on five cases of crush injury of the foot, all of which healed uneventfully.

Whatever means are utilized for management of open

wounds of the foot, either one-stage management as described by Ziv et al,[19] delayed split-thickness skin graft reported by Myerson,[12, 13] or the use of local or free tissue flaps, it is the early diagnosis and prompt decompression of a compartment syndrome that does the most to prevent the long-term deleterious effects of crush injuries and the resulting ischemia of the foot.

Author's Preferred Method of Treatment

I base the diagnosis of compartment syndrome and my decision to perform a fasciotomy on the history and clinical examination. I use tissue pressure measurements to confirm the clinical findings and diagnosis in cases with a confusing clinical picture. Patients with crush injuries, multiple foot fractures, or dislocations of the midtarsal or tarsometatarsal joints are considered to have a compartmental syndrome until proved otherwise. Swelling and pain not controlled by immobilization and worsened by stretching of the involved muscle are the key to the diagnosis. I base my decision to decompress the foot mainly on tissue pressure monitoring *only* in a comatose patient or a patient who has altered sensation in the limb. The diagnosis of clostridial myonecrosis must be considered in the differential diagnosis, particularly in open crush injuries of the foot.

I prefer to decompress the foot by using two dorsal incisions for the interosseous spaces and a medial incision for the medial, central, and the lateral compartments. All fractures and dislocations are rigidly stabilized at the time of fasciotomy. The wound is left open and debrided again every 24 to 48 hours until secondary closure or skin grafting is indicated. Prophylactic antibiotics and tetanus prophylaxis are instituted as for open fractures.

REFERENCES

Compartment Syndromes of the Foot

1. Barbari SS, Brevig K: Correction of claw toes by the Girdlestone-Taylor flexor-extensor transfer procedure, *Foot Ankle* 5:67–73, 1984.
2. Bonuti PM, Bell GR: Compartment syndrome of the foot. A case report, *J Bone Joint Surg [Am]* 68:1449–1451, 1986.
3. Chuinard EG, Baskin M: Claw-foot deformity, *J Bone Joint Surg [Am]* 55:151–162, 1973.
4. Cole WH: The treatment of claw foot, *J Bone Joint Surg [Am]* 22:895–908, 1940.
5. Grodinski M: A study of fascial spaces of the foot, *Surg Gynecol Obstet* 49:739–751, 1929.
6. Heckman JD, Champine MJ: New techniques in the management of foot trauma, *Clin Orthop* 240:105–114, 1989.
7. Jones R: An address on Volkman's ischemic contracture with special reference to treatment, *Br Med J* 2:639–642, 1928.
8. Kamel R, Salka BF: Anatomical compartments of the sole of the human foot, *Anat Rec* 140:57–64, 1961.
9. Loeffler RD, Ballard A: Plantar fascial spaces of the foot and a proposed surgical approach, *Foot Ankle* 1:11–14, 1980.
10. Matsen FA III: Compartmental syndrome. A unified concept, *Clin Orthop* 113:8–14, 1975.
11. Mubarak SJ, Hargens AR: *Compartment syndrome and Volkman's contracture*, Philadelphia, 1981, WB Saunders.
12. Myerson MS: Acute compartment syndromes of the foot, *Bull Hosp Jt Dis Orthop Inst* 47:261, 1987.
13. Myerson MS: Experimental decompression of the fascial compartments of the foot. The basis for fasciotomy in acute compartment syndrome, *Foot Ankle* 8:308–314, 1988.
14. Rorabeck CH, Castle GS, Hardie R, et al: Compartmental pressure measurements. An experimental investigation using the slit catheter, *J Trauma* 21:446–449, 1981.
15. Saraffian SK: *Anatomy of the foot and ankle*, Philadelphia, 1983, JB Lippincott.
16. Tsuge K: Treatment of established Volkman's contracture, *J Bone Joint Surg [Am]* 57:925–929, 1987.
17. Whitesides TE Jr, Harada H, Morimoto K: Compartment syndrome and the role of fasciotomy: its parameters and techniques, *Instr Course Lect* 25:179–196, 1977.
18. Wood-Jones F: *Structure and function as seen in the foot*, ed 2, London, Balliere, Tindall, & Cox, 1949.
19. Ziv I, Mosheiff R, Zeligowski A, et al: Crush injuries to the foot with compartment syndrome; immediate one stage management, *Foot Ankle* 9:185–189, 1989.

FRACTURES OF THE CALCANEUS

The calcaneus is the most frequently fractured of all the tarsal bones[96, 178] and constitutes 60% of all major tarsal injuries.[29] Of all patients with calcaneus fractures, 10% have associated fractures of the spine,[56, 103, 168] and 26% have other associated extremity injuries.[56, 106, 168] About 7% of these fractures are bilateral, and fewer than 2% are open.[114]

The economic importance of these fractures is apparent in that although they represent only 2% of all fractures, 90% occur in males between 41 and 45 years of age.* They occur most often in middle-aged industrial workers.[1, 18, 173, 202–204, 207] The economic impact becomes even more apparent when one considers that 20% of patients may be incapacitated for up to 3 years following the fracture and many are still partially incapacitated as long as 5 years after the fracture.[138]

Conn[32] in 1926 termed calcaneus fractures "serious and disabling injuries in which the end results are in-

**References 50, 85, 114, 129, 136, 142, 150, 173, 202–204, 207.*

credibly bad," and Mercer[130] called calcaneus fractures the most disabling of all injuries. The pessimism surrounding these fractures was echoed by Cotton and Henderson[36] and by Bankart, who termed the results of treatment of crush fractures of the calcaneus "rotten."[10]

Although some aspects of the treatment of calcaneus fractures are well accepted, a standard method of treatment is not agreed on by most authors.[175] The first written report of closed treatment was by Bailey[9] in 1880, while Morestein[135] in 1902 first reported open reduction and internal fixation of calcaneus fractures. Since these very early reports, the emphasis on treatment has vacillated between open and closed methods. There is no current concensus of opinion regarding the treatment of all calcaneus fractures. Additionally, a direct comparison of various treatment modalities is difficult for several reasons:

1. Different authors have used different methods of classification of calcaneal fractures, which makes comparisons difficult.[211]
2. There are no true prospective studies available that compare the various treatment modalities.
3. Methods of postfracture evaluation have varied greatly and make a comparison of results difficult.[154]

The purpose of this section is to present the logic and theory for each method of treatment and to combine in the section "Author's Preferred Method" the points of each method of treatment that I have found most useful.

Anatomy

The calcaneus transmits the weight of the body to the ground and forms a strong lever for the muscles of the calf.[3] The calcaneus consists of an internal structure of cancellous bone surrounded by an outer shell of cortical bone.[12, 137] This cortical shell is very thin except at the posterior tubercle, and the enclosed pattern of cancellous bone reflects the static and dynamic strains to which the calcaneus is exposed.[80] Traction trabeculae radiate from the inferior cortex of the calcaneus, while compression trabeculae converge to support the posterior and anterior articular facets. Soeur and Remy[184] have termed this condensation of bone trabeculae beneath the anterior and posterior facets "the thalamic portion of the calcaneus." According to Letournel,[112] however, Destot termed the posterior articular surface of the calcaneus "the thalamus."[112]

The so-called neutral triangle with its sparseness of trabeculae is located just beneath the crucial angle of Gissane (Fig 35–8). According to Harty,[80] the neutral triangle is where blood vessels reach the medullary cavity of the calcaneus and is therefore a common site for the early manifestations of blood-borne infection.

The calcaneus has six distinct surfaces: superior, inferior, lateral, medial, posterior, and anterior.[171]

Superior Surface

The superior surface of the calcaneus can be conveniently divided into three parts: posterior, middle, and anterior[171, 207] (Fig 35–9).

The posterior third of the superior surface is completely nonarticular. It is perforated by multiple vascular foramina.[171] This posterior nonarticular portion of the calcaneus joins with the middle surface and marks the highest portion of the bone, "the posterior peak."[206]

The middle third of the superior surface consists of the large posterior facet of the calcaneus. The articular surface of the posterior facet is convex along the longitudinal axis of the calcaneus.[171]

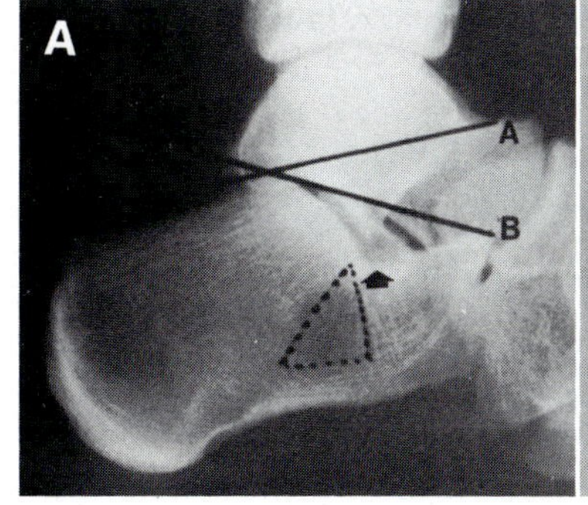

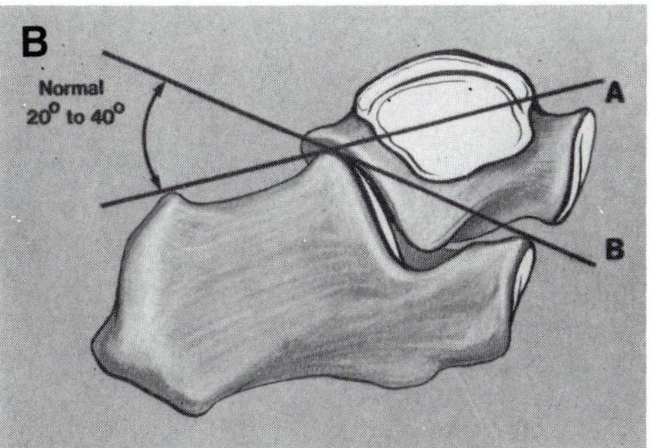

FIG 35–8.
A, "neutral triangle" *(dotted lines)* beneath the crucial angle of Gissane *(arrow).* Note the sparcity of trabeculae in the neutral triangle. **B,** Bohler's tuberosity joint angle. *Line A,* from the highest point on the posterior articular surface to the most superior part of the calcaneal tuberosity. *Line B,* from the highest point on the anterior process of the calcaneus to the highest part of the posterior articular surface. The intervening angle *(arrow)* is Bohler's tuberosity joint angle (20 to 40 degrees).

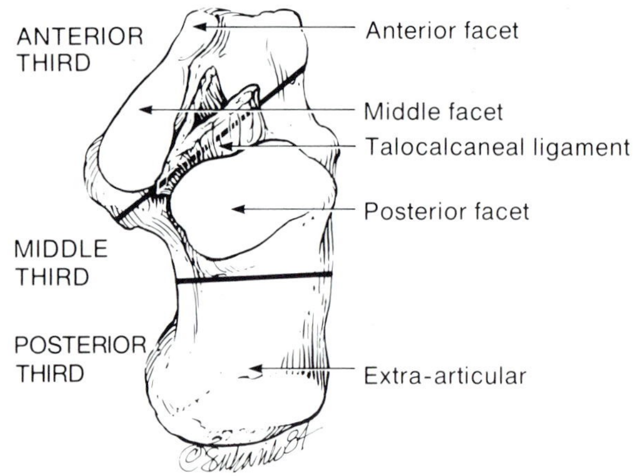

FIG 35–9.
The superior surface of the calcaneus is divided into thirds. The posterior third is extra-articular, the middle third contains the posterior facet, and the anterior third contains the articular surface of the middle and anterior facets.

The anterior third of the superior surface consists of the sinus tarsi, the sulcus calcanei, and the articular surfaces of the anterior and medial facets. The anterior and medial facets form a concavity that corresponds to the convexity of the talar head.[171] The anterior articular surface is supported by the beak of the os calcis, and the medial surface is supported by the sustentaculum tali.[171, 206] Variations occur in the contour and degree of separations of these two articular surfaces. The anterior and medial facets can be either separate or confluent.[171]

The tarsal canal separates the middle and posterior articular facets. This canal is narrow and is oriented obliquely forward, laterally, and inferiorly.[171] The intraosseous talocalcaneal ligament inserts in the floor of the canal, and it serves to separate the posterior facet from the anterior and middle facets[63] (Fig 35–9). Although the anterior, middle, and posterior talocalcaneal articular facets have separate synovial cavities and are curved in opposite directions, they function as a single reciprocal unit.[80]

Inferior Surface

The inferior surface of the calcaneus is triangular, with the base located posteriorly and the apex anteriorly.[171] The inferior surface is composed of a medial and a lateral tuberosity, with the medial tuberosity being the main weight-bearing structure.[171] The medial tuberosity gives origin to the abductor hallucis muscle, and the lateral tuberosity gives origin to the abductor digiti minimi. According to Sarrafian,[171] 36% of os calcis have a heel spur, which is a shelflike anterior bony projection originating from the medial tuberosity.

Lateral Surface

The lateral surface of the body of the calcaneus is flat and contains a shallow groove for the peroneal tendons.[171] A separate groove for the peroneus longus tendon is present on the lateral aspect of the os calcis in 85% of specimens,[171] while a definite groove for the peroneus brevis tendon is present in only about 3% of specimens.

Medial Surface

The configuration of the medial calcaneal surface is determined mainly by the sustentaculum tali, a large triangular projection with a posterior base and an anterior apex.[171] Its superior surface represents the middle articular facet of the calcaneus, and its inferior surface is curved into a groove for the flexor hallucis longus tendon and provides attachment for the fibrous tunnel of this tendon.[171] Additionally, the tibiocalcaneal component of the deltoid ligament and the superomedial calcaneonavicular ligament insert on the upper border of its medial surface.

Posterior Surface

The posterior surface of the calcaneus is also triangular in shape, with the apex superior and the base inferior. The overall contour of this surface is convex.[171] Sarrafian[171] stresses that the lower border of this posterior surface serves as the insertion for the Achilles tendon while the upper portion of the posterior surface is free from tendinous insertion (Fig 35–10).

Anterior Surface

The anterior surface of the calcaneus is entirely articular.[171] It is saddle shaped, convex transversely, and concave vertically. It serves as the articulation between the calcaneus and cuboid.

The Tuberosity Joint Angle

Bohler[18] in 1931 described the tuberosity joint angle, or "salient" angle, that is noted on the lateral radiographic projection (see Fig 35–8). This angle is formed by the intersection of two lines: (1) a line from the highest point on the posterior articular surface to the most superior point of the calcaneal tuberosity (see Fig 35–8,A) and (2) a line from the highest point on the anterior process of the calcaneus to the highest part of the posterior articular surface (see Fig 35–8,B). Bohler[18] considered the normal angle to be between 30 and 35 degrees, while Palmer[145] reported that the angle can vary from 10 to 40 degrees. Stephenson[185] also reports a great deal of variation in the tuberosity joint angle in the normal foot, from 25 to 40 degrees with an average of 35 degrees.[185] The angles in the right and left calcanei of the same individual are equal.[18]

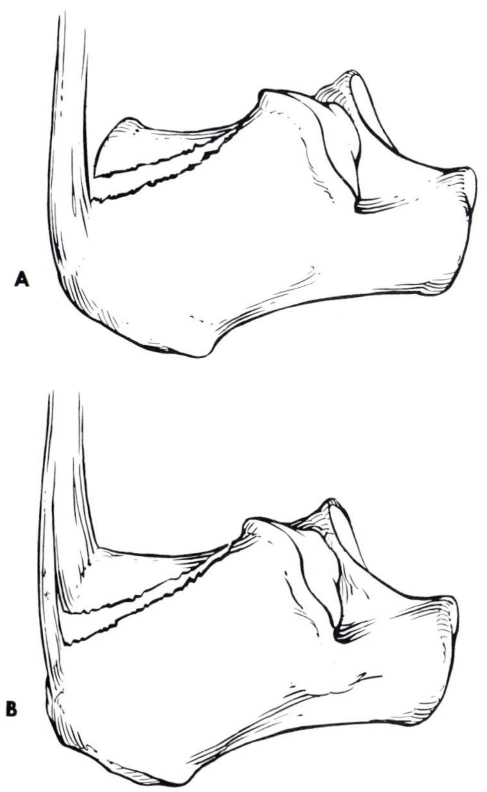

FIG 35–10.
A, according to Sarafian,[171] the upper portion of the posterior surface is free from attachment of the Achilles tendon. **B,** according to Lowy,[116] however, there is great variability at the point of insertion of the Achilles tendon. As indicated here, the Achilles tendon can insert very proximally on the calcaneus.

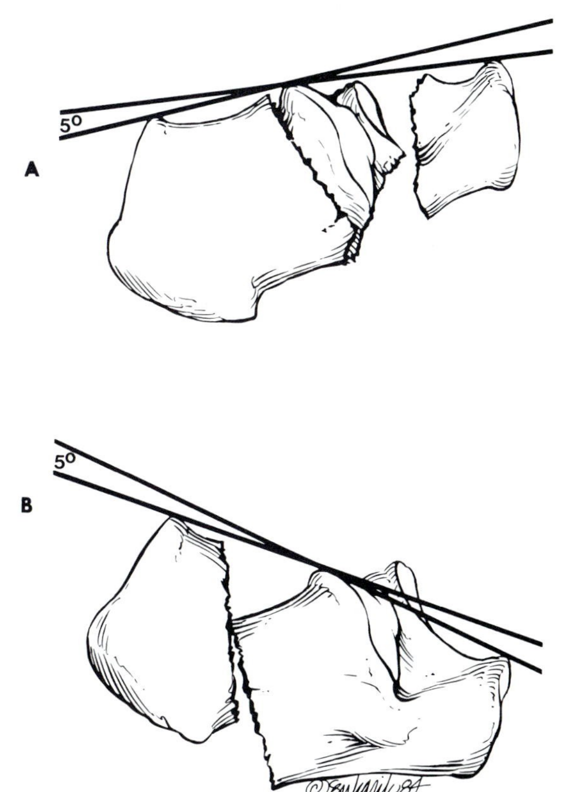

FIG 35–11.
A, intra-articular fracture with a decrease in Bohler's tuberosity joint angle. **B,** extra-articular fracture with a decrease in Bohler's tuberosity joint angle.

In severe fractures of the os calcis, this angle becomes smaller, straight, or even reversed.[142] The angle can therefore be taken as a relative measure of the degree of compression and deformity in calcaneus fractures.[160, 171] According to Bohler[18] the displacement evidenced by a change in the angle is maintained by the muscle pull of the gastrocnemius.

While Stephenson[185] stresses that the tuberosity joint angle is a measure of the height of the posterior facet, McLaughlin[118] pointed out that reduction or reversal of the tuberosity joint angle simply measures the degree of proximal displacement of the tuberosity and can therefore be decreased in both intra-articular and extra-articular fractures of the calcaneus (Fig 35–11). Rosendahl-Jensen[166] also stresses that the angle is simply an expression of the form of the calcaneus and that it gives no information on the position of the surfaces of the subtalar joint or the location of the bone in relationship to the other bones of the tarsus.

The tuberosity joint angle can therefore be an expression of both posterior facet involvement in an intra-articular fracture and simple proximal displacement of the tuberosity of the calcaneus in fractures that are entirely extra-articular[25, 30, 118, 166, 185] (Fig 35–11). This must be kept in mind when considering its value in evaluation of fractures of the calcaneus.

Crucial Angle of Gissane

A thick and strong cortical strut exists within the calcaneus and extends from the front of the bone to the posterior margin of the posterior subtalar facet. This strut is angled, and the angle supports the lateral process of the talus.[52] This angle was termed "the crucial angle" by Gissane in 1947 (see Fig 35–8,A).[52, 66] According to Stephenson,[185] the crucial angle also shows a great deal of individual variation that ranges from 120 to 145 degrees with an average of 130 degrees in the normal, uninjured foot. Again, the angle in the two normal feet of an individual should be approximately equal.[157] The densities on the lateral radiograph that make up the crucial angle consist of the subchondral bone of the posterior facet and the subchondral bone of the anterior and medial facets. The angle therefore gives some indication of the relationship of the posterior, anterior, and medial facets.

When axial compression forces are applied, the lateral process of the talus acts as a bursting wedge that points directly into the crucial angle in the floor of the calcaneal sulcus.[63, 80] This produces the primary fracture line in calcaneal fractures and extends from the crucial angle to the inferior surface of the calcaneus (see Figs 35–36,A and 35–37,A).[51] Secondary fracture lines may also emanate from the crucial angle.[51, 185]

Classification

Attempts to classify fractures of the calcaneus have been made by many authors.[18, 33, 51, 82, 168] However, no single classification system has been completely satisfactory, largely because of the implications of a statement by Cotton and Wilson[37] in 1908 that it was not possible to classify "the fracture in a nut subjected to the stresses of a nutcracker." Horn[86] also emphasized that any classification system is limited by the tremendous number of variations possible in fracture patterns.

For practical purposes, fractures of the calcaneus are usually divided into two general groups: intra-articular and extra-articular fractures.[76] Essex-Lopresti strongly emphasized the importance of simplifying these classification systems by dividing calcaneus fractures generally into those that involve the subtalar joint and those that do not.[52] This simple classification is based on the fact that an extra-articular calcaneus fracture tends to have a very good prognosis while the prognosis of an intra-articular fracture is much less predictable and satisfactory.[52]

Extra-articular fractures of the calcaneus are less common and compose from 25% to 35% of all calcaneus fractures.* Intra-articular fractures make up from 70% to 75% of all calcaneus fractures.[18, 52, 114, 211] Within the intra-articular fracture group, Essex-Lopresti identified two distinct fracture patterns: tongue and joint depression.[52] Essex-Lopresti further divided extra-articular fractures into tuberosity fractures and fractures involving the calcaneocuboid joint. Essex-Lopresti stressed the importance of long-term disability of associated subluxation of the talar head at the talonavicular joint in comminuted calcaneus fractures and of involvement of the calcaneocuboid joint.

References 18, 52, 105, 106, 114, 121.

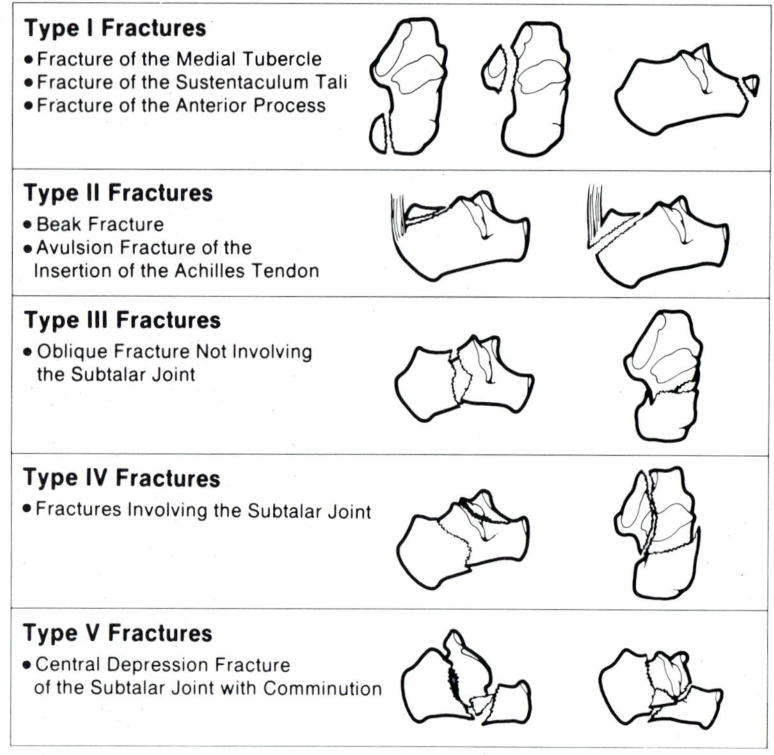

FIG 35–12.
Classification of calcaneal fractures by Rowe et al.[168] (Adapted from Rowe CR, Sakellarides HT, Freeman PA, et al: *JAMA* 184:920–923, 1963.)

Rowe et al.[168] presented a classification modified from the system presented by Watson-Jones.[200] They divided fractures of the calcaneus into five types (Fig 35–12). The first three types are separate from the last two in that they do not involve the subtalar joint. These extra-articular fractures are easier to treat and have a uniformly better prognosis than do fractures in which the subtalar joint is involved.[52, 142]

Stephenson[186] uses a classification modified from that of Warrick and Bremner[199] for intra-articular fractures. The mechanism of injury (shear, compression, or shear-compression), the primary sagittal fracture line location in relation to the posterior facet, the number of major displaced fracture fragments (two or three parts), and the shape of the thalamic fragment (tongue or joint depression type) are considered (Fig 35–13).

In this section I will use a classification system (Table 35–1) based primarily upon that of Rowe et al.[168]

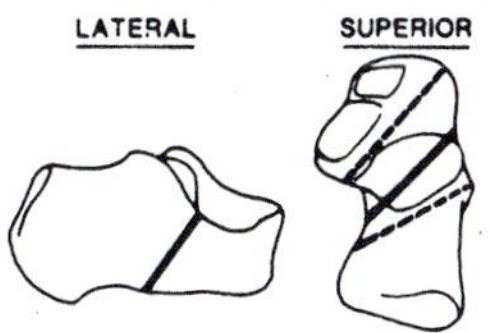

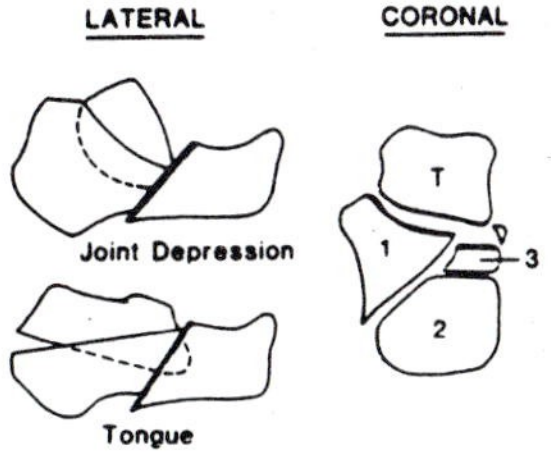

FIG 35–13.

Line drawings showing the types of fractures. The differences in the patterns of the fractures, moving from the top to the bottom of the figure, are the result of increasing injuring forces. The *thick solid lines* show the primary fracture, as described by Essex-Lopresti. This is an intra-articular fracture that involves the posterior facet. The *thick broken lines* show the other paths that the primary sagittal fracture may take, either lateral to the posterior facet or along the calcaneal sulcus medial to the facet. (The fracture line that goes through the calcaneal sulcus is through a nonarticulating portion of the subtalar joint, but this fracture is considered to be intra-articular.) The *thin broken lines* show the outlines and positions of the displaced fragments in the two-part and three-part fractures. Note that the two-part and three-part shear-compression fractures (shown only as lateral views and as coronal sections through the posterior facet of the talus and the posterior facet of the calcaneus) may be one of two types, either a joint depression or a tongue fracture. In the two-part compression fracture, the superomedial fragment *(1)* and the fragment of the tuberosity *(2)* are present, separated by the undisplaced sagittal fracture that is visible only in the coronal plane. However, they are considered as one fragment (of a two-part fracture) for purposes of classification and treatment. If greater force is applied to a supinated foot, the fragment of the tuberosity *(2)* may be displaced superiorly with respect to the superomedial fragment *(1),* and then there is a three-part compression fracture (not illustrated). *T* = talus; *1* = superomedial fragment; *2* = fragment of the tuberosity; *3* = fragment of the posterior facet. (From Stephenson JR: *J Bone Joint Surg [Am]* 69:115–130, 1987. Used by permission.)

TABLE 35–1.
Author's Classification of Calcaneus Fractures

I. *Extra-articular fractures*
 A. Anterior process fracture (This can occasionally be intra-articular, in which case the results may be poor.)
 B. Tuberosity fracture: beak and avulsion fractures
 C. Medial or lateral process fracture
 D. Fracture of the body without involvement of the subtalar joint
II. *Intra-articular fractures*
 A. Sustentaculum tali fracture
 B. Tongue fracture
 C. Joint depression fracture
 D. Comminuted fracture
III. *Stress fractures*

(Fig 35–12) for extra-articular fractures and on that of Essex-Lopresti[52] (Table 35–2) for intra-articular fractures. A discussion of the various fracture types will follow this classification system. I have considered sustentaculum tali fractures as intra-articular fractures because the sustentaculum contains the middle subtalar facet on its superior surface. Also, although anterior process fractures are considered to be extra-articular, they can involve the subtalar or calcaneocuboid joints, in which instance the prognosis is less favorable.

Mechanism of Injury

In addition to having distinctly different prognoses, extra-articular and intra-articular fractures of the os calcis are the result of different mechanisms of injury.

Cave stressed that many extra-articular fractures result from twisting injuries that avulse fragments of bone, such as the avulsion fracture of the Achilles tendon insertion that results from a violent contraction of the gastrocnemius-soleus muscle group (see Fig 35–30) or the avulsion of the anterior process of the calcaneus caused by inversion of the foot.[29] Dodson[49] also emphasizes that twisting injuries of the foot produce the relatively minor extra-articular fractures. A direct blow can also result in fracture of the medial tubercle or an extra-articular fracture of the body of the calcaneus without displacement.[49]

On the other hand, intra-articular fractures are most commonly the result of a fall from a height with the patient's weight concentrated on the heels on landing.* Dodson[49] stresses that any patient who falls over 2 ft should be suspected of having a calcaneus fracture.

Although intra-articular calcaneus fractures are usually secondary to a fall from a height in civilian life, in war they usually result from a force inflicted from below, such as an exploding land mine beneath a military vehicle.[77] These war fractures are usually even more comminuted than those caused by falls and are often open with extensive soft-tissue damage.[78]

It is important to emphasize that every degree of severity of fracture can result from a fall, depending upon the distance fallen, the quality of the bone in the calcaneus, the firmness of the surface on which the patient lands, and the position of the foot and leg when the foot strikes the ground.[79, 137, 149] It is the various combinations of bone quality, height of fall, and foot position that produce the varying degrees of comminution and fracture patterns that make classification of these fractures so difficult.[79] Also, Barnard[11] correctly emphasizes that such a fall with the patient landing on a hard surface dissipates force to the ankle joint, skin, fibrous tissue, bone, and soft-tissue structures about the ankle, midfoot, and forefoot. Therefore, the actual fracture of the calcaneus with resulting damage to the subtalar joint is only a small part of the overall injury. The severity of the soft-tissue injury associated with these fractures must be kept in mind when treatment and results are considered. Finally, because the usual mechanism is a fall from a height, these fractures are bilateral in up to 9% of patients.[105, 106, 142, 149, 190]

Since a fall from a height is the most common cause of these fractures, associated injuries in general are quite frequent.[52, 83, 106, 168, 173] Rowe et al.[168] noted associated injuries in 26% of all patients with calcaneus fractures, while associated injuries were reported in 60% of the patients reported by Lance et al.[105, 106] and

TABLE 35–2.
Classification of Essex-Lopresti

I. *Fractures not involving the subtalar joint*
 A. Tuberosity fractures
  1. Beak type
  2. Avulsion of the medial border
  3. Vertical fracture
  4. Horizontal fracture
 B. Fractures involving only the calcaneocuboid joint
  1. Parrot-nose type
  2. Various types
II. *Fractures involving the subtalar joint*
 A. Without displacement
 B. With displacement
  1. Tongue-type of displacement
  2. Central lateral depression of the joint
  3. Sustentaculum tali fracture
  4. Comminution from below (including severe tongue and joint depression types)
  5. From behind and forward with dislocation of the subtalar joint

**References 49, 54, 82, 114, 137, 189, 201.*

in nearly 70% of those reported by Slatis et al.[179, 180] These injuries include compression fractures of the lumbar spine, which have been reported in 3% to 12% of cases,[52, 83, 106, 168, 173] and associated lower-extremity fractures, which can occur in up to 10% of patients.[211]

Cotton and Henderson[36] noted that such falls result in vertical compression of the calcaneus, which then expands laterally and pushes bone out beneath the fibula. The body of the calcaneus is therefore reduced in height and spread out laterally so that a considerable mass of bone piles up beneath the lateral malleolus and may impinge on it later.[77] King stresses that the area beneath the posterior facet has a paucity of trabeculae and therefore a downward force on the fixed os calcis, such as occurs in a fall, can result in impaction of the outer two thirds of the posterior facet into the os calcis.[100]

Palmer[145] gave a very clear explanation of the mechanism of calcaneal fracture secondary to a fall. According to him, the tuber calcanei is forced upward by the impact when it strikes the ground while the articular portion of the calcaneus is driven downward by the talus, thus resulting in a vertical shearing fracture[15] (Fig 35–14). If the foot is in a marked varus position when it strikes the ground, an extra-articular fracture of the medial tubercle can result. However, if the foot is in valgus on impact, a lateral shearing fracture will result. In most cases, this lateral shearing fracture is not restricted to the tubercle.

Instead, the line of fracture starts on the medial side and runs laterally and upward to enter the posterior facet of the talocalcaneal joint (see Fig 35–14,A). This primary fracture line separates the calcaneus into a posterolateral body fragment and an anteromedial sustentaculum fragment. With continued force and impaction, a secondary fracture line exiting posteriorly creates the thalamic fragment containing the depressed posterior facet. If the secondary fracture line exits superiorly, the thalamic fragment has been classified as a central depression-type fracture. A tongue-type fracture is created when the secondary fracture line exits posteriorly. The anteromedial sustentacular fragment remains undisplaced under the talus. The thalamic fragment separates from the lateral wall as the talus drives it into the cancellous body of the calcaneus. This results in lateral displacement of the calcaneal body, which predisposes to fibulocalcaneal impingement and peroneal tendon entrapment. When the compression force is removed, the lateral fracture recoils downward to form a step-off in the joint space (Fig 35–14,C).

Radiographic Diagnosis

Proper radiographic visualization is essential in both evaluation and treatment of calcaneal fractures. For any classification system to be accurate, excellent radiographic visualization of all components of the fracture is essential.[2, 109, 142, 175] Most authors feel that any patient with a calcaneal fracture should be evaluated by a minimum of three radiographic views: an anteroposterior view (the so-called dorsoplantar view), a lateral view, and an axial view of the foot.[49, 81, 83, 112, 178] Should

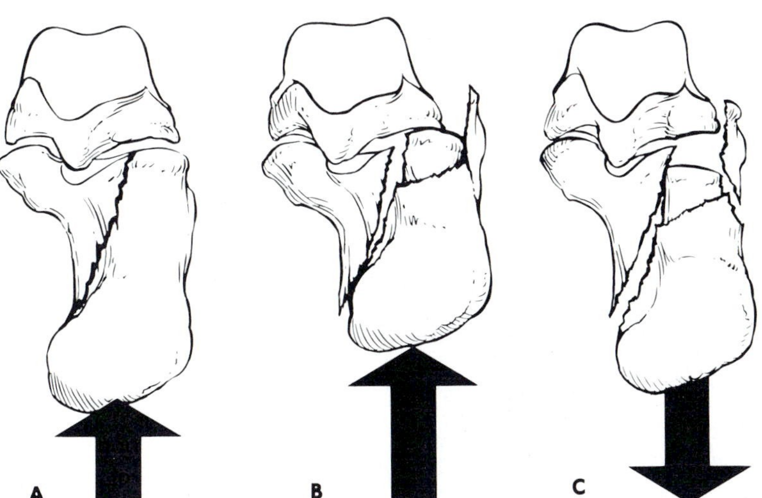

FIG 35–14.
Mechanism of a fracture of the calcaneus according to Palmer. **A,** the fracture line begins medially and runs laterally to exit into the posterior facet. **B,** the articular surface is maximally displaced at the time of injury. **C,** when the compression force is removed, the lateral surface recoils downward to form a step-off in the articular surface of the posterior facet. (Adapted from Palmer I: *J Bone Joint Surg [Am]* 30:2–8, 1948.)

these radiographs reveal an intra-articular fracture, CT evaluation is necessary to evaluate intra-articular extension, the degree of comminution, posterior facet depression, calcaneofibular impingement, and peroneal tendon entrapment. Additionally, an anteroposterior view of the ankle may be helpful.

Because fractures of the calcaneus may be bilateral, it may be advisable to take radiographs of both feet.[63] Also, Hazlett recommends taking radiographs of the uninjured foot to establish a baseline for Bohler's angle and to detect any congenital anomalies that may confuse the appearance of the contralateral fractured calcaneus.[81] Additionally, Horn,[86] Hermann,[83] and O'Connell et al.[142] all recommend routinely taking lumbar spine radiographs in patients with calcaneal fractures, whether or not they have back complaints, in an effort to detect mild compression fractures of the lumbar and lower thoracic vertebra that may go unnoted.

Standard Radiographic Views

The anteroposterior view of the midfoot (Fig 35–15) is taken with the foot flat on the cassette and the central ray directed vertically downward and centered over the calcaneocuboid joint. This view demonstrates the extent of involvement and degree of displacement of fractures into the calcaneocuboid joint.[2, 10, 190] Since Vestad[196] reports that 23% of calcaneal fractures involve the calcaneocuboid joint, this view is essential in evaluation. In addition, in severe fractures, medial subluxation of the talus at the talonavicular joint can occur and is well demonstrated on this anteroposterior view of the midfoot.[86, 141, 189] Finally, the amount of lateral spread of the lateral calcaneal surface is clearly visualized on the anteroposterior view.[86]

The lateral view (Fig 35–16) is useful in detecting the amount of vertical displacement of the tuberosity of the calcaneus as is reflected in Bohler's tuberosity joint angle.[2, 190] In addition, it may or may not demonstrate involvement of the posterior facet of the subtalar joint and/or the calcaneocuboid joint.[2]

The axial view (Fig 35–17) clearly demonstrates the medial concave and lateral convex surfaces of the body of the talus.[2, 190] Also, the articular margin of the posterior facet located on the lateral side of the foot and the sustentaculum tali and medial subtalar facet joint located on the medial side of the foot are clearly seen in this view.[2] Widening of the body of the calcaneus is also demonstrated on the axial view.[122, 123] According to McReynolds[122, 123] the axial view demonstrates the most significant deformity in calcaneal fractures, that being the marked depression and overriding of the superior medial fragment. It clearly demonstrates the main fracture line that begins in the medial cortex of the calcaneus and inclines upward and outward into the posterior facet joint.

Essex-Lopresti[52] cautions that interpretation of the axial view can be difficult. He stresses that in the axial view the appearance of the subtalar joint will depend upon the angle at which the central ray strikes it and often is not shown at all on this view. The main change in appearance obtained by altering the angle at which the tube is directed is one of lengthening or foreshortening

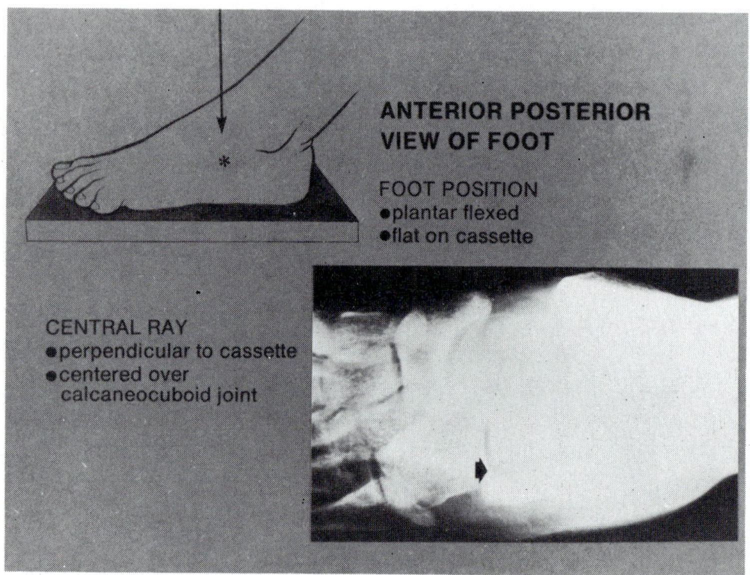

FIG 35–15.
Anteroposterior view of the foot. Note the fracture into the calcaneocuboid joint *(arrow)*.

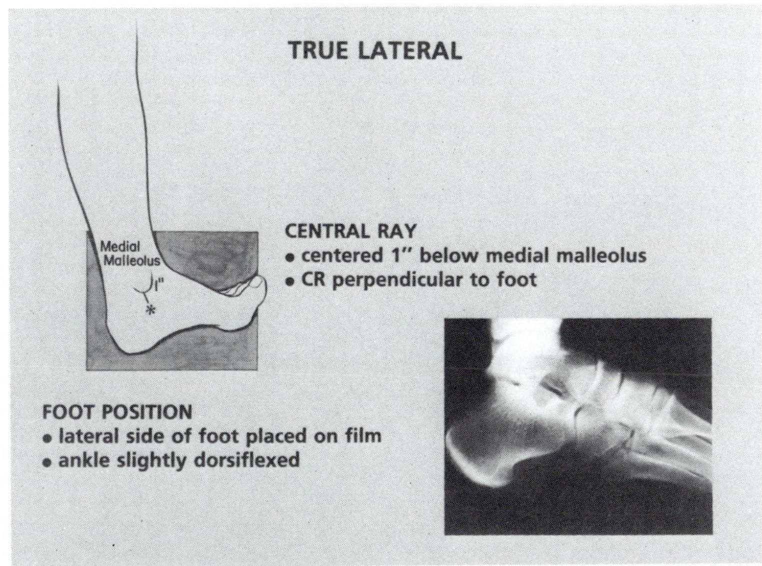

FIG 35–16.
Lateral view of the foot.

the body of the calcaneus. Unless the central x-ray strikes the subtalar joint tangentially, its outline will not show up against the mass of spongy bone anterior to it. Furthermore, Essex-Lopresti points out that if the joint is simply displaced downward and forward, that is, in the line of the central ray, no deformity will be present. Finally, Stephenson emphasizes the importance of the axial view being taken with the radiographic tube tangential to the posterior facet in order to delineate any step-off in the posterior facet joint.

An anteroposterior view of the ankle has been recommended by a few authors[110, 123, 190] because it demonstrates piling up of bone from the lateral cortex of the calcaneus beneath the fibular malleolus. Additionally, it will detect associated ankle injuries.[190] In addition to the routine views described above, special views that demonstrate the subtalar joint in detail may be helpful in correctly classifying these fractures and demonstrating the joint congruity present in intra-articular calcaneal fractures.[4, 22, 191, 196]

Radiographic Evaluation of the Subtalar Joint

The oblique radiographs of Broden and Anthonsen demonstrate the posterior articular facets. Anthonsen's oblique lateral, medial oblique axial, and lateral oblique axial views demonstrate the calcaneocuboid and anterior and posterior talocalcaneal joints. These special views have been replaced with CT evaluation because this allows a better evaluation of the fracture characteristics with less patient discomfort. CT evaluation can be accomplished without removing a splint. If a CT scan is not available, these views are useful.

Anthonsen's View.—Anthonsen[5] described a radiographic view in which the central ray is directed at a point just below the medial malleolus with the dorsiflexed foot in the lateral position on the film. The tube is tilted 25 degrees caudally and 30 degrees dorsoventrally (Fig 35–18).[195, 199] According to Anthonsen, this view is particularly useful in visualizing the posterior and middle facets of the subtalar joint.[4, 190] Schottstaedt,[175] Soeur and Remy,[184] and Warrick and Bremner[199] strongly recommend the use of Anthonsen's view. However, according to Isherwood[90] it is often difficult to produce these two roentgen tube tilts simultaneously. Although foot position can be adjusted to counter this problem, he believes that double angulation of the tube combined with foot positioning makes it difficult to reproduce the view. He therefore presented three additional oblique views for evaluating the subtalar joint: oblique lateral, medial oblique axial, and lateral oblique axial.

Oblique Dorsoplantar View (Oblique Lateral).—The inner border of the foot is placed on the film and the sole inclined 45 degrees to the film. The tube is centered 1 in. below and 1 in. anterior to the lateral malleolus. This view clearly demonstrates the anterior process of the calcaneus and the calcaneocuboid joint (Fig 35–19).[190]

Medial Oblique Axial View.—The foot is dorsiflexed and inverted, the position being maintained by a broad bandage held by the seated patient. The knee is rotated 60 degrees, and the foot rests on a 30 degree wedge. The tube is directed axially, tilted 10 degrees toward the head, and centered 1 in. below and 1 in. anterior to the lateral malleolus (Fig 35–20). This projection gives an "end-on" view of the tarsal canal as noted in An-

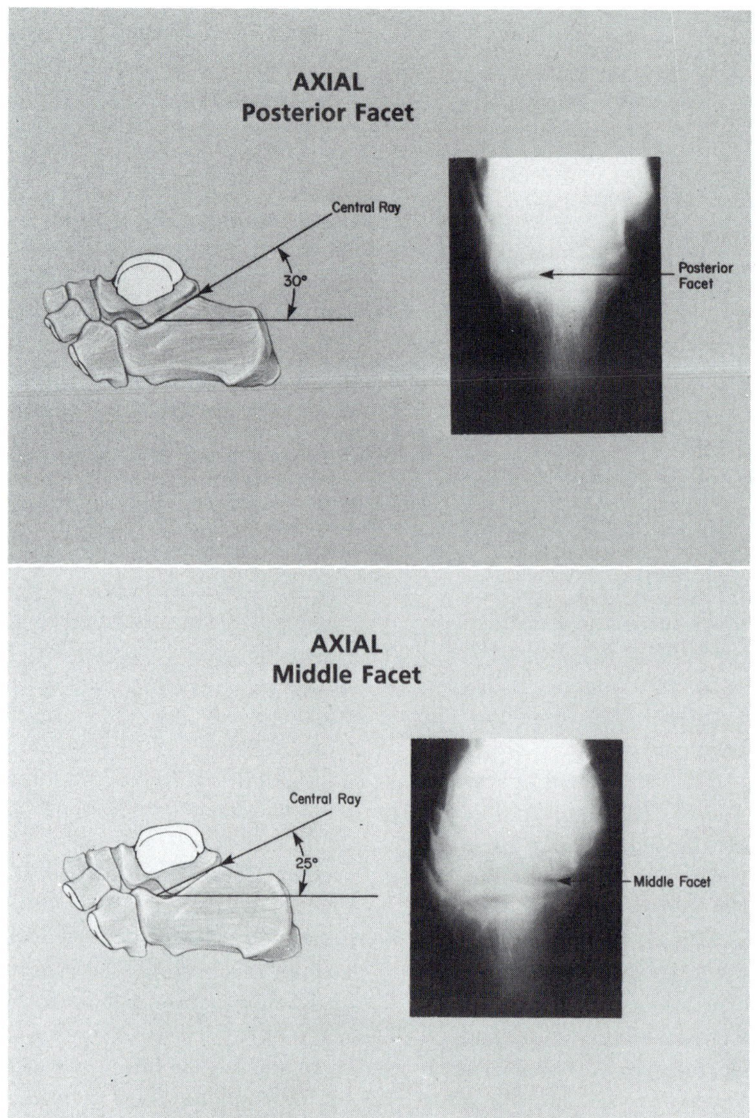

FIG 35–17.
Axial view of the heel. The variation in the angle of the central ray is necessary for visualization of the medial and posterior facets.

thonsen's view and has the added advantages of (1) placing the sustentaculum close to the film for bone detail and (2) being more easily reproduced by having a fixed angulation of the tube. The medial oblique axial view is used to demonstrate the medial joint and also to give a tangential view of the convexity of the posterior joint.

Lateral Oblique Axial View.—The foot is dorsiflexed and inverted, the position again being maintained by asymmetric pull on a broad bandage. The knee is laterally rotated 60 degrees and the foot rested on a 30-degree wedge. The tube is directed axially, tilted 10 degrees toward the head, and centered 1 in. below the medial malleolus. The tube direction and tilt are therefore fixed for both the medial and lateral oblique axial views (Fig 35–21). The lateral oblique axial view is excellent for demonstrating the posterior facet joint in profile.

Broden's Projections.—Broden's views (Fig 35–22) are helpful postoperatively to evaluate subtalar joint congruity. Any hardware used in fixation will cause radiation beam scattering in a CT scan. By using Broden's two projections, the entire posterior facet is evaluated from front to back.

Projection I.—The patient is supine. The leg and foot are rotated inward 45 degrees with the ankle joint

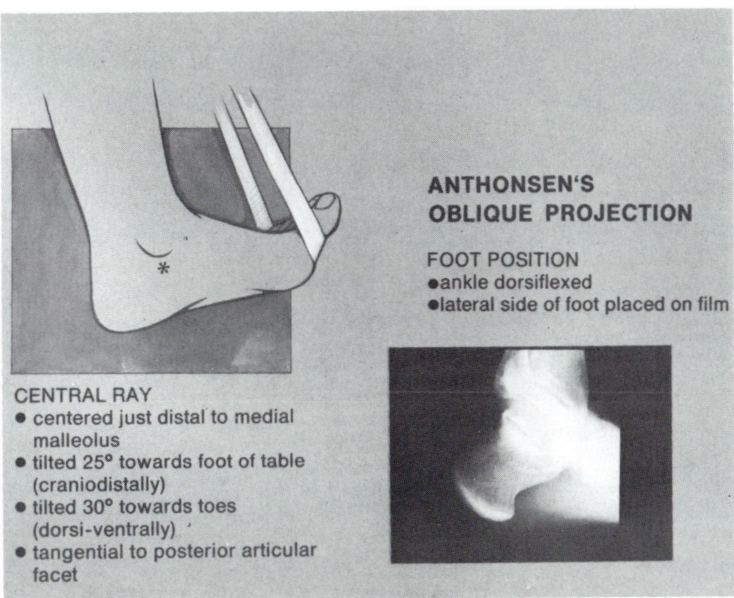

FIG 35–18.
Anthonsen's view of the calcaneus. This view demonstrates the posterior and medial facets of the subtalar joint.

at a right angle. The central ray is directed at a point 2 to 3 cm caudoventrally to the lateral malleolus. Four exposures are taken with the tube angled 40, 30, 20, and 10 degrees respectively toward the head. The picture taken with the tube angled at 40 degrees demonstrates the anterior part of the talocalcaneal joint, while the exposure with the tube angled at 10 degrees demonstrates the posterior aspect. Exposures with the tube angled at 30 or 20 degrees may demonstrate the articulation between the sustentaculum tali and the talus (Fig 35–22,A).[22]

Projection II.—The patient is supine. The foot and leg are turned 45 degrees outwards with the ankle joint at a right angle. The central ray is directed at a point 2 cm caudal-anterior to the medial malleolus with the tube angled 15 degrees toward the head. Three exposures with a difference of 3 or 4 degrees are then made

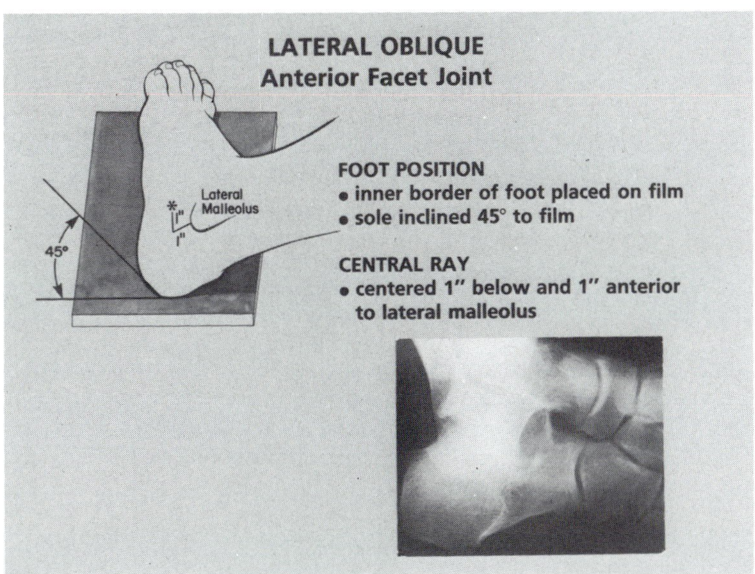

FIG 35–19.
Oblique dorsoplantar view (oblique lateral). Note the clarity of the anterior process and the calcaneocuboid joint.

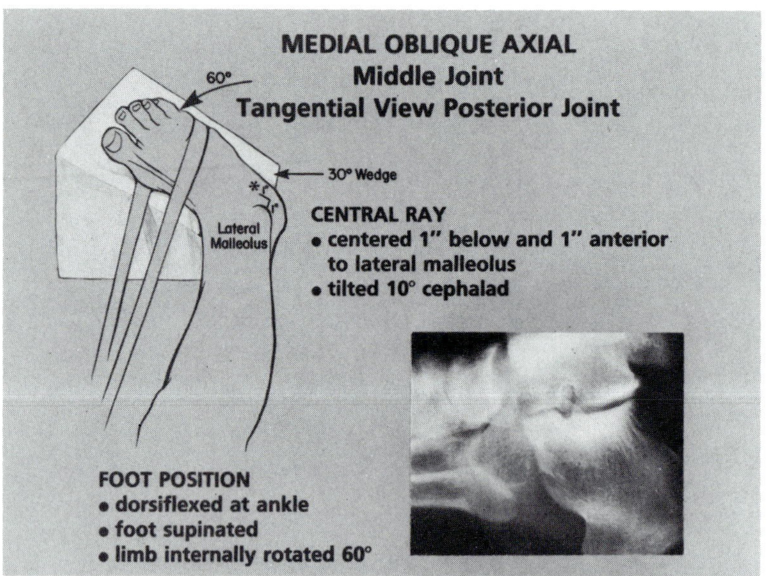

FIG 35–20.
Medial oblique axial view. Note the clarity of the medial and posterior facets of the subtalar joint.

(Fig 35–22). According to Broden, this view is useful in demonstrating the height of the articular cartilage and also in demonstrating dorsoplantar compression at the joint surface. Additionally, the sinus tarsi is distinctly visible.[22]

Conventional Tomography and Computerized Axial Tomography

The value of CT has been questioned by some authors in evaluating calcaneus fractures.[112, 182–184] From work presented by Gilmer,[65] Guyer,[72] and Lowrie et al,[115] it is clear that CT scanning is the best way to evaluate intra-articular calcaneus fractures. CT studies have also demonstrated that disruption of the articular surface is more common than previously recognized by plain radiographic evaluation. Lowrie[122] found that the best position for coronal imaging is with the foot in 20 degrees of plantar flexion by placing the knee in 50 degrees of flexion and the foot up to 30 degrees from the table, with the CT gantry angled 15 degrees toward the foot from vertical. This allows a 90-degree projection to

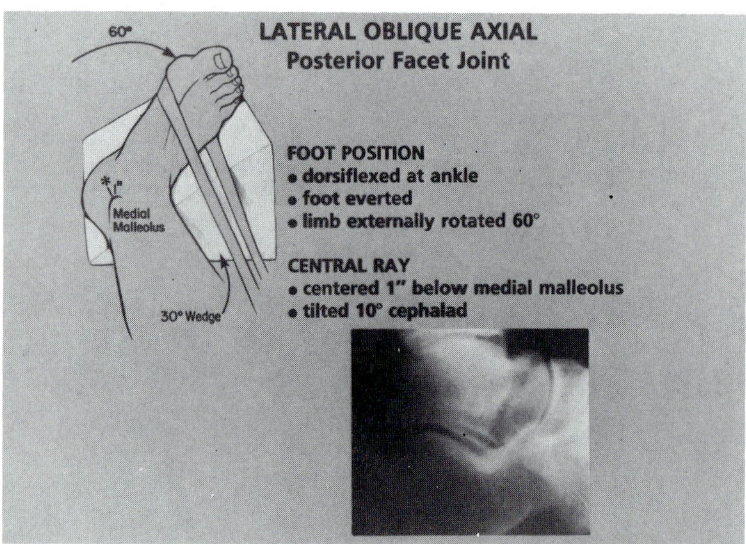

FIG 35–21.
Lateral oblique axial view. The posterior facet is seen in profile.

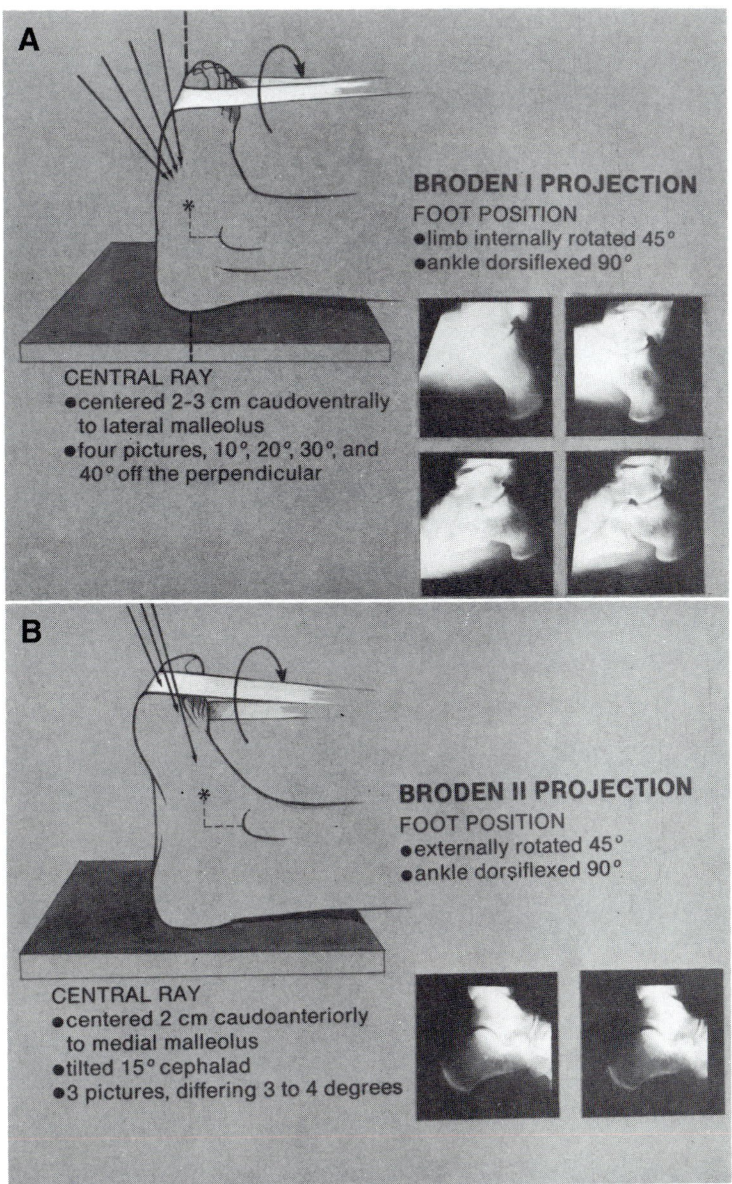

FIG 35–22.
Broden's radiographic views of the foot.[22] **A,** Broden's projection I. With this view one can see the entire posterior facet from front to back. **B,** Broden's projection II. This view demonstrates dorsoplantar compression at the joint surface and sinus tarsi.

the subtalar joint. Three-millimeter cuts are imaged at 3- to 5-mm intervals. The coronal image provides excellent evaluation of posterior facet disruption, comminution and depression of fragments, widening and loss of calcaneal height, and peroneal and flexor hallucis longus tendon impingement. Axial views allow further assessment of major fragments, calcaneal widening, and talonavicular and calcaneocuboid joint involvement.

Lowrie et al[122] found that intra-articular calcaneus fractures could be classified into four patterns based on CT evaluation:

1. Inverted Y.—The most common type of pattern revealed the posterior facet split into approximately two equal fragments diverging from each other and a large posterior fragment (Fig 35–23,A).
2. Large fragment type.—The posterior facet is complete or has a small fragment medially or laterally.
3. Longitudinal split.—A vertical fracture line through the posterior facet produces approximately equal fragments.
4. Comminuted.—The posterior facet is fractured into several fragments.

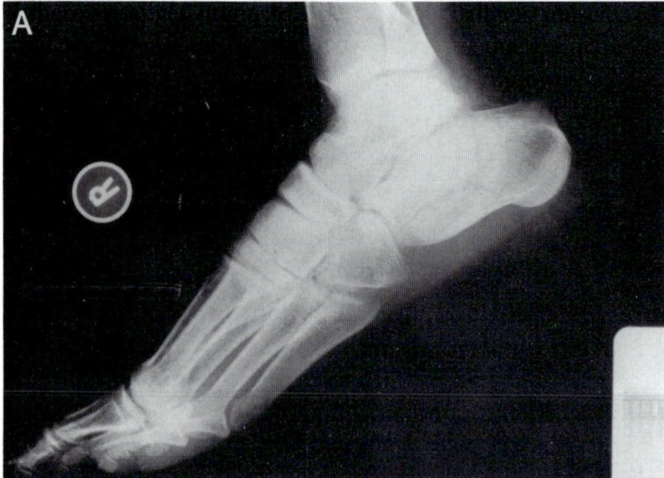

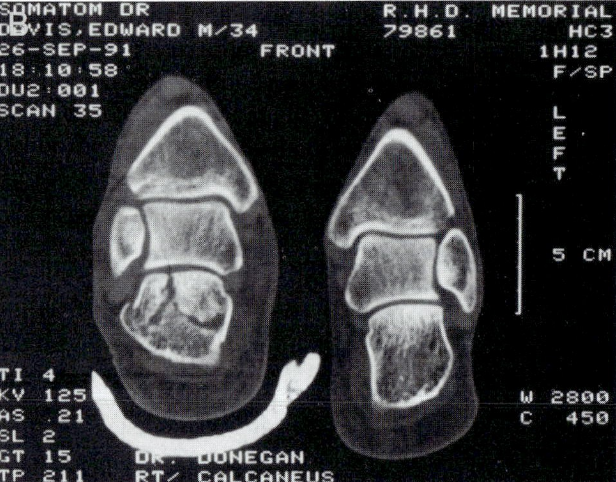

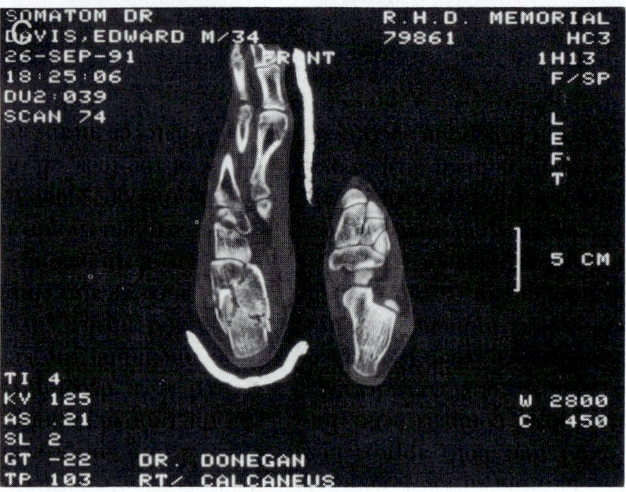

FIG 35–23.
A, lateral radiograph showing an intra-articular joint depression fracture. **B,** coronal CT clearly shows posterior facet disruption with a common inverted Y fracture pattern. **C,** axial CT demonstrates comminution and extension of the primary fracture line just medial to the calcaneocuboid joint. With minimal posterior facet depression and widening, this patient was treated conservatively.

Gilmer et al.[65] found that a large amount of the posterior facet is usually involved, contrary to the assertions of McReynolds and Bordeaux.

Allon and Mears[4] have found three-dimensional CT scans useful, especially in evaluating the rotational displacement of major fragments. In selected cases, computer-generated three-dimensional plastic models were helpful in preoperative planning. This requires high-quality three-dimensional hardware and software.

Zeiss et al.[212] found magnetic resonance imaging (MRI) for the evaluation of acute calcaneus fractures to be unsatisfactory. MRI is unable to image small fragments of cortical bone. The presence of small fragments is obscured by a change in normal marrow signal by contusion, hemorrhage, and edema.

Treatment

The variety of approaches to the treatment of calcaneal fractures that are presented in the literature are evidence of the frustration associated with managing this fracture. Standardization of treatment is nearly impossible because the damage sustained by the os calcis varies within such great limits as to present difficult problems in management.[78, 110] Little disagreement surrounds the treatment of extra-articular fractures, with good results reported in the majority of cases.[47, 53, 106, 168] It is the management of displaced intra-articular fractures (involving the subtalar joint) where the majority of controversy exists.* As emphasized by Dart et al.[42] most authors champion a particular technique, but fracture patterns vary so greatly that recommending a single technique for treatment is as rational as treating all fractures of the femur, regardless of location or type, in one particular way. Additionally, a comparison of one method of treatment with another is very difficult because so many variables are present that statistical significance becomes doubtful.[42]

The goal of treatment is solid union with normal motion in the talocalcaneal, calcaneonavicular, and calcaneocuboid joints.[87] All fractures of the calcaneus should be managed as severe injuries and consideration given to admission and elevation to avoid edema and discourage the spread of the fracture hematoma.[42] Pumping motion of the toes and early range of motion of the foot help prevent the development of stiffness and induration, which oftentimes is the overriding disability.[132] Although Horn[86] recommends restoration of the articular congruity, correction of widening of the calcaneus beneath the lateral malleolus, restoration of the height from the malleoli and the plantar surface of the heel pad, and early range of motion to restore function, other authors are not concerned about reduction, but instead encourage early activity and exercise in an effort to restore function to the foot.[13, 150, 169] When dealing with a fractured calcaneus, one must remember this controversy regarding the necessity of fracture reduction in the overall scheme of calcaneus fracture management. I strongly believe the recommendations of Miller,[132] who stresses that any treatment method *must* include early pumping action of the toes and early range of ankle, subtalar, and midfoot motion to prevent stiffness and induration.

One must remember that severe fractures may be less disabling than some of the more minor fractures because a severe fracture can damage the subtalar joint to the degree that it becomes virtually ankylosed.[79] In such cases there may be little pain even when the deformity is severe.[79]

Finally, the ideal method for managing fractures of the calcaneus that involve the subtalar joint has not been discovered.[11] One must remember, however, that the degree of accuracy of anatomic restoration of calcaneal contour may not parallel the excellence of the functional result in many cases.[128]

References 11, 18, 37, 47, 52, 81, 83, 106, 120–123, 128, 145, 152, 156, 168, 185, 190, 203, 210.

Extra-Articular Fractures

Extra-articular fractures (fractures *not* involving the subtalar joint) seem to do well with nearly any form of treatment.[30, 56, 57, 76, 83] Unfortunately, however, these extra-articular fractures constitute only about 25% of all calcaneal fractures.[26, 30, 56, 106]

Allan[3] reports that extra-articular fractures rarely produce disability. Essex-Lopresti[52] found that 92% of patients with extra-articular fractures were back to full work in under 6 months and that 93% had no or only trivial symptoms. Additionally, those extra-articular fractures treated by exercise alone had slightly better results than those treated in plaster.[52] Rosendahl-Jensen[166] reported bad results in only 5.6% of all extra-articular fractures. Pridie[156] also reports that early motion and freedom from weight bearing produces good results in extra-articular fractures and that the patients generally return to their preinjury occupations. Extra-articular fractures, then, as a group, seem to have a favorable long-term prognosis and, unless substantially displaced, can be treated in a conservative fashion. The various types of extra-articular fractures will now be considered.

Fractures of the Anterior Process of the Calcaneus

A fracture of the anterior process of the calcaneus is classified as an avulsion-type fracture of the calcaneus. [44, 168] Although historically this fracture has been considered an unusual injury, recent authors report that the fracture is more common than previously appreciated.[19, 61, 88, 153] This is secondary to the fact that in the past this fracture was often misdiagnosed as a sprain of the ankle. The true incidence of anterior process fractures is difficult to determine because the injury is often missed. Reports of the frequency have varied from 3% to 23% of fractures of the calcaneus.[91, 166, 168]

Anatomy

Anatomically, this portion of the calcaneus has been variously named the anterior lip,[19] the anterior process,[31] the anterosuperior portion,[40] the anterosuperior process,[113] the promontory,[153] and the anterior end of the calcaneus.[200] Whichever term is preferred, this anterior process forms a saddle-shaped promontory that varies in length and breadth.[44, 152] It can be completely absent or overhang the adjacent proximal superior portion of the cuboid similar to a parrot's beak.[92] The anterior process of the calcaneus is not seen roentgenographically before the age of about 10 years,[44, 92] and there is no physis in the area to cause confusion with the fracture. Rarely, however, an accessory ossicle, the calcaneus secundaris, occurs at this site and may be confused with a fracture.[44, 88]

Fractures of the anterior process of the calcaneus have previously been classified as nonarticular calcaneal fractures since they lack involvement of the subtalar joint.[44, 166, 168] However, the saddle-shaped promontory of the anterior process articulates inferiorly with the cuboid.[43, 44, 53, 88, 93] Additionally, when the anterior process is well developed, its medial surface may consist of a cartilaginous articular surface that articulates with the slightly flattened facet on the inferior portion of the neck of the talus and, hence, be involved in the subtalar joint.[92] Therefore, when the fracture includes a large portion of the anterior process, both the subtalar and calcaneocuboid joints may be involved (Fig 35–24). The significance of articular involvement of the calcaneocuboid joint has previously been noted only in relation to the uncommon compression fracture of the cuboid.[88] However, this process, irrespective of its size, articulates over its entire distal surface with the cuboid, and therefore, when it is fractured, the calcaneocuboid joint is usually involved.[93, 153] Thus, although it is conceivable that a small cortical avulsion from the *lateral* cortex of the anterior process could be extra-articular, it is more likely that most of these fractures are indeed intra-articular and involve the calcaneocuboid and oftentimes the anterior talocalcaneal joints.

Indeed, Jahss and Kay believe that the occasional poor results seen with this fracture are related to intra-articular involvement of the fractures.[92] Due to the variation in size of the anterior process and the size and/or presence of the variable anterior talocalcaneal facet, the size of the fracture fragment may determine the presence or absence of articular involvement.

Several ligaments have points of attachment along the calcaneal promontory. The most important of these is the strong bifurcate ligament.[92] It originates from the lateral aspect of the anterior calcaneal process. The calcaneonavicular portion inserts distally into the adjacent navicular, and the calcaneocuboid portion inserts distally into the cuboid.[92] Additionally, a small portion of the extensor digitorum brevis muscle may originate from this bony prominence.[9] Furthermore, the dorsal calcaneocuboid ligament connects the calcaneus and cuboid superiorly. Jahss and Kay[92] clearly delineated

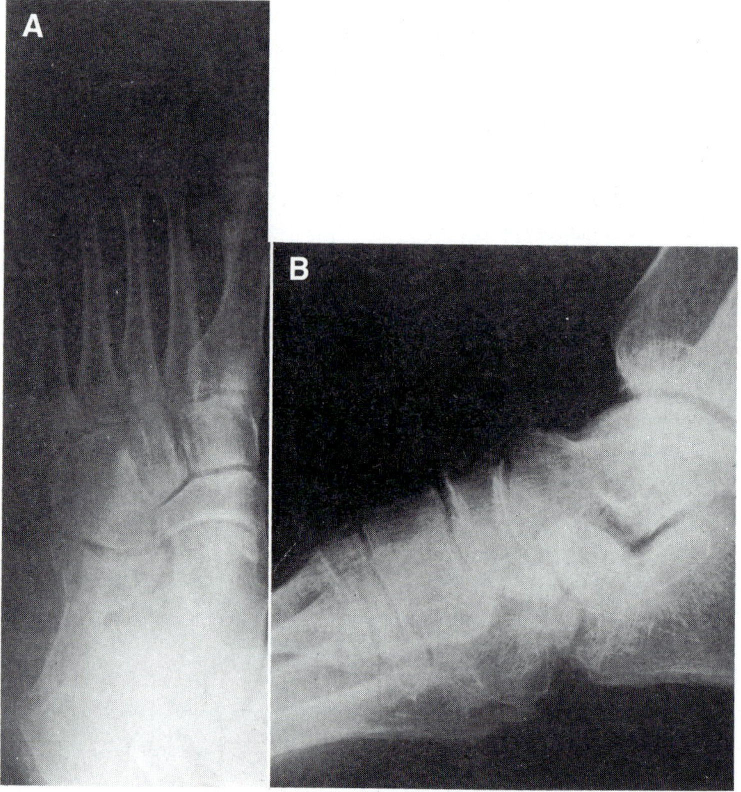

FIG 35–24.
A, displaced fracture of the anterior process of the calcaneus with involvement of the articular surface of the calcaneocuboid joint. Because of the size of the fracture, the anterior subtalar joint is also involved. **B,** degenerative arthritis in the calcaneocuboid, subtalar, and talonavicular joints following symptomatic treatment.

the presence of the anterior interosseous talocalcaneal ligament, which arises in the sinus tarsi from the posterior surface of the base of the anterior calcaneal process and extends dorsally to insert into the inferolateral margin of the neck of the talus. They theorize that the anterior interosseous ligament acts as a stabilizing point of fixation while the calcaneocuboid ligament avulses the anterior process fragment with flexion and inversion of the foot.

Mechanism of Injury

Three mechanisms of injury have been reported to cause a fracture of the anterior process of the calcaneus.[44]

1. Inversion and plantar flexion are the mechanism favored by most authors.[8, 31, 44, 61, 70, 153] This mechanism is felt to result in avulsion of the anterior process by the bifurcate ligament. Because this is the same mechanism that produces the more common sprain of the anterior talofibular ligament of the ankle, this latter entity is often confused with a fracture of the anterior process of the calcaneus. This has resulted in the fracture being termed the "fracture sprain" (Fig 35–25).[19]

Experimental studies on the production of these fractures confirms that the process may be fractured with forced flexion combined with inversion.[92] However, occasionally this mechanism may produce isolated rupture of the calcaneocuboid ligament.[8] Jahss and Kay were unable to determine experimentally whether the anterior interosseous ligament and/or the calcaneocuboid ligament were responsible for isolated fractures of the anterior calcaneal process.[92] They concluded, however, that since both are tight in inversion and plantar flexion, either or both may be responsible for the avulsion.[92]

2. Dachtler[40] described this fracture in association with a handcar injury in which the patient was struck just above the ankle posteriorly and suffered a violent

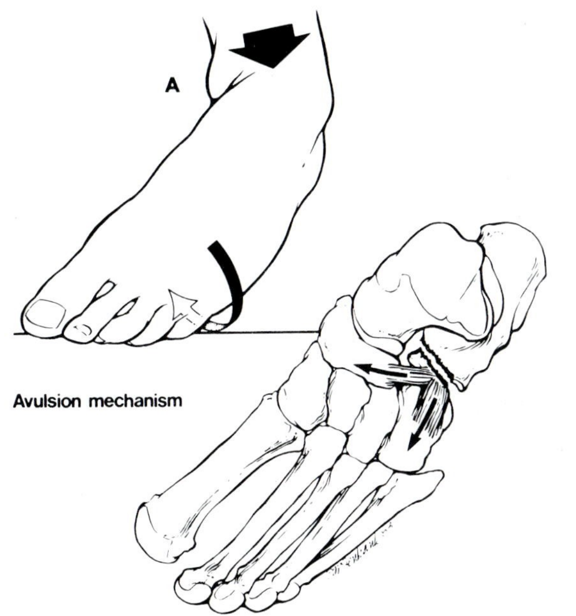

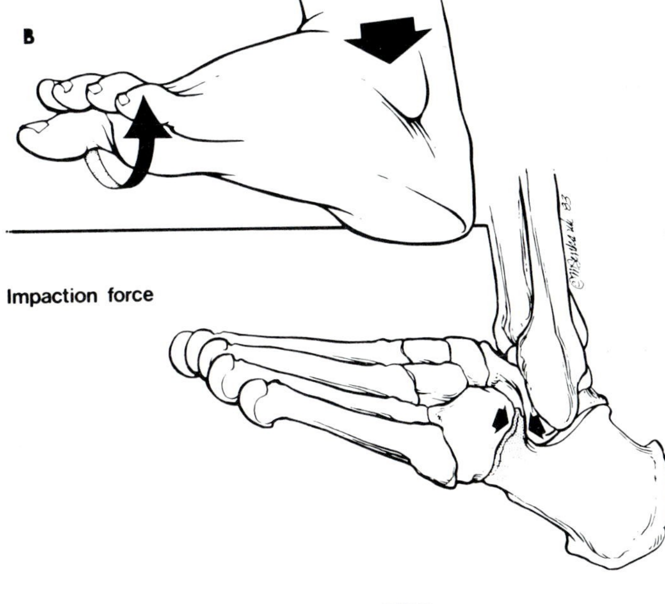

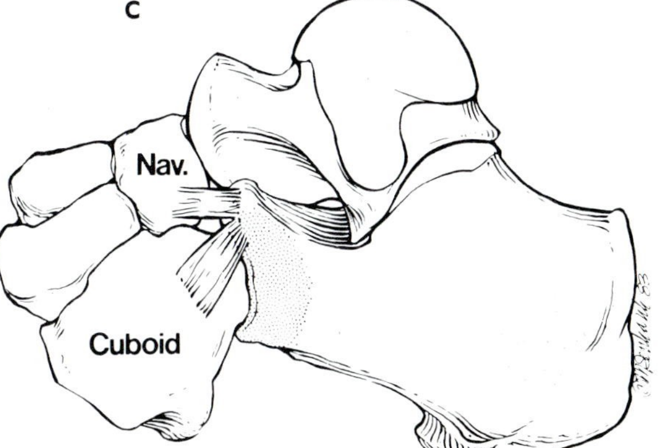

FIG 35–25.
A, inversion and plantar flexion result in avulsion of the anterior process by the bifurcate ligament. This is the same mechanism that produces a sprain of the anterior talofibular ligament, hence the term *sprain fracture.*[2] **B,** the anterior process is forced inward against the cuboid and produces an impaction force that fractures the anterior process. **C,** abduction and supination of the forefoot forces the cuboid against the inferior aspect of the calcaneus. This portion of the anterior process is compressed and posteriorly displaced.[13]

dorsiflexion injury to the foot. In this mechanism, the anterior process is forced downward into equinus against the cuboid to produce an impaction force that fractures the promontory (Fig 35–25).[19, 53, 70]

3. Finally, forceful abduction of the forefoot with a fixed hindfoot can result in a compression fracture of the anterior process of the calcaneus.[88] King[99] reported three cases of such a compression fracture in which the mechanism appeared to be sudden abduction of the forepart of the foot. Jaekle and Clark[91] also reported a similar fracture caused by a crushing injury. Hunt[88] emphasizes the importance of separating this type of fracture from the avulsion type due to the increased injury and more common displacement of the anterior process fracture by this mechanism.[88] He stresses that this results in severe derangement of the calcaneocuboid joint.[88] Gellman emphasizes that this mechanism may also result in damage to adjacent structures, particularly the cuboid articular surface. He theorizes that this may have contributed to the severe peroneal spasticity King noted in his patients (Fig 35–25).[61]

Diagnosis

History.—The history of a "cracking sensation" at the time of the injury is common.[8] The patient may complain of pain, but this is often not severe enough to be disabling.[19] The pain is located on the outer aspect of the midportion of the foot. In the non–weight-bearing position this pain is minimal,[70] and a considerable increase in pain occurs with weight bearing.[8, 19, 53, 61] This often leads patients to ignore the fracture and contributes to the large number of misdiagnoses and late diagnoses reported in the literature.[8, 19, 61]

Clinical Diagnosis.—Clinical examination of the foot reveals localized tenderness and swelling in a small, well-defined area 3 to 4 cm anterior and slightly below the lateral malleolus (Fig 35–26).[8, 44] This corresponds to an area on the dorsal surface of the calcaneocuboid joint.[19, 61] The location of tenderness and swelling should immediately suggest a differential diagnosis that includes injury to the lateral malleolus, the lateral ligaments of the ankle joint, and the base of the fifth metatarsal. *Careful* location of the point of maximal tenderness helps to differentiate these entities.[8, 19, 44, 70] Additionally, supination of the entire foot at the *ankle* does not reproduce pain as it does in a lateral ligamentous injury of the ankle.[8] Manipulation of the foot into inversion and adduction does increase the pain and spasm.[8, 19, 44]

This entity must be suspected when a patient with a history of trauma presents with a picture of marked peroneal spasm following a suspected ankle injury.[39, 99]

Radiographic Diagnosis.—The fracture cannot usually be seen on routine anteroposterior roentgenographs of the foot, and only occasionally is it visible on the lateral view.[19, 40, 44, 61, 153, 209] Although superoinferior views of the foot have been recommended to detect this fracture,[40] most authors agree that this area is best seen on an oblique projection of the foot in which the adjacent bones do not overlap.[53, 113, 209] These oblique views must be taken at several different angles in order to separate the shadow of the anterior process from that of the front and undersurface of the talus.[61] Bachman and Johnson[8] suggest that these radiographs be taken with a central beam directed 15 to 20 degrees superior and pos-

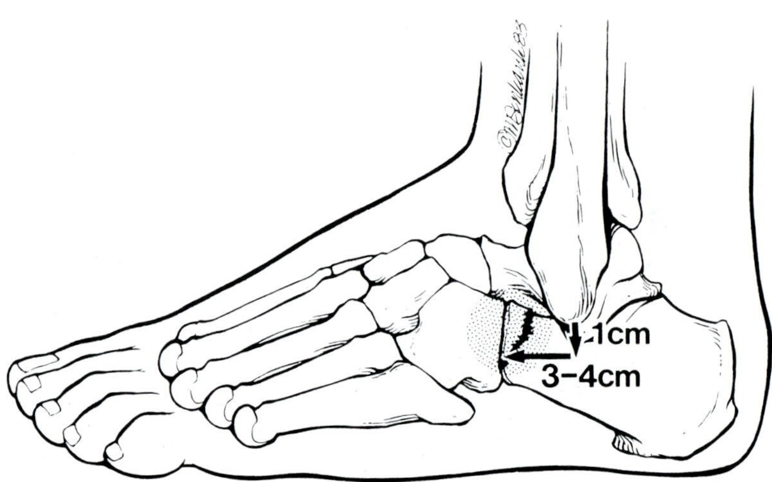

FIG 35–26.
The anterior process is located slightly below and 3 to 4 cm anterior to the lateral malleolus. Point tenderness in this area suggests an anterior process fracture.

terior to the midfoot. This projects the anterior process over the neck of the talus enough so that the fracture can be easily visualized (Fig 35–27).[44] Gellman[61] suggests a caudal and dorsal direction of the central ray so that it passes 15 to 25 degrees cranially and 10 to 15 degrees ventrally. However, the precise angles must be adjusted individually to meet the variations in the size and shape of the anterior calcaneal process in different patients.[8]

In spite of these special views, tomograms may be necessary to demonstrate the anterior process fracture and particularly to determine whether or not an anterior talocalcaneal facet is present and involved in the fracture.[35, 39] Conway and Cowell[35] have demonstrated the value of lateral tomography of the talocalcaneal joint to evaluate this anterior facet. Polytomography may also be useful to evaluate involvement of the calcaneocuboid joint. Finally, Jahss and Kay have suggested that subtalar arthrography combined with oblique radiographs may be important in evaluating the anterior talocalcaneal joint.[92]

When radiographs are evaluated, it is important to distinguish between an acute fracture of the anterior process (Fig 35–28,B), nonunion of this fracture (Fig 35–28,C), and an accessory ossicle, the calcaneus secundarius, which when present is located near the anterior process of the calcaneus (Fig 35–28,A).[209] The calcaneus secundarius, however, is usually round or ovoid

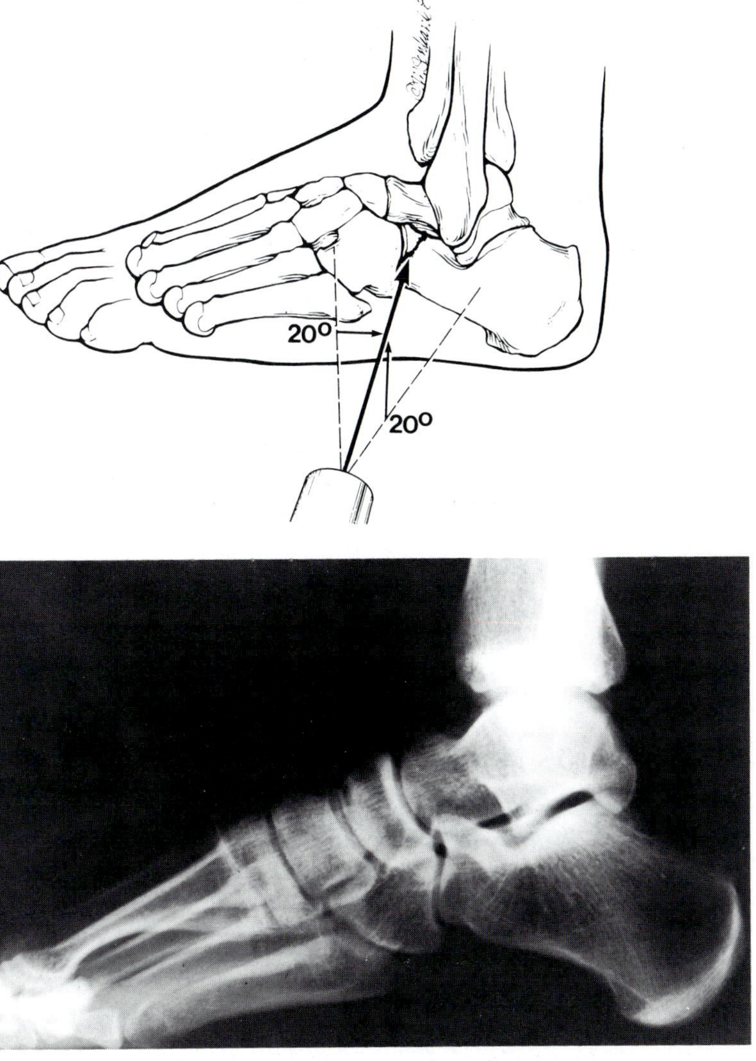

FIG 35–27.
The oblique view obtained by angling the central beam 20 degrees cephalad and 20 degrees to the posterior projects the anterior process over the neck of the talus to allow excellent visualization.[9]

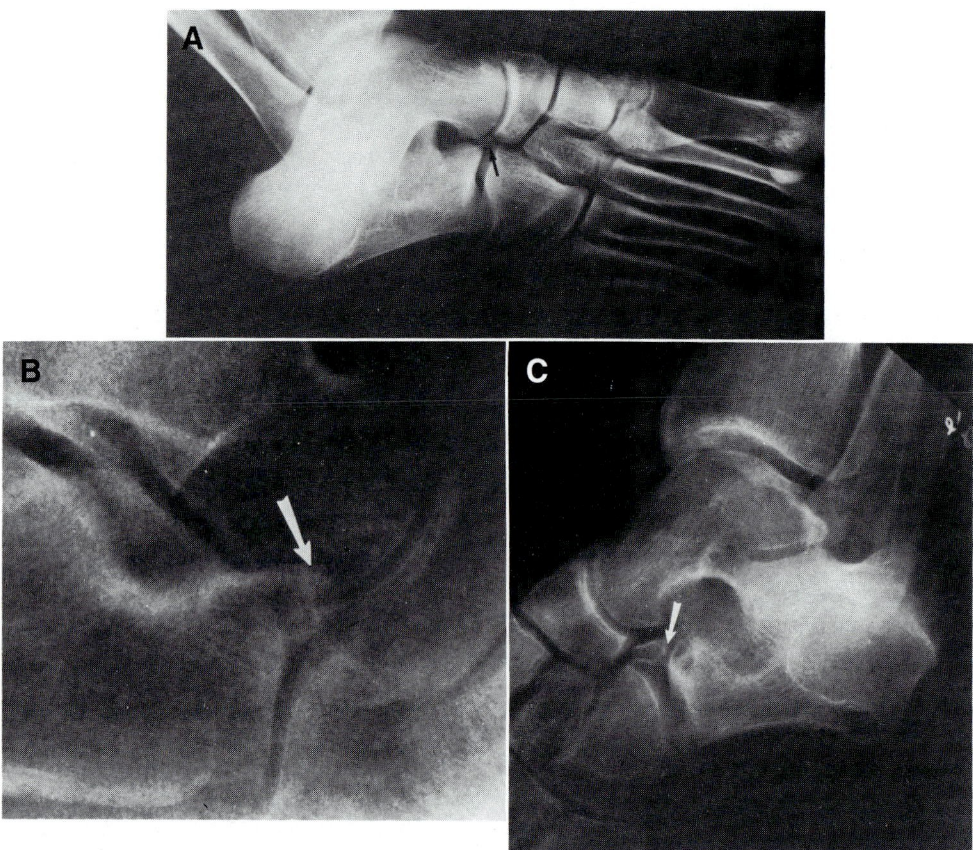

FIG 35–28.

A, os calcaneus secundarius, an accessory ossicle. Note the ovoid shape and irregular edges *(arrow).* **B,** fracture of the anterior process of the calcaneus. Note the triangular shape and irregular edges of the fracture surface *(arrow).* **C,** nonunion of the anterior process of the calcaneus. Sclerotic margins and a triangular shape help to differentiate it from an os calcaneus secondarius. (**B** and **C** from Degan TF, Morrey BF, Braun DP: *J Bone Joint Surg* 64:518–524, 1982. Used by permission.)

in shape with its cortex sheathing the bony density.[19, 153] The smooth edges and rounded appearance of this anomaly help to differentiate it from an acute fracture or a nonunion (Fig 35–28,A).[19] Although some authors have mentioned the possibility of confusing this fracture with an ununited epiphysis,[153] Piatt reports no such secondary epiphyseal center at this location, thereby excluding the possibility of an united epiphysis confusing the diagnosis.[153] In an acute fracture, the fragment is usually triangular in shape,[44] and the fracture surfaces are irregular (Fig 35–28,B). A nonunion is also triangular in shape, but the fracture surfaces are sclerotic (Fig 35–28,C).

To adequately outline a plan of treatment, the oblique views and/or tomograms must be *carefully* studied to determine (1) the size of the fracture fragment, (2) the degree of displacement, and (3) the presence of subtalar and calcaneocuboid joint involvement.

Treatment

A great deal of controversy surrounds the treatment of fractures of the anterior process of the calcaneus. Most authors report that the majority of these fractures unite in 2 to 3 months whether rigid or semirigid immobilization is utilized.[40, 43, 61, 92, 166] Gellman recommends a simple below-the-knee cast for severe cases and feels that an elastic bandage is sufficient for the less severe injuries.[61] He did not permit weight bearing for 4 weeks.[61] Backman and Johnson[8] recommend elastic bandage immobilization for 2 to 3 weeks unless the injury is severe, in which case a cast is applied. Bradford and Larsen also recommend either an elastic bandage or a short-leg plaster boot depending upon the degree of associated injury.[19] Likewise, Green recommends immobilizing the foot with either adhesive strapping or plaster in the neutral position with weight bearing only after 2 weeks.[70]

Debold and Stimson emphasize that maintaining function of the subtalar joint is more important that anatomic repositioning of the fracture.[43] They stress that prolonged immobilization and associated edema may lead to stiffness and weakness of the subtalar and other small joints of the foot.

Jahss and Kay also stress that although rigid immobilization gives more comfort, in their experience a cast has been associated with Sudeck's atrophy and extremely disabling stiffness of the entire foot and ankle.[92] They therefore recommend the use of an Unna boot as the treatment of choice for these fractures.

Although these fractures usually heal after 4 to 6 weeks of immobilization by either simple adhesive strapping or a plaster cast,[113] Degan et al. emphasize that they may not be completely asymptomatic after this period of immobilization.[44] In fact, 28% of their patients required *more* than a year to become aysmptomatic or to realize the final extent of recovery from this injury. Based on this experience, they recommend up to 1 year of nonoperative treatment before any consideration of further surgical treatment is entertained.[44]

The question of whether or not *immediate* surgical intervention in the form of excision would shorten the convalescence has often been raised.[19, 92] Due to the fact that the majority of these fractures heal without sequelae, both Jahss and Kay[92] and Bradford and Larsen[19] feel that such aggressive treatment is open to criticism. However, excision of a neglected fracture fragment that has progressed to nonunion with continuous pain and disability has been reported to be successful.[44, 53, 209] However, Finder et al.,[53] Degan et al.,[44] and Jahss and Kay[92] caution against performing such an excision before adequate time for recovery has elapsed. Excision of the nonunion may not result in permanent symptomatic relief, and recovery after the excision may be prolonged.[44, 53]

Likewise, the place of open reduction and internal fixation of *displaced* fractures of the anterior process of the calcaneus is not clear. Rowe et al.[168] report open reduction in two patients in whom the fracture fragments were large enough, and Watson-Jones[200] notes that when large fragments of the anterior process of the calcaneus are separated and tilted, operative intervention may be indicated. Hunt[188] reports a displaced fracture of the anterior process of the calcaneus secondary to an adduction force in which a good result was obtained following open reduction and internal fixation. It must be remembered that in this case, the fracture fragment was quite large and was associated with midtarsal subluxation. Open reduction in this situation not only restores the articular surface of the calcaneocuboid joint but also reduces and stabilizes the subluxation of the midtarsal joint.

Although Jahss and Kay[92] mention open reduction and internal fixation of larger fragments to correct a step-off on the articular surface of the calcaneocuboid joint, they caution against this procedure because of the good results reported with conservative treatment of most of these fractures.[92] However, Gould,[69] in discussing this article, recommends that large fragments undergo immediate surgical intervention. A determination is made whether the fracture should be firmly fixed and motion immediately initiated or whether the fragment should be excised. He emphasizes that whichever approach is utilized, *immediate* postoperative motion is essential since restoration of subtalar and midtarsal motion is as critical as restoration of joint surface alignment.[92]

Finally, in patients who have not had relief of symptoms following excision of the calcaneal fragment, Bradford and Larsen mention triple arthrodesis as a final attempt to relieve pain.[19]

Results

The prognosis following a fracture of the anterior process of the calcaneus is quite good, particularly if the fragment is *small* and minimally displaced. The large majority of these fractures unite without sequelae in 2 to 3 months.[40, 43, 92] Degan et al. report satisfactory results with no limitation of activity following conservative treatment of these fractures.[44] However, they stress that the time for recovery averaged 10 months and at follow-up fewer than half of the patients were completely pain free. The main factor associated with long-term disability and poor results is a delay in diagnosis and treatment.[19, 44, 113] Although Jaekle and Clark[91] report that involvement of the calcaneocuboid joint is unimportant and disability from this involvement practically nil, Hunt and Gould stress the importance of restoring the articular surface of the calcaneocuboid joint.[88, 92] The size of the fragment also affects results because the larger fragments have more involvement of the calcaneocuboid articular surface.[88]

Although they noted no loss of motion of the subtalar or Chopart joint following excision of the fragment, Degan et al, did report occasional ossification in the area of excision at follow-up.[44] They report that recovery is often prolonged following excision and that in patients in whom no early treatment had been rendered for 22 to 24 months postfracture an unsatisfactory result was obtained after fragment excision.[44]

Author's Preferred Method of Treatment

The author considers it extremely important to completely evaluate this fracture roentgenographically *before* deciding upon the method of treatment. Oblique radiographs and even polytomograms may be required to determine the size of the fracture fragment, the degree of displacement, *and* the presence or absence of anterior subtalar and calcaneocuboid joint involvement.

In patients with acute fractures of the anterior process of the calcaneus, treatment is based upon the size of the fracture fragment, associated soft-tissue injury, and the degree of displacement. For small, nondisplaced fragments in which involvement of the calcaneocuboid joint is minimal, the patient is immobilized in a short-leg fracture boot that is a commercially available or a removable short-leg cast. Elevation and a soft-tissue compression dressing are used to control edema. After the soft-tissue swelling decreases in 5 to 7 days, the patient starts range-of-motion exercises out of the boot three to four times daily. An elastic stocking is used to control swelling. Circumduction exercises using the foot to draw the alphabet in lukewarm water are useful exercises to maintain motion in the subtalar and Chopart joints. In addition, toe flexion exercises are instituted in an effort to help decrease edema in the foot. The patient's ambulatory status is non–weight bearing for 4 to 6 weeks in the boot and then gradually increasing to full weight bearing as pain allows. The boot is removed in 12 weeks if radiographs or tomograms demonstrate fracture healing.

In patients with a large displaced fracture fragment involving a major portion of the calcaneocuboid and/or anterior subtalar joint, consideration is given to open reduction and internal fixation or excision, depending upon the fragment size. I prefer a longitudinal incision over the calcaneocuboid joint and parallel to the sole of the foot. In my experience, this incision, parallel to the sural nerve fibers, results in less neuroma formation and less tender surgical incisions. It is important to stress that if either one of these methods is selected, the patient *must* initiate immediate range of motion so that subtalar and Chopart joint motion is not lost.

Excision of fracture fragments that represent a painful nonunion is withheld until at least a year postinjury in an effort to allow complete recovery prior to surgical intervention.

Tuberosity Fracture: Beak and Avulsion Fractures

Anatomy

Beak and avulsion fractures of the calcaneus, which involve the posterosuperior aspect of the calcaneus, are well recognized.[37, 157, 199] These fractures do not involve the subtalar joint unless the posterior fragment is unusually large.[174] Essex-Lopresti,[52] Bohler,[18] and Rothberg[167] report this injury to be extremely rare. Rowe et al[168] and Lyngstadaas[117] report that it accounts for 3% of all calcaneus fractures.

Classification of fractures of the posterosuperior aspect of the calcaneus is based on involvement of the insertion of the tendo Achillis into the calcaneus.[116, 117] Watson-Jones[200] and Bohler[18] have termed those fractures that do *not* involve the tendo Achillis insertion "beak fractures" (Fig 35–29,A). They term those fractures that do involve the tendo Achillis insertion into the calcaneus "avulsion fractures" (Fig 35–29,B). This avulsed fragment can vary in size from a small sliver of bone located beneath the tendo Achillis to a large mass consisting of the entire posterior tuberosity of the calcaneus.[142]

The posterior surface of the calcaneus has three distinct areas or subdivisions.[116] Most inferior on the posterior surface is a roughened area for the fibrofatty tissue of the heel pad. The middle surface, into which the tendo Achillis is inserted, joins the upper surface, which is smooth and is related to a bursa that lies deep to the tendo Achillis.[116] The tendo Achillis is separated

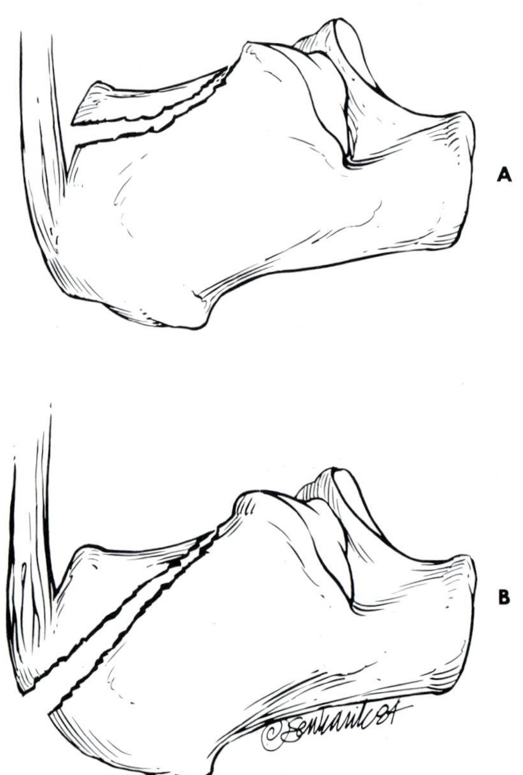

FIG 35–29.
Beak **(A)** and avulsion **(B)** fractures of the calcaneus.

from the proximal half of the posterior surface of the calcaneus by this bursa.[157] Fractures related to this bursa only are the so-called beak fractures, whereas those extending into the middle portion of the posterior surface involve the tendo Achillis insertion.

The Achillis tendon attachment is *usually* positioned in the middle third, but in 5% of patients it is located in the upper third of the posterior surface.[80, 86] Both Korn[103] and Lowy[116] demonstrated that the point of insertion of the tendo Achillis may cover a variable portion of the posterior aspect of the calcaneus.

Additionally, Sutro[187] has demonstrated degenerative changes at the point of insertion of the calcaneal tendon in persons over the age of 50 years. These changes, when present in an already high insertion, may produce the appearance of a "beak"-type fracture radiographically when, in fact, the entire insertion of the tendo Achillis has been avulsed.[187] Finally, Protheroe[157] casts doubt on the exact differentiation between "beak" and "avulsion" fractures on an anatomic basis. In two of the patients he reported, he found the tendo Achillis adherent to the *entire* posterior aspect of the calcaneus and, hence, inserted more proximally into the posterior surface of the calcaneus than has been classically described. One of these fractures was radiographically identical to a "beak" fracture but at surgery was found to be a true "avulsion."

Because of the variability in location of insertion of the tendo Achillis and the changes pointed out by Sutro[187] that are associated with aging, the only way to accurately differentiate "beak" and "avulsion" fractures is by clinical examination or surgical exploration, not by radiography.[157] Lowy[116] cautions that if the clinical diagnosis is in doubt, it is advisable to explore the heel because a failure to gain accurate reduction of the fracture (and, hence, tendo Achillis continuity) will produce substantial disability.

Mechanism of Injury

According to Watson-Jones[200] and Bohler,[18] "beak" fractures are caused by direct trauma to the posterior surface of the calcaneus, while "avulsion" fractures are secondary to a violent contraction of the tendo Achillis.[200] Parkes,[148] Korn,[103] and O'Connell et al.[142] also attribute avulsion fractures to a violent pull by the tendo Achillis with the foot in a fixed position. According to Lyngstadaas[117] and Rothberg,[167] the most frequent mechanism is a fall that causes the patient to strike his heel on a hard surface with the triceps surae tensed. Garcia and Parkes[58] believe that when a patient lands with the knee in full extension and the ankle in plantar flexion after a jump, it produces tension in the tendo Achillis that avulses the insertion.

Clinical Diagnosis

Patients give a history of a fall on the foot and of feeling a pop in the heel or a direct blow to the heel with sudden pain.[116, 148] They complain of pain in the heel and in "avulsion fractures" walk with a flat-footed, antalgic gait.[116, 148] In addition to pain in the heel and calf, there is commonly weakness of plantar flexion.[116 157] Clinically the heel is grossly swollen and after the first 12 to 24 hours may have ecchymosis and bulla formation in the area of the tuberosity.[48, 54, 113, 157, 167]

In avulsion fractures with displacement, there may be a palpable hollow between the calcaneus and the avulsed fragment that contains the tendo Achillis insertion.[157, 167] Also, in avulsion fractures, one can demonstrate a loss of function of the tendo Achillis by the absence of plantar flexion with calf compression. Lowy[116] emphasizes that the diagnosis of an "avulsion" fracture is based on the clinical examination and *not* on roentgenographs. As mentioned earlier, the variability of insertion of the tendo Achillis is responsible for "avulsion" fractures appearing radiographically as "beak"-type fractures. Careful *clinical* examination is essential to distinguish these two injuries and, hence, to permit correct treatment selection.

Radiographic Diagnosis

Radiographically both "beak" and "avulsion" fractures are best seen on a lateral roentgenograph of the foot and ankle, which demonstrates a fracture involving the posterosuperior aspect of the tuberosity of the calcaneus.[11, 123, 148, 157] Although "beak" fractures usually involve *less* than the upper half of the tuberosity of the calcaneus while "avulsion" fractures *never* involve less than half of the tuberosity, clinical examination is the *key* to distinguishing between these two injuries. Classically both of these fractures demonstrate separation at the fracture site with only minor comminution.[157] Displacement is the key to fracture evaluation because either beak or avulsion fractures that are displaced may require reduction.

Treatment

Treatment recommendations are based upon *clinically* distinguishing between "avulsion"- and "beak"-type fractures. Hence, it is essential to determine whether or not the fracture fragment contains the tendo Achillis insertion.

Beak Fractures.—Garcia and Parkes[58] recommend that nondisplaced "beak" fractures be treated by immobilization of the foot in the neutral position or slight plantar flexion for a period of 6 weeks of non–weight bearing. In displaced "beak" fractures (those that do not contain the tendo Achillis insertion), Schottstaedt[174] and Sisk[178] recommend closed reduction and immobilization in a plantar flexion cast for 6 weeks. Heck[82] reports that a displaced "beak"-type fracture can be repositioned by the surgeon applying direct pressure to the fragment with his thumb while the foot is in plantar flexion. Following reduction he recommends casting in a short-leg cast for 6 weeks. If these displaced "beak" fractures are not treated by closed reduction, the closeness of the skin overlying the displaced fracture fragment can produce skin necrosis.[157]

Avulsion Fractures.—Schottstaedt[174, 175] and Slatis et al[179] treat nondisplaced "avulsion" fractures of the calcaneus in a non–weight-bearing cast in the equinus position for 6 weeks, followed by non–weight bearing for an additional 2 weeks.[174, 175, 179]

The most important effect of displaced "avulsion" fractures of the calcaneus is impairment of heel cord function.[157] The greater the displacement of the avulsed fracture, the greater the functional loss, and hence, the more need for accurate reduction. There is general agreement that displaced "avulsion" fractures have to be repositioned,[82, 168] and the need for accurate reduction of the "avulsed" fracture is stressed by most authors.[116] Closed reduction by direct pressure over the displaced fragment with the foot in plantar flexion has been recommended.[48, 103] Following closed reduction, Key and Conwell recommended immobilization in a long-leg cast with the knee bent and the foot plantar-flexed.[97] Other authors recommend open reduction and internal fixation in all patients in whom the "avulsion" fracture is displaced.[156, 178]

Parkes[148] and Lowy[116] recommend open reduction and internal fixation with a screw followed by a cast with the foot in the equinus position for 6 weeks. The displaced fragment containing the tendo Achillis insertion can be fixed with a screw either from above through the fragment or from below through the calcaneus into the fragment (Fig 35–30).[116] Schottstaedt[174, 175] recommended open reduction using a medial or lateral incision paralleling the tendo Achillis. He stresses that the timing of surgery is dependent upon the degree of swelling present.[174, 175]

The choice of open vs. closed methods of reduction of "avulsion" fractures must take the patient and the displacement into consideration. According to McLaughlin,[118] if the insertion of the tendo Achillis is merely tilted upward, direct pressure over the fragment and casting in plantar flexion produce a good result. However, if the fracture is tilted *and* rotated with displacement, open reduction and internal fixation are necessary.[118] In elderly patients with impaired function or decreased demands and slightly displaced avulsion fractures, treatment by soft dressing immobilization and physical therapy will produce a good result.[157] However, younger patients with displacement of an "avulsion" fracture must have open reduction and internal fixation if normal function is to be expected.[157]

Results

According to Key and Conwell[97] and Parkes,[148] the prognosis for both fracture union and function are excellent when "avulsion" and "beak" fractures are reduced. Heck[82] and O'Connell et al[142] report excellent results if these fractures do not involve the posterior subtalar joint, which rarely occurs if the fragment is large.

Complications of persistent displacement of "avulsion" fractures include weak plantar flexion and difficulty climbing stairs.[157] Finally, skin slough over persistently displaced "beak" fractures has been reported.[157]

Author's Preferred Method of Treatment

In the author's opinion, the most important aspect in evaluating these patients is to *clinically* distinguish between beak and avulsion fractures. Weakness of ankle plantar flexion and loss of passive plantar flexion with squeezing the calf are signs I rely on to determine whether the fracture fragment contains the insertion of the tendo Achillis. If these tests are inconclusive in a young patient with a displaced fracture, I explore the fracture. If the Achillis tendon is attached to the fracture fragment, internal fixation of the fracture is performed.

Beak Fractures.—In beak fractures in which the displacement is minimal, that is, the fracture fragment does not pose any threat to the overlying skin, I use a short-leg walking cast for 4 to 6 weeks. I allow early weight bearing *only* if clinical examination confirms that the fracture is truly of the "beak" variety and that the insertion of the tendo Achillis is intact. If continuity of the tendo Achillis is not certain, non–weight bearing is selected because of the potential of activity of the tendo Achillis to produce displacement of the fracture.

In displaced fractures in which the overlying skin seems to be at risk, I perform a closed reduction. With the knee bent and the ankle in plantar flexion, I apply direct pressure to the displaced fragment. If the reduction is successful, I use a short-leg cast in plantar flexion for 6 weeks followed by progressive weight bearing. Early active motion of the metatarsophalangeal joints is encouraged. If the fracture is markedly displaced and cannot be reduced by closed methods, open reduction via an incision lateral to the tendo Achillis is recommended. I prefer AO cancellous screws for fixation. Postoperatively, if stable fixation is obtained, no immo-

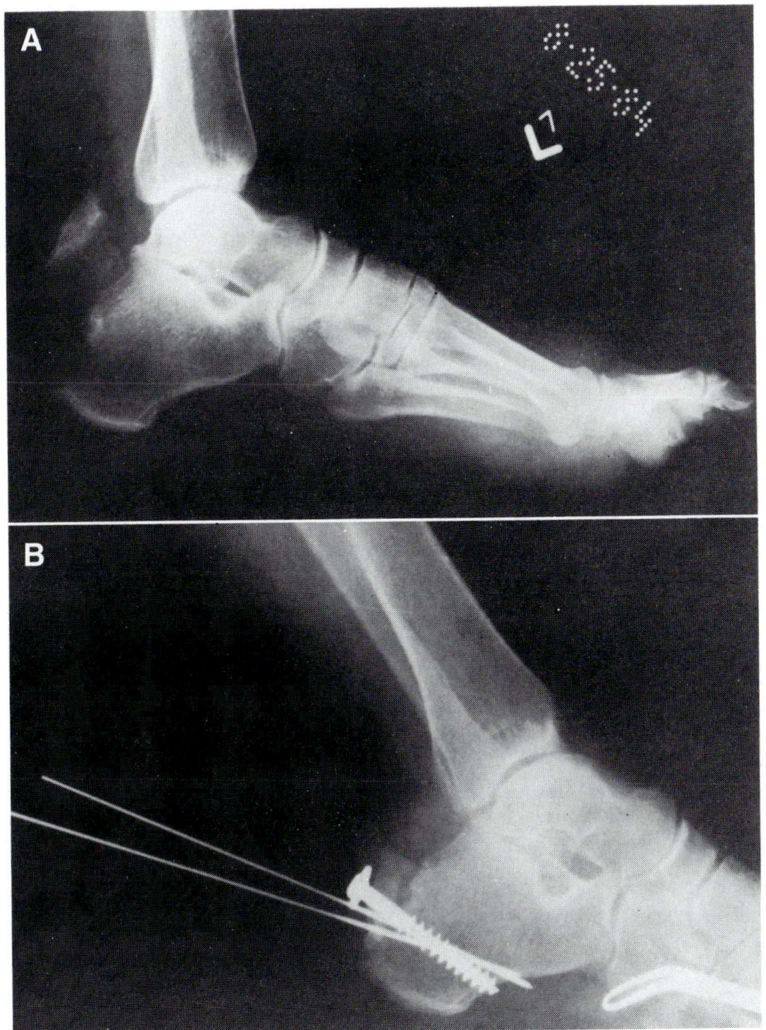

FIG 35–30.
A, avulsion fracture of the calcaneus. **B,** open reduction and internal fixation with an AO (Arbeitsgemeinschaft für Osteosynthese) 4-mm cancellous screw and washer.

bilization is used, and early motion of all foot joints is instituted. Progressive weight bearing is allowed at 4 to 6 weeks postoperatively.

Avulsion Fractures.—I believe that avulsion fractures of the calcaneus that are displaced to any degree must be reduced unless the patient is elderly and very inactive. Clinical examination is used to confirm the discontinuity of the tendo Achillis mechanism.

I prefer open reduction unless the local skin conditions are unacceptable. I use an incision lateral to the tendo Achillis. Once the reduction is obtained, fixation utilizing either 6.5 or 4.0 mm AO cancellous screws, depending on the fracture fragment size, is performed. Following open reduction and internal fixation, I place the foot in an equinus position with a built-up heel in a short-leg fracture boot. Following wound healing and suture removal at 2 weeks, the patient takes off the fracture boot three to fours times daily for active ankle and subtalar joint circumduction range-of-motion exercises. The patient's ambulatory status is non–weight bearing up to 4 weeks and then gradually increasing weight bearing in the fracture boot and weekly shaving down the built-up heel over the next 4 weeks. Progressive weight bearing is then begun out of the brace.

Finally, I emphasize the importance of careful evaluation of the lateral roentgenograph to make certain that neither "beak" nor "avulsion" fractures communicate with the posterior subtalar joint because of the adverse affect on long-term prognosis. If such communication is noted, accurate open reduction, stable internal fixation, and immediate range of motion is my choice of treatment.

Fractures of the Medial or Lateral Process of the Calcaneus

Anatomy and Mechanism of Injury

The medial process serves as the origin of the abductor hallucis and the medial portion of the flexor hallucis brevis and plantar fascia. The lateral process serves as the origin of the abductor digiti minimi. Fractures of the medial or lateral process of the tuberosity of the calcaneus are uncommon injuries,[49, 58] the medial tubercle being the most frequently fractured. These fractures are rarely significantly displaced (Fig 35–31).[118]

These fractures occur when an abduction or adduction force is exerted on the heel as it strikes the ground in eversion, which produces a fracture of the medial process, or in inversion, which leads to a fracture of the lateral process.[49, 58] A less common mechanism occurs when the medial aspect of the heel receives a glancing blow from below while the foot is held in a valgus position.[56, 118]

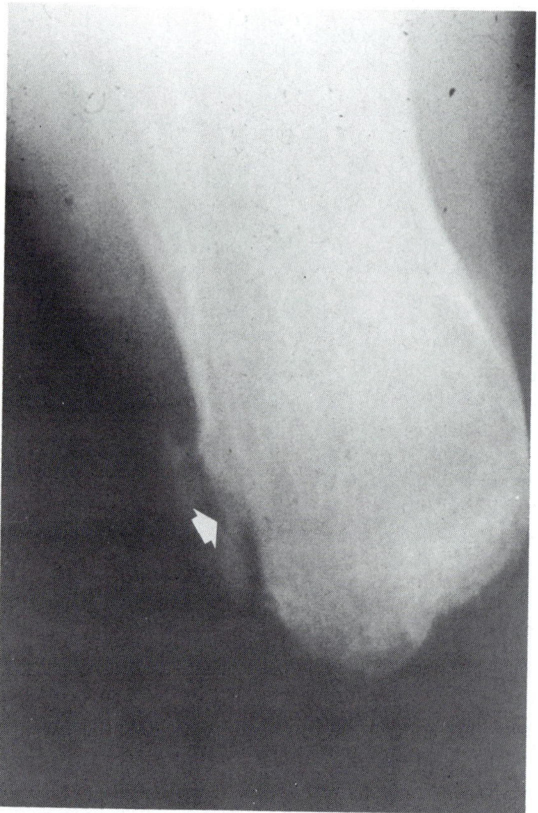

FIG 35–31.
Fracture of the medial process of the tuberosity of the calcaneus.

Clinical and Radiographic Diagnosis

Patients give a history of having fallen or jumped from a height and landing directly on the heel. The heel is thickened and swollen, and ecchymosis will appear within the first 24 hours.[118] In medial process fractures, the posteromedial sulcus of the heel is flattened, and the entire hindfoot may be tender.[118]

Tenderness may be localized to the posteromedial or posterolateral surface of the heel depending upon the location of the fracture.[58] Additionally, there may be tenderness on the plantar aspect of the heel.[58] Range of motion of the ankle, midfoot, and forefoot joints is usually within normal limits.[58]

Radiographically the diagnosis is confirmed on the axial view of the calcaneus or a posteroanterior view of the foot (Fig 35–31).[58, 91, 118]

Treatment

McLaughlin[118] recommends simple immobilization of these fractures in a walking cast until union occurs. Bohler[18] also recommends a short-leg cast for 6 weeks with immediate weight bearing.

Garcia and Parkes[58] recommend elevation in a pressure dressing. Ice is applied and early range of motion instituted. In displaced fractures, they recommend reduction by molding the heel and applying a well-padded plaster cast molded around the heel.[58] Since swelling usually decreases in 7 to 10 days, a cast change may be necessary. The cast is removed after 4 weeks and the patients begun on range-of-motion exercises. They are kept non–weight bearing for an additional 4 weeks. Schottstaedt[175] and Kalish[96] recommend a plaster cast for 5 to 6 weeks for undisplaced fractures of the tuberosities. Since displaced fractures can produce widening of the heel, they believe that consideration should be given to reduction by manipulation using the pressure of the heel of the hand or a compression clamp followed by a short-leg cast for 4 to 8 weeks.[96, 175]

Dodson[49] also bases treatment recommendations on fracture displacement. He recommends elevation and compression followed by non–weight bearing and range-of-motion exercises in nondisplaced fractures. If the fracture is displaced, he also recommends reduction by compression and application of a well-fitted non–weight-bearing cast that is worn for 8 weeks. Schofield[173] also recommends closed reduction following injection of the fracture site with an anesthetic agent.

Jaekle and Clark[91] report that fractures consisting of a longitudinal split with a slight medial to lateral separation produce minimal disability. However, if the medial or lateral tuberosity has any degree of proximal displacement, a painful heel will result unless it is reduced.

McLaughlin[118] mentions shoe modifications if malunion results in a painful prominence.

Results

Persistent tenderness in the heel managed by shoe modification or padding is the long-term problem that has been reported.[63, 118] Nonunion of the displaced fragment requiring excision has also been mentioned.[58]

Author's Preferred Method of Treatment

In nondisplaced fractures and those with only minimal separation of the fracture surfaces, I use a compression dressing with ice and elevation. Range of motion of the ankle, subtalar, midtarsal, and metatarsophalangeal joints is instituted immediately. Once pain and swelling have subsided, I place the patient in a well-molded short-leg walking cast for 3 to 4 weeks. A shoe with a well-padded heel is then recommended.

In fractures with proximal displacement and/or marked medial-lateral separation, I attempt closed reduction by applying medial-lateral compression on the heel with the heels of my hands. If this method is not successful in reducing the separation, compression with a Bohler clamp is utilized if the patient's local skin circulation is not compromised and the fracture is significantly displaced. After reduction of a displaced fracture, a well-padded short-leg nonwalking cast is applied with medial-lateral molding about the heel. The patient is kept non–weight bearing for 4 weeks. Weight bearing for an additional 2 weeks in a walking cast is then recommended.

If closed reduction is not successful, I treat these patients in the same manner as if the fracture were nondisplaced. This is because I have not seen long-term disability significant enough to warrant open reduction and internal fixation.

Fracture of the Body of the Calcaneus Not Involving the Subtalar Joint

Anatomy

Twenty percent of fractures of the body of the calcaneus do not involve the subtalar joint.[58, 168, 199] The only criteria for a fracture to be included in this group is a lack of involvement of the subtalar and calcaneocuboid joints. The fracture line usually extends from the posteromedial to the anterolateral aspect of the calcaneus, just behind the subtalar joint.[30] Even though the subtalar joint is not involved in the fracture, displacement of the fracture can occur in a proximal direction and result in reduction of the tuberosity joint angle or occur in a medial-lateral direction and produce widening of the heel.[169, 174]

Mechanism of Injury

The same mechanism that produces intra-articular fractures of the calcaneus can result in a fracture of the calcaneal tuberosity *without* involvement of the subtalar joint.[30] According to Chapman, the most common mechanism is that of landing on the heel after a fall or from a severe blow from below during standing.[30] Additionally, Garcia and Parkes[58] emphasize that a fall from a height with the heel in the neutral or valgus position produces this extra-articular fracture. Since the fall is usually not from a great height, there is often little comminution or displacement of this type of fracture.[148]

Clinical Diagnosis

The signs and symptoms of this fracture are similar to those present in an intra-articular fracture. The patient usually gives a history of a fall from a height with sudden severe pain and the inability to bear weight.[58] Shortly after the injury, swelling and ecchymosis of the heel are present.[58, 148] In addition to generalized pain and swelling about the heel, there is tenderness to pressure on both the medial and lateral aspects of the heel.[49, 58] If the fracture is displaced in a proximal-distal direction, weakness of plantar flexion may be present. Motion of the ankle and subtalar joint is usually painful.

Radiographic Diagnosis

Garcia and Parkes[58] emphasize that although this fracture is best seen on a lateral view of the foot, it is extremely important to obtain other views to make certain that there is no involvement of the subtalar joint.[49, 148] They recommend the axial view to rule out subtalar involvement.[58] On the lateral roentgenographic view Bohler's tuberosity joint angle can be determined and compared with the uninjured side (Fig 35–32).

Treatment

Controversy exists as to the best method of treatment of these fractures.[51] However, because fractures without subtalar involvement usually have good results, most authors recommend minimal treatment.[49, 58, 168, 174, 175] Garcia and Parkes[58] and Dodson[49] recommend ice, elevation, a compression dressing, and the institution of early range of foot motion for fractures without displacement. They recommend that patients be kept non–weight bearing for 12 weeks to prevent displacement of the fracture. Rowe et al.[168] recommend immobilization in a short-leg cast if the fracture is nondisplaced. Geckeler[60] recommends early protected weight bearing in an equinus cast for nondisplaced fractures. Early weight bearing is believed to prevent a loss of muscle tone and disuse changes in the joints of the foot.[60]

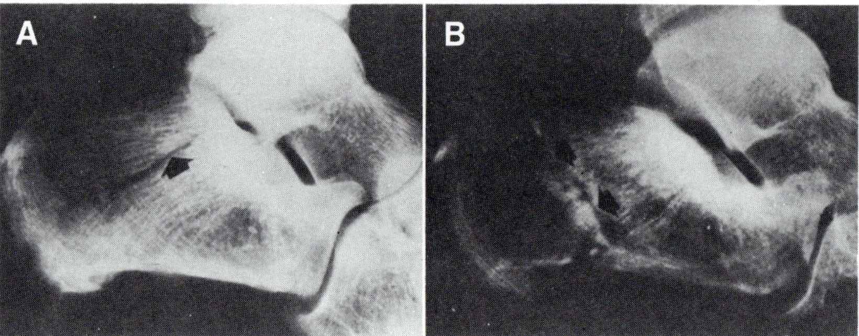

FIG 35–32.
A, extra-articular fracture of the body of the calcaneus, undisplaced. **B,** extra-articular fracture of the body of the calcaneus with proximal displacement of the tuberosity and a reduction in Bohler's tuberosity joint angle.

Rowe et al.[168] recommend closed reduction of displaced fractures. Schottstaedt[174, 175] recommends reduction by traction and immobilization in a cast molded with medial-lateral compression if the heel is widened.[175] Wilson[205] also recommends the use of a Bohler compression clamp followed by a short-leg cast in fractures with marked medial-lateral displacement (Fig 35–33).

According to Garica and Parkes[58] and McReynolds,[123] if the fracture exits posterior to the articular surface of the posterior facet and is displaced proximally, it should be reduced with a percutaneous Kirschner wire to pull the fragment down. Once reduction has been obtained in this manner, the traction wire is incorporated into a long-leg cast with the knee bent at 45 degrees to relax the tendo Achillis. Dodson[49] also recommends the use of a percutaneous Steinmann pin that is inserted into the main fragment to act as a lever to permit reduction of the fracture. This Steinmann pin is incorporated into a short-leg cast. The patient is kept non–weight bearing for 8 weeks.

According to Geckeler,[60] in severe fractures with loss of the tuberosity joint angle, reshaping of the calcaneus is often necessary.[60] A Steinmann pin used to restore Bohler's angle and a clamp to correct lateral spread are recommended.[60] Following the reduction, he recommends a short-leg, well-padded cast to incorporate the pin. The cast is changed at 4 weeks. At 8 weeks, a weight-bearing cast is applied for an additional 4 weeks. Finally, Heck[82] recommends attempted closed reduction followed by immobilization in a well-molded short-leg cast in equinus with varus or valgus of the heel as needed to maintain alignment. If closed reduction is not successful, he recommends open reduction and internal fixation of this fracture.

Prognosis

Most authors report that the prognosis in these fractures is good, particularly if the displacement is reduced.[30, 49, 58, 166, 175, 205] However, after healing of the fracture, patients may complain of pain around the heel and discomfort over the calcaneus for several months,

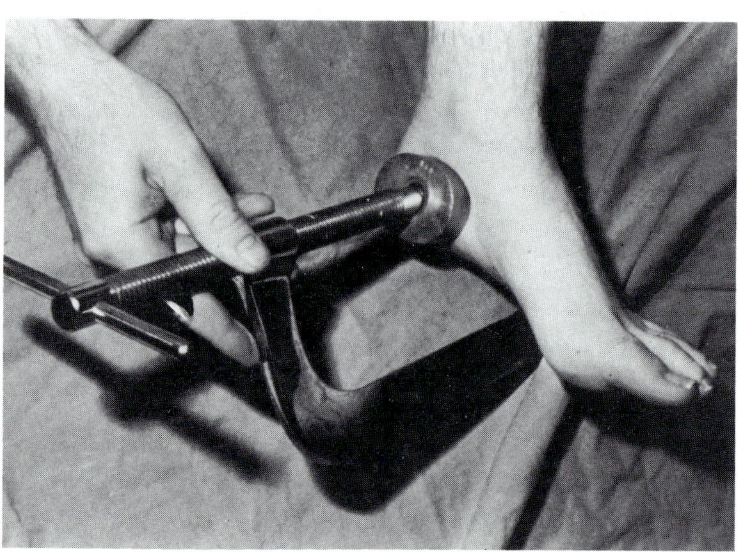

FIG 35–33.
Bohler-type clamp used to reduce mediolateral widening of the heel in a calcaneus fracture.

and Garcia and Parkes emphasize that swelling following this fracture may be slow to resolve.[58] The prognosis following these fractures depends upon the configuration of the heel following treatment. However, if the displacement is corrected, a good functional result should be expected.[30]

Although arthritis of the subtalar joint is not a complication of these fractures, soft-tissue injury and persistent broadening of the calcaneus secondary to medial-lateral displacement can occur if the fracture is not reduced.[30] Finally, a loss of push-off will result if the tuberosity joint angle is not restored in proximally displaced fractures.[30]

Author's Preferred Method of Treatment

I prefer closed treatment for fractures of the body of the calcaneus that do not involve the subtalar joint. In minimally displaced fractures, I apply a compression dressing and ice and elevate the foot. Range of motion of the ankle, subtalar joints, and metatarsophalangeal joints is begun immediately. Reliable patients are kept non–weight bearing on crutches for 4 to 6 weeks. Unreliable patients are placed in a short-leg cast in the equinus position (*after* motion is restored) for 4 to 6 weeks followed by progressive weight bearing.

In my experience, the critical displacements in these fractures are medial-lateral and/or proximal. If there is medial-lateral fracture displacement with widening of the heel or there is significant proximal displacement of the tuberosity fragment, I attempt closed reduction. If the calcaneus is widened, I apply manual compression to the calcaneus to decrease the medial-lateral spread. If manual compression does not reduce the medial-lateral spread in a young patient, consideration is given to the use of a Bohler clamp for compression. After the medial-lateral displacement is reduced by compression, motion is restored, and then a short-leg cast well-molded about the heel is applied and the patient kept non–weight bearing for 6 to 8 weeks until fracture union has occurred.

If the fracture is displaced proximally, I insert an axial Steinmann pin into the displaced fragment. The pin is used to lever the fragment into a reduced position. An axial pin is then driven into the main body of the calcaneus. When the fracture is reduced, the pin is incorporated into a slipper cast to allow early ankle and subtalar motion. The slipper cast and pin are removed after 4 to 6 weeks and a weight bearing cast is applied for an additional two weeks.

Finally, if the patient has altered sensation in the foot, such as a patient with diabetes, one must not initiate weight bearing until the fracture is completely healed. If early ambulation is allowed in these patients after a calcaneus fracture, progressive neuropathic changes can occur and result in complete disorganization of the heel (Fig 35–34). These changes can follow early resumption of weight bearing after *any* fracture of the foot in patients with altered sensation, a condition most commonly seen in the diabetic.

The amount of medial-lateral or proximal displacement that is clinically significant is dependent on the age and activity level of the patient. Medial-lateral displacement can produce widening and shortening of the heel with fibular abutment and problems in shoe fitting, while proximal displacement reduces Bohler's angle and, hence, results in weakness of plantar flexion. Generally speaking, the younger the patient, the more aggressive I am in reducing these displacements. If there is *complete* displacement with a lack of bony content at the fracture site (in either direction), I consider reduction essential.

Intra-articular Fractures

Intra-articular fractures, those fractures of the calcaneus involving the subtalar joint, make up 60% of all tarsal injuries and 75% of all calcaneal fractures.[29, 49] These fractures are commonly bilateral.[148] Recommendations concerning treatment vary from early motion without reduction to anatomic open reduction.[143] When considering intra-articular fractures of the calcaneus, one must remember that no single form of treatment is applicable to all patients.

Comminuted fractures of the body of the os calcis

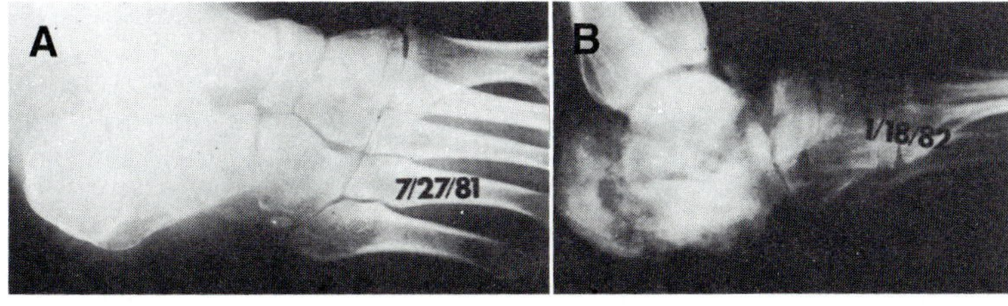

FIG 35–34.
A, nondisplaced fracture of the calcaneus in a severe diabetic. **B,** radiograph of the same patient 8 months later. The patient began bearing weight on the foot immediately. Note the neuropathic changes in the calcaneus.

with loss of vertical height, spreading, and involvement of the subtalar joint present difficult problems in treatment.[2] Chapman[30] recommends closed treatment and reports that of 100 os calcis fractures treated per year, he has to operate later for disability in only 1 or 2 patients. Other authors[110, 120–123, 145, 186] recommend open reduction and internal fixation of these fractures. However, McLaughlin[118, 119] compared attempts to maintain reduction of comminuted calcaneus fractures by internal or external methods with "nailing a custard pie to the wall."

Although Key and Conwell[97] recommended reduction of displacement in these fractures, they emphasized that inadequate reduction was not always followed by disability. Indeed, Rowe et al.[168] emphasize that 52% of fractures treated by casting, with or without manipulation, had good or excellent results, while 50% of those treated by accurate open reduction and internal fixation had good or excellent results.

McLaughlin[119] emphasized that attempts to classify intra-articular fractures of the calcaneus have failed to predict prognosis after these fractures. This is because the classifications are based only on subtalar joint involvement, which is just one of several factors that can produce pain and disability in the foot after these fractures.[119] Both Harris[79] and Miller[132] emphasize that disability following intra-articular fractures of the calcaneus results from a combination of (1) damage to the articular surface between the talus and os calcis, (2) deformity of the os calcis, and (3) damage to the surrounding soft tissues. Normally, ankle, subtalar, and midtarsal joint motion is necessary for the foot to adapt to the ground for walking. Pridie[156] emphasizes that when midtarsal and subtalar joint motion is limited, the patient has substantial disability.

In this chapter, intra-articular fractures are divided into four groups for purposes of discussion. These include fracture of the sustentaculum tali, tongue fracture, joint depression fracture, and comminuted fracture (see Table 35–2).

Fractures of the Sustentaculum Tali

Fractures of the sustentaculum tali account for fewer than 1% of all fractures of the calcaneus.[21, 77, 105, 106, 142, 200] Although fractures of the sustentaculum tali have often been included with extra-articular fractures of the calcaneus,[142] since the sustentaculum tali contains the medial subtalar facet, I have chosen to include it with intra-articular fractures.

Anatomy

The sustentaculum tali contains the middle facet of the subtalar joint on its superior surface. In a groove beneath the sustentaculum tali lies the tendon of the flexor hallucis longus, which serves as a sling to support the sustentaculum tali.[58] According to McLaughlin, this sling support is responsible for the fact that fractures of the sustentaculum tali are rarely displaced.[118] Additionally, the tibiocalcaneal components of the deltoid ligament attach to the sustentaculum and help to prevent its displacement when fractured.[171]

Mechanism of Injury

Several mechanisms have been implicated in the production of this fracture. A twisting injury less severe than what produces a fracture of the calcaneal tuberosity has been mentioned.[26, 104, 142] According to O'Connell et al.,[142] because less trauma is involved, the fracture is usually minimally displaced. McLaughlin[118] and Parkes[148] believe that this fracture is secondary to a fall on a strongly inverted foot that results in a downward impact of the talus against the sustentaculum tali. Gage and Premer[56] mention a force applied to the medial side of the foot with the heel in valgus as a mechanism of injury. Forceful inversion of the foot resulting in compression of the sustentaculum tali against the inferior surface of the talus has also been mentioned by O'Connell et al.[142]

Clinical Diagnosis

The patient gives a history of a fall on an inverted foot with a sudden pain on the medial aspect of the foot.[97] Point tenderness and swelling are located 1 in. inferior to the tip of the medial malleolus.[97, 148] There is usually little tenderness over the heel itself.[49] Pain located inferior to the medial malleolus with passive extension of the great toe (produced as the flexor hallucis longus slides beneath the fractured sustentaculum tali) has been mentioned as a diagnostic maneuver by Dodson.[49] Inversion of the foot may also produce pain below the medial malleolus.[54] Due to the location of tenderness and pain medially, one must avoid confusion with injury to the deltoid ligament.[58]

Subtalar motion is decreased and painful, while ankle motion is usually full and painless.[58]

Radiographic Diagnosis

Fracture of the sustentaculum tali is best visualized on an axial view of the calcaneus (Fig 35–35).[58, 148] It is important to obtain radiographs of the remainder of the calcaneus to rule out other calcaneal fractures.[58, 148]

Treatment

Fractures of the sustentaculum tali are rarely more than minimally displaced.[82, 118, 142] Brindley[21] and

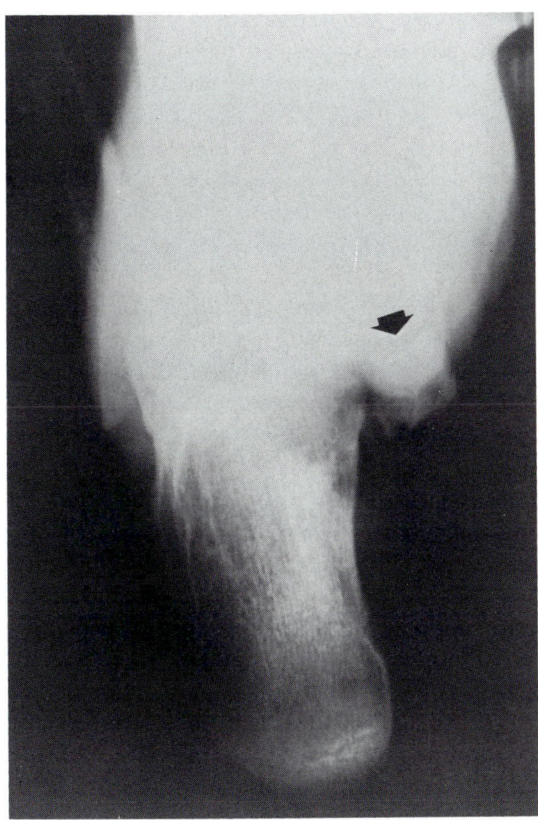

FIG 35–35.
Axial view of the calcaneus. Note the fracture of the sustentaculum tali *(arrow)*.

Carey et al.[26] recommend treating these fractures with a short-leg cast for 6 weeks and report that most patients return to work in 2 months with full weight bearing. O'Connell et al.[142] and Heck[82] recommend immobilization in a short-leg walking cast with the foot in slight varus to take stress off this fracture. In cases with minimal swelling and displacement, a comfortable shoe may suffice for treatment. Garcia and Parkes,[58] on the other hand, suggest treatment with ice, compression, elevation, and early range of motion. They strongly recommend avoiding plaster immobilization if possible.[58] They recommend non–weight bearing for 8 weeks because the sustentaculum tali is a weight-bearing structure and they believe that early weight bearing might cause fracture displacement. Dodson also recommends treating these fractures with ice, elevation, and non–weight bearing on crutches for 8 weeks without immobilization.[49]

If the fracture is displaced, Schottstaedt[174] recommends a walking cast without reduction, while Schofield[173] recommends closed reduction by digital pressure over the fragment. The foot is immobilized in a cast in inversion and dorsiflexion, and Reich[158] also recommends closed reduction using a compression clamp followed by immobilization in a cast.

According to Key and Conwell[97] displaced fractures of the sustentaculum tali should be reduced. The foot is inverted and plantar-flexed. The head of the first metatarsal is then pulled down in a plantar-flexed position and the forefoot pronated in order to restore the arch of the foot while digital pressure is applied upward against the sustentaculum tali. If the reduction is successful, the foot is held in a plantar-flexed and inverted position with the forefoot pronated in a short-leg cast for 6 weeks. Following cast removal, the patient is given a shoe with a heel elevation of ¼ in. on the inner border of the foot and a hard arch support.[97]

Prognosis

Carey et al.[26] report that most patients have a good result with only slight limitation of subtalar motion. However, one of their five patients developed subtalar arthritis.[26] McLaughlin[118] reports that union usually occurs after closed treatment and produces a good result. Nonunion of the sustentaculum tali, however, can produce pain on the medial aspect of the foot. If a painful nonunion is noted radiographically, excision of the fragment is the treatment of choice.[54] According to O'Connell et al.[142] and Heck[82] synovitis of the talocalcaneal joint may persist after cast removal and require the occasional use of anti-inflammatory agents and altered footgear.

Author's Preferred Method of Treatment

In my experience, fractures of the sustentaculum tali are most always only minimally displaced. I treat these patients with a compression dressing, ice, elevation, and early range of motion of the ankle, subtalar, midtarsal, and metatarsophalangeal joints. Active and passive motion of the great toe, which encourages immediate flexor hallus longus function, is recommended to prevent the flexor hallucis longus from scarring down beneath the sustentaculum tali. Once swelling has decreased and all motion restored, the patient is kept non–weight bearing on crutches for 4 weeks. This is followed by progressive weight bearing in a short-leg cast until painless weight bearing is possible.

If the fracture is displaced, I attempt closed reduction by inversion of the heel and upward digital pressure on the sustentaculum tali. If the fragment is successfully reduced, a short-leg cast with the toes free to allow metatarsophalangeal joint motion is applied for 4 weeks. Weight bearing in a short-leg cast is then allowed for the next 2 weeks. If no change in position of the fragment occurs, the patient is treated as though the fracture were nondisplaced, there being no indication, in my opinion, for open reduction of an isolated fracture of the sustentaculum tali. Should nonunion develop after a displaced fracture, excision will relieve the symptoms.

Tongue, Joint Depression, and Comminuted Fractures of the Os Calcis

Mechanism of Injury, Anatomy, and Classification

The usual mechanism of injury in intra-articular fractures is a fall from a height with the patient landing on his feet. Because of this mechanism, both heels are often involved.[60] As the heel strikes the ground, the talus acts as a wedge and compresses the posterior talocalcaneal joint into the body of the os calcis. According to McLaughlin,[118] this produces a fracture in the subtalar joint and results in two fragments: (1) a small superomedial fragment that includes the sustentaculum tali and medial portion of the posterior facet and (2) a large lateral plantar fragment that contains the tuberosity and the lateral aspect of the posterior facet of the subtalar joint. Since the calcaneus is made up entirely of cancellous bone, the entire posterior articular facet, or the lateral portion of it, can be easily driven or stamped into the underlying calcaneus.[174] The degree of fracture comminution and displacement depends on the weight and age of the patient, the height of the fall, and the mineral content of the bone.[58]

Aitken[2] emphasized that in these intra-articular fractures the tuberosity is usually displaced proximally, which reduces or reverses the tuberosity joint angle. Marked comminution and outward displacement of the lateral wall of the calcaneus obliterate the normal hollow beneath the lateral malleolus. According to Aitken, the main fracture line runs from the posteromedial wall of the calcaneus forward and outward toward the calcaneocuboid joint. This main fracture line may pass *lateral* to the posterior facet, in which case the joint is unharmed and a good result may be anticipated. However, the fracture line most often passes *through* the posterior facet, in which case the lateral joint fragment is displaced and rotated downward at its outer margin. Aitken believed that the medial half of the posterior facet in these fractures is usually not displaced. Displacement of the lateral half, however, results in a markedly irregular joint surface.

Essex-Lopresti[52] emphasized that the pattern of the fracture is remarkably constant. According to him, the biomechanics of this fracture involve vertical loading of the calcaneus by the talus at the crucial angle of Gissane.[52] The posterior subtalar joint is forced into eversion, with the lateral process of the talus being driven into the crucial angle. This produces a primary fracture line extending in the lateral cortex from the crucial angle to the plantar calcaneal surface (Figs 35–36,A and 35–37,A). If force is expended at this point, it results in a nondisplaced intra-articular fracture. However, if the force continues, a secondary fracture line is produced. The secondary fracture line extends from the crucial angle of Gissane posteriorly and produces two distinct types of displacement, tongue type and joint depression (Figs 35–36,B and 35–37,B). In the first, the tongue type, the secondary fracture line runs straight back from the crucial angle to the posterior border of the tuberosity. The anterior end of this large fracture fragment consists of the outer half of the subtalar articular surface and the upper border of the body (see Fig 35–36,B). As the force continues, the front end of the tongue is driven further down. While the tuberosity is still in contact with the ground, it is forced upward and backward. This results in the anterior end of the tongue being depressed *inside* the lateral wall of the body (Fig 35–36,C). An axial radiograph taken at this stage of the displacement demonstrates a step-off between the inner and outer components of the subtalar joint.

In the second, or joint depression, type the secondary fracture line runs across the calcaneal body to just *behind* the posterior facet of the subtalar joint. The lateral fragment consists of a well-defined unbroken piece of bone carrying the articular cartilage of the lateral half to two thirds of the posterior subtalar joint (see Fig 35–36,B). When the fracturing force continues, the lateral half joint fragment is depressed into the spongy bone of the calcaneus *inside* the lateral wall, which is driven outward. An axial radiograph of the calcaneus taken at this stage demonstrates the shearing fracture of the sustentaculum tali with displacement and bulging of the lateral wall. With further progression of the force, in addition to the inferior and posterior displacement of this articular fragment, the primary fracture line produced by the lateral process of the talus can open up and result in the tuberosity of the calcaneus being forced superiorly with a loss of the tuberosity joint angle and spreading of the primary fracture line (Fig 35–37,C).

Palmer believed that this shearing fracture was the primary force in calcaneal fractures.[145]

Soeur and Remy's classification[184] is similar to that of Essex-Lopresti,[52] with their "semilunar fracture" resembling the joint depression fracture and the "comet-shaped group" resembling the tongue fracture.

Essex-Lopresti emphasized that there is always a step-off with this displacement that varies from 3 to 10 mm between the outer and inner fragments of the posterior subtalar joint. At the moment of maximal compression, the medial (sustentacular) half of the posterior

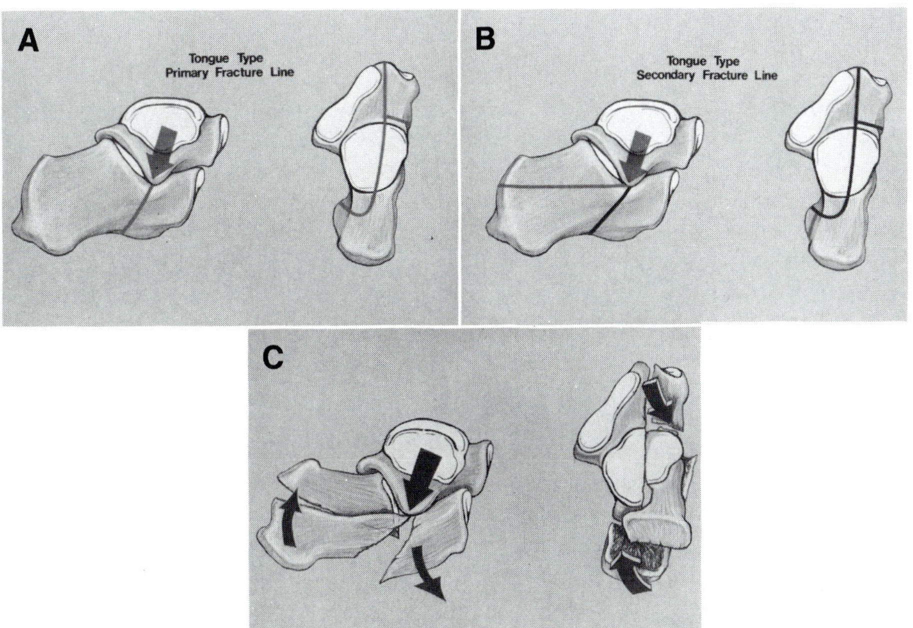

FIG 35–36.
Essex-Lopresti[52] tongue-type fracture. **A,** vertical loading of the calcaneus by the lateral process of the talus produces a primary fracture line from the crucial angle of Gissane to the plantar calcaneal surface. **B,** a secondary fracture line runs back to exit at the posterior border of the calcaneal tuberosity. The resulting tongue-shaped fragment contains the outer half of the posterior facet and the upper border of the body of the calcaneus. **C,** with further progression of force, the anterior end of the tongue is depressed inside the lateral wall of the body, and the tuberosity is displaced proximally. (Courtesy of BD Burdeaux, M.D., Houston.)

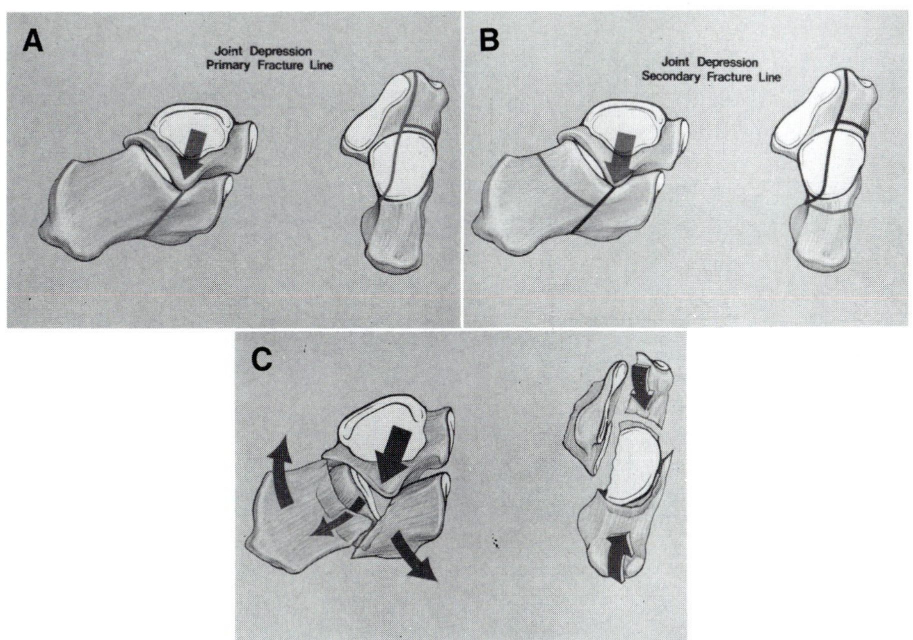

FIG 35–37.
Essex-Lopresti[52] joint depression–type fracture. **A,** vertical loading by the lateral process of the talus produces a primary fracture line from the crucial angle of Gissane to the plantar calcaneal surface. **B,** a secondary fracture line runs across the calcaneal body to exit *just* behind the posterior facet. The lateral fragment contains the lateral half to two thirds of the posterior facet with little soft-tissue attachment. **C,** with further progression of force, the lateral half of the joint fragment is depressed into the spongy bone of the calcaneus inside the lateral wall. The primary fracture line opens up and displaces the tuberosity proximally with loss of the tuberosity joint angle.

facet is depressed down to the level of the outer half. However, on release of the compression force, soft-tissue resilience of the foot causes the sustentacular half to be drawn up by its intact attachments to the talus. The outer half of the facet, buried inside the lateral wall, no longer has any attachments to the talus and therefore remains depressed. The height of the step-off is therefore a measure of the recoil that has occurred. Warrick and Bremner[199] and Stephenson,[186] on the basis of Thoren's work,[191] have noted that when the foot is in supination at impact, the primary sagittal fracture line passes along the calcaneal sulcus anterior to the posterior facet. If a secondary fracture line develops, the entire posterior facet remains intact but compressed. Supination of the foot also prevents the tuberosity fragment from being displaced laterally. The secondary fracture line creates a tongue or joint depression posterior facet fragment. Because this is the only displaced fragment, they are classified as compression, two part tongue, or compression, two-part joint depression fractures. The more common posterior facet intra-articular fractures are classified as shear compression, three-part tongue, or shear compression, three-part joint depression fractures, and occur with the foot in the neutral position. If the energy is dissipated after the primary fracture, two fracture fragments are created. The primary sagittal fracture line passes posterior to the posterior facet with the foot in pronation.

In cases in which the force is even greater, gross comminution of the remainder of the body of the calcaneus occurs and results in a severely comminuted fracture that does not fit in either the tongue-type or joint depression classification. These have been termed *comminuted fractures*[96] According to Stephenson[185] this mechanism produces a traumatic flatfoot deformity that has four components: (1) spread of the lateral wall; (2) depression of part of the posterior facet; (3) avulsion of the superomedial border of the calcaneus, which may include a portion of the posterior facet; and (4) shortening, which is a result of muscle forces crossing the bone. According to King,[100] 95% of fractures of the calcaneus that involve depression of the posterior facet can be classified into either the tongue or joint depression type as described by Essex-Lopresti.

McReynolds[123] on the other hand, believed that the oblique fracture originating in the medial cortex and extending upward, outward, and anteriorly to exit in some portion of the articular surface of the posterior facet is the primary fracture line. McReynolds emphasized that the point at which the oblique fracture line enters the posterior facet varies but that it is far more lateral than had been assumed by Essex-Lopresti. For this reason, the superomedial fragment often contains the sustentaculm tali and much more of the articular surface than the lateral fragment (Fig 35–38). There is medial displacement, overriding, and rotation of the superomedial fragment in 90% of both tongue-type and joint depression fractures. McReynolds found this to be the most constant significant deformity in these fractures.[123] He based his treatment on restoration of the position of this large superomedial fragment.

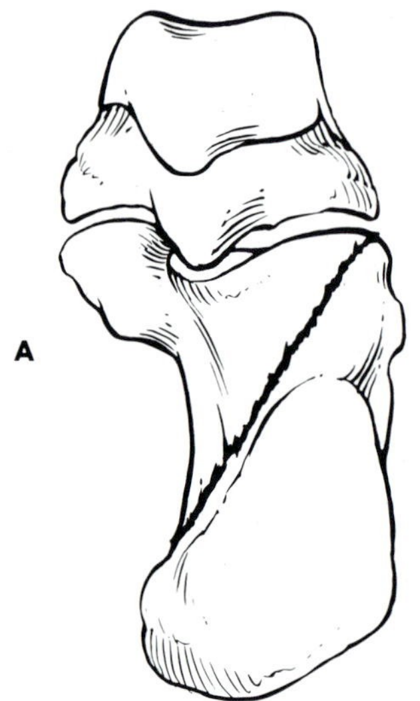

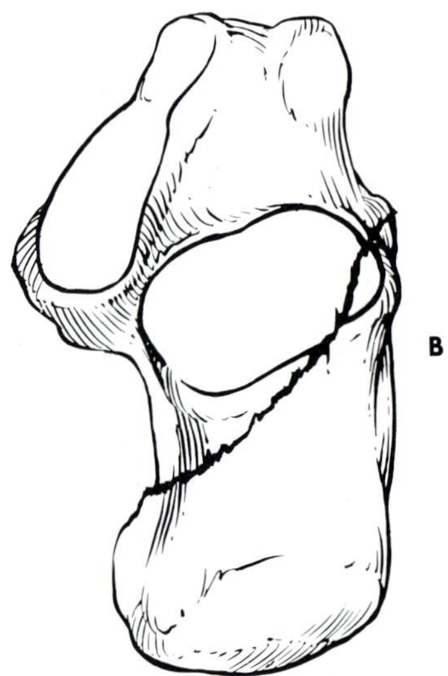

FIG 35–38.
A, According to McReynolds,[123] the main fracture line begins in the medial cortex and extends upward, outward, and anterior to exit in the posterior facet. **B,** the fracture line exits more laterally in the posterior facet than reported by Essex-Lopresti.[52] This fracture line produces a large superomedial fragment, reduction of which McReynolds believes is crucial.

In this section, I will use the Essex-Lopresti classification of intra-articular fractures of the calcaneus.

Clinical Diagnosis

The patient often gives a history of having fallen from a height.[97, 118] Indeed, according to Bohler,[18] the history of a vertical fall on the heel from a height of more than 5 m should suggest a calcaneus fracture. There is rapid swelling with severe pain in the heel.[91, 123] According to McReynolds, the pain is secondary to marked bleeding from the cancellous bone and to the fact that the heel is tightly enveloped in fascia, which prevents extravasation of the blood into the adjacent subcutaneous tissues.[123] Later, there is discoloration about the medial and lateral sides of the heel.[123] Occasionally the hemorrhage and discoloration may extend up the calf some distance away from the heel.[123] If treatment is delayed, severe swelling and blood collection in the skin over the medial and lateral aspects of the heel develops.

Objectively, there is tenderness and ecchymosis in the tissues surrounding the calcaneus.[58] Clinically the normal contour of the hindfoot is distorted.[58] The arch may also be flattened and the distance from the heel to the lateral malleolus shortened vs. the normal foot. According to Key and Conwell, the longitudinal arch of the foot is flattened by upward displacement of the tuberosity and sagging of the inner border of the foot, and the malleoli are lowered because of the upward displacement of the tuberosity.[97] Point tenderness is limited to the os calcis.[91] Subtalar motion is limited and painful, while ankle motion is painless.[58, 91, 97] One can usually palpate excess bone behind and below the external malleolus secondary to the bulge of the lateral calcaneal wall.[97] Upward and forward displacement of the tuberosity of the calcaneus in severely comminuted fractures tends to relax the Achilles tendon and decrease plantar flexion power, the so-called Hoffa sign.[97, 148] An inability to bear weight, broadening and swelling of the heel, and a hematoma that extends anteriorly toward the sole all help, according to Bohler,[18] to distinguish calcaneal fractures from fractures of the ankle.

If the mechanism of injury is a fall, one must look for associated compression fractures of the lumbar spine.[29, 58] Parkes emphasizes the importance of palpation of both the spine and the ankle to detect the tenderness that suggests these commonly associated fractures.[150]

Radiographic Diagnosis

A complete radiographic evaluation is essential in all patients with a history of a fall from a height and heel pain. Routine radiographs used to evaluate intra-articular fractures of the calcaneus include an anteroposterior, a true lateral, and an axial view. Anthonsen's view, Broden's projections I and II, the oblique dorsoplantar view, the medial oblique axial view, and the lateral oblique axial view can then be used to delineate the degree of involvement of the subtalar joint. A CT scan of the calcaneus is essential to evaluate these fractures. A complete description of these special radiographic views and their interpretation is found on pages 35-20 to 35-24.

Radiographs of the lumbar spine are mandatory in patients who suffer a significant fall and all patients who complain of back pain and have spine tenderness on physical examination.

Treatment

A review of the current literature reveals no universally accepted method for the treatment of intra-articular fractures of the calcaneus. According to Cave,[29] severely comminuted intra-articular fractures treated by expert fracture surgeons result in acceptable functional and economic results in no more than 50% of cases, no matter whether treatment is by manipulation and plaster fixation, wire traction, or open reduction.[29] He stresses that the surgeon *must* avoid overtreating the fracture while neglecting the remainder of the foot.[29]

Deyerle[46] reports that patients treated by open reduction and internal fixation or by immediate arthrodesis have no better results than those treated conservatively.[46] Thoren[191] stated that while in fractures with severe displacement open reduction may give a better result, in similar cases early physical therapy can give sufficient results to warrant the use of this method instead of open treatment.

In addition to conflicting reports regarding the best means of treatment of those fractures, there is difficulty in comparing the different reports in the literature because most evaluations depend on the patients' own concept of their results, an interpretation that is not always reliable.[74] Additionally, authors have used different objective evaluation systems in reporting their results.

At present there is no one method suitable for the treatment of all of these fractures. There are five basic methods of treatment of intra-articular fractures of the calcaneus: (1) closed treatment without reduction, (2) closed reduction with and without immobilization, (3) open reduction and internal fixation with and without bone grafting, (4) primary subtalar or triple arthrodesis, and (5) excision. Each of these methods will be discussed here, with the strengths and weaknesses of each emphasized in an effort to help the reader select the treatment modality most useful in each particular situation.

Closed Treatment Without Reduction.—Closed treatment of calcaneus fractures *without* an attempt at reduction has been advocated by many authors.* In 1946 Roberts and Sayle Creer emphasized the value of conservative treatment without reduction.[162] Trickey[192] emphasizes that this is *not* treatment by neglect; rather, the method must be learned and carefully supervised. Bankart,[10] Thoren,[191] and Essex-Lopresti[52] report good results with early motion and non–weight bearing. They report no loss of position with this method of treatment as long as early weight bearing is avoided.

McLaughlin[119] considered the physician treating a calcaneus fracture to be on the horns of a dilemma. By using early motion without reduction he accepts deformity in order to maintain motion. On the other hand, by attempting a reduction, he accepts the stiffness inherent in the immobilization necessary to maintain the reduction.[119] McLaughlin prefers early motion without reduction for the following reasons: (1) immobilization is not necessary for union, (2) these fractures will heal with or without treatment, (3) immobilization of these fractures invariably produces a stiffened foot, and (4) such a stiff foot is usually painful.

Since os calcis fractures will not be displaced by early active motion of the foot and ankle and because nonunion of the calcaneus is practically unheard of, Cave believed that early motion and partial weight bearing could be allowed without harm by using crutches and a well-fitting shoe soon after injury.[29] Early range of motion of the foot and toes helps to maintain muscle tone and to improve the circulatory status of the extremity.[29]

According to Lance et al.[105] stability of calcaneus fractures is secondary to bony impaction at the time of injury, and therefore, immobilization is not necessary. Their treatment consists of compression, early range of motion and non–weight bearing for 12 weeks. They emphasized that early weight bearing can result in a further loss of Bohler's angle.[106]

The disadvantage of this form of treatment is that the deformity present at the time of injury must be compatible with good function.[105] If the deformity is compatible with good function, good results can be obtained with early range of motion. Lance et al.[105] reported that fractures treated by compression dressing and early motion produced 55% satisfactory results while operative treatment produced only 48% satisfactory results with a staggering 17% complication rate. They set forth the following criteria for closed treatment: (1) proper weight-bearing alignment of the hindfoot, (2) freedom of the peroneal tendons of impingement from lateral bulge, (3) a congruent relationship between the posterior facets of the talus and calcaneus, and (4) an elderly patient. If patients meet these criteria, 99% return to their preactivity level of treatment.

Lapidus and Guidotti[109] also emphasize the importance of avoiding long-term immobilization. They believe that any attempt at reduction with either a compression clamp or skeletal traction will require prolonged immobilization of 6 to 8 weeks to maintain the alignment. This results in fibrous ankylosis of the subtalar joint *and* the remainder of the joints of the foot. A stiff, painful foot results. They therefore recommend the use of swimming pool exercises so that the buoyancy of the body in the water can unweight the injured limb. The patient initially begins in the deep water and progressively moves to shallower water as pain allows. Their patients returned to work in 3 to 5 months. Lapidus and Guidotti[107] believe that early range of motion helps to mold the articular surfaces of the involved joints and decrease swelling. On the other hand, Hazlett[81] does not believe that early range of motion does much to restore the irregular joint surfaces when congruity is marked.

Barnard[11, 12, 14] recommends elevation, ice packs, movement of the foot and ankle 5 minutes of every hour, and avoidance of weight bearing for 6 weeks. The first shoe used by the patient has the heel elevated to produce 45 degrees of ankle equinus. The heel is gradually decreased in height over the next 6 weeks until the foot is flat. If the patient cannot cooperate with this method of treatment, after the swelling has decreased, Barnard[11] recommends a walking cast with a sponge rubber pad about the heel and the foot in the equinus position. The height of the cast heel is decreased until the foot is in the normal position, usually after about 6 weeks.

Parkes[149, 150] also advocates early motion and non–weight bearing without reduction in the treatment of these fractures. The patient is admitted to the hospital, and a compression dressing is applied from the foot to the knee. Ice bags are applied to the heel and the foot elevated. After 24 hours, the patient is encouraged to move the foot and ankle in all directions. These exercises are performed once every waking hour. The whirlpool can be used to help the patient perform these exercises. After 3 to 5 days, when the pain begins to subside, the compression dressing is replaced by an elastic stocking. The patient is allowed to dangle his legs briefly over the side of the bed several times a day for 1 to 2 days and is then allowed up on crutches *with-*

**References 10, 12, 14, 16, 49, 56, 59, 102, 138, 139, 142, 177, 191.*

out weight bearing on the fractured heel. When not ambulatory on the crutches, the foot is kept elevated. The patient is then fitted with a walking oxford with a well-molded heel and built-in arch. The patient slowly increases the amount of pressure he applies to the foot. Between 4 to 8 weeks after injury, most patients are fully weight bearing, and many return to work after 6 to 12 weeks. Parkes emphasizes that if pain from arthritis or peroneal tenosynovitis develops following this mode of treatment, patients are treated as necessary later. He emphasizes that it may take up to 2 years to get an optimum result.[148] He recommends that this treatment be used particularly by those surgeons who have no experience in treating fractures of the calcaneus because it offers an acceptable result in most patients. Recently, Salama et al.[169] recommended early immediate elevation, ice, and early range of motion. Exercises are instituted within 24 hours. Resisted plantar flexion is emphasized to overcome the weakness of the gastrocnemius secondary to the shortened triceps surae resulting from proximal fracture displacement. They begin partial weight bearing at 4 to 6 weeks and patients are continued on partial weight bearing status for an additional 4 to 6 weeks. When this method of treatment is used, they report satisfactory results in 82% of fractures.[169]

When treating these fractures by early motion without reduction Vestad emphasizes the importance of avoiding cast immobilization.[196] Gage and Premer[56] report that the results of plaster immobilization without reduction are less satisfactory than early range of motion without immobilization. Dick[47] recognized the problem of stiffness in the foot following calcaneus fractures and recommended that a cast not be used postoperatively. Lindsay and Dewar[114] found that in conservatively treated patients, those that were manipulated had poorer results than those treated by early motion without reduction.

In reviewing the literature, good results are reported in a variety of fractures treated in this manner. The common theory is that early motion without immobilization avoids the stiff, painful foot that is often produced when cast immobilization is utilized.

However, the criteria for which patients should be treated in this fashion are not clear. Vestad[196] recommends this method of treatment in patients over 50 years of age and those with severely displaced fractures. Kalish[196] recommends this method for diabetics and patients with peripheral vascular disease due to the high incidence of complications in these patients following other forms of treatment. On the other hand, Burghele and Serban[425] report that since a valgus heel, flatfoot deformity, and painful arthrosis may occur following this method of treatment, reduction should be considered in those patients presenting with severe flatfoot deformity and a valgus heel. Finally, Harris[77] reports that even severely comminuted fractures of the calcaneus that result from war injuries and have marked displacement and soft-tissue injury often do fairly well after this treatment in spite of the marked deformity.

Closed Reduction.

Closed Reduction With Immobilization.—Since early motion without reduction necessitates that the surgeon accept the displacement present initially, reduction and maintenance of the reduction are recommended by some. Indeed, although McLaughlin prefers early motion without reduction as the main form of treatment, he does give three indications for reduction of calcaneus fractures: (1) if the tuberosity of the calcaneus is displaced proximally, it should be transfixed with a pin and pulled down to restore gastrocnemius-soleus length; (2) in grossly widened calcaneus fractures in which the lateral fragment is jammed up beneath the fibula, it should be reduced by compression either manually or with a clamp; (3) occasionally, if the displaced posterior articular facet is driven into the calcaneus without comminution, reduction is indicated.[118, 119]

The goals of closed reduction and fixation include (1) restoration of Bohler's angle, (2) restoration of the normal width of the calcaneus, and (3) an attempt to restore the congruity of the subtalar joint. Cotton and Wilson in 1908[37] emphasized the importance of decreasing the width of the heel following calcaneus fractures to prevent the lateral buildup of callus beneath the distal end of the fibula. Calcaneal width was reduced by pounding on the lateral surface of the calcaneus with a mallet, after which the foot was placed in plaster. However, Carothers and Lyons[27] found that when long-term immobilization was utilized following Cotton's reduction, lateral motion of the foot was entirely missing. The patients complained of the inability to walk on uneven terrain. They therefore modified Cotton's technique by removing the cast at the tenth postreduction day and instituting early motion while denying weight bearing for 8 weeks. They found that subtalar motion was restored relatively quickly. They report that this method resulted in a painless heel with good subtalar motion.

Wilson[206] also modified Cotton's technique for comminuted fractures. While one assistant maintains pull on the leg and another countertraction on the dorsum of the foot and the back of the heel, the lateral spread of the heel is reduced by a direct blow over a broomstick placed beneath the lateral malleolus. This results in decreasing the width of the calcaneus and restoring the proximal displacement of the tuberosity. If the reduction is acceptable, the patient is placed in a short-leg cast with sponge rubber padding placed beneath the medial and lateral malleoli. The foot is in moderate plantar flexion, and pressure is applied to the heel to maintain alignment and the decreased width. After 10 days the cast is removed and early motion begun. The patient is kept non–weight bearing for 8 weeks and is placed in a stiff-soled shoe.

Bohler's Method.—Bohler[18] in 1931 recommended closed reduction utilizing traction. His goal was to correct the axial deviation, flattening, and shortening of the calcaneus. Reduction is performed after 6 to 10 days to allow the swelling in the foot to subside. Under anesthesia, the fracture is disimpacted by placing the sole of the foot over a wooden wedge and forcing the foot into plantar flexion. The foot is then prepared and two pins inserted, one through the tibia four finger breadths above the ankle joint and a second, parallel to the first, through the posterior upper corner of the tuberosity of the calcaneus. Both of these pins are then connected to wire stirrups. By using these pins and stirrups, traction is applied first in the longitudinal axis of the leg in order to reduce the tuberosity joint angle and then in the axis of the body of the calcaneus to reduce shortening. Next, a screw vice is used to apply pressure medially and laterally beneath the malleoli to reduce the lateral spread. The reduction is then checked radiographically. An unpadded cast is applied from the toes to the popliteal fossa with the traction still in place. When the plaster hardens, the fracture alignment is maintained by the pins. The pins remain in for 3 to 5 weeks, at which time a walking plaster cast and stirrup are applied. When the fracture is healed, a Blucher-type shoe with a custom arch support is prescribed, and gradual weight bearing is permitted.

Aitken[2] utilized a modification of Bohler's pin traction and Cotton's reduction method for calcaneus fractures. He recommended immediate reduction to prevent further swelling and blood pooling since he believed that delaying reduction allows clot organization, which can prevent reduction. He placed the foot medial side down on padding and placed a rolled-up towel over the lateral aspect of the calcaneus. The towel was struck with a hammer. This corrected the lateral spread of the calcaneus. If it failed, a Bohler clamp was applied to reduce the residual displacement. If there was upper displacement of the tuberosity, it was grasped by tongs and a crutch placed in the arch of the foot, just distal to the calcaneocuboid joint. The tongs were pulled down and the crutch forced into the arch. This resulted in restoration of the arch and reduction and tuberosity displacement. If this method resulted in reduction, the patient was placed in a cast with pads placed beneath the medial and lateral malleoli. The cast was changed as swelling dictated, but the patient remained in the cast for 10 weeks. Following this the patient was placed in a stiff-soled shoe.

Olson[143] also modified Bohler's technique by using two turnbuckles to connect the pins in the tibia and os calcis. The turnbuckles were used to manipulate the fracture and maintain the reduction. According to Olson, the turnbuckles make fracture reduction and maintenance easier than casting.

Leonard[110] noted that since there are no fibrous structures passing between the adjacent articular surfaces of the posterior subtalar joint (which are necessary for traction to reduce depressed articular fragments), the logic behind Bohler's traction method is questionable. Allan[3] and Burghele and Serban[25] also report a failure of reduction of the displaced posterior facet with Bohler's method.

Schofield[173] reports good results with this technique and emphasized the importance of restoration of the normal weight-bearing alignment of the foot. However, Conn[33] reports that although alignment of the foot may be improved by traction methods, subtalar motion is often limited. Conn[33] recommends triple arthrodesis after reduction by Bohler's technique because of the stiffness present after traction treatment and casting. Gossett[68] reports that reduction by traction followed by early mobilization helps to decrease the incidence of stiff foot. However, according to Aitken, although the subtalar joint is often stiff after cast removal, it usually loosens up with ambulation, and 75% of patients treated in this manner return to gainful employment.[2]

Harris[77] found that while traction by Bohler's method would correct the gross alignment of the foot, it had no effect on restoring articular surface alignment. He therefore recommended fusion in conjunction with this reduction. Traction and heel compression are used to reduce the fracture. The traction pins are incorporated into a cast. If fracture reduction is not acceptable, fusion is carried out 10 days following reduction. According to Lindsay and Dewar,[114] reduction of calcaneus fractures is achieved in only 30% of patients when pin traction is used. Additionally, they report an 11% incidence of pin tract infection in patients when pins are used for reduction. Lance et al.[106] report that three fourths of patients treated by pin traction have unsatisfactory results, the group with the highest failure rate. They therefore suggest that pin traction be removed from the armamentarium of the surgeon treating calcaneus fractures.

Hermann's Method.—Hermann in 1937 reported a modification of Bohler's method of treatment.[83] After general or spinal anesthesia, the patient is turned on the side opposite the fracture, and a sandbag is placed under the medial aspect of the heel. A rolled towel is placed beneath the lateral malleolus and a hammer used to deliver a blow to the piled-up bone beneath the lateral malleolus. The blows are repeated until the normal depression beneath the lateral malleolus is restored. The heel is then molded by hand and subtalar motion tested. Hermann believes that unless subtalar motion is restored at this point, the lateral submalleolar bone block has not been sufficiently removed. After the lateral spread is reduced, tongs are used to grasp the upper posterior part of the calcaneus. Countertraction from a crutch placed in the arch of the foot just distal to the calcaneocuboid joint is then applied. Traction is applied through these tongs. This is done to overcome the posterior vertical pull of the calf muscles and the inferior horizontal pull of the intrinsic muscles of the foot. The tongs are then removed. A small roll of felt is placed obliquely beneath the medial and lateral malleoli and a plaster of paris cast applied with the foot in slight inversion and extreme plantar flexion. The cast is removed after 2 weeks and the submalleolar pads replaced. The foot is placed at a right angle and a new cast applied. New casts and pads are applied up to 10 or 12 weeks postfracture to maintain constant pressure beneath the malleoli. The patient is then fitted with a brace, and weight bearing is begun. Hermann reported 73% good results with this method of treatment. However, Giannestras and Sammarco[63] report that the end results of this method of treatment are no better than the nonreduction methods mentioned earlier in this section. McReynolds emphasizes that Hermann's method can be expected to do little more than change the tuberosity joint angle and does not offer any likelihood of reducing the displaced posterior facet.[121]

Modified Hermann's Method.—Giannestras and Sammarco recommend the use of a modified Hermann method for select displaced tongue-type fractures.[58, 63] The patient is placed on a fracture table under general anesthesia. A heavy, threaded Kirschner wire is inserted through the calcaneal tuberosity close to the superior cortex of the fragment. The knee is flexed 80 degrees over a knee support on the fracture table, thereby relaxing the gastrocnemius-soleus muscle complex. Traction is exerted on the calcaneus through a Kirschner bow incorporating the threaded pin with countertraction occurring at the knee. Traction is continued until the articular fragment is disimpacted and separated. According to Giannestras, by exerting sufficient traction on the intraosseous talocalcaneal ligament, the posterior articular fragment can be distracted from its bed.[58] When traction is released, the fragment will then settle into its original bed without any residual displacement. this traction force reestablishes the tuberosity joint angle of the calcaneus. The heel is palpated to be certain that the medial-lateral spread of the calcaneus has been reduced. In an acceptable reduction, the finger can be placed between each of the malleoli and the lateral or medial cortices of the calcaneus. If the normal width has not been restored by the traction, a compressive force is applied with a Bohler clamp.

A radiograph is taken to see whether the tuberosity joint angle has been reestablished and the tongue fragment has returned to its normal position. A long-leg cast is applied with molding about the heel and a roll of sheet wadding placed beneath the malleoli. The traction is released and a long-leg cast applied from the midthigh with the foot in the neutral position. Kirschner wires are incorporated into the cast. At the end of 3 weeks the cast and Kirschner wires are removed, and a new, well-molded long-leg cast is applied for 3 more weeks. When the cast is removed, the patient is begun on an exercise program to encourage range of motion. No weight bearing is permitted until there is radiographic evidence of union.

Essex-Lopresti Method.—Essex-Lopresti[52] credits William Gissane with introducing the method of closed reduction of intra-articular fractures of the calcaneus by means of a specially designed stainless steel spike introduced into the calcaneus and incorporated into a plaster cast.

According to Essex-Lopresti,[52] although both open and closed reduction using the spike for fixation achieves good reduction, they suffer from the disadvantage that postoperative fixation in plaster is necessary. After such immobilization some of the feet were quite stiff. For these reasons, he introduced a small shoe-shaped plaster slipper designed to hold the spike after reduction and yet enable ankle, subtalar, and midtarsal joint movement to begin the day after operation. He found the shoe-shaped plaster cast sufficient to hold the reduction in spite of early motion. This technique incorporates all the features of treatment that are necessary for a good result: exact reduction, minimal trauma, and immediate exercise of the joints to prevent stiffness.[52]

Essex-Lopresti[52] clearly distinguished between two types of displaced intra-articular calcaneal fractures, the tongue and joint depression types. He recommended closed reduction with a Gissane spike for the tongue-type fracture and open reduction using the Gissane spike to maintain reduction of the joint depression types.

For tongue-type fractures, the patient is anesthetized and placed in the prone position on the operating table. An incision is made over the displaced tuberosity of the calcaneus *lateral* to the insertion of the tendo Achillis. A Gissane spike or heavy Steinmann pin is introduced into the tongue fragment in the axis of the calcaneus and angled slightly toward its lateral wall (Fig 35–39). Radiographs are taken in the axial and lateral planes to determine the position of the pin. It must be in the tongue fragment but should not cross the fracture line. The knee is flexed to a right angle, and while holding the forefoot in one hand and the handle of the spike in the other, reduction is effected by lifting the knee just clear of the table. According to Essex-Lopresti, during this maneuver the fragment can be felt to click loose, and the handle of the spike will move upward as the tongue fragment rotates. The weight of the leg and thigh as they are lifted off the table exerts a sufficient force to pull the sustentacular fragment into alignment with the body of the os calcis. The displaced fragments are now lying in their correct relationship, and the depressed tongue fragment is once again clear of the

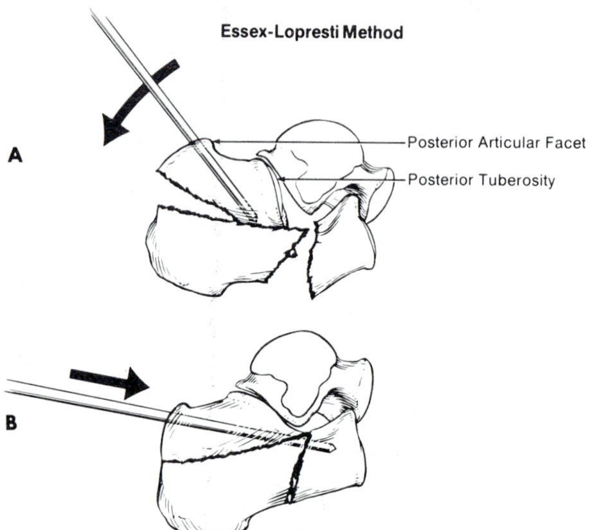

FIG 35–39.
Essex-Lopresti's method of reduction. **A,** in a tongue-type fracture, a Gissane spike or Steinmann pin is inserted into the calcaneal tuberosity, lateral to the Achilles tendon, while being careful not to cross the fracture site. A pin is then used to manipulate the tongue fragment into position. **B,** after radiographs confirm reduction of the fracture, the pin is driven into the anterior end of the calcaneus to maintain reduction.

bulged-out lateral wall. The heels of the surgeon's hands are then used to press the medial and lateral walls together and line up the tuberosity and sustentaculum tali. While the reduction is held by an assistant, a slipper cast is applied that incorporates the spike. The patient is kept at bed rest for 10 days.[52] The spike and plaster are removed in tongue fractures at the end of 4 weeks. Essex-Lopresti then recommends a protective below-the-knee plaster cast for 4 additional weeks. The patient is kept non-weight bearing for a total of 8 to 10 weeks, at which time radiographs indicate union. Weight bearing and walking exercises are then instituted.

In joint depression–type fractures, Essex-Lopresti[52] recommends exposure of the depressed fragment by open surgery, reduction of the fragment under direct vision, and maintenance of the reduction by a Gissane spike inserted from behind (see the section on open reduction).

King[100] has modified the Essex-Lopresti technique. He found that the slipper cast had occasionally resulted in a loss of reduction. Therefore, he places the patient immediately into a short-leg cast incorporating the axial spike. The cast and spike are left on for 4 weeks. The spike is then removed and a second short-leg cast applied for an additional 4 weeks. During the last 2 weeks of this period, the patient is allowed to bear weight via a walking heel applied to the cast. Although King recommended this method in both tongue- and joint depression–type fractures, he reported best results in the tongue type.

Both Essex-Lopresti[52] and King[100] report excellent results in patients treated by this method. Also, according to Aaron,[1] the results of patients treated by reduction with a spike are better than patients treated by early mobilization without reduction.

According to McReynolds,[123] however, this technique can result in overcorrection of the tuberosity joint angle. He also questions whether this technique will actually restore the displaced superomedial fragment and hence the intra-articular step-off. Finally, Slatis et al.[179] report that depression of the subtalar joint is not easily restored by utilizing a percutaneous Steinmann pin. Additionally, they believe that to restore Bohler's angle, one must reduce the posterior facet, not simply pull down a proximally displaced tuberosity. According to their report, reduction of the posterior facet by a percutaneous pin is rarely accomplished.

Closed Reduction Without Immediate Immobilization.—Omoto et al.[144] have recommended closed reduction without immobilization in calcaneal fractures. Their method of reduction is based on normal ligamentous anatomy of the foot. The talocalcaneal ligament inserting on the lateral side of the calcaneus, the medial talocalcaneal ligament inserting on the sustentaculum tali, and the interosseous ligament all have attachments to the subtalar joint. Additionally, the tibiocalcaneal fibers of the deltoid ligament, attached to the sustentaculum tali, and the calcaneofibular ligament, attached slightly posteriorly on the lateral side of the calcaneus, have attachments to the subtalar joint. If the calcaneofibular and tibiocalcaneal ligaments are intact, Omoto et al. believe that manual reduction can be performed.

In view of these anatomic facts, the patient, under spinal anesthesia, is placed in a prone position with the knee of the affected leg bent 90 degrees. The assistant holds the leg in this position, and the operating surgeon stands at the patient's feet. The surgeon then covers the medial and lateral sides of the calcaneus with both palms and crosses the fingers of both hands around the heel. The area is compressed with the palms, and the calcaneal tuberosity is repeatedly squeezed upward with strong traction and bending into varus and valgus (Fig 35–40). Anteroposterior, lateral, axial, and oblique radiographs are then obtained to confirm reduction.

According to the authors, a plaster cast is not necessary. The foot is kept elevated, and active motion exercises of the toes and ankle are started 1 day after reduction. When the swelling subsides, hot packs and baths are started. One month after reduction the patient begins weight bearing by walking in a swimming pool. Two months after reduction, the patient is allowed to walk with an arch support and crutches. At 3 months patients are allowed to walk without support

Finally, Rockwood[163] incorporates closed reduction, early motion, and *delayed* casting in the treatment of calcaneal fractures. The entire foot and heel are prepared, wrapped in a sterile dressing, and elevated. If the heel is widened or tilted into varus or valgus, he recommends the application of medial-lateral compression by utilizing the heels of the surgeon's palms beneath each malleoli. If the fracture is impacted, the compression force is combined with a shaking motion to break up the impaction. The heel is then molded into the correct position. The goal of this reduction is to decompress the lateral side of the heel by restoring normal width and place the weight-bearing surface of the heel *parallel* to the floor by correcting varus-valgus angulation of the calcaneus.

A sterile compression dressing is applied, and the limb is elevated with ice. The patient is immediately begun on range of toe, ankle, and subtalar joint motion under adequate pain medication coverage. The limb is left elevated until swelling decreases, usually around 7 to 10 days. According to Rockwood, this 7 to 10 days of early motion after manual reduction restores subtalar, ankle, and forefoot motion *before* casting. The patient is then placed in a well-molded "drop foot cast." This is a short-leg cast applied with the patient sitting and the leg hanging off of the bed. The foot thereby assumes a slight equinus position under the force of gravity only, *not* a full equinus position. After the cast is dried, a walking heel is applied to the cast *anterior* to the anterior border of the tibia. This location of the walking heel

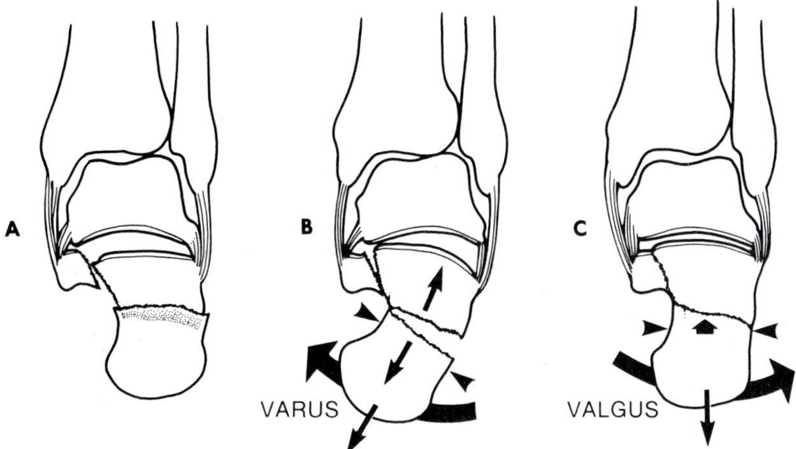

FIG 35–40.
Closed reduction of an intra-articular calcaneus fracture. **A,** depressed intra-articular fracture of the calcaneus. When the lateral fibulocalcaneal and medial talocalcaneal ligaments are intact, the joint will not open excessively with varus or valgus stress. **B,** when ligaments are intact, manipulation by traction and adduction opens up lateral compression *at the fracture site.* **C,** then valgus force is applied, which results in the distal fragment pushing the displaced fragment upward, thereby reducing the intra-articular displacement. (Adapted from Omoto H, Sakurada K, Sugi M, et al: *Clin Orthop* 177:104–111, 1983.)

permits early weight bearing under the theory that the vector of body weight passes from the tibia through the talus to the navicular, then to the metatarsals, and finally to the anteriorly placed walking heel to the floor. This permits early weight bearing with the calcaneus bypassed and its collapse thereby prevented. When the cast is dry, the patient begins to toe-touch with weight bearing as tolerated. This early weight bearing causes muscle contraction, which stimulates venous return. The cast is removed at 6 to 8 weeks. A tight lace-up boot is then applied for an additional 3 to 4 months. Rockwood reports good results even in severely comminuted fractures treated in this fashion.

Open Reduction.—Morestein[135] of Paris first recommended a direct approach to elevate the depressed posterior articular facet in a calcaneus fracture in 1902. Whittaker in 1947 first introduced open reduction of calcaneus fractures in the United States.[203] Since then many authors have advocated open reduction of intra-articular calcaneus fractures.* Most authors emphasize that open reduction of the joint depression–type fracture is the only accurate method of achieving an anatomic reduction of the posterior facet.

Hammesfahr and Fleming[76] believe that treatment of intra-articular fractures of the calcaneus should follow the same guidelines as the treatment of any other intra-articular fracture: restoration of the joint surface and joint incongruity. They believe that although a tongue fracture can be treated by the Essex-Lopresti method, all joint depression–type fractures should be treated by open reduction. They reported a positive correlation between facet reduction and successful results. According to Allan,[3] the indications for open reduction include (1) depression of the posterior articular facet noted on the lateral radiographic view and (2) depression of the lateral half of the posterior facet noted on the axial view.

Miller[132] prefers open reduction for patients in the median age range and reserves closed treatment for patients at either end of the age scale. He reports that although swelling and discomfort occur with equal frequency after open or closed treatment, shoe-fitting problems are much more frequent following the closed treatment of calcaneus fractures. His indications for open reduction include improvement in shoe wear (particularly if there is a loss in Bohler's angle), a decrease in os calcis height, and crowding of bone laterally, under the fibular malleolus. He does not recommend open reduction in older patients or patients who have excessive swelling, abrasions, skin blistering, or other local conditions that predispose to good wound healing.

Several methods of open reduction have been popularized. The technique and indications given for the use of each are presented below.

Palmer's Method.—Palmer[145] in 1948 reported a method of open reduction of calcaneal fractures that he credited to Lenormant and Wilmoth.[109] After attempting primary arthrodesis of the talocalcaneal joint in these injuries, he became convinced that open reduction was possible. The fracture is approached through a 6-cm-long incision located beneath the lateral malleolus. The peroneal tendon sheath is incised and the tendons displaced forward. The middle part of the fibulocalcaneal ligament is then incised to expose the talocalcaneal joint. The foot is carefully dislocated into a varus position over a medial wedge to enable the surgeon to look into the joint and visualize displacement of the posterior facet. Reduction of the depressed fragment is obtained by direct traction downward and backward on the tuber calcanei, combined with elevation of the depressed lateral fragment into position by utilizing a lever. Once the traction and the elevator were released, however, Palmer noted that the displacement often recurred. When the fragments were held in position, a large defect formed by compression of the spongy bone of the calcaneus was noted beneath the articular fragment. Palmer therefore recommended direct bone grafting of this defect. Once bone grafting was performed, the reduction was noted to be stable. The patient is then placed in a short-leg cast for 12 weeks. The cast is followed by a stocking and firm shoe with a longitudinal arch support. According to Palmer, the majority of patients maintained a fourth to a half the normal range of subtalar motion following this method of open reduction.

Maxfield and McDermott[128] report excellent or good functional results in nearly 70% of patients treated by Palmer's method. They noted, however, that the degree of excellence of anatomic restoration of the contour of the calcaneus did *not* necessarily parallel the functional result. Maxfield[125] recommends open reduction in all fractures of the calcaneus with displacement or depression of the posterior articular facet, with the possible exception of fractures with extreme comminution of the facet.[125, 126] He strongly emphasized the importance of bone grafting to prevent loss of reduction of the fracture. He recommends that the operation be performed as soon as possible after injury, but notes that satisfactory results have been obtained as long as 2 weeks postfracture. If skin compromise is present in the area of the incision, he recommends that the operation be delayed

**References 76, 81, 111, 120–123, 145, 158, 159, 176, 184, 203, 204.*

until the skin has recovered. Hammesfahr and Fleming[76] report that 25% to 50% of subtalar motion is maintained following treatment of calcaneal fractures by Palmer's method. Other authors have reported excellent results in 50% to 80% of cases treated.[56, 109, 110, 168, 204]

Allan[3] also recommends open reduction with bone grafting through a lateral approach for displaced fractures involving the posterior articular facet. Postoperatively the patients are kept in a non–weight-bearing cast for 6 weeks. Hazlett[81] also recommends open reduction through a lateral incision. He reports that the posterior facet is usually divided longitudinally by the fracture line. The depressed lateral half of the posterior facet is elevated and transfixed to the medial fragment with a transverse screw. The cavity left following reduction is then filled with bone graft. Hazlett recommends no postoperative immobilization and instead encourages early range of motion of the ankle, subtalar, and small joints of the foot in an effort to restore mobility. Weight bearing is allowed when there is radiographic evidence of fracture union.

Stephenson's Method.—Stephenson[185, 186] uses a modification of Palmer's technique in which he stresses reduction of the superomedial fragment. The patient is positioned prone. A lateral modified Kocher incision is extended down to the peroneal tendon sheath. The peroneal tendons are retracted anteriorly and the sural nerve posteriorly. The fibulocalcaneal ligament is detached distally and retracted anteriorly. The lateral portion of the calcaneus is denuded of soft tissue and the fracture fragments identified. The posterior facet fragment is disimpacted and reduced by using a Langenbeck elevator and temporarily transfixed with K-wires to the superomedial fragment. Axial and lateral radiographs are taken to evaluate the posterior facet articular surface, the tuberosity joint angle, and reduction of the tuberosity with the superomedial fragment. If the superomedial fragment shows significant overhang on the tuberosity fragment, a vertical medial incision is centered over the fracture site where skin tents on palpation. A retinacular incision is made in line with the skin incision, the neurovascular bundle is retracted anteriorly, and the abductor hallucis fragment is retracted inferiorly. The K-wires are backed out of the superomedial fragment to allow manipulation of this fragment. The tuberosity is reduced by using large bone-holding forceps, and the fragments are predrilled and fixed with a medium-size two-prong staple. This staple should be driven only half way in order to not interfere with subsequent reduction of the posterior facet laterally. Through the lateral incision, the posterior articular fragment is again reduced and temporarily transfixed with two K-wires. A small cancellous lag screw is inserted between the K-wires to fix the posterior facet fragment to the superomedial fragment. The K-wires are removed, and fixation of the lateral vertical fracture line is accomplished with a stone staple after predrilling for two prongs anterior and two prongs posterior to the fracture line. The medial staple is then driven down completely. Bone grafting was not used. On closure, the fibulocalcaneal ligament is sutured to its distal insertion. A bulky dressing and posterior splint are applied and the extremity elevated. At 5 to 7 days, subtalar motion exercises are begun. Four to 6 weeks postoperatively, gentle strengthening exercises are started. Partial weight bearing is allowed after evidence of radiographic union, usually 8 to 10 weeks.

Stephenson[186] reported 77% good results of 22 intra-articular calcaneus fractures, with a 75% rate of average restoration of subtalar joint motion. A medial incision was required in 32% of cases and was more often required in the three-part tongue fractures to correct the medial overhang. The calcaneocuboid joint was involved by fracture extension in 68% of cases. He reported a 45% complication rate, including a 27% wound necrosis rate.

Paley and Hall[146] have reported early good results in three cases treated with the Ilizarov external fixator. He theorizes that early weight bearing allows desensitization of the heel pad and may reduce the long-term disability created by dystrophic soft-tissue changes from non–weight bearing. The Ilizarov external fixator is applied and a closed reduction performed. Open reduction and screw fixation of the thalamic fragment are then performed through a lateral approach. The rest of the fixation is carried out through the external fixator. The fixation extends from the tibia to the midfoot and hindfoot to bypass the crushed middle part of the calcaneus. This rigid construct allows immediate, early weight bearing within 24 hours. The trade-off is immobilization of the subtalar joint during rehabilitation.

Soeur and Remy[184] recommend open reduction and internal fixation of fractures *without* bone grafting. This is followed by the use of a cast for 12 weeks. Weight bearing is not permitted for the first 4 weeks. Reduction of the lateral or semilunar fragment restores the tuberosity joint angle. They report good anatomic and functional results with their technique. Finally, Segal et al.[176] recommends open reduction and internal fixation with immediate mobilization of the subtalar joint to avoid the complications of fracture immobilization. He prefers a lateral approach with care taken to avoid the sural nerve. He stresses the importance of stable internal fixation with a Y-shaped Vitallium plate used for immediate stability. He does not bone-graft because he reports that the defects fill in rapidly when stability of the bone is achieved. He reports that 56% of his patients have acceptable results.

Essex-Lopresti Method.—For joint depression–type fractures, Essex-Lopresti[52] in 1951 recommended open reduction of the depressed fragment via a lateral approach. Once the reduction is performed under direct vision, it is maintained by the insertion of a Gissane spike passed through the tuberosity of the calcaneus from posterior. A slipper plaster cast is applied for 6 weeks. This is followed by a short-leg walking plaster cast for an additional 4 weeks. At 8 to 10 weeks both the Gissane spike and the plaster are removed. According to Essex-Lopresti, bone grafting is unnecessary if surgery is performed in the first 2 to 3 days since the cavity caused by the compression will later fill in with new bone.

McReynolds' Method.—The late Isaac McReynolds[120–123] long advocated open reduction and internal fixation of calcaneus fractures via a *medial* approach. According to McReynolds, reduction from the lateral side of the heel, as popularized by Palmer, must be combined in the vast majority of cases with a medial approach. This is due to the fact that in 90% of these fractures there is medial displacement, overriding, and rotation of the superomedial fragment, a deformity that if uncorrected will add considerably to the residual permanent disability.[122] According to McReynolds, although the tuberosity joint angle is of significance in reduction, it is the combination of displacement, overriding, and rotation of the superomedial fragment that is the *prime* deformity in intra-articular calcaneus fractures.[123] These fractures are approached through a 2- to 3-in. slightly oblique incision located medially in the midportion of the heel, somewhat in line with the long axis of the os calcis. The fascia is incised in the line of the incision while being careful to avoid injury to the neurovascular plexus crossing vertically just under the fascia. The underlying quadratus plantae and abductor hallucis muscles are separated in the line of their fibers by blunt dissection to expose the medial cortical surface of the os calcis and the displaced superomedial fragment. The superomedial fragment is gently reduced by inserting an instrument inside the fracture and elevating the superomedial component. Once reduction is obtained, staple fixation is carried out to restore the continuity of the medial cortex. Only occasionally can the deformity not be corrected through this medial approach, and a second approach, located laterally just superior to the peroneal tendons, is necessary to reduce the deformity in the lateral part of the posterior facet under direct vision (Fig 35–41).

The patient is placed in a bulky dressing supported with plaster of paris to immobilize the foot and ankle. In 7 to 10 days the bulky dressing is removed, and a snug-fitting short-leg walking cast is applied. In tongue-type fractures partial weight bearing is started when the cast is dry and the patient progressed to full weight bearing in 1 to 2 weeks. In joint depression–type fractures, the stability of the reduction is not as good as in tongue-type fractures. Exactly when weight bearing is

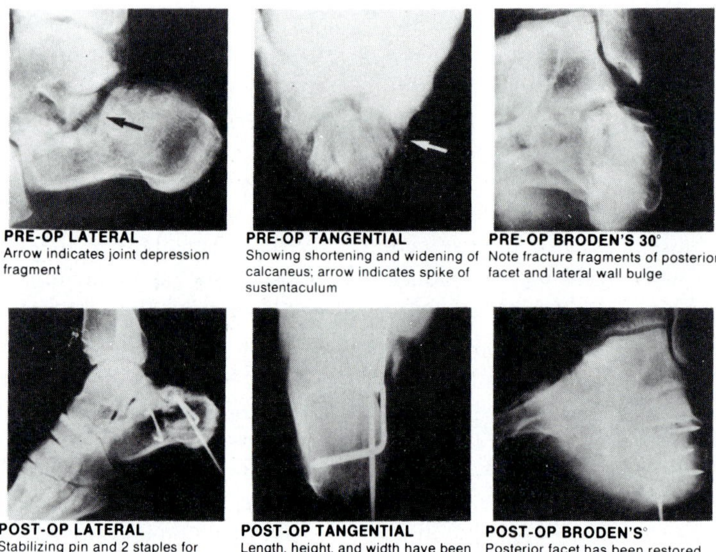

FIG 35–41.
McReynolds method of open reduction. (Courtesy of Dr. William Burdeaux, Houston.)

allowed in these fractures varies with each case. In some it can be started early; in others it must be delayed for 4 weeks or more. With this method, McReynolds reports excellent, good, or fair results in nearly 80% of cases, with only 16% of patients having poor results. Urowitz and Hall[194] also report open reduction and internal fixation with bone grafting via the medial approach. They report nearly 90% good results with this technique.

Romash[164] also believes that the key to intra-articular calcaneus fractures is accurate restoration of the medial wall. He advocates a medial approach to restore the medial wall with staple fixation. This is followed, however, by a lateral approach centered over the sinus tarsi to expose the posterior facet and lateral wall. The lateral portion of the posterior facet is then elevated to the level of the superomedial fragment and transfixed with cortical screws. The lateral wall is reduced and held to the previously restored medial wall with cortical screws. Restoration of the lateral wall will help support the articular fragment of the lateral posterior facet. The author cautions against what appears to be an "anatomic" reduction on the lateral view. It is possible to reconstitute Bohler's angle and yet still have a widened calcaneus with depression of a significant portion of the posterior facet.

Paley, Hall, and McMurty[147] reported 37% excellent, 25% good, 25% fair, and 7% poor results following open reduction and internal fixation through a medial approach. The 44 patients with 52 fractures had a minimum 4-year and average 8.9-year follow-up. The authors found that the factors associated with a poorer prognosis were heavy labor occupation, increased time off work, heavier patient weight, increased heel width, decreased fibulocalcaneal space, subtalar and calcaneocuboid incongruity and arthrosis, and ankle arthrosis.

Trickey[192] correctly states that there is nothing wrong with the idea of open reduction, it is the execution of the plan that is at fault. Although open reduction and internal fixation have the theoretical advantage of restoring joint anatomy, it is fraught with complications. Shannon and Murray[177] cite the risk of infection, tendon adhesion, and pain from further heel pad trauma as the primary drawbacks of open treatment. Gould[69] and Stephenson[185] stress the importance of placement of the incision and the technique of closure to prevent necrosis of skin edges in the lateral approach to calcaneus fractures. Lance et al.[105] reported complications in one of every six cases treated by open reduction and, more importantly, noted that 94% of patients with such complications had unsatisfactory end results.

Dart and Graham[42] believe that fractures involving the facet joint often result in crushed avascular fragments and, because of this, any attempt to restore the joint to a functioning unit is doomed to failure from the start. Finally, Sisk[178] reports that even after anatomic open reduction and internal fixation, traumatic arthritis of the subtalar joint may well occur. However, he does point out that arthrodesis is technically easier if the anatomy of the calcaneus has previously been restored.

Primary Arthrodesis.—Due to the fact that comminuted intra-articular fractures of the calcaneus often cause irreparable damage to the joint surfaces and result in a painful foot with minimal motion, some surgeons have advocated that primary subtalar or triple arthrodesis be performed in the first 2 to 3 weeks after injury in an effort to decrease the long-term disability.*

Subtalar Arthrodesis.—Von Stockum[198] first reported subtalar arthrodesis for fractures of the os calcis in 1912. Wilson[207] in 1927 also reported good results with this method of treatment. Gallie[57] introduced the posterior approach for subtalar arthrodesis following os calcis fractures. Its main limitations are the inability to correct heel malalignment secondary to the original fracture. Pennal and Yadav[152] reported excellent or good results in 75% of cases treated by primary subtalar fusion, while less than 50% satisfactory results were obtained when the subtalar fusion was performed secondarily. These authors recommend this method of treatment for severely comminuted and depressed fractures in patients who are not candidates for open reduction. Allan[3] also recommended primary fusion in comminuted fractures with severe joint involvement; however, he emphasized the importance of attempting to preserve motion in these joints if at all possible. Chapman[30] also cautions that while primary subtalar fusion is indicated in some instances, the results overall are not as good as those that have been reported following simple conservative management of these fractures.

Dick[47] recommends early subtalar fusion if the joint surfaces are distorted. He believes that early fusion shortens disability, decreases the amount of pain suffered by the patient, and prevents the development of a pain pattern in the cerebral cortex that can prevent later subtalar fusion from relieving the patient's symptoms. According to Dick, fusion is indicated in displaced fractures, not because the displacement cannot be reduced, but because a force great enough to displace the calcaneus almost certainly causes irreparable damage to the articular surface of the subtalar joint. He recommends initial elevation and range of motion of the foot. Three

---

**References 3, 33, 42, 74, 98, 158–161, 189, 190, 207, 210.*

weeks later, or after the initial swelling and ecchymosis have subsided, subtalar fusion is performed from a posterior approach. He makes *no* attempt to reduce the calcaneus fracture, and no cast is utilized following subtalar fusion; instead, he prefers early range of motion of the adjacent joints. Weight bearing is allowed in 8 to 10 weeks when radiographs show evidence of subtalar fusion. Recently, Noble and McQuillan[140] recommended early subtalar arthrodesis through a posterior approach in fractures of the os calcis with displacement of the articular surfaces and a reduction or reversal in Bohler's angle. They made no attempt to reduce the fracture. They report excellent, good, or satisfactory results in over 90% of patients.

Harris[79] reported disappointing results after intra-articular fractures of the calcaneus for two reasons. First, a good reduction is seldom possible; second, in comminuted fractures, fragments are often deprived of their blood supply and undergo aseptic necrosis. If these are isolated fragments of articular cartilage, their nourishment is often impaired. He therefore recommended early subtalar arthrodesis. However, Harris[79] emphasized that *any* heel deformity must be corrected before the subtalar fusion is performed. If the heel is fused in a position of valgus, undue pressure is transferred to the first metatarsal head. If it is fused in varus, undue pressure is transported to the fifth metatarsal head. With subtalar motion obliterated, there is no method for the patient to relieve these abnormal pressures, and hence, calluses develop. He corrects heel deformity in fresh fractures by traction through a pin placed through the posterosuperior corner of the os calcis with countertraction applied through a second pin in the tibia. The width of the heel is reduced by molding the heel by hand or with a Bohler clamp. A short-leg cast is then applied that incorporates the traction pins. Subtalar fusion, performed through a window in the cast, is performed 4 weeks later by using a tibial cortical strut for stability. According to Harris, even though the calcaneocuboid joint is occasionally involved in these fractures, it seldom causes trouble, and hence its inclusion in the fusion is not indicated. Additionally, he found that although radiographic evidence of traumatic talonavicular arthritis may develop following this method of treatment, it seldom causes disability. For these reasons he believed that triple arthrodesis was not necessary. He reported that 35 of 36 patients treated by early subtalar fusion returned to work in 6 months or less, and Hall and Pennal[74] reported 27 of 29 patients returning to work in a similar period.

Burghele and Serban,[25] also recommend early subtalar fusion for depressed fractures involving the subtalar joint. They too emphasize the importance of early restoration of the height and width of the calcaneus *prior* to subtalar fusion. They stress that the calcaneocuboid joint *must* be in the normal position at the time of subtalar fusion, or the position of the midfoot joints will be abnormal, and pain will result in these joints. These authors reported 87% good results with this method. They believe that triple arthrodesis used early in the course of calcaneal fracture treatment is indicated *only* if there is radiographic evidence of transverse tarsal joint involvement. Smith[181] recommends fusion of only the subtalar joints unless the calcaneocuboid and talonavicular joints are definitely involved. He reports that midtarsal joint motion usually increases following subtalar fusion and results in improved function.

Good results following early subtalar arthrodesis have ranged from 60% to over 90%.[140, 207, 211] Lindsay and Dewar[114] however, report only 60% good results after primary arthrodesis as compared with 76% good results in those fractures treated by simple conservative methods.

Triple Arthrodesis.—Bankart[10] reported unsatisfactory results after subtalar arthrodesis for calcaneal fractures. He believed that subtalar arthrodesis is incomplete because the unfused midtarsal joints remain painful and stiff. Additionally, the resulting foot is usually flat and ill-adapted for heel and toe walking. For these reasons, he recommended primary triple arthrodesis. He emphasized the importance of modifying the technique to restore the shape of the calcaneus at the time of arthrodesis.

Conn[33] and Geckeler[60] also emphasized the importance of triple arthrodesis because of the frequent involvement of the calcaneocuboid joints in these injuries. Conn reported that *one third* of patients treated by subtalar arthrodesis had unsatisfactory results while 23 of 26 patients treated by triple arthrodesis had good results.[32, 33] He recommended breaking up the impaction of the calcaneus by utilizing a lateral blow to the heel and then immobilization of the fracture with a modification of Bohler's technique. Five weeks later a triple arthrodesis was performed.[32, 33]

Thompson and Friesen[189, 190] advocate early triple arthrodesis following displaced intra-articular calcaneus fractures for two reasons: (1) unrecognized damage to the calcanealcuboid and talonavicular joints is often present, and (2) this three-joint complex is a single unit in which motion occurs, and fusion of only one of the three joints severely limits overall motion in the complex. They believe that the remaining motion in the unfused joints in the complex is painful. Arthrodesis is performed early, before swelling develops. They do not attempt reduction but fuse the foot in situ. Postoperatively the limb is immobilized in a cast and kept non–weight bearing for 8 weeks. Weight bearing is allowed in a cast at 8 weeks. Three to 4 weeks later the cast is removed and range of motion begun. Eighty-four percent of the patients in their series had good results.

Dart and Graham[42] also recommend early triple arthrodesis in grossly comminuted fractures involving the subtalar and calcaneocuboid joints. However, they emphasize the importance of restoring the external anatomy of the calcaneus, if possible, by using bone grafts during arthrodesis. Brattstrom[20] also reports good results after early triple arthrodesis in these injuries.

Not all authors have been favorably impressed with early arthrodesis. Essex-Lopresti[51] reports that the results after early arthrodesis are not as good as have been suggested. Additionally, he states that good results are often not possible after later arthrodesis because of the inherent deformity in the calcaneus that cannot be corrected.[52] Lance et al.[106] report only 50% to 60% of patients with satisfactory results after primary arthrodesis. Because of this, they recommend arthrodesis *only* as a salvage procedure. They emphasize, however, that salvage should be performed early and they favor triple over subtalar arthrodesis. Johansson et al.[94] and Thomas,[188] also prefer to wait 6 to 12 months before subtalar arthrodesis. According to them, not all intra-articular fractures are followed by the development of subtalar joint pain, and hence primary fusion is not indicated.

McReynolds[120, 121] also does not believe that there is a place for early triple arthrodesis in joint depression and certainly not in tongue-type fractures of the calcaneus. However, in certain irreducible intra-articular fractures he considers subtalar fusion an alternative. He too stresses, however, the importance of restoring normal heel alignment and shape before the arthrodesis is undertaken.

Excision.—According to Pridie,[156] although treatment of these fractures with early motion and protection from weight bearing produced occasional good results, subtalar arthritis develops out of proportion to radiographic findings in some cases, with the end result being worse than would be expected. Also he found that subtalar arthrodesis was difficult to perform and the results were unpredictable. For these reasons, in 1946 he reported early excision of the os calcis in the treatment of comminuted intra-articular fractures of the calcaneus. According to his method, the calcaneus is excised through a midline posterior approach. Following excision the patient is placed in a cast in plantar flexion. The foot is immobilized for 1 month.

The position of plantar flexion is important to allow relaxation of the Achilles tendon so that its new attachment is not strained. After 1 month, non–weight-bearing exercises commence. Patients are usually able to walk 6 weeks postinjury. Pridie reported 15 cases treated in this manner, with 13 good or acceptable results. According to Pridie, the advantages of this method include (1) freedom from pain, (2) good range of inversion and eversion, (3) maintenance of good mobility of the entire foot, and (4) good toe action. In spite of the results reported by Pridie, this method of treatment has not been reported by other authors dealing with calcaneus fractures.

Factors Affecting Prognosis

Since fracture classification and postoperative evaluation methods are different in most of the reported series of calcaneal fractures, the reader is left in a confused state as regards which method of treatment produces the best results. Because of these limitations, I will attempt to discuss factors in calcaneal fractures that *seem* to alter long-term prognosis. The reader must remember that the effect of a single factor on the result must be considered in conjunction with each of the other factors known to affect prognosis.

Fracture Displacement.—Persistent fracture displacement has been identified by many authors as adversely affecting function and results. Essex-Lopresti[52] reports that nondisplaced intra-articular fractures treated in a closed manner have good results in 80% of patients, with 95% returning to work in 12 months. In displaced fractures treated by closed reduction, 65% have good results with 91% returning to work. If the closed reduction was unsuccessful, however, 70% of patients had a poor result, thus stressing the importance of persistent displacement in these fractures.

Posterior Facet Displacement.—Dodson[49] reports that persistent displacement of the posterior facet is the prime cause in the development of degenerative joint disease. Gaul and Greenburg[59] also noted that persistent displacement, especially rotation of the posterior articular facet, was associated with a poor result in the majority of cases. Hammesfahr and Fleming[76] reported a positive correlation between persistent facet displacement and successful results, and Thoren[191] noted that persistent displacement of the posterior facet of the subtalar joint had the highest correlation with long-term poor results. Finally, Conn[33] reported that persistent subtalar joint displacement, particularly involving the sustentaculum tali, can allow subluxation of the talonavicular and calcaneocuboid joints and lead to degenerative arthritis in those joints.

Varus/Valgus Heel Displacement.—Persistent displacement of the heel in varus or valgus has also been identified as a poor prognostic indicator. According to Schottstaedt,[174] persistent valgus deformity of the heel secondary to incomplete reduction of the depressed lateral fracture fragment portends a poor prognosis. Rosendahl[165] also emphasized the importance of persistent displacement of the heel and found that *all* patients with residual heel valgus had a poor result. Lance et al[105] report that while persistent broadening of the heel does not alter the long-term outcome, significant displacement of the heel in valgus or varus often produces a poor result. The authors emphasize that such displacement can occur with early weight bearing, with or without plaster protection.

Proximal Displacement.—Finally, McLaughlin[119] and Harris[77] report that persistent displacement of the calcaneus in a *proximal* direction, which produces a decreased tuberosity joint angle, results in a shortened triceps surae and a decrease in push-off strength of the limb.

Widened Heel.—Displacement that results in persistent *widening* of the calcaneus may result in peroneal tendonitis because impingement of the tendons occurs between the lateral aspect of the calcaneus and the lateral malleolus.[49] This is discussed in greater detail in the section on complications.

It therefore appears that persistent displacement of the posterior facet, varus or valgus of the heel, widening of the heel, and proximal displacement of the calcaneal tuberosity can each adversely affect the long-term results.

However, Lindsay and Dewar[114] reported that 48 of 83 conservatively treated cases had marked persistent fracture displacement, but in this group 71% had good results while only 29% had poor results. This finding is in direct opposition to those who believe that persistent displacement leads uniformly to a poor result. Also, the excellent results reported by Parkes[148–150] Salama et al.[169] in which *no* attempt at reduction of any displacement was attempted make one question the true role of fracture displacement in determining long-term prognosis.

Persistent Reduction in Bohler's Angle.—Vestad[196] reports that while there is no definite relation between the size of the tuberosity joint angle at the time of injury and the final result, there is a tendency to better results when the tuberosity joint angle is 20 degrees or *greater* following reduction.

Gaul and Greenburg[59] also believe that the tuberosity joint angle is greatly overrated as a guide to long-term prognosis. They report that morbidity has little or no relationship to the final tuberosity joint angle. They found that there was no difference in results between those fractures with *both* a depressed tuberosity joint angle and a symmetric subtalar facet when compared with those in which the subtalar facet was not involved in the fracture. However, if there was *depression* of the subtalar facet, the results were poor. This suggests that it is subtalar facet displacement, not reduction in the tuberosity joint angle, that adversely affects the results. Rosendahl-Jensen[166] and Widen[204] also emphasized that they found no relationship between Bohler's tuberosity joint angle and prognosis in these injuries.

Arnesen[6] however, reports that results parallel the accuracy of reduction of the tuberosity joint angle, and Salama et al.[169] report that there were more unsatisfactory results in patients whose tuberosity joint angle posttreatment measured 10 degrees or less when compared with those in whom the angle was 10 degrees or greater. Dart and Graham[42] found that minor degrees of flattening of the tuberosity joint angle were well compensated for. However, if the angle is markedly decreased, the resulting flatfoot can be painful. They therefore recommend that severe displacements be corrected.

Thoren[191] reports that a persistent decrease in the tuberosity joint angle is the second most important factor in evaluating calcaneus fractures. He reports that in those patients with good results the angle measured an average of 17 degrees as compared with 5 degrees in patients with a poor result. Finally, Slatis et al.[180] found that subtalar motion was more restricted in fractures in which the Bohler angle measured −20 to +10 degrees than in fractures in which the angle was normal or only slightly reduced. Indeed, Letournel[112] suggests that anatomic reduction with rigid internal fixation should produce better subtalar motion postfracture. However, only 3% of his patients had normal joint motion, and 36% had very stiff subtalar joints in spite of restoring the tuberosity joint angle.

Fracture Comminution.—Severe comminution of a calcaneus fracture is one of the prognostic factors over which the physician has no control.[46] Such severe comminution, particularly when intra-articular, often results in poor function.[46, 52, 152] Deyerle[46] emphasizes that such comminution results in shortening of the os calcis and, in many cases, spreading of the os calcis under the fibula, displacements that have both been associated with a poor long-term prognosis. According to Essex-Lopresti[57] if the comminution is such that surgical open reduction is not possible, early motion, in an effort to retain some of the subtalar motion and possibly reshape joint surfaces, can produce a favorable result.

Early Range of Motion and Weight Bearing.—Essex-Lopresti[52] stressed that early range of motion has advantages over immobilization in all age groups. Parkes[149] also emphasized the importance of early active exercise to maintain subtalar motion and help decrease swelling in the soft tissues as the most important factor in the treatment of calcaneal fractures.

According to Pozo et al,[154] early range of motion provides the most effective treatment for soft tissue and also contributes to molding of a congruous subtalar joint. Deyerle[46] also believes that early range of motion of the foot helps prevent the peroneal tendons from becoming tethered to the lateral calcaneus.

Roberts and Sayle Creer[162] and Bertelsen and Hasner[16] report shorter periods of incapacitation following treatment by early range of motion than after reduction and casting. Finally, Rosendahl[165] recommends early exercise to maintain subtalar motion because restoration of subtalar motion paralleled good results in his patients. Most important, however, *no* authors have indicated that early motion has resulted in further displacement of calcaneal fractures.

Regarding the institution of weight bearing, most authors prefer to delay weight bearing 6 to 12 weeks to allow fracture healing and to prevent further fracture displacement. According to Rosendahl,[165] early weight bearing often produces poorer results due to secondary compression and fracture displacement, which result in an increased valgus deformity of the heel. Even though Rockwood[163] recommends early weight bearing, he carefully places the heel of the cast so that all weight is borne *anterior* to the calcaneus to prevent weight transference across the calcaneus and secondary fracture displacement. Additionally, he emphasizes the importance of restoring motion *prior* to casting and early weight bearing.

Overall, most authors agree that no matter what form of treatment is selected in these fractures, early motion to correct soft-tissue swelling and restore subtalar motion is the *cornerstone* of treatment. Early unprotected weight bearing with or without plaster fixation can lead to secondary displacement and is generally not recommended.

Damage to the Soft Tissues and Fat Pad of the Heel.—The complex structure of the heel pad, which is necessary for painless weight bearing, has been expertly described by Blechschmidt.[17] Essex-Lopresti,[52] Miller and Lichtblau,[133] and Schottstaedt[175] have all emphasized the importance of damage to the soft tissue of the heel pad in affecting long-term prognosis.

According to Miller, the columns of fat in the heel pad normally create a hydraulic effect that cushions the heel during weight bearing.[132] If this hydraulic action is lost, no salvage procedure, including arthrodesis, will relieve this cause of pain.[133] Harris[77] stresses that the weight-bearing function of the heel pad can be compromised by the impact of the acute injury or by long-term localized pressure from the bony prominences of a malunion. Either of these can result in a painful heel. Barnhart and Odegard[13] and Lance et al.[106] emphasize that plantar pain resulting from damage to the fibrofatty elements in the heel pad is a disaster and is not helped by any surgical treatment.

Although damage to the fibrofatty elements of the heel pad is a prognostic factor beyond the control of the surgeon, he must recognize this as a postinjury cause of pain that at the present time has no surgical treatment.

Age.—Essex-Lopresti[52] introduced the concept of a relationship between the age of the patient and results following calcaneus fractures. He believed that patients over the age of 50 years had lost some of the mobility of their subtalar joint. Since their feet had an age-related stiffness, better results were to be obtained by conservative treatment consisting of early exercise therapy. For these reasons, he suggested that patients over the age of 50 years did better with closed treatment consisting of early exercise while patients under the age of 50 years were better treated by open reduction. In spite of his recommendations, Gaul and Greenburg,[59] Pennal and Yadav,[152] and Lindsay and Dewar[114] could find no relationship between patient age and long-term results.

Associated Injury.—Gaul and Greenburg[59] emphasize the fact that associated fractures, particularly those involving the ipsilateral lower extremity, have a strongly adverse affect on the outcome of fractures of the calcaneus. This is likely due to constraints on treatment of the calcaneal fracture that ipsilateral injuries impose on the physician. Indeed, Vestad[196] stresses that *systemic* injury in itself does not have any effect on the long-term result after these fractures.

Involvement of the Midtarsal Joints.—Involvement of the calcaneocuboid and/or talonavicular joints by (1) communication with the original fracture or (2) subluxation secondary to original displacement of the calcaneal fracture can result in pain in the midfoot following a calcaneal fracture.

Conn[33] warns of prolonged disability following involvement of the calcaneocuboid joint in calcaneal fractures. Heck[82] also reports that involvement of the calcaneocuboid joint by the calcaneal fracture can result in pain in this joint. If pain in the calcaneocuboid joint persists after the primary fracture has healed and shoe modifications are not helpful, arthrodesis of the calcaneocuboid joint may be indicated.

Talonavicular joint subluxation secondary to a calcaneal fracture healing in a position of displacement has been reported and can be symptomatic.[97] If either of the midtarsal joints are symptomatic following a calcaneus fracture, consideration should be given to arthrodesis, either alone or in combination with subtalar fusion.[82]

Complications Following Calcaneal Fractures

Most authors have emphasized that results after calcaneus fractures can continue to improve for a long period of time. According to Gage and Premer,[56] a long period of slow improvement may last up to 2 years. Essex-Lopresti reports continued improvement over a 3- to 6-year period, while Lindsay and Dewar[114] report that results can improve up to 10 years following a fracture. Therefore, one must wait at least 18 to 24 months before assigning a disability and relating that disability to a specific complication of the fracture.

Complications following calcaneal fractures are mainly related to malunion, stiffness, and soft-tissue injury because nonunion of calcaneus fractures is extremely rare.[119] According to McLaughlin,[119] most of the complications following calcaneus fractures are contained in a clinical syndrome characterized by a gait abnormality resulting from a stiff and painful foot. Pain is the predominant feature of this syndrome, and there appears to be a tendency to attribute this symptom to mechanical disorders in the subtalar joint.[119] This presumption is strengthened by radiographic evidence of gross distortion of the joint by the fracture. The origin of pain following subtalar fractures, however, is debatable.[93] Indeed, McLaughlin taught that the *greater* the involvement of the talocalcaneal joint, the more likely it is for an eventual spontaneous fibrous ankylosis to occur that should eliminate pain in the area.

It is essential that the examiner delineate the exact cause of pain following a calcaneal fracture so that treatment can be directed to a specific cause. Pain following a calcaneal fracture can arise from the subtalar joint,[57] the midtarsal joint,[32] the ankle,[114] the malleoli,[89, 119] and the soft tissues of the heel pad.[134] However, difficulty in determining the exact cause of heel pain following calcaneal fractures led Sallick and Blum[170] to recommend sensory denervation of the heel for persistent pain following fractures of the calcaneus.

Heel Pain.—Heel pain following calcaneal fracture is usually located in one of three anatomic areas: laterally, over the point of the heel, and medially. According to O'Connell et al,[142] lateral heel pain is first, medial heel pain is second, and pain over the point of the heel is third in frequency of occurrence.

Lateral Heel Pain.—Lateral heel pain is usually due to an abnormality in the subtalar joint, peroneal tenosynovitis, fibular abutment, or calcaneocuboid joint involvement.

Subtalar Joint Pain.—Key and Conwell[97] and Reich[158] believe that pain from subtalar arthritis is the leading cause of disability after calcaneus fractures. On the contrary, Bankart[10] believed that undue importance had been placed on subtalar arthritis as a source of pain following calcaneal fracture.

According to Johansson et al.[94] and Thomas,[188] pain secondary to subtalar arthritis is usually located on the lateral and plantar aspects of the foot, is increased with walking or stressing the subtalar joint, and is relieved by injection of lidocaine (Xylocaine) into the joint. Garcia and Parkes[58] emphasize that pain on inversion or eversion of the foot that is referred to the area of the sinus tarsi suggests subtalar arthritis. If these clinical signs are present, the authors recommend injecting the joint with a local anesthetic. If the pain is relieved, subtalar fusion may be indicated. If the injection does not relieve the symptoms, the leg can be immobilized in a short-leg cast. If immobilization relieves the pain, it is another sign that arthrodesis may relieve the patient's pain. Dodson[49] recommends injecting the subtalar joint with steroids in an effort to *treat* subtalar arthritis. If this fails, again arthrodesis is indicated.

If subtalar arthritis is believed to be the etiology of the pain, Bankart,[10] Rosendahl-Jensen,[166] Sisk,[178] and McLaughlin[118] recommend subtalar arthrodesis. Isolated subtalar arthrodesis is adequate treatment for subtalar arthritis *provided* that subtalar steroid injection has completely relieved the patient's pain, thus indicating that the calcaneocuboid and talonavicular joints are not involved in pain production. If these joints are involved, triple arthrodesis should be performed. Subtalar arthrodesis in these situations usually produces better results if done within 1 year of fracture rather than waiting a prolonged period of time.[94]

McReynolds[122] stresses that while arthrodesis for malunited fractures may stop subtalar pain, it will do nothing for the widening, shortening, and valgus deformity of the calcaneus that results in a broad flatfoot and can potentially be a problem in shoe fitting. Kalamachi and Evans[95] report a technique of subtalar arthrodesis through a posterior approach in which a graft is taken from the lateral aspect of the heel in patients with old calcaneus fractures. By taking the graft from the calcaneus, the width of the heel is decreased, the valgus of the heel is corrected, and the peroneal tendons are decompressed.

Deyerle,[46] on the other hand, believes that stiffness and the inability to control the foot on uneven ground are more frequent causes of disability than subtalar pain from arthritis. Indeed, Slatis et al.[180] report a decreased range of motion of the subtalar joint in 74% of all patients following calcaneal fracture and in 89% of those with a depressed intra-articular fracture. Lance et al.[105] report that the loss of half of the subtalar motion resulted in unsatisfactory function in 75% of his patients. However, Letournel[112] reports that a normal life and sports participation are possible with a subtalar joint with half of the normal motion. Indeed, those patients who retain a fourth of the normal range of motion functioned better than did patients who underwent arthrodesis. However, Pozo et al.[154] report that neither the degree of stiffness of the subtalar joint nor the radiographic evidence of degenerative joint disease corresponded well with the patient's symptoms.

Peroneal Tendonitis and Fibular Abutment.—When the lateral cortex of the calcaneus bursts in severely comminuted fractures, fragments may be displaced in a medial-lateral plane and come to lie below the tip of the lateral malleolus. If they unite in this position, they produce a lateral bony prominence posterior and inferior to the lower end of the fibula.[123] The resulting permanent bony prominence can force the peroneal tendons against the fibula, entrap them in a callus, force them anteriorly, and occasionally actually result in abutment against the tip of the fibula.[122, 181] Magnuson in 1923 was the first to recognize this lateral piling up of bone beneath the external malleolus and recommended removing the mass to create a trough for the peroneal tendons. Key and Conwell[97] reported that excess bone behind and beneath the external malleolus is the second most frequent cause of heel pain following calcaneal fracture.

McLaughlin[118] and Barnard[11–14] report that crowding of the peroneal tendons under the lateral malleolus often produces peroneal tenosynovitis and spasm and results in a valgus forefoot and a painful spastic flatfoot. According to Parvin and Ford,[151] peroneal tendonitis should be suspected if there is pain below the tip of the malleolus that is aggravated by supination and pronation. McLaughlin[119] recommends that treatment of this should be a longitudinal incision of the peroneal tendon sheaths with the retinaculum left intact to prevent subluxation of the tendons from their fibular groove. Also, Lindsay and Dewar[114] caution that pain beneath the tip of the lateral malleolus may also be secondary to injury to the lateral ligaments of the ankle at the time of the original fracture.

Recently, Fitzgerald and Coventry[55] report that antalgic gait, limited subtalar motion, and point tenderness over the peroneal tendons at the inferior peroneal retinaculum are the physical findings suggestive of peroneal tenosynovitis. The diagnosis is further substantiated if the pain is relieved by the injection of 1 to 2 mL of local anesthetic into the tendon sheath. Peroneal tenography performed by the intrasynovial injection of Hypaque into the common peroneal tendon sheath proximal to the ankle will reveal a complete or partial block at the level of the inferior retinaculum.[55] Conservative treatment by the injection of steroids may relieve the symptoms. However, if injection fails, excision of the bony prominence beneath the peroneal tendon sheath[55] or release of the tendon sheath may be helpful.[58]

Deyerle reports that peroneal dysfunction can also result from the tethering of the peroneal tendons as they course behind the malleolus in the region of the fracture.[46] In some patients spreading of os calcis can actually push the peroneal tendons out of the tunnel behind the fibula, and they can become dislocated *anterior* to the fibula. Those patients with dislocated peroneal tendons have the inability to resist inversion and complain of instability and a lack of control of the foot. According to Deyerle, they are greatly improved by excision of the excess bone in the region of the old healed fracture and rerouting of the peroneal tendons beneath the fibula. He too emphasizes the importance of a peroneal synoviogram in the diagnosis and treatment of peroneal tenosynovitis to determine whether the tendon sheath is only obstructed or actually dislocated anteriorly.

In addition to peroneal tenosynovitis and spasm, Isbister[89] reports "abutment" of the tip of the fibula against the displaced lateral wall of the calcaneus as a cause of pain. Although Magnuson and Cotton recommended excision of the displaced lateral calcaneal bone, Isbister[89] believes that resection of the tip of the fibula is a simpler procedure. He recommends resection of 1 cm of the tip of the fibula subperiosteally. Interestingly, he reports that this procedure will relieve symptoms whether they are secondary to impingement, compression of the peroneal tendons, or direct bony abutment. He reports success following this method of treatment in 80% of patients so treated.

Both Deyerle[46] and Isbister[89] emphasize the importance of prevention in lateral peroneal tenosynovitis and fibular abutment. They recommend primary fracture treatment that tends to narrow the width of the heel immediately behind the fibula and that tends to lengthen the os calcis.[46, 89] Deyerle[46] also emphasizes the importance of regular vigorous contractions of the peroneal tendons in any form of treatment to prevent them from becoming tethered at the site of the lateral wall of the calcaneus.

On the contrary, Reich[159] believed that disability after a calcaneus fracture was secondary to degenerative joint disease of the subtalar joint, not to impingement of the peroneal tendons. Because of difficulty in delineating whether subtalar arthritis or peroneal tenosynovitis or "abutment" is responsible for lateral pain after calcaneus fractures, Mann[124] prefers to decompress the peroneal tendons at the time of subtalar fusion. The lateral calcaneal cortex beneath the peroneal tendons is removed intact. The cancellous bone beneath the lateral cortex is removed and used for grafting the subtalar joint. This decreases the width of the calcaneus. The intact cortex is then reinserted into the defect to decrease the potential of scarring between the exposed cancellous bone and the peroneal tendons.

Calcaneocuboid Arthritis.—Key and Conwell[97] believe that traumatic arthritis of the calcaneocuboid joint is the third most common cause of pain following calcaneal fracture. McLaughlin[118] also reports that derangement of the calcaneocuboid joint can be a significant source of pain. The pain may be secondary to actual involvement of the calcaneocuboid joint by the original fracture[118] or by stiffness or malposition of the joint resulting from a malunion of the calcaneus. Selective injection of the calcaneocuboid joint that relieves the patient's pain suggests that isolated calcaneocuboid fusion is indicated. If the injection relieves only part of the patient's pain, fusion of the calcaneocuboid and/or talonavicular joints in conjunction with subtalar arthrodesis should be considered.

Pain Over the Point of the Heel.

Bony Prominence.—A recognized cause of heel pain following calcaneus fractures is the plantar heel spur. Barnard,[11] Dodson,[49] Reich,[160] and Key and Conwell[97] all mention pain on the plantar surface of the calcaneus following a fracture. Bony projections secondary to persistent plantar displacement of fracture fragments or to exuberant callus formation on the plantar aspect of the calcaneus can produce localized tender areas or painful callosities.[49, 142, 175] According to McLaughlin,[118] particularly when the calcaneal arch is reversed, this tenderness results from the concentration of pressure on the plantar aspect of the fracture deformity. Garcia and Parkes[58] recommend initial treatment by local injection. However, such injections usually fail, and excision of the bone fragment may be required.[58] Although Garcia and Parkes,[58] Key and Conwell,[97] Barnard,[11] and Dotson[49] mention resection of the bony prominence of these malunions, McLaughlin[119] warns that such prominences should be approached only with great caution. He emphasizes that postoperative fibrosis in the area of bone excision may produce as much discomfort on weight bearing as did the original lesion, even though the skin incision is kept well away from the weight-bearing area. He prefers to use soft rubber heels and foam rubber donuts placed inside the shoe in a position to protect the tender area from pressure.

Finally, McReynolds[123] and Key and Conwell[97] mention pain on the plantar aspect of the foot resulting from malunion. This pain, located over the posterior end of an angulated fracture of the calcaneus just anterior to the tuberosity, occurs with weight bearing. If this pain is severe, they recommended excising the plantar fragment and using it as a bone graft in an opening wedge osteotomy of the calcaneus just anterior to the tuberosity in order to restore the normal contour of the plantar surface of the calcaneus. No results of this technique are given.

Heel Pad Damage.—In addition to exostoses, exuberant callus, and a plantar prominence secondary to malunion, many authors mention damage to the heel pad itself as contributing to heel pain. According to Barnard,[11, 13] Dodson,[49] and Pozo et al.[154] pain on the *plantar* surface of the heel with weight bearing is not pathognomonic of subtalar joint problems. Instead, this pain may arise from rupture of the fibrous septa and the fat-filled compartments in the soft tissue over the plantar aspect of the calcaneus. This results in a loss of the hydraulic buffer that protects the heel with weight bearing. Additionally, according to Barnard and Odegard, long-term immobilization favors fibrosis of these tissues.[13]

O'Connell et al.[134] note that pain over the heel that is reproduced with minimal pressure is usually related to disruption of the fibrofatty elements of the heel pad and to secondary scar formation. In their review of calcaneus fractures, Lance et al.[105] found that loss or atrophy of the heel pad is associated with an unsatisfactory result in every case. Obviously, if in addition to a plantar spur damage to the heel pad is present, simple excision of the spur will not result in relief of heel pain.

I have found xeroradiographs very useful in demonstrating a loss of thickness of the heel pad following calcaneus fractures, and use them frequently in evaluating heel pain after calcaneus fractures. If loss of the heel pad is present, Dodson[49] recommends treatment simply with a heel cushion or by orthotic relief in the shoe.

Medial Heel Pain.

Ankle Joint and Flexor Tenosynovitis.—According to Barnard[11, 12] and O'Connell et al.,[142] the second most common site of pain following calcaneus fractures is beneath the medial malleolus. This pain is not due to subtalar arthritis.[142] Although it may be secondary to spreading of the calcaneus, both Barnard[11, 12] and O'Connell et al.[142] suggest that it is most likely due to damage to the ankle joint itself and the flexor tendons that pass beneath the medial malleolus. O'Connell et al.[142] believe that this damage is compounded by immobilization, which results in further stiffness and arthrofibrosis of the ankle. Hence, these authors recommend active early mobilization of the ankle joint and the medial flexor tendons to prevent arthrofibrosis of the ankle and posttraumatic tenosynovitis of the flexor tendons.[10, 12, 142]

Nerve Entrapment.—Guillen-Garcia et al.[71] noted that the tarsal tunnel is bordered on its medial side by the os calcis and reported tarsal tunnel syndrome following fractures of the calcaneus, particularly when the medial wall is displaced into the tunnel. They reported a 10% incidence of tarsal tunnel syndrome following these fractures. The patients complain of medial heel pain and paresthesias in the distribution of the posterior tibial nerve. The pain is frequently worse at night or with walking or standing. According to these authors, the diagnosis is based on the clinical picture but can be assisted by a trial injection of a local anesthetic into the tarsal tunnel. They report that only 28% of patients require operative decompression of the posterior tibial nerve and its branches, but when performed the results are excellent.

Finally, Hall and Pennal reported six patients with sural nerve injury secondary to surgical exposure of the calcaneus.[74] These patients complained of an ache and pain in the area of the heel. In my experience, such pain from iatrogenic cutaneous nerve damage is extremely recalcitrant to treatment.

Weakness of Plantar Flexion.—McLaughlin[118] and Barnard[13] mention that malunion of the calcaneus with upward displacement of the tuberosity usually results in effective shortening of the tendo Achillis and a reduction in a calf power. The resulting disability is marked weakness and reduction in the ability to plantar-flex the foot (Fig 35–42). McLaughlin[119] believes that when there is severe upward displacement of the calcaneal tuberosity, primary treatment of the fracture should include measures to return the tuberosity to its normal level and to hold the calf muscles at normal length until the fracture unites. In this way, weakness of plantar flexion can be prevented.

Initially, patients whose fractures have *healed* with the tuberosity displaced superiorly walk with a flat-footed gait and are unable to take off from or stand on their toes. According to McLaughlin, however, eventually compensatory shortening of the calf muscles results in a satisfactory gait.[118] Surgical shortening of the Achilles tendon is not recommended[118] in these patients.[13, 118]

Fixed Flatfoot.—According to McLaughlin, upward displacement of the posterior half of the os calcis also results in elimination of the longitudinal arch of the foot[119] (Fig 35–42). The normal plantar arch of the hindfoot is reduced, eliminated, or reversed. If the upward displacement of the tuberosity is sufficient to reverse the plantar arch of the os calcis, it should be corrected.[119] Only by reducing the displacement can flatfoot deformity be minimized and painful weight bearing at the apex of a "rocker-bottom" heel be prevented.[119]

Stiffness of the Forefoot and Toes.—Barnard,[11, 13] O'Connell et al,[142] and Pozo et al.[154] mention stiffness and pain in the forepart of the foot and toes, areas not involved in the fracture, as a significant cause of disability. These authors relate this stiffness and pain to an initial injury to the ankle and midtarsal joints that is complicated by long periods of immobilization and disuse so often used to treat calcaneus fractures. According to Barnard, fibroblastic adhesions and thickening of the capsular elements around the midtarsal joints are responsible for this stiffness. Indeed, Pozo et al.,[154] report that in addition to the fact that 80% of their patients had less than 50% of normal subtalar motion, 20% had at least a 50% restriction of ankle motion, and 15% had at least a 50% reduction of midtarsal motion. I have also seen stiffness of the metatarsophalangeal joints after calcaneus fractures. According to Pozo et al.,[154] the combined stiffness of these joints produces a stiff foot and an unsatisfactory outcome. According to McLaughlin,[119] a stiff midfoot can produce a shuffling gait since attempts to step off from the forefoot are accompanied by midtarsal pain. Once established, high shoes with a well-fitted arch support rigid enough to relieve the midtarsal joints from the strain of ambulation may help to decrease symptoms.

These reports of stiffness of the forefoot further emphasize the importance of early motion of the ankle, subtalar, midtarsal, and metatarsophalangeal joints in an effort to produce a mobile foot following calcaneus fractures.

Reflex Sympathetic Dystrophy.—Reflex sympathetic dystrophy following fracture of the calcaneus has been reported.[118, 119] Severe pain burning in nature that is associated with shiny, cold, and discolored skin around the heel should suggest this diagnosis. Early motion, progressive weight bearing, and early use of the foot

A

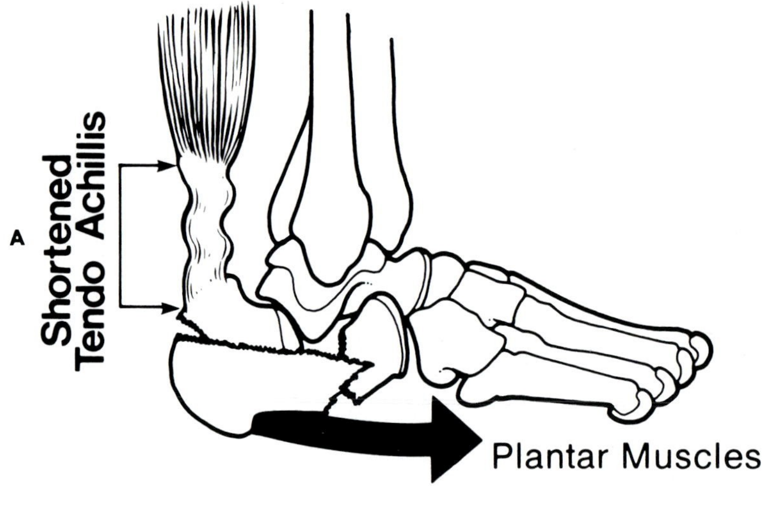

B

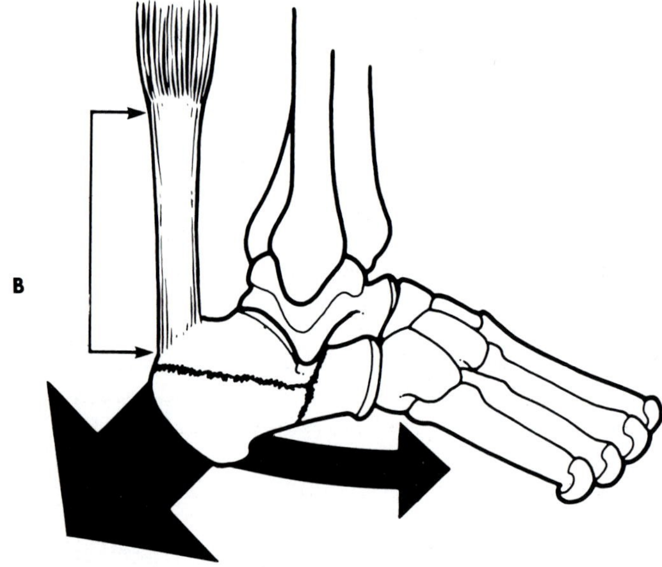

FIG 35–42.
A, upward displacement of the calcaneal tuberosity results in shortening of the Achilles tendon and weak plantar flexion. It also results in a loss of the longitudinal arch of the foot. **B,** reduction of the fracture restores Achilles tendon length and hence plantar flexion power. The longitudinal arch is also restored.

will prevent the development of reflex dystrophy. Indeed, Rockwood[163] notes that with his method of early motion and weight bearing, reflex dystrophy has not been noted.

The treatment of established reflex sympathetic dystrophy is beyond the scope of this text.

Infection.—Infection following the open reduction of intra-articular calcaneus fractures has been mentioned by many authors. The magnitude of the original injury, the precarious nature of the blood supply about the heel, and the gross swelling usually present in these fractures all predispose to infection after open reduction.[119] Letournel[112] reported a 10% incidence of skin necrosis following open reduction, with nearly half of these patients developing severe infection. Debridement of the infection followed by closure over suction drains was recommended to treat the infection. However, in all patients in whom an infection developed, the subtalar joint remained stiff, and a fair or poor result was recorded.

Author's Preferred Method of Treatment

As the review of the modes of treatment recommended for intra-articular fractures of the calcaneus reveals, many factors are believed to affect results. However, it is my opinion that *early active* range of motion of the subtalar, ankle, midtarsal, and metatarsophalangeal joints is the *key* to successful treatment of these fractures and *must* be stressed no matter which method is selected.

Nondisplaced Intra-articular Fractures.—I treat all nondisplaced, intra-articular fractures by the application of a compression dressing and elevation with ice. Pain medication adequate to control the patient's discomfort is essential. The use of a fracture boot allows immobilization for fracture healing, pain control, and reduction of soft-tissue edema while allowing daily range-of-motion exercises.

Active range of motion of all joints in the foot, especially the subtalar joint, is encouraged. I believe that the responsibility of prescribing and supervising range of motion is the physician's, *not* the physical therapist's. In my experience, subtalar motion is poorly understood by patients, and physician explanation is essential for patient understanding and cooperation.

Once swelling has subsided and the patient has demonstrated the ability to actively move the subtalar, ankle, midtarsal, and metatarsophalangeal joints, he is discharged on crutches. He is kept non–weight bearing on crutches for 4 to 6 weeks in well-fitting support hose. Partial weight bearing in the fracture boot is then instituted over the next 6 weeks. Weight bearing is progressed within the tolerance of pain. Range-of-motion exercises are continued until fracture union and painless weight bearing are achieved.

Alternatively, once motion has been restored, a short-leg "drop foot" cast with a weight-bearing heel placed anterior to the anterior border of the tibia is applied. Weight bearing is progressed and the cast discontinued in 4 to 6 weeks. This treatment scheme is useful in patients who cannot manage non–weight bearing for 4 to 6 weeks.

Displaced Intra-articular Fractures.—I treat displaced intra-articular fractures initially with sterile preparation of the foot, application of a compression dressing, elevation with ice, and early motion of the ankle, subtalar, midtarsal, and metatarsophalangeal joints. I instruct the patients in each of these motions myself, particularly subtalar motion. Routine radiographs consisting of anteroposterior, lateral and axial views are obtained. A CT scan in the coronal and axial planes is a necessity in assessing comminution, posterior facet involvement, depression, possible extension of the primary sagittal fracture line into the calcaneocuboid joint, loss of calcaneal height with heel widening, calcaneofibular impingement, and peroneal and flexor hallucis longus tendon entrapment (Fig 35–43,A). With an understanding of the primary and secondary fracture line characteristics and the number of major fracture fragments, I then classify the fracture as a tongue, joint depression, or comminuted type by using the terminology of Essex-Lopresti.

Tongue-Type and Joint Depression Fractures.—The goals of calcaneal fracture treatment include restoration of posterior articular facet congruity, restoration of Bohler's angle, positioning of the hindfoot in a neutral position in relation to the forefoot, restoration of calcaneal height, restoration of the normal calcaneal width to prevent calcaneofibular impingement or peroneal tendon entrapment, and maintenance of functional range of motion in the subtalar and midfoot joints. I believe that anatomic restoration of the posterior articular surface while accomplishing the rest of these goals is best achieved by open reduction and internal fixation. Factors in patient selection include adequate skin conditions without abrasions, fracture blisters, or severe edema preventing closure. Also, the articular fracture fragments must be large enough to hold screw fixation, and the patient must be young, motivated, and willing to accept the risks of wound necrosis or postoperative infection.

With the patient in the prone position, a lateral curvilinear incision is made posterior to the peroneal tendons and sural nerve. This is extended down to the lateral calcaneus with a thick anterior flap maintained. The peroneal tendons are decompressed with a longitudinal incision in the tendon sheath. The disimpaction of the posterior articular facet fragment, reduction, and fixation are performed in steps similar to that described by Stephenson.[186] I rarely have to make a separate medial incision but do not hesitate if this is required to correct a large medial overhang or varus or valgus angulation of a tuberosity fragment. Indications for bone grafting include a significant defect in the posterior facet or subchondral bone (Fig 35–44). Occasionally, the posterior facet articular surface is more comminuted than anticipated from preoperative studies and does not offer adequate screw fixation purchase. A reconstruction plate can be fashioned to run parallel and just beneath the articular surface, transfixed to the lateral wall, and extended toward the calcaneocuboid joint to act as a buttress plate. Postoperatively, the foot is elevated and immobilized in a fracture boot. Wound healing is the primary concern during this stage. After the postoperative edema decreases, sutures have been removed, and the wound has healed, usually at 10 to 14 days, the patient starts active range-of-motion exercises out of the brace four times daily. An elastic stocking is used to control edema. The ambulatory status remains non–weight-bearing for 6 weeks and then progressive weight bearing in the brace. After 10 to 12 weeks, if radiographic studies show satisfactory union, they are progressed to weight bearing to tolerance in a well-fitted shoe.

Patients with diabetes mellitus or arteriosclerotic vascular disease or other vascular compromise and debilitated patients are treated nonoperatively with early motion. Progression of ambulatory status in a fracture brace is the same as the postoperative protocol.

Superior Displacement of the Tuberosity.—Superior displacement of the tuberosity can usually be reduced

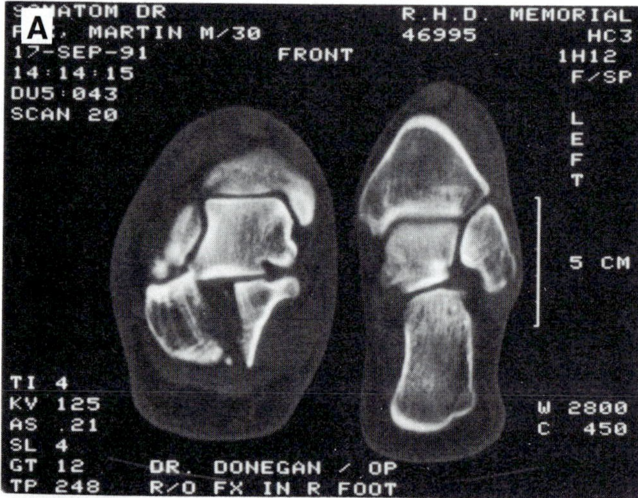

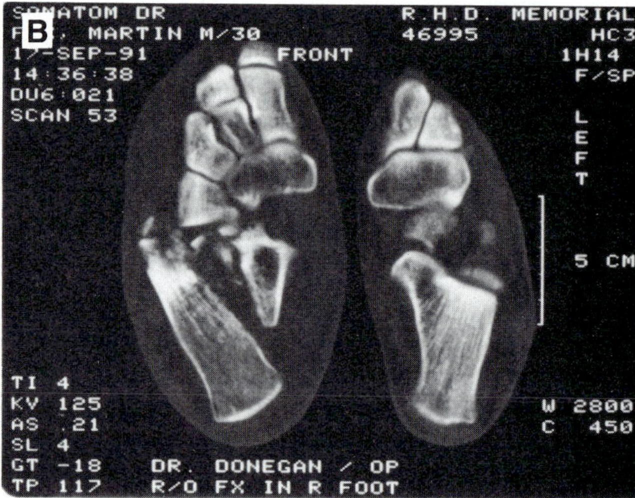

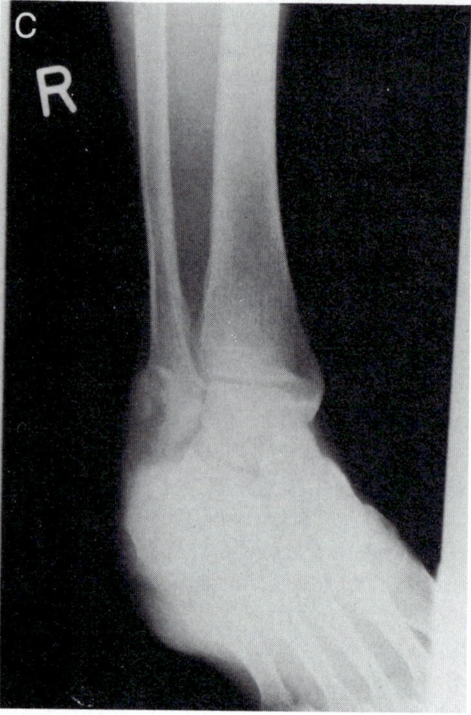

FIG 35–43.
A, a coronal CT view demonstrates dislocation of the lateral posterior facet under the distal fibula. **B,** an axial CT view demonstrates a primary sagittal fracture line with extension into the calcaneocuboid joint and comminution. **C,** a postoperative Broden's view demonstrates restoration of the posterior facet. The patient also suffered a comminuted distal fibula fracture secondary to the calcaneus fracture dislocation.

by simply plantar-flexing the foot. However, if successful, it requires casting to maintain the reduction, a fact that prevents early motion. Therefore, I use a ⅛-in. Steinmann pin inserted into the tuberosity of the calcaneus and driven across the fracture site into the anterior calcaneus to hold the reduction. If the anterior process is comminuted and does not provide adequate fixation, the pin is driven across the calcaneocuboid joint into the cuboid to stabilize its position. A slipper cast is applied to allow early range of motion of the ankle and subtalar joint.

Management, then, is just as following Essex-Lopresti's method of treating tongue-type fractures (see page 35-56).

Medial-Lateral Spread, Displacement, or Angulation.—Young patients with abrasions, fracture blisters, severe swelling, compromising closure, or severe posterior facet comminution precluding screw fixation are treated with closed reduction in an attempt to reduce the medial-lateral heel spread, restore some of the lost calcaneal height, and align the heel.

Medial-lateral spread of the calcaneus is reduced by using the heels of the surgeon's palms placed beneath the malleoli to compress the calcaneus and restore its width. The patient is placed in the prone position and the knee flexed 90 degrees. The heel is grasped between the heels of the surgeon's palms. The thigh is lifted off the table and the heel "shaken" to disimpact the frac-

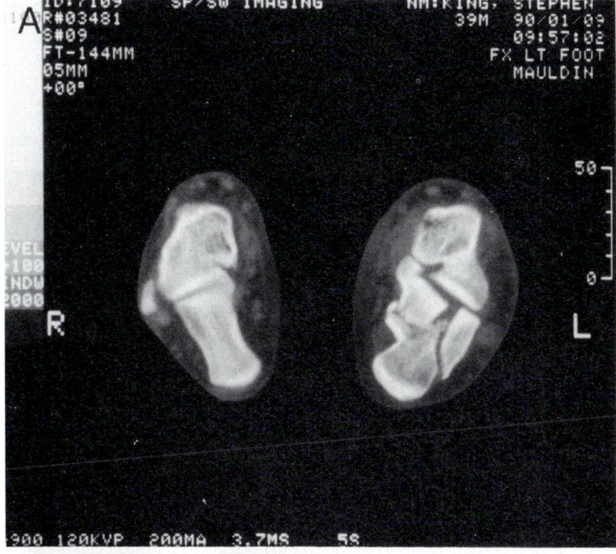

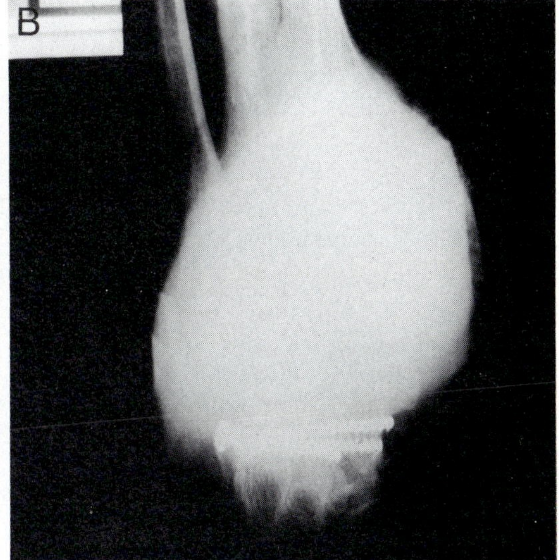

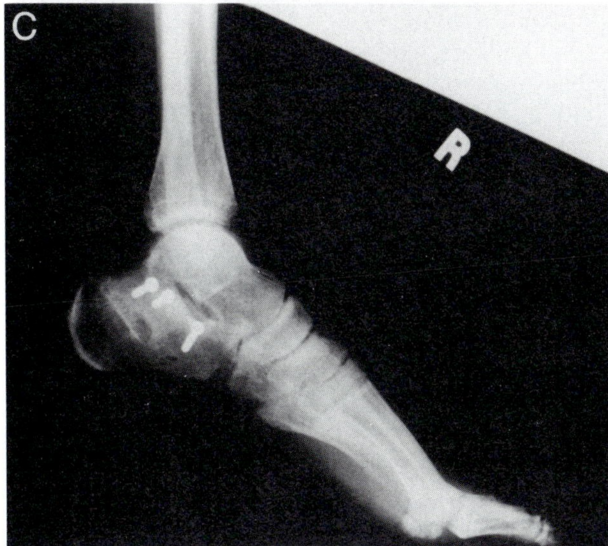

FIG 35–44.
A, coronal CT shows fracture extension through the posterior facet with significant calcaneal widening and medial cortex comminution. Postoperative axial **(B)** and lateral **(C)** views demonstrate restoration of the posterior facet and Bohler's angle.

ture. The heel is then compressed. If more compression is required, a Bohler clamp can be utilized.

If there is significant medial-lateral displacement or varus-valgus angulation of the tuberosity of the calcaneus (resulting in an abnormal weight-bearing alignment of the hindfoot), these displacements are reduced by applying a varus or valgus stress to the tuberosity of the calcaneus. The reduction is confirmed radiographically. This compression and molding decompress the lateral aspect of the heel and peroneal tendons and also place the heel parallel to the floor for weight bearing.

If the medial-lateral displacement or varus-valgus angulation recurs after closed reduction, a Steinmann pin can be inserted into the tuberosity fragment and driven across the fracture, thereby stabilizing it into the anterior process of the calcaneus in a reduced position. The foot is then placed in a slipper cast incorporating the pin, and early motion of the ankle and subtalar joint is instituted. The pin is removed at 4 to 6 weeks, the patient is placed in a "drop foot" cast, and weight bearing is instituted with the heel placed anterior to the tibia. The cast is removed at 8 to 10 weeks and the patient placed in a sturdy boot, the heel of which is slowly decreased in height.

If the closed reduction is stable, it does not require a pin for maintenance of the reduction. The patient is kept at bed rest with the foot elevated in a compression dressing with ice packs. Adequate pain medication is prescribed. Intensive ankle, subtalar, midtarsal, and metatarsophalangeal joint motion is instituted after swelling decreases, usually at 5 to 7 days. The progression of ambulatory status in a fracture boot is the same as the postoperative protocol above.

It is important to emphasize to the patient that continued improvement in function will occur for 18 to 24 months following the fracture. Only after this period of time has passed is consideration given to reconstructive surgery such as arthrodesis. Additionally, careful evaluation to determine the exact cause of postfracture disability is essential before *any* surgical treatment is instituted. I am particularly careful to evaluate heel pad damage, usually with xeroradiography, because in my experience this damage precludes a good result from any surgical treatment.

Stress Fractures of the Calcaneus

A stress or fatigue fracture is defined as a break in the continuity of normal bone due to repeated subthreshold stresses or a break in the continuity of abnormal bone because of repeated normal stresses.[42, 107, 108] The os calcis is the tarsal bone most commonly affected with stress fractures.[41] D'Ambrosia and Drez[41] suggest that gait variations play a role in the anatomic predisposition to stress fractures in certain tarsal bones.

According to Leabhart,[108] the first stress fractures were reported by Brehithaupt in 1855 in the painful feet of soldiers. Scheller[172] reported 590 stress fractures, 4 of which involved the calcaneus. Hullinger[87] in 1944 reported 53 stress fractures of the calcaneus in army recruits. Van DeMark and McCarthy[195] also noted that stress fractures of the calcaneus were a frequent cause of painful heels in soldiers. Finally, Leabhart in 1959 reported 134 stress fractures of the calcaneus in soldiers and stated that this fracture occurred in 0.45% of new recruits. Nearly three fourths of the patients in Leabhart's series had bilateral fractures, and fewer than 10% had been physically active prior to enlistment in the service. He found no relationship between abnormal foot structure and the incidence of calcaneal stress fractures.

Clinical Diagnosis

Calcaneal stress fractures have been misdiagnosed as tenosynovitis, tendonitis, arthritis, rheumatic fever, cellulitis with lymphangitis, and neurosis.[108] The clinical examination is essential in preventing such misdiagnosis.

The key to the diagnosis of a stress fracture of the calcaneus is a high index of suspicion.[41] Stress fractures usually occur in long-distance runners and army recruits. Patients complain of painful swelling of the heel that occurs within the first 7 to 10 days of increased training.[108] They do not give a specific history of trauma. According to Leabhart,[108] edema in the area of the precalcaneal bursa, anterior to the Achilles tendon, is highly suggestive of a stress fracture. Tenderness over the posterosuperior aspect of the calcaneus in the area of the stress fracture is diagnostic.[108] According to Leabhart, stretching the heel cord by dorsiflexion of the foot does not substantially increase the pain. Although the edema subsides with rest, the tenderness usually persists until the fracture is healed.[108] Pain on medial-lateral compression of the calcaneus and positive roentgenographic findings at 3 weeks confirm an os calcis stress fracture.[41]

Radiographic Diagnosis

Radiographic findings are negative until 10 to 14 days after the onset of symptoms, at which time a definite line or density is usually seen in the posterosuperior aspect of the calcaneus, perpendicular to the trabecular stress lines.[41, 108] The fracture line increases in density up to 6 weeks after the beginning of symptoms, and then the density gradually resolves.[108] The radiographic differential diagnosis of a stress fracture of the calcaneus includes osteogenic sarcoma, osteomyelitis, and osteoid osteoma.

Radionuclide bone scanning will substantiate the diagnosis as early as 2 to 8 days from the onset of symptoms.[155] Because it takes 2 to 3 weeks before roentgenographic changes are manifested, a positive bone scan permits early treatment that can forestall the development of the full clinical and radiographic syndrome of a stress fracture.[155] Prather et al.[155] found that patients with negative bone scan findings never subsequently developed radiographic changes in the bone, but there was a 24% incidence of false-positive bone scans. According to D'Ambrosia and Drez,[41] a false-positive bone scan is the result of accelerated bone remodeling in these highly active individuals. Standard radiographs, on the other hand, have a false-negative rate of 71% when performed early in the clinical syndrome.[154]

Treatment

According to D'Ambrosia and Drez[41] treatment is symptomatic, with symptoms resolving in 2 to 3 weeks.[41] Leabhart[108] found that weight bearing on crutches with a half-inch sponge rubber heel insert will decrease the symptoms. He reports that attempts to return patients to stressful ambulatory status before 8 weeks usually resulted in the recurrence of symptoms. Importantly, he reports that no calcaneal stress fracture underwent displacement.

Author's Preferred Method of Treatment

My experience with stress fractures is mainly in long-distance runners. These patients present with a gradual onset of pain in the heel. The symptoms must be distinguished from plantar fasciitis and Achilles tendonitis. Differentiating Achilles tendonitis and plantar fasciitis is most easily done on the basis of the specific area of point tenderness. If there is still confusion, a bone scan will help to distinguish these entities. I treat patients with calcaneal stress fractures by limitation of the inciting activity until the symptoms subside. Contrast baths using heat followed by ice help to decrease the symptoms. Once the symptoms have subsided, a heel pad and possibly an arch support in the running shoe are useful in preventing their recurrence. Resumption of the activity that caused the stress fracture is usually not possible before 4 to 6 weeks. If activity is resumed earlier, the symptoms usually recur. I have not seen a stress fracture of the calcaneus undergo displacement.

Dislocation of the Calcaneus

Dislocation of the calcaneus at the subtalar and calcaneocuboid joints is a rare injury with only eight cases reported in the recent literature.[26, 75, 197] According to Hamilton[75] the mechanism of injury is a large force against the lower part of the leg that causes the leg to be displaced backward against a fixed heel. Twisting injuries have also been implicated in causing this dislocation.[26] The calcaneus usually dislocates laterally[26, 75, 197], however, an inferior dislocation has also been reported.[197]

Treatment in all but one of the cases reported in the literature has been by closed reduction followed by cast immobilization in a short-leg cast[26, 75, 197] for 6 to 9 weeks.[75]

In a single case reported by Viswanath and Shephard,[197] closed reduction of a lateral dislocation of the calcaneus was unsuccessful. Open reduction was performed through a lateral approach but was unstable and required a Kirschner wire across the calcaneocuboid joint for stability. At follow-up, this patient had a persistent limp and slight varus deformity of the heel. However, most reports in the literature indicate that these patients recover a useful foot without significant disability.[75, 197]

None of the cases in the literature had intra-articular fractures associated with this dislocation. Such fractures could render the reduction unstable and require internal fixation. They can also lead to more severe long-term subtalar and midfoot stiffness and disability.

REFERENCES

Calcaneus

1. Aaron DAR: Intra-articular fractures of the calcaneus, *J Bone Joint Surg [Br]* 56:567, 1974.
2. Aitken AP: Fractures of the os-calcis—treatment by closed reduction, *Clin Orthop* 30:67–75, 1963.
3. Allan JH: The open reduction of fractures of the os calcis, *Ann Surg* 141:890–900, 1955.
4. Allon SM, Mears DC: Three dimensional analysis of calcaneal fractures, *Foot Ankle* 11:254–263, 1991.
5. Anthonsen W: An oblique projection for roentgen examination of the talo-calcanean joint, particularly regarding intra-articular fracture of the calcaneus, *Acta Radiol* 24:306–310, 1943.
6. Arnesen A: Fracture of the os calcis and its treatment, *Acta Chir Scand Suppl* 234:2–70, 1958.
7. Arnesen A: Treatment of fracture of the os calcis with traction and manipulation, *Acta Chir Scand* 132:566–573, 1966.
8. Backman S, Johnson SR: Torsion of the foot causing fracture of the anterior calcaneal process, *Acta Chir Scand* 105:460–466, 1953.
9. Bailey FA: *Proc Oregon Med* 7:68, 1880.
10. Bankart ASB: Fractures of the os calcis, *Lancet* 2:175, 1942.
11. Barnard L: Non-operative treatment of fractures of the calcaneus, *Instr Course Lect* 28:249–251, 1973.
12. Barnard L: Non-operative treatment of fractures of the calcaneus, *J Bone Joint Surg [Am]* 45:865–867, 1963.
13. Barnard L, Odegard JK: Conservative approach in the treatment of fractures of the calcaneus, *J Bone Joint Surg [Am]* 37:1231–1236, 1955.
14. Barnard L, Odegard JK: Conservative approach in the treatment of fractures of the calcaneus, *J Bone Joint Surg [Am]* 52:1689, 1970.
15. Bellenger M, Vander Elst E, Lorthior J: Les fractures du calcaneum: leur traitement des sequelles, *Acta Orthop Belg* 17:59–167, 1951.
16. Bertelsen A, Hasner E: Primary results of treatment of fracture of the os calcis by "foot-free walking bandage" and early movement, *Acta Orthop Scand* 21:140–154, 1951.
17. Blechschmidt E: The structure of the calcaneal padding. *Foot Ankle* 2:260–283, 1982.
18. Bohler L: Diagnosis, pathology, and treatment of fractures of the os calcis, *J Bone Joint Surg* 13:75–89, 1931.
19. Bradford CH, Larsen I: Sprain-fractures of the anterior lip of the os calcis, *N Engl J Med* 244:970–972, 1951.
20. Brattstrom H: Primary arthrodesis in severe fractures of calcaneum, *Nord Med* 50:1510–1511, 1953.
21. Brindley HH: Fractures of the os calcis: a review of 107 fractures in 95 patients, *South Med J* 59:843–847, 1966.
22. Broden B: Roentgen examination of the subtaloid joint in fractures of the calcaneus, *Acta Radiol* 31:85–91, 1949.
23. Brown JE: Early ambulation of os calcis fractures, *Clin Orthop* 63:252, 1963.
24. Burdeaux BD: Reduction of calcaneal fractures by the McReynolds medial approach technique and its experimental basis, *Clin Orthop* 177:87–103, 1983.
25. Burghele N, Serban N: Reappraisal of the treatment of fractures of the calcaneus involving the subtalar joint, *Ital J Orthop Traumatol* 2:273–279, 1976.
26. Carey EJ, Lance EM, Wade PA: Extra-articular fractures of the os calcis, *J Trauma* 5:362–372, 1965.
27. Carothers RG, Lyons JF: Early mobilization in treatment of os calcis fractures, *Am J Surg* 83:279–280, 1952.
28. Carr JB, Hamilton JJ, Bear LS: Experimental intraartic-

ular calcaneal fractures: anatomic basis for a new classification, *Foot Ankle* 10:81, 1989.
29. Cave EF: Fractures of the os calcis: the problem in general, *Clin Orthop* 30:64–66, 1963.
30. Chapman MW: Fractures and fracture-dislocations of the ankle and foot. In Mann RA, editor: *DuVries' surgery of the foot*, ed 4, St Louis, 1978, Mosby–Year Book.
31. Christopher F: Fracture of the anterior process of the calcaneus, *J Bone Joint Surg* 13:877–879, 1931.
32. Conn HR: Fractures of the os calcis: diagnosis and treatment, *Radiology* 6:228–235, 1926.
33. Conn HR: The treatment of fractures of the os calcis, *J Bone Joint Surg* 17:392–405, 1935.
34. Connolly NF: Persistent heel pain twenty years after calcaneal fracture and triple arthrodesis relieved by lateral decompression, *J Trauma* 27:809–810, 1987.
35. Conway JJ, Cowell HR: Tarsal coalition: clinical significance and roentgenographic demonstration, *Radiology* 92:799–811, 1969.
36. Cotton FJ, Henderson FF: Results of fracture of the os calcis, *Am J Orthop Surg* 14:290–298, 1916.
37. Cotton FJ, Wilson LT: Fractures of the os calcis, *Boston Med Surg J* 159:559–565, 1908.
38. Court-Brown CM, Boot DA, Kellam JF: Fracture dislocation of the calcaneus. A report of two cases, *Clin Orthop* 213:201–206, 1986.
39. Cowell HR: Talocalcaneal coalition and new causes of peroneal spastic flatfoot, *Clin Orthop* 85:16–22, 1972.
40. Dachtler HW: Fractures of the anterior superior portion of the os calcis due to indirect violence, *Am J Roentgenol* 25:629–631, 1931.
41. D'Ambrosia RD, Drez DJ: *Prevention and treatment of running injuries*, Thorofare, NJ, 1982, Charles B Slack, pp 25–31.
42. Dart DE, Graham WP: The treatment of fractured calcaneum, *J Trauma* 6:362–367, 1966.
43. DeBold C Jr, Stimson BB: Treatment of injuries involving the subtalar joint, *Am J Surg* 93:604–608, 1958.
44. Degan TJ, Morrey BF, Braun DP: Surgical excision for anterior-process fractures of the calcaneus, *J Bone Joint Surg [Am]* 64:519–524, 1982.
45. Devas M: *Stress fractures*, Edinburgh, Churchill Livingstone, 1975.
46. Deyerle WM: Long-term follow-up of fractures of the os calcis. Diagnostic peroneal synoviogram, *Orthop Clin North Am* 4:213–227, 1973.
47. Dick IL: Primary fusion of the posterior subtalar joint in the treatment of fractures of the calcaneum, *J Bone Joint Surg [Br]* 35:375–380, 1953.
48. Dieterle JO: A case of so-called "open-beak" fracture of the os calcis, *J Bone Joint Surg* 22:740, 1940.
49. Dodson CF Jr: Fractures of the os calcis. *J Ark Med Soc* 73:319–322, 1977.
50. Dragonetti L: A proposito del trattamento incruento delle fratture di calcagno, *Arch Orthop Suppl* 82:381–394, 1969.
51. Essex-Lopresti P: Results of reduction in fractures of the calcaneum, *J Bone Joint Surg [Br]* 33:284, 1951.
52. Essex-Lopresti P: The mechanism, reduction technique, and results in fractures of the os calcis, *Br J Surg* 39:395–419, 1952.
53. Finder JG, Hussussian JG, Levin B: Promontory fractures of the calcaneus, *J Int Coll Surg* 35:84–90, 1961.
54. Fisk GR: Fractures of the os calcis treated by open reduction and iliac crest grafting, *J Bone Joint Surg [Br]* 62:263, 1980.
55. Fitzgerald RH Jr, Coventry MB: Post-traumatic peroneal tendonitis. In Bateman JE, Trott AW, editors: *The foot and ankle*, New York, 1980, Brian C Decker.
56. Gage JR, Premer R: Os calcis fractures. An analysis of 37, *Minn Med* 54:169–176, 1971.
57. Gallie WE: Subastragalar arthrodesis in fractures of the os calcis, *J Bone Joint Surg* 25:731–736, 1943.
58. Garcia A, Parkes JC II: Fractures of the foot. In Giannestras NJ, editor: *Foot disorders: medical and surgical management*, ed 2, Philadelphia, 1973, Lea & Febiger.
59. Gaul JS Jr, Greenburg BG: Calcaneus fractures involving the subtalar joint: a clinical and statistical survey of 98 cases, *South Med J* 59:605–613, 1966.
60. Geckeler EO: Comminuted fractures of the os calcis, *Arch Surg* 61:469–476, 1950.
61. Gellman M: Fractures of the anterior process of the calcaneus, *J Bone Joint Surg [Am]* 33:382–386, 1951.
62. Giachino AA, Uhtoff HK: Current concepts review: Intraarticular fractures of the calcaneus, *J Bone Joint Surg [Am]* 71:784–787, 1989.
63. Giannestras NJ, Sammarco GJ: Fractures and dislocations in the foot. In Rockwood CA Jr, Green DP, editors: *Fractures*, vol 2, Philadelphia, 1975, JB Lippincott.
64. Gillette EP: An apparatus for treatment of fractures of the os calcis, *J Bone Joint Surg* 12:670–671, 1930.
65. Gilmer PW, Herzenberg J, Frank L, et al: Computerized tomographic analysis of acute calcaneal fractures, *Foot Ankle* 6:184–193, 1986.
66. Gissane W: Proceedings of the British Orthopaedic Association, *J Bone Joint Surg* 29:254–255, 1947.
67. Goff CW: Fresh fracture of the os calcis, *Arch Surg* 36:744–765, 1938.
68. Gossett J: Mobilisation precoce apres reduction et contention par broches des fractures du tarse posterieur, *Mem Acad Chir* 95:365–370, 1969.
69. Gould N: Lateral approach to the os calcis, *Foot Ankle* 4:218–220, 1984.
70. Green W: Fractures of the anterior-superior beak of the os calcis, *NY State J Med* 56:3515–3517, 1956.
71. Guillen-Garcia P, Garcia-Rubio M, Concejero-Lopez V, et al: Tarsal tunnel syndrome: a report of fifty-six cases, *J Bone Joint Surg [Br]* 61:123, 1979.
72. Guyer B, Levinsohn M, Fredrickson BE, et al: Computed tomography of calcaneal fractures: anatomy, pathology, dosimetry, and clinical revelance, *Am J Radiol* 145:911–919, 1985.
73. Hackenbroch M: Eine seltene Lokalisation der stenosierenden Tendovaginitis (An der Sehnenscheide bei Peroneen), *Munchen Med Wochnschr* 74:932, 1927.
74. Hall MC, Pennal GF: Primary subtalar arthrodesis in the treatment of severe fractures of the calcaneum, *J Bone Joint Surg [Br]* 42:336–343, 1960.
75. Hamilton AR: An unusual dislocation, *Med J Aust* 1:271, 1949.
76. Hammesfahr R, Fleming LL: Calcaneal fractures: a good prognosis. *Foot Ankle* 2:161–171, 1981.
77. Harris RI: Fractures of the os calcis, *Instr Course Lect* 9:375–379, 1952.
78. Harris RI: Fractures of the os calcis: their treatment by tri-radiate traction and subastragalar fusion, *Ann Surg* 124:1082–1100, 1946.

79. Harris RI: Fractures of the os calcis: treatment by early subtalar arthrodesis, *Clin Orthop* 30:100–110, 1963.
80. Harty M: Anatomic considerations in injuries of the calcaneus, *Orthop Clin North Am* 4:179–183, 1973.
81. Hazlett JW: Open reduction of fractures of the calcaneum, *Can J Surg* 12:310–317, 1969.
82. Heck CW: Fracture of the bones of the foot, *Surg Clin North Am* 45:108–117, 1965.
83. Hermann OJ: Conservative therapy for fracture of the os calcis, *J Bone Joint Surg* 19:709–718, 1937.
84. Hildebrand O: Tendovaginitis chronica deformans und Luxation der Peronealsehnen, *Dtsch Z Chir* 86:526–531, 1907.
85. Hoaglund FT: Fractures of the os calcis. Editor's comment. In Leach RE, Hoaglund FT, Riseborough EJ, editors: *Controversies in orthopaedic Surgery*, Philadelphia, 1982. WB Saunders.
86. Horn CE: Fractures of the calcaneus, *Calif Med* 108:209–215, 1968.
87. Hullinger CW: Insufficiency fracture of the calcaneus similar to march fracture of the metatarsal, *J Bone Joint Surg* 26:751–N757, 1944.
88. Hunt DD: Compression fracture of the anterior articular surface of the calcaneus, *J Bone Joint Surg [Am]* 52:1637–1642, 1970.
89. Isbister JFStC: Calcaneo-fibular abutment following crush fracture of the calcaneus, *J Bone Joint Surg [Am]* 56:274–278, 1974.
90. Isherwood I: A radiological approach to the subtalar joint, *J Bone Joint Surg [Br]* 43:566–574, 1961.
91. Jaekle RF, Clark AG: Fractures of the os calcis, *Surg Gynecol Obstet* 64:663–672, 1937.
92. Jahss MH, Kay BS: An anatomic study of the superior process of the os calcis and its clinical application, *Foot Ankle* 3:268–281, 1983.
93. James ETR, Hunter GA: The dilemma of painful old os calcis fractures, *Clin Orthop* 177:112–115, 1983.
94. Johansson JE, Harrison J, Greenwood FAH: Subtalar arthrodesis for adult traumatic arthritis, *Foot Ankle* 2:294–298, 1982.
95. Kalamachi A, Evans JG: Posterior subtalar fusion. A preliminary report on a modified Gallie's procedure, *J Bone Joint Surg [Br]* 59:287–289, 1977.
96. Kalish SR: The conservative and surgical treatment of calcaneal fractures, *J Am Podiatr Assoc* 65:912–926, 1975.
97. Key JA, Conwell HE: *Fractures of the Calcaneus in the management of fractures, dislocations, and sprains*, St Louis, 1951, Mosby–Year Book.
98. Kiaer S, Anthonsen W: Fracture of the calcaneus treated with arthrodesis, *Acta Chir Scand Suppl* 87:191, 1942.
99. King D: Correspondence club letter, Sept 22, 1949.
100. King RE: Axial pin fixation of fractures of the os calcis (method of Essex-Lopresti), *Orthop Clin North Am* 4:185–188, 1973.
101. Kohler A: *Borderlands of the normal and early pathologic in skeletal*, New York, 1956, Grune & Stratton, pp 626–630 (translated and edited by JT Case).
102. Kongsholm J, Egham L: Early mobilization of unilateral and bilateral fractures of the calcaneus, *Acta Orthop Scand* 52:702, 1981.
103. Korn R: Der Bruch durch das hintere Obere drittel des Fersenbeines, *Arch Orthop Unfallchir* 41:789, 1942.
104. Kuhns JG: Changes in elastic adipose tissue, *J Bone Joint Surg [Am]* 31:541–547, 1949.
105. Lance EM, Carey EJ Jr, Wade PA: Fractures of the os calcis: treatment by early mobilization, *Clin Orthop* 30:76–90, 1963.
106. Lance EM, Carey EJ, Wade PA: Fractures of the os calcis: a follow-up study, *J Trauma* 4:15–56, 1964.
107. Lapidus PW, Guidotti FP: Immediate mobilization and swimming pool exercises in some fractures of foot and ankle bones, *Clin Orthop* 56:197–206, 1968.
108. Leabhart JW: Stress fractures of the calcaneus, *J Bone Joint Surg [Am]* 41:1285–1290, 1959.
109. Lenormant C, Wilmoth P: Les fractures sous-thalamiques du calcaneum. Leur traitement par la reduction a ciel ouvert et la greffe osteo-periostique, *J Chir* 40:1–25, 1932.
110. Leonard MH: Treatment of fractures of the os calcis, *Arch Surg* 75:990–997, 1957.
111. Leriche R: Osteosynthese primitive pour fracture par ecrasement du calcaneum a sept fragments, *Lyon Chir* 19:559, 1922.
112. Letournel E: Open reduction and internal fixation of calcaneus fractures. In Spiegel PG, editor: *Techniques in orthopaedics: topics in trauma*, Baltimore, 1984, University Park Press.
113. Levine J, Kerim A, Spinner M: Nonunion of a fracture of the anterior process of the calcaneus, *J Bone Joint Surg [Am]* 41:178–180, 1959.
114. Lindsay WRN, Dewar FP: Fractures of the os calcis, *Am J Surg* 95:555–576, 1958.
115. Lowrie IG, Finlay DB, Brenkel IJ, et al: Computerized tomographic assessment of the subtalar joint in calcaneal fractures, *J Bone Joint Surg [Br]* 70:247–250, 1988.
116. Lowy M: Avulsion fractures of the calcaneus, *J Bone Joint Surg [Br]* 51:494–497, 1969.
117. Lyngstadaas S: Treatment of avulsion fractures of the tuber calcanei, *Acta Chir Scand* 137:579–581, 1971.
118. McLaughlin HL: *Trauma*, Philadelphia, 1959, WB Saunders.
119. McLaughlin HL: Treatment of late complications after os calcis fractures, *Clin Orthop* 30:111–115, 1963.
120. McReynolds IS: Fractures of the os calcis involving the subastragalar joint: treatment by open reduction and internal fixation with staples, using a medial approach, *J Bone Joint Surg [Am]* 58:733, 1976.
121. McReynolds IS: Open reduction and internal fixation of calcaneal fractures, *J Bone Joint Surg [Br]* 54:176–177, 1972.
122. McReynolds IS: The case for operative treatment of fractures of the os calcis. In Leach RE, Hoaglund FT, Riseborough EJ, editors: *Controversies in orthopaedic surgery*, Philadelphia, 1982, WB Saunders.
123. McReynolds IS: Trauma to the os calcis and heel cord. In Jahss MH, editor: *Disorders of the foot*, vol 2, Philadelphia, 1982, WB Saunders.
124. Mann RA: Personal communication, 1982.
125. Maxfield JE: Os calcis fractures: treatment by open reduction, *Clin Orthop* 30:91–99, 1963.
126. Maxfield JE: Treatment of calcaneal fractures by open reduction, *Instr Course Lect* 18:252–254, 1973.
127. Maxfield JE: Treatment of calcaneal fractures by open reduction, *J Bone Joint Surg [Am]* 45:868–871, 1963.
128. Maxfield JE, McDermott FJ: Experiences with the

Palmer open reduction of fractures of the calcaneus, *J Bone Joint Surg [Am]* 37:99–106, 1955.
129. Meberg E, Erfors CG: Primar terapi vid grava intra-articulara kalcaneus frakturer, *Nord Med* 9:150, 1953.
130. Mercer W: *Orthopaedic surgery*, London, 1944, Arnold.
131. Merrill V: *Atlas of roentgenographic positions and standard radiologic procedures*, ed 4, St Louis, 1975, Mosby–Year Book.
132. Miller WE: Pain and impairment considerations following treatment of disruptive os calcis fractures, *Clin Orthop* 177:82–86, 1983.
133. Miller WE, Lichtblau PO: The smashed heel, *South Med J* 58:1229–1237, 1965.
134. Miller WS: The heel pad, *Am J Sports Med* 10:19–21, 1982.
135. Morestein (1902): Quoted by Schwartz MA: *Bull Soc Nat Chir* 55:148, 1921.
136. Moretti O, Pivani C: Trattamento ed esiti in 90 osservazioni di fratture del calcagno, *Chir Organi Mov* 56:441, 1967.
137. Moseley HF: Traumatic disorders of the ankle and foot, *Clin Symp* 17:3–30, 1965.
138. Nade SML, Monahan PRW: Fractures of the calcaneum: a study of the long-term prognosis, *Injury* 4:200–207, 1973.
139. Nade SML, Monahan PRW: Results of non-operative treatment of calcaneal fractures: a study of long-term prognosis, *J Bone Joint Surg [Br]* 55:429–430, 1973.
140. Noble J, McQuillan WM: Early posterior subtalar fusion in the treatment of fractures of the os calcis, *J Bone Joint Surg [Br]* 61:90–93, 1979.
141. Nosny P, Bourrel P, Caron JJ: Mobilisation precoce apres reduction et contention par broches des fractures du tarse posterieur, *Mem Acad Chir* 95:365–370, 1969.
142. O'Connell F, Mital MA, Rowe CR: Evaluation of modern management of fractures of the os calcis, *Clin Orthop* 83:214–223, 1972.
143. Olson PF: The treatment of fractures of the os calcis, *J Bone Joint Surg* 21:747–751, 1939.
144. Omoto H, Sakurada K, Sugi M, et al: A new method of manual reduction for intra-articular fracture of the calcaneus, *Clin Orthop* 177:104–111, 1983.
145. Palmer I: The mechanism and treatment of fractures of the calcaneus. Open reduction with the use of cancellous grafts, *J Bone Joint Surg [Am]* 30:2–8, 1948.
146. Paley D, Hall H: Calcaneal fracture controversies. Can we put Humpty Dumpty together again? *Orthop Clin North Am* 20:665–677, 1989.
147. Paley D, Hall H, McMurty R, et al: Operative treatment of calcaneal fractures: a long term followup: calcaneal protocol score; and factors that affect outcome, *Orthop Trans* 11:484, 1987.
148. Parkes JC II: Injuries of the hindfoot, *Clin Orthop* 122:28–36, 1977.
149. Parkes JC II: The conservative management of fractures of the os calcis. In Leach RE, Hoaglund FT, Riseborough EJ, editors: *Controversies in orthopaedic surgery*, Philadelphia, 1982, WB Saunders.
150. Parkes JC II: The non-reductive treatment for fractures of the os calcis, *Orthop Clin North Am* 4:193–195, 1973.
151. Parvin RW, Ford LT: Stenosing tenosynovitis of the common peroneal tendon sheath, *J Bone Joint Surg [Am]* 38:1352–1357, 1956.
152. Pennal GF, Yadav MP: Operative treatment of comminuted fractures of the os calcis, *Orthop Clin North Am* 4:197–211, 1973.
153. Piatt AD: Fracture of the promontory of the calcaneus, *Radiology* 67:386–390, 1956.
154. Pozo JL, Kirwan EO'G, Jackson AM: The long-term results of conservative management of severely displaced fractures of the calcaneus, *J Bone Joint Surg [Brcb* 66:386–390, 1984.
155. Prather JL, Nusynowitz ML, Snowdy HA, et al: Scintigraphic findings in stress fractures, *J Bone Joint Surg [Am]* 59:869–874, 1977.
156. Pridie KH: A new method of treatment for severe fractures of the os calcis. A preliminary report, *Surg Gynecol Obstet* 82:671–676, 1946.
157. Protheroe K: Avulsion fractures of the calcaneus, *J Bone Joint Surg [Br]* 51:118–122, 1969.
158. Reich RS: End results in fractures of the calcaneus, *JAMA* 99:1909–1912, 1932.
159. Reich RS: Subastragaloid arthrodesis in the treatment of old fractures of the calcaneus, *Surg Gynecol Obstet* 42:420–422, 1926.
160. Reich RS: The present status of treatment of fractures of the calcaneus, *Int Abstr Surg* 68:302–310, 1939.
161. Roberts N: Fractures of the calcaneus, *J Bone Joint Surg [Br]* 50:884, 1968.
162. Roberts NW, Sayle Creer WN: Calcaneus fractures, *Lancet* 2:65, 1947.
163. Rockwood CA: Personal communications, 1976.
164. Romash MM: Calcaneal fractures: three-dimensional treatment, *Foot Ankle* 8:180–197, 1988.
165. Rosendahl SV: The significance of the valgus deformity in fracture of the calcaneus, *Acta Orthop Scand* 36:339, 1965.
166. Rosendahl-Jensen S: Fractura calcanei. Prognosis of an insurance material, *Acta Chir Scand* 112:69–78, 1956.
167. Rothberg AS: Avulsion fracture of the os calcis, *J Bone Joint Surg* 21:218–220, 1939.
168. Rowe CR, Sakellarides HT, Freeman PA, et al: Fractures of the os calcis: a long-term follow-up study of 146 patients, *JAMA* 184:920–923, 1963.
169. Salama R, Benamara A, Weissman SL: Functional treatment of intra-articular fractures of the calcaneus, *Clin Orthop* 115:236–240, 1976.
170. Sallick MA, Blum L: Sensory denervation of the heel for persistent pain following fractures of the calcaneus, *J Bone Joint Surg [Am]* 30:209–212, 1948.
171. Sarrafian SK: *Anatomy of the foot and ankle: descriptive, topographic, and function*, Philadelphia, 1983, JB Lippincott.
172. Scheller F: Uberlastungsschaden am Knochengerust junger Manner, *Med Welt* 13:1333–1336, 1939.
173. Schofield RO: Fractures of the os calcis, *J Bone Joint Surg* 18:566–580, 1936.
174. Schottstaedt ER: Introduction. Symposium on treatment of fractures of the calcaneus. *Instr Course Lect* 18:247–248, 1982.
175. Schottstaedt ER: Symposium: treatment of fractures of the calcaneus, *J Bone Joint Surg [Am]* 45:863–864, 1963.
176. Segal D, Malkin C, Pick RY, et al: Surgical treatment of joint depressed calcaneal fractures, *Foot Ankle* 2:356, 1982.
177. Shannon FT, Murray AM: Os calcis fractures treated

by non–weight bearing exercises. A review of 65 patients, *J R Coll Surg Edinb* 23:355–361, 1978.
178. Sisk TD: Fractures. In Edmonson AS, Crenshaw AH, editors: *Campbell's operative orthopaedics*, ed 6, vol 1, St Louis, 1980, Mosby–Year Book.
179. Slatis P, Kiviluoto O, Santavirta S, et al: Fractures of the calcaneum, *Acta Orthop Scand* 50:361, 1979.
180. Slatis P, Kiviluoto O, Santavirta S, et al: Fractures of the calcaneum, *J Trauma* 19:939–943, 1979.
181. Smith H: Malunited fractures. In Edmonson AS, Crenshaw AH, editors: *Campbell's operative orthopaedics*, ed 6, vol 1, St Louis, 1980, Mosby–Year Book.
182. Smith R, Staple T: CAT scan evaluation of the hindfoot—an anatomical and clinical study, *Foot Ankle* 2:346, 1982.
183. Smith RW, Staple TW: Computerized tomography (CT) scanning technique for the hindfoot, *Clin Orthop* 177:34–38, 1983.
184. Soeur R, Remy R: Fractures of the calcaneus with displacement of the thalamic portion, *J Bone Joint Surg [Br]* 57:413–421, 1975.
185. Stephenson JR: Displaced fractures of the calcaneus involving the subtalar joint: the key role of the superomedial fragment, *Foot Ankle* 4:91–101, 1983.
186. Stephenson JR: Treatment of displaced intra-articular fractures of the calcaneus using medial and lateral approaches, internal fixation, and early motion, *J Bone Joint Surg [Am]* 69:115–130, 1987.
187. Sutro CJ: The os calcis. The tendo Achillis and local bursae, *Bull Hosp Jt Dis* 27:76, 1966.
188. Thomas FB: Arthrodesis of the subtalar joint, *J Bone Joint Surg [Br]* 49:93–97, 1967.
189. Thompson KR: Treatment of comminuted fractures of the calcaneus by triple arthrodesis, *Orthop Clin North Am* 4:189–191, 1973.
190. Thompson KR, Friesen CM: Treatment of comminuted fractures of the calcaneus by primary triple arthrodesis, *J Bone Joint Surg [Am]* 41:1423–1436, 1959.
191. Thoren O: Os calcis fractures, *Acta Orthop Scand Suppl* 70:1–116, 1964.
192. Trickey EL: Treatment of fractures of the calcaneus, *J Bone Joint Surg [Br]* 57:411, 1975.
193. Trolle D: *Accessory bones of the human foot*, Copenhagen, 1948, Munksgaard, pp 1–272.
194. Urowitz E, Hall H: The medial approach to fracture of the os calcis, *J Bone Joint Surg [Br]* 62:131, 1980.
195. Van DeMark RE, McCarthy PV: March fracture, *Radiology* 46:496–501, 1946.
196. Vestad E: Fractures of the calcaneum: open reduction and bone grafting, *Acta Chir Scand* 134:617–625, 1968.
197. Viswanath SS, Shephard E: Dislocation of the calcaneum, *Injury* 9:50–52, 1978.
198. Von Stockum: Operative Behandlung der calcaneus und talus Fractur, *Z Chir* 39:1438, 1912.
199. Warrick CK, Bremner AE: Fractures of the calcaneum: with an atlas illustrating the various types of fracture. *J Bone Joint Surg [Br]* 35:33–45, 1953.
200. Watson-Jones R: *Fractures and joint injuries*, ed 4, vol 2, Baltimore, 1955, Williams & Wilkins.
201. Wells C: Fractures of the heel bones in early and prehistoric times, *Practitioner* 217:294–298, 1976.
202. Westhues H: Eine neue Behandlungmethode der Calcaneusfrakturen. Zugleich ein Vorschlag zur Behandlung der Talusfrakturen, *Z Chir* 62:995–1002, 1935.
203. Whittaker AH: Treatment of fractures of the os calcis by open reduction and internal fixation. *Am J Surg* 74:687–696, 1947.
204. Widen A: Fractures of the calcaneus: a clinical study with special reference to the technique and results of open reduction. *Acta Chir Scand Suppl* 188:1–119, 1954.
205. Wilson DW: Functional capacity following fractures of the os calcis, *Can Med Assoc J* 95:908–911, 1966.
206. Wilson GE: Fractures of the calcaneus, *J Bone Joint Surg [Am]* 32:59–70, 1950.
207. Wilson PD: Treatment of fractures of the os calcis by arthrodesis of the subastragalar joint, *JAMA* 89:1676–1683, 1927.
208. Wilson PD, editor: *Experience in the management of fractures and dislocations*, Philadelphia, 1938, JB Lippincott.
209. Zacharin D: Fracture of the anterior process (promontory) of the calcaneus, *Med J Aust* 50:737–738, 1963.
210. Zagra A, Bellistri D: L'artrodesi sottoastragalica immediata nelle fratture talamiche del calcagno, *Minerva Ortop* 21:574–577, 1970.
211. Zayer M: Fracture of the calcaneus, *Acta Orthop Scand* 40:530–542, 1969.
212. Zeiss J, Ebraheim N, Rusin J, et al: Magnetic resonance imaging of the calcaneus: normal anatomy and application in calcaneal fractures. *Foot Ankle* 11:264–273, 1991.

FRACTURE AND FRACTURE-DISLOCATIONS OF THE TALUS

Although fractures of the talus are not common,[30, 75] the frequency and disability resulting from the complications of these fractures serve to emphasize their importance.* Giannestras and Sammarco[48] report that injuries of the talus are second in frequency of all tarsal bone injuries.

The terms *talus* and *astragalus* are linked in antiquity with the manufacture of dice.[52, 74, 101, 138] The word "talus" is derived from the Roman word for dice, *taxillus*, because the Romans made dice from the heel bone of a horse.[52, 74, 138] The Greeks made their dice from the second cervical vertebra of the sheep. The word for this vertebrae in Greek is *astragalus*.

The importance of injuries to the talus lies in the fact that it transmits weight from the distal end of the tibia above to the calcaneus below.[61] According to Boyd and Knight[15] more weight is borne by the superior surface of the talus than by any other joint in the body. The talus also allows for extensive motion between the tibia and calcaneus through the ankle, subtalar, and midtar-

---

**References 13, 14, 27, 31, 50, 55, 65, 74, 84, 89, 93, 106, 112, 121, 151.*

sal joints.[48] Injuries to the talus can therefore result in a substantial loss of motion and arthritic changes in these three major joints of the foot. These factors contribute to the poor results following injury to the talus.

Finally, the fact that three fifths of the talus is covered with articular cartilage leads to increased risk of joint involvement when the talus is damaged.[87]

This section deals with the various types of fractures and dislocations of the talus. These include fractures of the head of the talus, fractures of the neck of the talus, and fractures of the body of the talus. Fractures of the body of the talus are subdivided into shearing fractures of the body, fractures of the dome, fractures of the lateral process, and fractures of the posterior process of the talus. Each fracture type is discussed individually in detail.

Vascular Anatomy

The blood supply to the talus has been studied in great detail because of the incidence of aseptic necrosis following fractures and dislocations.* Although early investigators reported a very poor blood supply to this bone,[141] more recent investigators note the presence of an extensive blood supply to the talus.[52, 83, 97, 155] However, because three fifths of the talar surface is covered with articular cartilage and because no muscles have their origin or insertions into the talus, there is very limited surface area to serve as a portal of entry for incoming vessels.[63, 97, 101] Therefore, a fracture with any degree of associated soft-tissue injury or displacement can result in a loss of blood supply to the talus. The blood supply of the talus will be discussed under two divisions: extraosseous and intraosseous.

Extraosseous Arterial Supply

The extraosseous arteries providing blood supply to the talus include branches from the posterior tibial, anterior tibial, and peroneal arteries.

The posterior tibial artery supplies the talus through two avenues. First, the posterior tibial artery gives rise to the artery of the tarsal canal about 1 cm proximal to the origin of the medial and lateral plantar arteries. The artery of the tarsal canal passes anteriorly between the sheaths of the flexor digitorum longus and flexor hallucis longus to enter the tarsal canal (Fig 35–45). About 5 mm from its origin, the artery of the tarsal canal gives rise to a branch to the medial surface of the body of the talus. This vessel passes between the talotibial and talocalcaneal portions of the deltoid ligament and supplies the medial periosteal surface of the body of the talus (Fig 35–45). This vessel has been termed "the deltoid branch."[52, 63, 97]

Second, the calcaneal branches of the posterior tibial artery form a network over the posterior medial tubercle of the talus (Fig 35–45). These vessels anastomose in this area with branches from the peroneal artery.[52, 63, 97]

The anterior tibial or dorsalis pedis artery also provides blood supply to the talus from two groups of vessels. First, it sends branches to the superior surface of the neck of the talus (Fig 35–46). These branches arise either directly from the dorsalis pedis artery as medial tarsal branches or indirectly as branches of the anteromedial malleolar artery.[63, 67, 114, 137] According to Kelly and Sullivan[63] these branches are important sources for circulation to the tarsal head.

Second, the anterior tibial artery gives rise to the anterolateral malleolar artery, which may anastomose with the perforating peroneal artery to become the artery of the tarsal sinus (Fig 35–46).

The peroneal artery also provides two sources of blood supply to the talus. First, tiny branches from the peroneal artery join with the calcaneal branches of the posterior tibial artery to form a vascular plexus over the posterior tubercle of the talus. Additionally, the perforating peroneal artery, as mentioned above, contributes to the vessel known as the artery of the tarsal sinus (Fig 35–46).

According to Wildenauer,[155] the talar vascular supply arising from these three main arteries reaches the talus through a vascular network that covers all of its cartilage-free surfaces. Wildenauer stressed the importance of two vessels, the artery of the tarsal canal and the artery of the tarsal sinus.[155] The tarsal canal, formed by the tarsal and calcaneal sulci, extends 1.5 cm laterally and opens abruptly into the funnel-shaped tarsal sinus.[52, 63, 97] The tarsal sinus faces anterolaterally and is bounded by the inferolateral surface of the neck of the talus above and in front, by the anterolateral surface of the body of the talus behind, and by the anterosuperior surface of the calcaneus below.[52] The artery of the tarsal canal lies in the dorsal half of the canal closer to the talus than the calcaneus.[97] It anastomoses with the artery of the tarsal sinus to form what is called the artery of the tarsal sling; this artery is located beneath the talus and passes through the tunnel formed by the tarsal sinus and the tarsal canal.[63] In this tunnel, it gives rise to branches that enter the inferior aspect of the neck of the talus (Fig 35–47).[63] Mulfinger and Truetta[97] found this anastomosis in all of their specimens. Wildenauer[155] believes that the arteries of the tarsal sinus and tarsal ca-

**References 52, 63, 73, 83, 93, 97, 114–116, 130, 141.*

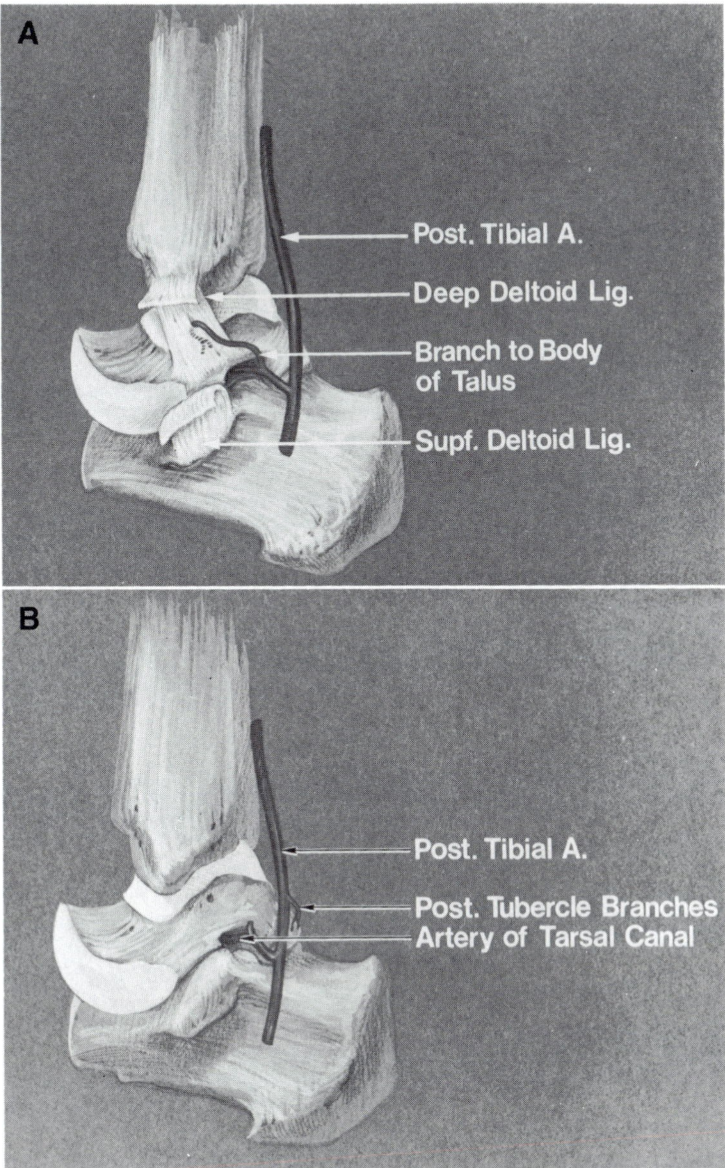

FIG 35–45.
A, the "deltoid branch" ("branch to the talar body") of the artery of the tarsal canal passes between the talotibial and talocalcaneal portions of the deltoid ligament to supply the medial aspect of the body of the talus. **B,** calcaneal branches from the posterior tibial artery form a network over the posteromedial tubercle of the talus. Note the artery of the tarsal canal as well as a branch of the posterior tibial artery entering the canal.

nal, together with the medial periosteal network, are the most important sources of blood supply to the talus.

Intraossseous Arterial Supply

The Head.—There are two sources of blood supply to the head of the talus. First, branches from the anterior tibial (or dorsalis pedis) artery supply the superior medial half, while the lateral and inferior half of the head is supplied directly from the arteries of the tarsal sling.[52, 63, 97] Inferiorly, the part of the talar neck that forms the anterior boundary of the tarsal sinus is the entry way for the intraosseous circulation to the head of the talus (Fig 35–48). According to Mulfinger and Trueta[97] this vascular pattern to the talar head is relatively constant.

Body of the Talus.—The body of the talus is supplied by vessels that enter through five of the talar surfaces[63]

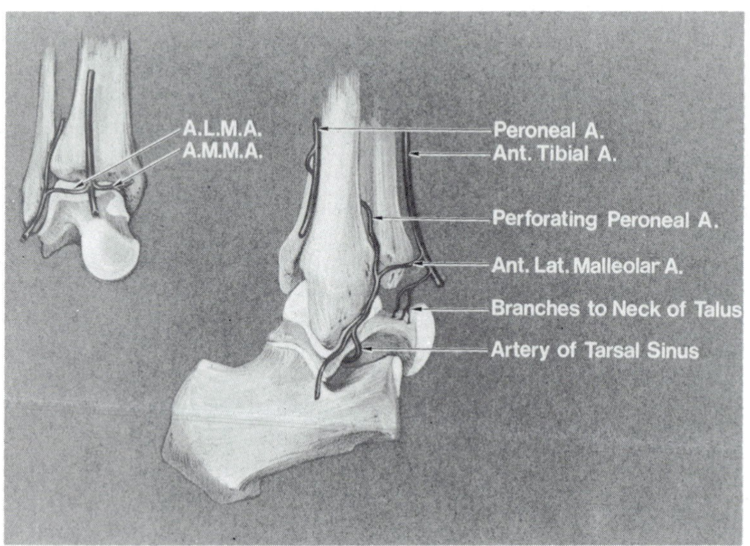

FIG 35–46.
The anterior tibial artery gives rise to the anterolateral malleolar artery *(A.L.M.A.),* which may anastomose with a perforating peroneal artery to form the artery of the tarsal sinus, anteromedial malleolar artery *(A.M.M.A.),* and direct branches to the superior aspect of the neck of the talus.

1. The superior surface of the neck
2. The anterolateral surface of the body
3. The inferior surface of the neck (the roof of the tarsal canal)
4. The medial surface of the body of the talus (deltoid ligament)
5. The posterior tubercle

The main supply of the body of the talus is from the anastomotic artery in the tarsal canal.[52, 67, 73, 114, 137] This artery provides four or five main branches onto the body of the talus that forms arcs curving posterolaterally into the body (Fig 35–48). According to Sarrafian[130] the artery of the tarsal canal and its anastomoses provide all the blood supply to the lateral two

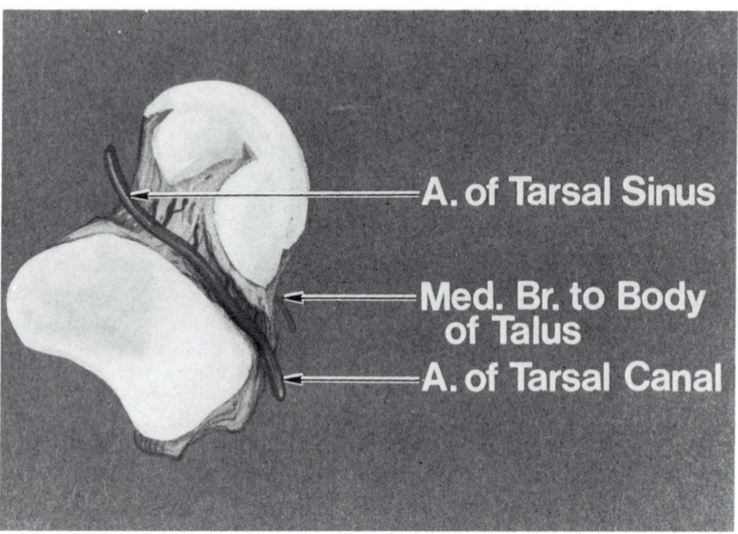

FIG 35–47.
The artery of the tarsal canal, which arises from the posterior tibial artery, anastomoses with the artery of the tarsal sinus, which arises from the dorsalis pedis, lateral malleolar, or perforating branch of the peroneal artery. This anastomotic vessel is known as the artery of the tarsal sling.

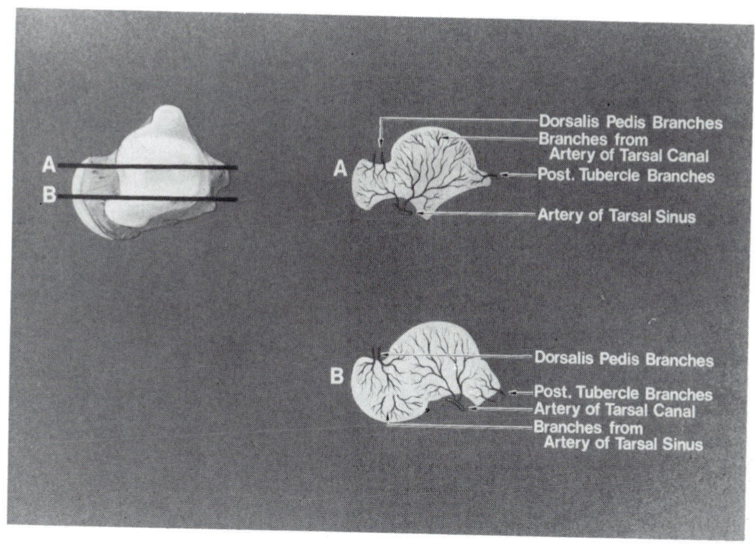

FIG 35–48.
Sagittal sections through the talus in planes *A* and *B*. Note that the body of the talus is supplied mainly by branches from the artery of the tarsal canal and posterior tubercle **(B)**, while the head of the talus is supplied from branches from the dorsalis pedis and tarsal sinus arteries **(A)**.

thirds of the talar body except for a small superior area in the middle third which is supplied by superior neck arteries. The medial third to fourth of the talar body is supplied by deltoid branches entering from the medial surface of the talus (Fig 35–49).

The arteries that enter the superior aspect of the neck usually send one or two branches into the middle of the anterosuperior aspect of the body (see Fig 35–48).

The posterior tubercle area is suppled by small branches from the posterior anastomotic network formed by the peroneal artery and posterior branches from the posterior tibial artery.[97] Peterson and Goldie[114] emphasize that these posterior vessels provide communication between the intraosseus blood supply of the tibia and that the talus via the anastomoses that occur through the posterior capsule of the talotibial joint.

Intraosseous Anastomoses

Anastomoses between the various intraosseous arteries of the talus occur and are responsible for survival of

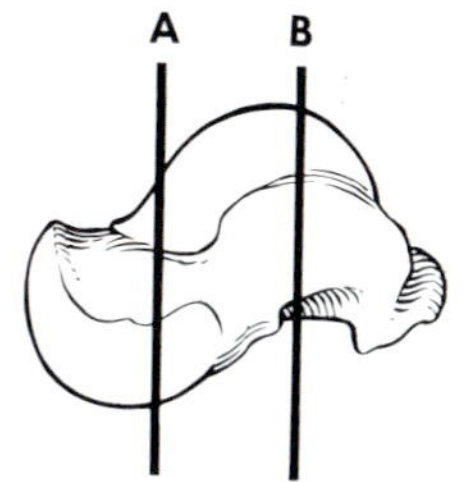

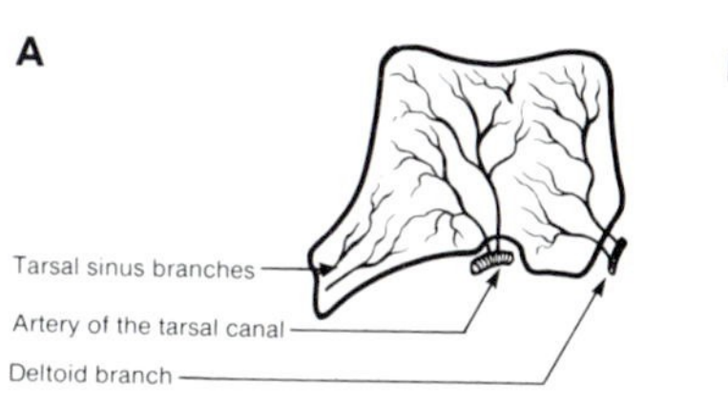

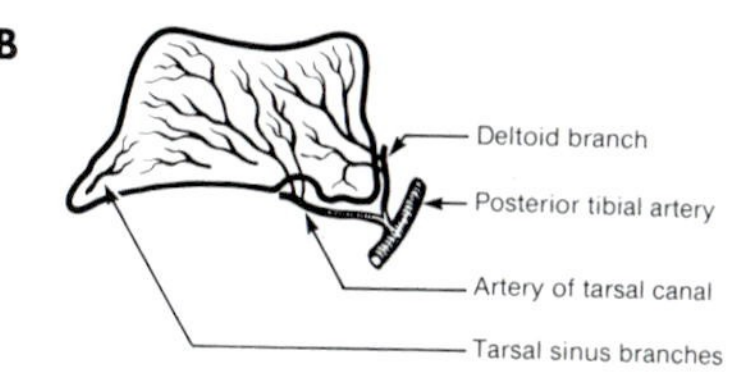

FIG 35–49.
In the coronal plane, the lateral two thirds of the talar body is supplied by branches from the artery of the tarsal canal, and the medial third is supplied by branches entering through the deltoid ligament insertion.

the talus in severe injuries.[52] The lack of these anastomoses in certain areas of the talus helps to explain avascular necrosis involving only a part of the talar body.[34] Mulfinger and Trueta[97] noted definite anastomoses *within* the talus in 18 of 30 specimens. Arteries entering the superior neck anastomoses with branches of the artery of the tarsal canal in 26% of cases, and anastomoses between the inferior and superior vessels of the talar head were noted in 13% of cases.[97] Anastomoses between branches of the artery of the tarsal sinus and the artery of the tarsal canal occurred *within* the talus in 13% while anastomoses between the posterior tubercle branches and branches arising from the artery of the tarsal canal occurred in 3% of specimens. Finally, the deltoid branches medially anastomosed with branches from the artery of the tarsal canal in 3% of patients. Thus, in approximately 60% of patients, there is some intraosseous anastomoses between the various vessels supplying blood to the talus (Figs 35–48 and 35–49). These intraosseous anastomoses may provide for adequate vascularity in some tali that have their major vascular source interrupted.[97]

The variation in contributions of the various vessels of the leg to the extraosseous vascular supply of the talus and the variation noted by Mulfinger and Trueta[97] in the frequency of intraosseous anastomoses are responsible for the variations reported in the incidence of aseptic necrosis following fracture-dislocation of the talus. Peterson and associates[114–116] demonstrated that while *non*displaced fractures of the talar neck disrupt some of the intraosseous branches from the arteries of the tarsal sinus and tarsal canal, the major portion of the vascular supply of the talus remains intact through the deltoid ligament and major branches from the artery of the tarsal sling. With displaced fractures of the talar neck, however, the branches arising through the deltoid ligament, those branches of the dorsalis pedis artery that entered the superior talar neck, and the artery of the tarsal sling can all be potentially disrupted and lead to an increased incidence of avascular necrosis. When one of these three major sources is spared injury, intraosseous anastomoses may permit the talus to survive. These findings underline the concept that loss of blood supply is directly related to fracture displacement.

Skeletal Anatomy

The talus has seven articular surfaces, all of which have a weight-bearing function. Since two thirds of the talar surface is covered with articular cartilage,[67] almost all fractures of this bone are intra-articular and hence, arthritis and disability are frequent complications.[15, 61, 101]

The talus is composed of three parts: the head, neck, and body. Sarrafian[130] defines the body as that part of the talus located posterior to a plane passing through the anterior border of the superior surface of the trochlea tali and the posterior calcaneal surface (Fig 35–50). The neck is that part of the bone anterior to this plane between the body and the head. The body and neck of the talus are not coaxial because in the horizontal plane the neck angles medially with a variable angle of declination.[130]

The Head

The head of the talus forms *articulations* with the navicular, the calcaneus, and the *calcaneonavicular ligament.* The articular surface for the navicular is the largest of these three surfaces. The important anterior calcaneal articular surface of the talar head is quadrilateral or oval in shape and provides articulation with the anterior subtalar facet of the calcaneus. It is flat and continuous anteriorly with the navicular articular surface.[130]

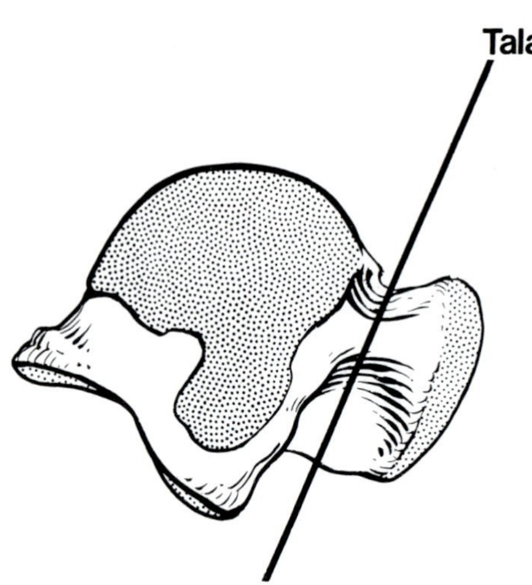

FIG 35–50.
The talar body lies posterior to a plane from the anterior edge of the trochlea tali to the anterior edge of the posterior subtalar facet. The fracture in the body therefore involves the articular surface of the posterior facet of subtalar and ankle joints.

The Neck

The neck of the talus has four surfaces, superior, lateral, medial, and inferior. The superior surface of the neck is limited posteriorly by the anterior border of the trochlea tali and anteriorly by the articular surface of the talar head. The talotibial capsule inserts along this superior surface just proximal to the insertion of the capsule of the talonavicular joint. The lateral surface of the neck provides an insertion of the medial aspect of the inferior extensor retinaculum.[130] The inferior surface of the neck forms the roof of the sinus tarsi and sinus canal (Fig 35–47). The medial surface provides an area for insertion of the talonavicular ligaments.[130]

The Body

The body of the talus is arbitrarily divided into five surfaces: lateral, medial, superior, inferior, and posterior, (Fig 35–51).

The lateral surface of the body of the talus consists of a large articular surface, the facies malleolaris lateralis (Fig 35–51).[130] The lateral talocalcaneal ligament inserts at the apex of the lateral process. Along the anterior border of the trigonal articular surface of the lateral surface are two tubercles for insertion of the anterior talofibular ligament. Along the posteroinferior border of the lateral malleolar surface lies a groove for attachment of the posterior talofibular ligament.

The medial surface presents two areas, superior and inferior (Fig 35–51). The superior portion is occupied by the articular facet, or facies malleolaris medialis.[130] This articular surface is shaped like a comma, with the long axis oriented anterioposteriorly. The inferior portion is nonarticular and consists in its anterior half of a depressed surface perforated by numerous vascular foramina. Under the tail of the superior surface, the posterior half of the inferior surface consists of a large oval area that provides insertion for the deep component of the deltoid ligament.[130]

The superior surface of the body is shaped like a pulley, with the groove of the pulley near the medial border (Fig 35–51,C). The transverse diameter of the superior surface is greater anteriorly than posteriorly.[130]

The inferior surface consists of the facies articularis calcanea posterior tali (Fig 35–51,D).[130] This articular surface is quadrilateral in shape and is concave in the long axis while being flat transversely. It articulates with the posterior facet of the calcaneus.

The posterior surface consists of posterolateral and

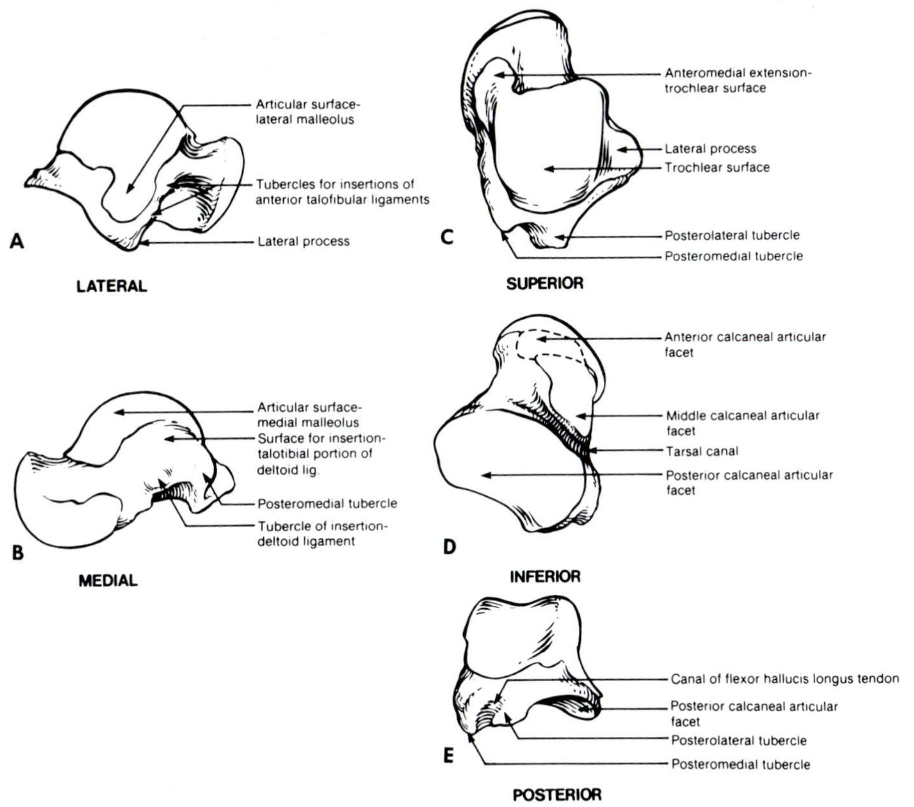

FIG 35–51.
Five surfaces of the talar body. **A,** lateral. **B,** medial. **C,** superior. **D,** inferior. **E,** posterior.

posteromedial tubercles that flank the sulcus for the flexor hallucis longus tendon (Fig 35–51,E).[130] The posterolateral tubercle is larger and more prominent than the posteromedial tubercle. This posterolateral tubercle contributes an inferior articular surface that is in continuity with the posterolateral aspect of the posterior calcaneal surface of the talus. An accessory bone, the os trigonum, may be found in connection with the posterolateral tubercle.[130]

Open Fractures of the Talus

Due to the trauma that results in fractures of the talus, these injuries often present with open wounds.[5, 10, 42, 45, 66, 89, 111] The wounds are often of the bursting type, and the wound margins are often ischemic.[27, 38] In open fractures and fracture-dislocations, antibiotic coverage is begun immediately upon the patient's arrival. An antibiotic providing both gram-positive and gram-negative coverage is recommended.[48, 109] One must consider these antibiotics therapeutic and not prophylactic because such wounds are known to be contaminated at the time of injury.[109] The choice of antibiotic is changed only after cultures taken in the emergency room and the operating room reveal microbial sensitivities that demand such a change. Immunization against tetanus by the use of tetanus toxoid and/or human immune globulin must be considered in light of the patient's history.[48]

Giannestras and Sammarco[48] recommend an attempt to reduce the open fracture-dislocation in the emergency room and the application of a simple sterile dressing. When the patient is taken to the operating room, the wound is completely debrided, including skin edges and all necrotic tissue, and irrigation is performed. Once a complete debridement is performed, these authors recommend a change of instruments to perform the open reduction and internal fixation. Following the open reduction, the skin is left open, and a plaster splint is applied to the leg. At 48 to 72 hours the patient is brought back to the operating room for wound examination and possible closure. These authors emphasize that if the wound cannot be closed at that time, surrounding ligamentous, capsular, and other soft tissues are utilized to cover the joint. The wound is reexamined in another 48 hours. If the wound still cannot be closed, plastic surgery consultation is obtained for skin grafting, a muscle pedicle flap, or a free flap to obtain joint closure.

Author's Preferred Method of Treatment

In open fracture-dislocations of the talus, the basic principles of the management of open fractures must be *strictly* followed.

Cultures are obtained in the emergency room immediately upon arrival. I prefer to not attempt reduction because this may result in further contamination of the ankle and subtalar joints if done before a complete soft-tissue debridement is performed. A sterile dressing is applied to the open wound after povidone-iodine (Betadine) preparation is performed. The patient is taken *immediately* to the operating room for debridement and reduction of the fracture-dislocation. Any delay at this point in treatment will result in significant soft-tissue necrosis due to the persistent dislocation.

I prefer a cephalosporin as the initial antibiotic, which is begun immediately upon arrival in the emergency room after the initial wound culture is taken. This antibiotic therapy is continued until culture and sensitivity reports from the cultures taken in the emergency room or in surgery dictate a change in antibiotic coverage. Antibiotic treatment is continued for 48 to 72 hours, depending upon the degree of initial contamination. The patient's tetanus immunization history is evaluated and tetanus toxoid and/or immune globulin administered as indicated.

The patient is brought to the operating room immediately and undergoes a routine 10-minute surgical preparation. Following draping, the edges of the open wound are debrided and a second set of cultures taken. The area from which the body of the talus has been subluxated or dislocated is thoroughly debrided. Any tissue with a suggestion of necrosis is sharply excised. Following extensive debridement of all tissue of questionable viability, a thorough irrigation is performed. I prefer to use a series of irrigating solutions, including Betadine solution diluted with normal saline, followed by a triple antibiotic solution containing polymyxin, neomycin, and bacitracin, and finally, normal saline. Following debridement and extensive irrigation, a sterile dressing is applied. The limb is then reprepared and redraped and new surgical instrumentation opened.

The particular talar fracture is then dealt with as indicated in the various sections of this chapter. Once reduction and internal fixation have been performed, the wound is left open and the patient placed in a short-leg splint. The patient is returned to the operating room in 48 to 72 hours. At this time the wound over the joint and the talus is closed if it is clean. If there is insufficient soft tissue or skin for closure or if the wound does not appear clean, a second debridement of necrotic tissue is performed, and the wound is again left open. The wound is reexamined 48 hours later, and a decision is made to utilize skin grafting, local muscle pedicle grafting, or a distant free flap to obtain coverage. It is my opinion that coverage of this wound within the first 5 to 7 days is essential (providing that the wound is clean) to prevent the long-term sequelae of talar osteomyelitis.[38]

Fractures of the Head of the Talus

Fractures of the head of the talus are rare injuries, less common than fractures of the neck or body.[15, 27] Coltart[27] reports that 5% and Pennal[111] states that 10% of all fractures and dislocations of the talus involve the talar head. The disability arising from these fractures can be severe.[15] The contusion and fibrillation of the articular cartilage of the talonavicular joint that are associated with these fractures may result in severe arthritis and pain on weight bearing and later require talonavicular fusion.[132]

Fractures of the head of the talus are of two varieties. First are compression fractures of the head of the talus as described by Pennal,[111] Schrock,[132] and Boyd and Knight.[15] These injuries represent simple impaction of the talar head and are often associated with compression fractures of the tarsal scaphoid.[15] The second variety consists of fractures of the talar head in the longitudinal or oblique plane, both of which result in two or more major fragments of the head of the talus.[132]

Mechanism of Injury

Two mechanisms of injury producing talar head fractures have been proposed. According to Pennal,[111] the compression-type fracture results from a longitudinal compression force that acts on the foot when it is in some degree of plantar flexion. Coltart[27] reports that the force of impaction is transmitted along the longitudinal axis of the foot through the metatarsals and navicular to compress the talar head. This force usually produces a fracture in the medial portion of the talar head.[111] Coltart[27] suggests that due to the association of talar head fractures with midtarsal joint dislocations, abduction and adduction may be important in addition to longitudinal compression in producing these injuries.

On the other hand, Garcia and Parkes[45] believe that this injury is due to a fall on the completely extended (dorsiflexed) foot. In this mechanism, the talar head is presumably compressed against the anterior edge of the tibia by the force transmitted from the forepart of the foot to the navicular.[45]

Clinical Diagnosis

These patients give a history of a fall or motor vehicle accident in which the foot is plantar-flexed at the time of impact. They present with complaints of pain over the dorsal aspect of the foot in the region of the talonavicular joint.[42, 45, 48] There is usually point tenderness and swelling located over the head of the talus. If the diagnosis is delayed, ecchymosis may be present.[45, 48] Attempted dorsiflexion and plantar flexion of the midtarsal joint will reproduce the pain.[45, 48] Additionally, inversion and eversion of the hindfoot will produce pain in the talonavicular area.[45] Ankle motion, if performed *without* stress at the midtarsal level, is not painful. Careful palpation of the calcaneocuboid and the subtalar joints for tenderness will detect an associated midtarsal subluxation that has spontaneously reduced, a finding that is important in planning treatment.

Radiographic Diagnosis

Fractures of the head of the talus may be demonstrated on anteroposterior, lateral, and oblique roentgenographs of the foot. Careful evaluation of the outline of the talar head and neck on the *lateral* roentgenograph may be particularly helpful in making the diagnosis and determining displacement.[42] Although fractures of the talar head are often comminuted, they are seldom displaced because the fragments are held in place by the strong intertarsal ligaments of the foot.[45, 48]

If routine roentgenographs do not give a clear indication of fracture location and size, particularly in longitudinal or oblique (nonimpaction type) fractures, polytomography may be useful. It is important to roentgenographically differentiate between a single displaced fracture fragment and a comminuted fracture for treatment purposes. Careful evaluation of the films, particularly for associated injury of the scaphoid and the calcaneocuboid joint, is important.

Treatment

Nondisplaced Fractures.—Dunn et al.[42] recommended that nondisplaced fractures be treated in a short-leg cast allowing partial weight bearing for a minimum of 3 weeks. Boyd and Knight[15] also recommended that compression fractures of the head of the talus be immobilized in a non–weight-bearing cast for 3 to 4 weeks followed by a walking cast until union has occurred. They suggested that if there is a tendency to flattening of the longitudinal arch of the foot, an arch support should be utilized after the walking cast is removed. Giannestras and Sammarco[48] recommended that a Whitman-type steel arch support be fitted in the shoe for a period of 3 months following cast removal in an effort to decrease the stress on the talonavicular joint. Pennal[111] noted that these fractures are usually located in the medial portion of the head and that although there may several fracture lines, significant displacement is not common. He recommended that these nondisplaced fractures be treated by mobilization in a walking cast for 4 to 6 weeks.

Displaced Fractures.—In those cases in which the fracture of the talar head is *displaced* and results in disruption of the talonavicular joint, Pennal suggested fragment excision.[111] According to Schrock,[132] a displaced fragment of the talar head may be excised *only* if more than half of the talar head remains intact.[132] On the other hand, Dunn et al.[42] recommended that displaced fractures of the talar head be treated by open reduction and internal fixation if the fracture fragments are large enough *and* if closed reduction is unsuccessful. Following open reduction they recommended partial weight bearing in a short-leg cast until healing occurs.

Boyd and Knight[15] report that distortion of the talonavicular joint following this injury is significant and may result in traumatic arthritis necessitating midtarsal arthrodesis for pain relief. Schrock[132] also reports that the associated contusion and fibrillation of the articular cartilage may result in traumatic arthritis requiring talonavicular fusion. Garcia and Parkes[45] state that although the prognosis is generally good, chondromalacia of the head of the talus or osteoarthritis of the talonavicular joint may develop and require arthrodesis of this articulation. However, before fusion, they recommend a steroid injection on one or two occasions in an effort to postpone arthrodesis.[45] Although Dunn et al.[42] prefer triple arthrodesis when there is isolated talonavicular arthritis, Garcia and Parkes[45] believe that isolated talonavicular fusion is the most conservative approach. Should this fail, a triple arthrodesis can be performed.

Author's Preferred Method of Treatment

I emphasize the importance of careful palpation to detect occult injury to the calcaneocuboid or subtalar joints. Careful radiographic examination of these areas for associated fractures is essential. If on clinical examination there is tenderness over the calcaneocuboid joint, one must consider that the talar head fracture has been associated with a midtarsal subluxation or dislocation that has spontaneously reduced. Stress roentgenographs are helpful in determining the degree of this subluxation or dislocation. If injury to these joints occurs, treatment is altered as indicated on pages 35-208 to 35-209.

Isolated talar head fractures of the impaction type that are comminuted but nondisplaced are treated in a short-leg non–weight-bearing cast for 3 weeks. This is followed by a weight-bearing cast for an additional 3 to 5 weeks depending upon the degree of comminution. The cast is well molded in the longitudinal arch. Cast immobilization is discontinued when union is present. The toes are left free in the cast to encourage early active range of motion to the metatarsophalangeal joint. After cast immobilization, the shoe is fitted with a firm longitudinal arch support.

For those fractures in which there is a displaced fracture involving the talonavicular joint I prefer open reduction–internal fixation or fragment excision, depending upon the size of the fragments. I prefer not to excise a fragment of the talar head if the remaining head of the talus covers less than half of the articular surface. Open reduction and internal fixation using Kirschner wires or AO small screws for the single large displaced fragment has been successful in my hands. Following open reduction, if fracture fixation is stable, the patient is begun on an early range-of-motion program while still in the hospital. Once motion has been restored to the midtarsal and subtalar joints, a short-leg cast is worn until union occurs. After union, a longitudinal arch support is recommended.

If the fracture fragments are excised, the foot is immobilized in a short-leg walking cast for 3 weeks followed by a rigorous range-of-motion exercise program. Once motion has been restored, a longitudinal arch support is recommended.

For those patients who develop traumatic arthritis of the talonavicular joint following these fractures, I prefer isolated talonavicular arthrodesis. Before this arthrodesis is performed, I inject local anesthetic into the talonavicular joint under fluoroscopic control as a diagnostic test. The patient is then allowed to be up walking about. If the injection produces pain relief, an isolated talonavicular fusion is performed. If the pain persists, sequential injection of the talonavicular, calcaneocuboid, and subtalar joints is performed to see which of these joints is responsible for the pain. Arthrodesis of one, two, or all three of the joints is performed based on the results of injection. Isolated arthrodesis of small joints in the foot have produced good results in my patients when this type of preoperative evaluation has been performed.

If the calcaneocuboid joint has been subluxated but not dislocated, the talar head fracture is managed as above, but weight bearing is delayed for 3 weeks to allow healing of the calcaneocuboid joint capsule. If there has been frank dislocation, consideration is given to percutaneous pinning of the calcaneocuboid joint. Such pins can be inserted under radiographic control, cut off, bent beneath the skin, and removed later. In these patients, weight bearing is delayed for 4 to 6 weeks, at which time the pins are removed.

Fractures of the Neck of the Talus

Fractures and fracture-dislocations of the neck of the talus account for 50% of all major injuries to the talus.[27, 55, 64, 111, 121, 146] The significance of these injuries is due to the frequency and severity of the complications and long-term disability they produce.[112]

Coltart[27] credits Fabricius of Hilden with the first account of an injury to the talus in 1608. Sir Astley Cooper[28, 111] first described the natural history of dislocation of the talus in 1818. Sir James Syme[147] in 1848 reported that of 13 patients admitted to the Royal Infirmary of Edinburgh with compound fracture-dislocation of the talus, only 2 survived. Therefore, he recommended below-the-knee amputation for these injuries, a procedure that still produced a mortality rate of 25% in his era. Stealy[145] in 1909 reviewed the literature to that date and noted a 50% mortality rate following open fracture-dislocation of the talus.

Anderson[2] in 1919, while serving as consultant surgeon to the Royal Flying Corps, collected 18 cases of fracture-dislocation of the talus resulting from airplane crashes and coined the term "aviator's astragalus" for this injury because of its occurrence in "belly landings" of small aircraft.[93] Coltart[27] in 1952, in an excellent and detailed review, described 228 injuries of the talus that he collected from the Royal Air Force.

Hawkins[55] in 1970 suggested a classification of vertical fractures of the neck of the talus. This classification is based on the roentgenographic appearance at the time of injury and divides these fractures into three groups. He noted that vertical fractures of the neck of the talus frequently enter a portion of the body; in these injuries, the fracture line involves the trochlea *and* the articular surface of the posterior facet of the subtalar joint. He included these fractures with fractures that only involved the talar neck in his classification. In my experience, those fractures that involve the body have an increased incidence of degenerative arthritis of both the ankle and the subtalar joint and also an increased incidence of aseptic necrosis. Indeed, Mindel et al.[89] reported that the incidence of satisfactory results in fractures of the talar *neck* with dislocation was 64% as compared with the 29% satisfactory results in fractures of the talar *body* with dislocation. Schrock[132] also reports that the level of fracture in the talus is of significance in predicting viability of the body. Therefore, I have chosen to separate fractures of the talar neck and body in this chapter because of this difference in prognosis.

In group I injuries the vertical fracture in the neck of the talus is undisplaced (Fig 35–52,A). The body of the talus maintains its normal relationship in both the ankle and subtalar joints. In group I injuries, only one of the three main sources of blood supply to the talus is interrupted: those vessels that enter the foramina on the dorsal and lateral aspect of the neck of the talus and progress proximally into the body.

In group II injuries (Fig 35–52,B), the vertical fracture of the neck of the talus is displaced, and the subtalar joint is either subluxated or dislocated. The associated subtalar dislocation may occur medially, secondary to an inversion force, or laterally if secondary to an eversion force. According to Penny and Davis,[112] medial dislocation is more frequent. If the subtalar dislocation is complete, the injuries are frequently open because of the thin subcutaneous layer of tissue at the level of the ankle joint. The relationship of the talus in the ankle joint is normal, and the head of the talus retains its normal relationship with the navicular and the anterior facet of the subtalar joint. In group II injuries, at least two of the three sources of blood supply to the talus are interrupted: first, the blood supply proceeding proximally from the talar neck (as in group I) and, second, that entering vascular foramina located inferiorly in the roof of the sinus tarsi and tarsal canal. The third main source of blood supply, that entering vascular foramina on the medial surface of the talar body, may also be injured.

In group III injuries, the vertical fracture of the neck of the talus is displaced, and the body of the talus is dislocated from *both* the ankle and subtalar joints (Fig 35–52,C). The body of the talus is often extruded posteriorly and medially and is thus located between the posterior surface of the tibia and the Achilles tendon. The head of the talus maintains its normal relationship with the navicular. All three of the main sources of blood supply to the body of the talus are damaged in group III injuries. The foot adopts a position of slight eversion and lateral dislocation.[112] More than half of group III fracture-dislocations are open injuries, and in the closed injuries, the overlying skin and occasionally the neurovascular bundle are in jeopardy.[101] Pantazopoulos et al.[107] presented an unusual group III fracture-dislocation of the talus in which there was a fracture of the neck of the talus with complete dislocation of the body that was difficult to detect. The body was displaced and rotated 180 degrees on its transverse axis so that it was lying upside down in the ankle joint.

Canale and Kelly[19] added a fourth type of dislocation, group IV, in which there is a fracture of the talar neck associated with dislocation of the body from the ankle or subtalar joint *and* dislocation or subluxation of the head of the talus from the talonavicular joint. In this injury, damage to the vascularity of *both* the body (as in group III injuries) and the head and neck fragments is possible (Fig 35–52,D).[76] Boyd and Knight[15] have also reported a fracture of the neck of the talus with dislocation of the head. Pantazopoulos et al.[106] reported a variation of a group IV injury in which there was a dislocation of the head of the talus while the body of the talus remained reduced.

Shelton and Pedowitz[135] believe that the main shortcoming of Hawkins' classification is the failure to emphasize slight subluxation as opposed to frank dislocation of the subtalar and tibiotalar joints. They emphasize the possibility of momentary subluxation or dislocation of these joints that spontaneously become reduced *prior* to radiographic studies. This can only be diagnosed on stress films.[135] Such spontaneously reduced fracture-dislocations may appear to be group I injuries but instead are group II or III injuries with their attendant increased morbidity.

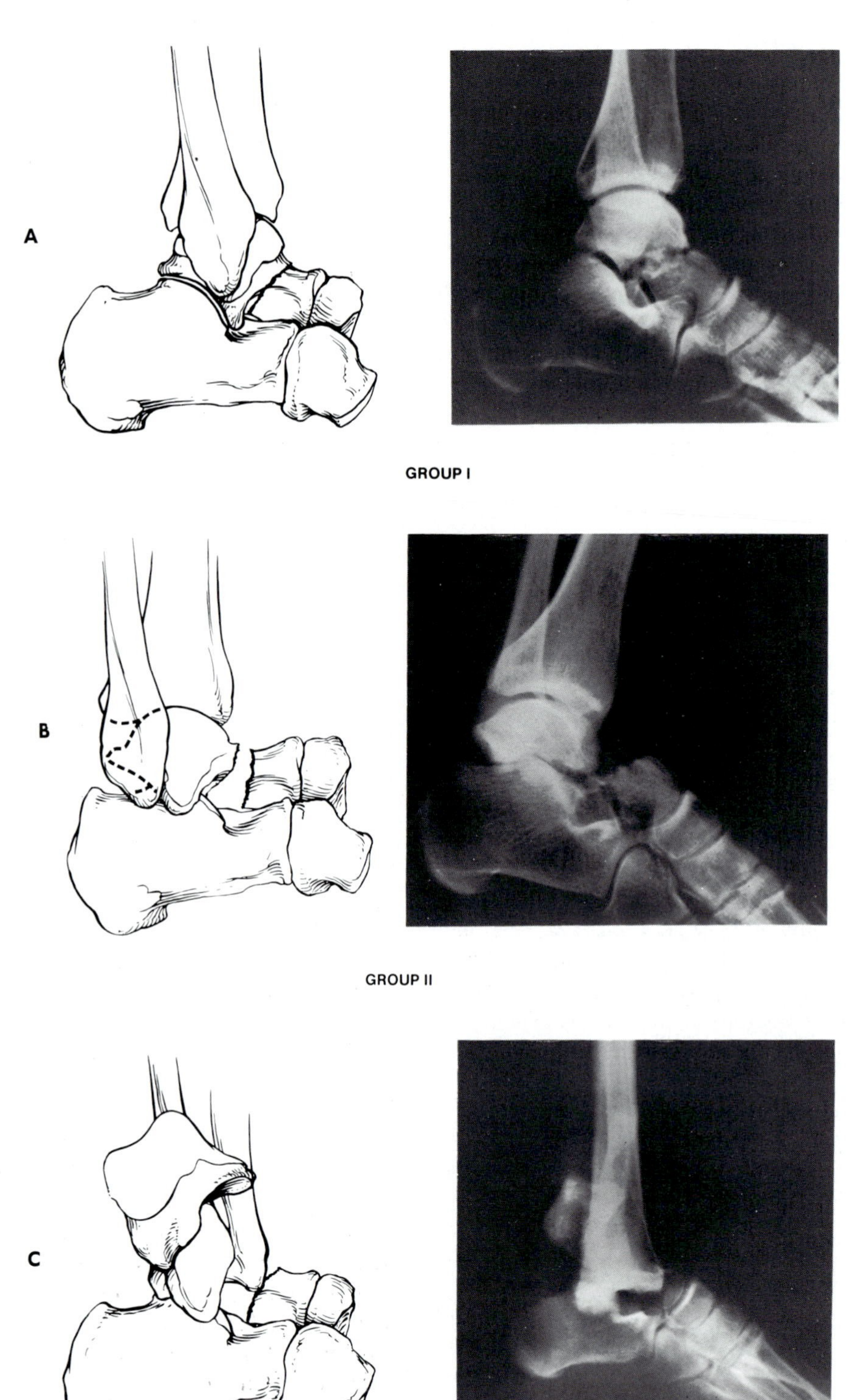

FIG 35–52.
A, group I[54]: nondisplaced fracture of the talar neck. Subtalar joint alignment is anatomic. **B,** group II[54]: displaced fracture of the talar neck with associated subluxation or dislocation of the subtalar joint. **C,** group III[54]: displaced fracture of the neck of the talus with the talar body dislocated from both the subtalar *and* the ankle joints. **D,** group IV[14, 19]: displaced fracture of the talar neck associated with dislocation of the body from the ankle or subtalar joint and with additional dislocation or subluxation of the head of the talus from the talonavicular joint. (From Canale ST, Kelly FB Jr: *J Bone Joint Surg [Am]* 60:143–156, 1978. Used by permission.)

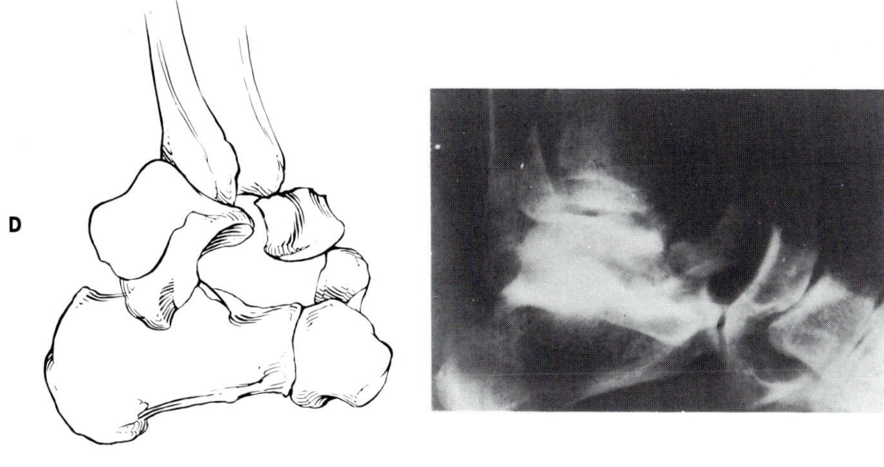

FIG 35–52 (cont.).

This discussion of fractures in the neck of the talus includes coronal fractures through the neck. Sagittal fractures that exit through the talonavicular joint and therefore involve the head of the talus are not included in this section (see page 35-83).

Anatomy

The neck of the talus represents the weakest portion of that bone and is located where the sulcus of the talus reduces the thickness of the bone considerably. The fracture line usually begins dorsally in the talar sulcus and exits inferiorly along the line of insertion of the interosseous talocalcaneal ligament (Fig 35–53). Fractures that occur more posteriorly and involve both the articular surface of the talocrural and posterior facet of the subtalar joint are discussed under fracture-dislocations of the body of the talus (see page 35-103).

Mechanism of Injury

Fractures of the talar neck are most common in motor vehicle accidents, airplane crashes, and falls from heights.* Anderson[2] identified the mechanism as a hyperdorsiflexion force exerted on the sole of the foot by the rudder bar of an aircraft upon impact, hence the

**References 9, 19, 43, 45, 55, 64, 66, 107, 132.*

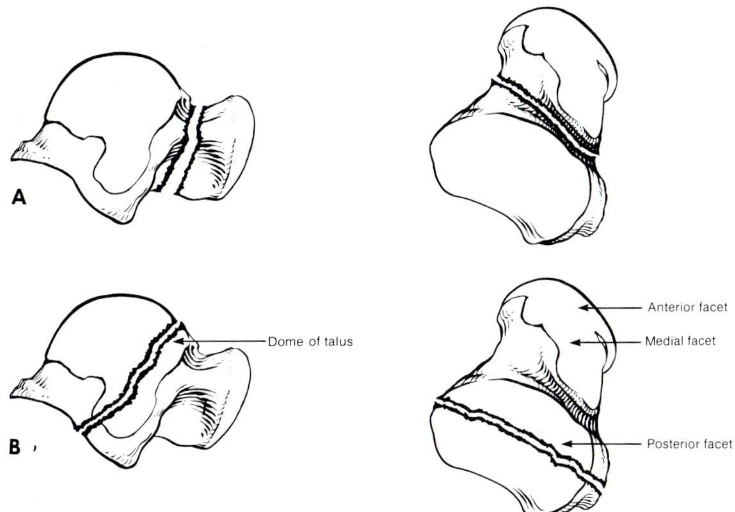

FIG 35–53.
A, this fracture of the talar neck exits inferiorly between the middle and posterior subtalar facets of the talus. **B,** this fracture of the talar body involves both the ankle joint and the articular surface of the posterior subtalar facet.

term "aviator's astragalus." Penny and Davis[112] emphasize that a hyperdorsiflexion injury produced by the clutch or brake pedal of an automobile reproduces this mechanism of the aviator's astragalus. The same mechanism occurs in a fall if the forepart of the foot strikes the rung of a ladder or some other object on the ground.[112] Pennal[111] reports that although the mechanism of a talar neck fracture is usually a force from below, the opposite force whereby a weight falls on the dorsum of the foot can produce a talar neck fracture.

With a dorsiflexion injury, the posterior capsular ligaments of the *subtalar* joint are the first structures to rupture. The neck of the talus then impacts against the anterior edge of the distal end of the tibia, and a fracture line develops through the neck and enters the nonarticular portion of the subtalar joint between the middle and posterior facets.[112] Jensenius[61] likens the anterior margin of the tibia to a wedge that is driven into the dorsal aspect of the neck of the talus (and occasionally into the anterior part of the trochlea) and results in a fracture with an angle opening to the dorsum.[61] If the force ceases at this point, a nondisplaced fracture of the talar neck (group I) occurs. With continuation of the dorsiflexion force, the calcaneus and remainder of the foot, including the head of the talus, subluxate or dislocate anteriorly. At this point, if there is an inversion component to the force, the foot may subluxate or dislocate medially, while a concomitant eversion force results in lateral dislocation of the foot.[112] If the dorsiflexion force subsides at this point, the body of the talus tips into equinus (being dislocated at the subtalar joint), and the fracture surface of the talar neck rides on the upper surface of the os calcis (group II).[111, 112] If the dorsiflexion force continues, however, rupture of the posterior capsular ligaments of the *ankle*, the strong posterior talofibular ligament, and the superficial and posterior portions of the deltoid ligament occurs.[28, 111, 112] The body of the talus is then forced backward out of the ankle mortise, follows the curve of the posterior facet of the os calcis, and rotates so that the undersurface of the talus faces downward and outward, while the neck of the talus points upward and outward.[111, 112] The body of the talus comes to lie in the interval between the posterior aspect of the medial malleolus and the anterior aspect of the tendo Achillis. The posterior tibial neurovascular structures may escape injury by this mechanism since they lie anterior to and are protected by the flexor hallucis longus tendon.[112]

According to Penny and Davis,[112] in group III fractures the talus pivots around the remaining intact fibers of the deltoid ligament. This produces a kinking of the deltoid ligament that may obstruct the only remaining vascular pathway to the body of the talus. According to Pennal,[111] if there is a fracture of the medial malleolus, the attachment of the deltoid ligament to the talus is protected. He stresses the importance of this anatomically as it protects the branch of the posterior tibial artery that passes deep to the deltoid ligament to enter the medial aspect of the talar body.

Schrock believes that the lack of damage to the anterior margin of the tibia and the dorsal cortex of the neck of the talus casts some doubt on the simplistic explanation of dorsiflexion as the mechanism of injury.[132] Also, Shelton and Pedowitz[135] stress that typical fractures of the talar neck are not produced experimentally by simple forced dorsiflexion, but only by eliminating ankle joint motion and fixing the talus as a cantilever between the tibia and calcaneus.[135] Only in this position does a blow to the sole of the foot produce a talar neck fracture.

Other authors suggest that supination may be important in the mechanism of talar neck fracture production.[43, 143] Indeed, Sneppen[142] emphasizes that the position of the foot at the moment of injury is of decisive importance in the frequency of talar fractures and dislocations. He noted that supination predisposed the neck and trochlea of the talus to fractures as well as to subtalar dislocation.[142]

Clinical Diagnosis

Although talar neck fractures have been reported from infancy to old age, most of these injuries occur in young adults,[50, 111, 112] with men outnumbering women 3 to 1.[112]

Associated injuries to the musculoskeletal system are common, being present in 64% of Hawkins' patients.[55] Of particular significance is fracture of the medial malleolus, which was present in 19% of cases reported by Canale and Kelly[19] and in 28% of the patients reported by Lorentzen et al.[79] According to Penny and Davis,[112] a fracture of the medial malleolus usually occurs when there is significant displacement at the talar neck fracture site, particularly if there has been posterior dislocation of the body of the talus. Penny and Davis also emphasize that with any fractured talar neck sustained in a fall from a height, injuries of the lumbar spine must also be suspected.[112]

The history of an injury that reproduces Anderson's "rudder bar mechanism" of the "aviator's astragalus" such as a motor vehicle accident, a motorcycle accident, or a fall from a height is usually present.[14, 48] Occasionally, there may be a history of a weight falling on the dorsum of the foot.[14, 111] Patients present with complaints of severe pain in the foot and ankle.[48] If there is displacement at the fracture site with associated dislocation of the talar body, there is a loss of the normal contour of the ankle.[48] In these instances, the rapid onset of swelling may prevent palpation of the displaced body of the talus in its subcutaneous location.[14] With a delay in presentation, discoloration extending to the knee may be present.[141]

If seen before swelling is marked, the body of the talus can be palpated either anterior or posterior to the ankle. In anterior dislocations, the skin is stretched tightly over the body of the talus.[14] There is less tissue anteriorly than posteriorly, and hence, open anterior dislocations are more common.[14] The distance between the malleoli and heel is shortened so that the foot appears to be increased in length and the ankle appears broader than usual.[14] In posterior dislocations, the body of the talus is palpable in the hollow on the lateral or medial side of the Achilles tendon where it forms a visible swelling.[14] In posterior dislocations, the toes are flexed, and there is pain with contraction of the flexor hallucis longus and flexor digitorum longus. Motion of the foot in any direction produces pain.[45]

Although Penny and Davis[112] report that the posterior tibial neurovascular structures usually escape injury in posterior dislocation, O'Brien[101] and Bonnin[14] warn that there may be pressure on the posterior tibial nerve and/or artery with accompanying pain, paresthesia, and paralysis. Also, in anterior dislocations, Bonnin reports that the dorsalis pedis artery can be disrupted.[14]

If significant dislocation of the talar body is present, the injury may be open. The incidence of open dislocations varies from 16 %[19] to 44%.[14] If the fracture is not open, the skin may be tented over the displaced fragment and be ischemic due to local tension and swelling.[101] Unless prompt reduction of the displaced fragment is performed, skin slough and subsequent infection will intervene.[14, 101] Indeed, Bonnin reports that in 56 irreducible dislocations occurring in earlier days, sloughing of the skin occurred in 41. Reduction of the dislocated bone is thus of extreme urgency.

Radiographic Diagnosis

Routine anteroposterior, lateral, and oblique radiographs are used in fracture evaluation.[17] The anteroposterior and oblique views demonstrate the relationship of the talus within the ankle mortise. The lateral projection of the foot and ankle, however, best demonstrates fractures in the talar neck.[48] The close association of medial malleolar fractures with talar neck fractures emphasizes the importance of searching for these lesions when one or the other is present.

The fracture may be displaced or nondisplaced. The lateral radiograph is carefully evaluated to classify the injury into one of the four groups.[55] Penny and Davis[112] emphasize that if there is *any* degree of displacement of the talar neck fracture, the injury is at least a group II injury because there must be associated subluxation of the subtalar joint (Fig 35–54). O'Brien[101] also cautions that a talar neck fracture with minimal dis-

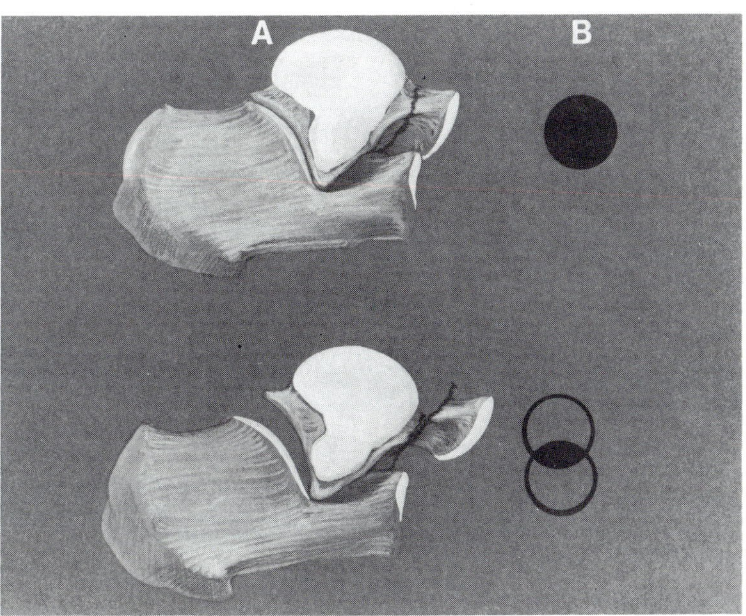

FIG 35–54.
A, in a nondisplaced talar neck fracture, the subtalar joint is congruous. If there is any displacement of the fracture, subtalar joint subluxation is also usually present (unless the talar head-neck fragment is dislocated). **B,** if a talar neck fracture is not reduced, the area for revascularization is greatly reduced. (See the dark area of overlapping circles.)

placement is a pitfall for the unwary because minimal subtalar subluxation may be missed unless it is suspected. He emphasizes the importance of looking for shortening of the heel clinically and of evaluating incongruity between the posterior facets of the talus and calcaneus on the lateral roentgenograph. Additionally, the invariably present plantar flexion of the talar body fragment in *displaced* fractures should be a tip-off that the subtalar joint is either subluxated or dislocated.[101] Failure to detect and treat subtalar subluxation or dislocation results in malreduction of the fracture and the subtalar joint, and this produces incongruity and arthritis.[101]

Canale and Kelly[19] point out that displacement of talar neck fractures can occur in two planes. Dorsal/plantar displacement, which is noted on the lateral roentgenograph, is well recognized. Varus displacement of a talar neck fracture, which is difficult to see on a routine anteroposterior roentgenograph, however, is less commonly appreciated. To evaluate this varus displacement and/or malreduction, Canale and Kelly introduced a modified view of the talar neck taken in the frontal plane. A cassette is placed directly under the foot. The ankle is placed in maximal equinus (this being the usual position following reduction of talar neck fractures). In order to obtain this position, the hip and knee must be maximally flexed. The foot is pronated 15 degrees and the roentgen tube directed cephalad at a 75-degree angle from the horizontal or tabletop (Fig 35–55). This radiograph is essential in determining the degree of initial displacement of a talar neck fracture for purposes of classification. It is also mandatory in evaluating talar neck reduction to prevent varus and/or dorsal malunion.[19]

The importance of postreduction roentgenographs to evaluate the *quality* of the reduction was noted by Dunn et al.,[42] who found that in 21% of displaced fractures, the reduction was rated unsatisfactory *retrospectively*. They believed that this was due to an incomplete x-ray examination following reduction, particularly the failure to obtain an anteroposterior view of the foot, which may be the only view that demonstrates residual angulation at the talar neck. These authors also emphasize the use of tomography to determine postreduction fracture alignment and in follow-up to determine the status of fracture union and the presence of avascular necrosis.

Treatment

The goal of management of fractures of the neck of the talus includes early *anatomic* reduction to (1) avoid incongruity of the ankle and subtalar joints (and hence, secondary osteoarthritis of these joints), (2) reduce the risk of aseptic necrosis after a talar fracture, and (3) help promote revascularization of the injured talus.

The best functional results occur when anatomic reduction is achieved whether by open or closed means.[9, 111] Boyd and Knight[15] emphasize that accurate reduction is essential in order to reestablish the ana-

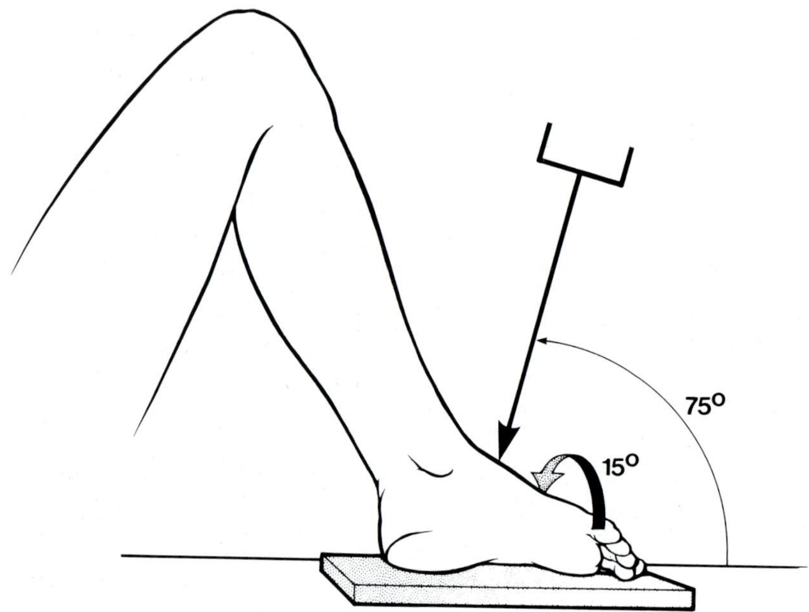

FIG 35–55.
View described by Canale and Kelly[19] to demonstrate talar neck alignment in the anteroposterior plane. The cassette is directly under the foot. The ankle is in maximum equinus with the foot pronated 15 degrees. The roentgen tube is directed at a 75-degree angle from the horizontal or the tabletop.

tomic position of the ankle and subtalar articular surfaces. Miller[88] stresses the accuracy of contact of the bone at the talus fracture, whether accomplished by open or closed means. He believes that bone healing is directly proportional to the accuracy of restoration of bone contact. Additionally, he emphasizes that restoration of circulation is directly proportional to the accuracy of reduction under the assumption that this restoration occurs reasonably close in time to the original injury. Also, anatomic reduction of talar neck fractures increases the surface area across which revascularization of the body can occur (see Fig 35–54,B).

The status of circulation to the entire foot must be evaluated before treatment is initiated.[48] Bonnin[14] and Schrock[132] emphasize prompt treatment of the dislocated talus to minimize damage to the circulation of both the overlying stretched skin and bone. The contused and stretched skin overlying the displaced talar fragment can soon become necrotic, which may lead to bony infection.[132] Also, persistent kinking of the remaining vessels to the displaced talar body, particularly those through the deltoid ligament, may produce thrombosis and an increased risk of aseptic necrosis (Fig 35–56). Treatment of displaced talar neck fractures must therefore be considered urgent.

If the fracture presents as an open injury, the open wound is managed as described in the section on open dislocation of the talus. After the open wound is managed, treatment of the specific type of talar fractures is carried out as outlined below.

Group I Injuries

O'Brien[101] and Penny and Davis[112] emphasize that only fractures in which there is displacement at the talar neck are classified as group I. Any displacement of the talar neck fracture results in subtalar subluxation or dislocation and, hence, a group II injury. O'Brien[101] emphasizes that group I, nondisplaced talar neck fractures are often missed and the patient treated for a simple sprained ankle.

The majority of authors recommend treatment of group I injuries by immobilization in a plaster cast until union is demonstrated radiologically.* Boyd and Knight[15] recommend immobilization in a boot cast for 5 to 6 weeks followed by a walking plaster until the fracture is united. O'Brien[101] and Hawkins[54] suggest a short-leg non–weight-bearing cast with the foot at a right angle until there is *roentgenographic* evidence of fracture union. Dunn et al.[42] also use a short-leg non–walking cast but place the foot in 30 degrees of equinus. When roentgenographic evidence of fracture healing is present, the equinus is slowly reduced. Hawkins[54] suggests that weight bearing prior to fracture union may lead to displacement of a previously nondisplaced fracture and the increased disability attendant with this complication.

**References 15, 27, 64, 83, 87, 88, 106, 156.*

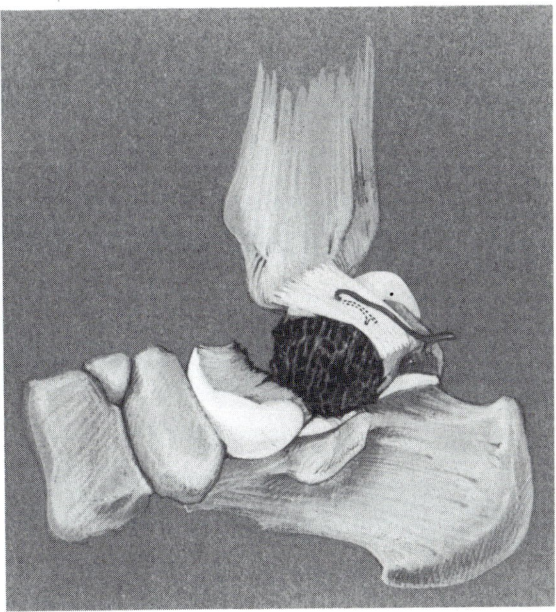

FIG 35–56.
Group III injury. The branch of the posterior tibial artery that enters the body through the deltoid ligament is kinked and may thrombose if reduction is delayed.

Penny and Davis[112] suggest that impacted fractures of the talar neck in *reliable* patients can be treated with early range of motion of the ankle and subtalar joint while keeping the patients non–weight bearing. This is an effort to decrease the subtalar joint stiffness that has been noted following type I fractures. They caution, however, against weight bearing until fracture union has occurred. In an unreliable patient, they suggest non–weight bearing while *hospitalized* until full range of motion of the ankle and subtalar joint is obtained. Then a cast is applied. It must be emphasized that these recommendations pertain to impacted and stable fractures.[112]

Nonunion following closed treatment of type I fractures has not been reported.[135] Although aseptic necrosis has been reported in up to 13% of type I injuries,[19] Shelton and Pedowitz[135] believe that these may indeed represent occult group II lesions that have reduced spontaneously.

Group II Injuries

Group II fractures of the talar neck are characterized by displacement of the talar neck fracture and associated dislocation or subluxation of the subtalar joint. It is important to emphasize that any persistent displacement at the fracture site that results in malunion of the neck of the talus may result in an inadequate reduction of the subtalar joint and, hence, an unacceptable result.[19]

Group II injuries are frequently associated with compromise of the skin about the ankle, and hence, prompt reduction is urgent.[135] Any skin slough that leads to wound infection places the underlying osseous structures at risk for deep infection.[135] Once osteomyelitis is established, it is difficult to eradicate, and the functional result is poor.[64, 66, 104, 111]

Pennal[111] and Giannestras and Sammarco[48] perform a closed reduction by manipulating the foot into full plantar flexion, thereby bringing the distal fragment, the head, in line with the proximal fragment, the body. Reduction of the subtalar joint is obtained by manipulating the heel into either inversion or eversion depending upon whether the subtalar component of the dislocation is medial or lateral. Pennal[111] and Dunn et al.[42] caution against repeated forceful attempts at closed reduction and encourage open reduction in these instances.

If reduction is obtained, Pennal[111] and Pantazopoulos et al.[106] recommend immobilization in plaster in full plantar flexion with slight inversion or eversion. Pennal[111] stresses the importance of good-quality roentgenographs to confirm an exact reduction of *both* the talar neck fracture and subtalar dislocation. Should closed manipulation fail, Pantazopoulos et al.[106] recommend open reduction and prefer a medial approach with fixation of the fracture by using Kirschner wires. Roentgenographs should be repeated at 24 to 48 hours post-reduction to detect early loss of reduction.[48] At 4 to 6 weeks the foot is brought into dorsiflexion from full plantar flexion. Care must be taken at this stage to prevent redisplacement of the neck fracture or the subtalar joint. Following this maneuver, cast immobilization is continued for another 6 weeks. O'Brien[101] suggests reduction by closed means followed by percutaneous pinning in the plantar-flexed position in an effort to maintain the reduction.

Penny and Davis[112] compare group II fractures in which the fracture line enters the subtalar joint in the nonarticular area between the medial and posterior facets, with the T-shaped intracondylar fracture of the distal end of the femur. Any displacement at the fracture site must result in joint incongruity and ultimately degenerative changes in the joint despite the fact that the articular surfaces of the joint remain intact (see Fig 35–54,A). They suggest reduction by manipulating the foot into equinus after the medial or lateral subluxation has been corrected. They report that union requires longer than in group I fractures, usually 10 to 12 weeks. They emphasize the use of the special anteroposterior x-ray view of Canale and Kelly[19] to evaluate reduction of the talar neck. The criteria of an adequate reduction recommended by Canale and Kelly[19] is less than 5 mm of displacement and less than 5 degrees of malalignment. If the closed reduction fails, Penny and Davis[112] utilize an open reduction by an *anterolateral* incision in an effort to avoid further devascularization of the talus. Internal fixation using two AO compression screws or one AO compression screw and a Kirschner wire to prevent rotatory displacement is recommended.

Shelton and Pedowitz[135] also recommend closed reduction. If closed reduction is not satisfactory or is unstable, they recommend open reduction and internal fixation from a medial approach with osteotomy of the medial malleolus. They take particular care to avoid damage to the arterial branches to the talus located in the deltoid ligament. Once an anatomic reduction of the talar neck is obtained, stabilization with interfragmentary compression screws is performed. If there is a defect at the fracture site, they recommend cancellous bone grafting from the distal tibial metaphysis.

Hawkins[54] reports that anatomic closed reduction was obtained in 40% of his group II patients. Even with adequate closed reduction, aseptic necrosis occurred in 40% of these injuries.[54] When closed reduction was not successful, open reduction through an anteromedial arthrotomy provided good visualization of the medial and superior aspects of the talar neck fracture. He suggests drilling two Steinmann pins from the navicular and head of the talus through the fracture site and into the body of the talus to secure fixation and maintain the reduction.

In 1970, Trillat et al.[149] recommended a unique method of treatment that combined closed reduction under fluoroscopic control and fixation with a lag screw inserted from the *posterior* tubercle of the talus to stabilize group II fractures. Lahaut[71] first utilized this posterior approach to insert a tibial graft through the posterior tubercle to stabilize a talar fracture. Lemaire and Bustin[75] recommend this technique in both group II and III fractures. Group II fractures are first reduced by manipulation under fluoroscopic control. Anatomic alignment is obtained and maintained by plantar flexion of the foot. In the group III fractures, open reduction is necessary. Once reduction is obtained, the posterior tubercle of the talus is approached through a posterolateral incision adjacent to the Achilles tendon. A Kirschner wire is introduced under fluoroscopic control from the posterior tubercle, along the longitudinal axis of the talus, and perpendicular to the fracture line.[75] An

AO cancellous screw is then inserted parallel to the Kirschner wire. Despite the fact that good fixation was obtained, the authors did not use early range of motion. Instead, they immobilized the foot and ankle for 4 to 6 weeks following surgery. The advantages of this approach in group II injuries are that (1) it avoids immobilization in the equinus position, (2) it shortens the time to union, and (3) it allows immediate mobilization if stable fracture fixation is achieved.[75] The authors emphasize that fixation achieved by means of Kirschner wires or a screw introduced from the *anterior* fragment into the body of the talus *rarely* achieves firm fixation with compression in the appropriate plane. The authors agree with Trillat et al.[149] that this technique is superior to closed reduction or to open reduction and fixation through an anterior approach for group II injuries. Also, the posterolateral approach may preserve some of the blood supply to the body of the talus that enters anteromedially. However, the method does not prevent osteonecrosis.[75]

Group III Injuries

Closed Group III Injuries.—In Hawkins' group III fractures, the talar body is displaced from both the ankle and subtalar joints. The talar body usually rests posteriorly and medially and rotates around the deep fibers of the deltoid ligament.[54] The blood supply to the body of the talus is completely disrupted with the possible exception of that through the deltoid ligament.[54] The Committee on Trauma of the American Orthopaedic Foot Society in 1983 recommended early *anatomic* reduction to decompress the remaining deltoid ligament vessels, to allow the maximum surface area for revascularization across the talar neck fracture, and to ensure an anatomic reduction of the subtalar joint.[34] Although McKeever[83, 84] and Boyd and Knight[15] suggest that early subtalar fusion in these patients with a denuded talus may hasten revascularization of the talus, this has not been shown to accelerate revascularization.[54]

Nearly 50% of the injuries are open[101]; however, if the injury is not open, the displaced body usually puts extreme tension on the overlying skin, which can result in necrosis unless prompt reduction is instituted.

Although closed reduction is recommended by most authors, it is usually not successful.[42, 101, 111, 135] Pennal[111] and Shelton and Pedowitz[135] recommend *immediate* closed reduction unless there is an open wound that demands debridement. This reduction is performed under general or spinal anesthesia because muscle relaxation is essential. A large Kirschner wire or Steinmann pin is inserted transversely through the calcaneus. The calcaneus is plantar-flexed and everted and the joint distracted by using this pin as a handle. Pressure is then applied from behind the body of the talus to force it forward into the mortise. Coltart[27] reports that Armstrong used a Steinmann pin inserted into the talar body to control the body while manipulating it into the mortise of the ankle joint. The subtalar dislocation, which is usually medial, is then reduced by applying traction to the forefoot and lateral pressure on the calcaneus with the ankle in equinus. A long-leg, bent-knee cast is applied with the foot in eversion and equinus. Routine postreduction roentgenographs are carefully reviewed to detect a varus angulation of the talar neck fracture that will lead to delayed union or malunion. If this occurs, immediate open reduction is recommended.

If closed reduction fails, Shelton and Pedowitz recommend open reduction through a medial approach sparing the deltoid ligament.[135] The talar neck fracture is anatomically reduced and fixed internally with an interfragmentary compression screw. A short-leg non–weight-bearing cast in the neutral position is recommended for 3 months, or until fracture union is present radiographically. Weight bearing is delayed until fracture healing is complete, usually in 12 weeks.

Pennal,[111] Penny and Davis,[112] and Giannestras and Sammarco[48] recommend a posteromedial approach for open reduction. They cite the following advantages for the posteromedial approach: (1) it is centered directly over the fractured body, which allows direct visualization of the neurovascular structures, and (2) it is easily extended to allow osteotomy of the medial malleolus, which protects the medial talar vascular supply.[112] Lemaire and Bustin[75] also recommend the posteromedial approach because it allows fixation of an associated malleolar fracture and also permits insertion of a screw from posterior to anterior for fixation of the talar neck fracture.

Deyerle and Burkhardt[39] emphasize the importance of osteotomy of the medial malleolus for better exposure in type III injuries. They believe that this technique completely protects the remnants of the deltoid ligament and its associated vascular supply to the talus. When this method is used for early anatomic reduction, they report aseptic necrosis in only 10% of group III injuries. Indeed, Hawkins[54] notes that revascularization of the necrotic talus begins medially and progresses laterally, which suggests that vessels persist in the deltoid ligament that supply the talar body. Dunn et al.[42] recommend a lateral approach to avoid further damage to these important medial arteries to the talar body.

Open Group III Injuries.—*Open* group III injuries present a particular challenge to the orthopaedist because the decision of whether or not to retain the contaminated body of the talus must be made. Removal of the talar body, particularly when it is open and devoid of soft-tissue attachment, has been suggested by some authors.[14, 49] Gibson and Inkster[49] reported that although partial talectomy was unsatisfactory, complete talectomy may indeed produce a satisfactory result. However, Miller and Baker[87] and Boyd and Knight[15] caution against talectomy because of poor results due to shortening, pain with weight bearing, instability, and lack of endurance. They suggest that if talectomy is necessary, it should be considered temporary and that tibiocalcaneal fusion should be performed later. Bohler[12] and Coltart[27] recommend that the talar body not be discarded because its removal causes severe and lasting disability. Winkler[156] also recommends against talectomy because an ankle without a talus is invariably painful and disabled and such patients are frequently incapable of any type of weight bearing.

Penny and Davis[112] believe that the best solution in a working man is to discard the body of the talus, wait for primary wound healing, and then proceed with an early Blair[10] fusion. In those patients in whom it is preferable to retain the body of the talus, they prefer primary rigid internal fixation with an AO cancellous screw. This allows easier management of associated soft-tissue injury without the problems associated with casting.

Percy[113] recommends that a completely dislocated talar body be cleansed and replaced because the bony stock it provides may be needed later for reconstruction. Indeed, Sneed[141] reported a case in which the talus was completely dislocated and replaced and revascularization proceeded with a good functional result. O'Brien et al.[101, 102] emphasize that in an open dislocation, the talus should not be discarded unless infection *or* late presentation prevent its salvage. In these instances, the talus is removed and tibiocalcaneal fusion performed at a later date.

Although it provides stability, tibiotalar fusion is difficult to achieve, results in some loss of heel height with difficulty fitting shoes, and allows no tibiopedal motion.[10, 15, 36, 93] As a result, Blair introduced a modified tibiotalar fusion for these injuries. In patients with fractures of the neck or body, neither the head nor the distal part of the neck of the talus are involved; therefore, the anterior and middle calcaneal articular facets of the talus remain intact. In a Blair fusion a sliding bone graft anteriorly from the tibia is inserted into the remaining neck of the talus (see Fig 35–60). This does not shorten the limb, and it maintains some subtalar motion through the retained anterior and medial subtalar facets; thus, late progressive deformity does not occur. Morris et al.[94] and Dennis and Tullos[36] have reported excellent results with the Blair modified tibiotalar arthrodesis. Poor results were noted only if a pseudarthrosis developed.[36] In an open injury, initial wound debridement and secondary closure are performed, with the Blair fusion performed later when the wounds are healed. A more complete discussion of the Blair fusion can be found in the section on complications.

Group IV Injuries

Group IV fractures in which there is a fracture of the talar neck and subluxation or dislocation of the talar body and a dislocation of the head of the talus have rarely been reported in the literature.[14, 19, 107] Shelton and Pedowitz[135] advise anatomic reduction and temporary fixation of the talonavicular joint. Boyd and Knight[15] and Canale and Kelly,[19] report that open reduction, with or without internal fixation, is necessary in the management of these injuries. In this group of patients aseptic necrosis of both the talar body and head fragments is possible.[76]

Prognosis and Complications

The prognosis in fractures of the neck of the talus is directly related to Hawkins' classification of the fractures. Lorentzen et al.[79] report that 46% of their group I patients had complications including aseptic necrosis, osteoarthritis, and painful subtalar joints. Despite union without aseptic necrosis, Penny and Davis note that 50% of patients with group I fractures have unsatisfactory results.[112] Group II injuries have an even less favorable prognosis. Penny and Davis[112] report aseptic necrosis in 20% and Hawkins in 42% of patients with group II injuries. Although union occurred in all fractures, persistent subtalar joint symptoms in spite of an anatomic reduction were noted. Also, delayed union occurs in up to 15% of group II fractures.[115] In group III fractures aseptic necrosis varies between 90% and 100%[54, 112] and nonunion occurs in 10% of patients.[54, 112] Group IV injuries have been too infrequently reported to give an accurate accounting of the prognosis.

The complications most frequently noted following fractures of the neck of the talus include (1) skin necrosis, (2) osteomyelitis, (3) delayed union or nonunion, (4) malunion, (5) traumatic arthritis, and (6) avascular necrosis of the talus. Although rarely mentioned, Dunn et al.[42] report that injury to the posterior tibial nerve and artery can occur particularly if the body is dislocated. According to McKeever,[84] the treatment of these complications is primarily prophylactic and depends upon prompt and accurate reduction at the time of initial treatment. He emphasizes that once the complications occur, any treatment must be considered salvage.

Early Complications

Skin Necrosis.—The lack of excess subcutaneous tissue and skin over the dorsum of the foot predisposes the skin in this area to pressure necrosis from underlying displaced talar fractures.[84] Indeed, Gillquist et al.[50] report that postoperative skin necrosis occurs in the majority of patients. Although skin necrosis was common in their series, Gillquist et al.[50] did not find a relationship between soft-tissue loss, infection, and the functional end results. They did note, however, that osteomyelitis changes the prognosis substantially.

If skin necrosis occurs, McKeever[84] recommends excision of the gangrenous skin and closure of the area of skin loss with a flap of skin and subcutaneous tissues. Garcia and Parkes[45] and Giannestras and Sammarco[48] have also emphasized the importance of early debridement and coverage of the necrotic skin areas in an attempt to prevent any superficial infection from contaminating the joint and the talar body. Septic arthritis or talar osteomyelitis, which may complicate skin necrosis, are catastrophic.[48]

Osteomyelitis.—If the fractured talus is contaminated and osteomyelitis develops, it is very recalcitrant to treatment.[84] According to Dunn et al.,[42] McKeever,[84] and O'Brien,[101] established osteomyelitis of the talus can only be eliminated by excision of the talus. Due to the disability after talar excision, tibiocalcaneal or Blair fusion is indicated later.[10, 15, 19, 27, 42, 156] Gillquist et al.[50] report uniformly poor results if infection occurs after these injuries. For these reasons, most authors recommend thorough debridement, delayed closure, and prophylactic antibiotic coverage to prevent this sequela.

Late Complications

Delayed Union and Nonunion.—Although delayed union is not uncommon[79] definite nonunion is unusual after talar neck fractures. The severity of disruption of the talar blood supply, particularly in group II and III injuries, the lack of thick periosteum on the talar neck, and the small fracture area available for repair (see Fig 35–46) are responsible for delayed union in these fractures. If weight bearing is not restricted until union is evident roentgenographically, the nonunion rate will be unacceptably high. Peterson et al.[114] believe that delayed union is present when no healing is radiographically evident within 6 months. They found this present in slightly over 10% of their patients, none of whom went on to develop a nonunion. Miller[88] reports no cases of nonunion in his patients. Mindel et al.[89] noted delayed union in over 10% of their cases and report that it is associated with an increased incidence of poor results.

Lorentzen et al.[79] noted nonunion in fewer than 5% of fractures, but report that all were symptomatic. Avascular necrosis was a contributory factor in only one case.

Hawkins[55] reports nonunions only in group III fractures and found that all had associated aseptic necrosis. Direct bone grafting of an established nonunion can be considered if union is not present 12 months postfracture.[19, 68] Talectomy as a salvage procedure for nonunion is suggested only if there is a lack of talar neck bone stock.

Malunion.—Malunion results from accepting a poor reduction or from the loss of an acceptable reduction. Persistent displacement at a talar neck fracture is likely to result in incongruity and degenerative arthritis in the ankle, subtalar, and/or midtarsal joints (see Fig 35–54). McKeever[83, 84] warns against loss of reduction during the first few weeks of cast immobilization as swelling subsides and the foot becomes less secure in the cast. To prevent displacement and malunion, he stresses the importance of open reduction or closed manipulative reduction secured by internal fixation.

Canale and Kelly[19] have stressed the frequency of malunion following talar neck fractures. They note that malunions can occur in the dorsal or varus position.[19] A dorsal malunion (one in the lateral plane) results in pain and restricted dorsiflexion of the ankle (Fig 35–57). Dunn et al.[42] mention a dorsal exostosis of the talar neck as a complication of these fractures. They are not certain whether this is secondary to injury to the anterior capsule of the ankle, to callus formation at the fracture site, or to malunion. They mention that removal of the exostosis has restored dorsiflexion in some cases.

Varus malunion of the talar neck produces varus positioning of the forefoot.[19] This causes excessive weight bearing on the lateral side of the foot, with plantar callus formation and pain. Also, almost half of the patients reported by Canale and Kelly[19] with varus malunion developed degenerative arthritis of the subtalar joint that required surgical treatment.

Traumatic Arthritis of the Subtalar and Talocrural Joints.—Fractures of the neck of the talus, even when not complicated by aseptic necrosis, are associated with subtalar arthrofibrosis and arthritis secondary to the original injury and the immobilization necessary until union occurs.[34, 84]

Lorentzen et al.[79] stress that the most important complication following fractures of the neck of the talus is not aseptic necrosis, but osteoarthrosis, particularly of the subtalar joint. One-third of their patients with talar neck fractures developed talotibial osteoarthritis, and over half developed subtalar osteoarthritis. Addition-

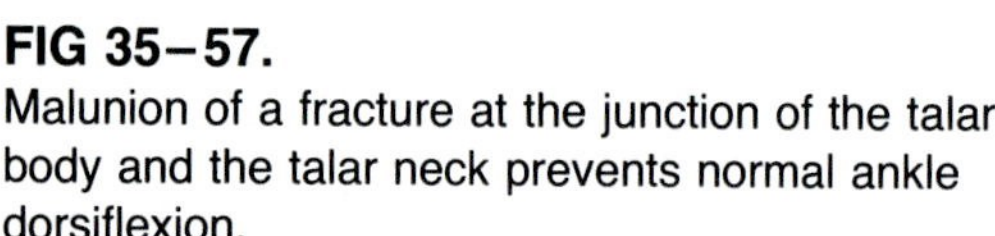

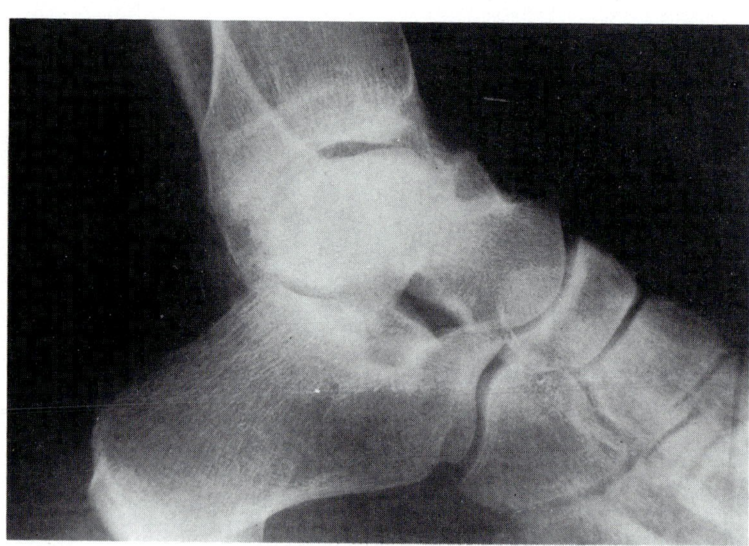

FIG 35–57.
Malunion of a fracture at the junction of the talar body and the talar neck prevents normal ankle dorsiflexion.

ally, 24% of their patients had *both* talotibial and subtalar osteoarthrosis. While the incidence of talotibial osteoarthritis increased from group I to III, the incidence of subtalar osteoarthritis was essentially the same in the two groups.

Dunn et al.[42] report that restricted ankle and subtalar motion was responsible for poor results in over half of their patients. They believe that restricted ankle dorsiflexion is due to prolonged immobilization in equinus and recommend that that position be avoided. They believe that the loss of subtalar motion is secondary to the damage to the articular surfaces at the time of the subtalar dislocation in type II and III injuries.

Canale and Kelly[19] used decreased range of motion in the involved joint along with roentgenographic evidence of arthritic changes as the definition for traumatic arthritis. With this definition, almost half of their talar neck fractures had traumatic arthritis in the subtalar joint. Importantly, one third of the patients who developed subtalar arthritis had malunion of their fractures. In the remainder, the etiology of the arthritis was believed to be the amount of initial disruption of the subtalar joint or possibly aseptic necrosis of the inferior aspect of the body.[19]

Lemaire and Bustin[75] also note a loss of subtalar motion and osteophyte formation in both the tibiotalar and subtalar joints even following anatomic reduction and stable internal fixation of group II and III fractures. However, these patients were not managed with early motion. McKeever[84] suggests the arthrofibrosis can be minimized by promoting venous drainage with elevation of the foot and by beginning early range of motion of the foot. This has been found effective by DeLee and Curtis[35] in restoring motion following subtalar dislocations.

Even though established subtalar arthrosis can be alleviated by subtalar or triple arthrodesis, McKeever[84] stresses that particularly in patients over the age of 40 years, the end results are not predictable. In addition, Canale and Kelly[19] caution against subtalar or triple arthrodesis in patients with subtalar arthritis following talar neck fractures due to the associated damage to the ankle joint. Since a moderate degree of stiffness in the subtalar joint can be tolerated, patients with stiffness and no degenerative changes should be treated with a rigid shoe before resorting to subtalar arthrodesis.[84]

Avascular Necrosis.—Lemaire and Bustin[75] emphasize that most if not all talar neck fractures are followed by a period of ischemia of the talar body and to some extent by necrosis of bone. The fate of the talar body after fracture of the neck is unpredictable in any given patient and is influenced by individual variations in blood supply of the talus, particularly the intraosseous anastomoses between the different vascular channels.[34] It is dependent upon the extent of damage, not only to the main blood supply in the tarsal canal but also to the periosteal network.[73] Peterson and Goldie[114] documented experimentally that with increasing degrees of displacement, the incidence of aseptic necrosis rises.

The Trauma Committee of the American Orthopaedic Foot Society[34] reported that total-body aseptic necrosis was certain only if the body were extruded and had no soft-tissue attachments or if there were a prolonged delay before treatment. They distinguished between aseptic necrosis involving the entire body and that involving only a part of the body of the talus. They noted that the medial aspect of the talus (near the blood supply through the deltoid ligament) was occasionally spared of these necrotic changes. They proposed that whether partial- or total-body aseptic necrosis developed was dependent upon individual variations in talar vascular supply.[34] Although actual disruption of the vessels supplying blood to the talus is generally believed to be the cause of aseptic necrosis following fractures of the talar neck, Cobey[25] reported a case of aseptic necrosis caused by concussion of the bone without dislocation of the surrounding joints.

Bobechko and Harris[11] correlated the radiographic and microscopic findings in aseptic necrosis. Microscopically, there appear to be two stages. First, there is rapid encapsulation of the necrotic bone by new bone, and second, slow resorption of the necrotic bone occurs. Indeed, the second stage may never be completed. Penny and Davis[112] report that a talus that appears dense, homogeneous, and sclerotic takes a long time, often in excess of 2 years, to revascularize completely. According to these authors, collapse of the dome of the talus rarely occurs during this sclerotic phase. They note that since revascularization of the sclerotic talus is slow and requires up to 2 to 3 years in the adult, collapse is unlikely to occur. On the other hand, if revascularization is rapid and occurs in a patchy distribution, gross collapse of the dome of the talus is more likely.[112] When late segmental collapse occurs, it is due to a fracture along the interface of the avascular trabeculae and the invading vascular granulation tissue.

Lorentzen et al.[79] emphasize the importance of distinguishing aseptic necrosis and late segmental collapse because in patients in whom no collapse occurs, the results are better. DeLee[34] also stresses the importance of distinguishing late segmental collapse and aseptic necrosis. It is late segmental collapse, secondary to aseptic necrosis, that leads to joint incongruity and pain.[34]

Aseptic necrosis has been reported to occur after 50% of all talar neck fractures.[19, 42] In group I injuries, aseptic necrosis rarely occurs because only one source of talar blood supply is injured. The incidence in group I varies from 0% to 13%.[19, 93] Indeed, Shelton and Pedowitz believe that if aseptic necrosis occurs in this group, the patient may have had a subluxated subtalar joint (i.e., an occult group II injury) that was missed. In group II fractures the incidence varies from 20% to 50%,[15, 55, 64, 89, 93] while in type III fractures, an incidence of from 80% to 100%* has been reported.

Deyerle and Burkhardt[39] report that the incidence of aseptic necrosis is decreased to 10% in group II and III fractures if open reduction utilizing medial malleolar osteotomy is elected to protect the remaining talar blood supply in the deltoid ligament. In addition, Miller[88] emphasizes the importance of an early, accurate reduction to ensure good contact at the fracture surfaces of the talar neck so that bone healing will occur and permit restoration of circulation to the talar body across the healed fracture. With stable internal fixation, rapid revascularization across the fracture site coupled with any remaining revascularity via the deltoid ligament may forestall the development of aseptic necrosis.[34] With inadequate internal fixation, motion at the fracture site will result in shearing of the granulation tissue buds as they attempt to cross the fracture site, thereby delaying revascularization.[34] Peterson et al.[115] documented that aseptic necrosis was less frequent in fractures that were internally fixed, thus suggesting that stabilization allows more rapid revascularization.

The Trauma Committee of the American Orthopaedic Foot Society[34] reports that late segmental collapse involving the ankle and/or subtalar joint occurs in one of three patients with total-body aseptic necrosis and is unusual in patients in whom only a portion of the body appears to be necrotic roentgenographically. It is important to emphasize that aseptic necrosis is only one of several complications that occur following a talar neck fracture. Indeed, Monkman et al.[92] noted that while aseptic necrosis with late segmental collapse is a poor prognostic sign, it is not incompatible with a reasonable functional result, and Dunn et al.[42] report that the development of necrosis does not guarantee a poor result. In fact, in over half of their cases of aseptic necrosis the end result was satisfactory.

Gillquist et al.[50] reported that aseptic necrosis did not influence to any significant degree the end result in their patients. They noted that even patients with minor late segmental collapse were free of pain and walked without a limp. Hawkins[54] too found that collapse of the dome was well tolerated in most patients and that it occurred in spite of prolonged non–weight bearing. Peterson et al.[115] noted that collapse of the talar dome, particularly if it occurred late in the disease, did not have much effect on the clinical result. In addition, both Hawkins[54] and Canale and Kelly[19] report that although aseptic necrosis is important in contributing to the poor result, only rarely do patients require reconstructive surgery for aseptic necrosis.

Finally, although the presence of aseptic necrosis may delay healing of a talar neck fracture,[54, 89, 112] both Pantazopoulos et al.[106] and Mindel et al.[89] noted that aseptic necrosis did not prevent union in their patients.

Detection of Aseptic Necrosis.—Classically, aseptic necrosis has been identified roentgenographically by an increase in bone density of the affected part. Bobechko

---

**References 15, 27, 54, 64, 66, 83, 84, 89, 93, 111, 112.*

and Harris[11] report that this increased density is in fact a sign of reossification and is secondary to three factors: (1) viable bone being laid down on necrotic bone with a resultant absolute increase in density; (2) osteoporosis from disuse of neighboring bone, which produces a relative increase in density; and (3) calcification of the necrotic bone marrow, which also produces an increase in density. This increase in density may not be noted for 3 months or more postinjury.

In 1970 Hawkins reported that the presence of subchondral atrophy in the dome of the talus on the anteroposterior view, particularly when a similar finding is present in the distal end of the tibia, excludes the possibility of aseptic necrosis. This has been termed "Hawkins' sign" and is usually visible 6 to 8 weeks postinjury. If instead of subchondral atrophy, the dome of the talus is sclerotic in relationship to the rounding structures, the body is assumed to be avascular (Fig 35–58). Hawkins stresses that although the same sign may be seen on the lateral view it is more difficult to see because of the overlying malleoli and, hence, is less reliable.[55] Peterson et al.[115] also note that a line of subchondral atrophy noted 6 to 8 weeks postinjury is a good indicator that vascularity remains in the talus. They emphasize that

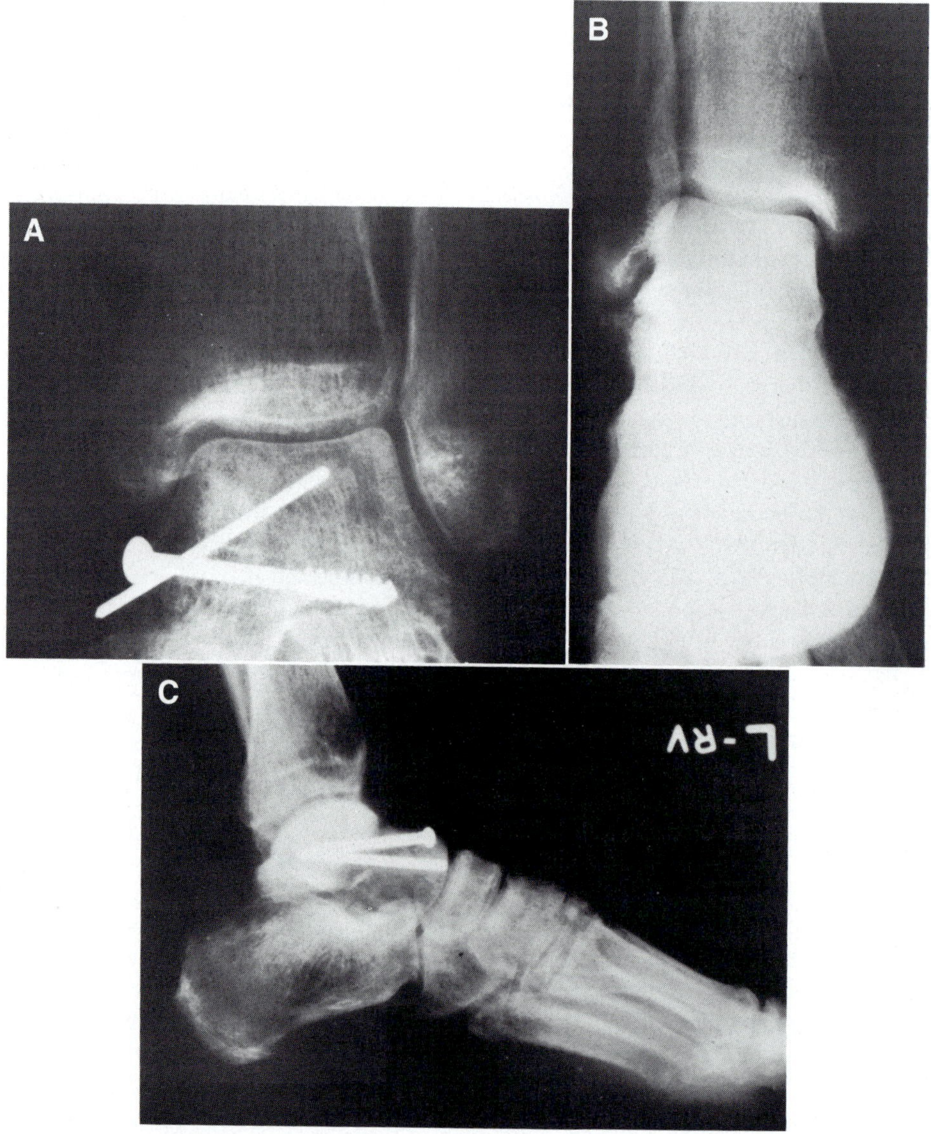

FIG 35–58.
A, subchondral atrophy 6 weeks after fracture suggesting vascularity of the talus is noted on this radiograph. **B,** sclerotic subchondral bone of the talus 6 weeks after injury suggests avascularity. **C,** lateral view demonstrating sclerotic bone with surrounding atrophy, again suggesting avascularity.

radiographs must be taken with the foot out of plaster to better detect the subchondral atrophy.

Canale and Kelly[19] found that the presence of a radiolucency in the subchondral area indicates that the body of the talus has not undergone aseptic necrosis. However, the absence of this radiolucency in their series was *not* a totally reliable indicator that aseptic necrosis was inevitable.

The value of Hawkins' sign is in its early detection of avascularity, which permits institution of treatment early in the course of the disease process. Recently, bone scanning with a pinhole collimator[19, 112] has been used in the early detection of aseptic necrosis. The exact place of bone scanning techniques in the detection of aseptic necrosis of the talus is at present unclear.

Treatment of Aseptic Necrosis.—The treatment of aseptic necrosis is controversial. Hawkins,[54] O'Brien et al.,[101, 102] Miller,[88] and Pantazopoulos et al.[106] recommend that weight bearing be delayed until there is solid union at the fracture site to prevent resorption, nonunion, and deformity.[54] Once union is established, even in the presence of aseptic necrosis, weight bearing is permitted. Because revascularization of the talus can take up to 36 months in the adult[83, 84, 101, 102] and because prolonged non–weight bearing may not prevent collapse,[101, 102] non–weight bearing is not a logical mode of treatment of aseptic necrosis in an adult. Hawkins notes that even collapse of the dome of the talus was well tolerated in most patients and occurred in some patients in spite of enforced non–weight bearing for several years.

On the other hand, in about half of their patients with aseptic necrosis who began early weight bearing, Mindel et al.[89] noted late segmental collapse of the talar body. They therefore recommended protection from weight bearing until the necrotic bone had been replaced. Pennal[111] believes that during the healing process of aseptic necrosis, the foot must be protected from full weight bearing.

Canale and Kelly[19] also reported that patients with aseptic necrosis who are kept non–weight bearing have a higher percentage of satisfactory results than do those patients in whom early weight bearing is allowed. Partial weight bearing in a patellar tendon–bearing brace (Fig 35–59) offers a suitable alternative to non–weight bearing and appears to be superior to unrestricted weight bearing.[19, 31, 39] Indeed, Davis et al.[31] documented a decrease in weight transmitted across the ankle joint when this brace was worn.

According to McKeever, Phemister demonstrated that by denuding the articular cartilage of the avascular talus, more rapid revascularization occurs because the

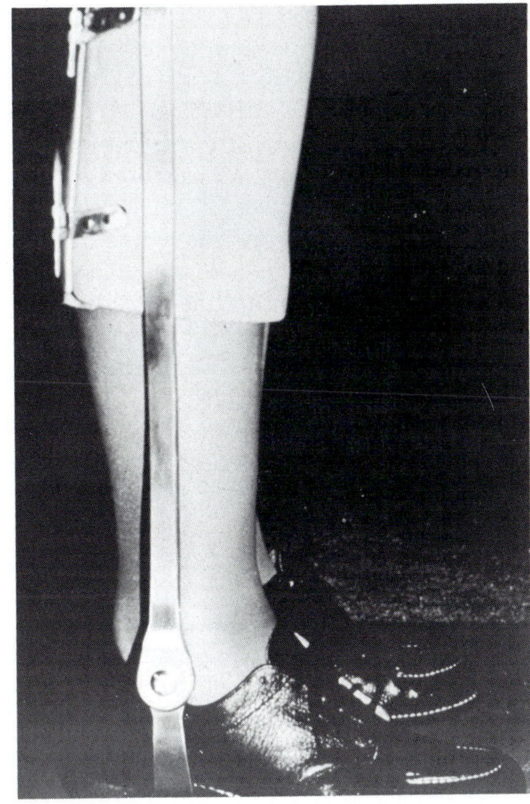

FIG 35–59.
Patellar tendon–bearing brace used to decrease weight transmission across the talus.

articular cartilage acts as a barrier to revascularization.[83, 84] From these findings, Boyd and Knight[15] and McKeever[83, 84] suggested that when displacement of the dislocated fragment of the talus has been such that its vascular supply is seriously injured, primary subtalar, talonavicular, and calcaneocuboid arthrodesis should be performed with excision of all overlying cartilage in an effort to speed up revascularization. Also, DePalma et al.[37] report that dowel fusion of the subtalar joint accelerates replacement of avascular bone. However, operative methods such as bone grafting or primary triple or subtalar arthrodesis to accelerate the process of replacement of necrotic bone have not been uniformly successful.[19, 54, 111]

In conclusion, although aseptic necrosis is an important complication of talar neck fractures, not all patients who develop aseptic necrosis are significantly symptomatic. Prevention is directed at early, anatomic reduction and stable internal fixation. Weight bearing is delayed only until there is union of the talar neck fracture. Early diagnosis of aseptic necrosis by radiography and/or bone scanning is encouraged. Since revascularization in the adult takes 2 to 3 years, non–weight bearing for this length of time is not practical. However, partial weight bearing in a patellar tendon–bearing brace is indicated.

Treatment of the Sequelae of Aseptic Necrosis.— Aseptic necrosis followed by late segmental collapse of the ankle and subtalar joints and pain presents a particularly difficult treatment problem. Simple ankle arthrodesis is difficult to achieve, and the foot is likely to remain painful due to collapse in the subtalar joint.[14] Miller and Baker[87] recommended triple arthrodesis and occasionally pantalar arthrodesis. Although Garcia and Parkes[45] mention pantalar arthrodesis, they report that it often results in a stiff, immobile foot and a limp.[45] Schrock[132] suggests that if the calcaneocuboid and talonavicular joints are not involved, these midtarsal joints should not be fused.

Coltart[27] reported good results after talectomy only *if* solid ankylosis occurred between the tibia and calcaneus. However, most authors recommend that simple excision of the talus as definitive treatment be avoided.[10, 19, 27, 36, 62] Talectomy results in an extremity 1½ in. short, a deformed foot that is difficult to fit with a shoe, and frequently persistent pain with weight bearing.[14]

Tibiocalcaneal fusion following aseptic necrosis has been reported by several authors.[19, 111, 122, 128] Canale and Kelly[19] and Pennal[111] report that tibiocalcaneal fusion is superior to ankle fusion or talectomy in these patients. Reckling[123] reports an average leg length discrepancy of 1¼ in. following tibiocalcaneal fusion. He recommends fusion in 5 to 10 degrees of equinus, removal of the medial and lateral malleoli to facilitate skin closure, use of the malleoli as a bone graft to ensure fusion, and fixation of the fusion with axial Steinmann pins or Charnley compression clamps.

The shortcomings of tibiocalcaneal fusion include (1) shortening and a decrease in height of the foot, and (2) an absence of motion in the anterior subtalar and tibiopedal joints. Because of these disadvantages, Blair introduced a modified tibiotalar fusion (Fig 35–60,A). Since neither the neck nor head of the talus is involved in the necrotic process, Blair recommends salvaging them. This preserves the anterior and middle articular facets of the subtalar joint. By fusing the tibia to the neck and head fragment by arthrodesis, some subtalar motion can be preserved. Through an anterolateral approach to the ankle a bone graft 1 in. wide and 2 in. long is taken from the anterior part of the tibia and slid into a trough in the neck of the talus. The foot is placed into 10 to 15 degrees of equinus, and cancellous bone is packed around the sliding graft. The Blair fusion has five advantages over other operations for aseptic necrosis of the talus[10, 36, 78]: (1) it retains the normal appearance of the foot, (2) the alignment of the foot relative to the ankle and leg is normal, (3) no shortening is produced, (4) the weight-bearing thrust is on normal tissue, and (5) the fusion allows some flexion and extension of the foot on the leg.

Morris et al.[93, 94] (Fig 35–60,B) modified this method by stabilizing the calcaneus on the tibia in the early postoperative phase by inserting a Steinmann pin through the os calcis into the tibia. They also use an AO screw through the graft and the tibia to prevent upward displacement of the graft. They recommended the modified Blair fusion for compound fractures of the talus with extrusion of the body and for aseptic necrosis. All of their patients maintained some motion at the subtalar joint because of preservation of the anterior and middle articular facets of the talus. Additionally, they report that the extremity is not shortened, the relation-

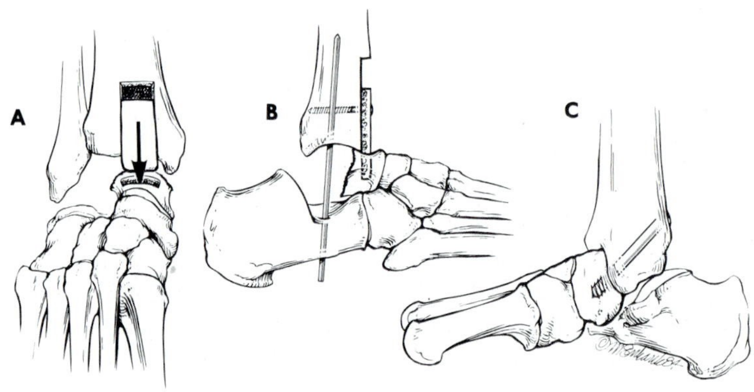

FIG 35–60.
A, Blair fusion as originally described. **B,** Morris, Hand, and Dunn[94] modified fusion by using an axial Steinmann pin for stability and fixing a sliding graft to the tibia with a screw. **C,** Lionberger et al.[78] used a compression screw from the posterior to the anterior to stabilize fusion.

ship of the foot and the ankle remains physiologic, and some tibiopedal flexion is preserved.

Dennis and Tullos[36] have reported good long-term results following Blair fusion. All patients had 15 to 20 degrees of motion about the long axis of the tibia. In addition, subtalar motion of some degree was present in all patients. They found that as long as some tibiopedal flexion-extension, subtalar, and talonavicular motion remained, a near-normal gait pattern resulted. However, when tibiopedal motion was not present, the results were poor.

Canale and Kelly[19] report poor results following a Blair fusion when a pseudarthrosis develops. In an effort to decrease the incidence of pseudarthrosis following the classic Blair fusion, Lionberger et al.[78] further modified the technique by utilizing a compression screw from the posterior portion of the tibia into the head and neck fragment. They report no nonunions and excellent function with this technique (Fig 35–60,C).

Author's Preferred Method of Treatment

Group I Injuries.—In patients with group I fractures of the neck of the talus, the lateral roentgenograph is *carefully* studied to ensure that a subtalar subluxation is not inadvertently overlooked. Additionally, I palpate along the subtalar joint to detect any tenderness that suggests a subtalar subluxation that has spontaneously reduced. This is important in that the patient may actually have a group II injury in which the subtalar joint injury is occult. The increased disability associated with group II injuries makes their detection important.

Patients with group I fractures in whom the fracture is impacted *and* is demonstrated to be stable under roentgenographic control are placed in a posterior splint. The splint is removed to allow early ankle and subtalar motion while the patient is hospitalized. Once motion of the ankle and subtalar joint has been restored, a non–weight bearing short-leg cast is applied for 6 weeks. A short-leg weight-bearing cast is then used until fracture union is evident. Lateral tomography may be required to determine fracture union.

Group I fractures that are not stable enough to allow early motion are treated in a short-leg non–weight-bearing cast for 6 weeks. If clinical signs of union are present, a short-leg walking cast is recommended until there is x-ray evidence of fracture union. In the initial cast, the toes are left free so that early range of motion of the metatarsophalangeal joints can be encouraged. Once union is documented roentgenographically, the cast is discontinued, and physical therapy is instituted to restore subtalar and ankle motion.

Group II Injuries.—All group II fractures must be *anatomically* reduced. My preference for treatment of these injuries is closed reduction under general or spinal anesthesia. The reduction is performed by manipulating the foot into plantar flexion followed by inversion or eversion to correct the associated medial or lateral displacement of the forefoot. Once the reduction is achieved, anteroposterior, modified anteroposterior[19] lateral, and oblique radiographs are taken to accurately evaluate the fracture reduction. If an anatomic reduction is achieved, internal fixation is recommended to avoid immobilization in plantar flexion. Two methods of fixation are considered. First, crossed Kirschner wires inserted percutaneously from an anterior direction can be utilized to stabilize the fracture.[148] These Kirschner wires pass from the head of the talus, across the fracture site, and into the body. This fixation allows the foot to be placed in a short-leg cast in the neutral position, avoids equinus casting, and is particularly useful in open fractures and those fractures associated with crushing in which rapid stabilization without further dissection is indicated. Recently I have combined closed reduction with insertion of a cancellous screw through a posterolateral approach as described by Lemaire and Bustin.[75] I have found that this provides quite stable fixation and permits early range of motion of the foot and ankle (Fig 35–61).

Once the fracture has been anatomically reduced and stabilized by percutaneous Kirschner wires, the patient is placed in a short-leg, non–weight-bearing cast for 6 weeks. The Kirschner wires are then removed, and a second short-leg non–weight-bearing cast is then applied. The patient is allowed to bear weight only when there is radiographic evidence of fracture union. If rigid fixation is obtained with a cancellous screw across the fracture site, the leg is placed in a posterior splint so that early range of motion of the subtalar and ankle joints can be instituted. After motion has been restored, a short-leg non–weight-bearing cast is recommended until fracture union is present. Weight bearing is not allowed until fracture union is demonstrated.

If an anatomic reduction of the subtalar joint or talar neck fracture is not achieved by closed manipulation, open reduction is performed. I prefer an anteromedial approach and am prepared to osteotomize the medial malleolus if the exposure is not adequate. A Kirschner wire inserted through the calcaneus may be helpful in the open manipulation. Once an anatomic reduction has been obtained, I stabilize this fracture by using a cancellous screw inserted posterolaterally, crossed Kirschner wires, or a cancellous screw inserted anteriorly, depending upon the situation. Postoperative management is the same following successful closed reduction.

Group III Injuries.—My efforts at closed reduction of group III fractures have been uniformly unsuccessful.

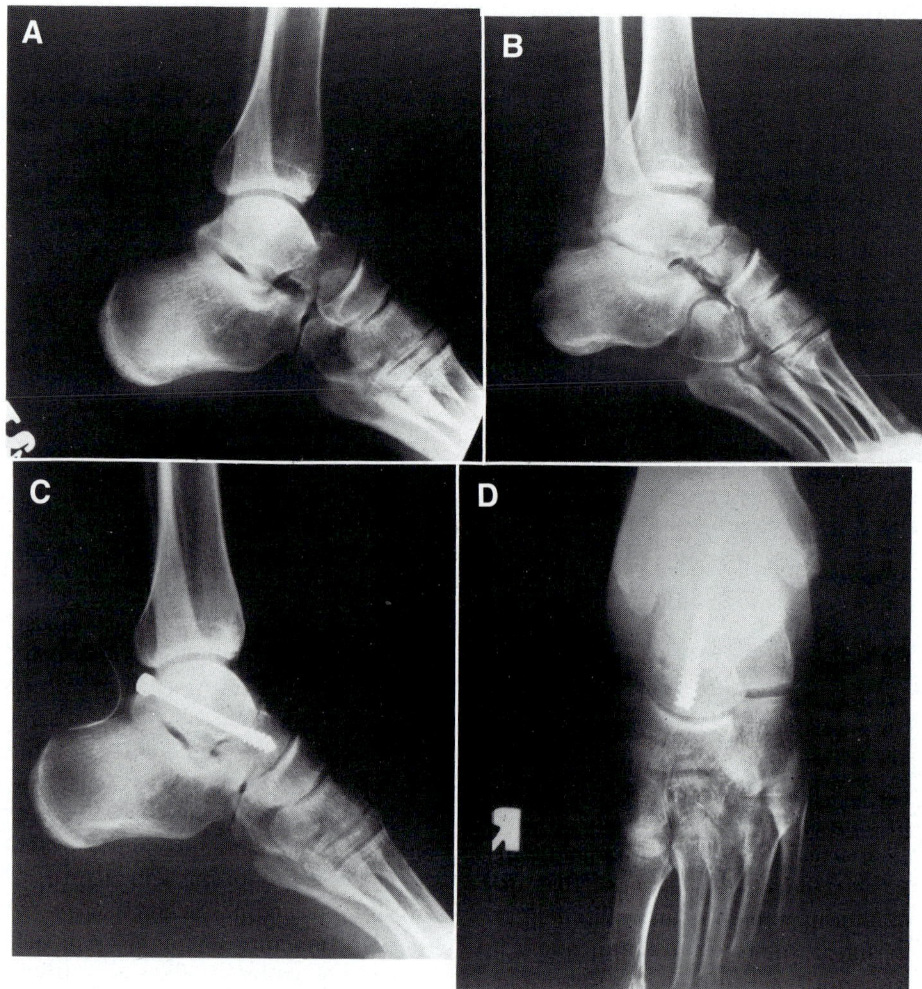

FIG 35–61.
A, displaced group II fracture of the neck of the talus with incongruity of the subtalar joint. **B,** anatomic closed reduction of *both* the talar neck fracture and the subtalar joint. **C,** stabilization of the fracture with an ASNIS cannulated screw inserted from the posterolateral direction. **D,** modified anteroposterior view of the foot demonstrating anatomic fracture reduction in this plane also.

For this reason, all patients with group III injuries are taken directly to the operating room.

Under general or spinal anesthesia the limb is prepared and draped. A temporary Kirschner wire is placed through the calcaneus and attached to a traction bow for manipulating the heel. At this point, a single attempt at closed reduction can be performed. If this fails, open reduction is indicated.

I prefer a posteromedial incision while being careful to not damage the overlying neurovascular bundle. The medial malleolus is osteotomized after being predrilled for insertion of an AO malleolar screw. I believe that osteotomy of the medial malleolus is essential to the approach of group III fractures because it maintains some of the intact deltoid ligament blood supply. The talar body is reduced in the mortise and into the subtalar joint. All osteocartilaginous fragments are debrided from both joints. Once an anatomic reduction has been obtained, the fracture is stabilized by utilizing either crossed Kirschner wires, AO screws from an anterior direction, or a cancellous screw inserted from the posterior aspect of the talus, again depending upon the situation. Cancellous bone grafting of the fracture site is performed in cases of severe comminution. The medial malleolus is then replaced with an AO malleolar screw.

In most group III injuries, the overlying skin is compromised. Therefore, I prefer a delayed primary closure at 3 to 5 days following the open reduction.

If the internal fixation is stable, early range of motion beginning after wound closure is instituted in the hospital. Once the range of motion has been restored, the limb is placed in a short-leg non–weight-bearing cast.

Weight bearing out of a cast is allowed only after fracture union is noted.

If the patient presents acutely with the talus completely extruded from the ankle joint, the talus is cleansed and replaced, and the wounds are left open and managed as described in the section on open dislocations of the talus. If the talus is an extruded fragment with severe contamination that presents 12 hours or more postinjury, consideration is given to talectomy, delayed wound closure, and Blair fusion as modified by Morris et al.[93, 94] when all wounds are healed.

Postoperative Care.—Patients with group I, II, and III fractures are followed with serial anteroposterior radiographs taken out of plaster at 6, 8, and 12 weeks postinjury to detect the presence of aseptic necrosis. We currently also follow these patients with an initial medullary bone scan repeated every 6 weeks. The results of bone scanning to detect aseptic necrosis are not yet conclusive. If aseptic necrosis becomes apparent roentgenographically, no change in treatment is planned until fracture union is obtained. When the talar neck fracture is healed, patients are placed in an active physical therapy program to restore range of motion of the ankle, midtarsal, and subtalar joints. Once union occurs and joint motion is restored, the patients are allowed to bear weight in a patellar tendon–bearing brace. This brace is recommended until the necrotic talus has been revascularized and replaced.

When aseptic necrosis results in late segmental collapse and *significant* pain and disability, I prefer Blair fusion to tibiocalcaneal arthrodesis because the tibiocalcaneal fusion shortens the foot and results in its decreased height, problems that make shoe fitting difficult. In addition. the lack of tibiopedal motion causes the patient to limp.

I reserve talocalcaneal fusion for those patients with a nonunion of the fracture of the neck of the talus and resorption of the majority of the neck in which no talar head is left to support the distal end of the tibia and in those in whom osteomyelitis of the talus erodes the head and neck fragment. I prefer the technique of tibiocalcaneal fusion described by Reckling.[123]

Fractures of the Body of the Talus

In addition to its critical weight-bearing function, the talar body is a central component of the talotibial and subtalar joints and therefore is of extreme importance in both rotation and hinge movements of the foot.[144] Due to these important functions, fractures of the talar body often result in significant disability, a problem further compounded by the unique vascular supply to the body of the talus that produces an increased risk of aseptic necrosis.[52, 73, 97, 114, 144]

TABLE 35–3.
Talar Body Fractures

Group I:	Transchondral or compression fractures of the talar dome. This type includes so-called osteochondritis dissecans of the talus (Fig 35–62, group I).
Group II:	Coronal, saggital, or horizontal[12, 33] shearing fractures involving the entire talar body (Fig 35–62, group II).
Group III:	Fractures of the posterior tubercle of the talus (Fig 35–62, group III).
Group IV:	Fracture of the lateral process of the talus (Fig 35–62, group IV).
Group V:	Crush fractures of the talar body (Fig 35–62, group V).

Fractures of the body of the talus are extremely uncommon and represent approximately 1% of all fractures.[27, 144] Due to their uncommon frequency, the prognosis of the various types of talar body fractures is not entirely clear. Sneppen et al[144] stressed the importance of classifying and studying the various morphologic types of talar body fractures with the goal of predicting a prognosis for each type.

To discuss the various types of talar body fractures, I have used a modification of the classification presented by Sneppen et al.[144] that divides talar body fractures into five groups (see Table 35–3).

It is essential when discussing talar body fractures that one distinguish between the various groups because the prognoses of each group vary significantly.[144] Each group will be discussed individually, with the exception of group V, crush fractures, which are considered under shearing fractures of the talar body (group II).

Group I: Osteochondral Fractures of the Talar Dome

An osteochondral fracture of the talar dome is an uncommon ankle injury that in the past has been considered under a variety of terms such as osteochondritis dissecans,* transchondral fractures,[6, 30, 135] osteochondral fractures,[18, 51, 98] talar dome fractures,[27, 96, 100, 128, 158] and flake fractures.[81]

Berndt and Harty[6] define a transchondral fracture as a fracture of the articular surface that is produced by a force transmitted from the articular surface of a contiguous bone across the joint surface, through the articular cartilage, and into the subchondral bony trabeculae of the fractured bone. Brendt and Harty[6] suggest that two types of fractures result: (1) a fracture consisting of a

**References 6, 7, 18, 77, 98, 122, 126, 131, 134, 152, 157.*

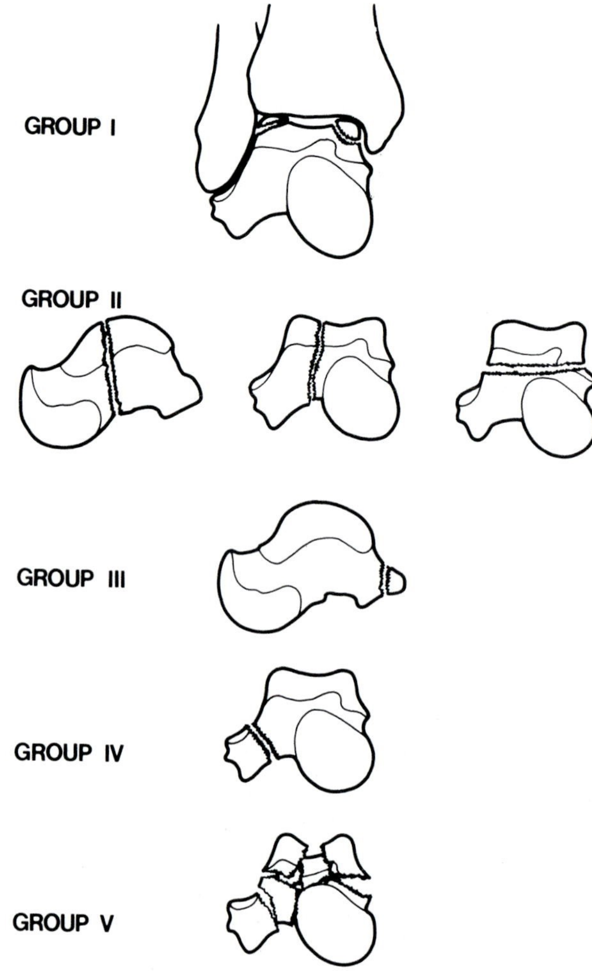

FIG 35–62.
Talar body fractures. **Group I,** transchondral fractures. **Group II,** coronal, sagittal, and horizontal shearing fractures. **Group III,** posterior tubercle fracture. **Group IV,** lateral process fracture. **Group V,** crush fracture.

small area of compressed trabeculae, with or without demonstrable damage to the overlying cartilage, and (2) a fracture consisting of an avulsion of an osteocartilaginous plate.[6] The compressed or avulsed fracture fragment has no soft-tissue attachments and, hence, no blood supply. Therefore it is susceptible to the development of aseptic necrosis.[6] According to Berndt and Harty, approximately 0.09% of all fractures are transchondral fractures of the talus.[6]

There is much confusion between the entities termed dome fractures, transchondral fractures, osteochondral fractures, etc., which are due to definite traumatic episodes, and osteochondritis dissecans, which suggests a vascular insult as the cause. Kappis in 1922[62] was the first to use the term "osteochondritis dissecans" as applied to the ankle joint, while Rendu in 1932[125] first reported a case of intra-articular fracture of the talus. Defects in the talar dome have, since these original descriptions, been reported with confusing terminology.[98] Lesions with identical roentgenographic characteristics have been classified by some as fractures and by others as osteochondritis dissecans.[6, 7] According to Anderson et al.,[3] these lesions are actually osteochondral fractures and can be produced by trauma to both the medial and lateral aspect of the talus.

The most recent concept is that the lesion termed osteochondritis dissecans of the talus is not due to idiopathic aseptic necrosis but, instead, to an injury.[6, 103, 122] Ray and Coughlin[122] report that the condition is due to trauma but stress that the trauma can be in the form of a single recognized episode or, more importantly, repeated minor unnoticed episodes. Such injuries result in a localized decrease in vascularity that leads to avascular separation of a loose fragment of cartilage and subchondral bone.[122]

Roden et al.[126] report that almost all such lesions that occur on the *lateral* aspect of the talus (Fig 35–63) are secondary to trauma, rarely heal spontaneously, and are frequently the source of continued symptoms. On the other hand, they found that the majority of lesions on the *medial* aspect of the talus (Fig 35–64) are not secondary to a *recognizable* episode of trauma, produce fewer symptoms, and frequently heal spontaneously. Canale and Belding[18] also noted that there were differences between the medial and lateral lesions: the lateral lesions seem to be traumatic in origin, while the medial lesions appear to be either traumatic or atraumatic. Additionally, the lateral lesions are wafer shaped while the medial lesions are cup shaped (Fig 35–65), and the lateral lesions are more frequently associated with persistent symptoms and degenerative changes. They were unable to state, however, that the lateral lesion was a transchondral or dome fracture and that the medial lesion represented a true osteochondritis dissecans. Indeed, Berndt and Harty[6] in 1959 demonstrated that both the medial and lateral talar dome lesions of osteochondritis dissecans were transchondral or osteochondral fractures secondary to trauma. O'Donoghue is also of the opinion that the majority of cases of so-called osteochondritis dissecans are in fact osteochondral or chondral fractures that arise from avulsion or shearing fractures or by direct compression.[103]

Marks in 1952[81] reported a patient in whom the progression of a simple flake fracture of the talus to definite osteochondritis dissecans was documented.[81] Alexander and Lichtman,[1] in an effort to combine the concepts of transchondral fracture and osteochondritis dissecans, report that the lesion referred to in the literature as osteochondritis dissecans in reality represents a "compression

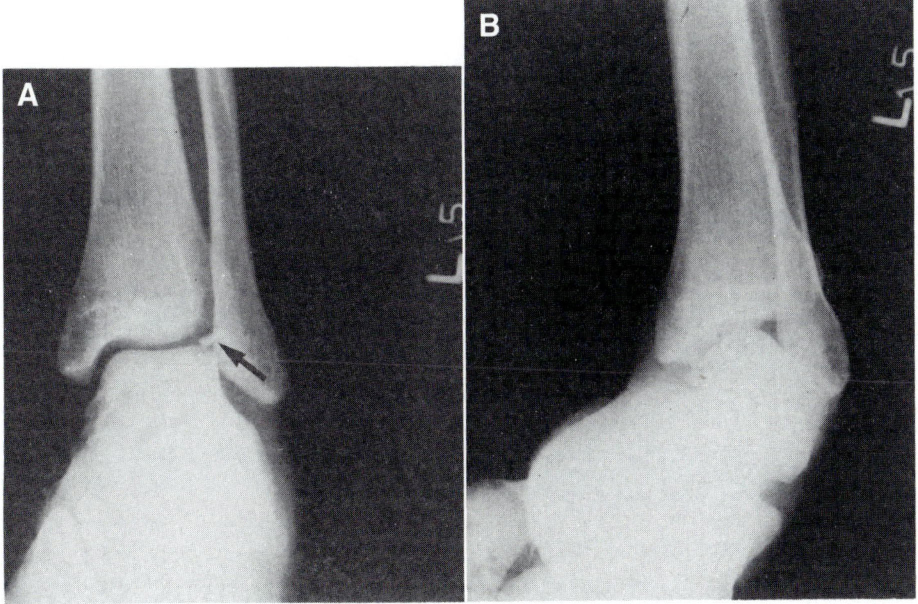

FIG 35–63.
A, transchondral fracture of the talar dome, completely displaced. **B,** a stress view shows associated lateral ligament disruption.

lesion" of the articular surface of the talus and that these lesions may progress to actual loose body formation and fragment separation. Alexander and Lichtman also note that the diagnosis of a transchondral fracture of the talar dome is often delayed because initial roentgenograms are negative or, because the injury is so trivial, roentgenographs are indeed not even taken.[1] Also, Shelton and Pedowitz[135] note that these fractures are commonly associated with more obvious injuries to the malleoli and/or the adjacent ligaments, which tends to obscure their detection (Fig 35–66).

In 1959 Berndt and Harty[6] classified lesions of the dome of the talus into four stages: stage I, a small area

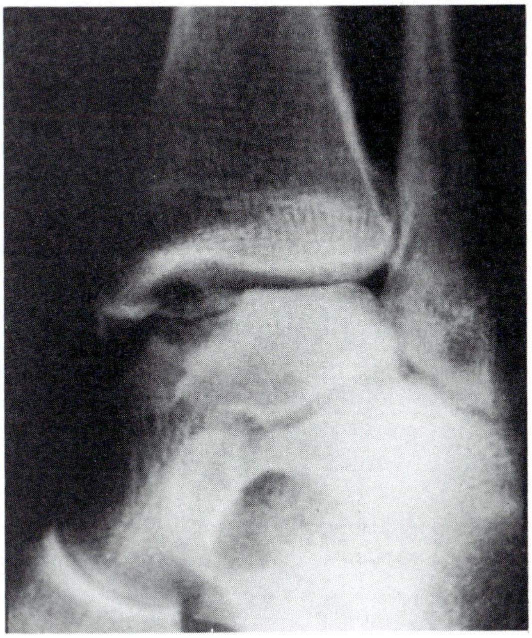

FIG 35–64.
Stage III lesion of the medial talar dome.

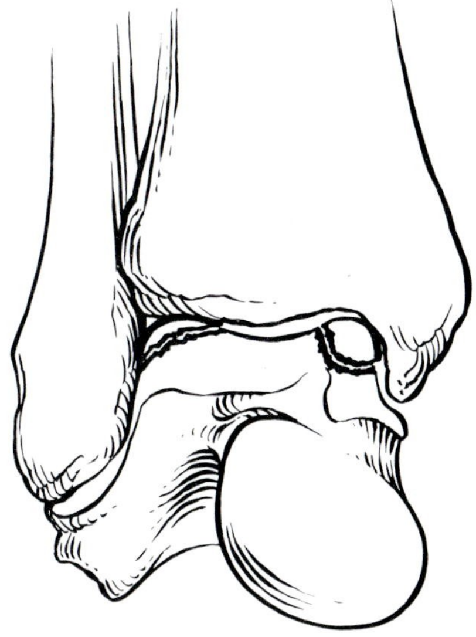

FIG 35–65.
Medial lesions are often cup shaped, while lateral lesions are waferlike or flakelike. (Adapted from Canale ST, Belding RH: *J Bone Joint Surg [Am]* 62:97–102, 1980.)

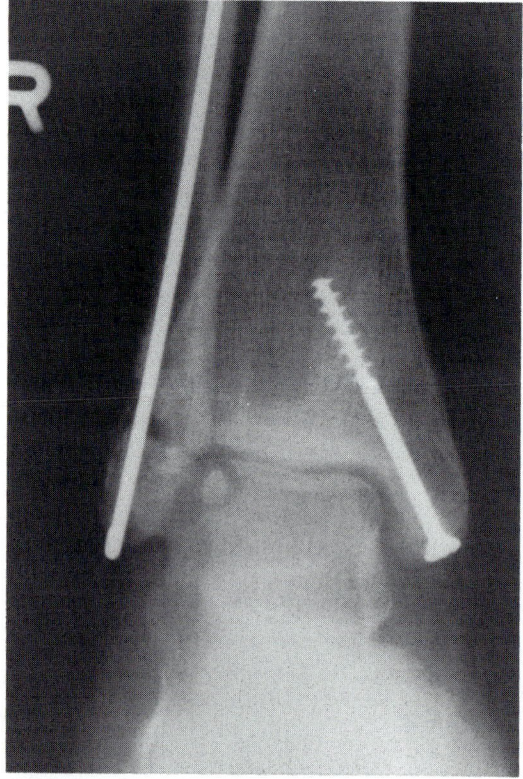

FIG 35–66.
Bimalleolar fracture of the ankle treated by open reduction and internal fixation. Note the lesion in the lateral dome of the talus, which was not detected at the time of open reduction.

of compression of subchondral bone; stage II, a partially detached osteochondral fragment; stage III, a completely detached osteochondral fragment that remains in the talar crater; and stage IV, a displaced osteochondral fragment (Fig 35–67). Alexander and Lichtman[1] believe that the lesion that has been termed osteochondritis dissecans, particularly in those patients in whom a history of trauma is indefinite, actually represents a Berndt and Harty stage I compression lesion that is painless at the onset because no ligaments are torn. It is with further weight bearing that this lesion progresses to a stage II or III lesion.

In spite of confusion regarding the terminology of fractures vs. the concept of osteochondritis dissecans, for the purpose of discussion in this chapter, these lesions are considered as one. The fact that treatment recommendations and prognosis are not dependent upon the etiology makes the discussion of these entities under one heading justified.

Anatomy

The dome of the talus is that part of the talus that articulates with the lower articular surface of the tibia and fibula.[96] A secure fit of the dome of the talus into the ankle mortise, particularly in dorsiflexion, predisposes it to the shearing forces necessary to produce transchondral fractures. The inversion or eversion of the foot and ankle that is necessary to produce these fractures may produce associated injuries of the medial or lateral collateral ligaments of the ankle (see Fig 35–63).[87]

Berndt and Harty[6] found that 43% of these lesions are in the lateral aspect of the talus while 57% of the fractures are located on the medial aspect of the dome of the talus. Canale and Belding[18] found an almost equal distribution of medial and lateral lesions. Those lesions on the medial aspect of the dome of the talus are usually located in the posterior third,[6, 18, 30] while lesions in the lateral portion are most commonly located in the middle third of the talus.[6, 18, 30]

Pathology

Berndt and Harty[6] believe that once an osteochondral fracture occurs, whether it be on the medial or lateral dome, it can heal like other fractures, but *only* if it is reduced *and* immobilized until union occurs. They emphasize that in stage I, II, and III fractures, the blood supply of the compressed or avulsed fragment has been cut off at the fracture line. The process of healing can occur only by the ingrowth of capillaries from the adjacent talus *across* the fracture line. The fracture fragment is avascular until a new blood supply arrives from the adjacent talus. These authors emphasize that if immobilization of the fracture in stages I, II, and III is incomplete or of too short duration, resultant motion at the fracture line will shear off ingrowing capillaries and prevent the reparative process. Also, unless stage I and II lesions are immobilized, continued weight bearing may rupture the remaining attachment of the fragment and convert it to a detached stage III or completely displaced stage IV lesion.[6]

The gross appearance of the dome of the talus will depend upon the stage of the lesion; it varies from the appearance of normal cartilage with slight softening and discoloration over the lesion to an actual defect in the articular surface of the affected bone in situations in which there is a displaced osteocartilaginous loose body.[122] In a stage I lesion[30] no damage may be evident on superficial examination of the talar dome due to the fact that this may entirely be a compression force that has caused microscopic injury to the bony trabeculae supporting the articular cartilage. The overlying articular cartilage does not become necrotic initially since it obtains the majority of its nutrition from the synovial fluid.

Once the fragment becomes displaced, its bed becomes covered with a fibrous coating of host tissue as a

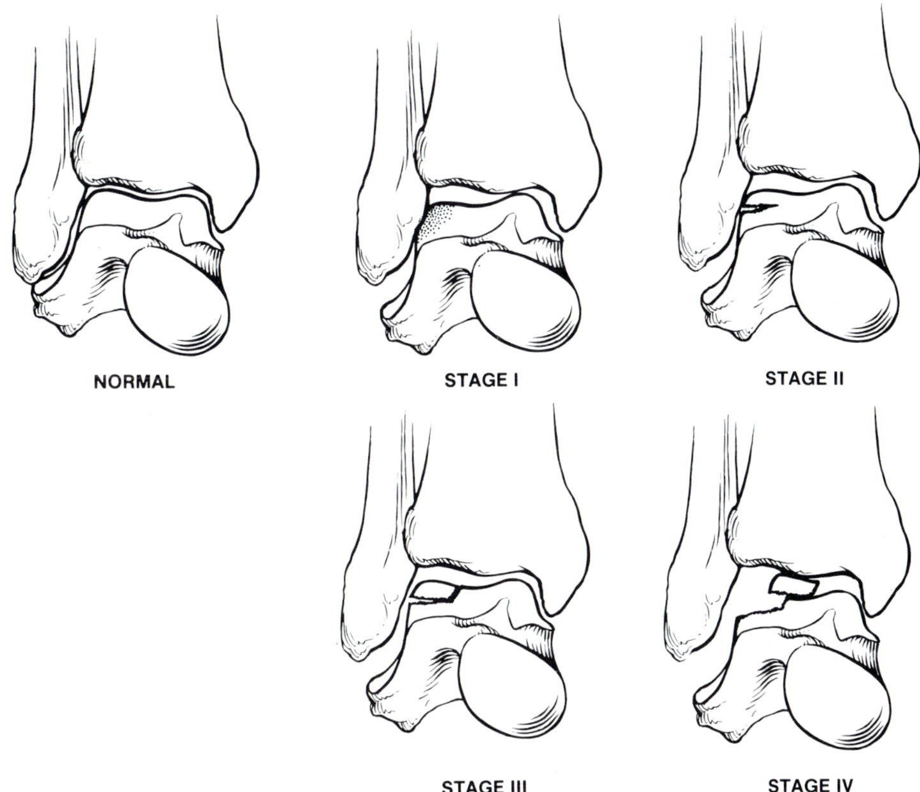

FIG 35–67.
Classification of osteochondral lesions of the talus by Berndt and Harty.[6] Stage I, small area of compressed subchondral bone. Stage II, partially detached fragment. Stage III, completely detached fragment remaining in the talar crater. Stage IV, fragment loose in the joint.

new reparative process begins. Once the fragment is removed, the defect can become filled with fibrous connective tissue that restores the original shape of the talus and is of sufficient firmness to act as satisfactory replacement for the missing bone.[6]

Mechanism of Injury

Although reports of lesions of the talar dome without a history of trauma are present in the literature, there is overwhelming agreement that the majority of these injuries are posttraumatic in nature.[127] Lindholm et al.[77] found that trauma such as a fall from a height or a twisting injury during a sporting activity was the main cause of these lesions.[77] Vaughan and Stapleton[152] stressed that even though trauma is a major factor, at least some patients have an underlying predisposition to the lesion, possibly a local area of decreased vascular supply to the subchondral bone that might produce a necrotic area with minimal injury.

The current literature suggests that osteochondral fractures of the talus are due to inversion injuries.[30, 81] O'Farrell and Costello[104] suggest that if the foot is plantar-flexed during inversion, a medial lesion results from compression of the medial talar dome by the tibia. On the other hand, if the foot is dorsiflexed, a lateral talar lesion results from shearing forces produced by striking the fibula.

The most detailed investigation into the mechanism of these injuries was that reported by Berndt and Harty.[6] They found that with strong inversion of the dorsiflexed foot, a lesion of the lateral border of the talar dome resulted. This fracture was located at the middle or anterior half of the lateral border of the talus. With ankle dorsiflexion, the wider anterior half of the talus fits tightly into the ankle mortise. Inversion then impacts the lateral dome against the articular surface of the fibula. It is for this reason that the injury may be accompanied by a tear of the lateral ankle ligaments.[81, 98] On the other hand, when the foot is in plantar flexion, the narrow posterior half of the talar dome occupies the mortise, and forceful inversion accompanied by medial rotation of the tibia on a fixed foot results in posteromedial talar impaction.

Rosenberg emphasizes a clinical correlation with the mechanism of injury. He notes that the lateral lesion is easily recognized as an acute fracture because it is elevated by the levering effect of the articular facet of the fibula.[128] On the other hand, the medial lesion occurs as a result of impaction against the medial malleolus and is rarely displaced. These medial injuries become demonstrable roentgenographically only when absorption of bone has occurred at the impaction fracture site.

Finally, Mukherjee and Young[96] report an unusual fracture of the *anterior* dome of the talus, the mechanism of which they ascribe to plantar flexion and vertical compression whereby the anterior edge of the lower articular surface of the tibia fractures the anterior aspect of the dome of the talus.

Clinical Diagnosis

The diagnosis of an osteochondral fracture of the talus is often missed in the early stages because many of these patients are originally treated as having sprains, the fracture being overlooked.[1, 98] VanBuecken et al.[151] report that 6.5% of patients with sprains have transchondral talar dome fractures. For this reason, the authors emphasize that any patient with persistent symptoms after conservative treatment of an ankle sprain should be suspected of having a transchondral talar dome fracture.

Alexander and Lichtman[1] reported that 28% of these patients have associated fractures, usually of the malleoli (see Fig 35–66). In these situations, clinical examination may divert one's attention from the possibility of an injury to the dome of the talus.

Canale and Belding[18] found that the majority of patients, and all patients with lateral lesions, had a history of trauma to the ankle.[1, 77, 122, 128] Other authors have also found a history of trauma in most patients, although in some instances it seems insignificant.[122] In most series, patients are predominantly athletic males in the second and third decades of life.[135]

Berndt and Harty[6] stress that there are no symptoms pathognomonic of a transchondral fracture. In fact, Roden et al.[126] stressed that lesions of the lateral talar dome are more frequently associated with definite symptoms while medial dome lesions usually have minimal symptoms. The symptoms vary depending upon the stage of the injury, i.e., acute or chronic.[30, 104, 122] Acute fractures are often misdiagnosed as sprains, while patients with chronic injuries are misdiagnosed as arthritics. The symptoms of acute transchondral fractures are those of an inversion sprain, that is, pain and tenderness in the torn lateral collateral ligaments, swelling of the ankle, ecchymosis, and limited motion.[6, 104] However, stage I lesions may be almost painless due to an absence of sensory fibers in the compressed articular cartilage and a lack of associated ligamentous change.[1, 30] In a chronic injury the symptoms depend to a large degree on the amount of healing of the associated torn ligaments and on the size and displacement of the fracture fragment. The symptoms suggest arthritis and include freedom of pain when the joint is at rest, but crepitus, stiffness, swelling, and limited motion after exercise also occur.[6, 103, 122] Tenderness, crepitation, recurrent swelling, clicking, or symptoms of "a weak ankle" should all suggest the possibility of a fracture of the dome of the talus.[32, 98, 158] In stage IV lesions, locking occurs in addition to the symptoms of osteoarthritis.[6]

The physical findings in acute injury include swelling and tenderness.[96] The location of point tenderness can often determine the location of the lesion in the talar dome. In midlateral lesions, tenderness is usually located between the talus and tibiofibular syndesmosis,[100, 122, 135] while in posteromedial lesions tenderness is usually present behind the medial malleolus.[135] Marks[81] noted that there was swelling beneath the lateral malleolus and tenderness over the whole insertion of the lateral collateral ligament of the ankle, most marked over the attachment of the anterior and middle fasciculi to the talus and calcaneus, respectively.

Flexion and extension of the ankle are normal, but in acute injuries there is marked limitation of inversion by pain, and limitation of eversion by swelling.[81, 100]

Limitation of motion, locking, instability (secondary to associated ligamentous injury or to a loose body), and a palpable loose body may be present in cases of longstanding injury.[122]

Radiographic Examination

Although the clinical history of an inversion sprain should suggest the diagnosis of an osteochondral fracture of the talus, roentgenographs are mandatory to establish the diagnosis. It is important to emphasize that when only the articular cartilage is damaged, i.e., a stage I injury, the fracture may not be noted radiographically. A medial lesion is, in particular, commonly the result of impaction against the medial malleolus and is rarely displaced; therefore, it may become demonstrable roentgenographically only when absorption of bone and/or sclerosis has occurred at the fracture site. Indeed, Shelton and Pedowitz,[135] Alexander and Lichtman,[1] and Vaughan and Stapleton[152] stress the importance of repeat radiographic examination in certain patients in an effort to prevent a delay in diagnosis, which often leads to chronic disability. If pain about the ankle persists following an injury (despite normal initial films), they recommend repeating the radiographs because they may detect a stage II or III lesion that has developed from an undetected stage I injury.

Roden et al.[126] stressed that anteroposterior and lateral roentgenographs of the ankle are not adequate for diagnosis. Berndt and Harty[6] recommend a minimum of three views of the ankle, anteroposterior, oblique (10 degrees of medial rotation), and lateral, all centered over the joint line and taken with the foot in the neutral position. The anteroposterior view usually demonstrates the medial margin of the dome of the talus clearly, but the lateral border of the talar dome is obscured by the lateral, malleolus, which is superimposed over the lateral talar dome.[30, 98] The oblique view with 10 degrees of medial rotation of the limb demonstrates the talofibular joint and gives a clear view of the lateral border of the talar dome. Newberg[98] and Yvars[158] stress that even anteroposterior, lateral, and oblique views may not demonstrate the lesion. They therefore recommend taking the internal oblique radiographs of the ankle in neutral, plantar flexion, and dorsiflexion. In addition, Davidson et al.[30] mention that to evaluate lateral dome lesions, views taken in 35 degrees of obliquity and full plantar flexion are useful. Also, Davis[32] and Alexander and Lichtman[1] suggest that inversion stress radiographs help to demonstrate these lesions, particularly of the superolateral aspect of the dome of the talus.

Finally, although part of the talar dome is obscured by the overlying medial and lateral malleoli on the lateral view, this view is important because it indicates whether the lesion is anterior or posterior on the talar dome, a finding necessary for preoperative planning.[6, 98]

Anderson et al.[3] report the use of bone scintigraphy of the ankle as a screening process to evaluate patients with undiagnosed posttraumatic disability of the ankle. The authors report that 57% of patients with normal radiographs and undiagnosed posttraumatic symptoms of the ankle had an osteochondral fracture of the dome of the talus detected by bone scintigraphy. The authors then utilized MRI in those patients with positive scintigrams to demonstrate the osteochondral fractures. Of those previously undiagnosed osteochondral fractures, 23% were of the medial aspect on the dome of the talus. The most remarkable feature of this report was the frequency with which osteochondral fractures of the talus were found in patients who complained of chronic disability after an ankle sprain.

The osteochondral fracture changes noted by MRI were altered signal intensity of the bone marrow. The change often involves a surprisingly large area of surrounding bone. The normal high-intensity signal of cancellous bone on T1- and T2-weighted images is due to fat in the marrow. Following an injury, there is decreased T1 signal intensity from the cancellous bone surrounding the fracture due to the edematous reaction in the acute and subacute stages and due to deposition of fibrous tissue and fibrocartilaginous tissue in more chronic injuries. This change is easily detected on MRI, thus allowing detection of the most subtle fractures (Fig 35–68). The authors report that although CT is adequate for assessing the progress of an osteochondral fracture, it was unable to detect lesions in the dome of the talus that were not visible on routine radiographs.

Mensor and Melody in 1941[86] first described the use of tomograms in evaluating lesions in the dome of the talus. Most authors believe that tomograms provide more accurate information as to the size and location of these lesions.[1, 6, 19, 26] Newberg[98] suggests the value of polytomography in both lateral and oblique planes when localizing the fracture fragment and notes that anteroposterior tomograms may obscure a small fragment due to overlapping shadows.

It is important to remember that radiographically the fragment appears much smaller than when seen at surgery because the chondral component is radiolucent.[98] Air-contrast arthography may be useful in better defining the size of a fragment and in determining whether it is completely detached.[135, 140] Additionally, air-contrast arthrography may demonstrate lesions that are purely chondral.[140] Recently, Reis et al.[124] clearly demonstrated the value of high-resolution computerized axial tomography (CAT) for lesions of the dome of the talus. I too have found CAT scan studies valuable in selecting the best surgical approach for these lesions.

The incidence of talar dome lesions is nearly equally distributed between the medial and lateral talar dome.[46, 122, 131] According to Canale and Belding,[18] medial lesions are usually deeper and cup shaped while lateral fragments are shallow and wafer shaped (see Fig 35–65). The radiographic appearance of the osteochondral lesion also depends upon its duration.[18, 51, 128, 158] In acute injuries, the osteochondral fragment has sharp edges demonstrable roentgenographically, and there is no resorption of the fracture site. When seen later in the course of the disease, the signs of nonunion may be present. These include a sclerotic margin lining the concave talar bed and fragmentation of the subchondral bone plate.[158] It is this chronic picture that suggests the term osteochondritis dissecans.[81, 158] Finally, secondary degenerative arthritis can be found either in the medial or lateral aspect of the ankle in cases with a long history.

Davidson et al.[30] emphasize the importance of follow-up radiographs to determine the progress of healing of these lesions. They stress that early healing is by fibrocartilage that is radiolucent. Therefore, the defect and the fragment may appear larger in the early follow-up films than initially.

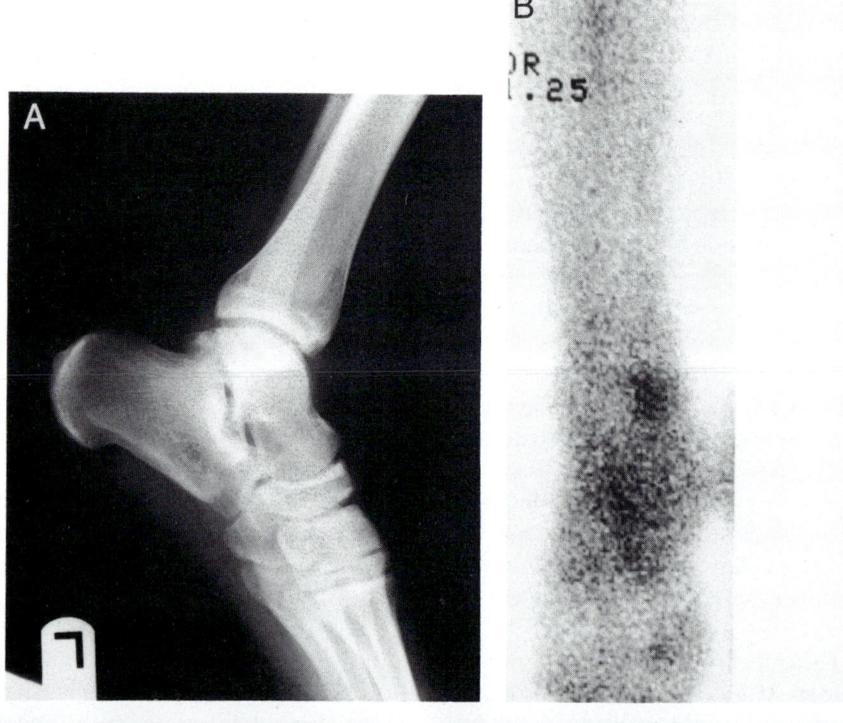

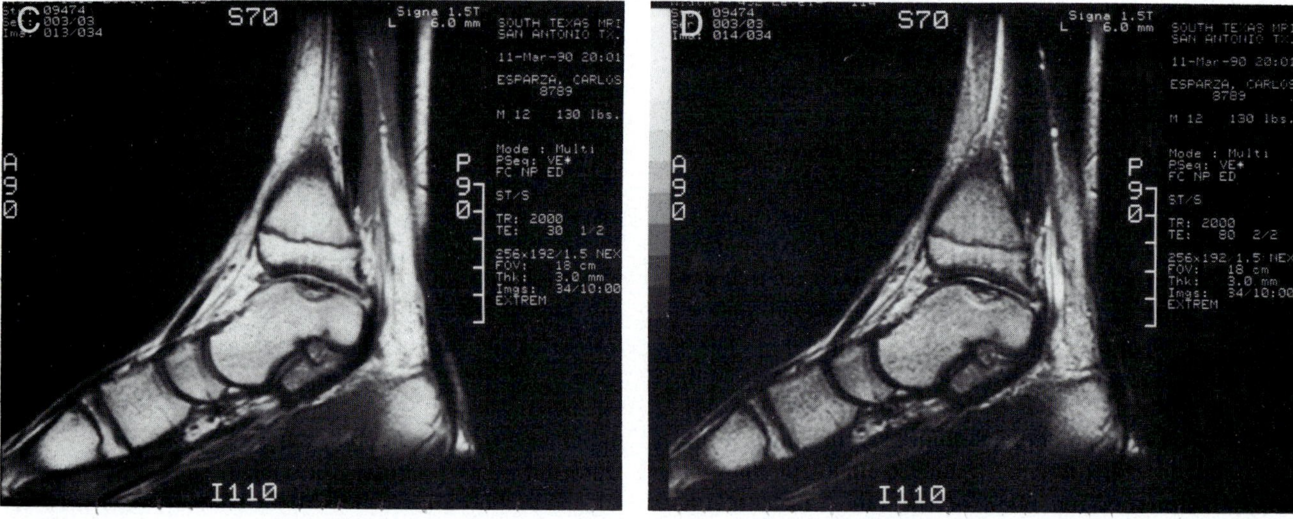

FIG 35–68.
Patient with persistent pain after an ankle sprain. **A,** Routine radiograph of the ankle interpreted as negative. **B,** a bone scan showing a lesion on the medial aspect of the talar dome. **C,** MRI (proton density) demonstrating the extent of the lesion in the talar dome. **D,** T_2 MRI image demonstrating fluid beneath the lesion, which indicates that the fragment is unstable.

Treatment

Acute Fractures.—Berndt and Harty[6] report that following an acute injury, treatment by reduction and adequate immobilization ordinarily results in healing, while Canale and Belding[18] found that with long-term follow-up few lesions united when treated nonoperatively.

Shelton and Pedowitz[135] stress the importance of correct staging and prompt and adequate treatment to produce the best results. For healing to take place, capillaries from the remaining talar body must cross the fracture site. If immobilization is inadequate, repetitive motion at the fracture site may transect these ingrowing capillaries and result in delayed union or nonunion.[6, 135] They recommend treating stage I, II, and III lesions without roentgenographic signs of an established nonunion (i.e., sclerosis, uneven joint surfaces, or arthritic changes) in a short-leg non–weight-bearing cast until union is demonstrated roentgenographically. They believe that stage IV displaced fractures are best treated by surgical removal of the fragment in order to prevent deterioration of the joint.[135] Newberg[98] recommends repair of associated ligamentous damage to improve results. In stage IV fractures with associated severe osteoarthritic changes in the ankle, simple removal of the loose body may be inadequate, and ankle fusion may be necessary.[135]

Canale and Belding[18] base treatment not only on displacement but also on location of the lesion. They recommend that stage I and II lesions, whether medial or lateral in location, be treated nonoperatively in a cast or patellar tendon–bearing brace. They believe that stage III lesions on the medial dome talar should be treated by the same method. If symptoms persist after this conservative treatment, surgical excision and curettage of the lesion is recommended. In stage III lesions involving the lateral dome of the talus and in both medial and lateral dome stage IV lesions, treatment by immediate excision of the fragment and curettage of the defect is recommended. Rosenberg,[128] on the other hand, reports that although prolonged immobilization has frequently been used, none of the lateral fractures he treated in this manner healed. He therefore believes that lateral lesions most always require surgical treatment and the decision of excision of the fragment, curettage, or replacement is dependent upon the size of the lesion.[128] Anderson et al.[3] recommend that all stage I and Stage II lesions be treated by immobilization for 6 weeks. The authors emphasize that although healing may appear to have occurred, patients need to be followed for a minimum of 3 years because the lesion may progress to a higher stage at a later date. In stage IIA lesions the authors recommend deroofing the cyst and drilling the base of the crater down to bleeding bone. In stage III and IV fractures, arthroscopic removal of the separated fragment followed by curettage or drilling of the fracture bed down to bleeding bone is recommended.

Pettine and Morrey[117] also demonstrated that a delay in diagnosis and treatment produced poor results only if the fracture was type III or type IV. The authors were unable to conclusively demonstrate that the results in patients following surgical treatment deteriorate with time. In fact, most of their patients seem to be stable 1 year following definitive treatment.

Management of the talar dome defect left after fragment excision is controversial. Ray and Coughlin[122] believe that the defect in the talus should be saucerized and all loose fragments from the joint excised. On the other hand, O'Donoghue[103] stresses that the articular cartilage at the edge of the defect should not be saucerized, but trephined by cutting the articular cartilage vertical to the articular surface. This minimizes the size of the articular cartilage defect that has to be filled. Also, to encourage revascularization of this denuded area, he recommends the use of fine drills or Kirschner wire holes as advocated by Smillie.[139]

Long-standing Lesions.—In dealing with long-standing lesions, Vaughan and Stapleton[152] and Nisbet[100] recommend operative removal of the fragment and curettage of the necrotic bone, while Lindholm et al.[77] recommend conservative treatment initially. However, if symptoms persist following conservative treatment, they recommend removal of the loose bodies. In those situations in which a large fragment from the weight-bearing dome is present, they suggest replacement of the fragment by using bone pegs for internal fixation. Ray and Coughlin recommend that in patients in whom the lesion is discovered accidently and who have no definite symptoms referable to the lesion, operative intervention be delayed until symptoms develop or until roentgenographs demonstrate progression of the lesion.[122] They note that once the diagnosis is established and the patient has symptoms referable to the site of the lesion, surgical intervention is the only satisfactory method of treatment. O'Farrell and Costello[104] report that results are better in patients in whom surgery is performed within 12 months of the onset of symptoms. They suggest drilling the base of the defect after excision of the osteochondritic fragment in an effort to promote fibrocartilage formation in the defect. Davidson et al.[30] also note that a delay in surgical removal of a loose fragment may result in or contribute to posttraumatic arthritis.

Recently, in patients in whom roentgenographs suggest an osteochondral defect, a small-caliber arthroscope has been used to evaluate the joint surface of the ankle[41, 77, 108] and, hence, to stage the lesions. Additionally, small loose bodies can be removed arthroscopically, thereby limiting the degree of postoperative rehabilitation necessary.[41] Arthroscopic curettage, debridement, and drilling of the defect after loose body removal is possible and greatly reduces postoperative morbidity.[41] VanBuechen et al.[151] reported 15 cases of transchondral talar dome fractures treated arthroscopically. They report that all patients with stage III or IV lesions had abnormal articular cartilage overlying the lesion. These lesions were treated by arthroscopic excision of fragments with abrasion and/or drilling of the remaining crater. The authors reported no complications. They also concluded, however, that if their patients treated arthroscopically are compared with a previous study of open treatment, the percentage of good to excellent results was virtually identical. The authors conclude that the arthroscopic management of transchondral fractures of the talar dome has the advantage of decreased morbidity and more rapid rehabilitation. The authors believe that this is especially true in medial lesions that have traditionally required osteotomy for adequate exposure when open techniques are used.

Operative Treatment.—Ray and Coughlin[122] recommend an anteromedial incision for lesions in the superomedial aspect of the talus. However, in some cases the lesion may be completely hidden beneath the medial malleolus. Exposure of these lesions can be obtained by an osteotomy of the medial malleolus across its base.[122] A standard anterolateral approach to the ankle is used for lesions involving the superolateral aspect of the talus.[122] For lesions located more posteriorly on the lateral border of the talus, a posterolateral incision may be utilized. Occasionally, exposure of a lateral lesion may be improved by a Gatellier fibular osteotomy, particularly in cases in which the lesion lies directly beneath the fibula.[122] The importance of using dorsiflexion and plantar flexion of the ankle to bring the defect into view at surgery cannot be overemphasized.

Ove et al.[105] suggest that surgical dissection of the distal end of the fibula to reach posterolateral lesions is extensive and devascularizing. They propose an alternative technique for the treatment of posterolateral talar dome lesions through a *medial* transmalleolar approach. The authors recommend approaching these posterolateral lesions by performing a medial malleolar osteotomy after the medial malleolus has been predrilled and tapped. A traction pin is then placed in the calcaneus to aid in distraction and valgus positioning of the ankle joint. This allows the ankle joint to be explored on both the tibial and talar surfaces. The posterolateral talar defects can then be debrided with small, straight and curved curettes. The medial malleolar osteotomy is reattached by utilizing two 4.0-mm AO cancellous screws.

Postoperative Care.—Postoperative treatment varies depending upon the surgical approach used. Early resumption of motion and partial weight bearing postoperatively are recommended for patients treated by simple arthrotomy, curettage, and drilling.[30, 135, 158] Alexander and Lichtman[1] recommend a short-leg cast for 7 to 10 days in patients who do not require an osteotomy. The patients then begin range-of-motion exercises to "mold" the new fibrocartilage after primary wound healing occurs. Weight bearing is not allowed for 8 to 12 weeks to allow the fibrocartilage to mature.

In patients in whom an osteotomy is performed, Davidson et al.[30] and Yvars[158] recommend plaster immobilization without weight bearing until malleolar union occurs. Alexander and Lichtman[1] recommend a non–weight-bearing long-leg cast for 6 weeks in these patients. At that point, the cast is removed, and radiographs are taken to ascertain whether the malleolar osteotomy has healed. Non–weight bearing is continued for 6 additional weeks while range of motion is encouraged. Finally, in patients treated by the internal fixation of dome fragments, no weight bearing is allowed until fracture union is demonstrated roentgenographically.[135]

Results and Prognosis

Yvars[158] stresses that although short-term results of fragment excision indicate relief of preoperative discomfort, the late results of removal of fragments has not been accurately documented. The long-term complications most commonly reported following this injury are posttraumatic arthritis and limited range of motion.[17, 30, 88, 96, 103, 126]

Davidson et al.,[30] O'Farrell and Costello,[104] and Newberg[98] emphasize that *early* operation and excision of most osteochondral fractures of the talus produce the best result and that any delay in removal of a loose fragment can result in posttraumatic arthritis. Pettine and Morrey[117] also demonstrated that a delay in diagnosis and treatment produced poor results only if the fracture was type III or type IV. The authors were unable to conclusively demonstrate that the results in patients following surgical treatment deteriorate with time. In fact, most of their patients seem to be stable 1 year following definitive treatment.

It is virtually impossible to accurately prognosticate the outcome in any given case.[30, 104] Davidson et al.[30] and O'Farrell and Costello[104] emphasize the lack of correlation between symptomatology and radiographic findings at follow-up. The rate and severity of arthritic deterioration are related to the size of the lesion, the location of the lesion, the weight and activity status of the patient, and finally, the associated ligamentous laxity.[135]

Conservative treatment of nondisplaced stage I fractures produces good results in about three fourths of patients.[5, 126, 140] Stage II and III lesions treated conservatively show satisfactory results in only about 25%.[135] According to Ray and Coughlin[122] the prognosis is excellent in patients diagnosed early, in those without actual separation of the osteochondral fragment, and in those without secondary degenerative change present at the time of diagnosis. According to VanBuecken et al.,[151] the stage of the lesion does seem to affect the clinical result. There is a greater tendency toward excellent results in stage II and III lesions as compared with stage IV lesions. The authors also concluded that the presence of healing radiographically had no bearing on the clinical outcome.

Canale and Belding[18] found that in 50% of their patients, the long-term sequelae of osteochondral lesions of the ankle was degeneration of the joint with resultant arthrosis, regardless of the type of treatment. They too stressed that although poor clinical results were uniformly associated with roentgenographic evidence of arthrosis, radiographic evidence of arthrosis did not alone guarantee a poor clinical result. They did stress, however, that in such patients further follow-up is necessary to distinguish the relationship. Scharling[131] reports that only half of his patients were free of pain and that limited ankle motion was often present. Angerman and Jensen[4] reported 20 patients with osteochondritis dissecans at a follow-up of 9 to 15 years following surgical treatment that included multiple drilling of the base of the lesion combined with excision of loose fragments. Eighty-five percent of the patients initially reported satisfactory results. At long-term follow-up, however, more than half the patients had some degree of pain and swelling of the ankle during activity, but only 1 patient (5%) developed generalized osteoarthritis. The authors conclude that early surgical treatment of complete or displaced talar osteochondral lesions is associated with better long-term results than late surgical treatment is.

Author's Preferred Method of Treatment

I must emphasize the importance of correlating roentgenographic findings with the symptoms of the patient. The incidental finding of a talar dome lesion in an asymptomatic patient should not be treated surgically. I base my treatment of osteochondral lesions of the talar dome on the classification of Berndt and Harty.[6] For this classification to be used, one *must* be certain of the location, size, and displacement of the osteochondral fragment. I place great emphasis on further investigation of patients with persistent disability in the ankle following an ankle sprain. Those patients who continue to have symptoms following adequate treatment of an ankle sprain undergo scintigraphy. If the scintigraphy results are positive, MRI is ordered to evaluate talar dome fractures. By this method, lesions not evident radiographically are detected. If a lesion is noted on routine radiographs, I use lateral polytomograms and/or CT or MRI to further evaluate the size of the lesion and to indicate the location anteriorly or posteriorly. Additionally, I have recently used arthroscopy to help in staging these talar lesions. I have found it particularly useful in stage II and III lesions to differentiate between an incomplete and completely detached but nondisplaced fragment. Also, improvement in instrumentation now permits an experienced arthroscopist to remove loose bodies, debride and curette the talar defect, and drill the bed without ankle arthrotomy.

The scheme for treating acute and chronic lesions is the same. Initially, I treat all stage I and stage II lesions, whether they are medial or lateral, acute or chronic, in a short-leg non–weight-bearing cast for 6 weeks. Stage III lesions located on the medial dome of the talus are also treated in a short-leg non–weight-bearing cast for 6 weeks. Roentgenographs are taken to evaluate healing, and further immobilization is recommended if healing is incomplete. If symptoms persist following conservative treatment, arthroscopy (or arthrotomy) is performed to see whether the fragment is loose. Small stage III lesions are then treated by curettage and drilling of the talar bed. Open reduction and internal fixation are performed if the fragment is large enough to be stabilized with Kirschner wires.

For stage III lesions involving the lateral talar dome and stage IV lesions involving either the medial or lateral dome of the talus, removal of the fragment, trephining, and drilling the bed are recommended. Open reduction and internal fixation of the fragment by using Kirschner wires or small AO screws are performed *only* in cases of acute injury in which the fracture represents at least one third of the medial or lateral dome of the talus.

The surgical approach for open reduction and internal fixation or fragment excision is based upon the lateral roentgenograph, tomograms, or CAT scan. For lesions located in the anterior aspect of the lateral talar dome, an anterolateral arthrotomy is utilized. Occasionally, a posterior lesion of the lateral dome can be more easily approached through a posterolateral arthrotomy. I have not found a lateral fibular osteotomy necessary to expose these lateral dome lesions since dorsiflexion and plantar flexion will usually bring them into view.

Lesions on the medial dome of the talus in the anterior half are approached through an anteromedial arthrotomy. Occasionally, lesions located at the midportion or posterior portion of the medial dome require osteotomy of the medial malleolus for exposure. In this instance, I prefer to predrill the malleolus for an AO malleolar screw prior to the osteotomy, which is performed just below the joint line.

Once the surgical exposure is obtained, all small loose fragments are removed. The articular cartilage at the edge of the articular defect is trephined and the bed of the lesion curetted and drilled with a 0.045-in. Kirschner wire. Postoperative treatment varies. If a malleolar osteotomy is not performed, the limb is placed in a short-leg splint for 3 to 5 days. Immediately following this, range-of-motion exercises are instituted. Patients are kept non–weight bearing for 8 to 12 weeks depending upon the size and location of the lesion. This allows time for fibrocartilaginous ingrowth to occur.

If a malleolar osteotomy is performed, the patients are kept in a short-leg cast for approximately 2 weeks. They then are given a posterior plaster splint that they can remove to encourage range-of-motion exercises on a daily basis. After the malleolar osteotomy has healed, progressive weight bearing is instituted at 8 to 12 weeks.

I have recently used the arthroscope, not only in evaluating the articular surface over the bony defect but also in treatment. In stage III lateral and all stage IV lesions, arthroscopy is initially performed on the ankle by using the portals outlined by Drez et al.[41] Lesions located in the anterior half of the medial or lateral talar domes are easily approached with arthroscopic instruments. The loose fragment can be removed arthroscopically, the bed prepared with a curet and drilling performed, without arthrotomy. Postoperative management is the same as though an arthrotomy had been performed. Lesions in the posterior aspect of the medial and lateral talar domes are accessible through posterior arthroscope portals; however, these are difficult and require considerable care and expertise.[41]

Groups II and V: Shearing and Comminuted Fractures of the Body of the Talus

The distinction between fractures involving the posterior aspect of the talar neck and coronal fractures involving the anterior portion of the talar body may, at times, be difficult. In this section a fracture of the talar body (either coronal, sagittal, or comminuted) is defined as a fracture that involves the superior *articular* surface or trochlea of the talus. Any fracture that lies anterior to this articular surface is classified as a talar neck fracture. Fractures of the neck of the talus tend to exit inferiorly through the insertion of the talocalcaneal interosseous ligament, an area that does not directly involve the articular *surfaces* of the subtalar joint.[29] On the other hand, fractures of the body of the talus exit more posteriorly and usually involve not only the trochlea of the ankle joint but also the posterior facet of the subtalar joint (see Fig 35–53,B).

It is well accepted that the prognosis for displaced fractures of the body of the talus is poor.[27, 89, 144] The importance of distinguishing fractures of the talar neck from fractures of the talar body rests in the poorer prognosis of the later.[27, 89, 144] Indeed, Mindel et al.[89] report a satisfactory result in 64% of fractures of the talar neck with dislocation as compared with only 29% of fractures of the talar body with dislocation.

Because talar body fractures are situated more posteriorly than talar neck fractures are, persistent displacement can result in incongruence in the talotibial joint and a block of dorsiflexion (see Fig 35–57).[143] Due to the fact that the literature does not always clearly distinguish between neck and body fractures, the discussion of the treatment and complications of the two entities will at times be repetitious.

Fractures of the body of the talus compose 13% to 20% of all talar injuries.[27, 45] Fractures of the body of the talus are of two main types: shearing fractures (group II) and compression or comminuted fractures (group V) (see Table 35–3).[144] Shearing fractures can be in either the coronal, sagittal, or horizontal planes (Fig 35–69,A–C). Bonnin[14] mentions the horizontal fracture of the talus, a series of which was first collected by Deetz.[33] In these injuries, a horizontal fracture through the body of the talus permits displacement similar to that present in a subtalar dislocation, with the body of the talus remaining anatomically between the malleoli. According to Bonnin, this displacement occurs either forward, imitating an anterior subtalar dislocation, or medial, which clinically presents as a medial subtalar dislocation.

I have chosen a classification of talar body fractures derived from that presented by Sneppen et al.[144] and by Boyd and Knight (see Tables 35–3 and 35–4).[15] Group II coronal, sagittal, and horizontal shearing fractures are broken into two types: type I, coronal or sagittal shear-

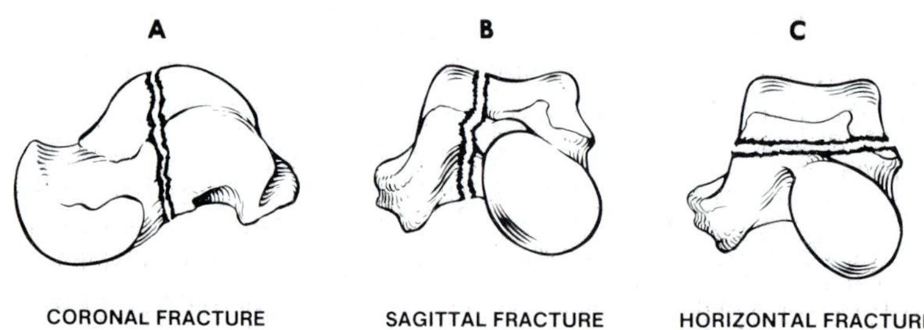

FIG 35–69.
Shearing fractures of the talar body are located in the coronal **(A)**, sagittal **(B)**, and horizontal **(C)** planes.

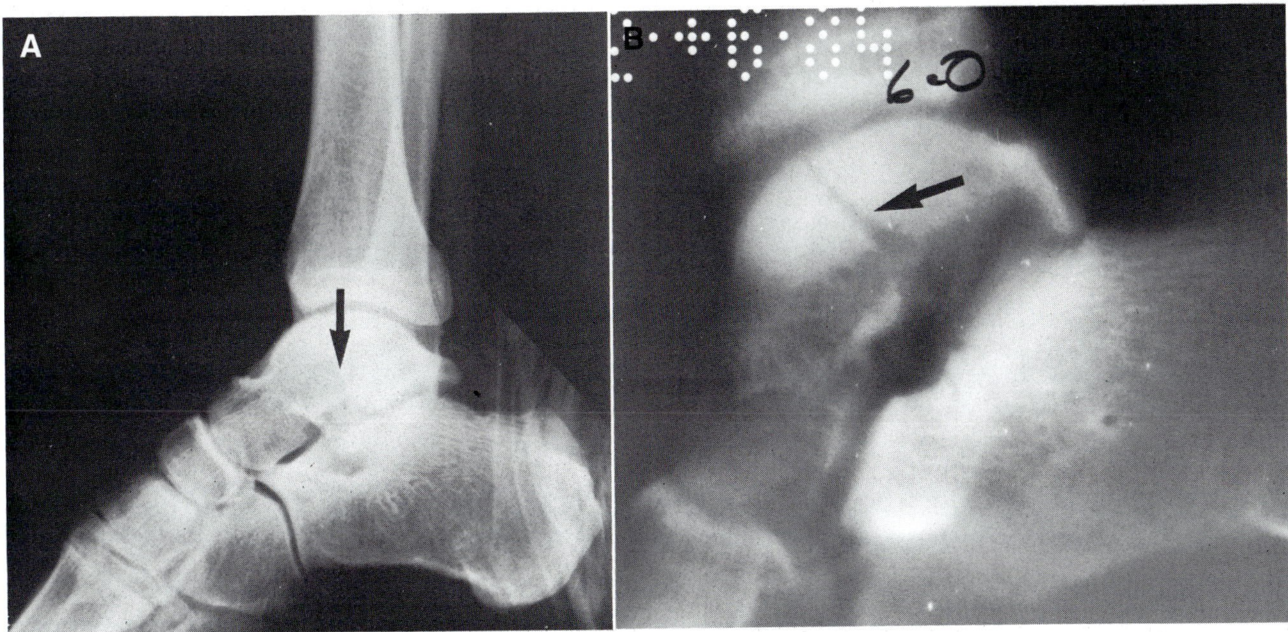

FIG 35–70.
A, coronal shearing fracture of the talar body. **B,** lateral polytomography is necessary to demonstrate the fracture.

ing fractures, and type II, horizontal shearing fractures. Coronal (Fig 35–70) and sagittal (Fig 35–71) fractures (type I) can be simple nondisplaced fractures (type IA), fractures in which there is displacement only at the trochlear articular surfaces (type IB), fractures in which there is displacement at the trochlear articular surface and a dislocation of the subtalar joint (type IC), and finally, displaced fractures in which the talar body fragment is dislocated from the subtalar and talocrural joints (type ID in Table 35–4) (Fig 35–72).

A horizontal shearing talar fracture (type II) can be nondisplaced (type IIA) or displaced (type IIB) (Fig 35–73). Displaced fractures are defined as those in which the fracture surfaces are displaced greater than 3

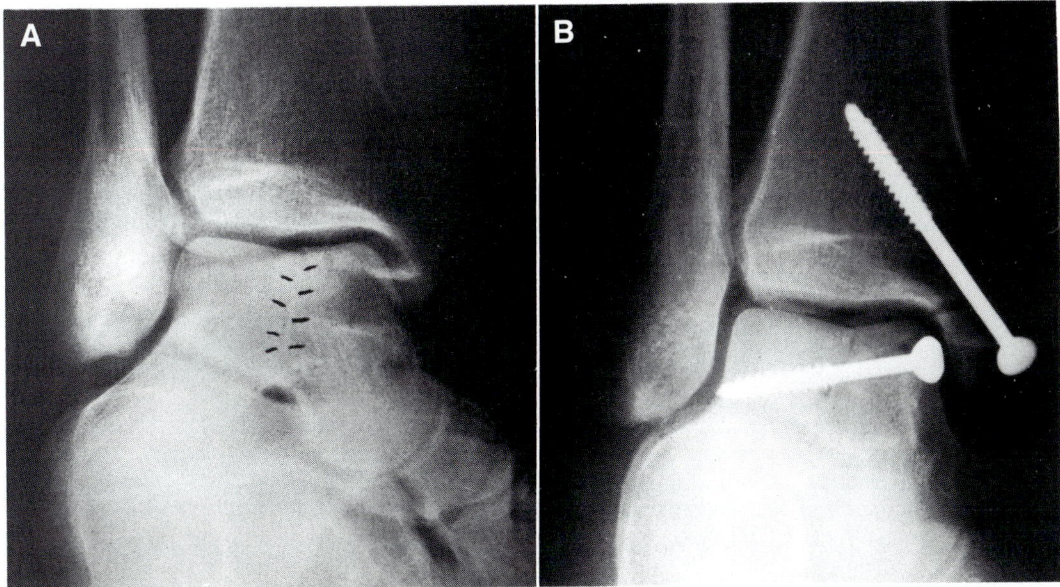

FIG 35–71.
A, sagittal shearing fracture of the talar dome; note the displacement of the articular surface. **B,** treatment by open reduction and internal fixation with a malleolar osteotomy used for exposure.

TABLE 35–4.
Group II: Shearing Fractures of the Talar Body*

Type I: Coronal or sagittal fractures
Type IA—Nondisplaced
Type IB—Fractures with displacement only at the trochlear articular surface
Type IC—Fractures with displacement of the trochlear articular surface plus associated subtalar dislocation
Type ID—Fractures with total dislocation of the talar body
Type II: Horizontal fractures
Type IIA—Nondisplaced
Type IIB—Displaced

*See Figure 35–72.

mm (see Table 35–4). Comminuted fractures, group V (see Table 35–3) on the other hand, can be either displaced or nondisplaced. Talar body fractures are classified as displaced if the trochlear articular surface has a displacement of 3 mm or greater.[144]

Mechanism of Injury

Giannestras and Sammarco[48] report that the mechanism in linear or shear fractures is similar to that encountered in talar neck fractures: an impact on the foot in the completely dorsiflexed position. It is important to emphasize that even though the mechanism for shear-

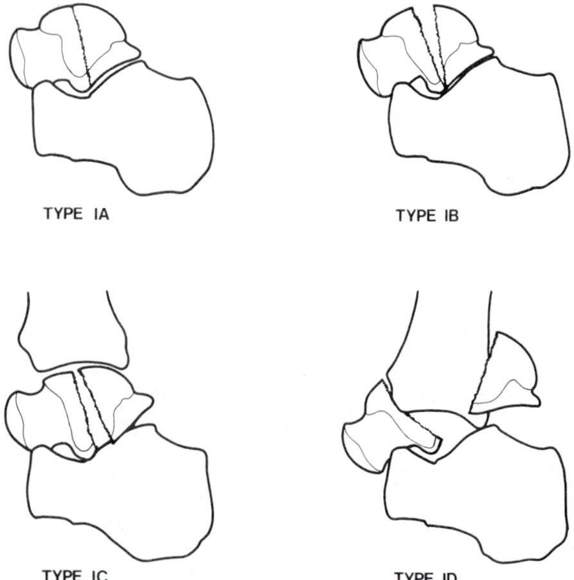

FIG 35–72.
Shearing fractures of the talar body. Type IA fractures are nondisplaced. Type IB fractures are displaced at the talocrural (ankle) articulation. Type IC fractures are displaced at *both* the talocrural (ankle) and subtalar articulations. In type ID fractures, the talar body fragment is completely dislocated.

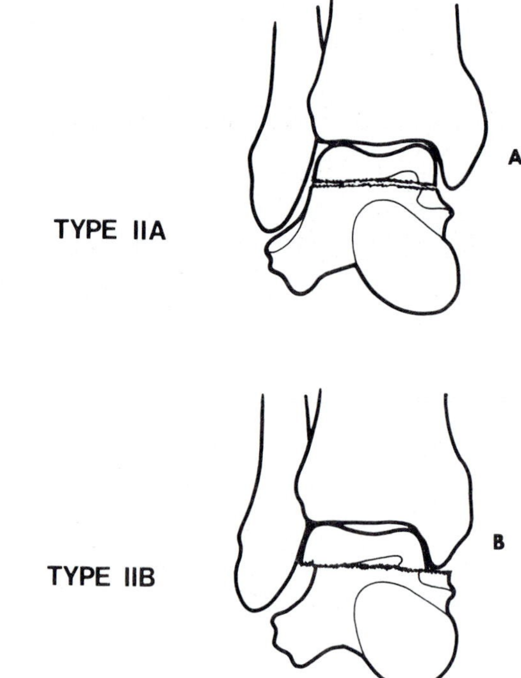

FIG 35–73.
Nondisplaced **(A)** and displaced, **(B)** horizontal shearing fractures of the body of the talus.

type fractures of the body of the talus and fractures of the neck are similar, talar body fractures are located more posteriorly. According to Kleiger,[66] as the foot goes into marked dorsiflexion, the anterior lip of the tibia acts as a wedge across the dome of the talus, which is fractured either in the neck or in the area of the body. As the dorsiflexion continues, dislocation of the talar body occurs in the posterior subtalar joint. As the heel is displaced forward, the posterior capsule of the ankle joint is ruptured. According to Watson-Jones[153] the sustentaculum tali then passes under the medial tubercle of the talus. When dorsiflexion stops and the foot returns to the neutral or equinus position, the medial tubercle of the talus is caught behind the sustentaculum tali, and the body of the talus is pushed posteriorly behind the tibia. This mechanism of injury was also demonstrated by Gibson and Inkster[49] for fractures of the neck of the talus.

When comminution of the talar body exists, it implies that in addition to the excessive dorsiflexion mechanism, a significant compression force is also exerted.[48] These injuries are usually the result of severe trauma such as a fall from a great height. Hence, they are associated with fractures of the calcaneus and the malleoli (Fig 35–74,A and B).[74]

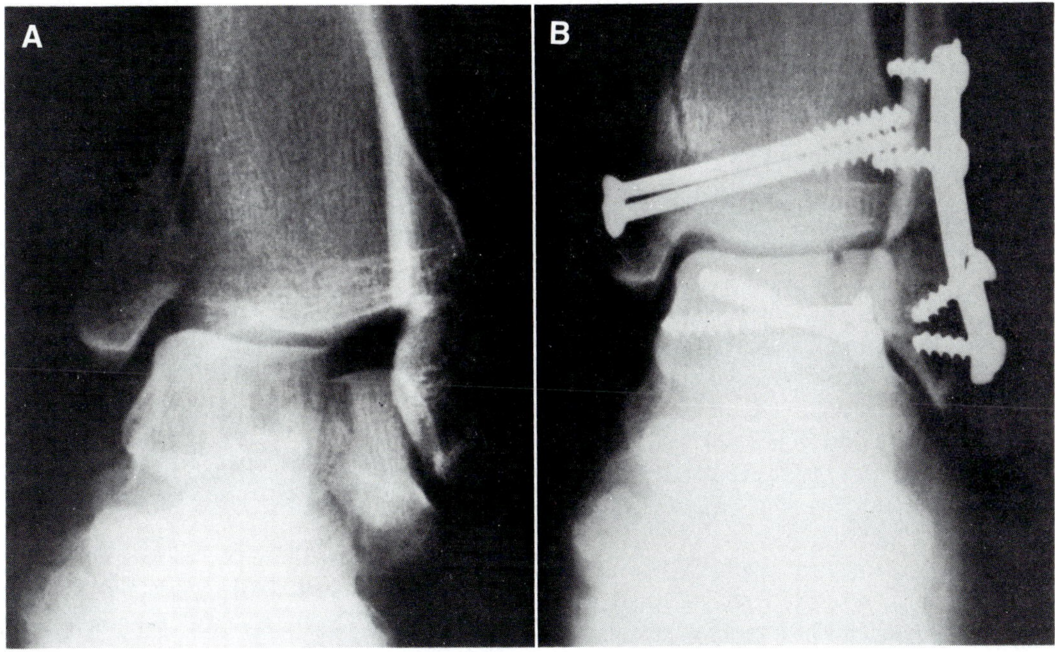

FIG 35–74.
A, sagittal shearing fracture of the talar body associated with a bimalleolar ankle fracture. **B,** treatment by open reduction and internal fixation of the talus with small AO cancellous screws.

Clinical Diagnosis

These patients present with a history of an injury in which the foot is acutely dorsiflexed.[45, 48] This often occurs in a fall from a height or a motor vehicular accident.[27] The patient will complain of pain in the region of the ankle joint, and if the joint capsule about the talus is not ruptured, the pain will be intense.[45]

On physical examination there is marked swelling and tenderness, particularly over the anterior aspect of the ankle.[15, 45, 89] Since these fractures involve both the ankle and the subtalar joints, inversion and eversion of the subtalar joint in addition to dorsiflexion and plantar flexion of the ankle are extremely painful. As with other injuries to the talus, the force dissipated at the time of injury is substantial, and it is not uncommon for these fracture-dislocations to be associated with open wounds.[45] If the injury is closed, however, circulation to the overlying skin is often compromised.[89]

Radiographic diagnosis

Routine anteroposterior, lateral, and oblique radiographs of the ankle are necessary to evaluate these injuries.[45, 48, 66] In all fractures of the talar body, particularly those that appear to be simple and nondisplaced, careful roentgenographic evaluation of the subtalar joint is essential to make certain that a subluxation of the subtalar joint is not missed.[66] Displacement at the site of a talar body fracture rarely occurs without an associated subtalar dislocation or subluxation.

Giannestras and Sammarco[48] note that the pain associated with these injuries may make it impossible to position the patient properly to obtain the necessary roentgenographs. Therefore, they suggest that final radiographs used for the evaluation of the fracture and for treatment planning be taken in the operating room with the patient under anesthesia in order that the correct views may be taken.

Minimally displaced fractures of the body of the talus may be difficult to detect on routine films, so polytomography (see Fig 35–70,B) or a CAT scan can be used to confirm the diagnosis and determine displacement.

Treatment of Group II Fractures

Type I: Coronal or Sagittal Fractures

Type IA & IB: Nondisplaced and Minimally Displaced Fractures.—Nondisplaced (type IA) or minimally displaced (type IB) coronal or sagittal shear fractures of the body of the talus (i.e., those with less than 2- or 3-mm displacement at the trochlear articular surface) are best treated conservatively with a short-leg non–weight-bearing cast for 6 to 8 weeks or until fracture union occurs.[15, 42, 45, 48, 111] Mindel et al.[89] report that union occurs in 2 to 3 months with this method of treatment.

Type IC: Displaced Fractures with Subtalar Dislocation.—In displaced shear fractures, associated subtalar dislocation is *usually* present and must be detected (type IC) (see Fig 35–72). In displaced fractures the goal of treatment is anatomic reduction of both the displaced fracture and the subtalar joint.[42] Results of displaced intra-articular fractures of the body of the talus are dependent upon exact reduction and stable internal fixation.[144] Kleiger[66] reports that in five of his eight patients with displaced fractures of the talar body, the posterior subtalar joint was also dislocated. Reduction by *closed* manipulation is attempted under general or spinal anesthesia with the knee flexed to 90 degrees and the foot held in equinus. Traction is exerted on the foot by grasping both the heel and the forepart of the foot, while countertraction is maintained at the thigh. While this traction is maintained, pressure is exerted with the thumb on the sole of the foot at the level of the displacement in an attempt to manipulate the fragments into position. Dunn et al.[42] caution against repeated forcible attempts at a closed reduction; instead they prefer open reduction as recommended by Boyd and Knight.[15]

Kleiger[66] cautions that the reduction of these fractures must be accurate because any remaining displacement in the superior articular surface may cause the distal fragment to abut against the anterior margin of the articular surface of the distal end of the tibia and thereby block dorsiflexion. For this reason he emphasizes the importance of an absolutely true lateral roentgenograph postreduction to evaluate talar body reduction.

Watson-Jones[153] advocated that the foot be kept in equinus following reduction to prevent recurrence of the subtalar displacement. Kleiger,[66] however, believes that once properly reduced, the fragments are stable in the neutral position. Following reduction, immobilization in a non–weight-bearing short-leg cast is recommended until union occurs.[66, 153]

Type ID: Fractures With Complete Dislocation of the Talar Body.—In fractures of the talar body in which there is complete dislocation of the body from both the subtalar and ankle mortise (type ID) (see Fig 35–72), Watson-Jones[153] recommended closed reduction. The calcaneus is distracted from the tibia by traction on the calcaneus with the foot in equinus. The displaced fragment is then replaced by pressure of the fingers on the displaced fragment. Watson-Jones suggested that a metal pin can be inserted into the talar fragment and used to manipulate it into position, while Kleiger[66] believes that using such a pin is not indicated because it might further damage the articular cartilage.

Giannestras and Sammarco[48] recommend open reduction of these fractures after one attempt at closed reduction. Garcia and Parkes[45] prefer a medial incision with an accompanying transverse osteotomy of the medial malleolus because it provides excellent exposure of the talus and facilitates internal fixation. Additionally, this approach does not violate the deltoid ligament with its accompanying vascular supply to the talar body.[42] Once the fracture is reduced, two Kirschner wires are driven from the talar neck into the body, and the medial malleolus is reattached with a screw.[44, 48] Following open reduction, a cast extending from the toes to the midthigh with the knee in 25 degrees of flexion and the foot in 25 degrees of equinus is applied. The Kirschner wires are removed at 4 weeks. Weight bearing is not permitted until there is x-ray evidence of fracture union, usually in 12 to 16 weeks.

Dunn et al.[42] and Kleiger[66] suggest a lateral approach to avoid further damage to the medial artery to the talar body and to avoid the traumatized skin medially that overlies the displaced fragment.[42, 66] A Kirschner wire in the calcaneus during open reduction to supply the distraction needed for the reduction is helpful.[66] Once the reduction is obtained, Kleiger recommends the use of screw fixation from the outer surface of the distal portion of the neck into the body of the talus, while Dunn et al.[42] use Kirschner wire fixation. Kleiger[66] suggests subtalar arthrodesis in these cases in addition to open reduction to eliminate later disability and also supply an additional source of circulation to the talus, which he feels most likely will undergo aseptic necrosis. However, subtalar arthrodesis to improve circulation has not been found to be successful by other authors.[18]

Type II: Horizontal Fractures.—Little is written regarding treatment of horizontal shear fractures (type II)[13, 33] According to Bonnin[13] these fractures can be best reduced by lateral pressure combined with skeletal traction. Immobilization in a short-leg cast is utilized until union is present. He reports that aseptic necrosis is more likely to occur in these fractures than in fractures of the talar neck.

Treatment of Group V: Comminuted Fractures of the Body of the Talus

Nondisplaced Fractures.—Pennal[111] recommends mobilization in a short-leg cast for 4 to 6 weeks for nondisplaced comminuted fractures. Boyd and Knight[15] also recommend cast immobilization for comminuted fractures of the body of the talus without displacement.

They caution, however, that even without displacement, later subtalar or ankle arthritis may necessitate arthrodesis.

Displaced Fractures.—Due to the mechanism of injury, most comminuted talar body fractures are severely displaced and rarely result in a good ankle.[48, 111] Treatment recommendations in this group depend upon the degree of comminution and displacement. Boyd and Knight[15] emphasize that it is impractical to attempt open reduction in a severely comminuted fracture and suggest talectomy as the only logical treatment. However, they emphasize that a talectomy alone usually results in poor function due to pain on weight bearing, instability, and a lack of endurance, and for this reason, they prefer a tibiocalcaneal fusion after talectomy. Dunn et al.[42] also recommend primary tibiocalcaneal fusion rather than talectomy because of the poor results following simple talectomy noted by other authors.[20, 83, 87, 111, 132]

Pennal[111] also prefers tibiocalcaneal fusion but waits until the third or fourth week postinjury in grossly comminuted and displaced fractures.[111] Giannestras and Sammarco[48] treat such patients initially with splint immobilization and elevation in bed. Once the acute reaction to injury has subsided and the soft tissues are able to safely tolerate an operative procedure, they recommend pantalar arthrodesis if the comminution is not too severe. Alternatively, they recommend tibiocalcaneal fusion in 5 degrees of plantar flexion for those patients in whom the fracture is extremely comminuted.

Blair,[10] Dennis and Tullos,[36] and Lionberger et al.[78] recommend the Blair fusion for patients with a comminuted fracture of the body of the talus. Because the head and neck of the talus, which contain the anterior middle facets of the subtalar joint, are usually not involved in these fractures, Blair recommends leaving the head and neck of the talus in situ. A sliding bone graft is taken from the anterior aspect of the tibia and placed into the neck of the talus to effect a tibiotalar fusion. The principal advantages of this procedure are that the foot has a more normal appearance and some motion remains in the talonavicular, calcaneocuboid, and anterior talocalcaneal joints. The patient is therefore not left with a completely rigid foot and a short limb as in a tibiocalcaneal fusion.[10, 36] Further discussion of the technique of the Blair fusion is in the section on talar neck fractures.

Results

The only chance for good long-term results following these fractures hinges upon early anatomic reduction and stable internal fixation.[144] Sneppen et al.[144] concluded that results in talar body fractures are directly related to the severity of the initial injury. They emphasize that if at the time of initial injury there had been subluxation and articular damage to the subtalar and talotibial joints, a grave long-term prognosis is likely. Kleiger[66] emphasizes that good results following talar body fractures decrease as one progresses from a nondisplaced fracture to a fracture with complete talar body dislocation.

Complications

The most important complications following fractures of the talar body are aseptic necrosis, nonunion, malunion, stiffness, and osteoarthritis involving the ankle and/or subtalar joint.

Aseptic Necrosis.—The incidence of aseptic necrosis following a coronal fracture of the talar body has been reported to be higher than that following talar neck fractures.[144] This might be explained by the fact that the fracture line occurs more posteriorly and may exit through the insertion of the deltoid ligament medially into the talus, thereby disrupting a source of blood supply to the body of the talus that may remain intact in most talar neck fractures.[90, 99, 133] Also, the more posterior in the body the fracture occurs, the more chance there is for disruption of intraosseous vascular anastomoses.[34]

The incidence of aseptic necrosis in the individual groups of coronal shearing fractures (i.e., nondisplaced [IA and IB], displaced with subtalar dislocation [IC], and displaced with a completely dislocated talar body [ID]) has not been documented in the literature. Mindel et al.[89] report that 25% of patients with nondisplaced shearing-type fractures developed aseptic necrosis. They also report that aseptic necrosis developed in 50% of patients with fractures of the talar body and dislocation. They did not, however, distinguish between dislocation of the subtalar joint and complete dislocation of the talar body. Sneppen et al.[144] report that aseptic necrosis occurred in 5 of 13 displaced shearing fractures.

Garcia and Parkes, quoting Hawkins, report an incidence of aseptic necrosis of 40% to 50% in patients with talar body fractures in which there is an associated subtalar dislocation, and if the talar body fragment is completely dislocated, the necrosis incidence rises to 90%. It must be remembered, however, that Hawkins' work is based upon fractures of the neck of the talus, fractures more distal than those being discussed here.

Finally, Bonnin[14] reports that particularly in horizontal shearing fractures of the body, the incidence of aseptic necrosis is much higher than in talar neck fractures.

The incidence of aseptic necrosis following crush-type fractures is not well documented, partly because so many of these fractures are treated primarily by excision. However, Sneppen et al.[144] reported that three of four patients with comminuted fractures developed aseptic necrosis.

It is important to remember that even though aseptic necrosis develops, up to 50% of patients may have little disability.[42, 45] The principles of the diagnosis, treatment, and prognosis of aseptic necrosis of the talus are more thoroughly discussed in the section on talar neck fractures.

Delayed Nonunion.—Mindel et al.[89] report that all of the patients with fractures of the body of the talus healed in an average of 3.4 months. However, union time was delayed in fractures with complete displacement and those that developed aseptic necrosis. Garcia and Parkes[45] also note a delay in union in displaced fractures of an average of 5 months as compared with 8 to 10 weeks when the talar body is undisplaced.[45]

Malunion and Osteoarthritis.—In a retrospective analysis, Sneppen et al.[144] report that one third of displaced talar body fractures were inadequately reduced. This suggests the need to more critically analyze postreduction roentgenographs. Indeed, Kleiger[66] stresses the importance of evaluating the reduction on a *true lateral* roentgenograph to determine whether or not the superior articular surface of the talus is satisfactorily aligned. If it is not, a malunion will result in limited dorsiflexion of the ankle. The malunion also results in a step-off on the trochlear articular surface that can lead to arthritic changes in the ankle. Additionally, any residual displacement at this fracture site suggests residual subtalar subluxation and, hence, long-term disability (see Fig 35–54,A).

Boyd and Knight[15] caution that traumatic arthritis involving the subtalar joint may develop following acceptable reduction and union. They compare this with the subtalar arthritis seen following a well-reduced os calcis fracture in which minor disturbances remain at the articular surface in spite of a good reduction. They emphasize that these minor disturbances in the subtalar joint may not be seen roentgenographically but may produce significant discomfort in the subtalar area. Coltart[27] also mentions late subtalar osteoarthritis following nondisplaced fractures of the talar body.

Sneppen et al.[144] documented that fractures that united with displacement resulted in osteoarthritis of the talocrural and/or subtalar joints. Additionally, 75% of fractures that united without displacement resulted in osteoarthritis changes. The importance of the direct relationship between osteoarthritis, malunion, and subluxation as documented by these authors must be emphasized.

Other complications that may occur following talar body fracture include persistent infection, skin loss, and scar sensitivity following open fractures. A detailed discussion of these complications is included in the section on fractures of the talar neck.

Author's Preferred Method of Treatment

For open fractures of the talar body, management of the open wound is performed as outlined under the section on open fractures of the talus. The fractures are then managed individually as described below.

Group II: Shear Fractures.—Shearing fractures of the talar body in the coronal or sagittal plane are evaluated roentgenographically to determine the degree of displacement at the ankle articular surface. I have found polytomography particularly useful in evaluating the degree of displacement at the articular surface (see Fig 35–70,B). In those fractures that are truly nondisplaced or in which the displacement is only 1 to 2 mm, I immobilize the ankle in the neutral position and keep the patient non–weight-bearing until fracture union is noted.

In fractures with minimal displacement at the ankle articular surface and no subtalar dislocation (i.e., in the range of 2 to 3 mm), I prefer closed reduction by the technique described later under image intensification. I consider percutaneous Kirschner wire fixation essential following reduction to maintain stability. Patients are kept non–weight-bearing in a short-leg splint. If stable fixation is obtained by percutaneous fixation, the posterior splint is removed and early range-of-motion exercises instituted. After motion has been restored, a short-leg non–weight-bearing cast is applied. Weight bearing is allowed only when union is present. The Kirschner wires are removed at 4 to 6 weeks.

Fractures of the body of the talus with more than 3-mm displacement but without associated subtalar dislocation are extremely rare, and displacement at the talar articular surface of this magnitude usually requires subluxation of the subtalar joint. These patients should be treated by closed reduction with critical evaluation of both the subtalar joint and the articular surface of the ankle joint in the post reduction radiographs. Percutaneous Kirschner wire fixation or compression screw fixation of these fractures is performed. If good stability is obtained with either type of fixation, early inversion and eversion exercises are encouraged with the patient in a posterior splint that is removed for these exercises. Once motion has been restored, immobilization in a non–weight-bearing short-leg cast at 90 degrees is used until union occurs.

Shearing fractures of the body of the talus with associated subtalar dislocation are reduced by closed reduction. General or spinal anesthesia is preferred. The knee is flexed 90 degrees over the patient's bed. Longitudinal traction on the heel and forefoot, plantar flexion, and an anterior force applied to the heel will usually reduce the fracture. The reduction is monitored under image intensification. It is important that the postreduction films be evaluated for residual subtalar and ankle joint displacement. Anatomic reduction is essential. Once the reduction has been obtained, percutaneous Kirschner wire fixation or fixation with an AO compression screw across the fracture site is utilized (see Figs 35–71,A and B and 35–74,A and B). Postoperative management is the same as mentioned above.

Patients who present with a talar body fracture and complete dislocation of the body are considered surgical emergencies. I do not attempt a closed reduction in these patients because this has been unsuccessful in my hands. In the operating room, after the limb has been prepared and draped, a sterile Steinmann pin is placed through the calcaneus to be used for traction during the open reduction. I prefer a medial surgical approach and osteotomize the medial malleolus to improve exposure. Due to the fact that the talar body is displaced and may be rotated on its deltoid pedicle, I consider these an emergency in an effort to reduce the fracture before the vessels remaining in the deltoid ligament thrombose (see Fig 35–56). After malleolar osteotomy, the talus is manipulated back into position. Once an anatomic reduction has been obtained, the fracture is stabilized by utilizing AO screws or Kirschner wires. The choice of internal fixation depends upon the associated soft-tissue injury. Crossed Kirschner wires are easier to insert and require less dissection. However, they do not provide the stability of an AO cancellous screw.

Following open reduction in these injuries, the limb is placed in a short-leg non–weight-bearing cast. If the fracture is stable, the cast is bivalved and the patient allowed to remove the cast and institute early range of motion of the ankle, subtalar, and midtarsal joints. Weight bearing is not allowed until there is x-ray evidence of fracture union. Once fracture union is obtained, weight bearing is begun.

After fractures of the talar body, patients undergo serial roentgenographs to detect aseptic necrosis as soon as possible. The diagnosis and treatment of aseptic necrosis after a fracture of the talus is discussed completely in the section on talar neck fractures.

Group V: Comminuted Fractures.—For comminuted fractures of the body of the talus in which displacement is minimal, I prefer closed treatment. A short-leg non–weight-bearing cast is utilized until there is evidence of fracture healing. If the fracture fragments are stable, early range of motion is instituted by using a removable posterior splint. These patients are kept non–weight-bearing until there is evidence of fracture healing.

In severely comminuted and displaced fractures of the body of the talus, I prefer the Blair fusion to a tibiocalcaneal arthrodesis. In my opinion, there is no place for a talectomy as a definitive form of treatment in these injuries. If the injury is open and severely contaminated or if the overlying skin is compromised, a talectomy is performed as an *initial* procedure. When the soft tissue has healed, a Blair fusion is performed by using the technique described in the section on talar neck fractures.

Group III: Fractures of the Posterior Process of the Talus

Fractures of the Lateral Tubercle of the Posterior Process

Cloquet in 1844 was the first to describe a fracture of the lateral tubercle of the posterior process.[24] Shepherd in 1882 described an additional three cases in the English literature, and the fracture has subsequently come to be known as "Shepherd's fracture."[136] Although Giannestras and Sammarco[48] report that this fracture is uncommon, Sneppen et al.[144] found fractures of the posterior tubercle to represent 20% of all fractures of the talar body.

Anatomy.—The posterior process of the talus is composed of the posterolateral and posteromedial tubercles, which are separated by the sulcus for the flexor hallucis longus tendon (see Fig 35–51,C and E).[130] The posterolateral tubercle is larger and more prominent than the posteromedial tubercle. The size of the posterolateral tubercle varies from a barely perceptible structure to a well-developed tubercle projecting posterolaterally from the talus (Fig 35–75,A and B).[130]

The superior surface of the posterolateral tubercle is nonarticular and provides insertion for the posterior talofibular ligament and the talar component of the fibuloastragalocalcaneal ligament.[130] The inferior surface is in continuity with the posterior calcaneal articular surface of the talus.

Os Trigonum.—An accessory bone, the os trigonum, can be found in association with the posterolateral tubercle. Howse[58] stresses that the os trigonum varies in size and one that appears to be small radiographically may indeed be much larger because of the cartilage present around the bony nucleus (see Fig 35–76,A and B).

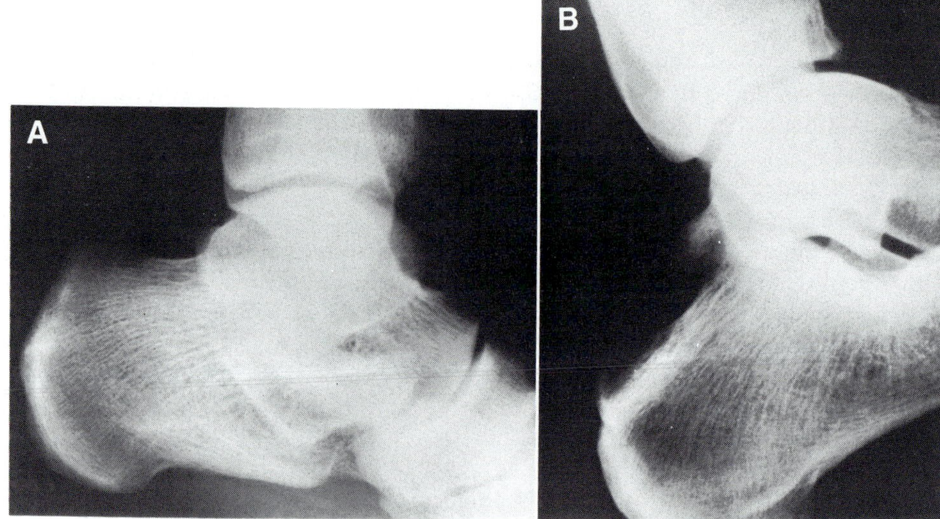

FIG 35–75.
The size of the posterolateral tubercle varies from being nearly absent **(A)**, to a large prominent process **(B)**.

Rosenmuller[129] was the first to describe the os trigonum in 1804. According to Sarrafian,[130] the frequency of occurrence varies from 1.7% to 7.7% in the literature. The os trigonum can be present unilaterally or bilaterally and can be fused to the talus or calcaneus.[62] Geist[47] found seven cases of unilateral os trigonum separated from the talus, with three of the seven having a large posterior process of the talus in the *opposite* foot. He also noted 12 cases of large posterior processes, 4 of which were bilateral. Burman and Lapidus[16] report that an os trigonum, either fused or separated, occurs in 50% of all feet. They found the os trigonum to be unilateral in 10% of cases. Fewer than 1% had a free os trigonum on one side and a fused os trigonum on the other, while 17% of patients had bilaterally fused ossa trigona (i.e., the trigonal process).

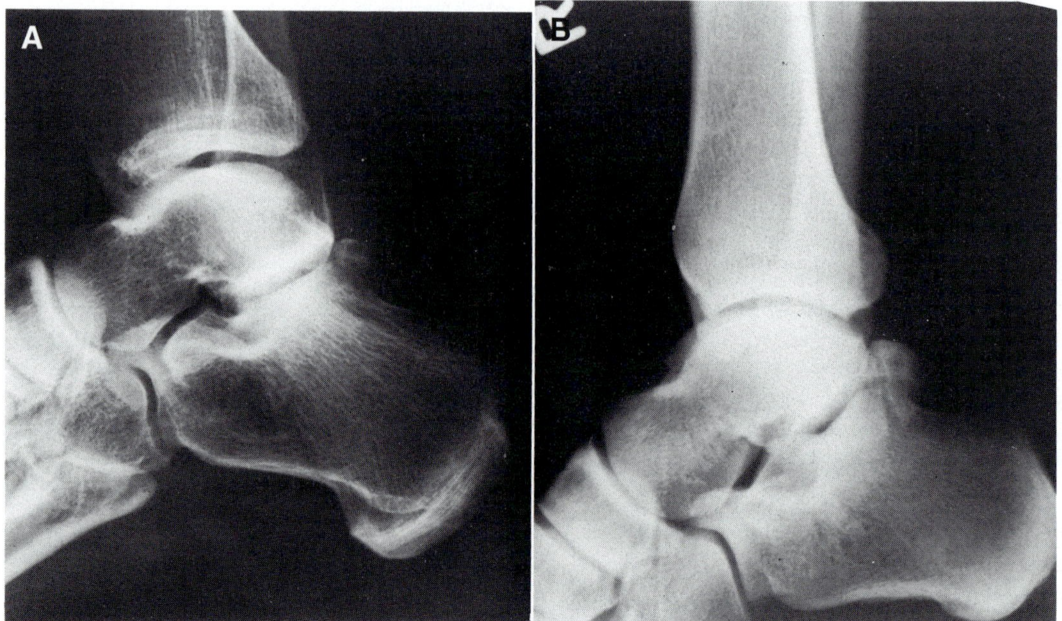

FIG 35–76.
The os trigonum varies greatly in size from a small oval structure with smooth surfaces **(A)** to a large structure involving more of the subtalar joint **(B)**.

According to Sarrafian 10.9% of tali have a separated ossicle in the region of the os trigonum.

This ossicle presents three surfaces: anterior, inferior, and posterior. The anterior surface connects with the posterolateral tubercle by fibrous, fibrocartilaginous, or cartilaginous tissue (Fig 35–77). The inferior surface of the os trigonum articulates with the os calcis.[130] The posterior surface is nonarticular and serves as the point of attachment for structures that insert on the posterior tubercle.

The relationship of the os trigonum to the posterior tubercle varies from complete separation to complete fusion. The separation can include a notch in the margin of the posterior lateral tubercle, a groove on the articular surface, or a complete separation. A fused os trigonum called the trigonal process, appears as a very large posterolateral tubercle (see Fig 35–75,B).[130]

The os trigonum has created a problem in differential diagnosis since its original description.[136] Indeed, Shepherd reported a talus fracture in which he described a fragment located posterior to the talus, lateral to the groove for the flexor hallucis longus.[136] He believed that this fragment of bone was torn off by the posterior fasciculus of the talofibular ligament. He did not believe that this could represent an ununited apophysis since he believed that there was only one ossific center for the talus. However, he was unable to reproduce this fracture

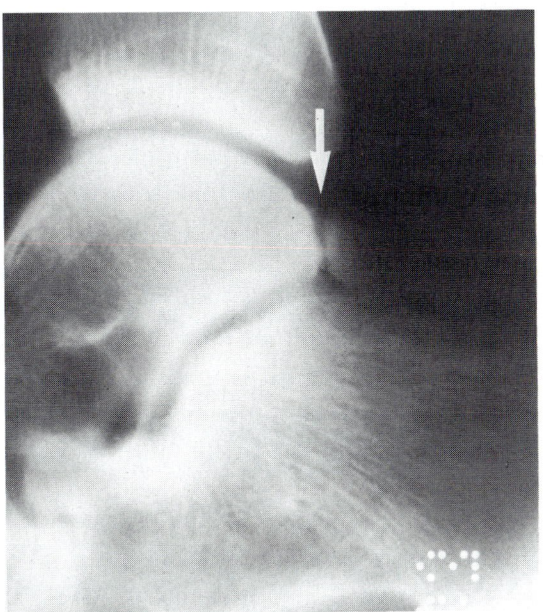

FIG 35–77.
A lateral tomogram clearly demonstrates a fibrous connection *(arrow)* between the posterolateral tubercle and the os trigonum. Note the sclerotic margin of the adjacent os trigonum and posterolateral tubercle of the talus. The width of the fibrous connection does not suggest disruption.

in cadavar specimens. Turner,[150] in the same year, presented the theory that the os trigonum was a secondary center of development and cited other references that agreed with his theory. Kohler and Zimmer,[70] noting the confusion among clinicians as to whether the free ossicle represents a fracture of a fused os trigonum or developmental failure of fusion of a secondary ossification center in the talus, reported that the os trigonum is actually embraced on both sides by the posterior process of the talus. They believed that the posterior process is actually made up of the lateral tubercle *and* the os trigonum, both of which may unite to form the trigonal process.

McDougall,[82] in an excellent anatomic study of the talus, reports that the lateral tubercle is usually the larger and is commonly referred to as the posterior process, although not infrequently the medial tubercle may be as large. He stresses that the tubercles vary considerably in size from small processes hardly discernible on a lateral radiograph to a prominent posterior projection. He found that in early childhood the posterior border of the talus is rounded without the projection seen in the adult talus. Secondary centers of ossification for the medial and lateral tubercles appear at the posterior margin of the talus between the ages of 8 and 11 years. These quickly unite with the main bone, usually within a year of their appearance. McDougall[82] notes that the lateral secondary center of ossification may be prevented from uniting with the main body of the talus and may thereby produce an os trigonum, but that this occurs infrequently. Instead, he notes an *increased* incidence of the so-called os trigonum associated with age. He believes that the os trigonum is secondary to repeated trauma that results in fracture of the fused os trigonum or posterior process of the talus. Indeed, Paulos et al.[110] suggest that athletic patients have an increased incidence of posterior process fractures, with a number of these progressing to asymptomatic nonunion that suggests an os trigonum.

Shelton and Pedowitz[135] attempt to distinguish a fracture of the posterior tubercle from the os trigonum. They too believe that the os trigonum arises from failure of fusion of a secondary center of ossification on the posterior aspect of the talus with the body of the talus. They believe that the os trigonum does not involve the subtalar or ankle joint and that its separation rarely causes symptoms. However, Sarrafian[130] points out that the inferior aspect of the os trigonum contains an articular surface for the posterior talocalcaneal joint.

Therefore, in the adult, the os trigonum may represent either a failure of fusion of the secondary center of ossification or a fracture of a the lateral tubercle of the posterior process that develops a nonunion.[82, 99, 110] To add to the confusion, a true os trigonum may become symptomatic due to disruption of its fibrous or fibrocartilaginous attachment to the posterior process of the talus.[61] Indeed, Moeller[91] has documented pain in the area of an established os trigonum secondary to increased activity.

The medial tubercle of the posterior process is also variable in size.[82] It provides attachment to the deep and superficial layers of the talotibial component of the deltoid ligament and forms a medial wall of the tunnel for the flexor hallucis longus.[21] According to Sarrafian,[130] this tubercle may rarely be very large, extended down over the os calcis, and contribute to a talocalcaneal coalition.

Mechanism of Injury.—Two mechanisms of injury to the lateral tubercle of the posterior process of the talus have been presented. First, forced plantar flexion of the foot causes direct impingement of the posterior tibial plafond on the posterolateral process. This forced plantar flexion may result in a fracture of the posterolateral process, separation through the fibrous attachment of an os trigonum, or if the os trigonum is attached to the talus by bone, a fracture of the resulting trigonal process.[53, 61, 66]

The second theory is that excessive dorsiflexion of the ankle that results in increased tension in the posterior talofibular ligament may avulse the lateral tubercle of the posterior facet.[85] The occurrence of this fracture in an athlete suffering twisting injuries of the ankle helps to support this mechanism.[85, 110]

Clinical Diagnosis.—A careful history and physical examination are important to differentiate a fracture of a lateral process or a fused os trigonum, a disruption of the fibrous attachment of an os trigonum to the body of the talus, and an asymptomatic os trigonum. Only if the physical examination correlates with the roentgenographic findings is damage or injury to the lateral tubercle or os trigonum confirmed.

The patient usually gives a history of sudden uncontrolled injury to the foot, such as catching the heel on a step when going down stairs.[82] McDougall[82] notes that forced equinus from kicking a football may be responsible for the injury. Moeller[91] emphasizes that a history of repetitive microtrauma secondary to a rapid increase in weight, activity, or change to a more strenuous routine may be present in the patient with a painful os trigonum. This microtrauma can lead to disruption of the fibrous attachment of the os trigonum to the body of the talus.

Patients usually complain of pain with mild swelling in the posterior aspect of the ankle.[29] The pain may be accentuated by running, jumping, or descending stairs, and symptoms of giving way may be present.[110] Schrock[132] emphasizes that pain aggravated by walking downhill or squatting on a plantar-flexed foot is suggestive of a posterior process fracture.

The clinical picture may be as helpful as the serrated edge of a fragment noted roentgenographically in diagnosing a fracture of the os trigonum or posterior process.[60] Clinically, tenderness is present anterior to the Achilles tendon and posterior to the talus.[61] A circumscribed area of ecchymosis just anterior to the Achilles tendon may be noted 24 to 48 hours following an acute injury.[85] Crepitation may be heard or felt with plantar flexion of the foot.[60] Pain is increased when plantar flexion stress is applied to the foot.[110] Pain can also be accentuated by resisted plantar flexion or dorsiflexion of the great toe due to the presence of the flexor hallucis longus tendon in the groove between the fractured lateral tubercle and the medial tubercle of the posterior process.[29, 61, 110, 130]

Associated ligamentous instability is usually not clinically detectable.[110] Hamilton utilizes an injection of 1 cc of lidocaine into the affected area for temporary relief of symptoms in an effort to confirm the diagnosis. This is particularly useful in a patient with the clinical findings of a posterior process fracture in a radiograph suggesting an os trigonum.

Radiographic Diagnosis.—A lateral radiographic view of the ankle best demonstrates the lateral tubercle of the posterior process of the talus and the os trigonum. It is well known that the os trigonum, following a plantar flexion injury, can become symptomatic due to disruption of its fibrous attachment to the main body of the talus.[99] Although many authors have emphasized the importance of differentiating the os trigonum (which can be a normal variant noted roentgenographically) from a fracture of the posterior process, if the patient has a history of injury and the clinical findings suggestive of an injury to the posterior process, this roentgenographic differentiation may not be so important. Indeed, Jensenius[61] stresses that differentiating between an os trigonum and a fracture in the symptomatic patient is of minor *practical* importance because the indications for excision in both instances are similar.

However, if roentgenographic differentiation is important because of a *lack* of clinical correlation, Kohler describes the os trigonum as a round, oval and three-cornered bone located behind the talus (see Fig 35–76,A).[69] On the other hand, in acute fracture of the posterior process of the talus, the fracture surfaces should be rough and irregular (Fig 35–78). Due to the fact that the os trigonum is reported to be unilateral in

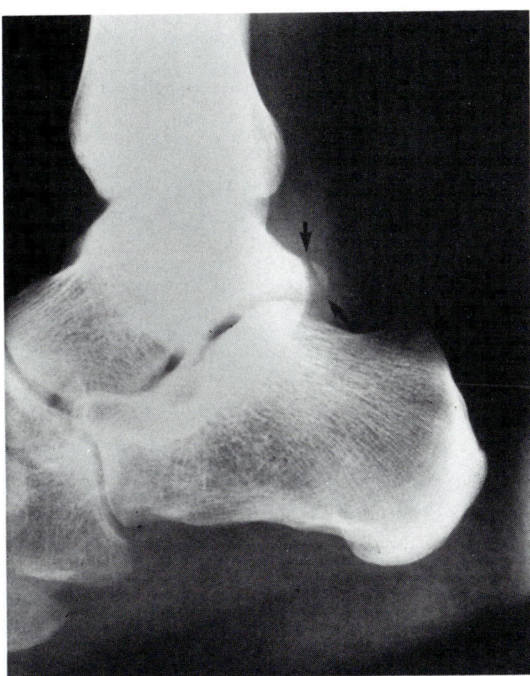

FIG 35–78.
Fracture of the posterior tubercle of the talus *(arrow)*.

over two thirds of cases,[47, 82] comparison radiographs may not be of value.

Paulos et al.[110] suggest the use of a special 30-degree subtalar oblique view to help distinguish between an acute fracture and an os trigonum. They find that a posterior process fracture is generally larger and extends further into the body of the talus. In an acute fracture they report that the fracture line is very different from the smooth, rounded, well-corticated os trigonum (see Fig 35–76,A).[110]

I have found lateral polytomograms useful to delineate the connection between the posterior lateral process of the talus and the os trigonum (see Fig 35–77). However, they rarely confirm disruption of the fibrous attachment of the os trigonum to the posterolateral process of the talus. Paulos et al.[110] were the first to show that the definitive distinction between a normal os trigonum, a traumatic separation of a normal os trigonum through its fibrous attachment to the talus, and a fractured posterior process of the talus can be made with a technetium bone scan. A positive technetium bone scan was present in all patients with fracture of the posterior process and in those with disruption of the fibrous attachment of the os trigonum to the talus. However, it was negative in patients with a normal, asymptomatic os trigonum (Fig 35–79,A and B). This can be quite helpful in determining whether the os trigonum is responsible for a patient's posterior ankle pain.

Treatment.—The recommended treatment of acute fractures of the posterior process of the talus is conservative.[29] Giannestras and Sammarco[48] suggest immobilization in a short-leg walking cast with the foot in 15 degrees of equinus for 4 to 6 weeks. Because the fracture involves the weight-bearing surface, Sneppen et

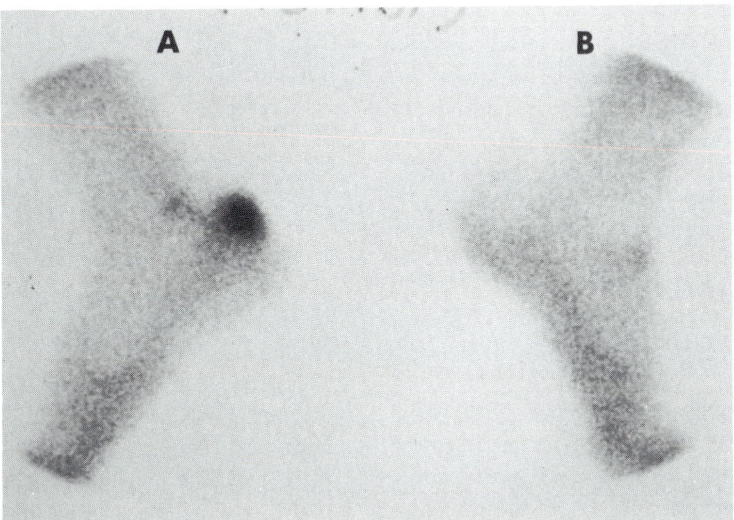

FIG 35–79.
Technetium bone scan of both feet of a patient with bilateral os trigonum on radiography. The bone scan is positive over the area of the right os trigonum **(A)** and negative over the left **(B).** This confirms the presence of disruption of the fibrous attachment between the talus and the os trigonum in the right foot. (From Paulos LE, Johnson CL, Noyes FR: *Am J Sports Med* 11:439–443, 1983. Used by permission.)

al.[144] do not permit weight bearing until the fracture has healed. Even if a nonunion results, the fragment should not be removed unless the patient complains of persistent pain in the region of the fragment.[48] Paulos et al.[110] recommend casting for 6 weeks following an acute injury. For a chronic injury, they also suggest conservative treatment in a short-leg cast initially. However, if symptoms persist for longer than 4 to 6 months after the initiation of conservative treatment in either acute or chronic injuries, they recommend surgical removal of the fragment.

Shelton and Pedowitz[135] suggest that anatomic reduction and rigid internal fixation by open methods followed by early range of motion would be the *ideal* treatment for a *large* fracture of the posterior process of the talus that involves a significant portion of the articular surface of the posterior facet of the subtalar joint. They concede, however, that this technique has not been reported and would be technically difficult. They therefore recommend plaster immobilization and non–weight bearing for 6 to 8 weeks until union occurs.

If symptoms of pain and decreased ankle motion persist following conservative treatment, Ihle and Cochran[60] and Paulos et al.[110] recommend surgical excision of the fracture fragment. The preferred surgical approach to the posterior process varies. Howse[58] recommends a medial rather than a lateral approach because the latter interferes with the peroneal tendons and may produce postoperative stiffness. However, posterolateral arthrotomy has been recommended by Ihle and Cochran,[60] McDougall,[82] and Weinstein and Bonfiglio.[154] Paulos et al.[110] state that either a posteromedial or posterolateral approach can be utilized for fragment excision. They stress that following surgical removal, the patient's ankle is splinted only briefly and then a vigorous stretching and strengthening program is instituted.

Results.—Most authors report that conservative treatment produces relief of symptoms.[48, 60, 72, 82, 85, 110] However, should conservative treatment fail, they believe that simple excision of the fragment will restore normal joint function.[48, 60, 72, 82, 85, 110] Paulos et al.[110] report that one third of their patients responded to conservative treatment and were only occasionally symptomatic. Two thirds of their patients failed initial conservative treatment consisting of 6 weeks of cast immobilization. These patients then underwent steroid injection into the os trigonum and 4 weeks of additional casting. This was successful in fewer than 10% of the patients, the remainder requiring surgical removal of the posterior bony fragment. Surgical excision was effective in relieving these patients' symptoms.[152]

On the contrary, some authors report that these fractures may not produce the excellent results associated with other avulsion fractures. Sneppen and Buhl[143] found that of 11 patients with fractures of the posterior process, 8 developed talocrural or subtalar arthritis and that *all* 8 of these persisted with complaints of pain in the foot and prolonged disability. Jensenius[61] also reports persistent disability and discomfort in over half of his patients following this fracture.

Author's Preferred Method of Treatment.—I routinely obtain anteroposterior, mortise, lateral, and 35-degree oblique radiographs in a patient presenting with pain in the posterolateral aspect of the ankle following injury. If the radiographs confirm a definite fracture of the lateral tubercle of the posterior process, the patients are treated with a short-leg non–weight-bearing cast for 4 weeks. The toes are left free in this cast, and early range of motion of the metatarsophalangeal joints of the great toe is initiated to prevent trapping of the flexor hallucis longus tendon in the groove of the posterior process. After 4 weeks a short-leg walking cast is worn for an additional 2 weeks. At this point, immobilization is discontinued. If radiographic nonunion results, no further treatment is recommended *unless* the patient is symptomatic. If symptoms persist, another 4- to 6-week period of immobilization is recommended. If symptoms persist for 6 to 8 months in patients with a nonunion, excision of the fragment is recommended (see below). If the posterior process fracture is very large and occupies a *substantial* portion of the posterior calcaneal facet of the talus, consideration can be given to open reduction and stable internal fixation. However, I have not seen this type of fracture in my practice.

In patients who present with a history and clinical examination suggestive of injury to the posterior process and who have roentgenographic evidence suggesting an os trigonum or nonunion of a posterior process fracture, I obtain a technitium bone scan to determine whether the nonunion or os trigonum is hot, which indicates a recent injury. These patients are treated exactly as outlined for acute fractures, with fragment excision being recommended only if conservative treatment fails.

In patients in whom conservative therapy fails and in whom significant pain on the posterolateral aspect of the ankle persists, consideration is given to surgical excision of the free fragment. Prior to surgical excision, injection of the area with lidocaine under roentgenographic control is utilized to confirm that the fragment is the actual cause of the persistent posterolateral pain. In these patients, positive technitium bone scan findings are considered contributory evidence that the fragment is responsible for the pain.

I prefer the posterolateral approach for fragment excision while being careful to avoid the sural nerve. The fragment is excised and the foot immobilized in a short-leg cast *only* for soft-tissue healing, usually 7 to 10 days. Immediately postoperatively, flexor hallucis longus function and range of motion of the metatarsophalangeal joints of all toes are instituted. After initial immobilization for 7 to 10 days stretching and range-of-motion exercises are encouraged, and weight bearing is allowed.

Fracture of the Medial Tubercle of the Posterior Process

Fractures of the medial tubercle of the posterior process of the talus are much more uncommon than fractures of the lateral tubercle of the posterior process. Cedell[21] in 1974 reported four cases of fracture of the medial tubercle that he believed were secondary to avulsion of the bone fragment by the posterior talotibial ligament when the ankle is dorsiflexed and pronated.

Clinically, there is obvious swelling behind the medial malleolus with loss of the normal contour of the posteromedial aspect of the ankle. Roentgenographic examination demonstrates a fragment of varying size situated medial and dorsal to the talus (Fig 35–80,A and B). All patients in Cedell's series were treated by immobilization and a soft bandage. Although the injuries seemed to heal, when patients resumed sporting activities, medial pain and swelling recurred. As a result of this, three of his four patients subsequently underwent excision of the fragment with restoration of normal function.[21]

Author's preferred method of treatment.—Pain posteromedially in the ankle following a pronation injury to the foot should suggest avulsion of the medial tubercle of the posterior process. In these patients, careful roentgenographic evaluation, including polytomography (Fig 35–80,B), may be necessary to document the fracture. If the fracture fragment is small and does not interfere with ankle or subtalar motion, I prefer immobilization in a short-leg non–weight-bearing cast for 4 to 6 weeks. If pain and swelling persist for 4 to 6 months following this conservative treatment, surgical excision through a posteromedial arthrotomy is recommended.

If the fragment is larger or it interferes with ankle or subtalar motion, consideration is given to open reduction and internal fixation, or excision management after excision through a posteromedial arthrotomy is as outlined above for a lateral tubercle excision.

Group IV: fractures of the lateral process of the talus

Fractures of the lateral process of the talus, first described in detail by Dimon in 1961,[40] account for 24% of fractures of the body of the talus.[135] Indeed, Hawkins[54] regards this to be the second most common fracture of the body of the talus. Mukherjee et al.[95] found 13 cases of fracture of the lateral process of the talus in 1,500 cases of fractures and sprains about the ankle. Several small series have been reported in the literature, with most authors stressing that this fracture occurs more commonly than is suspected and is often overlooked.*

**References 8, 23, 41, 44, 54, 67, 95, 111, 120, 135, 144.*

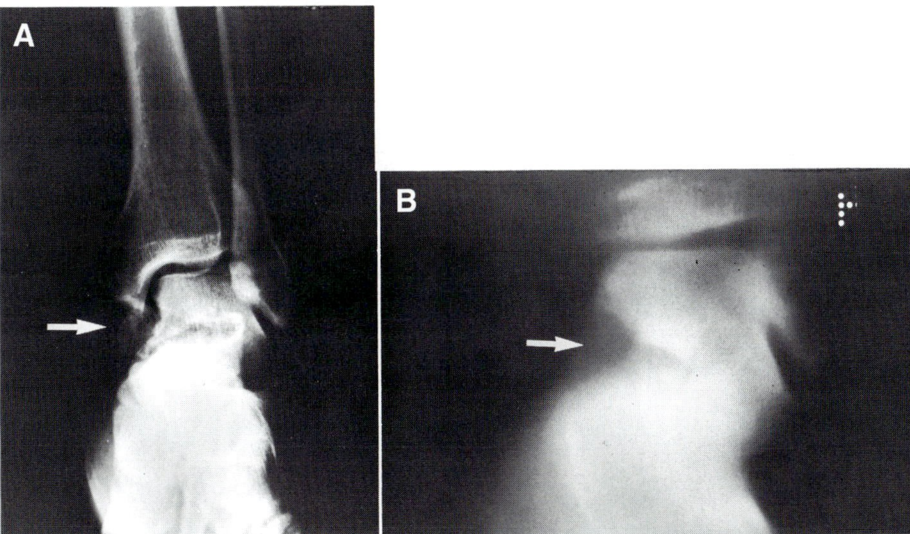

FIG 35–80.
A, fracture of the medial tubercle of the posterior process. A large medial tubercle fragment is located beneath the medial malleolus. **B,** an anteroposterior tomogram demonstrates the fracture communicating with the posterior subtalar facet.

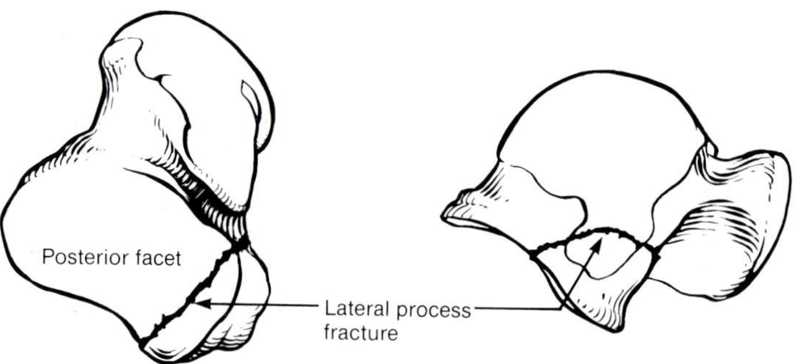

FIG 35–81.
Fracture of the lateral process of the talus involving the talofibular component of the ankle joint as well as the posterior facet of the talocalcaneal joint.

This fracture has been variously termed "fracture of the lateral process,"[8, 23, 44, 54, 119] "fracture of the posterior facet of the talus,"[40] and "fracture of the lateral tubercle."[135] The diagnosis of this fracture is frequently overlooked,[23, 54] and substantial disability can result.[135]

Anatomy

The lateral process of the talus is a wedge-shaped prominence that composes the most lateral aspect of body of the talus and extends from the lower margin of the talar articular surface for the fibula to the posteroinferior surface of the talus (Fig 35–81).[96] A fracture of the lateral process of the talus therefore involves both the talofibular articulation of the ankle joint and the posterior talocalcaneal articulation of the subtalar joint.[23, 40, 54] The degree of involvement of the talofibular and posterior talocalcaneal joints is dependent on fracture size. Shelton and Pedowitz[135] point out that the presence of heavy cancellous trabecular bone and its horizontal orientation within the lateral process emphasize its importance in weight bearing.[135]

Additionally, the lateral process serves as a point of attachment for the lateral talocalcaneal, cervical, bifurcate, and the anterior talofibular ligaments (Fig 35–82). The lateral process of the talus is therefore an important structure providing stability to the ankle mortise and also participates in the weight-bearing role of the distal end of the fibula.[135]

Mechanism of Injury

Several mechanisms of injury have been postulated.[23, 40]

1. The lateral process is sheared off the posterior facet of the talus by the lateral malleolus as the foot is forced into eversion.[40] Dimon states that because he has

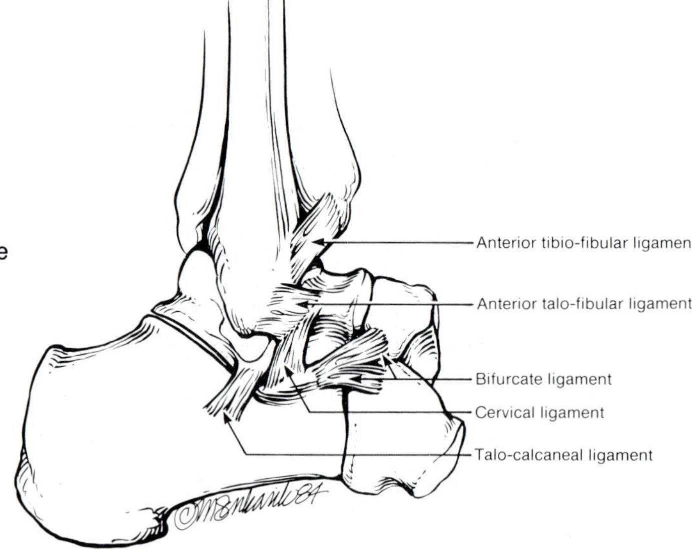

FIG 35–82.
The lateral process serves as a point of attachment for the anterior talofibular, cervical, bifurcate, and talocalcaneal ligaments.

not seen evidence of a deltoid ligament sprain or a fracture of the medial malleolus associated with this injury, this mechanism is unlikely.[40]

2. The lateral malleolar fragment could be avulsed by the anterior talofibular or talocalcaneal ligaments (Fig 35–82).[23, 40] However, Dimon again postulates that because inversion injuries of the ankle are so common, if this mechanism were a frequent cause of lateral process fractures, they should be seen more frequently.[40] Also, Hawkins[54] believes that since he has not noted this fracture in association with subtalar dislocations, which usually ruptures the strong talocalcaneal ligament, this mechanism is unlikely.

3. Cimmino[23] reports that a direct blow can produce this fracture.

4. Most authors agree that fractures of the lateral process are the result of acute dorsiflexion and inversion of the foot.[21, 44, 54, 95, 114] Huson[59] noted that the articular surfaces of the posterior talocalcaneal joints are congruous in the standing position. However, when the heel is inverted, a lateral shift of the head of the talus results in an upward shift of the lateral process of the talus on the posterior articular surface of the calcaneus.[95] This results in the posterior talocalcaneal joint being incongruous.[95] If the foot is then acutely dorsiflexed, force is concentrated on the lateral process of the talus (Fig 35–83). Compression of the lateral process of the talus in inversion and dorsiflexion therefore results in the fracture.[44, 95]

Mukherjee et al.[95] report that in all of their patients the injury resulted from inversion and dorsiflexion of the ankle. According to Shelton and Pedowitz,[135] the mechanism of inversion and dorsiflexion of the foot is supported by the association of this fracture with (1) anterior subtalar dislocations, (2) fractures of the talar neck, (3) adduction-type fractures of the medial malleolus, and (4) complete rupture of the lateral collateral ligament and avulsion fractures of the fibula.

Clinical Diagnosis

Because the mechanism of injury and the clinical findings following a lateral process fracture are identical to those of an inversion sprain of the ankle, careful evaluation of patients whose history suggests an ankle sprain is indicated if the diagnosis is to be made. Indeed, in every patient diagnosed as having an ankle sprain that is resistant to the usual conservative treatment, the roentgenographs must be reviewed and even repeated with a fracture of the lateral talar process in mind.[40]

These patients are usually young males who have fallen from a height, have been involved in a motor vehicle accident, or have stepped in a hole.[54] The physical findings are indistinguishable from those that occur with a sprain of the anterior talofibular ligament.[40] Immediate disability with swelling and tenderness located over the anterolateral aspect of the foot just anterior to the lateral malleolus is noted.[23, 23, 40, 54, 56] Ecchymosis in the same location may occur within 24 hours.[23] Although specific clinical signs may be masked by the associated soft-tissue injury, acute local tenderness over the lateral process of the talus just below the tip of the lateral malleolus is diagnostic.[95] Pain occurs with dorsiflexion and plantar flexion of the ankle and inversion or

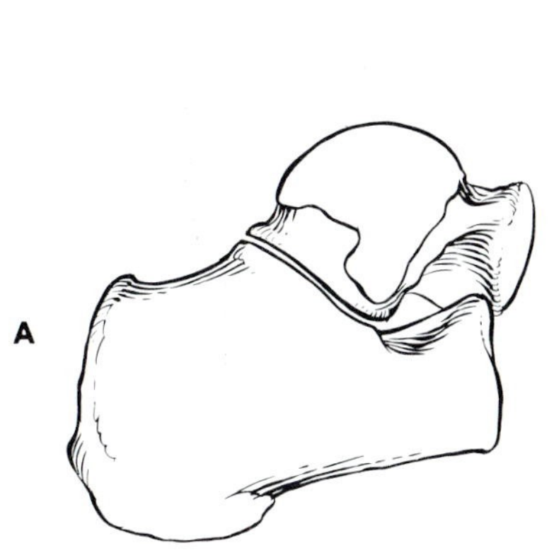

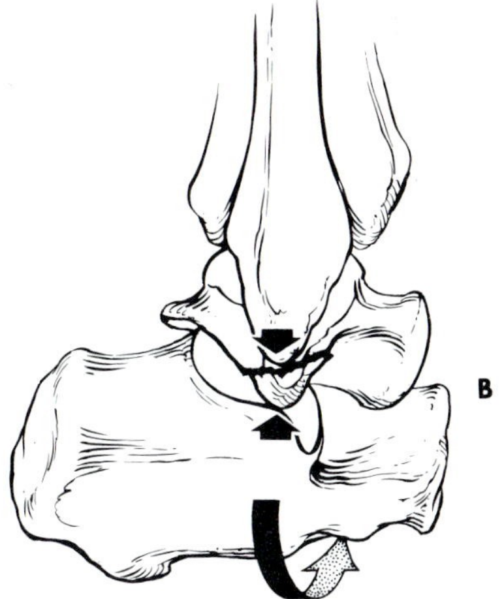

FIG 35–83.
A, normal talocalcaneal articulation. **B,** when the heel of the foot is inverted a lateral shift of the talar head results in an upward shift of the lateral process of the talus on the calcaneus. This produces an incongruity in the posterior talocalcaneal joint. Dorsiflexion of the foot then concentrates force on the lateral process of the talus and results in its fracture.

eversion of the subtalar joint.[23, 54] Crepitus is usually not present.[54]

Radiographic Diagnosis

Generally, fractures of the lateral process of the talus can be easily demonstrated on a standard ankle series that includes anteroposterior, lateral, and mortise views.[23, 95] The key to radiographic diagnosis is awareness of the injury rather than a specific roentgenographic view.[95]

Hawkins[54] emphasized the need for both anteroposterior and lateral radiographs to make the diagnosis. He pointed out that in some situations the fracture may only be demonstrable on the lateral roentgenograph. Mukherjee et al.[95] recommend the use of an anteroposterior view taken with the ankle in neutral and the leg rotated inward 20 degrees to demonstrate a fracture of the lateral process of the talus. This view, a variation of the mortise view, best demonstrates this fracture because the process lies almost in the frontal plane in this projection (Fig 35–84,A).[95] Dimon[40] recommended routine roentgenographs of the ankle but noted that in cases of doubt, oblique radiographs consisting of an anteroposterior view with the foot in 45 degrees of internal rotation and 30 degrees of equinus are helpful.[40] We too have found this view useful in cases in which the fracture is not clearly visualized. Cimmino[23] noted that the downward-directed apex of the lateral process of the talus and the upward-directed apex of the sustentaculum tali are superimposed on a lateral roentgenogram of the ankle. He stresses that one must differentiate the two processes on the lateral view to make the diagnosis of a lateral process fracture. He also emphasized that a posterior subtalar joint effusion noted on the lateral view suggests this injury.[23] Cimmino[23] mentions that a congenital "ununited process" may occur and should not be mistaken for a fracture. Shelton and Pedowitz[135] also stress that normal accessory ossicles occur in the area of the lateral process and must be differentiated from fractures.[135] I have noted an apparent accessory ossification center in one case that caused confusion with a fracture. The presence of this lesion bilaterally helped to exclude an acute fracture (Fig 35–85).

Evaluation of the size, amount of articular involvement, and degree of displacement of lateral process fractures can be greatly improved by the use of anteroposterior polytomograms of the talus (see Fig 35–74,B). High-resolution CAT scanning can also be helpful in

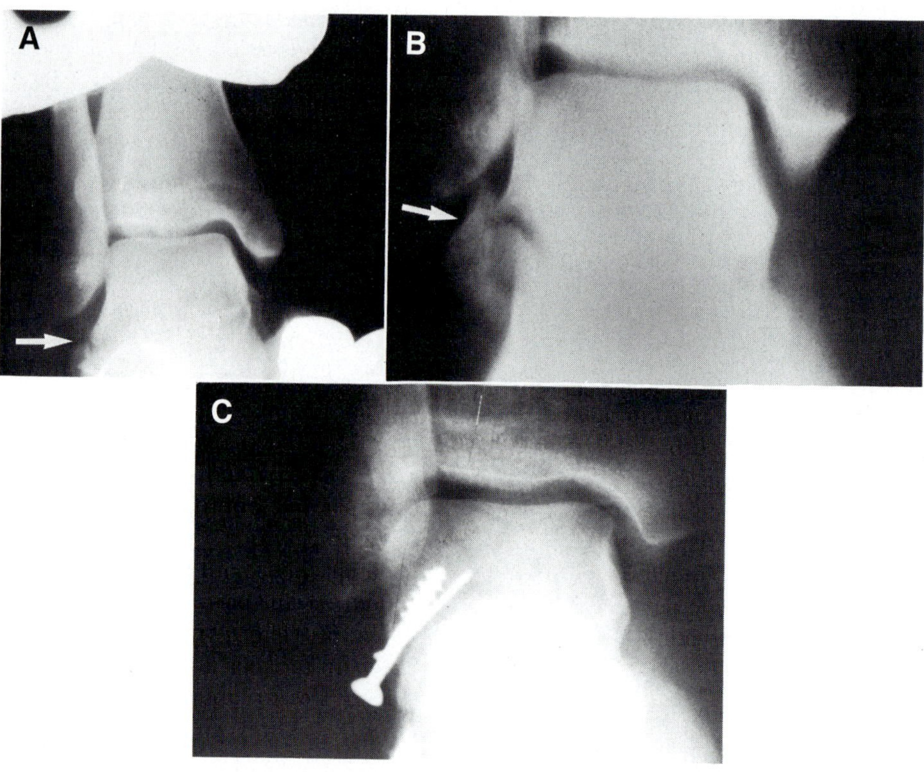

FIG 35–84.
A, this anteroposterior view of the ankle with the leg internally rotated 20 degrees suggests a large fracture of the lateral process *(arrow)*. **B,** polytomography more clearly denotes the fragment size and displacement. **C,** open reduction and stable internal fixation of the talar process fracture.

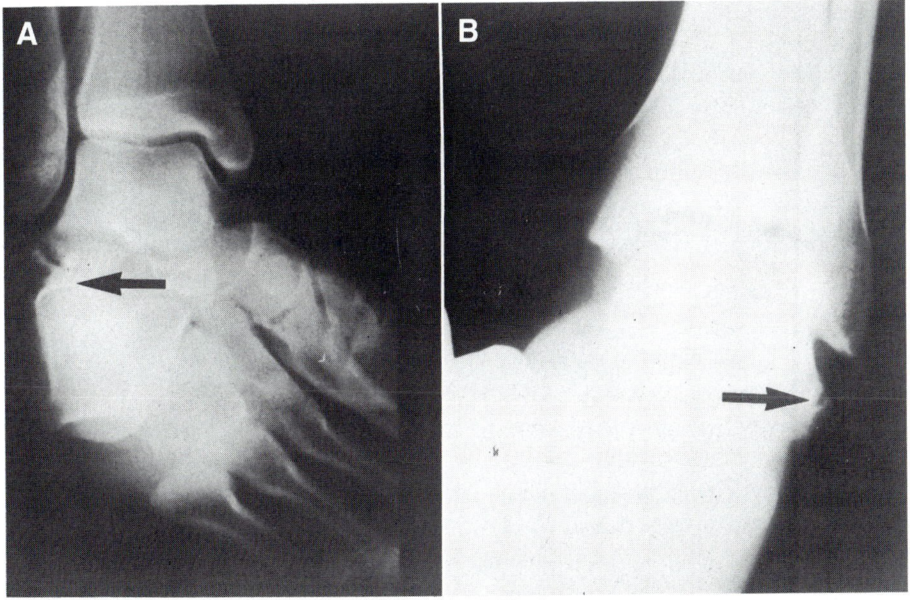

FIG 35–85.
Mortise views of the right **(A)** and left **(B)** ankles. Note the radiolucency in both lateral processes, which suggests a fracture *(arrows).* The right ankle was explored because a lesion was detected radiographically after an acute inversion sprain. No defect was noted in the lateral processes, thus suggesting an unfused accessory ossification center. Comparison views taken later demonstrated a similar lesion in the left ankle **(B).**

determining fracture location, size, and displacement.[124]

Hawkins[54] reports three types of lateral process fracture: type I, a simple fracture of the lateral process of the talus that extends from the talofibular articular surface to the posterior talocalcaneal articular surface of the subtalar joint; type II, a comminuted fracture involving both the fibular and posterior talocalcaneal articular surface of the talus and the entire lateral process; and type III, a chip fracture of the anterior and inferior portion of the posterior articular process of the talus. Type III fractures could be seen only on the lateral radiograph and are noted in the region of the sinus tarsi. This type III fracture does not extend into the talofibular articulation.

Treatment

The size of the lateral process fracture and the degree of comminution and displacement are the critical factors in determining treatment.[56] Heckman et al.[56] and Cimino[23] report that acute nondisplaced fractures will heal with immobilization but displaced fragments require open reduction and internal fixation or excision.

Hawkins[54] and Shelton and Pedowitz[135] recommend that closed reduction be attempted in all fractures of the lateral process of the talus. The lateral process is palpated and manipulated into an acceptable position with the foot in the neutral or everted position. Following reduction, a cast is applied from the toes to just below the knee with the foot in the neutral position. If the reduction is satisfactory, the cast is maintained for 4 weeks without weight bearing. An additional 2 weeks of cast immobilization with weight bearing is then recommended. Hawkins[54] and Shelton and Pedowitz[135] believe that this approach is also indicated for comminuted (type II) and chip (type III) fractures. Simple fractures (type I) that remain severely displaced, even after an attempted closed reduction, should be considered for open reduction and internal fixation with Kirschner wires or small compression screws.[23, 54, 135] Mallon et al.[80] report the use of a Herbert screw to internally fix a displaced fracture of the lateral process of the talus. The authors believe that the advantages of the Herbert screw over standard 4.0-mm AO screws are that the head of the AO screw, when used in interarticular fractures, removes a much larger portion of articular cartilage than does the Herbert bone screw. The authors believe that because it leaves no protruding screw head, the Herbert screw is ideal for fixation of lateral process fractures. Their biomechanical study also supports the use of the Herbert screw to stabilize these fractures. Mukherjee et al.[95, 120] believe that a large single fragment should be reduced accurately by open reduction in order to restore the congruity of the subtalar joint, while small and comminuted fractures are best treated by removal.

In fractures detected late, Cimino[23] prefers a trial of immobilization but stresses that eventually excision of the fragment will be necessary. Pringle and Mukherjee emphasize that simple plaster immobilization in fractures diagnosed late often produces a poor result.[120] Although Dimon[40] was unable to draw any definite conclusions regarding the best treatment, he did emphasize that if the fracture is not recognized initially, prolonged disability will usually occur and this disability is often *not* relieved by excision of the fragment. Mukherjee et al.[95, 120] also stressed the need for treatment soon after the injury to prevent long-term disability.

Sneppen et al.[144] stress that whatever treatment modality is utilized, it is *essential* to aim at rapid normalization of function of the talocrural and subtalar joints. This can best be accomplished by a brief period of immobilization that allows healing of the joint capsule and ligamentous structures. Thereafter, active foot movement is instituted. Because these fractures invariably involve a weight-bearing joint, they recommend that patients not be allowed to bear weight on the foot until there is solid union of the fracture.

Prognosis

All series reported in the literature emphasize the importance of *early* diagnosis followed by reduction or excision to prevent long-term sequelae.[17, 23, 54, 56, 135, 144] Pringle and Mukherjee[120] found that in their patients with poor results, the injury had not been recognized for 6 to 9 months postoperatively. Hawkins[54] also found that all patients who required subtalar fusion following this injury had inadequate initial treatment. Additionally, Dimon[40] and Shelton and Pedowitz[135] stress that not only does delayed diagnosis produce disability but delayed excision of the fragment may also not relieve the symptoms.

Sneppen et al.[144] and Mukherjee and Pringle[95, 120] emphasize that even nondisplaced fractures of the lateral process can result in long-term disability due to subtalar osteoarthrosis and moderate to severe discomfort on the lateral aspect of the ankle with weight bearing. Hawkins[54] reports that pain with walking or standing sufficient to warrant exploration was present in half of his patients. He also stresses the frequency of symptomatic nonunions in the untreated patient, a finding also noted by Heckman et al.[56]

Overgrowth of bone in the region of the sinus tarsi that impinges upon the calcaneus or the fibula has also been reported after this fracture.[54, 56, 135] Hawkins[54] and Shelton and Pedowitz[135] conclude that if there is evidence of nonunion, malunion, or overgrowth of the lateral process, excision of the fracture or subtalar fusion should be considered.

Author's Preferred Method of Treatment

Due to the disability resulting from a missed or delayed diagnosis, a high index of suspicion is *essential* in evaluating patients who present with a clinical history suggestive of a lateral ankle sprain because they may indeed have a lateral process fracture. I routinely use anteroposterior, lateral, and mortise roentgenographs to evaluate the lateral process. If these do not demonstrate a fracture but the clinical findings suggest one, 30-degree internal oblique films are taken. One must clearly see the lateral process in these patients before a fracture is excluded. If a fracture is noted on routine roentgenographs, polytomograms or a CAT scan may be necessary to determine fragment size, displacement, and comminution. I must again emphasize the importance of recognizing accessory ossicles in the region of the lateral process (see Fig 35–85)[57, 134] so that they are not interpreted as fractures.

In fractures that are truly nondisplaced, I use a short-leg non–weight-bearing cast for 4 weeks. This is followed by 2 weeks in a walking cast.

In my experience displaced fractures cannot be reduced anatomically by closed means. Also, displaced fractures are associated with more severe damage to the subtalar joint. If closed reduction and prolonged casting are used in these patients, subtalar stiffness and pain often result. Therefore, I choose either excision or open reduction and stable internal fixation so that early subtalar motion can be instituted. Open reduction and internal fixation are recommended if the fracture fragment is large enough to allow stable internal fixation (see Fig 35–84,C). I have found a modified anterolateral ankle arthrotomy very acceptable. The incision begins just anterior to the fibula, 5 cm above the ankle, progresses to the tip of the fibula, and curves slightly posteriorly beneath the fibula. This gives excellent exposure to the lateral process. If comminution or fracture size prevent stable internal fixation, immediate excision is performed.

Following open reduction and stable internal fixation, a short-leg cast is applied to allow the surgical wound to heal. Active range of motion of the metatarsophalangeal joints is encouraged in the cast to decrease swelling in the foot. The cast is removed at 2 to 3 weeks and replaced with a removable splint. Removal of the splint allows a physical therapy program stressing subtalar and midtarsal motion. Weight bearing is allowed when there is radiographic evidence of union, usually at 6 weeks.

If the lateral process fragments are small and excision is necessary, the patients are kept in a short-leg cast for 3 weeks. Following this, active subtalar and midtarsal motion is encouraged, and progressive weight bearing is allowed within the limits of pain.

For those patients who present late, that is, 12 weeks or longer postinjury, I have found that cast immobilization does not produce predictable results. Therefore, in these patients I proceed directly to excision of the fragment unless it is large and an anatomic reduction can be obtained. The likelihood of obtaining an anatomic reduction following any delay in treatment, however, is not good. The postoperative management following excision of these fractures in which the diagnosis is delayed is the same as that used for excision of an acute fracture.

REFERENCES

Body of the Talus

1. Alexander AH, Lichtman DM: Surgical treatment of transchondral talar-dome fractures (osteochondritis dissecans), *J Bone Joint Surg [Am]* 62:646–652, 1980.
2. Anderson HG: *The medical and surgical aspects of aviation*, London, 1919, Hodder.
3. Anderson JF, Crichton KJ, Grattan-Smith T, et al: Osteochondral fractures of the dome of the talus, *J Bone Joint Surg [Am]* 71:1143–1152, 1989.
4. Angerman P, Jensen P: Osteochondritis dissecans of the talus: long term results of surgical treatment, *Foot Ankle* 10:161–163, 1989.
5. Arcomano JP, Kamhi E, Karas S, et al: Transchondral fracture and osteochondritis dissecans of talus, *N Y State J Med* 78:2183–2189, 1978.
6. Berndt AL, Harty M: Transchondral fractures (osteochondritis dissecans) of the talus, *J Bone Joint Surg [Am]* 41:988–1020, 1959.
7. Besson J, Wellinger C: L'osteochondrite dissequante de l'astragale A propos de 12 observations, *Rev Rheum* 34:552–566, 1967.
8. Bigelow DR: Fractures of the processus lateralis tali, *J Bone Joint Surg [Br]* 56:587, 1974.
9. Birt D, Townsend R: Major talar fractures, *J Bone Joint Surg [Am]* 58:733, 1976.
10. Blair HC: Comminuted fractures and fracture dislocations of the body of the astragalus, *Am J Surg* 59:37–43, 1943.
11. Bobechko WP, Harris WR: The radiographic density of avascular bone, *J Bone Joint Surg [Br]* 42:626–632, 1960.
12. Bohler L: *Treatment of fractures*, ed 5, New York, 1956, Grune & Stratton.
13. Bonnin JG: Dislocations and fracture-dislocations of the talus, *Br J Surg* 28:88–100, 1940.
14. Bonnin JG: *Injuries to the ankle*, Darien, Conn, 1970, Hafner, pp 324–380.
15. Boyd HB, Knight RA: Fractures of the astragalus, *South Med J* 35:160–167, 1942.
16. Burman MS, Lapidus PW: The functional disturbances caused by the inconstant bones and sesamoids of the foot, *Arch Surg* 22:936–975, 1931.
17. Cameron BM: Osteochondritis dissecans of the ankle joint, *J Bone Joint Surg [Am]* 38:857–861, 1956.
18. Canale ST, Belding RH: Osteochondral lesions of the talus, *J Bone Joint Surg [Am]* 62:97–102, 1980.
19. Canale ST, Kelly FB Jr: Fractures of the neck of the talus, *J Bone Joint Surg [Am]* 60:143–156, 1978.
20. Carmack JC, Hallock H: Tibiotarsal arthrodesis after astragalectomy: a report of 8 cases, *J Bone Joint Surg* 29:476–482, 1947.
21. Cedell CA: Rupture of the posterior talotibial ligament with the avulsion of a bone fragment from the talus, *Acta Orthop Scand* 45:454–461, 1974.
22. Chapman MW: Fractures and fracture-dislocations of the ankle. In Mann RA, editor: *DuVries' surgery of the foot* ed 4, St Louis, 1978, Mosby–Year Book.
23. Cimmino CV: Fracture of the lateral process of the talus, *AJR* 90:1277–1280, 1963.
24. Cloquet: *Bull Soc Anat Paris* 19:131, 1844.
25. Cobey MC: Traumatic avascular necrosis of the talus, *Clin Orthop* 81:180–181, 1971.
26. Coker TP Jr, Arnold JA: Sports injuries to the foot and ankle. In Jahss MH, editor: *Disorders of the foot*, vol 2, Philadelphia, 1982, WB Saunders.
27. Coltart WD: "Aviator's astragalus," *J Bone Joint Surg [Br]* 34:545–566, 1952.
28. Cooper, Sir Astley: *A treatise on dislocations, and on fractures of the joints*, ed 2, Boston, 1832, Lilly, Wait, Carter & Hendee, pp 341–342.
29. Craig FS, McLaughlin HL: Injuries of the foot. In McLaughlin HL, editor: *Trauma*, Philadelphia, 1959, WB Saunders, pp 307–317.
30. Davidson AM, Steele HD, MacKenzie DA, et al: A review of twenty-one cases of transchondral fracture of the talus, *J Trauma* 7:378–415, 1967.
31. Davis FJ, Fry LR, Lippert FG, et al: The patellar tendon–bearing brace: report of 16 patients, *J Trauma* 14:216–221, 1974.
32. Davis MW: Bilateral talar osteochondritis dissecans with lax ankle ligaments, *J Bone Joint Surg [Am]* 52:168–170, 1970.
33. Deetz E: Ueber Luxatio Pedis Subtalo nach Vorn mit Talus-fraktur, *Dtsch Z Chir* 76:581–593, 1904.
34. DeLee JC: Talar neck fracture with total dislocation of the body, report of the Committee on Trauma of the American Orthopaedic Foot Society, Anaheim, Calif, February 1983.
35. DeLee JC, Curtis R: Subtalar dislocation of the foot, *J Bone Joint Surg [Am]* 64:433–437, 1982.
36. Dennis MD, Tullos HS: Blair tibiotalar arthrodesis for injuries of the talus, *J Bone Joint Surg [Am]* 62:103–107, 1980.
37. DePalma AF, Ahmed I, Flannery G, et al: Aseptic necrosis of the talus: revascularization after bone grafting, *Clin Orthop* 101:232–235, 1974.
38. Detenbeck LC, Kelly PJ: Total dislocation of the talus, *J Bone Joint Surg [Am]* 51:283–288, 1969.
39. Deyerle WM, Burkhardt BW: Displaced fractures of the talus: an aggressive approach. Presented at the Association of Bone and Joint Surgeons 33rd annual meet-

ing, Lexington, Kentucky, April 8–12, 1981, *Orthop Trans* 5:465, 1981.

40. Dimon JH: Isolated displaced fracture of the posterior facet of the talus, *J Bone Joint Surg [Am]* 43:275–281, 1961.
41. Drez DJ, Guhl JF, Gollehan DL: Ankle arthroscopy: technique and indications, *Foot Ankle* 2:138–143, 1981.
42. Dunn AR, Jacobs B, Campbell RD Jr: Fractures of the talus, *J Trauma* 6:443–468, 1966.
43. Fahey JJ, Murphy JL: Dislocations and fractures of the talus, *Surg Clin North Am* 45:79–102, 1965.
44. Fjeldborg O: Fracture of the lateral process of the talus. Supination-dorsal flexion fracture, *Acta Orthop Scand* 39:407–412, 1968.
45. Garcia A, Parkes JC II: Fractures of the foot. In Giannestras NJ, editor: *Foot disorders: medical and surgical management*, ed 2, Philadelphia, 1973, Lea & Febiger.
46. Gatellier J: Juxtoretroperoneal route in operative treatment of fracture of malleolus with posterior marginal fragment, *Surg Gynecol Obstet* 52:67–70, 1931.
47. Geist ES: Supernumerary bones of the foot—a roentgen study of the feet of one hundred normal individuals, *Am J Orthop Surg* 12:403–414, 1914.
48. Giannestras NJ, Sammarco GJ: Fractures and dislocations in the foot. In Rockwood CA Jr, Green DP, editors: *Fractures*, vol 2, Philadelphia, 1975, JB Lippincott.
49. Gibson A, Inkster RG: Fractures of the talus, *Can Med Assoc J* 31:357–362, 1934.
50. Gillquist J, Oretorp N, Stenstrom A, et al: Late results after vertical fracture of the talus, *Injury* 6:173–179, 1974.
51. Gustilo RB, Gordon SS: Osteochondral fractures of the talus, *Minn Med* 51:237–241, 1968.
52. Haliburton RA, Sullivan CR, Kelly PJ, et al: The extra-osseous and intra-osseous blood supply of the talus, *J Bone Joint Surg [Am]*, 40:1115–1120, 1958.
53. Hamilton WG: Stenosing tenosynovitis of the flexor hallucis longus tendon and posterior impingement upon the os trigonum in ballet dancers, *Foot Ankle* 3:74–80, 1982.
54. Hawkins LG: Fracture of the lateral process of the talus, *J Bone Joint Surg [Am]*, 47:1170–1175, 1965.
55. Hawkins LG: Fractures of the neck of the talus, *J Bone Joint Surg [Am]* 52:991–1002, 1970.
56. Heckman JD, McLean MR, DeLee JC: Fracture of the lateral process of the talus. Presented at the Association of Bone and Joint Surgeons 33rd Annual Meeting in Lexington, Kentucky, April 8–12, 1981, *Orthop Trans* 5:465, 1981.
57. Holland CT: *The accessory bones of the foot, with notes on a few other conditions. The Robert Jones Birth Volume*, New York, 1928, Oxford University Press, pp 157–182.
58. Howse AJG: Posterior block of the ankle joint in ballet dancers, *Foot Ankle* 3:81–84, 1982.
59. Huson A: *An anatomical and functional study of the tarsal joints*, Leiden, 1961, Drukkerij Luctor et Emergo.
60. Ihle CL, Cochran RM: Fracture of the fused os trigonum, *Am J Sports Med* 10:47–50, 1982.
61. Jensenius H: Fracture of the astragalus, *Acta Orthop Scand* 19:195–209, 1950.
62. Kappis M: Weitere Beitrage zur Traumatisch—mechanischen Entstehung der "spontanen" Knorpelablosungen (sogen. Osteochondritis Dissecans), *Dtsch Z Chir* 171:13–29, 1922.
63. Kelly PJ, Sullivan CR: Blood supply of the talus, *Clin Orthop* 30:37–44, 1963.
64. Kenwright J, Taylor RG: Major injuries of the talus, *J Bone Joint Surg [Br]* 52:36–48, 1970.
65. Key JA, Conwell HE: *The management of fractures, dislocations and sprains*, ed 4, St Louis, 1946, Mosby–Year Book.
66. Kleiger B: Fractures of the talus, *J Bone Joint Surg [Am]* 30:735–744, 1948.
67. Kleiger B, Ahmed M: Injuries of the talus and its joints, *Clin Orthop* 121:243–262, 1976.
68. Kleinberg S: Supernumerary bones of the foot, *Ann Surg* 65:499–509, 1917.
69. Kohler A: *Roentgenology*, ed 2, London, 1935, Bailliere, Tindall & Cox.
70. Kohler A, Zimmer EA: *Borderlands of the normal and early pathologic in skeletal roentgenology*, ed 11, New York, 1968, Grune & Stratton.
71. Lahaut M: Fracture du col de l'astragale traitee par autogreffe immediate, *Mem Acad Chir* 81:261–264, 1955.
72. Lapidus PW: A note on the fracture of os trigonum. Report of a case, *Bull Hosp Jt Dis* 33:150–154, 1972.
73. Larson RL, Sullivan CR, Janes JM: Trauma, surgery, and circulation of the talus—what are the risks of avascular necrosis? *J Trauma* 1:13–21, 1961.
74. Laughlin JE: Injuries of the talus: a review of the literature and case presentation, *J Am Osteopath Assoc* 71:334–341, 1971.
75. Lemaire RG, Bustin W: Screw fixation of fractures of the neck of the talus using a posterior approach, *J Trauma* 20:669–673, 1980.
76. Lieberg OU, Henke JA, Bailey RW: Avascular necrosis of the head of the talus without death of the body: report of an unusual case, *J Trauma* 15:926–928, 1975.
77. Lindholm TS, Osterman K, Vankka E: Osteochondritis of the elbow, ankle, and hip, *Clin Orthop* 148:245–253, 1980.
78. Lionberger DR, Bishop JO, Tullos HS: The modified Blair fusion, *Foot Ankle* 3:60–62, 1982.
79. Lorentzen JE, Christensen SB, Krogsoe O, et al: Fractures of the neck of the talus, *Acta Orthop Scand* 48:115–120, 1977.
80. Mallon WJ, Wombwell JH, Nunley JA: Interarticular talar fractures: repair using the Herbert screw, *Foot Ankle* 10:88–91, 1989.
81. Marks KL: Flake fracture of the talus progressing to osteochondritis dissecans, *J Bone Joint Surg [Br]* 34:90–92, 1952.
82. McDougall A: The os trigonum, *J Bone Joint Surg [Br]* 37:257–265, 1955.
83. McKeever FM: Fracture of the neck of the astragalus, *Arch Surg* 46:720–735, 1943.
84. McKeever FM: Treatment of complications of fractures and dislocations of the talus, *Clin Orthop* 30:45–52, 1963.
85. Meisenbach R: Fracture of the os trigonum: report of two cases, *JAMA* 89:199–200, 1927.
86. Mensor MC, Melody GF: Osteochondritis dissecans of ankle joint. The use of tomography as a diagnostic aid, *J Bone Joint Surg* 23:903–909, 1941.

87. Miller OL, Baker LD: Fracture and fracture-dislocation of the astragalus, *South Med J* 32:125–136, 1939.
88. Miller WE: Operative intervention for fracture of the talus. In Bateman JE, Trott AW, editors: *Foot and ankle*, New York, 1980, Brian C Decker.
89. Mindel ER, Cisek EE, Kartalian G, et al: Late results of injuries to the talus, *J Bone Joint Surg [Am]* 45:221–245, 1963.
90. Mitchell JI: Total dislocation of the astragalus, *J Bone Joint Surg* 18:212–214, 1936.
91. Moeller FA: The os trigonum syndrome, *J Am Podiatr Assoc* 63:491–501, 1973.
92. Monkman GR, Johnson KA, Duncan DM: Fractures of the neck of the talus, *Minn Med* 58:335–340, 1975.
93. Morris HD: Aseptic necrosis of the talus following injury, *Orthop Clin North Am* 5:177–189, 1974.
94. Morris HD, Hand WL, Dunn AW: The modified Blair fusion for fractures of the talus, *J Bone Joint Surg [Am]* 53:1289–1297, 1971.
95. Mukherjee SK, Pringle RM, Baxter AD: Fracture of the lateral process of the talus. A report of thirteen cases, *J Bone Joint Surg [Br]* 56:263–273, 1974.
96. Mukherjee SK, Young AB: Dome fracture of the talus: a report of ten cases, *J Bone Joint Surg [Br]* 55:319–326, 1973.
97. Mulfinger GL, Trueta J: The blood supply of the talus, *J Bone Joint Surg [Br]* 52:160–167, 1970.
98. Newberg AH: Osteochondral fractures of the dome of the talus, *Br J Radiol* 52:105–109, 1979.
99. Newcomb WJ, Brav EA: Complete dislocation of the talus, *J Bone Joint Surg [Am]* 30:872–874, 1948.
100. Nisbet NW: Dome fracture of the talus, *J Bone Joint Surg [Br]* 36:244–246, 1954.
101. O'Brien ET: Injuries of the talus, *Am Fam Physician* 12:95–105, 1975.
102. O'Brien ET, Howard JB, Shepard MJ: Injuries of the talus (abstract), *J Bone Joint Surg [Am]* 54:1575–1576, 1972.
103. O'Donoghue DH: Chondral and osteochondral fractures, *J Trauma* 6:469–481, 1966.
104. O'Farrell TA, Costello BG: Osteochondritis dissecans of the talus, *J Bone Joint Surg [Br]* 64:494–497, 1982.
105. Ove N, Bosse MJ, Reinert CM: Excision of posterolateral talar dome lesions through a medial transmalleolar approach, *Foot Ankle* 9:171–175, 1989.
106. Pantazopoulos T, Galanos P, Vayanos E, et al: Fractures of the neck of the talus, *Acta Orthop Scand* 45:296–306, 1974.
107. Pantazopoulos T, Kapetsis P, Soucacos P, et al: Unusual fracture-dislocation of the talus: report of a case, *Clin Orthop* 83:232–234, 1972.
108. Parisien JS: Arthroscopic treatment of osteochondral lesions of the talus, *Am J Sports Med* 14:211–217, 1987.
109. Patzakis MJ, Harvey JP, Ivler D: The role of antibiotics in the management of open fractures, *J Bone Joint Surg [Am]* 56:532–541, 1974.
110. Paulos LE, Johnson CL, Noyes FR: Posterior compartment fractures of the ankle—a commonly missed athletic injury, *Am J Sports Med* 11:439–443, 1983.
111. Pennal GF: Fractures of the talus, *Clin Orthop* 30:53–63, 1963.
112. Penny JN, Davis LA: Fractures and fracture-dislocations of the neck of the talus, *J Trauma* 20:1029–1037, 1980.
113. Percy EC: Open fracture of the talus, *Can Med Assoc J* 101:91–92, 1969.
114. Peterson L, Goldie IF: The arterial supply of the talus. A study on the relationship to experimental talar fractures, *Acta Orthop Scand* 46:1026–1034, 1975.
115. Peterson L, Goldie IF, Irstam L: Fracture of the neck of the talus. A clinical study, *Acta Orthop Scand* 48:696–706, 1977.
116. Peterson L, Goldie I, Lindell D: The arterial supply of the talus , *Acta Orthop Scand* 45:260–270, 1974.
117. Pettine KA, Morrey BF: Osteochondral fracture of the talus, *J Bone Joint Surg [Br]* 69:89–92, 1987.
118. Pinzur MS, Meyer PR Jr: Complete posterior dislocation of the talus. Case report and discussion, *Clin Orthop* 131:205–209, 1978.
119. Pirie AH: Extra bones in the wrist and ankle found by roentgen rays, *Am J Roentgenol* 8:569–573, 1921.
120. Pringle RM, Mukherjee SK: Fracture of the lateral process of the talus, *J Bone Joint Surg [Br]* 56:201–202, 1974.
121. Ray A: Fractures de l'astragale (a propos de 34 observations), *Rev Chir Orthop* 53:279–294, 1967.
122. Ray RB, Coughlin EJ: Osteochondritis dissecans of the talus, *J Bone Joint Surg* 29:697–706, 1947.
123. Reckling FW: Early tibiocalcaneal fusion in the treatment of severe injuries of the talus, *J Trauma* 12:390–396, 1972.
124. Reis ND, Zinman C, Besser MIB, et al: High-resolution computerized tomography in clinical orthopaedics, *J Bone Joint Surg [Br]* 64:20–24, 1982.
125. Rendu A: Fracture intra-articulaire parcellaire de la poulie astragalienne, *Lyon Med* 150:220–222, 1932.
126. Roden S, Tillegard P, Unander-Scharin L: Osteochondritis dissecans and similar lesions of the talus: a report of fifty-five cases with special reference to etiology and treatment, *Acta Orthop Scand* 23:51–66, 1954.
127. Rogers LF, Campbell RE: Fractures and dislocations of the foot, *Semin Roentgenol* 13:157–166, 1978.
128. Rosenberg NJ: Fractures of the talar dome, *J Bone Joint Surg [Am]* 47:1279, 1965.
129. Rosenmuller: Quoted in Holland CT: On rarer ossifications seen during x-ray examinations, *J Anat* 55:235–248, 1921.
130. Sarrafian S: *Anatomy of the foot and ankle*, Philadelphia, 1983, JB Lippincott, pp 47–54, 295–297.
131. Scharling M: Osteochondritis dissecans of the talus, *Acta Orthop Scand* 49:89–94, 1978.
132. Schrock RD: Fractures of the foot. Fractures and dislocations of the astragalus, *AAOS Instr Course Lect* 9:361–368, 1952.
133. Shahriaree H, Sajadiik AK, Silver C, et al: Total dislocation of the talus: a case report of a four-year follow-up, *Orthop Rev* 9:65–68, 1980.
134. Shands AR Jr, Wentz IJ: Congenital anomalies, accessory bones and osteochondritis in the feet of 850 children, *Surg Clin North Am* 33:1643–1666, 1953.
135. Shelton ML, Pedowitz WJ: Injuries to the talus and midfoot. In Jahss MH, editor: *Disorders of the foot*, vol 2, Philadelphia, 1982, WB Saunders.

136. Shepherd FJ: A hitherto undescribed fracture of the astragalus, *J Anat Physiol* 18:79–81, 1882.
137. Sisk TD: Fractures In Edmonson AS, Crenshaw AH, editors: *Campbell's operative orthopaedics,* ed 6, vol 1, St Louis, 1980, Mosby–Year Book.
138. Skinner HA: *The origin of medical terms,* ed 2, New York, 1970, Hafner.
139. Smillie IS: *Osteochondritis dissecans. Loose bodies in joints. Etiology, pathology, treatment,* Edinburgh, 1960, E & S Livingstone.
140. Smith GR, Winquist RA, Allan TNK, et al: Subtle transchondral fractures of the talar dome: radiological perspective, *Radiology* 124:667–673, 1977.
141. Sneed WL: The astragalus. A case of dislocation, excision and replacement. An attempt to demonstrate the circulation in this bone, *J Bone Joint Surg* 7:384–399, 1925.
142. Sneppen O: Fracture of the talus, a study of its genesis and morphology. Proceedings of the Danish Orthopaedic Society, *Acta Orthop Scand* 48:334, 1977.
143. Sneppen O, Buhl O: Fracture of the talus. A study of its genesis and morphology based upon cases with associated ankle fracture, *Acta Orthop Scand* 45:307–320, 1974.
144. Sneppen O, Christensen SB, Krogsoe O, et al: Fracture of the body of the talus, *Acta Orthop Scand* 48:317–324, 1977.
145. Stealy JH: Fracture of the astragalus, *Surg Gynecol Obstet.* 8:36–48, 1909.
146. Sullivan CR, Jackson SC: Fracture dislocations of the astragalus in children, *Acta Orthop Scand* 27:302–309, 1958
147. Syme J: *Contributions to the pathology and practice of surgery,* Edinburgh, 1848, Sutherland & Knox, p 126.
148. Taylor RG: Immobilization of unstable fracture dislocations by the use of Kirschner wires, *Proc R Soc Med* 55:499–501, 1962.
149. Trillat A, Bousquet C, Lapeyre B: Les fractures—separations totales du col ou du corps de l'astragale: interet du vissage par voie posterieure, *Rev Chir Orthop* 56:529–536, 1970.
150. Turner W: A secondary astragalus in the human foot, *J Anat Physiol* 17:82, 1882.
151. VanBuecken K, Barrach RL, Alexander AH, et al: Arthroscopic treatment of osteochondral talar dome fractures. *Am J Sports Med* 17:350–356, 1984.
152. Vaughan CE, Stapleton JG: Osteochondritis dissecans of the ankle, *Radiology* 49:72–79, 1947.
153. Watson-Jones R: *Fractures and joint injuries,* ed 4, vol 2, Baltimore, 1955, Williams & Wilkins.
154. Weinstein SL, Bonfiglio M: Unusual accessory (bipartite) talus simulating fracture. A case report, *J Bone Joint Surg [Am]* 57:1161–1163, 1975.
155. Wildenauer E: Die Blutversorgung der Talus, *Z Anat,* 115:32, 1950.
156. Winkler H: The treatment of trauma to the foot and ankle, *Instr Course Lect* 1:30, 1947.
157. Yuan HA, Cady RB, DeRosa C: Osteochondritis disseccans of the talus associated with subchondral cysts, *J Bone Joint Surg [Am]* 61:1249, 1979.
158. Yvars MF: Osteochondral fractures of the dome of the talus, *Clin Orthop* 114:185–191, 1976.
159. Zatzkin HR: Trauma to the foot, *Semin Roentgenol* 5:419–435, 1970.

FRACTURES OF THE MIDPART OF THE FOOT

Isolated fractures of the individual bones of the midfoot, the navicular, cuboid, and cuneiforms, are unusual.[17, 18, 29, 33] Due to the rigidity of the midpart of the foot, injuries to that portion of the foot are usually a combination of fracture and/or subluxation of the adjacent joints.[17, 18, 36, 43,] In this section, we will be dealing with apparent isolated injuries to the midtarsal bones. A discussion of associated midtarsal dislocations can be found in the section "Injuries of The Midtarsal Joint." However, one must keep in mind during this discussion that fractures of the midtarsal bones may be associated with sprains or complete disruption of the adjacent ligaments.

Fractures of the Tarsal Navicular

Fractures of the tarsal navicular are rare injuries.[1, 7, 11, 18, 22, 24, 29, 33] However, navicular fractures were noted more frequently by Wilson[48] than either cuboid or cuneiform fractures. Bonvallet reports that these fractures represent only about 26% of all fractures.[3, 4]

Both Watson-Jones[44] and Joplin[26] divided fractures of the tarsal navicular into three types: (1) fractures of the tuberosity, (2) chip fractures of the dorsal lip, and (3) fractures of the body with or without displacement.[3, 5, 33] Sangeorzan et al.[38] have classified *displaced* interarticular fractures of the tarsal navicular into three types based upon the direction of the fracture line, the direction of displacement of the fore and middle parts of the foot, and the pattern of disruption of the talonavicular joint (see Fig 35–92). Recently, attention has been directed to a fourth group of tarsal navicular injuries, stress fractures. I prefer to include these in a classification system that results in four types of navicular fracture (see Table 35–5).

Anatomy

The tarsal navicular has a convex proximal articular surface for articulation with the head of the talus and a

TABLE 35–5.
Classification of Navicular Fractures

1. Fractures of the tuberosity (Fig 35–89)
2. Chip fractures of the dorsal lip (Fig 35–87)
3. Fractures of the body
   a. Without displacement (Fig 35–90)
   b. With displacement (Fig 35–91)
      Type 1 (Fig 35–92,A)
      Type 2 (Fig 35–92,B)
      Type 3 (Fig 35–92,C)
4. Stress fractures of the navicular (Fig 35–94)

concave distal articular surface that is divided into three facets for articulation with each of the three cuneiforms.[15] There may be a fourth facet for articulation with a cuboid.[15] Eichenholtz and Levine[15] stress that due to the strategic location of the navicular in the medial longitudinal arch of the foot, this bone plays a major role in weight bearing during locomotion.[15] It is their opinion that the navicular rather than the talus acts as a keystone for vertical stress on the arch.

Lehman and Eskeles[29] emphasized that the ligaments connecting the navicular to the cuneiforms are weaker than those connecting the talus to the navicular. This difference in strength between the two sets of ligaments results in disruption of the naviculocuneiform ligaments with forced plantar flexion of the foot. Disruption of the naviculocuneiform ligaments permits naviculocuneiform subluxation which results in a compression fracture of the body of the navicular by the cuneiforms.

The blood supply of the navicular plays a major role in the prognosis of injury to this bone.[27] The navicular receives its blood supply from the dorsal and plantar aspects and from the tuberosity.[27, 39, 45] Sarrafian[39] emphasizes that direct branches enter the dorsum of the bone from the dorsalis pedis artery while the plantar surface receives vessels from the medial plantar artery. The tuberosity, on the other hand, receives vessels from an arterial network formed by the union of the two source arteries, the dorsalis pedis and the medial plantar arteries.

Torg et al.[41] stressed that because much of the surface area of the navicular is covered by articular cartilage, only a small area of cortical bone is available for vessels to enter and leave the bone. Their microangiographic studies showed that the medial and lateral thirds of the navicular body have a good blood supply but the central third is relatively avascular (Fig 35–86).[34]

Sarrafian[39] emphasizes that between the ages of 20 and 65 years the number of arteries supplying the navicular decreases. Due to this decreased vascularity with increasing age, pseudarthrosis and aseptic necrosis following injury to this bone, particularly when there is extensive displacement of the fracture, increase with the age of the patient.

Radiographic Diagnosis

Anteroposterior, lateral, and oblique roentgenographs are needed to evaluate the navicular for fractures. However, Eichenholtz and Levine[15] report that fractures of the navicular may be missed, even when the correct roentgenographic views are obtained. It was their opinion that such factors were missed either because the fracture was not suspected or because roentgenographs were not taken at the time of initial examination and were only obtained when persistent pain brought the patient back for a return visit. These authors report that the lateral roentgenograph was particularly important in demonstrating fractures of the navicular. They noted that that portion of the navicular that approximates the cuboid is particularly difficult to evaluate roentgenographically for a fracture.

Chip fractures of the navicular are most commonly

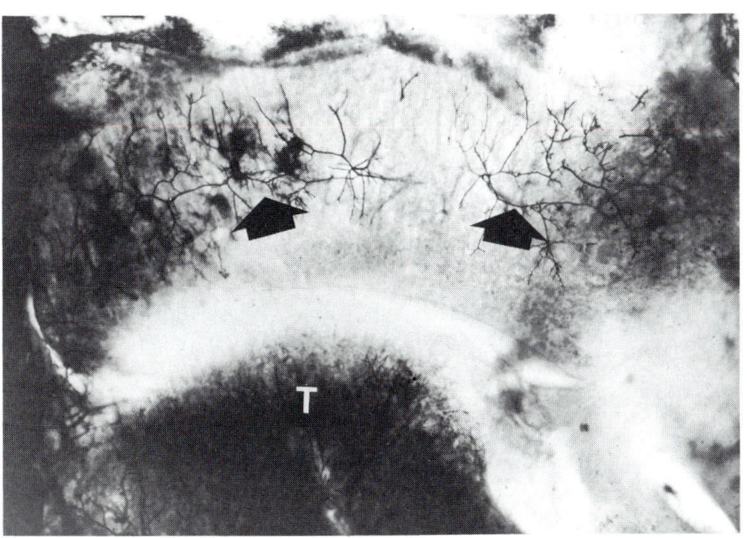

FIG 35–86.
Microangiogram of the tarsal navicular. Note that the medial and lateral thirds of the navicular are well vascularized *(arrows)* while the central third, over the dome of talus *(T),* is relatively avascular. (From Torg JS, Pavlou H, Cooley LH, et al: *J Bone Joint Surg [Am]* 64:700–712, 1982. Used by permission.)

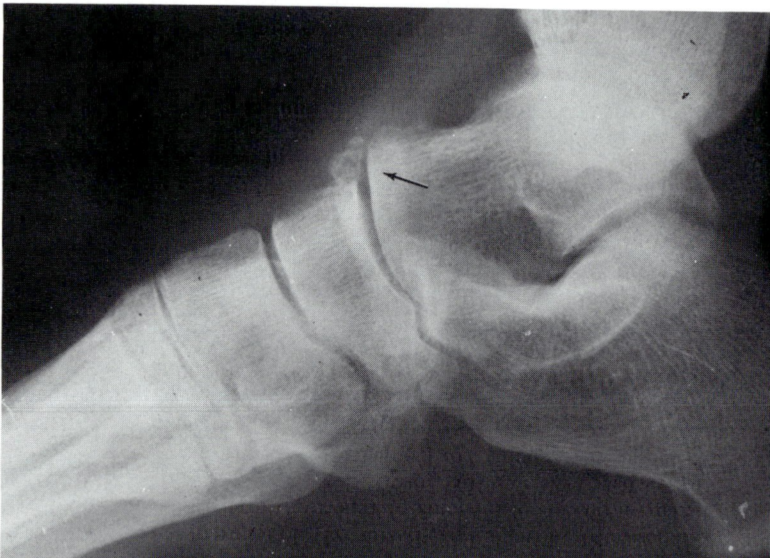

FIG 35–87.
Chip fracture of the dorsum of the navicular *(arrow)*.

noted roentgenographically on the lateral radiograph and are located near the talonavicular articular junction (Fig 35–87). Fractures of the tuberosity of the navicular are best demonstrated on anteroposterior and oblique roentgenographs of the foot with the foot in moderate equinus (see Fig 35–89).[17, 18] One must be certain to exclude the presence of an accessory scaphoid or an os tibiale externum, which may be confused with this fracture (Fig 35–88).[18] The line of separation in the os tibiale externum is usually smooth and regular, whereas a fracture surface should be rough and irregular (Figs 35–88 and 35–89). Additionally, the os tibiale externum is more commonly bilateral. Mygind[32] reports the condition to be bilateral in 90% of cases and unilateral only in about 10%. McKeever[30] reports that an os tibiale externum is present in 15% to 25% of all individuals. These authors, however, also suggest that adult patients with an accessory scaphoid can suffer disruption of the synchondrosis between the two bones, thereby producing an avulsion of the accessory bone.[30, 32]

Giannestras and Sammarco[18] stress that fractures of the body are best delineated by anteroposterior, lateral, and oblique radiographs of the foot (see Fig 35–91). Because of the strong ligamentous attachments of the navicular, the fracture is usually nondisplaced. In such instances, the fracture may be particularly difficult to delineate roentgenographically. In evaluating fractures of the body of the navicular, Morrison[31] and Penhallow[35] stress the importance not only of the fracture but also of the displacement of the fracture fragments. A failure to appreciate displacement of the fracture fragments can lead to a pressure phenomenon within the shoe or to a loss of medial longitudinal arch length of the foot and result in painful degenerative changes later.

Finally, persistent pain in the area of the navicular following traumatic injury, in the face of negative x-ray findings, may suggest the need for a bone scan or polytomography to clearly identify stress fractures of the navicular. This is discussed further under the section on stress fractures of the navicular.

Fractures of the Dorsal Lip of the Navicular

Fractures of the dorsal lip of the navicular are the most frequent type of navicular fractures encountered.[18] They accounted for 47% of fractures of the navicular in the series reported by Eichenholtz and Levine.[15] They are often associated with sprains of the midfoot. The mechanism of injury is usually an acute plantar flexion, inversion injury of the foot in which the talonavicular ligament avulses a portion of the navicular from the proximal dorsal aspect of that bone (see Fig 35–87).

Clinical Diagnosis

The signs and symptoms of dorsal chip fractures consist of pain, swelling, and point tenderness on the dorsal and dorsomedial aspect of the foot in the area of the talonavicular junction. Giannestras and Sammarco[18] emphasize the association of this injury with a lateral sprain of the ankle. A careful clinical search for point tenderness will help prevent confusing these injuries.

Treatment

Dorsal chip fractures should be treated conservatively. Chapman[5] recommends a short period of immobilization and states that usually little disability results. However, he suggests excision of the fragment if pain persists following immobilization. Giannestras and

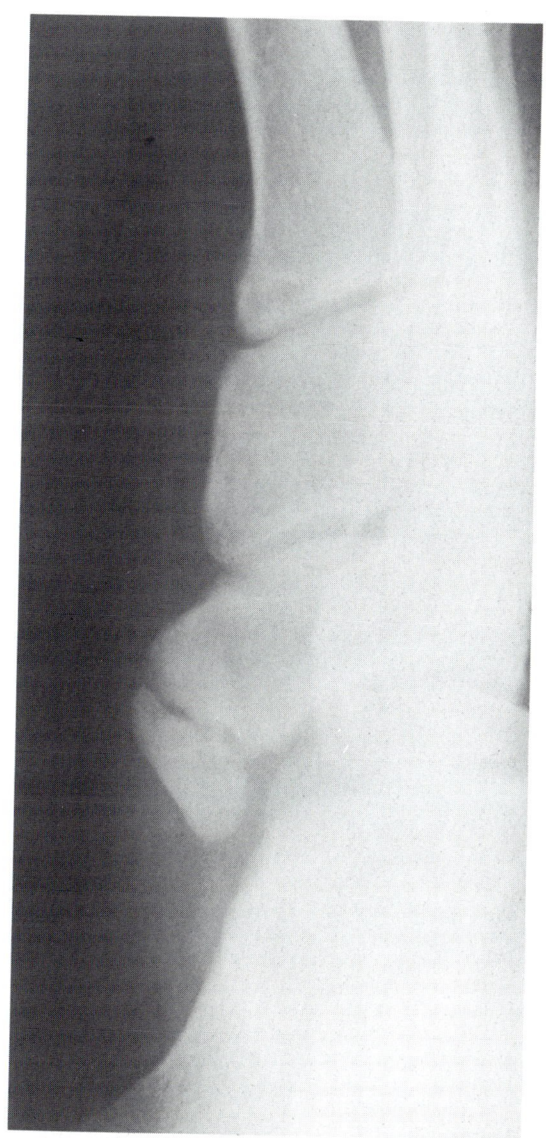

FIG 35–88.
Os tibiale externum (accessory scaphoid). Note that the line of separation is smooth and regular, not irregular as noted in a fracture.

Sammarco[18] recommend the use of an Elastoplast dressing similar to an Ace bandage. In cases in which the symptoms of pain are severe and the chip fragment is larger than a flake of bone, they recommend a below-the-knee walking cast for 3 to 4 weeks. If the fragment is large enough to be a symptomatic bony prominence, they recommend delayed excision of the fragment.

Hillegass[23] agrees with a short period of immobilization for these fractures. However, he suggests open reduction and internal fixation in cases in which the avulsed fragment is a major portion of the articular surface of the navicular. Watson-Jones[44] states that although results are usually excellent following short-term immobilization, these avulsion injuries may be a part of a midtarsal subluxation. If such a subluxation is present, he recommends immobilization for 6 weeks followed by the use of a molded longitudinal arch support.

Fractures of the Navicular Tuberosity

Fracture of the navicular tuberosity results from acute eversion of the foot that leads to increased tension on the tibialis posterior tendon. This increased tension results in an avulsion fracture of the navicular tuberosity.[18] Eichenholtz and Levine[15] suggest that the strong attachment of the deltoid ligament to the tuberosity of the navicular, by way of the spring ligament, is also a major contributing factor that transmits the stress resulting in the fracture.

The fracture is usually only minimally displaced due to the other insertions of the tibialis posterior tendon in the forefoot that prevent the fracture from marked displacement.[17, 47] Because this fragment is seldom widely displaced, operative treatment is usually not necessary.[47] As mentioned under roentgenographic examination, it is important to distinguish avulsion fractures of the tuberosity from an accessory bone, the os tibiale externum, when evaluating these patients acutely (see Figs 35–88 and 35–89,A).

Clinical Diagnosis

The patient usually gives a history of having twisted the foot. He complains of pain over the navicular tuberosity that is accentuated by weight bearing.[17, 18] There is point tenderness on the medial aspect of the navicular. With attempted eversion of the foot, pain is referred to the involved area.[17] This referred pain is due to the increased tension that is applied to the tibialis posterior tendon with eversion of the foot and thus to the fracture site.

Treatment

Most authors suggest that treatment should be symptomatic. In patients with mild pain who are not very active, Giannestras and Sammarco[18] recommend an Elastoplast dressing with guarded weight bearing on crutches. The crutches are discarded as the pain subsides. They recommend changing the dressing every 10 days and continuing support for 4 weeks. However, if the symptoms are severe, they recommend a below-the-knee walking cast with the foot in the neutral position and well molded under the longitudinal arch. These authors stressed that although nonunion may occur, it is usually asymptomatic. In such cases the nonunion is disregarded. However, if pain persists, surgical excision

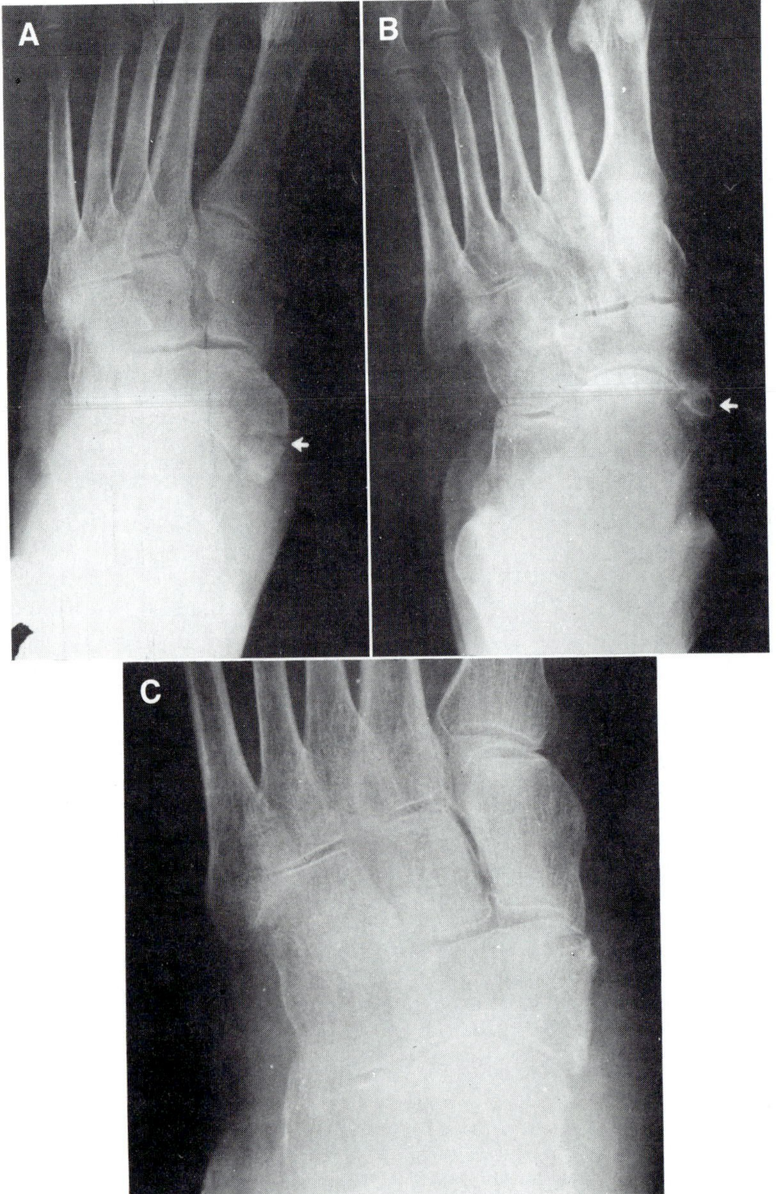

FIG 35–89.
A, nondisplaced fracture of the navicular tubercle. **B,** 1 year after conservative treatment, the patient had pain and peroneal spasm. **C,** fragment excised and pain relieved.

of the tubercle is performed through a slightly curved incision placed medially over the tuberosity of the navicular (see Fig 35–89,A–C). The navicular surface is freshened and the raw surfaces of the tendon sutured to the area under the same tension that existed prior to excision of the navicular tubercle. Following excision the patient is kept in a below-the-knee cast from the tibial tubercle to the toes for 3 to 4 weeks, at which time the cast is removed and weight bearing is gradually permitted.

Garcia and Parkes[17] recommend treating these injuries similar to the method used for a sprained ankle. They use a Gibney adhesive tape dressing with a superimposed elastic (Ace) bandage. If the symptoms are severe, however, they too agree with the use of a below-the-knee walking cast. In such cases immobilization is maintained for 4 weeks. They stress that in this type of fracture, therapy should not be generalized. Instead, each patient's injury should be treated individually. They reserve a short-leg walking cast for patients with severe pain, those who will be quite active during the healing phase, or those in whom walking or manual labor will be required during healing.

Coker and Arnold[6] recommend the use of an inversion cast for 3 weeks followed by inversion strapping for 3 weeks. They too recommend removal of the displaced fragment and repositioning of the posterior tibial tendon in those patients in whom conservative treatment results in a painful nonunion.

Fractures of the Body of the Navicular

Fractures of the body of the navicular are the least frequent of the acute fractures of the tarsal navicular. These fractures can result from direct or indirect force. A direct force due to a crushing injury or blow to the navicular often results in a comminuted fracture. The fragments, however, are usually not displaced since the navicular is well endowed with strong intertarsal ligaments that hold the fragments together (Fig 35–90).[17, 18]

Fractures of the tarsal navicular from indirect violence are usually the result of a fall onto the foot from a height with the foot in marked plantar flexion at the moment of impact.[15, 29] Such fractures are usually described as compression fractures resulting from a force transmitted down through the head of the talus and the cuneiforms.[29] Finsterer[16] believed that the indirect mechanism of fracture was first separation of the talonavicular joint so that the head of the talus lies in contact with the *lower* border of the convex proximal articular surface of the navicular. The application of body weight to the navicular over this limited area then results in fracture. However, Lehman and Eskeles[29] found that with the articulated foot plantar-flexed, the naviculocuneiform ligaments are disrupted and result in the inferior articular surface of the medial cuneiform being driven into the navicular, thereby causing its fracture. Eftekhar et al.[14] and Nadeau and Templeton[33] also suggest that the mechanism of vertical fracture-dislocation of the navicular is combined plantar flexion and abduction of the body of the midtarsal joint. This mechanism results in damage not only to the articular surface of the navicular but also to the articular cartilage at the head of the talus and/or the medial cuneiform.[30] Lehman and Eskeles[29] emphasize that due to the support given the navicular by its neighboring bones, it is hard to conceive of a fracture of the navicular occurring with intact ligaments. This emphasizes the close association between fractures and fracture-dislocations of the body of the navicular and the mechanism of indirect force.

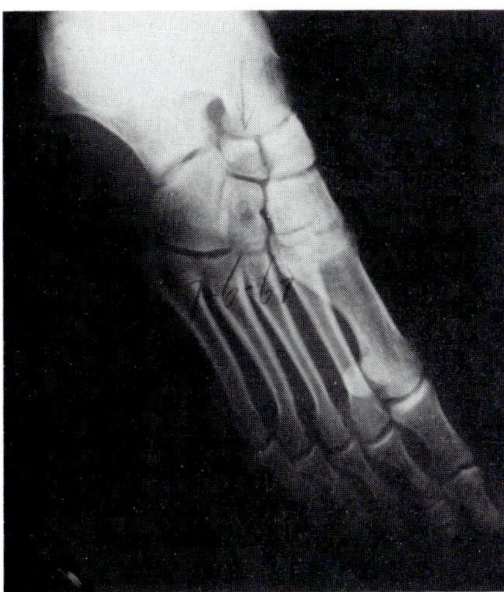

FIG 35–90.
Nondisplaced fracture of the body of the tarsal navicular.

The marked displacement of the fracture fragments resulting from this mechanism of indirect force can produce extensive ligament disruption, fracture displacement, and later, aseptic necrosis (Fig 35–91). The fractured navicular fragments are extruded between the talus and the cuneiforms into the medial or dorsal aspect of the foot. If such an extruded fragment is not reduced, it can produce a bony prominence and result in shortening of the inner border of the foot.[30]

Sangeorzan et al.[38] using radiographic evaluation, have classified fractures of the body of the navicular by the degree and direction of displacement, the number of articular fragments, the alignment of the forefoot, and the presence of associated injuries. In a type 1 fracture, the primary fracture line is transverse in the coronal plane with a dorsal fragment that consists of less than 50% of the body. On the anteroposterior radiograph, the medial border of the foot does not appear to be disrupted (Fig 35–92,A). In a type 2 fracture, the most common, the fracture line traverses dorsolaterally to plantar-medially across the body of the tarsal navicular. The major fragment is dorsal medial, with a small, often comminuted plantar lateral fragment. The calcaneonavicular joint is not disrupted (Fig 35–92,B). Type 3 injuries include fractures with central or lateral comminution. The major fragment is usually the medial one, and the medial border of the foot is disrupted at the calcaneonavicular joint. There may be lateral displacement of the foot with some disruption or subluxation of the calcaneocuboid joint (Fig 35–92,C).

Clinical Diagnosis

Patients usually present with pain localized to the navicular in the midtarsal aspect of the foot.[18] Marked tenderness over the medial aspect of the navicular is usually present.[35] Prior to the onset of swelling, the dis-

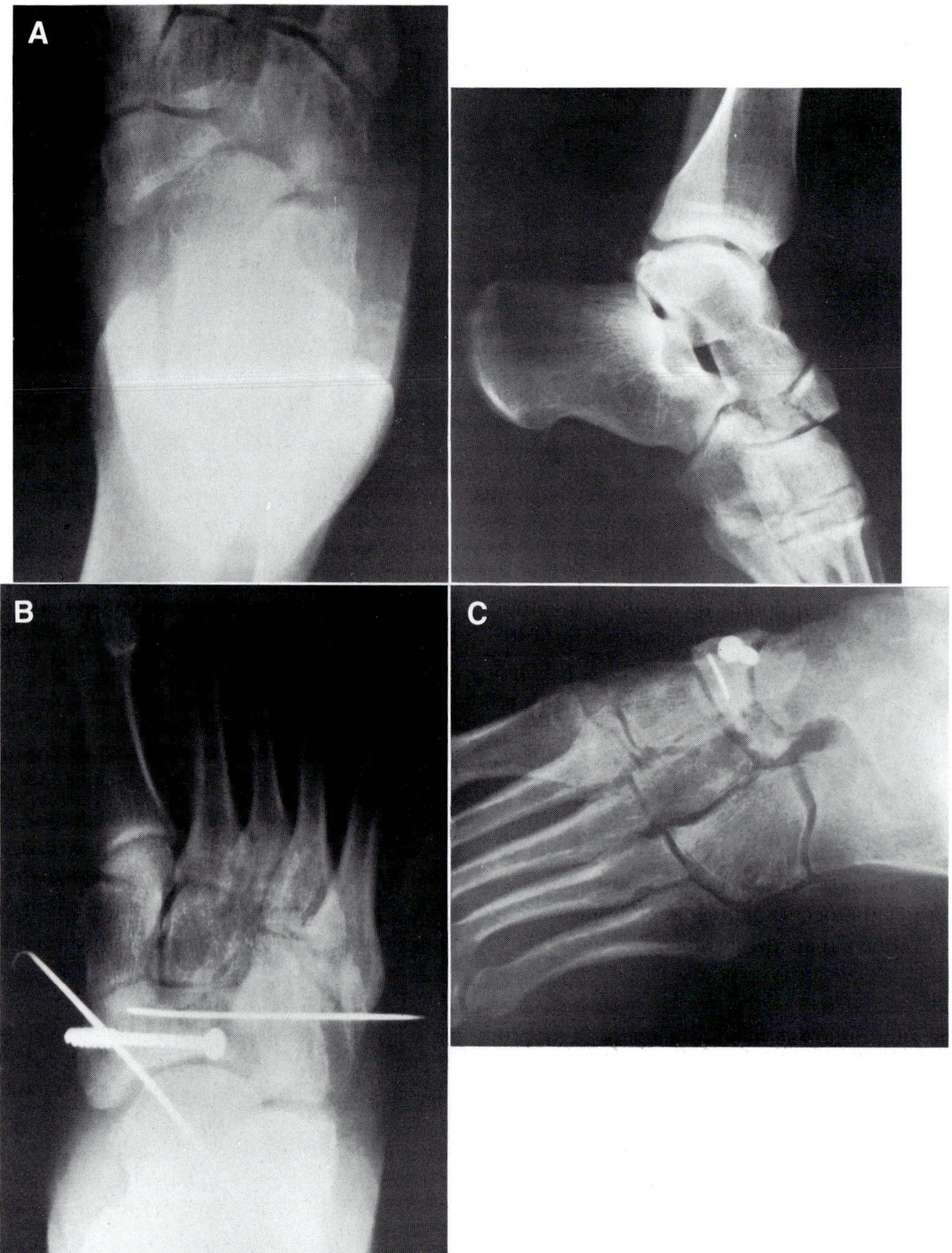

FIG 35–91.
A, anteroposterior and lateral radiographs of a displaced fracture of the tarsal navicular. Note the incongruity of the talonavicular and naviculocuneiform joints. **B,** open reduction and internal fixation of the fracture to restore joint congruity. **C,** follow-up 18 months later demonstrating increased density of the navicular suggesting aseptic necrosis. The patient is pain free.

placed fracture fragments may be palpated on the dorsal aspect of the foot. Motion of the foot, particularly inversion-eversion and abduction-adduction, produces localized pain.[18] Pain and tenderness located on the lateral aspect of the midtarsal joint should suggest a more extensive midtarsal joint injury that should be excluded by physical and roentgenographic evaluation.[18]

Treatment

Treatment of fractures of the body of the navicular is determined by the degree of comminution and displacement of the fracture fragments.[21, 40] Heck recommends a short-leg cast with the foot in equinus for 4 to 6 weeks if the fragments are minimally displaced.[21] Following cast immobilization he recommends the use of a good

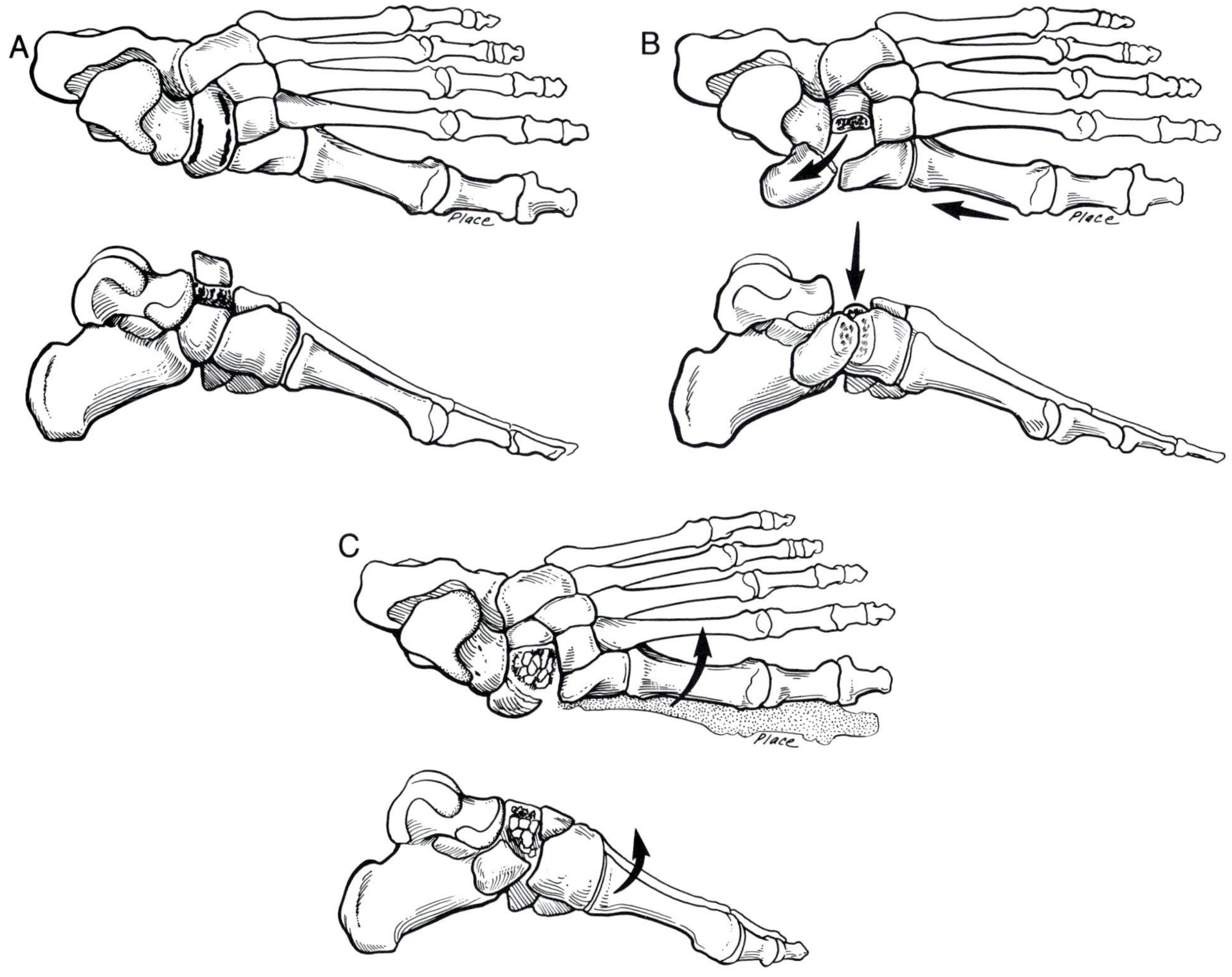

FIG 35–92.
Classification of tarsal navicular fractures described by Sangeorzan et al.[37] **A,** *type 1:* the fracture line is in the plane of the sole of the foot and separates the navicular into dorsal and plantar components. **B,** *type 2:* the fracture line passes from dorsolateral to plantar medial to create a large medial and a smaller lateral fragment. **C,** *type 3:* there is marked comminution in the body of the fracture, which makes anatomic reduction difficult. (From Sangeorzan BJ, Benirschke SK, Mosca V, et al: *J Bone Joint Surg [Am]* 71:1504-1510, 1989. Used by permission.)

shoe with a longitudinal arch support for an additional 6 weeks. Giannestras and Sammarco[18] recommend the use of a snug below-the-knee walking cast with the ankle in the neutral position for 6 to 8 weeks in undisplaced fractures whether or not comminution is present. This is followed by the use of a molded longitudinal arch support in the shoe.

Heck,[21] Speed,[40] and Greenberg and Levine[20] stressed the need for reduction in cases in which the fragments are displaced.[21] If the fracture is displaced, reduction is necessary for two reasons.[35, 40] First, in order to restore the articular surface of the talonavicular and naviculocuneiform joints, reduction is essential. Second, without reduction, shortening of the medial longitudinal arch of the foot can result in a fixed adduction deformity of the forefoot and, later, degenerative arthritis. In addition to resulting in articular incongruity, residual displacement of a navicular fracture may be associated with subluxation of the remainder of the midtarsal joint. Therefore, open reduction may also be necessary to restore the entire midtarsal joint stability. Finally, displaced fragments may produce pressure symptoms in a shoe.

In the presence of a displaced fracture of the navicular body, some authors recommend attempted closed reduction. Heck recommends manual reduction of the displaced fracture with the foot in plantar flexion and eversion.[21] Wilson[48] recommends closed reduction by opening the space between the talus and internal cuneiform by forced plantar flexion of the forefoot and ankle, combined with direct pressure over the dorsal surface of the fracture. A plaster cast extending to the knee and maintaining the position of plantar flexion is then applied. Penhallow[35] and Lehman and Eskeles[29] also reported methods of manipulation that produced good reduction. Following reduction, immobilization in a plaster cast produces a good functional result. Eichenholtz and Levine[15] recommend closed reduction of a dorsally dislocated fragment by manipulation of the forefoot over a plantar block combined with direct pressure over the displaced fragment. They stress, however, that redislocation or partial redisplacement of such a fracture fragment occurs with sufficient frequency to make closed treatment without stabilization uncertain. Coughlin et al.[8] reported a closed reduction under general anesthesia of a fracture-dislocation of the tarsal navicular. Under fluoroscopic control, the fracture was reduced by using a hyper–plantar flexion maneuver with direct pressure over the displaced tarsal navicular fracture fragment. The fracture reduced and was found to be stable. The patient was treated in a below-the-knee non–weight-bearing cast for 4 weeks. He was then begun on progressive weight bearing, and range-of-motion exercises. The authors report good results with this method of treatment.

Bonvallet[3] believed that the generally poor results of conservative therapy were due to a non-anatomic position of the navicular that, following inadequate reduction, acts like a sagging cornerstone in a vault construction. Secondary deformities become manifested following resumption of weight bearing and lead to painful traumatic flat feet with degenerative arthritis. This arthritis involving the talonavicular and naviculocuneiform joints is usually present 6 to 12 months following injury. Day[10] stressed that following closed manipulation, if some deformity of the navicular remains, traumatic arthritis is likely and may require an arthrodesis procedure. He also stressed that since the talonavicular joint is continuous with the subtalar joint, the motions of inversion and eversion of the foot are often disturbed by abnormalities of the surface of the talonavicular joint. Wilson believes that when complete reduction is not accomplished by a closed method or when the patient is seen late (8 to 10 days following injury), arthrodesis of the talonavicular joint is advisable.[10, 48]

Giannestras and Sammarco[18] and Garcia and Parkes[17] indicate that when the fractured navicular is displaced, closed reduction is of little or no value. Nadeau and Templeton[33] recommend open reduction, particularly when there are two major fragments with little or no comminution. The fracture is approached through a dorsal longitudinal incision beginning at the neck of the talus and descending to the distal articular surface of the medial cuneiform.[18] Giannestras and Sammarco stress that following reduction, internal fixation is essential to prevent fragment displacement. They recommended the use of threaded Kirschner wires rather than smooth ones in an effort to prevent fracture displacement. In situations in which the fracture is comminuted, they pass these wires into adjacent tarsal bones for additional stability. Following open reduction, they recommend non–weight-bearing treatment in a short-leg cast for approximately 8 weeks. Eftekhar et al.[14] report open reduction and internal fixation with a Sherman bone screw placed transversely across the fracture.

Recently, Sangeorzan et al.[38] reviewed patients who underwent open reduction and internal fixation of navicular fractures. The authors recommended open reduction and internal fixation of all displaced fractures. They recommended an anteromedial approach in which the interval between the anterior and posterior tibial tendons, beginning just distal to the medial malleolus, is opened. The periosteum over the navicular is not divided in order to protect the remaining blood supply to the bone. The articular surfaces of the talonavicular and calcaneonavicular joints are inspected. The authors recommend the use of a combination of direct and indirect reduction techniques to reduce the injury and occasionally, the utilization of bone grafting to fill central defects in the bone following elevation of joint surfaces. The authors recommend taking the bone graft from either the iliac crest or the distal end of the tibia.

The authors divided these fractures into three types and recommended open reduction and internal fixation depending upon the fracture pattern. In a type 1 fracture (see Fig 35–92,A), the fracture line and joint surfaces are easily seen through the incision. The joints are inspected, loose debris removed, and the dorsal and plantar fragments reduced and held with lag screws directed across the fracture. Reduction of a type 2 injury (see Fig 35–92,B) is more difficult. The fracture lines pass dorsolaterally to plantar-medially. The body of the navicular must be reduced to inspect the joints. The length of the medial border of the foot may be disrupted. In this case, it can be restored by insertion of a mini external fixator onto the talus and first metatarsal. All joints are then inspected for articular depression and loose bodies. When there is minimal comminution and the lateral fragment is large, the dorsomedial fragment is reduced and held with lag screws to the lateral fragment. If the lateral fragments are very comminuted, the defect can be spanned with a mini external fixator and screws passed through the navicular into the second and third cuneiforms or the cuboid to provide temporary stabilization during healing. Type 3 fractures (see Fig

35–92,C) can be treated similarly with additional fixation across the calcaneonavicular joint.

Following internal fixation, a short-leg cast is worn for 6 to 8 weeks. The smooth pins that cross joints are generally removed before weight-bearing or motion is begun. The patients do not bear weight until radiographs indicate that the fracture appears to be healed and manual stress on the medial border of the foot does not cause pain. When swelling in the foot diminishes, the patients are fitted with a shoe with a custom-made insole. The authors report good results in 70% of their patients treated in this manner.

If there is extensive damage to the articular cartilage, consideration should be given to primary arthrodesis.[18] Giannestras and Sammarco[18] emphasized that upon removal of articular cartilage fragments and comminuted cortical surfaces, shortening of the medial longitudinal arc will prevent good bony apposition. In such cases, multiple cancellous bone chips from the iliac crest may be needed to fill the defect.[18] Following such an arthrodesis, a non–weight-bearing cast is recommended for 6 weeks followed by a below-the-knee walking cast for another 6 weeks. Wilson[48] reports that painful function is the invariable result of unreduced fractures of the navicular. He found that primary arthrodesis of the talonavicular joint in cases in which complete reduction could be obtained results in an asymptomatic foot. Dick[13] advocates primary arthrodesis for all tarsal navicular body fractures with dorsally displaced fragments. Day,[10] using amputation specimens, found that localized arthrodesis, i.e., arthrodesis involving the talonavicular and naviculocuneiform joints, resulted in a loss of nearly all the inversion and eversion of the foot. He found that more extensive arthrodesis, including triple arthrodesis plus arthrodesis of the naviculocuneiform joint, produced superior results to those obtained following fusion of only the involved joint. Garcia and Parks[17] utilize the degree of damage to the articular cartilage surfaces as criteria for immediate arthrodesis of either the talonavicular and/or naviculocuneiform joints in younger patients. Both of these authors, however, believe that in the elderly patient in whom cast immobilization is detrimental, Elastoplast dressing and a well-fitted oxford shoe should be utilized until healing takes place.

Finally, Crossan[9] reports that removal of part or all of the fractured bone helps to relieve symptoms in cases in which open reduction is impossible and in those patients who report late for treatment.

Results

Eichenholtz and Levine[15] report that uniformly good results can be expected following the treatment of cortical avulsion fractures and undisplaced tuberosity and body fractures of the tarsal navicular. However, following the reduction of displaced fractures, Dick reports that degenerative changes in the talonavicular and/or naviculocuneiform joints will often result in a painful foot.[13]

Additionally, the development of aseptic necrosis of the navicular following open reduction and internal fixation can result in late segmental collapse and further degenerative changes (see Fig 35–91,C).[13, 46] Day also concluded that traumatic arthritis was a very common sequela to fracture-dislocation of the tarsal navicular.[10] Sangeorzan et al.[38] report that satisfactory reduction was obtained in all type 1 displaced fractures, in 67% of type 2 fractures, and in 50% of type 3 fractures. Of the 15 patients with a satisfactory reduction, 14 had a good result, and one had a fair result. The authors concluded that both the type of fracture and the accuracy of operative reduction directly correlated with the final outcome. The authors did report, however, that only 4 of their 21 patients with an injured foot were totally asymptomatic and fully functional at follow-up.

Stress Fractures of the Tarsal Navicular

Although stress fractures of the tarsal navicular are recognized by veterinarians as a common problem in greyhounds,[2] their occurrence in humans is less well recognized.[41] Towne et al.[42] first reported a stress or fatigue fracture in two patients in 1970. Devas[12] reported two additional cases in 1975, both in older women. Orva et al.[34] found only 1 such case in 142 stress fractures, an incidence of 0.7%. Goergen et al.[19] reported two additional cases in runners, one of which required open reduction and internal fixation.

Hunter in 1981 stressed that these injuries are probably more common than recognized.[25] She emphasized that the pain associated with tarsal navicular stress fractures may often be vague and diffuse. However, the fact that the pain in these patients increases during activity and *not* following it helps to differentiate this stress fracture from overuse syndromes in the foot. She also noted that these patients are usually involved in athletic activities, particularly track.[25, 42] Torg et al.[41] in a classic multicenter study reported 21 cases and carefully outlined diagnosis and treatment.

Clinical Diagnosis

The diagnosis in these patients is difficult because the symptoms may be diffuse and the physical examination nondiagnostic.[25] The patients usually give a history of the insidious onset of vague pain over the dorsum of the foot or the medial aspect of the longitudinal arch.[41]

The pain is an ill-defined soreness or cramping sensation.[41] It is accentuated with inversion or eversion of the forepart of the foot.[42] The tarsal navicular is tender in most cases.[41] There is usually little if any swelling or discoloration. Foot abnormalities including a short first metatarsal, metatarsus adductus, limited ankle dorsiflexion and subtalar motion are occasionally present and may concentrate stress on the navicular.[41]

Hunter[25] found that when these patients stand on their toes and exert downward pressure on the metatarsal heads, the symptoms of pain in the area of the navicular are reproduced. Hunter emphasizes the importance of being alert to this potential diagnosis in athletes with foot pain because a failure to recognize this entity and curtail the athletic activity may result in a displaced stress fracture of the navicular.[25, 42]

Radiographic Diagnosis

Towne et al.[42] found that initial roentgenographs may fail to reveal the fracture. However, roentgenographs taken 1 to 2 months following the development of symptoms may reveal a vertical radiolucent line in the tarsal navicular. Towne et al.[42] also point out that conventional radiographs are often negative but that laminagrams may reveal a vertical fracture of the tarsal navicular in cases of stress fracture (see Fig 35–94). Hunter[25] also emphasizes that in patients who present with pain in the foot suggestive of a navicular stress fracture, the roentgenographic findings may be negative. She suggests the use of bone scans or tomograms for verification of the stress fracture.

Torg et al.[41] also stress the need for appropriate radiographic studies to ensure a prompt diagnosis. They suggest standing anteroposterior, lateral, and oblique views if such a fracture is suspected. They emphasize that the tarsal navicular is often underpenetrated on these roentgenographs and that a coned-down anteroposterior view centered on the navicular may be required.[41] If the radiograph is normal, a radionuclide bone scan using technetium 99m will help to make the diagnosis (Fig 35–93).[37, 41] These authors stress that if radiographic findings are normal but the bone scan indicates a lesion of the navicular, tomograms of the navicular are required (Fig 35–94). The position of the foot for accurate tomographic examination is important. The tarsal navicular must be in the *true* anteroposterior position. To accomplish this the foot is inverted until the entire medial-to-lateral width of the foot is demonstrated. Additionally, the dorsal surface of the navicular must be parallel to the tomographic cut to avoid missing an incomplete stress fracture that is confined to the dorsal aspect of the bone (Fig 35–94,B). Any obliquity of the foot during tomography will obscure such a fracture.[41] Using these techniques the authors found all fractures to be located in the sagittal plane in the central third of the bone. Partial fractures located in the dorsal cortex involved the proximal articular surface in most cases.

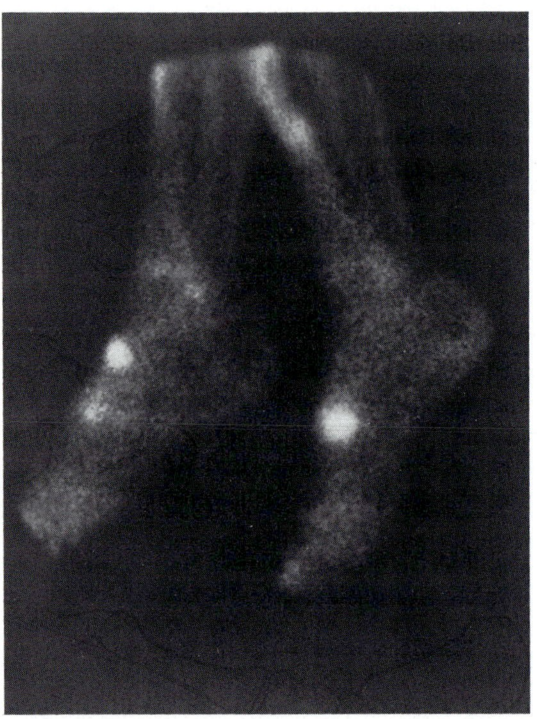

FIG 35–93.
Radionuclide bone scan demonstrating increased uptake in both tarsal naviculars.

Confusion of a fatigue fracture of the tarsal navicular with a bipartite navicular is possible.[25, 41, 42] Anteroposterior roentgenographs in cases of a bipartite navicular reveal the bone to be comma shaped and bent, and on the lateral roentgenograph a cleft is noted to run from the proximal plantar aspect to the distal dorsal margin and separate a triangular osseous structure located dorsal to the rest of the body of the navicular.[28] True stress fractures occur in the sagittal plane.[41] Bone scans and tomography can be also be used to distinguish between a bipartite navicular and a stress fracture.

Treatment

Hunter[25] recommends treating nondisplaced stress fractures by curtailing athletic activity to prevent the development of a displaced stress fracture. She reports open reduction and internal fixation of a stress fracture that displaced prior to diagnosis. In patients in whom repeated stress fractures of the navicular are noted in spite of an alteration in training techniques, she suggests that inherent abnormal anatomy may be a signifi-

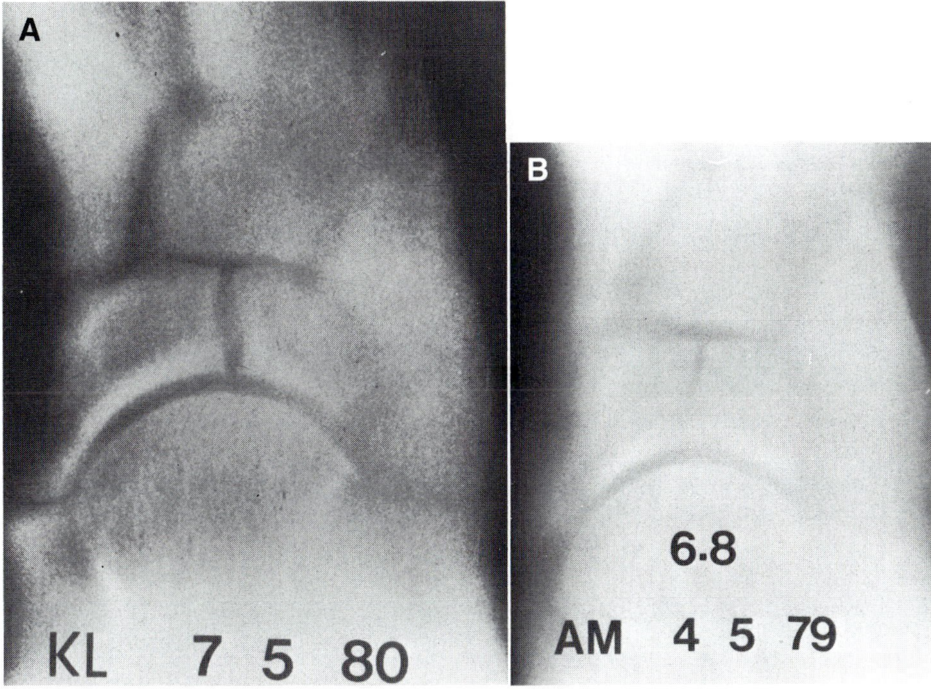

FIG 35–94.
A, polytomogram of the tarsal navicular demonstrating a complete stress fracture. **B,** polytomogram shows an incomplete stress fracture in the central third of the navicular. (From Torg JS, Pavlou H, Cooley LH, et al: *J Bone Joint Surg [Am]* 64:700–712, 1982. Used by permission.)

cant predisposing factor. In such cases she recommends the use of orthotics to correct the abnormal anatomy. Her main emphasis, however, is on the early recognition of stress fractures to prevent displacement.

Towne et al.[42] presented two cases. In the first, a vertical fracture of the navicular required open reduction and internal fixation with bone grafting followed by non–weight bearing for 3 months. In the second case, a nondisplaced stress fracture of the navicular was treated simply by crutches and non–weight bearing for 4 months. Healing without sequelae resulted.

Wiley and Brown[46] reported three patients with stiff, painful feet in which the tarsal scaphoid apparently separated to such a degree that the head of the talus became approximated to the cuneiforms. Although these authors termed this entity "listhesis of the tarsal scaphoid," it may well have represented a stress fracture of the navicular that became displaced. Two of the patients received some relief from conservative therapy, while the third required a triple arthrodesis.

Torg et al.[41] indicated that the result of treatment is not dependent on the type of fracture. However, a failure to treat these fractures with *non*–weight bearing seems to contribute to disability because of delayed union, nonunion, and refracture.[41] These authors recommend that uncomplicated partial stress fractures and nondisplaced stress fractures of the tarsal navicular be treated by immobilization in a plaster cast with non–weight bearing for 6 to 8 weeks. Displaced, complete fractures and ununited fractures should be treated with internal fixation and/or bone grafting followed by immobilization and non–weight bearing until union occurs. They stressed that treatment by limitation of activity but continued weight bearing or immobilization in a weight-bearing plaster cast may lead to prolonged disability.

Author's Preferred Method of Treatment

Dorsal Chip Fractures of the Navicular

In cases of dorsal chip fracture of the navicular, care is taken to ascertain whether these are isolated avulsion injuries or whether they represent part of a midtarsal subluxation. I treat isolated cases of avulsion fracture symptomatically. In patients with minimal pain and swelling, an Elastoplast dressing or Unna boot and crutch walking with partial weight bearing are recommended until symptoms subside. Dressings are changed when they become loose. If the initial pain is severe and the patient must be weight bearing during treatment, a below-the-knee walking cast is applied for 3 to 4 weeks. Following this a good shoe with a well-molded arch support is utilized. The author has not found these injuries to result in significant sequelae. However, if pain persists after treatment, excision of the fracture fragment is recommended.

Fractures of the Navicular Tuberosity

I prefer to treat these fractures symptomatically. If the patient is not active and the pain resulting from the injury not severe, an Elastoplast dressing or Unna boot is applied from the toes to above the ankle. This dressing is changed every 2 weeks and is maintained for approximately 4 weeks. If the pain is severe and the patient is active, a below-the-knee walking cast is applied with the foot and ankle in the neutral position. This is maintained for 3 to 4 weeks.

Following this initial treatment, nonunion of the fracture site may occur. In those instances in which it is asymptomatic, no treatment is recommended. However, if pain persists following initial treatment, consideration is given to excision of the navicular tuberosity. In such instances, a curved incision placed over the navicular tuberosity is utilized. The navicular tuberosity is removed from the posterior tibial tendon, the fracture surface is freshened, and the posterior tibial tendon is resutured to the area. Postoperatively the patient remains in a below-the-knee cast extending from the toes to the tibial tubercle with a well-molded longitudinal arch support. The cast is removed in 4 to 6 weeks, at which time gradually increased weight bearing is permitted.

Fractures of the Body of the Navicular

In nondisplaced fractures of the body of the navicular, I prefer a below-the-knee walking cast from the tibial tubercle to the toes with the foot and ankle in the neutral position. This cast is maintained for 6 weeks and is removed when there is x-ray evidence of union. The patient is then instructed in the use of a well-molded longitudinal arch support.

If the fracture is displaced, the author has found closed reduction rarely successful. The decision to perform open reduction is based upon the degree of comminution. I prefer to treat these fractures by open reduction through a dorsal longitudinal incision from the neck of the talus to the middle aspect of the medial cuneiform. The fracture is carefully reduced under direct vision in an effort to anatomically restore the articular surface of the talonavicular and naviculocuneiform joints. Initially internal fixation with Kirschner wires is utilized. If the fracture fragments are large enough, screws from the small-fragment AO set are used (see Fig 35–91,C).

In patients with severely comminuted fractures whose job will require prolonged weight bearing, open reduction and internal fixation with Kirschner wires through the fracture fragments into the adjacent tarsal bones are utilized in an effort to maintain the longitudinal and medial arches of the foot. Although anatomic reduction is not obtained, restoration of the arch may result in a functional foot, particularly when one considers the limited motion available in the talonavicular and naviculocuneiform joints. However, if there is severe damage to the head of the talus or to the articular surface of the medial cuneiform in conjunction with a comminuted navicular fracture, consideration is given to primary arthrodesis of the talonavicular and naviculocuneiform joints. In such cases, I have found it necessary to use a full-thickness iliac crest bone graft to replace the navicular and fuse the talonavicular and naviculocuneiform joints in order to prevent a loss of length of the medial arch of the foot. The bone graft is stabilized with Kirschner wires. Following bone grafting a short-leg non–weight-bearing cast for 8 weeks followed by a short-leg weight-bearing cast for an additional 4 to 6 weeks is recommended. I prefer to attempt an open reduction initially to restore medial arch alignment and reserve arthrodesis as a secondary procedure for cases in which the indications for arthrodesis are not certain at the time of initial treatment.

Stress Fractures of the Navicular

I agree with Hunter[25] and Torg et al.[41] that an early diagnosis of stress fractures of the navicular is the cornerstone of treatment. In the athletic individual, particularly the long-distance runner, pain in the arch of the foot with slight swelling and tenderness should suggest the presence of a tarsal navicular stress fracture. In these patients, the diagnosis is made by routine roentgenographs, laminagrams, and/or radionuclide bone scans. In cases in which the fracture is not displaced or is incomplete, treatment is by immobilization in a short-leg *non*–weight-bearing cast for 6 to 8 weeks.

In patients who present with a displaced stress fracture of the navicular and in those with an established nonunion, I prefer reduction and internal fixation with bone grafting through a dorsal approach. Following bone grafting and internal fixation, a short-leg non–weight-bearing cast is worn until union occurs.

In patients with repetitive stress fractures, custom orthotics are used in an effort to alter the cyclic forces on the foot. If this fails, such patients are encouraged to change their athletic activities.

REFERENCES

Midpart of Foot

1. Bohler L: *The treatment of fractures*, ed 5, vol 3, New York, 1958, Grune & Stratton.

2. Bateman JK: Broken hook in the greyhound. Repair methods and the plastic scaphoid, *Vet Rec* 70:621–623, 1958.
3. Bonvallet JM: The surgical treatment of recent scaphoid fractures of the foot, *Int Abstr Surg* 90:295, 1950.
4. Bonvallet JM: The surgical treatment of recent scaphoid fractures of the foot, *Semin Hop Paris* 59:2513, 1949.
5. Chapman MW: Fractures and fracture dislocations of the ankle and foot. In Mann RA, editor: *DuVries' surgery of the foot*, ed 4, St Louis, 1978, Mosby–Year Book.
6. Coker TP Jr, Arnold JA: Sports injuries to the foot and ankle. In Jahss MH, editor: *Disorders of the foot*, vol 2, Philadelphia, 1982, WB Saunders.
7. Conwell HE, Reynolds FC: *Key and Conwell's management of fractures, dislocations, and sprains*, ed 7, St Louis, 1961, Mosby–Year Book.
8. Coughlin L, Kwok D, Oliver J: Fracture dislocation of the tarsal navicular, *Am J Sports Med* 15:614–615, 1987.
9. Crossan ET: Fractures of the tarsal scaphoid and of the os calcis, *Surg Clin North Am* 10:1477, 1930.
10. Day AJ: The treatment of injuries to the tarsal navicular, *J Bone Joint Surg* 29:359–366, 1947.
11. DePalma AF: *The management of fractures and dislocations: an atlas*, Philadelphia, 1959, WB Saunders.
12. Devas M: *Stress fractures*, New York, 1975, Churchill Livingstone.
13. Dick IL: Impacted fracture-dislocation of the tarsal navicular, *Proc R Soc Med* 35:760, 1942.
14. Eftekhar NM, Lyddon DW, Stevens J: An unusual fracture-dislocation of the tarsal navicular, *J Bone Joint Surg [Am]* 57:577–581, 1969.
15. Eichenholtz SN, Levine DB: Fractures of the tarsal navicular bone, *Clin Orthop* 34:142, 1964.
16. Finsterer H: Ueber Verletzungen im bereiche de fusswurzelknochen mit besonderer berucksichtigung des os naviculare. *Beitr Klin Chir* 59:99, 1908.
17. Garcia A, Parkes JC: Fractures of the foot. In Giannestras NJ, editor: *Foot disorders: medical and surgical management*, ed 2, Philadelphia, 1973, Lea & Febiger.
18. Giannestras NJ, Sammarco GJ: Fractures and dislocations in the foot. In Rockwood CA Jr, Green DP, editors: *Fractures*, vol 2, Philadelphia, 1975, JB Lippincott.
19. Goergen TG, Venn-Watson EA, Rossman DJ, et al: Tarsal navicular stress fractures in runners, *AJR* 136:201–203, 1981.
20. Greenberg MJ, Levine DB: Vertical fracture of the tarsal navicular, *Orthopedics* 3:254–255, 1980.
21. Heck CV: Fractures of the bones of the foot (except the talus), *Surg Clin North Am* 45:103–117, 1965.
22. Henderson MS: Fractures of the bones of the foot—except the os calcis, *Surg Gynecol Obstet* 64:454, 1937.
23. Hillegass RC: Injuries to the midfoot: a major cause of industrial morbidity. In Bateman JE, editor: *Foot science*, Philadelphia, 1976, WB Saunders.
24. Hoffman A: Ueber die isolierte fraktur des os naviculare tarsi, *Beitr Klin Chir* 59:217, 1908.
25. Hunter LY: Stress fractures of the tarsal navicular, *Am J Sports Med* 9:217–219, 1981.
26. Joplin RJ: Injuries of the foot. In Cave EF, editor: *Fractures and other injuries*, St Louis, 1958, Mosby–Year Book.
27. Kelly PJ: Anatomy, physiology and pathology of the blood supply of bones, AAOS Instr Course Lectures, *J Bone Joint Surg [Am]* 50:766–783, 1968.
28. Kohler A, Zimmer EA, Case JJ: *Borderlands of the normal and early pathologic in skeletal roentgenology*, New York, 1956, Grune & Stratton, p 723.
29. Lehman EP, Eskeles IH: Fractures of tarsal scaphoid: with notes on the mechanism, *J Bone Joint Surg* 10:108, 1928.
30. McKeever FM: Fractures of the tarsal and metatarsal bones, *Surg Gynecol Obstet* 90:735–745, 1950.
31. Morrison GM: Fractures of the bones of the foot, *Am J Surg* 38:721, 1937.
32. Mygind HB: The accessory tarsal scaphoid, *Acta Orthop Scand* 23:142–151, 1954.
33. Nadeau P, Templeton J: Vertical fracture-dislocation of the tarsal navicular, *J Trauma* 16:669–671, 1976.
34. Orva S, Puranen J, Ala-Ketola L: Stress fractures caused by physical exercise, *Acta Orthop Scand* 49:19–27, 1978.
35. Penhallow DP: An unusual fracture-dislocation of the tarsal scaphoid with dislocation of the cuboid, *J Bone Joint Surg* 19:517, 1937.
36. Perriard M, Dieterli J, Jeannet E: Les lesions traumatiques recentes comprises entre les articulations de Chopart et de Lisfranc, incluses, *Z Unfallmed Berufskr* 63:318, 1970.
37. Prather JL, Nusynowitz ML, Snowdy HA, et al: Scintigraphic findings in stress fractures, *J Bone Joint Surg [Am]* 59:869–874, 1977.
38. Sangeorzan BJ, Benirschke SK, Mosca V, et al: Displaced intra-articular fractures of the tarsal navicular, *J Bone Joint Surg [Am]* 71:1504–1510, 1989.
39. Sarrafian SK: *Anatomy of the foot and ankle*, Philadelphia, 1983, JB Lippincott.
40. Speed K: *A textbook of fractures and dislocations covering their pathology, diagnosis and treatment*, ed 4, Philadelphia, 1942, Lea & Febiger.
41. Torg JS, Pavlov H, Cooley LH, et al: Stress fractures of the tarsal navicular, *J Bone Joint Surg [Am]* 64:700–712, 1982.
42. Towne LC, Blazina ME, Cozen LN: Fatigue fracture of the tarsal navicular, *J Bone Joint Surg [Am]* 52:376–378, 1970.
43. Waters CH Jr: Midtarsal fractures and dislocations. In *American Academy of Orthopaedic Surgeons: instructional course lectures*, vol 9, Ann Arbor, Mich, 1952, JW Edwards.
44. Watson-Jones R: *Fractures and joint injuries*, ed 4, vol 2, Baltimore, 1955, Williams & Wilkins.
45. Waugh W: The ossification and vascularization of the tarsal navicular and their relationship to Köhler's disease, *J Bone Joint Surg [Br]* 40:765–777, 1958.
46. Wiley JJ, Brown D: Listhesis of the tarsal scaphoid, *J Bone Joint Surg [Br]* 56:586, 1974.
47. Wilson JN: *Watson-Jones fractures and joint injuries*, ed 6, New York, 1982, Churchill Livingstone.
48. Wilson PD: Fractures and dislocations of the tarsal bones, *South Med J* 26:833, 1933.

FRACTURES OF THE CUBOID AND CUNEIFORM BONES

Isolated fractures of the cuboid and cuneiform bones are quite rare.[12, 14] McKeever[12] believed that this was secondary to the fact that both the cuboid and cuneiform bones occupy a protected and buttressed location in the metatarsus. When these fractures do occur, they are most frequently caused by a direct crushing force[12] or by a fall on the foot in plantar flexion with accompanying inversion or eversion.[14] Wilson[14] reported that fractures of the cuboid or cuneiform, either singly or in combination with other injuries, were of no serious significance. McKeever also reported that due to their protected and buttressed location, displacement was seldom present and, therefore, reduction was usually not required.

Fractures of the Cuboid

Chapman[4] reports that isolated fractures of the cuboid are quite rare and that they more commonly occur in conjunction with fractures of the cuneiforms or the bases of the lateral metatarsals. Garcia and Parks[6] emphasize that fractures of the cuboid, although usually comminuted, are seldom displaced due to the maintenance of position of the fracture fragments by the strong intertarsal ligaments. They stress that fractures of the cuboid are often associated with tarsometatarsal or midtarsal dislocations or subluxations and that the cuboid may also be involved in calcaneal fractures.

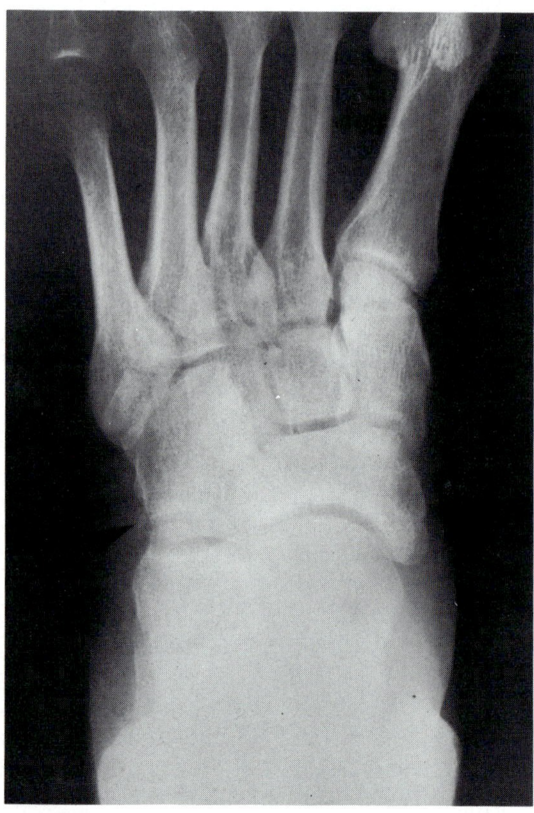

FIG 35–95.
Chip fracture of the cuboid *(arrow)*.

Hillegass[10] reports two types of cuboid injuries. The first and most frequent are avulsion fractures of the cuboid (Fig 35–95). Second are fractures that involve the entire body of the cuboid. Blazina and Westover[1] report an avulsion injury of the cuboid and emphasize that the location of such cortical avulsions on the lateral aspect of the foot causes them to be confused with a routine ankle sprain. Hermel and Gershon-Cohen[9] reported five cases of the so-called "nutcracker fracture of the cuboid" as an example of the second type of fracture. In these five cases the cuboid was caught "like a nut in a cracker" between the bases of the fourth and fifth metatarsals and the calcaneus. In each instance, the toes were fixed, and the weight of the body was transmitted by the calcaneus through the cuboid and the two lateral metatarsals.[9, 11] The cuboid was thus crushed and gave rise to an impacted and comminuted fracture (Fig 35–96). It is important to recognize that in two of the five patients reported by these authors there was an associated subluxation of Chopart's joint.

Clinical Diagnosis

The patient will give a history of either a direct blow to the lateral aspect of the foot or trauma to the foot following jumping or twisting the foot beneath the body.[7, 9] There is pain on the lateral border of the foot with point tenderness over the cuboid. Associated tenderness over the medial aspect of Chopart's joint suggests associated subluxation or actual dislocation of the entire midtarsal joint. Passive abduction and adduction or inversion and eversion of the foot will accentuate the pain in the midpart of the foot.

Radiographic Diagnosis

Anteroposterior, lateral, and oblique roentgenographs are useful in evaluating fractures of the cuboid.[7] In the author's experience, the oblique radiograph is most helpful in determining not only the direction of the fracture line but also the presence or absence of displacement of the calcaneocuboid or cuboid-metatarsal joint surfaces. Evaluation of this oblique roentgenograph is also essential to determine the presence or absence of associated fractures of the calcaneus or metatarsals. As emphasized by Hermel and Gershon-Cohen,[9] in patients with the "nutcracker fracture" *and* an associated avulsion fracture of the navicular tubercle, midtarsal subluxation must be considered.

Treatment

Bohler[2] and Conwell and Reynolds[5] both emphasize that fractures of the cuboid rarely demonstrate displacement and, hence, treatment need only be immobiliza-

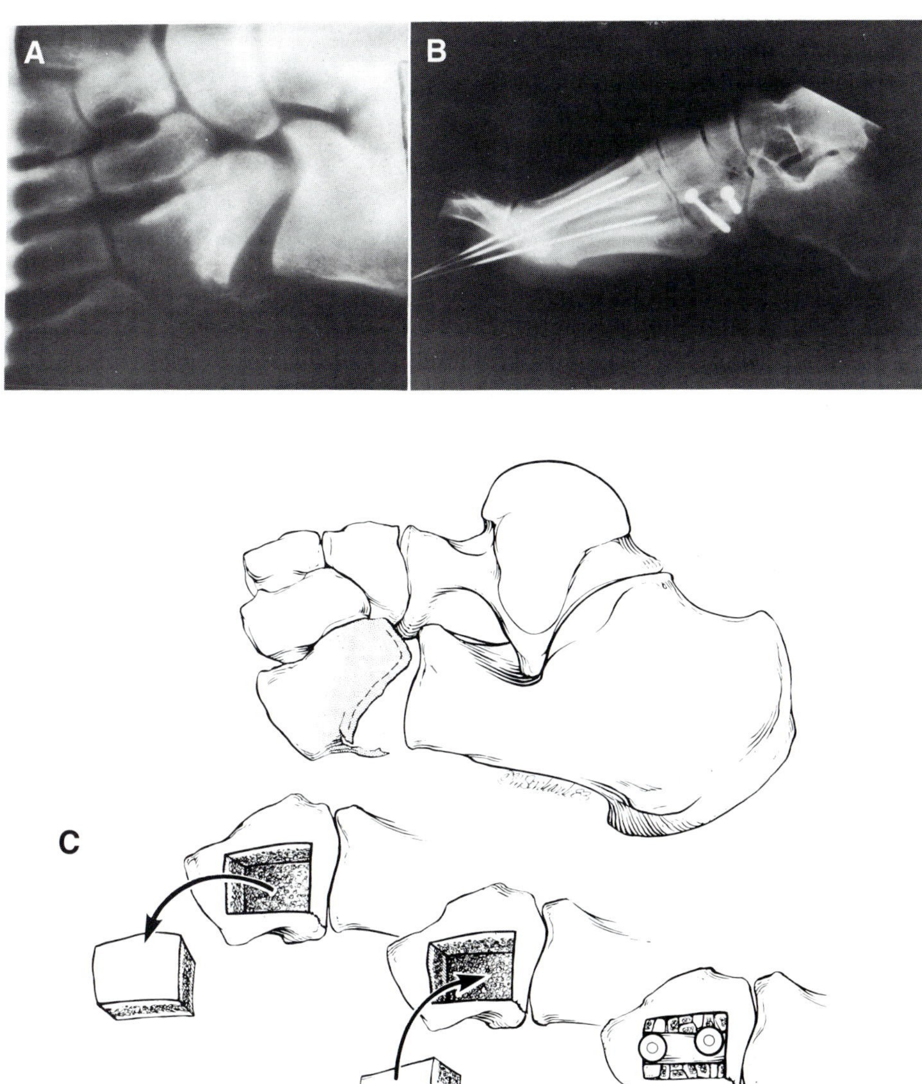

FIG 35–96.
A, impacted fracture of the cuboid involving the calcaneocuboid articular surface. **B,** open reduction and internal fixation of the cuboid. The joint surface has been restored. Kirschner wires are stabilizing the associated metatarsal shaft fractures. **C,** a corticocancellous strut graft was used to stabilize reduction of the articular surface. Cancellous bone was used to fill in the defect.

tion. Heck[8] also reports that displacement of such fractures is rare and healing occurs with few complications. He recommends early treatment with a short-leg cast for 3 to 4 weeks followed by an adequate shoe. He warns of the late complication of a bony prominence over the dorsum of the foot in the area of the fracture that may interfere with the wearing of shoes.

Giannestras and Sammarco[7] also prefer a well-padded and molded short-leg weight-bearing cast for 5 to 6 weeks following the injury. This is followed by a well-fitting longitudinal arch support for an additional 4 to 6 months. They report that although there may be some discomfort on weight bearing for several weeks after cast removal, long-term complications are unusual. Garcia and Parkes[6] recommend a below-the-knee walking cast for 6 to 8 weeks with progressive ambulation. These authors report that since there is little motion in these joints normally, little or no impairment of function of this part of the foot is noted following this injury. The authors, however, do stress that the mechanism of these injuries, a crushing-type trauma from heavy objects falling on the foot, can result in severe soft-tissue damage. Therefore they stress the importance of close observation of the soft tissues in the area of the fracture in the hospital until the period of danger to the soft tissues has passed.

Hermel and Gershon-Cohen[9] recommended early midtarsal fusion for severe fractures associated with subluxation or dislocation of the cuboid. Hillegass,[10] however, believes that these injuries might respond well to accurate open reduction and internal fixation if the cuboid articular surface is significantly displaced (see Fig 35–96).

Author's Preferred Method of Treatment

In patients with chip fractures of the cuboid, clinical and roentgenographic evaluation of the *medial* aspect of the midtarsal joint is essential. If there is no injury to the ligaments on the medial aspect of the midtarsal joint, treatment is based on the patient's requirements for weight bearing. If the patient needs to be ambulatory, I prefer a short-leg walking cast until the pain is relieved. If the pain is minimal, an Ace wrap or Unna boot is used until the pain has subsided. If an avulsion fracture of the navicular tubercle or medial midtarsal tenderness suggests an associated midtarsal sprain, short-leg cast immobilization for 4 to 6 weeks followed by the use of a good shoe with a longitudinal arch support is recommended.

In fractures involving the body of the cuboid, particularly those of the nutcracker variety as described by Hermel and Gershon-Cohen,[9] careful evaluation of the oblique roentgenographs is undertaken. In these injuries residual displacement of the articular surface of the cuboid can result in persistent subluxation of the midtarsal joint and long-term arthritic changes. If a large portion of the calcaneocuboid or cuboid-metatarsal joint is displaced, consideration is given to open reduction. A longitudinal incision parallel to the sole of the foot and located over the cuboid followed by open reduction and bone grafting is utilized. A corticocancellous bone graft used as a strut may be necessary due to compression of the cancellous bone of the cuboid that results from the "nutcracker" mechanism (see Fig 35–96). Following open reduction and reconstruction of the articular surface, range of motion of the foot is encouraged if fracture fixation is stable. Once range of motion of the foot has been restored, the patient is placed in a short-leg non–weight-bearing cast for 6 weeks. The patient is then placed in a good shoe with a longitudinal arch support.

If the comminution is too severe or if the fracture is not significantly displaced, a short-leg walking cast is applied for 4 to 6 weeks followed by the use of a shoe with an arch support. In the author's experience, such fractures have not resulted in long-term disability.

Cuneiform Fractures

Fractures of the cuneiform bones are quite rare.[7, 10] According to Heck,[8] displacement of these fractures is unusual, and healing with few complications is likely.

The mechanism of injury of cuneiform fractures is usually that of direct trauma.[7] Therefore, the treating surgeon must be cognizant of associated soft-tissue trauma that may not be appreciated initially.

Clinical Diagnosis

The patient usually presents with complaints of pain in the area of the specific cuneiform injury. The location of tenderness helps to delineate the particular cuneiform involved. As with fractures of the cuboid, inversion and eversion of the forefoot are distinctly painful.[6]

Radiographic Diagnosis

Anteroposterior, lateral, and oblique roentgenographs are useful in evaluating fractures of the cuneiform (Fig 35–97). Chip fractures are usually nondisplaced due to the fact that the associated intertarsal ligaments are strong and prevent their displacement.[12, 14]

Treatment

Avulsion fractures are usually treated symptomatically by immobilization in a short-leg weight-bearing cast until the pain subsides.[10] Hillegass[10] recommends that significant fracture displacement be reduced accurately and that internal fixation may be necessary to maintain the reduction. Due to the limited motion in the normal midtarsal joint, long-term complications are not common. Buchman[3] reported osteochondritis dissecans and bipartite cuneiforms, and these must be distinguished roentgenographically from fractures. The bipartite cuneiform is most easily distinguished because of its smooth articular surfaces, whereas the irregular surfaces of a fracture should be diagnostic.

Author's Preferred Method of Treatment

In the author's experience isolated fractures of the cuneiforms are rarely displaced. If a displaced fracture is present, one must be suspicious of an associated "silent" midtarsal joint dislocation. In a nondisplaced fracture, treatment is based on the patient's requirement for ambulation. If the patient's employment requires prolonged weight bearing, I prefer treatment with a short-leg walking cast until the pain is relieved, followed by a good shoe and longitudinal arch support. Long-term disability has not been a complication. If pain is minimal, an Unna boot or Ace wrap is used until the pain subsides. This is followed by a good shoe and longitudinal arch support.

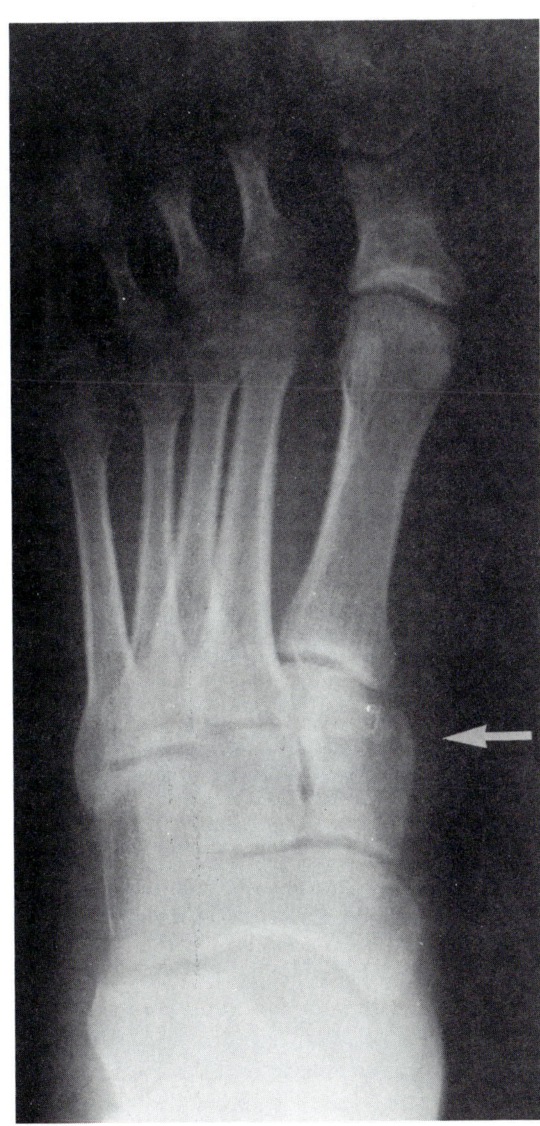

FIG 35–97.
Fractured cuneiform *(arrow)*.

In displaced fractures, consideration is given to open reduction, particularly if there is an associated subluxation or dislocation of the midtarsal joint that can be stabilized by restoring cuneiform anatomy. If the displaced fracture is not amenable to open reduction, a short-leg weight-bearing cast is used for 6 weeks. I emphasize that the midtarsal joint must be reduced to prevent long-term disability.

REFERENCES

Cuboid and Cuneiform Bones

1. Blazina ME, Westover JL: The ankle joints of college athletes, *Clin Orthop* 42:73–80, 1965.
2. Bohler L: *The treatment of fractures*, ed 5, vol 3, New York, 1958, Grune & Stratton.
3. Buchman J: Osteochondritis of the internal cuneiform, *J Bone Joint Surg* 15:225–232, 1933.
4. Chapman MW: Fractures and dislocations of the ankle and foot. In Mann RA, editor: *DuVries' Surgery of the Foot*, ed 4, St Louis, 1978, Mosby–Year Book.
5. Conwell HE, Reynolds FC: *Key and Conwell's management of fractures, dislocations, and sprains*, ed 7, St Louis, 1961, Mosby–Year Book.
6. Garcia A, Parkes JC: Fractures of the foot. In Giannestras NJ, editor: *Foot disorders: medical and surgical management*, ed 2, Philadelphia, 1973, Lea & Febiger.
7. Giannestras NJ, Sammarco GJ: Fractures and dislocations in the foot. In Rockwood CA Jr, Green DP, editors: *Fractures*, vol 2, Philadelphia, 1975, JB Lippincott.
8. Heck CV: Fractures of the bones of the foot (except the talus), *Surg Clin North Am* 45:103–117, 1965.
9. Hermel MB, Gershon-Cohen J: The nutcracker fracture of the cuboid by indirect violence, *Radiology* 60:850, 1953.
10. Hillegass RC: Injuries to the midfoot: a major cause of industrial morbidity, In Bateman JE, editor: *Foot Science*, Philadelphia, 1976, WB Saunders.
11. Jones FW: *Structure and fixation as seen in the foot*, Baltimore, 1944, Williams & Wilkins.
12. McKeever FM: Fractures of the tarsal and metatarsal bones, *Surg Gynecol Obstet* 90:735–745, 1950.
13. Wilson JN: *Jones fractures and joint injuries*, ed 6, New York, 1982, Churchill Livingstone.
14. Wilson PD: Fractures and dislocations of the tarsal bones, *South Med J* 26:833, 1933.

FRACTURES OF THE METATARSALS

Metatarsal fractures are relatively common and are frequently the cause of prolonged disability due to the fact that the fracture was either initially overlooked or unsuccessfully treated.[36, 37, 45, 48, 57] Many of these injuries occur as the result of direct crushing injuries, such as the dropping of a heavy object on the foot or the foot being run over by a heavy motorized vehicle.[22, 36] In such fractures multiple metatarsals are often involved, and the associated soft-tissue injury is of extreme importance.[22]

In Johnson's series[31] the most commonly fractured metatarsal was the third. First and second metatarsal fractures occurred with equal frequency, while the fourth metatarsal was the least commonly fractured. However, Johnson's was a study of industrial accidents.[31] When one considers inversion-type injuries that result in fractures of the base of the fifth metatarsal, the fifth metatarsal is by far the most commonly fractured.[30, 47]

In spite of the disability that arises from these fractures, Johnson stresses that very little in the way of scientific articles has been written about the management of metatarsal fractures and that most discussion has been brief and confined to textbooks where treatment has been similar and repetitive.[31]

Anatomy

Lindholm[42] emphasized that due to rigid ligamentous anchoring of the metatarsal bones to each other, particularly at the points of insertion on the tarsal and phalangeal bones, displacement of simple fractures of the metatarsals is usually minimal. Additionally, metatarsal shaft fractures are not likely to become displaced unless there is extensive damage to the interossei, lumbricals, and/or distal ligamentous attachments to the adjacent metatarsals. Lindholm notes that distal fractures near the neck of the metatarsal are the exception.[42] In these fractures the metatarsal heads are commonly dislocated and contact between the fracture surfaces totally lost. The head-neck fragment of the metatarsal is displaced *beneath* the distal metaphyses at the level of the anterior foot arch.[42] The anatomic reason for this tendency of the distal fracture fragments to become displaced is the arrangement of the extensor and flexor tendons of the toes. These tendons, passing near the metatarsophalangeal joints and terminating in the phalanges, exert a strong proximal and plantar dislocating force on the distal fragment.[42]

In the gait phase, each of the lesser metatarsals supports an equal load while the first metatarsal carries twice the load of each of the lateral four metatarsals. Displacement of a metatarsal fracture may therefore lead to a nonplantigrade foot.[55] Displacement of a distal fragment in a plantigrade direction results in increased loading of the metatarsal and may result in an intractable plantar keratosis at that site.[55] Dorsal displacement of the distal fragment decreases the load applied to that metatarsal and transfers greater pressure to the adjacent metatarsal heads.[55] Persistent medial-lateral displacement of the fracture fragment to an adjacent metatarsal can lead to mechanical impingement and interdigital neuroma formation.[55] In addition, medial displacement of the distal fragment of a first metatarsal fracture and lateral displacement of the distal fragment of a fifth metatarsal fracture may lead to a bony prominence that can produce difficulties with shoe wear in the toe box.[55]

Mechanism of Injury

Metatarsal fractures result from direct or indirect forces.[28, 30] Fractures of the second, third, and fourth metatarsals usually result from a direct force such as a crushing blow to the dorsum of the foot.[22] This mechanism often results in multiple metatarsal fractures. An indirect force such as a twisting injury in which the forepart of the foot is fixed as the patient turns produces a mediolateral torque that often fractures a metatarsal, particularly the fifth.[23] The direct mechanism of injury resulting in crushing is more common in industry, while the twisting injuries are more common in athletic endeavors. Fractures of the metatarsal head may result from direct crush injuries or occasionally from bullet or shell fragment wounds.[6]

Clinical Diagnosis

Anderson[2] emphasizes that fractures of metatarsals are frequently overlooked due to the fact that they occur in motor vehicle accidents in which severe trauma to major bones or visceral organs is more apparent, although the history and physical examination will help to avoid this error.

Giannestras and Sammarco[23] emphasize the importance of investigating, in the history, the intensity of the original blow that produced the fracture. They caution against casually reducing a metatarsal fracture, placing the foot in a cast, and allowing the patient to go home. Within 48 to 72 hours later the patient may return with a skin slough involving a large area of the dorsum of the foot and with tendon and intrinsic muscle damage. They therefore recommend that if there is soft-tissue damage, the patient be hospitalized irrespective of how minimal the underlying fracture appears to be.[23]

Patients usually complain of pain over the midfoot with an inability to bear weight.[23] The foot is swollen, particularly on the dorsal aspect.[22, 23] Ecchymosis over the fracture area will be present after the first 12 hours. If seen early, point tenderness may be present over the fracture site; however, due to the close proximity of adjacent metatarsals, exact localization of an individual bone may be difficult.[36] With gross displacement, particularly of the first or fifth metatarsals, palpation of the fracture site may be possible.[36] In fractures of the first and fifth metatarsal, grasping the distal fragment with the thumb and forefinger and flexing and extending the fragment will produce motion, potentially crepitus, and pain at the fracture site.[22] In the case of the second, third, and fourth metatarsals, relatively little false motion can be demonstrated. Garcia and Parks also emphasize that axial pressure may reproduce pain in the involved metatarsal.[22] Finally, care must be taken to evaluate the dorsalis pedis artery as it passes between the first and second metatarsals to determine whether or not circulation has been compromised.

Radiographic Diagnosis

Anderson[2] emphasizes that roentgenographs of the forefoot are often of poor quality and do not demonstrate the osseous structure of the forefoot adequately. Exposure for these roentgenograms is usually set to provide penetration of the large tarsal bones, and this results in overexposure of the smaller metatarsal and phalangeal bones. Adequate roentgenographic exposure of the metatarsals is an essential prerequisite.

Metatarsal fractures are visualized on routine anteroposterior, oblique, and lateral roentgenographs of the foot. The anteroposterior and oblique radiographs are *more* useful due to the fact that the shafts of the metatarsals are superimposed on the lateral view.[23] Fractures of the metatarsals may be either transverse, oblique, or segmental.[22, 23] Metatarsal fractures may be angulated dorsally at the fracture site due to pull of intrinsic muscles and the overpull of strong toe flexors.[22] The axial or sesamoid view is particularly helpful in detecting such plantar displacement of a metatarsal fracture, which if allowed to heal in this position, may result in a plantar callosity.[47] Fractures of the bases of the metatarsals may require polytomography to delineate fracture fragment size and the associated subluxation of the tarsometatarsal joint (Fig 35–98).

Treatment

Open Fractures

In injuries resulting from direct or crushing blows, the fractures may be open.[2]In such instances, initial irrigation and debridement with appropriate antibiotic coverage just as for other open long-bone fractures are indicated.[2, 31] All wounds are left open for delayed primary closure or skin grafting. Management of the fractured metatarsal in these cases is similar to that recommended for closed fractures below. However, axial Kirschner wire fixation is performed more routinely in open fractures to provide soft-tissue stability for healing.[2, 27] Shereff[55] emphasizes the importance of adequate fixation to hasten bony union and allow adequate treatment of the soft-tissue injuries in open fractures (Fig 35–99).

Closed Fractures

Undisplaced Fractures.—Garcia and Parks[22] recommend treating undisplaced fractures in a below-the-knee cast for 2 to 3 weeks without weight bearing followed by a walking cast for an additional 3 weeks. They believe that this treatment is particularly indicated for a *first* metatarsal fracture or when more than one metatarsal is involved. Heck agrees that fractures of the first metatarsal require immobilization in plaster of Paris, not a shoe, for support.[28] If the fracture is a solitary one involving the second, third, fourth, or fifth metatarsals with minimal or no displacement, Garcia and Parks prefer the application of a comma-shaped felt pad on the plantar aspect of the foot with gradual weight bearing in a shoe.[22]

Giannestras and Sammarco[23] recommend a short-leg walking cast for undisplaced fractures of the lateral four metatarsals for 4 to 6 weeks. During the first 24 hours the foot is elevated and the patient instructed to watch for edema and swelling of the toes with unrelenting pain. When the first metatarsal is involved, they recommend non–weight bearing in a short-leg cast for 2 to 3 weeks, followed by a short-leg walking cast for an additional 3 weeks. They prefer a comma-shaped metatarsal pad *only* in *undisplaced* fractures of the second, third, and fourth metatarsals with *minimal* soft-tissue damage. Such a pad is changed on a weekly basis so that the strapping required for its application does not become loose.

Lewin[40] recommended aggressive treatment of metatarsal fractures, including traction with a banjo splint if necessary to restore the longitudinal and transverse arch of the foot. In metatarsal fractures that are not open and not completely displaced, Johnson,[31] however, recommends simple treatment with compression dressings and several pairs of fluffy stockings. These patients are then fitted with an oversized snug-fitting work boot and allowed to return to work as *soon* as possible. He believes that immediate ambulation and weight bearing on the fractured foot are the key to a rapid return to work *and* minimal disability. The boot in this instance serves the same function as the short-leg walking cast.

Morrissey[48] recommended the application of a simple molded leather arch support with or without a metatarsal pad of sponge rubber. The leather arch is applied to the foot by means of adhesive strapping. Although initially he used strapping to the tibial tubercle in an effort to hold the foot in a neutral position (as regards inversion and eversion), Morrissey[48] subsequently determined that such a long stirrup was not necessary and that short strips of adhesive tape used only to approximate the leather arch to the foot were all that was necessary. The leather strapping is changed once a week for a period of about 4 weeks. In cases with marked swelling or with lacerations, the leather arch was held in place by means of an elastic bandage. This is removed for physiotherapy and whirlpool treatment until the swelling has subsided. Active weight bearing on the molded leather arch is begun early after injury. Morrissey found this method to be extremely valuable in getting patients back to work early. The condition of the associated soft tissues and the presence of multiple metatarsal fractures had the most direct effect on prolonging time off work. Morrissey found that by comparing this method of treatment with plaster of paris

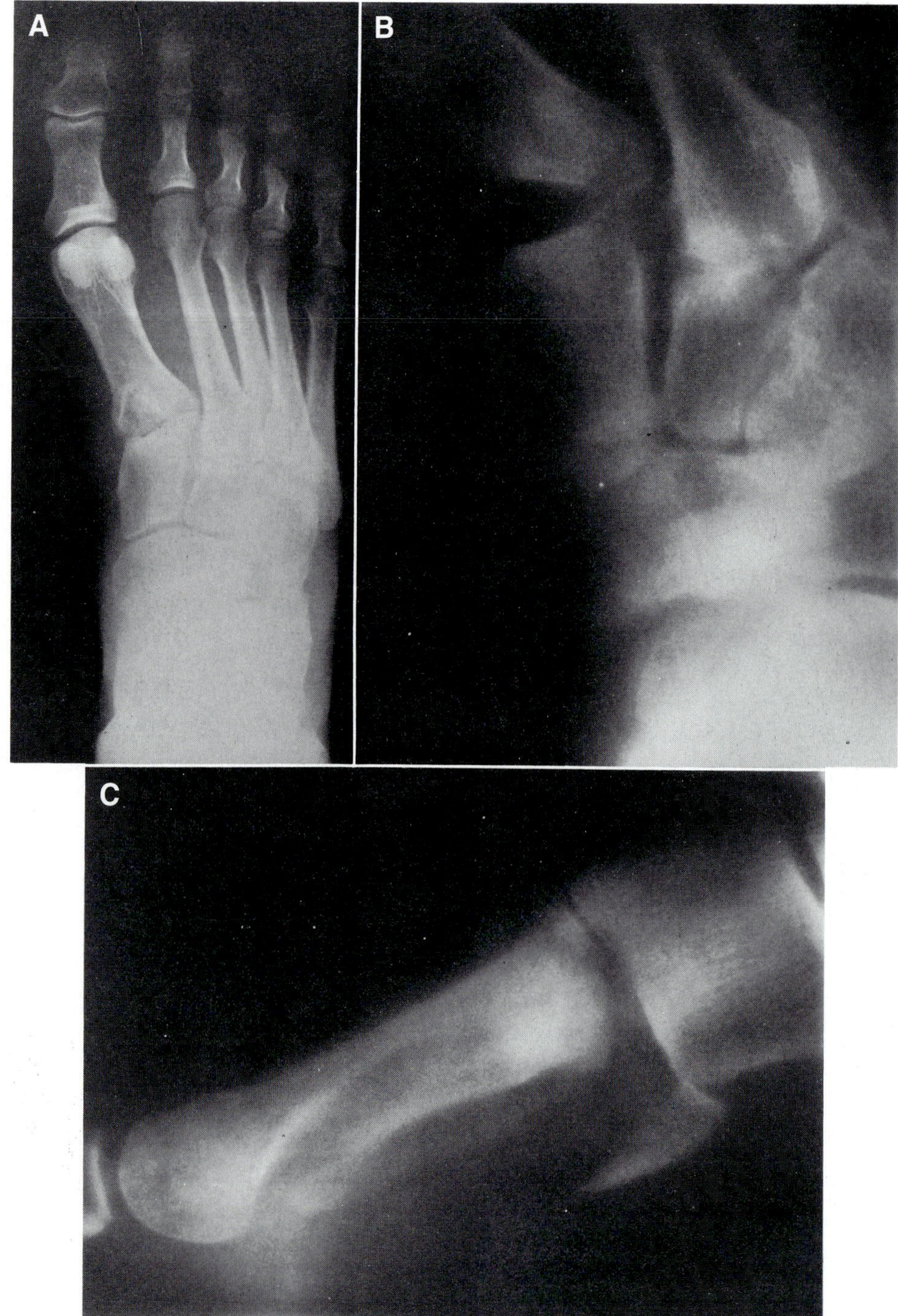

FIG 35–98.
A, fracture of the base of the first metatarsal. **B,** anteroposterior polytomogram demonstrating displacement of the articular surface of the base of the first metatarsal. **C,** lateral polytomogram demonstrating a fracture of the base of the first metatarsal. Fragment size and the absence of joint subluxation are noted.

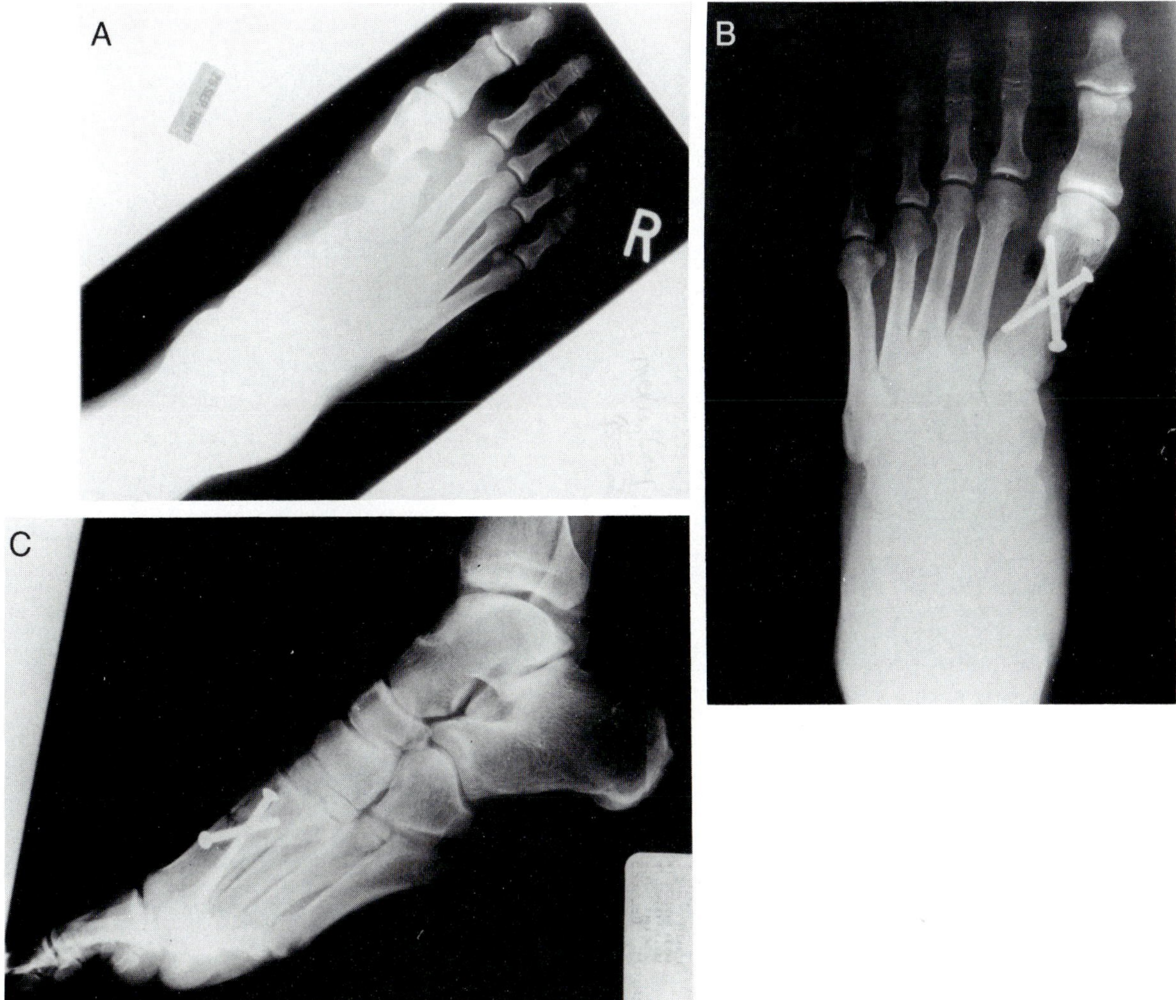

FIG 35–99.
A, anteroposterior radiograph of an open, displaced fracture of the first metatarsal shaft. **B** and **C,** anteroposterior and lateral radiographs after open reduction and rigid internal fixation with AO screws.

immobilization the average period of disability was remarkably decreased.[48]

Mann[43] uses one half-inch adhesive tape strapping about the foot combined with a hard-sole, bunion-type shoe for a period of 3 to 5 weeks in nondisplaced fractures (Fig 35–100).[43] Disability after this treatment scheme has been minimal.

Displaced Fractures.—Displaced fractures may require more aggressive treatment.[36] For displaced fractures of the first metatarsal shaft, closed reduction is attempted. If the reduction is acceptable, it is followed by cast immobilization for 6 weeks. Weight bearing is usually not permitted until healing is complete.[23] If the displacement can be reduced by closed means, Chapman prefers percutaneous Kirschner wire fixation to maintain the reduction.[8] If closed reduction is not successful, Garcia and Parkes emphasize the need for open reduction through a dorsal approach and transfixation with Kirschner wires.[22]

Anderson[2] reports that most displaced metatarsal fractures can be manipulated into satisfactory position under anesthesia and their position held by cast immobilization. Likewise, Garcia and Parkes[22] recommend attempted closed reduction of displaced metatarsal fractures. They use Chinese finger traps applied to each toe as soon as possible after the fracture is diagnosed. After the Chinese finger traps are applied to the toes, countertraction at the ankle usually results in satisfactory alignment of the fracture (Fig 35–101). Following reduction of the fractured metatarsal shaft, a well-molded plaster cast is applied. The cast is first applied from the tips of the toes to the midtarsal area. Once this is allowed to set, the countertraction on the ankle is released, and the

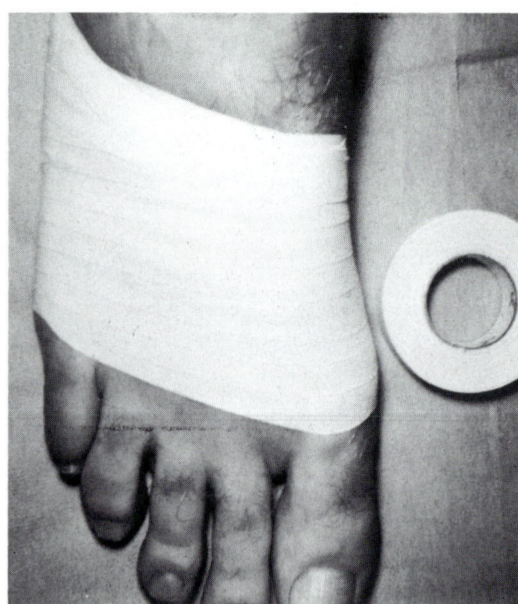

FIG 35–100.
Taping a foot with ½-in. adhesive tape for a nondisplaced metatarsal fracture. After taping, ambulation is begun in a postoperative shoe.

cast is extended to the level of the tibial tubercle. The patient remains non–weight bearing in this cast for a period of 4 weeks, at which time the cast is removed and radiographs obtained. Weight bearing in a short-leg walking cast is then permitted.

Giannestras and Sammarco[23] also recommend the use of Chinese finger traps in displaced metatarsal fractures. Following reduction, the patient is kept in a non–weight-bearing cast for 4 weeks. At this time the cast is changed, roentgenographs are taken, and the patient is allowed to begin weight bearing. If reduction by manipulation and traction is unsuccessful, open reduction and internal fixation with crossed Kirschner wires may be indicated in certain instances.[15, 23] Giannestras and Sammarco[23] believe that displacement of a metatarsal shaft fracture, with the exclusion of the first metatarsal, is of no great significance and does not require open reduction. Severe dorsal or plantar angulation, however, cannot be accepted.[2, 23, 47] Malalignment in this plane may result in abnormal pressure on the plantar aspect of the foot or in deformity of the toes with painful plantar callosities.[2, 23, 28]

Garcia and Parkes[22] believe that if closed reduction fails, open anatomic reduction and fixation with Kirschner wires are necessary. Open reduction of fractures of the metatarsals is carried out through one or more longitudinal dorsal incisions.[2, 42, 56] Usually two adjacent metatarsal necks or shafts can be exposed adequately through one incision placed midway between and parallel to the metatarsal shafts.[2]

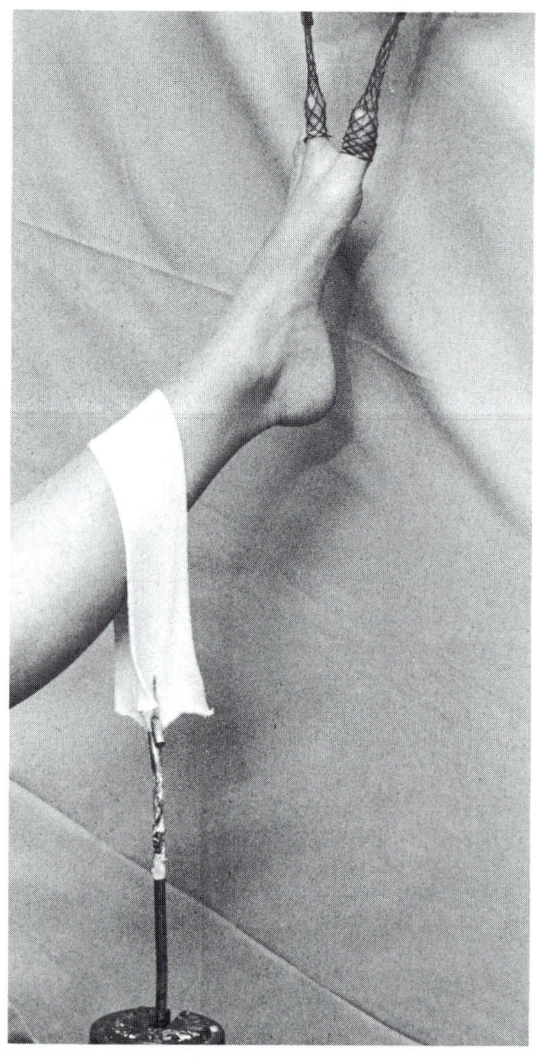

FIG 35–101.
Chinese finger traps with ankle countertraction are used to reduce a fracture of the forefoot.

Johnson [31] emphasizes that if after closed reduction the fragments are in any degree of apposition and not displaced toward the sole, conservative treatment can be continued. Shortening, particularly in single or multiple fractures of the middle three metatarsals, is not significant according to Johnson.[31] If an unacceptable reduction is obtained, he feels that open reduction under anesthesia with intramedullary Kirschner wire fixation and early ambulatory treatment postoperatively is indicated.[31] He stresses, however, that as long as the alignment is maintained by open or closed methods, axial shortening can be accepted rather than subjecting the foot to any form of fixed traction. He believes that such fixed traction devices lead to stiffness of the forefoot that results in more disability than the metatarsal fracture itself.

Sisk[56] recommends that isolated fractures in the metatarsal diaphysis, particularly if the adjacent metatarsals are intact, be treated conservatively. He emphasizes, however, that the more distal the fracture of a metatarsal, the more definite the indication for open reduction. Open reduction and internal fixation of such fractures in the distal end of the metatarsal are most often indicated when there is significant dorsal angulation of the fracture that is causing the metatarsal head to be prominent on the plantar aspect of the sole of the foot.[56] He recommends open reduction and intramedullary Kirschner wire fixation with the wire left protruding through the skin in the area of the metatarsophalangeal joint for 3 weeks. The wire thus crosses the articular surface of the head of the metatarsal. Sisk, however, reports no complications from infection and minimal problems due to stiffness of the metatarsophalangeal joint. In selected mid-shaft fractures undergoing open reduction, he recommends the use of a four- to five-hole plate contoured to the dorsolateral surface of the metatarsal and fixed to the bone with multiple screws.

Shereff[55] emphasizes that if left unreduced, metatarsal fractures may lead to a nonplantigrade foot and difficulties with ambulation. This is more important in the younger, more active patient. He recommends that an attempt be made to improve alignment in *any* metatarsal fracture displaying displacement of greater than 3 to 4 mm or angulation of more than 10 degrees. He recommends that displaced fractures be treated by reduction using Chinese finger traps. If adequate reduction is obtained, then a short-leg cast from the tips of toes to the tibial tubercle is applied. The patient is kept non–weight bearing on crutches for 4 to 6 weeks. After the cast is removed, the patient gradually resumes weight-bearing activity.

Following reduction, if the fracture is unstable, he recommends percutaneous pinning of the fracture fragments. For those fractures that are not successfully reduced by closed methods, he recommends open reduction and internal fixation. He prefers the use of a dorsal longitudinal incision centered over the metatarsal. His choice of fixation is 0.045 smooth Kirschner wires crossed at the fracture site. The patient is then placed in a short-leg cast and kept non–weight bearing on crutches. At 6 weeks, if union is present radiographically, the pins are removed, and a gradual return to weight bearing is allowed. He emphasizes that multiple displaced metatarsal fractures commonly require open reduction and internal fixation. The author also states that although transverse fractures are usually amenable to cross-pin fixation, oblique and spiral fractures may be better managed with interfragmentary lag screws.[55]

Metatarsal Neck Fractures

Fractures of the *necks* of the metatarsals are usually multiple and are often displaced.[2] Persistent displacement of the metatarsal head and neck into the plantar aspect of the sole and foot may result in plantar callosities or corns.[2, 23, 24, 47, 54] Anderson stresses the importance of an accurate reduction of these fractures to prevent such sequelae.[2] Such fractures can usually be reduced under anesthesia by using the Chinese finger trap technique[6] or by digital pressure under the metatarsal head with traction of the toe.[44] If a good reduction is obtained, closed treatment in a short-leg walking cast may be satisfactory.[6] However, Lindholm[42] warns that maintenance of a closed reduction of a completely dislocated metatarsal neck fracture without internal fixation is uncertain.

If complete displacement with a lack of apposition of the fracture surfaces and plantar displacement of the head and neck fragment persists following attempted closed reduction, open reduction is indicated.[31, 42] Sisk[56] and Goldstein and Dickerson[25] utilize a longitudinal dorsal incision because it will usually allow access to adjacent metatarsal necks.[56] In these more distal fractures, Sisk prefers the use of intramedullary Kirschner wire fixation. In this technique, the proximal end of the distal fragment is lifted out of the wound, and toes are held in hyperextension. The Kirschner wire is inserted into the medullary canal of the distal fragment and advanced distally until the point emerges through the skin in the area of the metatarsophalangeal joint. The wire is then withdrawn through the skin until its end is even with the fracture site. The fracture is then reduced and the wire drilled proximally until it meets resistance at the base of the metatarsal. The wire is left protruding through the skin, and a small dressing is applied over the ends of the wire. The patient is immobilized in a cast from the tibial tuberosity to the toes with protection of the wire to prevent it from coming in contact with the plaster. The wires are removed at 3 weeks, and a walking cast is applied.[25, 56]

Lindholm has modified intramedullary Kirschner wire fixation to prevent leaving the wire out of the skin and from going through the metatarsophalangeal joint.[42] The major drawback to leaving the Kirschner wires exiting the skin is that it exposes the metatarsophalangeal joint to infection and may result in impairment of motion of the metatarsophalangeal joint. In Lindholm's technique, the fracture is exposed through a dorsal incision and a Kirschner wire drilled into the proximal fracture fragment. Enough of the wire is left exposed from the distal end of the proximal fracture fragment to engage the distal fragment. The distal fragment, like a cup, is then pressed against the proximal fragment and Kirschner wire. The wound is closed and the patient placed in a well-fitting plaster cast. Weight bearing is permitted after 2 weeks. The cast is kept in place until bony union is ensured. The Kirschner wires in these instances are left permanently within the metatarsal. Lindholm has noted no problems with corrosion of the implants or other difficulty by leaving them in the metatarsals.[42]

Metatarsal Head Fractures

Fractures of the metatarsal heads are uncommon. Blodgett[6] recommends skeletal traction by use of a transverse Kirschner wire through the proximal or middle phalanx or by pulp wire traction for shatter-type fractures of the metatarsal head. The traction applied is maintained by a rubber band attached to an outrigger mounted on a below-the-knee cast. Such traction is maintained for 7 weeks with limited weight bearing on the forefoot for 10 to 12 weeks. Following this treatment, Blodgett states that only limited metatarsophalangeal flexion can be expected.

Dukowsky and Freeman[18] reported a fracture dislocation of the articular surface of the third metatarsal head. They believe that metatarsal head fractures are usually the result of direct trauma. However, in their patient, the mechanism of injury was a shear force on the metatarsal head at the time of dislocation of the third metatarsophalangeal joint. The authors recommend closed reduction under digital block anesthesia by applying longitudinal traction to the toe. Roentgenograms are taken to confirm an anatomic reduction. If reduction is obtained, the digit is treated by buddy-taping the toe to the adjacent toe and applying a short-leg cast with a toe plate. According to the authors, closed reduction of metatarsal head fractures (and even no reduction) seems to produce an acceptable result. The authors state, however, that if closed reduction is unsuccessful in obtaining reduction of the metatarsal head fragment, then open reduction and internal fixation are logical alternatives.

Heckman[29] states that fractures occur through the metatarsal head and produce a distal fragment that is intraarticular and without capsular attachments. He recommends manipulation and traction to obtain a stable reduction that is maintained in a walking cast with a toe plate. He also described a patient with an isolated osteochondral fracture that was not diagnosed or treated. The patient did well despite persistent dislocation of the metatarsal articular surface.

Author's Preferred Method of Treatment

I agree with Johnson[31] and Irwin[30] concerning the importance of early weight bearing in the treatment of metatarsal fractures to help minimize long-term disability. In nondisplaced fractures of the first metatarsal, I prefer a short-leg walking cast well molded beneath the first metatarsal. Weight bearing is begun in 7 to 10 days. This cast is removed when there is evidence of healing. The patient is then placed in a stiff-soled shoe with good arch support. In nondisplaced fractures of the lateral four metatarsals, I prefer either a short-leg walking cast or taping the foot with ½-in. adhesive tape and using a bunion-type shoe. The choice is dependent upon the patient's employment requirements. The patient is transferred to a stiff-soled walking shoe or boot with a good arch support when comfort allows.

Displaced Fractures of the Metatarsals.—In patients with displaced metatarsal fractures, I strongly recommend extensive evaluation of the soft tissues to determine the degree of associated damage. If soft-tissue damage is significant, consideration is given to placing the foot in a bulky dressing.

The foot is elevated and ice applied until subsidence of the swelling permits more aggressive fracture treatment.

In displaced fractures of the first metatarsal shaft I recommend reduction of all angulation in the dorsal-plantar plane. Additionally, comminution of fractures of the first metatarsal may result in shortening and can accentuate callosities beneath the second metatarsal. In displaced fractures of the first metatarsal, I attempt a closed reduction with the Chinese finger traps. If comminution has resulted in shortening of the metatarsal and the length can be restored, I use transfixing pins from the first to the the second metatarsal to maintain the length of the metatarsal. In displaced fractures that cannot be reduced by these closed methods, open reduction through a dorsal incision and fixation with crossed Kirschner wires or AO screws is utilized. Following reduction and internal fixation, patients are kept in a non–weight-bearing short-leg cast for 4 weeks followed by a walking cast for 2 additional weeks. The Kirschner wires are removed between the fourth and sixth weeks.

In displaced fractures of the shafts of the lateral four metatarsals closed reduction is attempted by using Chinese finger traps on the involved digit (see Fig 35–101). If a reduction is obtained, consideration is given to percutaneous Kirschner wire fixation to an adjacent intact metatarsal, particularly when the fifth metatarsal is fractured. Following reduction, patients are placed in a short-leg cast. Weight bearing is allowed after the second week of immobilization. In the author's opinion, an accurate reduction is more critical in the dorsal-plantar plane than in the medial-lateral plane. If dorsal-plantar angulation causing prominence of the metatarsal head plantarly persists following closed reduction, open reduction–internal fixation with either longitudinal intramedullary or crossed Kirschner wires is utilized for stability. In patients in whom there is more than one displaced metatarsal fracture, internal fixation either by percutaneous methods or by open reduction may be necessary because of the loss of the splinting effect of adjacent metatarsals.

Following open reduction and internal fixation of these metatarsal shaft fractures, patients are kept non–weight bearing in a short-leg cast for 2 weeks. Weight bearing is then initiated for an additional 6 weeks. The Kirschner wires are removed between 4 and 6 weeks.

Metatarsal Head Fractures.—Metatarsal head fractures are not common. I divide metatarsal head fractures into two groups. In the first group, the metatarsal head fracture fragment is small, and whether it is displaced does not affect the stability of the reduction of the metatarsophalangeal joint. This fracture is treated by closed reduction under digital block anesthesia by applying longitudinal traction to the tow. If the reduction is unsuccessful, open reduction with internal fixation is performed only if the intraarticular fragment results in limiting the range of motion of the joint. Otherwise, the toe is treated as if the reduction were successful.

In the second group of patients, the metatarsal head fracture consists of a large enough fragment that its displacement results in instability of the metatarsophalangeal joint. In this situation, I consider anatomic reduction and stable fixation to be essential. The fracture is treated by closed reduction under digital anesthesia. If an acceptable reduction is obtained and it is stable, it is treated by buddy-taping to the toe opposite the side of the metatarsal head fracture. The foot is then placed in a short-leg cast. If the reduction is not anatomic or if displacement occurs, traction is released and open reduction–internal fixation with smooth Kirschner wires is undertaken.

Metatarsal Neck Fractures.—In evaluating fractures of the necks of the metatarsals, the oblique and sesamoid views help to demonstrate the degree of plantar displacement of the metatarsal head. If the metatarsal head and neck fragment is displaced, I attempt closed reduction and use Chinese finger traps for traction and direct pressure beneath the metatarsal head to reduce the displacement. A short-leg cast with a toe plate and molding beneath the metatarsal heads is applied with traction in place. If the reduction is maintained in the cast, the patient is treated with weight bearing in the cast for 4 to 6 weeks followed by the use of a stiff-soled shoe. If the reduction is not acceptable by these methods or is unstable and redisplaces in the cast, percutaneous Kirschner wire fixation of the fracture while in the Chinese finger traps is attempted (Fig 35–102,A–C). If this fails, open reduction through a dorsal incision and intramedullary Kirschner wire fixation after the method of Sisk is utilized. It is important to emphasize that these Kirschner wires are left in place only *3* weeks and then removed. The patients are allowed to begin weight bearing in a short-leg cast when swelling subsides. Following removal of the wires, the patients are managed for an additional 2 weeks in a cast and then transferred to a stiff-soled shoe.

Metatarsal Base Fractures.—Fractures at the base of the metatarsals are not common. If the fracture fragments of the metatarsal base are displaced and large enough to permit internal fixation, I recommend attempted closed reduction. Care must be taken in evaluating the roentgenographs that an associated dislocation of the involved joint is not missed (see Fig 35–98). Traction using the Chinese finger traps is applied. If the articular surface reduces, percutaneous Kirschner wire fixation, either transarticularly or into an adjacent intact metatarsal, is performed. If the persistently displaced fracture fragments are large enough to permit internal fixation or if there is an associated dislocation of the involved joint (not the entire tarsometatarsal joint, only a single tarsometatarsal joint) that cannot be reduced closed, an open reduction is performed. The goal of open reduction is to restore dorsal-plantar displacement of the metatarsal to prevent later callosities beneath the forefoot and to restore the articular surface of the involved tarsometatarsal joint. This is particularly important in the first and fifth metatarsals. After open reduction patients are treated in a weight-bearing short-leg cast for 4 weeks and then transferred to a shoe with a molded arch. Due to the limited motion present in the tarsometatarsal joints prior to the injury, open reduction does not usually result in significant loss of motion. However, restoring the subluxation of the joint, in my experience, has helped to decrease the problem with painful degenerative arthritis in these joints.

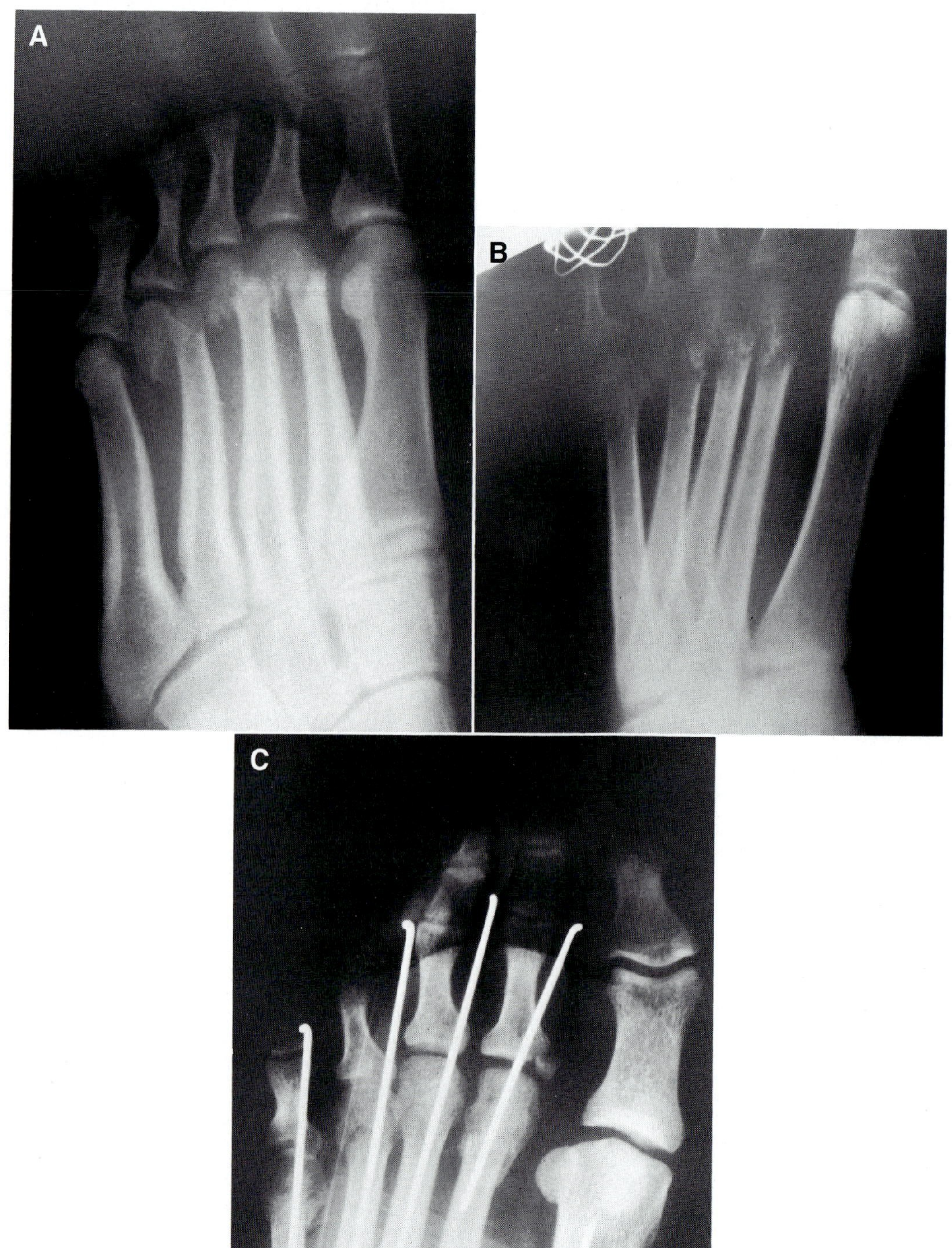

FIG 35–102.
A, displaced fractures of the second through fifth metatarsal necks. **B,** closed reduction with Chinese finger traps. **C,** percutaneous Kirschner wire fixation.

If the comminution is too severe to permit open reduction and internal fixation, closed reduction with application of a short-leg cast *well* molded in the arch to support the injured metatarsal base is applied. The patient is kept non–weight bearing for 2 to 4 weeks. Weight bearing in a similar cast is then instituted. The patient is then changed to a stiff-soled shoe with a good arch support. Later, arthrodesis of the injured joint may be required if pain persists.

Fractures of the Base of the Fifth Metatarsal

Fractures of the base of the fifth metatarsal are treated here as a separate group for two reasons: (1) they are the most common type of metatarsal fractures,[23] and (2) there is confusion in the literature as to their treatment. Fractures of the base of the fifth metatarsal have been classically termed "Jones fracture" after Sir Robert Jones described the injury in his own foot in 1902.[32] However, as stressed by Kavanaugh et al.,[34] there is confusion as to exactly which fracture Jones described. Jones actually described a transverse *diaphyseal* fracture of the fifth metatarsal, three fourths of an inch from the base. This fracture is a less common injury than avulsion of the fifth metatarsal tuberosity with which the Jones fracture has been confused.[32, 52] The transverse proximal diaphyseal fracture described by Jones often goes on to delayed union or nonunion.[3, 12, 34] In addition to confusion as to the anatomic location of the fracture, recently Zelko et al.[64] Kavanaugh et al.[34] and DeLee et al.[14] have reported difficulty treating fractures of the proximal fifth metatarsal in which the diagnosis was initially overlooked and also stress fractures in this area.

In an effort to clarify fractures of the base of the fifth metatarsal, Stewart[58] introduced a classification of these fractures (Table 35–6). Type 1 fractures are fractures at the junction of the metatarsal shaft and the base. This type is subdivided into two groups: noncomminuted fractures (1A) and fractures with comminution (1B). Type 2 fractures are those that involve only the styloid process. This type is also subdivided into two groups: those with (2B) and those without (2A) joint involvement. Stewart formulated treatment recommendations on the basis of this classification system.

Zelko et al. and Torg et al.[64, 64] divided fractures of the fifth metatarsal occurring at the metaphyseal-diaphyseal junction into four subgroups based upon their clinical history *and* initial roentgenographic findings.[64] Group 1 contains patients with an acute traumatic injury and no prior symptoms (Fig 35–103,A). Roentgenographs demonstrate an acute fracture line with no chronic changes. Group 2 includes patients who sustain an acute injury but who previously have had mild symptoms on the lateral border of the foot (Fig 35–103,B). Roentgenographs demonstrate a lucent fracture line with some periosteal reaction. Group 3 encompases patients who present with traumatic reinjury after one or more previous injuries. Radiographs in these patients demonstrate a lucent fracture line with periosteal reaction and often intramedullary sclerosis (Fig 35–103,C). Finally, Group 4 includes patients who present with a history of chronic pain or multiple injury episodes. Radiographs demonstrate a lucent fracture line with sclerotic margins (Fig 35–103,D).

In an effort to simplify the discussion of these injuries, I prefer to use a classification system that incorporates both that of Stewart[58] and Zelko et al.[64] (Table 35–7).

I view these fractures as being of three distinct types, I, II, and III. Type IA includes nondisplaced *acute* fractures at the junction of the shaft and base; type IB, *acute* comminuted fractures at the junction of the metatarsal shaft and base; and Type II, fractures at the junction of the metatarsal shaft and base with clinical and roentgenographic evidence of previous injury. To

TABLE 35–6.

Stewart's Classification of Fractures of the Base of the Fifth Metatarsal*

Type		Description
1	A	Fracture of the junction of the shaft and base (see Fig 35–103,A)
	B	Comminuted
2	A	Fracture of the styloid process without articular involvement (Fig 35–104)
	B	With joint involvement (Fig 35–105)

*Adapted From Stewart IM: *Clin Orthop* 16:190–198, 1960.

TABLE 35–7.

Author's Classification of Fractures of the Base of the Fifth Metatarsal

Type		Description
I		Acute fractures at the metaphyseal-diaphyseal junction
	A	Nondisplaced (Fig 35–103,A)
	B	Displaced and/or comminuted
II		Fractures at the metaphyseal-diaphyseal junction with clinical and/or radiographic evidence of previous injury (i.e., pain, sclerosis, etc.) (Fig 35–103,B–D)
III		Fractures of the styloid process of the fifth metatarsal
	A	*Without* involvement of the fifth metatarsocuboid joint (Fig 35–104)
	B	With involvement of the fifth metatarsocuboid joint (Fig 35–105)

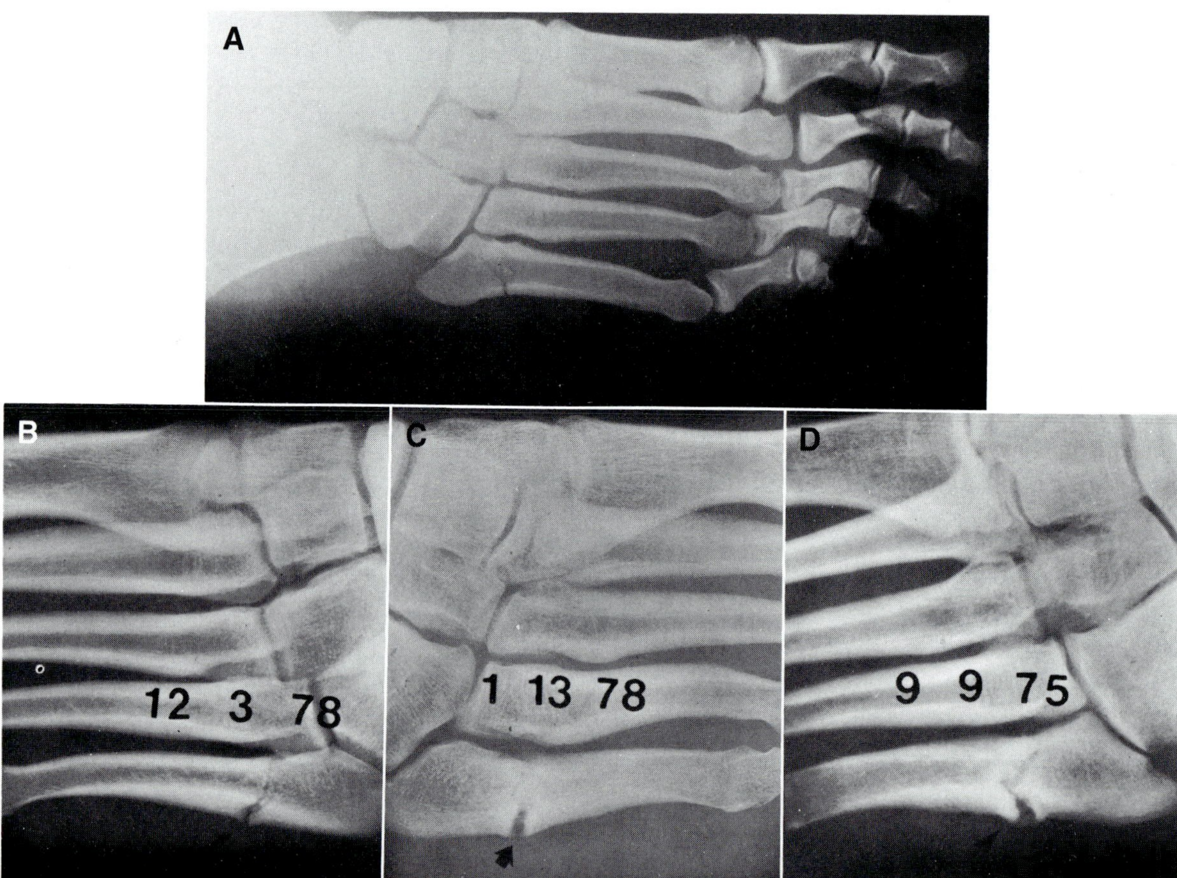

FIG 35–103.
Classification of Zelko et al.[64] for fractures of the base of the fifth metatarsal. **A,** group 1: acute fracture of the proximal diaphysis of the fifth metatarsal. **B,** group 2: acute fracture of the proximal diaphysis of the fifth metatarsal. Note the pre-existing periosteal reaction. **C,** group 3: fracture of the proximal diaphysis of the fifth metatarsal. Note the lucent fracture line and periosteal reaction. **D,** group 4: fracture of the proximal diaphysis of the fifth metatarsal. Note the lucent fracture line, periosteal reaction, and intermedullary sclerosis. See the text for a more complete description of each group. (From Zelko RR, Torg J, Rachun A: *Am J Sports Med* 7:95–101, 1979. Used by permission.)

be classified as having a type II fracture, patients must have a history of prodromal symptoms along the lateral aspect of the foot prior to their acute fracture and/or x-ray findings suggesting chronic reaction to stress, i.e., a radiolucent fracture line, periosteal reaction, heaped-up callus on the lateral cortical margin, and intramedullary sclerosis that obviously preceded the acute episode of pain[14] (see Fig 35–103,D). Type IIIA includes fractures of the styloid process without joint involvement, and type IIIB encompasses fractures of the styloid process with involvement of the fifth metatarsocuboid joint.

Stress fractures involving the proximal shaft of the fifth metatarsal distal to the tuberosity are different in their behavior from other metatarsal stress fractures. Zelko et al.[64] found them to be slow to heal, predisposed to reinjury, and often causing prolonged disability, particularly in the young athlete.[64] Kavanaugh et al.[34] also stressed that this injury frequently occurs in young athletes and may be the source of prolonged disability. Its occurrence in basketball players has been emphasized by several authors.[14, 34] Kavanaugh et al.[34] found that 41% of patients with fractures of the fifth metatarsal related a history of discomfort over the lateral aspect of the foot at least 2 weeks *prior* to the roentgenographic evidence of the fracture (type II). Zelko et al.[64] found roentgenographic evidence of a lucent fracture line with periosteal reaction in 14 of 21 patients at the time of the initial fracture.

Anatomy

Due to the articulation between the base of the fifth metatarsal and the cuboid and that between the bases of the fifth and fourth metatarsals, fractures of the base of

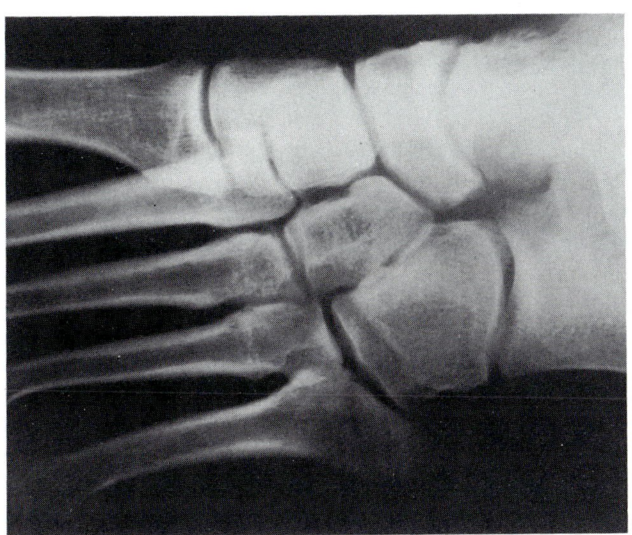

FIG 35–104.
Fracture of the styloid process of the base of the fifth metatarsal without articular involvement.

the fifth metatarsal can be intra-articular in either of these two joints.[58]

Jones[32] stressed that the base of the fifth metatarsal is closely bound to the cuboid and to the fourth metatarsal by strong ligaments on every side. He believed that since these ligaments are so strong, dislocation of the base at the time of fracture is "the rarest of accidents." He did not mention the function of the insertion of the peroneus brevis tendon in this fracture. Kavanaugh et al.[34], after anatomic dissection of five fresh specimens, confirmed Jones' observations on the thickness and strength of these ligaments. They stressed that the diaphyseal fracture reported by Jones occurs 0.5 cm distal to the splayed insertion of the peroneus brevis and almost invariably just distal to the joint between the fourth and the fifth metatarsals. It was their opinion that the firm capsular attachments of the metatarsocuboid joint helped to stabilize the joint, thereby concentrating fracture forces at the metaphyseal-diaphyseal junction. The strong tendon of the peroneus brevis inserts on the dorsolateral aspect of the base of the fifth metatarsal over a relatively large area. This insertion has given rise to the theory that avulsion fractures occur due to contracture of this muscle.[23, 51]

The base or proximal end of the fifth metatarsal presents a flair, the tuberosity, that protrudes down and laterally beyond the surfaces of the shaft of the metatarsal and the adjacent cuboid.[13] Dameron[13] emphasized the individual variations in the size and shape of this tubercle. Stewart noted that the amount the styloid process overhangs the metatarsocuboid joint appears to vary and invite isolated fractures when it is relatively long.[58]

Carp,[7] in discussing delayed union of fractures of the fifth metatarsal, presented the thesis that poor blood supply to the shaft of the fifth metatarsal was responsible for the tendency to delayed union.

Mechanism of Injury

Jones'[32, 33] original description clearly delineated the mechanism of his own injury: "While dancing, I trod on the outer side of my foot, my heel at the moment being off the ground. Something gave midway down my foot, and I at once suspected a rupture of the peroneus longus tendon." Since that description, both direct and indirect mechanisms of injury have been given responsibility for this fracture.[23] The marked prominence of the tuberosity of the fifth metatarsal beyond the lateral line of the shaft of the metatarsal on the lateral border of the anterior two thirds of the foot makes it particularly at risk to direct trauma.[23, 46]

Fractures of the tuberosity of the fifth metatarsal by indirect violence are more common, possibly secondary

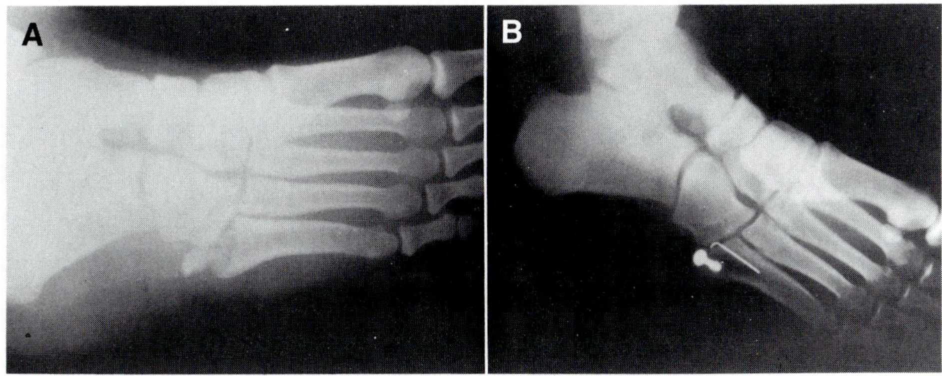

FIG 35–105.
A, fracture of the styloid process of the base of the fifth metatarsal with joint involvement. **B,** open reduction and internal fixation to restore articular congruity.

to the number of structures that attach to this prominence.[9] These include the peroneus brevis tendon, a portion of the adductor digiti quinti muscle, the outer portion of the plantar fascia, occasionally the abductor ossei metatarsi quinti muscle, and finally the flexor minimi digiti brevis muscle.[9] Lichtblau[41] has stressed the importance of the active role played by the peroneus brevis tendon in pulling the base of the metatarsal away from the shaft. According to Lichtblau, because the peroneus brevis muscle contracts during stance phase, it is already contracted when an inversion stress is applied to the weight-loaded and plantar-flexed foot. Due to its insertion into the base of the fifth metatarsal, the tendon of the peroneus brevis holds firmly as the shaft is pulled away from it. Avulsion of the base from the rest of the fifth metatarsal, is the result. Giannestras and Sammarco[23] also note that a plantar flexion, inversion stress placed on the forefoot, accompanied by contraction of the peroneus brevis muscle, avulses the styloid at the base of the fifth metatarsal where the tendon inserts. Pritsch et al.[53] believed that contraction of the peroneus brevis, occurring while the distal cuboid articular surface acts as a fulcrum, combines to cause lateral displacement *and* rotation of a free fragment of the base of the fifth metatarsal in their patient.

Kavanaugh et al.[34] used cinematography and force platform analysis in an effort to mimic the position of the foot at the time of the original injury. They concluded that either a vertical force, a medial-lateral force, or a combination of the two acts on the base of the fifth metatarsal in conjunction with a posterior ground (braking) force to bring the patient up on the metatarsal heads and concentrate the vertical and mediolateral forces on the lateral metatarsal. They postulated that an inability or failure of the foot to go into inversion at that moment produces the large vertical and mediolateral ground forces that are responsible for the injury.[34]

Finally, it has recently been demonstrated that increased stress on the foot secondary to increased activity, prolonged running, or participation in certain sports may produce stress fractures of the proximal diaphysis of the fifth metatarsal.[14, 34, 64]

Clinical Diagnosis

History.—Careful evaluation of the patient's history is essential to distinguish between fractures of acute onset and stress-type fractures.[14, 34, 64] Kavanaugh et al.[34] report that there may be no history of a specific injury and that an aching sensation on the lateral aspect of the foot may be the initial symptom of a roentgenographically diagnosable fracture. Zelko et al.[64] and Torg et al.[60] also emphasized the presence of prodromal symptoms of pain at the fracture site several weeks before any acute injury occurs. Patients with an *acute* fracture give a history of a twisting injury of the ankle or a sudden inversion of the foot. Jones reported that the patient will usually complain of pain when he endeavors to put pressure on his toes or the inner side of the foot or if he attempts to invert the foot.[32]

Physical Examination.—The clinical diagnosis is based upon the finding of point tenderness at the lateral aspect of the base of the fifth metatarsal.[62] Localized tenderness over the base of the fifth metatarsal and/or proximal metatarsal shaft helps to clinically distinguish this fracture from an injury to the lateral ligaments of the ankle.[23, 61, 63] Accentuation of the pain by inversion of the foot will help to confirm the diagnosis.[9, 23, 62] Initially, swelling may be minimal, but it increases, particularly if the foot is held dependent for any length of time.[23, 61, 63] Edema and ecchymosis in the area of the fracture will be present if the patient's diagnosis and treatment are delayed beyond the first 24 hours.[24]

Jones[32] noted that there was generally no crepitus, no deformity, and no mobility on manipulation. However, Stewart[58] emphasized the importance of searching for abnormal mobility at the fracture site. He felt that if such abnormal mobility were present, it suggested the need for operative treatment for fracture stabilization.[58]

Radiographic Diagnosis

Roentgenographs in the anteroposterior and oblique projections are the most valuable in demonstrating the fracture.[23, 58] On the lateral roentgenograph, displacement and intra-articular involvement may not be as clearly demonstrated. An oblique roentgenograph clearly demonstrating the joint space between the bases of the fourth and the fifth metatarsal and the cuboid is essential to detect both intra-articular involvement and displacement.

In evaluating fractures in the area of the base of the fifth metatarsal, congenital anomalies of ossification must be kept in mind.[62] Dameron[13] investigated the secondary center of ossification (apophysis) within the proximal end of the fifth metatarsal. He was unable to demonstrate this accessory ossification center in children under the age of 8 years and found that the apophysis was united to the shaft of the bone before the age of 12 years in girls and 15 in boys. He reported that 22% of the children he examined demonstrated such a secondary center of ossification. Clearly, a distinction between this accessory center of ossification and a fracture is essential in this age group. The roentgenographic characteristics of a normal apophysis that differentiate it from a fracture include the fact that (1) the apophyseal line traverses the tubercle in a direction *parallel* to the long axis of the shaft and (2) the apophysis does not extend proximally into the metatarsal joint or medially into the joint between the fourth and fifth metatarsals.[13] Fractures, on the other hand, are usually oriented at right angles to the shaft of the fifth metatarsal, and the fracture usually involves one or both articulations between the fifth metatarsal and the cuboid or between the fourth and fifth metatarsals (Fig 35–106).

Additionally, two accessory bones may be present near the base of the fifth metatarsal and must be distinguished from a fracture. The os peroneum, a sesamoid bone located within the tendon of the peroneus longus as it curves under the cuboid, and the os vesalianum, a secondary ossicle in the peroneus brevis, were both mentioned by Dameron (Fig 35–107).[13] The os peroneum was noted in 15% of roentgenographs.[13] The os vesalianum was present in only 1 of 1,000 feet in the study, and the location was proximal to the insertion of the peroneus brevis on the proximal tip of the fifth metatarsal. A smooth sclerotic opposing surface of this bone and most of the proximal portion of the fifth metatarsal should differentiate it from a fracture.[13] Additionally, O'Rahilly stresses that the os vesalianum is usually found bilaterally.[50]

When a fracture is diagnosed, evaluation of the roentgenograph is essential to determine whether the fracture is acute or whether a pre-existing stress reaction is present. Roentgenographic evidence of a radiolucent fracture line, periosteal reaction, and callus on the lateral cortical margin with intramedullary sclerosis present at the time of the initial complaint suggests a stress reaction to bone.[14] Zelko et al.[64] discovered a lucent fracture line with periosteal elevation in 14 of their 21 patients on *initial* roentgenographic evaluation.

Treatment

Treatment of fractures of the base of the fifth metatarsal is directed at the type of fracture present. Type I fractures (fractures at the junction of the shaft and base of the fifth metatarsal) have been reported to produce significant problems in treatment. Stewart[58] believes that when communication of these fractures is present and allows abnormal mobility between the shaft and the base of the fifth metatarsal, consideration should be given to open reduction and internal fixation to decrease motion and accelerate union.

Giannestras and Sammarco[23] believe that transverse fractures of the base of the fifth metatarsal should be treated with rest. They prefer short-leg walking cast immobilization for 5 to 6 weeks and state that such transverse fractures usually heal without complications. Dameron,[13] however, reported that patients with this fracture are generally younger than patients with fractures of the tuberosity. While he found that patients with fractures of the tuberosity (type II) uniformly respond well to conservative treatment, 5 of 20 fractures involving the proximal shaft (type I fractures) required bone grafts for nonunion, and the time elapsed before roentgenographic and clinical union was often prolonged. He was unable to determine, however, whether initial treatment of these fractures influenced the result. Therefore, he recommended that treatment of these fractures be individualized according to the demands of the patient and that early bone grafting be considered in high-performance athletes. Arangio[3] also emphasized the problem with healing in these fractures and recom-

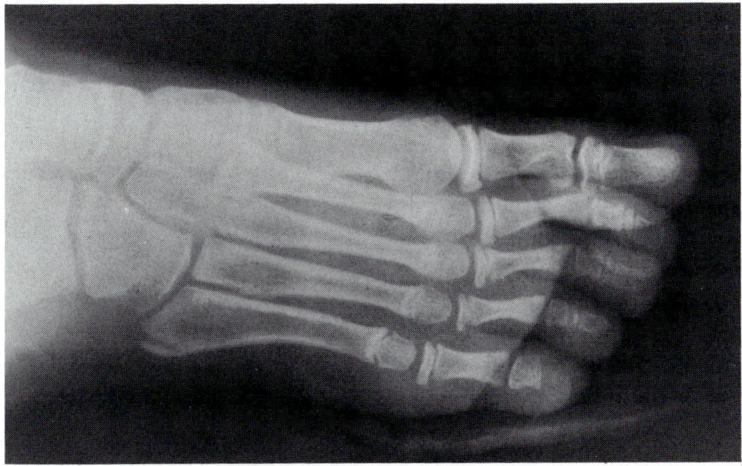

FIG 35–106.
Apophysis of the fifth metatarsal base. (See the text for a description.)

mended cross-pinning the fracture in an effort to accelerate union. He found, after an extensive review of the literature, that 38% of patients with acute fractures in this area developed delayed union and that 14% went on to develop definite nonunions.

In evaluating type IA fractures, that is, acute fractures at the junction of the metaphysis and diaphysis that are nondisplaced, one must distinguish between acute fractures and fractures with a delayed diagnosis or with evidence of long-standing stress reaction of bone.[14] I classify fractures at the metatarsal-diaphyseal junction with x-ray evidence of pre-existing stress reaction in bone as type II fractures. Kavanaugh et al.[34] reported 22 patients with fractures of the diaphysis of the fifth metatarsal, 9 of whom complained of discomfort over the lateral aspect of the foot at least 2 weeks prior to the time of injury. They found that in 41% of their patients, the clinical picture was consistent with the stress fracture evident on the initial roentgenographs. They found that no such fracture treated conservatively in varsity basketball players united and that two thirds of the patients treated conservatively in their series developed delayed union or nonunion. Even those patients whose fracture went on to union in a non–weight-bearing short-leg cast required 10 to 12 weeks of treatment. They therefore advocated the use of intramedullary screw fixation of this fracture in athletes on the professional level due to the time required for union. Following this treatment, athletic competition was allowed in 6 weeks. Zelko et al.[64] also stressed the importance of refractures in these patients. Carp[7] also cited delayed union in 5 of 20 patients with fractures of the fifth metatarsal and ascribed this to poor blood supply. Zelko et al.[64] classified fractures of the base of the fifth metatarsal into four groups for treatment purposes. Group 1 patients (see Fig 35–103,A), those patients who were classified as having an acute traumatic injury with no prior symptoms, do well following plaster immobilization. These correspond to our group 1 category. Patients with pre-existing clinical or x-ray evidence of stress reaction made up groups 2, 3, and 4. Group 2 patients, those with an acute traumatic injury but with minor prior symptoms, also do well when treated by plaster immobilization (see Fig 35–103,B). However, this group of fractures requires more aggressive treatment in athletes, particularly basketball players. In group 3 patients, those who suffered a reinjury and in whom there was a lucent fracture line with periosteal reaction, consideration is given to bone grafting (see Fig 35–103,C). In group 4 patients, those with chronic symptoms and multiple reinjuries, lucent lines at the fracture, dense sclerotic margins, and periosteal callus, direct primary bone grafting is the recommended means of treatment (see Fig 35–103,D). They found that although many of these fractures will heal in the athlete if he is willing to restrict his activities for a prolonged period of time, the incidence of refracture is relatively high. In their group 4 patients, bone grafting was done with a tibial corticocancellous inlay graft after thorough curettage of the sclerotic bone that had obliterated the medullary canal. Following this treatment, the patient returned to activity within 3 months.

Dameron[13] also recommended early bone grafting of these fractures in the professional athlete, while symptomatic treatment was usually effective in sedentary patients.

DeLee et al.[14] reported ten cases of stress fractures of the base of the fifth metatarsal in athletes.[14] All ten patients had prodromal symptoms and x-ray evidence of a pre-existing stress reaction of bone. These patients were treated by axillary screw fixation (Fig 35–108). In all ten, the fractures united within 6 weeks, and the patients returned to activity. They recommend this form of treatment because of shorter disability and the lack of refracture in their series. Minor discomfort over the screw head in the tuberosity of the metatarsal was decreased by countersinking the screw head. Slight discomfort underneath the fifth metatarsal head was eliminated by the use of shoe inserts.

Lehman et al.[38] concluded that although fractures with delayed union may eventually heal if treated conservatively, an active athlete with delayed union or established nonunion will benefit from operative intervention. Although these authors admit that intermedullary screw fixation has the advantages of not opening the fracture site, is a shorter procedure, and

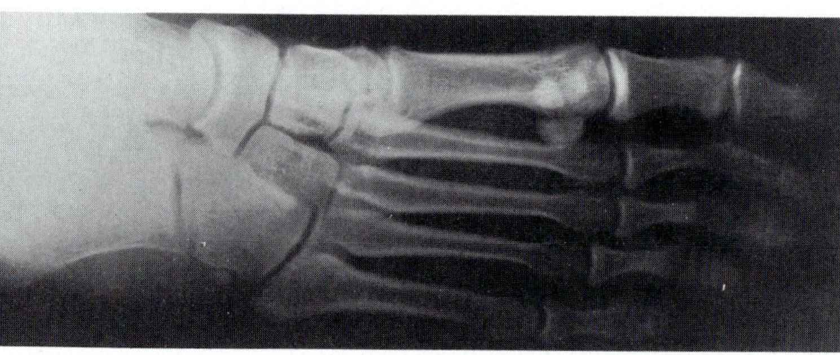

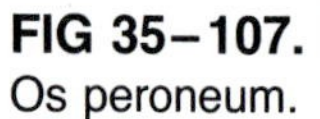

FIG 35–107.
Os peroneum.

has a decreased healing time, they believe that the complications are significant. These include screw fracture, the screw missing the medullary canal, and complaints of pain over the protruding screw head. They emphasize that complications were not reported by Torg et al.[60] following bone grafting. The authors conclude that fractures with no intermedullary sclerosis should be treated with non–weight-bearing casts for 6 to 8 weeks. Fractures with intramedullary sclerosis, particularly in the serious athlete, benefit from surgical treatment. Also, those patients with nonunion of a fracture and dense sclerotic bone adjacent to the fracture line require surgical treatment. These authors believe that the treatment of choice is medullary curettage and bone grafting or closed intermedullary screw fixation. The authors prefer medullary curettage and bone grafting because of the decreased risk of complications.

Recently, Zogby and Baker[65] reported ten patients with Jones fractures. These patients were treated conservatively in a short-leg non–weight-bearing cast. All competitive athletes returned to the preinjury level of competition within 12 weeks. The authors conclude that nonoperative treatment of chronic or subacute fractures *without* intermedullary sclerosis compares favorably with surgical treatment in returning athletes to play.

Acker and Drez[1] reported three patients with fractures of the fifth metatarsal diaphysis that fit the criterion of stress fractures. All roentgenograms demonstrated a lucent fracture line with periosteal reaction on the initial films. These patients were treated in short-leg walking casts until the pain subsided. Patients were allowed to return to athletic activity when roentgenograms demonstrated healing, which occurred within 6 weeks in all patients. The authors conclude that surgical treatment should be performed only in those patients in whom conservative treatment fails and recurrent pain develops.

In type III fractures, that is, fractures involving only the tuberosity of the base of the fifth metatarsal, two groups are present. The fracture may be extra-articular (type IIIA) or intra-articular (type IIIB). In undisplaced fractures of the styloid process seen within the first 48 hours of injury, Giannestras and Sammarco[23] recommend the use of a snug Elastoplast dressing or Gibney-type adhesive strapping. Patients are initially given crutches for partial weight bearing. They believe that a walking cast for such undisplaced fractures is unnecessary. In displaced extra-articular fractures of the styloid process, a below-the-knee walking cast is utilized for 4 to 6 weeks. The authors emphasize that even though union may not be present roentgenographically, as long as a fracture is asymptomatic, the cast is removed at 4 to 6 weeks.

Stewart[58] also believes that the treatment of these fractures should be largely symptomatic. Such symptomatic treatment includes the use of supporting footwear or strapping with or without padding around the tender prominence. He believes that unless the fracture is intra-articular, there is no indication for open reduction. Stone[59] suffered this fracture himself and recommends treatment by simple support of the foot. Stone found that after a Gibney basketweave strapping of the fracture, the foot became extremely painful with prolonged weight bearing. Even a walking cast did not stop the pain with prolonged weight bearing. He therefore recommended the use of a padded metal foot splint incorporated into a short-leg cast. After about a week, the cast is removed, and the padded metal foot splint is applied to the foot with a snug Ace bandage. The patient then walks in a canvas boot. He found that after 2 weeks of this treatment, the fracture was usually pain free. Stone's basic concept was to treat the fracture with the goal of relieving pain. He stressed that a reduction in the period of disability could be obtained by avoiding the use of a short-leg cast for periods as prolonged as 6 weeks. He also stressed that even though the fracture heals with a fibrous union roentgenographically, such a fibrous union is usually *not* symptomatic.

Pearson[51] found that treatment of these fractures by infiltration of the fracture site with procaine followed by strapping of the foot produced much better results (with less time off work) than did treatment by strapping alone or with plaster. Christopher[9] also recommends that treatment be simplified and suggested immobilization in a plaster cast for 2 to 3 weeks followed by massage.

Coker and Arnold[11] report that fractures of the tuberosity heal quickly both clinically and roentgenographically. They state that symptomatic treatment alone suffices and that plaster immobilization is not required. Giannestras and Sammarco[23] distinguished between displaced and nondisplaced avulsion fractures of the styloid process and recommended 4 to 6 weeks of short-leg cast immobilization *only* for displaced fractures.

In type IIIB fractures, that is, fractures of the tuberosity of the fifth metatarsal that are intra-articular, Stewart[49] suggests open reduction and internal fixation in an effort to reconstruct the fifth metatarsocuboid joint, especially when these avulsion fractures consist of a large fracture fragment (see Fig 35–105). However, he emphasizes a problem of tenderness in the healed skin incision overlying the bony prominence on the foot after these open reductions. Pritsch et al.[53] presented a case in which there was marked lateral and rotational displacement of the tuberosity fragment. He stressed the need for accurate open reduction and internal fixation to restore the articular surface of the fifth metatarsocuboid joint. He mentions that with this degree of displacement, an alternative would be removal of the fragment and reinsertion of the peroneus brevis tendon into the metatarsal shaft.

Pearson[51] stressed that the presence of bony union is not considered important and that the final roentgenograph demonstrates a 19% rate of nonunion in these fractures. However, all of his nonunions were painless. Although the literature implies that avulsion fractures of the fifth metatarsal heal with little difficulty or residua (whether by fibrous or bony union), Lichtblau[41] reported a case of painful nonunion of a fracture of the base of the fifth metatarsal. He believes that activity of the peroneus brevis muscle is not only important in causation of the fracture but may also assist in the production of a nonunion. For this reason he recommends restriction of weight bearing for the initial 3 weeks to avoid nonunion. In addition, Gould and Trevenio[26] reported three cases of sural nerve entrapment following avulsion fractures of the base of the fifth metatarsal. They emphasize that the sural nerve is stressed over the displaced fragment and produces pain, both at the fracture site and distally along the course of the sural nerve. Clinically, the patients note bulging of the skin, local pain increasing with shoe wear, a positive Tinel sign, and dysesthesias distal to the fracture in the distribution of the sural nerve. They report prompt recovery following removal of the ununited fragment and neurolysis of the sural nerve.

Author's Preferred Method of Treatment

I stress the need for careful evaluation of anteroposterior, lateral, and oblique roentgenographs of the foot to detect the presence of stress changes in the bone that antedate any acute fracture. In those patients in whom no evidence of stress is present, treatment is undertaken as follows.

In acute type IA fractures involving the metaphyseal-diaphyseal junction, I prefer short-leg cast immobilization with early weight bearing. The patient is kept immobilized, usually for 4 to 6 weeks or until union is present. It is important to remember that in these cases 8 to 12 weeks are often required before there is roentgenographic and clinical evidence of union. In type IB fractures in which there is comminution and increased mobility at the fracture site, I give consideration to cross-pinning to stabilize the fracture and promote union, especially in active patients. In older, less active patients, a short-leg non–weight-bearing cast for 4 to 6 weeks followed by weight bearing in a good shoe is recommended.

The treatment of type II fractures (fractures at the metaphyseal-diaphyseal junction with evidence of pre-existing stress reaction of bone) is based upon the patient's level of activity. In a high-performance athlete with a pre-existing stress reaction in the bone but no evidence of intramedullary sclerosis, I consider an attempt at conservative treatment with a non–weight-bearing cast until the pain subsides. Cast immobilization is maintained until there is evidence of bony union. The patient is then fitted with a molded arch support in a snug-fitting shoe and is allowed to return to sports if radiographs reveal healing of the fracture. If the patient has recurrent pain following resumption of activities, operative treatment is recommended. The risk in this form of treatment is loss of time from athletic activities if conservative treatment fails.

In a high-performance athlete in whom there is a pre-existing stress reaction of bone *including* intramedullary sclerosis or in whom a loss of time from athletic participation due to failed conservative treatment is not acceptable, I prefer to proceed directly to intermedullary screw fixation as demonstrated in Figure 35–108. Following axial screw fixation, the patient is treated in a short-leg nonwalking cast for 2 weeks. The cast is then removed, and the foot is placed in a hard-soled shoe. Either a wooden shoe of the postbunionectomy type or a standard tennis shoe with a semiflexible steel sole insert is utilized to protect the foot. Progressive weight bearing is then begun. Patients are usually allowed to return to competitive sports when pain over the fifth metatarsal and the incision is gone. A soft-soled insert with protective padding over the lateral border of the foot at the base of the fifth metatarsal will prevent pressure over the screw head or under the fifth metatarsal head when the patient returns to activity.

In patients whose activity level is minimal, I utilize a period of immobilization in a short-leg walking cast. Following casting the decision for intramedullary screw fixation is then based upon progression toward union. I have not used bone grafting of the fracture site in treating type II fractures.

In type IIIA fractures (the fracture is extra-articular and involves the tuberosity of the base of the fifth metatarsal), I prefer symptomatic treatment. Strapping the foot with or without a sturdy arch support is utilized until the patient becomes asymptomatic. In patients with marked displacement of the fracture, a short-leg walking cast is used until pain allows treatment by strapping. In all cases, plaster immobilization is utilized

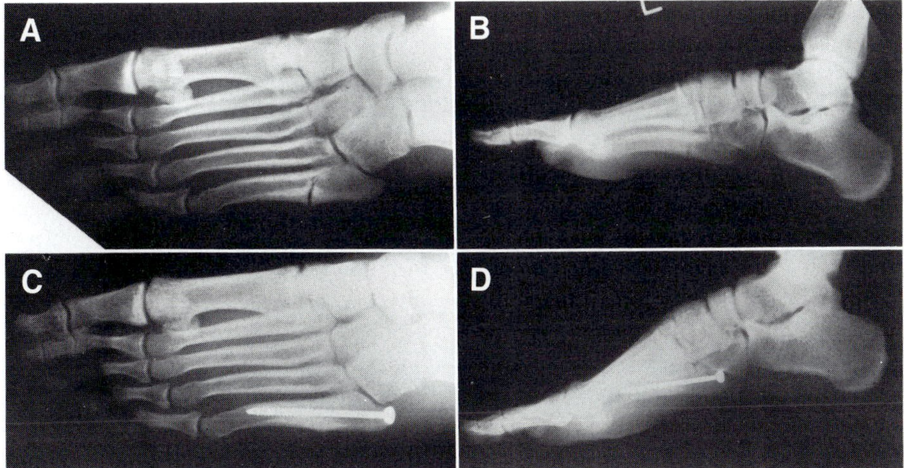

FIG 35–108.
Oblique **(A)** and lateral **(B)** radiographs of a stress fracture of base of the fifth metatarsal. Lateral **(C)** and oblique **(D)** radiographs demonstrate an intramedullary axial screw and a healed fracture.

only in patients in whom strapping or arch supports do not alleviate pain. Weight bearing is begun as soon as the pain allows.

In patients with type IIIB fractures (fractures of the tuberosity involving the fifth metatarsocuboid joint), treatment is based on the patient's level of activity. In a highly competitive athlete, open reduction to restore articular congruity is recommended (Fig 35–105). However, in the majority of patients, I have found very little disability from allowing these fractures to heal in the displaced position (Fig 35–109). Should such a malunion produce symptoms, excision of the displacement fragment and advancement of the peroneus brevis tendon are undertaken.

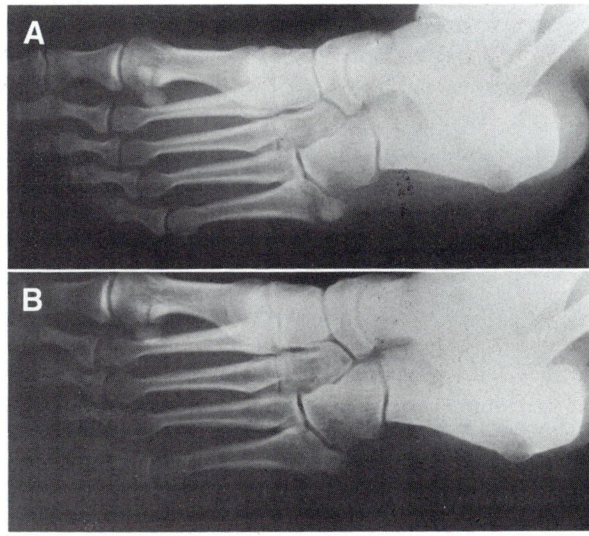

FIG 35–109.
A, displaced intra-articular fracture of the styloid process of the base of the fifth metatarsal. **B,** the fracture healed in a displaced position. The patient is asymptomatic.

Stress Fractures of the Metatarsal Diaphysis

Stress fractures are defined as spontaneous fractures of normal bone that result from a summation of stresses, any one of which by itself is harmless.[19, 39] These fractures occur in the normal bones of healthy people involved in everyday activities.[16, 19] Devas notes that these patients do not report with a history of a specific injury.[16] Although stress fractures have been reported at many different sites, the metatarsals are among the best known of the stress fractures.[16] These fractures have been termed "march fractures" due to their frequent occurrence in military personnel.[5, 22]

The distribution of stress fractures of the metatarsal diaphysis is variable, but they are noted most commonly in the second and third metatarsals.[21, 46] Bernstein and Stone[5] found the second metatarsal most frequently involved, followed closely by the third metatarsal. The first, fourth, and fifth metatarsals were less frequently involved. Levy, however, found the order of frequency of stress fractures to be the second, third, first, fourth, and finally the fifth metatarsal.[39] Levy notes that the reason first metatarsal stress fractures are so rarely reported is their different appearance roentgenographically.[39]

The etiology of these fractures is not completely understood, but it is felt to be recurrent microfractures of the involved bone.[23] As with stress fractures in other locations, force is applied to the bone in a normal physiologic manner, but the frequency and magnitude of the force are increased.[23] The physiologic response of the bone to this stress on a microscopic level is increased osteoclastic and osteoblastic activity. If such altered stress is given time to heal, the bone will remodel to accommodate the forces according to Wolfe's law.[23] However, repetitive microfractures that are not given an opportunity to heal will produce a stress fracture across the shaft of the bone.

Predisposing Conditions and Activities

Congenital shortening of the first metatarsal has been suggested as a predisposing condition in the development of stress fractures of the second and third metatarsals.[4, 62] However, Drez et al. were unable to show that the length of the first metatarsal in patients with stress fractures differed significantly from that in a randomly selected control group.[17] The occurrence of metatarsal stress fractures of the lateral metatarsals following Keller or Mayo bunion operations has been reported by Ford and Gilula.[20] Battey[4] theorized that a shortened first metatarsal, the posterior displacement of the sesamoids due to the loss of insertion of the flexor hallucis brevis, and hypermobility of the first ray following the Keller procedure all predisposed the foot to stress fractures of the lesser metatarsals[24, 35] (Fig 35–110).

Stress fractures are also commonly noted in new military recruits who undergo intensive training to which the bones of the foot are not adapted.[5, 16] With the current enthusiasm in sports, particularly jogging, metatarsal stress fractures are seen with increasing frequency in normal healthy young patients.[10, 11]

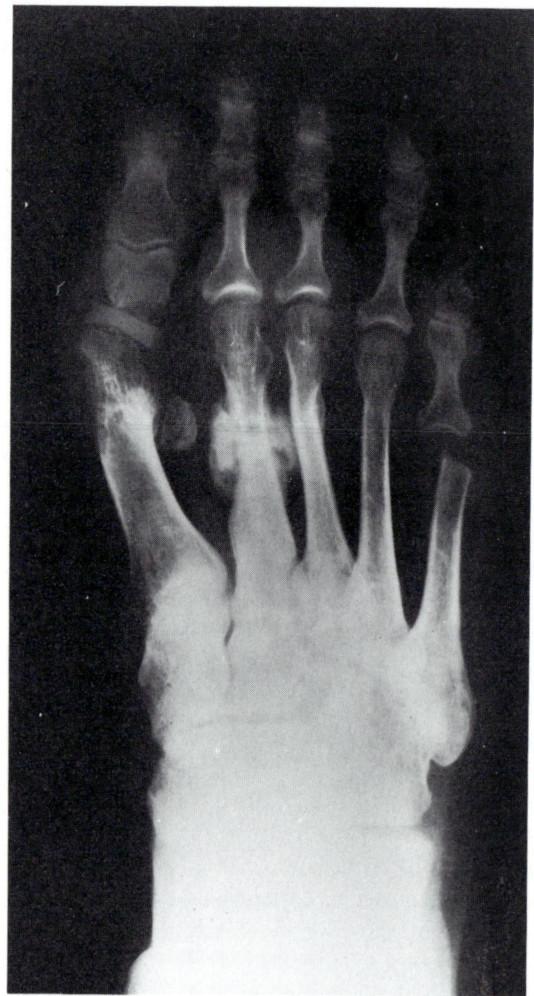

FIG 35–110.
Stress fractures of the second and third metatarsal shafts after Keller bunionectomy with a Silastic implant.

Clinical Diagnosis

History.—The most common presenting complaint is pain on a long march or with increased running on hard pavement.[22] The pain is usually described as an aching or soreness in the foot.[39, 46, 62] Although the pain is described as an ache, stiffness, or tiredness, there is always a direct relationship to activity.[16] The patient usually states that relief of the pain occurs only when the foot is elevated and protected from activity.[22] The pain is initially vague and may be difficult to localize.[22] As the pain increases in intensity, a limp usually develops.[5, 16, 39] Devas also notes that if activity is continued, pain comes on earlier each day until it ultimately prevents the activity concerned.[16]

Physical Examination.—Early after the onset of symptoms, there may be no swelling present.[23] However, after 10 to 15 days, as the pain becomes more disabling, definite clinical findings begin to appear.[23] These include tenderness, swelling, and ecchymosis over the shaft of the involved metatarsal.[22, 62] On examination, pain on dorsiflexion of the involved metatarsal is present.[39] Direct point tenderness over the location on the metatarsal shaft where the fracture has occurred is diagnostic. The patient will often have a limp. Bernstein and Stone[5] stress the importance of a limp on the involved side due to pain with weight bearing. They note that the forefoot is held in either the inverted or everted position depending upon which metatarsal is fractured. Swelling on the dorsal aspect of the foot may obliterate the spaces normally seen between the extensor tendons.[5] Crepitus is rarely if ever elicited due to the rarity of a completely displaced stress fracture.[5] In the author's experience, grasping the involved metatarsal by the head while forcing it in a dorsal and plantar direction recreates the pain the patient has with weight bearing. There may also be pain on forced plantar flexion or traction of the corresponding toe.[5] It is important to note, as Devas stresses,[16] that metatarsal stress fractures represent a continuum of disease and that the physical findings become more diagnostic as the pain, disability, and duration from the actual moment of stress fracture increase.

Radiographic Diagnosis

Devas emphasizes that stress fractures must be diagnosed clinically because radiologic confirmation is usually delayed.[16] Roentgenograms taken within 10 to 14 days of the onset of symptoms usually do not demonstrate a metatarsal stress fracture.[5, 22, 23] Two to 3 weeks following the development of pain, a fine line in the metatarsal shaft secondary to bone resorption along the fracture surface is noted.[22, 23] Anteroposterior and oblique roentgenographs are the most useful in detecting metatarsal stress fractures due to the overlap of metatarsals present on the lateral radiographs.[22, 23]

Several authors have reported the varying roentgenographic characteristics of metatarsal stress fractures.[16, 39, 62] Levy[39] found two distinct types of stress fractures. First, fractures form in the *shafts* of long bones and usually produce tiny cortical interruptions on early films. Later, a dense accumulation of callus forms in the fractures and is easily visible. He reports that this type of fracture is most commonly noted in the second through fifth metatarsals (Fig 35–111). Second, fractures in the ends of long bones in areas of predominantly cancellous bone produce a different roentgenographic appearance. Initially, the films are normal, but 10 to 14 days after the onset of pain there is linear sclerosis perpendicular to the direction of the stress. He reports that this second type of fracture is the one noted in first metatarsal stress fractures (Fig 35–112). Levy noted that a lack of familiarity with the roentgenographic appearance of this second type of stress fracture has led to a decrease in first metatarsal stress fractures being diagnosed.

Devas[16] also reports two main types of stress fractures: distraction types and compression types. The distraction types are so named because of an apparent crack located on one cortex of the bone. The compression types, on the other hand, are noted by an area of increased density within the confines of the cortex. Devas reports that distraction-type stress fractures are the ones most commonly noted in the metatarsals, with the exception of the first metatarsal, which classically demonstrates compression-type fractures. Meurman[46] notes that compression fractures appear as internal transverse callus, while distraction fractures appear as periosteal

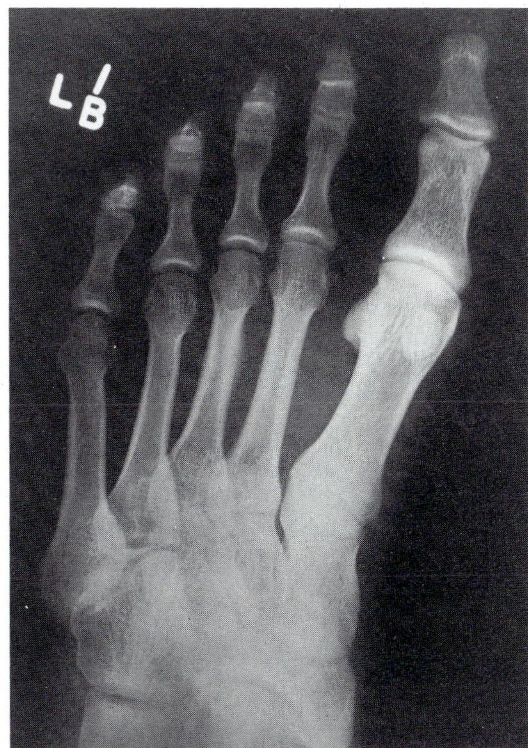

FIG 35–111.
Stress fracture of the shaft of the third metatarsal.

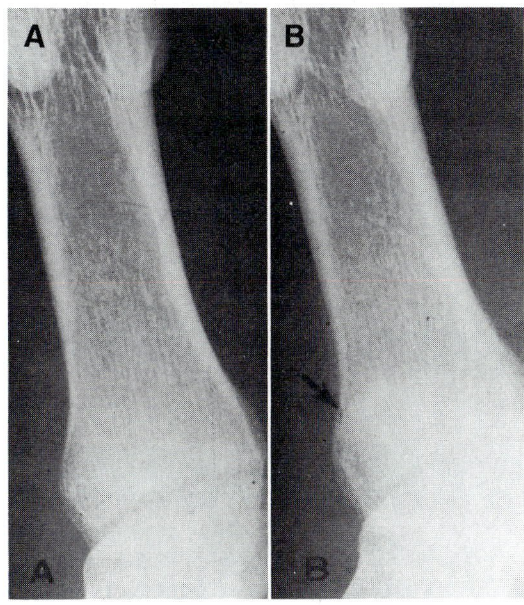

FIG 35–112.
Stress fracture of the first metatarsal in an area of predominantly cancellous bone. **A,** radiograph taken at the onset of symptoms. No stress fracture was noted. **B,** radiograph taken 3 weeks later. Note the linear slcerosis *(arrow)* in the base of the first metatarsal. (From Levy JM: *AJR* 130:679–681, 1978. Used by permission.)

callus indicating a cortical fissure or break.[16, 46] Wilson and Katz[62] noted four basic x-ray patterns, the dominant pattern depending not so much on the particular bone involved but on the period in the evolution of the process when the roentgenograph was first obtained. The importance in noting the differing roentgenographic appearances of stress fractures is not in categorizing the fractures as compression or distraction types, but in recognizing their different roentgenographic presentations so that they are not overlooked.

During the period when pain is present and x-ray findings are negative, newer bone scanning techniques may be utilized to diagnose stress fractures.[46] However, since it is the clinical syndrome that makes the diagnosis, patients are treated as though they have a fracture whether or not the roentgenographs are positive. Therefore, except in unusual instances, bone scans to confirm the diagnosis of a metatarsal stress fracture seem unnecessary.

In the first metatarsal, stress fractures are classically in the proximal portion of the bone.[16, 46] Fractures of the second and third metatarsals usually occur in the middle of the shaft or in the neck of the bone.[16] Meurman[46] reports that stress fractures of the fourth metatarsal occur in the distal part of the diaphysis. Fifth metatarsal stress fractures, according to Devas, may be of two types.[16] The most common is a fracture at the base of the metatarsal in which the fracture line opens up on the lateral side and runs transversely across the bone (see the section on fractures of the base of the fifth metatarsal). This is the more common type. Rarely, there may be a stress fracture of the *shaft* of the fifth metatarsal in the same location as other metatarsal shaft fractures.[16] Devas also reports that multiple stress fractures may occur and involve several metatarsals either at the same time or in sequence.[16]

Displacement of metatarsal stress fractures is distinctly unusual.[22, 23] Meurman reported only a single completely displaced stress fracture in his series.[46]

Treatment

The type of treatment selected depends upon the pain and disability with which the patient presents. Giannestras and Sammarco[23] suggest a short-leg walking cast only in patients with severe pain and an inability to walk. Garcia and Parkes[22] agree that unless severe pain is present, plaster cast immobilization is unnecessary. Bernstein and Stone[5] believe that plaster of paris immobilization is not indicated due to the fact that this is not a complete fracture and there is no loss of position. They feel that such rigid immobilization leads to bone and muscle atrophy of the involved limb.

Most patients can be treated with a molded arch support combined with snugly wrapping the forefoot in two or three layers of Elastoplast dressing.[22, 23] This dressing is changed weekly. At the end of 3 to 6 weeks sufficient callus is usually present to permit removal of support and allow increasing activity within the limits of pain.[22, 23] Bernstein and Stone[5] emphasize that patients with stress fractures of the metatarsals complain of pain during the push-off phase of gait, that is, when weight is on the heads of the metatarsals with the toes dorsiflexed and the heel off the ground. Therefore, these authors believe that by eliminating metatarsophalangeal joint motion, pain can be markedly decreased. They accomplish this by the use of a steel bar countersunk into the sole of a shoe. They used these steel bars in the boots of military recruits and were able to decrease their period of disability. Wilson et al.[62] also emphasize a conservative approach. They feel that the majority of metatarsal stress fractures respond favorably to limited weight bearing while only the more symptomatic fractures require plaster immobilization.

Author's Preferred Method of Treatment

My treatment of metatarsal stress fracture is based on the degree of severity of the patient's pain. Stress fractures of the first through the fourth metatarsals are treated similarly. For those patients with minimal pain, forefoot strapping, using either Elastoplast or an adhesive dressing, combined with a molded arch support worn in the shoe for 4 to 6 weeks is recommended. If the stress fracture is the result of increased activity, the responsible activity is limited until pain subsides. After 4 to 6 weeks or when the pain has subsided, the taping is stopped. All activities are increased within the limits of pain. The molded arch support is continued until the patient has returned to his normal activities.

Only in those patients with severe pain do I use a short-leg walking cast in which the arch has been well molded. This weight-bearing cast is utilized for 4 to 6 weeks. Following removal of the cast, a molded arch support is placed in the patient's shoe, and the forefoot is taped for an additional 3 weeks. Activity is then progressed within the limits of pain.

Due to the problems associated with stress fractures of the fifth metatarsal, they are considered in the section on fractures of the base of the fifth metatarsal. In patients with recurrent stress fractures, evaluation for a biomechanical or metabolic abnormality is essential.

REFERENCES

Metatarsals

1. Acker JH, Drez D: Nonoperative treatment of stress fractures of the proximal shaft of the fifth metatarsal: Jones fracture, *Foot Ankle* 7:152–155, 1986.

2. Anderson LD: Injuries of the foot, *Clin Orthop* 122:18–27, 1977.
3. Arangio GA: Proximal displaced fractures of the fifth metatarsal (Jones fracture): two cases treated by cross pinning with review of 100 cases, *Foot Ankle* 3:293–296, 1983.
4. Battey MA: The lesser metatarsal stress fracture as a complication of the Keller procedure, *J Am Podiatr Assoc* 70:182–186, 1980.
5. Bernstein A, Stone JR: March fracture: a report of three hundred and seven cases, and a new method of treatment, *J Bone Joint Surg* 26:743, 1944.
6. Blodgett WH: Injuries of the forefoot and toes. In Jahss MH, editor: *Disorders of the foot*, vol 2, Philadelphia, 1982, WB Saunders.
7. Carp L: Fracture of the fifth metatarsal bone, with special reference to delayed union, *Ann Surg* 86:308–320, 1927.
8. Chapman MW: Fractures and fracture-dislocations of the ankle and foot. In Mann RA, editor: *DuVries' surgery of the foot*, ed 4, St Louis, 1978, Mosby–Year Book.
9. Christopher F: Fractures of the fifth metatarsal, *Surg Gynecol Obstet* 37:190–194, 1923.
10. Clancy WG Jr: Lower extremity injuries in the jogger and distance runner, *Phys Sports Med* 2:47, 1974.
11. Coker TP Jr, Arnold JA: Sports injuries to the foot and ankle, In Jahss MH, editor: *Disorders of the foot*, vol 2, Philadelphia, 1982, WB Saunders.
12. Crenshaw AH: Delayed union and nonunion of fractures. In Edmonson AS, Crenshaw AH, editors: *Campbell's operative orthopaedics*, ed 6, St Louis, 1980, Mosby–Year Book.
13. Dameron TB: Fractures and anatomical variations of the proximal portion of the fifth metatarsal, *J Bone Joint Surg [Am]* 57:788–792, 1975.
14. DeLee JC, Evans JP, Julian J: Stress fracture of the fifth metatarsal, *Am J Sports Med* 11:349–353, 1983.
15. DePalma A: *The management of fractures and dislocations*, vol 2, Philadelphia, 1959, WB Saunders.
16. Devas M: *Stress fractures*, New York, 1975, Churchill Livingstone.
17. Drez D Jr, Young JC, Johnston RD, et al: Metatarsal stress fractures, *Am J Sports Med* 8:123–125, 1980.
18. Dukowsky J, Freeman BL: Fracture dislocation of the articular surface of the third metatarsal head, *Foot Ankle* 10:43–44, 1989.
19. Engh CA, Robinson RA, Milgram J: Stress fractures in children, *J Trauma* 10:532–541, 1970.
20. Ford LT, Gilula LA: Stress fractures of the middle metatarsals following the Keller operation, *J Bone Joint Surg [Am]* 59:117–118, 1977.
21. Frieberg AH: Infraction of the second metatarsal bone, a typical injury, *Surg Gynecol Obstet* 19:191–193, 1914.
22. Garcia A, Parkes JC: Fractures of the foot. In Giannestras NJ, editor: *Foot disorders: medical and surgical management*, ed 2, Philadelphia, 1973, Lea & Febiger.
23. Giannestras LJ, Sammarco GJ: Fractures and dislocations in the foot. In Rockwood CA Jr, Green DP, editors: *Fractures*, vol 2, Philadelphia, 1975, JB Lippincott.
24. Giannestras NJ: Shortening of the metatarsal shaft in the treatment of plantar keratosis, *J Bone Joint Surg [Am]* 40:61–71, 1958.
25. Goldstein LA, Dickerson RC: *Atlas of orthopaedic surgery*, St Louis, 1974, Mosby–Year Book.
26. Gould N, Trevenio S: Sural nerve entrapment by avulsion fracture of the base of the fifth metatarsal bone, *Foot Ankle* 3:153–155, 1981.
27. Hansen ST: Severe trauma to the forefoot: initial management, American Orthopedic Association Third International Symposium: "Musculoskeletal trauma," San Francisco, May 17–21, 1982.
28. Heck CV: Fractures of the bones of the foot (except the talus), *Surg Clin North Am* 45:103–117, 1965.
29. Heckman JD: Fractures and dislocations of the foot, In Rockwood CA, Green DP, editors: *Fractures*, Philadelphia, 1954, JB Lippincott, 1984, pp 1808–1809.
30. Irwin CG: Fractures of the metatarsals, *Proc R Soc Med* 31:789–793, 1938.
31. Johnson VS: Treatment of fractures of the forefoot in industry, In Bateman JE, editor: *Foot science*, Philadelphia, 1976, WB Saunders.
32. Jones R: Fracture of the base of the fifth metatarsal bone by indirect violence, *Ann Surg* 35:697–700, 1902.
33. Jones R: Fractures of the fifth metatarsal bone, *Liverpool Med Surg J* 42:103–107, 1902.
34. Kavanaugh JH, Brower TD, Mann RV: The Jones fracture revisited, *J Bone Joint Surg [Am]* 60:776–782, 1978.
35. Kelikian H: *Hallux valgus, allied deformities of the forefoot and metatarsals*, Philadelphia, 1965, WB Saunders.
36. Key JA, Conwell HE: *The management of fractures, dislocations and sprains* ed 3, St Louis, 1942, Mosby–Year Book.
37. Klenerman L: *The foot and its disorders*, Oxford, 1976, Blackwell.
38. Lehman RC, Torg JS, Pavlov H, et al: Fractures of the base of the fifth metatarsal distal to the tuberosity: a review, *Foot Ankle* 7:245–252, 1987.
39. Levy JM: Stress fractures of the first metatarsal, *AJR* 130:679–681, 1978.
40. Lewin R, editor: *The foot and ankle*, Philadelphia, 1940, Lea & Febiger.
41. Lichtblau S: Painful nonunion of a fracture of the 5th metatarsal, *Clin Orthop* 59:171–175, 1968.
42. Lindholm R: Operative treatment of dislocated simple fracture of the neck of the metatarsal bone, *Ann Chir Gynaecol Tenn* 50:328–331, 1961.
43. Mann RA: Personal communication, 1980.
44. McKeever FM: Fractures of the tarsal and metatarsal bones, *Surg Gynecol Obstet* 90:735–745, 1950.
45. McKeever FM: Injuries of the forefoot. In *American Academy of Orthopaedic Surgeons instructional course lectures*, vol 2, Ann Arbor, Mich, 1944, JW Edwards, pp 120–129.
46. Meurman KOA: Less common stress fractures in the foot, *Br J Radiol* 54:1–7, 1981.
47. Morrison GM: Fractures of the bones of the feet, *Am J Surg* 38:721–726, 1937.
48. Morrissey EJ: Metatarsal fractures, *J Bone Joint Surg* 28:594–602, 1946.
49. Moseley HF: Traumatic disorders of the ankle and foot, *Clin Symp* 17:29–30, 1965.
50. O'Rahilly R: A survey of carpal and tarsal anomalies, *J Bone Joint Surg [Am]* 35:626–642, 1953.
51. Pearson JB: Fractures of the base of the fifth metatarsal, *Br Med J* 1:1052–1054, 1962.
52. Peltier LF: Eponymic fractures: Robert Jones and Jones's fracture, *Surgery* 71:522–526, 1972.
53. Pritsch M, Heim M, Tauber H, et al: An unusual fracture of the base of the fifth metatarsal bone, *J Trauma* 20:530–531, 1980.
54. Sammarco GJ: Biomechanics of the foot. In Frankel

VH, Nordin M, editors: *Basic biomechanics of the skeletal system*, Philadelphia, 1980, Lea & Febiger, pp 193–220.
55. Shereff MJ: Fractures of the forefoot, *Instr Course Lect* 29:133–140, 1990.
56. Sisk TD: Fractures. In Edmonson AS, Crenshaw AH, editors: *Campbell's operative orthopaedics*, ed 6, vol 1, St Louis, 1980, Mosby–Year Book.
57. Speed K: *Fractures and dislocations*, ed 2, Philadelphia, 1928, Lea & Febiger.
58. Stewart IM: Jones's fracture: fracture of base of fifth metatarsal, *Clin Orthop* 16:190–198, 1960.
59. Stone MM: Avulsion fracture of the base of the fifth metatarsal, *Am J Orthop Surg* 10:190–193, 1968.
60. Torg JS, Balduini FC, Zelco RR, et al: Fractures of the base of the fifth metatarsal distal to the tuberosity: classification and guidelines for nonsurgical and surgical management, *J Bone Joint Surg* 66A:209–214, 1984.
61. Wharton HR: Fractures of the proximal end of the fifth metatarsal bone, *Ann Surg* 47:824–826, 1908.
62. Wilson ES Jr, Katz FN: Stress fractures. An analysis of 250 consecutive cases, *Radiology* 92:481–486, 1969.
63. Young JK: Fracture of the proximal end of the fifth metatarsal bone, *Ann Surg* 47:824–826, 1908.
64. Zelko RR, Torg JS, Rachun A: Proximal diaphyseal fractures of the fifth metatarsal—treatment of the fractures and their complications in athletes, *Am J Sports Med* 7:95–101, 1979.
65. Zogby RB, Baker B: A review of nonoperative treatment of Jones fracture, *Am J Sports Med* 15:304–307, 1987.

FRACTURES OF THE PHALANGES

Fractures of the phalanges represent the most common fractures of the forefoot.[2, 3, 6, 13, 14] The most common of all the phalangeal injuries is the so-called night walker fracture of the proximal phalanx of the fifth toe.[2] However, injuries to the first digit are also frequent and more commonly lead to periods of long-term disability following their occurrence.[8, 14] Although open fractures of the phalanges are not common, they can occur, particularly when the fracture is secondary to a crushing injury.

The hallux phalanges are larger and functionally much more important than the phalanges of the lesser toes.[3] Of the hallux phalanges, the proximal one is fractured most frequently.[3] When the distal phalanx is fractured, it is often comminuted or dislocated.[3] Also, an avulsion fracture involving the dorsal aspect of the distal phalanx of the hallux, similar to that seen in the hand, can occur.[3] Fractures of the lesser toes usually occur through the proximal phalanx, the longest of the phalanges, while the middle and distal phalanges are less frequently fractured.[3]

Fractures of the proximal phalanx of the lesser toes are prone to plantar angulation secondary to the combined action of the toe extensor, flexor, interosseous, and lumbrical muscles.[2, 5] Angulation of middle and distal phalangeal fractures is more dependent upon the direction of the trauma that produced the fracture.

Excluding the hallux, the range of motion of the interphalangeal and metatarsophalangeal joints of the toes is not of much functional significance.[2] However, should malunion at the fracture site in a toe occur, it may be a persistent source of pain while wearing a constricting shoe.[2] Should such a painful malunion of a lesser toe persist, Morrison mentions amputation of a part or all of the toe.[12]

Mechanism of Injury

Fractures of the toes are usually caused by direct trauma to the involved toe.[9, 12] The patient may relate to a history of dropping a heavy object on the toe that results in a crushing injury to the soft tissue and a fracture of a phalanx, most commonly the middle or distal phalanx.[5, 6, 7, 9, 12, 13] Jahss[10] emphasized unique "stubbing" injuries to the hallux that result in fracture-dislocations that are often missed. A fracture of the proximal phalanx of the lateral four digits is most commonly produced by an abduction injury such as occurs when the toe strikes a table leg and results in the classic "night walker fracture."[2, 7]

Yokoe and Mannoji[15] reported three cases of stress fracture of the proximal phalanx of the great toe. In all three patients, the fracture occurred on the medial aspect of the base of the proximal phalanx, and all patients had significant hallux valgus. The authors believe that hallux valgus leads to the extensor hallucis longus and adductor tendons having a bowstringing effect on the hallux. This bowstringing effect on the big toe and the medial collateral ligament resulted in strain that produced an avulsion-type stress fracture of the proximal phalanx.

Clinical Diagnosis

Jahss[10] emphasized that the relatively mild discomfort associated with certain fractures of the hallux phalanges may cause them to be interpreted as simple sprains. This can result in the diagnosis being overlooked by the physician or in the patient not seeking early medical care. Similarly, fractures of the lesser toes are often dismissed as sprains.

The patient will most commonly relate symptoms of acute pain, swelling, and difficulty in wearing a shoe or in walking.[2, 6, 7] Clinically, the toe is swollen and tender to palpation, and crepitus is usually present.[2, 6, 7] There is often a subungual hematoma when the distal phalanx is involved.[2, 6, 7] *Any* movement of the toe produces pain. If the patient is seen very soon after the injury, no ecchymosis will be present. However, within 12 to 24 hours marked swelling and ecchymosis of the involved digit are present.[6]

Open fractures of the phalanges usually occur from direct trauma. In these situations the neurovascular status of the toe distal to the open fracture may be in jeopardy due to the fracture and the crushing of the soft tissues that occurs with the fracture.

Radiographic Diagnosis

Anteroposterior, oblique, and lateral roentgenograms of the *toe* (not the foot) are necessary to delineate the fracture location and displacement of the fracture. Although comminution is frequently present, unlike fractures of the fingers, most of these fractures are not significantly displaced.[6, 7, 9]

Fractures of the hallux phalanges, however, are most commonly displaced. Jahss emphasizes that fractures of the great toe vary from a mildly displaced fracture of the medial or lateral margin of the distal portion of the proximal phalanx to a frank fracture-dislocation.[10] He stresses the importance of critically evaluating roentgenographs of the great toe to distinguish between simple fractures and fracture-dislocations involving the proximal phalanx. In these fractures, it is essential to have a *true* lateral radiograph of the hallux. Jahss also points out the value of magnification of x-ray films to demonstrate fractures of the toes.[10] Roentgenographs taken with traction applied to hallux are often helpful in further evaluating the fracture (see Fig 35–114).

Treatment

If an open fracture of the lesser toes is present, the wounds should be irrigated and debrided just as with any other open fracture.[5, 6] Consideration is given to the use of intramedullary Kirschner wire fixation in cases in which severe soft-tissue damage is present. Antibiotics are given for 48 hours after initial irrigation and debridement. If the hallux is involved, the indications for internal fixation of the articular surface are the same as listed below.

In closed fractures, treatment recommendations depend upon the digit involved.

Hallux Phalangeal Fractures

Fractures of the distal phalanx of the great toe are most often secondary to dropping heavy objects on the toe.[12, 14] This often results in comminution.[5] Subungual hematomas are usually present and can be relieved by drilling the nail bed.[7, 11] Avulsion of the nail to decompress the subungual hematomas is not warranted.[2]

In simple fractures of the phalanges of the great toe without displacement (Fig 35–113), Cobey recommends treatment with a metatarsal bar.[4] Alternatively, the great toe can be bound to the adjacent two toes for stability and ambulation initiated in a stiff-soled shoe.[3] Johnson stresses the necessity for simple treatment of nondisplaced phalangeal fractures by protective splinting (usually to an adjacent toe), symptomatic medication, and immediate ambulation.[11] The stress fractures reported by Yokoe et al.[15] were treated by a simple decrease in the athletic activity that produced the fracture. This resulted in healing of the stress fracture.

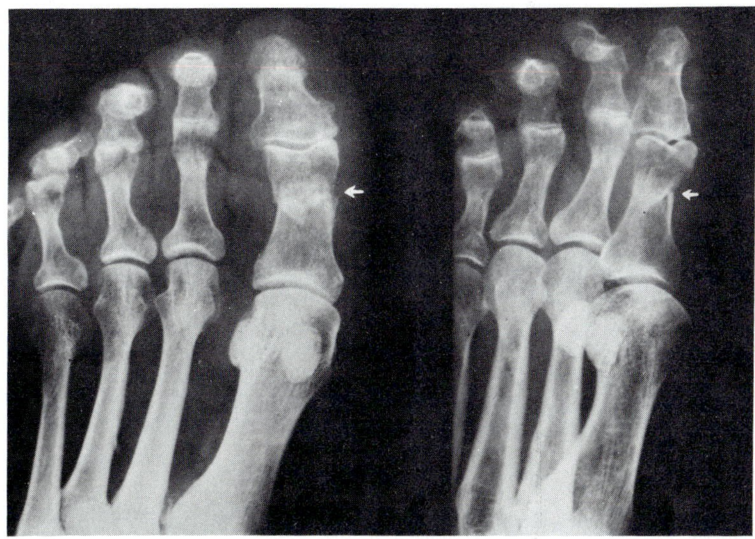

FIG 35–113.
Nondisplaced fracture *(arrows)* of the proximal phalanx of the great toe.

Jahss[10] reports that displaced fractures of the hallux phalanges (when treated *early*) can usually be reduced by closed means with traction under local anesthesia and that the reduction can usually be maintained in a plaster boot. He recommends treatment by adhesive strapping of minor angulation or minor displacement of fractures through the condylar neck.

When hallux phalangeal fractures are displaced and reduction cannot be obtained by manipulation, Chapman suggests open reduction.[3] Taylor[14] stresses the importance of maintaining the nail in treating fractures of the distal phalanx of the hallux. He believes that it serves as an important splint to the broken phalanx and also that its removal exposes a tender area that will prevent the patient from returning to work for some weeks.[14] He recommends the use of a plaster of paris "thimble" enclosing the whole toe to provide immobilization of these fractures. Blodgett[2] recommends treating crush fractures of the terminal phalanx of the great toe with elevation and ice, followed by a cut-out shoe with a stiff sole. Heck[8] stresses that in such comminuted fractures reduction is not always possible, but care should be taken to place the toe in a functional position. If a crushing-type fracture of the great toe is severely comminuted and open and involves the majority of the distal phalanx with extensive soft-tissue loss, debridement of the wound, nail excision, and a terminal Syme amputation may be indicated.[7]

If there is displacement of single fractures of the proximal or distal phalanx of the great toe, every attempt should be made to correct the displacement.[6, 10] Isolated medial or lateral condylar fractures or fracture-dislocations typically seen in stubbing injuries are unstable. Zrubecky[17] recommended open reduction and Kirschner wire stabilization of these unstable fractures (Fig 35–114,A–C). Jahss[10] stresses that displaced fractures of the great toe phalanges, particularly those associated with dislocations of the adjacent joint, require *anatomic* reduction. Although outrigger pulp or skeletal traction has been advised in the presence of instability of these fractures,[5, 8, 9] Zorzi considers this unnecessary and potentially dangerous because it can lead to infection or vascular impairment of the digit.[16] Johnson[11] also cautions against such overtreatment of these injuries.

Lesser Toe Phalangeal Fractures

In fractures involving the second, third, fourth, and fifth toe phalanges, Giannestras and Sammarco[7] believe that moderate displacement is of no great significance. Although they recommend attempted reduction, they believe that if an anatomic reduction is not obtained, one need not be concerned as long as the general alignment of the toe is satisfactory.[7] They treat these injuries by placing a single layer of sheet wadding between the involved toe and two adjacent toes. The toes are then strapped together with adhesive tape while being careful not to compromise the circulation.[5] Ambulation is permitted in a stiff-soled shoe with the toe cut out. They emphasize that if the displacement is gross or if dislocation of the adjacent joint is present, closed reduction with or without Kirschner wire fixation may be indicated.[7] Chapman[3] emphasizes that displacement of a fracture of the phalanges, particularly of the middle three toes, is rare but that when it does occur, it can usually be reduced even without anesthesia (Fig 35–115,A–C). He, too, recommends adhesive strapping to the adjacent two toes for approximately 4 weeks and stresses *immediate* ambulation in a shoe with a semi-rigid sole.

Cobey[4] felt that most of the pain associated with a fractured toe results from dorsiflexing the toes with walking. In his opinion, neither taping adjacent toes together nor a hard leather sole will prevent this dorsiflexion. He therefore recommended the use of a metatarsal bar made from tongue blades and taped to the bottom of the shoe. The patient then begins early ambulation. He found that this method functionally immobilized the toes and the metatarsophalangeal joint without permanently altering the shoe. The use of tongue blades also eliminates the need for an expensive metatarsal bar.

On the contrary, Blodgett stressed that fractures of the proximal phalanx of the second through the fourth toes are prone to plantar angulation.[2] If this angulation persists, painful plantar pressure areas may develop under the toe and require operative correction.[2] He emphasized that aggressive treatment of the fractures of the proximal phalanx of the lesser toes was essential to prevent such deformity.[2] He suggests immobilization in flexion with Kirschner wire fixation or traction obtained by skin traction, pulp traction, or skeletal traction through the middle or distal phalanx. When severe comminution occurs, however, Blodgett recommends the use of adhesive taping to adjacent toes.[2] He stresses that such fractures need only be held in alignment by the tubular soft tissue of the toe and that full recovery of joint motion in the toe is not required for full walking function and shoe wearing. Johnson[11] strongly emphasizes the danger in overtreating and overprotecting patients with fractures of the phalanges, a practice that may result in long-term complications.

Long-term sequelae from phalangeal fractures of the lesser toes are rarely reported. Angulation at the fracture site with malunion may result in a painful plantar pressure area under a toe, particularly when a fractures

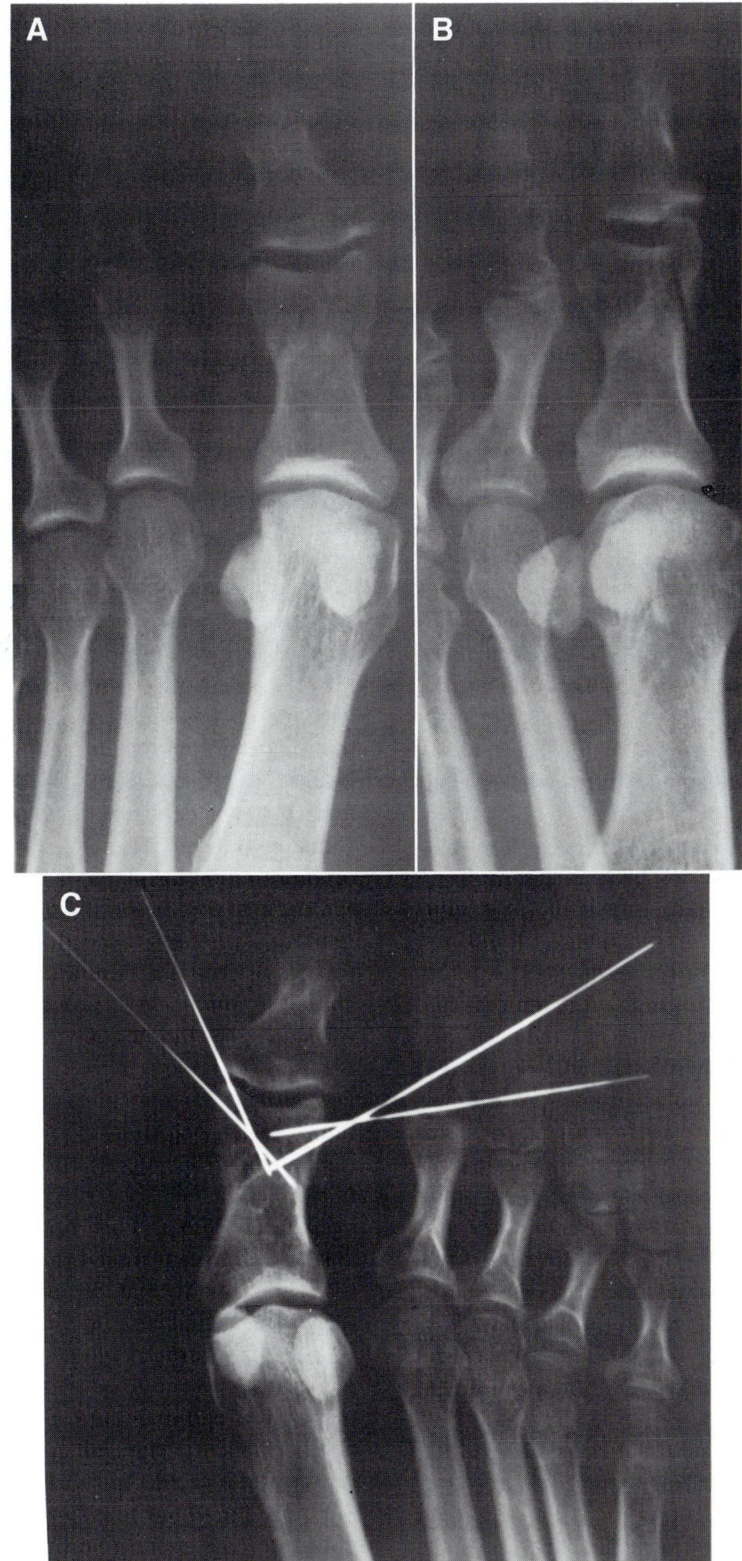

FIG 35–114.
A, displaced fracture of both condyles of the proximal phalanx of the hallux. **B,** radiograph taken with traction applied to better demonstrate the fracture anatomy. **C,** open reduction and internal fixation of the fracture with Kirschner wires. Wires are cut off beneath the skin and removed between 4 and 6 weeks. Note the restoration of the articular surface.

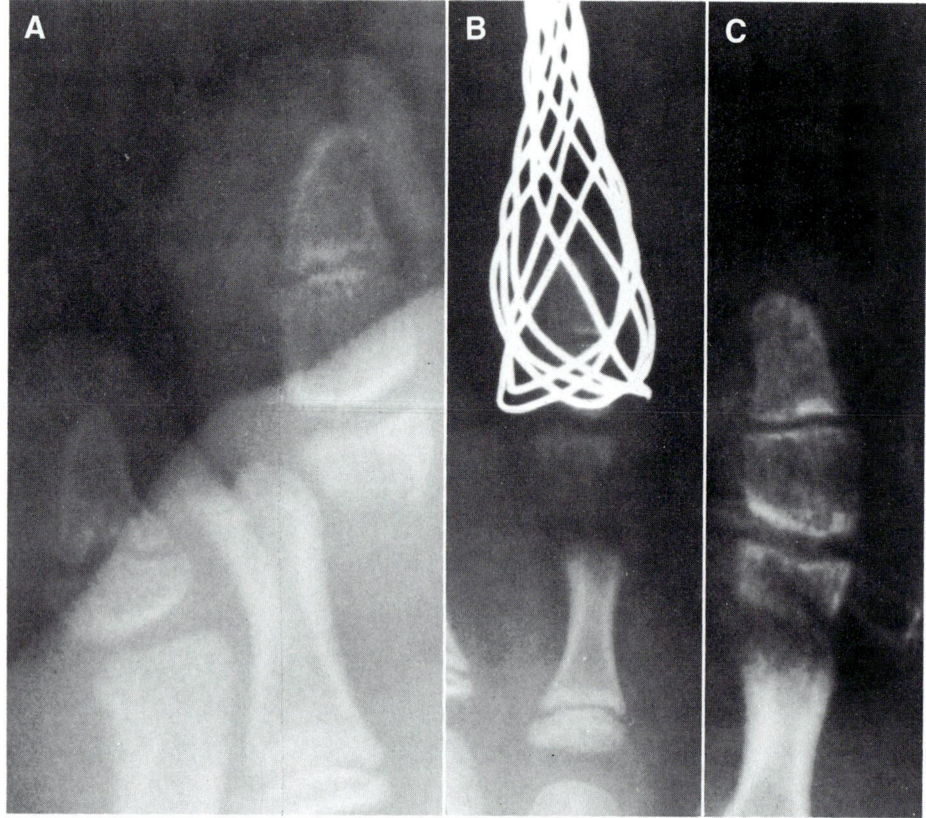

FIG 35–115.
A, displaced fracture of the proximal phalanx of the third toe. **B,** closed reduction using Chinese finger traps. Note the distraction at the fracture site. **C,** stabilization was achieved by taping to the adjacent toe. Alignment of the fracture is excellent.

involves the proximal phalanx of the second through the fourth toe.[2] Such plantar pressure areas may require later operative correction.[2, 12] However, according to Johnson, disability from stiffness, swelling, and occasional Sudek's atrophy resulting from the more aggressive types of therapy are more significant in regard to long-term disability.[11]

Author's Preferred Method of Treatment

In patients with open fractures involving the toes, thorough irrigation and debridement as indicated in open fractures of the major bones are performed. With extensive soft-tissue damage, I prefer axial Kirschner wire fixation as a splint to provide stability for soft-tissue healing. If such open fractures involve the metatarsophalangeal or interphalangeal joint of the great toe, anatomic reduction and Kirschner wire fixation are performed at the time of initial debridement. The patient is treated initially in a short-leg cast and transferred to a stiff-soled shoe when swelling and pain permit.

Fractures of the Hallux Phalanges

In nondisplaced simple fractures of the great toe, the patient is placed in a short-leg walking cast with a toe plate until swelling and pain allow the use of a stiff-soled shoe with a high toe box.

In crushing injuries of the hallux phalanges in which there is comminution and no involvement of the interphalangeal joint, most attention is directed to care of the soft tissues. The subungual hematoma is drained after sterile preparation, and the patient is placed in a short-leg cast with *immediate* ambulation.

In displaced fractures of the hallux, an attempted closed reduction is performed. If this is unsuccessful, open reduction and internal fixation are recommended. This is particularly true in fractures involving the interphalangeal and metatarsophalangeal joints. In the author's experience, residual displacement of these fractures has resulted in arthritic changes and pain with ambulation. The author has found the use of Chinese finger traps applied to the toe with the patient in a supine position and weights draped over the ankle occasionally useful in reducing these fractures (see Fig

35–114,A–C). When such a reduction is obtained, percutaneous pin fixation, possibly utilizing a Blalock clamp,[1] is performed. Following fixation the patient is treated in a walking cast for 4 to 6 weeks, at which time the Kirschner wires are removed. A stiff-soled shoe is recommended for an additional 4 to 6 weeks.

If open reduction is required in these injuries, timing is critical. Unless this can be done very early, swelling of the great toe resulting from the fracture makes soft-tissue compromise following surgery commonplace. If open reduction cannot be performed within 24 to 48 hours, I prefer to wait 7 to 14 days after the fracture to allow the swelling to subside. Following open reduction of great toe fractures, patients are immobilized in a short-leg cast with immediate ambulation. The cast is removed at 4 to 6 weeks, and then ambulation in a stiff-soled shoe is initiated. Kirschner wires are removed between the fourth and sixth weeks.

Fractures of the Lesser Toe Phalanges

I prefer to treat fractures of the middle and distal phalanges of the lateral four toes by adhesive taping to the adjacent toe and using sheet wadding between the toes to prevent maceration. Ambulation is begun immediately in a stiff-soled shoe with an adequate toe box.

Treatment of proximal phalangeal fractures of the lateral four toes is done in a similar fashion. In my experience moderate displacement of the phalanges of the lateral four toes is usually of no consequence. If complete displacement is present, and attempt at closed reduction under local anesthesia is made by using Chinese finger traps (see Fig 35–115,A–C). The toe is then strapped to the adjacent toes with half-inch adhesive tape while being careful to use sheet wadding between the toes. Only with gross displacement in which closed reduction is not successful is any consideration given to open reduction. In my experience, such displacement is extremely unusual. When open reduction is considered, one must remember that minimal disability results from these injuries. Therefore, I prefer to treat all these fractures in a closed manner by adhesive strapping and weight bearing. Morbidity following malunion of these fractures has not been a significant problem in my practice. If it does occur, simple exostosectomy results in relief of symptoms.

REFERENCES

Phalanges

1. Blalock S, Pearce HL, Kleinert H, et al: An instrument designed to help reduce and percutaneously pin fractured phalanges, *J Bone Joint Surg [Am]* 57:792–794, 1975.
2. Blodgett WH:Injuries of the forefoot and toes. In Jahss MH, editor: *Disorders of the foot*, vol 2, Philadelphia, 1982, WB Saunders.
3. Chapman MW: Fractures and fracture-dislocations of the ankle and foot, In Mann RA, editor: *DuVries' surgery of the foot*, ed 4, St Louis, 1978, Mosby–Year Book.
4. Cobey JC: Treatment of undisplaced toe fractures with a metatarsal bar made from torque blades, *Clin Orthop* 103:56, 1974.
5. DePalma A: *The management of fractures and dislocations*, vol 2, Philadelphia, 1959, WB Saunders.
6. Garcia A, Parkes JC: Fractures of the foot. In Giannestras LJ, editor: *Foot disorders: medical and surgical management*, ed 2, Philadelphia, 1973, Lea & Febiger.
7. Giannestras NJ, Sammarco GJ: Fractures and dislocations in the foot. In Rockwood CA Jr, Green DP, editors: *Fractures*, vol 2, Philadelphia, 1975, JB Lippincott.
8. Heck CV: Fractures of the bones of the foot (except the talus), *Surg Clin North Am* 45:103–117, 1965.
9. Henderson MS: Fractures of the bones (except the os calcis), *Surg Gynecol Obstet* 64:454–457, 1937.
10. Jahss MH: Stubbing injuries to the hallux, *Foot Ankle* 1:327–332, 1981.
11. Johnson VS: Treatment of fractures of the forefoot in industry. In Bateman JE, editor: *Foot science*, Philadelphia, 1976, WB Saunders.
12. Morrison GM: Fractures of the bones of the feet, *Am J Surg* 38:721–722, 1937.
13. Moseley HF: Traumatic disorders of the ankle and foot, *Clin Symp* 17:30, 1965.
14. Taylor GN: Treatment of the fractured great toe, *Br Med J* 1:724–725, 1943.
15. Yokoe K, Mannoji T: Stress fracture of the proximal phalanx of the great toe, *Am J Sports Med* 14:240–242, 1986.
16. Zorzi C, Grisostomi E: Le fratture dell'alluce, *Riv Infort Mal Prof* 49:317–330, 1962.
17. Zrubecky G: Bruche der Grosszehe, deren Behandlung und Behandlungsergebnisse, *Arch Ortop Unfallchir* 47:591–611, 1955.

FRACTURES OF THE SESAMOID

The function of the sesamoids was addressed by the very early practitioners.[28] The ancients believed that the medial sesamoid was the one "unbreakable, uncombustible, and indestructible" bone of the body that remains on the earth after death as the germ from which the whole body is later resurrected.[11] Additionally, the name *sesamoid* denotes the similarity in the size and shape of these bones to the flat oval seeds of *Sesamum indicum*, an ancient East Indian plant that was used by the Greeks for purging.[10]

Fractures of the sesamoids were observed and reported earlier in animal than in man. Bizarro credits Schunke (1901) as the first author to describe a case of a fractured sesamoid in man.[2, 15] Since that original description, most authors have found sesamoid fractures quite rare.[9, 10, 23, 28] Recently, however, the marked increase in popularity of jogging, long-distance running, and ballet has caused injuries to the sesamoids to be more common.[3]

The sesamoids are termed by location as either tibial (medial) or fibular (lateral). The hallux sesamoids are fractured most frequently.[12] Of those occurring under the first metatarsal head the tibial (medial) sesamoid is more frequently fractured.[12, 19] Indeed, most reports have found fractures of the fibular sesamoid to be *extremely* rare.[7, 23] Most authors believe that the fibular sesamoid is less frequently fractured because of its position slightly lateral to the head of the first metatarsal.[12, 13] The tibial sesamoid is more frequently involved because it receives most of the weight transmitted by the first metatarsal.[12, 13]

Anatomy

Sesamoids in the hallux metatarsophalangeal joint are a constant feature of the foot.[2] However, sesamoids of the metatarsophalangeal joint of the fifth digit are present in only 10% of cases, in the fourth in 2%, and the second in 1%.[2]

The hallux sesamoids have a dorsal cartilaginous facet that articulates with the metatarsal head, while fibers of the flexor hallucis brevis tendon cover their rough, nonarticular plantar surface. The sesamoids are separated from each other by the flexor hallucis longus tendon as it traverses to its insertion into the distal phalanx. They are invested by the deep tendons of the short flexor of the great toe and are joined to each other by a strong, short transverse ligament.[3] The concave articulating surfaces of the sesamoids contact the plantar aspect of the first metatarsal head and provide a gliding surface for the weight-bearing functions of the first metatarsal.[3]

The tibial sesamoid is situated directly beneath the medial half of the first metatarsal head where it is frequently subjected to mechanical trauma. The fibular sesamoid, however, extends well beyond the lateral margin of the metatarsal head and assumes a relatively protected position in the soft tissues between the first and second metatarsal heads.[22, 23]

The sesamoids begin as islands of undifferentiated connective tissue in their normal location during the 8th week, are precartilaginous by the 10th week, and develop chondrification centers by the 12th week. They attain their adult shape by the 5th month.[10] Ossification of the sesamoid is variable and occurs between the 8th and 14th years, usually earlier in girls than in boys.[10]

The sesamoids can have one or more ossification centers that may or may not unite. The incomplete coalition of the primordial chondrification centers may result in a bipartite or tripartite sesamoid that may be confused with a fracture.[3, 21] The sesamoids are reported to be multipartite in 5% to 30% of normal asymptomatic persons.[2, 5, 16, 23, 30] Such multiple centers of ossification and incomplete fusion are more common in the tibial sesamoid, which is usually the larger of the two.[10] Bipartite sesamoids may be bilateral; therefore, the presence of a divided sesamoid in the contralateral foot may help in distinguishing it from a fracture.[3] However, Inge and Ferguson[18] found sesamoid partitions to be unilateral in 75% of cases and bilateral in only 25%. Therefore, unilaterality does not *confirm* a fracture. In the bilateral cases, Inge and Ferguson[18] report that 85% show the same type of division in the corresponding bone of the opposite foot.[18]

Mechanism of Injury

The hallux sesamoids are particularly vulnerable to injury because of their biomechanical function and anatomic location.[28] The sesamoids elevate the first metatarsal head so that it is level with the adjacent metatarsal heads, and hence they are important weight-bearing structures. They also serve as a fulcrum to increase the mechanical advantage of the flexor hallucis brevis tendons.[28] Some authors believe that the medial sesamoid is more prone to injury because it lies directly under the head of the first metatarsal.[10, 14, 18, 28, 30] Additionally, Scranton and Rutkowski[25] believe that malalignment of the first metatarsal may predispose patients to sesamoid fractures.

Direct and indirect trauma has been shown to produce sesamoid fractures in cadavers.[10] Direct trauma is more common and may result from a crushing injury, an object falling onto the foot, a fall from a height and landing on the head of the first metatarsal, or direct trauma beneath the head of the first metatarsal bone.[7, 10, 13, 21, 23] When a person lands directly on the ball of his foot after a fall, most of the force is borne by the first metatarsal head. This compresses the sesamoids, particularly the tibial one, against the first metatarsal head and leads to the fracture.[12] The mechanism of a fall also explains the frequency of this fracture in ballet dancers because of the repeated trauma they inflict on the first metatarsal head during leaping.[3, 13]

These fractures may also be caused by indirect trauma. This mechanism has been documented experimentally.[22] The indirect type of fracture arises when the toe undergoes sudden marked hyperextension of the phalanx on the metatarsal head. Such forced dorsiflexion of the great toe can occur in football and has been implicated in causing this injury.[8] In cadavers it has been shown that forcible dorsiflexion and abduction of the great toe may produce fractures of the tibial sesamoid.[2, 28] This mechanism usually produces a simple separation fracture, while marked comminution of the sesamoid is secondary to a direct force on the foot with or without a shoe on.[15]

Clinical Diagnosis

It is important to remember that a history of trauma is paramount to the diagnosis of an acute fracture.[10] Most patients are able to recall a specific episode of trauma with the sudden onset of sharp pain.[2, 15] Although the onset of symptoms may be sudden, patients often do not seek immediate medical care.[7] The pain is located in the region of the sesamoid bones and is associated with any movement of the metatarsophalangeal joint. Although the pain may be reduced or absent at rest, it uniformly returns with walking.[15] The pain with walking occurs at the end of each step when the metatarsophalangeal joint is in hyperextension and the body weight is thrown forward onto the ball of the foot.[10, 23]

Sir Robert Jones was the first to suggest that there may be an association between the presence of hallux valgus and symptoms following injury to the sesamoids.[2] Point tenderness is located on the plantar aspect of the foot beneath the first metatarsal head on the tibial or fibular side depending on which sesamoid is involved.[8, 13, 26] Swelling of the periarticular structures on the plantar aspect of the foot may be present.[7, 13]

Dorsiflexion of the metatarsophalangeal joint accentuates pain in the area of the fracture on the plantar aspect of the foot[7, 13] secondary to the increased tension in the tendons of the flexor hallucis brevis muscle that

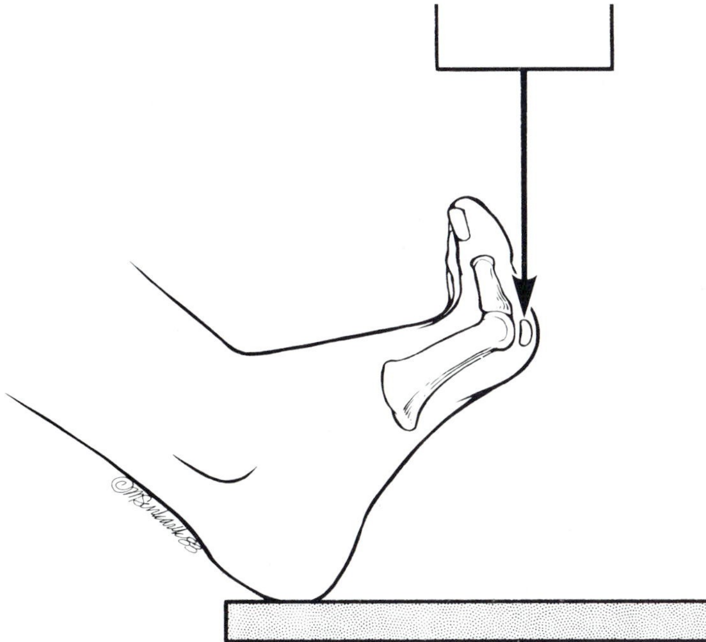

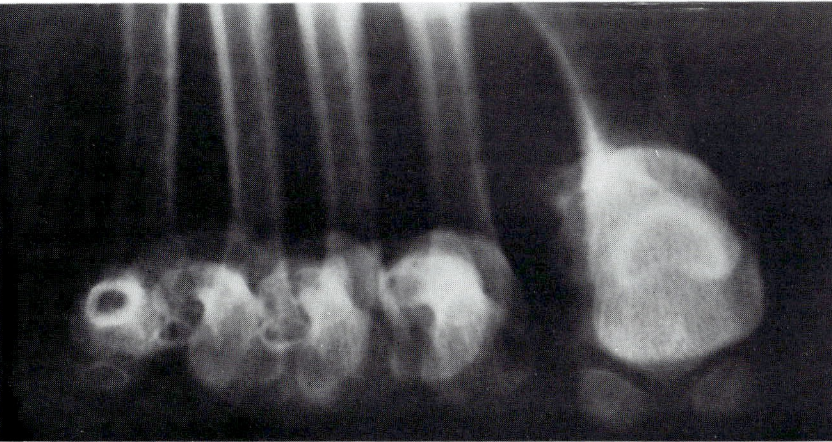

FIG 35–116.
Axial view of the sesamoids. The hallux metatarsophalangeal joint is dorsiflexed and the roentgen tube aligned vertically.

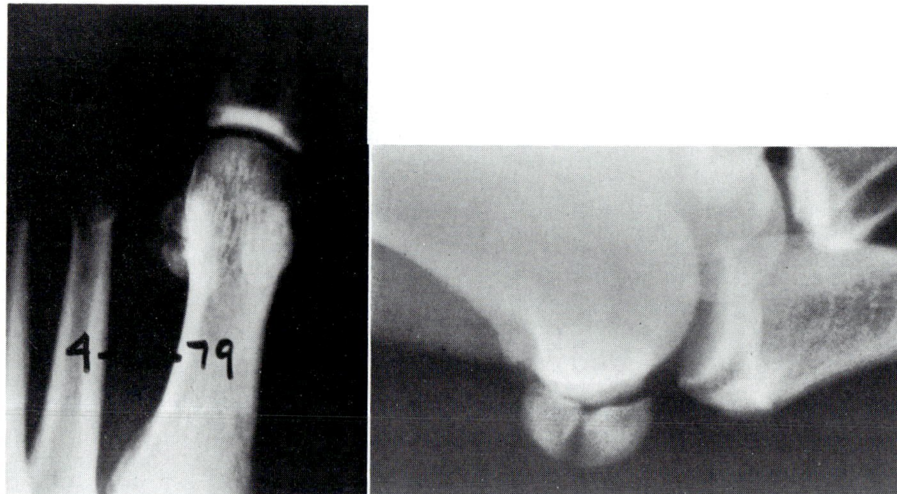

FIG 35–117.
Fracture of the fibular sesamoid. Note the irregular, jagged edges of the fracture line.

enclose the fractured sesamoid.[7, 12, 13] Additionally, passive adduction and abduction of the toe may reproduce the pain.[1] Crepitus is rarely palpable.[22]

Radiographic Diagnosis

The presence of a fractured sesamoid is confirmed by roentgenographic examination. Complete roentgenographic evaluation includes an anteroposterior view of the forefoot, a lateral view, and a tangential or axial view of the plantar aspect of the first metatarsal head.[10, 23, 30] The tangential or axial view beautifully demonstrates the articular surface of the sesamoids.[10, 12] This sesamoid view is made in a plane from toe to heel with the toe dorsiflexed (Fig 35–116). A sesamoid fracture is usually transverse or comminuted (Fig 35–117).

Roentgenographically, the differential diagnosis of a fractured sesamoid includes (1) fracture of the sesamoid (Fig 35–117), (2) a bipartite or multipartite sesamoid (Fig 35–118),[7] and (3) osteochondritis dissecans of the sesamoid (Fig 35–119).[1, 7, 30]

Sundt[27] stressed that clinically silent bilateral division of the sesamoid is congenital in origin. If a true fracture is present, the line of division should be jagged and irregular, and the fragments are usually of equal size, whereas in a bipartite sesamoid, the outline is usually regular and the division smooth.[7, 10, 13, 26] In addition, a bipartite sesamoid is usually larger than a single sesamoid; however, a fractured sesamoid may appear larger than its normal partner.[10] The absence of similar roentgenographic findings in the opposite foot is not diagnostic of a fracture since a bipartite sesamoid is unilateral in 75% of patients.[9, 10, 14, 18] Golding[14] stressed the importance of the presence of a history of injury in trying to distinguish between a bipartite sesamoid and a fracture. Kewenter[20] mentions the importance of demonstrating callus formation in distinguishing a bipartite from a fractured sesamoid. In addition to the tangential view, Colwill suggests the use of tomography to help in the diagnosis of these injuries.[9] It is also important to note that a bipartite sesamoid, although nontraumatic in its *primary* etiology, can separate through its synchondrosis and thereby represent a variety of fractures.[11]

Finally, a fractured sesamoid must be distinguished from osteochondritis dissecans of the first metatarsal sesamoid.[17, 30] The roentgenographic findings in this condition are those of fragmentation, irregularity, and modeling of the sesamoid.[17] An axial view of the metatarsal head shows these changes, which may not be visible on standard anteroposterior projections[14, 17] (Fig 35–119). It is the medial sesamoid that is most commonly involved with osteochondritis and by fracture, and therefore differentiation between the two is critical.[14]

Treatment

Nonoperative Treatment

Initially, it is important to inform the patient that fractures of the sesamoids may be resistant to treatment and that symptoms are apt to persist for a long time.[10, 23]

The treatment most frequently recommended following this injury is rest and protection of the first metatarsal head from weight bearing.[2, 12, 22]

Chapman immobilizes the fracture for 3 weeks with

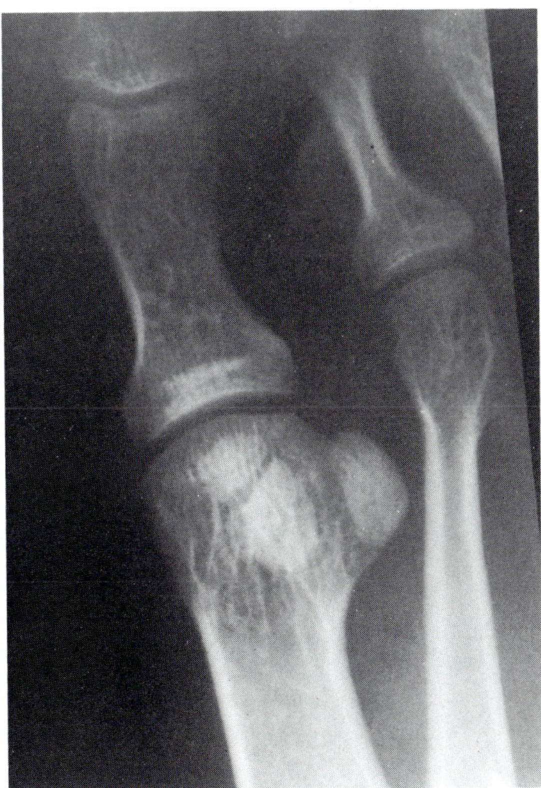

FIG 35–118.
Bipartite tibial sesamoid. A bipartite tibial sesamoid is larger than a fibular sesamoid, and the line of division is smooth and regular. Also, note that the fragments are not same size.

the metatarsophalangeal joint in a flexed position.[7] If this fails to relieve the symptoms, excision is recommended.[7] Coker and Arnold[8] also use cast immobilization for 3 weeks. If symptoms persist after 8 weeks of treatment, the fractured sesamoid may be excised.[8] Hobart[15] recommends that the patient be kept off the injured foot and that it be immobilized until the fracture is healed, a period of time that he believes to be between 3 and 6 weeks. He recommends immobilization in a plaster of paris cast that includes the great toe during this period. However, Giannestras and Sammarco[13] believe that only in cases with severe pain is a short-leg weight-bearing cast necessary.

Other authors have not recommended cast immobilization. Bizarro recommended the use of a metatarsal bar on the sole of the shoe, a trick he learned from Sir Robert Jones.[2] Morrison recommended an anterior arch support to remove the weight from the tender area for 1 to 2 months.[21] If symptoms persist, he recommends excision. Garcia and Parkes[12] also recommended the use of a comma-shaped metatarsal pad in the shoe to relieve pressure on the plantar aspect of the first metatarsal head or the use of a transverse metatarsal bar for a period of 6 to 8 weeks postinjury.

Orr[22] cautions that unless rest is prolonged, the patient may remain symptomatic. He therefore recommends a shoe with a depression on the inner sole designed to relieve pressure under the first metatarsal head for prolonged periods of time. He states that if after a reasonable period of conservative treatment the area is still tender, the sesamoid fragments should be excised. Giannestras and Sammarco[13] recommend a stiff-soled shoe and metatarsal pad with an elevation behind the head of the metatarsal to relieve pressure on the plantar aspect of the first metatarsal head.[12] Although this fracture may unite with bony union if treated for an extended period of time, Brugman[4] believes that the resulting callus may be a source of pain for some time after use of the foot has been resumed unless protective pads are utilized.

Surgical Treatment

Although Brugman mentions immediate removal of the fractured sesamoid in an effort to decrease the morbidity from this fracture, no other authors recommend such aggressive initial treatment.[4] However, in cases with persistent disability after a reasonable period of conservative therapy, most authors recommend excision of the involved sesamoid.[7, 8, 12, 13, 22] The indications commonly given for sesamoid excision include (1) painful nonunion, (2) prolonged pain in spite of conservative treatment, and (3) the development of posttraumatic degenerative changes on the sesamoid articular surface.

Although Orr[22] credits Speed with suggesting that *both* sesamoids be removed in these situations because of subsequent degenerative changes in the remaining sesamoid,[22] Blodgett confirms my experience that excision of only the fractured sesamoid is indicated.[3]

Several authors have emphasized the importance of placing the surgical incision so as to avoid painful scar formation.[21, 28] Van Hal et al.[28] report the use of a medial longitudinal plantar incision to remove the medial sesamoid. However, care must be taken that the digital nerve be visualized and protected. Although Van Hal et al.[28] approach the fibular sesamoid through a plantar incision between the first and second metatarsal heads, a dorsal web-splitting incision between the first and second metatarsal heads will avoid a plantar scar and is safer. McBride recommends division of the the strong intersesamoid ligament as early as possible in the procedure to allow easier mobilization and removal of the sesamoid.[3] Additionally, the sesamoid must be carefully shelled out of the tendon of the flexor hallucis brevis to

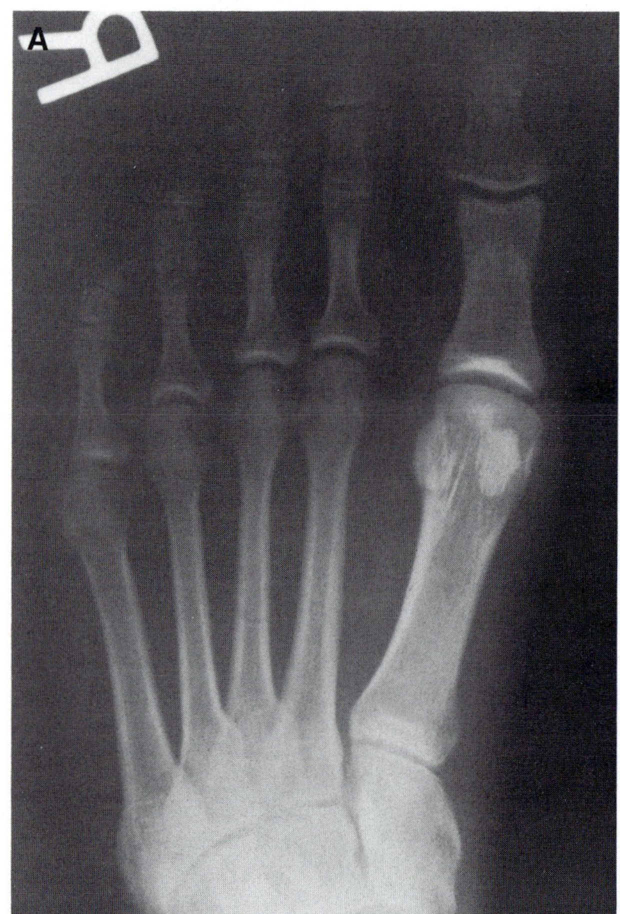

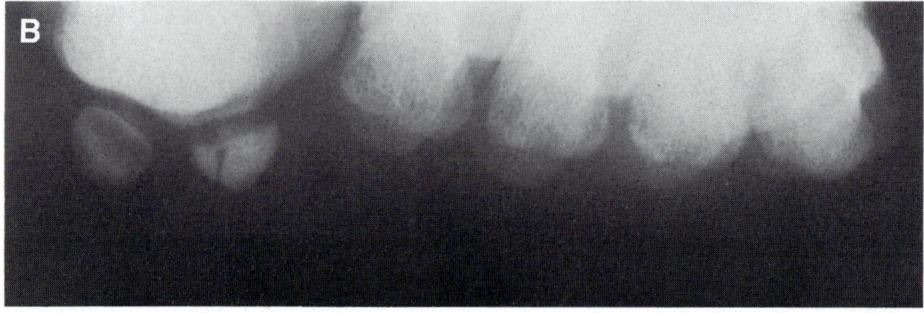

FIG 35–119.
Anteroposterior **(A)** and axial **(B)** views of a patient with osteochondritis dissecans of the fibular sesamoid. Note the increased density. The patient is nonathletic and had a spontaneous onset of pain.

prevent the later development of a cockup or varus/valgus deformity of the hallux.[13, 25]

Author's Preferred Method of Treatment

A complete set of roentgenographs including anteroposterior, oblique and axial views of the sesamoid are essential in evaluating injuries to these bones. The axial views are particularly helpful in distinguishing between osteochondritis dissecans, a bipartite sesamoid, and a fracture with displacement. Although I strive to distinguish between an acute fracture and a bipartite sesamoid, in reality the conservative treatment I use for a painful bipartite sesamoid and for a fractured sesamoid is similar.

For patients who suffer a fracture of the sesamoid, I prefer a short-leg walking cast with the walking heel placed so that all weight is transferred from beneath the first metatarsal head to a more posterior location. This cast is usually worn for a period of 2 to 3 weeks. The patients are then placed in a stiff-soled shoe with a metatarsal pad placed behind the head of the first metatarsal to relieve pressure from the plantar aspect of the first metatarsal head. The patients are warned that total relief of symptoms may require 4 to 6 months, during which time a metatarsal support is essential.

If after 6 months of conservative treatment significant symptoms persist, excision of the involved sesamoid is recommended. I prefer a medial longitudinal approach for tibial sesamoid excision and a dorsal incision between the first and second metatarsals for fibular sesamoid excision. Care is taken to protect the digital nerves with both incisions.

Stress Fractures of the Sesamoids

Although Golding in 1960 alluded to hallux sesamoid stress fractures,[14] he did not provide histologic documentation of his cases. Scranton and Rutkowski[25] in 1980 reported the histology of a sesamoid excised from a runner, but they concluded that the microscopic findings were indistinguishable from a nonunion or bipartite sesamoid. Van Hal et al.[28] in 1982 reported four cases of stress fractures of the hallux sesamoids with histologic confirmation of the diagnosis. According to these authors, theirs were the first histologically documented cases of sesamoid stress fractures. Van Hal et al.[28] stressed that patients have a history of an insidious onset of pain in the area of the first metatarsophalangeal joint during and/or after athletic activity. The pain is usually relieved by rest. The pain is accentuated by palpation and hyperextension of the first metatarsophalangeal joint. Importantly, there is no history of a specific episode of foot trauma. Richardson[24] also states that a single traumatic event resulting in fracture of a sesamoid is distinctly uncommon in the athlete. In the athlete, Richardson reports that there is usually a several-week history of pain that is poorly localized until the examiner elicits tenderness under the sesamoid with palpation. In these patients, he feels that the mechanism of injury is repetitive stress. The clinical differential diagnosis includes sesamoiditis, metatarsalgia, chondromalacia, and sesamoid-metatarsal degenerative arthritis.[24, 25, 28] Failure to recognize and treat a sesamoid stress fracture can lead to prolonged disability.[27]

If a stress fracture is suspected, Van Hal et al.[28] suggest weight-bearing anteroposterior, lateral, and axial radiographs at 3-week intervals. They emphasize that a delay in diagnosis is likely if roentgenographs initially interpreted as being negative are not repeated. The authors also emphasize the importance of distinguishing stress fractures from a multipartite sesamoid.[14, 16, 28] A bone scan will demonstrate characteristic increased bony activity in the area of the first metatarsophalangeal joint, while a multipartite or bipartite sesamoid will be "cold" on scans.[24, 28]

Although most stress fractures heal when the precipitating activity is limited, sesamoid stress fractures seem to behave differently.[28] None of the patients presented by Van Hal et al.[28] healed their fractures despite 6 weeks of casting and/or 4 to 6 months of inactivity. The authors report that persistent symptoms often lead to excision of the involved sesamoid before relief is obtained. However, following excision all of their patients returned to athletic activities. The authors believe that the anatomic location and biomechanical function of the sesamoids lead to the failure of nonoperative treatment.

The authors recommend that all stress fractures of the sesamoids be treated immediately in a cast for 6 weeks at which time new roentgenographs are taken and the fractures are recasted if necessary. Excision of the involved sesamoid is reserved for those patients in whom the fracture does not heal with casting or in whom the athlete does not desire further casting.[28] Three patients returned to prefracture activities without symptoms at an average of 10 weeks after excision. None of the patients had a loss of great toe flexion power as the result of sesamoid excision.[28]

Richardson[24] reports that prolonged conservative treatment either in a short-leg cast or with molded supports is not effective in the athlete. He believes that the indications for excision of the involved sesamoid include the following

1. Displaced fractures of the sesamoid
2. Nondisplaced fractures of the sesamoid not responding to cast immobilization and shoe inserts over a 12-week period
3. Sesamoiditis and osteochondritis if symptoms are not relieved by the use of inserts for a period of 6 weeks
4. Recurrent bursitis overlying the tibial sesamoid
5. Osteomyelitis of the sesamoid

For displaced fractures of both sesamoids, Richardson recommends removal of only the tibial sesamoid. He states that even though the fibular sesamoid does not bear weight to the same extent as the tibial sesamoid, it is technically difficult to repair the flexor hallux brevis if both sesamoids are removed. Removal of both sesamoids oftentimes violates flexor hallucis function and results in an intrinsic minus or cockup toe. This is often just as disabling to the athlete as the fracture.[24]

He recommends the use of a straight medial incision for excision of either the tibial or fibular sesamoid. He prefers this approach because it is an "internervous plane" between the medial plantar digital branch of the medial plantar nerve and the most medial branch of the superficial peroneal nerve dorsally. Postoperatively, patients are placed in a bulky soft-tissue dressing surrounded by a nonwalking cast with dorsal and plantar toe plates extending distal to the hallux. Seven to 9 days after the surgery, this cast is removed, and the patient is allowed to begin motion. The dressing is removed at 14 days after surgery, and the patient begins toe stands and toe curls. Acceleration and deceleration sports such as racquet sports are not allowed until after 6 weeks postsurgery.

Author's Preferred Method of Treatment

In patients at risk for a sesamoid stress fracture, early diagnosis is essential. If initial roentgenographs are negative, they are repeated in 3 weeks. If the second set of roentgenographs is negative, a bone scan is recommended.

Once the diagnosis has been confirmed, I prefer to treat these patients in a shortleg cast with a toe plate to relieve the stresses on the metatarsophalangeal joint for 6 weeks. If the fracture is not healed, a second 6-week period is recommended. Following casting, a soft insert placed behind the sesamoids in the arch of the foot is utilized to relieve the stress of weight bearing on the first metatarsophalangeal joint. If symptoms persist following this sequence of conservative therapy, excision is recommended.

Dislocation of the Sesamoids

Intersesamoid ligament disruption with dislocation of the sesamoid is distinctly unusual as an isolated entity not associated with metatarsophalangeal dislocation. Capasso et al.[6] in 1990 reported a traumatic dislocation of the lateral sesamoid secondary to disruption of the intersesamoid ligament. Barnett et al.[1] had previously reported an intraarticular dislocation of the sesamoid in a patient with a supernumerary hallucal sesamoid. The lateral dislocation of the sesamoid was suggested by the presence of pain and tenderness around the first metatarsophalangeal joint.[6] Routine radiographs revealed lateral dislocation of the lateral sesamoid. An axial view of the sesamoids demonstrated the sesamoid in the lateral intermetatarsal space.

The authors did not relate a mechanism of injury in their patient but suspected a kick to the ground with the great toe as the probable cause of total rupture of the intersesamoid ligament.

Open reduction and repair of the intersesamoid ligament through a plantar longitudinal incision in the first intermetatarsal web space was successful. The patient resumed normal activities 2 months later and had no further disability. Although sesamoidectomy is an alternative to repair of the intersesamoid ligament in a sporting population, excision of the sesamoid may limit sporting activities.[6]

REFERENCES

Sesamoid

1. Barnett JC, Crespio A, Daniels VC: Interarticular assessory sesamoid dislocation of the great toe, *J Bd Florida Med Assoc* 66:613–615, 1979.
2. Bizarro AH: On the traumatology of the sesamoid structures, *Ann Surg* 74:783–791, 1921.
3. Blodgett WH: Injuries of the forefoot and toes. In Jahss MH, editor: *Disorders of the foot*, vol 2, Philadelphia, 1982, WB Saunders.
4. Brugman JC: Fractured sesamoids as a source of pain around the bunion joint, *Milit Surgeon* 49:310–313, 1921.
5. Burman MS, Lapidus PW: The functional disturbance caused by the inconstant bones and sesamoids of the foot, *Arch Surg* 22:936–975, 1931.
6. Capasso G, Maffulli N, Testa V: Rupture of the intersesamoid ligament of a soccer player's foot, *Foot Ankle* 10:337–339, 1990.
7. Chapman MW: Fractures and dislocations of the ankle and foot. In Mann RA, editor: *DuVries' surgery of the foot*, ed 4, St Louis, 1978, Mosby–Year Book.
8. Coker TP Jr, Arnold JA: Sports injuries to the foot and ankle. In Jahss MH, editor: *Disorders of the foot*, vol 2, Philadelphia, 1982, WB Saunders.
9. Colwill M: Disorders of the metatarsal sesamoids, *J Bone Joint Surg [Br]* 52:390, 1970.
10. Feldman F, Pochaczevsky R, Hecht H: The case of the wandering sesamoid and other sesamoid afflictions, *Radiology* 96:275–284, 1970.
11. Freiberg AH: Injuries to the sesamoid bones of the great toe, *J Bone Joint Surg* 2:453–465, 1920.
12. Garcia A, Parkes JE: Fractures of the foot. In Giannestras NJ, editor: *Foot disorders: medical and surgical management*, Philadelphia, 1973, Lea & Febiger.
13. Giannestras NJ, Sammarco GJ: Fractures and dislocations in the foot. In Rockwood CA Jr, Green DP, *editors: Fractures*, vol 2, Philadelphia, 1975, JB Lippincott.
14. Golding C: Museum pages, V. The sesamoids of the hallux, *J Bone Joint Surg [Br]* 42:840–843, 1960.
15. Hobart MH: Fracture of sesamoid bones of the foot, *J Bone Joint Surg* 11:298–302, 1929.
16. Hubay CA: Sesamoid bones of the hands and feet, *Am J Roentgenol* 61:493–505, 1949.
17. Ifeld FW, Rosen V: Osteochondritis of the first metatarsal sesamoid, *Clin Orthop* 85:38–41, 1972.
18. Inge GL, Ferguson AB: Surgery of the sesamoid bones of the great toe, *Arch Surg* 21:456–489, 1933.
19. Kelikian H: *Hallux valgus, allied deformities of the forefoot and metatarsalgia*, Philadelphia, 1965, WB Saunders.
20. Kewenter Y: Die sesameine des metatarso-phalangeal gelenks des menschen, *Acta Orthop Scand* 2, 1936.
21. Morrison GM: Fractures of the bones of the feet, *Am J Surg* 38:721–726, 1937.
22. Orr TG: Fracture of the great toe sesamoid bones, *Ann Surg* 67:609–612, 1918.

23. Powers JH: Traumatic and developmental abnormalities of the sesamoid bones of the great toes, *Am J Surg* 23:315–321, 1934.
24. Richardson EG: Injuries to the hallucil sesamoids in the athlete, *Foot Ankle* 7:229–244, 1987.
25. Scranton PE, Rutkowski R: Anatomic variations in the first ray—part B. Disorders of the sesamoids, *Clin Orthop* 151:256–264, 1980.
26. Sisk TD: Fractures. In Edmonson AS, Crenshaw AH, editors: *Campbell's operative orthopaedics*, ed 6, vol 1, St Louis, 1980, Mosby–Year Book.
27. Sundt H: On partition of the sesamoid bones of the lower extremities, *Acta Orthop Scand* 15:59–138, 1944.
28. Van Hal ME, Keene JS, Lange TA, et al: Stress fractures of the sesamoids, *Am J Sports Med* 10:122–128, 1982.
29. Wilson DW: Fractures of the foot. In Klenerman L, editor: *The foot and its disorders*, ed 2, Oxford, 1982, Blackwell.
30. Zimmer EA: *Borderlands of the normal and early pathologic in skeletal roentgenology*, New York, 1968, Grune & Stratton, pp 531–534.

DISLOCATIONS ABOUT THE TALUS

Dislocations about the talus without fracture are classified into three types (see Table 35–8): first, talocrural dislocation in which the talus is dislocated from the ankle mortise but the subtalar and midtarsal joints remain intact (Fig 35–120) (the talocrural dislocation is not discussed in this chapter but is included in the chapter on fractures of the ankle); second, subtalar dislocation in which the calcaneus is dislocated from the intact talus but the relationship of the talus with the ankle mortise and midtarsal joints remains intact; and third, total dislocation of the talus in which the relationship of the talus with both the ankle and the subtalar joints is disrupted. The last two types of talar dislocations will be discussed in this chapter.

TABLE 35–8.
Dislocations About the Talus Without Fracture

Type 1—Talocrural dislocation
Type 2—Subtalar dislocation
Type 3—Total dislocations of the talar body

Subtalar Dislocations

Subtalar dislocation of the foot is an injury in which both the talocalcaneal and talonavicular joints are simultaneously dislocated without a fracture of the neck of the talus.[9, 12] The tibiotalar and calcaneocuboid joints remain intact.[37, 44] Barber et al.[2] felt that the term "peritalar dislocation of the foot" more accurately describes this condition. These dislocations have also been designated subastragalar,[45] subastragaloid,[43] and talocalcaneal-navicular dislocations.[14]

Subtalar dislocations unassociated with regional fractures are uncommon injuries.[1, 3, 9, 10, 44, 46, 49] Leitner[29, 30] and Smith[45] reported that these dislocations account for 1% of all traumatic dislocations. Additionally, Pennal[41] reported that they total only 15% of all injuries of the talus.

Judcy[24] and Dufaurest[11] were the first to report subtalar dislocations in 1811. Broca[4] in 1953 classified subtalar dislocations as medial, lateral, and posterior. Malgaigne[33] in 1856 added anterior dislocations to this classification. However, Fahey and Murphy[14] stated that while posterior and anterior dislocations have been described, they are usually considered as part of the displacement

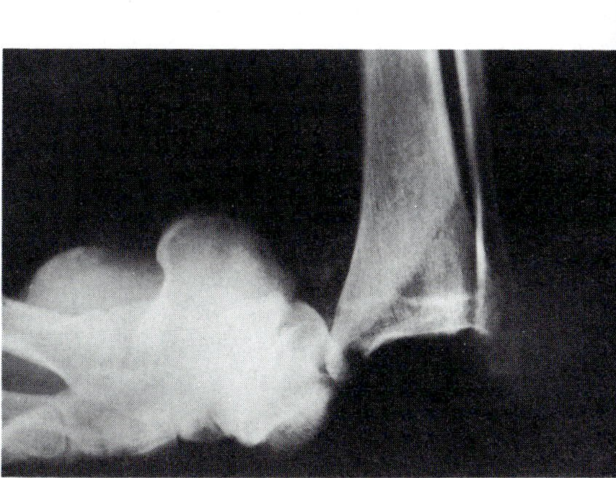

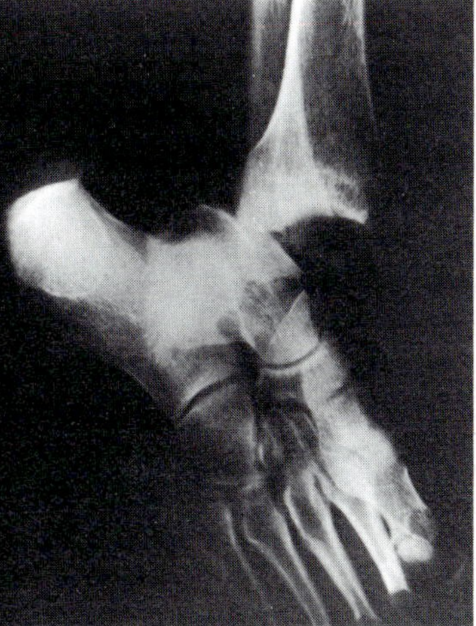

FIG 35–120.
Type I: talocrural dislocation.

present in the more common medial or lateral dislocations. Most authors, however, have preferred to use the classification of Broca and Malgaigne.[9, 17, 32, 44] Medial dislocations by far represent the majority of subtalar dislocations.[9, 12, 14, 17, 25, 30] According to Dunn,[12] Smith,[45] and Vincenti,[48] the frequency of occurrence in decreasing order is medial, lateral, posterior, and finally, anterior dislocation. Larsen[28] reports that medial dislocations account for 59%; lateral dislocations, 23%; posterior dislocations, 11%; and anterior dislocations, 7% of all subtalar dislocations. Patients suffering from this injury vary in age from 10 to 70 years with men being affected from three to ten times more frequently than women.[44]

Anatomy

The subtalar joint consists of three facets, anterior, medial, and posterior, through which the talus and calcaneus articulate.[5] The talus and calcaneus are united by the strong interosseous talocalcaneal ligament in the sinus tarsi.[5, 44] A fibrous capsule also connects the adjacent articular margins of the three talocalcaneal facets.[44] Medially, the superficial portions of the deltoid ligament and, laterally, the calcaneofibular ligament supplement talocalcaneal stability.[5, 44] Finally, the talus and navicular are united by a weak talonavicular capsule. All of these structures must be disrupted in order for a subtalar dislocation to occur. Additionally, the closely contoured surfaces of the subtalar joint afford significant stability to the joint, particularly regarding anteroposterior displacement.[44] Due to this bony stability, fractures involving the lateral process and posterior tubercles of the talus are often associated with subtalar dislocations.[9, 44]

Buckingham reports that in medial subtalar dislocations the head of the talus appears between the extensor hallucis longus and the long toe extensors and rests on either the navicular or cuboid bone.[5] In lateral dislocations, the prominent head of the talus is palpable over the medial aspect of the foot while the heel is displaced laterally.[5] Buckingham termed a medial dislocation in which the forepart of the foot is dislocated medially the "acquired clubfoot," while a lateral dislocation is occasionally called the "acquired flatfoot."[5]

Mechanism of Injury

The mechanism of a medial subtalar dislocation is plantar flexion of the foot with forceful inversion of the forepart of the foot.[5] This results in the neck of the talus pivoting with the sustentaculum tali as a fulcrum. This movement produces a dislocation of the talonavicular joint followed by dislocation of the subtalar joint.[5, 14–16, 28, 36] The less common lateral dislocation occurs with plantar flexion of the foot accompanied by forceful eversion of the forefoot. This results in the anterior lateral corner of the talus pivoting over the anterior calcaneal process as a fulcrum.[14, 36, 38] The head of the talus is forced through the talonavicular capsule, and the calcaneus is dislocated laterally.[44]

Giannestras and Sammarco[16] emphasized that the actual forces required to produce subtalar dislocations are not necessarily great. However, Kleiger and Ahmed[26] emphasize that even with minor injuries, the cartilage of the articular surfaces may be fractured or contused along with *or* independent of fractures involving the subchondral bone. This concept is particularly important when considering long-term sequelae. However, as the amount of force producing the dislocation increases, so too does the incidence of poor results due to increased soft-tissue and bony damage.

Grantham[17] termed medial subtalar dislocation "basketball foot" because the majority of the patients he reported were injured while playing basketball. This mechanism, involving plantar flexion and inversion, is less forceful as is evidenced by the excellent range of motion of the subtalar joint and minimal roentgenographic evidence of subtalar arthritis at follow-up. On the other hand, injuries secondary to motor vehicle accidents or falls from heights are more often associated with more initial trauma, a higher incidence of associated intra-articular fractures, and usually a poorer clinical result.[9]

Clinical Diagnosis

Although the patient may give a history of severe trauma to the foot,[15, 44] Grantham[17] and DeLee and Curtis[9] emphasized that subtalar dislocations, particularly medial ones, can occur secondary to minor trauma such as a missed step. The patient usually complains of pain about the hind part of the foot.[16] The entire foot is swollen, and any motion of the ankle and subtalar joint is painful.[15, 16] There is a complete loss of the normal bony contours of the foot in the region of the ankle joint.[15]

The clinical appearance of the foot is an excellent key to the type of subtalar dislocation. In medial subtalar dislocations the foot is plantar-flexed, adducted, and supinated, and the head of the talus is prominent over the dorsolateral aspect of the foot (Fig 35–121,A).[14, 44, 47] The overlying skin may appear blanched.[14] The heel is noted to be displaced medially in relation to the long axis of the leg.[44, 47] Additionally, the toes may be dorsiflexed.[14] The lateral border of the foot appears long, while the medial border appears short.[14] In lateral subtalar dislocations the foot appears pronated and abducted,[14] and the toes may appear in the plantar-flexed position.[14] The prominent talar head is palpable medi-

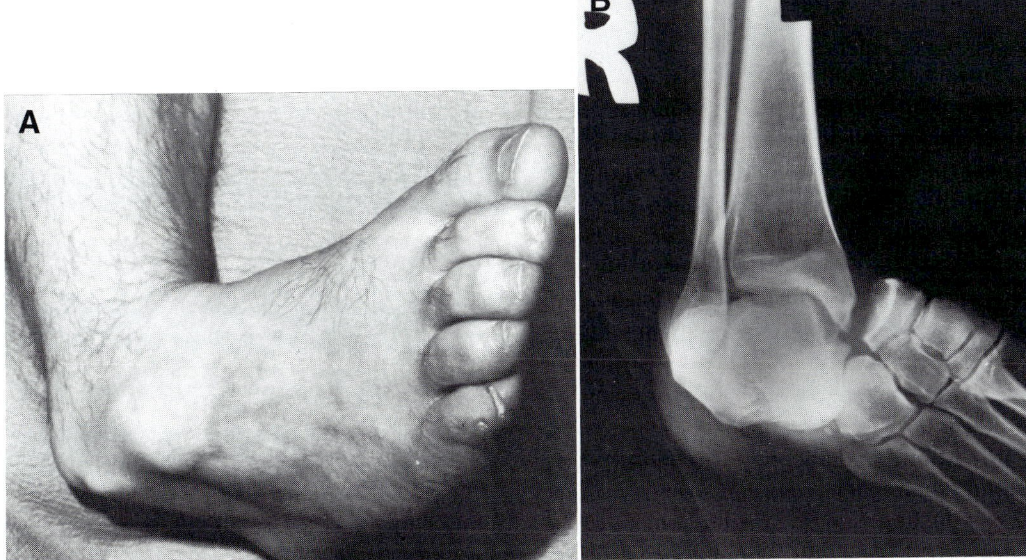

FIG 35–121.
A, medial subtalar dislocation. **B,** radiograph of a medial subtalar dislocation. (From DeLee JC, Curtis R: *J Bone Joint Surg [Am]* 64:433–437, 1982. Used by permission.)

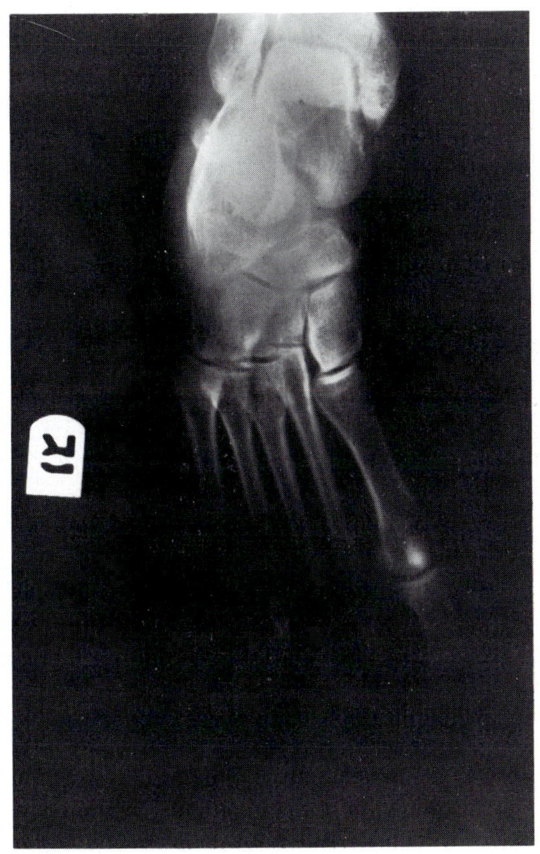

FIG 35–122.
Lateral subtalar dislocation. (From DeLee JC, Curtis R: *J Bone Joint Surg* 64:433–437, 1982. Used by permission.)

ally, and the heel is present lateral to the long axis of the leg (Fig 35–122).[44, 47] In posterior dislocations, the foot is shortened, and the heel projects posteriorly, but the normal longitudinal axis of the foot with the lower part of the leg is maintained.[28, 44] In anterior dislocations, the heel is flattened, and the foot appears to be extended while maintaining its normal longitudinal orientation[28, 44] (Fig 35–123). Any of the four types of subtalar dislocation may present as an open injury. Additionally, displacement of the dislocation may result in compromise of circulation to the overlying skin[14, 16, 44]

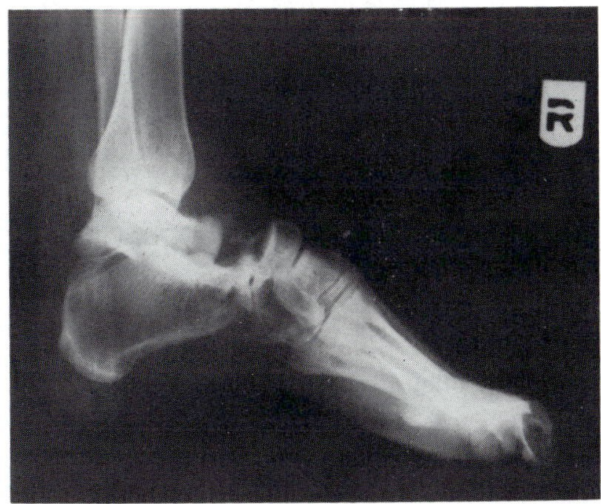

FIG 35–123.
Anterior dislocation demonstrated on a lateral radiograph. As emphasized by Fahey and Murphy,[14] the dislocation also had a component of lateral displacement.

and necessitate immediate reduction to prevent necrosis.

Radiographic Diagnosis

Anteroposterior, lateral, and oblique roentgenographs of the foot are the *minimum* studies required for complete evaluation of a subtalar dislocation.[15, 16, 44] Routine roentgenographs reveal the talus to be in a flexed position and the forefoot and os calcis to be displaced medially, laterally, anteriorly, or posteriorly depending upon the particular type of dislocation.[9, 15, 16] Barber et al.[2] stressed the use of a superoinferior view of the foot to clearly demonstrate the absence of the head of the talus in the cup of the navicular.

In a medial dislocation, the foot is displaced medially so that the plantar articulations of the talus are revealed without the calcaneus beneath it (see Fig 35–121). In lateral dislocations, the anteroposterior roentgenograph reveals the calcaneus to be displaced laterally (see Fig 35–122). Anterior and posterior dislocations are most easily diagnosed on a lateral roentgenograph of the foot in which the foot is displaced anteriorly and posteriorly, respectively (see Fig 35–123).

It is extremely important because of their detrimental effect on results to carefully scrutinize the initial roentgenographs for associated fractures that may be masked by the obvious deformity (Fig 35–124).[9, 15, 16, 44] Intra-articular fractures associated with subtalar dislocations have been mentioned by several authors.[2, 42, 44, 48] Smith was the first to emphasize that such associated tarsal fractures may complicate treatment and produce permanent disability.[45] Fahey and Murphy[14] reported impacted fractures of the medial portion of the head of the talus produced by the navicular (Fig 35–124), fracture of the posterior process of the talus, or a fracture of the navicular are associated with medial dislocations, while fractures of the lateral malleolus, calcaneus, or cuboid occur in conjunction with lateral dislocations. Anteroposterior, lateral, and oblique roentgenographs *must* be taken following reduction and *prior* to cast application in order to determine that an accurate reduction of the subtalar dislocation has been obtained and to further evaluate the possibility of associated fractures that may have been missed on the initial roentgenographs (Fig 35–124,B).[9]

Dunn[12] reported associated fractures in five of seven

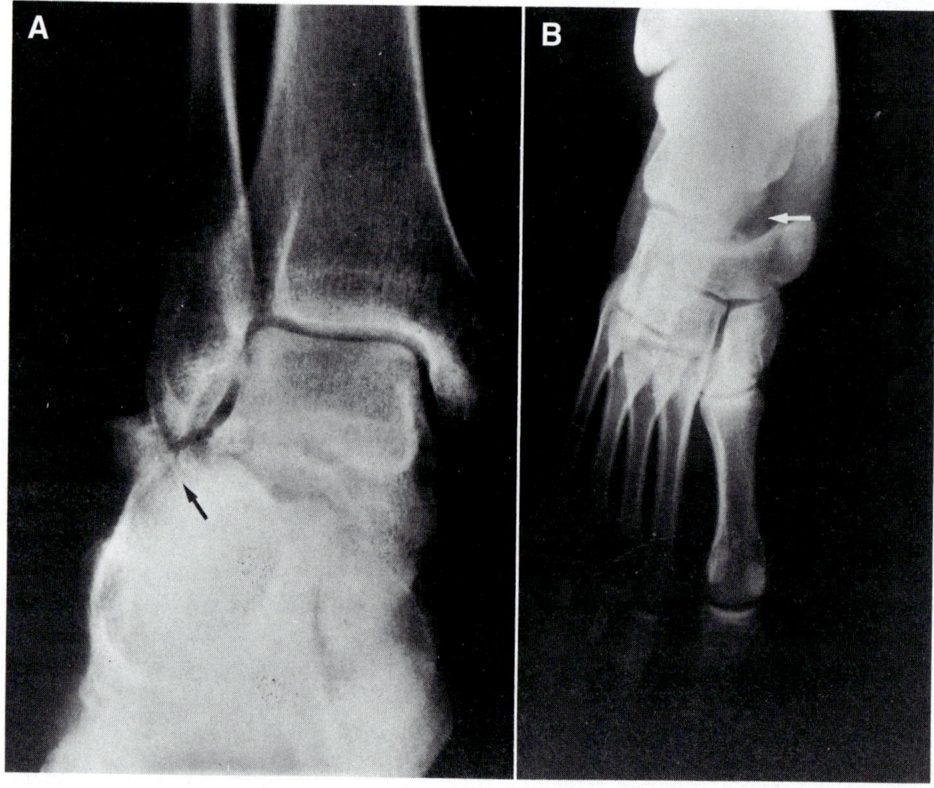

FIG 35–124.
A, lateral subtalar dislocation with an associated fracture of the lateral process of the talus *(arrow).* **B,** postreduction radiograph of a medial subtalar dislocation demonstrating an associated fracture of the talar head *(arrow).* (From DeLee JC, Curtis R: *J Bone Joint Surg [Am]* 64:433–437, 1982. Used by permission.)

and Barber et al.[2] in five of six subtalar dislocations. DeLee and Curtis reported that over half of their patients had associated fractures and that lateral subtalar dislocations have a higher incidence of associated intra-articular fracture than do medial dislocations.[9] The high incidence of associated intra-articular fractures noted in lateral dislocations has also been reported by Christensen et al.[7] and Heppenstall et al.[21] Kleiger and Ahmed[26] believed that lateral subtalar dislocations are associated with fractures near the lateral subtalar joint due to the limited subtalar eversion present in the normal foot. Curtis and DeLee[9] also emphasized that because patients with associated fractures had the most limited subtalar motion at follow-up, detecting these fractures was important for prognosis. They also suggested the use of polytomography postreduction in a further effort to diagnose intra-articular fractures, particularly those involving the subtalar joint. In their series, of the six patients with intra-articular fractures involving the subtalar joint, in two the diagnosis was only possible with polytomography.

Pavlov,[40] in discussing arthrography of the posterior subtalar joint, suggests that this technique may be helpful in evaluating the articular cartilage of the subtalar joint. The author has no experience with arthrography in evaluating subtalar dislocations.

Treatment

Subtalar dislocations should be treated promptly by reduction to avoid skin breakdown and distal circulatory compromise.[9, 39] Barber et al.[2] emphasized that due to increased tension in the skin over the side of the foot and ankle opposite to the direction of displacement, blistering and subsequent necrosis of the skin may occur if reduction is delayed. Coltart[8] and Wilhelm and Komanov[50] also emphasize the importance of the risk of skin slough over the projecting head of the talus in a neglected subtalar dislocation.

Subtalar dislocations occasionally present as open injuries.[9, 31, 50] DeLee and Curtis reported that 3 of their 17 subtalar dislocations were open.[9] Wilhelm and Komanov[50] emphasized that following open subtalar dislocation, infection of the wound is very likely and that accompanying circulatory compromise is more frequent in open injuries. They suggest that to prevent the development of either infection or circulatory compromise, reduction be done as soon as possible with adequate wound management, immobilization, and antibiotic therapy.[50] DeLee and Curtis[9] recommend that open dislocations be treated by extensive debridement and irrigation *prior* to reduction. The reduction is then performed and a second irrigation and debridement completed. All wounds are left open and closed secondarily at 5 to 7 days. Patients are placed in a short-leg cast for 3 weeks. Following this scheme of treatment, they had no cases of chronic infection.[9] However, these authors do report that all patients with open dislocations had decreased range of subtalar motion and pain when walking on uneven ground. They also emphasized that the skin scarring resulting from open dislocations is frequently tender and painful. Kenwright and Taylor[25] also noted uniformly poor functional results following open dislocations.

In closed subtalar dislocations, a closed reduction is performed as soon as possible. McKeever[34] emphasizes that subtalar dislocations may present a pressing surgical emergency. He believes that prompt reduction of the dislocation is mandatory to relieve pressure and tension if there is any evidence of circulatory embarrassment to the skin. He stresses that if the skin necrosis is irreversible, the gangrenous area of the skin should be excised and the area of skin loss closed by plastic techniques. The mode of anesthesia should be selected to provide adequate muscle relaxation.

O'Brien[38] recommends the use of general or spinal anesthesia to provide adequate muscle relaxation. Giannestras and Sammarco[16] and Shelton and Pedowitz[44] also recommend general or spinal anesthesia for complete muscle relaxation before attempted closed reduction. Fahey and Murphy[14] believe that when encountered within a few hours of the time of injury, most subtalar dislocations require only intravenous analgesia to affect reduction.

To reduce a medial dislocation, the foot is grasped, and an assistant applies countertraction. The thigh is flexed to relax the triceps surae.[14, 17] The deformity is then accentuated and the mechanism of injury reversed by pronating, abducting, and finally, dorsiflexing the foot.[9, 14, 17, 38, 39, 44] Direct pressure over the talar head may assist in the reduction technique.[16]

Lateral dislocations are reduced by applying traction on the foot and heel in line with the deformity. Countertraction is applied to the thigh with the knee in flexion to relax the triceps surae.[9, 14, 17, 38, 39, 44] Traction reduces the talocalcaneal joint,[5, 9, 14, 38] and the talonavicular joint is reduced by manual pressure on the head of the talus while the foot is held pronated.[5, 14, 38, 44] Alternatively, DeLee and Curtis recommend reduction of a lateral dislocation by traction in the line of the deformity, followed by adduction and dorsiflexion of the foot.[9]

In the more unusual posterior dislocations, the forefoot is first plantar-flexed, thereby releasing the neck of the talus from the superior edge of the navicular. The heel is then pulled plantarward and the entire foot dorsiflexed.[44] Anterior dislocations are reduced by pulling the foot distally so that the posterior surface of the calcaneus is free from the talar sulcus. The foot is then redirected backward to conclude reduction.[44]

Following closed reduction, roentgenographs are carefully evaluated to ascertain that *anatomic* reduction of the subtalar joint has been obtained and to detect associated fractures.[9] Dislocations that are irreducible by closed means have been reported by many authors.* The incidence of irreducible dislocation varies from 10% to 20%.[9, 30] Obstructions to the closed reduction of medial subtalar dislocations include (1) buttonholing of the talar head through the extensor retinaculum[19, 44] or the extensor digitorum brevis muscle,[19] (2) impaction of the lateral aspect of the navicular into the medial aspect of the head of the talus,[30, 44] (3) the dorsal talonavicular ligament,[30] and (4) the peroneal tendons.[44] In an irreducible medial dislocation, the surgical incision for open reduction should be placed laterally, parallel to the long axis of the foot, and directly over the talar head.[19] This will expose the area of the talar head about which the obstruction is usually located.[32, 44]

Obstructions to the closed reduction of lateral dislocations include (1) a tibialis posterior tendon that has been pulled from its groove behind the medial malleolus and passes forward to the lateral aspect of the talar neck,[5, 30, 31, 37, 44] (2) the flexor digitorum longus around the talar neck, and (3) marginal fractures involving the talar head.[5, 9, 44] Fahey and Murphy[14] and DeLee and Curtis[9] emphasized that lateral dislocations are more likely to have obstructions to closed reduction. If the posterior tibial tendon prevents reduction, Leitner[29] reports that extreme dorsiflexion and medial displacement of the foot may assist in freeing the posterior tibial tendon and permit a closed reduction. If this is not successful, an open reduction should be carried out immediately.[9, 44] Shelton and Pedowitz[44] suggest the use of an oblique anterolateral incision over the sinus tarsi that extends from the long extensor tendon sheath to the peroneal tendon sheaths. This exposes both the subtalar and midtarsal joints and allows the surgeon to free the neck of the talus of all obstructions. Alternatively, Mac and Kleiger[32] suggest exploration on the medial aspect of the foot to reduce an irreducible lateral dislocation.

Shelton and Pedowitz[44] suggest that irreducible anterior and posterior dislocations be approached through an incision placed under the lateral malleolus. Following this incision, the talus and calcaneus are separated by an elevator and reduced. It must be emphasized that following all open reductions excellent-quality roentgenographs be taken to ensure that anatomic reduction of the subtalar joint has been obtained.

Following reduction by either open or closed means, these dislocations are usually stable. Recommendations for immobilization after reduction vary from 3 weeks[9, 34] to 4 months.[45] Christensen et al.[7] recommended immobilization for 8 weeks postreduction in a long-leg cast. However, the majority of their patients had pain with walking following treatment by this method. Buckingham[5] reported that the majority of patients immobilized for 6 weeks had limited subtalar motion. Although Leitner[30] believed that poor results secondary to pain and limited movement of the subtalar joint were caused by a short period of immobilization, McKeever[34] strongly encouraged *early* mobilization of the foot to prevent subtalar fibrosis. Both McKeever[34] and DeLee and Curtis[9] stress that subtalar dislocations unassociated with fractures are extremely stable, thereby allowing early range of motion without fear of recurrent subluxation. These authors therefore recommend cast removal and range-of-motion exercises at 3 weeks and stress the importance of active assisted motion of *both* the subtalar and midtarsal joints. Neither article reported recurrent dislocation or instability of the subtalar joint following this short period of immobilization. In addition, DeLee and Curtis stressed the importance of leaving the metatarsophalangeal joints of the toes free in the cast to enable immediate metatarsophalangeal motion in an effort to prevent tendon scarring at the ankle and stiffness of these joints.

Results

Subtalar dislocations can often be easily reduced and produce good functional results.[5] However, this is not uniformly true.[9, 26, 29, 32] Most authors relate poor results to open injuries and to delayed reductions.[9, 20, 35] Smith,[45] Gross,[18] and DeLee and Curtis[9] have emphasized the increased disability produced by intra-articular fractures associated with subtalar dislocations. Christensen et al.[7] have also emphasized the relationship of subtalar arthrosis to associated fractures involving the subtalar joint. DeLee and Curtis[9] emphasized the direct association of poor functional results with open injuries and associated fractures involving the subtalar joint.

Aseptic necrosis of the talus following simple subtalar dislocation is rare.[39, 51] No cases of aseptic necrosis following subtalar dislocation were noted in the series reported by Buckingham,[5] Pennal,[41] Kenwright and Taylor,[25] Monson and Ryan,[36] DeLee and Curtis,[9] or Plewes and McKelvey.[42] Also, Grantham[17] noted that avascular necrosis had not been reported as a long-term

---

**References 5, 6, 9, 12, 14, 18, 19, 30, 32, 37, 44, 50.*

complication of this injury. However, recently Dunn[12] reported aseptic necrosis in two of seven patients following subtalar dislocation. In one, however, sepsis required removal of the bone and may have played a role in the development of aseptic necrosis. Additionally, Mindell et al.[35] reported aseptic necrosis in two of ten patients. The majority of authors, however, support the thesis that aseptic necrosis following this injury is extremely unusual.

Loss of motion of the subtalar joint following subtalar dislocation is common.[2, 8, 9, 13, 21, 28, 29, 36] Barber et al.[2] also emphasized that residual limitation of inversion and eversion should be expected following subtalar dislocation. DeLee and Curtis[9] measured the range of the subtalar joint following subtalar dislocation by using the method of Inman and Mann[22, 23] (see Chapter 2). They found that 9 of 17 patients had a greater than 50% loss of subtalar motion. These authors were able to correlate this loss of motion to (1) associated fractures involving the subtalar joint and (2) immobilization for longer than 6 weeks.

Monson and Ryan[36] introduced a simple *clinical* method of determining subtalar motion. With the ankle in the neutral position and the patient standing, a line is drawn down the Achilles tendon to the callosity of the heel. The patient is then asked to invert the foot maximally. The deviation in the line from the perpendicular is measured with a goniometer. Although this angle is not exactly equal to the arc of subtalar motion, the authors believed that it is a good approximation.[36] Using this technique, the authors found that all patients suffering a subtalar dislocation demonstrated a loss of subtalar motion. However, in pure subtalar dislocations without a major fracture, this loss is minimal.[36] Buckingham[5] also reported a substantial loss of subtalar motion, the majority of cases varying from the complete loss of motion to maintenance of 50% of the normal range.

Degenerative joint disease involving the subtalar joint has been reported by several authors.[7, 9, 28, 41] Pennal noted degenerative joint changes involving the subtalar joint in 9 of 15 patients.[41] These degenerative changes produced varying degrees of disability and were all associated with marginal fractures. However, Christensen et al.[7] noted arthrosis of the subtalar joint in 6 of 13 patients in whom associated subtalar fractures were *not* present. These authors also noted a higher incidence of arthrosis in open fractures and in fractures requiring immobilization for more than 8 weeks. DeLee and Curtis[9] found roentgenographic evidence of arthrosis of the subtalar and/or talonavicular joints in 7 of 17 cases. In all cases with arthrosis there was an intra-articular fracture involving the joint, or there was an open injury. These authors reported that pain associated with weather changes was present in all patients with roentgenographic evidence of arthritis and that 4 of the 7 had pain when walking on uneven ground.[9, 13] Due to the *direct* relationship of loss of range of motion and degenerative arthritis in the subtalar joint to the presence of associated fractures of the subtalar and talonavicular joints, these authors stress the use of polytomography post-reduction to delineate these fractures for prognosis purposes. They also suggest that open reduction and internal fixation or excision of these small intra-articular fractures be considered in an effort to reduce the incidence of poor functional results.

Finally, due to the inherent stability of the subtalar joint following reduction, recurrent dislocation rarely if ever occurs following subtalar dislocation.[9, 39] In my experience, the only case of recurrent subtalar dislocation that I have seen was in a patient with generalized ligamentous laxity. In this patient immobilization was for 6 weeks following initial reduction, but in spite of this prolonged immobilization, recurrent dislocation occurred.

Author's Preferred Method of Treatment

In patients with closed subtalar dislocations, anteroposterior, lateral, and oblique roentgenographs are obtained. The importance of good-quality roentgenographs cannot be overemphasized. One should search for intra-articular fractures involving the subtalar or talonavicular joints because of their direct effect on prognosis. Once a diagnosis of subtalar dislocation has been made, closed reduction is attempted. If this is an isolated injury and it presents early following injury, intravenous analgesia is used. However, in cases presenting late, I prefer general anesthesia.

The method of manipulation of all subtalar dislocations includes flexion of the knees to relax the gastrocnemius-soleus muscle group and traction on the heel in the line of the deformity. In a medial dislocation, the foot is then everted and the forefoot abducted followed by dorsiflexion. In lateral dislocations, the heel is inverted and the forefoot adducted followed by dorsiflexion. In a pure posterior dislocation the forefoot is plantar-flexed, the heel pulled plantarward, and the foot dorsiflexed as a unit. In a pure anterior dislocation the foot is plantar-flexed, the heel is pulled forward, and the entire foot is then pushed posteriorly as a unit. Following closed reduction, a repeat set of roentgenographs is obtained, and a careful evaluation of the subtalar joint for accurate reduction is performed. In those cases in which no associated intra-articular fractures are seen on routine films, polytomography is recommended. If large intra-articular fractures are present, consideration is given to open reduction and internal fixation or to excision. In patients with small intra-articular fractures that prevent an anatomic reduction of the subtalar joint, excision is recommended.

If closed reduction under general anesthesia fails, I proceed directly to open reduction. In an irreducible medial dislocation I utilize a surgical incision placed parallel to the long axis of the foot and over the talar head, which is easily palpated. This allows direct access to the extensor retinaculum and extensor digitorum brevis, which are most likely to be the obstacles to reduction. In an irreducible lateral dislocation, I prefer an incision over the sustentaculum tali. This allows exposure of both the subtalar and midtarsal joints and direct visualization of the neck of the talus. This incision allows access to the neck of the talus and the commonly obstructing posterior tibial tendon. In patients with irreducible anterior or posterior dislocations, a longitudinal incision parallel to the sole of the foot and just below the distal end of the fibula is utilized. This allows direct access to the subtalar joint, which can then be reduced under direct vision.

Following reduction of the dislocations and careful roentgenographic evaluation, the patient is placed in a short-leg nonwalking cast for a period of 3 weeks. The cast is well molded in the arch of the foot but extends only to the metatarsophalangeal joints. The patients are begun on immediate range-of-motion exercises of the metatarsophalangeal joint. At 3 weeks the casts are removed, and subtalar and ankle motion is initiated by utilizing both active and active-assisted methods. Intermittent soaking or swimming pool exercises may be added.[27] If associated fractures are present, I prefer a short period of immobilization, 3 to 4 weeks, followed by early range of motion as mentioned above. The only indication I have for a longer period of immobilization is in a patient in whom excision or comminution of fracture fragments has rendered the joint unstable. This determination is made at the time of the initial reduction and may require immobilization from 4 to 6 weeks.

During the rehabilitation phase, if subtalar or midtarsal motion does not appear to be progressing satisfactorily, I have utilized manipulation under anesthesia up to 3 months postinjury. I have noted a significant improvement in range of motion following this regime.

In patients in whom an open dislocation is present, extensive irrigation and debridement are carried out prior to reduction of the fracture. Performing irrigation and debridement *prior* to reduction allows access to the subtalar and talonavicular joints. Once the irrigation and debridement are completed, reduction under direct vision is performed. A second series of irrigation and debridement of equal thoroughness is then performed. The wounds are left open and a delayed primary closure performed at 5 to 7 days. The period of immobilization and postoperative management is identical to those patients with closed injuries.

REFERENCES

Dislocations About the Talus

1. Atsatt RF: Subastragalar dislocation of the foot, *J Bone Joint Surg* 13:574–577, 1931.
2. Barber JR, Bricker JD, Haliburton RA: Peritalar dislocation of the foot, *Can J Surg* 4:205–210, 1961.
3. Bohler L: *The treatment of fractures*, ed 5, vol 3, New York, 1958, Grune & Stratton.
4. Broca P: Memoire sur les luxations sous-astragaliennes, *Mem Soc Chir* 3:566–656, 1853.
5. Buckingham WW: Subtalar dislocation of the foot, *J Trauma* 13:753–765, 1973.
6. Chapman MW: Fractures and fracture-dislocations of the ankle and foot. In Mann RA, editor: *DuVries' surgery of the foot*, ed 4, St Louis, 1978, Mosby–Year Book.
7. Christensen SB, Lorentzen JE, Krogsoe O, et al: Subtalar dislocation, *Acta Orthop Scand* 48:707–711, 1977.
8. Coltart WD: "Aviator's astragalus," *J Bone Joint Surg [Br]* 34:545–566, 1952.
9. DeLee JC, Curtis R: Subtalar dislocation of the foot, *J Bone Joint Surg [Am]* 64:433–437, 1982.
10. Detenbeck LC, Kelly PJ: Total dislocation of the talus, *J Bone Joint Surg [Am]* 51:283–288, 1969.
11. Dufaurest P: Luxation du pied, en dehors, compliquee de l'issue de l'astragale a travers la capsule et les tequmens dechires, *J Med Chir Pharm* 22:348–355, 1811.
12. Dunn AW: Peritalar dislocation, *Orthop Clin North Am* 5:7–18, 1974.
13. Dwyer FC: Causes, significance and treatment of stiffness of the subtaloid joint, *Proc R Soc Med* 69:97–102, 1976.
14. Fahey JJ, Murphy JL: Dislocations and fractures of the talus, *Surg Clin North Am* 45:79–102, 1965.
15. Garcia A, Parkes JC: Fractures of the foot. In Giannestras NJ, editor: *Foot disorders: medical and surgical management*, ed 2, Philadelphia, 1973, Lea & Febiger.
16. Giannestras NJ, Sammarco GJ: Fractures and dislocations in the foot. In Rockwood CA, Green DP, editors: *Fractures*, Philadelphia, 1975, JB Lippincott.
17. Grantham SA: Medial subtalar dislocation: five cases with a common etiology, *J Trauma* 4:845–849, 1964.
18. Gross RH: Medial peritalar dislocation—associated foot injuries and mechanism of injury, *J Trauma* 15:682–688, 1975.
19. Haliburton RA, Barber JR, Fraser RL: Further experience with peritalar dislocation, *Can J Surg* 10:322–324, 1967.
20. Hauser EDW: Management of lesions of the subtalar joint, *Surg Clin North Am* 25:136–160, 1945.
21. Heppenstall RB, Farahvar H, Balderston R, et al: Evaluation and management of subtalar dislocations, *J Trauma* 20:494–497, 1980.
22. Inman VT: The joints of the ankle, Baltimore, 1976, Williams & Wilkins.
23. Inman VT, Mann RA: Principles of examination of the

foot and ankle. In Mann RA, editor: *DuVries' surgery of the foot*, ed 4, St Louis, 1978, Mosby–Year Book.
24. Judcy P: Observation d'une luxation metatarsienne, *Bull Fac Med Paris* 11:81–86, 1811.
25. Kenwright J, Taylor RG: Major injuries of the talus, *J Bone Joint Surg [Br]* 52:36–48, 1970.
26. Kleiger B, Ahmed M: Injuries of the talus and its joints, *Clin Orthop* 121:243–261, 1976.
27. Lapidus PW, Guidotti FP: Immediate mobilization and swimming pool exercises in some fractures of the foot and ankle bones, *Clin Orthop* 56:197–206, 1968.
28. Larsen HW: Subastragalar dislocation (luxatio pedis sub talo). A follow-up report of eight cases, *Acta Chir Scand* 113:380–392, 1957.
29. Leitner B: Behandlung und Behandlungsergebnisse von 42 frischen Fallen von Luxatio pedis sub talo im Unfallkrankenhaus Wien in den Jahren 1925–1950. *Ergeb Chir Orthop* 37:501–577, 1952.
30. Leitner B: Obstacles to reduction in subtalar dislocations, *J Bone Joint Surg [Am]* 36:299–306, 1954.
31. Loup J: Luxation ouverte sous-astragalienne, *Ann Chir* 27:993–995, 1973.
32. Mac SS, Kleiger B: The early complications of subtalar dislocation, *Foot Ankle* 1:270–274, 1981.
33. Malgaigne JF, Burger CG: *Du Knochenbruche and Verrenkungen*. Stuttgart, 1856, Reiger.
34. McKeever FM: Treatment of complications of fractures and dislocations of the talus, *Clin Orthop* 30:45–52, 1963.
35. Mindell ER, Cisek EE, Kartalian G, et al: Late results of injuries to the talus, *J Bone Joint Surg [Am]* 45:221–245, 1963.
36. Monson ST, Ryan JR: Subtalar dislocation, *J Bone Joint Surg [Am]* 63:1156–1158, 1981.
37. Mulroy RD: The tibialis posterior tendon as an obstacle to reduction of a lateral anterior subtalar dislocation, *J Bone Joint Surg [Am]* 37:859–863, 1955.
38. O'Brien ET: Injuries of the talus, *Am Fam Physician* 12:95–105, 1975.
39. Parkes JC II: Injuries of the hindfoot, *Clin Orthop* 122:28–36, 1977.
40. Pavlov H: Ankle and subtalar arthrography, *Clin Sports Med* 1:47–69, 1982.
41. Pennal GF: Fractures of the talus, *Clin Orthop* 30:53–63, 1963.
42. Plewes LW, McKelvey KG: Subtalar dislocation, *J Bone Joint Surg* 26:585–588, 1944.
43. Shands AR Jr: The incidence of subastragaloid dislocation of the foot with a report of one case of the inward type, *J Bone Joint Surg* 10:306–313, 1928.
44. Shelton ML Pedowitz WJ: Injuries to the talus and midfoot. In Jahss MH, editor: *Disorders of the foot*, vol 2, Philadelphia, 1982, WB Saunders.
45. Smith H: Subastragalar dislocation, *J Bone Joint Surg* 19:373–380, 1937.
46. Soustelle J, Meyer P, Sauvage Y: Luxation sous-astragalienne fermee, *Lyon Chir* 60:119, 1964.
47. Straus DC: Subtalus dislocation of the foot—with report of two cases, *Am J Surg* 30:427–434, 1935.
48. Vincenti FR: Subtalar dislocations, Western Orthopaedic Association meeting, Houston, 1975.
49. Von Vogt H: Drei seltene Verrenkungsformen im talusbereich, *Schweiz Med Wochenschr* 89:1005, 1959.
50. Wilhelm B, Komanov I: Subtalus luxation of the foot, *Lijec Vjesn* 94:283–286, 1972.
51. Wright PE: Dislocations. In Edmonson AS, Crenshaw AH, editors: *Campbell's operative orthopaedics*, ed 6, vol 1, St Louis, 1980, Mosby–Year Book.

Total Dislocation of the Talus

Total dislocation of the talus, an injury in which the talus is dislocated both from the ankle joint and from the rest of the foot, is extremely unusual and accounts for no more than 10% of all major talus injuries.[13] Indeed, Coltart[2] was able to find only 9 cases of total dislocation in 228 major talar injuries. Two thirds of these were open injuries, and all were the result of aircraft accidents. Detenbeck and Kelley[4] reported an additional nine cases, seven open, in 1969. Most of the literature consists of isolated case reports,* with no one author having extensive experience with these injuries.

Mechanism of Injury

Leitner[9] believed that total dislocation of the talus actually represents the end point in the spectrum of supination or pronation injury to the ankle. According to Leitner[9] a first-degree supination injury to the ankle results in a medial subtalar dislocation, while a second-degree supination injury results in medial subtalar dislocation and talocrural subluxation. Finally, a third-degree supination injury results in total *lateral* dislocation of the talus. A first-degree pronation injury, on the other hand, results in a lateral subtalar dislocation, while a second-degree pronation injury results in lateral subtalar dislocation *and* talocrural subluxation.[9] A third-degree pronation injury results in total *medial* dislocation of the talus. Therefore, the position of the talus in a total talar dislocation gives an indication as to whether supination or pronation was the mechanism of injury.[9] Leitner reports that supination injuries are much more common than pronation injuries, thus resulting in lateral talar dislocations being more common than those that occur medially.[9]

Pinzur and Meyer[15] in 1978 reported a case of complete posterior dislocation of the talus. The posterior location of the talar body in this case suggests that neither pronation nor supination is the mechanism of injury. Instead, this injury was accompanied by diastasis of the ankle and a fracture of the anterior process of the calcaneus, which suggests that severe dorsiflexion and forward displacement of the foot onto the leg were the mechanism of injury.

Finally, Pennal[14] reports that total dislocation of the talus is a result of a severe plantar flexion and inversion force on the foot. He believes that extreme plantar flex-

---

**References 1, 4, 7, 9, 10, 12–14, 16, 17.*

ion causes a forward dislocation of the foot at ankle joint with complete rupture of the collateral ligaments. As this force continues, an additional inversion stress will cause disruption of the talocalcaneal ligaments. As the displaced foot recoils, the detached talus remains rotated and lies anterior to the lateral malleolus.[14]

Clinical Diagnosis

According to Coltart[2] and Detenbeck and Kelley,[4] 75% of these injuries are open. The open wound consists of an irregular laceration, and the patient may actually present with his talus wrapped in his handkerchief.[13]

In those patients with a closed injury, physical examination will reveal marked inversion of the foot with a prominence located *anterior* to either the lateral or medial malleolus or posteriorly.[9, 12, 15, 19] The skin over the prominence of the talus is tented and blanched.[12, 14] The posterior and anterior neurovascular bundle may be compromised by the dislocation, thus leading to signs and symptoms of ischemia in the foot upon presentation.[1, 4]

Radiographic Diagnosis

Total dislocation of the talus is usually visualized on anteroposterior, lateral, and oblique roentgenographic views of the foot. However, Segal and Wasilewski[17] documented a complete talar dislocation that initially presented only as a talocrural dislocation. Only after stress roentgenographs were taken was it apparent that the connections of the talus to the calcaneus and midtarsal joints had been disrupted, but the associated dislocations apparently spontaneously reduced. These authors therefore emphasize the need for stress roentgenograms to test the integrity of the ligaments of the talonavicular and talocalcaneal articulations when a talocrural dislocation is evident roentgenographically.[16]

Treatment

Following total dislocation of the talus, most authors prefer open or closed reduction in an effort to preserve function of the joint and length of the extremity.[5, 11–13, 20, 22] On the other hand, Detenbeck and Kelley advocated primary excision of the talus and tibiocalcaneal fusion in an effort to prevent the long-term sequelae of infection that may follow open reduction.[4]

In total dislocation of the talus, all major vascular connections to the talus are usually disrupted, thereby leaving it completely avascular. However, incomplete dislocations and occasionally total dislocations may spare some ligamentous attachments to the talus, particularly the deltoid ligament, which explains why aseptic necrosis does not occur in all of these patients.[11, 12, 18] Segal and Wasilewski[17] found that in spite of total dislocation of the talus in their patient, the lateral malleolus remained attached by ligamentous tissue to the talus, thereby providing a blood supply to the talus and preventing the development of aseptic necrosis.

In closed injuries, immediate reduction is essential to remove pressure on the overlying skin. Pennal[14] reports a successful closed reduction of a total dislocation of the talus; however, aseptic necrosis later developed and required tibial calcaneal fusion. Newcomb and Brav[12] also reported successful closed reduction of a complete dislocation of the talus. They recommend spinal anesthesia for muscle relaxation, followed by the insertion of a Kirschner wire through the calcaneus to be used as a traction pin. Countertraction is obtained through a Steinmann pin inserted through the distal end of the tibia. These two pins are utilized to achieve the distraction of the ankle joint space that is necessary to allow reduction of the talus.[11, 12, 14] Once this distraction is obtained, pressure in a posteromedial direction over the laterally dislocated talus may force the displaced bone back into the ankle mortise. Newcomb and Brav[12] recommend removal of the Kirschner wires following the reduction. Following closed reduction, the talus is usually stable. The authors recommend a long-leg cast for 4 weeks. Shelton and Pedowitz[20] caution against attempting ligamentous repair, particularly of the deltoid ligament, following successful closed reduction for fear of further compromise to the damaged overlying skin.[20]

If closed reduction of a total dislocation of the talus is unsuccessful, open reduction is indicated. Shelton and Pedowitz[20] recommend the use of skeletal traction provided by Kirschner wires through the calcaneus and tibia in a similar manner as is used for closed reduction. An incision is made over the displaced talus, and the reduction is performed under direct vision. They strongly recommend capsular repair in an effort to cover exposed joint surfaces since skin necrosis may later develop.[20] They suggest leaving the skin open and delaying primary closure in an effort to minimize skin necrosis. When closure cannot be obtained within 5 days, they encourage coverage by a myocutaneous or a free flap because wounds left open more than 7 days may become infected.[20]

Up to 75% of these cases present as open injuries, with the open wounds being of a crushing, bursting type.[2, 4] The margins of the wound are often ischemic with early necrosis and are usually severely contaminated. O'Brien[13] cautions against discarding the talus in these open dislocations. He recommends that the wound and the talus be extensively cleansed and the talus replaced in its proper position by using Kirschner wires to maintain the reduction. He recommends that the skin be left open and closed secondarily. O'Brien[13] believes that the talus should not be discarded unless an infection intervenes or unless primary treatment is extremely delayed. Following extensive debridement of the fracture edges, Shelton and Pedowitz[20] also recommend replacement of the talus and leaving the wounds open for delayed closure. If delayed closure is not possible, either free or regional myocutaneous flaps may be necessary to cover the skin defect in an effort to prevent the development of talar osteomyelitis. After reduction, Shelton and Pedowitz[20] recommend a long-leg cast for 4 weeks followed by further immobilization in a short-leg cast. They recommend that patients be followed closely for the development of Hawkin's sign indicating talar aseptic necrosis.[6] A more complete discussion of the diagnosis and treatment of aseptic necrosis is found in the section on fractures of the neck of the talus.

Detenbeck and Kelley[4] reported nine cases of total dislocation of the talus in which there were *no* successful closed reductions. In spite of open reduction, infection occurred in eight of their nine patients, with the result that seven of the nine required talectomy. As a result of this experience, these authors recommend a more aggressive approach to this injury that includes talectomy and tibiocalcaneal arthrodesis as initial treatment. These authors[4] and Pennal[14] report that talectomy alone is not satisfactory because of progressive pain, varus deformity, and the weakness of the foot that results after talectomy.[4] Shelton and Pedowitz[20] caution that tibiocalcaneal fusion results in significant shortening of the limb and a decrease in foot height and therefore suggest that pantalar arthrodesis be performed as a salvage procedure for posttraumatic arthritis.

Complications

Soft-Tissue Infection.—Shelton and Pedowitz[20] stress the importance of wound debridement and leaving skin open primarily to avoid infection. If early soft-tissue infection occurs, prompt debridement and closure when the soft-tissue infection is controlled will help to prevent septic arthritis and talar osteomyelitis, which usually require talectomy for salvage.[20]

Osteomyelitis.—The fact that eight of nine patients reported by Detenbeck and Kelley[4] became infected following total dislocation of the talus emphasizes the importance of *early* adequate debridement and reduction. If the patient presents with an infection involving the talus following this injury, excision of the body of the talus and tibiocalcaneal arthrodesis are an acceptable salvage procedure.[4] Only rarely can the talar body be salvaged if it is infected. Even though tibiocalcaneal fusion resulted in a shortened extremity, it did not cause significant disability in their patients.[4] However, when talectomy alone was utilized, pain and giving way were a significant complication.

Aseptic Necrosis.—Aseptic necrosis may occur following total dislocation of the talus. Shelton and Pedowitz[20] emphasize that revascularization following this injury may be slow because of the large area covered with articular cartilage that limits access for revascularization. However, the medial talar attachment of the deltoid ligament is an important route of talar revascularization. The fact that revascularization often begins medially supports the importance of this soft-tissue attachment.[4, 8, 14] It is essential to emphasize that even though a patient develops aseptic necrosis (particularly if it is without collapse), good to fair function may result. (For a further discussion of talar aseptic necrosis see the section on talar neck fractures.)

Posttraumatic Arthritis.—Posttraumatic arthritis may occur in the subtalar, midtarsal, and/or ankle joint depending upon the severity of the initial injury, whether the initial injury was open or closed, and the presence or absence of aseptic necrosis.[4, 8, 14] Degenerative arthritis following this injury is best treated by arthrodesis of the involved joints, whether this be a triple or pantalar arthrodesis. Management of posttraumatic arthritis of the subtalar, midtarsal, and ankle joints is discussed in the section on complications of talar neck fractures.

Author's Preferred Method of Treatment

A closed total dislocation of the talus is considered a surgical emergency. The patient is brought to the operating room and sterilely prepared for an open reduction. A Kirschner wire is placed through the calcaneus and a Steinmann pin inserted in the distal end of the tibia to apply traction. Traction is applied under image intensification to distract the joint. One attempt at a closed reduction by manipulating the displaced talus in a posteromedial or posterolateral direction (depending on whether the talar body displacement is anteromedial or anterolateral) is performed. If this attempt is unsuccessful, immediate open reduction utilizing an incision directly over the displaced talus is carried out. Once the talus is exposed, distraction is again achieved by use of the pins in the tibia and calcaneus, and the talus is manipulated back into the ankle mortise.

Following closed reduction, the patient is placed in a long-leg bent-knee cast for 4 weeks. This is followed by a short-leg cast for an additional 2 weeks. Weight bearing in a patellar tendon–bearing brace is begun at 6 weeks, if swelling allows. Although these injuries have a high incidence of aseptic necrosis, the fact that revascularization of the talus may require more than 2 years makes prolonged non–weight bearing impractical.

If an open reduction is performed, the capsule is closed over the displaced talus, but the skin and subcutaneous tissues are left open. The patient is brought back to the operating room in 3 to 5 days for a delayed primary closure. Delayed wound closure is recommended in an effort to decrease the degree of skin edge necrosis. Following secondary closure, the patient is managed as following a closed reduction.

Patients who present with an open total dislocation of the talus are also considered surgical emergencies. An extensive debridement of the skin edges and dead space left by the displaced talus is performed. If the talar body has no soft-tissue attachments, it is removed from the wound so that a thorough debridement of the dead space is possible. If there is any soft-tissue attachment remaining on the talus, it is carefully preserved. Once a thorough debridement has been performed, traction wires are placed in the distal end of the tibia and the calcaneus to achieve distraction of the joint. The joint is distracted and a second thorough debridement carried out. At this point the talus is reduced into the ankle mortise. The overlying capsule is closed and the rest of the incision left open. The patient is kept on a regimen of intravenous antibiotics, usually a cephalosporin, for 48 hours postsurgery. Cultures taken in the operating room before debridement are observed to make certain that any organism cultured is sensitive to the cephalosporin. The patient is taken back to the operating room in 3 to 5 days, and closure of the wound is attempted. If closure is not possible, consideration is given to split-thickness skin grafting if an acceptable graft bed is available or to free or rotational flaps to obtain early closure over the talus if skin grafting is not possible. Following closure of the open dislocation, patients are treated as outlined in the section on closed dislocations.

Those patients who present late or in whom the talus is severely contaminated and detached are candidates for a primary talectomy. The talectomy is considered a staged procedure. After the wound heals, a tibial-calcaneal fusion using the method of Pennal[14] or Reckling[16] is performed.

REFERENCES

Total Dislocation of the Talus

1. Bonnin JG: Dislocations and fracture-dislocations of the talus, *Br J Surg* 28:88–100, 1940.
2. Coltart WD: "Aviator's astragalus," *J Bone Joint Surg [Br]* 34:545–566, 1952.
3. Craig FS, McLaughlin HL: Injuries of the foot. In McLaughlin HL, editor: *Trauma*, Philadelphia, 1959, WB Saunders, pp 307–319.
4. Detenbeck LC, Kelley PJ: Total dislocation of the talus, *J Bone Joint Surg [Am]* 51:283–288, 1969.
5. Fahey JJ, Murphy JL: Dislocations and fractures of the talus, *Surg Clin North Am* 45:79–102, 1965.
6. Hawkins LG: Fractures of the neck of the talus, *J Bone Joint Surg [Am]* 52:991–1002, 1970.
7. Kenwright J, Taylor RG: Major injuries of the talus, *J Bone Joint Surg [Br]* 52:36–48, 1970.
8. Klieger B: Fractures of the talus, *J Bone Joint Surg [Am]* 30:735–744, 1948.
9. Leitner B: The mechanism of total dislocation of the talus, *J Bone Joint Surg [Am]* 37:89–95, 1955.
10. Mindel ER, Cisek EE, Kartalian G, et al: Late results of injuries to the talus, *J Bone Joint Surg [Am]* 45:221–245, 1963.
11. Mitchell JI: Total dislocation of the astragalus, *J Bone Joint Surg* 18:212–214, 1936.
12. Newcomb WJ, Brav EA: Complete dislocation of the talus, *J Bone Joint Surg [Am]* 30:872–874, 1948.
13. O'Brien ET: Injuries of the talus, *Am Fam Physician* 12:95–105, 1975.
14. Pennal GF: Fractures of the talus, *Clin Orthop* 30:53–63, 1963.
15. Pinzur MS, Meyer PR Jr: Complete posterior dislocation of the talus. Case report and discussion, *Clin Orthop* 131:205–209, 1978.
16. Reckling FW: Early tibiocalcaneal fusion in the treatment of severe injuries of the talus, *J Trauma* 12:390–396, 1972.
17. Segal D, Wasilewski S: Total dislocation of the talus—case report, *J Bone Joint Surg [Am]* 62:1370–1372, 1980.
18. Schrock RD: Fractures of the foot. Fractures and dislocations of the astragalus. *Instr Course Lect* 9:361–368, 1952.
19. Shahriaree H, Sajadiik AK, Silver C, et al: Total dislocation of the talus: a case report of a four-year follow-up, *Orthop Rev* 9:65–68, 1980.
20. Shelton ML, Pedowitz WJ: Injuries to the talus and midfoot. In Jahss MH, editor: *Disorders of the foot*, vol 2, Philadelphia, 1982, WB Saunders.
21. Sisk TD: Fractures. In Edmonson AS, Crenshaw AH, editors: *Campbell's operative orthopaedics*, ed 6, vol 1, St Louis, 1980, Mosby–Year Book.
22. Sneed WL: The astragalus. A case of dislocation, excision and replacement. An attempt to demonstrate the circulation in this bone, *J Bone Joint Surg* 7:384–399, 1925.

INJURIES TO THE MIDTARSAL JOINT

The midtarsal joint, which consists of the talonavicular and calcaneocuboid joints, lies transversely across the medial and lateral longitudinal arches of the foot.[21, 26] Complete dislocation of this joint unassociated with a fracture is extremely unusual.[4, 5, 14, 15, 17, 29] Although isolated reports have appeared in both the French and German literature,[2, 12, 29, 32, 33] textbooks concerned with fractures and dislocations of the musculoskeletal system have mentioned them only superficially.[1, 3, 4, 11, 22, 31] However, if one considers injury to the midtarsal joint as a continuum of displacement that begins with a simple sprain of the midtarsal joint, progresses to a sprain-fracture, and culminates in complete dislocation, the incidence of injuries to these joints is much more common.[30, 31]

Fractures or dislocations of the navicular, talar head, cuboid, or anterior process of the calcaneus are commonly seen in association with these injuries.[7, 9, 26, 30] Indeed, Waters[30] reports that dislocations without such associated fractures are the exception. Kenwright and Taylor[19] reported ten midtarsal dislocations, eight of which were associated with fractures of the tubercle and body of the navicular or the head of the talus.

Dewar and Evans[5] reported five cases of "occult fracture-subluxation" of the midtarsal joint and stressed that this entity is commonly missed and may progress to severe disability. The injury they reported, which consisted of an avulsion fracture of the tubercle of the navicular accompanied by a fracture of the cuboid and subluxation of the midtarsal joint, was not previously considered with dislocations of this joint. Tountas[28] added fractures of the anterior articular surface of the calcaneus to this injury complex. Previously, all of these injuries had been misdiagnosed simply as ankle sprains.[5] Indeed, Dewar and Evans[5] and Stark[27] stressed the importance of not confusing these injuries with simple sprains. Main and Jowett[21] and Tountas[28] concluded that fractures of the navicular should not be considered isolated injuries and stressed that although avulsions of the tuberosity have occurred without damage to the midtarsal joint, this should suggest a fracture-subluxation of this joint. They also stressed that since these injuries occur predominantly in young patients, the economic loss produced by a bad result and permanent disability is critical.[14, 21]

In considering these injuries as a continuum of displacement from sprain to complete dislocation, a classification is essential. Main and Jowett[21] outlined a very complete classification based on the direction of the deforming force *and* the resulting displacement. They classified these injuries into six groups: I, medial; II, longitudinal; III, compression; IV, lateral; V, plantar; and VI, crush.

I. *Medial injuries* are divided into three subgroups:
   A. *Fracture-sprains*— Fracture-sprains include an inversion sprain of the foot with associated avulsion or a flake fracture of the dorsal surface of the talar head or navicular and avulsion or a flake of the lateral margins of the cuboid or calcaneus. No dislocation is present, and the bone fragments are usually small and minimally displaced. Therefore, no formal reduction is required.
   B. *Fracture subluxation and dislocation* (Fig 35–125).— In this injury the forefoot is displaced medially, which leaves the hindfoot in a normal relationship with the tibia. The mechanism of injury is the same as that for a fracture-sprain; however, a formal reduction is required due to displacement of the forefoot.
   C. *Swivel dislocations* (Fig 35–126,A and B).— This injury was first reported by Main and Jowett.[21] In this injury, the foot rotates medially, and the talonavicular joint is dislocated while the calcaneocuboid joint and interosseous talocalcaneal ligament are left intact. This should be contrasted to the situation in which the talocalcaneal ligament ruptures and produces a subtalar dislocation (Fig 35–127,A and B).[9, 21]

II. *Longitudinal injuries*, according to Main and Jowett, account for the largest percentage of midtarsal joint injuries.[21] In this injury a force is applied at the metatarsal heads to the plantar-flexed foot. The navicular is thereby compressed between the cuneiforms and head of the talus, with resultant fractures of either the navicular or the head of the talus (Fig 35–128,A and B). The pattern of the navicular fracture and degree of displacement are related to the following:
   A. The degree of the force.

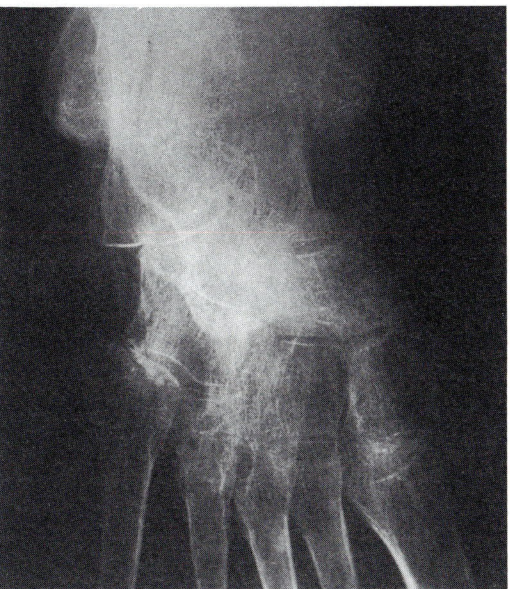

FIG 35–125.
Medial fracture-subluxation. Note the medial displacement of the forefoot at the talonavicular and calcaneocuboid joints. (From Main BJ, Jowett RL: *J Bone Joint Surg [Br]* 57:89–97, 1975. Used by permission.)

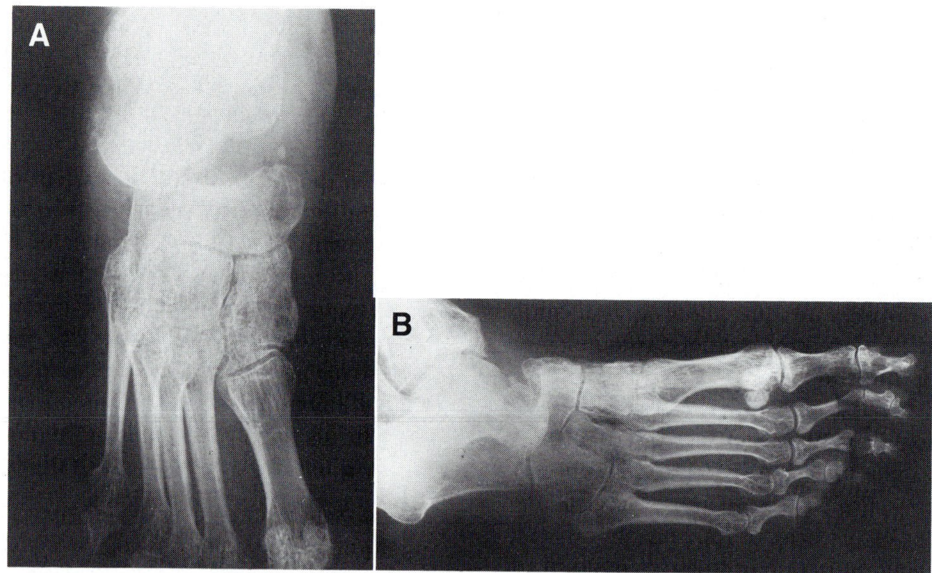

FIG 35–126.
Medial swivel dislocation. **A,** anteroposterior view showing talonavicular dislocation. **B,** an oblique view shows the calcaneocuboid joint to be intact. (From Main BJ, Jowett RL: *J Bone Joint Surg [Br]* 57:89–97, 1975. Used by permission.)

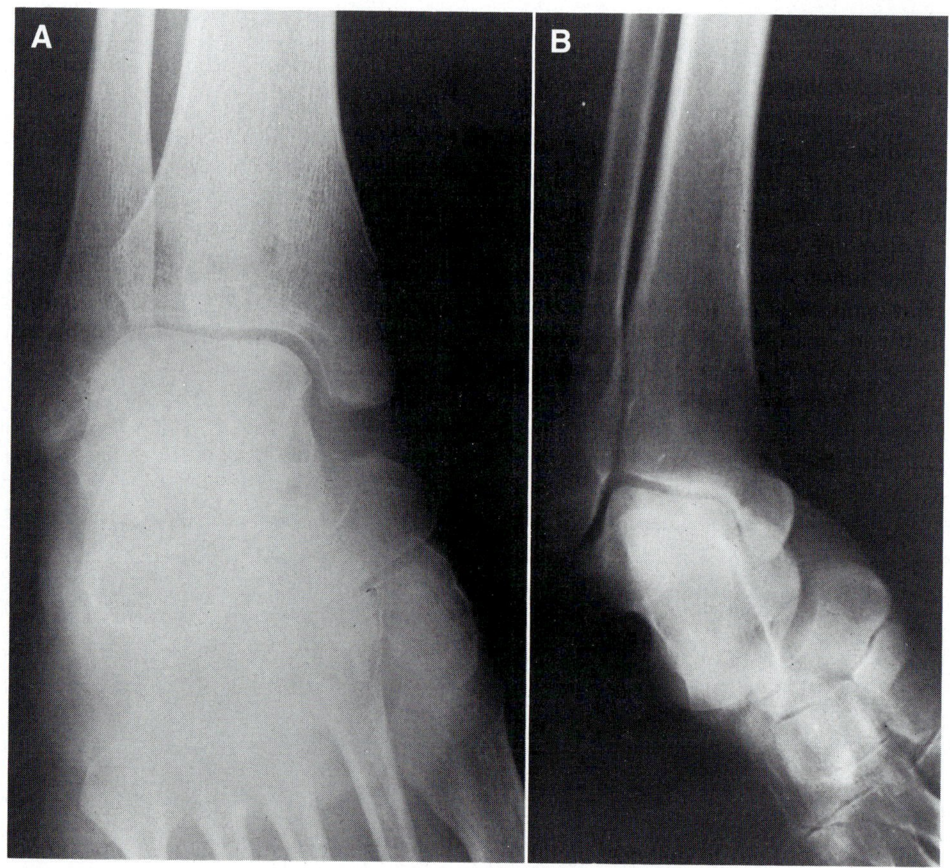

FIG 35–127.
Medial swivel dislocation. **A,** anteroposterior view of medial *swivel* dislocation. Note the vertical alignment of the calcaneus. **B,** anteroposterior view of medial *subtalar* dislocation. Note the tilting of the calcaneus. (From Main BJ, Jowett RL: *J Bone Joint Surg [Br]* 57:89–97, 1975. Used by permission.)

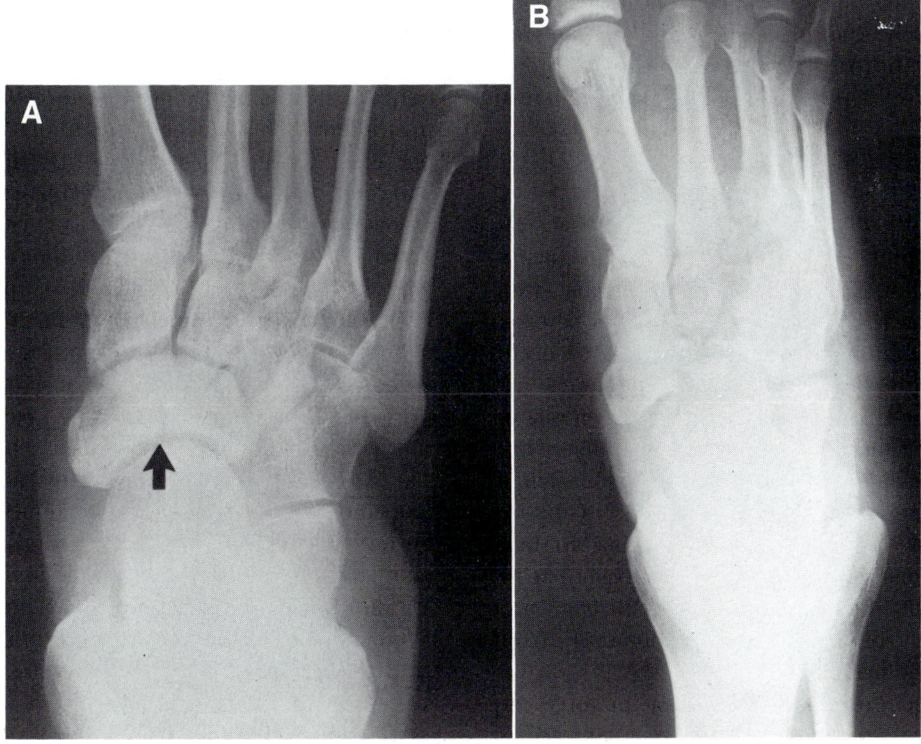

FIG 35–128.
Longitudinal injuries. **A,** nondisplaced longitudinal compression fracture of the navicular. **B,** severely comminuted longitudinal compression fracture of the navicular. (From Main BJ, Jowett RL: *J Bone Joint Surg [Br]* 57:89–97, 1975. Used by permission.)

B. Which metatarsal (1, 2, or 3) transmits the majority of the force.

III. Laterial injuries are divided into three subgroups:

A. *Fracture-sprain* (Fig 35–129,A).—In lateral fracture-sprains, an eversion sprain of the foot is associated with avulsion of the navicular tuberosity or a flake of bone from the dorsum of the navicular or medial talus. On the lateral side, the abduction force may produce an impaction fracture of the cuboid and/or calcaneus.

B. *Fracture-subluxations* (Fig 35–129,B).—In this injury associated with lateral subluxation of the talonavicular joint, the lateral column of the foot collapses because of comminution in the area of the calcaneocuboid joint. This mechanism is said to produce the "nutcracker" fracture of the cuboid[13] and also possibly total dislocation of this bone.[8]

C. *Lateral swivel dislocation* (Fig 35–129,C).—In this injury, there is a lateral dislocation of the talonavicular joint, but the calcaneocuboid and talocalcaneal joints remain intact.

IV. *Plantar injuries* are divided into two subgroups (Fig 35–130):

A. *Fracture-sprains.*—Avulsion fractures occur from the dorsum of the navicular or talus and from the anterior process of the calcaneus. These are stable injuries that respond well and produce good results with plaster immobilization.

B. *Fracture-subluxations and dislocations.*—In addition to avulsion fractures from the dorsum of the navicular or talus, impacted fractures occur at the calcaneocuboid dislocation. Complete dislocation of this joint, which may result from a plantar injury, is the so-called Chopart dislocation (Fig 35–130).

V. In *crush injuries* the entire midtarsal joint is crushed. There is no constant pattern of displacement, and the degree of comminution is variable (Fig 35–131).

Although discussions of fractures of individual tarsal bones, including the navicular, cuboid, and cuneiforms, are presented in this chapter, it is important to remember that *isolated* fractures of these bones without associated midtarsal ligamentous disruption and, hence, instability are distinctly unusual.[7] One must therefore remember to *always* associate these fractures with a mid-

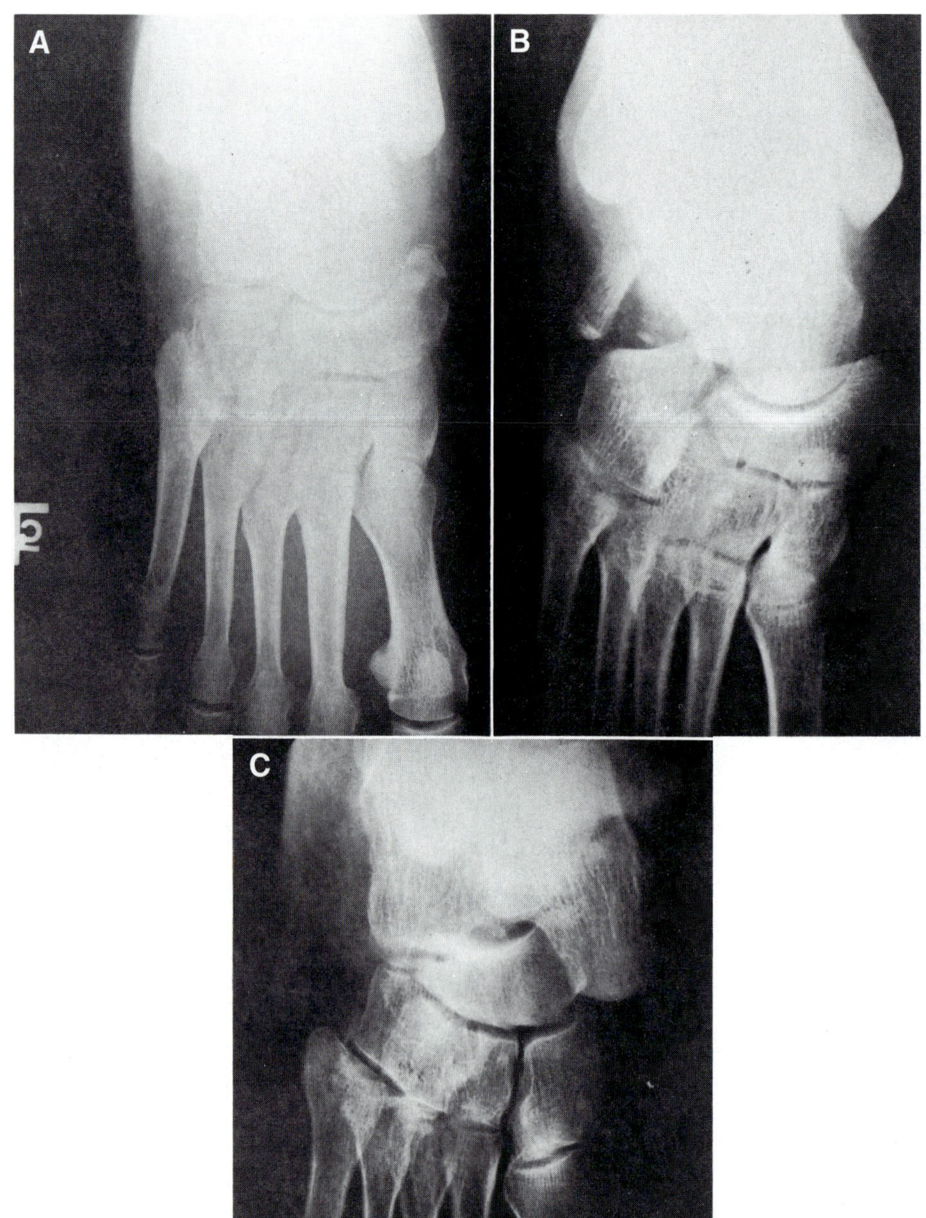

FIG 35–129.
Lateral injuries. **A,** lateral fracture-sprain. Note the avulsion of the navicular tuberosity and the impaction fracture of the cuboid. **B,** lateral fracture-subluxation. Note the comminution of the anterior process of the os calcis and subluxation of the midtarsal joint. **C,** lateral swivel dislocation of the talonavicular joint with the calcaneocuboid joint intact. (From Main BJ, Jowett RL: *J Bone Joint Surg [Br]* 57:89–97, 1975. Used by permission.)

tarsal joint sprain, subluxation, or a spontaneously reduced dislocation.

Anatomy

The midtarsal joint consists of the talonavicular and calcaneocuboid joints.[26] The calcaneocubiod joint is saddle shaped, while the talonavicular joint is condyloid.[24] Motion through the calcaneocuboid joint includes supination-adduction-flexion. This motion is stopped when the inferior medial portion of the cuboid impinges on the end of the coronoid fossa of the os calcis.[24] The motion of pronation-abduction-extension is blocked when the anterior process or beak of the os calcis impinges upon the cuboid.[24]

Motion through the talonavicular joint includes pronation with minimal abduction-extension and supination with minimal adduction-flexion.[24] The talonavicu-

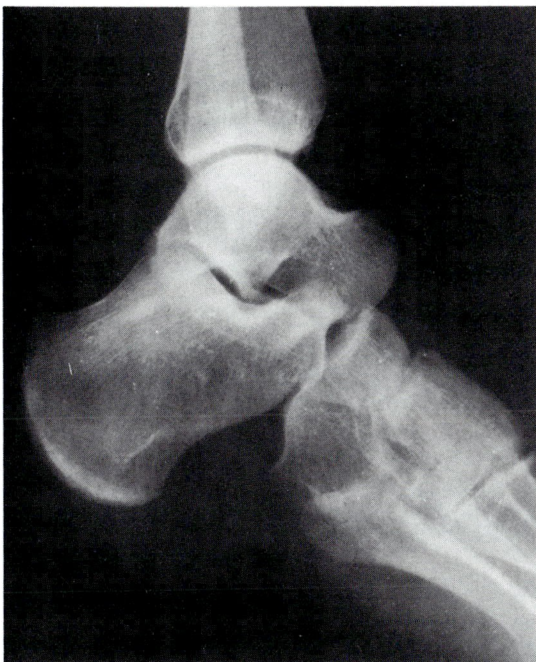

FIG 35–130.
Plantar dislocation. The subtalar joint is intact. (From Main BJ, Jowett RL: *J Bone Joint Surg [Br]* 57:89–97, 1975. Used by permission.)

lar and calcaneocuboid joints function in unison with the subtalar joint to produce inversion and eversion.[26]

The calcaneocuboid joint is stabilized by the medial calcaneocuboid ligament, the dorsolateral calcaneocuboid ligament, and the inferior calcaneocuboid ligament.[24] The talonavicular joint is stabilized by the talonavicular ligament, which occupies the interval between the superior medial calcaneonavicular ligament and the lateral calcaneonavicular ligament. These ligaments help to stabilize the midtarsal joint and are responsible for the avulsion fractures that occur in association with subluxation or dislocation of this joint.[24]

Jones[18] stressed that the medial longitudinal arch of the foot consists of elements articulating with each other through curved surfaces, a fact that provides elasticity to the medial longitudinal arch due to its ability to "give and bend." However, toward the lateral border of the foot, the arch becomes less elastic, which results in a more static, rigid relationship, important to foot stability. Hence, although the medial longitudinal arch permits elasticity, lateral arch rigidity is responsible for the fact that these injuries are relatively uncommon.

Mechanism of Injury

Dewar and Evans[5] believe that the mechanism of occult fracture-subluxation of the midtarsal joint is forced abduction that results in an avulsion fracture of the navicular with the fragment remaining attached to the posterior tibial tendon. The forefoot, freed on the medial arch, swings further into abduction and produces a compression fracture involving the calcaneocuboid joint. Fractures of the tubercle or body of the navicular associated with midtarsal dislocations were also noted by Kenwright and Taylor,[19] a fact that supports this mechanism. This mechanism results in an unstable fracture-subluxation of the midtarsal joint.[5, 19] Tountas[28] stressed that in an occult fracture-subluxation of the midtarsal joint, a trivial accident was usually the culprit. He described twisting of the foot in falling or missing a step as the mechanism of injury.

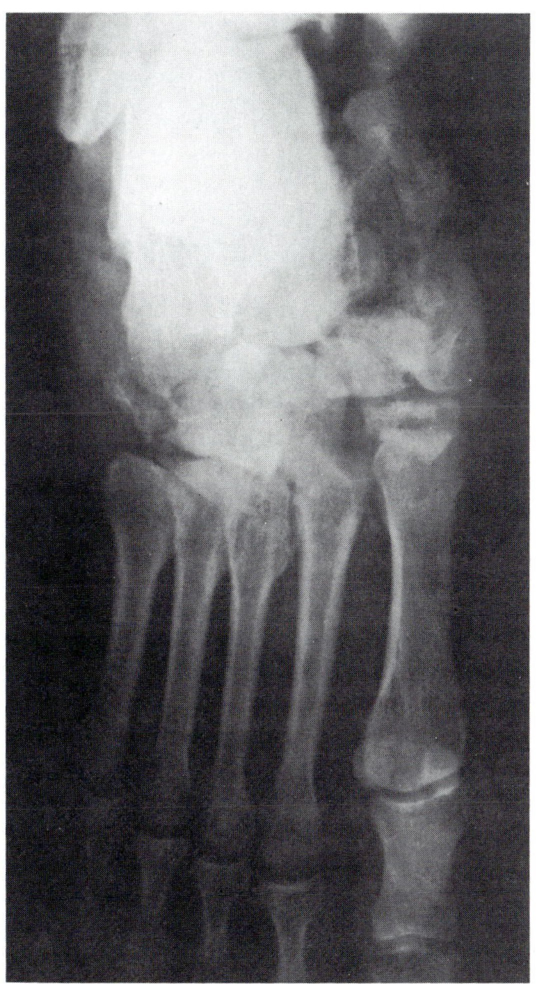

FIG 35–131.
Crush injury with severe comminution of the tarsal bones. (From Main BJ, Jowett RL: *J Bone Joint Surg [Br]* 57:89–97, 1975. Used by permission.)

Main and Jowett[21] used the direction of the deforming force and resultant displacement to formulate their classification. Therefore, the mechanism of injury is considered in the treatment of each type of midtarsal injury. Medial fracture-sprains, subluxations, and dislocations are produced by inversion strains or adduction stress to the forefoot. Medial swivel dislocations are produced by a medial force to the forefoot (secondary to a fall) that disrupts the talonavicular joint and leaves the calcaneonavicular joint intact. The foot rotates medially on the calcaneocuboid joint but does not invert or evert.

Longitudinal injuries result from forces being applied to the metatarsal rays with the ankle in fixed plantar flexion. This compresses the navicular between the head of the talus and the cuneiforms. The exact fracture pattern is dependent on the magnitude of the force and the degree of ankle plantar flexion.

Lateral fracture-sprains and subluxations result from valgus forces being applied to the forefoot (usually in a fall). This mechanism is the same as that proposed by Dewar and Evans.[5] Lateral swivel dislocations are produced by a valgus and rotational force (i.e., a missed step) that causes a lateral dislocation of the talonavicular joint while the calcaneocuboid joint remains intact.

Plantar fracture-sprains and fracture-subluxations or dislocations result when plantarly directed forces are applied to the dorsum of the forefoot such as occur when the foot is twisted beneath the body in a fall.

Finally, crush injuries of the midtarsal joint result when direct crushing forces are applied to the plantigrade foot.

Clinical Diagnosis

Although severe crushing often produces midtarsal joint injury,[21] the history of a minor injury to the foot, either a missed step or an inversion sprain, should suggest a midfoot injury. The inability to bear weight on the injured foot is a frequent complaint.[13] In patients who present with a complete dislocation, the forefoot deformity is easily noted.[23] The clinical appearance of the foot (i.e., fixed inversion and equinus of the forefoot, plantar flexion of the forefoot, etc.) is dependent upon the type of dislocation present.[21] An open laceration on the dorsum of the foot following a crushing injury should suggest the possibility of midtarsal joint involvement.[7]

In patients with pain in the midtarsal area but no overt clinical deformity, a physical examination is mandatory to evaluate occult midtarsal fracture-subluxations.[5, 13] There is usually slight swelling on the dorsum of the midtarsal joint.[9, 13, 27] Ecchymosis on the medial and lateral aspects of the foot with encroachment on the sole strongly suggests this injury.[5] Pain is elicited with any attempt at midtarsal motion.[27] Point tenderness over the calcaneocuboid and talonavicular joint is absolute evidence that midtarsal joint injury has occurred and makes further roentgenographic evaluation of the joint essential.[5, 13] Localization of the exact point of tenderness helps to differentiate this injury from an ankle sprain, an entity with which it is often confused.[5] Palpation may reveal a prominence of the talar head, navicular tubercle, or cuboid.[9] Stress applied to the midtarsal joint will usually produce severe pain.

Dewar and Evans[5] report that cases seen late present with pain on weight bearing, a fullness on the medial side of the foot, and depression of the midtarsal joint.

Radiographic Diagnosis

Roentgenographic diagnosis of injuries to the midtarsal joint can be difficult due to their rarity and a lack of familiarity with these injuries.[26] Good-quality anteroposterior, lateral, and oblique roentgenographs of the foot and ankle are essential in confirming the diagnosis.[6, 7] As with other injuries of the foot, frank dislocation is easily recognized; however, an occult midtarsal fracture-subluxation, stressed by Dewar and Evans, may be overlooked unless it is considered when reviewing the films.[5, 7] Because midtarsal fracture-subluxation is often mistaken for an ankle sprain, Dewar and Evans[6] believe that oblique radiographs of the foot should be taken in addition to routine views of the ankle in order to avoid missing this lesion.

When evaluating the radiographs to plan treatment, one must consider two points: first, the degree of subluxation or displacement of the midtarsal joint and, second, the degree of involvement of the articular surfaces of the talonavicular and/or calcaneo cuboid joint.

London[20] describes a special view of the midtarsal joint to diagnose fracture-subluxation in this area. In this special oblique view, the roentgen beam is centered on the talonavicular joint in the plane of the metatarsals and at right angles to the long axis of the foot. He finds this view helpful in more clearly delineating the talonavicular joint.[20] Polytomography and CAT scanning may be useful in delineating the degree of displacement of the articular surface of either the navicular or cuboid that is associated with these subluxations.[26]

When routine radiographs reveal avulsion or flake fractures of the cuboid, navicular, or talus or injuries of the anterior articular surface of the calcaneus, one should not assume that these are isolated injuries but consider them as *definite* evidence of injury (subluxation or a spontaneously reduced dislocation) to the midtarsal joint.[5, 21, 28] Tountas[28] emphasizes that if there is strong clinical suspicion of an injury to the midtarsal joint but plain roentgenographic findings are negative, a bone scan or possibly a CAT scan should be utilized to detect these occult injuries. Stress radiographs taken with the forefoot first in abduction and then in adduction may also be helpful in confirming an associated fracture-subluxation or a spontaneously reduced dislocation. If the pain is severe, anesthesia may be required for these stress radiographs.

Finally, careful evaluation of the postreduction roentgenographs to ensure reduction of *all* components of the midtarsal injury is critical to avoid minor degrees of persistent subluxation.

Treatment

Treatment of injuries to the midtarsal joint has classically been by closed methods. Kenwright and Taylor[19] recommend closed reduction and immobilization in a below-the-knee cast with the foot in a plantigrade position. Weight bearing is allowed after an average of 5 weeks, and immobilization is discontinued after 8 weeks. They recommend open reduction in cases in which closed reduction is not successful. In severe fracture-dislocations that are unstable, they recommend open reduction and fixation with a Kirschner wire.

Dewar and Evans[5] in discussing the occult fracture-subluxation of the midtarsal joint recommend, if patients are seen early, reduction of the subluxation, reattachment of the avulsed navicular fragment, and calcaneocuboid arthrodesis. Treatment by plaster immobilization alone following closed reduction resulted in persistent disability in their series.[5] Tountas,[28] Howie et al.[16] and Stark[27] also stress that with early diagnosis occult fracture-subluxations of the midtarsal joint can be effectively managed by conservative means. Tountas[28] recommends that for sufficient soft-tissue and osseous healing, the period of cast immobilization should be extended for at least 6 weeks, during which time weight bearing is restricted. These authors believe that a shorter period of immobilization and unrestricted weight bearing are often associated with unsatisfactory results.

On the contrary, Stark[27] recommended that occult fracture-subluxations of the midtarsal joint, when associated with a fracture of the navicular tubercle, be treated conservatively *if* the patient is seen early and is able to invert the foot against resistance. He used a short-leg cast and allowed walking after the first week. The cast was removed at 3 weeks and the patient allowed to bear weight. He believes that a fracture of the navicular tubercle can be ignored if the patient is able to invert the foot adequately, a fact that suggests that the remaining slips of the tibialis posterior tendon are intact.

Hillegass[14] emphasized that accurate reduction is the key to successful treatment. He recommends internal fixation when instability is present following the reduction. In patients with severe fractures, Hillegass gives consideration to early midtarsal arthrodesis.[14]

Friedmann[10] reported primary arthrodesis in a patient in whom a tibial strut graft was used in the midtarsal area to bridge a gap between the anterior portion of the talus and the first cuneiform that resulted from comminution of the talus and navicular. Although this case was not a simple midtarsal dislocation, the use of a graft to restore the length of the medial longitudinal arch is an important principle.

Both Main and Jowett,[21] and Shelton and Pedowitz[26] stressed the importance of the accuracy of reduction of all midtarsal injuries to prevent long-term sequelae. By far the most complete discussion of treatment of midtarsal joint injuries is that of Main and Jowett.[21] In medial fracture-sprains and fracture-subluxations or dislocations, they recommend empiric treatment with strapping or a plaster cast *after* reduction of dislocation. Their only failures occurred when reduction was not obtained. Shelton and Pedowitz[26] believe that these injuries are potentially unstable and therefore recommend plaster immobilization in a short-leg cast for 6 weeks, followed by 2 weeks in a walking plaster cast. They recommend percutaneous Kirschner wire stabilization when swelling, circulatory problems, or skin conditions prevent adequate plaster immobilization. Medial swivel dislocations are treated by closed reduction and immobilization by Main and Jowett.[21] Shelton and Pedowitz[26] recommend treating these medial swivel dislocations by anatomic reduction, which usually requires an open reduction because of interposed soft tissue. Following open reduction, a non–weight-bearing cast is used for 6 weeks with or without Kirschner wire fixation.

In longitudinal injuries, Main and Jowett[21] demonstrated that the clinical result is directly related to the displacement on standard radiographs, the severity of the injury, and the failure to achieve reduction. In undisplaced fractures, simple plaster immobilization produced a good result. In displaced fractures, reduction by closed or open means followed by plaster immobilization was utilized.[21] Main and Jowett[21] did not recommend early arthrodesis in these patients. Shelton and Pedowitz[26] recommend prompt anatomic reduction of displaced fractures followed by temporary Kirschner wire fixation.

In lateral injuries, Main and Jowett[21] utilized closed reduction and cast immobilization or strapping. They noted that the prognosis after lateral fracture-sprains, fracture-subluxations, and dislocations is worse than that following medial injuries due to involvement of the lateral stabilizing arch of the foot and the calcaneocuboid joint. Shelton and Pedowitz[26] believe that lateral fracture-sprains are potentially unstable and recommend treatment by plaster immobilization for 6 weeks. In fracture-subluxations and dislocations, the injury usually produces a subluxation of the talonavicular joint and comminution of the anterior column of the calcaneus or the cuboid that result in collapse of the lateral longitudinal arch.[26] Comminution of the calcaneocuboid joint in these instances is a major problem. They recommend open reduction but state that it does not guarantee restoration of a smooth and stable articulation. In lateral swivel dislocations they suggest closed reduction and cast immobilization.

Plantar injuries are treated by closed reduction and plaster immobilization by Main and Jowett.[21] Shelton and Pedowitz[26] recommend closed reduction followed by immobilization for 6 to 8 weeks for plantar fracture-subluxations and dislocations. If closed reduction is not successful, open reduction and temporary fixation of the talonavicular joint with Kirschner wires is recommended.[26]

In crushing injuries of the midtarsal joint, anatomic fixation of the comminuted fractures is not possible or practical. Despite persistent displacement, Main and Jowett found that none of their patients required secondary surgery.[21]

Main and Jowett[21] do not recommend early arthrodesis as has been recommended by Watson-Jones[31] and Dick[6] following midtarsal injuries. However, for persistent symptoms following medial or longitudinal injuries, they found triple arthrodesis better than talonaviculocuneiform arthrodesis or midtarsal arthrodesis for this injury. A naviculocuneiform arthrodesis in addition to the triple arthrodesis, as suggested by Friedmann[10] did not seem warranted in their experience.[24, 25]

Complications

Pennal[23] clearly documented that midtarsal dislocations unassociated with fractures had minimal disability at late review. However, dislocations associated with even marginal fractures resulted in varying degrees of disability.

Dewar and Evans[5] stressed the importance of early recognition and treatment of the occult fracture-subluxation to avoid long-term disability. In their series only one patient was seen in the first week of injury, the remaining patients being initially misdiagnosed as having ankle sprains. In the cases diagnosed late, it was necessary to correct the deformity, fuse the calcaneocuboid joint, and elongate the lateral side of the foot to correct length lost due to the compression fracture involving the calcaneocuboid joint. Early diagnosis and correct treatment should prevent these problems.

Hooper and McMaster[15] reported a case of recurrent subluxation of the midtarsal joint *in spite of* adequate immobilization. Recurrent subluxation has previously been associated with inadequate immobilization and hypermobility of the joints,[15] but in their case, the patient was adequately immobilized, and there were no signs of systemic ligamentous laxity.

Due to the direct relationship of inadequate reduction and poor results,[5, 21, 26] obtaining *and* maintaining an anatomic reduction are necessary to obtain a good result. Fahey and Murphy[9] reported recurrent subluxation requiring triple arthrodesis in a patient treated by open reduction *without* internal fixation. Therefore, percutaneous fixation should be considered in cases where stability is in question.[26]

Shelton and Pedowitz[26] report that both medial and lateral fracture-sprains, when treated correctly, seldom produce long-term disability. However, medial and lateral fracture-subluxation or dislocation are associated with a greater degree of articular damage to both the talonavicular and calcaneocuboid joints and may therefore result in persistent long-term disability, even with adequate treatment. Similarly, their patients with longitudinal and crush injuries, both representing increasing degrees of articular cartilage damage at the midtarsal joint, were noted to have increased disability. They reported midtarsal thickening, stiffness, swelling, and a loss of the longitudinal arches following crush injuries that may require shoe modifications on a long-term basis.[26] They mentioned the possibility of avascular necrosis of the navicular following this type of injury. Kenwright and Taylor[19] also report that these navicular fractures can lead to talonavicular arthritis and possibly require arthrodesis. They stress, however, that the development of aseptic necrosis of the navicular may not preclude a good result.[19]

Main and Jowett[21] distinguish between pure longitudinal and longitudinal medial injuries. In pure longitudinal injuries, unreduced severe displacement produced a poor result, while in longitudinal medial injuries, severe displacement may be compatible with a satisfactory result. This is because in the longitudinal medial group, although displaced medially, the arch is usually preserved.

Dewar and Evans[5] and Main and Jowett[21] stress that the disability following lateral fracture-subluxations or dislocations is best treated by calcaneocuboid arthrodesis rather than a triple arthrodesis. However, following medial or longitudinal injuries, they suggest triple arthrodesis rather than naviculocuneiform[25] arthrodesis.

Author's Preferred Method of Treatment

Grossly evident midtarsal dislocations and fracture-dislocations should be obvious to any examiner. However, a high index of suspicion is essential in diagnosing fracture-sprains and fracture-subluxations involving the midtarsal joint. A clinical examination that documents tenderness in the area of the talonavicular and/or calcaneocuboid joints following a twisting injury to the foot *demands* clear anteroposterior, lateral, and oblique radiographs of the foot.

Avulsion or marginal fractures in the area of the talonavicular or calcaneocuboid joint noted on routine roentgenographs suggest the diagnosis of a midtarsal fracture-sprain, fracture-subluxation, or a spontaneously reduced fracture-dislocation. I have found the special oblique radiograph demonstrated by London helpful in documenting the degree of associated damage to the navicular and cuboid. Additionally, polytomography and/or CT scanning are occasionally utilized to evaluate associated intra-articular fractures.

In cases of fracture-sprain, subluxation, or suspected spontaneously reduced dislocation, I consider evaluation of midtarsal joint stability *essential* because the degree of stability determines my treatment decision. Stress roentgenographs are helpful in demonstrating the degree of associated ligamentous injury. If pain or swelling prevents this stress examination, I consider examination under anesthesia to document the presence or absence of instability. I will discuss specific treatment recommendations by using the classification of Main and Jowett.[21]

Medial Injuries

Medial fracture-sprains, although clinically stable, have the potential to become displaced. Therefore, I treat these injuries in a short-leg walking cast with the foot in the neutral position for 4 weeks. Following this, a hard-soled shoe with a longitudinal arch support is recommended until the patient is pain free. In medial fracture-subluxation or dislocation, I take great care to ensure that an anatomic reduction is obtained. Due to the instability inherent in these injuries, I prefer percutaneous Kirschner wire stabilization and immobilization in a short-leg cast. These patients are kept non–weight bearing for 3 weeks, followed by 3 weeks in a weight-bearing cast. In medial swivel dislocations, I attempt a closed reduction. If the reduction is not anatomic, I proceed directly to open reduction. Following closed or open reduction, percutaneous Kirschner wire fixation of the talonavicular joint is performed. The foot is immobilized in a short-leg non–weight-bearing cast for 6 weeks. A hard-soled shoe and good arch support are then recommended.

Longitudinal Injuries

In longitudinal injuries, nondisplaced fractures are treated with immobilization in a short-leg walking cast for 4 to 6 weeks. In cases with displaced fractures of the navicular, open reduction and internal fixation with AO screws or Kirschner wires are considered, depending on the degree of comminution. This is followed by immobilization in a short-leg cast for 6 weeks. The patients are advised of the possibility of aseptic necrosis of the navicular and of degenerative arthritis of the talonavicular joint after these injuries. A longitudinal arch support is usually needed on a long-term basis. Aseptic necrosis of the navicular without collapse may not require later treatment. I am unaware of any *documented* successful method of preventing collapse once aseptic necrosis is noted.

Lateral Injuries

Lateral fracture-sprains are treated in a short-leg walking cast for 4 to 6 weeks. Fracture-subluxations, on the other hand, are usually associated with comminution of the lateral column of the foot, i.e., either the anterior portion of the calcaneus or the cuboid. In these injuries, comminution of the calcaneocuboid joint, in my experience, has led to long-term disability. Therefore, careful evaluation by polytomography is undertaken to see whether reconstruction of the articular surface of the cuboid is possible. If open reduction is possible, it is followed by short-leg non–weight bearing cast immobilization for 6 weeks. This is followed by an intensive period of physical therapy and ambulation in a stiff-soled shoe. If comminution of the articular surface is too severe, closed reduction and immobilization in a short-leg non–weight-bearing cast for 3 to 6 weeks are utilized. Long-term disability may require calcaneocuboid fusion.

Lateral swivel dislocations are treated by closed reduction followed by immobilization in a short-leg cast for 6 weeks. Progressive weight bearing is then instituted.

Plantar Injuries

Plantar fracture-subluxations and dislocations are treated by closed reduction and plaster immobilization for 6 weeks. In those cases in which closed reduction is not possible, I proceed to open reduction and percutaneous Kirschner wire fixation of the talonavicular and calcaneocuboid joints. A short-leg non–weight-bearing cast is used for 6 weeks, at which time the Kirschner wires are removed, and weight bearing and a stiff-soled shoe or short-leg cast are then instituted.

Crushing Injuries

In crushing injuries of the midfoot, I attempt a closed reduction. Due to instability, I prefer Kirschner wire stabilization. Any swelling is allowed to subside before a cast is applied. My decision to attempt an open reduction is based upon the ability to achieve anatomic reduction of the fracture fragments. Usually this is not possible due to severe comminution. Therefore, immobilization of these comminuted injuries with attention to molding of the arch in a non–weight-bearing cast for 4 to 6 weeks followed by a stiff-soled shoe with a longitudinal arch support is recommended.

The use of percutaneous Kirschner wires to prevent the redislocation of these injuries that may occur in a cast as swelling subsides should be considered in all cases. In all midtarsal injuries, the short-leg cast leaves the metatarsophalangeal joints free to allow early metatarsophalangeal motion. After cast immobilization, range-of-motion exercises and swimming pool or hydrotherapy may be useful. The long-term use of a stiff-soled shoe with a longitudinal arch support may be necessary.

REFERENCES

Midtarsal Joint

1. Bohler L: *The treatment of fractures*, ed 5, vol 3, New York, 1958, Grune & Stratton.
2. Boidard CAN: Contributiona l'etude des luxations astragalo— scaphoidiennes (thesis), University of Bordeaux, 1939.
3. Chapman MW: Fractures and fracture-dislocations of the ankle and foot. In Mann RA, editor: *DuVries' surgery of the foot*, ed 4, St Louis, 1978, Mosby–Year Book.
4. Conwell HE, Reynolds FC: *Key and Conwell's management of fractures, dislocations and sprains*, ed 7, St Louis, 1961, Mosby–Year Book.
5. Dewar FP, Evans DC: Occult fracture-subluxation of the midtarsal joint, *J Bone Joint Surg [Br]* 50:386–388, 1968.
6. Dick IL: Occult fracture-dislocation of the tarsal navicular, *Proc R Soc Med* 35:760.
7. Dixon JH: Letter to the editor, *Injury* 10:251, 1979.
8. Drummond PS, Hastings DE: Total dislocation of the cuboid bone, *J Bone Joint Surg [Br]* 51:716–718, 1969.
9. Fahey JJ, Murphy JL: Dislocations and fractures of the talus, *Surg Clin North Am* 45:79–102, 1965.
10. Friedmann E: Key graft fixation in mid-tarsal fracture dislocation, *Am J Surg* 96:81–83, 1958.
11. Giannestras NG, Sammarco GJ: Fractures and dislocations in the foot. In Rockwood CA Jr, Green DP, editors: *Fractures*, Philadelphia, 1975, JB Lippincott.
12. Gilland FAE: Les luxations isolees du scaphoid tarsien (thesis), University of Nancy, 1936.
13. Hermel MB, Gershon-Cohen J: The nutcracker fracture of the cuboid by indirect violence, *Radiology* 60:850–854, 1953.
14. Hillegass RC: Injuries to the mid foot: a major cause of industrial morbidity. In Bateman JE, editor: *Foot science*, Philadelphia, 1976, WB Saunders.
15. Hooper G, McMaster M: Recurrent bilateral mid-tarsal subluxations, *J Bone Joint Surg [Am]* 61:617–619, 1979.
16. Howie CR, Hooper G, Hughes SPF: Occult midtarsal subluxation, *Clin Orthop* 209:206, 1986.
17. Jaslow IA: Fracture-dislocation of the mid-tarsal and cuboideonavicular joints, *J Bone Joint Surg* 28:386–388, 1946.
18. Jones FW: Structure and fixation as seen in the foot, London, 1944, Bailliere, Tindall, Cox, p 246.
19. Kenwright J, Taylor RG: Major injuries of the talus, *J Bone Joint Surg [Br]* 52:36–48, 1970.
20. London PS: Wrinkle corner. A special view for midtarsal fracture-subluxation, *Injury* 5:65, 1973.
21. Main BJ, Jowett RL: Injuries of the mid-tarsal joint, *J Bone Joint Surg [Br]* 57:89–97, 1975.
22. McLaughlin HL: *Trauma*, Philadelphia, 1959, WB Saunders.
23. Pennal GF: Fractures of the talus, *Clin Orthop* 30:53–63, 1963.
24. Sarrafian SK: *Anatomy of the foot and ankle. Descriptive, topographic, functional*, Philadelphia, 1983, JB Lippincott.
25. Seymour N: The late results of naviculo-cuneiform fusion, *J Bone Joint Surg [Br]* 49:558–559, 1967.
26. Shelton ML, Pedowitz WJ: Injuries to the talus and midfoot. In Jahss MH, editor: *Disorders of the foot*, vol 2, Philadelphia, 1982, WB Saunders.
27. Stark WA: Occult fracture-subluxation of the midtarsal joint, *Clin Orthop* 93:291–292, 1973.
28. Tountas AA: Occult fracture-subluxation of the midtarsal joint, *Clin Orthop* 243:195–199, 1989.
29. Van Hove R: Luxation partielle de l'articulation de Chopart, *Acta Orthop Belg* 23:67–72, 1957.
30. Waters CH: Midtarsal fractures and dislocations, *Instr Course Lect* 9:368–374, 1952.
31. Watson-Jones R: *Fractures and joint injuries*, ed 4, vol 2, Baltimore, 1955, Williams & Wilkins.
32. Weh R: Ueber die isolierte luxation in talonaviculargelenk (thesis), University of Munich, 1939.
33. Willigens JEF: Contribution a l'etude de la luxation du scaphoid tarsien (thesis), University of Nancy, 1936.

TARSOMETATARSAL DISLOCATIONS

The tarsometatarsal joint, which consists of the bases of the five metatarsals and their articulation with the three cuneiforms and the cuboid, is named after Lisfranc, a French surgeon in the army of Napoleon who originally described an amputation through that joint.[14, 30, 39, 56] According to Cassebaum,[14] Lisfranc never actually wrote on the subject of fracture-dislocation of the tarsometatarsal joint, his name being attached to the dislocation simply because he described the amputation.

Dislocations and fracture-dislocations of the tarsometatarsal joint are rare injuries and are reported to occur at the rate of 1 person per 55,000 per year.[2, 23, 26, 39, 59] English reports that only 0.2% of all fractures involve this joint.[26] However, Del Sel[22] feels that this injury is more common than is generally supposed. Lenczner et al.,[48] Bassett,[8] and O'Regan[58] report that the injury was more common when the horse was the major means of transportation. In those days, being dragged by a horse with a foot caught in the stirrup was the common method of the injury. Today, motorcycle accidents produce a similar mechanism of injury.[23] Also, an increase in the incidence of motor vehicle accidents is believed by Lenczner et al.[48] to be responsible for an increasing incidence of injuries to the tarsometatarsal joint today. Wilson[71] reports that now 64% of all tarsometatarsal joint injuries are the result of road traffic accidents. According to Myerson et al.,[55] 81% of patients had sufficient additional major injuries to be considered polytrauma patients. Additionally, Coker and Arnold[17] and O'Donoghue[57] report that injuries to the tarsometatarsal joints are occurring with increasing frequency in athletic events.

Due to the fact that the metatarsals may be displaced with or without an associated fracture and that they may be displaced in a dorsal, ventral, medial, lateral, or any combination of these directions in relation to the hindfoot, a working classification is essential in understanding the diagnosis and treatment of these injuries.[59] It is important that one distinguish between a total dislocation in which all the metatarsals are dislocated and partial dislocations in which some but not all of the metatarsals are dislocated from the tarsometatarsal joint.[56, 72]

Although these dislocations present with a great deal of individual variation, in general, they have similar patterns of displacement.[15] Various classifications of tarsometatarsal dislocations have been presented.[16, 24, 39, 58–60] Quenu and Kuss[60] proposed a classification that is both simple and useful. They divided all these injuries into three types of dislocations: (1) homolateral dislocations in which all five metatarsals are displaced in the coronal plane, (2) isolated dislocations in which one or two metatarsals are displaced in the coronal plane, and (3) divergent dislocations in which there is a separation between the first and second metatarsals and the displacement occurs in the sagittal as well as the coronal plane. The simplicity of this classification system has made it attractive to many authors reporting tarsometatarsal injuries.[3, 33, 47]

Alternatively, O'Regan[58] utilizes a very simple classification system based upon displacement. Uniform dislocations are those in which all the metatarsals are displaced in the same direction, while divergent dislocations are those in which the first metatarsal moves medially away from the remaining four metatarsals. He emphasizes that the deformity may involve one, all, or any combination of the metatarsals.[58] O'Regan[58] and Granberry and Lipscomb[37] emphasized that fractures involving the tarsometatarsal joint are usually present with these dislocations.

Hardcastle et al.[39] used the classification of Quenu and Kuss as a basis for a classification that they developed and upon which they believe treatment can be based (Fig 35–132).

Type A: Total.—In these injuries there is incongruity of the entire tarsometatarsal joint. The displacement is in one plane, which may be sagittal, coronal, or combined.

Type B: Partial.—In these injuries there is incongruity of a part of the tarsometatarsal joint. The displaced segment is in one plane, which may be sagittal, coronal, or combined. There are two types of partial dislocations whose treatment and prognosis differ:

1. Medial dislocations.—Displacement affects the first metatarsal either in isolation or combined with displacement of one or more of the second, third, or fourth metatarsals.
2. Lateral dislocations.—Displacement affects one or more of the lateral four metatarsals. The first metatarsal is not affected.

Type C: Divergent.—In these injuries there may be partial or total incongruity. On the anteroposterior radiograph the first metatarsal is displaced medially while any combination of the lateral four metatarsals is displaced laterally. Sagittal displacement also occurs in conjunction with coronal displacement.

I prefer to use the classification of Hardcastle et al.[39] because of its relationship to the indicated treatment.

Anatomy

The tarsometatarsal joint consists of the five metatarsal bones, three cuneiforms, and the cuboid. The medial three metatarsals articulate individually with one of the three cuneiforms. The cuboid articulates with the fourth and fifth metatarsals. The second metatarsal is the longest of all metatarsals, while the second cuneiform is the shortest of the cuneiforms. This produces an indentation in the line of the cuneiforms into which the long second metatarsal fits (Fig 35–133,A).[31, 47] Lenczner et al.[48] emphasize that the stability of the second metatarsal base is the key to the structure of the tarsometatarsal joint. The second metatarsal has a broader dorsal surface and a narrow ventral surface, which makes this bone resemble the keystone of a Roman arch in shape, position, and function (Fig 35–133,B).[8, 48] Because of its recessed position between the medial and lateral cuneiforms, the second metatarsal articulates with all three cuneiforms.[12] Cain and Seligson[12] also report that the second metatarsal holds the keystone position of the tarsometatarsal joint and that no significant dislocation of the metatarsals or cuneiforms can occur unless this keystone is disrupted.

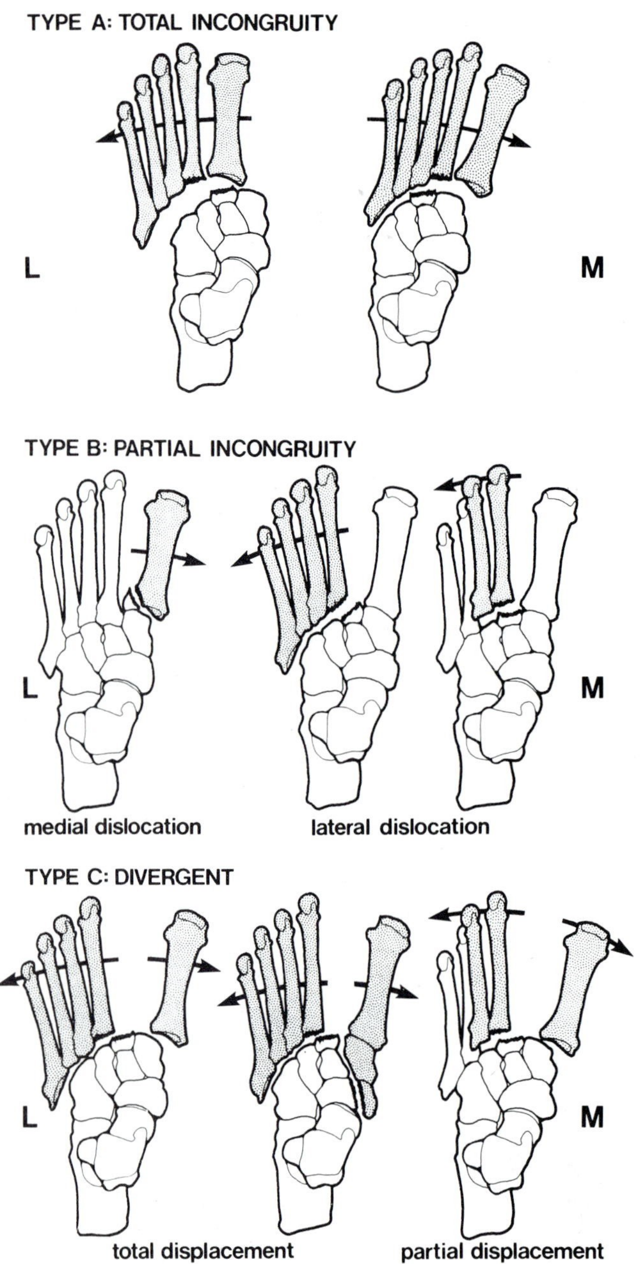

FIG 35–132.
Classification of Lisfranc fracture-dislocations. (Adapted from Hardcastle PH, Reschauer R, Kutscha-Lissberg E, et al: *J Bone Joint Surg [Br] 64:349–359, 1982.)*

Anderson[3] reports that it is indeed rare to see a tarsometatarsal dislocation without a fracture of the base of the second metatarsal, and Aitken and Poulson[2] emphasize that only if this recess is unusually shallow can a dislocation occur without a fracture of the second metatarsal. Additionally, Cain and Seligson[12] believe that the second cuneiform is an important element in the integrity of the transverse arch of the foot. Along with its nonmobile articulation with the second metatarsal, it constitutes the longitudinal axis of the foot.

In addition to the stability provided by the bone anatomy, the ligmentous structures of the tarsometatarsal joint are instrumental in instability. The second, third, fourth, and fifth metatarsal bases are bound to each other by transverse ligaments located on both the dorsal and plantar aspects of the joint. The plantar liga-

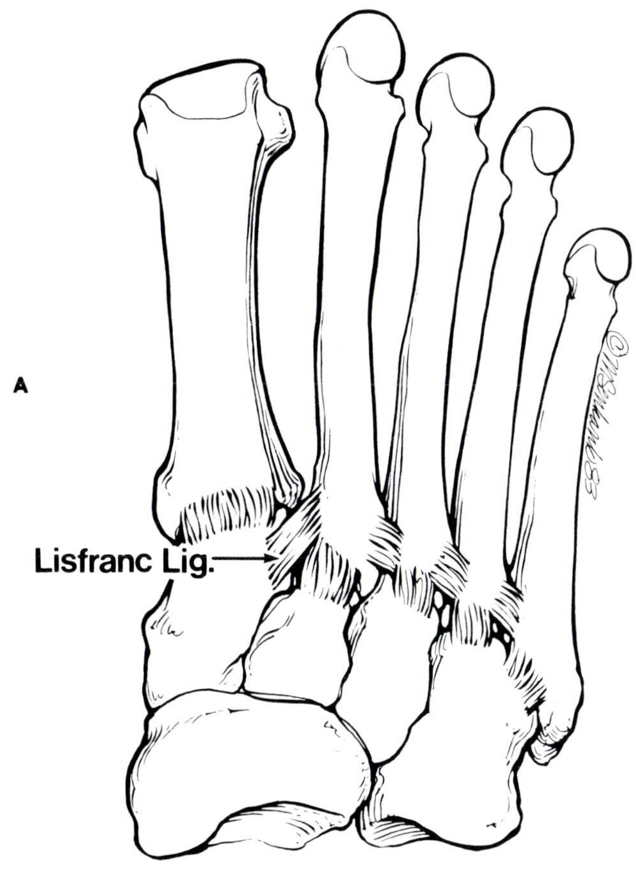

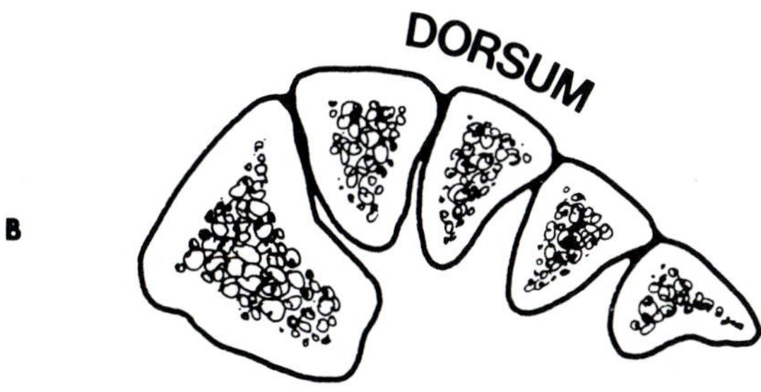

FIG 35–133.
A, diagram of the dorsal aspect of the foot. The base of the second metatarsal is mortised between three cuneiforms. The second, third, and fourth metatarsals are connected to each other by dorsal and plantar transverse ligaments. There is no transverse ligament between the bases of the first and second metatarsals. The lateral four metatarsals are attached to the first cuneiform by an obliquely placed Lisfranc ligament. **B,** transverse section of the metatarsals. Note that the dorsum of the second metatarsal is wider than the plantar aspect.

ments support the arch and are much stronger than the dorsal ligaments.[18] There is no ligament between the bases of the great and second metatarsals; instead, the metatarsal is attached primarily to the first cuneiform by an obliquely placed plantar and dorsal ligament. This oblique ligament, termed Lisfranc's ligament,[44] is important in that it is responsible for the avulsion fractures of the base of the second metatarsal so frequently seen in these fracture-dislocations.[3] The oblique ligament of Lisfranc is so placed that when an abduction force is applied to the metatarsus, it results in rupture or avulsion of the ligamentous insertion or fracture of the base of the second metatarsal, which permits lateral dislocation of the foot.[18]

The great toe metatarsal is secured to the medial cuneiform by ligaments placed in an axial direction (Fig 35–133,A). These ligaments permit marked abduction before yielding, and great force is necessary to disrupt their attachments.[18] The insertion of the anterior tibial tendon on the medial aspect of the proximal first metatarsal and the insertion of the peroneus longus tendon into the lateral aspect of the proximal first metatarsal are both factors adding to the security of the first metatarsal cuneiform joint.

The structures on the sole of the foot, including the plantar fascia, the intrinsic foot muscles, and the stronger plantar tarsometatarsal ligaments, make plantar dislocation unlikely. On the other hand, the soft tissue overlying the dorsal aspect of these joints is rather scant.[2, 3] These anatomic facts are responsible for displacements being most always dorsal and lateral.[9] Finally, the location of the junction of the dorsalis pedis artery with the plantar arterial arch at the proximal end of the space between the first and second metatarsals places this artery at risk for injury with any type of tarsometatarsal dislocation.[34]

Mechanism of Injury

The forces responsible for tarsometatarsal dislocation can be classified as direct and indirect.* A direct force such as a truck running over the foot or a heavy weight being dropped directly on the foot[47] results in plantar dislocation[41, 47, 58, 61] of the metatarsal bases. Secondary medial or lateral displacement may occur depending upon the exact nature of the applied force.[39] The mechanism of direct force produces extensive soft-tissue damage, and multiple associated fractures may be common.

**References 33, 39, 41, 44, 47, 58, 69, 71.*

The application of indirect force can also produce tarsometatarsal dislocations.[14, 44, 69, 71] Jumping onto a plantar-flexed foot or the application of a force up through the toes of an equinus-positioned foot can also result in the most common displacement, dorsal and lateral.[14] Jeffreys reported two patterns of indirect injury.[44] First, simple lateral dislocation of the forefoot can be produced by pronation of the hindfoot with a fixed forefoot position. Second, a medial dislocation of the first metatarsocuneiform joint can be produced by supination of the hindfoot with a fixed forefoot; this mechanism is followed by complete dislocation of the forefoot after fracture of the second metatarsal.[44]

Wiley[69] believes that the pattern of the fractured metatarsals and the configuration of the tarsometatarsal joint suggest that the mechanism involved in producing tarsometatarsal dislocations is either violent abduction or plantar flexion of the forefoot. When the forefoot is violently abducted, the brunt of the force is concentrated on the fixed base of the second metatarsal. As the remaining metatarsals slide in mass, the second metatarsal cannot move until it fractures. If lateral displacement of the metatarsals of a significant degree occurs, the cuboid bone may be crushed. Fractures of the cuboid and second metatarsal bones are therefore pathognomonic signs of this abduction type of tarsometatarsal disruption[41, 69] (Fig 35–134). According to Wiley,[44] plantar flexion injuries occur in two ways. First is a force applied to the heel along the axis of the foot when the toes are fixed. This mechanism, described in the early literature, occurred when cavalrymen were thrown from their horses. As the horse tumbles to the ground, it falls on the soldier and pins his foot to the ground. Second, plantar flexion of the foot is commonly noted in motor vehicle accidents, a situation that is far more common in today's society.[44] In this instance, the ankle is in a plantar-flexed position, and the foot becomes part of a long lever arm consisting of the entire lower portion of the leg. With the lower part of the leg and the foot in the same linear axis, a force applied to the end of the foot is transmitted up this axis. If the line of this force is dorsal to the tarsometatarsal joint, the weak dorsal ligament of the joint is disrupted as the force increases. This is also the mechanism of injury seen in Lisfranc stress fractures in female ballet dancers due to standing en pointe.[53] The entire joint complex may dislocate with or without associated fractures. Associated rotation at the time of application of this plantar flexion force can result in various combinations of associated fractures.[34, 44]

Adelaar[1] describes a mechanism common in today's football and rugby competition in which the plantar-flexed foot is planted on the ground and struck from a posterior direction by an opposing player. He describes a similar injury occurring in the performing arts when the loaded foot collapses in the extreme pointe position.[1]

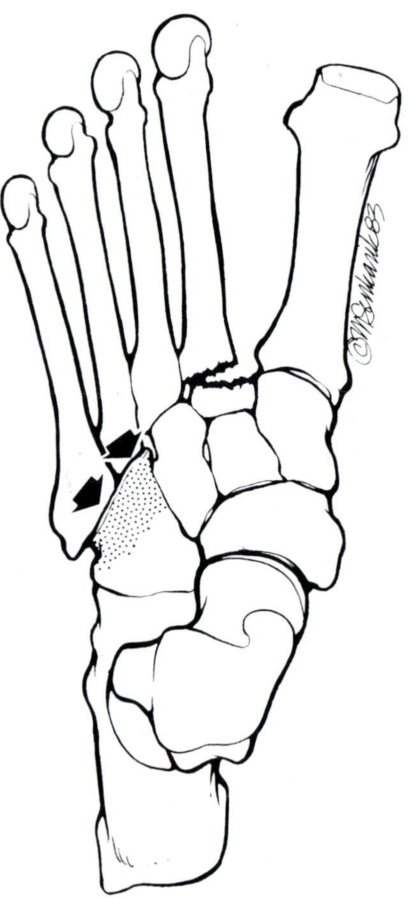

FIG 35–134.
Fractures of the cuboid and second metatarsal bones are pathognomonic signs of tarsometatarsal disruption.

Finally, Wilson demonstrated that tarsometatarsal injuries can result from eversion, inversion, and plantar flexion.[71] Forefoot eversion (pronation) produces two stages of tarsometatarsal injury.[71] The first stage is medial dislocation of the first metatarsal bone alone (the so-called isolated dislocation). The second stage, produced by more eversion, consists of medial dislocation of the first metatarsal *and* dorsolateral dislocation of the four lesser metatarsal bones (the "divergent dislocation"). Forefoot inversion (supination) also produces two stages of injury. Stage 1 injury consists of dorsolateral dislocation of up to four lesser metatarsal bones. The second stage consists of dorsolateral dislocation of all five metatarsal bones. Finally, pure plantar flexion force without rotation produces variable fracture patterns.

In summary, it is important to recognize that these

injuries are not the result of simple inversion, eversion, or plantar flexion mechanisms. They result from a combination of these forces plus rotation along the axis of the foot. Therefore, the injuries may occur with or without fractures depending upon the twisting forces simultaneously applied.[33] The importance in understanding these various mechanisms of injury is that at times the dislocation may have spontaneously reduced and the only clue to the extent of the injury may be the fracture pattern of the tarsal and metatarsal bones.[33]

Clinical Diagnosis

In two groups of patients injuries to the tarsometatarsal joints may be overlooked. First, in the multiply injured patient with severe trauma to other organ systems, closed injuries of the forefoot frequently go undiagnosed.[3, 8, 9] In cases of gross displacement of the metatarsals, the diagnosis is evident. However, the less severely displaced subluxations and those dislocations that spontaneously reduce are likely to be overlooked without a careful physical examination.[5, 68] This may result in considerable disability.[14] In less severely displaced subluxations, the clinical and roentgenographic findings may be subtle and go unrecognized, particularly when attention is focused on more severe injuries and other parts of the body.[68] Finally, simple sprains of the tarsometatarsal joints with or without minimal widening between the first and second metatarsal bases do occur, and their recognition is essential for proper treatment.[17]

The signs and symptoms of tarsometatarsal dislocation vary greatly depending upon the degree of displacement.[3] As mentioned, spontaneous reduction is not unusual and can complicate the diagnosis.[3] The patient usually presents with complaints of severe pain in the midpart of the foot and at times relates a feeling of paresthesia.[3, 33] The patient complains of the inability to bear weight on the foot.[9]

Swelling and associated deformity of the foot are obvious in complete dislocation.[4, 49, 56, 57] The deformity of the foot consists of forefoot equinus, forefoot abduction, and prominence of the medial tarsal area.[9] If the patient is not seen until 2 or more hours after the accident, gross ecchymosis and swelling of the foot are present.[8, 33] Giannestras and Sammarco[33] report that swelling of the foot may occur as soon as 2 hours following the injury. If the injury is seen early before swelling, shortening and displacement of the forefoot may be noticeable.[3, 33] There is diffuse tenderness across the tarsometatarsal joint, and marked pain is experienced upon passive motion.[3, 8] According to Anderson,[3] almost all of these injuries are closed unless they are associated with a crushing blow as the direct mechanism of injury.

The dorsalis pedis pulse may or may not be palpable.[33] Both Gissane,[34] and Groulier and Pinaud[38] reported cases of tarsometatarsal dislocation that required amputation. Although the dislocation occurs at the point of communication between the dorsalis pedis artery and the plantar arch and can result in damage to this communication, Gissane and Del Sel believed that this arterial injury does not endanger the life of the foot unless the posterior tibial or lateral plantar artery is also damaged.[22, 34] However, one must consider these injuries as orthopaedic emergencies requiring prompt reduction to prevent further swelling and vascular compromise.

Radiographic Diagnosis

Radiographs taken in three planes, anteroposterior, lateral, and 30-degree oblique, are essential in order to diagnose the initial displacement and to assess whether or not the reduction is anatomic.[33, 39] It is important to include the entire foot and ankle so that associated injuries are not missed.[39] Granberry and Lipscomb[37] reported that in only 8 of 25 cases were tarsometatarsal dislocations not associated with significant fractures. The authors stress the fact that associated fractures are probably present in all tarsometatarsal dislocations, even though they cannot be demonstrated roentgenographically.[37]

Aitken and Poulson[2] report that fractures of the base of the second metatarsal and compression fractures of the cuboid are the most commonly associated fractures with tarsometatarsal dislocations. Indeed, LaTourette et al.[47] report that fractures of the base of the second metatarsal, consisting of either a large or small fragment, are present in 90% of all tarsometatarsal disclocations. Due to the possibility that a fracture-dislocation has spontaneously reduced and due to the existence of subluxations in which the dislocation is not complete, roentgenographic hints that suggest tarsometatarsal injury are important to note. A fractured base of the second metatarsal with any displacement should suggest an injury to Lisfranc's joint.[33] Myerson et al.[55] described a small bone fragment that represents an avulsion fracture of the medial base of the second metatarsal or lateral base of the first metatarsal as a clue to this injury. They use the term "fleck sign" and found that it was radiographically evident in 90% of their patients with tarsometatarsal injuries. Cain and Seligson[12] report that the presence of an avulsion fracture of the medial pole of the navicular suggests a tarsometatarsal joint injury. Schiller and Ray suggest that the presence of an isolated medial cuneiform dislocation should also suggest that the presence of an unrecognized spontaneously reduced tarsometatarsal injury.[63] Coker and Arnold[17] suggest that a fracture of the base of the second metatarsal, a fracture of a cuboid, and the loss of a few degrees of varus of the first metatarsal are all clues that a tarsometatarsal dislocation has occurred. If one suspects a spontaneously reduced dislocation by the presence of such associated fractures, further evaluation by the use of comparative or stress roentgenographs is essential.

Anderson[3] initially emphasized the importance of evaluating both the relationship of the metatarsals to the cuneiforms and fractures of the base of the second metatarsal in patients with tarsometatarsal injuries. An evaluation of the relationship of the metatarsal bases with the cuneiforms and cuboid is essential, not only in detecting the subluxations of this joint but also in evaluating the quality of reduction. Giannestras and Sammarco[33] stated that the lateral two or three metatarsals tend to be somewhat variable in their relation to the lateral cuneiform and cuboid and that this relationship is less reliable in diagnosing dislocations.[33] In 1976, Foster and Foster[30] reviewed the roentgenographs of 200 feet. They found that the most consistent relationship at the tarsometatarsal joint was the alignment of the medial edge of the base of the second metatarsal with the medial edge of the second cuneiform on the frontal or oblique views. They felt that a space between the first and second metatarsal is, of itself, not evidence of a dislocation unless there is a step-off at the base of the second metatarsal and second cuneiform. Although the medial aspect of the base of the fourth metatarsal is usually aligned with the medial edge of the cuboid, these authors found a slight step-off (1 to 2 mm) in several cases without injury. They found that the base of the first metatarsal usually aligns with the lateral edge of the first cuneiform, but variations occur, particularly when the diameter of the metatarsal base is smaller than that of the third cuneiform. The authors stressed that the base of the third metatarsal usually aligns with the medial aspect of the third cuneiform, but this junction may be difficult to see on routine views. Foster and Foster[30] also emphasized that the position of the fifth metatarsal is often difficult to assess.

Stein[64] reported in 1983 that when all four lateral metatarsals move as a group, dislocation can be readily appreciated. However, he stresses that it is not unusual to see intermetatarsal ligamentous disruption. In these instances, evaluation of the position of only one metatarsal can lead to a missed diagnosis. Stein[64] therefore believes that it is essential for the clinician to assess the anatomic position of *all five* metatarsal shafts as they articulate with the tarsal bones. He reviewed 100 radiologic studies of the foot and observed the following constant anatomic relationships:

1. The medial border of the fourth metatarsal always forms a continuous straight line with the medial border of the cuboid on the medial oblique view (Fig 35–135).
2. The intermetatarsal space between the third and fourth metatarsals is continuous with the intertarsal space between the lateral cuneiform and the cuboid. Therefore, the lateral border of the third metatarsal shaft forms a straight line with the lateral border of the lateral cuneiform (see Fig 35–135).
3. On the medial oblique view, the intermetatarsal space between the second and third metatarsals is continuous and in a straight line with the intertarsal space between the lateral and middle cuneiforms (see Fig 35–135).
4. On the anteroposteior view, the medial border of the second metatarsal forms a continuous straight line

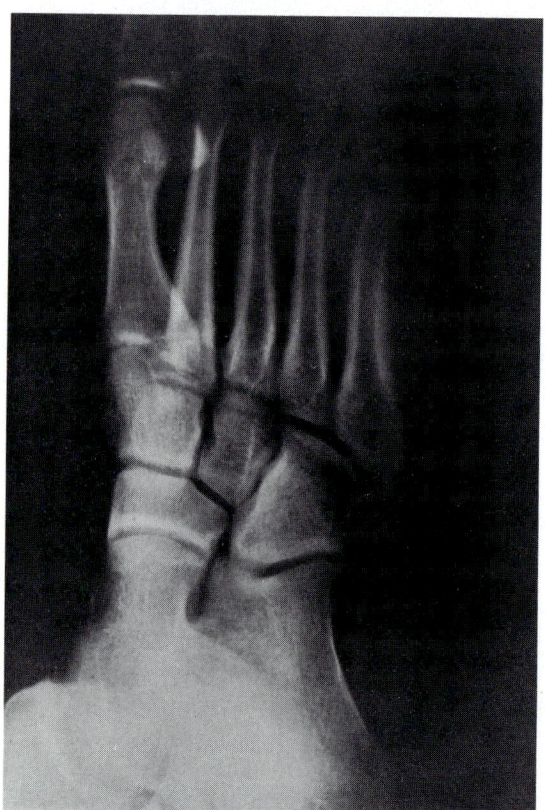

FIG 35–135.
Medial oblique view of the foot. The medial border of the cuboid and fourth metatarsal form a continuous line. The lateral border of the third metatarsal forms a continuous line with the lateral border of the third cuneiform. The intermetatarsal space between the second and third metatarsals is continuous with the intertarsal space between the middle and lateral cuneiforms.

with the medial border of the middle cuneiform (Fig 35–136).

5. Therefore, the intermetatarsal space between the first and second metatarsals is continuous with the intertarsal space between the medial and middle cuneiform (Fig 35–136).

6. The first metatarsal aligns itself with the medial cuneiform medially and laterally (Fig 35–136).

Stein stressed that these relationships are constant regardless of the rotation of the foot when the roentgenographs are taken.

Stein also emphasizes that it is difficult to assess the position of the fifth metatarsal in relation to the cuboid. However, the fourth and fifth metatarsals almost always move as a unit in their relationship to the cuboid, even if there is a disruption of the intermetatarsal ligaments between the third and fourth metatarsals. Therefore, an evaluation of the position of the fourth metatarsal will be satisfactory in assessing the position of the fifth.[64]

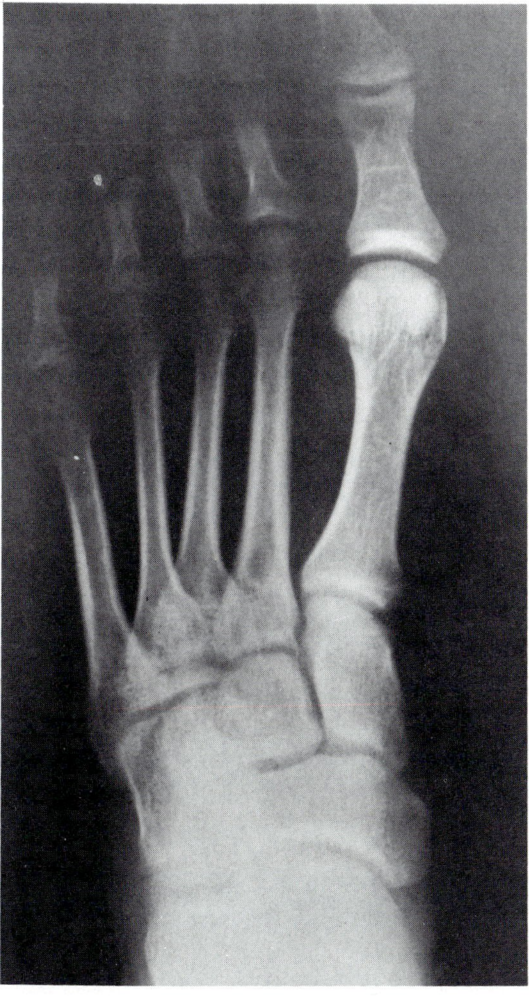

FIG 35–136.
Anteroposterior view of the foot. The medial border of the second metatarsal forms a continuous straight line with the medial border of the middle cuneiform. The intermetatarsal space between the first and second metatarsals is continuous with the intertarsal space between the medial and middle cuneiforms. The first metatarsal is aligned with the medial cuneiform medially and laterally.

Stein stresses that a lateral view of the foot is essential to complete the radiologic evaluation since dorsal subluxation of the metatarsal bases (particularly metatarsals 2 and 3) may not be readily apparent on the anteroposterior or oblique views of the foot.

Faciszewski[27] found that the measurement of the distance between the plantar surfaces of the medial cuneiform and the fifth metatarsal base on the weight-bearing lateral radiograph is a reliable indicator of how much flattening of the longitudinal arch has occurred. Normally, the medial cuneiform is dorsal to the base of the fifth metatarsal. With flattening of the longitudinal arch, these relationships become reversed, with the medial cuneiform plantar to the fifth metatarsal base. Foster[29] reported that the normal talometatarsal angle from the lateral weight-bearing radiograph measures 0 to 10 degrees.

Additionally, Brown and McFarland[10] emphasized that in most tarsometatarsal dislocations the naviculocuneiform joint remains intact while the metatarsals are displaced. However, occasionally the naviculocuneiform joint is disrupted in conjuction with tarsometatarsal fracture-dislocations. This results in complete dislocation of the medial cuneiform with a Lisfranc dislocation.[10] Cain and Seligson[12] stressed the importance of recognizing this variation of a tarsometatarsal dislocation because it is essential to reduce the medial cuneiform *before* the tarsometatarsal dislocation can be reduced.

Finally, English[26] emphasizes the importance of evaluating the metatarsophalangeal joints on the roentgenographs of patients with tarsometatarsal dislocations. One is likely to overlook a dislocation of the metatarsophalangeal joint due to the more impressive appearing dislocation of the tarsometatarsal joint. English refers to this injury combination as the "linked-toe dislocation of the metatarsal bone." He stresses the importance of recognizing the metatarsophalangeal joint dislocation because reduction of this dislocation is dependent upon accurate reduction of the fracture-dislocation of the base of the metatarsal.

Treatment

Treatment of tarsometatarsal dislocations is dependent upon the nature of any associated wound and the amount of swelling present. Care must be taken to rule out significant arterial injury and also compartment syndromes of the foot, which are oftentimes associated with tarsometatarsal dislocations.[54]

The goal of treatment of fracture-dislocations of the tarsometatarsal joints is restoration of a painless and stable plantigrade foot.[36] Geckeler[32] emphasized that unless reduced early and completely, these injuries cause permanent pain and disability. Although there have been reports of minimal symptoms following minimal or no treatment and persistent subluxation,[2, 11, 44, 48] most recent authors emphasize that reduction of the dislocation is essential for a good result.* Key and Conwell[46] stress that an anatomic reduction is a prerequisite for a painless, functioning foot.[46]

Closed reduction should be attempted as soon as possible.[36] If manipulation is carried out immediately, the reduction may be accomplished easily unless a chip fracture interferes with the reduction.[14, 15] Cain and Seligson[12] carefully outlined the technique of manipulative reduction of these injuries. The first step is to restore the length of the foot. Cain and Seligson[12] accomplish this by manually pulling on the metatarsals while the heel is fixed. Once the length is restored, the second metatarsal is reduced into its mortise, thereby reestablishing the transverse arch of the midfoot.[12] Collett et al.[18] also emphasize the importance of applying uniform traction as an essential part of the reduction. They recommend the use of woven wire traps (Chinese finger traps) placed over the toes. The patient is placed in the *prone* position with the foot projecting beyond the end of the table. Anderson[3] also recommends the use of Chinese finger traps applied to the toes to obtain traction. Once the metatarsals are out to length, manipulation of the metatarsals into their proper position is performed. Fitte and Garacotche[28] also use traction, which they obtain with pins through the metatarsals and calcaneus.

Anderson[3] believes that although most of these dislocations can be reduced by closed means, they are unstable. In patients in whom the reduction is not stable, he recommends percutaneous pin fixation to maintain the reduction. He prefers two Steinmann pins, one pin fixing the first metatarsal to the medial cuneiform and a second fixing the fifth metatarsal to the cuboid. He recommends that roentgenographs be taken prior to cast application to be certain that the reduction and the percutaneous pin fixation are accurate. Bassett also recommends Kirschner wire stabilization to prevent displacement after initial reduction.[8] Foster and Foster[30] believe that if anatomic or near-anatomic alignment is achieved by closed means, then cast immobilization can be utilized. They recommend the use of percutaneous Kirschner wire fixation only in cases of unstable reduction. Following successful reduction with or without percutaneous fixation, the patient is placed in a short-leg cast. Cassebaum[14] recommends non–weight bearing for 6 to 8 weeks following reduction. A loss of reduction may also develop when weight bearing is initiated too early.[9] Anderson,[3] Hardcastle et al.[39] and Myerson et al.[55] believe these reductions are inherently unstable and should be secured with percutaneous Kirschner wire fixation.

Adelaar[1] recommends closed treatment by means of placing traction on the second metatarsal, which he feels is the keystone of the foot. After reduction of the second metatarsal complex is achieved, the first metatarsal and the lateral four metatarsals are reduced. He recommends the use of two 0.062 Kirschner wires inserted from the first metatarsal to the second cuneiform. The lateral four metatarsals also require two to three Kirschner wires. Adelaar has experienced good results when using percutaneous wires with no loss of the reduction if the wires are kept in place 6 to 8 weeks. The patient is placed in a non–weight-bearing cast for 3 months. Following this, a semirigid full-length orthotic with metatarsal support is used for a year.

Hardcastle et al.[39] recommend attempted closed reduction by longitudinal traction. If the reduction is adequate, they recommend stabilization with percutaneous Kirschner wires. In their type A injuries (those with total incongruity), two Kirschner wires are necessary for stability. One from the first metatarsal to the medial cuneiform and the second laterally from the fifth metatarsal to the cuboid. In their type B injuries (partial displacements), those of the lateral segment need only a single Kirschner wire for stability. However, if the first metatarsal is displaced, the injury is inherently unstable, and two wires are required. In their type C injuries (divergent displacements), one or two Kirschner wires are necessary to stabilize the medial fragment, with another single wire used for the lateral displacement. Fixation by percutaneous Kirschner wires and external immobilization are both often necessary. This is due to both the initial instability of the reduction and the subsequent loss of position that may develop when the decrease in swelling invalidates the support of the cast.

After the manipulation is performed, a careful roentgenographic evaluation to ascertain that an anatomic reduction has been obtained is undertaken. Collett et al.[18] emphasize that the reduction must be anatomic on the anteroposterior, lateral, *and* oblique views since the dis-

**References 5, 8, 14, 22, 27, 33, 36, 37, 55.*

location occurs in all three planes. Evaluation of the relationship of the base of the metatarsals to the cuneiform and cuboids as outlined under "Radiographic Diagnosis " is *essential* (Figs 35–135 to 35–137). Wilson[71] found that of 14 patients who had undergone a closed reduction and were subsequently treated conservatively, only 1 had an *anatomic* reduction and that in half of the patients a residual displacement of 5 mm or more was present. This stresses the importance of an accurate roentgenographic evaluation of the closed reduction. Anderson,[3] Wilson,[71] and Myerson et al.[55] recommend open reduction and Kirschner wire internal fixation in cases in which an anatomic closed reduction is not obtained.

Mauldin[52] advocates immediate open reduction with cross screw fixation. A straight medial incision extends over the medial cuneiform 3 cm distal to the first tarsometatarsal joint. The anterior tibialis tendon must be identified and retracted. A second incision is centered over the second tarsometatarsal joint. The second and

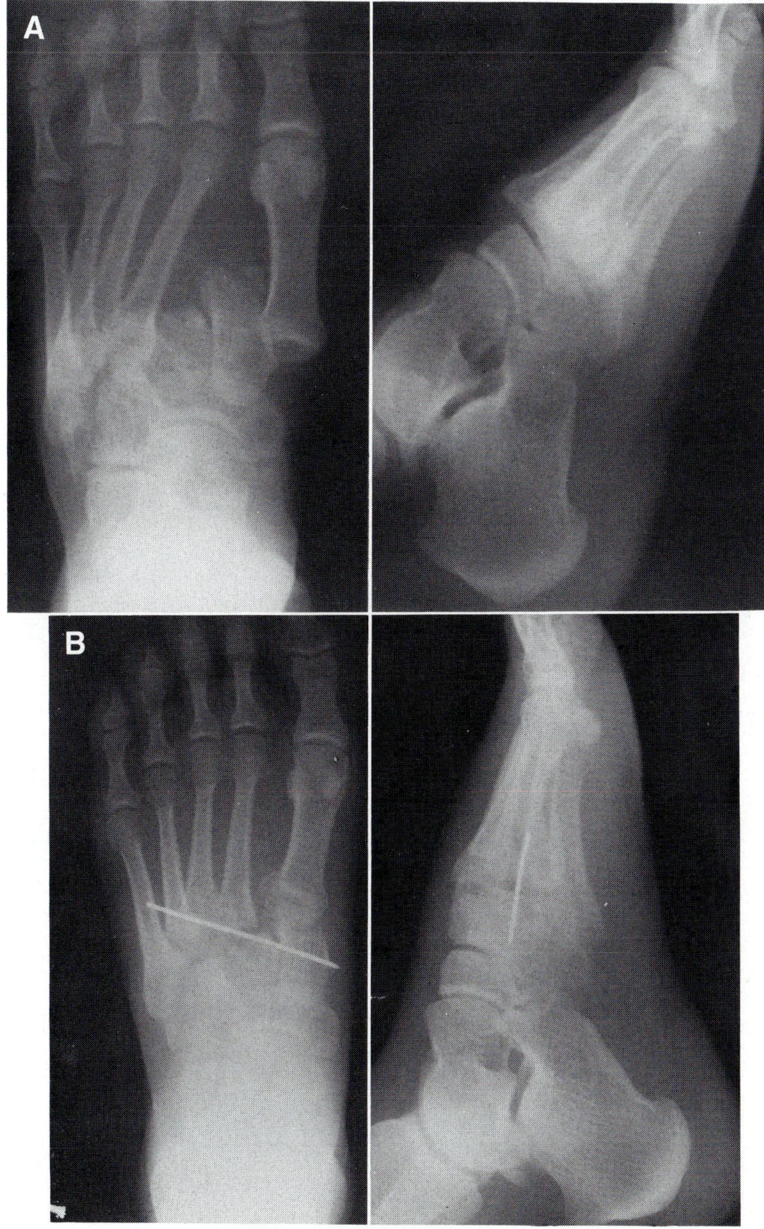

FIG 35–137.
A, tarsometatarsal dislocation. **B,** inadequate reduction. Note the persistent lateral subluxation of the second, third, fourth, and fifth metatarsal bases.

third metatarsal bases are held reduced as a guide pin is passed from the superomedial border of the medial cuneiform across the base of the second metatarsal and into the third metatarsal base. In a divergent type of fracture dislocation, the base of the first metatarsal is then reduced and provisionally stabilized with another guidewire. This is passed from the medial border of the base of the first metatarsal and crosses underneath the previously placed guidewire, through the middle cuneiform, and into the lateral cuneiform. Care should be taken to start the guidewire at least 1.0 cm from the joint line so as not to split the base of the first metatarsal on screw placement. An intraoperative radiograph confirms correct location of the guidewires. A cannulated drill and 4.0-mm cannulated Richards self-tapping screw of appropriate length are directed over each guidewire in the sequence in which the guidewires were placed Fig 35–138. Securing the second and third metatarsal bases usually stabilizes the fourth and fifth metatarsals.

Postoperatively, patients are non–weight bearing in a fracture boot for 8 weeks, followed by 4 weeks of weight bearing to tolerance. Postoperative rehabilitation includes removing the fracture boot daily and using the toes to pick up objects. The hardware is removed electively 12 weeks postoperatively through the medial incision when there is radiographic and clinical evidence of union.

Faciszewski et al.[27] recommend basing treatment on the weight-bearing lateral radiograph. Patients without flattening of the longitudinal arch are treated in a short-leg non–weight-bearing cast for 6 weeks, followed by a short-leg walking cast for 2 weeks. Patients with flattening of the longitudinal arch on their standing radiographs are treated with open reduction and internal fixation with either K-wires or screws.

Tarsometatarsal fracture-dislocations that are irreducible by closed means have been reported by several authors.[20, 25, 50] Lowe and Yosipovitch[50] reported an irreducible tarsometatarsal dislocation in which the closed

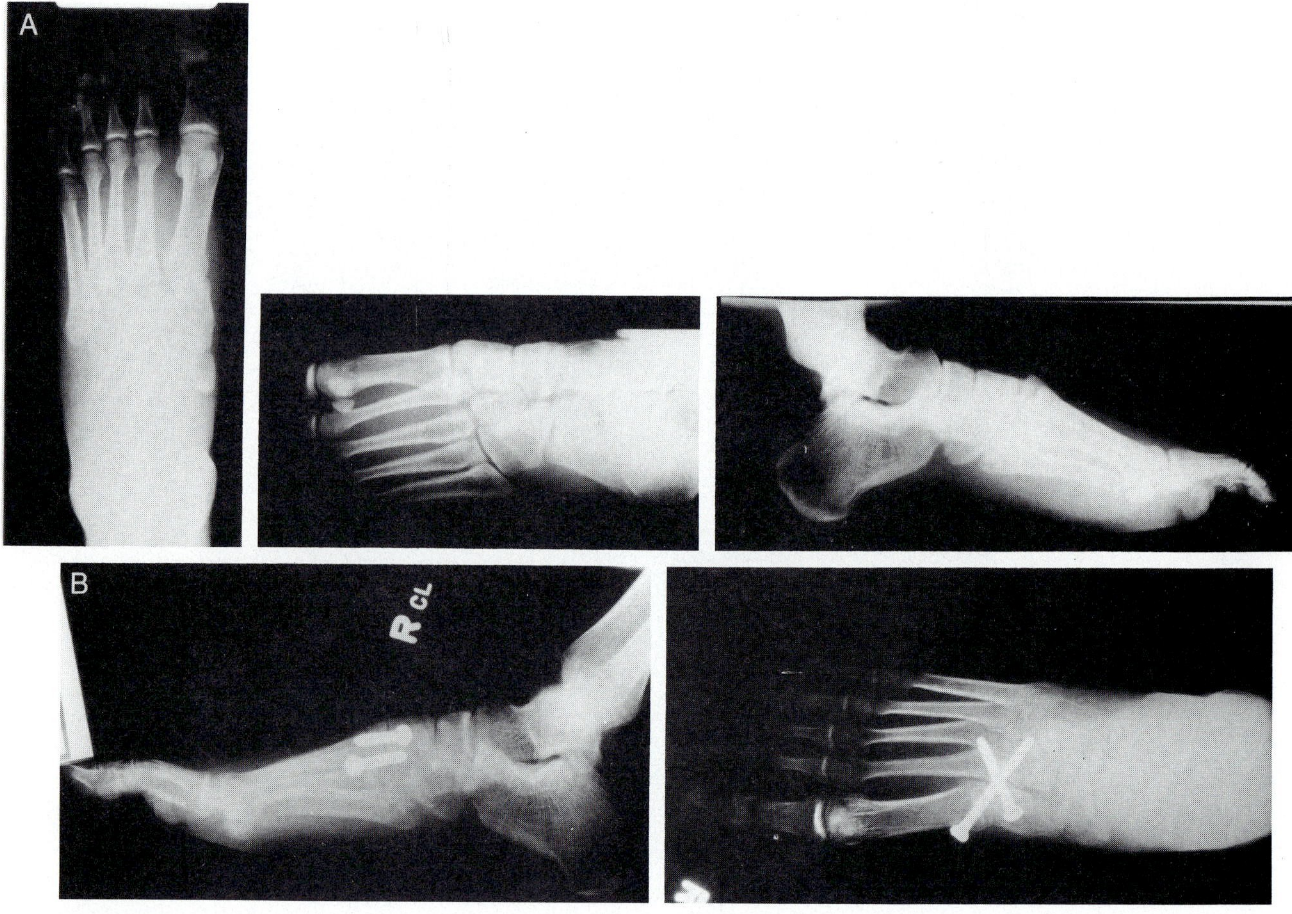

FIG 35–138.
A, anteroposterior, lateral, and oblique radiographs demonstrating a tarsometatarsal fracture-dislocation. **B,** anteroposterior and lateral radiographs following reduction of the tarsometatarsal fracture-dislocation by utilizing the technique of Mauldin.

reduction was blocked by a slip of the tibialis anterior tendon trapped between the medial and middle cuneiform. Holstein and Joldersma[42] also reported a case in which the tibialis anterior had become displaced between the first and second cuneiforms. DeBenedetti et al.[20] emphasized that irreducible dislocation secondary to the interposition of the tibialis anterior tendon occurs only with lateral dislocations of the first metatarsal. The presence of such a dislocation on preoperative roentgenographs might therefore suggest the need for an open reduction. Engber and Roberts,[25] Ballerio,[7] and Huet and Lecoeur[43] report that a superiorly dislocated peroneus longus tendon may act as an obstruction to reduction of the lateral tarsometatarsal joints in a tarsometatarsal fracture-dislocation. Open reduction to remove the trapped tibialis anterior or peroneus longus tendon is the treatment of choice.[20, 25]

Lenczner et al.[48] noted that in cases of dorsolateral dislocation with an avulsion fracture of the base of the second metatarsal, the avulsed fragment may act to prevent an anatomic reduction of the metatarsal base within the cuneiform mortise and result in persistent subluxation of the metatarsal. In their opinion, the avulsion fracture remained attached to Lisfranc's ligament and was therefore held firmly within the mortise and could not be displaced by closed manipulation in order to allow the metatarsal base access to the mortise. In such cases, they recommend that the fragment be excised at open reduction.

Geckeler[32] believed that it was nearly impossible to reduce dislocations of the tarsometatarsal joint by manipulation and therefore recommended operative treatment. He was the first to recommend the use of Kirschner wires for stabilization of the dislocation following open reduction. After open reduction he recommended the use of a short-leg cast. The Kirschner wires were removed after several weeks when soft-tissue stability permitted. Wilson[71] also found manipulative reduction not dependable. He therefore recommended that unless anatomic reduction is achieved, open reduction along with Kirschner pin transfixation is the treatment of choice. He recommended leaving the wires in for 6 weeks after which time the patient begins weight bearing. Anderson[3] also recommended open reduction and internal fixation with Kirschner pins in cases in which an anatomic closed reduction was not obtained. The patient was kept in a non-weight-bearing cast for 6 weeks followed by a short-leg walking cast for an additional 3 to 4 weeks. He recommended longitudinal arch support for an additional 6 to 12 months. Percutaneous Kirschner wire fixation is used to stabilize grossly unstable dislocations and also to allow maintenance of reduction during the period of time swelling decreases and in which a cast might not supply necessary stability to prevent redislocation.

In those patients in whom there is a dislocation of the medial cuneiform bone in conjunction with a tarsometatarsal fracture-dislocation,[10, 42] Brown and McFarland recommend primary open reduction through a dorsal incision centered between the first and second cuneiforms because of the lack of success with closed reduction. Following open reduction, Giannestras and Sammarco[33] recommend a short-leg cast molded well about the foot. The cast and pins are removed at 6 to 8 weeks, and weight bearing with a properly fitted arch support is permitted. These authors also stress that they have not seen a single patient who had any persistent dislocation that did not subsequently require an arthrodesis of the involved joint.

Del Sel in 1955[22] recommended primary open reduction and temporary internal fixation by percutaneous wires in patients with tarsometatarsal fracture-dislocations. He recommended the use of an incision in the first interosseous space with evacuation of the blood clot located there. In some cases a second incision was necessary to reduce the second and third metatarsals. He recommended debridement of the tarsometatarsal joint of bits of cartilage, soft-tissue, and bone and then stabilizing the reduction by using percutaneous Kirschner wires. The wires were left in place for 2 to 4 weeks. After the wires were removed, the patients were encouraged to walk in a below-knee cast. Tondeur[66] also advised open reduction and internal fixation of tarsometatarsal dislocations.

Wright[73] recommends longitudinal incisions on the dorsum of the foot for open reduction. He cautions, however, against the use of multiple incisions, particularly in patients in whom crushing has been extensive. After debridement of the joint, he uses multiple Kirschner wires or staples to stabilize the dislocation. If Kirschner wires are utilized, they are left long enough to allow palpation and subsequent removal. Patients are treated in a short-leg cast from the tip of the toes to the tibial tuberosity and are kept non–weight bearing for 3 weeks. Following this a short-leg walking cast is applied. The Kirschner wires are removed at 4 to 6 weeks. The foot is maintained in a cast for a total of 8 weeks, after which time an arch support is used for an additional 3 months. Wilppula[70] also recommends the use of a longitudinal incision between the first and second metatarsals on the dorsum of the foot. He found that when the first and second metatarsals are reduced, the remainder of the metatarsals easily fall into place. He also utilized Kirschner wire fixation from the metatarsals into the tarsal bones for stability.

Hardcastle et al.[39] believe that an *absolute* indication

for open reduction is vascular insufficiency that does not improve after closed reduction. In this situation, he agrees with Gissane[34] that both the dorsalis pedis and posterior tibial arteries must be explored at the time of open reduction. For open reduction, Hardcastle et al.[39] recommend the use of longitudinal incisions, the first between the first and second metatarsals with accessory incisions located more laterally over the tarsometatarsal joint.

They found that following reduction and stable internal fixation, weight bearing as soon as the swelling subsided did not affect the final outcome, provided that the foot was protected in a plaster cast and the reduction was stabilized with internal fixation. It was their opinion that such early weight bearing decreased the period of disability.

Arntz et al.[5] reported multiple problems with Kirschner wire fixation including pin migration, infection of pin tracts, and loss of reduction. Because of these difficulties, the authors recommend open reduction of fractures and fracture-dislocations of the tarsometatarsal joint followed by temporary internal fixation with AO screws. The authors recommend open reduction and internal fixation as quickly as possible. Exposure is achieved through one or more longitudinal incisions. The capsules of the tarsometatarsal joints are opened through a single dorsal incision. Comminuted interarticular fragments are reduced when possible, while smaller, irreducible fragments are excised. Once a precise reduction of each tarsometatarsal joint has been achieved, a notch is made on the dorsum of the metatarsal approximately 15 to 20 mm distal to the joint.

A drill bit 3.2-mm in diameter or smaller is then used to make a hole beginning in the proximal edge of the notch and directed across the base of the metatarsal into the body of the respective cuneiform. A 4.0-mm-diameter screw or malleolar screw is used to fix the joint with slight compression while holding the reduction anatomically (Fig 35–139). According to the authors, when the first metatarsal cuneiform joint had been reduced and stabilized, there was a simultaneous reduction of the second metatarsal that was stabilized in a similar manner. When the third metatarsal is also dislocated, a second dorsal incision is made between the third and fourth metatarsals and the third metatarsal cuneiform joint was similarly stabilized. Once the third metatarsal cuneiform joint is stabilized, the fourth and fifth metatarsal joints are usually fully reduced. Occasionally, a single screw is placed through a small stab incision across the base of the fifth metatarsal into the cuboid. Postoperatively, the patients are treated by partial weight bearing for 6 weeks. They are then placed in a weight-bearing cast, and full weight bearing is allowed for the initial 4 to 6 weeks. Internal fixation was maintained until radiographs showed evidence of osseous union. In their series, the screws were removed an average of 16 weeks following injury. The authors report no evidence of redisplacement or recurrent subluxation when they compared radiographs that had been made postoperatively, after removal of the screws, and at final follow-up.

The authors report patients whose apparently healed dislocations displaced following the removal of Kirschner wires 6 weeks after fixation. For these reasons, the authors recommend that the screws be left in place for a minimum of 12 weeks. According to the authors, fixa-

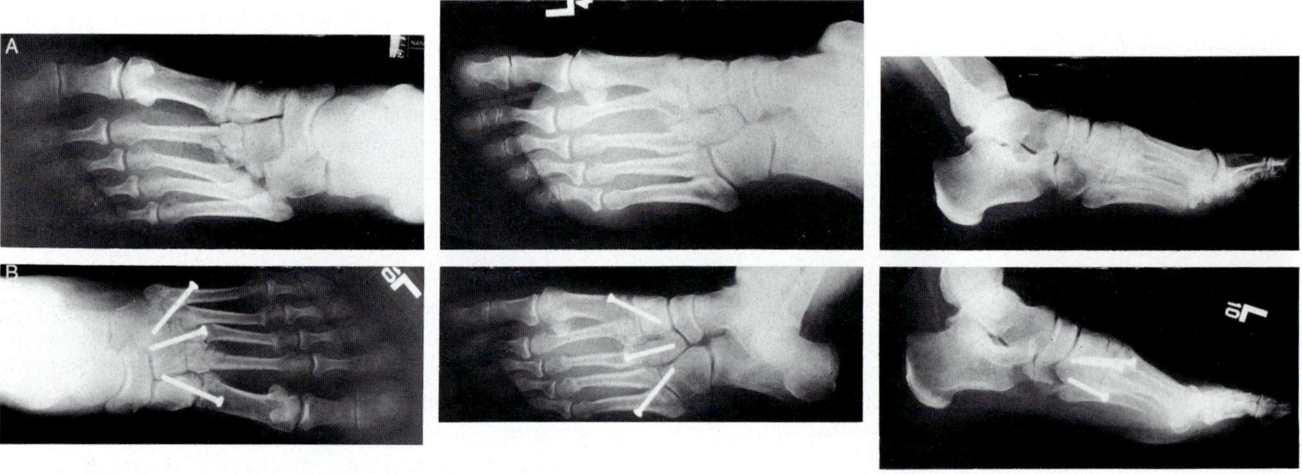

FIG 35–139.
A, anteroposterior, oblique, and lateral radiographs of a fracture-dislocation of the tarsometatarsal joint. **B,** anteroposterior, oblique, and lateral radiographs following open reduction and internal fixation of the tarsometatarsal joint by using the technique described by Arnzt et al.[5]

tion of the tarsometatarsal joints with AO screws had no apparent influence on the development of arthritic change in the affected tarsometatarsal joints. They found no discernible radiographic differences between adjacent joints, some of which had been stabilized with screws and others which had not. It was the authors' opinion that the tarsometatarsal joints, because of their normally limited range of motion, tolerate this method of stable internal fixation quite well. According to these authors, injury to the articular cartilage and failure to achieve and maintain an anatomic reduction proved to be the most important factors in the development of posttraumatic arthritis.

Granberry and Lipscomb[37] also recommend open reduction and internal fixation if an anatomic reduction is not obtained by closed means. Additionally, they suggest fusion of the involved joints in patients who require open reduction. This is because 11 of their 25 patients eventually required arthrodesis. Hardcastle et al.[39] suggest that primary arthrodesis may have a place in injuries where there is considerable comminution and where maintenance of reduction is difficult. However, the authors had no experience with the technique. Primary arthrodesis, however, is not supported by other authors.

Carr et al.[13] reviewed the concept of indirect reduction techniques for fractures involving the foot and ankle. Indirect reduction refers to the use of distractive forces to effect the bony reduction by means of ligamentotaxis. In this method, appropriately sized half pins are inserted into bone proximal and distal to the tarsometatarsal joints. A distractor is then applied to these half pins, and traction is exerted. The involved area is directly monitored radiographically or visually through an open incision to determine the amount of distraction necessary. Once a reduction is obtained, temporary fixation is performed. This technique combines the advantages of both the open and closed methods of treatment of Lisfranc's injuries. It allows lengthening of the contracted soft tissues, correction of angulation, a reduction in the amount of soft-tissue dissection for exposure, and a means of maintaining temporary stability prior to definitive fixation.

If the internal fixation following reduction is not stable, the half pins used for the distractor can be converted to an external fixation frame. This method seems to have most use in patients in whom treatment has been delayed and soft-tissue contractures have developed.

Similarly, DeCoster et al.[21] mention the use of a triangular external fixation frame utilizing 3-mm pins for Lisfranc's fractures. The pins are placed dorsally in the medial cuneiform, second metatarsal, and other affected bones depending upon the fracture pattern. The authors suggest that external fixation be considered for fractures and dislocations with associated soft-tissue injury and closed midfoot fracture-dislocations with significant joint disruption.

Results

Aitken and Poulson[2] report that although posttraumatic arthritis and ankylosis of the tarsometatarsal joints were common, they are not a source of discomfort and disability in the majority of their patients. Indeed, they did not see the need for a tarsometatarsal fusion in their patients at follow-up. Myerson et al.[55] found that degenerative changes were found in almost every patient following tarsometatarsal dislocation but there was a low level of correlation between the degree of degenerative changes and clinical results. Similarly, Brunet and Wiley[11] report that despite a variety of treatment methods, foot comfort usually progressed to a stable level by about 1.3 years after injury. The authors report that neither the initial fracture type nor treatment had any apparent bearing on the subsequent function. The authors also report that there was no correlation between radiographic assessment of the injury and the patient's symptoms. Almost 80% of their patients were able to return to their original occupations, and the majority were pain free. The authors believe that the relative absence of pain, even with persistent gross subluxation and radiographic evidence of advanced arthritis, may be secondary to a stable ankylosis or to disruption of sensory fibers of the torn capsular and ligamentous structures of the joint. On the contrary, LaTourette et al.[47] found that all patients complain of some degree of discomfort in the foot following tarsometatarsal injury. Additionally, the majority of patients complained of swelling. Hesp et al.[40] in 1984 reviewed 22 cases with 52 months' follow-up. A significant number of their patients developed late degenerative arthritis of the tarsometatarsal joint. They believe that the severity of the initial injury was *the* determining factor in late degenerative arthritis.

Goossens and DeStoop[35] reported that 35% of their patients developed degenerative arthritis following tarsometatarsal dislocation. Three of their patients underwent tarsometatarsal arthrodesis, and all had good results and returned to work. Johnson and Johnson[45] reported a Dowell graft arthrodesis technique used in 15 patients with posttraumatic degenerative arthritis after tarsometatarsal fracture dislocation. Thirteen of their 15 patients had excellent pain relief, and only 2 were dissatisfied. Sangeorzan et al.[62] report 15 patients who following fracture-dislocation of the tarsometatarsal joint had persistent pain requiring arthrodesis. The patients complained of pain and progressive flatfoot deformity with forefoot abduction. The authors describe a technique involving exposing Lisfranc's joint, denuding articular cartilage, and reducing the dislocation with fixation by lag screws. The authors recommend that when significant persistent displacement is present, reduction be performed before arthrodesis. The authors report good to excellent results in 70% of their patients. Poor reduction, a delay in treatment, and injuries occurring in the workplace all portend a bad prognosis following tarsometatarsal dislocations.

Obtaining and maintaining an anatomic reduction are believed to be of major importance in avoiding the degenerative changes that may require surgery at a later date.[33] LaTourette et al.[47] evaluated their results by using gait analysis with foot switches attached to the sole of the patient's shoes.[19, 51, 61] They concluded that anatomic reduction and early ambulation produce better results. Myerson et al.[55] concluded that the major determinant of unacceptable results was the quality of the initial reduction. According to these authors, open anatomic reduction and internal fixation using Kirschner wires yielded the best results. Wilson[71] also found that the most critical factor in preventing late deformity, stiffness, and degenerative arthritis is an anatomic reduction obtained by either closed or open means. Wilppula[70] demonstrated that although an anatomic result was no guarantee of a symptom-free foot, in general, a good anatomic result usually produced a good functional result. Additionally, Wilppula[70] reported that symptoms of degenerative arthritis in the tarsometatarsal joint tended to subside gradually during a period of several years' follow-up. He found no need for arthrodesis as a salvage procedure in his patients, although he suggested that early arthrodesis might have accelerated their recovery. Wilppula also found that limitation of motion in the foot was present in half of his patients and suggested that intensifying the mobilizing exercises during treatment could reduce this disability. According to Adelaar, although anatomic reduction does produce the best results, forefoot stiffness, unequal metatarsal plantar pressure, and intrinsic contractures may still produce a symptomatic foot, particularly when sympathetic dystrophy complicates these severe crushing injuries.[1]

Lenczner et al.[48] reported that the majority of their poor results were secondary *either* to failure to *obtain* an adequate reduction or to failure to *maintain* the reduction of the tarsometatarsal injury. This stresses the importance of stable fixation after reduction to prevent redislocation during the period of immobilization.[8] Arntz et al.[5] believed that the results following tarsometatarsal dislocations were most dependent upon the accuracy of the reduction and the presence of associated osteochondral fractures in the tarsometatarsal joint. Finally, Jeffreys[44] emphasizes that although accurate reduction is essential to prevent long-term disability, the late development of osteoarthritis may be determined by the damage sustained by the articular cartilage at the time of the injury. Therefore, in certain cases osteoarthritis may develop in spite of the method of treatment selected.

Author's Preferred Method of Treatment

The importance of early diagnosis and treatment of injuries to the tarsometatarsal joints cannot be overemphasized. Anteroposterior, oblique, and lateral roentgenographs will demonstrate frank dislocation of the tarsometatarsal joints. However, a careful evaluation of roentgenographs of the foot is essential to detect the subtle signs of a subluxation of the tarsometatarsal joint or of a complete tarsometatarsal dislocation that has spontaneously reduced. When the clinical examination indicates tenderness at the tarsometatarsal joint, a full roentgenographic evaluation of the joint is essential. In those cases in which such an injury is suspected, I use stress roentgenographs, possibly with anesthesia, to determine the degree of instability.

Once the diagnosis of tarsometatarsal dislocation is confirmed, evaluation of the foot for compartment syndrome and circulatory compromise is undertaken. If a foot compartment syndrome is present, I proceed directly to forefoot decompression through a combined medial incision and dorsal incisions between the second and third and between the fourth and fifth metatarsals. These dorsal incisions are also used for direct access to the tarsometatarsal dislocations, which are reduced and stabilized as an open procedure.

If the patient's medical condition or skin damage over the dislocation prevents open reduction, I proceed to closed reduction. In my experience, the earlier a reduction is attempted, the more likely that an anatomic reduction will be obtained by closed methods.

Traction is obtained with the patient in the supine position by suspending the leg with Chinese finger traps applied to the toes. A counterweight is placed over the ankle. Once the tarsometatarsal joints have been restored to length by traction, manipulation in the dorsal-plantar plane is performed. Roentgenographic evaluation is then performed to ascertain the quality of the reduction. Anatomic reduction of the relationship of *each* of the metatarsals to their respective cuneiform or cuboid is necessary. If such a reduction is achieved, the author uses two percutaneous Kirschner wires, one from the first metatarsal into the medial cuneiform and the second from the fifth metatarsal into the cuboid, to stabilize the dislocation (Fig 35–140). The question of whether or not a closed reduction is stable or not is *not* considered in determining whether or not Kirschner wire fixation is needed. In my opinion, all of these injuries that were *dislocated* initially require Kirschner wire stabilization. In patients with minor degrees of subluxation of the tarsometatarsal joint, Kirschner wire fixation is reserved only for those in whom cooperation with the postreduction regimen is questionable.

Following reduction and stabilization the foot is placed in a short-leg fracture boot for 4 weeks with toe touch weight bearing. The toes are left free at the end of the cast to encourage exercises of the metatarsophalangeal joints. After 4 weeks when the swelling is decreased, the fracture boot is removed to allow range-of-motion exercises. Partial weight bearing is allowed.

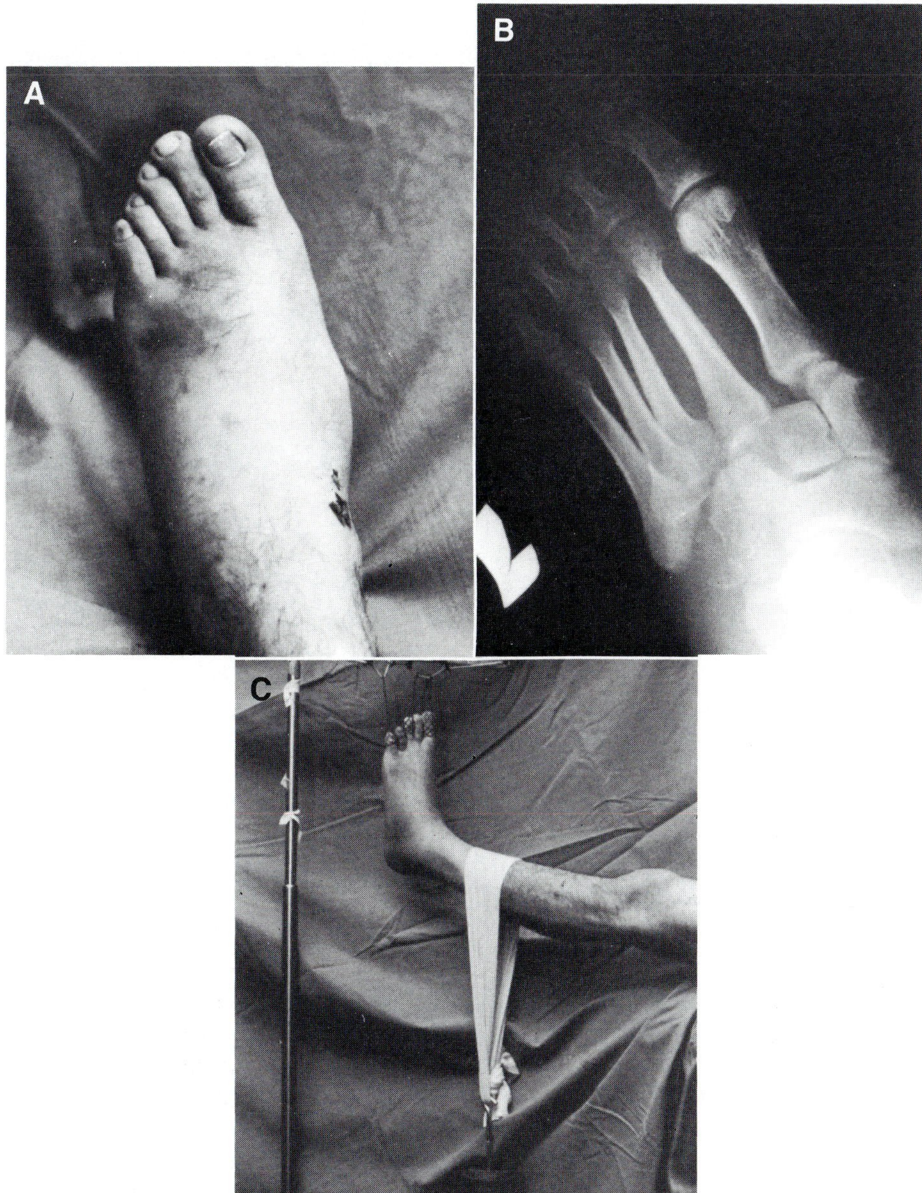

FIG 35–140.
Tarsometatarsal dislocation. **A,** clinical appearance of an injured foot. **B,** anteroposterior radiograph demonstrating dislocation of the tarsometatarsal joint. **C,** method of closed reduction with Chinese finger traps for fixed traction. **D,** radiograph of the foot in traction after manipulative reduction. The tarsometatarsal joint is restored. **E,** percutaneous Kirschner wire fixation to stabilize the tarsometatarsal reduction.

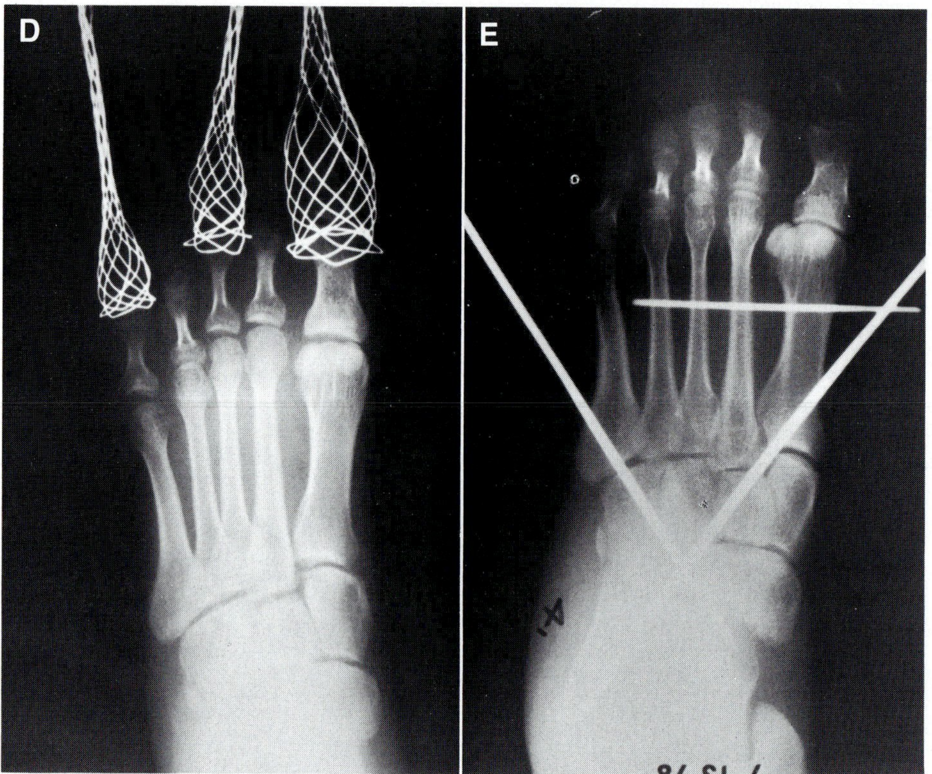

FIG 35–140 (cont.).

This fracture boot and the pins are removed at 12 weeks. At this point the foot is placed in a good shoe with a longitudinal arch support for an additional 9 to 12 months.

If skin and medical conditions permit, I prefer open reduction and internal fixation. In my experience, the best results are obtained with an anatomic reduction. The most predictable way for me to obtain an anatomic reduction and allow secure fixation is through open reduction and internal fixation. I have used both Kirschner wire and screw fixation and prefer the latter. Difficulty in achieving anatomic reduction through closed reduction and percutaneous pinning has led to this protocol. At the time of open reduction, it is important to remember that the reduction must be anatomic in all three planes. It is important to remember that the transverse "Roman arch" at the base of the metatarsals as well as the contralateral talometatarsal angle must be reconstituted during open reduction.

I prefer an incision over the first tarsometatarsal joint. Subsequent parallel longitudinal incisions are utilized, usually between the third and fourth metatarsals, to expose the remainder of the tarsometatarsal joint. Usually, debridement of small articular cartilage and osseous fragments is necessary to effect the reduction. In patients in whom there is a gross amount of swelling at the time of open reduction, interosseous decompression fasciotomies are performed between each of the metatarsals in an effort to decrease fibrosis in the foot. The cross screw fixation technique[52] or straight leg compression technique of Arntz et al.[5] gives equally good results. Postoperatively, the limb is placed in a short-leg fracture boot and elevated. When edema allows, usually after 48 hours, the patient starts toe touch weight bearing for 8 weeks. After the soft tissues have quiesced and sutures are removed at 2 weeks, the patient can take the fracture boot off several times during the day to perform active range of motion and pick objects up with the toes. After 8 weeks, the patient progresses to weight bearing to tolerance. After 12 weeks, the patient is allowed to wear a crepe-soled shoe with an arch support. When radiographs and clinical examination show evidence of fracture union, the hardware is removed, usually at 14 to 16 weeks.

If there is vascular compromise, I consider reduction of the dislocation an emergency. If clinical signs of insufficiency persist after anatomic reduction by open or closed means, an arteriogram is performed to evaluate the posterior tibial and lateral plantar arteries. I obtain vascular surgery consultation in these instances. Consideration is given to interosseous fasciotomy if the arteriograms show patency of the vessels.

Open dislocations are treated by irrigation and debridement before reduction. Anatomic reduction is then obtained under direct vision. A second debridement and irrigation are performed in 48 hours. Screw fixation is then performed, and the wounds are left open. The patient undergoes daily sterile dressing changes, and the wounds are closed secondarily at 5 to 7 days. Postoperative management is then identical to that following closed injuries.

In the author's experience, early mobilization and an early exercise program help to reduce edema and speed the return of the patient to his normal activities. It is not uncommon for the patient to complain of persistent aching in the tarsometatarsal joint for prolonged periods of time despite an anatomic reduction. Good arch support and a stiff-soled shoe are utilized to control these symptoms.

REFERENCES

Tarsometatarsal Dislocations

1. Adelaar RS: The treatment of tarsometatarsal fracture dislocation, *Instr Course Lect* 39:141–145, 1990.
2. Aitken AP, Poulson D: Dislocations of the tarsometatarsal joint, *J Bone Joint Surg [Am]* 45:246–260, 1963.
3. Anderson LD: Injuries of the forefoot, *Clin Orthop* 122:18–27, 1977.
4. Arenberg AA: Vyvikhi v sustave lisfranka (dislocation of Lisfranc's joint), *Vestn Khir* 102:126, 1969.
5. Arntz CJ, Veith RG, Hansen SJ Jr: Fractures and fracture-dislocations of the tarsometatarsal joints, *J Bone Joint Surg [Am]* 70:173–181, 1988.
6. Ashurst APC: Divergent dislocation of the metatarsus, *Ann Surg* 83:132–136, 1926.
7. Ballerio A: Un caso raro di lussazione tarso metatarsale isolata, *Chir Organi Mov* 38:286, 1953.
8. Bassett FH: Dislocations of the tarsometatarsal joints, *South Med J* 57:1294–1302, 1964.
9. Blodgett WH: Injuries of the forefoot and toes. In Jahss MH, editor: *Disorders of the foot*, vol 2, Philadelphia, 1982, WB Saunders.
10. Brown DC, McFarland GB: Dislocation of the medial cuneiform bone in tarsometatarsal fracture-dislocation, *J Bone Joint Surg [Am]* 57:858–859, 1975.
11. Brunet JA, Wiley JJ: The late results of tarsometatarsal joint injuries, *J Bone Joint Surg [Br]* 69: 437–440, 1987.
12. Cain PR, Seligson D: Lisfranc's fracture-dislocation with intercuneiform dislocation: presentation of two cases and a plan for treatment, *Foot Ankle* 2:156–160, 1981.
13. Carr JB, Hansen ST, Benirschke SK: Surgical treatment of foot and ankle trauma: the use of indirect reduction techniques, *Foot Ankle* 9:176–178, 1989.
14. Cassebaum WH: Lisfranc fracture-dislocations, *Clin Orthop* 30:116–129, 1963.
15. Chapman MW: Fractures and dislocations of the ankle and foot. In Mann RA, editor: *DuVries' surgery of the foot*, ed 4, St Louis, 1978, Mosby–Year Book.
16. Cherkes-Zade DI: Pepelomy-vyvikhi v sustave lisfranka (Fracture-dislocation of the Lisfranc's joint), *Vestn Khir* 103:102, 1969.
17. Coker TP Jr, Arnold JA: Sports injuries to the foot and ankle. In Jahss MH, editor: *Disorders of the foot*, vol 2, Philadelphia, 1982, WB Saunders.
18. Collett HS, Hood TK, Andrews RE: Tarsometatarsal fracture dislocations, *Surg Gynecol Obstet* 106:623–626, 1958.
19. Curry CL: Stride characteristics of normal adults (thesis), University of Southern California School of Physical Therapy, March 1976.
20. DeBenedetti MJ, Evanski PM, Waugh TR: The unreducible Lisfranc's fracture, *Clin Orthop* 136:238–240, 1978.
21. DeCoster T, Alvarez R, Trevino S: External fixation of the foot and ankle, *Foot Ankle* 17:40–48, 1986.
22. Del Sel JM: The surgical treatment of tarsometatarsal fracture-dislocations, *J Bone Joint Surg [Br]* 37:203–207, 1955.
23. Detlefsen M: Die luxation im Lisfrancschen gelenk als typischi verletzung des Montorrad fahrers, *Beitr Orthop Traumatol* 15:242, 1968.
24. Easton ER: Two rare dislocations of the metatarsals at Lisfranc's joint, *J Bone Joint Surg* 20:1053–1056, 1938.
25. Engber WD, Roberts JM: Irreducible tarsometatarsal fracture-dislocation, *Clin Orthop* 168:102–104, 1982.
26. English TA: Dislocations of the metatarsal bone and adjacent toe, *J Bone Joint Surg [Br]* 46:700–704, 1964.
27. Faciszewski T, Burks RT, Manaster BJ: Subtle injuries of the Lisfranc joint, *J Bone Joint Surg [Am]* 72:1519–1522, 1990.
28. Fitte M, Garacotche I: Luxation-fracture de l'articulation de Lisfranc, *J Chir* 56:367, 1940.
29. Foster SC: Lisfranc tarsometatarsal fracture dislocations, *Radiology* 21:988, 1981.
30. Foster SC, Foster RR: Lisfranc's tarsometatarsal fracture-dislocation, *Radiology* 120:79–83, 1976.
31. Funk FJ: Tarsometatarsal fracture-dislocations, closed (Lisfranc): early diagnosis and treatment, American Orthopedic Association Third International Symposium: "Musculoskeletal trauma," San Francisco, May 17–21, 1982.
32. Geckeler EO: Dislocations and fracture-dislocations of the foot: transfixion with Kirschner wires, *Surgery* 25:730–733, 1949.
33. Giannestras NJ, Sammarco GJ: Fractures and dislocations in the foot. In Rockwood CA Jr, Green DP, editors: *Fractures*, vol 2, Philadelphia, 1975, JB Lippincott.
34. Gissane W: A dangerous type of fracture of the foot, *J Bone Joint Surg [Br]* 33:535–538, 1951.
35. Goossens M, DeStoop N: Lisfranc's fracture-dislocations: etiology, radiology and results of treatment, *Clin Orthop* 176:154–162, 1983.
36. Graham J, Waddell JP, Lenczner E: Tarsometatarsal (Lisfranc) dislocation, *J Bone Joint Surg [Br]* 55:666, 1973.
37. Granberry WM, Lipscomb PR: Dislocation of the tarsometatarsal joints, *Surg Gynecol Obstet* 114:467–469, 1962.
38. Groulier P, Pinaud J-C: Les luxations tarsometatarsiennes (a proper de dix observations), *Rev Chir Orthop* 56:303, 1970.
39. Hardcastle PH, Reschauer R, Kutscha-Lissberg E, et al: Injuries to the tarsometatarsal joint: incidence, classifica-

tion and treatment, *J Bone Joint Surg [Br]* 64:349–356, 1982.
40. Hesp WLEM, VanderWerken Ch, Goris RJA: (Lisfranc's) dislocations: fractures and/or dislocations through the tarsometatarsal joints, *Injury* 15:261–266, 1984.
41. Hillegass RC: Injuries to the midfoot: A major cause of industrial morbidity. In Bateman JE, editor: *Foot science*, Philadelphia, 1976, WB Saunders.
42. Holstein A, Joldersma RD: Dislocation of the first cuneiform in tarsometatarsal fracture-dislocation, *J Bone Joint Surg [Am]* 32:419–421, 1950.
43. Huet P, Lecoeur P: Sur 4 cas de luxation tarsometarsienne, *Acad Chir Mem* 72:124, 1946.
44. Jeffreys TE: Lisfranc's fracture-dislocation. A clinical and experimental study of tarso-metatarsal dislocations and fracture-dislocations, *J Bone Joint Surg [Br]* 45:546–551, 1963.
45. Johnson JE, Johnson KA: Dowel arthrodesis for degenerative arthritis of the tarsometatarsal Lisfranc's joints, *Foot Ankle* 6:243–253, 1986.
46. Key JA, Conwell HE: *The management of fractures, dislocations and sprains*, ed 6, St Louis, 1956, Mosby–Year Book.
47. LaTourette G, Perry J, Patzakis MJ, et al: Fractures and dislocations of the tarsometatarsal joint. In Bateman JE, Trott AW, editors: *The foot and ankle*, New York, 1980, Brian C Decker.
48. Lenczner EM, Waddell JP, Graham JD: Tarsal-metatarsal (Lisfranc) dislocation, *J Trauma* 14:1012–1020, 1974.
49. London PS: Major injuries of the foot, *J Bone Joint Surg [Br]* 58:385, 1976.
50. Lowe J, Yosipovitch Z: Tarsometatarsal dislocation: a mechanism blocking manipulative reduction, *J Bone Joint Surg [Am]* 58:1029, 1976.
51. Manter JT: Distribution of compression forces in joints of the human foot, *Anat Rec* 96:313–321, 1946.
52. Mauldin D: Personal communication.
53. Micheli LJ, Sohn RS, Solomon R: Stress fractures of the second metatarsal involving Lisfranc's joint in ballet dancers, *J Bone Joint Surg [Am]* 67:1372–1375, 1985.
54. Myerson M: Acute compartment syndromes of the foot, *Bull Hosp Jt Dis Orthop Inst* 47:251–261, 1987.
55. Myerson MS, Fisher RT, Burgess AR, et al: Fracture dislocations of the tarsometatarsal joints: end results correlated with pathology and treatment, *Foot Ankle* 6:225–242, 1986.
56. Narat JK: An unusual case of dislocation of metatarsal bones, *Am J Surg* 6:239–241, 1929.
57. O'Donoghue DH: *Treatment of injuries to athletes*, ed 3, vol 1, Philadelphia, 1976, WB Saunders.
58. O'Regan DJ: Lisfranc dislocations, *J Med Soc N J* 66:575–577, 1969.
59. Perriard M, Deterle J, Jeannet E: Les lesions traumatiques recentes comprises entre les articulations de Chopart et de Lisfranc, incluses, *Z Unfallmed Berufskr* 63:318, 1970.
60. Quenu E, Kuss G: Etude sur les luxations du metatarse, *Rev Chir* 39:1, 1909.
61. Rousek R: Stride characteristics of normal adults (thesis), University of Southern California School of Physical Therapy, November 1976.
62. Sangeorzan BJ, Veith RG, Hansen ST: Salvage of Lisfranc's tarsometatarsal joints by arthrodesis, *Foot Ankle* 4:193–200, 1990.
63. Schiller MG, Ray RD: Isolated dislocation of the medial cuneiform bone—a rare injury of the tarsus, *J Bone Joint Surg [Am]* 52:1632–1636, 1970.
64. Stein RE: Radiological aspects of the tarsometatarsal joints, *Foot Ankle* 3:286–289, 1983.
65. Taussig G, Hautier S: Les fractures-luxations de l'articulation de Lisfranc, *Ann Chir* 23:1131–1141, 1969.
66. Tondeur G: Un cas de luxation-fracture tarsometatarsienne, *Acta Orthop Belg* 27:286, 1961.
67. Tountas AA: Occult fracture-subluxation of the midtarsal joint, *Clin Orthop* 243:195–199, 1988.
68. Turco VJ, Spinella AJ: Tarsometatarsal dislocation—Lisfranc injury, *Foot Ankle* 2:362, 1982.
69. Wiley, JJ: The mechanism of tarso-metatarsal joint injuries, *J Bone Joint Surg [Br]* 53:474–482, 1971.
70. Wilppula E: Tarsometatarsal fracture dislocation, *Acta Orthop Scand* 44:335–345, 1973.
71. Wilson DW: Injuries of the tarso-metatarsal joints: etiology, classification and results of treatment, *J Bone Joint Surg [Br]* 54:677–686, 1972.
72. Wilson PD: Fractures and dislocations of the tarsal bones, *South Med J* 26:833–845, 1933.
73. Wright PE: Dislocations. In Edmonson AS, Crenshaw AH, editors: *Campbell's operative orthopaedics*, vol 1, St Louis, 1980, Mosby–Year Book.

ISOLATED TALONAVICULAR DISLOCATIONS

Isolated talonavicular dislocations are extremely unusual.[1–4] Dixon[1] suggests that "isolated talonavicular dislocations are associated with momentary midtarsal subluxation or dislocation. Indeed, Fahey and Murphy[2] report two cases of "talonavicular dislocations" that subsequently subluxed after open reduction, thus suggesting associated midtarsal joint damage that was not appreciated at the time of treatment.

Giannestras and Sammarco[4] recommended closed reduction, Chinese finger traps to apply traction to the forefoot, and a muslin sling over the ankle joint to apply countertraction. With this method, these authors are able to gently manipulate the head of the talus into the navicular socket. Once the reduction is obtained, a below-knee non–weight-bearing cast is applied, and traction on the toes is removed. The authors stress that if there is an associated fracture of the navicular, open reduction with careful regard for the articular surfaces is indicated. In addition to reconstructing the navicular articular surface, a transfixing Kirschner wire from the navicular into the talus is often indicated.

In my experience, when talonavicular dislocations occur, they are rotational or swivel dislocations in which the axis of rotation is the calcaneocuboid joint. They are therefore midtarsal joint dislocations and are considered more completely in that section of this chapter.

REFERENCES

Talonavicular Dislocations

1. Dixon JH: Letter to the editor, *Injury* 10:251, 1979.
2. Fahey JJ, Murphy JL: Dislocations and fractures of the talus, *Surg Clin North Am* 45:79–102, 1965.
3. Garcia A, Parkes JC: Fractures of the foot. In Giannestras NJ, editor: *Foot disorders: medical and surgical management*, ed 2, Philadelphia, 1973, Lea & Febiger,
4. Giannestras NJ, Sammarco GJ: Fractures and dislocations in the foot. In Rockwood CA Jr, Green DP, editors: *Fractures*, vol 2, Philadelphia, 1975, JB Lippincott.

DISLOCATIONS OF THE CUNEIFORMS AND CUBOID

Isolated dislocation of the bones of the midfoot are exceedingly uncommon.[1–8] A review of the literature reveals that such dislocations are more common on the medial border of the foot involving the cuneiforms[1, 3, 6, 8] as compared with those involving the outer side of the foot.[4] Drummond and Hastings[4] believe that this is secondary to the relative elasticity of the medial border of the foot as compared with the outer border. In support of this concept they quote Jones'[7] description of the medial border of the foot as "a weed which bends before the wind" while the lateral border of the foot is likened to a "rigid oak which breaks before the force of the wind." Despite their rarity, awareness of these injuries is essential to prevent a delay in diagnosis.

Dislocations of the Cuneiforms

Dislocations of the cuneiforms have been reported both as isolated injuries[3, 8] and in association with tarsometatarsal fracture-dislocations.[1, 6] Schiller and Ray[8] reported a case of isolated dislocation of the medial cuneiform secondary to a crushing injury. These authors stressed the difficulty in interpreting standard anteroposterior, lateral, and oblique roentgenographs of the foot in making this diagnosis. In the normal anteroposterior roentgenograph, the navicular shadow will slightly overlap all of the cuneiforms equally.[8] There should be no gap between the first and second metatarsal bases. In the normal lateral roentgenograph, all the cuneiforms overlap and lie directly in line with the navicular.[8] The metatarsals are all superimposed, the shafts should be parallel to each other, and the first ray should be the most dorsal. These relationships make evaluation of the naviculocuneiform joints difficult.[8] The authors stressed the importance of a detailed history of the injury as an aid in the roentgenographic evaluation. In their patient, the medial cuneiform and first metatarsal were depressed plantarly with the dislocation having occurred at the naviculocuneiform joint. The only roentgenographic clue to the injury was persistent separation of the bases of the first and second metatarsals. Due to the fact that the diagnosis was delayed for 4 weeks, they performed arthrodesis on the navicular–medial cuneiform joint. The patient recovered with minimal discomfort in the foot.

Clark and Quint[3] reported an isolated dislocation of the middle (second) cuneiform. In their patient a closed reduction was attempted but was unstable. The patient subsequently underwent open reduction following partial excision of the cuneiform. These authors stressed the importance of making the diagnosis to prevent loss of the longitudinal arch of the foot.

More recently, the dislocation of a cuneiform associated with tarsometatarsal fracture-dislocations has been recognized. Brown and McFarland[1] emphasized that in most tarsometatarsal dislocations, the naviculocuneiform joint remains intact. However, occasionally the medial cuneiform bone is completely dislocated secondary to a disruption of the naviculocuneiform joint. They reported a case in which the medial cuneiform was dislocated laterally between the first and second metatarsals. They believe that with the foot in the equinus position, a force from the navicular forces the medial cuneiform to dislocate forward and laterally, which they believe is the anatomic path of least resistance. Treatment by open reduction of the medial cuneiform in conjunction with reduction of the tarsometatarsal joint was performed. Holstein and Joldersma[6] emphasized the increased difficulty of reduction of tarsometatarsal fracture-dislocations in patients in whom there is an associated dislocation of the first cuneiform. In these patients, there is disruption of the articulation between the first cuneiform and first metatarsal, with outward rotation of the first cuneiform separating it from the second cuneiform. The portion of the anterior tibial tendon that remains attached to the first metatarsal slips between the first and second cuneiforms and often prevents closed reduction.[6]

Isolated Dislocations of the Cuboid

Drummond and Hastings[4] have reported an isolated dislocation of the cuboid bone. They stressed that such a dislocation can be missed on plane roentgenographs because in two dimensions it may be difficult to appreciate displacement of a single bone or disruption of one of its articulations. Additionally, they emphasized that such isolated tarsal dislocations are so uncommon that unfamiliarity contributes to their misdiagnoses. In their case, there was inferomedial dislocation of the cuboid secondary to a fall. The cuboid was displaced downward and medially. Open reduction and internal fixation of the cuboid with Kirschner wires followed by immobilization in a below-the-knee cast resulted in a pain-free foot with the patient returning to work. These authors stressed that such isolated cuboid dislocations are extremely rare due to the fact that the cuboid has a very stable relationship to the five bones with which it articulates and, therefore, crushing fractures rather than dislocations are more common.

Clinical Diagnosis

Most patients give a history of either a direct crushing injury or an injury secondary to a fall.[1, 3, 4, 5, 8] Due to the degree of injury, gross swelling is usually present. Tenderness occurs at the midtarsal joint and is usually most concentrated in the area of the particular tarsal dislocation.

Radiographic Diagnosis

Although isolated tarsal dislocations are apparent on routine anteroposterior, lateral, and oblique radiographs of the foot, a lack of familiarity with these injuries has led to the diagnosis being frequently missed and difficult to confirm roentgenographically.[4, 8] Careful correlation of the history and clinical examination is essential in x-ray interpretation.[8]

Treatment

Due to the degree of soft-tissue injury and swelling associated with these injuries, prompt reduction is essential.[5] Because these injuries are secondary to extreme force, they are usually quite unstable and require the use of crossed Kirschner wires to maintain their reduction. A delay in reduction can result in blistering and vascular compromise of the overlying skin. If this occurs, open reduction should be undertaken only after the skin has healed.[5]

Author's Preferred Method of Treatment

A careful evaluation of the roentgenographs of the foot that takes into consideration the anatomic relationships recognizable roentgenographically and the patient's description of the injury is essential to prevent overlooking these dislocations. Once dislocation of either a cuneiform or the cuboid is recognized, open reduction is performed. A skin incision directly over the dislocated tarsal bone is utilized. In my experience these injuries are extremely unstable and require crossed Kirschner wire fixation for stability. Following reduction, patients are placed in a short-leg non–weight-bearing cast with the toes free to allow early range of motion of the metatarsophalangeal joints. The Kirschner wires are removed at 4 to 6 weeks. Weight bearing is then begun in a hard-soled shoe with a good arch support.

Although the articular surfaces of the cuneiforms or cuboid may be damaged in these injuries, due to the minimal amount of motion present in these joints I have not relied upon primary arthrodesis in these cases. Should pain persist in the area after open reduction and internal fixation of the dislocation, intertarsal fusions are considered.

REFERENCES

Cuneiforms and Cuboid

1. Brown DC, McFarland JB Jr: Dislocation of the first cuneiform in tarsometatarsal fracture-dislocation, *J Bone Joint Surg [Am]* 57:858–859, 1975.
2. Chapman MW: Fractures and dislocations of the ankle and foot. In Mann RA, editor: *DuVries' surgery of the foot*, ed 4, St Louis, 1978, Mosby–Year Book.
3. Clark DF, Quint HA: Dislocation of a single cuneiform, *J Bone Joint Surg* 15:237–239, 1933.
4. Drummond DS, Hastings DE: Total dislocation of the cuboid bone: report of a case, *J Bone Joint Surg [Br]* 51:716, 1969.
5. Giannestras NJ, Sammarco JJ: Fractures and dislocations in the foot. In Rockwood CA Jr, Green DP, editors: *Fractures*, vol 2, Philadelphia, 1975, JB Lippincott.
6. Holstein A, Joldersma RD: Dislocation of the first cuneiform in tarsometatarsal fracture-dislocation, *J Bone Joint Surg [Am]* 32:419–421, 1950.
7. Jones FW: Structure and fixation as seen in the foot, London, 1944, Bailliere, Tindall & Cox, p 246.
8. Schiller MG, Ray RD: Isolated dislocation of the medial cuneiform bone—a rare injury of the tarsus, *J Bone Joint Surg [Am]* 52:1632, 1970.

DISLOCATIONS OF THE METATARSOPHALANGEAL JOINTS

Dislocations of the metatarsophalangeal joints are uncommon injuries.[33] Although they are the most common of the metatarsophalangeal dislocations, traumatic dislocations or fracture-dislocation of the first metatarsophalangeal joints are still quite rare.* Indeed, Mouchet[24] found only 50 cases reported prior to 1931. Isolated dislocation of the metatarsophalangeal joints of

**References 5, 8, 13 14, 18, 19, 22, 30, 35.*

the second through the fifth toes are even more unusual.[16, 27, 29]

Metatarsophalangeal joint injuries are usually associated with motor vehicle accidents.[8, 9, 14, 18, 21] However, Coker et al.[6, 7] have reported injuries to the first metatarsophalangeal joint in football. Indeed, these are seen now with more frequency due to the combination of non–leather-soled shoes and artificial turf.[2, 6, 7]

Anatomy

Hallux Metatarsophalangeal Joint

The metatarsophalangeal joint of the hallux is composed of the concave base of the proximal phalanx which articulates with the convex head of the first metatarsal.[31] A fibrous capsule lined with synovial membrane surrounds this joint. The plantar surface of the joint capsule consists of a heavy ligament attached to both the metatarsal head and the proximal phalanx. This volar fibrous ligament blends laterally with the deep transverse metatarsal ligament that runs transversely between the heads of the metatarsals.[31] The plantar aspect of the capsule contains the sesamoids, which serve as points of insertion of the tendons of the flexor hallucis brevis. The medial (tibial) sesamoid serves as a point of insertion for the medial head of the flexor hallucis brevis and the abductor hallucis brevis, while the lateral (fibular) sesamoid serves as a point of insertion of the lateral head of the flexor hallucis brevis and both heads of the adductor hallucis.[30] The tendons of the lateral head of the flexor hallucis brevis and the adductor hallucis insert into the lateral sesamoid joint proximal and dorsal to the deep transverse metatarsal ligament (Fig 35–141,A).[31]

This volar fibrous plate is firmly attached to the volar aspect of the base of the phalanx, while proximally it is loosely attached to the subcapital area of the metatarsal neck.[14, 17, 31] Giannikas et al.[14] state that with hyperextension of the toe the plantar part of the capsule is avulsed from the head and neck of the metatarsal. The base of the first proximal phalanx then slides over the head of the metatarsal, followed by the fibrocartilaginous plate, which becomes locked in this position (Fig 35–141,A and B). The collateral ligaments remain intact and hold the locked fibrocartilaginous plate over the dorsum of the head of the metatarsal.[14] When this occurs, the first metatarsal head becomes trapped between the tendons of the two heads of the flexor hallucis brevis.[30] The fact that some of these dislocations are irreducible by closed means has led some authors to call these complex or buttonhole dislocations.[1]

Lesser Toe (II to V) Metatarsophalangeal Joints

Although reports of metatarsophalangeal dislocations of the lesser toes (II to V) are unusual, Rao and Banzon[29] found that the fibrocartilaginous volar plate was interposed between the metatarsal head and the base of the proximal phalanges in metatarsal dislocations of the third and fourth digits. They also noted that the flexor digitorum longus and flexor digitorum brevis tendons were located on the lateral side of the metatarsal necks

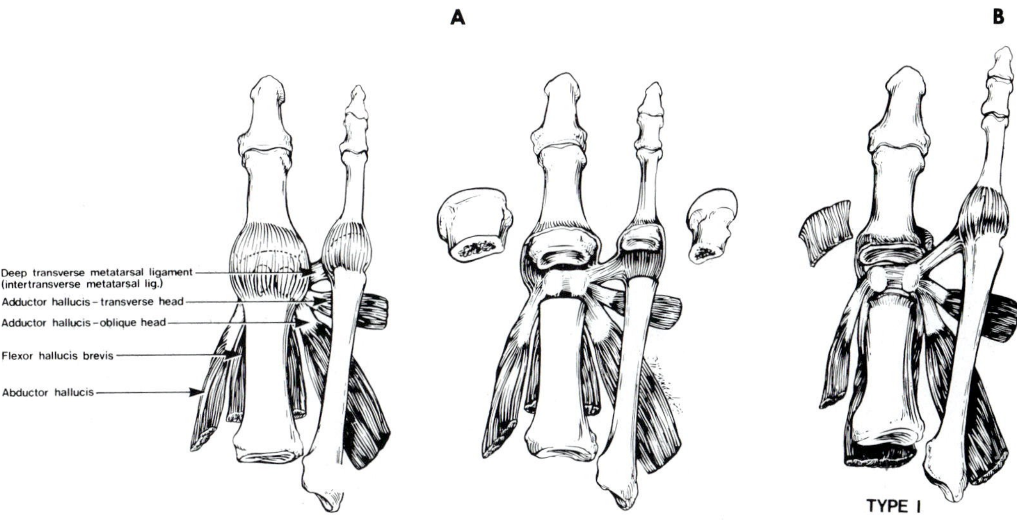

FIG 35–141.
A, normal anatomy of the first metatarsophalangeal joint. Note the relationship of the deep transverse metatarsal ligament and the conjoined tendon of the adductor hallucis and lateral head of the flexor hallucis brevis. **B,** type I dorsal dislocation of the first metatarsophalangeal joint. Note that the sesamoids are not fractured nor is the intersesamoid ligament disrupted.

while the lumbrical tendons were located on the medial aspect of the metatarsal necks. Murphy[27] also reported that the main obstacle to reduction in a dorsal dislocation of the second metatarsophalangeal joint was the plantar fibrocartilaginous plate.

Classification

Jahss,[18] in a detailed study of the pathomechanics of dorsal dislocations of the first metatarsophalangeal joint, classifies these dislocations into two types. In type I, the volar plate, which consists of the sesamoid mass and the thick plantar capsule that is attached proximally to the plantar aspect of the neck of the first metatarsal, ruptures at its attachment beneath the metatarsal neck. The hallux, with the sesamoids still attached to the base of the proximal phalanx, rides over the dorsum of the metatarsal head and locks the head in a plantar position (Fig 35–142,A and B). The medial and lateral conjoined tendons (consisting of the medial head of the flexor hallucis brevis and abductor hallucis medially and the lateral head of the flexor hallucis brevis and the adductor hallucis laterally) come to rest tightly on either side of the metatarsal neck (see Fig 35–141,B). This is a so-called type I dislocation.[18] Such cases in the literature have been irreducible by closed manipulation.[8, 14, 18, 21] Several authors have compared the type I dislocation to that of the complex metacarpophalangeal joint dislocation noted in the hand.[21, 30]

With more dorsiflexion force, the intersesamoid ligament will rupture and result in wide separation of the sesamoids (type IIA), or a transverse fracture of one or both sesamoids will occur (type IIB)[3, 18] (Fig 35–143,A and B). These are the so-called type II dislocations.[18] If the mechanism is a fall from a height, the sesamoid fracture may be due to a crushing against the metatarsal condyles that results in comminution of the sesamoid fracture.[24] If pure hyperextension is the force responsible for the dislocation, the fracture more often resembles an avulsion. In either situation, the more proximal fragment of the fractured sesamoid remains in a normal position in relation to the adjacent sesamoid via the remaining intact intersesamoid ligament. The distal fragment widely separates from its proximal fragment because it is not only forcibly separated from its attachment to the intersesamoid ligament but is also pulled distally into the joint space by its peripheral attachments at the base of the proximal phalanx. This fragment essentially acts as a loose body and may require removal.[9, 19] In a situation in which there is rupture of the volar plate through the intersesamoid ligament or through a fracture of one or both sesamoids, reduction is usually easily accomplished by closed means. Henderson and Denno[15] recently reported simultaneous open dislocation of the metatarsophalangeal and interphalangeal joints of the hallux. The metatarsophalangeal and interphalangeal joints were easily reduced by closed means due to the severe disruption of the capsule.

The importance in classifying these injuries as type I or type II injuries lies in being able to predict whether closed reduction will be successful.

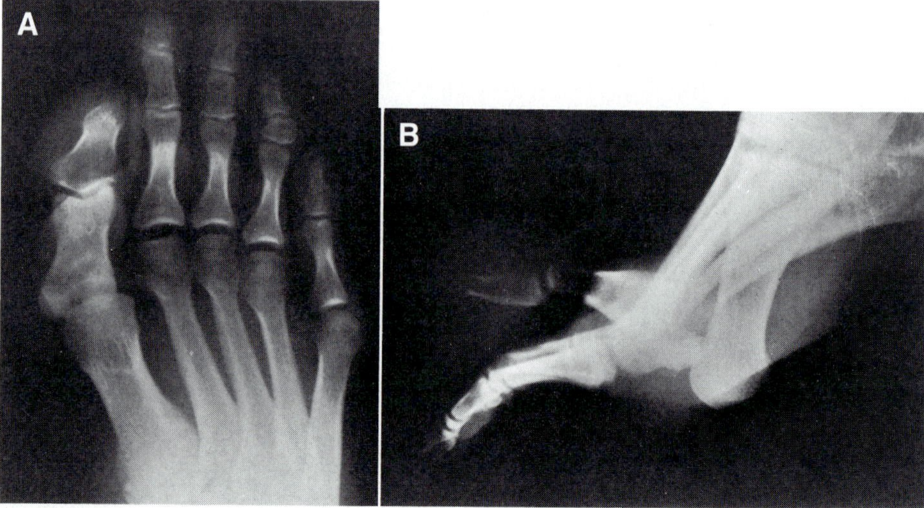

FIG 35–142.
A, anteroposterior radiograph of a type I dislocation with a slight medial displacement. The sesamoids are neither fractured nor separated on this view. **B,** lateral radiograph of a type I metatarsophalangeal joint dislocation. Both sesamoids are dorsal to the first metatarsal head, and there is marked plantar angulation of the first metatarsal shaft.

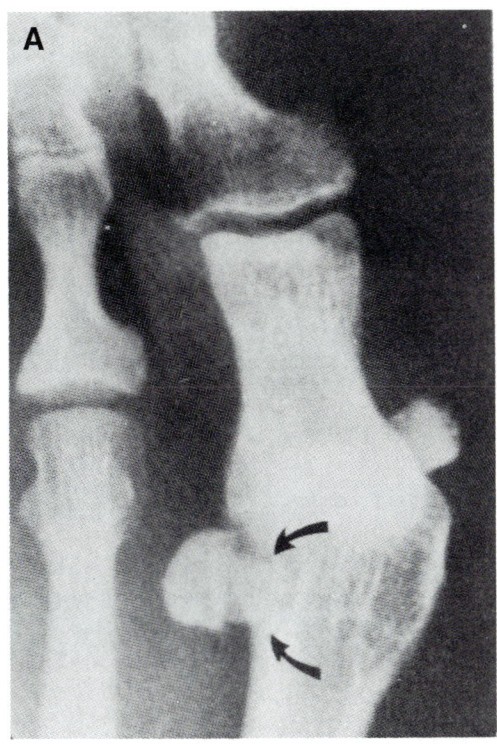

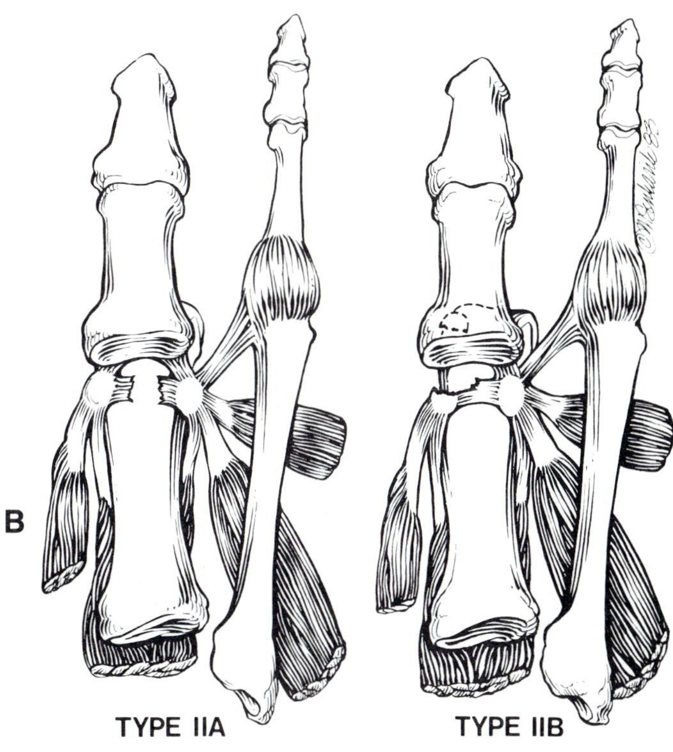

FIG 35–143.
A, anteroposterior radiograph of a type II metatarsophalangeal dislocation. The hallux metatarsophalangeal joint is dislocated, and the medial sesamoid is fractured. *Arrows* denote a displaced fragment of the *medial* sesamoid. **B,** type II dislocations. In type IIA; the intersesamoid ligament is ruptured. In type IIB; a transverse fracture of the medial sesamoid is noted. The proximal fragment remains in its normal relationship to the adjacent sesamoid via the intact intersesamoid ligament. The distal fragment is separated from the proximal fragment and remains attached to the base of the proximal phalanx. (**A** from Jahss MH: *Foot Ankle* 1:15–21, 1980. Used by permission.)

Mechanism of Injury

Hallux Metatarsophalangeal Dislocations

The dislocation is usually the result of forces that hyperextend the great toe and cause displacement of the proximal phalanx onto the dorsum of the first metatarsal neck.[14, 35] Hyperextension of the proximal phalanx of the hallux on the first metatarsal, such as occurs when the toes are forcibly dorsiflexed against the floorboard of an automobile, results in the metatarsal head being pushed through the plantar capsule between the medial head of the flexor hallucis brevis, the abductor hallucis, and the associated medial sesamoid and the lateral head of the flexor hallucis brevis, the adductor hallucis and the lateral sesamoid. The plantar capsule is disrupted at its proximal attachment to the neck of the metatarsal, similar to the volar capsular avulsion noted in dorsal dislocation of the metacarpophalangeal joints in the hand.[30] Coker et al.[6, 7] note that in pileups in a football game, when one player lands on the back of the leg of another, such hyperextension of the metatarsophalangeal joint can occur. Changes in the playing surfaces, the decreased support of footgear used in football today, and finally, poor shoe fitting are reported as explanations of the increased incidence of such metatarsophalangeal injuries noted in football today.[6, 7]

Konkel and Muehlstein[19] suggest that in dislocations of the first metatarsophalangeal joint with a displaced fracture of the medial sesamoid, an alternative mechanism of injury is crushing of the medial sesamoid at the time the great toe is forced dorsally and dislocated. When the displacing force is relieved, the medial sesamoid returns to its normal position and leaves a displaced fragment in the joint. Jahss stresses that in the pure hyperextension mechanism, any associated sesamoid fractures are avulsion in nature[18] while comminution of the sesamoid suggests crushing against the metatarsal condyles due to a fall from a height.[18, 24]

Lesser Toe (II to V) Metatarsophalangeal Dislocations

Rao and Banzon[29] report that forcible dorsiflexion of the proximal phalanx over the metatarsal head is also the most common mechanism of injury in dislocations of the metatarsophalangeal joints of the lesser toes. This results in the metatarsal head being forced through the plantar fibrocartilaginous plate. Murphy also documents forcible dorsiflexion as the mechanism of injury in this dislocation.[27] In both of these patients there was an associated fracture of the second metatarsal neck due to a similar mechanism.[27, 29]

Jahss has reported chronic lateral dislocations of the fifth toe metatarsophalangeal joint.[16] The mechanism of injury in these cases is forced abduction such as occurs when the small toe catches on a piece of furniture. Reports of lateral dislocations of the other toes are not noted in the literature.

Clinical Diagnosis

In dislocations of the first metatarsophalangeal joint physical examination reveals marked distortion of the anatomic contour of the great toe (Fig 35–144). Swelling and tenderness are usually present, and the patient cannot walk or bear weight on the foot.[13] The most impressive finding is the prominence of the metatarsal head on the plantar aspect of the foot.[14, 18, 22] Pressure from the metatarsal head may result in blanching of the plantar skin.[21] The proximal phalanx rests on the dorsum of the metatarsal head in extension with slight outward deviation.[14, 21] If there is a lateral component to the dislocation, there will be an increase in the interdigital space between the toes.[13] The distal phalanx of the great toe is usually flexed and the extensor tendons relaxed. Rao and Banzon[29] report that the important clinical findings in dislocations of the lesser toe metatarsophalangeal joints include swelling and hyperextension deformity with corresponding prominences on the sole of the foot. Murphy[27] reports that swelling of the forefoot and shortening of the involved toe are also important clinical findings. Again, a palpable tender bony prominence on the sole of the forefoot representing the displaced metatarsal head is classic.

Jahss[16] mentions abduction deformity with widening of the interdigital space as the classic clinical finding in lateral dislocation of the fifth metatarsophalangeal joint.

Radiographic Diagnosis

Hallux Metatarsophalangeal Dislocations

Anteroposterior, lateral, and oblique views of the metatarsophalangeal joints are essential in confirming the diagnosis. Garcia and Parkes[12] believe that the injury is best visualized roentgenographically on lateral and oblique radiographs of the foot. Giannestras and Sammarco[13] stress that anteroposterior roentgenographs demonstrate a double density of the proximal phalanx overlying the metatarsal head in a pure dorsal dislocation. In evaluating the roentgenographs, it is important to specifically analyze each sesamoid. Fractures of the sesamoid that may be associated with these injuries need to be identified *prior* to reduction. Additionally, a careful evaluation of postreduction radiographs is essential to rule out the presence of a fracture fragment within the joint.[9, 14, 19] Finally, careful evaluation of these roentgenographs is necessary to classify these as type I or type II injuries. If there is frank separation of the sesamoids to either side of the metatarsal head on the anteroposterior roentgenograph, there is a complete disruption of the intersesamoid ligament and a type II injury. Additionally, if a fracture of the sesamoids is present, this can be seen on anteroposterior and oblique radiographs and also represents a type II lesion (see Fig

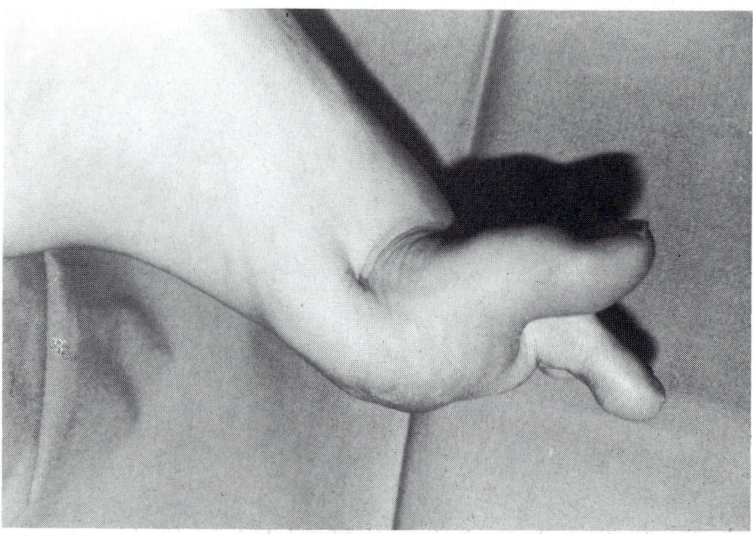

FIG 35–144.
Clinical appearance of first metatarsophalangeal joint dislocation. Notice the skin dimple, which suggests irreducibility.

35–143,A and B). As mentioned by Jahss,[18] these are usually reducible by closed methods. If, however, the sesamoids are not separated or fractured on the anteroposterior view and, on the lateral view, they appear to be riding dorsal to the metatarsal head, a type I dislocation that is usually irreducible by closed methods is present (see Fig 35–142,A and B). It is important to note that the involved metatarsal is plantar-flexed at the tarsometatarsal joint in this injury (see Fig 35–142,B). According to Giannikas et al.,[14] a lateral radiograph demonstrating the head of the first metatarsal depressed into the sole of the foot and the proximal phalanx resting on the dorsum of the head of the metatarsal is the most important roentgenograph.

Lesser Toe Metatarsophalangeal Dislocations

Murphy[27] emphasizes that in dislocations of the lesser (II to V) metatarsophalangeal joints the anteroposterior x-ray view may be diagnostic. He stresses the finding of widening of the metatarsophalangeal joint on the anteroposterior view. The plantar location of the metatarsal head may be visualized on the lateral roentgenograph. However, an overlap of the metatarsal heads may obscure this finding. Rao and Banzon[29] demonstrated widening of the metatarsophalangeal joints of the third and fourth digits with lateral displacement of the phalanges with respect to the metatarsals as findings suggesting dislocation of these joints (Fig 35–145).

Treatment

Hallux Metatarsophalangeal Dislocations

Dislocations of the metatarsophalangeal joint of the hallux can initially be approached by closed reduction. The closed reduction is first attempted under local anesthesia.[12] This can be augmented by intravenous analgesia.[12, 13] The method of manipulation includes hyperextension of the phalanx with plantar angulation of the metatarsal so that the inferior edge of the articular surface of the phalanx contacts the superior aspect of the articular surface of the metatarsal head.[5, 12, 23] Traction and then direct plantar pressure and flexion of the phalanx are used to complete the reduction.[5, 12, 23] Following reduction, most dislocations are stable.[5, 23] As emphasized by Deluca and Kenmore[9] it is essential to obtain adequate postreduction radiographs to identify loose bony fragments remaining in the metatarsophalangeal joint that may require subsequent surgical excision. After a stable reduction, Garcia and Parkes[12] recommend immobilization for 2 to 3 weeks by the use of a dorsal metallic splint to prevent extension of the metatarsophalangeal joint. The patient is allowed to begin weight bearing within the limits of pain.[13] Moseley believes that a metatarsal bar to protect the foot from plantar pressure during the early postreduction period is all that is necessary.[23] Chapman recommends the use of minimal external fixation by strapping following reduction.[5] Coker et al. recommend the use of a 0.5-mm-thick spring steel splint within the shoe extending from just anterior to the heel to the forward edge of the inner sole to protect the metatarsophalangeal joint from further hyperextension.[6, 7]

If following reduction there is even a slight tendency toward redislocation, a walking cast extending to the tip of the toes should be applied.[13] Giannestras and Sammarco[13] emphasize that in those dislocations with a component of lateral displacement, the damage to the collateral ligaments may prevent a stable closed reduction. In this instance, a percutaneous K-wire across the joint is used to help maintain the reduction.[13]

If an attempt at closed reduction under local anesthesia is unsuccessful, a second attempt under general anesthesia is warranted.[8] If closed reduction is unsuccessful under general anesthesia, a complex or irreducible dislocation requiring open reduction is present.[13] Open reduction may also be necessary if in addition to being irreducible, the post reduction radiographs reveal an intra-articular loose body in the metatarsophalangeal joint that must be removed.[9] Daniel et al.[8] recommend a dorsomedial approach to the metatarsophalangeal joint through which a "Z-plasty" tenotomy is performed on the extensor hallucis longus tendon. The metatarsophalangeal joint capsule is opened via an inverted L-shaped capsulotomy. Following this arthrotomy, manipulative reduction is performed under direct vision. Wright[35] also recommends the use of a medial approach to the first metatarsophalangeal joint to perform this open reduction.

Salamon et al.[30] compare this dislocation of the metatarsophalangeal joint with the complex dislocation of the index finger and recommend the use of a plantar approach for the best visualization of the pathologic anatomy and the most direct means of reduction. Giannikas et al.[14] also recommend the use of a plantar incision, transverse in nature, under the first metatarsophalangeal joint.

Lewis and DeLee[21] recommend the use of a dorsal incision in the web space between the first and second metatarsal heads to surgically reduce this irreducible dislocation. The advantages of the dorsal approach include the lack of an incision over the plantar aspect of the foot with the attendant risk of formation of a painful plantar scar, better visualization of the pathologic anatomy, and finally a decreased risk of damage to the plantar digital nerves, which are at risk through the plantar approach. These authors also emphasize the importance of surgically releasing both heads of the adductor hallucis and the deep transverse metatarsal ligament from the lateral sesamoid to allow enough mobility to easily reduce the volar fibrocartilaginous plate from its location dorsal to the neck of the metatarsal.

Following surgical reduction, these dislocations are usually stable.[21, 30, 35] Wright[35] recommends the use of a splint for 2 weeks to allow soft-tissue healing followed by progressive weight bearing in a good shoe. Daniel et al.[8] recommend non–weight bearing for a short period of time followed by progressive weight bearing within the limits of pain. The total period of cast immobilization is 3 to 4 weeks. Following cast removal, they recommend hydrotherapy and an exercise program to regain the range of motion.[8] Lewis and DeLee recommend the use of a short-leg cast for 2 weeks followed by weight bearing in a shoe. It is essential to begin early hydrotherapy and toe exercises to restore range of metatarsophalangeal motion.[8, 21] Although Wright[35] recommends the use of a toe splint for 4 to 6 weeks following cast removal to prevent an extension contracture, other authors have not found this to be necessary.[21]

Lesser Toe (II to V) Metatarsophalangeal Dislocations

In dislocations of the lesser metatarsophalangeal joints, closed reduction is attempted first.[27, 29] Rao and Banzon[29] attempted closed reduction by hyperextension of the phalanx, pressure against the base of the phalanx, and then flexion. They were able to reduce one of three lesser toe dislocations by this method. Murphy,[27] however, found a dislocation of the second metatarsophalangeal joint to be irreducible by this method. If the manipulation is unsuccessful, open surgical reduction is performed. Rao and Benzon[29] utilized a dorsal incision between the dislocated third and fourth metatarsophalangeal joints. They found that this provided excellent exposure to demonstrate the plantar fibrocartilaginous plate that was interposed between the metatarsal head and the base of the phalanges. Once the surgical exposure was obtained, they again attempted a manipulative reduction, which was unsuccessful. They found that release of the dorsal capsule and deep transverse metatarsal ligament was necessary for the reduction to be successful.

Like dislocations of the first metatarsophalangeal joint following closed or open reduction, these dislocations are usually stable.[27, 29] Following reduction Rao and Benzon[29] protected the dislocations in a short-leg walking cast for 6 weeks. Rao and Benzon[29] and Murphy[27] found at follow-up that their patients were able to dorsiflex their toes without pain and radiographs showed no evidence of metatarsophalangeal joint degenerative arthritis.

Jahss[16] mentions abduction instability at the metatarsophalangeal joint following inadequate treatment of lateral metatarsophalangeal joint dislocations of the fifth metatarsophalangeal joint. The instability is demonstrated by abduction of the fifth toe on weight bearing. Such abduction instability is quite symptomatic because it results in catching the fifth toe on the sock, shoe, etc., and may require later reconstructive surgery.[16] He recommended adequate immobilization of this joint following a lateral dislocation to allow the medial joint capsule to heal.

Results

Usually no permanent disability results from these dislocations.[13] Lewis and DeLee report restoration of essentially a normal range of motion of the metatarsophalangeal joint following this dislocation.[21] Garcia and Parkes[12] also report in the majority of instances that there is no permanent disability following this injury. They do caution that occasionally a patient may return 4 to 5 years postinjury with symptoms of early osteoarthritis of the first metatarsophalangeal joint as evidenced by the slight restriction of motion often noted in patients with hallux rigidus.[12] Garcia and Parkes[12] stress that in dislocations that remain unreduced, the long extensors and flexors of the toe produce a clawing deformity that leads to severe metatarsalgia and plantar callosities beneath the involved metatarsal head. In this instance, roentgenographic evidence of degenerative arthritis is present, and clinically the patients present with restricted joint motion. Reconstructive surgery of the metatarsophalangeal joint is then necessary.

Author's Preferred Method of Treatment

Hallux Metatarsophalangeal Dislocations

I have found Jahss' classification most helpful in predicting reducibility of dislocations of the first metatarsophalangeal joint. Radiographs clearly demonstrating both sesamoids are essential before closed reduction is attempted. Patients in whom the sesamoids are not separated on the anteroposterior view and are not fractured have type I injuries in Jahss' classification and usually require an open reduction. I have also noted that the presence of a skin dimple located *medially* on the metatarsophalangeal joint may be associated with irreducibility by closed methods (see Fig 35–145) Even in patients with type I dislocations I attempt a closed reduction. All type II dislocations initially undergo an attempted closed reduction.

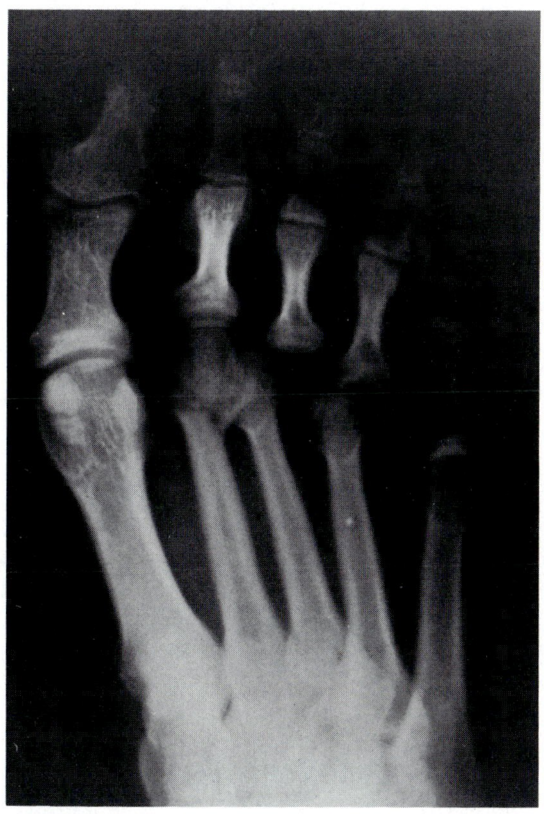

FIG 35–145.
Anteroposterior radiograph of dislocations of the third and fourth metatarsophalangeal joints. Joint spaces are widened, and the phalanges are displaced laterally with respect to the metatarsals. (From Rao JP, Banzon MT: *Clin Orthop* 145:224–226, 1979. Used by permission.)

I attempt the closed reduction first under local anesthesia augmented by intravenous analgesia. Longitudinal traction, hyperextension of the metatarsophalangeal joint, and plantar pressure on the dorsal aspect of the base of the involved proximal phalanx are attempted in an effort to obtain a reduction. Post reduction radiographs are carefully evaluated to make certain that the reduction is anatomic and there are no intra-articular bone fragments that require surgical removal. If closed reduction under local anesthesia is unsuccessful, the patient is taken to the operating room, and a second closed reduction under general anesthesia is attempted with the same manipulation.

If the closed reduction is successful, the patient is placed in a short-leg walking cast that extends past the toes to prevent their hyperextension. Weight bearing is encouraged as soon as the pain is tolerable. Cast immobilization is used for 2 to 3 weeks. Following this a stiff-soled shoe with a metatarsal bar is recommended. After the cast is removed, toe flexion exercises and hydrotherapy are instituted in an effort to regain a complete range of metatarsophalangeal joint motion. In my experience, the most frequent disability following simple dislocation of this joint is a loss of metatarsophalangeal joint motion.

If closed reduction is unsuccessful under general anesthesia or if bony fragments are trapped in the joint, open reduction is performed through a *dorsal* incision placed between the first and second metatarsal heads. Following exposure of the joint, a second closed reduction is attempted to demonstrate the pathologic anatomy. In my experience, detachment of both heads of the adductor hallucis from the fibular sesamoid followed by transection of the deep transverse metatarsal ligament allows one to return the fibrocartilaginous plate to the plantar aspect of the metatarsal head. Following this reduction the joint is irrigated, and documentation of articular cartilage damage to the metatarsal head and base of the proximal phalanx is made. The adductor and the deep transverse metatarsal ligament are reattached to the lateral sesamoid. Following open reduction, in the author's experience, these dislocations are stable. The postoperative immobilization is similar to that following closed reduction.

Lesser Toe Metatarsophalangeal Dislocations

I treat dislocations of the lesser toe metatarsophalangeal joints similar to the method used for the hallux. Closed reduction is attempted first by using the same hyperextension maneuver. If this is unsuccessful, open reduction through a dorsal longitudinal incision placed adjacent to the involved metatarsophalangeal joint is preferred. After open reduction, a short-leg walking cast with a toe plate is used for 2 weeks followed by the use of a stiff-soled shoe. Range-of-motion exercises are begun after 3 weeks.

DISLOCATIONS OF THE INTERPHALANGEAL JOINTS

Dislocations of the interphalangeal joints of the toes are extremely unusual, those of the great toe being by far the most common.[10] Giannestras and Sammarco[13] report that these dislocations are most commonly associated with other trauma to the foot. The anatomy of the interphalangeal joint shows little anatomic variation.[21] The extensor hallucis longus tendon crosses the joint dorsally and inserts into the distal phalanx. The capsule of the interphalangeal joint is strengthened medially and laterally by collaterals that provide medial and collateral stability. The flexor hallucis longus is beneath the volar surface and inserts into the distal phalanx. The volar plate, a thickening in the volar capsule, forms a plantar accessory ligament. Invagination of this ligament into the joint with or without an accompanying sesamoid has been shown to produce an irreducible dislocation of the interphalangeal joint.[21] Approximately 13% of the population has an interphalangeal sesamoid in the great toe.[4]

Anteroposterior, oblique, and lateral radiographs reveal the loss of integrity of the interphalangeal joint. Care must be taken to evaluate the joint surfaces for associated fractures. This injury is oftentimes open and may be associated with comminuted fractures at the base of the distal phalanx.[13]

Eibel,[10] Laczay and Csapo.[20] Murakawami and Tokuyasu,[26] Yasuda et al.,[36] and Wolfe and Goodhart[34] reported dislocations of the interphalangeal joints of the great toe with interposition of the plantar sesamoid. Muller[25] is credited by Eibel as first reporting this dislocation.[10] In Eibel's case[10] the interphalangeal joint was dislocated dorsally. He reported marked swelling dorsally and an open laceration on the plantar surface of the interphalangeal joint. Although closed reduction was successfully accomplished, it required considerable force, and the reduction was not stable. Post-reduction radiographs revealed an osseous body within the interphalangeal joint that proved to be an interphalangeal sesamoid. Following open reduction a splint was applied to the great toe for 3 weeks, following which ambulation was initiated. Recovery was reported to be complete at 5 weeks. In the cases reported by Yasuda et al.[36] and Wolfe and Goodhart[34] the interphalangeal joint dislocations of the great toe were closed injuries that did not reduce upon attempts at closed reduction. Yasudo et al.[36] recommended a plantar approach with repair of the plantar plate and preservation of the sesamoid bone. Alternatively, Wolfe and Goodhart[34] report using the dorsal approach to remove the entrapped sesamoid.

Interphalangeal joint dislocations of the lesser toes have been reported to occur following abduction stresses to the interphalangeal joints, particularly of the fifth toe.[18] These dislocations are usually stable if reduction is performed in the early postinjury period. If following reduction there is any sign of instability because of capsular damage, a Kirschner wire from the distal phalanx into the proximal phalanx may be necessary to hold the reduction. If such a pin is utilized, it usually remains in place for 3 weeks to allow the soft tissues to heal. If closed reduction is successful, simple taping to the adjacent digit is all the immobilization that is necessary.

Fugate et al.[11] reported an irreducible fracture dislocation of the proximal interphalangeal joint of the third toe. Closed reduction was unsuccessful because the flexor tendon was entrapped between the middle and proximal phalanges. A dorsal longitudinal arthrotomy was used to remove the interposed tissue. The toe was apparently stable post-reduction, and at follow-up a good functional result was obtained.

Author's Preferred Treatment

For interphalangeal joint dislocations of the hallux, I prefer closed reduction by traction, hyperextension, and plantar pressure on the distal phalanx. If the reduction is stable, the patient is placed in a short-leg walking cast for 2 to 3 weeks followed by a stiff-soled shoe or a stainless steel insert, as has been recommended by Coker et al.[6, 7] This is used for a period of 4 to 6 weeks. If closed reduction is unsuccessful or unstable, careful x-ray analysis is performed to detect an interphalangeal sesamoid or other incarcerated bone fragment preventing a stable reduction. An open reduction through a dorsal incision is then performed with removal of the offending sesamoid or fragment. Postoperative management is similar to that after closed reduction.

In the lesser toes (II to V), if the dislocation is stable, the author prefers to tape the involved toe to the adjacent toe until the swelling and pain have subsided. In the event that the dislocation is unstable, a Kirschner wire across the interphalangeal joint is utilized for 3 weeks to provide stability.

Late complications following interphalangeal or distal interphalangeal dislocations are not common. If they do occur, however, I have found that excisional arthroplasty or arthrodesis usually results in pain relief.

REFERENCES

Metatarsophalangeal and Interphalangeal Joints

1. Blodgett WH: Injuries of the forefoot and toes. In Jahss MH, editor: *Disorders of the foot*, vol 2, Philadelphia, 1982, WB Saunders.
2. Bowers KD Jr, Martin RB: Impact absorption, new and old Astroturf at West Virginia University, *Med Sci Sports* 6:217, 1974.
3. Brown TIS: Avulsion fracture of the fibular sesamoid in association with dorsal dislocation of the metatarsophalangeal joint of the hallux, *Clin Orthop* 149:229–231, 1980.
4. Burman MS, Lapidus PW: The functional disturbances caused by the inconstant bones and sesamoids of the foot, *Arch Surg* 22:936–975.
5. Chapman MW: Fractures and dislocations of the ankle and foot. In Mann RA, editor: *DuVries' surgery of the foot*, ed 4, St Louis, 1978, Mosby–Year Book.
6. Coker TP, Jr, Arnold JA: Sports injuries to the foot and ankle. In Jahss MH, editor: *Disorders of the Foot*, vol 2, Philadelphia, 1982, WB Saunders.

7. Coker TP Jr, Arnold JA, Weber DL: Traumatic lesions of the metatarsophalangeal joint of the great toe in athletes, *J Arkansas Med Soc* 74:309, 1978.
8. Daniel WL, Beck EL, Duggar GE, et al: Traumatic dislocation of the first metatarsophalangeal joint. A case report, *J Am Podiatr Assoc* 66:97–100, 1976.
9. DeLuca FN, Kenmore PI: Bilateral dorsal dislocations of the metatarsophalangeal joints of the great toes with a loose body in one of the metatarsophalangeal joints, *J Trauma* 15:737–739, 1975.
10. Eibel P: Dislocation of the interphalangeal joint of the big toe with interposition of a sesamoid bone, *J Bone Joint Surg [Am]* 36:880–882, 1954.
11. Fugate DS, Thomson J, Christansen KP: An irreducible fracture dislocation of a lesser toe: a case report, *Foot Ankle* 11:317–319, 1991.
12. Garcia A, Parkes JC: Fractures of the foot. In Giannestras NJ, editor: *Foot disorders: Medical and surgical management*, ed 2, Philadelphia, 1973, Lea & Febiger.
13. Giannestras NJ, Sammarco GJ: Fractures and dislocations in the foot. In Rockwood CA Jr, Green DP, editors: *Fractures*, vol 2, Philadelphia, 1975, JB Lippincott.
14. Giannikas AC, Papachristou G, Papavasiliou N, et al: Dorsal dislocation of the first metatarsophalangeal joint, *J Bone Joint Surg [Br]* 57:384–386, 1975.
15. Henderson CE, Denno G: Simultaneous open dislocation of the metatarsophalangeal and interphalangeal joint of the hallux: a case report, *Foot Ankle* 6:305–308, 1986.
16. Jahss MH: Chronic and recurrent dislocations of the fifth toe, *Foot Ankle* 3:275–278, 1981.
17. Jahss MH: LeLievre bunion operation, *Instr Course Lect* 21:295–310, 1972.
18. Jahss MH: Traumatic dislocations of the first metatarsophalangeal joint, *Foot Ankle* 1:15–21, 1980.
19. Konkel KF, Muehlstein JH: Unusual fracture-dislocation of the great toe: case report, *J Trauma* 15:733–736, 1975.
20. Laczay V, Csapo K: Interphalangeal Luxation der Grobzehe mit Interposition eines Sesambeiwes, *Fortschr Rontgenstr* 116:571–572, 1972.
21. Lewis AG, DeLee JC: Type I complex dislocation of the first metatarsophalangeal joint, reduction through a dorsal approach, *J Bone Joint Surg* 66A:1120–1123, 1984.
22. McKinley LM, Davis GL: Locked dislocation of the great toe, *J La State Med Soc* 127:389–390, 1975.
23. Moseley HF: Traumatic disorders of the ankle and foot, *Clin Symp* 17:30, 1965.
24. Mouchet A: Deux cas de luxation dorsale complete du gros orteil avec lesions des sesamoides, *Rev Orthop* 18:221–227, 1931.
25. Muller GM: Dislocation of sesamoid of hallux, *Lancet 1:789, 1944.*
26. Murakawami Y, Tokuyasu Y: A case of dislocation of the first toe with the sesamoid bone interfering with orthopaedic manipulation, *Orthop Surg (Tokyo)* 22:751–753, 1971.
27. Murphy JL: Isolated dorsal dislocation of the second metatarsophalangeal joint, *Foot Ankle* 1:30–32, 1980.
28. Nelson TL, Uggen W: Irreducible dorsal dislocation of the interphalangeal joint of the great toe, *Clin Orthop* 151:256–264, 1980.
29. Rao JP, Banzon MT: Irreducible dislocation of the metatarsophalangeal joints of the foot, *Clin Orthop* 145:224–226, 1979.
30. Salamon PB, Gelberman RH, Huffer JM: Dorsal dislocation of the metatarsophalangeal joint of the great toe. A case report, *J Bone Joint Surg [Am]* 56:1073–1075, 1974.
31. Sarrafian SK: *Anatomy of the foot and ankle: Topographical, functional and descriptive*, Philadelphia, 1983, JB Lippincott.
32. Scranton PE, Ruthowski R: Anatomic variations in the first ray. Part II: disorders of the sesamoids, *Clin Orthop* 151:256–264, 1980.
33. Wilson JL, editor: *Watson-Jones fractures and joint injuries*, ed 5, New York, 1976, Longman.
34. Wolfe J, Goodhart C: Irreducible dislocation of the great toe following sports injury, *Am J Sports Med* 17:695–696, 1989.
35. Wright PE: Dislocations. In Edmonson AS, Crenshaw AH, editors: *Campbell's operative orthopaedics*, ed 6, vol 1, St Louis, 1980, Mosby–Year Book.
36. Yasuda T, Fujio K, Tumra K: Irreducible dorsal dislocation of the interphalangeal joint of the great toe: report of two cases, *Foot Ankle* 10:331–336, 1990.

Index

A

Abduction/external rotation stress test, 1146
Abductor digiti quinti, compression or entrapment of nerve to, heel pain from, 838, 839, 841, 1231–1232
Abductor hallucis tendon
  lengthening for metatarsus adductus, 1331
  sesamoids and, 469
Abscess, in diabetic foot, 914, 915
Accessory anterior tibiofibular ligament, 1144
Accessory bones of foot and uncommon sesamoids, 499–535
  anatomy, 528–532, 535
Accessory navicular, 521–523, 741
  clinical significance, 523–525
  flatfoot associated, 522, 1338, 1340
    in adults, 764–765
    clinical significance, 523–525
    clinical symptoms, 741
    diagnosis, 742
    discussion, 743–744
    treatment
      author's preferred method, 743
      conservative, 742
      Kidner procedure, 522–523, 525
      surgical, 742–743
  navicular fracture vs., 1602, 1603
  painful, in dancers, 1254
  types, 741, 742
  variations, 521, 523
Accessory scaphoid, navicular fracture vs., 1602, 1603
Accessory soleus muscle, in dancers, 1273
Achilles tendinitis
  in dancers, 1271–1272
  retrocalcaneal bursitis associated with, surgical treatment, 854–855
  in runners, 1233–1234
  superior heel pain from, 848
Achilles tendinitis and ruptures in athletes, 1181–1184
  clinical evaluation, 1182–1183
  epidemiology, 1181–1182
  etiology, 1182
  nonoperative treatment, 1183
  surgical treatment, 1183–1184
Achilles tendon
  bursitis, 809–810
  in calcaneal fractures, 1498–1499
  in Charcot collapse of arch, 931, 932
  contracture
    flatfoot from, 1339
    hallux valgus from, 173
  dancing injuries, 1271–1273
  lengthening
    for equinus deformity in cerebral palsy, 594, 596
    for flatfoot, 731, 735, 736
  magnetic resonance imaging, 100, 101, 103, 121
  peritendinitis treatment, 811–812
  ruptured
    results of treatment, 814, 816–817
    treatment, 812–816
  ultrasound, 90–91
Achilles tendon disease
  physical findings, 810
  radiographic examination, 810–811
Achilles tenodesis
  for calcaneus foot, 588
  for valgus foot, 590, 591
Acquired immune deficiency syndrome
  Kaposi's sarcoma in, 1084
  Reiter's syndrome and psoriasis and, 619
Acromegaly, 1027, 1028
Acute inflammatory polyradiculoneuropathy, 580
Adductor hallucis tendon, sesamoids and, 469
Adventitious bursa, surgical treatment, 853–854
AFO (ankle-foot orthoses), 145–146
AIDS
  Kaposi's sarcoma in, 1084
  Reiter's syndrome, psoriasis, and, 619
Aircast ankle brace, 1133, 1160, 1161
Air-contrast arthrography, in osteochondral fracture evaluation, 1573
Akin procedure
  for adult hallux valgus, 239
    complications, 240, 242
    contraindications, 239
    indications, 239
    postoperative care, 240
    radiographs, 198
    recurrent deformity after, 282
    results, 240, 241–242, 243
    surgical technique, 239–240
  for juvenile bunions, 312
    postoperative care, 312
    results and complications, 312, 314
    technique, 312, 313
Alban-Grace hindfoot stabilization, 598
Allescheria boydii, 1082
Allografts, 1393, 1396
Ambulatory surgery
  discussion, 153
  follow-up care, 153
  peripheral anesthesia, 151–164
  postoperative management, 152–153
  preoperative management, 151–152
  Amputation
  in diabetic patient, 878, 888, 891
    osteomyelitis and, 915–921
  of hallux or digits, skin coverage, 1384–1386, 1387–1389
  second toe, hallux valgus from, 173, 356, 357
Amputation surgery, 959–990
  below-knee, 989
  Chopart amputations, 978, 979, 1395, 1400
    aftercare, 978, 980
    pitfalls and complications, 980
    technique, 978, 980
  general considerations, 960
  great toe, 966–967
  indications, 960, 1369

Amputation surgery *(cont.)*
lesser toes
pitfalls and complications, 969–970
technique, 967
Pirigoff amputation, 988, 989
ray and partial forefoot, 967–968, 969, 970–973, 974
pitfalls and complications, 973, 974
Syme amputation, 980–981
aftercare, 984–987
pitfalls and complications, 987–989
technique, 981–984, 985–986
terminal, 964–966
techniques
determination of amputation level, 964
drains, 963
skin grafting and flap coverage, 963
soft-tissue preservation, 960–962
tourniquets, 960
vascular reconstruction, 963–964
wound closure, 962–963
terminal amputation of toe and nail, 964
aftercare, 966
pitfalls and complications, 966
technique, 965–966
transmetatarsal, 973–974
aftercare, 977–978
pitfalls and complications, 978
technique, 975–977
Anatomy
for imaging ankle, 76–77
for imaging foot, 62–66, 69
for peripheral anesthesia, 154–157
Anesthesia, peripheral, 151
anatomy, 154–157
digital block, 157–158, 1061–1062
nerve block of foot, 158–163
Aneurysmal bone cysts, 1004–1006
Angiography, 106–108
popliteal artery entrapment syndrome, 1119
tarsal navicular, 1601
Angiopathy, in diabetes, 883–884
Angioplasty, 108
Angiosarcomas, Kaposi's sarcoma, 1002–1003, 1048, 1083–1084
Angular and linear relationships of foot, 69
Animal bites, antibiotic treatment, 861
Ankle
anatomy, 1280, 1441
dancing injuries
anterior, 1256–1264
lateral, 1258–1264
medial, 1255–1256
posterior, 1265–1271
impingement syndromes, 1235
lateral instability, arthroscopic treatment, 1299–1300
limited dorsiflexion, 1101
osteomyelitis in diabetic foot, 923
posteromedial stenosis, 823–824
surface examination, 50
Ankle arthrodesis, 674, 676
arthroscopic, 1300–1303
avascular necrosis of body of talus and, 680–681
biomechanical considerations, 33–34, 35
complications, 680
desired position, 676
for failed total ankle replacement, 681–683
indications, 676
postoperative care, 680
surgical approach, 676
technique, 676–680
Ankle arthroscopy
anterior impingement syndrome in dancers, 1257
arthrodesis, 1300
discussion, 1302–1303
postoperative care, 1302
results, 1302
surgical technique, 1300–1302
author's preferred technique
ankle distractor, 1283–1284
anterior portal establishment, 1284
external anatomic landmark, 1283
patient positioning, 1283
posterior portals, 1284–1285
chondral and osteochondral lesions of ankle, 1295
chondral lesions, 1298–1299
loose bodies, 1296–1297
osteophytes, 1297–1298
complications, 1307–1308
congenital plicae, 1285
equipment and setup
ankle distractors, 1281–1282
arthroscope, 1280–1281
instruments, 1281
leg holder, 1282
pumps, 1282
fifteen-point examination, 1280
fractures, 1299
future directions, 1308
lateral ankle instability, 1299–1300
normal anatomy, 1280
osteochondral lesions of talus, 1290–1295
CAT scan staging, 1291, 1292, 1293
diagnosis, 1291
incidence, 1290–1291
operative techniques, 1293–1294, 1295, 1296
postoperative care, 1294
surgical treatment, 1291–1293
terminology, 1290
portals, 1279–1280
soft-tissue lesions, 1285
synovectomy technique, 1289
trauma
anterior soft-tissue impingement, 1286–1287
nonspecific generalized synovitis, 1285
nonspecific localized synovitis, 1285–1286
posterior soft-tissue impingement, 1287–1289
syndesmotic impingement, 1289
traumatic and degenerative arthritis, 1299
Ankle braces, 1160, 1161
for lateral ankle sprain, 1130–1131, 1133
Ankle diastasis, 1142
classification, 1149–1150
radiographic evaluation, 1146–1147
Ankle-foot orthoses, 145–146
Ankle fractures, 1439–1464
arthroscopic treatment, 1299
classification, 1440–1444
compartment syndrome, 1463
criteria for treatment, 1439–1440
epiphyseal injuries in children, 1462
fracture-dislocations, 1450–1453
Tillaux fractures, 1462
triplane fractures, 1462–1463
vertical compression fractures, 1444
diagnosis and emergency treatment, 1445–1446
surgical technique, 1454–1462
treatment, 1446–1454
Ankle joint
anteroposterior projection, 1448
ball-and-socket, 33, 750
biomechanics, 15–19, 20
impingement syndrome, 1235
range of motion examination, 51, 52
in rheumatoid arthritis, 644, 646
treatment, 664–667
rotation and musculature about, 36
traumatic arthritis after talar neck fracture, 1559–1560
Ankle joint and flexor tenosynovitis, after calcaneal fracture, 1528–1529
Ankle ligaments
anatomy, 1121–1123
biomechanics, 36–42, 1123–1124
Ankle ligaments and muscular structures, examination, 54–56
Ankle pain
lateral
as residual of lateral ankle ligament sprain, 817
sequence of, 1288
medial, in dancer, differential diagnosis, 1255
Ankle replacement, failed total, arthrodesis for, 681–683
Ankle sprains, 817, 1286–1287
Ankle sprains in athletes
lateral
anatomy, 1121–1123

biomechanics, 1123–1124
chronic sprains and instability
diagnosis, 1134–1135
sources of pain and instability, 1134
treatment, 1135–1139
classification, 1126, 1128–1129, 1130
diagnosis
clinical evaluation, 1124–1125
radiographic evaluation, 1125–1126, 1127
pathology, 1124
treatment of acute sprain, 1129–1134
complications, 1134
nonoperative, 1129–1133
postoperative care, 1134
surgical, 1131, 1133–1134
medial
anatomy, 1139, 1140
biomechanics, 1139–1140
chronic instability, 1141–1142
diagnosis
clinical evaluation, 1140
radiographic evaluation, 1140, 1141
treatment, 1140–1141
operative repair, 1141
postoperative care, 1141–1142
syndesmotic
anatomy, 1143–1144
biomechanics, 1144–1145
classification, 1149–1150
definition, 1142
diagnosis
clinical evaluation, 1145–1146
radiographic evaluation, 1146–1149
incidence, 1142–1143
mechanism of injury, 1145
treatment, 1150
acute injury, 1150–1152
chronic injury, 1152–1153
results, 1153
subacute injury, 1152
tarsal coalition and, 750
Ankle sprains in dancers, lateral, 1258
classification, 1259–1260
conditions simulating or accompanying, 1258–1259
nonhealing, 1263–1264
treatment
conservative, 1260–1261
surgical, 1261–1263
Ankle swelling, 817
Ankylosing spondylitis, 617, 618
Anonychia, 1036, 1059
Anterior ankle dancing injuries, 1256–1258
Anterior compartment syndrome, surgical treatment, 1109–1110, 1111
Anterior drawer test, 1125, 1126, 1128, 1129
Anterior impingement syndrome, in dancers, 1256–1258
Anterior inferior tibiofibular ligament
accessory, 1144
anatomy, 1143, 1144
biomechanics, 1144–1145
as impingement site, 1286, 1287, 1289
Anterior talofibular ligament
anatomy, 1121, 1122
biomechanics, 37–38, 42, 1123
Anterior tibial artery, talar blood supply from, 1540, 1541, 1542, 1543
Anterior tibial tendon
rupture, 824–825
sesamoid of, 500, 501
Anterior tibial tendon transfer, 828–829
for calcaneus foot, 586–587, 588
for metatarsus adductus, 1331–1333
for stroke and traumatic brain injury, 606–607
for varus deformities in cerebral palsy, 594, 596, 597
Anthonsen's view, for subtalar joint, 1485–1486, 1487
Antibiotics, 872–873
aminoglycosides, 875
aztreonam, 874
cephalosporins, 874
clindamycin, 874–875
for diabetic foot infections, 909–912
imipenem, 874
metronidazole, 875
in open fractures of talus, 1546
for osteomyelitis in diabetic foot, 914–915
penicillins, 874
quinolones, 875
selection, 873–874
in traumatic wound treatment, 1372
trimethoprim-sulfa, 875
Antidepressants, in reflex sympathetic dystrophy syndrome, 1417–1418
Antimicrobial sensitivities, 873
A-O classification of ankle fractures, 1442, 1444, 1446
Appliances
felt pads, 146–148
for toes, 146
UCBL insert, 148–149
Arm swing, examination, 47
Arteriography, 106–107
popliteal artery entrapment syndrome, 1119
Arteriovenous fistula, 1081–1082
Arthritides
crystal-induced arthritis, 615–617
degenerative joint disease, 620–637
rheumatoid arthritis, 637–667
seronegative spondyloarthropathies, 617–620
Arthritis
algorithmic approach to imaging, 127–129
calcaneocuboid, 1528
first metatarsocuneiform, 634–636
interphalangeal joint, 258, 620–622
metatarsal sesamoid, 480–481, 483
psoriatic, toenail abnormalities in, 1037
rheumatoid (*see* Rheumatoid arthritis)
subtalar and talocrural joints, 1559–1560, 1659
after talar fractures and dislocations, 1559–1560, 1584, 1663
talonavicular joint, 517, 521, 636–637
after tarsometatarsal dislocation, 1687–1688
traumatic and degenerative, ankle arthroscopy, 1299
Arthrodesis, 673–713
ankle, 676–683
arthroscopic, 1300–1303
for calcaneal fractures, 1521–1523
for Charcot foot, 943–944
complications, 675–676
double, 688–694
first metatarsocuneiform, 702–705, 707
for flatfoot, 739
in rheumatoid arthritis, 661
first metatarsophalangeal joint, for hallux valgus, 250
complications, 255, 257–258
contraindications, 250
fixation with Steinmann pins, 253, 255–257
indications, 250
postoperative care, 253
radiographs, 204, 252
results, 253–255, 258
surgical technique, 250–252
surgical technique with curved surfaces, 253, 254
for hallux rigidus, 628–629, 634, 635
interphalangeal joints, 712–713
pantalar, 581, 674
principles, 674
soft-tissue swelling after, 675
subtalar, 674, 683–687
for calcaneal fractures, 57
for flatfoot, 731, 779
for valgus foot, 591–592
talonavicular, 661–662, 664, 674, 687–690
complications, 675–676, 688
for degenerative arthritis, 636–637
for flatfoot, 779
tarsometatarsal, 674, 701–711
technical considerations, 674–675

Arthrodesis *(cont.)*
tibiocalcaneal, 680, 681, 1583
triple (*see* Triple arthrodesis)
types, 674–675
Arthroereisis for flatfoot, 731–732
Arthrofibrosis
after distal soft tissue realignment procedure, 215
of first metatarsophalangeal joint, from hallux valgus surgery, 278–279
Arthrography
air-contrast, in osteochondral fracture evaluation, 1573
ankle, 1126
syndesmosis sprains, 1148
subtalar, 1159, 1166
Arthrogryposis multiplex congenita, 1346–1347
talectomy, 1348, 1349
treatment options, 1347, 1349
Arthroscopes, 1280–1281
Arthroscopy, 1277–1310
advantages and disadvantages, 1278
ankle (*see* Ankle arthroscopy)
great toe, 1305–1307
history, 1278
indications and contraindications, 1278–1279
subtalar joint, 1303–1305
Arthrosis, flatfoot from, 780–783
Aseptic necrosis
after talar body fracture, 1583–1584
after talar dislocation, 1663
after talar neck fracture, 1560–1561, 1560–1565
detection, 1561–1563
treatment, 1563–1564
treatment of sequelae, 1564–1565
Athletes
retrocalcaneal bursitis, treatment, 851–852
subcalcaneal pain syndrome, treatment, 843–844
tarsal coalition, 749–750
Athlete's foot, 1077
Athletic soft-tissue injuries, 1095–1224
Achilles tendinitis and ruptures, 1181–1184
ankle sprains
lateral, 1121–1139
medial, 1139–1142
syndesmotic, 1142–1153
bunions, 1200–1206
chronic leg pain, 1105
chronic compartment syndrome, 1106–1112
differential diagnosis, 1105
exercise-induced muscle pain, 1120–1121
gastrocnemius-soleus strain, 1116–1117
incidence, 1105–1106
medial tibial stress syndrome, 1112–1115
nerve entrapment syndromes, 1117–1118
stress fractures of tibia and fibula, 1115–1116
vascular problems, 1118–1120
epidemiology, 1097–1099
etiology, 1096–1105
biomechanical abnormalities, 1100
flexibility, 1100–1102
playing surfaces, 1105
shoe wear and orthoses, 1102–1105
strength, 1102
forefoot sprains, 1191–1200
historical perspective, 1097
midfoot sprains, 1184–1191
peroneal tendinitis and ruptures, 1177–1179
peroneal tendon subluxation and dislocation, 1167–1177
posterior tibial tendinitis and tendon rupture, 1180–1181
sinus tarsi syndrome, 1165–1167
subtalar sprains, 1153–1165
Atopic dermatitis, 1074
Atrophy of nail matrix, 1059–1060
Autoimmune diseases, dermatologic problems from, 1077
Autonomic nervous system, sympathetic division, 1412–1414
Avascular necrosis
algorithmic approach to imaging, 122, 124–125
from hallux valgus surgery
metatarsal head, 233, 235, 272–273, 274
proximal phalanx, 274, 276
after talar neck fracture, 1560–1565
of talus, 1029–1030
ankle fusion and, 680–681
Avulsion fracture, impaction fracture vs., 1442
Avulsion injury of foot, 1371, 1372
Avulsion of nail plate
complete, 1063–1064
partial, 1062–1063
Aztreonam, 874
for diabetic foot infections, 910, 911

B

Bacterial infections
bone, 865–868 (*see also* Osteomyelitis)
dermatologic aspects, 1077
diabetic foot, 868
joint, 864–865
Lyme disease, 869
soft tissue, 859–860
deep infections, 861–864
puncture wounds, 860
surgical treatment of felon, 860
trauma, 860–861
Bacteroides fragilis, 911
Baker osteotomy of os calcis, 727
Ball-and-socket ankle joint, 33, 750
Ballet dancers, flexibility in, 1101–1102
Ballet dancing
bunions from, 1201, 1202
posterior ankle in, 1264
Bandages, elastic, in fracture and dislocation treatment, 1470
Basal cell carcinoma, 1085
Bassett's ligament, 1257
Baxter's nerve, entrapment in dancers, 1274
Beau's lines, 1036, 1039, 1040, 1060
Below-knee amputations, 989
Bicycling, femoral or external iliac arterial occlusion in, 1120
Bimalleolar fractures and fracture-dislocations, surgical treatment, 1450
Biomechanics, 3–43
ankle joint ligaments, 36–42
athletic soft-tissue injuries, 1100
axes of rotation
ankle joint, 15–19, 20
metatarsophalangeal break, 24–26
plantar aponeurosis, 26–27
subtalar joint, 19–23
talonavicular joint, 27–28
transverse plane rotation, 28
transverse tarsal articulation, 23–24
keratotic lesions, 413
kinematics of human locomotion, 5–9
kinetics of human locomotion, 9–10
lateral ankle sprain, 1123–1124
locomotor system, 4–5
running mechanics, 31–33
surgical implications, 33
ankle arthrodesis, 33–34, 35
forefoot principles, 35–36
hindfoot alignment, 34
midfoot alignment, 35
tendon transfers, 36, 825–826
walking cycle, 15
walking cycle events, 28–31
weight bearing, 10–15
Bipartite first cuneiform, 527
Bipartite navicular, 525, 1610
Bipartite sesamoids and fractures, 471, 473–474, 475–476
Bipartite talus, os trigonum vs., 509, 510–511
Bites, animal, antibiotic treatment, 861
Black heel, 1081
Blair tibiotalar fusion, 1558, 1564, 1565, 1583
Blastomyces dermatitidis, 872
Blisters
in dancers, 1244
in runners, 1237
Blood supply
to metatarsal head, 175, 177, 178
plantar, 459
to sesamoids, 470
Blue nail/blue-gray nail, 1042
Blue nevus, 1079
Bohler's method of intra-articular calcaneal fracture treatment, 1514

Bohler's tuberosity joint angle, 1477, 1478–1479, 1504, 1524
Bone cysts
  aneurysmal, 1004–1006
  epidermoid, 1004
  solitary, 1003–1004
Bone fibromas, 1009, 1011–1012
Bone infections, 865 (*see also* Osteomyelitis)
Bone islands, 1011–1012, 1014
Bone scanning, 86–89
  diabetes, 892–893
  forefoot pain, 377, 380
  infection, 129, 133, 865–867
  medial tibial stress syndrome, 1114
  osteochondral fractures, 1573, 1574
  osteomyelitis, 865–867
  osteoporosis, 1020–1021
  subcalcaneal pain syndrome, 840–841, 842
  syndesmosis sprains of ankle, 1148, 1149
  tarsal navicular stress fracture, 1610
  tibial stress fracture, 1115
  tumors, 992–993
Bone spurs, 1006
Bone tumors and cysts of foot, 991–992
  benign, 1003–1012
  general considerations and staging process, 992–993
  malignant, 1012–1018
Bony stabilization, in pes cavus, 798–801
Borrelia burgdorferi, 869
Bosworth fractures, 1453
Bowen's disease, 1048, 1085
Braces/bracing
  ankle, 1160, 1161
    for lateral sprain, 1130–1131, 1133
  for Charcot joints in diabetes, 938
  double-upright, 146
  patellar tendon bearing, 1563
  for tibial torsion, 1357
Brain injury, traumatic, 607–608
Broden's views, for subtalar injuries, 1155, 1157, 1486–1488, 1489
Broström procedure, modified, 1136–1138, 1261–1263
Bunnell suture technique, in Achilles tendon repair, 813
Bunionette deformity, 441
  clinical evaluation, 443
  conservative treatment, 443–444
  discussion, 462–463
  lateral keratosis, 443
  plantar keratosis, 444
  recurrence after lateral condylectomy, 446
  surgical treatment, 444
    diaphyseal osteotomy, 455–457
    fifth metatarsal head resection, 447–449
    fifth metatarsal osteotomy, 449–455
    lateral condylectomy, 444–447
    proximal fifth metatarsal osteotomy, 457–462
  types, 441–443
Bunionettes, in dancers, 1254
Bunions (*see also* Hallux valgus deformity)
  in athletes, 1200
    clinical evaluation, 1202, 1204
    differential diagnosis, 1205
    etiology, 1200–1202
    radiographic evaluation, 1204–1205
    treatment, 1205–1206
  in dancers, 1247
  definition, 168
  juvenile (*see* Juvenile bunions)
  surgery, patient expectations, 195
Burns, 1426–1428
  classification, 1428
  treatment, 1428–1432
Bursae, 808
  adventitious, surgical treatment, 853–854
  classification of pathology, 809
  infections, 861
Bursitis, 808–809
  Achilles tendon and retrocalcaneal, 809–810
  in dancers
    plantar calcaneal, 1273–1274
    sesamoid, 1249
  heel inflammation terminology, 810
  intermetatarsal phalangeal, 809
  posterior aspect of heel, 809
  sesamoid associated, 478–479, 481
    treatment, 479

C

Calcaneal apophysitis, 1029, 1030
  heel pain from, 844–845
Calcaneal dislocation, 1535
Calcaneal fibular ligament, biomechanics, 37–42
Calcaneal fractures, 1476–1477
  anatomy, 1477–1480
  classification, 1480–1482
  compartment syndrome and, 1379–1380
  evaluation by computed tomography, 98
  extra-articular, 1491
    anterior process, 1259, 1491
      anatomy, 1491–1493
      author's preferred treatment, 1498
      diagnosis, 1494–1496
      mechanism of injury, 1493–1494
      results of treatment, 1497
      treatment, 1496–1497
    body, not involving subtalar joint
      anatomy, 1503
      author's preferred treatment, 1505
      clinical diagnosis, 1503
      mechanism of injury, 1503
      prognosis, 1504–1505
      radiographic diagnosis, 1503
      treatment, 1503–1504
    medial or lateral process, 1502–1503
    tuberosity (beak and avulsion fractures)
      anatomy, 1498–1499
      author's preferred treatment, 1500–1502
      clinical diagnosis, 1499
      mechanism of injury, 1499
      radiographic diagnosis, 1499
      results of treatment, 1500
      treatment, 1499–1500
  flatfoot from, 782–783
  intra-articular, 1505–1506
    stress fractures, 1534–1535
    sustentaculum tali, 1506
      anatomy, 1506
      author's preferred treatment, 1507–1508
      clinical diagnosis, 1506
      mechanism of injury, 1506
      prognosis, 1507
      radiographic diagnosis, 1506, 1507
      treatment, 1506–1507
    tongue, joint depression, and comminuted
      anatomy, 1508–1510
      author's preferred treatment, 1530–1534
      classification, 1508–1510
      clinical diagnosis, 1511
      closed reduction, 1513–1518
      closed treatment without reduction, 1512–1513
      complications, 1526–1530
      excision, 1523
      factors affecting progress, 1523–1526
      mechanism of injury, 1508–1510
      open reduction, 1518–1521
      primary arthrodesis, 1521–1523
      radiographic diagnosis, 1511
      treatment methods, 1511
  mechanism of injury, 1482–1483
  radiographic diagnosis, 1483–1484
    conventional and computerized axial tomography, 1485, 1488–1490
    standard radiographic views, 1484–1485, 1486
    subtalar joint, 1485–1488, 1489

Calcaneal fractures *(cont.)*
subtalar arthrodesis and, 687
treatment
differences, 1477, 1490–1491
goals, 1491
Calcaneal nerve, medial, in subcalcaneal pain syndrome, 838, 839
Calcaneal osteotomy
for excessive eversion, 737–738
for flatfoot, 725–728, 732, 735, 737–738
for pes cavus
crescentic or sliding osteotomy, 797–798
Dwyer procedure, 794, 796–798
Samilson osteotomy, 593, 798, 799
Calcanectomy, partial, in diabetic patient, 922, 923
Calcaneocuboid arthritis, after calcaneal fracture, 1528
Calcaneocuboid articulation, examination, 56–57
Calcaneocuboid joint anatomy, 1668, 1669
Calcaneofibular ligament
anatomy, 1121
biomechanics, 1123–1124
Calcaneonavicular coalition, 748, 1341
radiographic evaluation, 748
treatment, 748–749
excision of calcaneonavicular bar, 752–753
Calcaneus
anatomy, 73, 840, 1477
anterior surface, 1478
crucial angle of Gissane, 1477, 1479–1480
superior tuberosity, 847, 848
tuberosity joint angle, 1477, 1478–1479
anterior process fracture, 1259
bone cyst, 1004
diagnostic and roentgenographic studies, for heel pain, 840–842
imaging, 72, 73
radiographic landmarks, 848, 849
spur, 837–838
in transverse tarsal articulation, 23
Calcaneus accessorius, 513–514
Calcaneus foot, in myelodysplasia, 586, 587
surgical management, 586–588, 589
Calcium pyrophosphate dihydrate deposition disease, 616
Calf pseudotumor, in dancers, 1273
Calluses
in dancers, 1243–1244
dermatologic aspects, 1085–1087
in diabetes, trimming instruments, 957
differentiated from other lesions, 1085–1087, 1090
formation in hallux valgus, 185, 186
plantar (*see* Plantar keratoses)
in runners, 1237
with significant scar tissue formation, 435, 436
from subhallux sesamoid, 433
treatment, 1086–1087
Candida albicans, 872
Candida onychomycosis, 1054, 1055
Cardiovascular disorders, toenail pathology from, 1040
Carville sandal, 947–948
Casting
external rotation-eversion injury, 1449
metatarsus adductus, 1329–1331
myelodysplasia, 581–582
talipes equinovarus, 1323
total-contact cast in diabetes, 898, 900–901, 938
CAT scans (*see* Computed tomography)
Causalgia, 1411, 1414–1415
Cavus foot, callus formation from, 415
Cavus foot (*see* Pes cavus)
Cellulitis
in diabetes, 914
treatment, 860
Central nervous system disorders, 604–608
Cerebral palsy, 594–599
assessment of foot deformities, 594
equinus deformities, 594
Achilles tendon lengthening for, 594, 596
EMG tracings of gait, 595
forefoot deformities, 598–599
valgus deformities, 597–598
varus deformities, 594–597
Cerebral vascular accident, 604
orthotic management, 604–605
surgical treatment, 605
postoperative management, 607
SPLATT procedure, 605–607
Cervical ligament
anatomy, 1122–1123
biomechanics, 1123
Chambers osteotomy of os calcis, 727
Charcot foot
flatfoot from, 783, 784
"rocker-bottom," 931, 932
Charcot joints, arthrodesis and, 581
Charcot joints in diabetes, 879, 925–927, 928, 929
anatomic classification, 934–937, 938, 939
clinical signs and symptoms, 931–932
complications, 940–942
developmental stages, 928, 930, 931
diagnostic evaluation, 884–885, 932–934
epidemiology, 930–931
histology, 933, 934
imaging, 892, 893, 932–934
pathophysiology, 927–931
treatment
flowchart, 941
nonoperative, 937–940
surgical, 937, 942–944
ulcerations over, 900
surgical treatment, 907–908
Charcot-Marie-Tooth disease, 578, 580, 609
muscle imbalance in, 790
treatment, 609
Cheilectomy for hallux rigidus
indications, 625
postoperative management, 632
results, 625, 628, 632–634
technique, 630–631, 632
Chemical burns, 1430
Chevron osteotomy
for adult hallux valgus, 196, 202, 227
complications, 233, 234–235
contraindications, 227
dorsiflexion deformity from, 266
hallux varus after, 288, 289
indications, 227
metatarsal head avascular necrosis from, 233, 235, 273, 274
metatarsal head displacement from, 270, 272
metatarsal nonunion from, 270
metatarsal shortening from, 262, 263
plantar flexion deformity from, 267
postoperative care, 231
radiographs, 197, 200
recurrent deformity after, 282
results, 231–233
surgical technique, 227–231
distal fifth metatarsal, for bunionette deformity, 449, 450–452, 461
for juvenile bunions, 314
postoperative care, 315
results and complications, 319–320
technique, 314–315
for plantar keratosis, 423, 425
Chilblain, 1426
Children
congenital foot deformities, 1313–1363
epiphyseal injuries of ankle, 1462
examination principles for neonates and toddlers, 45–46
flatfoot, 717–756
juvenile bunions, 297–339
Chinese finger traps
for metatarsal fractures, 1622, 1626
for phalangeal fractures, 1644, 1645
for tarsometatarsal dislocations, 1688
Chondral fractures, in hallux rigidus, 624
Chondral lesions of ankle, arthroscopy, 1298–1299

Chondroblastomas, 1009, 1010
Chondrocalcinosis, 616
Chondrodysplasia punctata, 1011
Chondromas, 1008–1009, 1010
Chondromyxoid fibromas, 1009, 1012
Chondrosarcomas, 1017–1018//
Chopart amputations, 978, 979, 1395, 1400
  aftercare, 978, 980
  pitfalls and complications, 980
  technique, 978, 980
Chrisman-Snook procedure, 1162
  modified, 1136, 1138–1139, 1162, 1164
Chromoblastomycosis, 1082
Chrondrocalcinosis, 616
Chrondrodysplasia punctata, 1011
Cincinnati incision, 583, 584, 1325
Circulation
  to metatarsal head, 175, 177, 178
  plantar, 459
  to sesamoids, 470
Clawtoe, 341–342, 363, 366, 367
  from crush injury, 1405–1406
  definition, 341–342
  in diabetes, 883, 904
  etiology, 342, 344–345
  hammer toe differentiated from, 363
  in myelodysplasia, 593–594
  after partial forefoot amputation, 973
  in pes cavus, surgical treatment, 793–794
  treatment, 366–367
    algorithm, 366
    postoperative care, 370–371
    results and complications, 371–372
    technique for repair of fixed clawtoe, 368–370
Cleating of athletic shoes, 1104
Closing wedge osteotomy
  dorsiflexion deformity from, 263–264
  for hallux rigidus, 629
  for juvenile hallux valgus, 325
  for plantar-flexed first metatarsal, 494, 497
Cloward plug, 598
Clubbing of toenails, 1036, 1050–1051, 1053–1054
Clubfoot (*see* Talipes equinovarus)
Coalitions (see Tarsal coalitions)
Coccidioides immitis, 871
Cockup fifth toe deformity, 395, 400
  Ruiz-Mora procedure, 401, 402
  syndactylization of lesser toes, 401, 403
Cold injuries, 1420–1421
  classification by severity, 1421
  frostbite, 1421–1422
    chilblain, 1426
    immersion and trench foot, 1424, 1426
    treatment, 1422–1424, 1425
  mechanism, 1420
  stages, 1423
Cole osteotomy, for pes cavus, 801
Compartments of foot, 1378, 1472
Compartments of leg, 1106
Compartment syndrome in athletes, chronic
  clinical features, 1106–1107, 1108
  definition, 1106
  diagnosis
    physical examination, 1107–1108
    pressure measurements, 1108, 1110
    radiologic evaluation, 1108, 1109
  incidence, 1106
  mechanism of injury, 1107
  runners, 1230–1231
  treatment
    nonoperative, 1108–1109
    results, 1111–1112
    surgical, 1109–1111, 1112, 1113
Compartment syndrome of foot, 1471–1472
  acute, 1377–1383
    anatomy, 1378
    calcaneus fractures and, 1379–1380
    from crush injury, 1378–1379
    diagnosis, 1380–1381
    pain in, 1380
    pathophysiology, 1377–1378
    treatment, 1381–1383
  anatomy, 1378, 1472
  author's preferred treatment, 1476
  chronic, 1405–1406
  clinical presentation, 1472–1473, 1474
  surgical decompression, 1473, 1474, 1475–1476
Compartment syndrome of leg or foot, 1463
Computed tomography
  advantages, 91
  anatomic imaging planes, 93
  axial scan of feet, 92
  calcaneal fractures, 1485, 1488–1490, 1532, 1533
  coronal foot positioning, 94
  diabetes, 893
  foreign body localization, 95, 97, 110
  fractures, 95, 98
  gantry positioning, 93–95
  indications, 95
  mechanism, 93
  osteochondral fractures, 1573
  patient positioning, 93, 94
  peroneal tendon injury, 121
  scanners, 91, 93
  section thickness, 93
  SPECT, 86
  subtalar joint, 95, 96
  syndesmosis sprains of ankle, 1148
  talocalcaneal coalition, 95, 97
  tumors, 992
  two-dimensional reconstruction images, 92
Condylectomy
  for bunionette deformity, 444, 446
    dislocation of fifth metatarsophalangeal joint from, 463
    postoperative care, 446
    results, 446–447
    surgical technique, 444–445, 446
  for diabetic ulcerations, 906–907
  for fifth toe keratotic deformity, 407–408
  for localized intractable plantar keratosis
    Coughlin's modified, 422–423, 424
    DuVries technique, 421–422, 424
Congenital foot deformities
  arthrogryposis multiplex congenita, 1346–1349
  classification, 1315
  embryology, 1313–1314
  flatfoot, 1335–1346
  genetic basis, 1314
  growth and development, 1314
  in neonate and preambulatory infant, examination principles, 45
  talipes deformities, 1314–1335
  toe abnormalities, 1349–1354
  torsional deformities of lower extremities, 1354–1360
Connective tissue disorders, toenail pathology from, 1041
Conradi's disease, 1011
Conservative treatment of foot, 141–149
Contact dermatitis, 1074–1075
  of toenail folds, 1038
Convex pes valgus, in myelodysplasia, 592–593
Cooling stages, 1423
Corns
  in dancers, 1243
  differentiated from other lesions, 1086
  hard, 403, 404
    treatment, 405, 407–408
  seed, 418
  soft, 403, 404, 406
    treatment, 407, 409–410
Cornuate navicular, 1338, 1340 (*see also* Accessory navicular)
Corticosteroids
  for interdigital plantar neuroma, 549
  in reflex sympathetic dystrophy syndrome, 1418
  for retrocalcaneal bursitis, 853
  for subcalcaneal pain, 845–846

Coughlin's modified metatarsal condylectomy, for localized intractable plantar keratosis, 422–423, 424CPPD deposition disease, 616
Crescentic or sliding osteotomy, for pes cavus, 797–798, 799
Crescentic osteotomy
  for adult hallux valgus, 202, 217–222, 223, 224
    dorsiflexion deformity from, 266
    metatarsal nonnion from, 270
  for juvenile hallux valgus, 325–328
Cross-leg flaps, in soft-tissue trauma, 1403–1405
Crossover second toe, 379, 386
Crush-amputation injury, skin coverage, 1397–1398, 1401
Crush injuries of foot, 1368, 1369–1371
  associated deformities, 1405–1406
  compartment syndrome from, 1378–1379, 1383
  equinovarus from, 1406
  soft-tissue coverage, 1388–1389, 1404, 1405
  zone of injury, 1373, 1374
Crush injuries of midtarsal joint, 1667, 1669, 1673–1674
Cryptococcus neoformans, 871–872
Crystal-induced arthritis, 615
  CPPD disease, 616
  gouty arthritis, 616–617
CT (*see* Computed tomography)
Cuboid dislocations, 1693–1694
Cuboid fractures, 1613–1614
  author's preferred treatment, 1616
  clinical diagnosis, 1614
  radiographic diagnosis, 1614
  tarsometatarsal dislocations and, 1678, 1679
  treatment, 1614–1616
Cuboid osteotomy for forefoot abduction, 738
Cuneiform, first
  bipartite, 527
  osteotomy for juvenile bunions, 329–332
Cuneiform-cuboid wedge osteotomy, for equinovarus deformity, 584–586
Cuneiform dislocations, 1693, 1694
Cuneiform fractures, 1613–1614, 1616
  author's preferred treatment, 1616–1617
  clinical diagnosis, 1616
  radiographic diagnosis, 1616, 1617
  treatment, 1616
Cuneonavicular articulation, examination, 56–57
Curly toe deformity, 362–363, 365
  congenital, 1354
Cutaneous nerves, entrapment or severance from hallux valgus surgery, 261
Cyclists, femoral or external iliac arterial occlusion in, 1120
Cysts
  bone, 1003–1006
  epidermal inclusion, 1080
  ganglionic, hallux valgus from, 173
  rheumatoid, 660

D

Dancers, flexibility in, 1101–1102
Dancer's foot, 1242–1243
  radiographic evaluation, 1252, 1253
Dancing injuries, 1241–1276
  Achilles tendon, 1271
    pseudotumor of calf, 1273
    rupture, 1272–1273
    tendinitis, 1271–1272
  anterior ankle
    impingement syndromes, 1256–1258
    tendinitis, 1258
  biomechanical abnormalities and, 1100
  bunions, 1201, 1202
  heel pain, 1273–1274
  interphalangeal joint of hallux, 1247
  lateral ankle sprains, 1258
    classification, 1259–1260
    conditions simulating or accompanying, 1258–1259
    nonhealing, 1263–1264
    treatment
      conservative, 1260–1261
      surgical, 1261–1263
  leg pain, 1274–1275
  lesser metatarsophalangeal joints
    acute dislocation, 1250–1251
    Freiberg's disease, 1250
    idiopathic synovitis, 1251
    instability, 1251
  medial ankle, 1255–1256
  metatarsals
    bunionettes, 1254
    fifth, 1253–1254
    "pseudotumor" of first web space, 1252
    stress fractures, 1252–1253
    third and fourth, 1253
  metatarsophalangeal joint of hallux
    bunions, 1247
    hallux rigidus, 1247–1249
    lateral instability of first MTP joint, 1247
    sesamoid injuries, 1249–1250
  midtarsal area, 1254–1255
  posterior ankle, 1264–1265
    flexor hallucis longus tendinitis, 1270–1271
    impingement syndrome, 1265–1266
      treatment, 1266–1270
    pain syndromes, 1265
  toes
    blisters, 1244
    calluses, 1243–1244
    chronically unstable fifth proximal interphalangeal joint, 1245
    corns, 1243
    fractures and dislocations, 1244–1245
    mallet toes, 1246
    painful fifth toenails, 1246–1247
    "proud" fourth toe, 1246
    subungual exostoses, 1246
    subungual hematomas, 1246
Dancing shoes, 1244
  bunions and, 1203
Darier's disease/Darier-White disease, 1042, 1043
Debridement
  burn injury, 1429–1430
  deep infections, 861, 863–864
  soft-tissue trauma, 1373, 1376, 1377
Deep peroneal nerve
  anatomy, 156, 157
  entrapment, 569–571
Deep posterior compartment syndrome, surgical treatment, 1110–1111, 1113
Degenerative joint disease
  conservative treatment, 620
  first metatarsocuneiform arthritis, 634–636
  general concepts, 620
  hallux rigidus, 622–634
  interphalangeal joint arthritis, 620–622
  subtalar joint, 1659
  surgical treatment, 620
  talonavicular joint arthritis, 636–637
  after tarsometatarsal dislocation, 1687–1688
Degloving injury of foot, 1371, 1372, 1374
Deltoid ligament, anatomy and biomechanics, 1139–1140
Denis-Browne bar, 1357
Dermatitis, 1073–1074
  atopic, 1074
  contact, 1038, 1074–1075
Dermatofibromas, 1080
Dermatofibrosarcoma protuberans, 995
Dermatology, 1073–1091
  autoimmune diseases, 1077
  calluses, 1085–1087
  common infections, 1077–1078
  corns, 1087–1088
  diabetes, 944–946
  discrete lesions, 1079–1083
    malignant, 1083–1085
  inflammatory problems of feet, 1073–1077
  keratoses of soles, 1088
  plantar warts, 1088–1091
  primary vs. secondary lesions, 1073
  toenail abnormalities, 1036
    eczema and contact dermatitis, 1038
    psoriasis, 1036–1038
    pyodermas, 1038–1040
Dermatomyositis, 1077
Diabetic foot, 877–958
  background and history, 877–878
  callus trimming instruments, 957
  over Charcot joints, surgical treatment, 907–908
  Charcot joints (*see* Charcot joints in diabetes)
  classification systems, 893–894, 896
  complications, 878, 879

diagnosis
imaging
bone scans and MRI, 892–893
computed tomography, 893
gallium scans, 893
radiographs, 888, 891–892
neurologic evaluation, 885–886, 956
physical examination, 884–885
vascular evaluation, 886–888, 889–891, 956
evaluation and treatment flow chart, 895
infections, 868–869
abscess, 914, 915
antibiotic regimens and selections, 909–912
cellulitis, 914
gas in soft tissue, 912
microbiology, 908–909
osteomyelitis, 914–923, 932–933, 934
surgical treatment, 912–914
nail care instruments, 957
pathophysiology
angiopathy, 883–884
limited joint mobility syndrome, 884
metabolic control, 884
neuropathy, 878–883
nutrition, 884
patient care instructions, 958
shoe wear and shoe insoles, 946–948
insole materials, 949–952, 957
nomenclature, 947, 948–952
skin and nail problems, 944–946
team approach, 948–952
ulcers, 896–898
over Charcot joints, 900
diagnostic evaluation, 885, 887
grade 1 and 2, 896, 897, 898
on heel, 901
nonhealing, 902
pathophysiology, 880–882
soft-tissue coverage, 908
surgical treatment
chronic and recurrent ulceration, 902–908
fifth metatarsal head, 906–907
first metatarsal head, 904
hallux, 902–904
lateral border of foot, 908
beneath middle three metatarsal heads, 904–906
toes, 902
total-contact cast, 898, 900–901, 956
weight-relieving devices, 897, 899
wound care, 901–902
wound closure and foot reconstruction principles, 923–925, 926, 927
Diaphyseal osteotomy for bunionette deformity, 455
postoperative care, 455
results, 457
surgical technique, 455, 456
variations, 455, 457
Diaphysectomy, for hammer toe deformity, 357–358
Diastasis of ankle, 1142
classification, 1149–1150
radiographic evaluation, 1146–1147
Digital amputation and closure, 1384–1386, 1387–1388
Digital anesthetic block, 157–158
for toenail procedures, 1061–1062
Digital nerve, lateral proper, entrapment in dancers, 1249–1250
Digital nerve compression, sesamoid associated, 471, 479–480, 482
Discoid lupus erythematosus, 1077
Dislocation and fractures of foot *(see also specific anatomic areas)*
diagnosis, 1467
treatment, 1471
Distal calcaneal osteotomy for forefoot abduction, 738
Distal fifth metatarsal osteotomy, for bunionette deformity, 449–450, 463
chevron, 450–452
oblique, 452–455
Distal metatarsal articular angle, 177, 179
Distal phalanx, anatomy for lesser toe deformities, 345, 346
Distal soft tissue procedure with proximal crescentic osteotomy, for adult hallux valgus, 216–217
complications, 226–227, 228
contraindications, 217
indications, 217
postoperative care, 222
results, 222, 225–226, 227
surgical technique, 217–222, 223–224
Distal soft tissue realignment for adult hallux valgus, 204–205
complications, 215–216
contraindications, 206
indications, 205–206
metatarsocuneiform arthrodesis and, 244–245, 248–250
postoperative care, 211–212, 213
radiographs, 197, 200, 201, 202, 203
recurrent deformity, 282
results, 212–215
surgical technique, 206–211
for juvenile bunions, 320–321
postoperative care, 321
results and complications, 321, 323
technique, 321, 322
Distal tendon transfer, 829–830
DOOR syndrome, 1042
Doppler ultrasound imaging, 89–90
arterial
in diabetes, 886–887, 888, 889–890, 956
in evaluation for amputation, 964
Dorsalis pedis artery, talar blood supply from, 1540, 1541, 1542, 1543
Dorsiflexion osteotomy
for diabetic ulceration, 903, 904, 906
of first metatarsal, 494, 497
for juvenile hallux rigidus, 625, 629
Double arthrodesis, 688, 691
complications, 693
desired position, 691
indications, 691
postoperative care, 691, 693
special considerations, 693–694
surgical approach, 691
technique, 691, 692
Double-crush syndrome, 559
Double-upright brace, 146
Drains, in amputation surgery, 963
Drawer test of metatarsophalangeal joint, 373
Duchenne pseudohypertrophic muscular dystrophy
correction of equinus deformity, 576
correction of varus and adductus deformity, 576–577
early and late walking phases, 576
postsurgical management, 577
wheelchair patients, 577–578
Durham procedure, 728, 729
DuVries metatarsal condylectomy, for localized intractable plantar keratosis, 421–422, 424
DuVries procedure
for deltoid imbrication, 1141
for dislocating peroneal tendons, 1173
for fifth toe exostosis, 405, 407
for mild overlapping fifth toe deformity, 395–396
results, 397
technique, 395
Dwyer calcaneal osteotomy, 728, 794
postoperative care, 798
results, 798
technique, 794, 796–798
triple arthrodesis and, 701
Dyskeratosis congenita, 1042

E

Eccrine poroma, 1080
Ecthyma, 1038–1039
Ectopic ossification, 1000, 1001
Eczema, 1038, 1073–1075
Ehlers-Danlos syndrome, 766–767
Elastic bandages, in fracture and dislocation treatment, 1470
Electrical burns, 1430–1431
Electrodiagnostic testing, in tarsal tunnel syndrome, 555–556
Electromyography, of gait in cerebral palsy, 594, 595, 596

Elmslie procedure with fascia lata graft, for lateral ankle sprain and instability, 1137, 1162
Embolization of vascular malformations, 109
Enchondromas, 1008–1009
Endocrine disorders, toenail pathology from, 1040
Enterococcus, 909, 911
Epidermoid cysts, 1004, 1080
Epidermolysis bullosa, 1076–1077
Epiphyseal injuries of ankle in children, 1462
Epithelioma cuniculatum, 1085
Equinovalgus deformity, in myelodysplasia, 592–593
Equinovarus deformity
  from crush injury, 1406
  in myelodysplasia, 582–583
    cuneiform-cuboid wedge osteotomy for, 584–586
    surgical management, 583–584, 585
Equinovarus posturing, after stroke, 604
Equinus deformities
  callus formation from, 415
  in cerebral palsy, 594
    Achilles tendon lengthening for, 594, 596
    EMG tracings of gait, 595
  forefoot, in pes cavus, 787
Equinus deformity, in myelodysplasia, 582
Erythema multiforme, 1077
Erythrasma, 1039
Escharotomy, 1428–1429
Essex-Lopresti classification of calcaneal fractures, 1482, 1508–1510
Essex-Lopresti method of intra-articular calcaneal fracture treatment, closed reduction, 1515–1516
Essex-Lopresti's method of intra-articular calcaneal fracture treatment, open reduction, 1520
Evans osteotomy of os calcis, 725, 728, 732, 735
Evans procedure for lateral ankle sprain and instability, 1136
Ewing's sarcoma, 1015–1017
Examination principles
  neonatal and infant congenital abnormalities, 45
  older children and adults, 46–60
    calcaneocuboid, talonavicular, and cubeonavicular articulations, 56–57
    interphalangeal joints, 58
    ligamentous and muscular structures, 54–56
    metatarsophalangeal articulations, 57–58, 59
    peripheral nerves, 58, 60
    range of motion, 50–53
    relationship of forefoot to hindfoot, 53–54
    sequence of examination, 47–50
    tarsometatarsal articulations, 57
    viewpoints, 46–47
  toddlers, 45–46
Exercise-induced muscle pain, 1120–1121
Exercises, in fracture and dislocation rehabilitation, 1469, 1470–1471
Exostectomy, for Charcot foot, 942–943
Extensor digitorum longus
  in clawtoe deformity, 344
  in hammertoe deformity, 346, 348
Extensor digitorum longus tendon, rupture, 825
Extensor hallucis longus, in clawtoe deformity, 345
Extensor hallucis longus tendon
  irritated in dancers, 1258
  rupture, 825
  transfer for correction of hallux varus, 288, 290, 291
    postoperative care, 290, 292, 293
Extensor mechanism of lesser toes, 345, 346
Extensor tendon disorders, 824–825
External fixation of severely comminuted fracture, 1452
External iliac arterial occlusion, in cyclists, 1120

F

Fallen arches
  acquired, 767–784
  classification, 757–758
  congenital, 758–767
Fascia lata strips, in Achilles tendon repair, 815
Fascial spaces, 863
Fasciotomy, for compartment syndrome, 1381–1383
Fat pad trauma, in runners, 1231
Felon, 860–861
Felt pad supports, 146–148
Femoral anteversion, 1358–1359
  supracondylar femoral derotational osteotomy, 1359–1360
Femoral arterial occlusion, in cyclists, 1120
Fibrinolysis, 108–109
Fibromas, 993, 994
  of bone, 1009, 1011–1012
  periungual, 1057
Fibromatosis, plantar, 994–995
Fibrosarcomas, 1000, 1002, 1017, 1018
Fibula
  distal isthmus, stress fracture in dancers, 1274
  stress fracture, in runners, 1230
Fibular abutment, after calcaneal fracture, 1527–1528
Fibular epiphysis injuries in children, 1462
Fibular fracture, ankle injury with, 1450
Fibular problems, after ankle sprain in dancers, 1263
Fibular sesamoid
  excision technique
    dorsal approach, 492–493
    plantar approach, 493–494, 495
  osteochondritis dissecans, 1650
  percentage of bipartite sesamoids, 471
  radiography, 471, 472
Fibular syndesmosis, distal, injuries, 55
Fifth metatarsal, fractures of base, 1627–1628
  anatomy, 1628–1629
  author's preferred treatment, 1634–1635
  classification, 1627–1628, 1629
  clinical diagnosis, 1630
  mechanism of injury, 1629–1630
  radiographic diagnosis, 1630–1631
  treatment, 1631–1634
Fifth metatarsal base
  ossifying apophysis, 533, 535
  ununited apophysis, 534–535
Fifth metatarsal head
  bunionette deformity, 441–444
    surgical treatment, 444–462
  diabetic ulceration, surgical treatment, 906–907
  resection for bunionette deformity, 447–449
Fifth metatarsal head resection for bunionette deformity, 447–449
Fifth metatarsal osteotomy
  for bunionette deformity, 449–450
    distal chevron osteotomy technique, 450–452
    distal oblique osteotomy technique, 452–455
    distal osteotomies, 449–450, 463
  proximal, 449, 457–458
    anatomy for, 459
    postoperative care, 459
    results, 459, 461–462
    surgical technique, 458–459, 460
    Fifth proximal interphalangeal joint, chronically unstable, in dancers, 1245
  Fifth toe deformities
  anatomy, 394–395
  cockup deformity, 395, 400
    Ruiz-Mora procedure, 401, 402
    syndactylization of lesser toes, 401, 403
  etiology, 394
  flail toe from excessive bony resection, 406
  hammer toe, 361
  mild overlapping, 395
    DuVries procedure, 395–396, 397
    Wilson procedure, 396–397
  physical examination, 394–395
  severe overlapping, Lapidus procedure, 397–400
  underlapping, 400, 401

First cuneiform, bipartite, 527
First cuneiform osteotomy, for juvenile bunions, 329
  indications, 329–330
  postoperative care, 330
  results and complications, 330–332
  technique, 330, 331
First metatarsal
  anatomy, 174–181
  fracture of base, 1620
  length of, hallux valgus and, 172
  osteotomy for pes cavus, 794, 795
  plantar-flexed, dorsiflexion osteotomy for, 494, 497
  position of, 722, 723
  tuberculosis of, 870
First metatarsal head
  blood supply to, 175, 177, 178
  bursa beneath, 481
  diabetic ulcerations, surgery for, 904
  sesamoids and, 468
  tendons in normal articulation and hallux valgus, 186
  variations in shape, 177, 178
First metatarsal osteotomy, proximal
  for adult hallux valgus
    crescentic osteotomy, 217–222, 223, 224
    radiographs, 200, 203
    recurrent deformity after, 282, 283
  for juvenile bunions, 323–324
    indications, 325
    postoperative care, 328
    postoperative radiographs, 329, 330
    results and complications, 328–329
    technique, 325–328
  metatarsal nonunion from, 270
First metatarsocuneiform joint
  arthrodesis, 702–705, 707
    for flatfoot, 739
    for midfoot deformity in rheumatoid arthritis, 661
  degenerative arthritis, 634–635
    conservative treatment, 635–636
    surgical treatment, 636
First metatarsophalangeal joint
  anatomy, 168, 174–175, 176, 1193, 1695
  arthrodesis
    in hallux rigidus, 628–629, 634, 635
    for hallux valgus, 250
      complications, 255, 257–258
      contraindications, 250
      fixation with Steinmann pins, 253, 255–257
      indications, 250
      postoperative care, 253
      radiographs, 204, 252
      results, 253–255, 258
      surgical technique, 250–252
      surgical technique with curved surfaces, 253, 254
    in rheumatoid arthritis, 650–651, 661
  arthrosis, 194
  capsular tissue, hallux valgus and, 278–279
  cockup deformity in hallux valgus surgery, 280–281, 285
  dancing injuries, 1247–1250
  dislocations
    anatomy, 1695
    author's preferred treatment, 1700–1701
    mechanism of injury, 1695, 1697
    radiographic diagnosis, 1696–1697, 1698–1699
    treatment, 1699–1700
  in gouty arthritis, 616, 617
  in hallux rigidus, 622–624, 625, 629
  hyperextension deformity, 792
  impingement syndrome, 1235
  in juvenile bunions, 299–301, 303
  lateral instability in dancers, 1247
  normal joint and intermetatarsal angulation, 179, 181
  osteomyelitis in diabetic foot, 917–919
  pain from hallux valgus surgery, 292
  in rheumatoid arthritis, 638, 639, 640, 651, 652
  sesamoidectomy and, 498
  sesamoids (*see* Sesamoids of first metatarsophalangeal joint)
  sprain (turf toe), 1191–1200
  surgical implications of biomechanics, 35–36
  unstable from excessive excision in hallux valgus surgery, 271
First toe Jones procedure, in pes cavus, 792–793
Fistula, arteriovenous, 1081–1082
Flake fractures, 1290, 1567–1578
Flaps
  in amputation surgery, 961, 962, 963
    rays, 967, 971, 972
  in soft-tissue trauma
    cross-leg, 1403–1405
    free tissue, 1400–1403
    skin coverage, 1385–1386, 1387, 1389, 1392
    split-thickness skin excision and, 1394, 1397
    transpositional and island pedicle, 1399–1400
Flatfoot
  after calcaneal fracture, 1529, 1530
  callus formation from, 415
  flexible, 758–760, 1336–1338, 1339
  hallux valgus from, 170–172
  plantar fascia and, 839–840
  rigid, 760–762, 1338, 1340
    congenital convex pes valgus, 1343–1346
    peroneal spastic flatfoot, 1340–1343
  types, 48, 50
Flatfoot in adults, 757–784
  acquired
    arthrosis, 780–782
      traumatic, 782–783
    Charcot foot, 783, 784
    nature of deformity, 767
    neuromuscular imbalance, 783
    posterior tibial tendon dysfunction, 767–780
    tumors in foot, 783–784
  classification, 757–758
  congenital
    accessory navicular, 764–765, 1338, 1340
    flexible, 758–760, 1336–1338, 1339
    generalized dysplasia, 766–767
    peroneal spastic flatfoot, 760, 762–764, 1340–1343
    residual deformity, 765–766
    rigid, 760–762, 1338, 1340–1346
Flatfoot in children and young adults, 717–756
  accessory navicular, 741
    clinical symptoms, 741
    diagnosis, 742
    discussion, 743–744
    treatment
      author's preferred method, 743
      conservative, 742
      surgical, 742–743
    types, 741, 742
  conservative care, 724–725, 732, 733
  evaluation, 719
    physical, 720–723
    radiographic, 723–724
    terminology, 719–720
  foot as functional unit, 717–719
  incidence, 724
  surgical treatment, 725
    ages 3 to 8, 736
    ages 9 to 15, 736–737
      calcaneal osteotomy for excessive eversion, 737–738
      cuboid osteotomy for forefoot abduction, 738
      distal calcaneal osteotomy for forefoot abduction, 738
      medial soft-tissue repair, 739
      metatarsal cuneiform fusion, 739
      navicular cuneiform fusion, 738–739
      plantar flexion osteotomy of first metatarsal, 739
    arthroereisis, 731–732
    author's preferred method, 732–736
    fusion of subtalar joint complex, 731
    implants, 732
    infants and young children, 736
    medial column stabilization, 728–731
    osteotomy of os calcis, 725–728, 737–738

Flatfoot in children and young adults *(cont.)*
tendo Achilles lengthening, 731
young adults, 740–741
tarsal coalition, 744
in athletes, 749–750
author's preferred treatment, 750–751
calcaneonavicular coalition, 748–749, 752–753
discussion, 753
excision of calcaneonavicular bar, 752–753
incidence, 744–745
multiple and other coalitions, 749
pathomechanics, 745
talocalcaneal coalition, 745–748, 751–752
talonavicular coalition, 745
types, 718
Flexibility
athletic soft-tissue injuries and, 1100–1102
in dancers, 1101–1102
Flexor digitorum longus
in clawtoe deformity, 344
in hammertoe deformity, 348
Flexor digitorum longus tendon transfer
in Achilles tendon repair, 816
in posterior tibial tendon reconstruction, 775–779
in stroke treatment, 605–606
Flexor hallucis brevis
sesamoids and, 468
tendon of, 185
Flexor hallucis longus, in clawtoe deformity, 345
Flexor hallucis longus tendon
adhesions from hallux valgus surgery, 274
disorders, 823
tendinitis in dancers, 1267, 1270–1271
posterior impingement of ankle vs., 1266
tenolysis in dancers, 1267–1269
Flexor tendon transfers
for flexible or dynamic hammer toe, 358–361
results and complications, 371–372
in stroke treatment, 605–606
Flexor tenotomy
for curly toe deformity, 362–363, 365
with hammer toe repair, 351
Fluorescein testing, 1377, 1398
Fonsecaea compactum, 1082
Fonsecaea pedrosi, 1082
Football shoes, bunions and, 1203
Foot exercises, in fracture and dislocation rehabilitation, 1469, 1470–1471
Foot orthoses, 144–145
Foot surface, examination, 50
Footwear (*see* Shoes)
Forefoot
amputations, 971–973, 974
osteomyelitis in diabetic foot, 915–917
relationship to hindfoot, examination, 53–54, 55
stiffness after calcaneal fracture, 1529
varus and valgus, 55
Forefoot deformities in cerebral palsy, 598–599
Forefoot disorders in runners, 1235–1237
Forefoot reconstruction in rheumatoid arthritis, 653
complications, 659–660
postoperative care, 659
results, 659
technique, 653–659
Forefoot sprains in athletes, 1191
anatomy and biomechanics, 1193–1194
clinical evaluation, 1195–1196
epidemiology, 1191
etiologic factors, 1194–1195
historical perspective, 1191
mechanism of injury, 1192
radiographic evaluation, 1196–1198
severity of injury, 1191–1192
treatment
nonoperative, 1198, 1199
results, 1199–1200
surgical, 1198–1199
Forefoot surgery, biomechanical considerations, 35–36
Foreign bodies, 1432–1436
localization, 1432, 1434
algorithmic approach to imaging, 119, 122, 123–124
computed tomography, 95, 97
interventional radiology, 110
magnetic resonance imaging, 104
ultrasound, 123
of sole, 1080–1081
Fowler and Philip angle, 850
Fractures
ankle (*see* Ankle fractures)
avulsion vs. impaction, 1442
computed tomography, 95, 98
in diabetes, 878, 879
stress (*see* Stress fractures)
toe, in dancers, 1245
Fractures and dislocations of foot *(see also specific anatomic areas)*
diagnosis, 1467
treatment, 1467–1471
Free tissue flaps, in soft-tissue trauma, 1400–1403
Freiberg's infraction, 435, 1029, 1250
diagnosis, 435, 437
radiographs, 438–439
treatment, 437
postoperative care, 437
results, 437, 441
surgical technique, 437, 440
Frostbite, 1421–1422
risk factors, 1422
treatment, 1422–1424
Fungal infections, 871–872
dermatologic aspects, 1077–1078
of toenails, 1054–1055

G

Gait cycle
events, 15, 28
first interval, 29
second interval, 29–30
third interval, 30–31
phases, 15
Gait training, in outpatient surgery center, 153
Gallium scans, 87
of bone infections, 129, 133, 866
in diabetes, 893
Ganglionic cyst, hallux valgus from, 173
Ganglions, 127, 997
Gas gangrene, 861, 862
Gas in soft tissue, in diabetic infections, 912
Gastrocnemius-soleus strain in athletes, 1116–1117
Gastrointestinal disorders, toenail pathology from, 1041
Genetics and foot, 1314 (*see also* Congenital foot deformities)
Giant-cell tumors
of bone, 1006
of tendon sheath, 997–998
Girdlestone transfer, 593
Gissane's crucial angle, 1477, 1479–1480
Glass, embedded in foot, 1435–1436
Gleich osteotomy of os calcis, 726
Glomus tumors, 1000, 1001, 1079–1080
of toenails, 1044
Gout, 616–617, 1025–1026, 1028
Gram-negative bacteria, dermatologic aspects, 1077
Granuloma annulare, 1076
Great toe
amputation surgery, 966–967, 1384–1386, 1387–1389
arthroscopy, 1305–1307
bifurcated (*see* Accessory navicular)
deviation in sesamoid disruption, 471
diabetic ulcerations, surgery for, 902–904
dorsiflexion and arch elevation, 51
gouty arthritis, 616
hammered, 343
repair of, 370–371
interphalangeal joint
arthrodesis in degenerative arthritis, 621
dancing injuries, 1247
interphalangeal sesamoid, 498–499
metatarsophalangeal joint (*see* First metatarsophalangeal joint)
osteomyelitis, 868
paresthesias from hallux valgus surgery, 261
phalangeal fractures, treatment, 1641–1642, 1644–1645
in rheumatoid arthritis, 638

sesamoids
interphalangeal, 498–499
osteomyelitis in diabetic foot, 917–919, 920
shoe modifications, 143
silicone arthroplasty, weight bearing biomechanics in, 13, 14
stenosis, 824
weight bearing after amputation, 12
Grice procedure, 731
Griseofulvin, for onychomycosis, 1056
Guanethidine, in reflex sympathetic dystrophy syndrome, 1418
Gunshot, embedded in foot, 1432
Gymnasts, flexibility in, 1101

H

Haemophilus influenzae, 864, 865
Haglund deformity, 847, 848
Achilles tendinitis and, 1233, 1234
surgical treatment, 851, 854
Half-and-half nail, 1042
Hallux (*see* Great toe)
Hallux flexus, 622, 624
Hallux rigidus
in athletes, 1200
clinical findings, 625
congenital, 1350
conservative treatment, 625
in dancers, 1247–1249
etiology, 622–624
juvenile, 622, 625
radiographic findings, 625
in runners, 1236
shoe modification, 143
surgical treatment
arthrodesis of first metatarsophalangeal joint, 628–629, 634, 635
cheilectomy, 625, 628, 630–631, 632–634
decision making, 625, 628–629, 630
proximal phalangeal osteotomy, 625, 629, 632
Hallux saltans, 1270
Hallux valgus angle, radiographic evaluation, 192
Hallux valgus deformity, 167–296
adult vs. juvenile, 297–298
anatomic considerations, 168
anatomic relationships, 174–175, 176
blood supply to metatarsal head, 175, 177, 178
distal metatarsal articular angle, 177, 179
normal first metatarsophalangeal joint and intermetatarsal angle, 179, 181
relationship of proximal phalanx to metatarsal head, 179, 180
shape of first metatarsal head and metatarsocuneiform joint, 177, 178
in athletes, 1200–1206
causes, 168–169
first metatarsal length, 172
heredity, 169–170
hypermobility of metatarsocuneiform joint, 172–173
metatarsus primus varus, 172
miscellaneous factors, 173–174
pes planus, 170–172
predisposing factors, 168–169
shoes, 142, 168–169
in cerebral palsy, 598, 599
classification, 189–191
complications of surgery, 258–259
causes of failure, 259–260
hallux varus, 284–292, 293
intractable plantar keratosis, 281–282
metatarsal head problems, 267–273
metatarsal shaft problems, 262–267
pain about first metatarsophalangeal joint, 292
problems with capsular tissue of first metatarsophalangeal joint, 278–279
proximal phalanx problems, 273–278
recurrent deformity, 282–284
sesamoid problems, 279–281
soft-tissue problems, 260–262
conservative treatment, 195
in dancers, 1247
definition, 168
juvenile (*see* Juvenile bunions)
pain in runners from, 1236–1237
pathophysiology, 181–189
effect of lateral drift on lesser toes, 187, 189
joint capsule changes, 184
medial eminence, 187, 188, 194
metatarsophalangeal articulation, 181–183
progression over 10 years, 182
relationships of sesamoids to metatarsal head, 185
severe end-stage deformity, 187
patient evaluation
history and physical examination, 191–192
radiographs, 192–194
progression after second toe amputation, 356, 357
prostheses, 292, 294
radiographs of stages of deformity, 190, 191
recurrent
after distal soft tissue realignment procedure, 215
after hallux valgus surgery, 282–284
in rheumatoid arthritis, 639–640, 643–644, 645
second metatarsophalangeal joint dislocation and, 372, 373, 377, 378
from sesamoid excision, 494
with sesamoid subluxation, 481–482, 484–486
surgical treatment
Akin procedure, 239–242, 243
algorithms, 196, 199
arthrodesis of first metatarsophalangeal joint, 250–258
chevron osteotomy, 196, 202, 227–235
decision making, 195–202
distal soft tissue procedure, 204–216
distal soft tissue procedure with proximal crescentic osteotomy, 216–227
goals of procedures, 202, 204, 259
Keller procedure, 242, 244, 246–247
metatarsocuneiform arthrodesis and distal soft tissue procedure, 244–245, 248–250
Mitchell procedure, 233–239
procedures for congruent joint, 196
procedures for incongruent joint, 196, 199
Hallux valgus interphalangeus, 181
Hallux varus deformity
causes, 284–287
congenital, 284, 1349–1350
after distal metatarsal osteotomies, 288, 289
after distal soft tissue procedure with proximal crescentic osteotomy, 216, 218, 275, 277
after distal soft tissue realignment procedure, 216
extensor hallucis longus transfer for, 288, 290–292, 293
after McBride procedure, 323, 324
after proximal first metatarsal osteotomy, 329
in rheumatoid arthritis, 638, 640
with sesamoid dislocation, 486
from sesamoid excision, 494
Hammer toe, 341, 342
anatomy and pathophysiology, 345–348
clawtoe vs., 363
congenital, 1352
definition, 341
etiology, 342, 343–344
treatment, 349–351, 352, 377, 378
algorithm, 353
fifth toe, 361
flexible or dynamic hammer toe, 358–361
postoperative care, 355
results and complications, 355–358
technique, 351, 354–355
Hapalonychia, 1036
Harris mat, 58, 59
Harris mat prints, for plantar keratoses, 415, 416, 417, 420
Heat generation and conservation by body, 1420

Heat injuries, 1426–1428
classification, 1428
treatment, 1428–1432
Heat transfer mechanisms, 1420
Heel
bursitis, 809–810
strike and rise, examination, 47
ulcerations in diabetes, 901
varus in pes cavus, 787
Heel of shoe, modifications, 142–143, 144
Heel pain
after calcaneal fracture, 1526–1529
in dancers, 1273–1274
in runners, 1231–1233
subcalcaneal pain syndrome, 837–838
anatomy, 838–839, 840, 841
diagnosis, 839–842
treatment, 842–847
superior
anatomy, 848, 849
diagnosis, 848–850
etiology, 847–848, 850
treatment, 850–855
Heel spur
in dancers, 1273
subcalcaneal pain syndrome and, 837–838
Heifetz procedure, 1065–1067
Hemangiomas, 999, 1000
Hematologic disorders, toenail pathology from, 1040
Hematomas, subungual, 1057–1058, 1246
Hemophilus influenzae, 864, 865
Hemorrhage
splinter, 1039
under toenail, 1036
Hepatic disorders, toenail pathology from, 1041
Heredity and foot, 1314 (*see also* Congenital foot deformities)
Hermann's method of intra-articular calcaneal fracture treatment, 1515
Herpetic whitlow, 1058
Heterotopic bone formation, in heel cord, after trauma, 1000, 1001
Hindfoot
alignment, surgical implications of biomechanics, 34
ligaments
anatomy, 1121–1122
biomechanics, 1123
osteomyelitis in diabetic foot, 921–923
radiographic evaluation, 63, 65, 73–74
relationship to forefoot, examination, 53–54, 55
Histoplasma capsulatum, 872
HIV-associated Reiter's syndrome or psoriasis, 619
Hoke-Miller procedure, 730, 731
Hoke procedure, 729, 730, 731
Howard technique, in Achilles tendon repair, 814
Human immunodeficiency virus, Reiter's syndrome or psoriasis and, 619
Hypercholesterolemia, 1027, 1028
Hyperkeratosis, skin grafting and, 1391, 1393
Hyperkeratosis subungualis, 1036, 1038, 1057
Hyperparathyroidism, 1023, 1024
Hyperthyroid osteoporosis, 1020
Hypertrophy of nail matrix, 1059–1060
Hypertrophy of ungualabia, 1049
Hypothyroid osteoporosis, 1020

I

Imaging, 61–139
algorithmic approach, 110
arthritis, 127–129
avascular necrosis, 122, 124–125
chronic undiagnosed posttraumatic pain, 113–117
foreign body localization, 119, 122, 123–124
ligamentous injury, 113, 117–118
neoplasm, 122, 125–127
osteochondral injury, 111–113
reflex sympathetic dystrophy, 111, 112
tendon injury, 119–122
angiography, 106–108
popliteal artery entrapment syndrome, 1119
tarsal navicular, 1601
ankle fractures, 1445, 1447, 1448
arthrography, 83–84
air-contrast, in osteochondral fracture evaluation, 1573
ankle, 1126, 1148
subtalar, 1159, 1166
bunions in athletes, 1204–1205
bursography, 83
calcaneal anatomy, 73
calcaneal fractures, 1483–1484
conventional tomography and computerized axial tomography, 1485, 1488–1490
extra-articular, 1494–1496, 1499, 1502, 1503, 1504
intra-articular, 1506, 1507, 1511, 1534
standard radiographic views, 1484–1485, 1486
subtalar joint, 1485–1488, 1489
Charcot foot, 932–934
compartment syndrome, 1108, 1109
computed tomography (*see* Computed tomography)
congenital convex pes valgus, 1344
cuboid dislocations, 1694
cuboid fractures, 1614
cuneiform fractures, 1616, 1617
diabetes, 888, 892–893
fifth metatarsal base fractures, 1630–1631
flatfoot, 723–724
of foot fractures and dislocations, 1467
foreign bodies, 1433–1436
hallux rigidus, 625, 626–628
hallux valgus, 192–194
interventional radiology, 108–110
lateral ankle sprain, 1125–1126, 1127
lesser toes, 349, 350
magnetic resonance imaging (*see* Magnetic resonance imaging)
metatarsal fractures, 1618–1619, 1620
metatarsophalangeal joint dislocations, 1696–1697, 1698–1699, 1701
midfoot sprains, 1186–1187, 1188, 1189
nuclear medicine, 86–89
peroneal spastic flatfoot, 1341–1342
peroneal tendinitis and ruptures, 1178–1179
peroneal tendon subluxation and dislocation, 1171
phalangeal fractures, 1641, 1643
radiographic evaluation of ankle
anteroposterior projection, 75, 76, 81
internal oblique (mortise) projection, 75, 77–78
lateral projection, 75, 77
stress views, 75, 79, 80
weight-bearing views, 79, 81
radiographic evaluation of foot
anatomy, 62, 63
anteroposterior projection, 62, 64, 67, 68, 69
calcaneus, 72, 73
hindfoot, 63, 65, 73–74
lateral oblique projection, 62–63, 65
lateral projection, 65, 68
medial oblique projection, 62, 65
phalanges, 63, 70
sesamoid bones, 63, 71
talocalcaneal medial oblique special projections, 74
weight-bearing views, 63, 67–69
radionuclide bone scanning (*see* Bone scanning)
rheumatoid foot, 639–645
second metatarsophalangeal joint, 375, 376–377, 378, 379
sesamoid fractures, 1647–1648, 1649, 1650
sesamoids of first metatarsophalangeal joint, 471, 472
sinus tarsi syndrome, 1166–1167
soft corns, 406
stress fractures of metatarsal diaphysis, 1637–1638
subcalcaneal pain syndrome, 840–842
subtalar instability, 1155–1158
superior heel pain, 849–850
syndesmosis sprains of ankle, 1146–1149

talar dislocations, 1655, 1656–1657, 1662
talar fractures and fracture-dislocations, 1547, 1553–1554
lateral process, 1594–1595
osteochondral fractures, 1572–1574, 1577
posterior process, 1586, 1587, 1588–1589
shearing and comminuted fractures, 1581
talipes equinovarus, 1317–1320
tarsal navicular fractures, 1601–1602, 1603, 1604, 1605
stress fractures, 1610, 1611
tarsometatarsal dislocations, 1679–1681, 1683
tenography, 83, 84
thermography, 85–86
tomography, 79, 82
computed (*see* Computed tomography)
partial volume effect, 81
polytomography of fractures, 1573, 1610, 1611, 1620
of tumors, 122, 125–127, 992–993
turf toe, 1196–1198
ultrasound, 89–91
diabetes, 886–887, 888, 889–890, 956
evaluation for amputation, 964
foreign body localization, 123
Immobilization of fractures or dislocations, 1468
Impaction fracture, avulsion fracture vs., 1442
Impetigo, 1038
Impingement (syndromes)
in dancers, 1256–1258
after ankle sprain, 1263
posterior, 1265–1266, 1266–1270
in runners, 1235
soft-tissue, arthroscopy for, 1286–1289
Implant arthroplasty
for degenerative joint disease, 620
for hallux rigidus, 629
Inclusion cyst, epidermal, 1004, 1080
Inconstant sesamoids, 499–500
Indium scans, 87–88, 866, 933
Infants, preambulatory, examination for congenital abnormalities, 45
Infections
algorithmic approach to imaging, 129–133
in ankle fractures, 1453
antibiotics, 872–875
after arthrodesis, 675
bacterial, 860–869, 1077
after calcaneal fracture treatment, 1530
in Charcot foot, 941
classification, 859
in diabetic foot, 868–869, 909–923
fungal, 871–872, 1077–1078
in hallux valgus surgery, 260
joint, 864–865
magnetic resonance imaging, 104, 131–132
mycobacterial, 869–871
nail plate trimming and, 1051, 1052
of sesamoids, 484–485, 487
in soft-tissue trauma, 1372, 1373
after talar dislocation, 1663
toenail pathology from, 1041
Inferior extensor retinaculum of hindfoot, 1121–1122
Inflammation of tendons, 807
Inflammatory skin problems of feet, 1073–1077
Ingrown toenails, 1049–1054
differential diagnosis, 1052
soft-tissue wedge resection for, 1065
stages, 1051–1052
treatment, 1052–1053
types, 1050
Innervation of foot, by musculature, 587
Insoles
for diabetic foot, 946–947, 948–952, 957
partial amputation, 919, 921
for forefoot amputation, 973
for midfoot sprain, 1190
Interdigital neuromas
clinical symptoms, 560
conservative treatment, 560–561
diagnosis, 560
etiology, 560
incidence, 560
in runners, 1237
surgical treatment, 561–562
Interdigital plantar neuromas
anatomic factors, 544–545, 546
clinical results, 551
conservative treatment, 549
diagnosis, 548
differential diagnosis, 548–549
etiology, 544
extrinsic causes, 546–547
history, 544
postoperative care, 550–551
recurrent, 552–553
surgical treatment, 549–550
technique for excision, 550–551
symptom complex, 547–548
traumatic causes, 545–546
uncommon findings, 551
Intermetatarsal angle
in bunionette deformity, 441, 442
radiographic evaluation, 192
Intermetatarsal phalangeal bursitis, 809
Interosseous ligament anatomy, 1144
Interosseous talocalcaneal ligament, 1123
Interphalangeal joint arthrodesis
in clawtoe, 369–370, 371
great toe, 712, 713
in rheumatoid arthritis, 660
lesser toes, 712–713
Interphalangeal joint dislocations, 1244–1245, 1701–1702
Interphalangeal joints
arthritis, 258, 620–622, 640
examination, 58
great toe, dancing injuries, 1247
proximal
dislocations in dancers, 1244–1245
fifth, chronic instability in dancers, 1245
stiff from hammer toe, 1102
Interphalangeal sesamoid of hallux, 498–499
Intertrigo, infected, 1039
Interventional radiology, 108–110
Ischemia
in crush injury, 1405–1406
in diabetes, 887–888
Island pedicle flaps, 1399–1400

J

Jadassohn-Lewandowsky syndrome, 1042, 1043
Japas osteotomy, for pes cavus, 801
Jogger's foot, 845
Jogging, running and walking vs., variations in gait cycle, 32
Joints
hyperelasticity, hallux valgus and, 174
infections, 864–865
instability, 1102
limited mobility in diabetes, 884
Jones fracture of fifth metatarsal, 1253, 1254
Jones procedure for superior peroneal retinaculum reconstruction, 1173–1174
Jones procedure of great toe, 792–793
Joplin's neuroma, 1249
Juvenile bunions, 297–339
adult vs., 297–298
age of onset, 297
algorithm for severe deformity, 311
algorithms for mild deformity, 310
anatomy
first metatarsophalangeal joint, 299–301, 303
metatarsocuneiform joint, 301–302, 304–306, 307
open ephiphysis, 306–308
etiology, 299
radiographs, 309
treatment
Akin procedure, 312–314
conservative care, 308–309
decision making, 309–311
discussion, 335–337
distal metatarsal osteotomy, 314–320
distal soft tissue realignment, 320–323, 324
double osteotomy, 335–337
first cuneiform osteotomy, 329–332

Juvenile bunions *(cont.)*
metatarsocuneiform arthrodesis, 332–335
operative repair, 311–312
postsurgical complications, 337–338
proximal first metatarsal osteotomy, 323, 325–329, 330
Juxta-articular chondromas, 1009, 1010

K

Kallassey ankle brace, 1161
Kaposi's sarcoma, 1002–1003, 1048, 1083–1084
Keller procedure
for adult hallux valgus, 242, 244
complications, 244, 247
contraindications, 244
indications, 244
instability after resection of base of proximal phalanx, 276–278
postoperative care, 244
recurrent deformity after, 282
results, 244, 246
surgical technique, 244, 245
hallux clawing after resection arthroplasty, 483
for hallux rigidus, 629
modified (resection of base of proximal phalanx), for diabetic ulcerations, 903
in rheumatoid forefoot, 648, 650
Kelly bone block procedure, 1173
Keloids, 993–994, 1081
Keratinization, pathologic, of nail matrix, 1060–1061
Keratoacanthoma, 1085
Keratoses, plantar (*see* Plantar keratoses)
Keratotic lesser toe deformities
crossover, of second toe, 386
etiology, 403–404
hard corns, 403, 404
treatment, 405, 407–408
physical examination, 404–405
soft corns, 403, 404, 406
treatment, 407, 409–410
Ketoconazole, for onychomycosis, 1056
Köhler's disease, 1028–1029
Kidner procedure, 524–525, 731, 741, 742
technique, 525
Kirschner wires
malleolar fracture fixation, 1456, 1458
metatarsal fractures, 1625, 1626
midfoot sprain, 1190
phalangeal fractures, 1642, 1643, 1644, 1645
tarsometatarsal dislocations, 1682, 1685, 1686, 1688–1690
Kite's angle, in clubfoot evaluation, 1317–1319
Koilonychia, 1036, 1060, 1061
Koutsogiannis osteotomy of os calcis, 726

L

Landry-Guillain-Barré-Strohl syndrome, 580
Lapidus procedure for severe overlapping fifth toe deformity
modified, 399
postoperative care, 399
results and complications, 399–400
technique, 397–399
Larsen procedure for lateral ankle sprain and instability, 1136
Lateral ankle sprains
in athletes, 1121–1139
chronic residual, 817
in dancers, 1258–1264
Lateral border of foot, diabetic ulcerations, surgical treatment, 908
Lateral compartment syndrome, surgical treatment, 1110, 1112
Lateral condylectomy, for bunionette deformity, 444, 446
dislocation of fifth metatarsophalangeal joint from, 463
postoperative care, 446
results, 446–447
surgical technique, 444–445, 446
Lateral gutter impingement, arthroscopy, 1286
Lateral malleolus, surgical treatment of fractures, 1449, 1451, 1455–1458
Lateral plantar nerve
anatomy, 155
compression, in runners, 1231–1233
entrapment of first branch
anatomy, 562
clinical symptoms, 563
diagnosis, 563
etiology, 563
incidence, 562–563
postoperative care, 564
surgical treatment, 563–564
Lateral proper digital nerve, entrapment in dancers, 1249–1250
Lateral talocalcaneal ligament, 1122
Lateral tendon transfer, 829
Latissimus dorsi flap, 1400, 1401, 1403
Lauge-Hansen classification of ankle fractures, 1440
Leg
gross abnormalities, examination, 48, 49, 50
nonoperative, labeling, 152
surface examination, 50
Leg length discrepancy, in runners, 1229
Leg pain
in athletes, 1105–1121
in dancers, 1274–1275
in runners, 1230–1231
Lesser toe deformities (*see also* Clawtoe; Hammer toe), 341–411
congenital abnormalities
hammer toe, 1352
macrodactyly, 1352, 1353
overlapping toes, 1352–1354
polydactyly, 1350–1352
syndactyly, 1352
underlapping toes (curly toe), 1354
crossover of second toe, 379, 386
curly toe, 362–363, 365, 1354
in dancers, 1246
fifth (*see* Fifth toe deformities)
fracture or dislocation, soft corns from, 409
keratotic
etiology, 403–404
hard corns, 403, 404
hard corn treatment, 405, 407–408
physical examination, 404–405
soft corns, 403, 404, 406
soft corn treatment, 407, 409–410
mallet toe, 341, 342, 361–364
metatarsophalangeal joint
author's preferred treatment, 1701
dislocations, anatomy, 1695–1696
mechanism of injury, 1695–1696
radiographic diagnosis, 1699, 1701
treatment, 1700
pathophysiology, 345–348
phalangeal fractures, treatment, 1642, 1644, 1645
physical examination, 348–349
radiographic examination, 349, 350
syndactylization, 401–403
Lesser toes
amputation surgery, 967
pitfalls and complications, 969–970
technique, 967
anatomy, 345–347
interphalangeal joint fusion, 712–713
metatarsal head osteomyelitis in diabetes, 919, 921
metatarsophalangeal joints
dancing injuries, 1250–1251
in hallux valgus, 187, 189
Leukonychia, 1036, 1060, 1061
Lichen planus, 1076
Ligamentous and muscular structures, examination, 54–56
Ligamentous injury, algorithmic approach to imaging, 113, 117–118
Ligament ruptures, with ankle fracture, 1454
Ligaments, ankle
anatomy, 1121–1123
magnetic resonance imaging, 102, 103
Limited joint mobility syndrome, in diabetes, 884
Linear and angular relationships of foot, 69

Lipomas, 996
Lisfranc dislocations/fracture-dislocations (*see* Tarsometatarsal dislocations)
Lisfranc's ligament, 1186
Local flaps, in soft-tissue trauma, 1399–1400
Locomotion
kinematics
horizontal body displacements, 6, 9
lateral body displacements, 7–8, 9
vertical body displacements, 5–6
kinetics, 9–10
Locomotor system of foot, 4–5
Loose bodies of ankle, arthroscopy, 1296–1297
Looser's zones, in first metatarsals of osteomalacic bone, 1021, 1022
Lord osteotomy of os calcis, 726
Lower extremity
gross abnormalities, examination, 48, 49, 50
nonoperative, labeling, 152
surface examination, 50
Lower extremity discrepancy, in runners, 1229
Lower extremity pain
in athletes, 1105–1121
in dancers, 1274–1275
in runners, 1230–1231
Lowman procedure, 731
Lumbar sympathetic blocks, in reflex sympathetic dystrophy syndrome, 1417, 1418
Lupus erythematosus, discoid, 1077
Lyme disease, 619, 869
Lymphangitis, treatment, 860

M

Macrodactyly, 1352, 1353
Madura foot/maduromycosis, 871, 872, 1082–1083
Magnetic resonance imaging
Achilles tendon injury, 810–811
ankle ligaments, 101, 103
ankle tendons, 100, 101, 103
diabetes, 892, 893
foreign bodies, 104, 1435
indications, 101, 103, 105–106
mechanism, 98–100
osteochondral fractures, 1573, 1574, 1577
osteomyelitis, 104
running injuries, 1227
scanners, 100–101
soft-tissue masses, 103, 105
stress fractures, 104, 106
syndesmosis sprains of ankle, 1148–1149
tissue signal intensities, 99–100
tumors, 992
Malignant melanoma, 1003, 1083
of toenails, 1046–1047, 1048
Malleolar fractures
closed reduction, 1448–1449
lateral, surgical treatment, 1449, 1451, 1455–1458
medial, surgical treatment, 1449–1450, 1454–1455, 1456
open reduction with internal fixation, 1449–1451
posterior, surgical treatment, 1458
Mallet toe, 341, 342, 361, 362
in dancers, 1246
definition, 341
etiology, 342–343
treatment, 361
algorithm, 363
postoperative care, 362
results and complications, 362–363
technique, 361–362, 364
Marfan's syndrome, 766–767
Matrisectomy, phenol/alcohol, 1068–1070
McBride procedure, 320–323, 324
hallux varus after, 284
McReynold's method of intra-articular calcaneal fracture treatment, 1520–1521
Medial ankle dancing injuries, 1255–1256
Medial ankle sprains in athletes, 1139–1142
Medial calcaneal nerve, in subcalcaneal pain syndrome, 838, 839
Medial column stabilization, for flatfoot, 728–731
Medial epiphyseal stapling, for valgus foot, 590, 591
Medial malleolus, surgical treatment of fractures, 1449–1450, 1454–1455, 1456
Medial plantar nerve
anatomy, 154–155
entrapment
anatomy, 566
clinical symptoms, 566–567
diagnosis, 567
etiology, 566
incidence, 566
postoperative care, 567
surgical treatment, 567
neuropraxia, heel pain from, 845
third branch, 546
Medial soft-tissue repair, for flatfoot, 739, 740
Medial tibial stress syndrome in athletes
classification, 1112
clinical features, 1112–1113
definition, 1112
diagnosis, 1113–1114
runners, 1230
treatment, 1114–1115
Mee's lines, 1040, 1042
Melanoma, malignant, 1083
of toenails, 1003, 1046–1047, 1048
Melanotic whitlow, 1046–1047, 1048
Melorheostosis, 1010, 1013
Metabolic bone disease, 1018
acromegaly, 1027, 1028
gout, 1025–1026, 1028
hypercholesterolemia, 1027, 1028
osteomalacia, 1021–1025
osteoporosis, 1018–1021
Paget disease, 1024, 1025
Metabolism, in diabetes, 884
Metaphyseal dysostosis, 1022–1023
Metastatic tumors to foot, 1018
Metatarsal articular angle, distal, 177, 179
Metatarsal base, fifth (*see* Fifth metatarsal base)
Metatarsal condylectomy, for localized intractable plantar keratosis
Coughlin's modified, 422–423, 424
DuVries technique, 421–422, 424
Metatarsal fractures, 1617–1618
anatomy, 1618
base, author's preferred treatment, 1625, 1627
clinical diagnosis, 1618
fifth metatarsal base, 1627–1628
anatomy, 1628–1629
author's preferred treatment, 1634–1635
classification, 1627–1628, 1629
clinical diagnosis, 1630
mechanism of injury, 1629–1630
radiographic diagnosis, 1630–1631
treatment, 1631–1634
mechanism of injury, 1618
radiographic diagnosis, 1618–1619, 1620
second metatarsal base, tarsometatarsal dislocations and, 1678, 1679, 1680
stress fractures of metatarsal diaphysis, 1635–1636
author's preferred treatment, 1638
clinical diagnosis, 1636–1637
predisposing conditions and activities, 1636
radiographic diagnosis, 1637–1638
treatment, 1638
treatment
author's preferred methods, 1624–1627
closed fractures
displaced, 1621–1623, 1624–1625
undisplaced, 1619, 1621
head fractures, 1624, 1625
neck fractures, 1623–1624, 1625
open fractures, 1619, 1621
Metatarsalgia
in dancers, 1251
examination, 58, 59
in runners, 1235
weight bearing biomechanics, 11, 12
Metatarsal head complications, of hallux valgus surgery, 267, 269–273, 274, 275

Metatarsal heads
complications of hallux valgus surgery
avascular necrosis, 233, 235, 272–273, 274, 275
displacement, 269–272
excessive excision, 269, 271
fifth
bunionette deformity, 441–444
surgical treatment, 444–462
diabetic ulceration, surgical treatment, 906–907
first
blood supply to, 175, 177, 178
bursa beneath, 481
diabetic ulcerations, surgery for, 904
in hallux rigidus, 623, 624
relationship of sesamoids to, in hallux valgus, 185
relationship to proximal phalanx, 179, 180
sesamoids and, 468
tendons in normal articulation and hallux valgus, 186
variations in shape, 177, 178
flat vs. round, 181, 182
lesser heads, osteomyelitis in diabetic foot, 919, 921
osteochondrosis
diagnosis, 435, 437, 438–439
treatment, 437, 440–441
resection for intractable plantar keratosis, 432, 433
Metatarsal osteotomy
closing wedge
dorsiflexion deformity from, 263–264
for juvenile hallux valgus, 325
crescentic osteotomy
for adult hallux valgus, 202, 217–222, 223, 224
dorsiflexion deformity from, 266
metatarsal nonunion from, 266
for juvenile hallux valgus, 325–328
for diffuse intractable plantar keratosis, 426–433
distal
chevron procedure, 314–316, 319–320
Mitchell procedure, 316–320
fifth (*see* Fifth metatarsal osteotomy)
first (*see* First metatarsal osteotomy)
oblique
for bunionette deformity, 452–455
for diffuse intractable plantar keratosis, 427–431
to relieve metatarsalgia, 432
opening wedge, for juvenile hallux valgus, 324–325, 329–331
Metatarsal shaft complications of hallux valgus surgery, 262
dorsiflexion, 262–266
excessive valgus of first metatarsal, 266–267, 268–269
nonunion of metatarsal, 267, 270
plantar flexion, 266, 267
shortening, 262, 263
Metatarsals (*see also* Fifth metatarsal; First metatarsal)
anatomy
dorsal aspect, 1677
radiography, 1680–1681
dancing injuries, 1252–1254, 1255
deformities in pes cavus, 786, 788
shoe modifications in region of, 143–144
shoe pads, 147
Metatarsal supports, 418, 419
Metatarsocuneiform arthrodesis, 332
for arthritis, 636, 661
dorsiflexion deformity from, 266
first, 636, 661, 702–705, 707, 739
for flatfoot, 739
indications, 332
postoperative care, 332
results and complications, 332, 334–335
technique, 332, 333
Metatarsocuneiform arthrodesis and distal soft tissue procedure, for adult hallux valgus, 244–245
complications, 250
contraindications, 245, 248
indications, 245
results, 248–250
surgical technique, 248
Metatarsocuneiform joint
anatomy, 174–175
examination, 57, 191, 192
first
arthrodesis, 702–705, 707
for flatfoot, 739
for hallux valgus, 244–245
for midfoot deformity in rheumatoid arthritis, 661
degenerative arthritis, 634–635
conservative treatment, 635–636
surgical treatment, 636
hypermobility and hallux valgus, 172–173
in juvenile bunions, 301–302, 304–306, 307
in rheumatoid arthritis, 638, 641–642, 661
second, arthrodesis, 706, 707
unstable with medial deviation, 184, 193
variations in shape, 177, 178
Metatarsophalangeal angle, in bunionette deformity, 441
Metatarsophalangeal articulations, examination, 57–58, 59
Metatarsophalangeal break, biomechanics, 24–26
Metatarsophalangeal bursitis, 809
Metatarsophalangeal joint deformity, with hammer toe deformity, 357
Metatarsophalangeal joint dislocations, 1694–1695
anatomy, 1695–1696
author's preferred treatment, 1700–1701
classification, 1696–1697
clinical diagnosis, 1698
mechanism of injury, 1697–1698
radiographic diagnosis, 1696–1697, 1698–1699, 1701
results, 1700
treatment, 1699–1700
Metatarsophalangeal joints
abnormal alignment, callus formation from, 415
anatomy for lesser toe deformities, 346–348
arthroscopic normal examination, 1306–1307
collateral ligaments, 174, 175
congruent vs. incongruent, 181, 183, 192–193
surgical decision making, 195–196
deformities in pes cavus, 788–789
drawer test, 373
fifth, dislocation after lateral condylectomy, 463
first (*see* First metatarsophalangeal joint)
hyperextension deformity
in clawtoe, 369
flexor tendon transfer for, 385
lesser toes
dancing injuries, 1250–1251
in hallux valgus, 187, 189
range of motion
examination, 53
in rheumatoid arthritis, 638, 639, 640, 648, 649
arthrodesis, 650–651
subluxation or dislocation, 660
second (*see* Second metatarsophalangeal joint)
subluxation after later condylectomy, 446
Metatarsus adductus, 1327–1328
anatomy, 1328
etiology, 1328–1329
juvenile bunions and, 307
primary problems, 1315
radiographic appearance, 1328
treatment, 1329
cast application, 1329–1331
operative, 1331–1334

Metatarsus primus varus
first cuneiform osteotomy for, 329, 331
hallux valgus and, 172
recurrent, 308
Metatarsus varus, 1327–1328
anatomy, 1328
etiology, 1328–1329
resistant in older child, treatment, 1334, 1335
Methylmethacrylate, in flatfoot surgery, 732
Metronidazole, 875
Midfoot
alignment, surgical implications of biomechanics, 35
anatomy, 65
ligaments and tendons, 1186
osteomyelitis in diabetic foot, 921
Midfoot fractures
author's preferred treatments, 1611–1612
body of navicular, 1605–1609
dorsal lip of navicular, 1602–1603
navicular tuberosity, 1603–1605
tarsal navicular, 1600–1602
stress fractures, 1609–1611
Midfoot sprains in athletes
definition, 1184
diagnosis
anatomic considerations, 1185
clinical findings, 1185–1186
radiographic evaluation, 1186–1187, 1188, 1189
incidence, 1184–1185
mechanism of injury, 1185
treatment
acute injury, 1187–1189
chronic injury, 1189–1191
Midtarsal area, dancing injuries, 1254–1255
Midtarsal joint injuries, 1664–1665
anatomy, 1668–1669
author's preferred treatment, 1672–1674
clinical diagnosis, 1670
complications, 1672
crush, 1667, 1669, 1673–1674
lateral, 1667, 1668, 1673
longitudinal, 1665, 1667, 1673
mechanism of injury, 1669–1670
medial, 1665–1666, 1673
plantar, 1667, 1669, 1673
radiographic diagnosis, 1670–1671
treatment, 1671–1672
Midtarsal osteotomies for pes cavus, 801
Miller procedure, 728–729, 730
Mitchell procedure
for adult hallux valgus, 202, 233, 235
complications, 237–239
avascular necrosis of metatarsal head, 238, 239, 273
dorsiflexion deformity, 239, 266
hallux varus, 288, 289
metatarsal head displacement, 270, 272
metatarsal shortening, 237–238, 262, 263
plantar flexion deformity, 239, 267
contraindications, 235
indications, 235
postoperative care, 236
radiographs, 201
results, 236–237
surgical technique, 235–236
for juvenile bunions, 316
postoperative care, 318–319
postoperative radiographs, 318, 319
results and complications, 319–320
technique, 316–318
Moberg procedure, for hallux rigidus, 625, 629, 632
Mobility, in athletic injuries, 1101
Morton extension, 1228
Morton's foot/syndrome, 423, 544
shoe pads for neuroma, 147
Motor unit disease, 575–580
Charcot-Marie-Tooth disease, 578, 580, 609, 790
Duchenne pseudohypertrophic muscular dystrophy, 576–578
Landry-Guillain-Barré-Strohl syndrome, 580
myotonic dystrophy, 578, 579
spinal muscular atrophy, 580
treatment goal, 576
Movable units of foot, 720–721
MRI (*see* Magnetic resonance imaging)
Muehreke's lines, 1042
Muscle action, in clawtoe deformity, 344–345
Muscle flaps, 1400
Muscle function about foot and ankle, 826–827
Muscle imbalance, 826, 827
diagnosis, 828
patient evaluation, 827–828
in pes cavus, 790
treatment, 828–830
Muscle injuries
classification, 806
etiology, 806
pathology, 806–808
Muscle pain, exercise-induced, 1120–1121
Muscles about ankle, relative strengths, 826, 827
Muscle strength, athletic injuries and, 1102
Muscular and ligamentous structures, examination, 54–56
Mycetoma, 871, 872, 1082–1083
Mycobacterial infections
atypical, 870–871
tuberculosis, 869–870
Mycotic infections of toenails, 1054–1055
Myelodysplasia, 580–594
arthrodesis, 581
calcaneus foot, 586, 587
surgical management, 586–588, 589
casting, 581–582
cavus foot and clawtoes, 593–594
convex pes valgus (paralytic vertical talus), 592–593
equinovarus deformity, 582–583, 585
cuneiform-cuboid wedge osteotomy for, 584–586
surgical management, 583–584
equinus deformity, 582
incisions, 581
orthoses, 582
principles of care, 580–582
protection for foot, 581
surgical evaluation, 581
valgus foot, 588–590
surgical management, 590–592
Myopathies, 576
Myotonic dystrophy, 578, 579

N

Nail-patella syndrome, 1042, 1043
Nails (*see* Toenails)
Navicular
accessory (*see* Accessory navicular)
bipartite, 525, 1610
Naviculare secondarium (*see* Accessory navicular)
Navicular fractures (*see* Tarsal navicular fractures)
Naviculocuneiform fusion for flatfoot, 738–739
Naviculocuneiform joint, in rheumatoid arthritis, 641
Necrosis
aseptic
after talar dislocation, 1663
after talar fracture, 1583–1584
after talar neck fracture, 1560–1565
avascular
algorithmic approach to imaging, 122, 124–125
from hallux valgus surgery
metatarsal head, 233, 235, 272–273
proximal phalanx, 274, 276
after talar neck fracture, 1560–1565
of talus, 1029–1030
skin, after talar neck fracture, 1559
Needle aspiration, 109–110
Needles, embedded in foot, 1432, 1433, 1434
Neisseria gonorrheae, 864
Neonates, examination for congenital abnormalities, 45
Neoplasms (*see* Tumors)
Nerve block of foot
choice of agents, 158
complications, 163
considerations after, 161, 163

Nerve block of foot *(cont.)*
deep peroneal nerve, 12, 160
posterior tibial nerve, 158–159, 160
saphenous nerve, 160, 162
superficial peroneal nerve, 159, 161
sural nerve, 160–161, 163
Nerve compression, sesamoid associated, 471, 479–480, 482
treatment, 480
Nerve disorders, 543–544
acquired, of adult foot, 603
central nervous system disorders, 604–608
Charcot-Marie-Tooth disease, 609
postpolio syndrome, 610
congenital
cerebral palsy, 594–599
motor unit disease, 575–580
myelodysplasia, 580–594
in diabetes, 878–883
functional, 559–560
deep peroneal nerve entrapment, 569–571
interdigital neuromas, 560–562
lateral plantar nerve entrapment, first branch, 562–564
medial plantar nerve entrapment, 566–567
superficial peroneal nerve entrapment, 567–569
sural nerve entrapment, 571–572
tarsal tunnel syndrome, 564–566
static
interdigital plantar neuromas, 544–551
recurrent neuromas, 552–553
tarsal tunnel syndrome, 554–558
traumatic and incisional neuromas, 558–559
Nerve entrapment
in athletes, 1117–1118
after calcaneal fracture, 1529
in dancers
Baxter's nerve, 1274
around sesamoids, 1250
or disruption, after arthrodesis, 675
after distal soft tissue realignment procedure, 215–216
examination, 58, 60
proximal, in runners, 1236
or severance, from hallux valgus surgery, 261
Nerve fibers, 1412–1413
Nerve injuries, 609–610
Nerves
anatomy for subcalcaneal pain syndrome, 838, 839, 840
evaluation of diabetic foot, 885–886, 956
plantar, 545
Nervous system, autonomic, sympathetic division, 1412–1414
Neurapraxia, medial plantar, heel pain from, 845
Neurilemomas, 995
Neuroarthropathy, 926
Neurofibromas, 995–996
Neurofibromatosis, 996
Neurologic disorders (*see* Nerve disorders)
Neuromas
on dorsum of foot, surgical treatment, 559
interdigital, 560–562, 1237
interdigital plantar, 544–551
Joplin's, 1249
recurrent, 552
clinical symptoms, 552
conservative treatment, 552
diagnosis, 552
postoperative care, 553
surgical treatment, 552–553
uncommon findings, 553
in tarsometatarsal arthrodesis, 708
traumatic and incisional, 558–559
Neuromuscular imbalance, flatfoot from, 783
Neutral position of foot, 721, 722
determined by palpation, 720–721
Nevus, benign pigmented, 1079
Nocardia, 872, 1082
Nodule, heel pain from, 845
Nonoperative extremity, labeling, 152
Nonunion of attempted arthrodesis site, 675–676
Nuclear medicine, 86–89 (*see also* Bone scanning)
Nutrition, diabetic wound healing and, 884

O

Oblique metatarsal osteotomy
for bunionette deformity
postoperative care, 454
results, 454–455
technique, 452–454
for diffuse intractable plantar keratosis, 427–428, 429
postoperative care, 429
results, 429, 431
technique, 428–429, 430
to relieve metatarsalgia, 432
Onychauxis, 1036, 1050–1051, 1053–1054, 1060
Onychectomy
complete, 1067, 1068
partial, 1065–1067
Onychia, 1036, 1056, 1058
Onychitis, 1036
Onychoclasis, 1036
Onychocryptosis, 1036, 1049–1052
treatment, 1052–1053
Onychogryphosis, 1036, 1053–1054, 1060
Onycholysis, 1036, 1037–1038, 1056
Onychoma, 1036
Onychomadesis, 1036, 1056
Onychomalacia, 1036
Onychomycosis, 1036, 1037, 1054–1056
classification, 1054
organisms cultured in, 1054–1055
treatment, 1056
Onychopathy (*see* Toenail abnormalities)
Onychophosis, 1058
Onychorrhexis, 1036
Onychoschizia, 1036, 1060–1061
Onychosis, 1036
Onychotrophia, 1036
Open epiphysis, in juvenile bunions, 306–308
Opening wedge osteotomy, for juvenile hallux valgus, 324–325, 329–331
Orthoses
ankle-foot, 145–146
athletic injuries, 1103
bunions, 1205
Charcot joints in diabetes, 939–940
dancers, 1244
degenerative joint disease, 620
diabetes, 886, 887, 922, 946–952
first metatarsocuneiform joint degenerative arthritis, 635
flatfoot, 732, 733
foot, 144–145
forefoot amputation, 973
hallux rigidus, 625
miscellaneous, 146
myelodysplasia, 581–582
peroneal nerve injury, 610
rheumatoid arthritis, 646–647, 661
runners, 1237–1238
stroke management, 604–605
subcalcaneal pain, 845, 846
superior heel pain, 853
turf toe, 1198
Orthotics, use of term, 948–949
Os aponeurosis plantaris, 515, 517
Os calcaneus secundarius, 512–513, 514, 1496
clinical significance, 513
Os calcis (*see* Calcaneus)
Os cuboides secundarium, 517, 518
Os cuneo-I metatarsale-I dorsali, 525–526
clinical significance, 526–527
Os cuneo-I metatarsale-I plantare, 525, 526
clinical significance, 526–527
Os cuneometatarsale I tibiale, 523, 524
Os intercuneiforme, 525, 526
Os intermetatarseum, 527–530
clinical significance, 530, 531
Os paracuneiforme, accessory navicular vs., 523, 524
Os peroneum, 500–502, 1632
clinical significance, 502, 505
osteochondritis dissecans, 503
postoperative care, 502
proximal migration, 504
surgical technique, 502
Os retinaculi, 507
Os subcalcis, 515, 517

Os subfibulare, 505–507
  clinical significance, 507
Os subtibiale, 502–505, 506
  clinical significance, 505
Os supranavicular, 517
Os supratalare, 517, 520, 521
  clinical significance, 521
Os sustentaculi, 514, 515
  clinical significance, 514–515, 516
Os talocalcaneare laterale, 513
Os talonaviculare dorsale, 517, 519–521
  clinical significance, 521
Osteoarthritis (*see* Arthritis)
Osteoblastomas, 1008
Osteochondral fractures, 1290
Osteochondral injury, imaging, 111–113
Osteochondral lesions of talus, arthroscopy for
  CAT scan staging, 1291, 1292, 1293
  diagnosis, 1291
  incidence, 1290–1291
  operative techniques, 1293–1294, 1295, 1296
  postoperative care, 1294
  surgical treatment, 1291–1293
  terminology, 1290
Osteochondritis dissecans, 1290, 1567, 1568–1569
  fibular sesamoid, 1650
  os peroneum, 503
  talus, 1255–1256
Osteochondritis of sesamoids, 487–488
  treatment, 488–489
Osteochondromas, 1006, 1007
  subungual exostosis vs., 1045
Osteochondroses, 1028
  avascular necrosis of talus, 1029–1030
  Freiberg's infraction, 1029
  Köhler's disease, 1028–1029
  metatarsal head
    diagnosis, 435, 437, 438–439
    treatment, 437, 440–441
  Sever's disease, 1029, 1030
Osteoid osteomas, 1007–1008, 1258
Osteomalacia, 1021–1025
Osteomyelitis
  algorithmic approach to imaging, 129–133
  in Charcot foot, 941
  diagnosis, 865–867
  magnetic resonance imaging, 104, 131–132
  of sesamoids, 484–485
    treatment, 487
  after talar dislocation, 1663
  after talar neck fracture, 1559
  treatment
    acute, 867
    chronic, 867–868
Osteomyelitis in diabetes, 914–915
  ankle, 923
  Charcot joint vs., 932–933, 934
  first metatarsophalangeal joint and sesamoids of hallux, 917–919, 920
  forefoot, 915–917
  hindfoot, 921–923
  lesser metatarsal heads, 919, 921
  midfoot, 921
  toes, 917, 918
Osteophytes of ankle, arthroscopy, 1297–1298
Osteopoikilosis, 1014
Osteoporosis, 1018–1021
Osteosarcomas, 1012, 1014–1016
  Ewing's sarcoma, 1015–1017
  imaging, 126
Osteotomy *(see specific types)*
Os tibiale externum (*see* Accessory navicular)
Os trigonum, 507, 509
  in dancers, 1265–1267
    excision, 1267–1270
  surgical procedure for removal, 510, 512
  talar fractures and, 1585–1588
  talus partitus vs., 509, 510–511
  variations, 507, 508
Os versalianum, 530, 532
  clinical significance, 533–535

P

Pachyonychia, 1036
Pachyonychia congenita, 1042, 1043
Paget disease of bone, 1024, 1025
Pain, chronic undiagnosed posttraumatic, algorithmic approach to imaging, 113–117
Painful arc sign, 1183
Palmer's method of intra-articular calcaneal fracture treatment, 1518–1519
Pantalar arthrodesis, 581, 674
Paralytic vertical talus, in myelodysplasia, 592–593
Paresthesias, from hallux valgus surgery, 261
Paronychia, 1036, 1057, 1058
Partial proximal phalangectomy
  for hammer toe deformity, 357–358
  syndactylization and, 392–394
Pasteurella multocida, 861
Patellar tendon bearing brace, 1563
Peabody procedure, 586–587
Pediatric patients
  congenital foot deformities, 1313–1363
  epiphyseal injuries of ankle, 1462
  examination principles for neonates and toddlers, 45–46
  flatfoot, 717–756
  juvenile bunions, 297–339
Pelvic tilt, examination, 49
Percutaneous transluminal angioplasty, 108
Periosteal chondromas, 1009
Peripheral anesthesia, 151
  anatomy, 154–157
  digital block, 157–158, 1061–1062
  nerve block of foot, 158–163
Peripheral nerves (*see* Nerves)
Peritendinitis, 807
  Achilles tendon, 1183
    treatment, 811–812
  differential diagnosis, 812
  extensor tendons, 824
  nonoperative treatment, 812
  peroneal tendons, 817–818, 1177–1179
Periungual verruca, 1058–1059
Peroneal artery, talar blood supply from, 1540
Peroneal nerve
  deep
    anatomy, 156, 157
    entrapment, 569–571
      anatomy, 569
      clinical symptoms, 570
      diagnosis, 570
      etiology, 569–570
      incidence, 569
      postoperative care, 571
      surgical treatment, 570–571
  superficial
    anatomy, 155–156, 157
    anesthesia, 159, 161
    entrapment, 567–569, 1117
      anatomy, 567
      clinical symptoms, 568
      conservative treatment, 568–569
      diagnosis, 568
      etiology, 567–568
      incidence, 567
      postoperative care, 569
      surgical treatment, 569
Peroneal nerve injury, 609
Peroneal spastic flatfoot, 1340–1342
  tarsal coalition and, 760, 762–764
  treatment, 1342–1343
Peroneal tendinitis
  fibular abutment and, after calcaneal fracture, 1527–1528
  in runners, 1234–1235
Peroneal tendinitis and ruptures in athletes, 1177
  diagnosis, 1178–1179
  etiologic factors, 1177–1178
  treatment, 1178–1179
Peroneal tendon injury, computed tomography, 121
Peroneal tendons, 817
  anatomy, 817
  dislocations in dancers, 1264
  peritendinitis, 817–818, 1177–1179
  rupture, 818–819, 1177–1179
  traumatic dislocation, 819
    classification, 819, 820
    clinical findings, 819–820
    treatment, 820–823
Peroneal tendon subluxation and dislocation in athletes, 1167
  acute
    author's operative technique, 1171–1172
    nonoperative treatment, 1171
    postoperative care, 1172
  anatomy, 1168–1169
  chronic, surgical treatment, 1172–1173
    author's technique, 1176–1177
    bone block procedures, 1173

Peroneal tendon subluxation and dislocation in athletes *(cont.)*
  groove-deepening procedures, 1175–1176
  postoperative care, 1177
  rerouting procedures, 1174–1175
  soft-tissue reconstruction, 1173
  tissue transfer procedures, 1173–1174
 classification, 1170, 1171
 diagnosis, 1170–1171
 etiology, 1167–1168
 historical perspective, 1168
 mechanism of injury, 1169–1170
 rim fracture associated with, 1171
Peroneus brevis tendon
 in Achilles tendon repair, 815
 in ankle reconstruction in dancers, 1261
 longitudinal tear, 1178
Peroneus longus tendon
 degenerative mass of previously torn, 1179
 sesamoid of, 500–505
Pes cavus, 415, 718, 719, 785–801
 clawtoes and, in myelodysplasia, 593–594
 clinical symptoms, 791
 conservative treatment, 791
 etiology, 789–790
 forefoot deformity, 786–788
 hindfoot deformity, 786, 787
 metatarsophalangeal joint deformity, 788–789
 overview, 785–786
 physical examination, 791
 plantar fascia and, 840
 soft-tissue deformity, 789
 surgical treatment
  bony stabilization by triple arthrodesis, 798–801
  decision making, 791
  osteotomies, 794
   crescentic or sliding calcaneal, 797–798
   Dwyer calcaneal, 794, 796–797
   first metatarsal, 794, 795
   midtarsal, 801
  soft-tissue procedures
   clawtoe deformities, 793–794
   first toe Jones procedure, 792–793
   plantar fascial release (Steindler stripping), 791–792
Pes planus (*see* Flatfoot)
Pes valgus, congenital convex, 1343–1344
 physical findings, 1344
 radiographic findings, 1344
 treatment, 1344–1346
Phalangeal fractures, 1640
 clinical diagnosis, 1640–1641
 mechanism of injury, 1640
 radiographic diagnosis, 1641, 1643
 treatment
  author's preferred methods, 1644–1645
  hallux, 1641–1642, 1644–1645
  lesser toes, 1642, 1644, 1645
Phalangeal osteotomy, proximal, for hallux rigidus, 625, 629, 632
Phalangectomy, partial proximal
 for hammer toe deformity, 357–358
 syndactylization and, 392–394
Phalanges
 buckling from restrictive shoes, 342, 343
 distal, anatomy for lesser toe deformities, 345, 346
 proximal
  anatomy for lesser toe deformities, 345, 346, 347, 348
  avascular necrosis after Mitchell procedure, 242, 243
  complications of hallux valgus surgery, 273–278
  relationship to metatarsal head, 179, 180
 radiographic evaluation, 63, 70
Phenol/alcohol matrisectomy, 1068–1070
Phenol injection, into tibial nerve, after traumatic brain injury, 608
Phialophora verrucosa, 1082
Physical therapy, for rheumatoid arthritis, 645–646
Pigmented villonodular synovitis, 998, 1000
Pins, embedded in foot, 1432, 1433, 1434
Pirie's bone, 517
Pirigoff amputation, 988, 989
Pitted keratolysis, 1077
Plantar aponeurosis
 anatomy, 838, 839
 biomechanics, 26–27
 examination, 56
Plantar calcaneal bursitis, in dancers, 1273–1274
Plantar calcaneonavicular (spring) ligament, examination, 56
Plantar circulation, 459
Plantar fascia
 physical examination, 839–840
 release in pes cavus, 791–792
 rupture in dancers, 1273, 1274
Plantar fasciitis
 in athletes, 843, 844
 in dancers, 1273
 in runners, 1231
 seronegative spondyloarthropathies and, 841–842
Plantar fibromatosis, 994–995
Plantar flap, for soft-tissue coverage, 1385, 1387, 1399
Plantar flexion of first metatarsal, from hallux valgus surgery, 266, 267
Plantar flexion osteotomy of first metatarsal, for flatfoot, 739
Plantar flexion weakness, after calcaneal fracture, 1529, 1530
Plantaris tendon, in Achilles tendon repair, 1273
Plantar keratoses
 anatomic considerations, 414–415
 in bunionette deformity, 444
 conservative treatment, 418, 419
 diagnosis, 415–417
 etiology, 414
 of first metatarsal, dorsiflexion osteotomy, 494, 497
 from hallux valgus surgery, 281–282
 with significant scar tissue formation, 435, 436
 from subhallux sesamoid, 433–435
 surgical treatment
  diffuse intractable plantar keratosis, 426–432
  discrete callus beneath tibial sesamoid, 425–426, 427
  localized intractable plantar keratosis, 421–423, 424
  metatarsal head resection for intractable keratosis, 432, 433
  other metatarsal osteotomies, 432–433
  vertical chevron procedure, 423, 425
 beneath tibial sesamoid, 425–426, 427, 477–478, 480
 types of callosities
  diffuse, 420–421
  discrete, 418, 419, 420
Plantar nerves, 545
 lateral
  anatomy, 155
  compression in runners, 1231–1233
  entrapment of first branch, 562–564
 medial
  anatomy, 154–155
  entrapment, 566–567
  neurapraxia, heel pain from, 845
 third branch, 546
Plantar neuromas, interdigital (*see* Interdigital plantar neuromas)
Plantar scars, 435, 437
Plantar spaces, 863
Plantar ulcerations, in diabetes, 880–881, 882
Plantar warts, 416, 417, 1088–1090
 in dancers, 1243
 differential diagnosis, 1090
 treatment, 1090–1091
Plastazote shoe, 947–948
Plastic reduction of nail lip, 1064–1065
Plating, for malleolar fractures, 1457
Platzgummer reconstruction for dislocating peroneal tendons, 1174
Playing surfaces
 athletic injuries and, 1105
 turf toe and, 1191, 1195
Pneumatic arthrography, in osteochondral fracture evaluation, 1573

Polio, postpolio syndrome, 610
Polydactyly, 1315, 1350–1352
Polyonychia, 1043, 1044
Polyostotic fibrous dysplasia, 1009, 1011
Polytomography
  metatarsal fractures, 1620
  osteochondral fractures, 1573
  tarsal navicular stress fractures, 1610, 1611
Pompholyx, 1074
Popliteal artery entrapment syndrome in athletes
  classification, 1118
  definition, 1118
  diagnosis, 1119
  historical perspective, 1118
  prevalence, 1118
  treatment, 1120
Posterior ankle, dancing injuries, 1264–1271
Posterior impingement syndrome in dancers, 1265–1266
  treatment, 1266–1270
Posterior inferior tibiofibular ligament
  anatomy, 1143–1144
  biomechanics, 1145
Posterior malleolus, surgical treatment of fractures, 1458
Posterior talofibular ligament
  anatomy, 1121, 1122
  biomechanics, 1123
Posterior tendon transfers, 829
Posterior tibial artery, talar blood supply from, 1540
Posterior tibial nerve
  anatomy, 154
  anesthesia, 158–159, 160
  entrapment, 838–839
Posterior tibial tendon
  laceration, flatfoot from, 783
  pain, magnetic resonance imaging, 117
  sesamoid of, 500, 501
  tendinitis, 1180–1181
    in dancers, 1255
    in runners, 1234–1235
    rupture and, 1180–1181
  transfer for calcaneus foot, 587–588
Posterior tibial tendon dysfunction, 767
  clinical presentation, 768, 769
  conservative treatment, 771, 774
  etiology, 767–768
  pathophysiology, 767
  physical examination, 768, 770–771
  radiographic evaluation, 771, 772–773
  surgical treatment
    criteria for reconstruction, 774
    decision making, 774
    goals, 774
    reconstruction with flexor digitorum longus, 775–779
    synovectomy, 774–775
Postganglionic nerve fibers, 1412–1413
Postmenopausal osteoporosis, 1020
Postpolio syndrome, 610
Pozo and Jackson method for rerouting peroneal tendons, 1175
Preganglionic nerve fibers, 1412–1413
Prehallux (*see* Accessory navicular)
Prescription Footwear Association, 948, 958
Pronated, 720
Pronation
  in early stance phase, examination, 47
  in hallux valgus, 170–172
Prostheses
  in bunion surgery, 292, 294
  Syme, 985–987
Proximal fifth metatarsal osteotomy, for bunionette deformity, 449–450, 457–458
  anatomy, 459
  postoperative care, 459
  results, 459, 461–462
  surgical technique, 458–459, 460
Proximal first metatarsal osteotomy
  for adult hallux valgus
    crescentic osteotomy, 217–222, 223, 224
    radiographs, 200, 203
    recurrent deformity after, 282, 283
  for juvenile bunions, 323–324
    indications, 325
    postoperative care, 328
    postoperative radiographs, 329, 330
    results and complications, 328–329
    technique, 325–328
  metatarsal nonunion from, 270
Proximal interphalangeal joint
  dislocations in dancers, 1244–1245
  fifth, chronically instability in dancers, 1245
  stiff, from hammer toe, 1102
Proximal nerve entrapment, in runners, 1236
Proximal phalangeal osteotomy (Moberg procedure), for hallux rigidus, 625, 629, 632
Proximal phalanx
  anatomy for lesser toe deformities, 345, 346, 347, 348
  avascular necrosis after Akin procedure, 242, 243
  complications of hallux valgus surgery, 273–278
    adhesions of flexor hallucis longus, 274
    avascular necrosis, 242, 243, 274, 276
    instability after resection of base, 276–278
    malunion, 273–274
    nonunion, 273
    violation of metatarsophalangeal joint, 276
  relationship to metatarsal head, 179, 180
Proximal plantar subcutaneous plexus, flaps based on, 1399
Pseudogout, 616
Pseudohypoparathyroidism, 1023, 1024–1025
Pseudomonas aeruginosa, 860, 868
  diabetic foot infection, 911, 912
Pseudotumors
  of first web space, in dancers, 1252
  of hemophilia, 1015, 1016
  stress fracture, 1015, 1016
Psoriasis, 1075–1076
  AIDS and Reiter's syndrome and, 619
  of toenails, 1036–1038
Psoriatic arthritis, 617, 618
Pterygium, 1036, 1059, 1060
Pulmonary disorders, toenail pathology from, 1041
Puncture wounds, 860
Pyodermas, 1038–1039
Pyogenic granulomas, 1058, 1080

Q

Quinolones, 875

R

Radial forearm fasciocutaneous flap, 1400
Radiation burns, 1430–1431
  classification, 1432
Radiology (*see* Imaging)
Radionuclide bone scanning (*see* Bone scanning)
Range of motion examination, 50–51
  ankle joint, 51, 52
  metatarsophalangeal joints, 53
  subtalar joint, 51–53
  transverse tarsal joint, 53
Ray amputations, 967–968, 969, 970–971
  pitfalls and complications, 973
Reflex sympathetic dystrophy (syndrome)
  algorithmic approach to imaging, 111, 112
  anatomy and physiology, 1411–1414
  after calcaneal fracture, 1529–1530
  classification, 1414–1415
  clinical symptoms, 1415–1417
  diagnosis, 1417
  etiology, 1414, 1416
  management algorithm, 1419
  stages, 1415
  treatment, 1417
    discussion, 1419
    first level, 1417–1418
    second level, 1418
    surgical, 1418–1419
Regional anesthesia
  anatomy, 154–157
  digital block, 157–158
Rehabilitation
  fractures and dislocations, 1469–1471
  running injuries, 1238–1239
Reiter's syndrome, 617, 618–619, 620
Renal osteodystrophy, 1021–1022
Replantation of foot, 1371
Reserpine, in reflex sympathetic dystrophy syndrome, 1418

Retrocalcaneal bursa, 848, 849
Retrocalcaneal bursitis, 809–810, 847, 848–849
  in athletes, treatment, 851–852
  etiology and diagnostic tests, 850
  surgical treatment, 851, 852–854
Rheumatoid arthritis, 637
  ankle joint, 644, 646
  clinical course, 644–645, 646
  conservative treatment, 645
    drug therapy, 645
    orthotic devices, 646–647
    physical therapy, 645–646
  diagnosis, 637
  etiology, 637
  flatfoot from, 780, 782
  foot radiograph, 129
  pathophysiology of rheumatoid foot, 637–638
    forefoot changes, 638, 639–640
    hindfoot changes, 638, 642–644, 645
    midfoot changes, 638, 641–642
  seronegative spondyloarthropathies vs., 617–618
  surgical treatment, 647
    ankle joint, 664–667
    forefoot deformity, 647–651
      reconstruction, 653–660
      synovectomy, 651–653
      uncommon associated problems, 660–661
    hindfoot, 667
    midfoot deformity
      subtalar joint, 664
      talonavicular joint, 661–664
      tarsometatarsal joint, 661
    stress fracture, 667
  weight bearing biomechanics, 11, 12
Rheumatoid nodule or cyst, 660
Rheumatologic conditions, spontaneous fusion in, 1101
RICE treatment, for lateral ankle sprain, 1130
Rickets, 1021–1022
"Rocker-bottom" Charcot foot, 931, 932
Rotatory slippage of shoe on floor at lift-off, examination, 47–48
Rowe classification of calcaneal fractures, 1480
Ruiz-Mora procedure for cockup fifth toe deformity, 401, 402
Running injuries, 1225–1240
  biomechanical abnormalities and, 1100
  bunions, 1201
  diagnostic studies, 1227
  etiology, 1225, 1228
  forefoot disorders, 1235–1237
  heel pain, 1231–1233
  history, 1225–1226
  impingement syndromes, 1235
  incidence, 1225
  leg pain, 1230–1231
  orthoses and complications of rigid orthoses, 1237–1238
  physical examination, 1226–1227
  primary and secondary, 1227–1228
  rehabilitation, 1238–1239
  shoes and, 1238
  short-leg syndrome, 1229
  stress fractures, 1229–1230
  surface and, 1228
  tendinitis, 1233–1235
  torsional joint, 1228–1229
Running biomechanics, 31–33
Rupture of tendons, 807–808
  Achilles, 1181–1184
    in dancers, 1272–1273
    treatment, 812–816
    treatment results, 814, 816–817
  extensor, 824
  peroneal, 818–819, 1177–1179
  posterior tibial, 1180–1181

S

SACH heel, 143
Salter-Harris classification of ankle injuries, 1462
Samilson calcaneal osteotomy, 593, 798, 799
Saphenous nerve
  anatomy, 156–157
  anesthesia, 160, 162
Sarcoidosis, 1009–1010, 1012
  heel pain in, 845
Sarcomas
  chondrosarcoma, 1017–1018
  Ewing's sarcoma, 1015–1017
  fibrosarcoma, 1000, 1002, 1017, 1018
  Kaposi's sarcoma, 1002–1003, 1048, 1083–1084
  osteosarcoma, 1012, 1014–1015
  synovial cell, 126, 1001–1002
Sarmiento and Wolf method for rerouting peroneal tendons, 1175
Scaphoid, accessory, navicular fracture vs., 1602, 1603
Scapular flap, 1400, 1402
Scars
  adherent to underlying tissue, from hallux valgus surgery, 261
  plantar, 435
Schmid form of metaphyseal chondrodysplasia, 1022–1023
Sciatic nerve palsy, lower extremity management, 610
Scintigraphy (*see also* Bone scanning), syndesmosis sprains of ankle, 1148, 1149
Scottish-Rite procedure, 730, 731
Scurvy, osteoporosis and, 1021
Second metatarsal, fractured base, tarsometatarsal dislocations and, 1678, 1679, 1680
Second metatarsocuneiform joint, arthrodesis, 706, 707
Second metatarsophalangeal joint
  differential diagnosis of pain, 375
  evaluation of congruity, 376
  mild subluxation, 380
    soft tissue release, 380, 382, 383
    treatment algorithm, 381
  moderate subluxation, 382
    reefing of joint capsule, 382, 385, 386
    treatment algorithm, 384
  rupture of lateral collateral ligament, 374
  severe subluxation and dislocation, 385
    arthroplasty, 385, 388–392
    treatment algorithm, 387
  subluxation and dislocation, 372–394
    etiology, 372, 373
    physical examination, 372–376
    radiographic examination, 376–377, 378, 379
    treatment, 377–378, 380–394
Second toe
  amputation, hallux valgus from, 173, 356, 357
  mallet and hammer toe, 343, 344
Seed corn, 418
  in dancers, 1243–1244
Selakovich osteotomy of os calcis, 727
Semmes-Weinstein monofilaments, 885–886, 956
Seronegative spondyloarthropathies, 617–618
  AIDS, Reiter's syndrome, and psoriasis, 619
  ankylosing spondylitis, 617, 618
  Lyme disease in foot and ankle, 619
  psoriatic arthritis, 617, 618
  Reiter's syndrome, 617, 618–619, 620
  subcalcaneal pain syndrome and, 841–842
  superior heel pain in, 850
  treatment, 619–620
Sesamoid complications of hallux valgus surgery, 279
Sesamoid complications of hallux valgus surgery
  cockup deformity of first metatarsophalangeal joint, 280–281
  medial subluxation or dislocation of tibial sesamoid, 279–280
  uncorrected sesamoids, 279
Sesamoids
  fibular, osteochondritis dissecans, 1650
  uncommon, and accessory bones of foot, 499–535
  Sesamoid dislocation, 1652
  Sesamoid excision
  decision making, 489
  postoperative results
    hallux migration, 494
    motion and strength, 494, 497–498
    pain relief, 494, 495
  surgical approach, 26, 489

technique for fibular sesamoid
dorsal approach, 492–493
plantar approach, 493–494, 495
technique for tibial sesamoid, 490–491, 492
Sesamoid fractures, 1645–1646
anatomy, 1646
clinical diagnosis, 1647–1648
mechanism of injury, 1646–1647
radiographic diagnosis, 1647–1648, 1649, 1650
stress fractures, 1651–1652
treatment
author's preferred method, 1650–1651
nonoperative, 1648–1649
surgical, 1649–1650
Sesamoid injuries
in dancers, 1249–1250
in runners, 1236
Sesamoiditis, causes, 1249
Sesamoid of peroneus longus tendon, 500–502
clinical significance, 502, 505
osteochondritis dissecans, 503
postoperative care, 502
proximal migration, 504
surgical technique, 502
Sesamoid of tibialis anterior tendon, 500, 501
Sesamoid of tibialis posterior tendon, 500, 501
Sesamoids, 467–499
anatomy, 63, 174, 1646
arterial circulation, 470
conservative care, 489
fibular
excision technique, 492–495
percentage of bipartite sesamoids, 471
radiography, 471, 472
frequency of occurrence, 500
inconstant, 499–500
pressure on, felt pads for, 147
radiographic evaluation, 63, 71
relationship to metatarsal head, in hallux valgus, 185
resection in diabetic ulceration, 904
shape, 473
surgical implications of biomechanics, 36
tibial
callus beneath, 478
excision technique, 490–491, 492
intractable plantar keratosis and, 478–479, 480
percentage of bipartite sesamoids, 471
radiography, 471, 472
shaving for discrete callus, 425–427, 492–494
weight bearing and, 170, 171
Sesamoid shaving
for discrete callus, 425–427, 492–494
postoperative results, 494
technique for prominent tibial sesamoid, 492, 493
Sesamoids of first metatarsophalangeal joint, 468
anatomy, 468–470
arthritis, 480–481, 483
treatment, 481, 483
bipartite sesamoids and fractures, 471, 473–474, 475–476
bursitis, 478–479, 481
treatment, 479
congenital absence, 474, 477
distorted or hypertrophied, 477, 478, 479
treatment, 477
infection, 484–485
treatment, 487
intractable plantar keratoses, 477–478, 480
treatment, 478
nerve compression, 471, 479–480, 482
treatment, 480
osteochondritis, 487–488
osteomyelitis in diabetic foot, 917–919, 920
treatment, 488–489
physical examination, 471
radiographic examination, 471, 472
sesamoiditis, 489
subluxation and dislocation, 481, 484
treatment, 481–482, 484–486
Sever's disease, 1029, 1030
heel pain from, 844–845
Shank of shoe, modifications, 143
Shaver blades for arthroscopy, 1290
Shear avulsion injury of foot, 1397
Shinsplints, 1230, 1274–1275
Shoe dermatitis, 1074–1075
Shoe insoles
in diabetes, 946–947, 948–952, 957
partial amputation, 919, 921
for forefoot amputation, 973
for midfoot sprain, 1190
Shoes
athletic injuries and, 1102–1105
bunions and, 1201, 1203, 1204, 1205
for dancers, 1244
for degenerative joint disease, 620
in diabetes, 940, 946–948
felt pads in, 146–148
for forefoot amputation, 971, 973
hallux valgus deformity from, 142, 168–169
hammer and mallet toe from, 342, 343, 348
modifications, 142
combination of heel and sole lifts, 144
heel, 142–143, 144
shank, 143
sole, 143–144
proper fit, 141–142
rotatory slippage on floor at lift-off, examination, 47–48
for runners, 1238
for transmetatarsal amputation, 978
turf toe and, 1194
type of shoe and height of heel, examination, 48–49
Short-leg syndrome, 1229
Siffert triple arthrodesis, for pes cavus, 798–801
Silastic
in flatfoot surgery, 732
implant arthroplasty in rheumatoid forefoot, 647–648, 650
Silver osteotomy of os calcis, 726
Single-photon emission computed tomography (SPECT), 86
Sinus tarsi syndrome in athletes, 1165
diagnosis, 1166–1167
historical perspective, 1165–1166
treatment and results, 1167
Skeletal shortening and primary closure, in soft-tissue trauma, 1384–1386, 1387–1389
Skeletal structures, examination, 50
Skewfoot, 1328, 1335
Skin excision, split-thickness, in soft-tissue trauma, 1393–1394, 1397–1399
Skin grafting
in amputation surgery, 963
in soft-tissue trauma, 1374, 1375, 1377, 1381, 1383, 1386, 1388–1395, 1400
Skin necrosis, after talar neck fracture, 1559
Skin problems (*see* Dermatology)
Skin slough
after arthrodesis, 675
in hallux valgus surgery, 260
in tarsometatarsal arthrodesis, 708
Sliding or crescentic osteotomy, for pes cavus, 797–798, 799
Soft tissue, gas in, in diabetic infections, 912
Soft-tissue deformity, in pes cavus, 789
Soft-tissue infection, after talar dislocation, 1663
Soft-tissue infections, bacterial, 859–864
Soft-tissue injuries
athletic (*see* Athletic soft-tissue injuries)
foreign bodies, 1432–1436
heat and cold injuries, 1420–1432
reflex sympathetic dystrophy syndrome, 1411–1419
Soft-tissue masses, magnetic resonance imaging, 103, 105, 126, 127
Soft-tissue preservation
in amputation surgery, 960–962
in fracture treatment, 1468
Soft-tissue problems, from hallux valgus surgery, 260–262
Soft-tissue realignment, distal for adult hallux valgus, 204–216

Soft-tissue realignment, distal *(cont.)*
  for juvenile bunions, 320–323
Soft-tissue trauma, 1367–1410
  acute compartment syndromes of foot, 1377–1383
  chronic compartment syndromes, 1405–1406
  coverage options, 1383–1384
    cross-leg flaps, 1403–1405
    free tissue flaps, 1400–1403
    skeletal shortening and primary closure, 1384–1386, 1387–1389
    skin grafting, 1374, 1375, 1377, 1381, 1383, 1386, 1388–1395, 1400
    split-thickness skin excision, 1393–1394, 1397–1399
    transpositional and island pedicle flaps, 1399–1400
  initial evaluation and determination of salvageability, 1367–1371
  initial treatment, 1372
  zone of injury, 1372–1377
Soft-tissue tumors of foot, 991–992
  benign, 992–993
  general considerations and staging process, 992–993
  malignant, 1000–1003
Sole of foot
  foreign body, 1080–1081
  keratoses, 1088
Sole of shoe, modifications, 143, 144
Soleus muscle, accessory, in dancers, 1273
Soleus syndrome, in dancers, 1256, 1275
Solid ankle, cushion heel (SACH), 143
Sorbitol, in diabetic neuropathy, 880
Spasticity, after traumatic brain injury, 607–608
Spinal muscular atrophy, 580
SPLATT procedure, 829
  for metatarsus adductus, 1331–1333
  for traumatic brain injury or stroke, 605–607
  for varus deformities in cerebral palsy, 594, 596, 597
Splaying in rheumatoid foot, 660–661
Splinter hemorrhages, 1039
Splinters, 1434–1435
Split anterior tibial tendon transfer, 829
  for metatarsus adductus, 1331–1333
  for traumatic brain injury or stroke, 605–607
  for varus deformities in cerebral palsy, 594, 596, 597
Split-thickness skin excision
  in crush injury, 1370, 1371
  in soft-tissue trauma, 1393–1394, 1397–1399
Split-thickness skin grafts, in soft-tissue trauma, 1374, 1375, 1377, 1381, 1383, 1386, 1388–1395, 1400
Spondyloarthropathies, seronegative, 617–618
  AIDS, Reiter's syndrome, and psoriasis, 619
  ankylosing spondylitis, 617, 618
  Lyme disease in foot and ankle, 619
  psoriatic arthritis, 617, 618
  Reiter's syndrome, 617, 618–619, 620
  subcalcaneal pain syndrome and, 841–842
  superior heel pain in, 850
  treatment, 619–620
Sporothrix schenkii, 872
Sports medicine (*see also* Athletes; Athletic soft-tissue injuries), historical perspective, 1097
Sprain fractures, 1493
Sprains in athletes
  forefoot, 1191–1200
  lateral ankle, 1121–1139
  medial ankle, 1139–1142
  midfoot, 1184–1191
  subtalar, 1153–1165
  syndesmotic ligaments of ankle, 1142–1153
Sprains in dancers
  base of fourth and fifth metatarsals, 1255
  medial ankle, 1255–1256
Squamous cell carcinoma, 1084–1085
Squeeze test, in sprain diagnosis, 1145, 1146
Staphylococcus aureus, 860, 864, 865, 868
Staphylococcus diabetic foot infection, 911, 912
Steindler stripping, in pes cavus, 791–792
Steinmann pins, in arthrodesis for hallux valgus, 253, 255–257
Stenosing tenosynovitis, 823–824
Stenosis at great toe, 824
Stenosis at posteromedial ankle, 823–824
Stephenson's method of intra-articular calcaneal fracture treatment, 1519–1520
Steroid osteoporosis, 1020
Steroids
  for interdigital plantar neuroma, 549
  in reflex sympathetic dystrophy syndrome, 1418
  for retrocalcaneal bursitis, 853
  for subcalcaneal pain, 845–846
Stewart's classification of fractures of base of fifth metatarsal, 1627
Stiffness of forefoot and toes, after calcaneal fracture, 1529
Stippled epiphyses, 1011, 1014
Strength, athletic soft-tissue injuries and, 1102
Streptococci, 860
  dermatologic aspects, 1077
  diabetic foot infection, 909
Streptokinase, 109
Streptomyces, 1082
Stress fractures
  biomechanical abnormalities and, 1100
  in dancers, 1273, 1274, 1275
    distal isthmus of fibula, 1274
    heel pain from, 1273
    second metatarsal base, 1252–1253
    tarsal navicular, 1254
    tibia, 1275
  magnetic resonance imaging, 104, 106, 115, 116
  metatarsal diaphysis, 1635–1636
    author's preferred treatment, 1638
    clinical diagnosis, 1636–1637
    predisposing conditions and activities, 1636
    radiographic diagnosis, 1637–1638
    treatment, 1638
  phalangeal, 1640, 1641
  as pseudotumor, 1015
  in rheumatoid arthritis, 667
  in runners, 1229–1230
  sesamoids, 1651–1652
  tarsal navicular, 1609
    clinical diagnosis, 1609–1610
    radiographic diagnosis, 1610–1611
    treatment, 1611–1612
  of tibia and fibula, in athletes, 1114–1115
Stress tomography of subtalar joint, 1157–1158
Stretch box, for tendinitis in dancers, 1272
Stroke, 604
  orthotic management, 604–605
  surgical treatment, 605
    postoperative management, 607
    SPLATT procedure, 605–607
Subcalcaneal pain syndrome, 837–838
  anatomy, 838–839, 840, 841
  diagnosis
    history, 839
    imaging and laboratory studies, 840–842
    physical examination, 839–840
  etiology, 837
  treatment, 842–843
    in athletes, 843–844
    author's method, 845–847
    conservative, 845–847
    other causes of inferior heel pain, 844–845
    surgical, 845, 846, 847
Subhallux sesamoid, 433, 434, 498–499
  in dancers, 1247
  postoperative care, 433, 435
  results, 433
  surgical technique, 433
Subtalar arthrodesis, 664, 666, 674, 683

for calcaneal fractures, 1521–1522
complications, 687
desired position, 683
for flatfoot, 731, 779
indications, 683
postoperative care, 687
special considerations, 687
surgical approach, 683
for talocalcaneal coalition, 763
technique, 683–687
for valgus foot, 591–592
Subtalar dislocations, 1653–1654
anatomy, 1654
author's preferred treatment, 1659–1660
clinical diagnosis, 1654–1656
mechanism of injury, 1654
radiographic diagnosis, 1655, 1656–1657
results, 1658–1659
treatment, 1657–1658
Subtalar joint
anatomy, 1122, 1154, 1303, 1654
Anthonsen's view, 1485–1486, 1487
arthroscopy, 1303–1305
arthrosis, flatfoot from, 780, 781
biomechanics
axis of rotation, 19–23
ligaments, 37–38, 42
rotation and musculature, 36
surgical implications, 34–35
Broden's projections, 1486–1488, 1489
computed tomography, 95, 96
in dancers, 1264
deformity, hallux valgus and, 173–174
examination of stability, 49–50
lateral ligamentous support, 1154
motion, clinical determination, 1659
pain, after calcaneal fracture, 1526–1527
range of motion examination, 51–53
in rheumatoid arthritis, treatment, 663, 664, 666, 667
traumatic arthritis after talar neck fracture, 1559–1560
Subtalar sprains in athletes, 1153
anatomy, 1153–1154
diagnosis
clinical evaluation, 1154–1155
radiographic evaluation, 1155–1158
historical perspective, 1153
treatment
acute vs. chronic, 1159
historical perspective, 1158–1159
nonoperative, 1159–1160, 1161
results, 1163–1165
surgical, 1160, 1162–1163
Subungual clavus, 1036, 1057
Subungual exostosis, 1006–1007, 1044–1045, 1057
in dancers, 1246
nail plate deformity from, 1052
osteochondroma vs., 1045
treatment, 1045–1046, 1047
Subungual hematomas, 1057–1058, 1246
Subungual melanoma, 1003
Subungual tumors, 1057
Subungual verruca, 1058
Suction sign, 1125
Sudeck's atrophy, 1020, 1415
Superficial peroneal nerve
anatomy, 155–156, 157
anesthesia, 159, 161
entrapment, 567–569, 1117
Superior heel pain
anatomy, 848, 849
diagnosis, 848
examination and laboratory studies, 850
physical examination, 848–849
radiographic studies, 849–850
etiology, 847–848, 850
treatment, 850–853
author's method, 853–855
Superior peroneal retinaculum, in subluxation and dislocation, 1169
Supracondylar femoral derotational osteotomy, 1359–1360
Supramalleolar osteotomy, for valgus foot, 590–591
Supramalleolar tibial derotational osteotomy, 1358
Sural nerve
anatomy, 155, 156
anesthesia, 160–161, 163
entrapment, 571–572
Surface injuries in runners, 1228
Surfer's knobs, 993, 994
Surgical procedures
abductor hallucis tendon lengthening for metatarsus adductus, 1331
accessory navicular excision, 742–743
Achilles tendinitis and rupture, 1183–1184
Achilles tendon lengthening for flatfoot, 731, 735, 736
Achilles tendon repair, 813–816
Achilles tendon repair using plantaris tendon, 1273
acute dislocation of lesser metatarsophalangeal joints, 1250–1251
acute operative repair for lateral ankle sprain, 1133–1134
acute peroneal tendon dislocation, 1171–1172
Akin procedure
for adult hallux valgus, 239–243
for juvenile bunions, 312–314
Alban-Grace hindfoot stabilization, 598
ankle arthrodesis, 664–666, 667, 676–683
arthroscopic, 1300–1302
ankle arthroscopy, 1283–1285
ankle synovectomy, 1289–1290
anterior compartment fasciotomy, 1109–1110, 1111
anterior tibial stress fracture, 1116
arthrodesis for hallux rigidus, 628–629
arthrodesis for tarsal coalition, 1343
arthrodesis of first metatarsophalangeal joint, 650–651
for hallux rigidus, 634, 635
for hallux valgus, 250–258
arthroscopy
ankle arthrodesis, 1300–1302
chondral and osteochondral lesions of ankle, 1297, 1298, 1299
osteochondral lesions of talus, 1291–1296
stabilization of ankle, 1300
basal metatarsal osteotomy for diffuse intractable plantar keratosis, 429, 432
Broström procedure, modified, 1136–1138, 1261–1263
bunions in athletes, 1205–1206
calcaneal fractures
extra-articular, 1497, 1498, 1500, 1501, 1504, 1505
intra-articular, 1512–1523, 1531–1533
calcaneal osteotomy
flatfoot, 725–728, 732, 735, 737–738
pes cavus, 794, 796–798
calcaneus foot in myelodysplasia, 586–588, 589
Charcot foot, 942–944
cheilectomy for hallux rigidus, 625, 628–634
chevron osteotomy
adult hallux valgus, 196, 202, 227–235
juvenile bunions, 314–320
Chopart amputations, 978–980
Chrisman-Snook procedure, modified, 1136, 1138–1139
Chrisman-Snook procedure and modifications, 1136, 1138–1139, 1162, 1164
chronic medial ligament instability, 1142
chronic peroneal tendon dislocation, 1172–1177
clawtoe deformities in pes cavus, 793–794
clawtoe repair, 368–372
closed reduction of ankle fractures, 1448–1449

Surgical procedures *(cont.)*
closing wedge metatarsal osteotomy for juvenile hallux valgus, 325
clubfoot correction, 1325–1327
complete nail plate avulsion, 1063–1064
complete onychectomy, 1067, 1068
congenital convex pes valgus, 1345–1346
congenital curly toe, 1354
congruent joint in hallux valgus, 196
Coughlin's modified metatarsal condylectomy, 422–423, 424
coverage of hallux and digital amputations, 1385–1386, 1387–1389
crescentic or sliding osteotomy for pes cavus, 797–798, 799
crescentic osteotomy
adult hallux valgus, 217–224
juvenile hallux valgus, 325–328
cross-leg flaps in soft-tissue trauma, 1403–1405
cuboid fractures, 1615, 1616
cuboid osteotomy for forefoot abduction, 738
cuneiform and cuboid dislocations, 1694
cuneiform-cuboid wedge osteotomy for equinovarus deformity, 584–586
decompression for compartment syndrome, 1473, 1474, 1475–1476
diabetic foot infections, 912–914
diabetic ulcerations, 902–908
diaphyseal osteotomy for bunionette deformity, 455–457
diaphysectomy for hammer toe deformity, 357–358
distal calcaneal osteotomy for forefoot abduction, 738
distal metatarsal osteotomy for juvenile bunions, 314–320
distal soft tissue procedure with proximal crescentic osteotomy for adult hallux valgus, 216–224
distal soft tissue realignment
adult hallux valgus, 204–216
juvenile bunions, 320–323
dorsiflexion osteotomy, 494, 497
double arthrodesis, 688, 691–694
double osteotomy for juvenile bunions, 335–337
Durham procedure, 728, 729
DuVries procedure
deltoid imbrication, 1141
dislocating peroneal tendons, 1173
fifth toe exostosis, 407
localized intractable plantar keratosis, 421–422, 424
mild overlapping fifth toe deformity, 395–397
Dwyer calcaneal osteotomy, 701, 728, 794, 796–798
Elmslie procedure, 1137, 1162
equinovarus deformity in myelodysplasia, 583–586
equinus deformity in Duchenne muscular dystrophy, 576
Evans osteotomy for flatfoot, 725, 728, 732, 735
excisional arthroplasty in rheumatoid forefoot, 647, 649, 650
excision of calcaneonavicular bar, 752–753
excision of os trigonum by lateral approach, 1269–1270
extensor hallucis longus transfer for adult hallux varus, 288–293
extensor tendons repair, 825
extra-articular subtalar fusion for valgus foot, 591
fasciotomy
compartment syndrome, 1381–1383
medial tibial stress syndrome, 1114–1115
fifth metatarsal base fractures, 1631–1635
fifth metatarsal head resection for bunionette deformity, 447–449
fifth metatarsal osteotomy for bunionette deformity, 449–455
first cuneiform osteotomy, 329–332
first metatarsal osteotomy for pes cavus, 794, 795
first metatarsocuneiform arthrodesis, 636, 702–705, 707, 739
first metatarsophalangeal joint arthrodesis, 661
first toe Jones procedure in pes cavus, 792–793
flexor digitorum longus transfer in stroke treatment, 605–606
flexor tendon transfer for flexible or dynamic hammer toe, 358–361
flexor tenotomy
for curly toe deformity, 362–363, 365
with hammer toe repair, 351
forefoot reconstruction in rheumatoid arthritis, 653–660
forefoot sprains, 1198–1199
free tissue flaps in soft-tissue trauma, 1400–1403
Girdlestone transfer, 593
great toe amputation, 966–967
great toe arthroscopy, 1306, 1307
Grice procedure, 731
hallux rigidus in dancers, 1248–1249
hammer toe repair, 351, 354–355
Heifetz procedure, 1065–1067
Hoke-Miller procedure, 730, 731
Hoke procedure, 729, 730, 731
implant arthroplasty
degenerative joint disease, 620
hallux rigidus, 629
incongruent joint in hallux valgus, 196, 199
interdigital neuroma treatment, 561–562
interdigital plantar neuroma treatment, 549–551
interphalangeal joint arthrodesis, 369–371, 712–713
interphalangeal joint dislocations, 1702
Jones procedure of superior peroneal retinaculum reonstruction, 1173–1174
Keller procedure
hallux rigidus, 629
hallux valgus, 242–247
Kelly bone block procedure, 1173
Kidner procedure, 524–525, 741, 742
Lapidus procedure, 523–526
lateral compartment fasciotomy, 1110, 1112
lateral condylectomy for bunionette deformity, 444–447
lateral malleolus fracture repair, 1455–1458
lesser toes amputation, 967, 969–970
mallet toe treatment, 361–362, 364
McBride procedure, 320–323, 324
medial ankle sprain repair, 1141
medial column stabilization for flatfoot, 728–731
medial malleolus fracture repair, 1454–1455, 1456
medial plantar nerve entrapment treatment, 567
medial soft-tissue repair for flatfoot, 739, 740
metatarsal fractures, 1619, 1621–1627
metatarsal head resection for plantar keratosis, 432, 433
metatarsal osteotomies for plantar keratosis, 432–433
metatarsocuneiform arthrodesis and distal soft tissue procedure for hallux valgus, 244–245, 248–250
metatarsocuneiform arthrodesis for juvenile bunions, 332–335

metatarsocuneiform arthrodesis with mobile metatarsal cuneiform joint, 739
metatarsophalangeal instability, 1251
metatarsophalangeal joint arthrodesis for hallux valgus, 250–258
metatarsophalangeal joint dislocations, 1699–1701
midtarsal joint injuries, 1671–1672, 1673–1674
midtarsal osteotomies for pes cavus, 801
Miller procedure, 728–729, 730
Mitchell procedure
  adult hallux valgus, 233, 235–239
  juvenile bunions, 316–320
Moberg procedure, 625, 629, 632
navicular cuneiform fusion for flatfoot, 738–739
navicular fractures, 1603–1604, 1607–1609, 1612
neuromas on dorsum of foot, 559
oblique metatarsal osteotomy
  bunionette deformity, 452–455
  diffuse intractable plantar keratosis, 427–431
  distal, to relieve metatarsalgia, 432
opening wedge metatarsal osteotomy for juvenile hallux valgus, 324–325, 329–331
open reduction with internal fixation of ankle fractures, 1449–1454
os trigonum removal, 510, 512
overlapping toes, 1353–1354
pantalar arthrodesis in myelodysplasia, 581
partial nail plate avulsion, 1062–1063
partial onychectomy, 1065–1067
partial proximal phalangectomy for hammer toe deformity, 357–358
Peabody procedure, 586–587
peroneal tendon repair, 821–823
peroneal tenosynovitis, 1179
phalangeal fractures, 1642–1645
phenol/alcohol matrisectomy, 1068–1070
plantar fascial release (Steindler stripping) in pes cavus, 791–792
plantar flexion osteotomy of first metatarsal, 739
plantaris tendon in lateral ankle ligament reconstruction, 1163
plantar keratosis treatment, 423–433
plastic reduction of nail lip, 1064–1065
Platzgummer reconstruction for dislocating peroneal tendons, 1174
popliteal artery entrapment syndrome, 1120
posterior compartment fasciotomy, 1110–1111, 1113
posterior malleolus fracture repair, 1458
posterior tibialis tendon transfer for calcaneus foot, 587–588
posterior tibial tendon reconstruction, 775–779
Pozo and Jackson method of rerouting peroneal tendons, 1175
proximal fifth metatarsal osteotomy for bunionette deformity, 449, 457–462
proximal first metatarsal osteotomy
  adult hallux valgus, 217–224
  juvenile bunions, 323–330
ray and forefoot amputation, 967–968, 969, 970–973, 974
recurrent neuromas, 552–553
resection of medial facet talocalcaneal coalition, 751–752
Ruiz-Mora procedure, 401, 402
Samilson crescentic osteotomy, 593, 798, 799
Sarmiento and Wolf method of rerouting peroneal tendons, 1175
Scottish-Rite procedure, 730, 731
second metatarsocuneiform arthrodesis, 706, 707
sesamoid excision
  fibular, 492–494, 495
  tibial, 490–491, 492
sesamoid fractures, 1649–1652
sesamoids of first metatarsophalangeal joint, 471–489
Silastic implant arthroplasty in rheumatoid forefoot, 647–648, 650
sinus tarsi syndrome, 1167
skin grafting in soft-tissue trauma, 1386, 1389–1393, 1394, 1395–1396
SPLATT procedure
  metatarsus adductus, 1331–1333
  stroke, 605–607
  varus deformities in cerebral palsy, 594, 596, 597
split-thickness skin excision in soft-tissue trauma, 1393–1394, 1397–1399
stabilization of syndesmosis separation, 1458–1459
subcalcaneal pain syndrome, 843, 844, 846, 847
subhallux sesamoid, 433
subluxation and dislocation of second metatarsophalangeal joint, 380–394
subtalar arthrodesis, 683–687
  flatfoot, 731, 779
  valgus foot, 591–592
subtalar instability, 1160, 1162–1163
subtalar joint arthroscopy, 1304–1305
subungual exostosis resection, 1046, 1047
superior heel pain, 851, 852–855
supracondylar femoral derotational osteotomy, 1359–1360
supramalleolar osteotomy for valgus foot, 590–591
supramalleolar tibial derotational osteotomy, 1358
Syme amputation, 980–989
  toenails, 1067–1068, 1069
syndactylization of lesser toes, 401, 403
syndesmosis injury, 1151–1153
synovectomy
  posterior tibial tendon, 774–775
  rheumatoid forefoot, 651–653
talar dislocations, 1657–1658, 1659–1660, 1662–1664
talar fractures and fracture-dislocations
  body of talus, 1575–1578, 1582–1585, 1590–1591, 1595–1597
  head of talus, 1547–1548
  neck of talus, 1554–1558, 1564, 1565–1567
  open fractures, 1546
talectomy for arthrogryposis, 1348, 1349
talonavicular arthrodesis, 687–690, 779
tarsal tunnel syndrome treatment, 556–557, 565–566
tarsometatarsal arthrodesis, 701–711
tarsometatarsal dislocations, 1682–1687, 1688–1691
tarsometatarsal joint mobilization for metatarsus adductus, 1331
tendon transfers, 825–830
tenolysis of flexor hallucis longus and excision of os trigonum from medial side, 1267–1269
terminal amputation of toe and nail, 964–966
Thompson procedure for underlapping fifth toe, 400, 401
Thompson-Terwilliger procedure, 1067–1068, 1069

Surgical procedures *(cont.)*
tibial pilon fracture repair, 1459–1460, 1461
tibial sesamoid
excision technique, 490–491, 492
shaving discrete callus, 425–427
shaving prominent sesamoid, 492–494
tibial tendon transfer
calcaneus foot, 586–587, 588
stroke, 606–607
varus deformities in cerebral palsy, 594, 596, 597
toe deformities in compartment syndrome, 1406
toenail abnormalities, 1061–1069
transmetatarsal amputations, 973–977
transpositional and island pedicle flaps in soft-tissue trauma, 1399–1400
triple arthrodesis, 694–701
cerebral palsy valgus deformity, 597
myelodysplasia, 581
triple arthrodesis (Siffert procedure) for pes cavus, 798–801
valgus foot in myelodysplasia, 590–592
varus and adductus deformity in Duchenne muscular dystrophy, 576–577
vertical chevron procedure for plantar keratosis, 423, 425
V-Y gastroplasty in Achilles tendon repair, 815
Wilson osteotomy for adult hallux valgus, complications, 266, 271–272
Wilson V-Y plasty for mild overlapping fifth toe deformity, results, 396–397
Wiltberger and Mallory procedure, 1142
Winograd procedure, 1065–1067
Sustentaculum tali fractures, 1506–1508
Suturing, in Achilles tendon repair, 813, 814
Syme amputation, 980–981
aftercare, 984–987
pitfalls and complications, 987–989
technique, 981–984, 985–986
terminal, 964–966
toenails, 1067–1068, 1069
Syme prosthesis, 985–987
Sympathetic nervous system, 1412–1414
Syndactylization
lesser toes, 401, 403
partial proximal phalangectomy and, 392–394
Syndactyly, 1315, 1352
Syndesmosis separations, stabilization, 1457, 1458–1459
Syndesmosis sprains of ankle in athletes, 1142–1153
Syndesmotic impingement, arthroscopy for, 1289
Synovectomy
ankle, 1289–1290
posterior tibial tendon, 774–775
for rheumatoid forefoot, 651–652
postoperative care, 653
results and complications, 653
technique, 652–653
Synovial chrondromatosis of ankle, 1296
Synovial irritation, sources, 1285
Synovial sarcomas, 1001–1002
magnetic resonance imaging, 126, 1002
Synovitis
idiopathic, in dancers, 1251
nonspecific generalized, arthroscopy, 1285
nonspecific localized, 1285–1286
Systemic lupus erythematosus, 1077
Systemic nail disorders, 1036, 1040–1042

T

Tailor's bunion (*see* Bunionette deformity)
Talar beaking, 1342
Talar compression syndrome, in dancers, 1265–1270
Talar dislocations
classification, 1653
subtalar, 1653–1654
anatomy, 1654
author's preferred treatment, 1659–1660
clinical diagnosis, 1654–1656
mechanism of injury, 1654
radiographic diagnosis, 1655, 1656–1657
results, 1658–1659
treatment, 1657–1658
total, 1661
author's preferred treatment, 1663–1664
clinical diagnosis, 1662
complications, 1663
mechanism of injury, 1661–1662
radiographic diagnosis, 1662
treatment, 1662–1663
Talar fractures and fracture-dislocations, 1539–1540
body of talus, 1567
classification, 1567, 1568
lateral process, 1591–1592
anatomy, 1592
author's preferred treatment, 1596–1597
clinical diagnosis, 1593–1594
mechanism of injury, 1592–1593
prognosis, 1596
radiographic diagnosis, 1594–1595
treatment, 1595–1596
lateral tubercle of posterior process, 1585
anatomy, 1585, 1586
author's treatment, 1590–1591
clinical diagnosis, 1588
mechanism of injury, 1588
os trigonum, 1585–1588
radiography, 1586–1589
results, 1590
treatment, 1589–1590
medial tubercle of posterior process, 1591
osteochondral fractures, 1567–1570
anatomy, 1570
author's preferred treatment, 1577–1578
classification, 1569–1570, 1571
clinical diagnosis, 1572
mechanism of injury, 1571–1572
pathology, 1570–1571
postoperative care, 1576
radiographic examination, 1572–1574, 1577
results and prognosis, 1576–1577
treatment, 1574–1576
shearing and comminuted fractures, 1578
author's treatment, 1584–1585
classification, 1578–1580
clinical diagnosis, 1581
complications, 1583–1584
mechanism of injury, 1580
radiographic diagnosis, 1581
results, 1583
treatment, 1581–1583
dome fractures, arthroscopy, 1290, 1295
head of talus, 1547–1548
neck of talus, 1548–1549
anatomy, 1551
author's preferred treatment
group I injuries, 1565
group II injuries, 1565, 1566
group III injuries, 1565–1567
classification, 1549–1551
clinical diagnosis, 1552–1553
complications, 1558
arthritis of subtalar and talocrural joints, 1559–1560
aseptic necrosis, 1560–1565
delayed union and nonunion, 1559
malunion, 1559, 1560
osteomyelitis, 1559
skin necrosis, 1559
mechanism of injury, 1551–1552
postoperative care, 1567
prognosis, 1558
radiographic diagnosis, 1553–1554
treatment, 1554–1555
group I injuries, 1555

group II injuries, 1555–1557
group III injuries, 1557–1558
group IV injuries, 1558
open, 1546
skeletal anatomy, 1544–1546
vascular anatomy, 1540–1544
Talar (*see also* Talus)
Talar tilt view, 1125–1126, 1127
Talectomy
for arthrogrypotic foot, 1348, 1349
for equinovarus deformity, 583–584
Talipes calcaneovalgus, 1334–1335
Talipes calcaneus, primary problems, 1315
Talipes cavus, primary problems, 1315
Talipes deformities, 1314–1335
Talipes equinovarus, 1314
etiology, 1317
incidence, 1315
in newborn arthrogrypotic, 1347
pathologic anatomy, 1316–1317
primary problems, 1315
radiographic evaluation, 1317–1320
residual congenital deformity, 765, 766
in older child, 1327
treatment, 1320
at birth, 1320–1321
surgical, 1323–1327
tape application, 1321–1323
Talipes equinus deformities
in cerebral palsy, 594
Achilles tendon lengthening for, 594, 596
EMG tracings of gait, 595
in myelodysplasia, 582
Talipes planovalgus, primary problems, 1315
Talipes varus, primary problems, 1315
Talocalcaneal angle, in clubfoot evaluation, 1317–1319
Talocalcaneal coalition, 745, 1342, 1343
computed tomography, 95, 97
diagnosis, 745–746
subtalar arthrodesis for, 764
treatment, 746–748
resection of medial facet talocalcaneal coalition, 751–752
Talocalcaneal ligament, anatomy and biomechanics, 1122–1123
Talocalcaneal medial oblique special projections, 74
Talocrural joint (*see* Ankle joint)
Talofibular ligament
anterior
anatomy, 1121, 1122
biomechanics, 37–38, 42, 1123
posterior
anatomy, 1121, 1122
biomechanics, 1123
tear, magnetic resonance imaging, 118
Talonavicular arthrodesis, 636–637, 661–662, 664, 674
complications, 675–676, 688
desired position, 688
for flatfoot, 779
indications, 687
postoperative care, 688
surgical approach, 687–688
technique, 688, 689–690
Talonavicular articulation, examination, 56–57
Talonavicular coalition, 745
Talonavicular joint
anatomy, 1668–1669
arthritis, 517, 521
arthrosis, flatfoot from, 780
biomechanics, 27–28
breaking from subtalar coalition, 34
degenerative arthritis, 636–637
flatfoot and, 783
in rheumatoid arthritis, 643, 644
treatment, 661–662, 664
Talonavicular ossicle, 517
Talus (*see also* Talar *entries*)
avascular necrosis, 1029–1030
ankle fusion and, 680–681
congenital vertical, 765, 1343–1344
physical findings, 1344
radiographic findings, 1344
treatment, 1344–1346
curvature of trochlear surface, 37
in dancers, 1264–1265
imaging, 73
normal tomography, 82
lateral subluxation, 1453
osteochondral lesions, arthroscopy for, 1290–1295
paralytic vertical, in myelodysplasia, 592–593
plantar-flexed, 49
skeletal anatomy, 1544
body, 1545–1546
head, 1544–1545
neck, 1545
in talipes equinovarus, 1316–1317
vascular anatomy, 1540
extraosseous arterial supply, 1540–1541, 1542
intraosseous anastomoses, 1543–1544
intraosseous arterial supply, 1541–1543
vertical talus deformity in myelodysplasia, 592–593
Talus partitus, os trigonum vs., 509, 510–511
Talus secundarius, 517, 521
Taping
lateral ankle sprains, 1131–1132
after metatarsophalangeal arthroplasty, 391
nondisplaced metatarsal fracture, 1622
turf toe, 1199
Tarsal articulation, transverse, biomechanics, 23–24
Tarsal bones, spontaneous fusion in rheumatologic conditions, 1101
Tarsal canal, artery of, 1540, 1541, 1542–1543, 1544
Tarsal coalition, 744, 1340–1342
in athletes, 749–750
author's preferred treatment, 750–751
calcaneonavicular coalition, 748–749, 752–753, 1341
discussion, 753
excision of calcaneonavicular bar, 752–753
incidence, 744–745
multiple and other coalitions, 749
pathomechanics, 745
with resulting peroneal spastic flatfoot, 760, 762–764
talocalcaneal coalition, 745–748, 1342, 1343
computed tomography, 95, 97
resection of medial facet, 751–752
talonavicular coalition, 745
treatment, 1342–1343
Tarsal joint
slot graft for disruption, 693
transverse
evaluation of instability, 1190
range of motion examination, 53
surgical implications of biomechanics, 35
Tarsal navicular, osteoid osteoma, 1258
Tarsal navicular fractures, 1600
anatomy, 1600–1601
body, 1605
author's preferred treatment, 1612
classification, 1605, 1607
clinical diagnosis, 1605–1606
results, 1609
treatment, 1606–1609
classification, 1600
dorsal lip, 1602–1603
author's preferred treatment, 1611–1612
flatfoot from, 783
radiographic diagnosis, 1601–1602, 1603, 1604, 1605
stress fractures, 1609
author's preferred treatment, 1612
clinical diagnosis, 1609–1610
radiographic diagnosis, 1610, 1611
treatment, 1610–1611
tuberosity, 1603, 1604
author's preferred treatment, 148
clinical diagnosis, 1602, 1603
treatment, 1603–1605
Tarsal sinus, artery of, 1540, 1542, 1543, 1544
Tarsal tunnel anatomy, 554, 564
Tarsal tunnel syndrome, 554, 562, 564
clinical results, 557–558

Tarsal tunnel syndrome *(cont.)*
clinical symptoms, 555, 564–565
conservative treatment, 556, 565
case history, 565
diagnosis, 565
differential, 556
electrodiagnostic studies, 555–556
physical examination, 555
etiology, 554–555, 564
incidence, 564
postoperative care, 557, 566
surgical treatment, 556
case histories, 565–566
technique, 556–557, 565
Tarsoephiphyseal aclasis, 1010, 1013
Tarsometatarsal arthrodesis, 674, 701–702
complications, 708
desired position, 702
indications, 702
postoperative care, 708
surgical approach, 702
techniques
isolated first metatarsocuneiform arthrodesis, 702–705, 707
isolated second metatarsocuneiform arthrodesis, 706, 707
multiple tarsometatarsal arthrodesis, 707–711
Tarsometatarsal articulations
anatomy, 175, 177
examination, 57
Tarsometatarsal injuries in athletes, 1185
radiographic evaluation, 1189
Tarsometatarsal joint
anatomy, 1675
arthrosis, flatfoot from, 780, 781
degeneration in dancers, 1254–1255
mobilization for metatarsus adductus, 1331
in rheumatoid arthritis, treatment, 661
Tarsometatarsal (Lisfranc's) dislocations, 1674–1675
anatomy, 1675–1677
author's preferred treatment, 1688–1691
classification, 1675, 1676
clinical diagnosis, 1679
isolated, 1692–1693
mechanism of injury, 1677–1679
radiographic diagnosis, 1679–1681, 1683
results, 1687–1688
treatment, 1681–1687
Tarsometatarsal (Lisfranc's) dislocations
in dancers, 1255
flatfoot from, 783
Technetium 99 bone scan
diabetes, 892–893
subcalcaneal pain syndrome, 840, 842
Technetium 99m methylene diphosphonate imaging, 87
Tendinitis
Achilles
Achilles ruptures and, in athletes, 1181–1184
in dancers, 1271–1272
retrocalcaneal bursitis associated with, surgical treatment, 854–855
in runners, 1233–1234
superior heel pain from, 848
in dancers
Achilles, 1271–1272
anterior ankle, 1258
flexor hallucis longus tendon, 1270–1271
posterior tibial, 1255
magnetic resonance imaging, 117
peroneal, 1177–1179
after calcaneal fracture, 1527–1528
posterior tibial tendon, 1180–1181, 1255
in runners, 1233–1235
ultrasound, 91
Tendinosis, 807, 1177
differential diagnosis, 812
Tendo Achillis (*see* Achilles tendon)
Tendon disorders, 805–835
Achilles tendon
physical findings, 810
radiographic examination, 810–811
results of treatment, 814, 816–817
treatment, 811–816
algorithmic approach to imaging, 119–122
bursitis, 808–810
classification, 806
etiology, 806
extensor tendons, 824–825
flexor hallucis longus, 823
inflammation classification, 807
pathology, 806–808
peritendinitis, 807
peroneal tendons, 817
anatomy, 817
peritendinitis, 817–818
rupture, 818–819
traumatic dislocation, 819–823
posterior tibial tendon (*see* Posterior tibial tendon dysfunction)
rupture, 807–808
sequential changes of healing, 807
stenosing tenosynovitis, 823–824
tendinitis (*see* Tendinitis)
tendon transfers about foot and ankle, 825–830
Tendons
anatomy, 805–806
ankle, magnetic resonance imaging, 100, 101, 103, 119, 120, 121
Tendon sheath, giant-cell tumor, 997–998
Tendon transfers, 825
anterior, 828–829
biomechanics, 36, 825–826
diagnosis, 828
distal, 829–830
for flexible or dynamic hammer toe, 358–361
lateral, 829
muscle function principles, 826–827
patient evaluation, 827–828
for peroneal nerve injury, 609–610
posterior, 829
results and complications, 371–372
split-tendon transfer, 829
for calcaneus foot, 586–587, 588
for metatarsus adductus, 1331–1333
in stroke treatment, 606–607
surgical principles, 828
for varus deformities in cerebral palsy, 594, 596, 597
Tennis injuries, 1203, 1205
Tenography, 83, 84
Tenosynovitis (*see also* Peritendinitis), 861
Tenotomy, flexor
for curly toe deformity, 362–363, 365
with hammer toe repair, 351
TENS, in reflex sympathetic dystrophy syndrome, 1418
Terminal Syme amputation, 964
aftercare, 966
pitfalls and complications, 966
technique, 965–966
Terminology, for foot positions, 719–720
Terry's nail, 1042
Thawing-rewarming stages, 1425
Thermal injuries, 1426–1428
classification, 1428
treatment, 1428–1432
Thermography, 85–86
Thompson procedure for underlapping fifth toe, 400, 401
Thompson "squeeze test," 810
Thompson-Terwilliger procedure, 1067–1068, 1069
Tibial arteries
fibrinolysis, 109
percutaneous transluminal angioplasty, 108
talar blood supply from, 1540, 1541, 1542, 1543
Tibial epiphysis injuries in children, 1462
Tibial fractures
anterior lip, 1449, 1451
posterior lip, 1450
stress fracture
in dancers, 1275
in runners, 1229–1230
Tibialis anterior tendon (*see* Tibial tendon, anterior)
Tibialis posterior tendon (*see* Tibial tendon, posterior)
Tibial nerve
entrapment, 838–839
identification of motor branches with stimulator, 608
phenol injection into, after traumatic brain injury, 608
posterior
anatomy, 154
anesthesia, 158–159, 160
Tibial pilon (plafond) fractures
classification, 1446
surgical treatment, 1459–1460, 1461

Tibial sesamoid
callus beneath, 478
excision technique, 490–491, 492
intractable plantar keratosis and, 478–479, 480
percentage of bipartite sesamoids, 471
radiography, 471, 472
shaving prominent
postoperative results, 494
technique, 492, 493
Tibial sesamoid shaving, for discrete callus, 425, 426
complications, 426
postoperative care, 425
results, 425–426
surgical technique, 425, 427
Tibial stress syndrome in athletes
medial
classification, 1112
clinical features, 1112–1113
definition, 1112
diagnosis, 1113–1114
treatment, 1114–1115
runners, 1230
Tibial tendon
anterior
rupture, 824–825
sesamoid of, 500, 501
transfer
for calcaneus foot, 586–587, 588
in stroke treatment, 606–607
for varus deformities in cerebral palsy, 594, 596, 597
posterior
dysfunction (*see* Posterior tibial tendon dysfunction)
laceration, flatfoot from, 783
pain, magnetic resonance imaging, 117
sesamoid of, 500, 501
tendinitis, 1180–1181
in dancers, 1255
in runners, 1234–1235
Tibial torsion, 1357–1358
supramalleolar tibial derotational osteotomy, 1358
Tibiocalcaneal arthrodesis, 680, 681, 1583
Tibiofibular articulation
anatomy, 1143
radiographic relationships, 1147
Tibiofibular ligament
anterior inferior
accessory, 1144
anatomy, 1143, 1144
biomechanics, 1144–1145
as impingement site, 1286, 1287, 1289
posterior inferior
anatomy, 1143–1144
biomechanics, 1145
Tibiofibular syndesmosis, distal, "high" ankle sprain of, in dancers, 1263–1264
Tibiotalocalcaneal tunnel, proximal segment, 159
Tillaux fracture, 1462
Tinea pedis, 871
dermatologic aspects, 1077–1078
Tissue biopsy, 993
Toddlers, examination principles, 45–46
Toe-in and toe-out, examination, 47
Toeing in, 1356
Toeing out, 1355–1356
Toenail abnormalities, 1033–1071
anatomy, 1034–1035
causes, 1049
classification, 1035–1036
in dancers, 1246–1247
dermatologic disorders, 1036
eczema and contact dermatitis, 1038
psoriasis, 1036–1038
pyodermas, 1038–1039
etiology, 1033
genetic disorders with nail changes, 1042–1044
incidence, 1034
ingrown nails, 1049–1054, 1065
nail bed disorders, 1056–1058
nail fold disorders, 1058–1059
nail matrix disorders, 1059–1061
nail plate disorders, 1049–1056
in runners, 1237
systemic diseases, 1036, 1040–1042
terminology, 1036
trauma, 1044
treatment
complete nail avulsion, 1063–1064
complete onychectomy, 1067, 1068
conservative, 1061
digital anesthetic block, 1061–1062
partial nail plate avulsion, 1062–1063
partial onychectomy, 1065–1067
phenol/alcohol matrisectomy, 1068–1070
plastic reduction of nail lip, 1064–1065
tumors, 1044
glomus tumor, 1044
melanotic whitlow, 1046–1047, 1048
other tumerous conditions, 1047–1049
subungual exostosis, 1044–1046
Toenails
anatomy, 1034–1035
avulsion, complete, 1063–1064
in diabetes, 944–946, 957
Toes
amputation and closure, 1384–1386, 1387–1388
anesthesia, 157–158
appliances, 146
after calcaneal fracture, 1529
congenital abnormalities, 1349
great toe, 1349–1350
lesser toes, 1350–1354
dancing disorders, 1243–1247
diabetic foot
amputation, 917
osteomyelitis, 917, 918
surgery for ulcerations, 902
digital nerve compression, sesamoid associated, 471, 479–480, 482
great (*see* Great toe)
lesser (*see* Lesser toes)
limited motion, 1101
patient rising on, examination, 49
second
amputation, hallux valgus from, 173, 356, 357
mallet and hammer toe, 343, 344
Toe shoes, 1204, 1244
ribbon burn from, 1271
Tomography, 79, 82
computed (*see* Computed tomography)
partial volume effect, 81
polytomography of fractures, 1573, 1610, 1611, 1620
stress, subtalar joint, 1157–1158
Torsional deformities of lower extremities, 1354
physical examination and normal parameters, 1354–1355, 1356, 1357
treatment
femoral anteversion, 1358–1360
tibial torsion, 1357–1358
toeing in, 1356
toeing out, 1355–1356
Torsional joint injuries, 1228–1229
Total ankle replacement, failed, arthrodesis for, 681–683
Total-contact cast, in diabetes, 898, 900–901, 938
Tourniquets, in amputation surgery, 960
Transchondral fractures, 1290, 1567–1578
Transcutaneous electrical nerve stimulation, in reflex sympathetic dystrophy syndrome, 1418
Transcutaneous oxygen measurements, in evaluation for amputation, 964
Transmetatarsal amputation, 973–974, 1384, 1385
aftercare, 977–978
pitfalls, 978
technique, 975–977
Transpositional flaps, 1399–1400
Transverse plane rotation, biomechanics, 28
Transverse tarsal joint
biomechanics, 23–24
evaluation of instability, 1190
range of motion examination, 53
surgical implications of biomechanics, 35
Trauma
antibiotic treatment, 860–861
soft-tissue (*see* Soft-tissue trauma)

Trauma *(cont.)*
toenail abnormalities from, 1044
Traumatic arthrosis, flatfoot from, 782–783
Traumatic brain injury, 607–608
Trench foot, 1424, 1426
Trichophyton mentagrophytes, 871, 1077, 1078
Trichophyton rubrum, 871, 1077, 1078
Trichophyton toenail infection, 1054, 1055
Tricyclic antidepressants, in reflex sympathetic dystrophy syndrome, 1417–1418
Trimalleolar fractures and fracture-dislocations, surgical treatment, 1450–1451
Triplane fractures, 1462–1463
Triple arthrodesis, 674, 694, 698
calcaneal fractures, 1522–1523
cerebral palsy valgus deformity, 597
complications, 700–701
indications, 698
myelodysplasia, 581
pes cavus, 798
postoperative care, 801
technique, 798–801
postoperative care, 700
radiographs, 694–697
special considerations, 701
technique, 698–700
Tuberculosis, 869–870
Tumors, 991–992
algorithmic approach to imaging, 122, 125–127
benign soft-tissue tumors, 993–1000
benign tumors and cysts of bone, 1003–1012
classification, 993
diagnostic studies, 993
flatfoot from, 783–784
history and physical examination, 992
magnetic resonance imaging of soft-tissue masses, 103, 105, 126, 127
malignant soft-tissue tumors, 1000–1003
malignant tumors of bone, 1012–1018
metastatic to foot, 1018
radiographic evaluation, 992–993
subungual, 1057
toenail disorders from, 1041, 1044–1049
vascular, 999, 1000
Turf toe, 1191
diagnosis
clinical evaluation, 1195–1196
radiographic evaluation, 1196–1198
epidemiology, 1191
etiologic factors, 1194
historical perspective, 1191
mechanism of injury, 1192
severity of injury, 1191–1192
treatment
nonoperative, 1198, 1199
results, 1199–1200
surgical, 1198–1199
Two-joint muscle test, 594

U

UCBL insert, 148–149
Ulcerations
in Charcot foot, 900, 907–908, 941
in diabetes (*see* Diabetic foot, ulcers)
of fibula after Syme amputation, 987
Ultrasonography
arterial Doppler
in diabetes, 886–887, 888, 889–890, 956
in evaluation for amputation, 964
diagnostic, 89–91
foreign body localization, 123
Unguis incarnatus, 1049
Unna-Thost disease, 1088
Urokinase, 109

V

Valgus foot
callus formation from, 415, 416
in cerebral palsy, 597–598
in myelodysplasia, 588–590
surgical management, 590–592
Varus foot
callus formation from, 415, 416
in cerebral palsy, 594–597
talipes varus, primary problems, 1315
Vascular disease in diabetes, 883–884
Vascular evaluation of diabetic foot, 886–888, 956
Vascular malformations, embolization, 109
Vascular problems in athletes
femoral or external iliac arterial occlusion, 1120
popliteal artery entrapment syndrome, 1118–1120
venous disease, 1120
Vascular reconstruction, in amputation surgery, 963–964
Vascular tumors, 999, 1000
Venography, 107–108
Venous disease in athletes, 1120
Verruca, periungual and subungual, 1058–1059
Vertical compression fractures of the ankle, 1444
classification, 1444, 1446
emergency treatment, 1446
history, 1445
physical diagnosis, 1445
radiographic findings, 1445, 1447, 1448
surgical technique, 1454
lateral malleolus, 1455–1458
medial malleolus, 1454–1455, 1456
posterior malleolus, 1458
postoperative care, 1460, 1462
syndesmosis separations, 1458–1459
tibial pilon fractures, 1459–1460, 1461
treatment
closed reduction, 1448–1449
closed vs. open, 1447–1448
open reduction with internal fixation, 1449–1454
soft-tissue considerations, 1446–1447
Vertical talus deformity, in myelodysplasia, 592–593
V-Y gastroplasty, in Achilles tendon repair, 815
V-Y plasty for mild overlapping fifth toe deformity, 396–397

W

Wagner classification for diabetic foot, 893–894
Walking
ground reaction to, 7–8, 9
jogging and running vs., variations in gait cycle, 32
kinematics, 5–9
kinetics, 9–10
limp, examination, 47
weight bearing biomechanics, 10–15
Walking cycle
events, 15, 28
first interval, 29
second interval, 29–30
third interval, 30–31
phases, 15
Warts, plantar, 416, 417, 1088–1090
differential diagnosis, 1090
treatment, 1090–1091
Watson-Jones procedure for lateral ankle sprain and instability, 1136
Weak foot
acquired, 767–784
classification, 757–758
congenital, 758–767
Weight bearing
biomechanics, 10–15
in fracture and dislocation treatment, 1468–1469
Harris mat and, 58, 59
pronation and supination in, 171–172
Weitlaner retractor, 493
Wilson osteotomy, for adult hallux valgus
dorsiflexion deformity from, 266
metatarsal malunion and elevation from, 271–272
Wilson V-Y plasty for mild overlapping fifth toe deformity, 396–397
Wiltberger and Mallory procedure for chronic medial ankle ligamentous instability, 1142

Windlass action/mechanism
examination, 49, 51
loss of, 14
Winograd procedure, 1065–1067
Wound, in diabetes, closure and foot reconstruction, 923–925, 926, 927
Wounds
classification, 1453
closure in amputation surgery, 962–963
contraction, 916
in diabetes, care, 901–902
in hallux valgus surgery
delayed breakdown, 261–262
delayed healing, 260

X

Xenografts, 1393, 1429, 1430

Y

Yellow nail syndrome, 1039
Young procedure, 731

Z

Zadik procedure, 1067, 1068

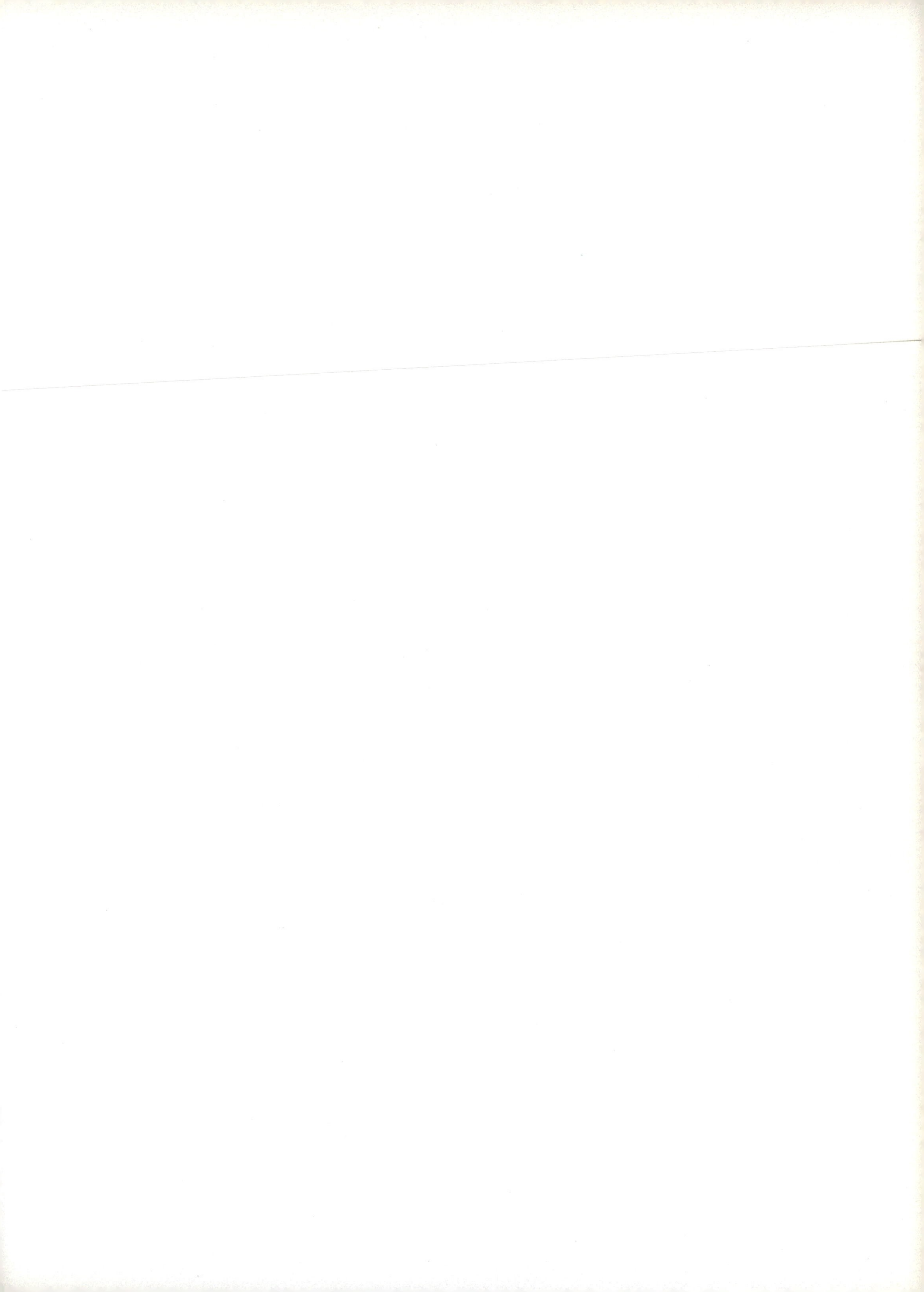